Critical Care Nursing

4e

Critical Care Nursing

4e

Leanne Aitken
RN, PhD, BHSc(Nurs)Hons, GCertMgt, GDipScMed(ClinEpi), FACCCN, FACN, FAAN, Life Member – ACCCN
Professor of Critical Care, School of Health Sciences, City, University of London, UK
Professor of Critical Care Nursing, School of Nursing and Midwifery, and Menzies Health Institute Queensland, Griffith University, Qld, Australia

Andrea Marshall
RN, PhD, MN(Research), BN, Grad Cert Ed Studies (Higher Ed), IC Cert, FACCCN, FACN, Life Member – ACCCN
Professor of Acute and Complex Care Nursing, School of Nursing and Midwifery and Menzies Health Institute Queensland, Griffith University, Qld, Australia
Intensive Care Unit, Gold Coast Hospital and Health Service, Qld, Australia

Wendy Chaboyer
RN, PhD, MN, BSc(Nu)Hons, Crit Care Cert, FACCCN, FAAN, Life Member – ACCCN
Professor and Deputy Head of School (Research), School of Nursing and Midwifery and Person-Centred Health Services Group Leader, Menzies Health Institute Queensland, Griffith University, Qld, Australia

ELSEVIER

ELSEVIER

Elsevier Australia. ACN 001 002 357
(a division of Reed International Books Australia Pty Ltd)
Tower 1, 475 Victoria Avenue, Chatswood, NSW 2067

Reprinted 2020

ISBN: 978-0-7295-4297-5

National Library of Australia Cataloguing-in-Publication Data

NATIONAL LIBRARY OF AUSTRALIA

A catalogue record for this book is available from the National Library of Australia

Content Strategist: Natalie Hunt
Content Project Manager: Shravan Kumar
Edited by Lynn Watt
Proofread by Sarah Newton-John
Cover by Georgette Hall
Internal design: Non-Standard
Permissions by Sarah Thomas & Regina Remigius
Index by Innodata Indexing
Typeset by Toppan Best-set Premedia Limited
Printed in China by 1010

Last digit is the print number: 9 8 7 6 5 4 3 2

Contents

Foreword

It is a great privilege and with respectful pride that I introduce the fourth edition of *Critical Care Nursing* endorsed by the Australian College of Critical Care Nurses (ACCCN). As the current President of the ACCCN, I have been observing the impact and flow this work has and will have on improving critical care nursing practice.

There is a strong and enduring collaborative relationship between the College, the Publisher and the Editors that has sustained a reputation of excellence and legacy for critical care nursing. The editors, who are committed to excellence, are acknowledged expert practitioners, educators and researchers in critical care nursing.

This fourth edition of *Critical Care Nursing*, endorsed by the ACCCN, continues to be the reference book for nurses caring for critically ill patients and their families. Since the first edition there have been significant advances in most areas of critical care nursing as the specialty has continued to evolve. This has included continued insights into both normal biology and disease, translation of this to the bedside and the results of large clinical trials, alongside a plethora of quality nursing and multidisciplinary research that contributes to current evidence-based practice. The text tailored for practice in the international arena is underpinned by the quality of Australian and New Zealand nursing practice whose reputation is supported and sustained by some of the best patient care outcomes worldwide. The ACCCN Practice Standards for the Specialist Critical Care Nurses is central to these outcomes and features as part of the text. As in previous editions, the translation of research to practice continues, with several pedagogical features such as summary tables, illustrative figures, case studies and research vignettes, which provide several options for preferred learning styles. There are three sections and 29 chapters to this edition:

Section One: Includes chapters on the scope of critical care nursing, quality and safety, recovery and rehabilitation and ethical issues in critical care.

Section Two: The focus is on the principles and practice of critical care. Essential nursing care, psychological care and family and cultural care are scientifically and creatively presented. Further chapters are aligned around physiological systems concluding with multi-organ dysfunction syndrome.

Section Three: Here specialty practice is detailed including paediatric, pregnancy and postpartum considerations. Emergency presentations, trauma management, resuscitation, postanaesthetic recovery and organ donation and transplantation are essential inclusions.

The fourth edition continues the tradition of excellence in nursing care found in the previous editions by having all chapters written by scholarly clinical experts. Critical care nursing colleagues worldwide are becoming more connected and the world is becoming smaller. Hence there is considerable broadening of evidence and practice recommendations in this edition to reflect international practice.

The fourth edition of *Critical Care Nursing* endorsed by ACCCN provides a comprehensive international resource for critical care nurses, students and educators seeking to develop and renew their knowledge and skills for the best patient-centred care and outcomes in critical care nursing.

Diane Chamberlain RN MN MPH PhD
FRCNA FACCCN MAICD
Associate Professor Critical Care Nursing,
Higher Degree Research Coordinator,
College of Nursing & Health Sciences,
Flinders University, Adelaide, Australia
National President: Australian College of
Critical Care Nurses

Preface

Critical care as a clinical specialty is over half a century old. With every successive decade, advances in the education and practices of critical care nurses have been made. Today, critical care nurses are some of the most knowledgeable and highly skilled nurses in the world, and ongoing professional development and education are fundamental elements in ensuring we deliver the highest quality care to our patients and their families.

This book is intended to encourage and challenge nurses to further develop their critical care nursing practice. Since the first edition in 2007, with a focus on Australasian practice, we have now expanded the text to reflect international practice and expertise in the field. Our authors come from many countries including Australia, Canada, England, the Netherlands, New Zealand, Northern Ireland, Scotland, Sweden, Switzerland, United Arab Emirates and the USA.

This fourth edition of ACCCN's *Critical Care Nursing* has 29 chapters that reflect the collective talent and expertise of 55 contributors – a strong mix of academics and clinicians with a passion for critical care internationally. All contributors were carefully chosen for their current knowledge, clinical expertise and strong professional reputations.

The book has been developed primarily for use by practising critical care clinicians, managers, researchers and graduate students undertaking a specialty critical care qualification. In addition, senior undergraduate students studying high acuity nursing subjects will find this book a valuable reference tool, although it goes beyond the learning needs of these students. The aim of the book is to be a comprehensive resource, as well as a portal to an array of other important resources, for critical care nurses. The nature and timeline of book publishing dictate that the information contained in this book reflects a snapshot in time of our knowledge and understanding of the complex world of critical care nursing. We therefore encourage our readers to continue to also search for the most contemporary sources of knowledge to guide their clinical practice. A range of website links have been included in each chapter to facilitate this process.

This fourth edition is divided into three broad sections: the scope of critical care nursing, core components of critical care nursing and specialty aspects of critical care nursing. Revisions to existing chapters were based on our reflections and suggestions from colleagues and reviewers as well as on evolving and emerging practices in critical care.

Section 1 introduces a broad range of professional issues related to practice that are relevant across critical care. Initial chapters provide contemporary information on the scope of practice, systems and resources and ethical issues, with expanded information on quality and safety, and recovery and rehabilitation in critical care.

Content presented in Section 2 is relevant to the majority of critical care nurses, with a focus on concepts that underpin practice such as essential physical, psychological, social and cultural care. Remaining chapters in this section present a systems approach in supporting physiological function for a critically ill person. This edition has multiple linked chapters for some of the major physiological systems – four chapters for cardiovascular, three for respiratory and two for neurological. Chapters on support of renal function; nutrition assessment and therapeutic management; gastrointestinal, metabolic and liver alterations; management of shock; and multi-organ dysfunction complete this section.

Section 3 presents specific clinical conditions such as emergency presentations, trauma, resuscitation, postanaesthesia recovery, paediatric considerations, pregnancy and postpartum considerations and organ donation, by building on the principles outlined in Section 2. This section enables readers to explore some of the more complex or unique aspects of specialty critical care nursing practice.

Chapters have been organised in a consistent format to facilitate identification of relevant material. Where appropriate, each chapter commences with an overview of the relevant anatomy and physiology and the epidemiology of the clinical states. Nursing care of the patient, delivered independently or provided collaboratively with other members of the healthcare team, is then presented. Pedagogical features include a case study that elaborates relevant care issues and a critique of a research publication that explores a related topic. Tables, figures and practice tips have been used extensively throughout each chapter to identify areas of care that are particularly pertinent for readers. Each chapter also has specific learning activities, and model responses to these questions to further support learning can be found online. It is not our intention that readers progress sequentially through the book, but rather explore chapters or sections that are relevant for different episodes of learning or practice.

The delivery of effective, high-quality critical care nursing practice is a challenge in contemporary healthcare. We trust that this book will be a valuable resource in supporting your care of critically ill patients and their loved ones.

Leanne **Aitken**
Andrea **Marshall**
Wendy **Chaboyer**

About the **Australian College of Critical Care Nurses** (ACCCN)

The Australian College of Critical Care Nurses, with over 2400 members, is the peak professional organisation representing critical care nurses in Australia. Membership types include standard members, international members, associate members, life members, and corporate members. All individual members are eligible and are encouraged to participate in the activities of the College. Members receive the College journal, plus discounts for ACCCN conference registration, education events and for ACCCN publications. Life memberships are awarded to individuals in recognition of their outstanding contribution to ACCCN and/or to critical care nursing excellence in Australia.

ACCCN is a company limited by guarantee and has branches in each state of Australia. Two members from each state branch management committee form the ACCCN National Board of Directors. Each committee facilitates the activities of the College at a local/state level providing local and, at times, national representation. The ACCCN Editorial Committee and Editorial Board, under the leadership of the editor of the *Australian Critical Care (ACC)* journal, are responsible for College publications including the journal *Australian Critical Care* and the digital newspaper *Critical Times*.

There are a number of national advisory panels and special interest groups dedicated to providing the organisation with expert opinion on issues relating to critical care nursing. These include:

Resuscitation Advisory Panel, which consists of 12 members representing each branch of the ACCCN, plus a paediatric nurse representative. It has developed a complete suite of contemporary advanced life support and resuscitation educational materials and offers its ACCCN National ALS Courses throughout Australia

Research Advisory Panel, which, in addition to providing expert advice to ACCCN, is responsible for evaluating and making recommendations on research strategy. Additionally, this panel assesses grant submissions to ACCCN, and evaluates abstracts submitted to the ANZICS/ACCCN Annual Scientific Meeting on Intensive Care

Education Advisory Panel, which advises ACCCN on all matters relating to education specific to critical care nursing. This panel has developed a position paper on critical care nursing education and written submissions on behalf of ACCCN to national reviews of nursing education

Workforce Advisory Panel, which has represented ACCCN on a number of national health workforce and nursing committees. The panel has also developed position statements on nurse staffing for intensive care and high dependency units in Australia. This panel annually reviews the dataset design for national workforce data collection in conjunction with ANZICS

Organ and Tissue Donation and Transplantation Advisory Panel, which advises the board and developed a position statement on organ donation and transplantation as it relates to intensive care. It disseminates related information to critical care nurses regarding the promotion and national reform objectives of organ and tissue donation in Australia

Quality Advisory Panel, which provides expert knowledge, advice and information to ACCCN on matters relevant to critical care nursing practice relating specifically to patient management

Paediatric Advisory Panel, which provides expert knowledge, advice and information to ACCCN on matters relevant to paediatric critical care nursing in addition to recommending content and speakers for the annual ACCCN conferences.

In addition to branch educational events and symposiums, ACCCN conducts three national conferences each year: ACCCN Institute of Continuing Education (ICE) and, in conjunction with our medical colleagues from The Australian and New Zealand Intensive Care Society (ANZICS), the ANZICS/ACCCN Annual Scientific Meeting on Intensive Care plus the Australian and New Zealand Paediatric and Neonatal Intensive Care Conference.

ACCCN has a representative on the Australian Resuscitation Council (ARC) and has representation at a federal government advisory level through the Nursing and Midwifery Stakeholder Reference Group (NMSRG) chaired by the Chief Nurse of Australia. ACCCN is also a member of the Coalition of National Nursing Organisations (CoNNO). The founding Chairperson of the World Federation of Critical Care Nurses (WFCCN) continues to represent ACCCN on the WFCCN Council, and the College also has representatives on the World Federation of Paediatric Intensive and Critical Care Societies and is a member of the Intensive Care Foundation.

More information can be found on the ACCCN website: www.acccn.com.au.

About the editors

Leanne Aitken is Professor of Critical Care at City, University of London, United Kingdom and also a Professor of Critical Care Nursing at Griffith University, Queensland, Australia. She has had a long career in critical care nursing, including practice, education and research roles. In all her roles, Leanne has been inspired by a sense of enquiry, pride in the value of expert nursing and a belief that improvement in practice and resultant patient outcomes is always possible. Research interests include developing and refining interventions to improve long-term recovery of critically ill and injured patients, decision-making practices of critical care nurses and a range of clinical practice issues within critical care, such as sedation management.

Leanne has been active in the Australian College of Critical Care Nurses (ACCCN) for more than 30 years and was made a Life Member and Fellow of the College in 2006 after holding positions on a range of state and national boards, panels and working groups, as well as been an Associate Editor with *Australian Critical Care*. Leanne is an Ambassador for the World Federation of Critical Care Nurses.

Leanne is a Fellow of both the American Academy of Nursing and the Australian College of Nursing. She is also a Fulbright Alumnus after receiving a Fulbright Senior Scholarship to undertake research at the University of Pennsylvania, Philadelphia, USA. Leanne has published more than 130 original publications in peer-reviewed journals. She is also a peer reviewer for a number of national and international journals and reviews grant applications for a range of organisations internationally.

Andrea Marshall is Professor of Acute and Complex Care Nursing at Griffith University and Gold Coast Health, Queensland, Australia. She has been working in critical care as a clinician, educator and researcher for more than two decades. Andrea has a strong interdisciplinary focus on research, translation of research into clinical practice and implementing patient- and family-centred approaches to clinical care and research. Her program of research focuses on improving nutrition delivery to acute and critically ill patients during hospitalisation and following discharge.

Andrea has been actively involved with the ACCCN for over two decades in a variety of state- and nationally-based leadership roles. In 2014 her contribution to the College was recognised with Life Membership. She is currently Editor-in-Chief of *Australian Critical Care* and has played a key editorial role in this journal since 2003. She is an active contributor to grant reviews for a number of national and international funding bodies and serves as a reviewer on several international journals, many of which have an interdisciplinary focus.

Wendy Chaboyer is Professor of Nursing at Griffith University, the Deputy Head of School (Research) in the School of Nursing and Midwifery and the Group Lead for Patient-Centred Health Services in Menzies Health Institute Queensland (Griffith University), Australia. Wendy has 30 years of experience in the critical care area, as a clinician, educator and researcher, and she is passionate about the contribution nurses can make to the hospital experience for patients and their families. Her early research examined ICU patients' experiences and the role nurses can play to assist in their transition from ICU to the ward. She has subsequently focused on patient safety, undertaking research into adverse events after ICU, clinical handover and 'transforming care at the bedside'. Three recent areas of work have been in relation to patient participation in care, pressure injury (ulcer) prevention and surgical dressings to prevent surgical site infections. Wendy has over 250 peer-reviewed publications and has been awarded over $9 million in competitive external grants.

Wendy has been active in ACCCN since her arrival in Australia in the early 1990s and was awarded Life Membership in 2006. She has been a National Board member and member of the Queensland Branch Management Committee. Wendy is a past Chair of the Research Advisory Panel and past Chair of the Quality Advisory Panel of the ACCCN. She played a role in the formation of the World Federation of Critical Care Nurses and continues to support their activities. Wendy reviews for a number of journals and funding bodies such as the National Health and Medical Research Council (NHMRC) and the Australian Research Council. She was inducted into the Sigma Theta Tau International Nurse Researcher Hall of Fame in 2015 and became a Fellow of the American Academy of Nursing in 2017.

List of contributors

Leanne Aitken RN, PhD, BHSc(Nurs)Hons, GCertMgt, GDipScMed(ClinEpi), FACCCN, FACN, FAAN, Life Member – ACCCN
Professor of Critical Care, School of Health Sciences, City, University of London, UK
Professor of Critical Care Nursing, School of Nursing and Midwifery, and Menzies Health Institute Queensland, Griffith University, QLD, Australia

Ian Baldwin RN, PhD, FACCCN
Clinical Educator, Department of Intensive Care, Austin Health, Melbourne, VIC, Australia

Jayne Bancroft RN
Clinical Nurse Consultant, Mechanical Circulatory Support & Recipient Transplant Coordinator, The Prince Charles Hospital, QLD, Australia

Catherine Bell RN, MN(CritCare), PostGradDip, AdvNsg Crit Care, DipApSc-Nsg, Cert of Nursing
ICU Clinical Nurse Consultant – Trauma, Alfred Hospital, Melbourne, VIC, Australia

Suzanne Bench PhD, MSc Advanced Practice (Crit Care), PGDipHE, BSc(Hons), ENB 100 (Intensive Care), RGN
Associate Professor of Nursing and Deputy Director of Research (nursing), London South Bank University and the Royal National Orthopaedic Hospital, London, UK

Lina Bergman RN, MN(ICU), PhD candidate
Institute of Health and Care Sciences, University of Gothenburg, Sweden

Thomas Buckley RN, MN, PhD, CertICU, GCertHpol
Associate Professor and Academic Leader Research Education, Susan Wakil School of Nursing and Midwifery, Faculty of Medicine and Health, The University of Sydney, NSW, Australia

Pauline Calleja RN, PhD, MAdvNursPrac, GradCert HigherEd, BNSc, DipManagement, MACN, FCENA
Director of Post Graduate Nursing and Infection Prevention and Control programs, Senior Lecturer, School of Nursing and Midwifery, Griffith University, QLD, Australia

Wendy Chaboyer RN, PhD, FAAN, FACCCN
Professor and Deputy Head of School (Research), School of Nursing and Midwifery and Menzies Health Institute, Griffith University, QLD, Australia

Maureen A Coombs MBE, PhD, RN
Professor in Clinical Nursing, School of Nursing and Midwifery, University of Plymouth, Plymouth, UK

Fiona Coyer RN, Dip Nsg (Dist), PGCEA, MSc Nsg, PhD
Professor of Nursing, Royal Brisbane and Women's Hospital, Metro North Hospital Health Services and School of Nursing, Queensland University of Technology, Brisbane, QLD, Australia

Jennifer Dennett RN MN BAppSc (Nursing Ed), CritCareCert, Dip Management, MCNA
Nurse Unit Manager, Critical Care, Oncology, Cardiology, Renal Dialysis, Central Gippsland Health, VIC, Australia

Malcolm Dennis RN, Critical Care Cert, BEd, IBHRE-Certified Cardiac Device Specialist
Field Technical Expert, Cardiac Rhythm Management and Heart Failure, Abbott Medical, Melbourne, VIC, Australia

Susan Dirkes RN, MSA, CCRN
University of Michigan Health System: Educator, Staff Nurse, Surgical ICU, Intermediate Care Unit, Ann Arbor, MI, USA

Andrea Driscoll RN, NP, MN, MEd, MHEconomics, PhD, FAHA, FACNP, FCSANZ
Professor of Nursing, Deakin University and Austin Health, Melbourne, VIC, Australia

Trudy Dwyer RN, Nr Cert, ICU Cert, BHlthScn, GDipFlex Ed, MClinEd, PHD, FACCCN
Professor, CQ University, Rockhampton, QLD, Australia
Visiting Research Fellow Central Queensland Hospital and Health Service, QLD, Australia

Rosalind Elliott RN, PhD
Clinical Nurse Specialist (ICU) and Clinical Nurse Consultant – translational research co-ordinator, Northern Sydney Local Health District, Sydney, NSW, Australia

Ruth Endacott PhD, MA, DipN (Lond), Cert Ed, RN
Professor of Clinical Nursing, University of Plymouth, Plymouth, UK
Professor of Clinical Nursing, Monash University, VIC, Australia

Anne Flodén RN, PhD, CRNA, ICCN
Clinical Researcher in organ donation and Director of Research, Development and Education, Södra Älvsborg Hospital, Borås, Sweden
Assistant Professor, University of Gothenburg, Sweden

Paula Foran RN, GC Perianaesthesia, Master Professional Education and Training, PhD
Education Officer, Australian College of Perioperative Nurses (ACORN), Australia
Academic (Casual), School of Health Sciences, Faculty of Health, University of Tasmania, TAS, Australia

Deb Friel RN, BA, HSc, GC Critical Care, GC Clinical Nursing, GC Management, GCTE, JP (Qual)
Manager, Centre for Professional Development, CQ University, Rockhampton, QLD, Australia

Sher Michael Graan MNursPrac, GradDipNurs (CritCare), BHlthSc(Nurs)
Lecturer in Nursing, Faculty of Health, School of Nursing and Midwifery, Deakin University, VIC, Australia

Bernadette Grealy RN, RM, GradDip CritCare, MN, FACCCN
Nursing Director, Intensive Care Services and Hyperbaric Medicine, Central Adelaide LHN, Adelaide, SA, Australia

Carol Grech RN, BN(Ed), GradDipNsg(Crit Care), MN, PhD
Pro Vice Chancellor: Student Engagement and Equity, University of South Australia, SA, Australia

Melanie Greenwood RN, PhD, MNurs, GradCert UniLearnTeach, Cert Intensive Care, Cert Neurological Nursing
Senior Lecturer, Director Postgraduate Nursing Courses, School of Nursing, University of Tasmania, TAS, Australia

Janice Gullick RN, PhD, MArt, BFA, Cardiothoracic cert
Associate Professor, Coordinator of Intensive Care Nursing, Susan Wakil School of Nursing and Midwifery, Faculty of Medicine and Health, University of Sydney, NSW, Australia

Alister Hodge RN, NP, MN (Nurse Prac), MN (Emerg), PGCert (Crit Care), BN
Nurse Practitioner, Sutherland Hospital Emergency Department, Clinical Lecturer, School of Nursing, The University of Sydney, Sydney, NSW, Australia

Anastasia Hutchinson RN, BN, GradCert Crit Care, GradDipl, Clinical Epidemiology, PhD
Associate Professor Nursing (Research), Deakin University, Centre for Quality and Patient Safety Research Epworth/Deakin Partnership, Melbourne, VIC, Australia

Alison James RM, PhD, MSc, BSc (Hons), PG Cert Education
Associate Professor Midwifery (Education), University of Plymouth, Plymouth, UK

Lotta Johansson CCRN, PhD, Head Nurse
Care Unit Manager, Department of Intensive Care, Sahlgrenska University Hospital, Sweden

Alison Juers RN, BN, MClinicalNg (Crit Care)
Nurse Educator, Brisbane Private Hospital, Brisbane, QLD, Australia

Tina Kendrick RN, GradCert PIC Nursing, BNurs(Hons), MNurs
Clinical Nurse Consultant – Paediatrics
NSW Newborn and paediatric Emergency Transport Service (NETS)
Clinical Lecturer, School of Nursing, University of Tasmania, TAS, Australia

Ruth Kleinpell PhD, RN, FCCM, FAAN, FAANP
Assistant Dean of Clinical Scholarship; Professor, Vanderbilt University School of Nursing, Nashville, TN, USA

Leila Kuzmiuk RN, BN CPIT, DipAdvClinNursing, MN, GradCert Hlth Serv Mgt
Nurse Educator, Intensive Care Services, John Hunter Hospital, Hunter New England Health, NSW, Australia

Frances Lin RN, BMN, MN(Hons), PhD, FACCCN
Senior Lecturer, School of Nursing and Midwifery, Griffith University, QLD, Australia

Andrea P Marshall RN PhD
Professor of Acute and Complex Care Nursing, Gold Coast Health and Griffith University, Southport, QLD, Australia

Jennifer McGaughey RGN, RMN, ENB 100, RNT, BSc (Hons), MSc, PhD
Senior Lecturer in Critical Care Nursing, Queen's University Belfast, Belfast, UK

Elaine M[c]Gloin RN, Cert Crit Care, Cert Neonatal Intensive Care
Clinical Nurse Consultant, Royal Prince Alfred Hospital, Sydney, NSW, Australia

Marion Mitchell RN, BN(Hon), GradCert (Higher Ed), PhD
Professor of Critical Care and Higher Degree Research Convenor, School of Nursing and Midwifery, Menzies Health Institute Queensland, Griffith University and Princess Alexandra Hospital, Intensive Care Unit, Brisbane, QLD, Australia

Margherita Murgo BN, MN (Crit Care), Dip Proj Man
Senior Nursing Advisor, Australian Commission on Safety and Quality in Health Care, Honorary Clinical Lecturer, University of Sydney, Sydney, NSW, Australia

Ulrica Nilsson RNA, PhD
Professor, School of Health Sciences, Faculty of Medicine and Health, Orebro University, Orebro, Sweden

DaiWai M Olson PhD RN CCRN FNCS
Professor of Neurology and Neurotherapeutics, Professor of Neurosurgery, University of Texas Southwestern, Dallas, TX, USA

Frederique Paulus RN, PhD
Senior Researcher Department of Critical Care, Amsterdam University Medical Centers, Associate Professor Amsterdam University of Applied Sciences, Amsterdam, the Netherlands

Wendy Pollock RN, RM, GradCert Adv Learning and Leadership, GradDip Crit Care Nsg, Grad Dip Ed (tertiary), PhD
Director, Maternal Critical Care, Melbourne, VIC, Australia

Anne-Sylvie Ramelet, PhD, PICU Certificate
Professor, Institute of Higher Education and Research in Healthcare, Faculty of Biology and Medicine, University of Lausanne, Lausanne, Vaud, Switzerland

Janice Rattray RGN, SCM, DipN, MN, PhD,
Reader in Acute and Critical Care Nursing (Hon) School of Nursing and Health Sciences, University of Dundee, Dundee, UK

Adam Riedlinger RN, FHEA, BSc (Hons), PGCert (Clin Ed)
Lecturer and Practice Development Nurse, Florence Nightingale School of Nursing, Midwifery and Palliative Care, King's College London University and King's College Hospital, London, UK

Mona Ringdal RN (Crit Care) MN PhD
Professor (Associate) Nursing, Director of Studies, PhD program in Health and Care Sciences, Institute of Health and Care Sciences, Sahlgrenska Academy, Gothenburg University, Gothenburg, Sweden
Senior Nurse Consultant, Department of Anesthesiology, Kungälvs Hospital, Kungälvs, Sweden

Louise Rose RN, BN, GradCert ICU Nursing, GradCert Adult Ed, MN, PhD
Professor of Critical Care Nursing, Florence Nightingale Faulty of Nursing, Midwifery and Palliative Care, King's College London, London, UK

Michael Sampson RN, BSc (Hons), MA, NMP, FHEA
Senior Lecturer in Cardiac Nursing, London South Bank University, London, UK
Arrhythmia Nurse Specialist, St George's Hospital, London, UK

Kerstin Prignits Sluys PhD, APRN Intensive Care Trauma
Senior Lecturer, Associated Researcher, Karolinska Institutet, Stockholm, Sweden

Karen Smith RGN, PhD, BSc, PG cert HE
Nurse Consultant Cardiology, NHS Tayside and School of Nursing and Health Sciences, University of Dundee, Dundee, UK

Ged Williams RN, RM, Crit Care Cert, MHA, LLM, FACHSM, FACN, FAAN
Chief Nursing Officer, Al Mafraq Hospital, United Arab Emirates
Adjunct Professor of Nursing, Griffith University, QLD, Australia
Founding President, Australian College of Critical Care Nurses
Founding President, World Federation of Critical Care Nurses

Teresa Williams PhD(Distinction), MHSci(Res), PGDip ClinEpi, BN, RN
Adjunct Appointment Clinical Research, Intensive Care Unit, Royal Perth Hospital, Perth, WA, Australia

Denise Wilson RN, PhD, MA(Hons), BA(SocSc)
Professor Māori Health, Auckland University of Technology, Auckland, New Zealand

List of reviewers

Adeniyi O Adeleye RN, GCertHServMgt, GradDipCritCareNurs, GradDipHL, MPH, PhD Candidate
Lecturer, School of Nursing, Midwifery and Social Sciences, CQ University, Mackay City, QLD, Australia

Anthony Cignarella RN, MN(Hons), BN(Hon), BAppSci(OT), GradCertIntCareN, GradCertHE
Lecturer Practitioner (ICU), La Trobe University Alfred Clinical School, VIC, Australia
Clinical Nurse Educator, Intensive Care Unit, Alfred Hospital, VIC, Australia

Elyse Coffey RN, BaNurs(Hon), MNurs (Perianaesthesia)
Lecturer, School of Nursing and Midwifery, Deakin University, Melbourne, VIC, Australia

Lorna A Davies RN, MA, BA(Hons), PGDip Periop, DTLT
Senior Nursing Lecturer, Ara Institute of Canterbury, Christchurch, New Zealand

Lori Delaney RN, PhD Candidate, MIHM, MN, GradDip CritCare, GradCert Ed, BN
Lecturer in Nursing, Queensland University of Technology, Brisbane, QLD, Australia

Rachel Euler RN, BHSc(Nurs), GCert RIPRN, Master ANP(Emerg)
Associate Lecturer, School of Nursing, CQ University, Mackay, QLD, Australia

Lyn Francis RN, MHM, CM, LLB, LLM, PhD
School of Nursing and Midwifery, Western Sydney University, NSW, Australia

Malcolm Green RN, BN, MN (Critical Care)
Senior Manager, Adult Patient Safety Program, Clinical Excellence Commission, NSW, Australia

Rebecca J Jarden RN, MN, PhD candidate
Lecturer and Course Coordinator Graduate Certificate in Critical Care, Department of Nursing, University of Melbourne, Melbourne, VIC, Australia

Rose Jaspers RN, MN(Crit Care)
Lecturer/Course Coordinator in Master of Advanced Clinical Nursing (Intensive Care), Monash University, VIC, Australia

Rita Maurice RN, BSc Nursing (General), GradCert Critical Care Nursing
Clinical Nurse, Intensive Care Unit, Fiona Stanley Hospital, Murdoch, WA, Australia

Linda McKean, RN, Neonatal Trained, PGradDipNsg, GradDipHeath Professional Education, MNsg
University Associate: Stream Coordinator Graduate Certificate in Critical Care Nursing, School of Nursing, Midwifery and Paramedicine, Curtin University, Perth, WA, Australia

Anne McLeod RGN, BSc(Hons), MSc Crit Care, PGDip Teaching and Learning
Senior Lecturer in Critical Care, City, University of London, London, UK

Claire Minton, RN, MN, PhD
Senior Lecturer/Clinical Lead, School of Nursing, Massey University, Palmerston North, New Zealand

Blake Mulraney Masters Nursing Practice, BA, Grad Cert Clin Nursing, RN
National representative WA branch ACCCN, Perth, WA, Australia

Georgina Neville RN, BN, MN(Crit Care), GC Higher Ed, GradCert (Crit Care)
Lecturer, Bachelor of Nursing Program, School of Nursing and Midwifery, Griffith University, QLD, Australia

Miles Peters BNS, Med, GradCert (Crit Care), Grad Dip Leadership
Nurse Educator, Intensive Care Unit, Canterbury District Health Board, Christchurch, New Zealand

Evan Plowman RN, MN, GradCert Crit Care (ICU), BN/BClinPrac(Paramedics)
Lecturer in Nursing, School of Nursing, Midwifery and Indigenous Health, Charles Sturt University, NSW, Australia

David Thomas RN, MHA, Grad Cert in Critical Care, Grad Dip in Nurs
Nurse Unit Manager, Austin Health, Victoria, Australia

Ylona Chun Tie RN, BNSc, PGCertNsgSc(Int Care), MAdvNsgPrac, GCertHlthProfEd, PhD
Lecturer, Nursing and Midwifery, College of Healthcare Sciences, James Cook University, Townsville, Qld, Australia

Virginia Vandall-Walker CTN, CCD, PhD, RN
Associate Professor, Faculty of Health Disciplines Athabasca University, Athabasca, Canada
Adjunct Associate Professor, Faculty of Nursing University of Alberta, Alberta, Canada

Cindy Weatherburn MN, ICU, RN
Clinical Nurse Consultant, Royal Hobart Hospital, Tasmania, Hobart, TAS, Australia

Acknowledgements

A project of this nature and scope requires many talented and committed people to see it to completion. The decision to publish this fourth edition was supported enthusiastically by Elsevier Australia. To our chapter contributors for this edition, both those returning from the previous editions and our new collaborators – thank you for accepting our offer to write, for having the courage and confidence in yourselves and us to be involved in the text, and for being committed in meeting writing deadlines while developing the depth and quality of content that we had planned. We also acknowledge the work of chapter contributors from our previous edition – Denise Harris, Karena Conroy, Robyn Aitken, Robyn Gallagher, David Glanville, Judy Currey, Sharon Wetzig, Bronagh Blackwood, Rand Butcher, Diane Chamberlain, Gavin Leslie, Christopher Gordon, Julia Crilly, David Johnson, Ian Jacobs (deceased) and Emma Kingwell.

We acknowledge support from the staff at Elsevier Australia, our publishing partner. Thanks to our Content Strategist, Natalie Hunt, for guiding this major project; our Content Development Specialist, Martina Vascotto; and to Lynn Watt, our editor. To others who produced the high quality figures, developed and executed the marketing plan and undertook myriad other activities, without which a text such as this would never come to fruition, thank you. We acknowledge our external reviewers who devoted their time to provide insightful suggestions in improving the text and contributed to the quality of the finished product. We also acknowledge the role of ACCCN in reviewing the chapters and endorsing this text as a valuable resource for critical care nurses.

Finally, and most importantly, to our respective loved ones – Steve; David, Abi and Hannah; and Michael – thanks for your belief in us, and your understanding and commitment in supporting our careers.

Leanne **Aitken**
Andrea **Marshall**
Wendy **Chaboyer**

Detailed contents

Abbreviations

AACN	American Association of Critical-Care Nurses
ABG	arterial blood gas
A/C	assist control ventilation
ACCCN	Australian College of Critical Care Nurses
ACCESS	assistance, coordination, contingency, education, supervision, support
ACEI	angiotensin-converting enzyme inhibitor
ACh	acetylcholine
ACPO	acute cardiogenic pulmonary oedema
ACS	abdominal compartment syndrome
ACS	acute coronary syndrome
ACT	activated clotting time
ACTR	Australian Clinical Trial Registry
ADAPT	Australasian Donation Awareness Program
ADH	antidiuretic hormone
ADL	activities of daily living
AE	adverse event
AED	automatic external defibrillator
AF	atrial fibrillation
AFE	amniotic fluid embolism
AHF	acute heart failure
AIS	Abbreviated Injury Score
AIVR	accelerated idioventricular rhythm
AKI	acute kidney injury
ALF	acute liver failure
ALI	acute lung injury
ALS	advanced life support
ALT	alanine amino transferase
AMI	acute myocardial infarction
AMR	antimicrobial resistance
ANP	atrial natriuretic peptide
ANS	autonomic nervous system
ANZBA	Australia and New Zealand Burns Association
ANZICS	Australian and New Zealand Intensive Care Society
ANZOD	Australia and New Zealand Organ Donation
AoCLF	acute-on-chronic liver failure
AODR	Australian Organ Donor Register
AOTA	Australian Organ and Tissue Authority
AP	anteroposterior
APACHE	Acute Physiology And Chronic Health Evaluation (score)
APC	activated protein C
APH	antepartum haemorrhage
APRV	airway pressure release ventilation
APTT	activated partial thromboplastin time
AQoL	Assessment of Quality of Life
ARAS	ascending reticular activating system
ARB	angiotensin receptor blocker
ARC	Australian Resuscitation Council
ARDS	acute respiratory distress syndrome
ARF	acute renal failure
ARNI	angiotensin receptor neprilysin inhibitor
ARP	absolute refractory period
aSAH	aneurysmal subarachnoid haemorrhage
ASL	arterial spin labelling
AST	aspartate aminotransferase
ATN	acute tubular necrosis
ATP	adenosine triphosphate
ATP	anti-tachycardia pacing
ATS	Australasian Triage Scale
AV	arteriovenous
AV	atrioventricular
AVPU	awake verbal pain unresponsiveness score
AVNRT	atrioventricular nodal reentry tachycardia
AVRT	atrioventricular reentrant tachycardia
AWS	alcohol withdrawal syndrome
BACCN	British Association of Critical Care Nurses
BACPR	British Association for Cardiovascular Prevention and Rehabilitation
BAEDP	balloon-assisted end-diastolic pressure
BBB	blood–brain barrier
BBV	blood-borne viruses
BE	base excess
BiPAP	bi-phasic positive airways pressure
BIS	bispectral index
BLS	basic life support
BMI	body mass index
BNP	B-type natriuretic peptide
BP	blood pressure
BPS	Behavioural Pain Scale
BSLTx	bilateral sequential lung transplantation
BTF	Brain Trauma Foundation
BURP	backwards, upwards, rightward pressure
CABG	coronary artery bypass graft
CACCN	Canadian Association of Critical Care Nurses
CAM-ICU	Confusion Assessment Method for the Intensive Care Unit
CAP	community-acquired pneumonia
CAUTI	catheter-associated urinary tract infection

CAV cardiac allograph vasculopathy
CAVH continuous arteriovenous haemofiltration
CBF cerebral blood flow
CBV cerebral blood volume
CCRN critical care registered nurse
CCU coronary/cardiac care unit
CDSS clinical decision support systems
CHD congenital heart disease
CHD coronary heart disease
CHF congestive heart failure
CHF chronic heart failure
CI cardiac index
CICM College of Intensive Care Medicine of Australia and New Zealand
CIM critical illness myopathy
CINM critical illness neuromyopathy
CIP critical illness polyneuropathy
CK creatine kinase
CLAB central line-associated bacteraemia
CLABSI central line associated blood stream infection
CMV controlled mandatory ventilation
CMV cytomegalovirus
CN cranial nerve
CNC clinical nurse consultant
CNE clinical nurse educator
CNM clinical nurse manager
CNPI Checklist of Non-verbal Pain Indicators
CNS central nervous system
CO cardiac output
CO_2 carbon dioxide
CONSORT Consolidated Standards of Reporting Trials
COPD chronic obstructive pulmonary disease
COPE Committee of Publication Ethics
CPAP continuous positive airway pressure
CPB cardiopulmonary bypass
CPG clinical practice guidelines
CPOE computerised provider order entry
CPOT Critical-care Pain Observation Tool
CPP cerebral perfusion pressure
CPR cardiopulmonary resuscitation
CR cardiac rehabilitation
CRE carbapenem-resistant Enterobacteriaceae
CRRT continuous renal replacement therapy
CRT cardiac resynchronisation therapy
CSF cerebral spinal fluid
CT computerised tomography
CTA computed tomography angiography
CTAS Canadian Triage and Acuity Scale
CTG cardiotocograph
CUSP Comprehensive Unit-Based Safety Program
CVAD central venous access device
CVC central venous catheter
CVP central venous pressure
CVR cerebrovascular resistance
CVVH continuous venovenous haemofiltration
CVVHDf continuous venovenous haemodiafiltration
CX circumflex coronary artery
CXR chest X-ray
DAVID Dual Chamber and VVI Implantable Defibrillator (trial)
DCD donation after cardiac death
DCM dilated cardiomyopathy
DCR damage-control resuscitation
DCR direct current reversion
DCS damage-control surgery
DES drug eluting stents
DIC disseminated intravascular coagulation
DIEP deep inferior epigastric perforators
DKA diabetic ketoacidosis
DLT double lumen endotracheal tubes
DN dicrotic notch
DNA deoxyribonucleic acid
DNAR do not attempt resuscitation
DPL diagnostic peritoneal lavage
DRG Diagnostic Related Groups
DTS Davidson Trauma Scale
DVT deep vein thrombosis
EAR expired air resuscitation
EBN evidence-based nursing
EC extracorporeal circuit
ECC external cardiac compressions
ECG electrocardiography
ECMO extracorporeal membrane oxygenation
ED emergency department
EDIMCU emergency department intermediate care unit
EDP end-diastolic pressure
EE energy expenditure
EEG electroencephalogram/ electroencephalography
EfCCNa European federation of Critical Care Nursing associations
EGDT early goal-directed therapy
EMS emergency medical service
EMSB early management of severe burns
EN enteral nutrition
EPAP expiratory positive airway pressure
EPUAP European Pressure Ulcer Advisory Panel
EoL end-of-life
ER emergency room
ERC European Resuscitation Council
ESI emergency severity index
ESICM European Society of Intensive Care Medicine
ESRD end-stage renal disease
ET endothelin

$ETCO_2$	end-tidal carbon dioxide
ETT	endotracheal tube
ETT	exercise tolerance testing
EU	European Union
EVD	external ventricular drain
EVLW	extravascular lung water
EVLWI	extravascular lung water index
F	frequency
FAST	focused assessment with sonography in trauma
FBC	full blood count
FCC	family-centred care
FES	fat embolism syndrome
FFP	fresh frozen plasma
FH	fetal heart
FIM	Functional Independence Measure
FiO_2	fraction of inspired oxygen
FLACC	Faces Legs Activity Cry Consolability (scale)
FMEA	failure mode and effect analysis
FOUR	Full Outline of Unresponsiveness scale
FPDR	family presence during resuscitation
FRC	functional residual capacity
FTE	full time equivalent (staff)
f/V_T	frequency/tidal volume
FVC	forced vital capacity
FWR	free wall rupture
GABA	gamma-aminobutyric acid
GBS	Guillain–Barré syndrome
GCS	Glasgow Coma Scale
GEDV	global end-diastolic volume
GEDVI	global end-diastolic volume index
GFR	glomerular filtration rate
GGT	gamma-glutamyl-transpeptidase
GOAT	Galveston orientation amnesia test
GP	general practitioner
GRACE	Global Registry of Acute Events
GRV	gastric residual volume
GTN	glyceryl trinitrate
H^+	hydrogen ion
H_2CO_3	carbonic acid
H_2RA	histamine-2 receptor antagonist
HADS	Hospital Anxiety and Depression Scale
HAI	hospital-acquired/healthcare-acquired infection
Hb	haemoglobin
HCM	hypertrophic cardiomyopathy
HCO_3^-	bicarbonate ion
HD	haemodialysis
HDU	high dependency unit
HE	hepatic encephalopathy
HELLP	haemolysis, elevated liver enzymes and low platelets
HEPA	high-efficiency particulate air
HFO	high-flow oxygen
HFOV	high-frequency oscillation ventilation
HFpEF	heart failure with preserved ejection fraction
HFrEF	heart failure with reduced ejection fraction
HHS	hyperosmolar hyperglycaemic state
Hib	*Haemophilus influenzae* type b
HIV	human immunodeficiency virus
HLA	human leucocyte antigen
HME	heat and moisture exchanger
HOB	head of bed
HR	heart rate
HRC	Health Research Council
HRECs	Human Research Ethics Committees
HRQOL	health-related quality of life
HRS	hepatorenal syndrome
HSV	herpes simplex virus
I	inspiration
IABP	intra-aortic balloon pump
IAC	interposed abdominal compression
IAD	incontinence-associated dermatitis
IAH	intraabdominal hypertension
IAP	intraabdominal pressure
ICC	intercostal catheter
ICD	implantable cardioverter defibrillator
ICDSC	Intensive Care Delirium Screening Checklist
ICH	intracerebral haemorrhage
ICN	International Council of Nurses
ICON	Intensive Care Over Nations
ICP	intracranial pressure
ICS	Intensive Care Society (UK)
ICU	intensive care unit
ICU-AW	intensive care unit-acquired weakness
IDC	indwelling catheter
I:E	inspiratory/expiratory ratio
IE	infective endocarditis
IES	Impact of Event Scale
IHCA	in-hospital cardiac arrests
IHPA	Independent Hospital Pricing Authority
IL	interleukin
ILCOR	International Liaison Committee on Resuscitation
ILV	independent lung ventilation
IM	intramuscular
IMA	internal mammary artery
IMD	invasive meningococcal disease
INR	international normalised ratio
IP	inflation point
IPAP	inspiratory positive airway pressure
i-PARIHS	integrated Promoting Action on Research Implementation in Health Services
IPAT	Intensive Care Psychological Assessment Tool

IPC intermittent pneumatic compression
ISS injury severity score
ITBV intrathoracic blood volume
ITBVI intrathoracic blood volume index
IV intravenous
IVC inferior vena cava
JVP jugular venous pressure
KDIGO Kidney Diseases Improving Global Outcomes
kPa kilopascals
KT knowledge translation
LAD left anterior descending
LAP left atrial pressure
LBBB left bundle branch block
LDB load-distributing band
LiDCO lithium dilution cardiac output
LMA laryngeal mask airway
LMW low molecular weight
LMWH low molecular weight heparin
LN liaison nurse
LOS length of stay
LP lumbar puncture
LV left ventricle
LVAD left ventricular assist device
LVEDV left ventricular end-diastolic volume (preload)
LVEF left ventricular ejection fraction
LVF left ventricular failure
LVSWI left ventricular stroke work index
MAC mid-arm circumference
MAMC mid-arm muscle circumference
MAP mean arterial pressure
MARSI medical adhesive-related skin injuries
MASD moisture-associated skin damage
MCA middle cerebral artery
MCS mechanical circulatory support
MEDSAFE Medical Devices Safety Authority (New Zealand)
MELD model of end-stage liver disease
MERS Middle East respiratory syndrome
MERS-CoV Middle East respiratory syndrome coronavirus
MET medical emergency team
MERS Middle East respiratory syndrome
MI myocardial infarction
MIDCABG minimally invasive direct coronary artery bypass grafting
mmHg millimetres of mercury
MMSE Mini-Mental Status Examination
MODS multiple organ dysfunction syndrome
MRC Medical Research Council
MRI magnetic resonance imaging
MRO multi-resistant organism
MRSA methicillin-resistant *Staphylococcus aureus*
MTS Manchester Triage Scale
MV mechanical ventilation
MV minute ventilation
MVA motor vehicle accident
MVE Murray Valley encephalitis
NAS Nursing Activities Score
NAVA neurally adjusted ventilatory assist
NEMS Nine Equivalents of nursing Manpower use Score
NETS newborn emergency transfer service
NEXUS National Emergency X-radiography Utilization Study
NFkB nuclear factor kappa B
NFR not for resuscitation
NGAL neutrophil gelatinase-associated lipocalin
NHBD non-heart-beating donor
NHMRC National Health and Medical Research Council
NHS National Health Service (UK)
NICE National Institute for Health and Care Excellence
NICU neonatal intensive care unit
NIPPV non-invasive positive pressure ventilation
NIPSV non-invasive pressure support ventilation
NIRS near-infrared spectroscopy
NIV non-invasive ventilation
NMDA N-methyl-D-aspartate
NO nitric oxide
NOC nurses' observation checklist
NOK next of kin (legally authorised representative)
NP nurse practitioner
NPC nurse practice coordinator
NPUAP National Pressure Ulcer Advisory Panel
NRT nicotine replacement therapy
NSAID non-steroidal anti-inflammatory drug
NTS National Triage Scale
NTS non-technical skills
NUM nursing unit manager
NUTRIC NUTritional RIsk in the Critically ill score
NYHA New York Heart Association
NWAU national weighted activity unit
O_2 oxygen
OHCA out-of-hospital cardiac arrest
OPCAB off pump coronary artery bypass
ONS oral nutrition supplements
ORIF open reduction internal fixation
OT operating theatre
OUD opioid use disorder
Pa arterial pressure
P_A alveolar pressure
PA phlebostatic axis
PA posterioanterior
PAC pulmonary artery catheter

P_aCO_2 partial pressure of carbon dioxide in arterial blood
PACU post-anaesthesia care unit
PAH pulmonary arterial hypertension
PaO_2 partial pressure of oxygen in arterial blood
$P_{BT}O_2$ partial pressure of brain tissue oxygen
PAOP pulmonary artery occlusion pressure
PAP pulmonary artery pressure
PAT Paediatric Assessment Triangle
PAV proportional assist ventilation
Paw airway pressure
PAWP pulmonary artery wedge pressure
PAWSS Prediction of Alcohol Withdrawal Severity Scale
$PbtO_2$ brain tissue oxygenation
PCA patient-controlled analgesia
PCI percutaneous coronary intervention
PCM protein-calorie malnutrition
PCP phencyclidine
PCR polymerase chain reaction
PCV pressure-controlled ventilation
PCWP pulmonary capillary wedge pressure
PD peritoneal dialysis
PDH pulmonary dynamic hyperinflation
PDP peak diastolic pressure
PE pulmonary embolism
PEA pulseless electrical activity
PEEP positive end-expiratory pressure
PELD paediatric end-stage liver disease
PEP Professional Education Package
PER passive external re-warming
PET positron emission tomography
$PetCO_2$ partial pressure of end-tidal carbon dioxide
PFIT Physical Function ICU Test
PGD primary graft dysfunction
pH acid–alkaline logarithmic scale
PI pressure injury
PI pulsatility index
PiCCO pulse-induced contour cardiac output
PICS post-intensive care syndrome
PICU paediatric intensive care unit
PIH pregnancy-induced hypertension
PIP peak inspiratory pressure
P_{insp} inspiratory pressure
PLR pupillary light reflex
PMCS perimortem caesarean section
PMIP post-MI pericarditis
PN parenteral nutrition
PND paroxysmal nocturnal dyspnoea
PNS peripheral nervous system
PPE personal protective equipment
PPH postpartum haemorrhage
PPI proton pump inhibitors
PR pulse rate
pRIFLE paediatric risk, injury, failure, loss and end-stage kidney disease criteria
PRO patient-reported outcomes
PROM patient-reported outcome measures
PROQOLID Patient-reported Outcome and Quality of Life Instruments Database
PS pressure support
PSG polysomnography
PSI Pneumonia Severity Index
PSP peak systolic pressure
PSV pressure support ventilation
PT prothrombin
PTA post-traumatic amnesia
PTCA percutaneous transluminal coronary angioplasty
PTSD post-traumatic stress disorder
PTSS post-traumatic stress symptoms
PTT partial thromboplastin time
PV per vagina
Pv venous pressure
PVC premature ventricular contraction
PVI pulmonary vein isolation
PVR pulmonary vascular resistance
R respiration
RAAS renin–angiotensin–aldosterone system
RAP right atrial pressure
RASS Richmond Agitation Sedation Scale
RBANS Repeatable Battery for the Assessment of Neuropsychological Status
RBC red blood cells
RCA right coronary artery
RCM restrictive cardiomyopathy
RCSQ Richards–Campbell Sleep Questionnaire
RCT randomised controlled trial
RDC regional donor coordinator
REE resting energy expenditure
REM rapid eye movement
RICA right internal carotid artery
RCA root cause analysis
REBOA resuscitative endovascular balloon occlusion of the aorta
RHD rheumatic heart disease
RM recruitment manoeuvres
RN registered nurse
ROSC return of spontaneous circulation
RR respiratory rate
RRP relative refractory period
RRS rapid response system
RRT rapid response team
RRT renal replacement therapy
RSV respiratory syncytial virus
RV right ventricular
RVEDV right ventricular end-diastolic volume

RVEDVI	right ventricular end-diastolic volume index
RVEF	right ventricular ejection fraction
RVESV	right ventricular end-systolic volume
RVF	right ventricular failure
RVSWI	right ventricular stroke work index
SA	sinoatrial node
SAB	*Staphylococcus aureus* bacteraemia
SAFE	Saline versus Albumin Fluid Evaluation
SAH	subarachnoid haemorrhage
SAI	State Anxiety Inventory
SAQ	Safety Attitudes Questionnaire
SaO_2	saturation of oxygen in arterial blood
SAPS	Simplified Acute Physiology Score
SARS	severe acute respiratory syndrome
SAS	Sedation-Agitation Scale
SBP	systolic blood pressure
SBS	State Behavioural Scale
SBT	spontaneous breathing trial
SCA	sudden cardiac arrest
SCD	sudden cardiac death
SCI	spinal cord injury
SCUF	slow continuous ultrafiltration
SE	status epilepticus
SEIPS	Systems Engineering Initiative for Patient Safety
SGA	subjective global assessment
SIADH	syndrome of inappropriate antidiuretic hormone
SICQ	Sleep in Intensive Care Questionnaire
SIMV	synchronised intermittent mandatory ventilation
SIRS	systemic inflammatory response syndrome
SjO_2	jugular venous oxygen saturation
SLED	slow low efficiency dialysis
SLS	sodium lauryl sulfate
SLTx	single lung transplantation
SNS	sympathetic nervous system
SOB	shortness of breath
SOBOE	shortness of breath on exertion
SOFA	sequential organ failure assessment
SOMANZ	Society of Obstetric Medicine of Australia and New Zealand
SPECT	single photon emission computed tomography
SpO_2	saturation of oxygen in peripheral tissues
SR	sinus rhythm
SSD	subglottic secretion drainage
ST	sinus tachycardia
STEMI	ST-elevation myocardial infarction
SV	stroke volume
SVG	saphenous vein graft
SvO_2	saturation of oxygen in venous system
SVR	systemic vascular resistance
SVT	supraventricular tachycardia
SWS	slow wave sleep
T_3	triiodothyronine
TAD	thoracic aortic dissection
TAVI	trans-catheter aortic valve implantation
TBI	traumatic brain injury
TBSA	total body (or burn) surface area
TBW	total body weight
TCD	transcranial Doppler
TdP	torsades de pointes
TEG	thromboelastograph
TENS	transcutaneous electrical nerve stimulation
TEVAR	thoracic endovascular aortic repair
TGA	Therapeutic Goods Administration
TIMI	thrombolysis in myocardial infarction
TIPS	transjugular intrahepatic portosystemic shunt/stent
TISS	Therapeutic Intervention Scoring System
TNF-α	tumour necrosis factor alpha
TOE	transoesophageal echocardiography
TPM	Transplant Procurement Management
TRALI	transfusion-related acute lung injury
TRAM	transverse rectus abdominis myocutaneous
TSANZ	Transplant Society of Australia and New Zealand
TST	total sleep time
TT	tube thoracostomy
UH	unfractionated heparin
ULR	underlying rhythm
UO	urine output
URTI	upper respiratory tract infection
VAD	ventricular assist device
VAE	ventilator-associated event
VAP	ventilator-associated pneumonia
VAS	visual analogue scale
VATS	video-assisted thorascopic surgery
VCA	vascularised composite allotransplantation
VCV	volume-controlled ventilation
VE	expired minute volume
VF	ventricular fibrillation
V/Q	ventilation/perfusion
VRE	vancomycin-resistant enterococci
V_T	tidal volume
VT	ventricular tachycardia
VTE	venous thromboembolism
WBC	white blood cells
WCC	white cell count
WFCCN	World Federation of Critical Care Nurses
WFSICCM	World Federation of Societies of Intensive and Critical Care Medicine
WHO	World Health Organization
WPW	Wolff–Parkinson–White (syndrome)
XeCT	xenon-enhanced computed tomography

Section 1

Scope of critical care

Chapter 1

Scope of critical care practice

Leanne Aitken, Wendy Chaboyer, Andrea Marshall

KEY WORDS

advanced practice nursing
clinical competence
clinical leadership
critical care education
critical care nursing
critical care research
evidence-based nursing
knowledge translation
nurse practitioner
roles of critical care nurses

Learning objectives

After reading this chapter you should be able to:

- describe the development of critical care nursing practice, education, research and professional activities
- discuss the influences on the development of critical care nursing as a discipline and the professional development of individual nurses
- discuss the education and professional development of critical care nurses
- outline the various roles available to nurses within critical care areas or in outreach services and examine how these roles influence the standard of care
- discuss the role of research in the development of critical care nursing, including strategies to achieve evidence-based practice
- analyse the leadership attributes and strategies that are likely to be effective in the critical care practice setting.

Introduction

For over 50 years critical care services have been supporting the sickest of patients and today they are available in most countries in the world.[1] Although the focus was originally at local, regional and national levels, there is now an imperative for a strong international focus for the delivery of critical care services. International collaborations are necessary for responding to events that result in a sudden increased need for critical care services, including pandemics and disasters.[2,3] The term 'critical care' is used in different ways in different contexts; although critical care can be considered to include practice in the emergency department in some contexts, in this text we are primarily focusing on practice in intensive care (including all specialties) and coronary care settings.

There is unprecedented demand for critical care services globally. Increasing population sizes and extended life expectancies mean that the projected need for critical care beds will continue to increase.[4] The number of intensive care unit (ICU) beds available varies between countries. When considering only high-income countries, a range of 3 beds per 100,000 population in the

UK up to 25 beds per 100,000 in Germany has been reported.[1] Similar data related to low to middle-income countries is not available, but it is recognised far fewer resources exist. These figures frequently do not include patients admitted to coronary care, paediatric or other specialty units, so the overall clinical activity for 'critical care' is much higher in many countries. Survival in critically ill patients is high, with approximately 80% of patients surviving to be discharged out of acute hospital.[5] Importantly, critical care treatment is a high-expense component of hospital care. Various cost estimates have been conducted over the past 6–8 years, with European costs estimated to be between €1168 and €2025 per day for direct ICU costs[6] with very similar costs reported in the USA at $US2636 (approximately €2100) per ICU day.[7] Approximately two-thirds of these costs are for staff, with the remainder spread between clinical consumables, diagnostic procedures, hotel and nutritional costs.[6] In European countries a direct cost analysis suggests the daily ICU cost is approximately €1425,[8] while in developing countries such as India the cost is substantially less (approximately US$200 per day),[9] although this continues to represent a substantial cost relative to the cost of living. The cost of critical care is, however, difficult to determine because there is no internationally agreed methodology, there is a wide variation in resource consumption by patients in different settings, and there are different models of care.[10] Further, survivors of critical illness continue to require healthcare resources at a higher rate than non-critically ill hospitalised patients for up to 5 years, and this ongoing cost to individuals and the healthcare system is not always recognised.[11]

This chapter provides a context for subsequent chapters, outlining some key principles and concepts for studying and practising nursing in a range of critical care areas. Development of the specialty is discussed, along with the professional development and evolving roles of critical care nurses in contemporary health care. The scope of critical care nursing is described including advanced practice roles and, specifically, the nurse practitioner role. Leadership, as it pertains to the practice and development of critical care nursing, is also reviewed.

Critical care nursing

Critical care as a specialty in nursing has developed significantly since its inception.[12] Importantly, the development of the specialty has occurred in concert with the development of intensive care medicine as a defined clinical specialty.[13] Critical care nursing is defined by the World Federation of Critical Care Nurses as:

> *Specialised nursing care of critically ill patients who have manifest or potential disturbances of vital organ functions and who need assistance, support and restoration to health or the delivery of pain management preparation for a dignified death.*[14]

Critically ill patients are those at high risk of actual or potential life-threatening health problems, and may be separated into different categories based on the severity of their health problems. Care of the critically ill can occur in a number of different locations in hospitals. Critical care is generally considered a broad term, incorporating subspecialty areas of emergency, coronary care, high-dependency, cardiothoracic, paediatric, surgical, neurological and general intensive care units.

Developing critical care nursing knowledge and practice

Critical care as a specialty emerged in the 1950s and 1960s in Australasia, North America, Europe and South Africa.[12,15-18] During these early stages, critical care consisted primarily of coronary care units for the care of cardiology patients, cardiothoracic units for the care of postoperative patients and general intensive care units for the care of patients with respiratory compromise. Later developments in renal, metabolic and neurological management led to the principles and context of critical care that exist today. Development of critical care nursing has been characterised by a number of features,[12] including:

- the development of a new, comprehensive partnership between nursing and medical staff
- the collective experience of a steep learning curve for nursing and medical staff
- the courage to work in an unfamiliar setting, caring for patients who are extremely sick – a role that required the development of higher levels of competence and practice
- a high demand for education specific to critical care practice, which was initially difficult to meet owing to the absence of experienced nurses in the specialty
- the development of technologies such as mechanical ventilators, cardiac monitors, pacemakers, defibrillators, dialysers, intra-aortic balloon pumps and cardiac assist devices, which prompted development of additional knowledge and skills.

There was also recognition that improving patient outcomes through optimal use of these technologies was linked to nurses' skills and staffing levels.[19] The role of adequately educated and experienced nurses in these units was recognised as essential from an early stage,[15] and led to the development of the nursing specialty of critical care. Although not initially accepted, nursing expertise, ability to observe patients and appropriate nursing intensity are now considered essential elements of critical care.[19,20]

As the practice of critical care nursing evolved, so did the associated areas of critical care nursing education and specialty professional organisations, of which there are at least 40 organisations across six continents.[21] The combination of adequate nurse staffing, observation of the patient and the expertise of nurses to consider the complete needs of patients and their families is essential to optimise the outcomes of critical care. As critical care continues to evolve, the challenge remains to combine excellence in nursing care with judicious use of technology to optimise patient and family outcomes.

Research

Research is fundamental to the development of nursing knowledge and practice. Research is a systematic inquiry using structured methods to understand an issue, solve a problem or refine existing knowledge. Qualitative research involves in-depth examination of a phenomenon of interest, typically using interviews, observation or document analysis, to build knowledge and enable depth of understanding. Qualitative data analysis is in narrative (text) form and involves some form of content or thematic analysis, with findings generally reported as narrative (words rather than numbers describe the research findings). In contrast, quantitative research involves the measurement (in numeric form) of variables of interest and the use of statistics to test hypotheses. Results of quantitative research are often reported in tables and figures, identifying statistically significant findings. One particular type of quantitative research, the randomised controlled trial (RCT), is used to test the effect of a new nursing intervention on patient outcomes. In essence, RCTs involve:

1. randomly allocating patients to receive either a new intervention (the experimental or intervention group) or an alternative or standard intervention (the control group).
2. delivering the intervention or alternative treatment measuring an a priori identified patient outcome.
3. statistical analyses are used to determine whether the new intervention is better for patients than the alternative treatment.

Mixed methods research has now emerged as an approach that integrates data from qualitative and quantitative research at some stage in the research process.[22] In mixed methods approaches, researchers decide on both the priority and sequence of qualitative and quantitative methods. In terms of priority, equal status may be given to both approaches. Priority is indicated by using capital letters for the dominant approach, followed by the symbols + and → to indicate either concurrent or sequential data collection, for example:

- QUAL + QUANT: both approaches are given equal status and data collection occurs concurrently.
- QUAL + quant: qualitative methods are the dominant approach and data collection occurs concurrently.
- QUAL → quant: the qualitative study is given priority and qualitative data collection will occur before quantitative data collection.

There are other mixed-methods classifications used. For example, Pluye and Hong[23] describe terms such as sequential exploratory, sequential explanatory and convergent mixed methods designs. For more details refer to their publication.

Irrespective of which type of research design is used, there are several common steps in the research process (Table 1.1), consisting of three phases: planning for the research, undertaking the research and analysing and reporting the research findings.

While not all nurses are expected to conduct research, it is a professional responsibility to use research in practice.[24] Each chapter in this text contains a research critique to assist nurses in developing critical appraisal skills, which will help to determine whether research evidence should change practice.

Evidence-based nursing

Evidence-based nursing (EBN) is the 'application of valid, relevant, research-based information in nurse decision-making'.[27] Research evidence, however, is only one of four considerations in making a clinical decision. Three other considerations include: 1) knowledge of patients' conditions (i.e. preferences and symptoms); 2) the nurses' clinical expertise and judgement; and 3) the context in which the decision is taking place (i.e. setting, resources). Fig. 1.1 provides a schematic representation of EBN, using an example of a decision about weaning a patient from a mechanical ventilator. EBN has emerged as a way to improve nursing practice by considering the care that nurses give to patients, and whether this care results in the best possible outcomes for patients. Over the past few decades, recognition that EBN is more complex than simply focusing on knowledge to inform clinical decision making has emerged. This has led to a focus on better understanding about the challenges in changing clinical practice in order to use this evidence. As a result, knowledge translation has emerged as a means to bridge the evidence-practice gap.

Knowledge translation

Clinicians, quality improvers and researchers have identified that, despite high quality evidence, it is very difficult to get this evidence into practice (i.e. change clinicians' behaviour). As a result of this, knowledge translation (KT) and implementation science have developed to try to guide this process. KT has been defined by the Canadian Institutes of Health Research as a dynamic and iterative process that includes the synthesis, dissemination, exchange and ethically sound application of knowledge to improve health, provide more effective health services and products, and strengthen the healthcare system.[28] This definition has been widely adopted including by the World Health Organization.[28] KT is recognised as integral to incorporate evidence into clinical practice. Some authors distinguish between KT and implementation science, which has been defined as the scientific study of methods to promote the systematic

TABLE 1.1
Steps in the research process

PHASE	STEP	DESCRIPTION
Planning the research	Identify a clinical problem or issue	Clinical experience and practice audits are two ways that clinical issues or problems can be identified.
	Review the literature	A comprehensive literature review is vital to ensure that the issue or problem has not yet been solved and that the proposed research builds on what is already known, and extends it to fill a gap in knowledge
	Develop a clear research question	A precise question may follow either of two approaches: 1 PICO (population, intervention, comparator, outcome)[25] 2 SPIDER (sample, phenomenon of interest, design, evaluation, research type)[26]
	Write a research proposal	Write a clear description of the proposed research design and sample and a plan for data collection and analysis. Ethical considerations and the required resources (i.e. budget and personnel) for the research should be identified
	Secure resources	Resources such as funding for supplies and research staff, institutional support and access to experienced researchers are needed to ensure a study can be completed. Plans for how to access the relevant type and number of study participants should also be considered.
	Obtain ethics and governance approvals	Approval of the proposed research by a human research ethics committee (HREC) is required before the study can commence. Some jurisdictions also require institutional governance approval
Undertaking the research	Conduct the research	Adequate time for recruitment of participants, data collection and analysis are crucial to ensure that valid and relevant data are obtained
Analysing and reporting the research	Data analysis	Ensure the analyst has the appropriate skills to conduct the analysis. The data analysis plan developed in the first phase (write the research proposal) should be followed. If there are deviations, there should be a clear rationale for these deviations
	Disseminate the research findings	Discussion of the results and implications for practice with clinicians within the study site should occur as soon as possible. Distribution of a brief summary of the results is also frequently provided to study participants. Conference presentations and journal publications are two additional ways that research findings are disseminated and are vital to ensure that both nursing practice and nursing knowledge continue to be developed

uptake of research findings and other evidence-based practices into routine practice, and hence, to improve the quality and effectiveness of health services and care.[29] Thus, KT is often viewed as the process used to bridge the evidence–practice gap, and implementation science is viewed as the formal study of how this can be done.

Over the past 10–15 years, there has been a plethora of theories, models and frameworks developed to guide KT.[30] Some have come from disciplines such as psychology, sociology and marketing while others have been developed by researchers focusing their work on KT and implementation science. As one example, the integrated Promoting Action on Research Implementation in Health Services (i-PARIHS) framework was developed by a group of nurse researchers in the late 1990s[31] and has continued to evolve.[32] According to i-PARIHS, successful implementation of evidence into practice results from facilitation of an evidence-based innovation with the intended recipients of the implementation in their local, organisational and health system context.[32] *Innovation* refers to a change in clinical practice informed by research evidence. *Context* is defined as the environment or setting in which the proposed change is to be implemented. The *Recipients* are people affected by and influence implementation. *Facilitation* is defined as the techniques (coaching, managing group processes and conflict etc.) used by individuals (facilitators) to help people understand what they need to change and how they change to achieve a desired outcome.[32]

Another very practical approach to KT is the four-step process,[33] which consists of a series of guiding questions, to select the implementation strategy. In essence, this implementation strategy is the 'intervention' that will be used to change clinicians' behaviour. These four steps and associated tasks are displayed in Table 1.2 and are considered very useful and straightforward.[34]

FIGURE 1.1 Schematic representation of evidence-based nursing including an example of weaning from mechanical ventilation.

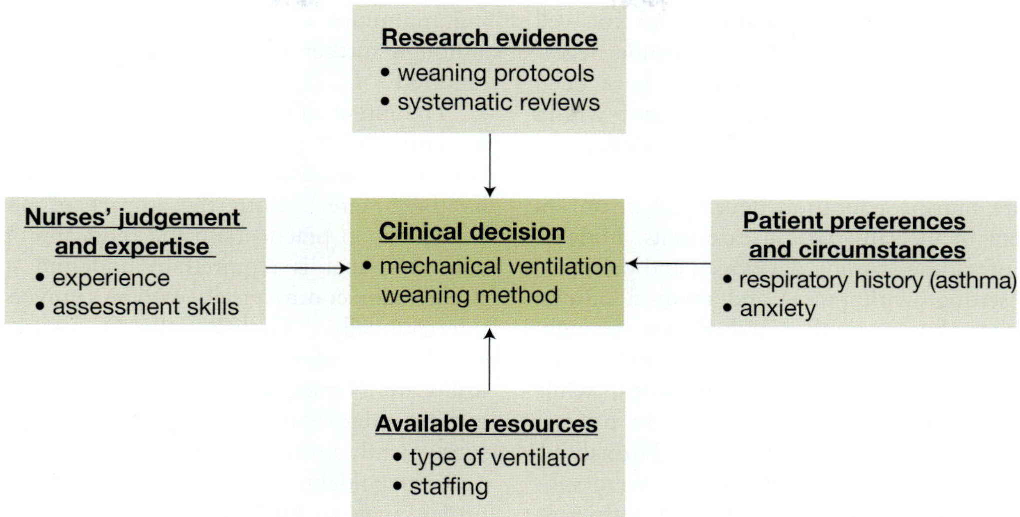

TABLE 1.2
Steps for developing a theory-informed implementation intervention[33]

STEP	TASKS
STEP 1: Who needs to do what, differently?	• Identify the evidence–practice gap • Specify the behaviour change needed to reduce the evidence–practice gap • Specify the health professional group whose behaviour needs changing
STEP 2: Using a theoretical framework, which barriers and enablers need to be addressed?	• From the literature, and experience of the development team, select which theory(ies), or theoretical framework(s) are likely to inform the pathways of change • Use the chosen theory(ies), or framework, to inform the pathways of change and the possible barriers and enablers to that pathway • Use qualitative and/or quantitative methods to identify barriers and enablers to behaviour change
STEP 3: Which intervention components (behaviour change techniques and model(s) of delivery) could overcome the modifiable barriers and enhance the enablers?	• Use the chosen theory, or framework, to identify potential behaviour change techniques to overcome the barriers and enhance the enablers • Identify evidence to inform the selection of potential behavior change techniques and modes of delivery • Identify what is likely to be feasible, locally relevant, and acceptable and combine identified components into an acceptable intervention that can be delivered.
STEP 4: How can behaviour change be measured and understood?	• Identify mediators of change to investigate in the proposed pathways of change • Select appropriate outcome measures • Determine feasibility of outcomes to be measured

Reproduced with permission from French SD, Green SE, O'Connor DA, et al. Developing theory-informed behaviour change interventions to implement evidence into practice: a systematic approach using the Theoretical Domains Framework. Implement Sci 2012;7(1):38. doi:10.1186/1748-5908-7-38.

There are many more theories, models and frameworks that can be used when trying to bridge the evidence-practice gap.[30,35,36] Importantly, research evidence has shown how difficult this task is and the need to use some theoretical foundation upon which to base implementation strategies.[35] Simply educating health care professionals is not enough to change practice.

Education

Appropriate preparation of specialist critical care nurses is a vital component in providing quality care to patients and their families.[37] A central tenet within this framework of preparation is the formalised education of nurses to practise in critical care areas.[38] Formal education – in conjunction with experiential learning, continuing professional development and training and reflective clinical practice – is required to develop competence in critical care nursing, although how this is achieved across different international contexts is inconsistent and not well understood.[39] The knowledge, skills and attitude necessary for quality critical care nursing practice have been articulated in competency statements[37,40–42] and within certification processes that recognise the knowledge and expertise of critical care nurses.[43,44]

Critical care nursing education developed in unison with the advent of specialist critical care units. Initially, this consisted of ad hoc training developed and delivered in the work setting, with nurses and medical officers learning together. For example, medical staff brought expertise in physiology, pathophysiology and interpretation of electrocardiographic rhythm strips, while nurses brought expertise in patient care and how patients behaved and responded to treatment.[19] Formalised, post-registration critical care nursing courses were subsequently developed from the early 1960s in both Australasia and the UK.[12,15] Today there are a number of different approaches to educating critical care nurses. For example, in the USA nurses are required to work in a critical care area providing direct patient care for a minimum of 1750 hours before they are eligible to sit the Critical Care Registered Nurse (CCRN) exam.[44] In Australia and New Zealand, postgraduate qualifications in critical care are provided through tertiary education providers.[39] Although variability within these programs is recognised, many incorporate clinical components and are conducted in conjunction with healthcare providers.

In the UK, similar provisions for postgraduate critical care nursing education at multiple levels are available, although some universities also offer critical care specialisation at the undergraduate level (for example, City, University of London). In Europe, The World Health Organization has published a curriculum for critical care nursing which specifies completion of a postgraduate specialty qualification in critical or intensive care nursing as necessary for qualification as a critical care nurse.[45] In the European setting education has also undergone significant change over the last decade as the framework articulated under the Bologna Process has become a more widespread strategy to ensure comparability in the standards and quality of higher education qualifications.[46] In relation to critical care nursing, this has led to the expansion of programs, primarily at the postgraduate level, for specialist nursing education. Critical care nursing education in North America maintains a slightly different focus, with most postgraduate studies being generic in nature, including a focus on advanced practice roles such as clinical nurse specialists and nurse practitioners, while specialty education for critical care nurses is undertaken as continuing education[47] or is completed through college- or hospital-based short courses.[48]

The diversity of critical care programs internationally has led to significant variability in programs and outcomes.[39] The recent development of the Standard of Practice and Evaluation of Critical-Care-Nursing Tool may be one strategy for assessing outcomes of critical care programs internationally by means of standardising minimum criteria for critical care qualifications,[49] although further international validation of this tool is required.

The intent of such programs is to improve outcomes for critically ill patients and their families yet, to date, consumer consultation to inform curricula development has been rare.[50] Both the impact of post-registration education on practice and the most appropriate level of education that is required to underpin specialty practice remain controversial, with no universal acceptance internationally.[39] Globally, the Declaration of Madrid, which was endorsed by the World Federation of Critical Care Nurses, provides a baseline for critical care nursing education. Originally developed in 1993 and subsequently updated in 2005, the Declaration of Madrid presents guidelines accepted worldwide by critical care professionals to guide education of critical care nurses. With the rapid changing of health delivery and critical care nursing practice, it would be timely to again revisit this position statement.

A range of factors continue to influence critical care nursing education provision, including government policies at national and state levels, funding mechanisms and resource implications for organisations and individual students, education provider and healthcare sector partnership arrangements, and tensions between workforce and professional development needs.[39,48]

Although postgraduate specialty specific education is recognised as a foundation for developing a strong knowledge base, it is also expected that critical care nurses engage in ongoing education and professional development. This is especially important given the rapidly developing nature of critical care practice and the plethora of research generated which is specific to the care and management of critically ill patients and their families. Ongoing learning may continue to occur through formal postgraduate education but the value of workplace learning,[51] continuing education in the form of short courses, and independent, self-directed learning is also recognised.[52] In our digital age, there are also many web-based education opportunities and resources to support learning. Many countries now incorporate requirements for continuing professional development into their annual licensing processes. Specific requirements include elements such as minimum hours of required professional development and/or ongoing demonstration of competence against predefined competency standards.

How we approach lifelong learning within the critical care context is an important consideration. Innovations in health professional education such as interprofessional and interdisciplinary learning,[53] simulated learning,[54] and use of innovative technologies including social media[55] are strategies to consider in the delivery of going education to critical care nurses.

Specialist critical care competencies

Critical care nursing involves a range of skills, classified as psychomotor (or technical), cognitive or interpersonal and performance of these skills requires special training and practice to enable proficiency. Clinical competence is a combination of personal traits, professional clinical practice, legal and ethical practice, ensuring safety and quality, communication, management of nursing care, leadership, teaching-coaching, cooperation and therapeutics practice, critical thinking and innovation, and professional development.[56] Although the concepts of competence are broad, they do need to be applied to the specific context in which the nurse is working.[57] Assessing the level of competency of a critical care nurse is challenging although ways of measuring competency are being explored.[58] All elements comprising the notion of competence are equally important in promoting quality critical care nursing practice.

Worldwide there are a number of practice standards published which are specific to critical care nursing.[41,59-61] Most practice standards build upon respective national registered nurse entry-to-practice standards[39] and although there are some differences in approaches, the common tenet of each set of practice standards is the goal of promoting the delivery of quality care to critically ill patients and their family. Common elements include patient and family-focused care, recognition of scope of practice and reflection, professional development, planning of care, leadership and evidence-based practice.[39]

Professional organisations

Professional leadership of critical care nursing has undergone considerable development in the past three decades. On an international level the World Federation of Critical Care Nurses (WFCCN) was formed in 2001 to provide professional leadership for the specialty so as to strengthen the influence and contribution that critical care nurses make globally through improved nursing practice.[14] Professional bodies that represent critical care nurses around the world are eligible to join the WFCCN. The role of the WFCCN is supported by regional bodies such as those that exist in Europe, South America, Asia and Africa.

At the country level more than 40 organisations exist to represent the interests of critical care nurses through improving education, communication and professional standards. The first of these professional organisations was formed in 1969 in the USA with the formation of the American Association of Cardiovascular Nurses, which, 2 years later, changed its name to the Association of Critical-Care Nurses (AACN).[62]

Within Australia, the Australian College of Critical Care Nurses (ACCCN, formerly the Confederation of Australian Critical Care Nurses) was formed from a number of preceding state-based specialty nursing bodies (e.g. the Australian Society of Critical Care Nurses, the Clinical Nurse Specialists Association) that had provided professional leadership for critical care nurses since the early 1970s. Similar organisations that have been formed for many years include the British Association of Critical Care Nurses (BACCN) and the Canadian Association of Critical Care Nurses (CACCN).

The professional bodies that exist to represent critical care nurses also have strong links with professional bodies representing their medical and allied health colleagues, including the World Federation of Societies of Intensive and Critical Care Medicine (WFSICCM) and various regional and country specific bodies. (See *Online resources* for further details about professional bodies and activities.)

Advanced practice nursing

'Advanced practice nursing' has been used as an umbrella term to designate various roles such as clinical nurse specialists, clinical nurse consultants and nurse practitioners (NPs).[63] In fact, recently, the distinction has been made between advanced *nursing practice* and *advanced practice* nursing. Advanced nursing practice is viewed as registered nurses who develop their professional knowledge and skills along a continuum from novice to expert in some area of practice such as critical care.[64] *Advanced practice* nursing reflects registered nurses who are legislated to practice at an advanced level, generally known as a NP.[64] The ICU Liaison/Outreach Nurse role exemplifies these related, and somewhat confusing, terms. Many papers have been published about the ICU Liaison/Outreach Nurse advanced practice role, reflecting it as an 'expert' nurse[65-67] (i.e. an example of *advanced nursing* practice) but over a decade ago, a paper was also published about the NP Outreach service[68] (i.e. an *advance practice* nursing role). This latter paper identified the legislated scope of practice for this NP role.

The International Council of Nursing (ICN) defines the nurse practitioner/advanced practice roles as a 'registered nurse who has acquired the expert knowledge base, complex decision-making skills and clinical competencies for expanded practice, the characteristics of which are shaped by the context and/or country in which she/he is credentialled to practice'.[69] The ICN notes that the education of nurse practitioners/advanced practice nurses is at an advanced level and is accredited or approved, with some form of licensure, registration, certification or credentialling. This description of nurse practitioners/advanced practice nurses should not be confused with specialist critical care nurses who are credentialled (i.e. *advanced nursing* practice). In some countries, including Australia, Canada and the USA, the nurse practitioner role is legislated.

The ICN[69] describes the nature of practice of nurse practitioners/advanced practice nurses as including a high degree of autonomy and independent practice. While the ICN acknowledges country specific regulation, it suggests nurse practitioners/advanced practice

TABLE 1.3
Global characteristics of the APRN role[74]

Right to diagnose
Authority to prescribe medication
Authority to prescribe treatment
Authority to refer clients to other health professionals
Authority to admit patients to hospital
Legislation to confer and protect the title 'Nurse Practitioner/ Advanced Practice Nurse'
Officially recognised titles for nurses working in advanced practice roles

Reproduced with permission from Kleinpell R, Scanlon A, Hibbert D, et al. Addressing issues impacting advanced nursing practice worldwide. Online J Issues Nurs 2014;19(2):1–13.

TABLE 1.4
Global challenges to the APRN role[74]

Limited access to educational programs
Insufficient nursing education
Focus on the medical model
Lack of understanding of the APRN role
Lack of respect towards the nursing profession
Dominance of the medical profession
Issues related to credentialling

Reproduced with permission from Kleinpell R, Scanlon A, Hibbert D, et al. Addressing issues impacting advanced nursing practice worldwide. Online J Issues Nurs 2014;19(2):1–13.

nurses will be able to diagnose, prescribe medications and treatments, refer clients to other health professionals and admit patients to hospital. Skills such as advanced health assessment and decision making are required. In Australia, new standards for practice for NP came into effect in 2014.[70] These standards encompass assessment using diagnostic capabilities, planning of care and engaging others in this planning, prescribing and implementing therapeutic interventions and evaluation of outcomes and improvements to practice.[71]

There are a number of nurse practitioner/advanced practice nursing roles in critical care. A review described three nurse practitioner roles: 1) adult, 2) paediatric and 3) neonatal.[72] The author described aspects of the role including direct patient management, assessment, diagnosis, monitoring and procedural activities.[72] Retrieval and trauma nurse practitioners have also emerged.[72,73] As part of her review, Fry[72] described the historical developments of the nurse practitioner role in critical care. She noted that the role was established in the USA in the 1960s, in the UK in the 1980s, in Canada and New Zealand in around 2000 and to some extent in Australia in 1995, although formal recognition of the nurse practitioner role did not occur in Australia until somewhat later.[72] More recently, Kleinpell and colleagues have described *advanced practice* nursing and advanced *nursing practice* roles from an international perspective.[74] Table 1.3 provides their summary of the global characteristics of the advanced practice nursing role, which is based on the International Council of Nursing's work in the area. Kleinpell and colleagues also provide a description of the global challenges to the advanced practice role in nursing, as shown in Table 1.4.

Nurse practitioners

There is a growing body of research on the NP role, which is generally distinguished by the legislated right to diagnose, prescribe medications and treatments, refer clients to other health professionals and admit patients to hospital. One recent observational study conducted in the USA compared patient outcomes when a nurse practitioner or a resident provided care to ICU patients.[75] All patients were overseen by an attending physician and a critical care fellow. The researchers found that there was no difference in 90-day survival or hospital mortality and ICU length of stay; however, ICU mortality and hospital length of stay were shorter for patients who were cared for by NPs.[75] Other US observational research has found that patient outcomes have not been negatively affected by the use of NPs,[76,77] although the latter study did find ICU length of stay was longer in the NP group. In addition to research focusing on patient outcomes associated with the NP role, there are numerous other studies published about the various aspects of NPs. For example, over a decade ago, a study of the services provided by a NP outreach nurse in New Zealand was published.[68] It described the activities the NP undertook during outreach visits to the wards, as well as an evaluation of the role, which showed that the NP outreach nurse was associated with fewer ICU readmissions within 72 hours.[68] UK authors provide a description of the activities undertaken by advanced NP in critical care.[78] They noted that NP time was most frequently spent on three activities: ward rounds 46%, documentation 19% and patient assessment 12% of their time. Other less time-consuming activities included data input, lines, blood and other.[78] Given these activities do not reflect extended role activities such as diagnosing, prescribing medications, and treatments and referrals to other health professionals, it is clear the NP role in the UK does not reflect the NP in the USA, Australia and New Zealand. A recent paper provides guidance on how one US hospital integrated the NP role into ICU, focusing on establishing the NP resources, recruitment and training, start-up preparation implementation, evaluation and feedback.[76] These authors note that neonatal, paediatric and adult ICUs had employed NP since the mid-1990s. Thus, there is a long history of NP in the ICU in the USA, but its adoption in other countries is more recent. For more information, see an overview of the developments in the advanced nursing practice role in various countries such as Australia, Canada, China (Hong Kong and Mainland China), Israel, the UK and Saudi Arabia, published in 2014.[74]

Leadership in critical care nursing

Effective leadership within critical care nursing is essential at several organisational levels, including the unit and hospital levels, as well as within the specialty on a broader professional scale. The leadership required at any given time and in any specific setting reflects the surrounding environment and the prevailing culture. Regardless of the setting, effective leadership involves having and communicating a clear vision – particularly one that represents excellence, motivating a team to achieve a common goal, communicating effectively with others, role modelling, meaningful recognition, creating and sustaining the critical elements of a healthy work environment and implementing change and innovation.[79-81] Leadership at the unit and hospital levels is essential to ensure excellence in practice, retention of a skilled and satisfied body of staff and adequate clinical governance. In addition to the generic strategies described above, it is essential for leaders in critical care units and hospitals to demonstrate a patient focus, establish and maintain excellence in standards of practice, and foster collaboration with other members of the multidisciplinary healthcare team. There is also recognition of the need for clinical leaders to have strong knowledge of the evidence base, and to use that knowledge to inform decisions and practices within the clinical environment.[82]

Leadership is essential to achieve growth and development in our specialty and is demonstrated through such activities as conducting research, producing publications, delivering conference presentations, representation on relevant government and healthcare councils and committees and participation in organisations such as the WFCCN, ACCCN, BACCN, AACN and the European federation of Critical Care Nursing associations (EfCCNa). As outlined earlier, we have seen the field of critical care grow from early ideas and makeshift units to a well-developed and highly organised international specialty in the course of a generation. Such development would not have been possible without the vision, enthusiasm and commitment of many critical care leaders throughout the world.

Leadership styles vary and are influenced by the mission and values of the organisation as well as the values and beliefs of individual leaders. These styles of leadership are described in many different ways, sometimes by using theoretical underpinnings such as 'transactional' and 'transformational' and sometimes by using leadership values and characteristics. Regardless of the terminology in use, some common principles can be expressed. Desired leadership characteristics include the ability to:

- articulate a personal vision and expectations
- inspire a shared vision that represents excellence
- act as a catalyst for change and be prepared to challenge the status quo
- establish and implement organisational standards
- model effective leadership behaviours through both change processes and stable contexts
- monitor practice in relation to standards and take corrective action when necessary
- recognise the characteristics and strengths of individuals, and stimulate and support individual development and commitment
- empower staff to act independently and interdependently.[79,80,83]

Personal characteristics of an effective leader, regardless of the style, include honesty, integrity, respect, commitment, credibility, courage and wisdom, as well as the ability to be approachable and supportive.[82,84] Effective leaders inspire their team members to take the extra step towards achieving the goals articulated by the leader and to feel that they are valued, independent, responsible and autonomous individuals within the organisation. Members of teams with effective leaders are not satisfied with maintaining the status quo but believe in the vision and goals articulated by the leader and are prepared to work towards achieving a higher standard of practice.

Although all leaders share common characteristics, some elements vary according to leadership style. Different styles – for example, transactional, transformational, authoritative or laissez faire – incorporate different characteristics and activities. Having leaders with different styles or a range of strengths and characteristics ensures that there is leadership for all stages of an organisation's operation or a profession's development. A combination of leadership styles also helps to overcome team member preferences and problems experienced when a particularly visionary leader leaves. The challenges often associated with the departure of a leader from a healthcare organisation are generally reduced in the clinical critical care environment, where a nursing leader is usually part of a multidisciplinary team, with resultant shared values and objectives.

Clinical leadership

Clinical leaders are those who provide leadership specifically within a clinical area; such leadership is an essential component of any effective team. It is generally accepted that effective clinical leaders require a combination of clinical expertise and leadership characteristics to perform this role to a high level.[85,86] Leadership characteristics that are considered particularly important for clinical leaders include creating a culture of collaboration, role modelling and creating a work environment that is conducive to delivering the highest quality of care to patients and their family.[82,87] Clinical leaders may or may not have formal authority vested in them, but are ultimately responsible for the quality and safety of patient care that is delivered within their clinical area. It is therefore essential that clinical leaders work within an effective interdisciplinary model, so that all aspects of patient care and family support, as well as the needs of all staff, are met.[86,88] Effective clinical leadership of critical care is essential in achieving:

- effective and safe patient care
- high quality, evidence-based healthcare
- satisfied patients and family members
- satisfied staff, with a high level of retention
- development of staff through an effective coaching and mentoring process.[82,89,90]

Effective clinical leaders build cohesive and adaptive work teams, and improve interdisciplinary collaboration.[88] They also promote the intellectual stimulation of individual staff members, which encourages the analysis and exploration of practice that is essential for evidence-based nursing.[90] Clinical leadership is particularly important in contemporary critical care environments in times of dynamic change and development. We are currently witnessing significant changes in the organisation and delivery of care, with the development of new roles such as the nurse practitioner (see this chapter) and liaison nurse (see Chapter 3), the introduction of services such as rapid response systems, including medical emergency teams (see Chapter 3) and the extension of activities across the care continuum (see Chapter 8). Effective clinical leadership ensures that:

- critical care personnel are aware of, and willing to fulfil, their changing roles
- personnel in other areas of the hospital or outside the hospital recognise the benefits and limitations of developments, are not threatened by the developments and are enthusiastic to use the new or refined services provided by critical care
- Staff are satisfied in their work setting, improving staff retention and reducing the need for high levels of staff turnover and the challenges associated with orientating large numbers of new staff
- patients receive optimal quality of care.[81,91]

The need to provide educational opportunities to develop effective clinical leadership skills is recognised.[80] Although not numerous in number or variety, programs are beginning to be available internationally that are designed to develop clinical leaders, both within the clinical environment and in partnership with higher education institutions.[92-94] Factors that influence leadership ability include the external and internal environment, demographic characteristics such as age, experience, understanding, stage of personal development including self-awareness capability and communication skills.[80,94] In relation to clinical leadership, at least some of the development of these factors must be in a clinical setting, so the development of clinical leaders should be based in that environment. Development programs based on mentorship, with strong academic support, are superbly suited to developing those that demonstrate potential for such capabilities.[93,95]

Mentorship has received significant attention in the healthcare literature and has been specifically identified as a strategy for clinical leadership development.[95-97] Although many different definitions of mentoring exist, common principles include a relationship between two people that incorporates mutual sharing, learning and acquisition of knowledge, usually for the purpose of helping one person in the relationship to develop new skills related to their career.[95] A related process might also be referred to as coaching.[96] Mentoring programs can be either formal or informal and either internal or external to the work setting. Mentorship involves a variety of activities directed towards facilitating new learning experiences for the mentee, guiding professional development and career decisions, providing emotional and psychological support and assisting the mentee in the socialisation process both within and outside the work organisation to build professional knowledge and networks.[96,97] Role modelling of occupational and professional skills and characteristics is an important component of mentoring that helps develop future clinical leaders.[95]

Summary

This chapter has provided a context for subsequent chapters, outlining some key issues, principles and concepts for practising and studying nursing in a range of critical care areas. Critical care nursing now encompasses a broad and ever-expanding scope of practice. The previous focus on patients in ICU only has given way to a broader concept of caring for an individual located in a variety of clinical locations across a continuum of critical illness.

The discipline of critical care nursing, in collaboration with multidisciplinary colleagues, continues to develop to meet the expanding challenges of clinical practice in today's healthcare environment. Critical care clinicians also continue their professional development individually, focusing on education and training and on practice improvement and research activities, to facilitate quality patient and family care during a time of acute physiological derangement and emotional turmoil. The principles of decision making and clinical leadership at all levels of practice serve to enhance patient safety in the critical care environment.

Case study

Assessment of central line-associated blood stream infections (CLABSI) is a core component of quality assessment processes in the ICU. CLABSI is a contributor to *Staphylococcus aureus* bacteraemia (SAB) infections and accounts for approximately one-third of hospital-acquired and preventable infections that can contribute to significant morbidity.[98] There is a significant cost implication for CLABSI rates with an estimated cost of AUD$14,886 per patient and extended hospital stay by 10 days. Worldwide, the development of CLABSI can contribute significantly to health system and patient costs.[99]

To minimise infection risk, clinical practice guidelines (CPG) from professional organisations are available and can be adapted to local requirements.[100] Although such guidelines are available and may be implemented within the ICU, variability in adherence to guideline recommendations can result higher rates of CLABSI.

Local surveillance of CLABSI is routinely undertaken in most ICUs and can often be benchmarked at a national level. In one ICU CLABSI rates were reported as 2.1 per 1000 line days – four times higher than the national average of 0.51 per 1000 line days and twice that of the national benchmark.[101] This increase in CLABSI rates led to the formation of a clinical–academic partnership designed to explore which factors were contributing to the increased CLABSI rate in this ICU.

An integrated knowledge translation approach[102] to this clinical issue allowed for a collaborative, context-specific approach to be used. For the 12-month period preceding the evaluation, we obtained baseline data including patient demographics, number of central lines inserted, CLABSI rates and service outcomes such as length of stay. Following the Ottawa Model of Research use, we first undertook a clinical audit of CVC insertion and management practices. Individual and group interviews were then undertaken to determine what factors either helped or hindered adherence to recommendations within current clinical practice guidelines. A summary of the process and actions is included in Table 1.5.

In summary, by using an integrated KT approach which incorporated multidisciplinary expertise of clinicians and academics we were able to undertake a systematic, data and theory-informed approach to practice change which ensured that interventions were developed to target key area of improvement. Ongoing evaluation through regular clinical audits will be undertaken to ensure adherence to guideline recommendations. The local guideline will continue to be revised to ensure it continues to reflect the most current and best evidence.

CASE STUDY QUESTION

1 Reflect on a recent approach to a change in your own clinical practice setting and consider what strategies were effective or not, and consider how these strategies could be improved using knowledge translation strategies in the future.

TABLE 1.5

Process and actions to improve adherence to CVC insertion and management recommendations

STEP	WHAT WE DID	FINDINGS
Step 1: Who needs to do what, differently?	• An audit of clinical practice on CVC insertion and management was undertaken to identify the evidence–practice gap • We were able to identify which recommendations for CVC insertion and management were done well and which needed to be improved, and by whom	Things done well • Daily chlorhexidine bath (100%); Flushing CVC port before and after giving medications (95.8%); using dedicated ports for PN (100%); blood transfusion management (100%); giving set changes (100%); CVC dressing change (100%); documentation (94%) Areas for improvement • CVC access ports cleaning time for 15 sec (8%); CVC ports allowed to air dry (68%); spare CVC ports flushed with normal saline (37%); crystalloid solutions changed every 24 hours (62.5%); lipid containing solutions changed every 12 hours (87.5%); propofol administration set changed every 6–12 hours (72.7%); labels changed for add-on solutions (70%), administration set change (82%), single infusion line (72%); documenting CVC depth at the skin (12%), CVC site appearance (24%); staff assisting with insertion wearing a hat (24%)

Continued

TABLE 1.5
Process and actions to improve adherence to CVC insertion and management recommendations—cont'd

STEP	WHAT WE DID	FINDINGS
Step 2: using a theoretical framework, which barriers and enablers need to be addressed?	• The Theoretical Domains Framework informed the development of specific questions to staff to help us identify what was helping and hindering adherence to specific recommendations	Facilitators 1 Explicit statement in protocol 2 Education 3 Reinforcement from senior staff including CNC and ACCESS nurse 4 Regular assessment and audit were effective strategies which facilitated good compliance and promoted evidence-based practice. Same were suggested by participants in relation to improving current practice in the areas that need improvement Barriers Barriers to good compliance to recommended clinical practice guidelines were the: 1 Lack of knowledge on evidence 2 Lack of clarity in protocol 3 Time constraints and patient clinical condition (such as in emergency situations) 4 Lack of education 5 Rapid growth of the unit in relation to providing adequate education to a large number of staff 6 Problems with access to products in patient rooms
Step 3: Which intervention components (behaviour change techniques and model(s) of delivery) could overcome the modifiable barriers and enhance the enablers?	• Using audit and interview data together with published literature we were able to identify strategies which could support adherence to CVC insertion and management recommendations.	• Review and update ICU CVC policy and ensure that this is consistent with the hospital-wide policy • Establish change champions • Review electronic medical record system to streamline documentation and provide on-the-spot training/reinforcement on documentation CVC-related information • Establish a formal education process to target areas where improvement is needed • Communicate audit findings through ICU newsletter • Review contents of the CVC insertion and management packs to ensure all relevant equipment is included (e.g. eye shields) • Communicate changes to policy internally to ICU staff and externally through the hospital to relevant stakeholders (emergency department, anaesthetics, infusion therapy team, infection control)
Step 4: How can behaviour change be measured and understood?	• Evaluation of the implementation strategies was undertaken to ensure that they were feasible and delivered as intended	• Standardised education was developed through an online PowerPoint presentation • A record of staff completing the education was maintained by the ICU education team

RESEARCH VIGNETTE

Lima EC, Bernardes A, Baldo PL, Maziero VG, Camelo SHH, Balsanelli AP. Critical incidents connected to nurses' leadership in Intensive Care Units. Rev Bras Enferm 2017; 70(5): 1018–1025

Abstract

Objective: The goal of this study is to analyse nurses' leadership in intensive care units at hospitals in the state of São Paulo, Brazil, in the face of positive and negative critical incidents.

Method: Exploratory, descriptive study, conducted with 24 nurses using the Critical Incident Technique as a methodological benchmark.

Results: Results were grouped into 61 critical incidents distributed into categories. Researchers came to the conclusion that leadership-related situations interfere with IC nurses' behaviours. Among these situations they found: difficulty in the communication process; conflicts in the daily exercise of nurses' activities; people management; and the setting of high quality care targets.

Final considerations: Researchers identified a mixed leadership model, leading them to the conclusion that nurses' knowledge and practice of contemporary leadership theories/styles are crucial because they facilitate the communication process, focusing on behavioural aspects and beliefs, in addition to valuing flexibility. This positively impacts the organization's results.

Critique

Exploratory research examining perceived leadership characteristics has been described in this paper. Leadership can be viewed from several perspectives including from those who are in management positions and have a formal leadership role as well as those who provide informal leadership. Leadership can also be considered from the perspective of providing or receiving leadership. In this study, leadership appears to have been considered from all perspectives as participants were in both formal and informal leadership roles and talked about their leadership experience from the perspective of both providing and receiving leadership. A more specific focus may have been useful to consolidate findings in this study.

The method used to conduct this exploratory study involved interviewing 24 nurses including 4 who had a management role, and therefore held a formal position of leadership and 20 who did not hold a formal leadership position. This mix of participants is useful in helping to understand the different perspectives on leadership, although unfortunately the number of participants in the group who held a management role was small and therefore may have limited the strength of their voice in the results. In addition, it appears that analysis has not been conducted in a manner that recognises the different roles of the participants, although it is not clear how analysis was approached – only that content analysis was conducted.

Despite the limitations of the analysis method, three themes have been identified including *interventions in the work environment*, *establishing targets for the quality of care* and *nurses' performance in people management*. Based on the authors' description of these themes, the first of these themes appear to have been raised by participants not in management roles while the latter two appear to have come predominantly from the four participants in management roles. These differences suggest it is imperative to explore these themes further, with sufficient participants in different roles to enable more detailed analysis and description.

Although it is not possible to suggest categories based only on the quotes provided in the paper rather than the full set of data, the reader is left to wonder if more depth was available in the data. For example, within the theme of '*interventions in the work environment*' strategies related to showing initiative, delegating and encouraging the team to work collaboratively for the benefit of the patient are evident; however, it is not known if these categories were apparent throughout the data or only the specific quotes presented.

Despite the methodological limitations of this study, some important considerations related to characteristics or strategies that are important for effective leadership are raised. All critical care practitioners, whether in management positions or not, should consider how they achieve leadership in their role.

Learning activities

1 As the nurse educator in an ICU, you have recently become aware of the high-quality research evidence for the benefits of early mobilisation of mechanically ventilated patients. But, in your unit, this does not occur. Describe a process you could use to try to bridge this evidence–practice gap.

2 An experienced critical care nurse, Beverly, has recently been hired in your unit. At a break, when describing her background, Beverly claims to be a NP but lets slip that her highest education qualification is a certificate in critical care. As nurse manager, what how would you respond to Beverly's claim?

3 As an intensive care nurse educator you are approached by one of the more senior staff members for some advice about ongoing professional development. The staff member has completed an 8-week intensive care specialty program delivered by a hospital-based education service approximately 8 years ago. What suggestions would you provide?

4 Observe the leaders within your critical care practice environment and reflect on the attributes they have and strategies they use to provide leadership to the team. Consider what you consider to be their strengths and how you could develop similar characteristics and abilities.

Online resources

American Association of Critical-Care Nurses, www.aacn.org

ANZICS/ACCCN Annual Scientific Meeting on Intensive Care, www.intensivecareasm.com.au

ANZICS Clinical Trials Group, www.anzics.com.au/clinical-trials-group

Australia and New Zealand Intensive Care Society, www.anzics.com.au

Australian College of Critical Care Nurses, www.acccn.com.au

British Association of Critical Care Nurses, baccn.org.uk

Canadian Association of Critical Care Nurses https://www.caccn.ca/

Canadian Critical Care Trials Group, www.ccctg.ca/Home.aspx

College of Intensive Care Medicine (CICM), www.cicm.org.au

European federation of Critical Care Nursing associations (EfCCNa), http://www.efccna.org/

European Society of Intensive Care Medicine, www.esicm.org

Intensive Care Foundation (Australia and New Zealand), www.intensivecarefoundation.org.au

Intensive Care National Audit and Research Centre, www.icnarc.org

Intensive Care Society, www.ics.ac.uk

Life in the FastLane, https://lifeinthefastlane.com/

NHS Leadership Academy, The Healthcare Leadership Model, www.leadershipacademy.nhs.uk/resources/

New Zealand College of Critical Care Nurses, https://www.nzno.org.nz/groups/colleges_sections/colleges/new_zealand_college_of_critical_care_nurses

Royal College of Nursing (UK) Critical Care and In-Flight Nursing Forum community, www.rcn.org.uk/get-involved/forums/critical-care-and-in-flight-nursing-forum

Scottish Intensive Care Society, www.scottishintensivecare.org.uk/

World Federation of Critical Care Nurses, wfccn.org/

World Federation of Societies of Intensive and Critical Care Medicine, www.world-critical-care.org

Further reading

Grol R, Wensing M, Eccles M, et al, editors. Improving patient care: the implementation of change in health care. 2nd ed. Oxford: Wiley Blackwell; 2013.

Malloch M, Cairns L, Evans K, et al. The SAGE handbook of workplace learning. Thousand Oaks: SAGE; 2010.

Straus SE, Tetroe J, Graham ID, editors. Knowledge translation in health care: moving from evidence to practice. 2nd ed. Oxford: Wiley Blackwell; 2013.

References

1. Murthy S, Wunsch H. Clinical review: international comparisons in critical care – lessons learned. Crit Care 2012;16(2):218.
2. Devereaux AV, Tosh PK, Hick JL, et al. Engagement and education: care of the critically ill and injured during pandemics and disasters: CHEST consensus statement. Chest 2014;146(4 Suppl.):e118S–33S.
3. Sprung CL, Zimmerman JL, Christian MD, et al. Recommendations for intensive care unit and hospital preparations for an influenza epidemic or mass disaster: summary report of the European Society of Intensive Care Medicine's Task Force for intensive care unit triage during an influenza epidemic or mass disaster. Intensive Care Med 2010;36(3):428–43.
4. Rhodes A, Moreno RP. Intensive care provision: a global problem. Rev Bras Ter Intensiva 2012;24(4):322–5.
5. Intensive Care National Audit and Research Centre (ICNARC). Key statistics from the Case Mix Programme – adult, general critical care units. London: ICNARC; 2017.
6. Tan SS, Bakker J, Hoogendoorn ME, et al. Direct cost analysis of intensive care unit stay in four European countries: applying a standardized costing methodology. Value Health 2012;15(1):81–6.
7. Gershengorn HB, Garland A, Gong MN. Patterns of daily costs differ for medical and surgical intensive care unit patients. Ann Am Thorac Soc 2015;12(12):1831–6.
8. Lefrant J-Y, Garrigues B, Pribil C, et al. The daily cost of ICU patients: a micro-costing study in 23 French intensive care units. Anaesth Crit Care Pain Med 2015;34(3):151–7.
9. Shweta K, Kumar S, Gupta AK, et al. Economic analysis of costs associated with a Respiratory Intensive Care Unit in a tertiary care teaching hospital in Northern India. Indian J Crit Care Med 2013;17(2):76–81.
10. Prin M, Wunsch H. International comparisons of intensive care: informing outcomes and improving standards. Curr Opin Crit Care 2012;18(6):700–6.
11. Lone NI, Gillies MA, Haddow C, et al. Five-year mortality and hospital costs associated with surviving intensive care. Am J Resp Crit Care Med 2016;194(2):198–208.
12. Wiles V, Daffurn K. There's a bird in my hand and a bear by the bed - i must be in ICU. In: The pivotal years of Australian Critical Care Nursing. Melbourne: Australian College of Critical Care Nurses; 2002.
13. Vincent JL. Critical care – where have we been and where are we going? Crit Care 2013;17(Suppl. 1):S2.
14. World Federation of Critical Care Nurses. Constitution Brisbane, Australia World Federation of Critical Care Nurses (WFCCN), 2016.
15. Gordon IJ, Jones ES. The evolution and nursing history of a general intensive care unit (1962–1983). Intensive Crit Care Nurs 1998;14(5):252–7.
16. Grenvik A, Pinsky MR. Evolution of the intensive care unit as a clinical center and critical care medicine as a discipline. Crit Care Clin 2009;25(1):239–50.
17. Prien T, Meyer J, Lawin P. Development of intensive care medicine in Germany. J Clin Anesth 1991;3(3):253–8.
18. Scribante J, Schmollgruber S, Nel E. Perspectives on critical care nursing: South Africa. Connect: The World of Critical Care Nursing 2005;3(4):111–15.
19. Fairman J, Lynaugh JE. Critical care nursing: a history. Philadelphia: University of Pennsylvania Press; 1998.
20. Scholes J. Developing expertise in critical care nursing. Oxford: Blackwell Publishing; 2006.
21. World Federation of Critical Care Nurses. World Federation of Critical Care Nurses Website: World Federation of Critical Care Nurses; 2014 [Accessed 19 May 2014].
22. Bergman MM, editor. Advances in mixed methods research: theories and applications. Los Angeles: Sage; 2008.
23. Pluye P, Hong QN. Combining the power of stories and the power of numbers: mixed methods research and mixed studies reviews. Annu Rev Public Health 2014;35(1):29–45.
24. Swenson-Britt E, Reineck C. Research education for clinical nurses: a pilot study to determine research self-efficacy in critical care nurses. J Contin Educ Nurs 2009;40(10):454–61.
25. Higgins J, Green S. Cochrane handbook for systematic reviews of interventions. www.handbook.cochrane.org: The Cochrane Collaboration; 2011. Available from: http://handbook.cochrane.org/. [Accessed 3 September 2017].
26. Cooke A, Smith D, Booth A. Beyond PICO: the SPIDER tool for qualitative evidence synthesis. Qual Health Res 2012;22(10):1435–43.
27. Cullum N, Cilicska D, Haynes RB, et al. Evidence-based nursing: an introduction. Oxford: Blackwell; 2008.
28. Straus SE, Tetroe J, Graham I. Defining knowledge translation. CMAJ 2009;181(3–4):165–8.
29. Eccles MP, Mittman BS. Welcome to implementation science. Implement Sci 2006;1(1):1.
30. Nilsen P. Making sense of implementation theories, models and frameworks. Implement Sci 2015;10(1):53.
31. Kitson A, Harvey G, McCormack B. Enabling the implementation of evidence based practice: a conceptual framework. Qual Health Care 1998;7(3):149–58.
32. Harvey G, Kitson A. PARIHS revisited: from heuristic to integrated framework for the successful implementation of knowledge into practice. Implement Sci 2016;11(33):1–13.
33. French SD, Green SE, O'Connor DA, et al. Developing theory-informed behaviour change interventions to implement evidence into practice: a systematic approach using the Theoretical Domains Framework. Implement Sci 2012;7(1):38.
34. Marshall A. Mind the gap – why is implementing research into practice so challenging? Aust Crit Care 2017;30(6):2.

35. Davidoff F, Dixon-Woods M, Leviton L, et al. Demystifying theory and its use in improvement. BMJ Qual Saf 2015;24(3):228–38.
36. Flottorp SA, Oxman AD, Krause J, et al. A checklist for identifying determinants of practice: a systematic review and synthesis of frameworks and taxonomies of factors that prevent or enable improvements in healthcare professional practice. Implement Sci 2013;8.
37. Forum CCNER. National standards for adult critical care nurse education. London: Critical Care Networks – National Nurse Leads; 2016. p. 20.
38. Australian College of Critical Care Nurses. ACCCN position statement on critical care nurse education. Melbourne: ACCCN; 2017.
39. Gill FJ, Leslie GD, Grech C, et al. A review of critical care nursing staffing, education and practice standards. Aust Crit Care 2012;25(4):224–37.
40. Gill FJ, Kendrick T, Davies H, et al. A two phase study to revise the Australian practice standards for specialist critical care nurses. Aust Crit Care 2017;30(3):173–81.
41. American Association of Critical Care Nurses. AACN scope and standards for acute and critical care nursing practice. Aliso Viejo, CA: AACN; 2015. p. 40.
42. Committee EFoCCNAE. EfCCNa competencies for European critical care nurses. EfCCNa; 2013.
43. Canadian Association of Critical Care Nurses. Certification London, ON: CACCN; 2018. Available from: https://www.caccn.ca/certification/index.html [Accessed 16 March 2018].
44. American Association of Critical Care Nurses. Certification Aliso Viejo, CA: AACN; 2018 [Accessed 16 March 2018].
45. Organisation WH. WHO Europe critical care nursing curriculum. Copenhagen, Denmark: WHO Regional Office for Europe; 2003. Available from: http://www.euro.who.int/. [Accessed 16 March 2018].
46. European Commission – Education and Training. The bologna process – towards the European higher education area. Brussels: European Commission; 2010.
47. American Association of Critical Care Nurses. Education. Aliso Viejo, CA: AACN; 2018. Available from: https://www.aacn.org/education [Accessed 16 March 2018].
48. Rose L, Goldsworthy S, O'Brien-Pallas L, et al. Critical care nursing education and practice in Canada and Australia: a comparative review. Int J Nurs Stud 2008;45(7):1103–9.
49. Gill FJ, Leslie GD, Grech C, et al. Developing and testing the standard of practice and evaluation of Critical-Care-Nursing tool (SPECT) for critical care nursing practice. J Contin Educ Nurs 2014;45(7):312–20.
50. Gill FJ, Leslie GD, Grech C, et al. Health consumers' experiences in Australian critical care units: postgraduate nurse education implications. Nurs Crit Care 2013;18(2):93–102.
51. Billett S. Learning through health care work: premises, contributions and practices. Med Educ 2016;50(1):124–31.
52. Kleinpell R, Ely EW, Williams G, et al. Web-based resources for critical care education. Crit Care Med 2011;39(3):541–53.
53. Daley BJ, Cervero RM. Adult, continuing and health professions education: moving forward together. New Directions for Adult and Continuing Education 2018;157:97–101.
54. Leclair LW, Dawson M, Howe A, et al. A longitudinal interprofessional simulation curriculum for critical care teams: exploring successes and challenges. J Interprof Care 2017;1-5.
55. O'Connor S, Jolliffe S, Stanmore E, et al. A mixed study systematic review of social media in nursing and midwifery education: protocol. J Adv Nurs 2017;73(8):1989–96.
56. Liu Y, Aungsuroch Y. Current literature review of registered nurses' competency in the global community. J Nurs Scholarsh 2018;50(2):191–9.
57. Lakanmaa RL, Suominen T, Perttila J, et al. Basic competence in intensive and critical care nursing: development and psychometric testing of a competence scale. J Clin Nurs 2014;23(5–6):799–810.
58. Franklin N, Melville P. Competency assessment tools: an exploration of the pedagogical issues facing competency assessment for nurses in the clinical environment. Collegian 2015;22(1):25–31.
59. Australian College of Critical Care Nurses. Practice standards for specialist critical care nurses. 3rd ed. Melbourne Australian College of Critical Care Nurses; 2015.
60. Canadian Association of Critical Care Nurses. Standards for critical care nursing practice. 5th ed. CACCN; 2017.
61. New Zealand Nurses Organisation. Philosophy and standards for nursing practice in critical care. Wellington: NZNO; 2002.
62. American Association of Critical-Care Nurses. Complete History of AACN: American Association of Critical-Care Nurses (AACN); 2018. [Accessed 4 April 2018].
63. Gardner G, Duffield C, Doubrovsky A, et al. Identifying advanced practice: a national survey of a nursing workforce. Int J Nurs Stud 2016;55:60–70.
64. Nursing and Midwifery Board of Australia. Fact sheet: advanced nursing practice and specialty areas within nursing. Melbourne: Nursing and Midwifery Board of Australia; 2016.
65. Chaboyer W, Foster MM, Foster M, et al. The intensive care unit liaison nurse: towards a clear role description. Intensive Crit Care Nurs 2004;20(2):77–86.
66. Endacott R, Chaboyer W. The nursing role in ICU outreach: an international exploratory study. Nurs Crit Care 2006;11(2):94–102.
67. Alberto L, Gillespie BM, Green A, et al. Activities undertaken by intensive care unit liaison nurses in Argentina. Aust Crit Care 2017;30(2):74–8.

68. Pirret AM. The role and effectiveness of a nurse practitioner led critical care outreach service. Intensive Crit Care Nurs 2008;24(6):375–82.
69. ICN Nurse Practitioner/Advanced Practice Nursing Network. Definition and characteristics of the role – nurse practitioner and advanced practice roles. Geneva: International Council of Nurses (ICN); 2014. Available from: https://international.aanp.org/Practice/APNRoles. [Accessed 30 November 2017].
70. Cashin A, Heartfeild M, Cox D, et al. Standards for practice for registered nurses in Australia. Collegian 2017;24:255–66.
71. Nursing and Midwifery Board of Australia. Nurse practitioner standards for practice – effective from 1 January, 2014. Melbourne: Nursing and Midwifery Board of Australia; 2013.
72. Fry M. Literature review of the impact of nurse practitioners in critical care services. Nurs Crit Care 2011;16(2):58–66.
73. Herring S. Retrieval nurse practitioners: the role and the challenges. Aust Crit Care 2013;26(3):102–3.
74. Kleinpell R, Scanlon A, Hibbert D, et al. Addressing issues impacting advanced nursing practice worldwide. Online J Issues Nurs 2014;19(2):1–13.
75. Landsperger JS, Semler MW, Wang L, et al. Outcomes of nurse practitioner-delivered critical care: a prospective cohort study. Chest 2016;149(5):1146–54.
76. Simone S. Integrating nurse practitioners into intensive care units. Crit Care Nurse 2016;36(6):59–69.
77. Costa DK, Wallace DJ, Barnato AE, et al. Nurse practitioner/physician assistant staffing and critical care mortality. Chest 2014;146(6):1566–73.
78. Jackson A, Carberry M. The advance nurse practitioner in critical care: a workload evaluation. Nurs Crit Care 2015;20(2):71–7.
79. Moneke N, Umeh OJ. How leadership behaviors impact critical care nurse job satisfaction. Nurs Manage 2013;44(1):53–5.
80. Hargett CW, Doty JP, Hauck JN, et al. Developing a model for effective leadership in healthcare: a concept mapping approach. J Healthc Leadersh 2017;9:69–78.
81. Nayback-Beebe AM, Forsythe T, Funari T, et al. Using evidence-based leadership initiatives to create a healthy nursing work environment. Dimens Crit Care Nurs 2013;32(4):166–73.
82. Larsson IE, Sahlsten MJ. The staff nurse clinical leader at the bedside: Swedish registered nurses' perceptions. Nurs Res Pract 2016;2016:1797014.
83. Cantarella Lima E, Bernardes A, Lapaz Baldo P, et al. Critical incidents connected to nurses' leadership in intensive care units. Rev Bras Enferm 2017;70(5):1018–25.
84. Stanley D. Clinical leadership characteristics confirmed. J Res Nurs 2014;19(2):118–28.
85. Stanley D, Stanley K. Clinical leadership and nursing explored: a literature search. J Clin Nurs 2017.
86. Richardson J, West MA, Cuthbertson BH. Team working in intensive care: current evidence and future endeavors. Curr Opin Crit Care 2010;16(6):643–8.
87. Chavez EC, Yoder LH. Staff nurse clinical leadership: a concept analysis. Nurs Forum 2015;50(2):90–100.
88. Bender M, Connelly CD, Brown C. Interdisciplinary collaboration: the role of the clinical nurse leader. J Nurs Manag 2013;21(1):165–74.
89. Bender M, Connelly CD, Glaser D, et al. Clinical nurse leader impact on microsystem care quality. Nurs Res 2012;61(5):326–32.
90. Wilson L, Orff S, Gerry T, et al. Evolution of an innovative role: the clinical nurse leader. J Nurs Manag 2013;21(1):175–81.
91. Shanafelt TD, Noseworthy JH. Executive leadership and physician well-being: nine organizational strategies to promote engagement and reduce burnout. Mayo Clin Proc 2017;92(1):129–46.
92. Aduddell KA, Dorman GE. The development of the next generation of nurse leaders. J Nurs Educ 2010;49(3):168–71.
93. Omoike O, Stratton KM, Brooks BA, et al. Advancing nursing leadership: a model for program implementation and measurement. Nurs Admin Q 2011;35(4):323–32.
94. Dierckx de Casterle B, Willemse A, Verschueren M, et al. Impact of clinical leadership development on the clinical leader, nursing team and care-giving process: a case study. J Nurs Manag 2008;16(6):753–63.
95. McCloughen A, O'Brien L, Jackson D. Journey to become a nurse leader mentor: past, present and future influences. Nurs Inq 2014;21(4):301–10.
96. McNamara MS, Fealy GM, Casey M, et al. Mentoring, coaching and action learning: interventions in a national clinical leadership development programme. J Clin Nurs 2014;23(17–18):2533–41.
97. Leggat SG, Balding C. Schiftan D. Developing clinical leaders: the impact of an action learning mentoring programme for advanced practice nurses. J Clin Nurs 2015;24(11–12):1576–84.
98. Bassetti M, Trecarichi EM, Mesini A, et al. Risk factors and mortality of healthcare-associated and community-acquired *Staphylococcus aureus* bacteraemia. Clin Microbiol Infect 2012;18(9):862–9.
99. Halton KA, Cook D, Paterson DL, et al. Cost-effectiveness of a central venous catheter care bundle. PLoS ONE 2010;5(9).
100. Control CfD. Bloodstream infection event (central line-associated blood stream infection and non-central line-associated blood stream infection). Atlanta: Center for Disease Control; 2018.
101. Australian Council on Healthcare Standards (ACHS). Australian clinical indicator report 2006–2013. 15th ed. Sydney: Australian Council on Healthcare Standards; 2014.
102. Gagliardi AR, Kothari A, Graham ID. Research agenda for integrated knowledge translation (IKT) in healthcare: what we know and do not yet know. J Epidemiol Community Health 2017;71(2):105–6.

Chapter 2

Systems and resources

Ged Williams, Ruth Endacott

Learning objectives

After reading this chapter, you should be able to:

- describe historical influences on the development of critical care and the way this resource is currently viewed and used
- explain the organisational arrangements and interfaces that may be established to govern a critical care unit
- identify resources and supports that assist in the governance and management of a critical care unit
- describe factors that impact on planning for the physical design and equipment requirements of a critical care unit
- describe the human resource requirements, supports and training necessary to ensure a safe and appropriate workforce
- explain common risks and the appropriate strategies, policies and contingencies necessary to support staff and patient safety
- discuss leadership and management principles that influence the quality, efficacy and appropriateness of the critical care unit
- discuss critical care considerations in responding to the threat of a pandemic.

KEY WORDS

budget
business case
competence
critical care
credentialling
governance
pandemic
patient dependency
resource management
risk management
skill mix
staff

Introduction

Critical care services are multifaceted and highly complex with very expensive human and technical resources needed to meet the expectations of an ever-growing sophisticated and informed community.[1] The provision of expensive technical and human resources requires prudent, rational and justified financial investments in a healthcare system burdened by growing cost and limited budgets. This chapter explores historical development of critical care and the way this resource is currently viewed and used, describes various organisational, staffing and training arrangements that need to be in place, considers the planning, design and equipment needs of a critical care unit, covers other aspects of resource management including the budget and financial modelling; and finishes with a description of how critical care staff may respond to a pandemic or other acute and dramatic demands on resources. First, however, important ethical decisions in managing the resources of a critical care unit are discussed. Chapter 5 explores ethical issues more broadly.

> **Practice tips**
>
> Ethical decision making related to managing resources at the unit level is as critical as ethical decision making at the individual patient level. Open and transparent decision making is key.

Ethical allocation and utilisation of resources

In management, as in clinical practice, careful consideration of the pros and cons of various decisions must be made on a daily basis. The interests of the individual patient, extended family, treating team, the organisation and the broader community are not always congruent, nor are they usually consistent. Decisions surrounding the provision of critical care services are often governed by a compromise between conflicting interests and ethical theories. Two main perspectives on ethical decision making, *deontological* and *utilitarian*, are explored briefly.[2]

The *deontological* principle suggests that a person has a fundamental duty to act in a certain way – for example, to provide full, active medical treatment to all persons. The rule of rescue, or the innate desire to do something – anything – to help those in dire need, may be a corollary to the deontological principle. These two concepts, the duty to act and the rule of rescue, tend to sit well with many trained and skilled clinicians and the Hippocratic Oath. In critical care there are some families and some clinicians who, for personal and/or religious reasons, take a strong stand and demand treatments and actions based on a deontological view (i.e. the fundamental belief that a certain action is the only one that should be considered in a given situation).

At the other extreme is the *utilitarian* view, which suggests an action is right only if it achieves the greatest good for the greatest number of people. This concept tends to sit well with pragmatic managers and policy makers. An example of a utilitarian view might be to ration funding allocated to heart transplantation and to utilise any saved money for prevention and awareness campaigns. A heart disease prevention campaign lends a greater benefit to a greater number in the population than does one transplant procedure.

The appropriate provision and allocation of critical care services and resources tend to sit somewhere between these two extreme ethical principles. This dilemma is true of all health services, but critical care, because of its high-technology, high-cost, low-volume outputs, is under particular scrutiny to justify its resource usage within a healthcare system. Therefore, not only do critical care managers need to be prudent, responsible and efficient guardians of this precious resource, they need to be seen as such if they are to retain the confidence of, and legitimacy with, the broader community values of the day.

Historical influences

The 1950s and early 1960s saw the development of the first critical care units in many parts of the developed world. If a hospital was to be relevant, it had to have one. In fact, what distinguished a tertiary referral teaching hospital from other hospitals was at its fundamental conclusion, the existence of a critical care unit.[3] Over time, practical reasons for establishing critical care units have led to their spread to most acute hospitals with more than 100 beds. Reasons for the proliferation of critical care services include, but are not limited to:

- economies of scale by cohorting critically ill patients to one area
- development of expertise in doctors and nurses who specialise in the care and treatment of critically ill patients
- an ever-growing body of research demonstrating that critically ill patient outcomes are better if they are cared for in a specifically equipped and staffed critical care unit.[4]

Funding for critical care services has evolved over time to be somewhat separate from mainstream patient funding, owing to the unique requirements of critical care units. Critical care is unique because patients are at the severe end of the disease spectrum. For instance, the funding provided for a patient admitted for chronic obstructive airway disease in an ICU on a ventilator is very different from that provided for a patient with the same diagnosis, but treated in a medical ward only. Each country/jurisdictional health department tends to create its own unique approach to funding ICU services. For instance, the Research and Development Corporation study[4] examined funding methods in many countries and concluded that there was no obvious example of 'best practice' or a dominant approach used by a majority of systems. Each approach had advantages and disadvantages, particularly in relation to the financial risk involved in providing intensive care. While the risk of underfunding intensive care may be highest in systems that apply Diagnostic Related Groups (DRGs) to the entire episode of hospital care, including intensive care, concerns about potential underfunding were voiced in all systems reviewed. Arrangements for additional funding in the form of co-payments or surcharges may reduce the risk of underfunding critical care episodes of care. However, these approaches also face the difficulty of determining the appropriate co-payment amount to be paid.[4]

As an example, Australia has established the Independent Hospital Pricing Authority (IHPA) whose task it is to harmonise the variations in funding processes across all states and territories and to establish a common and consistent and transparent funding process to be agreed by all.[5] All price weights are expressed as a single unit of measure being the national weighted activity unit (NWAU). It provides a scale that identifies the relative measure of resource use of each public hospital service and guides the Commonwealth contribution to funding such services. In 2016–17 NEP per NWAU is $4883.[5]

Critical care is an area that requires significant resources to the treatment of patients, which an AR-DRG alone does not reflect. Therefore, additional funding over and above the acute inpatient payment is made where a patient is admitted to an eligible ICU, NICU or PICU.[5]

The IHPA has developed a list of ICUs that are eligible to receive an ICU adjustment based on a measure of the size of the ICU and the overall complexity mix of patients.[5] IHPA is also exploring analysis of APACHE score, inotrope usage and AORTIC data, all indirect measures of criticality, acuity and expected outcomes, to determine if these measures can be further adapted to provide a patient level indicator of ICU need and patient complexity for potential implementation in future years.[5]

The actual number of ICU beds funded or available to the community is also a complex issue throughout the world. In a study of 11 countries,[6] there was a strong correlation between the number of ICU beds available per 1 million people and the national healthcare expenditure per capita. However, there was poor correlation between the number of ICU beds per million people and the number of hospital beds per million people. For instance, USA, Canada and UK have around 180, 100 and 40 ICU beds per million people, respectively, yet all have approximately 3–4000 hospital beds per million. Looking at these three countries alone, we know their health and ICU services and outcomes are relatively similar yet the way their ICUs are provided and resourced show substantial differences. There are many policy and political reasons for these differences, the discussion of which is beyond the scope of this chapter. Suffice to say, clinical evidence is not the only parameter on which government policy and resourcing decisions are made!

At the hospital level, most critical care units have capped and finite budgets that are linked to 'available beds' – that is, beds that are equipped, staffed, funded and ready to be occupied by a patient, regardless of whether they are actually occupied.[7] This is one crude yet common way that hospitals can control costs emanating from the critical care unit. The other method is to limit the number of trained and experienced nurses available to the specialty; consequently, a shortage of qualified critical care nurses results in a shortage of critical care beds, resulting in a rationing of the service available. The capping of beds and qualified critical care nurse positions can be convenient mechanisms to limit access and cost of this expensive service – critical care.

Funding based on achieving positive patient outcomes would be ideal, as it would ensure that critical care units were using their resources only for those patients who were most likely to achieve positive outcomes in terms of morbidity and mortality. However, funding based on health outcomes only does raise the risk of encouraging clinicians to 'cherry-pick' only the most 'profitable' or 'successful' patient groups at the expense of others. In private (for-profit) hospitals or countries with very poor health systems, 'cherry-picking' only those patients for whom a successful outcome is guaranteed is likely to be more common, whereas in the public hospitals of most Western countries an educated and informed prediction is often applied to the decision as to whether a patient should enter the critical care unit or not.

It is vital to note the very important role played by rural and isolated health services and, in particular, critical care units and outreach services in these regions. Many of the contemporary activity-based funding formulas are difficult to apply to rural and isolated settings. There are diseconomies of scale in such settings as a result of small bed numbers, limited but highly skilled nurses and doctors, and unpredictable peaks and troughs in demand, which make workforce planning and the management of call-in/overtime and fatigue difficult for small teams to manage. The professional isolation and limited access to education, training and peer support can also create morale problems for some members of the team. Furthermore, the diseconomies and isolation require empathetic funding processes to recognise the difficulties unique to rural and isolated critical care services. If such units are to remain viable and capable of delivering levels of safe and effective care equivalent to those expected in larger metropolitan hospitals, then additional support is required to compensate for the cost and limitations that result from being remote and isolated. To compensate further for these challenges, the use of tele-ICU;[8] artificial intelligence[9] and robotics[10] are beginning to show promise in helping to improve the quality and sustainability of treatment options in rural and isolated settings and these are areas of contemporary research that hope to overcome the tyranny of distance and isolation.

Practice tips

The capping of beds and qualified critical care nurse positions can be convenient mechanisms to limit access to and the cost of critical care services.

Economic considerations and principles

Almost 30 years ago, a comprehensive study of costs found that 8% of patients admitted to the ICU consumed 50% of resources but had a mortality rate of 70%, while 41% of patients received no acute interventions and consumed only 10% of resources.[11] More recent studies show that critical care services are increasingly being provided to patients who are older and with a higher severity of acute and chronic illnesses, despite higher mortality rates compared to matched younger patients.[12-14] However, a global snap shot of ICU services in 730 centres across 84 countries showed that on average mortality in ICU remains around 16% and total in hospital mortality of ICU patients is 22%.[15] Scrutiny of the costs and benefits of ICU services remain an ongoing activity.

Some authors provide scenarios as examples of poor economic decision making in critical care and argue for less extreme variances in the types of patients who are admitted to ICU in order to reduce the burden of cost on the health dollar.[16-17] Others have suggested that if all healthcare provided were appropriate, rationing would not be required.[18] Defining what is 'appropriate' can be subjective, although not always. The Research and Development Corporation[4,19] group suggests that there are at least three approaches that can be used to assess appropriateness of care. These include the benefit–risk, benefit–cost and implicit approaches. The first two approaches are considered to be explicit approaches, while the third tends to be subjective. However, all approaches have a subjective element. A benefit risk approach focuses on the benefit of treatment and the inherent risks to the patient are assessed to inform a decision; this approach excludes monetary costs. A benefit cost approach evaluates the benefit and cost of the decision to proceed; this approach incorporates cost to patient and society, while the implicit approach allows the medical practitioner to provide the service and judges its appropriateness. Irrespective of the approach taken, those responsible for admitting patients should involve the patient/family in their deliberations and ultimate decisions. Similar discussions have been advocated by the Taskforce on Values, Ethics and Rationing in Critical Care, who suggest rationing is not only unavoidable but essential to ensuring the ethical distribution of medical goods and services.[20] In end-of-life care situations, Medical Emergency Teams and ICU outreach nurses can facilitate early intervention, discussion and decision making to reflect the views of family, patient and the care team.[21,22]

What is best for the patient is not just the opinion of the treating doctor and needs to be considered in much broader terms such as the patient's previous expressed wishes and the family's opinion as de facto patient representatives. The quality of the decision and the quality of the expected outcome require many competing considerations.

Proponents of the 'quality' agenda in healthcare have argued for 'best practice' and 'best outcomes' in the provision of health services, although it may be more pragmatic to consider 'value' when discussing what is and what is not an appropriate decision in critical care. The following equation expresses the concept 'value' simply:

$$\text{Value} = \frac{\text{Quality}}{\text{Cost}} = \frac{\text{Benefit} \times \text{Sustainability}}{\text{Price} \times \text{Suffering}}$$

The quality of the outcome is a function of the benefit to be achieved and the sustainability of the benefit. The benefit of critical care is associated with such factors as survival, longevity and improved quality of life (e.g. greater functioning capacity and less pain and anxiety). The benefit is enhanced by sustainability: the longer the benefit is maintained, the better it is.[23]

Cost is separated into two components, monetary (price) and non-monetary (suffering). Non-monetary costs include such considerations as morbidity, mortality, pain and anxiety in the individual, or broader societal costs and suffering (e.g. opportunity costs to others who might have used the resources but for the current occupants, and what other health services might have been provided but for the cost of this service).[23]

Ethico-economic analyses of services like critical care and expensive treatments like organ transplantation are the new consideration of this century and are as important to good governance as discussions of medico-legal considerations. Sound ethical principles to inform and guide human and material resource management and budgets ought to prevail in the management of limited health resources.[2]

Practice tips

What is best for the patient is not just the opinion of the treating doctor and needs to be considered in much broader terms such as the patient's previous expressed wishes and the family's opinion as de facto patient representatives.

Budget and finance

This section provides information on types of budget, the budgeting process, and how to analyse costs and expenditure to ensure resources are utilised appropriately and in line with the service management plan, that is the operational and service goals of the critical care team expected by the hospital and broader community. As noted by one author, 'Nothing is so terrifying for clinicians accustomed to daily issues of life and death as to be given responsibility for the financial affairs of their hospital division!'.[18] Yet, in essence, developing and managing a budget for a critical care unit follows many of the same principles as managing a family budget. Consideration of value for money, prioritising needs and wants, and living within a relatively fixed income is common to all. This section in no way attempts to undermine the skill and precision provided by the accounting profession, nor will it enable clinicians to usurp the role of hospital business managers. Rather, the aim is to provide the requisite knowledge to empower clinicians to manage the key components of budget development and budget setting, and to know what questions to ask when confronted by this most daunting responsibility of managing a service budget.

> **Practice tips**
>
> Nothing is so terrifying for clinicians accustomed to daily issues of life and death as to be given responsibility for the financial affairs of their hospital division!

Types of budget

There are essentially three types of budget that a manager must consider: personnel, operational and capital. Within these budget types, there are two basic cost types: fixed and variable. Fixed costs are those essential to the service and are relatively constant, regardless of the fluctuations in workload or throughput (e.g. nurse unit manager salary, security, ventilators). Variable costs change with changing throughput (e.g. casual or agency nurses' salary, medicines or other clinical consumable items).

Personnel budget

Healthcare is a labour-intensive service, and critical care epitomises this fact with personnel costs being the most expensive component of the unit's budget. The staffing requirement for critical care generally follows a formula of *x* nurses per open (funded) bed. This figure is expressed in full-time equivalents (FTEs), i.e. the equivalent of a person working a 40-hour week if the standard full-time working week is 40 hours. This may equate to 5 × 8-hour shifts per week or 20 × 12-hour shifts in a 6-week period, or any other variable measure as determined by local employment law and custom.

Personnel costs include productive and non-productive hours. Productive hours are those utilised to provide direct work. A manager will determine the minimum or optimum number of nurses to be scheduled per shift and then calculate the nursing hours per day, multiplied by the hourly rate of pay and any penalties that are to be attributed to work done during the after-business-hours period. Non-productive hours include sick leave, holiday leave, education hours, maternity leave and any other paid time away from the actual job that staff are employed to do.

Personnel budgets tend to be fixed costs, in that most staff are employed permanently, based on an expected or forecast demand. Prudent managers tend to employ 5–10% less than the actual forecast demand and use casual staff to 'flex-up' the available FTE staff establishment in periods of increasing demand, hence contributing a small but variable component to the personnel budget.[24]

Operational budget

All other non-personnel costs (except major capital equipment) tend to be allocated to the operational budget. This includes fixed costs such as minor equipment, maintenance contracts, utility costs (e.g. electricity), and variable costs that fluctuate with patient type and number (e.g. pharmaceuticals, meals, consumable supplies such as gloves and dressings, laundry).

Compared with personnel costs, operational costs in critical care tend to be relatively small, but they can be managed and rationed with the help of good information and cooperation. For example, there is a range of dressing materials available on the market, and a simple dressing that requires less expensive materials should always be used unless a more expensive product is indicated and a protocol exists to inform staff of this clinical need/justification.

Fixed costs can also be turned into variable costs and hence encourage efficient usage. For example, pressure-reduction mattresses traditionally purchased as a fixed asset with variable (and unpredictable) repair and maintenance costs, can now be leased on a per-day or per-week basis, with no need for storage, cleaning or maintenance costs. Further, critical care managers can work with other hospital managers to create 'purchasing power' by cooperating to standardise the range and volume of products used to obtain a better price for a product that will benefit all users.

> **Practice tips**
>
> Compared with personnel costs, operational costs in critical care tend to be relatively small and can be managed and rationed with the help of good information and cooperation.

Capital budget

Capital budget items are generally expensive and/or large fixed assets that are considered long-term investments, such as building extensions, renovations and large equipment purchases. Capital budget items tend to be considered as assets that are depreciated over time. Most hospitals consider these items as a global asset – that is, as a group of investment items and activities for the hospital – rather than attributing these costs to an individual unit or department.

To request a capital budget item, a written proposal (Business case – see later) is generally required describing the item, its expected benefits, whether it replaces an existing item's service or function, the cost, possible revenue and cost-mitigating benefits. This analysis does not always have to demonstrate a profit, although the value and benefit of the service needs to be established/justified through a business case.

Budget process

The budget includes three fundamental steps: budget preparation and approval, budget analysis and reporting, and budget control and action.

> **Practice tips**
>
> The budget includes three fundamental steps: budget preparation and approval, budget analysis and reporting, and budget control and action.

Budget preparation and approval

A budget plan essentially runs in parallel with a unit or service management plan, forecasting likely activity and resulting financial costs. In most circumstances the preceding year's activity and costs are a good benchmark on which to base the next year's budget. However, hospital expectations in terms of new services, greater patient throughput or changes to staff salary entitlements will need to be factored into the new budget.

The budget period is generally a financial year, but developing monthly budgets (cash flowing) to coincide with predictable variations allows for a more realistic representation of how costs are incurred and paid throughout the financial year period. If the budget plan is well constructed, one always hopes and expects the final budget allocation (i.e. the approved budget) to be close to achievable.

Budget analysis and reporting

Most critical care managers analyse their expenditure against budget projections on a monthly basis to identify variances from planned expenditure. Information should not merely be financial: a breakdown of the monthly and year-to-date expenditures for personnel (productive and non-productive), and operational (fixed and variable) costs, should be matched against other known measurable indicators of activity or productivity (e.g. patient bed-days, patient diagnosis types/groups and staffing hours, including overtime and other special payments).[18] Ideally such measures should be matched against other quality outcome measures, such as pressure injuries, invasive device infections, length of stay, mortality index etc.

One common management maxim is: if it cannot be measured, then it cannot be controlled. Clinical managers therefore need to work closely with finance managers to develop consistent data measurements and reports to inform themselves and staff about where they should focus their efforts to achieve the approved budget target.

Budget control and action

When signs of poor performance or financial overrun are evident, managers cannot merely analyse the financial reports, hoping that things will sort themselves out. Every variance of a sizeable amount requires an explanation. Some will be obvious: an outbreak of community influenza among staff will increase sick leave and casual staff costs for a period of time, concurrently the same epidemic may increase demands on ICU beds. Other overruns can be insidious but no less important: overtime payments, although sometimes unavoidable, can also reflect poor time management or a culture of some staff wanting to boost their income surreptitiously.[24]

An effective method of controlling the budget is to actively engage staff in the process of managing costs. Managers can explain to staff how the budget has been developed and how their performance against budget is progressing, and identify areas for potential improvement. Seeking ideas from staff on how to improve efficiency and productivity and giving them some responsibility for the budget performance can encourage an esprit de corps and improvements from the whole team that a single manager cannot achieve alone.[25]

Developing a business case

The most common reason for writing a business case is to justify the resources and capital expenditure to gain the support and approval for a change in-service provision and/or purchase of a significant new piece of equipment/technology. This section provides an overview of a business case and a format for its presentation. The business case can be a valuable tool in the strategic decision-making process, particularly in an environment of constrained resources.[26]

A business case is a management tool that is used in the process of explaining and meeting a strategic goal of an organisation. Within a setting such as healthcare, the business case is required to outline clearly the clinical need and implications to be understood by leaders. Financial imperatives, such as return on investment (ROI), must also be defined and identified.[27,28] A business case is a document in which all the facts relevant to the case are identified and linked cohesively. Various templates are available (see *Online resources*) to assist with the layout. Key questions are generally the starting point for the response to a business case: why, what, when, where, who and how, with each question's response adding additional information to the process (Table 2.1). Business cases can vary in length from many pages to just a couple. Most organisations will have standardised headings and formats for the presentation of these documents. If the document is lengthy, inclusion of an executive summary is recommended to summarise the salient points of the business case (Box 2.1).

In summary, the business case is an important tool that is increasingly required at all levels of an organisation to clearly define a proposed service change or equipment purchase. This document should include clear goals and outcomes, a cost–benefit analysis, quality and safety considerations and timelines for achievement of the solution. While such a document is often developed towards the end of a formal multi-professional collaboration, the questions in Table 2.1 can also be used to structure early discussions about changes in nursing practices or roles in ICU.

TABLE 2.1
Key questions in writing a business case

QUESTION	EXAMPLE
Why?	What is the background to the project, and why is it needed: PEST (political, economic, sociological, technological) and SWOT (strengths, weaknesses, opportunities and threats) analysis?
What?	Clearly identify and define the project and the purpose of the business case and outline the solution. Clearly defined goals, outcomes and measurable benefits should be documented.
What if?	A risk assessment of the current situation, including any controls currently in place to address/mitigate the issue, and a risk assessment following the implementation of the proposed solution.
When?	What are the timelines for the implementation and achievement of the project/ solution?
Where?	What is the context within which the project will be undertaken, if not already included in the background material?
Who?	Who will be affected by this change, positively and negatively? Who will be responsible for overseeing and managing of the project/change?
How?	How much money, people and equipment, for example, will be required to achieve the benefits? A clear cost–benefit analysis should be included in response to this question.

BOX 2.1

Business case: sample headings

- Title
- Purpose
- Background
- Key issues
- Cost–benefit analysis
- Recommendations
- Risk assessment

Practice tips

A business case is a management tool that is used in the process of explaining and meeting a strategic goal of an organisation.

Critical care environment

A critical care unit is a distinct unit within a hospital that should have easy access to the emergency department, operating theatre and medical imaging. It provides care to patients with a life-threatening illness or injury and concentrates the clinical expertise, technological and therapeutic resources required. The College of Intensive Care Medicine[29] and the UK Faculty of Intensive Care Medicine[30] define three levels of intensive care to support the role delineation of a particular hospital, dependent upon staffing expertise, facilities and support services. A Level I ICU provides immediate resuscitation and short-term CPR support for critically ill patients; Level II ICU should be capable of providing complex multi-system life support for an indefinite period if appropriate specialty support is available within the hospital and a Level III ICU is a tertiary referral unit capable of providing comprehensive critical care including complex multi-system life support for an indefinite period. Access to a Level III ICU is by referral only.[29] Critical care facilities vary in nature and extent between hospitals and are dependent on the operational policies of each individual facility. In smaller facilities, the broad spectrum of critical care may be provided in combined units (e.g. a unit that admits intensive care, high-dependency, coronary care patients) to improve flexibility and aid the efficient use of available resources.[31]

Environmental design

The functional, organisational and unit designs are governed by available finances, an operational brief and the building and design standards of the state or country in which the hospital is located. A critical care unit should have access to minimum support facilities, which include staff station, clean utility, dirty utility, store room(s), education and teaching space, staff amenities, patients' en suites, patients' bathroom, relatives' room (with lockers for personal items), a room for bereaved families, linen storage, disposal room, pathology area and offices. Most notably, the actual bed space/care area for patients needs to be well designed.[31,32]

The design of the patient's bed space has received considerable attention in recent years. Most governments have developed minimum guidelines to assist in the design process. Each bed space should be a minimum of 20–25 square metres and provide for visual privacy from casual observation. At least one hand basin per single room or per two beds should be provided to meet minimum infection control guidelines.[31-33] Each bed space should have piped medical gases (oxygen and air), suction, adequate electrical outlets (essential and non-essential), data points and task lighting sufficient for use during the performance of bedside procedures. Further detailed descriptions are available in various health department documents.[31,32]

Equipment

Since the advent of critical care units, healthcare delivery has become increasingly dependent on medical technology to deliver that care. Equipment can be categorised into several funding groups: capital expenditure (generally in excess of $10,000 AUD or £5000), equipment expenditure (all equipment less than $10,000 AUD or £5000), and the disposable products and devices required to support the use of equipment. This section examines how to evaluate, procure and maintain that equipment.

Initial set-up requirements

Critical care units require baseline equipment that allows the unit to deliver safe and effective patient care. The list of specific equipment required by each individual unit will be governed by the scope of that unit's function. For example, a unit that provides care to patients after neurosurgery will require the ability to monitor intracranial pressure. Changes in practice such as early mobilisation[34] have an impact both on equipment requirements and storage space, although financial modelling has demonstrated considerable costs savings.[35] Table 2.2 lists the basic equipment requirements for a critical care unit. Information technology and communications options and requirements are growing rapidly in health and in particular in the critical care environment, with instant access to patient's physiological data at the bedside becoming standard practice. The rapid pace of innovation and change in this area requires the managers to think carefully when setting up information technology infrastructure and to be careful not to over capitalise on technology that might not be easily upgradeable when new and more efficient or more effective substitutes come on to the market. Envisioning what might be available in the future is difficult but it is important to consider such matters carefully to avoid very expensive upgrades in the future.[36] Further detail regarding information and communication technology can be found in Chapter 3.

TABLE 2.2
Basic equipment requirements

MONITORING	THERAPEUTIC
Monitors (including central station)	Ventilators (invasive and non-invasive)
End-tidal CO_2 monitoring	Infusion pumps
Arterial blood gas analyser (± electrolytes)	Syringe drivers
Invasive monitoring	CVVHDF
• arterial	EDD-f
• central venous pressure	Resuscitators
• intracranial pressure	Temporary pacemaker
Access to image intensifier	Defibrillator
Ultrasound	Suctioning apparatus
Access to CT/MRI	

Practice tips

Envisioning what might be available in the future is difficult but it is important to consider such matters carefully to avoid very expensive upgrades in the future.

Purchasing

The procurement of any equipment or medical device requires a rigorous process of selection and evaluation. This process should be designed to select functional, reliable products that are safe, cost-effective and environmentally conscious[37] and that promote quality of care while avoiding duplication or rapid obsolescence. In most healthcare facilities, a product (or medical devices) evaluation committee exists to support this process.

The product evaluation committee should include members who have an interest in the equipment being considered and should comprise, for example, biomedical engineers and representatives from the central sterile supply unit administration, infection control, end users and other departments that may have similar needs. Once a product evaluation committee has been established, clear, objective criteria for the evaluation of the product should be determined (Box 2.2). Ideally, the committee will screen products and medical devices before a clinical evaluation is conducted to establish its viability, thus avoiding any unnecessary expenditure in time and money.

The decision to purchase or lease equipment will, to some extent, be governed by the purchasing strategy approved by the hospital or health authority. The advantages of leasing equipment include the capital expenditure being defrayed over the life of the lease, with ongoing servicing and product upgrades built into the lease agreement and price structure. Any final presentation from the product evaluation committee should therefore include a recommendation to purchase or lease, based on a cost–benefit analysis of the ongoing expenditure required to maintain the equipment.

Many healthcare jurisdictions now have detailed 'sunshine' policies that have been implemented to guide and regulate potential conflicts of interest, especially in relation to the purchasing of products and services and the perception or actual conflict of interest than can be created between the various players in such

BOX 2.2

Example criteria for product evaluation

- Safety
- Performance
- Quality
- Use
  - purpose
  - ease of
- Cost–benefit analysis
  - include disposables
- Cleaning
  - central sterilising supply unit
  - infection control
- Regulatory control
  - Therapeutic Goods Administration
  - Australian Standards
- Adaptability to future technological advancements
- Service agreements
- Training requirements

Adapted from Association of Operating Room Nurses. Recommended practices for product selection in perioperative practice settings. AORN J 2004;79:678–82. Elliott D, Hollins B. Product evaluation: theoretical and practical considerations. Aust Crit Care 1995;8 (2):14–9.

transactions.[38,39] Experience shows that any participant in the product or service evaluation processes needs to be extremely careful and fully transparent in their dealings with companies and their representatives, especially outside the work environment. Gifts, such as free product samples, meals, conference attendance and any other activities that may be perceived as inducements, must be resisted or formally documented and submitted to higher management for scrutiny and approval. As a general rule, it is best to have a more senior manager approve or deny any such offers to ensure impartiality in accepting such offers.

Replacement and maintenance

The process for replacement of equipment is closely aligned with the process for the purchase of new equipment. The stimulus for the process to begin can be either the condemning of equipment by biomedical engineers or the planned replacement of equipment nearing the end of its life cycle. In general, most capital equipment is deemed to have a life cycle of 5 years. This time frame takes into account both the longevity of the physical equipment and its technology.

Ongoing maintenance of equipment is an important part of facilitating safety in the unit. Maintenance may be provided in-house by individual facility biomedical departments or as part of a service contract arrangement with the vendor company. The provision of a maintenance/service plan should be clearly identified during the procurement phase of the equipment purchase process. While equipment maintenance is not the direct responsibility of the nurses in charge of the unit, they should be aware of the scheduled maintenance plan for all equipment and ensure that timely maintenance is undertaken.

Routine ongoing care of equipment is outlined in the product information and user manuals that accompany devices. This documentation clearly outlines routine care required for cleaning, storage and maintenance. All staff involved in the maintenance of clinical equipment should be trained and competent to carry it out. As specialist equipment is a fundamental element of critical care, effective resourcing includes consideration of the purchase, set-up, maintenance and replacement of equipment. Equipment is therefore an important aspect of the budget process.

Practice tips

The provision of a maintenance/service plan should be clearly identified during the procurement phase of the equipment purchase process.

Staff

Staffing critical care units is an important human resource consideration. The focus of this section is on nursing staff, although the important role that other members of the multi-professional team provide is acknowledged. Nurses' salaries consume a considerable portion of any unit budget and, owing to the constant presence of nurses at the bedside, appropriate staffing plays a significant role in the quality and safety of care delivered. Nurse staffing levels influence patient outcomes both directly through the initiation of appropriate nursing care strategies and indirectly by mediating and implementing the care strategies of other members of the multidisciplinary healthcare team.[40] Therefore, ensuring an appropriate skill mix is an important aspect of unit management. This section considers how appropriate staffing levels are determined and factors, such as nurse–patient ratios and skill mix, which influence them.

Staffing roles

There are several different nursing roles in the ICU nursing team, and various guidelines determine the requirements of these roles. Some critical care nursing organisations have documented position statements surrounding the critical care workforce and staffing.[41–43] A designated nursing manager (nursing unit manager/

nurse practice coordinator/clinical nurse manager, or equivalent title) to direct and guide clinical practice is required for each unit. The nurse manager must possess a post-registration qualification in critical care or in the clinical specialty of the unit.[29,30,41–43] A clinical nurse educator should be available in each unit.[30] In Australia, the ACCCN recommends a minimum ratio of one FTE clinical nurse educator for every 50 nurses on the roster, to provide unit-based education and staff development.[41] Registered nurses (RNs) within the unit are generally nurses with formal critical care postgraduate qualifications and varying levels of critical care experience. However, this varies across countries, with the UK specifying a minimum of 50% of RNs nurses with a post-registration award in critical care nursing.[30]

In many developed economies, specialist critical care nurse education has moved from largely hospital-based certificates[42] into the tertiary education sector, although a recent survey identified wide variation in the regulation, assessment, program duration and qualification awarded for specialist critical care nurse education across Europe.[44] Since the move to tertiary education, postgraduate, university-based programs at the graduate certificate, postgraduate diploma or Masters level are now available, although some hospital-based courses that articulate to formal university programs may also be accessible. Some critical care organisations have developed position statements on the provision of critical care nursing education.[33,45,46] The consistent messages across these documents are: the requirement for at least 50% of RNs to have a specialist critical care qualification and at least one FTE senior ICU nurse dedicated to managing the education and competency evaluation. In addition, the World Federation of Critical Care Nurses (WFCCN)[46] make recommendations about topics to be included in education programs and the requirement for flexible pathways including recognition of prior learning. They also recommend that critical care education programs should be delivered by a higher education provide, for example a university. Various support staff are also required to ensure the efficient functioning of the department, including, but not limited to, administrative/clerical staff, domestic/ward assistant staff and biomedical engineering staff.

Staffing levels

A staff establishment refers to the number of nurses required to provide safe, efficient, quality care to patients. Staffing levels are influenced by many factors, including the economic, political and individual characteristics of the unit in question. Other factors, such as the population served, the services provided by the hospital and by its neighbouring hospitals, and the subspecialties of medical staff working at each hospital also influence staffing. Specific issues to be considered include nurse-to-patient ratios, nursing competencies and skill mix.

The starting point for most units in the establishment of minimum, or base, staffing levels is the patient census approach. This approach uses the number and classification (ICU or high-dependency unit (HDU), sometimes referred to as level 2 and level 3 patients[30] or patients within the unit to determine the number of nurses required to be scheduled on duty on any given shift. In many countries a registered nurse-to-patient ratio of 1:1 for ICU patients and 1:2 for HDU patients has been accepted for many years..[41–43] Other countries, such as the USA, have lower nurse staffing levels, but in those countries nursing staff is augmented by other types of clinical or support staff, such as dialysis and respiratory technicians.[47] A major limitation of the patient dependency approach to staffing is the lack of flexibility to respond to changing patient demand. Once the base staffing numbers per shift have been established, the unit manager is required to calculate the number of FTE that are required to implement the roster. One FTE is equivalent to the number of hours worked in one week by a full-time employee.

The development of the nursing establishment is dependent on many factors. Historical data from previous years of patient throughput and patient acuity assist in the determination of future requirements.

Nurse-to-patient ratios

Nurse-to-patient ratios refer to the number of nursing hours required to care for a patient with a specific set of needs. ICUs can be identified as combined units incorporating intensive care, coronary care and high-dependency patients;[48] different nurse-to-patient ratios are required for these, often diverse, groups of patients. It is important to note that nurse-to-patient ratios may be provided merely as a guide to staffing levels, and implementation should depend on patient acuity, local knowledge and expertise.

The WFCCN states that critically ill patients require one RN to be allocated at all times.[43] The College of Intensive Care Medicine in Australia and Faculty of Intensive Care Medicine in the UK also identified the need for a minimum nurse-to-patient ratio of 1:1 for intensive care patients and 1:2 for high-dependency patients.[29,30]

The ACCCN,[41] British Association of Critical Care Nurses (BACCN)[42] and the Critical Care Nurses Section – New Zealand Nurses Organisation, now named the New Zealand College of Critical Care Nurses,[49,50] have outlined the appropriate nurse staffing standards for ICUs within the context of accepted minimum national standards and evidence that supports best practice. The ACCCN statement identifies key principles to meet the expected standards of critical care nursing (Table 2.3). Key additional points in the BACCN standards relate to the role of healthcare assistants, who can work under direct supervision, and assistant practitioners, who work under indirect supervision of registered nurses.[42] The New Zealand College of Critical Care Nurses documents also emphasise the role of critical care nurses in negotiating to ensure staffing levels and skill mix are adequate to provide safe and effective care.[50]

TABLE 2.3
Ten key points of intensive care nursing staffing[45]

POINT	DESCRIPTION
1 Ventilated patients and any other patient that the nurse-in-charge deems to be clinically unstable or at risk	Require a standard nurse-to-patient ratio of at least 1:1.
2 Patients requiring a high complexity level of care (e.g. non-ventilated patients recovering from critical illness)	Require a standard nurse-to-patient ratio of at least 1:2
3 Clinical coordinator (team leader)	There must be a designated critical-care-qualified senior nurse per shift who is supernumerary and whose primary role is responsibility for the logistical management of patients, staff, service provision and resource utilisation during a shift
4 ACCESS nurses	These are nurses in addition to the bedside nurses, clinical coordinator, unit manager, educators and non-nursing support staff. They provide **A**ssistance, **C**oordination, **C**ontingency, **E**ducation, **S**upervision and **S**upport
5 Nursing manager	At least one designated Masters-prepared nursing manager (NUM/CNC/NPC/CNM or equivalent) who is formally recognised as the unit nurse leader is required per ICU
6 Clinical nurse educator	At least one designated Masters-prepared CNE should be available in each unit. The recommended ratio is one FTE CNE for every 50 nurses on the ICU roster.
7 ICU Liaison nurse services	A liaison nurse service must be provided to optimise the use of the ICU within the hospital, with one liaison nurse per 10 ICU beds.
8 Critical care nurses	The ACCCN recommends an optimum specialty qualified critical care nurse proportion of 75%.
9 Resources	These are allocated to support nursing time and costs associated with quality assurance activities, nursing and multidisciplinary research, and conference attendance.
10 Support staff	ICUs are provided with adequate administrative staff, ward assistants, manual handling assistance/equipment, cleaning and other support staff to ensure that nursing staff can focus on the delivery of care for critically ill patients.

Source: Chamberlain et al., 2017.

These recommendations serve merely to guide nurse-to-patient ratios, as extraneous factors such as the clinical practice setting, patient acuity and the knowledge and expertise of available staff will influence final staffing patterns that may be adapted to suit the requirements of individual countries or units. The requirement to provide continuity of care for patients and families should also be considered when appropriate. Patient-based tools either use dependency scoring models or activity-based models to guide these staffing decisions; the differences between these approaches are discussed below.

Practice tips

The WFCCN states that critically ill patients require one registered nurse to be allocated at all times.

Patient dependency models

Patient dependency refers to an approach to quantify the care needs of individual patients, to match these needs to the nursing staff workload and skill mix.[51] For many years, patient census was the commonest method for determining the nursing workload within an ICU. That is, the number of patients dictated the number of nurses required to care for them, based on the accepted nurse-to-patient ratios of 1:1 for ICU patients and 1:2 for HDU patients. This reflects the unit-based workload, and is also the common funding approach for ICU bed-day costs.

The nursing workload at the individual patient level; however, is also reflective of patient acuity, the complexity of care required and both the physical and the psychological status of the patient.[51] Strict adherence to the patient census model leads to the inflexibility of matching nursing resources to demand. For example, some ICU patients receive care that is so complex that more than one nurse is required, and an HDU patient may require less medical care than an ICU patient, but conversely may require more than 1:2 nursing care level secondary to such factors as physical care requirements, patient confusion, anxiety, pain or hallucinations.[51] A patient census approach therefore does not allow for the varying nursing hours required for individual patients over a shift, nor does it allow for unpredicted peaks and troughs in activity, such as multiple admissions or multiple discharges.

Activity-based models

Activity-based models calculate the time spent by nurses on patient activities. The prime purpose of these models is to classify patients into groups requiring similar nursing care and to attribute a numerical score that indicates the amount of nursing care required. Patients may also be classified according to the severity of their illness. The therapeutic intervention scoring system (TISS) was developed to determine severity of illness, to establish nurse-to-patient ratios and to assess current bed utilisation.[52] This system attributes a score to each procedure/intervention performed on a patient, with the premise that the greater the number of procedures performed, the higher the score, the higher the severity of illness, the higher the intensity of nursing care required.[51] Since its development in the mid-1970s, TISS has undergone multiple revisions but still captures the therapeutic requirements of the patient. It does not, however, capture the entirety of the nursing role. Another example of an activities-based model is the Nursing Activities Score (NAS),[53] developed from TISS with fewer items but capturing a wider range of activities relating to nursing roles, such as activities relating to family members and monitoring activities. NAS captures a greater portion of nurses' time than TISS-28[53] and has also been used to examine workload of different shifts.[54] However, it is also criticised for the subjective nature of some items, reportedly making the score less reliable.[55] Therefore, while these scoring systems may provide valuable information on the acuity of the patients within the ICU, they are not accurate indicators of total nursing workload. Other specific nursing measures have been developed but have not gained universal clinical acceptance or application.

Skill mix

Skill mix refers to the ratio of caregivers with varying levels of skill, training and experience in a clinical unit. In critical care, skill mix also refers to the proportion of RNs possessing a formal specialist critical care qualification. The ACCCN recommends an optimum qualified critical care nurse to unqualified critical care nurse ratio of 75%.[41] In Australia and New Zealand, approximately 60% and 40%, respectively, of the nurses employed in critical care units currently have some form of critical care qualification.[48]

Much of the original research fuelling the debate about optimum skill mix was undertaken in the general ward setting, but evidence is now mounting of the impact of ICU nurse staffing on patient outcomes. Quality of care outcomes that have been shown to worsen with lower numbers of RNs in ICU include pressure injuries,[56,57] healthcare-acquired infection[56,58] and critical incidents.[56]

Researchers have examined the substitution of one grade of staff with a lesser skilled, trained or experienced grade of staff, using adverse events as the outcome measure. Study results demonstrate that a rich registered nurse skill mix reduces the occurrence of adverse events.[59-61] Longitudinal studies of hospital nurse staffing and patient outcomes note that there should be better understanding of the effects of skill mix dilution, and justification of the need for greater numbers of skilled professionals at the bedside.[62] Recent studies have started to examine aspects of workload such as patient turnover and the number of life-sustaining procedures undertaken for the patient, and their impact on mortality. A prospective study conducted in eight ICUs over a calendar year found both of these indicators were associated with increased mortality.[63] Further, researchers undertook a retrospective analysis of nursing workload, severity of illness and hospital survival in two ICUs in Hong Kong and found that patients exposed to a higher workload/nurse ratio for ≥ 1 day had lower risk-adjusted odds of survival to hospital discharge than patients who were never exposed to a high ratio.[64]

Professional organisations have developed position statements on the use of staff other than RNs in the critical care environment.[41,65] The BACCN asserts that healthcare assistants employed in a critical care setting must undertake only direct patient care activities for which they have received training and for which they have been assessed competent and under the supervision of a registered nurse.[42]

Staffing levels and skill mix within critical care units should therefore be based on individual unit needs (e.g. unit size, layout and location) and patient clinical presentations/acuity, and be guided by the best available evidence to ensure safe, quality care for their patients within the context of national standards, expectations and resources.

Practice tips

Unit-specific orientation should be a formal, structured program of assessment, demonstration of competence and identification of ongoing educational needs, and should be developed to meet the needs of all staff new to the unit.

Rostering

Once the nursing establishment for a unit is determined and skill mix considered, the rostering format is decided.

FIGURE 2.1 Calculating staff requirements.

The following example is for a 6-bed intensive care unit. A roster has been determined to employ 6 nurses using a 3-shift/day approach (morning, evening, night [10 h]). A 2-hour morning (a.m.) to afternoon (p.m.) shift handover period and a 30-minute afternoon to night (ND) shift handover period are included. Local shift times and practices can be substituted.

Step 1 Calculate the number of working hours needed:

a.m. shift	0700 to 1530	= 7.6 h × 6 nurses × 7 days	319.2 h
p.m. shift	1330 to 2200	= 7.6 h × 6 nurses × 7 days	319.2 h
Night shift	2130 to 0730	= 10 h × 6 nurses × 7 days	420 h
Total			1058.4 h

These initial figures do not include sick leave or annual leave. An additional adjustment is therefore required to factor in paid, unpaid, sick and study leave. A 22% 'leave allowance' is included to accommodate these aspects. A locally derived figure may be substituted here, usually available from the finance or personnel department.

Step 2 Add the leave allowance:
1058.4 h × 1.22 (leave allowance) = 1291.2 h/38 h (1 FTE) = 33.9 FTEs

With a staffing pattern of 6 staff per shift, this unit requires an establishment of 33.9 full-time equivalents (FTEs) to meet the needs of this roster. This figure does not include positions such as the nurse unit manager, team leader/shift coordinator and clinical nurse educator, as outlined in the ACCCN guidelines[41]

In times of nursing shortages, one of the factors identified as affecting the retention of staff is the ability to provide flexibility in rostering practices. To some extent rostering practices are governed by government, hospital and industrial policies and these should be considered when deciding the roster format for individual units.

The traditional shift patterns are based on 3 × 8-hour shifts per day (Fig. 2.1) or 2 × 12-hour shifts or a combination of the two including the option of a 4-hour shift to accommodate expected new admissions. The implementation of a 12-hour roster requires careful consideration of its risks and benefits, with full consultation of all parties, unit staff, hospital management and the relevant nurses' union. Perceived benefits of working a 12-hour roster include improvement in personal/social life, reduction in overtime shifts, reduced carbon emissions, enhanced work satisfaction, improved patient care continuity and a better recovery time between shifts.[66] Perceived risks, such as an alteration in the level of sick-leave hours, decreased reaction times and reduced alertness during the longer shift, have not been found to be significant and a recent review of the evidence showed there was no clear evidence for implementing or withdrawing 12-hour shifts.[67] A reported disadvantage of 12-hour shifts is the loss of the shift overlap time, which has traditionally been used for providing in-unit educational sessions. A consideration, therefore, for units proposing the implementation of a 12-hour shift pattern is to build formal staff education sessions into the proposal.

Rostering should be structured in such a way as to promote continuity of care for patients and families and may also need to take account of additional staffing requirements to allow early rehabilitation. Staff availability has been reported as a key barrier to implementing or sustaining early rehabilitation for critically ill patients;[68] in another study rehabilitation therapy was not provided for 50% of ICU days per patient because of limited staffing.[69]

Education and training

During the latter half of the 20th century, specialist critical care nursing education made the transition from hospital-based courses in to the tertiary education sector. While some hospitals maintain in-house critical care courses, these are generally designed to meet the tertiary requirements of postgraduate education and to articulate with higher-level university programs.

Some organisations, both private and public, continue to offer a variety of short continuing education courses as well, generally at a fairly basic level of knowledge and skills, but which play a role in providing an introduction for a novice practitioner.[45] Position statements on the preparation and education of critical care nurses have been developed by professional societies;[45,46,70] these present frameworks to ensure that the course curricula provide adequate content to prepare nurses for this specialist nursing role.

Nursing has always been a profession that has required currency of knowledge and clinical skills through continuing education input, because of the rapidly changing knowledge base and innovative treatment regimens. These changes are occurring at an increasingly rapid rate, particularly in critical care. The need for critical care nurses to maintain current, up-to-date knowledge across a broad range of clinical states has therefore never been more important. Specific issues related to orientation and continuing education programs are briefly discussed below.

Orientation

The term orientation reflects a range of activities, from a comprehensive unit-based program, attendance at a hospital induction program covering the mandatory educational requirements of that facility, through to familiarisation with the layout of a department. The aim of an orientation program is the development of safe and effective practitioners. There may be other benefits. For example, a study evaluating an orientation program for new RN graduates in critical care reported significantly improved retention rates at 3, 6 and 12 months, and financial savings as a result of reduced nurse turnover.[71]

Unit-specific orientation should be a formal, structured program of assessment, demonstration of competence and identification of ongoing educational needs, and should be developed to meet the needs of all staff who are new to the unit. Competency-based orientation is learner-focused and based on the achievement of core skills that reflect unit needs and enable new employees to function in their role at the completion of the orientation period.[72] A number of professional organisations internationally have developed competency standards for specialist critical care nurses,[50,73,74] which may be used as a framework on which to build competency-based orientation programs.

Practice tips

It is alarming that many health practitioners do not acknowledge their own vulnerability to error.

Continuing education

Continuing education is a term used to reflect the education nurses undertake after their initial qualifications. While professional development has long been a requirement of continuing registration to practice, a formal requirement for continuing education or professional development is now mandated in some countries. The Nursing and Midwifery Board of Australia clearly identifies the standard for continuing professional development of nurses and midwives.[75] In New Zealand there is a requirement for nurses to complete a minimum of 60 hours professional development and 450 hours of clinical practice over a 3-year period for the purposes of registration renewal.[76] Conversely, North American nursing associations have for many years had formal programs for recognising continuing education and awarding continuing education points. These continuing education points have often been required to support continued registration.

Risk management

Managing risk is a high priority in health, and critical care is an important risk-laden environment in which the manager needs to be on the lookout for potential error, harm and medico-legal vulnerability. The Sentinel Events Evaluation study[77] has given an indication of this risk for critical care patients. The authors undertook a 24-hour observational study of 1913 patients in 205 ICUs worldwide; 584 errors were identified, causing harm or potential harm to 391 patients. The study authors concluded there was an urgent need for development and implementation of strategies for prevention and early detection of errors.[77] A second study by the same team specifically targeted errors in administration of parenteral drugs in ICUs.[78] In this study 1328 patients in 113 ICUs worldwide were studied for 24 hours; 861 errors affecting 441 patients occurred, or 74.5 parenteral drug administration errors per 100 patient days. The authors concluded that organisational factors such as error reporting systems and routine checks would reduce the risk of such errors.[78]

What is more alarming is that many health practitioners do not acknowledge their own vulnerability to error. In one study, airline flight crews (30,000) and health professionals (1033 ICU/operating room doctors and nurses, of whom 446 were nurses) from five different countries were asked a simple question, 'Does fatigue affect your (work) performance?', with fascinating results.[79] Of those responding, the following replied in the affirmative to the question: pilots and flight crew, 74%; anaesthetists, 53%; surgeons, 30% (a figure for nurses' responses to this question was not provided in the study). The study also found that only 33% of hospital staff thought errors were handled appropriately in their hospital and that over 50% of ICU staff found it hard to discuss errors.[79] Another source of risk to the safety and/or quality of patient care, specifically related to ICU nurses, is alarm fatigue, resulting in reduced attention or delayed response.[80] Interventions such as changing default alarm parameters, in order to reduce the number of false alarms, and providing in-service training for nurses, have not had a significant impact on nurses' attitudes to alarms.[81] Chapter 3 provides more information in the area of risk management including a description of non-technical skills and how training can help make critical care units safer for patients and staff.

Managerial activities that affect quality, safety and risk performance have been systematically reviewed highlighting the need to: establish goals and strategy to improve care; set a quality agenda; engage in quality activities; promote a quality improvement culture; manage those resistant of change; and procurement of organisational resources for quality.[82] In addition, the review authors advocate for positive actions, such as establishment of a quality committee, with a specific item on quality at the meeting, a quality performance measurement report and a dashboard with national quality and safety benchmarks, performance evaluation attached to quality and safety, and an infrastructure for staff–manager interactions on quality strategies.[82] Such activities are equally pertinent at the ICU management level.

Governance and management of the critical care environment requires a multidisciplinary team of senior clinician managers who understand both the clinical risk and the quality cycles of the environment as well as the executive requirements for financial and organisational viability. An astute and careful balance between good clinical governance (patient care and clinician practices) and good corporate governance (finance, information technology and other support services) is required to ensure sustainable and appropriate healthcare for all users. The take-home message in all this is that managers in hospitals manage enormous risks with patients, staff and visitors but often do not appreciate their own level of vulnerability to error and risk. Yet claims of negligence and charges of incompetence can be as threatening to the manager as they are to the clinician.

Practice tips

The ACCCN recommends an optimum qualified critical care nurse ratio of 75%.

Negligence

Negligence is a legal term that can be proven only in a court. In tort law four aspects to the charge of negligence are generally accepted:

1. The provider owed a duty of care to the recipient.
2. The provider failed to meet that duty, resulting in a breach of care.
3. The recipient sustained damages (loss) as a result.
4. The breach by the provider caused the recipient to suffer reasonably foreseeable damages.[83]

Courts use a multifactorial assessment of all the facts to determine the level of liability or otherwise of the defendant. The greatest impact of this is on the quantum of damages. Therefore, while health professionals can be held liable for negligence, the damages are reduced because of statutory limits like thresholds and caps.[84]

Critical to reducing liability in this area is the need for health services and managers to have in place policies, procedures and supervision processes that reflect best evidence in order to ensure contemporary and safe practices among its workforce.

The role of leadership and management

Managers must also be leaders, and the need to have good leaders and managers is as relevant to critical care as it is to any other business or clinical entity. Seminal research studies on organisational structures in ICUs across the US in the 1980s[85] and 1990s[86] demonstrated the important role leadership plays in patient care and risk management in the ICU. Using APACHE scoring, organisational efficiency and risk-adjusted survival were measured. High-performing ICUs demonstrated that actual survival rates exceeded predicted survival rates.[85,86]

Further investigation and analysis of the higher-performing units noted that these units had well-defined protocols, a medical director to coordinate activities, well-educated nurses and collaboration between nurses and doctors.[85,86] Clear and accessible policies and procedures to guide staff practice in the ICU setting were also highlighted. These policies and procedures need to be in written or electronic form, simple to read and in a consistent format, evidence-based, easy to understand and easy to apply and easy to access.

The latter study by Zimmerman et al[86] showed similar characteristics: they had a patient-centred culture, strong medical and nursing leadership, effective communication and coordination, and open and collaborative problem-solving and conflict management. One cannot underestimate the value of strong, dedicated and collaborative leadership from managers as the key to organisational success in the critical care setting. These factors are as pertinent now as they were when first studied over 30 years ago and remind us of the important role of leadership to ensure the safety of patients, visitors and staff alike in this complex health setting.[87,88] Chapter 1 contains a discussion about leadership.

Managing injury: staff, patient or visitor

When staff members are injured, the response must be swift and deliberate. Injury can come in many forms, involving physical injuries or biological exposures, for example. More often, the problems are grievances, such as missing out on an opportunity afforded to others (e.g. a promotion), feeling marginalised by others, or not getting a preferred roster. For patients, an injury can be physical, such as a drug error or an iatrogenic infection; however, the injury can also be non-physical and can affect patients, visitors and staff members, as with complaints about lack of timely information, misinformation or rudeness of staff. In all circumstances a manager needs to intervene proactively to minimise or contain the negativity or harm felt by the 'victim'. Some authorities have established frameworks to govern safety and risk management in health care.[89,90] Regardless of the cause of the injury, the principles governing good risk management are common to many situations and are summarised in Box 2.3.

If an incident occurs, it should be documented as soon as possible afterwards and when it is safe to do so. The clinician who discovers and follows up an incident must document the event, asking the questions that a manager, family member, police officer, lawyer or judge might wish to ask. The written account provided soon after the event or incident by a person closely involved, or witness to it, will form a very important testimonial in any subsequent investigation. Key points to document are identified in Table 2.4.

BOX 2.3

Defensive principles to minimise risk after an incident (patient or staff)[21]

- Those persons encouraged to participate in decision making are more inclined to 'own' the decisions made; therefore, involve them in deciding how the issue is to be tackled and help to make the expectations realistic.
- Education of the person in the various aspects of the incident/activity will reduce fear and anxiety.
- Explain the range of possible outcomes and where the affected person is currently situated on that continuum.
- Provide frequent and accurate updates on the person's situation and what is being done to improve that situation.
- Maintain a consistent approach and as far as possible the same person should provide such information/feedback.

Source: Guo, 2018.

Contemporary wisdom in modern health agencies advocates open disclosure: telling the truth to the patient or family about why and how an adverse event has occurred.[91,92] This practice may be contrary to informed legal advice and may not preclude legal action against the staff or institution.[93–95] However, openly informing the patient/family of what has occurred can regain trust and respect, and may help to resolve anger and frustration. The open disclosure process can also provide learning and education on how such events can be prevented in the future, a right for which many consumer advocates are now lobbying.[96]

The process of root cause analysis (RCA) can also assist the team to explore in detail the sequence of events and system failures that precipitated an incident and help to inform future system reforms to minimise harm. An RCA is a generic method of 'drilling down' to identify hospital system deficiencies that may not immediately be apparent, and that may have contributed to the occurrence of a 'sentinel event'. The general characteristics of an RCA are that it:[97]

- focuses on systems and processes, not individual performance
- includes a review of the relevant literature
- examines the event extensively for underlying contributing causes
- enables procedure and system modifications.

TABLE 2.4

Key points when documenting an incident in a patient's file notes[23]

QUESTION	EXPLANATION
Where did the incident occur?	For example, bedside, toilet, drug room
Were there any pre-event circumstances of significance?	For example, short-staffed, no written protocol, medications with side effects that could have contributed.
Who witnessed the event?	Including staff, patient, visitors
What was done to minimise negative effects?	For example, extra staff brought to assist, spill wiped up, sign placed on front of patient chart warning of reaction/sensitivity etc
Who in authority was notified of the incident?	Involving a senior, experienced manager/authority should help expedite immediate and effective action.
Who informed the victim of the event? What was the victim told? What was the response?	Clear, concise and non-judgemental explanations to victim or representative are necessary as soon as possible, preferably from a credible authority (manager/director).
What follow-up support, counselling and revision occurred?	This is important for both victim and perpetrator; ascertain when counselling occurred and who provided it.
What review systems were commenced to limit recurrence of the event?	Magistrates and coroners, in particular, want to know what system changes have occurred to limit the recurrence of the event.

Source: Williams et al., 2003.

Practice tips

If an incident does occur, it is always prudent to document the event as soon as possible afterwards and when it is safe to do so.

Management of disease outbreaks and pandemics

The World Health Organisation (WHO) defines a pandemic as the worldwide spread of a new disease.[98] A disease outbreak, on the other hand, is the occurrence of cases of disease in excess of what would normally be expected in a defined community, geographical area or season. An outbreak may occur in a restricted geographical area, or may extend over several countries. It may last for a few days or weeks, or for several years. A single case of a communicable disease long absent from a population, or caused by an agent (e.g. bacterium or virus) not previously recognised in that community or area, or the emergence of a previously unknown disease, may also constitute an outbreak and should be reported and investigated.[99]

Planning for the impact, or potential impact, of a disease outbreak/pandemic is required at the global (WHO), national (Federal Government), regional (state/province), organisational (hospital), department (ICU) and individual (health professional) level. All healthcare staff have an obligation to be aware of their roles and responsibilities if called upon to respond to a disease outbreak in our community. This section highlights the areas to be considered at the individual facility level (i.e. hospital) with an emphasis on the considerations common to the ICU service during such events.

Intensive care beds and their associated resources (space, equipment and staffing) are finite resources and an organisational response is required to maximise potential ICU capacity during outbreaks. Lessons can be learnt from the global H1N1 pandemic in 2009 and the recent Australian disease outbreak of H3N2 in 2017.[100] The knowledge gained from these experiences clearly identifies the need to plan for the potential increased demand on critical care services.[101] While it is beyond the scope of this chapter to cover this subject comprehensively, the aim is to outline the areas for further examination, touching on the concept of the development of a surge plan. Chapter 14 contains a description of critical care responses to respiratory pandemics.

In earlier experiences[101-106] critical care units play a key role in an organised response to a pandemic, particularly an airborne one such as influenza, where critical care units are often more severely affected than other clinical areas of a hospital. Demand for these services will at these times, exceed normal supply.

Development of a surge plan

Hota et al.[101] describe the preparations for a surge to service under the three headings 'staff, stuff and space', and we add 'command and communication'. The resources required in such a plan are examined under these headings.

Staff

The ability to provide additional staff for a potentially expanded critical care bed base should examine the following:

- staff with critical care skills who do not currently work in this area
- staff from other areas with critical care-based skills, such as recovery, anaesthetics, coronary care
- provision of training and education to support less experienced staff
- development of critical care nursing teams in which critical care expertise is spread across the teams to manage the patient load appropriately, i.e. in satellite units
- planning for critical care staff sick leave
- provision to redeploy pregnant staff, staff with chronic health conditions and/or emotionally vulnerable staff.
- emotional support in the form of team debriefing, and occasionally individual counselling, is essential during and after the event. Anxiety, panic, burnout, compassion fatigue and posttraumatic stress are all possible sequelae of an intense and sustained pandemic. One cannot underestimate the importance of experienced, emotionally intelligent leadership during such events.

Stuff

The ability to manage supplies at times of uncertain demand is a key element for examination, as is the knowledge and understanding of the processes for accessing additional equipment such as ventilators and medications from state emergency stockpiles, for example:

- Ensure supplies of appropriate personal protective equipment
- Develop plans/policies for the rational use of personal protective equipment
- Ensure supplies, and access to supplies, of required medications
- Plan ability to boost ventilator capacity, such as with increased use of BiPAP or accessing state emergency stockpile, or short-term leasing options with company providers.

Space

Examine and plan strategies to functionally increase the available critical care bed capacity, as follows:

- Defer elective surgery and other elective procedures
- Explore the ability of local private hospitals to assist with service provision for non-deferrable surgical case.
- Identify alternative clinical areas within the hospital that may provide additional critical care beds as a satellite unit, such as recovery and coronary care
- Triaging access to limited ventilation and/or critical care resources.[102,106]

Command and communication

- Identification of a clear chain of command is essential to facilitate fast and efficient decision making, communication and action. The person in command must have authority, experience and maturity to guide and make decisions during very dynamic changing circumstances. In addition, they must be precise in their communication ensuring orders are correct, understandable and implementable. While these qualities are essential in all leadership roles, they are particularly necessary during intense situations such as these.
- Hospital signage and communication to a) restrict visitor entrance and b) minimise person-to-person contact and c) appropriate use of personal protective equipment. Consideration should be given to the use of international symbols as well as common languages in the community.
- Provision of training and education of all staff to avoid panic and concern and to communicate appropriate messaging to others. For example, domestic and catering staff can play an important role in containing spread of disease/panic if informed and confident in their knowledge and role during an outbreak.
- Regular information circulars to keep all staff and the community abreast of what is being done to contain the disease and to keep people safe.

Developing a critical care surge plan

Templates to assist in the development of a critical care surge plan are available.[102] The following example is formatted in a graduated approach and is shown as a percentage (%) of current unit capacity:

- pre-surge
- minor surge: 5–10%
- moderate surge: 11–20%
- major surge: 21–50%
- large scale emergency >50%

The use of such a template, which can be populated with locally appropriate definitions and information, can provide the basis for a comprehensive unit/facility specific response to the requirement for a graduated response to a pandemic. Planning for events such as a pandemic require a coordinated, collaborative approach from all members of the healthcare team, resulting in scalable, flexible plans that are underpinned by the normal management structure and ensure effective lines of communication.[104]

Summary

The management of all resources in the critical care unit is key to meeting the needs of the patients in a safe, ethical, timely and cost-effective manner. Many factors influence not only the resources available but also how these resources are allocated. Managers of critical care units are required to be knowledgeable in the design and equipping of units; human resource management, including the make-up of the nursing workforce; and the fundamentals of the budget – how it is determined, monitored and managed. Understanding the principles of risk management and tools such as those that measure nursing workload help nurse managers in their planning and decision making. Having good structures and processes in place facilitate the delivery of care during times of crisis, such as what is experienced when pandemics occur.

Case study

The City Hospital is a 350-bed, metropolitan, public hospital that is planning to expand their intensive care unit from 20 to 30 beds. Five of the additional 10 beds will have negative pressure/isolation capacity. As the nurse unit manager you are required to determine the additional nursing and equipment resources required to make this a functional unit once it is fully commissioned. The hospital is geographically located close to a 100-bed private hospital and 25 km from an international airport. This hospital also has a separate 10-bed CCU and 12-bed post-anaesthetic care unit (PACU).

Among other things you must consider the following tasks and make recommendations to the Director of Nursing of The Royal Hospital (see *Learning activities* 1–8). Utilise information contained in this chapter to inform your work and recommendations.

RESEARCH VIGNETTE

Lee A, Cheung YS, Joynt GM, Leung CC, Wong WT, Gomersall CD. Are high nurse workload/staffing ratios associated with decreased survival in critically ill patients? A cohort study. Annals of Intensive Care. 2017; (7):146.

Abstract

Background: Despite the central role of nurses in intensive care, a relationship between intensive care nurse workload/staffing ratios and survival has not been clearly established. We determined whether there is a threshold workload/staffing ratio above which the probability of hospital survival is reduced and then modelled the relationship between exposure to inadequate staffing at any stage of a patient's ICU stay and risk-adjusted hospital survival.

Methods: Retrospective analysis of prospectively collected data from a cohort of adult patients admitted to two multidisciplinary intensive care units was performed. The nursing workload [measured using the therapeutic intervention scoring system (TISS-76) for all patients in the ICU during each day to average number of bedside nurses per shift on that day (workload/nurse) ratio, severity of illness (using Acute Physiology and Chronic Health Evaluation III) and hospital survival were analysed using net-benefit regression methodology and logistic regression.

Results: A total of 894 separate admissions, representing 845 patients, were analysed. Our analysis shows that there was a 95% probability that survival to hospital discharge was more likely to occur when the maximum workload-to-nurse ratio was <40 and a more than 95% chance that death was more likely to occur when the ratio was >52.

Patients exposed to a high workload/nurse ratio (≥52) for ≥1 day during their ICU stay had lower risk-adjusted odds of survival to hospital discharge compared to patients never exposed to a high ratio (odds ratio 0.35, 95% CI 0.16–0.79).

Conclusions: Exposing critically ill patients to high workload/staffing ratios is associated with a substantial reduction in the odds of survival.

Critique

This study was a retrospective observational cohort study designed to test the hypothesis that exposure to an inadequate workload/staffing ratio during a patient's ICU stay is independently associated with increased mortality. This was tested through a two-stage cohort study: firstly to identify a threshold/workload ratio above which staffing would be considered inadequate and, secondly, to determine whether exposure to inadequate staffing at any stage of the patient's ICU stay was associated with increased mortality.

The study was undertaken in two ICUs in Hong Kong of contrasting size (12 bed and 22 bed) in two different hospitals. The two ICUs had different staffing profiles; 28% of RNs in one unit and 67% RNs in the second unit had a post-registration critical care qualification. The ICUs are described as multidisciplinary but no explanation of this term is provided. However, the authors provide detail regarding key factors in each ICU that may impact on workload: unit layout; nursing, physician and allied health professional staffing; and the roles undertaken by nursing assistants. Sufficient detail is provided to allow the reader to interpret the results in the context of their own setting.

Study design, methods and statistical analysis are appropriate and sufficient detail is provided to allow replication in future studies. The study design is not intended to test cause and effect relationships; the correlational design also does not allow us to rule out other confounding factors that may account for the statistical association. Ethics approval was obtained from a University Clinical Research Ethics Committee. The accuracy of the data cannot be assured, which is an acknowledged limitation of retrospective studies. However, the TISS-76 data were collected prospectively by a dedicated audit nurse, reducing the likelihood of measurement variability.

The results are based on 894 ICU admissions (n=845 individual patients) and the researchers were able to identify a workload threshold beyond which patients had lower risk-adjusted odds of survival. Patients exposed to a workload/staffing ratio beyond this threshold for one day or more had lower odds of survival to hospital discharge.

The authors acknowledge the limitations of the two-site study, which may mean the results cannot be generalised. They also acknowledge that 'limitation of therapy orders', which were not recorded for the study, may have confounded the findings.

Learning activities

Learning activity relates to the case study.

1 Calculate the additional staffing numbers in FTEs that you will require to staff the increase in beds.

2 Identify the major equipment needs for the additional 10 beds and develop an estimated budget plan for these items based on your knowledge of costs in your region. List the criteria that should be included in the evaluation of new consumable products for this expansion.

3 Identify the three fundamental steps in the budget process and the important considerations for each in this project.

4 In preparation for writing a Critical Care Surge Plan calculate the surge capacity required for an additional 10- and 25-bed ICU beyond the capacity of the newly expanded (30-bed) ICU.

5 Your ICU receives three patients with a highly contagious and deadly disease. Despite staff education and training in appropriate handling of infectious patients, two of your staff have contracted the disease and are admitted to your hospital. What actions will you take?

6 Identify one major equipment item new to your department, e.g. ECMO machine. Develop a business case to explain the benefits of this item using the business case framework in this chapter.

Online resources

Australian Commission on Safety and Quality in Health Care. Australian safety and quality framework for healthcare. 2011. Available from: https://www.safetyandquality.gov.au/wp-content/uploads/2011/01/ASQFHC-Guide-Healthcare-team.pdf

Ettelt S, Nolte E. Funding intensive care: approaches in systems using diagnosis-related groups. Available from:

http://www.rand.org/content/dam/rand/pubs/technical_reports/2010/RAND_TR792.pdf

Frankel A, Haraden C, Federico F, Lenoci-Edwards JA. Framework for Safe, Reliable, and Effective Care. White Paper. Cambridge, MA: Institute for Healthcare Improvement and Safe & Reliable Healthcare 2017. Available from: http://www.ihi.org/resources/Pages/IHIWhitePapers/Framework-Safe-Reliable-Effective-Care.aspx

NHS. Managing Conflict in the NHS. 2017 Available from: https://www.england.nhs.uk/ourwork/coi/

NHS National Innovation Centre. Business Case Template. Available from: http://knowledge.nic.nhs.uk/documentDetails.aspx?docId=40

Parliament of Australia: Australia's capacity to respond to an infectious disease outbreak. Available from: https://www.aph.gov.au/About_Parliament/Parliamentary_Departments/Parliamentary_Library/pubs/rp/rp0405/05rp03

Tasmanian Government business case (small) template and guide. Available from: http://www.egovernment.tas.gov.au/__data/assets/word_doc/0013/15520/pman-temp-open-sml-proj-bus-case.doc

Further reading

Durbin CG. Team model: advocating for the optimal method of care delivery in the intensive care unit. Crit Care Med 2006;34(3 Suppl.):S12–17.

Gill FJ, Leslie GD, Grech C, et al. An analysis of Australian graduate critical care nurse education. Collegian 2015;22: 71–81.

Manojlovich M, Saint S, Forman J, et al. Developing and testing a tool to measure nurse/physician communication in the intensive care unit. J Patient Saf 2011;7(2):80–4.

Parker MM. Critical care disaster management. Crit Care Med 2006;34(3 Suppl.):S52–5.

Redden PH, Evans J. It takes teamwork ... the role of nurses in ICU design. Crit Care Nurs Q 2014;37(1):41–52.

Robnett MK. Critical care nursing: workforce issues and potential solutions. Crit Care Med 2006;34(3 Suppl.):S25–31.

Valentin A, Ferdinande P. Recommendations on basic requirements for intensive care units: structural and organizational aspects. Intensive Care Med 2011;37:1575–87.

References

1. Ristagno G, Weil MH. History of critical care medicine: the past, the present and the future. In: Gullo A, Lumb PD, Besso J, et al, editors. Intensive and critical care medicine. Milano: Springer; 2009. p. 3–9.
2. Johnston MJ. Bioethics: a nursing perspective. Sydney: Elsevier; 2009.
3. Wiles V, Daffurn K There is a bird in my hand and a bear by the bed – I must be in ICU. Sydney: Australian College of Critical Care Nurses, 2002.
4. Ettelt S, Nolte E Funding Intensive Care – approaches in systems using diagnosis-related groups. RAND California; 2010. Available from: http://www.rand.org/content/dam/rand/pubs/technical_reports/2010/RAND_TR792.pdf. [Accessed 30 December 2017].
5. Independent Hospital Pricing Authority. The Pricing Framework for Australian Hospitals Services 2015-16 Australia: Commonwealth of Australia; 2013. Available from: https://www.ihpa.gov.au/sites/g/files/net636/f/publications/final-2015-16-pricing_framework_for_australian_public_hospital_services_d14-43339.pdf. [Accessed 30 December 2017].
6. Murthy S, Leligdowicz A, Adhikari NKJ. Intensive care unit capacity in low-income countries: a systematic review. PLoS ONE 2015;10:e0116949.
7. ANZICS centre for outcome and resource evaluation annual report, ANZICS Melbourne; 2017. Available from: http://www.anzics.com.au/Downloads/ANZICS%20CORE%20Annual%20Report%202017.pdf. [Accessed 30 March 2018].
8. Kleinpell R, Barden C, Rincon T, et al. Assessing the impact of telemedicine on nursing care in intensive care units. Am J Crit Care 2016;25(1):e14–20.
9. Cismondi F, Celi LA, Fialho AS, et al. Reducing unnecessary lab testing in the ICU with artificial intelligence. Int J Med Inform 2013;82:345–58.
10. Halpern NA, Anderson DC, Kesecioglu J. ICU design in 2050: looking into the crystal ball! Intensive Care Med 2017;43:690–2.
11. Oye RK, Bellamy PE. Patterns of resource consumption in medical intensive care. Chest 1991;99:685–9.
12. Blot S, Koulenti D, Dimopoulos G, et al. Prevalence, risk factors, and mortality for ventilator-associated pneumonia in middle-aged, old, and very old critically ill patients. Crit Care Med 2014;42:601–9.
13. Williams TA, Ho KM, Dobb GJ, et al. Changes in case-mix and outcomes of critically ill patients in an Australian tertiary intensive care unit. Anaesth Intensive Care 2010;38:703–9.
14. Sim YS, Jung H, Shin TR, et al. Mortality and outcomes in very elderly patients 90 years of age or older admitted to the ICU. Respir Care 2015;60:347–55.
15. Vincent JL, Marshall JC, Ñamendys-Silva SA, et al. Assessment of the worldwide burden of critical illness: the Intensive Care Over Nations (ICON) audit. Lancet Respir Med 2014;2:380–6.
16. Wunsch H, Linde-Zwirble WT, Harrison DA, et al. Use of intensive care services during terminal hospitalizations in England and the United States. Am J Respir Crit Care Med 2009;180:875–80.
17. Pastores SM, Dakwar J, Halpern NA. Costs of critical care medicine. Crit Care Clin 2012;28:1–10.
18. Lawson JS, Rotem A, Bates PW. From clinician to manager. Sydney: McGraw-Hill; 1996.
19. Strosberg M, Wiener J, Baker R. Rationing America's medical care: the Oregon plan and beyond. Washington DC: The Brookings Institute Press; 1992.
20. Truog RD, Brock DW, Cook DJ, et al. Rationing in the intensive care unit. Crit Care Med 2006;34:958–63.
21. Guo C, Elliot S, Soso M. The role of Medical Emergency Team in end of life care planning for hospitalised patients. Aust Crit Care 2018;31:118.
22. Donohue LA, Endacott R. Track, trigger and teamwork: communication of deterioration in acute medical and surgical wards. Intensive Crit Care Nurs 2010;26:10–17.
23. Williams G. Quality management in intensive care. In: Gullo A, editor. Anesthesia, pain, intensive care and emergency medicine. Berlin: Springer-Verlag; 2003. p. 1239–50.
24. Gan R. Budgeting. In: Crowther A, editor. Nurse managers: a guide to practice. Sydney: Ausmed; 2004.

25. Donahue L, Rader S, Triolo PK. Nurturing innovation in the critical care environment: transforming care at the bedside. Crit Care Nurs Clin North Am 2008;20:465–9.
26. Capezio P. Manager's guide to business planning. Madison: McGraw-Hill; 2010.
27. Weaver DJ, Sorrells-Jones J. The business case as a strategic tool for change. J Nurs Adm 2007;37:414–19.
28. Paley N. Successful business planning – energizing your company's potential. London: Thorogood; 2004.
29. College of Intensive Care Medicine. Minimum standards for intensive care units. Australia.: CICM; 2011. Available from: http://www.cicm.org.au/CICM_Media/CICMSite/CICM-Website/Resources/Professional%20Documents/IC-1-Minimum-Standards-for-Intensive-Care-Units.pdf. [Accessed 14 January 2018].
30. The Faculty of Intensive Care Medicine/Intensive Care Society. Guidelines for the provision of intensive care services; 2015. Available from: https://www.ficm.ac.uk/sites/default/files/gpics_-_ed.1_2015_v2.pdf. [Accessed 14 January 2018].
31. Australian Health Infrastructure Alliance. Australasian health facility guidelines: Part B – health facility briefing and planning 360-intensive care-general. North Sydney: AHIA; 2016. Available from: https://aushfg-prod-com-au.s3.amazonaws.com/HPU_B.0360_6_0.pdf. [Accessed 14 January 2018].
32. Department of Health. Health building note 04-02 - critical care units: crown; 2013. Available from: https://www.gov.uk/government/uploads/system/uploads/attachment_data/file/147865/HBN_04-02_Final.pdf. [Accessed 14 January 2018].
33. Valentin A, Ferdinande P, the Esicm Working Group on Quality Improvement. Recommendations on basic requirements for intensive care units: structural and organizational aspects. Intensive Care Med 2011;37:1575–87.
34. Hashem MD, Parker AM, Needham DM. Early mobilization and rehabilitation of patients who are critically ill. CHEST J 2016;150:722–31.
35. Lord RK, Mayhew CR, Korupolu R, et al. ICU early physical rehabilitation programs: financial modelling of cost savings. Crit Care Med 2013;41:717–24.
36. Mahbub R. Technology and the future of intensive care unit design. Crit Care Nurs Q 2011;34:332–3.
37. Huffling K, Schenk E. Environmental sustainability in the intensive care unit: challenges and solutions. Crit Care Nurs Q 2014;37(3):235–50.
38. Grundy Q, Habibi H, Schnier A, et al. Decoding disclosure: comparing conflict of interest policy among the United States, France, and Australia. Health Policy. Available from: https://doi.org/10.1016/j.healthpol.2018.03.015. [Accessed 5 May 2018].
39. National Health Service. Managing conflicts of interest in the NHS. Available from: https://www.england.nhs.uk/commissioning/pc-co-comms/coi/. [Accessed 5 May 2018].
40. Kelly DM, Kutney-Lee A, McHugh MD, et al. Impact of critical care nursing on 30-day mortality of mechanically ventilated older adults. Crit Care Med 2014;42:1089–95.
41. Australian College of Critical Care Nurses. ICU staffing position statement (2003) on Intensive Care Nursing Staffing. Melbourne: ACCCN; 2003. Available from: http://www.acccn.com.au/documents/item/20. [Accessed 30 March 2018].
42. British Association of Critical Care Nurses. Standards for nurse staffing in critical care BACCN; 2009. Available from: http://www.baccn.org.uk/about/downloads/BACCN_Staffing_Standards.pdf. [Accessed 30 March 2018].
43. World Federation of Critical Care Nurses. Declaration of Buenos Aires: position statement on the provision of critical care nursing workforce; 2005. Available from: http://wfccn.org/publications/workforce. [Accessed 29 July 2014].
44. Endacott R, Jones C, Bloomer MJ, et al. The state of critical care nursing education in Europe: an international survey. Intensive Care Med 2015;41(12):2237–40.
45. Chamberlain D, Pollock W, Fulbrook P, the ACCCN Workforce Standards Development Group. ACCCN Workforce Standards for Intensive Care Nursing: systematic and evidence review, development, and appraisal. Aust Crit Care 2017;Available from: https://doi.org/10.1016/j.aucc.2017.08.007.
46. World Federation of Critical Care Nurses. Declaration of Madrid: position statement on the provision of critical care nursing education; 2005. Available from: http://wfccn.org/publications/education. [Accessed 29 July 2014].
47. Haupt MT, Bekes CE, Brilli RJ, et al. Guidelines on critical care services and personnel: recommendations based on a system of categorization of three levels of care. Crit Care Med 2003;31:2677–83.
48. Australia and New Zealand Intensive Care Society. Intensive care resources and activity in Australia and New Zealand – activity report 2015/16 Melbourne, Australia: ANZICS; 2017. Available from: http://www.anzics.com.au/Downloads/2015-16%20CCR%20Activity%20Report.pdf. [Accessed 22 January 2018].
49. Critical Care Nurses' Section: New Zealand Nurses Organisation. Minimum guidelines for intensive care nurse staffing in New Zealand Wellington: NZNO; 2005. Available from: http://www.nzno.org.nz/Portals/0/CCNSMin guidelinesforIntensiveCareOct 05.pdf. [Accessed 22 January 2018].
50. Critical Care Nurses' Section: New Zealand Nurses Organisation. New Zealand Standards for critical care nursing practice. Wellington: NZNO; 2014. Available from: http://www.nzno.org.nz/Portals/0/publications/New Zealand standards for critical care nursing practice, 2014.pdf. [Accessed 22 January 2018].
51. Adomat R, Hewison A. Assessing patient category/dependence systems for determining the nurse/patient ratio in ICU and HDU: a review of approaches. J Nurs Manag 2004;12:299–308.
52. Miranda DR, de Rijk A, Schaufeli W. Simplified Therapeutic Intervention Scoring System: the TISS-28 items - results from a multicenter study. Crit Care Med 1996;24:64–73.
53. Miranda DR, Nap R, de Rijk A, et al. System TWGTIS. Nursing activities score. Crit Care Med 2003;31:374–82.

54. Debergh DP, Myny D, Van Herzeele I, et al. Measuring the nursing workload per shift in the ICU. Intensive Care Med 2012;38:1438–44.
55. Carmona-Monge FJ, Rodríguez GM, Herranz CQ, et al. Evaluation of the nursing workload through the Nine Equivalents for Nursing Manpower Use Scale and the Nursing Activities Score: a prospective correlation study. Intensive Crit Care Nurs 2013;29:228–33.
56. Schubert M, Clarke SP, Aiken LH, et al. Associations between rationing of nursing care and inpatient mortality in Swiss hospitals. Int J Qual Health Care 2012;24(3):230–8.
57. Cremasco MF, Wenzel F, Zanei SS, et al. Pressure ulcers in the intensive care unit: the relationship between nursing workload, illness severity and pressure ulcer risk. J Clin Nurs 2013;22:2183–91.
58. Venier AG, Leroyer C, Slekovec C, et al. Risk factors for *Pseudomonas aeruginosa* acquisition in intensive care units: a prospective multicentre study. J Hosp Infect 2014;88:103–8.
59. Duffield C, Roche M, Diers D, et al. Staffing, skill mix and the model of care. J Clin Nurs 2010;19:2242–51.
60. Cho E, Sloane DM, Kim EY, et al. Effects of nurse staffing, work environments, and education on patient mortality: an observational study. Int J Nurs Stud 2015;52:535–42.
61. Aiken LH, Sloane DM, Bruyneel L, et al. Nurse staffing and education and hospital mortality in nine European countries: a retrospective observational study. Lancet 2014;383:1824–30.
62. Jianghua H, Staggs VS, Bergquist-Beringer S, et al. Nurse staffing and patient outcomes: a longitudinal study on trend and seasonality. BMC Nurs 2016;Available from: https://doi.org/10.1186/s12912-016-0181-3.
63. Neuraz A, Guérin C, Payet C, et al. Patient mortality is associated with staff resources and workload in the ICU: a multicenter observational study. Crit Care Med 2015;43:1587–94.
64. Lee A, Cheung YS, Joynt GM, et al. Are high nurse workload/staffing ratios associated with decreased survival in critically ill patients? A cohort study. Ann Intensive Care 2017;7:46.
65. Australian College of Critical Care Nurses. Position statement on the use of healthcare workers other than division 1 registered nurses in intensive care. Melbourne: ACCCN; 2006. Available from: http://www.acccn.com.au/documents/item/21. [Accessed 23 January 2018].
66. Costa G, Anelli MM, Castellini G, et al. Stress and sleep in nurses employed in "3× 8" and "2 × 12" fast rotating shift schedules. Chronobiol Int 2014;31:1169–78.
67. Harris R, Sims S, Parr J, et al. Impact of 12h shift patterns in nursing: a scoping review. Int J Nurs Stud 2015;52:605–34.
68. Dafoe S, Stiller K, Chapman M. Staff perceptions of the barriers to mobilizing ICU patients. Int J Allied Health Sci Pract 2015;13(2):Article 8.
69. Zanni JM, Korupolu R, Fan E, et al. Rehabilitation therapy and outcomes in acute respiratory failure: an observational pilot project. J Crit Care 2010;25:254–62.
70. Critical Care Nurses' Section: New Zealand Nurses Organisation. Critical care nurses' section position statement (2010) on the provision of critical care nursing education. Wellington: NZNO; 2010. Available from: http://www.nzno.org.nz/Portals/0/Docs/Groups/Critical Care Nurses/CCNS Position Statement on the Provision of Crticial Care Nursing Education 2010.pdf. [Accessed 23 January 2018].
71. Friedman MI, Cooper AH, Click E, et al. Specialized new graduate RN critical care orientation: retention and financial impact. Nurs Econ 2011;29(1):7–14.
72. Harper JP. Preceptors' perceptions of a competency-based orientation. J Nurses Staff Dev 2002;18:198–202.
73. American Association of Critical Care Nurses. Institute for Credentialing Excellence (ICE) and National Commission for Certifying Agencies (NCCA): AACN; 2014. Available from: https://www.aacn.org/nursing-excellence/standards/aacn-scope-and-standards-for-acute-and-critical-care-nursing-practice. [Accessed 23 January 2018].
74. European Federation of Critical Care Nursing Associations. EfCCNa Comptency Tool for European Critical Care Nurses; 2013. Available from: http://www.efccna.org/education/publications. [Accessed 23 January 2018].
75. Nursing and Midwifery Board of Australia. Registration standard: Continuing Professional Development; 2016. Available from: http://www.nursingmidwiferyboard.gov.au/Registration-Standards/Continuing-professional-development.aspx. [Accessed 23 January 2018].
76. Nursing Council of New Zealand. Guidelines for competence assessment Wellington: NZNO; 2008. Available from: http://www.nursingcouncil.org.nz/Nurses/Continuing-competence. [Accessed 23 January 2018].
77. Valentin A, Capuzzo M, Guidet B, et al. Patient safety in intensive care: results from the multinational Sentinel Events Evaluation (SEE) study. Intensive Care Med 2006;32:1591–8.
78. Valentin A, Capuzzo M, Guidet B, et al. Errors in administration of parenteral drugs in intensive care units: multinational prospective study. BMJ 2009;338:b814.
79. Sexton JB, Thomas EJ, Helmreich RL. Error, stress, and teamwork in medicine and aviation: cross sectional surveys. BMJ 2000;320:745–9.
80. Cho OM, Kim H, Lee YW, et al. Clinical alarms in intensive care units: perceived obstacles of alarm management and alarm fatigue in nurses. Healthc Inform Res 2016;22:46–53.
81. Sowan AK, Gomez TM, Tarriela AF, et al. Changes in default alarm settings and standard in-service are insufficient to improve alarm fatigue in an intensive care unit: a pilot project. JMIR Hum Factors 2016;3(1).
82. Parand A, Dopson S, Renz A, et al. The role of hospital managers in quality and patient safety: a systematic review. BMJ Open 2014;4(9):e005055.
83. MacFarlane PJM, Reid SJ. 2006 Queensland health law book. 16th ed. Brisbane: Federation Press; 2006.
84. Yule J. Defences in medical negligence: to what extent has tort law reform in Australia limited the liability of health professionals? JALTA 2011;4:53–63.

85. Knaus WA, Draper EA, Wagner DP, et al. An evaluation of outcome from intensive care in major medical centers. Ann Intern Med 1986;104:410–18.
86. Zimmerman JE, Shortell SM, Rousseau DM, et al. Improving intensive care: observations based on organizational case studies in nine intensive care units: a prospective, multicenter study. Crit Care Med 1993;21:1443–51.
87. Curtis JR, Cook DJ, Wall RJ, et al. Intensive care unit quality improvement: a 'how-to' guide for the interdisciplinary team. Crit Care Med 2006;34:211–18.
88. Thomas EJ, Sexton JB, Helmreich RL. Discrepant attitudes about teamwork among critical care nurses and physicians. Crit Care Med 2003;31(3):956–9.
89. Frankel A, Haraden C, Federico F, et al. Framework for safe, reliable, and effective care. White Paper. Cambridge, MA: Institute for Healthcare Improvement and Safe and Reliable Healthcare; 2017. Available from: http://www.ihi.org/resources/Pages/IHIWhitePapers/Framework-Safe-Reliable-Effective-Care.aspx. [Accessed 5 May 2018].
90. Australian Commission on Safety and Quality in Health Care. Australian safety and quality framework for healthcare; 2011. Available from: https://www.safetyandquality.gov.au/wp-content/uploads/2011/01/ASQFHC-Guide-Healthcare-team.pdf. [Accessed 5 May 2018].
91. Australian Commission on Safety and Quality in Healthcare. Australian Open Disclosure Framework Sydney: Commonwealth of Australia; 2013. Available from: http://www.safetyandquality.gov.au/wp-content/uploads/2013/03/Australian-Open-Disclosure-Framework-Feb-2014.pdf. [Accessed 30 March 2018].
92. Iedema RA, Mallock NA, Sorensen RJ, et al. The National Open Disclosure Pilot: evaluation of a policy implementation initiative. Med J Aust 2008;188:397–400.
93. Gold M. Is honesty always the best policy? Ethical aspects of truth telling. Intern Med J 2004;34:578–80.
94. Madden B, Cockburn T. Bundaberg and beyond: duty to disclose adverse events to patients. J Law Med 2007;14:501–27.
95. Johnstone M. Clinical risk management and the ethics of open disclosure. Part I. Benefits and risks to patient safety. AENJ 2008;11:88–94.
96. Harrison R, Birks Y, Hall J, et al. The contribution of nurses to incident disclosure: a narrative review. Int J Nurs Stud 2014;51:334–45.
97. Department of Human Services Victoria. Clinical risk management, root cause analysis; 2014. Available from: http://www.health.vic.gov.au/clinrisk/investigation/root-cause-analysis.htm. [Accessed 30 March 2018].
98. WHO. What is a pandemic? 2010. Available from: http://www.who.int/csr/disease/swineflu/frequently_asked_questions/pandemic/en/. [Accessed 30 December 2017].
99. WHO. Disease outbreaks. Available from: http://www.searo.who.int/topics/disease_outbreaks/en/. [Accessed 30 December 2017].
100. Department of Health, Australia. 2017 influenza season in Australia: a summary from the National Influenza Surveillance Committee. Information Brief, Update: 22 November 2017. Available from: http://www.health.gov.au/internet/main/publishing.nsf/Content/cda-surveil-ozflu-flucurr.htm/$File/2017-season-summary-22112017.pdf. [Accessed 30 December 2017].
101. Hota S, Fried E, Burry L, et al. Preparing your intensive care unit for the second wave of H1N1 and future surges. Crit Care Med 2010;38(4 Suppl.):e110–19.
102. Daugherty EL, Branson RD, Deveraux A, et al. Infection control in mass respiratory failure: preparing to respond to H1N1. Crit Care Med 2010;38(4 Suppl.):e103–9.
103. Funk DJ, Siddiqui F, Wiebe K, et al. Practical lessons from the first outbreaks: clinical presentation, obstacles, and management strategies for severe pandemic (H1N1) 2009 influenza pneumonitis. Crit Care Med 2010;38(4 Suppl.):e30–7.
104. Duggal A, Pinto R, Rubenfeld G, et al. Global variability in reported mortality for critical illness during the 2009-10 influenza A (H1N1) pandemic: a systematic review and meta-regression to guide reporting of outcomes during disease outbreaks. PLoS ONE 2016;11(5):e0155044.
105. World Health Organisation. Pandemic influenza risk management – interim guidance. Geneva: WHO; 2013. Available from: http://www.who.int/influenza/preparedness/pandemic/influenza_risk_management/en/.
106. New South Wales Health. Influenza pandemic – providing critical care: PD2010_28. Sydney: NSW Health; 2010. Available from: http://www0.health.nsw.gov.au/policies/pd/2010/PD2010_028.html. [Accessed 29 July 2014].

Chapter 3

Quality and safety

Wendy Chaboyer, Lina Bergman

Learning objectives

After reading this chapter, you should be able to:

- describe different approaches to quality and safety monitoring
- identify the steps in developing clinical practice guidelines
- explain the role care bundles and checklists have in promoting quality and safety in critical care nursing practice
- discuss the use of national quality indicators in intensive care
- describe the use of information and communication technologies in critical care
- identify techniques used to understand situations that place patients at risk of adverse events in critical care
- discuss rapid response systems used to respond to deteriorating patients
- explain the safety culture in ICUs
- identify strategies to improve the non-technical skills in critical care.

KEY WORDS

care bundles
checklists
clinical practice guidelines
information and communication technology
patient safety
quality improvement
quality indicators
rapid response systems
safety culture
Systems Engineering Initiative for Patient Safety

Introduction

Today's critical care units are both busy and complex, where nurses, doctors and other health professionals use their knowledge, skills and technology to provide patient care. The Institute of Medicine in the USA defines quality of health care as 'the degree to which health services for individuals and populations increase the likelihood of desired health outcomes and are consistent with current professional knowledge'.[1] Critical care nurses are well known for their skills in ongoing surveillance of a patient's condition, which means nurses are ideally positioned to prevent, discover and correct healthcare errors.[2] Thus, nurses play a key role in improving quality and safety in critical care, the focus of this chapter. First, approaches to quality are considered. Included in this section are the topics of quality monitoring, quality indicators, clinical practice guidelines (CPGs), care bundles, checklists and information and communication technologies. Finally, patient safety, including the noteworthy problem of medication errors, safety culture, rapid response systems and non-technical skills, is described. In Chapter 2 risk management, clinical governance and the role of clinical leaders and managers in delivering critical care services were addressed; this information is complementary to what is discussed in Chapter 3.

Approaches to quality

Healthcare quality is commonly described in terms of Donabedian's three major domains:[3]

1. Structure – the way the healthcare setting and/or system is organised to deliver care (e.g. staffing, beds, equipment)
2. Process – the practices involved in the delivery of care (e.g. pressure ulcer prevention strategies)
3. Outcomes – the results of care in terms of recovery, restoration of function and/or survival (e.g. mortality, health-related quality of life).

In addition to Donabedian's quality model, the Systems Engineering Initiative for Patient Safety (SEIPS) model has been developed.[4] The model provides a framework for understanding how the above-described domains (e.g. structures, processes and outcomes) and their relationships, can be used in clinical practice and research. Fig. 3.1 graphically presents the SEIPS model. The general structure of the model is that the work system (left), in which care is provided, affects clinical processes (middle), which further influences patient, employee and organisational outcomes (right).[5] Specifically, it expands Donabedian's first domain 'structure' (e.g. how care is organised) to include five components, referred to as the 'work system'.[5] The SEIPS model defines five work system components as, a) person(s) (i.e. patient, healthcare provider or the team), b) tasks, c) tools and technologies, d) environment, and e) organisation. Accordingly, a *person* performs *tasks* using *tools and technologies*. These performances occur in a physical *environment* influenced by *organisational* conditions.[4] The SEIPS model has been applied in various healthcare settings to guide quality and safety assessments, often providing recommendations for safety improvements[5] such as identifying contributing factors for medical errors in intensive care unit (ICU) setting,[6] and evaluating the intrahospital transfer process of critically ill patients.[7]

The overall aim of quality improvement is to provide safe, effective, patient-centred, timely, efficient and equitable health care.[8] Quality improvement activities identify and address gaps between knowledge and practice. Importantly, these activities need to reflect the most recent and robust clinical evidence to improve patient care and reduce harm. A common approach used for rapid improvement in health care is the plan–do–study–act (PDSA)[9] method where four essential steps are carried out in a continuous fashion to ensure processes are continually improved:

1. Plan – identify a goal, specify aims and objectives to improve an area of clinical practice, and how that might be achieved (i.e. how to test the intervention).
2. Do – implement the plan of action, collect relevant information that will inform whether the intervention was successful and in what way, taking

FIGURE 3.1 Systems Engineering Initiative for Patient Safety Improvement model.

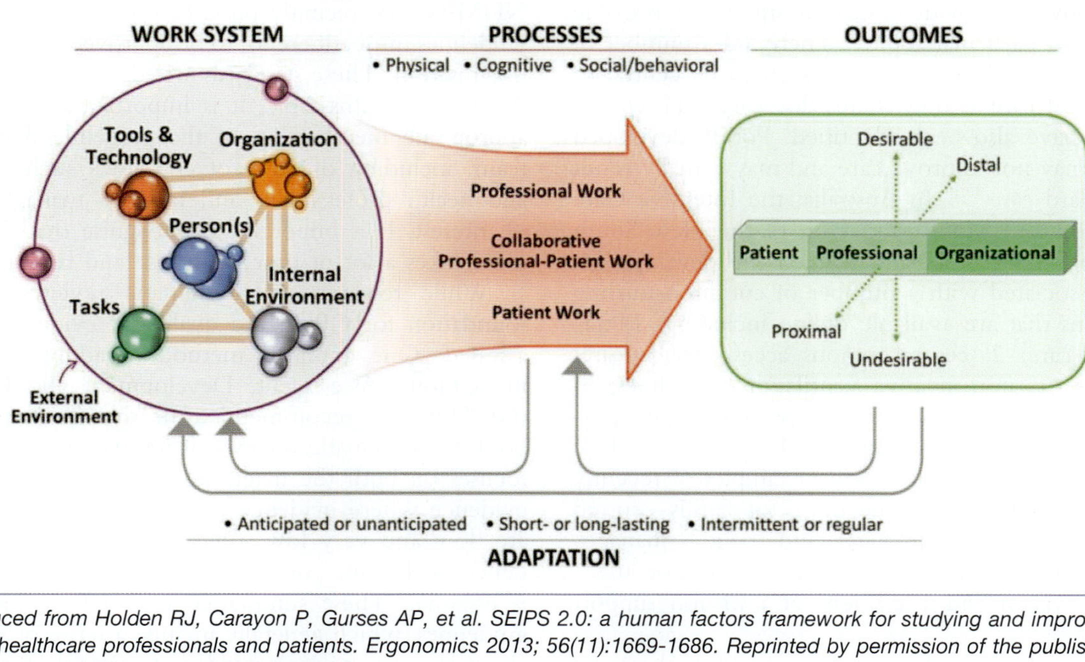

Reproduced from Holden RJ, Carayon P, Gurses AP, et al. SEIPS 2.0: a human factors framework for studying and improving the work of healthcare professionals and patients. Ergonomics 2013; 56(11):1669-1686. Reprinted by permission of the publisher Taylor & Francis Ltd, http://www.tandfonline.com

note of problems and unexpected observations that arise.

3 Study – evaluate the results of the intervention, particularly its impact on practice improvement, noting any strengths and limitations of the intervention.

4 Act – determine whether the intervention should be adopted, abandoned or adapted for further rapid cycle testing recommencing at the plan phase.

Quality monitoring includes measurement of, and response to, the incidence and patterns of adverse events (AEs). The rate of AEs varies greatly; retrospective studies from various countries have revealed that AEs occur in about 10% of hospitalisations.[10] In critical care settings, it is estimated that around 20% of patients experience AEs.[11] In an international study encompassing 29 countries, serious AEs were shown to occur in ICUs at a rate of 39 events per 100 patient days with those related to indwelling lines, prescription or administration of medications, equipment failure (e.g. infusion devices, ventilators) and airway (e.g. unplanned extubation) the most frequently reported.[12] Similar categories were also reported as highly prevalent in a more recent study in the UK;[13] however, there was also a high rate of incidents related to patient transfers, pressure injuries, and infection control issues.

Clinical practice guidelines

The development and use of CPGs is one strategy to improve the quality and safety of healthcare.[14] CPGs are statements about appropriate health care for specific clinical circumstances that assist practitioners in their day-to-day practice. They are systematically developed to assist clinicians, consumers and policy makers in healthcare decisions and provide critical summaries of available evidence on a particular topic.[15] There are a number of benefits of using CPGs. They are seen to be central to quality patient care as they standardise care.[15] However, limitations have also been identified. Poorly developed guidelines may not improve care and may actually result in substandard care.[15,16] In Australia, the Intensive Care Coordination and Monitoring Unit of the New South Wales Department of Health has led the development of CPGs associated with a number of common nursing interventions that are available online including: 1) tracheostomy care; 2) central venous access device care; 3) eye care; 4) non-invasive ventilation guidelines; 5) physical activity and movement; 6) pressure injury prevention; 7) suctioning an adult ICU patient; and 8) temperature measurement.[16] Other examples of recently developed ICU CPGs include those for family-centred care,[17] ICU admission, discharge and triage,[18] management of sepsis and septic shock,[19] safe medication use,[20] and the provision and assessment of nutrition support therapy.[21]

Clinical audits are often used to establish the need to develop new CPGs and protocols at the local unit level. Clinical audits generally involve chart reviews, but may also use direct observation or surveys of practice. Clinical audits often reveal variations in practice that are without adequate justification. A two-part 'how to' series focuses on the use of clinical audits to improve critical care.[22,23] The authors note audits involve the following 11 steps:[22,23]

1 Identify appropriate audit topics
2 Engage relevant stakeholders
3 Develop appropriate methods and audit criteria
4 Determine effective sample sizes
5 Develop reliable data collection tools
6 Establish consistent data collection procedures
7 Identify appropriate techniques for analysing audit data
8 Identify internal and external audit data for benchmarking
9 Feedback to clinical areas and management
10 Plan targeted strategies and processes for continuous improvement
11 Repeat the audit cycle; re-identify areas for improvement.

If clinical audits or other methods establish a need for improving practice, adopting, adapting or developing CPG may be the desired approach.

Developing, implementing and evaluating clinical practice guidelines

A number of steps are undertaken when developing CPGs. Organisations such as the Australian National Health and Medical Research Council (NHMRC) provide detailed descriptions for various aspects of the CPG development and reporting process.[24] The NHMRC has recently published a set of standards that guidelines must adhere to, to be approved by this national organisation. These standards are identified in Table 3.1. As shown in this table, it is important to consider the appropriate membership of the guideline development team, including the role of end users such as patients and health professionals and how to manage conflicts of interest. It is important to recognise that developing CPG takes a lot of time, expertise and resources.

While research and systematic reviews form the foundation for CPGs, the quality of evidence must be assessed. One appraisal method, Grading of Recommendations, Assessment, Development and Evaluation (GRADE), is recommended in the Cochrane handbook for systematic reviews of interventions.[25] GRADE focuses on both the magnitude of effect and quality of evidence where evidence is graded from high, moderate, low and very low. Overall summaries of the evidence with some quality assessment such as GRADE is essential. These summaries are used to develop the guidelines, which generally include a series of statements about the care to be provided, a rationale for this care and both the quality of evidence and strength of the recommendation.

TABLE 3.1
National Health and Medical Research Council standards for guidelines

STANDARD		SUB-ITEMS	
1	To be relevant and useful for decision making guidelines will:	1.1	Address a health issue of importance
		1.2	Clearly state the purpose of the guideline and the context in which it will be applied
		1.3	Be informed by public consultation
		1.4	Be feasible to implement
2	To be transparent guidelines will make publicly available:	2.1	The details of all processes and procedures used to develop the guideline
		2.2	The source evidence
		2.3	The declarations of interest of members of the guideline development group and information on how any conflicts of interest were managed
		2.4	All sources of funding for the guideline
3	The guideline development group will:	3.1	Be composed of an appropriate mix of expertise and experience, including relevant end users
		3.2	Have clearly defined, documented processes for reaching consensus
4	To identify and manage conflicts of interest guideline developers will:	4.1	Require all interests of all guideline development group members to be declared
		4.2	Establish a process for determining if a declared interest represents a conflict of interest, and how a conflict of interest will be managed
5	To be focused on health and related outcomes guidelines will:	5.1	Be developed around explicitly-defined clinical or public health questions
		5.2	Address outcomes that are relevant to the guideline's expected end users
		5.3	Clearly define the outcomes considered to be important to the person/s who will be affected by the decision, and prioritise these outcomes.
6	To be evidence-informed guidelines will:	6.1	Be informed by well-conducted systematic reviews
		6.2	Consider the body of evidence for each outcome (including the quality of that evidence) and other factors that influence the process of making recommendations including benefits and harms, values and preferences, resource use and acceptability.
		6.3.	Be subjected to appropriate peer review
7	To make actionable recommendations guidelines will:	7.1	Discuss the options for action
		7.2	Clearly articulate what the recommended course of action is, and when it should be taken
		7.3	Clearly articulate what the intervention is so it can be implemented
		7.4	Clearly link each recommendation to the evidence that supports it
		7.5	Grade the strength of each recommendation
8	To be up-to-date guidelines will:	8.1	Ensure that the recommendation is based on an up-to-date body of evidence
		8.2	Propose a date by which the evidence and the guideline should be updated. This may be specific to each recommendation
9	To be accessible guidelines will:	9.1	Be easy to find
		9.2	Ideally be free of charge to the end user
		9.3	Be clearly structured, easy to navigate and in plain English
		9.4	Be available online

Source: National Health and Medical Research Council (2016) Standards for Guidelines, https://nhmrc.gov.au/about-us/publications/2016-nhmrc-standards-guidelines. CC BY 3.0.

Once the guidelines are developed, a group of experts and users should assess the guidelines for accuracy, clinical utility and comprehension. International experts developed and have subsequently revised a 23-item appraisal instrument, termed the Appraisal of Guidelines for Research and Evaluation II (AGREE II), that assesses six domains: 1) scope and purpose of the CPG (three items); 2) stakeholder involvement in CPG development (three items); 3) rigour of development (eight items); 4) clarity of presentation (three items); 5) applicability (four items); and 6) editorial independence (two items).[26] Instruments such as AGREE II can be used to assess the quality of CPG.

Based on the assessment of the CPG, revisions may be required. Next, strategies for disseminating and implementing the guidelines should be developed along with a plan for their future updates. Importantly, simply publishing and circulating CPGs will have a limited impact on clinical practice, so specific activities must be undertaken to promote CPG adherence.[27] A systematic review of implementation strategies used to get ICU guidelines into practice identified multifaceted strategies that appear to be more effective than single strategies.[28] The most frequently used strategies included printed educational materials, information sessions, audit, feedback, use of champions, educational outreach visits and computer or internet usage.[28] A Canadian study identified the following factors as important for adherence to CPGs: characteristics of the CPG, implementation process, institutional characteristics, provider intent and patient characteristics.[27] Finally, a process for regularly evaluating and updating the guidelines must be developed, which may involve quality improvement activities or clinical research. In summary, by developing, using and evaluating CPGs, nurses may improve patient care and outcomes. Additionally, use of CPGs should ensure that nursing practice is based on the best available evidence.

Quality indicators

The true incidence of both errors and AEs has been found to be higher than what was reported[29,30] and, in the absence of evidence to the contrary, this is likely to have remained unchanged. Fortunately, most healthcare errors do not result in patient harm because of safety-net processes.[31] In the last two decades, there has been growing interest in quality management, including in ICU settings. Quality indicators, sometimes referred to as quality standards or clinical indicators, is a specified quantitative measure to assess clinical performances (on a hospital or unit level). One of the aims with quality indicators is to identify and prevent differences in quality of care, but also to initiate and facilitate quality improvement projects.[32,33]

Donabedian's structure-process-outcome model is commonly used as a framework when developing and classifying quality indicators.[34] Quality indicators measuring structural prerequisites includes how the ICU is integrated into the hospital, type and amount of technology available, and the number, roles and responsibilities of ICU staff. Process-related quality indicators refer to what we do, or fail to do, for patients and their families; for example, adherence to guidelines or transfers of patients between ICUs. Outcome-related quality indicators focus on the results achieved such as standardised mortality ratios, AEs, and patient satisfaction.[32,34] Moreover, quality indicators should be valid (i.e. both empirical research and clinical expertise supports that the indicator measures quality of care), reliable, responsive, interpretable, and feasible.[32,34]

The choice of quality indicators varies among countries. Comparing quality indicators in 10 countries, in 2016 Flaatten identified that those most commonly used were standardised mortality ratio followed by the availability of an intensivist in the ICU.[33] Some countries, for example Sweden, provide open access to the results even at individual hospital level. This enhances comparison between hospitals as well as benchmarking. For example, units with good results can be used as learning examples to inform others.[33] Table 3.2 provides a list of examples of quality indicators used in Australia, Sweden, Scotland, by the Society of Critical Care Medicine (US), and by the European Society for Intensive Care Medicine (Europe).

Practice tip

Adhering to the practices included in a ventilator care bundle (where appropriate) may lead to improved patient and service efficiency outcomes.

Care bundles

One quality improvement approach to the optimal use of best practice guidelines at the bedside is the development of 'care bundles'. A care bundle is a set of evidence-based interventions or processes of care applied to selected patients in order to standardise and ensure appropriate delivery of care. A number of bundles have been developed for critical care (Table 3.3). One systematic review and meta-analysis comparing care bundles with usual care concludes that the effect of care bundles on patient outcome is uncertain. However, this might be explained by low quality of evidence among the included studies.[42] In ICU settings, studies examining the process of care delivery using the ventilator care bundle revealed that increased bundle compliance was associated with decreased ICU length of stay, reduced ventilator days and increased ICU patient throughput,[43] in addition to decreased rates of ventilator-associated pneumonia.[44,45] Another care bundle used in research and clinical practice is the ABCDE bundle (Awakening and Breading Coordination of daily sedation and ventilator removal trials, Choice of sedatives and analgesic exposure, Delirium monitoring and management, and Early mobility and Exercise).[46] By focusing on five evidence-based steps of care, the bundle aims to optimise patient recovery and outcome from critical illness. One prospective before-and-after study in the USA concluded that critically ill patients managed with the ABCDE bundle experienced fewer days breathing with assistance, less delirium and were more likely to be mobilised during their ICU stay. Importantly, no differences were noted in self-extubation and re-intubation rates between groups.[47] However, despite recommendations, adoption of the ABCDE bundle remains limited. One survey in ICUs across the USA concluded that increased workload burden and perceived difficulties in carrying out the bundle reduced adherence to the ABCDE bundle.[48] On

TABLE 3.2
Examples of quality indicators used in intensive care

QUALITY INDICATORS	AUSTRALIA[35]	SWEDEN[32]	SCOTLAND[36]	SCCM (USA)[34]	ESICM (EUROPE)[37]
Standardised mortality ratio	✘	✓	✓	✓	✓
ICU fulfils national requirements to provide intensive care	✘	✓	✘	✘	✓
24 h availability of a consultant intensivist	✘	✘	✘	✘	✓
Clinical ward round (multidisciplinary and/or intensivist lead)	✘	✘	✓ (twice a day)	✓	✓
Use of patient assessment systems (participation in national databases and comparative audits)	✓	✘	✓	✘	✘
Rates of AEs or ADEs and/or multidisciplinary clinical meeting to discuss in-unit deaths and significant AEs	✘	✘	✓	✓	✓
Management plan for patient in the ICU	✘	✓ (within 48 h of admission)	✓ (daily review)	✘	✘
Appropriate nurse staffing and skill level	✘	✘	✓	✘	✘
Availability of pharmacist in ICU	✘	✘	✓ (minimum 5 days/week)	✘	✘
Availability of physiotherapist in ICU	✘	✘	✓ (24 h/day)	✘	✘
Unavailability of ICU beds (i.e. inadequate resources) measured by 1) transfer of patients to another facility; 2) inability to admit patient to ICU; or 3) deferral or cancellation of elective surgery	✓	✓	✘	✘	✘
Delays on discharging patients from the ICU	✓ (more than 12 h)	✘	✘	✓	✘
Discharge of patients from the ICU after hours	✓ (between 6 p.m. and 6 a.m.)	✘	✓ (between 10 p.m. and 8 a.m.)	✘	✘
Unplanned readmission to ICU, early unplanned discharge, or rapid response team called after discharge	✓ (within 48 h)	✓ (within 72 h)	✓	✓ (within 24–48 h)	✓ (within 48 h)
VTE prophylaxis	✓ (within 24 hours of admission)	✘	✘	✓	✘

Continued

TABLE 3.2
Examples of quality indicators used in intensive care—cont'd

QUALITY INDICATORS	AUSTRALIA[35]	SWEDEN[32]	SCOTLAND[36]	SCCM (USA)[34]	ESICM (EUROPE)[37]
Stress ulcer prophylaxis	✘	✘	✘	✓	✘
Assessment of communication and swallowing needs in patients with tracheostomy	✘	✘	✓	✘	✘
Rate of unplanned endotracheal extubations	✘	✘	✘	✓	✓
Use of care bundles or infection prevention strategies for VAP, IAP, CVC and PVC	✘	✘	✓	✓	✘
Adherence to best practices (i.e. care bundles, clinical practical guidelines, such as protocol-driven ventilator weaning, severe sepsis treatment, sedation scales, delirium screening, early enteral feeding etc)	✘	✓ (use of sedation scales)	✓ (delirium screening once per day)	✓	✘
ICU infection rates (i.e. CLASBI, HAI, VAP, or multiple resistant organism)	✓	✘	✓	✓	✓
Isolation of patients with multiresistant bacteria	✘	✓	✘	✘	✘
Empathetic practice towards families	✓	✘	✓ (annual survey)	✓	✘
End of life care policies and/or identification of possible organ donors	✘	✓	✓	✓	✘
Standardised handover procedure for ICU discharge	✘	✘	✘	✘	✓
Assessment of rehabilitation needs after ICU discharge	✘	✘	✓	✘	✘

AEs: adverse events; ADEs: adverse drug events; CLASBI; central line bloodstream infection; CVC: central venous catheter; ESICM: European Society of Intensive Care Medicine; HAI: healthcare-associated infections; IAP: intubation-associated pneumonia, ICU: intensive care unit; PVC: peripheral venous cannula; SCCM: Society of Critical Care Medicine; VAP: ventilator-associated pneumonia; VTE: venous thromboembolism.

the other hand, protocol attributes, role clarity, training/understanding, coordination and well-functioning teamwork were associated with less difficulties performing the ABCDE bundle.[49]

Checklists

Checklists have the potential to prevent omissions in care by serving as reminders to healthcare providers for the delivery of appropriate quality care for every patient, every time, in complex clinical environments. A checklist typically contains a list of action items or criteria arranged in a systematic way, allowing the person completing it to record the presence or absence of individual items to ascertain that all are considered or completed.[50]

In critical care settings, checklists have been used to facilitate staff training, detect errors, check compliance with safety standards and evidence-based processes of care (such as those outlined previously), increase knowledge of patient-centred goals and prompt clinicians to review certain practices on morning rounds in the ICU.

TABLE 3.3
Examples of care bundles

BUNDLE NAME	AIM	BUNDLE COMPONENTS
Central line[38]	Prevent central line-associated bloodstream infections	• Hand hygiene • Maximal barrier precautions • Chlorhexidine skin antisepsis • Optimal catheter site selection with avoidance of the femoral vein for central venous access in adult patients • Daily review of line necessity with prompt removal of unnecessary lines
Ventilator care[39]	Prevent ventilator-associated pneumonia	• Elevating the head of the patient's bed to between 30–45° • Daily assessment of the patient's readiness to extubate or wean from the ventilator • Daily 'sedation vacations' or gradually lightening sedative use each day • Delivering both PUD and DVT prophylaxis • Daily oral care with chlorhexidine
Severe sepsis 3-h resuscitation[40]	Reduce mortality due to severe sepsis	• Serum lactate measured • Blood cultures obtained prior to antibiotic administration • Administer broad-spectrum antibiotics • Administer crystalloid 30 mL/kg for hypotension or lactate ≥4 mmol/L
6-h septic shock[40]	Reduce mortality due to severe sepsis	• Apply vasopressors (for hypotension that does not respond to initial fluid resuscitation) to maintain a MAP ≥65 mmHg • In the event of persistent arterial hypotension despite volume resuscitation (septic shock) or initial lactate ≥4 mmol/L (36 mg/dL): • Measure CVP • Measure $ScvO_2$ • Re-measure lactate if initial lactate was elevated
ABCDE care bundle[46]	Optimise patient recovery and outcome	• Perform awakening and spontaneous breathing controlled trials • Perform delirium screening and apply appropriate treatment plan • Provide early mobilisation and exercise
eCASH[41]	Optimal patient comfort with minimal sedation	• Effective analgesia and minimised sedation – secondary to pain relief, sedation that preferably can be titrated to a predefined target – minimise routine use of benzodiazepines • Promote and facilitate humane person/family-centred care – sleep promotion – apply early mobilisation strategies – facilitate patient communication with staff and relatives – promote family engagement

ABCDE: Awakening and Breathing coordination of daily sedation and ventilator removal trials, Choice of sedatives and analgesic exposure, Delirium monitoring and management, and Early mobility and Exercise; CVP: central venous pressure; DVT: deep vein thrombosis; eCASH: early Comfort using Analgesia, minimal Sedatives and maximal Humane care; MAP: mean arterial pressure; PUD: peptic ulcer disease; $ScvO_2$: central venous oxygen saturation.

Studies suggest checklists contributed to improved outcomes such as reduced AEs and improved patient and care partner satisfaction;[51] improved delivery of essential daily care processes (such as pain management and physical therapy);[52,53] and reduced mean monthly rates of ventilator-associated pneumonia.[54] Another study has also suggested decreased infection rates (for central line-associated bloodstream infections (CLABSI), ventilator-associated pneumonia, urinary tract infections) in a trauma ICU.[55] However, one randomised multicentre study, including 118 ICUs in Brazil, that tested the effectiveness of checklist, daily goals assessment and clinical prompts as a multifaceted quality improvement found the intervention did not reduce in-hospital mortality.[56] Moreover, the lack of methodological rigour in studies prevents inferring causal links between checklist use and improved outcomes.[57] Careful consideration of both checklist design and implementation is required when planning to incorporate checklists into the clinical setting.[58] Based on the results of a qualitative multicentre study in 32 ICUs in the USA, a framework for adapting a round checklist in clinical practice has been developed. They suggest that development of a checklist should include attention to brevity and relevance to the specific ICU. Consistent and integrated use is needed when implemented. Moreover, review of the checklist should include updates accordingly to change in ICU practice, including item reduction, item rotation and revisiting goals.[59]

Practice tip

When developed in line with published guidelines, checklists may improve practice delivery by serving as an aide-mémoire.

Information and communication technologies

Health departments continue to develop systems and processes that will result in a complete electronic medical record. Critical care in particular is at the forefront of these developments, with bedside clinical information systems, order-entry strategies, decision support, handheld technologies and telehealth initiatives continuing to evolve and influence practice. Digital innovations are changing medicine, for example, the way in which information is delivered, where graphical displays and visualisation makes it possible to absorb large amount of data quickly.[60] In the future, medical devices that communicate and integrate information will probably be used to predict AEs, prevent errors, and propose the most rational therapy for the patient.[60] This section examines the current and future impacts that these technologies will have on patient care and safety, and on clinician workflows and practices, as clinical information fully assimilates with evidence-based practice and clinical decision support systems.

Clinical information systems

Clinical information systems may enable improved data collection, storage, retrieval and reporting of patient-based information; and facilitate unit-based outcomes research and quality improvement activities.[61] Patient-based bedside clinical information systems offer increasingly sophisticated functionality and device interfaces,[61] enabling real-time data capture, trending and reporting and linkage to relational databases.[62] In fact, a recent review identified computerised clinical decision support systems that were associated with better patient outcomes.[63]

The introduction of intravenous 'smart pump' technology is one application aimed at reducing adverse drug events and improving patient care by supporting evidence-based guidelines for medication management.[64] The operator-error prevention software is based on a device-based drug library with institution-established concentrations/dosage limits incorporated in the function of the pump. Resulting software functions include clinician alerts (for keystroke errors)[65] and transaction log data (post-incident analysis).[64] Medication errors and adverse drug events can be detected by this software. There is evidence to suggest, however, that despite the use of smart pumps, errors related to administration of intravenous medication remain.[66] This highlights the need for promotional and quality improvement activities targeting compliance in using smart pumps, including actions to increase usability such upgrading drug libraries, decrease the number of unnecessary warnings, and developing approaches to minimise workarounds.[67]

Although the proportion of ICUs using a clinical information system is not known, there are indications that uptake is on the increase.[68] Numerous benefits to healthcare systems that lead to enhanced quality of care have been reported such as improved documentation, legibility, increased access to data, evidence-based decision support, interdisciplinary communication and reduced duplication and medical errors.[61] In intensive care they have reduced documentation time and increased the proportion of time spent on direct care activities.[69] Implementation of a clinical information system has been shown to reduce ICU length of stay.[70] Moreover, it facilitates the use of real-time measurements of care processes and can be used for continuous quality improvements.[71] End-user support has been identified as an important factor in the success of clinical information system implementation.[72] Barriers that have been identified include integration issues with other software systems; poor usability; insufficient technical support; lack of knowledge and training; limited experience and confidence in using clinical information systems; time due to increased work demands; and lack of consultation with end users.[73]

Accuracy of data (correctness and completeness of the data set) from both manual and automated inputs to the information system requires further evaluation. While automated entry eliminates transcription errors from other data sources,[74] the use of 'carry-over' data to fields that require updating by clinicians, finding the right sampling frequency (i.e. the rate at which a clinical information system can record and display patient data) and human interaction such as clinician acceptance of monitor-generated data can all affect data accuracy. For example, if the pulmonary artery waveform is measured at a high-frequency rate and displays large variability because of 'noise' and is not checked, erroneously high systolic blood pressure readings will be recorded.[75] Improvements to systems, however, have reportedly led to increased accuracy of data collections,[60] suggesting that perhaps developments in technology and the implementation strategies used have mitigated these problems. Errors can also arise, however, if systems are not designed to enhance communication between healthcare workers and facilitate coordination of work processes.[76,77]

Clinical alert functions are designed to improve delivery of care; however, they may compromise patient safety when used excessively in clinical settings. For example, one study demonstrated 49–96% of drug safety alerts were overridden by clinicians.[78] Exposure to excessive alarms can lead to alarm fatigue, which is a global patient safety concern.[79] Researchers examining factors influencing ICU nurses' response to alarms concluded that visual access to physiological data, experience, teamwork, and false alarms are important determinants.[80] A systematic review revealed improvements in prescribing behaviours as a result of computerised alerts and prompts; however, among those studies investigating patient outcomes, no significant improvements were found.[81] A recent study of 250 nurses in 10 Irish ICUs in six hospitals found about 90% of respondents thought many alarms did not require an action but disrupted patient care.[82] In intensive care, computerised alerts have been used to improve glucose control in patients[83] and by using electronic blood 'tags' that support nurses in preventing, identifying and reporting adverse transfusion events.[84] The features that might make alerts and prompts more effective, however, are generally unknown and require further research.

Computerised order entry and decision support

Computerised provider order entry (CPOE) is a system that allows orders for medications, intravenous fluids, diagnostic tests and procedures to be entered then rapidly communicated to pharmacies. It can also be used for results management, treatment orders and clinical decision support.[85] CPOE is viewed as an important innovation in reducing medical errors, through minimising transcribing, dispensing and administration errors.[86]

A systematic review and meta-analysis of the impact of CPOE and clinical decision support systems on medication errors, length of stay and mortality in ICU found that the transition from paper-based ordering to CPOE systems were associated with an 85% reduction of medical prescribing errors and 12% reduction in ICU mortality rates. However, no significant changes in hospital mortality and length of stay were found.[87] Furthermore, implementation of CPOE and related clinical decision support systems demonstrate significant reductions in redundant or unnecessary order requests.[88] Decision support systems interface with hospital databases to retrieve patient-specific and other relevant clinical data to support medical decisions and other tasks. Importantly, clinical decision making at the bedside can be enhanced by providing clinicians with a readily available tool that incorporates relevant clinical information and evidence-based medicine. Clinician alerts (e.g. allergies or interaction effects) or prompts (e.g. to check coagulation when prescribing warfarin) can be generated. Yet, there is limited evidence that these systems reduce clinical adverse drug events.[89] This might be explained by implementation issues, failure to adequately tailor alarm resulting in alert fatigue, or system design problems.[89]

As with clinical information system implementation, detailed planning including examination of clinician workflow and care delivery patterns is required for successful implementation of a CPOE process.[90] A number of potentially important features of clinical decision support systems have been identified that cover communication content (e.g. provide recommendations with justifications in addition to assessment), clinician–system interaction (e.g. incorporate into clinical workflow, provide at the time and location it is required and request reason for not following recommendations) and improving usability, in particular facilitating the ease-of-use.[86,91,92]

Additional developments involving wireless communication, handheld technologies and closed-loop delivery systems may improve the efficiency, effectiveness and adoption of this innovation in clinical practice.[93] Closed-loop delivery systems offers automated treatment using feedback principles and are designed to maintain a given variable around a desired set point (e.g. inotropic dosages adjusted to a range for mean arterial pressure). Compared with manual control, automated systems can improve stability of target parameters and reduce workload in clinical practice.[94] An example in ICU settings is automated weaning systems using closed-loop controls to adapt ventilator output to the individual need of the patient. Compared with non-automated weaning strategies, it significantly decreased weaning time and length of stay in the ICU.[95]

Handheld technologies

Wireless applications enable clinical information access, portability and mobility within a critical care environment at the point of care. Handheld computers and devices use operating systems and pen-like styluses that enable touchscreen functionality, handwriting recognition and synchronisation with other hospital-based computer systems. Handheld devices provide easy access to information and enables timely documentation. They can provide healthcare professionals with evidence-based decision support and improves information seeking, adherence to guidelines, and clinical decision making.[96,97]

In critical care, handheld devices have been used to document clinical activities, such as logging critical care procedures, which was demonstrated as feasible and useful.[98] They have also been used to improve communication and pain assessment of critically ill patient with mechanical ventilation,[99] to improve documentation during resuscitation,[100] as well as to facilitate communication and shared decision making between surrogates and health care professionals.[101]

An increasing array of clinical applications and content is available for downloading to these devices. Specific applications for healthcare professionals in the ICU have been developed, for example an application for delirium assessment and decision-making assistance,[102] and for pressure injury/ulcer lesion monitoring and decision making in patients with mechanical ventilation.[103] Mobile technology and smartphone use has also been reported as a helpful nursing education tool,[104] where the use of mobile technology has improved nursing students' learning and performance in the clinical setting.[105]

The benefits of this mobile computing also create concerns over confidentiality. Health services, designers and developers therefore need policies that recognise individual's rights regarding information collected on them. Researchers and developers should design new methods that address security issues such as authentication, identification, data anonymisation, and software assurance.[106] As these issues are addressed, these technologies will form an integral component of routine clinical practice in critical care.

Practice tip

Although handheld devices can assist nurses in their practice, with a range of helpful clinical applications now available, it is necessary to ensure patient confidentiality is not breached and the devices are secure.

Telehealth initiatives

Remote critical care management (tele-ICU) using telemedicine/telehealth technologies is expanding as the necessary high bandwidths for transmitting large amounts of data and digital imagery become available between partner units or hospitals. Videoconferencing functions enable direct visualisation and communication of patients and on-site staff with the 'virtual' critical care clinician or team. Review of real-time physiological data, patient flowcharts and other documents (e.g. electrocardiograms, laboratory results) or images (e.g. radiographs) provides a comprehensive data set for patient assessment and management.

One recent systematic review of telemedicine and clinical decision support for ICU found a reduction in hospital mortality. However, they concluded that most studies investigating tele-ICU were of poor methodological quality, highlighting the need for further studies to determine the effectiveness of tele-ICU.[107] Another recent systematic review and meta-analysis of the literature concluded that tele-ICU may reduce ICU and hospital mortality and shorten ICU length of stay. But no significant effect was found in hospital length of stay and its long-term cost-effectiveness is still unclear.[108]

There are also characteristics of tele-ICU that are likely to impact on both the process and outcomes of care. Benefits are likely to be generated from the availability of extra resources and the ability of the tele-ICU to serve as a quality improvement trigger (e.g. checking compliance with evidence-based medicine) and to provide medication management support, software alerts and prompts, and real-time patient monitoring by camera.[109,110] For these benefits to be realised, however, the technology needs to be accepted and used appropriately by ICU staff. Further studies that include detailed descriptions of system implementation are required to determine the most effective elements of this technology in critical care settings as well as their impact on care processes and outcomes.[111] For instance, one study examining how tele-ICU nurses and organisational characteristics influenced trust and satisfaction among bedside ICU nurses concluded that optimised communication is an important aspect to establish trust between tele-ICU and bedside nurses.[112]

In addition to remote patient assessment and management, telecommunications have been used to deliver continuing education to rural healthcare professionals for many years via audio, video and computer. E-learning, defined as education mediated electronically via the internet has steadily increased among health care professionals'.[113] One Cochrane review, including 16 randomised trials, concluded that there were little or no differences in patient outcomes or healthcare professionals' behaviours, skills and knowledge between e-learning and traditional learning.[113] E-learning training platforms and tools has been used, for example, to increase the use of tools for neurological monitoring in ICU,[114] to prevent healthcare-associated infections,[115] and to increase nurses' skills in assessing and classifying pressure injuries.[116] The potential impact of online communities and social media in nursing education and clinical practice has also been systematically examined.[117] Online professional development courses are also available, but more trials are needed to assess the superiority of e-learning over traditional learning methods.[113]

The constantly evolving nature of technology and innovative ideas from healthcare workers can bring about novel approaches to healthcare delivery. One example is 'smart glasses', web-connected glasses that can present data onto the lenses and record images or videos through a camera. Smart glasses have been adopted in healthcare and can be used for different purposes such as electronic health record retrieval and input, diagnostic test analysis, and live broadcasting.[118] In intensive care, smart glasses are suggested as a complement to existing monitoring that could facilitate healthcare professionals' work.[119] The smart glass is depicted in Fig. 3.2.

Patient safety

The signing of the Declaration of Vienna in 2009[120] committed critical care organisations around the world, including the World Federation of Critical Care Nurses, to patient safety. Patient safety is viewed as a crucial component of quality.[121] Over the years, numerous definitions of patient safety have emerged in the literature. The Institute of Medicine described it as the absence of preventable harm to a patient during the process of healthcare.[8] The World Health Organisation has focused its patient safety efforts on: providing global leadership

FIGURE 3.2 Smart glass technology.

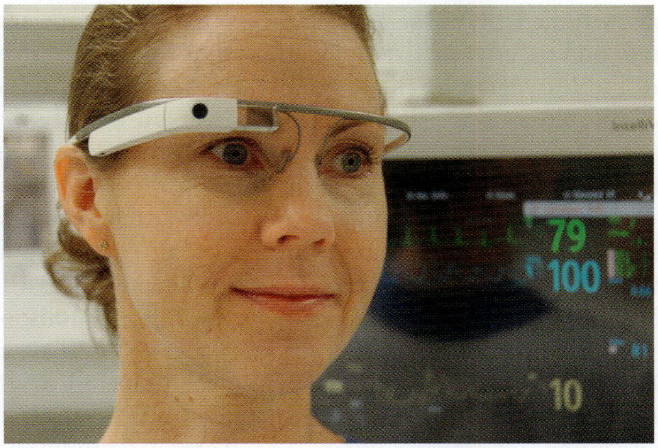

Courtesy Marcus Romare.

and fostering collaboration; developing guidelines and tools, and building capacity; engaging patients and families for safer health care and monitoring improvements in patient safety.[121] They have also identified a number of global safety challenges, including the one announced in 2017 to reduce the level of severe, avoidable harm related to medications by 50% over 5 years globally.[121]

Three techniques used to understand patient risk are: 1) analysing reports of clinical incidents and AEs, 2) root cause analyses and 3) failure mode and effect analysis. Research on AEs in critical care has helped to better understand patient risks and target improvement activities. For example, medications, indwelling lines and equipment failure were the three most frequent types of AEs in a study of 205 ICUs worldwide.[12] Focusing on analysing the narratives written about AEs is viewed as an important way to learn from errors. But, a recent systematic review of incident and reporting systems in the ICU found that none of the 36 papers reviewed completely met the World Health Organisation's criteria for AE reporting.[122] Root cause analysis is a structured process generally used to analyse catastrophic or sentinel events.[123] In root cause analysis, the various situations that led to the event are documented and analysed in order to identify contributing factors to the event and make recommendations for system changes to prevent the event from occurring again. Learning from both incident reporting and root cause analyses is based on the premise that the information they contain is of sufficient quality to allow accurate analysis, interpretation and detection of the root causes of problems and, even more importantly, the formulation and implementation of corrective actions. In one recent publication, the Veterans Health Administration in the United States analysed 70 ICU root cause analyses and found that delays in care, and medication errors were the most common types of events, with the root causes identified as predominantly related to policies and procedure processes, equipment or supply issues and knowledge deficit.[124] Failure mode and effect analysis identifies potential failures and their effects, calculating their risk and prioritising potential failure modes based on risk.[125] In addition to examining patient risk, another strategy has focused on understanding the safety culture of a unit or organisation, with subsequent activities aimed at improving components of this culture. A recent Spanish study used failure mode and effect analysis as part of their approach to improving the use of strategies to prevent venous thromboembolic disease in ICU patients.[126] Thus, it appears that contemporary techniques to understand patient safety risks are being used in critical care.

Practice tip

By undertaking a root cause analysis, the contributing factors to the event can be identified and strategies to mitigate future AEs can be implemented.

Medication errors

Medication administration is the most common intervention in healthcare, but the medication management process in the acute hospital setting is complex, and creates risk for patients. As a result, medication-related events are one of the most common AEs for critically ill patients[12] and the rationale for a focus on it. A Japanese study of adverse drug events in 459 patients found 99 AEs occurred in 70 patients (i.e. 15% of patients).[127] Although the rates of medication errors and adverse drug events vary greatly between settings despite geographical location, they are common in critical care units,[128] with higher rates of harmful errors than non-ICU settings, and those errors are more likely to be associated with requiring life-sustaining intervention, permanent harm or death.[129]

How medication incidents are defined and measured impact on reported error/adverse event rates and their interpretation. The way in which medication errors, for example, are calculated requires careful consideration of both the numerator (e.g. count of any error in the medication process) and the denominator (this could be the number of patients, patient days, medication days, administered doses – depending on the aim or purpose of the measure).[130]

One observational study found that an average of 2.9 preventable or potential adverse drug events occurred in each ICU admission,[131] and in Australia, research suggests that errors occur in 9% of all medications administered in hospitals.[132] Although it is estimated that only one out of 10 medical errors results in AEs,[130] such errors can lead to costly additional treatments and prolonged hospital stays as well as other implications for patients, families and healthcare providers.[130,133] Approximately 5% of medication errors relate to infusion pumps. These pumps are used to administer high-impact medications, such as inotropes, heparin or antineoplastics.[58] Analysis of a database describing 537 hospitals with ICUs showed main medication errors were errors of omission, improper dose or quantity and incorrect administration technique.[129] The leading sources of errors that caused harm in ICUs were knowledge and performance deficits (57%), not following procedure or protocol (26%), communication (15%) and dispensing device errors (14%).[129] Using the SEIPS model, one literature review revealed human factors (i.e. stress, high workload, knowledge and performances deficits) were associated with medical errors in the ICU.[6] Factors contributing to medication errors were frequent interruptions, communication problems and poor usability of health information technologies.[6] The occurrence of medical errors in ICUs has also been correlated with an increased task volume and with increased workload for nurses.[30] In response to this body of evidence pertaining to medication error, a number of strategies have been instituted; for example, in Australia under the auspices of the National Medicines Policy, the Quality Use of Medicines map is a searchable online database of related projects to assist health practitioners and researchers plan and carry out their work, and help policy makers evaluate quality use of medicines activity for potential use in policy development (see *Online resources*).

Practice tip

Given the high frequency and consequences of medication errors, it is important to be cognisant of the potential for error and be aware of strategies that can be used to prevent such errors, such as limiting interruptions.

It is important to evaluate interventions that can reduce the incidence and impact of adverse intravenous drug events, particularly in critical care settings.[6] Since most medication errors in the ICU occur in the administration phase,[129] critical care nurses play a key role in detection and prevention of errors before patient harm results. Evidence suggests that nurses who are interrupted while administering medications may have an increased risk of making medication errors.[134] Reducing interruptions to medication administration in ICU requires interventions that consider the complexity of working in an imperfect environment, in multidisciplinary teams, and under uncertain circumstances.[135]

Safety culture

Measurement of the baseline safety culture facilitates an action plan for improvement. Safety culture has been defined as 'the product of individual and group values, attitudes, perceptions, competencies, and patterns of behaviour that determine the commitment to, and the style and proficiency of, an organisation's health and safety management.'[136] It is commonly referred to as 'the way we do things around here.'[137] A systematic review found evidence for a relationship between safety culture and patient outcomes at both the hospital and unit level.[138] In addition to patient outcomes, researchers have studied the association between safety culture and staff outcomes. For example, in a study of ICU nurses in six Norwegian hospitals, researchers showed a positive safety culture was associated with lower burnout scores and a stronger sense of coherence, a construct reflecting how people cope with stressful situations.[139]

A widely used instrument to measure safety culture, the Safety Attitudes Questionnaire (SAQ), focuses on six domains: teamwork climate, safety climate, job satisfaction, perceptions of management, working conditions and stress recognition.[140] Interestingly, two studies in the US[141,142] and one Australian study conducted in 10 ICUs[143] showed that nurses and doctors differed in their perceptions of safety culture. The Australian study also identified some differences between bedside nurses and nursing leaders.[143] Using the SAQ, a Palestinian neonatal ICU study found a wide variation in the perceptions of the safety culture held by 164 nurses and 40 physicians in 16 hospitals.[144] Another European study of 378 patients in 57 ICUs showed a relationship between positive safety culture and fewer errors.[145] One recent study conducted in one Brazilian ICU found nursing staff in adult, paediatric and neonatal ICUs scored 75 (viewed to be a strong area of patient safety) on only two of the SAQ dimensions; job satisfaction and teamwork climate.[146]

Practice tip

A positive safety culture is associated with better patient outcomes.

One strategy to improve the safety culture has been to identify factors that make organisations safe, which in turn allows initiatives to be developed that target areas of specific need. For example, five characteristics of organisations that have been able to achieve high reliability include:[147]

1. safety viewed as a priority by leaders
2. flattened hierarchy that promotes speaking up about concerns
3. regular team training
4. use of effective methods of communicating
5. standardisation.

There are a number of other resources available to those interested in improving patient safety. For example, WHO has published a patient safety curriculum guide to assist organisations in this endeavour.[148] Leadership, teamwork and behavioural change strategies provide a foundation for improvements in safety culture.[149] In the USA, the Comprehensive Unit-Based Safety Program (CUSP) has emerged as one specific safety intervention.[150] Recent publications about the CUSP program support its benefits.[151,152] Another American critical care quality improvement program found that a nurse-led safety program that included executive walkrounds and a multidisciplinary team tasked with identifying and resolving safety issues were effective.[153] The three top safety issues identified related to nursing, supplies and daily unit operations with 36–70% of the issues being resolved. In summary, understanding the various dimensions of safety culture in a unit can be used as a foundation for the development and implementation of programs targeted at specific aspects that may benefit from improvements. To be successful, safety programs have to be supported by the leaders as well as other members of the unit.

Rapid response systems

Rapid response systems (RRS) have developed to recognise and provide emergency response to patients who experience acute deterioration.[154] A 2015 review and meta-analysis of 29 studies of RRS found that they were associated with an overall reduction in hospital mortality in both adults and paediatric patients. It was also associated with fewer cardiopulmonary arrests in adults.[155] While papers about RRS often reflect experiences in Australia, the USA and the UK, the 2015 review included studies from Canada, Pakistan, Portugal, Saudi Arabia, South Korea, Sweden and The Netherlands. One study not included in this review, which was set in 12 hospitals in The Netherlands, found RRS had positive effect on the composite outcome of cardiopulmonary arrest, unplanned ICU admission or death.[156] More recently, the New South Wales, Australia statewide adoption in over 230 hospitals of an RRS called 'Between the Flags' was associated with decreases in cardiac arrests, deaths from cardiac arrests, hospital mortality and failure to rescue.[157]

Although there has been a proliferation of papers on RRS, one recent and promising US innovation has been the development of an airway RRS, which focuses on airway emergencies.[158] The Australian Commission on Safety and Quality in Health Care identified eight essential elements in an RRS (Table 3.4).[159] And, McGaughery et al's realist review of over 270 papers on RRS identified that they were beneficial when there was a sufficient skill mix of experienced staff, when a scoring system for the identification of the deteriorating patient was used flexibly, alongside clinical judgement, and when staff had access to ongoing, multi-professional competency-based education.[160] Realist reviews focus on understanding the underlying theory of an intervention like RRS, including how the context, mechanism of action and outcomes interact. McGaughery et al's theory, which underpins RRS, is displayed in Fig. 3.3.

TABLE 3.4
Essential elements of a rapid response system (RRS)

DOMAIN	ELEMENT	DESCRIPTION
Clinical processes	Measurement and documentation	Vital signs, oxygen saturation and level of consciousness should be undertaken regularly on all acute care patients
	Escalation of care	A protocol for the organisation's response in dealing with abnormal physiological measures and observations including appropriate modifications to nursing care, increased monitoring, medical review and calling for assistance
	Rapid response systems	When severe deterioration occurs, medical emergency teams, outreach teams or liaison nurses are available to respond
	Clinical communication	Structured communication protocols are used to hand over information about the patient
Organisational prerequisites	Organisational supports	Executive and clinical leadership support and a formal policy framework for recognition and response systems should exist
	Education	Education should cover clinical observation, identification of deterioration, escalation protocols, communication strategies and skills in initiating early interventions
	Evaluation, audit and feedback	Ongoing monitoring and evaluation are required to track changes in outcomes over time and to check that the RRS is operating as planned
	Technological systems and solutions	As relevant technologies are developed, they should be incorporated into service delivery, after considering evidence of their efficacy and cost as well as potential unintended consequences

Adapted from Australian Commission on Safety and Quality in Health Care: National Consensus Statement: Essential Elements for Recognising and Responding to Clinical Deterioration. Sydney: ACSQHC; 2010.

FIGURE 3.3 Rapid response program theory.

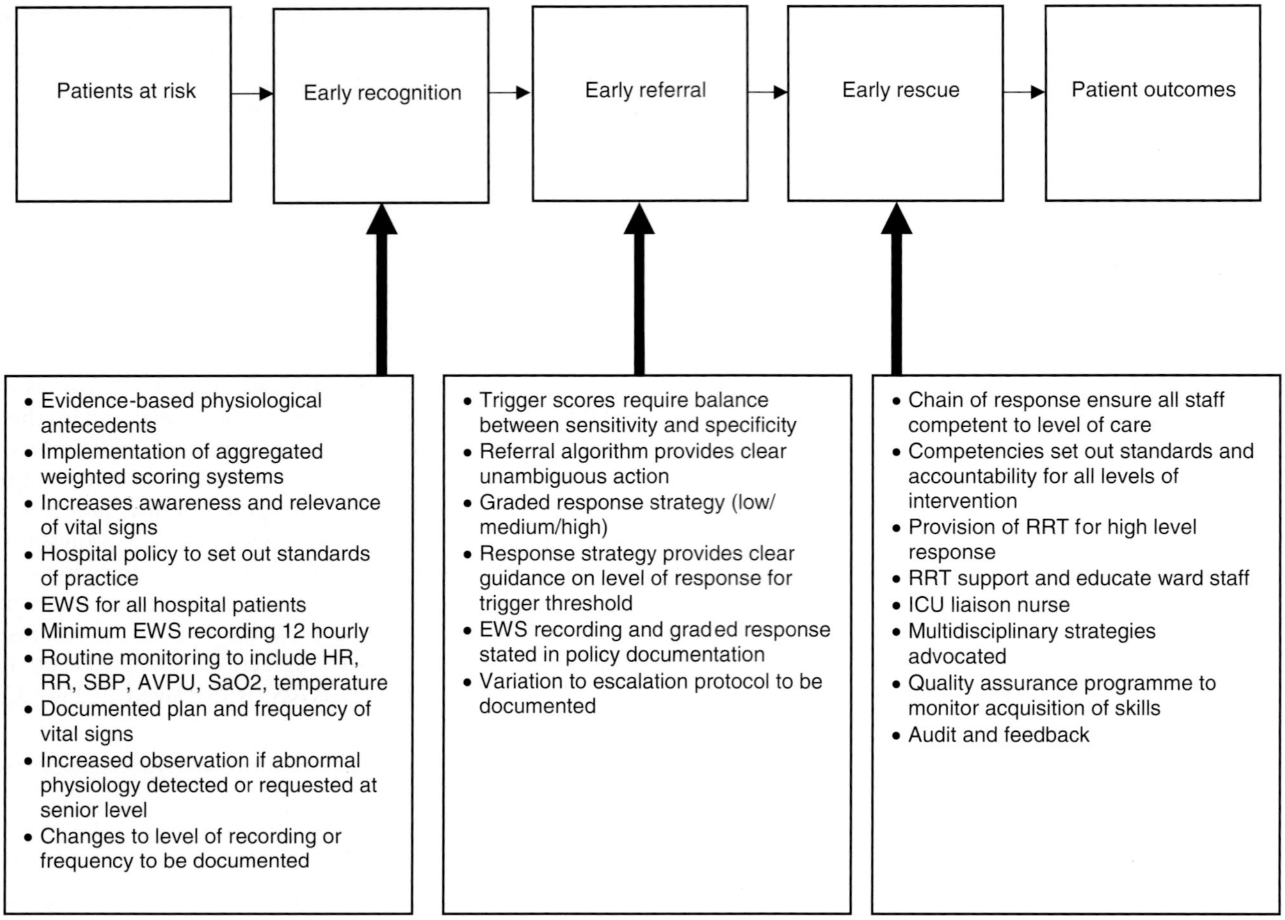

Reproduced from Figure 2: RRS programme theory; McGaughey J, O'Halloran P, Porter S, Blackwood B. Early warning systems and rapid response to the deteriorating patient in hospital: A systematic realist review. J Adv Nurs 2017;73(12): 2877-2891. doi:10.1111/jan.13398

RRS were originally conceptualised to have three components.[161] First, there are some criteria and a system for identifying and activating the rapid response team, often referred to as the afferent limb.[154] Second, there is the response, also termed the efferent limb.[161] Finally, there is an administrative and quality improvement component,[161] which is now referred to as two separate limbs, administrative and quality improvement.[162] Each of these limbs is briefly described.

Afferent limb

Recognising the deteriorating patient, the afferent limb has focused on measuring clinical signs including vital signs, level of consciousness and oxygenation as well as acting on abnormalities in these measurements.[161] They may also include concerns expressed by clinicians[163] and families.[164] Various scoring systems to identify ward patients with clinical deterioration have evolved as part of the development of critical care outreach[165] and the Medical Emergency Team (MET).[163] Authors of a 2017 scoping review of 21 studies on the use of early warning and track and trigger systems note a combination of parameters including respiratory rate, oxygen saturation, supplementary oxygen flow rates, systolic blood pressure, heart rate, temperature and level of consciousness continue to be used.[166] Two recent variations of early warning scoring systems are HOTEL (hypotension, oxygen saturation, temperature, electrocardiograph abnormalities, loss of independence) and TOTAL (tachypnoea, oxygen saturation, temperature, alert, loss of independence); both were found to be better for their particular populations than the modified early warning system.[166] All systems identify abnormalities in commonly measured parameters.

Early warning systems include calling criteria for contacting the admitting medical team, ICU staff, the critical care outreach team or the MET, depending on the severity of the patient's clinical deterioration and the resources available in the local clinical environment. In a 2017 review of 30 papers, activation of the RRS was influenced by perceptions and clinical experiences of ward nurses and physicians, accuracy of the activation criteria and monitoring technology.[167] Impediments included seeking further justification, deliberating over reactions from the RRT and the impact of workload and staffing.[167] In an Australian study of factors that influenced RRS in one hospital, organisational barriers were identified: that RRT medical responsibility was inversely proportional to clinical experience, system flexibility contributed to protocol deviation, misdistribution of resources led to perceptions of inadequate staffing, which prevented full optimisation of the RRS and poor communication and documentation increased clinician workload.[168] Patients and/or families calling the RRT is becoming more commonplace. A 2016 review of 10 studies focusing on family initiation of escalation of care for deteriorating patients found all of the 436 calls were appropriate, and stemmed from communication or system breakdowns.[164] Families viewed this calling positively but staff found the introduction of family activation to be stressful.[164]

Efferent limb

The efferent limb involves the team responding to clinical deterioration.[161] Some teams will include physicians and nurses, known as MET or RRT, whereas others, such as critical care outreach teams[161] and ICU liaison nurses, are nurse-led.[169] In some organisations, a graded response occurs, depending on how abnormal the early warning score is. One paper reported on a three-tiered response system as follows.[168] The first tier is a clinical review by two registered nurses within 30 min. The second tier is a rapid response by the patient's admitting medical team /medical registrar and an RRS resident medical officer within 30 min. The third tier is a code blue attended to immediately by an ICU-led team of registrars and critical care nurses. Irrespective of the title of the model used, the RRTs generally assess deteriorating patients and then initiate emergency treatments. A 2014 systematic review of critical care transition programs in general found they were associated with a reduced risk of ICU readmission.[170] This positive association was also found when the only service considered was an ICU liaison nurse.[170] One group reports that nurses on the MET undertake technical tasks related to airway (suctioning, inserting naso-pharyngeal airways etc) breathing (physical examination of the chest, increasing/adding oxygen etc), circulation (clinically examining circulation, performing ECGs etc), nervous system (assessing with the Glasgow Coma Scale etc) and various other tasks.[171] Non-technical tasks performed include reviewing investigations, contributing to information about patient history and plans for care, reassuring other healthcare professionals, educating staff, documenting care, application of monitoring equipment and supervising patient transport.[171] This study indicates the wide variety of activities that nurse members of a RRT undertake, which suggests the need for advanced knowledge and skills in a number of areas. Chapter 1 provides an overview of advanced nursing practice.

Administrative and quality improvement limbs

The third and fourth component of an RRS focuses on administration and quality improvement.[161] Generally, this involves both a governance plan and the collection and analysis of RRS data including the reason for the call, the treatments administered and patient outcomes. Analysing RRS data provides managers, clinicians and policy makers with guidance for future improvements. These activities are linked to previous information in this chapter on clinical audits, the PDSA cycle etc. In summary, RRS have evolved to provide emergency care to patients whose condition is deteriorating, and who are not already in the critical care unit. RRS involve a mechanism to identify these patients and call for help, as well as a response team. They also generally involve some administrative and quality improvement components to improve the service. RRT rely on team members working together, which leads to the next section on non-technical skills.

Non-technical skills

Nurses need to have current knowledge and skills in critical care to ensure safe, high quality care, but these technical skills are not sufficient. They also need to possess other, non-technical skills (NTS) to ensure patient safety. NTS have been described as the cognitive, social and personal skills that compliment technical skills.[172] This section provides an overview of four inter-related non-technical skills: situational awareness, decision making, communication and teamwork. Another important non-technical skill, leadership, is described in Chapters 1 and 2. Understanding the importance of NTS in providing safe, high quality care, has led to the development of a number of training programs, which are briefly described in this section.

Situational awareness

Situational awareness is the awareness and understanding of a situation and its possible outcomes.[173] Situations may be categorised on a continuum from routine and easily managed to confusing and dangerous, requiring specific skills and expertise.[174] Endsley,[175] whose work has been particularly influential, describes three levels of situational awareness. Level 1, *perception*, involves gathering data about the current situation. Level 2, *comprehension*, reflects interpretation and understanding the data. Level 3, *projection*, is concerned with predicting what can happen in the future. Fig. 3.4 demonstrates application of these three levels of situational awareness using the scenario of a postoperative patient whose blood pressure has dropped. Importantly, situational awareness is

FIGURE 3.4 Situational awareness example.

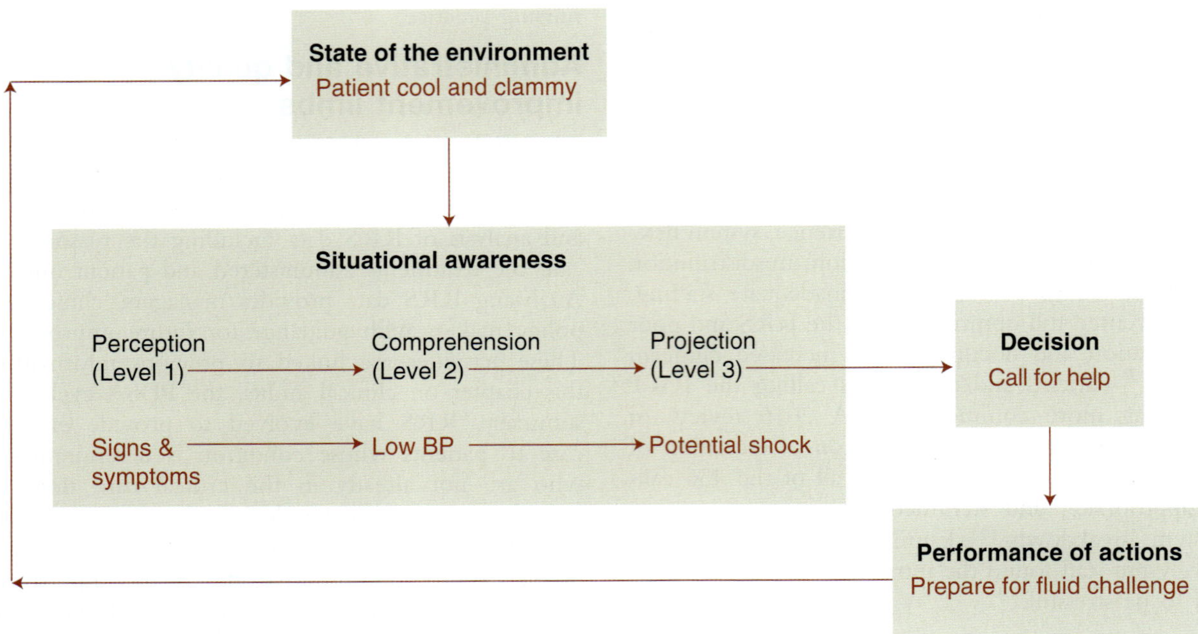

viewed as a necessary precursor for good quality decision making.[173]

Team situational awareness is a term applied to teams and reflects the notion that team members possess the situational awareness needed to perform their tasks in the team.[173] This team situational awareness has also been termed shared situational awareness.[175] In the critical care environment, nurses and physicians will have some unique but related tasks to undertake including during procedures such as central line insertions, intubations and bronchoscopies, and these tasks will require both complementary and shared situational awareness. The extent of team or shared situational awareness will influence the quality of decisions and subsequent team performance.[173]

Practice tip

Team briefings before undertaking a complex procedure can help to develop team situational awareness.

One review identified that both individual factors and interpersonal behaviours influenced situational awareness.[176] Lapses in situational awareness can occur because of issues such as distractions, fatigue, time pressures and team dynamics such as assertive authority figures. A number of strategies are recommended to overcome these lapses. They include thorough briefings about the nature and risk of a given activity, minimising distractions and interruptions during critical tasks, receiving regular updates, good time management, being physically and mentally fit for work and speaking up when not sure of a goal, procedure or next step.[175,177,178]

Decision making

Decision making involves a judgement or choosing an option (i.e. a course of action) to meet the needs of a given situation.[175] In critical care, multiple, complex decisions are made in rapid succession.[179] Decision making entails defining a problem, generating and considering one or more alternatives, selecting and implementing an option and reviewing the outcome. Clinical decision making is a complex process and is influenced by a number of factors. For example, environmental factors such as the team, the patient and resources can influence decision making as can situational awareness. Individual factors such as fatigue, affective state interruption in work and distractions can also influence decision making.[180,181] Authors of a systematic review on cognitive biases associated with medical decision making describe a decision-making framework that suggests two ways decisions are made.[182] In the first, unconscious, automatic or intuitive decisions are made quickly and effortlessly. In the second, decisions are deliberate, slower and require effort. Over-reliance on the first method can lead to cognitive biases, which influence decision making.[182]

Critical care nursing practice has been the focus of many studies on decision making in the early-mid 2000s. One study demonstrated that critical care nurses generate one or more hypotheses about a situation prior to decision making.[179] Other studies indicated that experienced and inexperienced nurses differ in their decision-making skills,[180,181,183] and that role models or mentors are

TABLE 3.5
Strategies to develop clinical decision making

STRATEGY	DESCRIPTION
Iterative hypothesis testing[186] (Narayan and Corcoran-Perry, 2008)	Description of a clinical situation for which the clinician has to generate questions and develop hypotheses; with additional questioning the clinician will develop further hypotheses. Three phases: 1 asking questions to gather data about a patient 2 justifying the data sought 3 interpreting the data to describe the influence of new information on decisions
Interactive model[186] (Narayan and Corcoran-Perry, 2008)	Schema (mental structures) used to teach new knowledge by building on previous learning. Three components: 1 advanced organisers – blueprint that previews the material to be learned and connects it to previous materials 2 progressive differentiation – a general concept presented first is broken down into smaller ideas 3 integrative reconciliation – similarities and differences and relationships between concepts explored
Case study[187] (Rivett and Jones, 2008)	Description of a clinical situation with a number of cues followed by a series of questions. Three types: 1 stable – presents information, then asks clinicians about it 2 dynamic – presents information, asks the clinicians about it, presents more information, asks more questions 3 dynamic with expert feedback – combines the dynamic method with immediate expert feedback
Reflection on action[186] (Narayan and Corcoran-Perry, 2008)	Clinicians are asked to reflect on their actions after a particular event. This pondering focuses on clinical judgements made, feelings surrounding the actions and the actions themselves. Reflection on action can be undertaken as an individual or group activity and is often facilitated by an expert
Thinking aloud[186] (Narayan and Corcoran-Perry, 2008)	A clinical situation is provided and the clinician is asked to 'think aloud' or verbalise their decisions. Thinking aloud is generally facilitated by an expert and can be undertaken individually or in groups

important in assisting to develop decision-making skills.[184] A Greek study classified ICU nurses' decisions as urgent or non-urgent and as independent or dependent.[185] The researchers observed that 75% (962/1281) of decisions were non-urgent and 60% (220/368) were independent.[185] It is clear that good quality clinical decisions, irrespective of what they are about, will likely improve patient care and outcomes.

Recommendations for developing clinical decision-making skills

Several strategies that can be used to help critical care nurses to develop their clinical decision making abilities are identified in Table 3.5.[186,187] These strategies can be used by nurses at any level to develop their own decision-making skills or by educators in planning educational sessions. It is important to note, however, that a review of interventions to improve decision making concluded that most studies in this area were of relatively poor quality.[188]

Communication

Communication has been described as 'the exchange of information, feedback or response, ideas and feelings'.[172] Good quality communication is viewed as a two-way sharing of information, whereby the sender encodes some idea into a message and transmits it to a receiver. The receiver then decodes the message to gain an understanding of it. Next, the receiver becomes the sender, encoding and transmitting a subsequent message.[172] There are various types of communication including verbal and non-verbal. Non-verbal communication includes written communication and body cues or gestures.

Reason,[189] a well-known safety researcher, suggests that there are three kinds of communication failure that contribute to accidents. The first, system failure, occurs when there are either no channels of communication or the channels that exist are not working or are not used. The second, message failure, happens when necessary information is not communicated. And finally, reception failure occurs when the information is misinterpreted or arrives too late.

Practice tip

Using closed-loop communications, where the receiver acknowledges the message was heard, can prevent miscommunication.

Experts recommend that communication be explicit, efficient and closed-loop.[190] By being explicit, a person is being clear in what they are saying. Being efficient means that the message is conveyed using only as many words as necessary. And closed-loop communication is a term used to signify that a receiver acknowledges or responds to the sender of information. This response lets the initiator know that the message was heard. Other strategies to improve communication include ensuring it is timely and assertive.[190] Timely communication means that the sender is cognisant of the other activities that the receiver may be doing and, because of this, provides information at a relevant time. Assertiveness involves standing up for yourself while respecting others.

In the critical care setting two specific communication situations have been the focus of recent research – clinical handover and rounds. Handover is more than the transfer of patient information; it has been described as the transfer of professional responsibility and accountability for some or all aspects of care for a patient, or group of patients, from one care provider to another.[191] Besides sharing patient information, handovers provide nurses with opportunities for social bonding, coaching and educating, and team building.[192,193] One Australian study focused on the content of ICU nursing handover.[194] The researchers found that while >95% of observed handovers included identifying nursing care needs, vital sign observations, changes in patient condition and the medical management of the patient, <40% included a discussion of discharge or long-term plans, cross-checking and reporting on resuscitation status.[194] A second study of 157 nursing shift-to-shift handovers conducted in seven ICUs in three countries (Australia, Israel and the UK)[195] found handovers were more comprehensive when: 1) the oncoming nurse did not know the patient; 2) the patient was expected to die during the shift; or 3) the family were present. Over 70% of nurses in Israel had cared for the patient in the previous 48 hours, in comparison to only 29% and 20% of UK and Australian nurses. Over 75% of the handover communication included the goals for care and 73% included pain management, but legal issues such as advance directives and identification of a health proxy were mentioned in less than 10% of the handovers. In recent years there have been many other studies of ICU handovers. For example, research focuses on shift-to-shift nursing[196] or medical handover,[197,198] handover from ICU to the wards[199,200] or the operating room[201] and handover from the operating room to the ICU.[202] A recent systematic review of eight studies of the handover from the ICU to the ward identified most studies were conducted in Australia, and examined various processes and interventions including the use of the ICU Liaison Nurse or critical care outreach service as a handover tool.[203] However, all but one meta-analysis was at a moderate or high risk of bias, suggesting there is a need for high quality research in this area.

A 2013 review identified three important features of good quality handover including: 1) face-to-face, two-way communication; 2) standardised templates or checklists that incorporate a minimum dataset; and 3) content that includes the patient's current diagnosis and clinical situation.[204] In order to improve the quality of handovers, a group of Australians has developed an interactive, 3D computer simulation (virtual world) for training intensive care nurses in shift-to-shift handover.[205]

Multidisciplinary rounds are seen to be one way to promote shared situational awareness. A 2013 systematic review of ICU rounds concluded that 'rounds conducted using a standardised structure and a best practice checklist by a multidisciplinary group of providers, with explicitly defined roles and a goal-orientated approach, had the strongest supporting evidence'.[204] Table 3.6 provides more specific details of the recommendations from this review. One notable cluster-randomised study undertaken in 118 Brazilian ICUs tested the effect of the use of a checklist and daily goal setting during multidisciplinary rounds.[56] Over 6750 patients were enrolled in the trial. The researchers found no difference in in-hospital mortality between the intervention and control groups although significant improvements were found in some specific secondary outcomes such as the use of low tidal volumes, avoidance of heavy sedation, use of central venous and urinary catheters, and perceptions of teamwork and safety climate.

Teamwork

Teams have been described as two or more individuals with specialised roles and responsibilities who act interdependently to achieve some common goal,[206] although in their systematic review Dietz et al noted teamwork is a broad term with varying definitions.[207] High performing teams share an understanding of the activity they are working on; they understand the aim or mission of that activity, and they know each other's roles and expectations. They are also trained and skilled in leadership, conflict resolution, back-up behaviour and closed-loop communication. Important aspects of leadership include coordinating the team, distributing workloads equitably and monitoring the team's performance. Conflict resolution often requires clarification of roles and responsibilities, fostering useful debate and assertive communication. Back-up behaviour is when one team member can step in to assist another in their role, providing support to other team members. In essence, teamwork is dependent on each member being able to anticipate the needs of others, adjust to others' actions and the changing environment and have a shared understanding of how a task should be performed. Dietz and colleagues found standardised protocols (such as using checklists), implementing daily rounds and training were the three main solutions used to improve ICU teamwork.[207] The findings from a more recent study focused on ICU teamwork in North America suggested it was more accurate to describe this work as interprofessional work, rather than teamwork.[208] They found that various relational factors, such as professional cultures, medical dominance and

TABLE 3.6
Recommendations for ICU rounds

BEST PRACTICE	STRENGTH OF RECOMMENDATION
Implement multidisciplinary rounds (including at least a medical doctor, registered nurse and pharmacist)	Strong – definitely do it
Standardise location, time and team composition	Strong – definitely do it
Define explicit roles for each HCP participating on rounds	Strong – definitely do it
Develop and implement structured tool (best practices checklist)	Strong – definitely do it
Reduce non-essential time-wasting activities	Strong – definitely do it
Minimise unnecessary interruptions	Strong – definitely do it
Focus discussions on development of daily goals and document all discussed goals in health record	Strong – definitely do it
Conduct discussions at bedside to promote patient-centredness	Weak – probably do it
Conduct discussions in conference room to promote efficiency and communication	Weak – probably do it
Establish open collaborative discussion environment	Weak – probably do it
Ensure clear visibility between all HCP	Weak – probably do it
Empower HCP to promote team-based approach to discussions	Weak – probably do it
Produce visual presentation of patient information	No specific recommendation

HCP = health care professional.
Adapted from Lane D, Ferri M, Lemaire J, et al. A systematic review of evidence-informed practices for patient care rounds in the ICU. Crit Care Med 2013;41(8):2015–29.

hierarchies, both within and between professions, influenced how work was undertaken. In another recently published grounded theory study of ICU teamwork in Sweden, balancing intertwined responsibilities was the core category identified.[209] Contextual conditions associated with this core category included the dynamic nature of the ICU and the number of team members in the ICU. Conditions that resulted in this balancing act included the need to be prepared and flexible, and the inter-dependence with others associated with overlapping roles. Intervening conditions that influenced team processes included the organisational and workplace culture and staff characteristics. As a result, staff adopted both active and passive approaches to clinical activities. Another term closely related to teamwork is interprofessional care, which in ICU is described as 'care provided by a team of healthcare professionals with overlapping expertise and an appreciation for the unique contribution of other team members as partners in achieving a common goal'.[210]

Non-technical skills training

Increasing recognition of the importance of NTS has led to the development of a number of training programs. These programs recognise that, while human error cannot be eliminated, it can be minimised, trapped or mitigated.[172] A systematic review of NTS training to enhance patient safety documented both the content of and training methods used in NTS training.[211]

Fig. 3.5 demonstrates the content covered in the team training studies reviewed by Gordon and colleagues.[211] In addition to the core NTS described in this section, the review also identified training programs focused on understanding error and systems such as the human/technology interface. Two well-known teamwork experts noted that factors such as how the team training is implemented, the method of its delivery and leadership all influence the effectiveness of team training on both processes and outcomes.[212]

Fig. 3.6 provides an overview of these training methods.[211] Most of the team training studies reviewed took a multidisciplinary approach, reflecting contemporary clinical practice. Simulation has attracted a lot of attention recently as a team training strategy. Simulation allows clinicians to practise skills and reflect on their performance in a simulated environment. That is, it increases both knowledge and performance. In their 2013 systematic review, Schmidt and colleagues[213]

FIGURE 3.5 Analysis of non-technical skills training teaching methods.

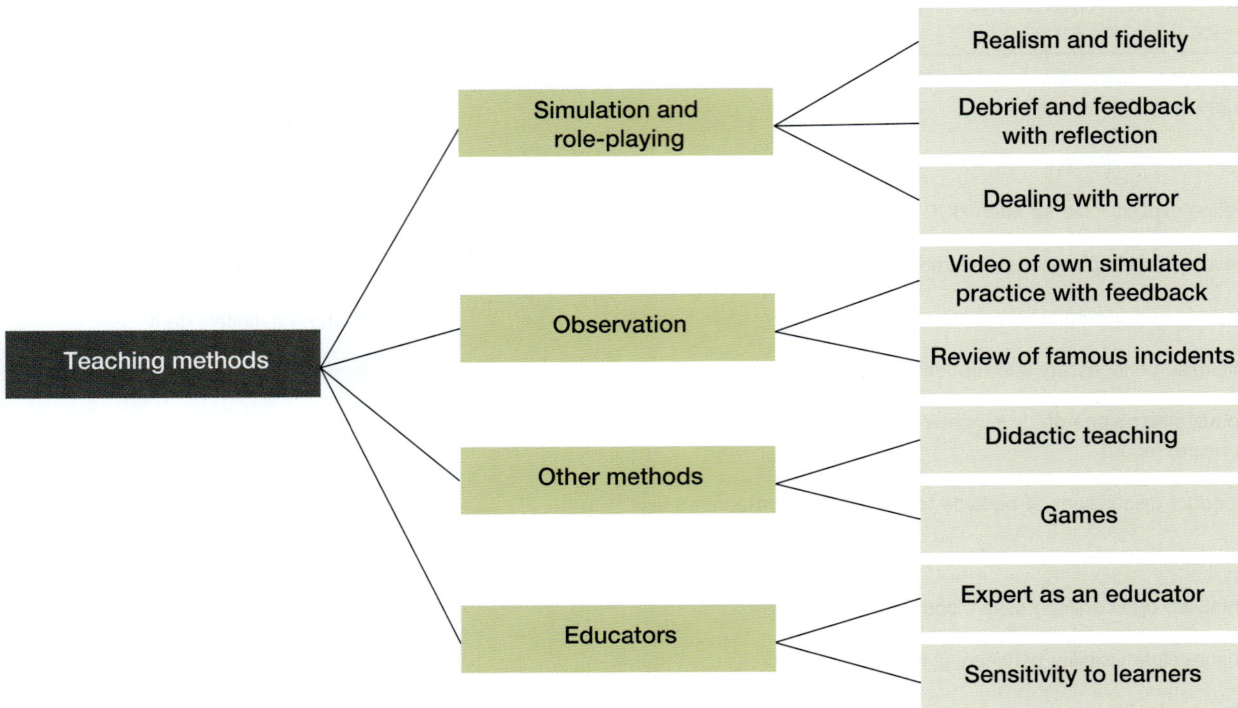

Reproduced from Gordon M, Darbyshire D, Baker P. Non-technical skills training to enhance patient safety: a systematic review. Med Educ 2012;46(11):1042-54, with permission.

asserted that simulation as a patient safety strategy had four purposes: 1) education; 2) assessment; 3) research; and 4) health system integration. It is evident that teamwork and NTS team training are core components of patient safety. One study of the use of a 2-day team training intervention, called crew resource management, in six ICUs in The Netherlands identified participants were positive about the training, and that participants recognised the importance of situational awareness.[214] Compared to the control group, participants reported enacting situational awareness and teamwork more but there was no statistically significant differences in communication between the two groups and no changes in patient outcomes were identified. In another study undertaken in two ICUs in Hong Kong, blended learning (both online and in person) and the flipped classroom approach where didactic teaching occurs prior to face-to-face teaching, were used to improve patient safety culture.[215] The researchers found that in the intervention site there were significant improvements in both perceptions of teamwork and perceptions of management support for patient safety. Intervention participants also reported greater improvements than control participants in other aspects of patient safety. A third study in six ICUs, three of which received a two-day crew resource management training course, identified that while participants were positive about the course, and self-reported behaviour aimed at improving situational awareness improved, no changes were found in observed communication or patient outcomes.[214] In summary, patient safety involves understanding the risks to patients and developing strategies to minimise these risks. Safety culture and non-technical skills are two important aspects of patient safety, with a number of strategies and programs available to enhance both.

FIGURE 3.6 Analysis of non-technical skills training content themes.

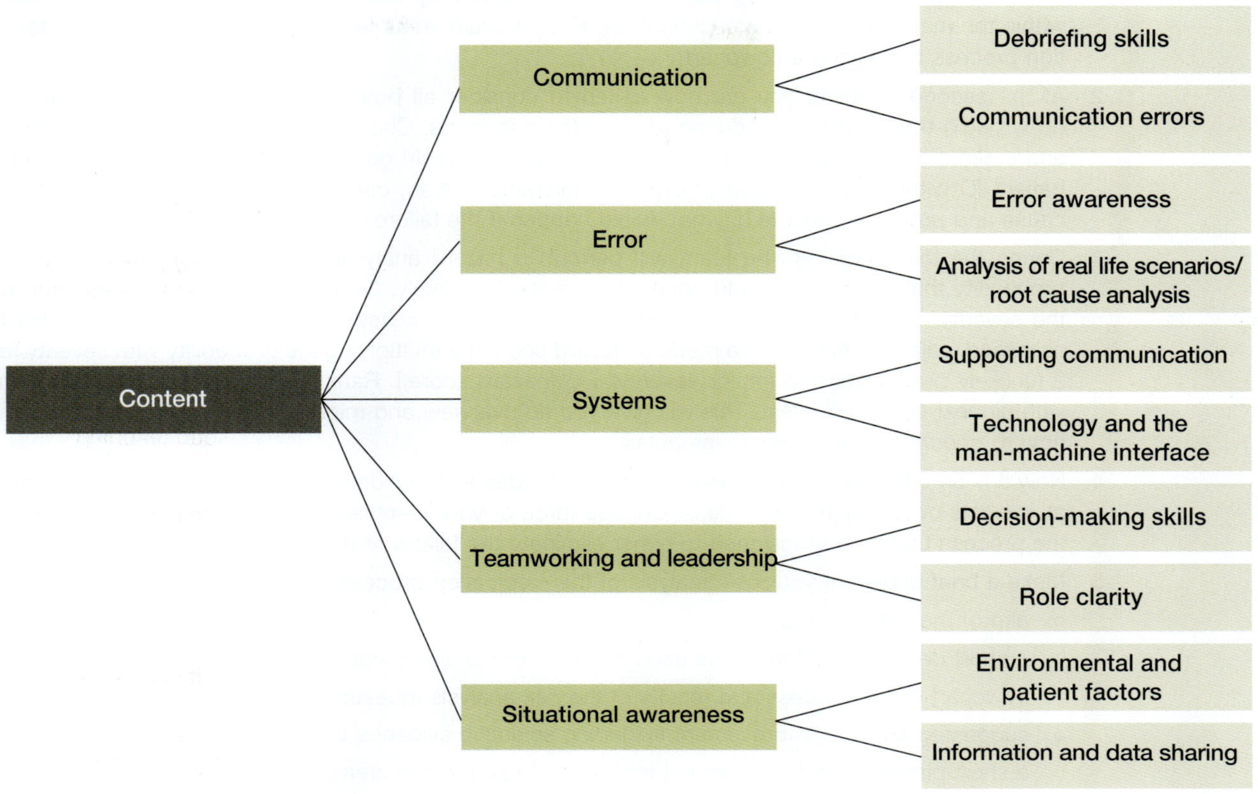

Reproduced from Gordon M, Darbyshire D, Baker P. Non-technical skills training to enhance patient safety: a systematic review. Med Educ 2012;46(11):1042–54, with permission.

Summary

In summary, this chapter has provided an overview of safety and quality in critical care. The development and use of good quality CPGs is an important foundation to promote quality and reduce variation in care. Quality and safety monitoring underpin understanding the risks that patients face in critical care. The use of care bundles, checklists and information and communication technologies may improve quality of care. Improving patient safety is multifaceted, but often includes understanding the safety culture as well as the risks faced by patients in a particular clinical area. Techniques such as the analysis of clinical incidents, root cause analyses and failure mode and effects analysis help in understanding situations that place patients at risk of AEs. One particular high-risk scenario is the deteriorating patient, with a number of RRS now being implemented to respond to this scenario. Other initiatives to improve patient safety include NTS training. Understanding situations that place patients at risk of harm as well as the safety culture of a unit or organisation provides the foundation to improve safety culture.

Case study

You have just been asked to participate in a multidisciplinary group to perform a risk analysis of the medication process at your ICU. The group consists of one additional critical care nurse, one physician, and one clinical pharmacist. The team is assigned to perform a risk analysis using the Failure Mode and Effect Analysis (FMEA) model. As a newly graduated critical care nurse, you are asked to contribute with your own experiences of the medication process, as well as thoughts and ideas regarding improvements. The questions below ask you to plan your contribution to this working group.

CASE STUDY QUESTIONS

1. At the first meeting, the group begins with mapping and graphically describing the process. Main areas are identified (e.g. drug administration), followed by sub-areas; that is, all steps performed within the main area (e.g. check patient ID). Identify main areas followed by sub-areas in the medication process by making a flowchart.
2. At the second meeting, you are now asked to consider all possible failure modes (i.e. what could go wrong?) that might occur during each of the sub-areas. Choose three of the sub-areas identified and make a list of all possible failure modes (e.g. what could go wrong in the sub-process checking patient ID within the main area of drug administration). Also, consider each failure mode's possible cause and potential effect (e.g. what would happen if the failure mode occurred).
3. During the third meeting, the team will perform a hazard analysis for each failure mode. Rate the probability that the failure would occur (1= remote; 2=unlikely; 3= likely; 4=frequent). Thereafter, rate the severity of harm (1= minor; 2=moderate; 3= major; 4=catastrophic). When all failure modes are assessed, calculate each failure mode's 'hazard score' by multiplying the probability with severity [e.g. 2 (unlikely probability) × 3 (major severity) = 6 (hazard score)]. Rank all failure modes from the ones with highest score to lowest. This will give you an overview and might guide the group's decision on how to prioritise areas of improvements.
4. Now it is time for the group to review all failure modes and decide whether to accept the failure mode as it exists or redesign the process. Choose three of your identified failure modes and consider *how* the process could be redesigned to either eliminate the failure or mitigate potential patient harm.
5. Make a brief outline of your risk analysis of the medication process. The report should include:
   - aim of the risk analysis
   - a short description of methods used and how the analysis was performed
   - flowchart of the process and results of the risk analysis (question 1–4)
   - suggested areas of improvement (including scientific evidence that supports your findings)
   - a short plan on how to implement and evaluate suggested areas of improvement.

Recommended reading for this case study:

Paparella S. Failure mode and effects analysis: a useful tool for risk identification and injury prevention. J Emerg Nurs 2007;33(4):367-71.

RESEARCH VIGNETTE

Abstract

Background: Use of the interprofessional Awakening and Breathing Coordination, Delirium Monitoring and Management, and Early Mobility (ABCDE) bundle is recommended practice in intensive care, but its adoption remains limited.

Objective: To examine the relationship between intensive care unit provider attitudes regarding the ABCDE bundle and ABCDE bundle adherence.

Methods: A 1-time survey of 268 care providers in 10 intensive care units across the country who had worked at least 4 shifts per month to examine their attitudes towards workload burden, difficulty carrying out the bundle, perceived safety, confidence, and perceived strength of evidence. Logistic regression models were used to examine the relationship of unit-level provider attitudes with ABCDE bundle adherence in 101 patients, adjusted for patients' age, severity of illness, and comorbidity.

Results: For every unit increase in workload burden, adherence to the ABCDE bundle decreased 53% (odds ratio [OR], 0.47; 95% CI, 0.28–0.79; *P* =.0040). Bundle difficulty (OR, 0.29; 95% CI, 0.08–1.07), perceived safety (OR, 0.51; 95% CI, 0.10–2.65), confidence (OR, 0.37, 95% CI, 0.10–1.35), and perceived strength of evidence (OR, 0.69; 95% CI, 0.14–3.35) were not associated with ABCDE bundle adherence. For every unit increase in perceived difficulty carrying out the bundle, adherence with early mobility was reduced 59% (OR, 0.41; 95% CI, 0.19-0.90; *P* =.03). In addition, ABCDE bundle adherence (i.e., ventilator bundle) was less than DE bundle adherence (i.e., ventilator-free bundle((97% vs 72%, z =5.47; *P* <.001).

Conclusions: Focusing interventions on workload burden and factors influencing bundle difficulty may facilitate ABCDE bundle adherence.

Critique

This study focused on understanding factors that influence the use of the ABCDE care bundle. The researchers provide a clear and strong rationale for undertaking the study; despite its wide endorsement, evidence shows the care bundle was not consistently used in practice. The study was set in 10 ICUs in six US hospitals, a strength because of the multiple sites. But, little description beyond the name of the hospitals makes it difficult to understand characteristics of the settings and thus the generalisability of the findings is difficult to judge. Data were collected from variety of health professional groups as well as patients enrolled in an ongoing clinical trial. Because of a low response rate from health professionals (25%) and because patient data reflected those recruited to a clinical trial suggesting they may be unique in some way, generalisability of the findings are also questionable. The researchers provide clear definitions for the variables they measure, which they showed were generally reliable. Self-report was used to collect data on adherence to the ABCDE care bundle, which may have resulted in some inaccuracies in this data, as clinicians may hesitate to state they did not follow a widely endorsed practice. Their logistic regression results are based on a sample of 101 patients, which is a small sample size for this multivariate analytic technique. Small samples affect the extent to which the findings are reproducible; that is, the extent to which similar results would be found if the study were repeated. Small sample sizes also affect the power of the study. Studies with low power are unlikely to identify statistically significant results even if the results are 'true' in reality. The researchers acknowledge a number of other limitations of their research including that the ABCDE care bundle evolved during their data collection, adherence data were not collected on all patients in the ICU and the potential for non-response bias with only 25% of healthcare professionals completing the surveys. However, this study provides some insight on the various issues that may impact on ABCDE care bundle adherence including the perceived ease and safety of its use, healthcare professional confidence and the perceived strength of evidence for its use.

Learning activities

1 Using each domain of quality and safety as headings (i.e. structure, process, outcome), list some of the key considerations for a quality improvement project targeting shift-to-shift nursing handover in your unit.

2 After identifying a CPG that guides nurses in providing care in your unit, assess it against the NHMRC standard displayed in Table 3.1.

3 Examine the patterns of high-frequency adverse event in your unit over the past 12 months. What were the causes of incidents? What targeted strategies could be used to reduce the incidence of these AEs?

4 Identify and provide a rationale for an aspect of care that might benefit from the use of a checklist in your unit. Develop some specific checklist items that you think should be included.

5 Describe how technology is used in your unit to improve care delivered to patients. Using the information outlined in the section on information and communication technologies, identify where there is potential to use technology to improve care delivery further. Use examples specific to your unit.

6 Describe how participants in multidisciplinary rounds can contribute to the activity.

7 Consider the NTS skills training teaching methods identified in Fig. 3.5 (simulation and role-playing, observation, other methods such as didactic teaching and gaming and the use of educators) and reflect on the ways you think you learn best. Then, identify three recent education/training sessions you have attended and comment on the extent to which the teaching methods were congruent with how you learn.

Online resources

Agency for Healthcare Research and Quality, www.ahrq.gov

Australian Commission on Safety and Quality in Health Care (ACSQHC), www.safetyandquality.gov.au

Australian Council on Healthcare Standards (ACHS), www.achs.org.au

Institute for Healthcare Improvement (IHI), USA, www.ihi.org/Pages/default.aspx

Intensive Care Coordination and Monitoring Unit (ICCMU), New South Wales Health, http://intensivecare.hsnet.nsw.gov.au

Joint Commission (USA), www.jointcommission.org

National E-Health Transition Authority, www.digitalhealth.gov.au/

National Health and Medical Research Council, www.nhmrc.gov.au

National Institute for Health and Care Excellence, https://www.nice.org.uk/

National Quality Forum, www.qualityforum.org/Home.aspx

Patient Safety Network, https://psnet.ahrq.gov/

Quality Use of Medicines, www.health.gov.au/internet/main/publishing.nsf/Content/nmp-quality.htm

World Health Organization Patient Safety, www.who.int/patientsafety/en

Further reading

Ausserhofer D, Schubert M, Desmedt M, et al. The association of patient safety climate and nurse-related organizational factors with selected patient outcomes: a cross-sectional survey. Int J Nurs Stud 2013;50(2):240–52.

Australian Commission on Safety and Quality in Health Care. Safety and Quality Improvement Guide Standard 9: Recognising and responding to clinical deterioration in acute health care. Sydney: ACSQHC; 2012.

Browne M, Cook P. Inappropriate trust in technology: implications for critical care nurses. Nurs Crit Care 2011;16(2): 92–8.

Craze L, McGeorge P, Holmes D, et al Recognising and responding to deterioration in mental state: a scoping review. Sydney: ACSQHC; 2014.

Donabedian A. Evaluating the quality of medical care. Milbank Mem Fund Q 2005;44(3):691–729.

Flin RH, O'Connor P, Crichton M. Safety at the sharp end: a guide to non-technical skills. Aldershot: Ashgate; 2008.

Nemeth CP. Improving healthcare team communication: building on lessons from aviation and aerospace. Aldershot: Ashgate; 2008.

Odell M. Human factors and patient safety: changing roles in critical care. Aust Crit Care 2011;24(4):215–17.

Reason JT. The human contribution: unsafe acts, accidents and heroic recoveries. Aldershot: Ashgate; 2008.

Rossi PJ, Edmiston CE Jr. Patient safety in the critical care environment. Surg Clin North Am 2012;92(6):1369–86.

Vincent C. Patient safety. 2nd ed. Chichester: Wiley-Blackwell; 2010.

World Health Organization Patient safety tool kit. World Health Organization Regional Office for the Eastern Mediterranean. Cairo, 2015.

References

1. Lohr K, Schroeder S. A strategy for quality assurance in medicine. New Engl J Med 1990;322:1161–71.
2. Henneman EA, Gawlinski A, Giuliano KK. Surveillance: a strategy for improving patient safety in acute and critical care units. Crit Care Nurse 2012;32(2):e9–18.
3. Donabedian A. Evaluating the quality of medical care. Milbank Mem Fund Q 2005;44(3):691–729.
4. Carayon P, Schoofs Hundt A, Karsh BT, et al. Work system design for patient safety: the SEIPS model. Qual Saf Health Care 2006;15(Suppl. 1):i50–8.
5. Holden RJ, Carayon P, Gurses AP, et al. SEIPS 2.0: a human factors framework for studying and improving the work of healthcare professionals and patients. Ergonomics 2013;56(11):1669–86.
6. Frith KH. Medication errors in the intensive care unit: literature review using the SEIPS model. AACN Adv Crit Care 2013;24(4):389–404.
7. Bergman LM, Pettersson ME, Chaboyer WP, et al. Safety hazards during intrahospital transport: a prospective observational study. Crit Care Med 2017;45(10):e1043–9.
8. Institute of Medicine. Crossing the quality chasm: a new health system for the 21st century. Washington, DC: National Academy Press; 2001.
9. Speroff T, O'Connor GT. Study designs for PDSA quality improvement research. Qual Manag Health Care 2004;13(1):17–32.
10. Schwendimann R, Blatter C, Dhaini S, et al. The occurrence, types, consequences and preventability of in-hospital adverse events – a scoping review. BMC Health Serv Res 2018;18:521.
11. Nilsson L, Pihl A, Tågsjö M, et al. Adverse events are common on the intensive care unit: results from a structured record review. Acta Anaesthesiol Scand 2012;56(8):959–65.
12. Valentin A, Capuzzo M, Guidet B, et al. Patient safety in intensive care: results from the multinational Sentinel Events Evaluation (SEE) study. Intensive Care Med 2006;32(10):1591–8.
13. Thomas AN, MacDonald JJ. A review of patient safety incidents reported as 'severe' or 'death' from critical care units in England and Wales between 2004 and 2014. Anaesthesia 2016;71(9):1013–23.
14. Eccles MP, Grimshaw JM, Shekelle P, et al. Developing clinical practice guidelines: target audiences, identifying topics for guidelines, guideline group composition and functioning and conflicts of interest. Implement Sci 2012;7:60.
15. Miller M, Kearney N. Guidelines for clinical practice: development, dissemination and implementation. Int J Nurs Stud 2004;41(7):813–21.
16. Intensive Care Coordination and Monitoring Unit. HSNet - human services network: New South Wales Department of Health; 2017 Available from: https://www.aci.health.nsw.gov.au/networks/icnsw/intensive-care-manual/statewide-guidelines. [Accessed 19 February 2019].
17. Davidson JE, Aslakson RA, Long AC, et al. Guidelines for family-centered care in the neonatal, pediatric, and adult ICU. Crit Care Med 2017;45(1):103–28.
18. Nates JL, Nunnally ME, Kleinpell R, et al. ICU admission, discharge, and triage guidelines: a framework to enhance clinical operations, development of institutional policies, and further research. Crit Care Med 2016;44(8):1553–602.
19. Rhodes A, Evans LE, Alhazzani W, et al. Surviving sepsis campaign: international guidelines for management of sepsis and septic shock: 2016. Intensive Care Med 2017;43(3):304–77.
20. Kane-Gill SL, Dasta JF, Buckley MS, et al. Clinical practice guideline: safe medication use in the ICU. Crit Care Med 2017;45(9):e877–915.
21. McClave SA, Taylor BE, Martindale RG, et al. Guidelines for the provision and assessment of nutrition support therapy in the adult critically ill patient: Society of Critical Care Medicine (SCCM) and American Society for Parenteral and Enteral Nutrition (A.S.P.E.N.). JPEN J Parenter Enteral Nutr 2016;40(2):159–211.
22. Ullman AJ, Ray-Barruel G, Rickard CM, et al. Clinical audits to improve critical care: part 1 prepare and collect data. Aust Crit Care 2017;31(2):101–5.
23. Ray-Barruel G, Ullman AJ, Rickard CM, et al. Clinical audits to improve critical care: part 2: analyse, benchmark and feedback. Aust Crit Care 2017;31(2):106–9.
24. National Health and Medical Research Council (NHMRC). Information for guideline developers Canberra: Commonwealth of Australia; 2017. Available from: https://nhmrc.gov.au/research-policy/guideline-development. [Accessed 19 February 2019].
25. Higgins J, Green S Cochrane handbook for systematic reviews of interventions: The Cochrane Collaboration; 2011. Available from: http://handbook.cochrane.org/. [Accessed 9 March 2017].
26. Brouwers MC, Kho ME, Browman GP, et al. AGREE II: advancing guideline development, reporting and evaluation in health care. CMAJ 2010;182(18):E839–42.
27. Cahill NE, Suurdt J, Ouellette-Kuntz H, et al. Understanding adherence to guidelines in the intensive care unit: development of a comprehensive framework. JPEN J Parenter Enteral Nutr 2010;34(6):616–24.
28. Jordan P, Mpasa F, Ten Ham-Baloyi W, et al. Implementation strategies for guidelines at ICUs: a systematic review. Int J Health Care Qual Assur 2017;30(4):358–72.
29. Henneman EA. Unreported errors in the intensive care unit: a case study of the way we work. Crit Care Nurse 2007;27(5):27–34, quiz 5.
30. Xu J, Reale C, Slagle JM, et al. Facilitated nurse medication-related event reporting to improve medication management quality and safety in intensive care units. Nurs Res 2017;66(5):337–49.
31. Reason J. Understanding adverse events: human factors. Qual Health Care 1995;4(2):80–9.

32. Pettersson JP, Lindgren P, Hillgren J. SIR:s & SIS:s national quality indicators for intensive care: Swedish Intensive Care Registry; 2016. Available from: https://www.icuregswe.org/riktlinjer2/riktlinjer-gallande-registrering-lista/nationella-kvalitetsindikatorer/. [Accessed 19 February 2019].
33. Flaatten H. National quality indicators revisited. ICU Manag Pract 2016;16(4).
34. Curtis JR, Cook DJ, Wall RJ, et al. Intensive care unit quality improvement: a 'how-to' guide for the interdisciplinary team. Crit Care Med 2006;34(1):211–18.
35. Standards ACoH. Intensive Care Clinical Indicator User Manual (version 5). [Consultation document]. In press 2018.
36. Scottish Intensive Care Society Quality Improvement Group. Minimum standards and quality indicators for critical care in Scotland. Edinburgh: NHS National Services Scotland; 2015.
37. Rhodes A, Moreno RP, Azoulay E, et al. Prospectively defined indicators to improve the safety and quality of care for critically ill patients: a report from the Task Force on Safety and Quality of the European Society of Intensive Care Medicine (ESICM). Intensive Care Med 2012;38(4):598–605.
38. Institute for Healthcare Improvement. How-to guide: prevent central line-associated bloodstream infections (CLABSI). Cambridge, MA: Institute for Healthcare Improvement; 2012.
39. Institute for Healthcare Improvement. How-to guide: prevent ventilator-associated pneumonia. Cambridge, MA: Institute for Healthcare Improvement; 2012.
40. Institute for Healthcare Improvement. Severe sepsis bundles. Cambridge, MA: Institute for Healthcare Improvement; 2013.
41. Vincent JL, Shehabi Y, Walsh TS, et al. Comfort and patient-centred care without excessive sedation: the eCASH concept. Intensive Care Med 2016;42(6):962–71.
42. Lavallee JF, Gray TA, Dumville J, et al. The effects of care bundles on patient outcomes: a systematic review and meta-analysis. Implement Sci 2017;12(1):142.
43. Crunden E, Boyce C, Woodman H, et al. An evaluation of the impact of the ventilator care bundle. Nurs Crit Care 2005;10(5):242–6.
44. Morris AC, Hay AW, Swann DG, et al. Reducing ventilator-associated pneumonia in intensive care: impact of implementing a care bundle. Crit Care Med 2011;39(10):2218–24.
45. Parisi M, Gerovasili V, Dimopoulos S, et al. Use of ventilator bundle and staff education to decrease ventilator-associated pneumonia in intensive care patients. Crit Care Nurse 2016;36(5):e1–7.
46. Pandharipande P, Banerjee A, McGrane S, et al. Liberation and animation for ventilated ICU patients: the ABCDE bundle for the back-end of critical care. Crit Care 2010;14(3):157.
47. Balas MC, Vasilevskis EE, Olsen KM, et al. Effectiveness and safety of the awakening and breathing coordination, delirium monitoring/management, and early exercise/mobility (ABCDE) bundle. Crit Care Med 2014;42(5):1024–36.
48. Boehm LM, Dietrich MS, Vasilevskis EE, et al. Perceptions of workload burden and adherence to ABCDE bundle among intensive care providers. Am J Crit Care 2017;26(4):e38–47.
49. Boehm LM, Vasilevskis EE, Dietrich MS, et al. Organizational domains and variation in attitudes of intensive care providers toward the ABCDE bundle. Am J Crit Care 2017;26(3):e18–28.
50. Hales BM, Pronovost PJ. The checklist–a tool for error management and performance improvement. J Crit Care 2006;21(3):231–5.
51. Dykes PC, Rozenblum R, Dalal A, et al. Prospective evaluation of a multifaceted intervention to improve outcomes in intensive care: the promoting respect and ongoing safety through patient engagement communication and technology study. Crit Care Med 2017;45(8):e806–13.
52. Ali R, Cornelius PJ, Herasevich V, et al. Effect of daily use of electronic checklist on physical rehabilitation consultations in critically ill patients. J Crit Care 2017;38:357–61.
53. Conroy KM, Elliott D, Burrell AR. Testing the implementation of an electronic process-of-care checklist for use during morning medical rounds in a tertiary intensive care unit: a prospective before–after study. Ann Intensive Care 2015;5:20.
54. DuBose JJ, Inaba K, Shiflett A, et al. Measurable outcomes of quality improvement in the trauma intensive care unit: the impact of a daily quality rounding checklist. J Trauma 2008;64(1):22–7.
55. Chua C, Wisniewski T, Ramos A, et al. Multidisciplinary trauma intensive care unit checklist: impact on infection rates. J Trauma Nurs 2010;17(3):163–6.
56. Cavalcanti AB, Bozza FA, Machado FR, et al. Effect of a quality improvement intervention with daily round checklists, goal setting, and clinician prompting on mortality of critically ill patients: a randomized clinical trial. JAMA 2016;315(14):1480–90.
57. Ko HC, Turner TJ, Finnigan MA. Systematic review of safety checklists for use by medical care teams in acute hospital settings – limited evidence of effectiveness. BMC Health Serv Res 2011;11:211.
58. Burian BK, Clebone A, Dismukes K, et al. More than a tick box: medical checklist development, design, and use. Anesth Analg 2018;126(1):223–32.
59. Hallam BD, Kuza CC, Rak K, et al. Perceptions of rounding checklists in the intensive care unit: a qualitative study. BMJ Qual Saf 2018.
60. Michard F. Hemodynamic monitoring in the era of digital health. Ann Intensive Care 2016;6(1):15.
61. Mason C, Leong T. Clinical information systems in the intensive care unit. Anaesth Intensive Care 2016;17(1):13–16.
62. Dziadzko MA, Thongprayoon C, Ahmed A, et al. Automatic quality improvement reports in the intensive care unit: one step closer toward meaningful use. World J Crit Care Med 2016;5(2):165–70.

63. Varghese J, Kleine M, Gessner S, et al. Effects of computerised decision support systems implementations on patient outcomes in inpatient care: a systematic review. J Am Med Inform Assoc 2018;25(5):593–602.
64. Kirkbride G, Vermace B. Smart pumps: implications for nurse leaders. Nurs Adm Q 2011;35(2):110–18.
65. Malashock CM, Shull SS, Gould DA. Effect of smart infusion pumps on medication errors related to infusion device programming. Hosp Pharm 2004;39(5):460–9.
66. Schnock KO, Dykes PC, Albert J, et al. The frequency of intravenous medication administration errors related to smart infusion pumps: a multihospital observational study. BMJ Qual Saf 2017;26(2):131–40.
67. Ohashi K, Dalleur O, Dykes PC, et al. Benefits and risks of using smart pumps to reduce medication error rates: a systematic review. Drug Saf 2014;37(12):1011–20.
68. NSW Goverment. Electronic record for intensive care (eRIC); 2018. Available from: http://www.ehealth.nsw.gov.au/programs/clinical/eric. [Accessed 19 February 2019].
69. Bosman RJ. Impact of computerized information systems on workload in operating room and intensive care unit. Best Pract Res Clin Anaesthesiol 2009;23(1):15–26.
70. Levesque E, Hoti E, Azoulay D, et al. The implementation of an intensive care information system allows shortening the ICU length of stay. J Clin Monit Comput 2015;29(2):263–9.
71. Wall RJ, Ely EW, Elasy TA, et al. Using real time process measurements to reduce catheter related bloodstream infections in the intensive care unit. Qual Saf Health Care 2005;14(4):295–302.
72. Qin Y, Zhou R, Wu Q, et al. The effect of nursing participation in the design of a critical care information system: a case study in a Chinese hospital. BMC Med Inform Decis Mak 2017;17(1):165.
73. Saleem JJ, Plew WR, Speir RC, et al. Understanding barriers and facilitators to the use of clinical information systems for intensive care units and anesthesia record keeping: a rapid ethnography. Int J Med Inform 2015;84(7):500–11.
74. Ward NS, Snyder JE, Ross S, et al. Comparison of a commercially available clinical information system with other methods of measuring critical care outcomes data. J Crit Care 2004;19(1):10–15.
75. Ward NS. The accuracy of clinical information systems. J Crit Care 2004;19(4):221–5.
76. Plumb JJ, Hains I, Parr MJ, et al. Technology meets tradition: the perceived impact of the introduction of information and communication technology on ward rounds in the intensive care unit. Int J Med Inform 2017;105:49–58.
77. Leslie M, Paradis E, Gropper MA, et al. An ethnographic study of health information technology use in three intensive care units. Health Serv Res 2017;52(4):1330–48.
78. van der Sijs H, Aarts J, Vulto A, et al. Overriding of drug safety alerts in computerized physician order entry. J Am Med Inform Assoc 2006;13(2):138–47.
79. Ancker JS, Edwards A, Nosal S, et al. Effects of workload, work complexity, and repeated alerts on alert fatigue in a clinical decision support system. BMC Med Inform Decis Mak 2017;17:36.
80. Despins LA. Factors influencing when intensive care unit nurses go to the bedside to investigate patient related alarms: a descriptive qualitative study. Intensive Crit Care Nurs 2017;43:101–7.
81. Page N, Baysari MT, Westbrook JI. A systematic review of the effectiveness of interruptive medication prescribing alerts in hospital CPOE systems to change prescriber behavior and improve patient safety. Int J Med Inform 2017;105:22–30.
82. Casey S, Avalos G, Downing M. Critical care nurses' knowledge of alarm fatigue and practices towards alarms: a multicenter study. Inten Crit Care Nurs 2018;https://doi.org/10.1016/j.iccn.2018.05.004. in press.
83. Colpaert K, Oeyen S, Sijnave B, et al. Influence of smart real-time electronic alerting on glucose control in critically ill patients. J Crit Care 2015;30(1):216.e1-6.
84. Henneman EA, Andrzejewski C Jr, Gawlinski A, et al. Transfusion-associated circulatory overload: evidence-based strategies to prevent, identify, and manage a serious adverse event. Crit Care Nurse 2017;37(5):58–65.
85. Maslove DM, Rizk N, Lowe HJ. Computerized physician order entry in the critical care environment: a review of current literature. J Intensive Care Med 2011;26(3):165–71.
86. Carayon P, Wetterneck TB, Cartmill R, et al. Medication safety in two intensive care units of a community teaching hospital after electronic health record implementation: sociotechnical and human factors engineering considerations. J Patient Saf 2017.
87. Prgomet M, Li L, Niazkhani Z, et al. Impact of commercial computerized provider order entry (CPOE) and clinical decision support systems (CDSSs) on medication errors, length of stay, and mortality in intensive care units: a systematic review and meta-analysis. J Am Med Inform Assoc 2017;24(2):413–22.
88. Curtis CE, Al Bahar F, Marriott JF. The effectiveness of computerised decision support on antibiotic use in hospitals: a systematic review. PLoS ONE 2017;12(8):e0183062.
89. Ranji SR, Rennke S, Wachter RM. Computerised provider order entry combined with clinical decision support systems to improve medication safety: a narrative review. BMJ Qual Saf 2014;23(9):773–80.
90. Holden RJ. Physicians' beliefs about using EMR and CPOE: in pursuit of a contextualized understanding of health IT use behavior. Int J Med Inform 2010;79(2):71–80.
91. von Dincklage F, Suchodolski K, Lichtner G, et al. Investigation of the usability of computerized critical care information systems in Germany. J Intensive Care Med 2017.

92. Kannry J, McCullagh L, Kushniruk A, et al. A framework for usable and effective clinical decision support: experience from the iCPR randomized clinical trial. EGEMS (Wash DC) 2015;3(2):1150.
93. Belard A, Buchman T, Forsberg J, et al. Precision diagnosis: a view of the clinical decision support systems (CDSS) landscape through the lens of critical care. J Clin Monit Comput 2017;31(2):261–71.
94. Brogi E, Cyr S, Kazan R, et al. Clinical performance and safety of closed-loop systems: a systematic review and meta-analysis of randomized controlled trials. Anesth Analg 2017;124(2):446–55.
95. Burns KE, Lellouche F, Nisenbaum R, et al. Automated weaning and SBT systems versus non-automated weaning strategies for weaning time in invasively ventilated critically ill adults. Cochrane Database Syst Rev 2014;(9):CD008638.
96. Mickan S, Atherton H, Roberts NW, et al. Use of handheld computers in clinical practice: a systematic review. BMC Med Inform Decis Mak 2014;14:56.
97. Mickan S, Tilson JK, Atherton H, et al. Evidence of effectiveness of health care professionals using handheld computers: a scoping review of systematic reviews. J Med Internet Res 2013;15(10):e212.
98. Rezende LC, Santos SR, Medeiros AL. Assessment of a prototype for the systemization of nursing care on a mobile device. Rev Lat Am Enfermagem 2016;24:e2714.
99. Shiber J, Thomas A, Northcutt A. Communicating while receiving mechanical ventilation: texting with a smartphone. Am J Crit Care 2016;25(2):e38–9.
100. Grundgeiger T, Albert M, Reinhardt D, et al. Real-time tablet-based resuscitation documentation by the team leader: evaluating documentation quality and clinical performance. Scand J Trauma Resusc Emerg Med 2016;24:51.
101. Ernecoff NC, Witteman HO, Chon K, et al. Key stakeholders' perceptions of the acceptability and usefulness of a tablet-based tool to improve communication and shared decision making in ICUs. J Crit Care 2016;33:19–25.
102. Yang F, Ji M, Ding S, et al. The development and evaluation of delirium assessment and nursing care decision-making assistant mobile application for intensive care unit. Stud Health Technol Inform 2016;225:668–72.
103. Loudet CI, Marchena MC, Maradeo MR, et al. Reducing pressure ulcers in patients with prolonged acute mechanical ventilation: a quasi-experimental study. Rev Bras Ter Intensiva 2017;29(1):39–46.
104. Mackay BJ, Anderson J, Harding T. Mobile technology in clinical teaching. Nurse Educ Pract 2017;22:1–6.
105. Raman J. Mobile technology in nursing education: where do we go from here? A review of the literature. Nurse Educ Today 2015;35(5):663–72.
106. Kotz D, Fu K, Rubin A. Security for mobile and cloud frontiers in healthcare. Commun ACM 2015;58(8):21–3.
107. Mackintosh N, Terblanche M, Maharaj R, et al. Telemedicine with clinical decision support for critical care: a systematic review. Syst Rev 2016;5(1):176.
108. Chen J, Sun D, Yang W, et al. Clinical and economic outcomes of telemedicine programs in the intensive care unit: a systematic review and meta-analysis. J Intensive Care Med 2017.
109. Khunlertkit A, Carayon P. Contributions of tele-intensive care unit (Tele-ICU) technology to quality of care and patient safety. J Crit Care 2013;28(3):315.e1-12.
110. Rincon TA, Manos EL, Pierce JD. Telehealth intensive care unit nurse surveillance of sepsis. Comput Inform Nurs 2017;35(9):459–64.
111. Goedken CC, Moeckli J, Cram PM, et al. Introduction of tele-ICU in rural hospitals: changing organisational culture to harness benefits. Intensive Crit Care Nurs 2017;40:51–6.
112. Hoonakker PLT, Pecanac KE, Brown RL, et al. Virtual collaboration, satisfaction, and trust between nurses in the tele-ICU and ICUs: results of a multilevel analysis. J Crit Care 2017;37:224–9.
113. Vaona A, Banzi R, Kwag KH, et al. E-learning for health professionals. Cochrane Database Syst Rev 2018;(1):CD011736.
114. Mistraletti G, Umbrello M, Anania S, et al. Neurological assessment with validated tools in general ICU: multicenter, randomized, before and after, pragmatic study to evaluate the effectiveness of an e-learning platform for continuous medical education. Minerva Anestesiol 2017;83(2):145–54.
115. Labeau SO, Rello J, Dimopoulos G, et al. The value of e-learning for the prevention of healthcare-associated infections. Infect Control Hosp Epidemiol 2016;37(9):1052–9.
116. Bredesen IM, Bjoro K, Gunningberg L, et al. Effect of e-learning program on risk assessment and pressure ulcer classification - a randomized study. Nurse Educ Today 2016;40:191–7.
117. Asiri H, Househ M. The impact of twitter and Facebook on nursing practice and education: a systematic review of the literature. Stud Health Technol Inform 2016;226:267–70.
118. Mitrasinovic S, Camacho E, Trivedi N, et al. Clinical and surgical applications of smart glasses. Technol Health Care 2015;23(4):381–401.
119. Romare C, Hass U, Skar L. Healthcare professionals' views of smart glasses in intensive care: a qualitative study. Intensive Crit Care Nurs 2017;45:66–71.
120. Moreno RP, Rhodes A, Donchin Y. Patient safety in intensive care medicine: the declaration of Vienna. Intensive Care Med 2009;35(10):1667–72.
121. World Health Organization. Patient safety: making health care safer. Geneva: World Health Organization; 2017.
122. Brunsveld-Reinders AH, Arbous MS, De Vos R, et al. Incident and error reporting systems in intensive care: a systematic review of the literature. Int J Qual Health Care 2016;28(1):2–13.

123. Bagian JP, Gosbee J, Lee CZ, et al. The veterans affairs root cause analysis system in action. Jt Comm J Qual Improv 2002;28(10):531–45.
124. Corwin GS, Shanawani H, Hemphill RR. Root cause analysis of ICU adverse events in the veterans health administration. Jt Comm J Qual Patient Saf 2017;43(11):580–90.
125. McDonough JE. Proactive hazard analysis and health care policy. New York: Milbank Memorial Fund; 2002.
126. Viejo MR, Sanchez-Izquierdo RJA, Molano AE, et al. Improvement of the safety of a clinical process using failure mode and effects analysis: prevention of venous thromboembolic disease in critical patients. Med Intensiva 2016;40(8):483–90.
127. Ohta Y, Sakuma M, Koike K, et al. Influence of adverse drug events on morbidity and mortality in intensive care units: the JADE study. Int J Qual Health Care 2014;26(6):573–8.
128. Valentin A, Capuzzo M, Guidet B, et al. Errors in administration of parenteral drugs in intensive care units: multinational prospective study. BMJ 2009;338:b814.
129. Latif A, Rawat N, Pustavoitau A, et al. National study on the distribution, causes, and consequences of voluntarily reported medication errors between the ICU and non-ICU settings. Crit Care Med 2013;41(2):389–98.
130. Moyen E, Camire E, Stelfox HT. Clinical review: medication errors in critical care. Crit Care 2008;12(2):208.
131. Carayon P, Wetterneck TB, Cartmill R, et al. Characterising the complexity of medication safety using a human factors approach: an observational study in two intensive care units. BMJ Qual Saf 2014;23(1):56–65.
132. Roughead EE, Semple SJ, Rosenfeld E. The extent of medication errors and adverse drug reactions throughout the patient journey in acute care in Australia. Int J Evid Based Healthc 2016;14(3):113–22.
133. Foster MJ, Gary JC, Sooryanarayana SM. Direct observation of medication errors in critical care setting: a systematic review. Crit Care Nurs Q 2018;41(1):76–92.
134. Westbrook JI, Woods A, Rob MI, et al. Association of interruptions with an increased risk and severity of medication administration errors. Arch Intern Med 2010;170(8):683–90.
135. Bower RA, Coad JE, Manning JC, et al. A qualitative, exploratory study of nurses' decision-making when interrupted during medication administration within the paediatric intensive care unit. Intensive Crit Care Nurs 2018;44:11–17.
136. Sorra JS, Nieva VF Hospital survey on patient safety culture. Rockville: Westat; 2004.
137. Davies HT, Nutley SM, Mannion R. Organisational culture and quality of health care. Qual Health Care 2000;9(2):111–19.
138. Dicuccio MH. The relationship between patient safety culture and patient outcomes: a systematic review. J Patient Saf 2015;11(3):135–42.
139. Vifladt A, Simonsen BO, Lydersen S, et al. The association between patient safety culture and burnout and sense of coherence: a cross-sectional study in restructured and not restructured intensive care units. Intensive Crit Care Nurs 2016;36:26–34.
140. Sexton JB, Helmreich RL, Neilands TB, et al. The safety attitudes questionnaire: psychometric properties, benchmarking data, and emerging research. BMC Health Serv Res 2006;6:44.
141. Huang DT, Clermont G, Sexton JB, et al. Perceptions of safety culture vary across the intensive care units of a single institution. Crit Care Med 2007;35(1):165–76.
142. Thomas EJ, Sexton JB, Helmreich RL. Discrepant attitudes about teamwork among critical care nurses and physicians. Crit Care Med 2003;31(3):956–9.
143. Chaboyer W, Chamberlain D, Hewson-Conroy K, et al. CNE article: safety culture in Australian intensive care units: establishing a baseline for quality improvement. Am J Crit Care 2013;22(2):93–102.
144. Hamdan M. Measuring safety culture in Palestinian neonatal intensive care units using the safety attitudes questionnaire. J Crit Care 2013;28(5):886.e7-14.
145. Steyrer J, Schiffinger M, Huber C, et al. Attitude is everything? The impact of workload, safety climate, and safety tools on medical errors: a study of intensive care units. Health Care Manage Rev 2013;38(4):306–16.
146. Santiago TH, Turrini RN. Organizational culture and climate for patient safety in intensive care units. Rev Esc Enferm USP 2015;49:123–30.
147. Clarke JR, Lerner JC, Marella W. The role for leaders of health care organizations in patient safety. Am J Med Qual 2007;22(5):311–18.
148. World Health Organization. Patient safety curriculum guide: multi-professional edition Geneva: WHO; 2011. Available from: https://www.who.int/patientsafety/education/mp_curriculum_guide/en/. [Accessed 19 February 2019].
149. Weaver SJ, Lubomksi LH, Wilson RF, et al. Promoting a culture of safety as a patient safety strategy: a systematic review. Ann Intern Med 2013;158(5):369–74.
150. Morello RT, Lowthian JA, Barker AL, et al. Strategies for improving patient safety culture in hospitals: a systematic review. BMJ Qual Saf 2013;22(1):11–18.
151. Hsu YJ, Marsteller JA. Influence of the comprehensive unit-based safety program in ICUs: evidence from the keystone ICU project. Am J Med Qual 2016;31(4):349–57.
152. Thornton KC, Schwarz JJ, Gross AK, et al. Preventing harm in the ICU-building a culture of safety and engaging patients and families. Crit Care Med 2017;45(9):1531–7.
153. Saladino L, Pickett LC, Frush K, et al. Evaluation of a nurse-led safety program in a critical care unit. J Nurs Care Qual 2013;28(2):139–46.
154. Winters BD, Weaver SJ, Pfoh ER, et al. Rapid-response systems as a patient safety strategy: a systematic review. Ann Intern Med 2013;158(5 Pt 2):417–25.
155. Maharaj R, Raffaele I, Wendon J. Rapid response systems: a systematic review and meta-analysis. Crit Care 2015;19:254.

156. Ludikhuize J, Brunsveld-Reinders AH, Dijkgraaf MG, et al. Outcomes associated with the nationwide introduction of rapid response systems in the Netherlands. Crit Care Med 2015;43(12):2544–51.
157. Chen J, Ou L, Flabouris A, et al. Impact of a standardized rapid response system on outcomes in a large healthcare jurisdiction. Resuscitation 2017;107:47–56.
158. Atkins JH, Rassekh CH, Chalian AA, et al. An airway rapid response system: implementation and utilization in a large academic trauma center. Jt Comm J Qual Patient Saf 2017;43(12):653–60.
159. Australian Commission on Safety and Quality in Health Care (ACSQHC). National consensus statement: essential elements for recognising and responding to clinical deterioration. Sydney: ACSQHC; 2010.
160. McGaughey J, O'Halloran P, Porter S, et al. Early warning systems and rapid response to the deteriorating patient in hospital: a systematic realist review. J Adv Nurs 2017;73(12):2877–91.
161. DeVita MA, Braithwaite RS, Mahidhara R, et al. Use of medical emergency team responses to reduce hospital cardiopulmonary arrests. Qual Saf Health Care 2004;13(4):251–4.
162. DeVita M, Hillman KM. Expanding the scope of the rapid response system. Jt Comm J Qual Patient Saf 2017;43(12):651–2.
163. Lee A, Bishop G, Hillman KM, et al. The medical emergency team. Anaesth Intensive Care 1995;23(2):183–6.
164. Gill FJ, Leslie GD, Marshall AP. The impact of implementation of family-initiated escalation of care for the deteriorating patient in hospital: a systematic review. Worldviews Evid Based Nurs 2016;13(4):303–13.
165. Morgan R, Lloyd-Williams F, Writght MM, et al. An early warning scoring system for detecting developing critical illness. Clin Intens Care 1997;8:100.
166. Le Lagadec MD, Dwyer T. Scoping review: the use of early warning systems for the identification of in-hospital patients at risk of deterioration. Aus Crit Care 2017;30(4):211–18.
167. Chua WL, See MTA, Legio-Quigley H, et al. Factors influencing the activation of the rapid response system for clinically deteriorating patients by frontline ward clinicians: a systematic review. Int J Qual Health Care 2017;29(8):981–98.
168. Rihari-Thomas J, DiGiacomo M, Phillips J, et al. Clinician perspectives of barriers to effective implementation of a rapid response system in an academic health centre: a focus group study. Int J Health Policy Manag 2017;6(8):447–56.
169. Eliott S, Chaboyer W, Ernest D, et al. A national survey of Australian intensive care unit (ICU) liaison nurse (LN) services. Aust Crit Care 2012;25(4):253–62.
170. Niven DJ, Bastos JF, Stelfox HT. Critical care transition programs and the risk of readmission or death after discharge from an ICU: a systematic review and meta-analysis. Crit Care Med 2014;42(1):179–87.
171. Topple M, Ryan B, Baldwin I, et al. Tasks completed by nursing members of a teaching hospital medical emergency team. Intensive Crit Care Nurs 2016;32:12–19.
172. Flin RH, O'Connor P, Crichton M. Safety at the sharp end: a guide to non-technical skills. Burlington: Ashgate Publishing; 2008.
173. Wright MC, Endsley MR. Building shared situation awareness in healthcare settings. In: Nemeth CP, editor. Improving healthcare team communication: building on lessons from aviation and aerospace. Burlington: Ashgate Publishing; 2008. p. 97–116.
174. Bucknall TK. Critical care nurses' decision-making activities in the natural clinical setting. J Clin Nurs 2000;9(1):25–35.
175. Endsley MR. Toward a theory of situation awareness in dynamic systems. Hum Factors 1995;37(1):32–64.
176. Stubbings L, Chaboyer W, McMurray A. Nurses' use of situation awareness in decision-making: an integrative review. J Adv Nurs 2012;68(7):1443–53.
177. Croskerry P, Singhal G, Mamede S. Cognitive debiasing 1: origins of bias and theory of debiasing. BMJ Qual Saf 2013;22(Suppl. 2):ii58–64.
178. Sendelbach S, Funk M. Alarm fatigue: a patient safety concern. AACN Adv Crit Care 2013;24(4):378–86, quiz 87-8.
179. Aitken LM. Critical care nurses' use of decision-making strategies. J Clin Nurs 2003;12(4):476–83.
180. Currey J, Botti M. The influence of patient complexity and nurses' experience on haemodynamic decision-making following cardiac surgery. Intensive Crit Care Nurs 2006;22(4):194–205.
181. Thompson C, Dalgleish L, Bucknall T, et al. The effects of time pressure and experience on nurses' risk assessment decisions: a signal detection analysis. Nurs Res 2008;57(5):302–11.
182. Saposnik G, Redelmeier D, Ruff CC, et al. Cognitive biases associated with medical decisions: a systematic review. BMC Med Inform Decis Mak 2016;16:138.
183. Hoffman KA, Aitken LM, Duffield C. A comparison of novice and expert nurses' cue collection during clinical decision-making: verbal protocol analysis. Int J Nurs Stud 2009;46(10):1335–44.
184. Hough MC. Learning, decisions and transformation in critical care nursing practice. Nurs Ethics 2008;15(3):322–31.
185. Karra V, Papathanassoglou ED, Lemonidou C, et al. Exploration and classification of intensive care nurses' clinical decisions: a Greek perspective. Nurs Crit Care 2014;19(2):87–97.
186. Narayan S, Corcoran-Perry S. Teaching clinical reasoning in nursing education. In: Higgs J, Jones MA, Loftus S, et al, editors. Clinical reasoning in the health professions. 3rd ed. Philadelphia: Butterworth-Heinemann; 2008. p. 405–30.
187. Rivett DA, Jones MA. Using case reports to teach clinical reasoning. In: Higgs J, Jones M, editors. Clinical reasoning in the health professions. Philadelphia: Butterworth-Heinemann; 2008. p. 477–84.

188. Thompson C, Stapley S. Do educational interventions improve nurses' clinical decision making and judgement? A systematic review. Int J Nurs Stud 2011;48(7):881–93.
189. Reason JT. Managing the risks of organizational accidents. Aldershot: Ashgate Publishing; 1997.
190. Orasanu J, Fischer U. Improving healthcare communication: lessons from the flightdeck. In: Nemeth CP, editor. Improving healthcare team communication: building on lessons from aviation and aerospace. Burlington: Ashgate Publishing; 2008. p. 23–46.
191. Australian Commission on Safety and Quality in Health Care (ACSQHC). OSSIE guide to clinical handover improvement. Sydney, NSW: ACSQHC; 2010.
192. Chaboyer W, McMurray A, Wallis M. Bedside nursing handover: a case study. Int J Nurs Pract 2010;16(1):27–34.
193. Halm MA. Nursing handoffs: ensuring safe passage for patients. Am J Crit Care 2013;22(2):158–62.
194. Spooner AJ, Chaboyer W, Corley A, et al. Understanding current intensive care unit nursing handover practices. Int J Nurs Pract 2013;19(2):214–20.
195. Ganz FD, Endacott R, Chaboyer W, et al. The quality of intensive care unit nurse handover related to end of life: a descriptive comparative international study. Int J Nurs Stud 2015;52(1):49–56.
196. Spooner AJ, Aitken LM, Corley A, et al. Developing a minimum dataset for nursing team leader handover in the intensive care unit: a focus group study. Aust Crit Care 2017;31(1):47–52.
197. Nanchal R, Aebly B, Graves G, et al. Controlled trial to improve resident sign-out in a medical intensive care unit. BMJ Qual Saf 2017;26(12):987–92.
198. Lane-Fall MB, Collard ML, Turnbull AE, et al. ICU attending handoff practices: results from a national survey of academic intensivists. Crit Care Med 2016;44(4):690–8.
199. Bunkenborg G, Bitsch Hansen T, Holge-Hazelton B. Handing over patients from the ICU to the general ward: a focused ethnographical study of nurses' communication practice. J Adv Nurs 2017;73(12):3090–101.
200. Graan SM, Botti M, Wood B, et al. Nursing handover from ICU to cardiac ward: standardised tools to reduce safety risks. Aust Crit Care 2016;29(3):165–71.
201. Caruso TJ, Marquez JLS, Gipp MS, et al. Standardized ICU to OR handoff increases communication without delaying surgery. Int J Health Care Qual Assur 2017;30(4):304–11.
202. Salzwedel C, Mai V, Punke MA, et al. The effect of a checklist on the quality of patient handover from the operating room to the intensive care unit: a randomized controlled trial. J Crit Care 2016;32:170–4.
203. Wibrandt I, Lippert A. Improving patient safety in handover from intensive care unit to general ward: a systematic review. J Patient Saf 2017.
204. Lane D, Ferri M, Lemaire J, et al. A systematic review of evidence-informed practices for patient care rounds in the ICU. Crit Care Med 2013;41(8):2015–29.
205. Brown R, Rasmussen R, Baldwin I, et al. Design and implementation of a virtual world training simulation of ICU first hour handover processes. Aust Crit Care 2012;25(3):178–87.
206. Brannick MT, Prince C. An overview of team performance measurement. In: Brannick MT, Salas E, Prince C, editors. Team performance assessment and measurement: theory, methods, and applications. Mahwah: Lawrence Erlbaum Associates; 1997. p. 3–16.
207. Dietz AS, Pronovost PJ, Mendez-Tellez PA, et al. A systematic review of teamwork in the intensive care unit: what do we know about teamwork, team tasks, and improvement strategies? J Crit Care 2014;29(6):908–14.
208. Alexanian JA, Kitto S, Rak KJ, et al. Beyond the team: understanding interprofessional work in two north American ICUs. Crit Care Med 2015;43(9):1880–6.
209. Bjurling-Sjoberg P, Wadensten B, Poder U, et al. Balancing intertwined responsibilities: a grounded theory study of teamwork in everyday intensive care unit practice. J Interprof Care 2017;31(2):233–44.
210. Donovan AL, Aldrich JM, Gross AK, et al. Interprofessional care and teamwork in the ICU. Crit Care Med 2018.
211. Gordon M, Darbyshire D, Baker P. Non-technical skills training to enhance patient safety: a systematic review. Med Educ 2012;46(11):1042–54.
212. Salas E, Rosen MA. Building high reliability teams: progress and some reflections on teamwork training. BMJ Qual Saf 2013;22(5):369–73.
213. Schmidt E, Goldhaber-Fiebert SN, Ho LA, et al. Simulation exercises as a patient safety strategy: a systematic review. Ann Intern Med 2013;158(5 Pt 2):426–32.
214. Kemper PF, de Bruijne M, van Dyck C, et al. Crew resource management training in the intensive care unit. A multisite controlled before-after study. BMJ Qual Saf 2016;25(8):577–87.
215. Ling L, Gomersall CD, Samy W, et al. The effect of a freely available flipped classroom course on health care worker patient safety culture: a prospective controlled study. J Med Internet Res 2016;18(7):e180.

Chapter 4

Ethical issues in critical care

Carol Grech, Maureen Coombs

Learning objectives

After reading this chapter, you should be able to:

- understand key ethical and legal principles in healthcare and how to apply them in everyday practice as a critical care nurse
- appreciate the complex ethical challenges inherent within today's critical care nursing practice
- identify and access additional resource material that may inform and support ethical professional conduct in critical care
- discuss ethical decision making involved when managing complex clinical situations such as may arise during admission and discharge, end-of-life care, working with families, and operating as a member of multidisciplinary clinical team
- describe the ethical conduct of human research in critical care, in particular issues of patient risk, protection and privacy, and how to apply ethical principles within research practice.

KEY WORDS

admission and discharge to critical care
autonomy
Clinical Ethics Committees
consent
end-of-life care
family-centred care
Human Research Ethics Committee
justice
multidisciplinary team working
patient rights
privacy
quality of life

Introduction

Nursing work, regardless of the context, will always involve an ethical dimension, and therefore nursing care should be guided by ethical principles. This has long been recognised with the International Council of Nurses (ICN) adopting a Code of Ethics for Nurses,[1] which, since its development in 1953, has undergone many iterations, in many languages. This code informs the ethical standards and guidelines developed by nursing authorities across the world. As a result, nurses are expected to provide compassionate and ethically coherent care, meet professional standards as stated by their regulatory authority and act in accordance with relevant codes of ethics at all times (see Box 4.1). In March 2018, the ICN *Code of ethics for nurses* was adopted by the Nursing and Midwifery Board of Australia (NMBA)[2] replacing the previous code that had been in effect since 2008.

Why is ethics so important? And why is ethics so important in critical care? Critical care nurses regularly encounter clinical situations that require them to employ ethical reasoning. However, the application of ethical reasoning to inform clinical decision making can be challenging and

BOX 4.1

Codes of ethics from selected countries

Australia: From 1 March 2018, the International Council of Nurses Code of ethics for nurses is in effect for all nurses in Australia, http://www.nursingmidwiferyboard.gov.au/Codes-Guidelines-Statements/Professional-standards.aspx

Nursing and Midwifery Board of Australia Code of Professional Conduct for Nurses (2018), http://www.nursingmidwiferyboard.gov.au/Codes-Guidelines-Statements/Professional-standards.aspx

Canada: Canadian Nurses Association – Code of Ethics for Registered Nurses (revised 2017), https://www.cna-aiic.ca/-/media/cna/page-content/pdf-en/code-of-ethics-2017-edition-secure-interactive.pdf

European Union: European Federation of Nursing Regulators – The Code of Ethics and Conduct for European Nursing (2007), http://journals.sagepub.com/doi/abs/10.1177/0969733008095390

Hong Kong: The Nursing Council of Hong Kong Code of Professional Conduct and Code of Ethics for Nurses in Hong Kong (2015), http://www.nchk.org.hk/en/code_of_conduct_and_practice/code_of_professional_conduct_and_code_of_ethics_for_nurses_in_hong_kong/index.html

India: Indian Nursing Council Code of Ethics & Professional Conduct, http://hmis.ap.nic.in/APNMC/pdfs/ethics.pdf

International Council of Nurses (ICN): Code of Ethics for Nurses (2012), http://www.icn.ch/who-we-are/code-of-ethics-for-nurses/

Ireland: Nursing and Midwifery Board of Ireland, Code of Professional Conduct and Ethics (2014), https://www.nmbi.ie/Standards-Guidance/Code.

Japan: Japanese Nursing Association Code of Ethics for Nurses (2003), https://www.nurse.or.jp/jna/english/activities/index.html

Malaysia: Nursing Board Malaysia Code of Professional Conduct for Nurses (1998), http://nursing.moh.gov.my/acts-guidelines/

New Zealand: Nursing Council of New Zealand Code of Conduct for Nurses (2012), http://www.nursingcouncil.org.nz/Nurses/Code-of-Conduct

UK: Nursing and Midwifery Council (NMC) The Code: Professional standards of practice and behaviour or nurses and midwives (2015), https://www.nmc.org.uk/standards/code./

USA: American Nurses Association Code of Ethics for Nurses with Interpretive Statements (2015), https://www.nursingworld.org/practice-policy/nursing-excellence/ethics/code-of-ethics-for-nurses/

demanding. Some of the routine challenges encountered in critical care include: developing clinical care plans for unconscious patients who lack capacity; working with family members who may be surrogate decision makers; managing conflict about the use or omission of life-sustaining technologies; and making decisions about equitable allocation of resources. Identifying the 'best' course of action in the face of opposing choices requires nurses to utilise rational and logical reasoning.

Working in contemporary healthcare, where health technology is constantly evolving and life expectancy increasing, requires increasingly complex decisions to be made about patient and health resource management. Difficult situations now arise where no consensus has been developed about ethical decision making or where all alternatives in a given situation have specific shortcomings. These types of situations are referred to as 'ethical dilemmas'. Ethical dilemmas are different from ethical problems in that no solutions have been identified.[3] It is in this world of ethical dilemmas that critical care nurses often find themselves.

This chapter therefore seeks to provide a resource to understand some of the current ethical issues across the continuum of critical care services. The chapter has three sections. The first section outlines the broad principles that underpin ethical decision making. The distinction between ethics, morality and values, and of key ethical concepts is explored. In linking ethics with the law, legal positions that inform healthcare are also described. The second section describes the application of ethical principles in critical care, with particular emphasis on decision-making processes that inform admission and discharge to critical care, and end-of-life care. The challenges of making decisions with others, and of developing resilience to maintain professional and ethical competence are also explored. The third and final section examines key ethical issues that arise from clinical research in the context of critical care.

Ethics and the law

When a dilemma evolves in critical care practice that calls into question how, as a health practitioner, one should or ought to respond to the issue, the need to consider the legal and ethical dimensions of the situation inevitably arises. Ethics and law are now fundamental components of nursing and medical education internationally. However, it is important to recognise that while ethical theories and principles have universal currency, laws and societal norms may differ between countries. While it is beyond the scope of this chapter to cover health laws pertaining to all countries and jurisdictions, increasingly the relationship between ethics and the law affecting health professionals in the workplace is shifting and adapting globally. This has been driven in part by: 1) the application of digital technologies in healthcare; and, 2) a series of widely published medical misadventures exposed by whistleblowers.

Digital technologies including the use of smart phones in the workplace, access to clinical diagnostic applications, computers at the bedside and electronic patient record systems have resulted in the need for government departments, hospitals and health professional regulation authorities to implement dedicated policies on the use of social media and access to patient e-records. Similarly, public expectations following the release of inquiries into systemic failures in some hospitals and health services identified the need to protect whistleblowers from bullying and reprisals through strengthening laws in this area.[4] Aligning with international best practice, Australia, for example, passed the *Public Interest Disclosure Act 2013*,[5] which has provided a comprehensive framework for protecting whistleblowers working in the public sector. This *statute* arose from the Parliamentary Standing Committee on Legal and Constitutional Affairs and during the Committee's Inquiry it was recognised that whistleblowers can play an important role in ensuring accountability and those making disclosures needed to be protected under the law from retribution.

Ethics, morality and values

Ethics in healthcare is concerned with clinical situations that invite reflection and raise questions about health professionals' inherent values informing decision making, as distinct from specific diagnostic or technical questions. Ethics involves the study of rational processes to inform a course of action in response to a particular situation where conflicting options exist.[6] Morality, however, can be understood as the norms widely shared by a community or among a professional group about what is 'right' or 'wrong' about human conduct, the widely held views then forming stable social consensus.[7] Values are the beliefs and attitudes that individuals hold about what is important and therefore influence individual actions and decision making.[8] It is important that critical care nurses remain attuned to, and reflect on, their personal and professional ethical, moral and value positioning to understand how they will approach ethical decision making in clinical practice.

Where personal ethics can be described as a personal set of moral values that an individual chooses to live by, professional ethics refer to agreed standards and behaviours expected of members of a particular professional group.[9] The value statements developed to underpin nursing and medical practice were originally informed by the moral traditions of Western civilisations with the resultant standards intended to guide and justify professional conduct. Interest in ethical practice in healthcare has now developed to such an extent that bioethics has emerged as a subject area concerned with moral issues raised by biological science developments and health service delivery.

Although this section has delineated the differences in definitions of ethics and morality, these concepts are sometimes used interchangeably when professional organisations articulate codes of professional conduct, for example in the *Code of professional conduct for nurses in Australia*.[10]

Ethical principles

Key ethical principles often used to explore healthcare ethics include autonomy, beneficence, non-maleficence, justice, veracity and fidelity.[7] While these are important in understanding the ethical dimensions of care, there are other ethical concepts important to understanding healthcare including integrity, best interests, informed consent and advance directives. All are applicable to critical care practice. These are explored individually in the following paragraphs or incorporated as part of the discussion of clinical issues, such as treatment withdrawal.

Autonomy

An autonomous person is an individual who is capable of deliberation, self-determination and action without the influence of external coercion. To respect autonomy is to give weight to, and respect, the autonomous person's considered opinions and choices and to not obstruct their actions unless these are detrimental to themselves or others. To show lack of respect for an autonomous agent or to withhold information necessary for that person to make a considered judgement when there are no reasons to do so, is to reject that person's judgement. To deny a competent individual their autonomy is to treat that person paternalistically. All individuals, including critical care patients, should be treated as autonomous agents and be able to self-determine, unless otherwise indicated. However, individuals with diminished autonomy, for example an unconscious person, are entitled to protection and, depending on the risk of harm and likely benefit of protecting them, paternalism may be considered justifiable.[7,11] In such cases, healthcare professionals should act to respect the autonomy of the individual as much as possible, for example by attempting to discover what the patient's preferences and decisions would have been in the circumstances.

Practice tip

A competent person has a right to make an informed choice about his or her treatment. When giving information about care options to a patient, keep the discussion accurate and factual. Do not direct or influence the patient's decision making. Respect the right of the person to make self-determining decisions.

Beneficence and non-maleficence

The principle of beneficence (i.e. to do good) requires that actions are undertaken to promote the wellbeing of another person. This incorporates the actions of doing no harm and maximising possible benefits while minimising possible harm (non-maleficence).[12] In healthcare practice, treatment is focused on 'doing no harm'. However, there may be times where, to 'maximise benefits' for health outcomes, it may be ethically justifiable to expose the patient to a 'higher risk of harm'. For example, consider a common clinical situation in the intensive care unit (ICU) where a patient requires a central venous catheter (CVC) to optimise fluid and drug therapy. This intervention is not without its own inherent risks (e.g. infection, pneumothorax on insertion). To minimise possible harm to the patient, evidence-based procedures are therefore developed to ensure safe insertion and subsequent care.

Justice

Justice may be defined as fair, equitable and appropriate treatment in light of what is due or owed to an individual. The fair, equitable and appropriate distribution of healthcare, as determined by justified rules or 'norms', is termed distributive justice.[7] There are well-regarded theories of justice in healthcare including egalitarian theories that propose people are provided with an equal distribution of particular goods or services. However, it is recognised that justice does not always require equal sharing of all possible social benefits. In situations where there are insufficient resources to be equally distributed, guidelines (e.g. ICU admission policies) may be developed in order to ensure treatment is as fair and equitable as possible.

Conditions of scarcity and competition for resources often lead to problems associated with fair and equitable allocation of resources (distributive justice). For example, a shortage of intensive care beds may result in critically ill patients having to 'compete' for access to the ICU. There is considerable debate about ICU admission criteria that varies across institutions, jurisdictional boundaries and countries with differing health funding structures. Such resource limitations can impact on distributive justice if decisions about access are influenced by economic factors as distinct from clinical need.[13]

Veracity and fidelity

The principle of veracity is concerned with telling the truth and is based on respect for persons and the concept of autonomy. To provide the opportunity for patients, or those authorised by law to act on their behalf, to make informed decisions about treatment options they must be provided with full and honest disclosure so that they can weigh up the risks and benefits of treatments.[6] It is also important to note that the principle of veracity can be violated through omission of important information – deliberately withholding information or using medical jargon or language that may camouflage or mislead the patient or their legal guardian. Critical care environments are highly complex, as are the technologies and procedures patients are exposed to. Patients and their families can easily feel overwhelmed by the critical care environment and by the choices that they may be faced with during critical illness.[14] Ensuring patients and families are informed and fully involved in the decision making is pivotal. Nurses and medical staff need to be vigilant in ensuring they convey information to patients and their families using language that can be readily understood and ensuring support services are drawn on (e.g. social workers, religious and spiritual advisers) to provide additional help to augment understanding so that patients or their legal guardian can make informed choices about care.

> **Practice tip**
>
> If you know a person's treatment is not working for them, you must help get their voice heard. This means having the courage to raise the matter with a more senior nurse or the doctor in a way that will be heard and considered in a timely way.

Fidelity refers to the concepts of keeping promises and honouring contracts and commitments[15] and is based upon the fundamental nursing virtue of caring with compassion and kindness. This principle encompasses qualities including loyalty, fairness, providing compassionate care to patients, advocacy and being responsible and accountable for the standard of nursing practice provided.

The principles of veracity and fidelity underpin the practice of every nurse. These values relate to professional ethics and the expectation that nurses are honest in all professional interactions, and demonstrate compliance with the professional codes of conduct, practice standards and regulatory reporting requirements.

> **Practice tip**
>
> Communicate with patients honestly and respectfully. If you tell a patient that you will be back in 10 minutes, mean it. However, if you know that you are busy and unlikely to meet that timeline, explain this to the patient instead of making false assurances.

Ethics and the law

Although distinct, ethics and the law overlap in many important ways. Moral rightness or wrongness may be quite distinct from legal rightness or wrongness and, while ethical decision making will always require consideration of the law, there may be conflict about the morality of the law. Ethically based nursing practice, such as confidentiality, respect for human rights, diversity and consent, are also legal requirements for health practice.[9,16]

The law enforces rules that are desirable for social good in every country. The terms 'legislation' and 'law' are used to refer generically to statutes, regulation and other legal instruments that may be the forms of law used in a particular country. A general distinction can be made between civil law jurisdictions (e.g. in France, Germany, Spain), which codify laws and in which the law is almost entirely based on legislative enactments and considered binding for all, and common law systems (e.g. in England, the USA, Australia and New Zealand (NZ)), where the law continually evolves in addition to being amended by laws passed by parliament.[6] In some countries, religion informs law, such as Sharia or Islamic law that specifically influences the legal code in some Muslim countries.

Laws related to healthcare are often created on the basis of what is considered morally right and of benefit to members of society. Statute law, i.e. written law set down by a legislature (e.g. parliament), has particular relevance to ethics in the critical care context. An example of how a statute law in one jurisdiction might be applied in practice pertaining to, for example, consent for life-sustaining measures is the *Consent to Medical Treatment and Palliative Care Act 1995* (SA).[17] This Act at s17 (2) states that: 'in the absence of an express direction by the patient or the patient's representative to the contrary, [the doctor is] under no duty to use, or to continue to use, life sustaining measures'.[17]

In some countries such as Australia, each state and territory has many different Acts pertaining to healthcare practices, and this can be confusing when practitioners work across jurisdictional borders. This is less problematic in countries such as NZ where health Acts are applicable across the whole country. Therefore, when sourcing laws relevant to healthcare in specific countries, it is important to use validated sources such as government websites.

Privacy and confidentiality

Although not an ethical principle as such, privacy and confidentiality are fundamental human entitlements recognised in all major international treaties and agreements on human rights. Nearly every country in the world acknowledges privacy as a fundamental human right in their constitution, either explicitly or implicitly. The right to privacy has been involved in new areas of debate given technology's increasing erosion of privacy, for example via video surveillance cameras, the internet and harvesting and sharing of data captured from social media sites. There is a growing trend towards comprehensive privacy and data protection legislation around the world. Many countries are adopting such laws to ensure compatibility with international standards developed by the European Union, the Council of Europe and the Organization for Economic Cooperation and Development. In NZ, privacy legislation is described in the *Privacy Act 1993*[18] and in Australia in the *Commonwealth Privacy Act 1988*.[19] In addition, each state and territory in Australia has additional jurisdictional regulatory guidelines that apply to privacy matters and disclosure of health information.[20]

Practice tip

Details about a patient's personal circumstance, condition and medical treatment must always be kept private and confidential. Do not discuss patients in inappropriate environments (e.g. in corridors and elevators where others could overhear). Do not take handover sheets or papers that have recorded patient details outside the unit where unauthorised personnel or members of the public could find them. When using electronic records systems, ensure you log in and out appropriately and don't leave the computer unattended when patient records are visible. Never discuss patients, colleagues or work-related matters on social media.

Patients' rights

Patients' rights arise from human rights law that universally recognises that everyone is born free and with equal rights irrespective of nationality, place of residence, gender, ethnic origin, race or religion.[21] Statements with a focus on patients' rights relate to the particular moral interests that a person might have in a healthcare context and any particular protection required when a person assumes the role of a patient.[9] Institutional-based charters (position statements), such as those in hospitals, are helpful in developing a shared understanding among patients/consumers, families and carers of the rights of people receiving healthcare and of the entitlements and special interests to be respected. Such charters also emphasise to health professionals that relationships with patients are constrained ethically and bound by certain associated duties.[9] The World Federation of Critical Care Nurses has recognised the importance of this and developed a position statement on the rights of the critically ill patient (see the World Federation of Critical Care Nurses website, http://wfccn.org).

To further protect patients' rights, attention should be paid to cultural differences in the provision of healthcare and to ensure cultural safety of both patients and the healthcare team. Clinical situations are culturally safe when patients and their families feel that cultural and spiritual needs are acknowledged and that those needs are met without prejudice.[22,23] In Australia, the impact of colonisation on the cultural, social and spiritual lives of Aboriginal and Torres Strait Islander peoples has contributed to significant health inequities in this population. Therefore, cultural safety has been enshrined in the *Registered nurse standards for practice*[24] and other key documents relevant to healthcare delivery.[25,26] Professional codes of conduct also incorporate an understanding of patients' rights and acknowledge that nurses accept the rights of individuals to make informed choices about their treatment and care. Box 4.2 provides some useful

BOX 4.2

Needs of diverse population groups in critical care

To cater for the needs of diverse population groups in critical care it is important to:

- organise and use qualified interpreters and cultural advisers when required
- create care environments that facilitate optimal patient and family control of decisions
- work collaboratively with other healthcare workers in a culturally sensitive and competent manner to ensure optimal outcomes
- identify and address bias, prejudice and discrimination in healthcare service delivery
- integrate measures of patient satisfaction into improvement programs

tips to ensure that the needs of diverse populations in critical care may be met.

Consent

Any procedure that involves intentional contact by a healthcare practitioner with the body of a patient is considered an invasion of the patient's bodily integrity and requires patient consent. A healthcare practitioner must not assume that a patient provides a valid consent purely on the basis that the individual has been admitted to a hospital.[24] All health professionals are expected to give information on management, care and alternative options to the patient to enable informed consent and decision making to occur.[25,26] The responsibility for obtaining consent for medical procedures generally rests with the medical practitioner and may not be delegated to a nurse. However, as advanced practice nurse roles develop in specialties like critical care, delegated consent for some procedures are being explored through position statements.[27]

Patients have the right, as autonomous individuals, to discuss any concerns or raise questions at any time with staff. Hospitals should provide detailed patient admission information, including information regarding 'patients' rights and responsibilities' and a broad explanation of the consent process within that institution. In many countries there is no distinction between the obligation to obtain valid consent from the patient and the overall duty of care that a practitioner has in providing treatment to a patient. Obtaining consent is part of the overall duty of care.[17]

In order to provide safe care where patients are able to make choices with informed consent, clear systems and processes are required. Critical care nurses need to be aware of relevant professional, organisational and unit-based policies and understand their individual obligations and responsibilities in this area. While the treating medical officer is most often legally regarded as the person who informs the patient about associated risks,[28] it is incumbent on all critical care nurses to be aware of the potential risks in critical care and ensure that informed consent is gained and when necessary advocate for the patient and family. Due to the nature of critical illness, direct informed consent is often difficult in critical care and surrogate consent may be the only option in emergency situations. Consent issues in critical care may be concerned with health treatment or, as discussed later, participation in human research and the use and disclosure of personal health information.[29]

Practice tip

Make sure that informed consent is consistently applied in every healthcare encounter. As such, consent is required for turning a patient and making them comfortable, for making sure that the patient understands the procedure that they are undergoing or that they understand what is involved in the research study that they have recently enrolled in. If a patient does not understand, stop and ensure appropriate information is given by the person whose responsibility it is before continuing your intervention further.

Consent to treatment

A competent individual has the right to decline or accept healthcare treatment. This right is enshrined in common law in Australia (with some variation across state or territory jurisdictions) and in the *Code of Health and Disability Consumers' Rights in New Zealand (1996)*.[30] With the introduction of human rights Acts (for example in the UK)[31] there is global awareness of the individual rights of patients in healthcare and of patients being actively encouraged to participate in treatment decisions.

Informed consent provides assurance that patients and others are neither deceived nor coerced in decision making; this recognises the person's autonomy. Consent procedures should minimise the potential for deception and coercion and should be designed to give patients control over the amount of information received and the opportunity to rescind consent already given.[32] However, clinical information can be complex and confusing for patients and obtaining informed consent can be problematic. Improved communication skills for doctors and nurses go some way toward resolving this problem. Shared decision making in clinical care can best be achieved by framing the relevant information in a comprehensible way to the patient, while understanding that some patients may not wish to make such choices themselves, preferring to have decisions made by clinicians.[33] Box 4.3 lists key criteria that describe valid consent.

Patients must have the mental capacity and be competent in order to give informed consent in healthcare decisions. To be competent, an individual must be able

BOX 4.3

Criteria for consent

Consent is considered VALID if:

- informed (the patient must understand the broad nature and effects of the proposed intervention and the material risks it entails)
- voluntarily given
- it encompasses the act to be performed
- given by a person legally competent to do so

to comprehend and retain information, must not be impervious to reason or incapable of judgement after reflection and must be able to weigh that information up (i.e. consider the effects of having or not having the treatment). Many jurisdictions around the world have legislation that addresses situations where adults lack the capacity to give consent. In emergencies, health-care treatment may be provided without the consent of a person. However, consent should be obtained for all procedures that involve 'doing' to a patient (e.g. administering an injection). Consent should never be implied irrespective of the situation of the person or the place of care, e.g. critically ill in ICU.[34] In many countries, if patients perceive that informed consent was not obtained, a civil court case can be actioned on the grounds of battery (deliberate touching without their consent) or negligence (receiving insufficient information about risk). Doctors and nurses therefore need to make clear what they are proposing to do to a patient and why they need to do it, with a 'reasonable' amount of information about any risks involved.[35]

If a person is assessed as not having capacity, consent must be sought from someone who has lawful authority to consent on his or her behalf. If the courts have appointed a person to be guardian for an individual, then the guardian can provide consent on behalf of that individual. However, even for legally appointed guardians, consent cannot be given for certain procedures and the consent of a guardianship statutory authority may be required. Some states have legislated to allow this authority to be delegated to a 'person responsible' or 'statutory health authority' without prior formal appointment. This person would usually be a spouse, next of kin or unpaid carer of the individual. As with formally appointed guardians, the powers of a 'person responsible' are limited by statute.[29]

Disclosure

It is important for all health professionals to recognise their obligations for disclosing information that may put the public at risk. This may include physical illnesses, mental health or addiction conditions that call into question a practitioner's fitness to practice to perform safely and effectively. Codes of conduct like those in the UK for nurses and midwives[36] identify what good nursing (and midwifery) practice looks like and clearly outline the obligation for disclosure of self and others when patient safety is at risk. In Australia and NZ this is outlined within legislation[37,38] governing health practitioners.

Nurses working in critical care may undertake exposure-prone procedure; however, the risk for transmission of blood-borne viruses (BBVs) should be low if correct infection control protocols are followed (see Chapter 5). Nonetheless, there are mutual obligations by health practitioners and patients concerning the risk of BBV transmission during treatment and therefore reasonable disclosure policies must be in place to protect health workers and the public.[39] It is also the responsibility of employers and health workers to operate in a way that minimises the risk of occupational exposure to BBVs and ensure that the use of the information must comply with relevant anti-discrimination, privacy, industrial relations and equal employment opportunity legislation.

Application of ethical principles to the care of the critically ill

Any health professional working with critically ill patients knows that the number and complexity of decisions made about clinical interventions are ever increasing. Given this, it is important that questions raised about medical and nursing care should be underpinned by consideration of the ethical dimensions involved.[40]

With the expanding number of technological developments, critical care nursing has evolved in scope and practice. Critical care nurses are more autonomous in their role, using more developed assessment and diagnostic skills, and managing more advanced patient interventions. With such increased autonomy comes increased responsibility;[41] this re-enforces the need for greater ethical awareness in practice. As demonstrated in findings from a Portuguese study,[42] ethical issues now pervade many aspects of day-to-day nursing care from admission to critical care (equality, distributive justice) through to end-of-life decision making (respecting autonomy). Faced with operating in such a difficult environment, nurses in clinical practice can feel vulnerable managing their ethical responsibilities.[43] This is an important issue to recognise as the ongoing challenge of navigating practice while upholding professional values, responsibilities and duties can lead to nurses experiencing moral distress. This can result in increased levels of emotional distress, withdrawal from patient care, decreased job satisfaction and, ultimately, increased attrition in nursing.[44] This section explores some of the key ethical challenges current in critical care practice, namely: admission and discharge decisions in critical care; end-of-life decision making; making decisions with others; and developing resilience to maintain professional and ethical competence.

Admission and discharge decisions in critical care

Critical care is an expensive healthcare resource.[45] Given the changing population health needs, the increased profile of chronic health illnesses, and greater use of technological diagnostics and intervention, it is not unreasonable to expect greater demand on use of critical care services. It is therefore likely that clear decision-making processes about use of critical care facilities, that is, who will be admitted into, and who will be discharged from, critical care will become even more important in the future.[46] Chapter 2 (Systems and resources) provides a description of the ethical allocation and utilisation of critical care resources, but when faced with excessive demand on critical care beds, patients who would benefit most from critical care are generally admitted. Indeed, this is the model most frequently cited during discussions on meeting unprecedented need, as in recent H1N1 influenza pandemics.[47]

Another area prompting debate regarding critical care admission concerns the age of the referred patient. Admitting very premature babies into neonatal care,[48] or very elderly patients[49] into critical care, has always been challenging, raising ethical issues related to the value or quality of life, and care that is in the patient's best interest. There are many examples of neonatal unit admission policies, electronically available, that state prematurity and weight of the neonate as key considerations for referral to a neonatal unit. There is also evidence that a decision to admit an elderly patient to critical care should be based on factors such as patient comorbidities, severity of illness and pre-hospital functional status, rather than chronological age.[50] However, decision making about admission to critical care should be based on more than physiological variables. We would suggest that a combination of a clear understanding of the ethical challenges raised, comprehension of the current evidence on patient management and outcomes, and an awareness of what the patient/family wishes are will enable full appreciation of the context and consequences for each case.

Less attention has been focused on discharge of patients from critical care to other units, or to ward areas. The subject of which patient to discharge is usually raised when critical care areas are at full bed capacity with referrals for admission being made. To date, literature in this area mainly focuses on family needs/experiences during discharge or tools to facilitate decision making,[51] with little exploration of the ethical challenges that discharge from critical care can invoke. However, there is an ethical challenge for patients and staff in the premature or sub-optimal discharge from intensive care.[52] Misunderstandings and irritation can occur between intensive care and general ward during discussions about transferring patients out of intensive care. Ward staff perceive that intensive care staff overestimate technical capabilities of ward staff, as well as the amount of time ward staff can give each patient. Clinical areas can operate independently and use 'lifeboat' ethics,[53] a metaphor for resource distribution, to prioritise care. Staff across clinical areas need to come together to understand how they can make decisions interdependently with each other, cognisant of the full pressures experienced in the system.

Admission to critical care will continue to challenge healthcare and using best clinical and ethical evidence to inform development of policies, and guide decision making is important.[50] Finally, it must be recognised that much of our understanding about critical care has historically been informed by the Western world and by developed countries. Globally, not all countries have the same level of critical care provision, and this brings its own unique ethical and resource challenges with regards to admission and discharge in ways that some of us may find difficult to comprehend.[54]

End-of-life decision making

With advances in healthcare, it is now possible to restore, sustain and prolong life with use of technology, for example extracorporeal oxygenation and ventricular assist devices. Each new medication or treatment on the market seems to promise added benefits to patients with improved outcomes and fewer side effects. However, critical care still remains more concerned with provision of supportive therapies until recovery occurs (or does not occur), rather than offering curative treatments.[55]

While this leads to many patients surviving their critical illness, it also results in some patients receiving life-sustaining therapies for prolonged periods with limited evidence about survival rates or impact on long-term quality of life. Therefore, a common ethical dilemma experienced by doctors and nurses in critical care concerns how to work through the opposing decision-making positions of 'maintaining life at all costs' and 'relieving suffering associated with the prolongation of life'. These are complex, emotive and much debated areas that often surface during decision making about withdrawal and withholding of life supporting treatment.[56]

While the following section explore these through the lens of intensive care, similar end-of-life challenges occur in emergency departments,[57] high dependency units, and on ward areas where critically ill patients may deteriorate, requiring support from critical care practitioners.[58] Whilst the contexts are different, the ethical principles and key decision-making approaches apply across all environments.

Withdrawing and withholding treatment

The incidence of withholding and withdrawal of life support from critically ill patients has increased to the extent that these practices now precede most deaths in intensive care[59] with evidence that the majority of clinicians in the USA[60-63] and Europe[64,65] have been involved in the withholding or withdrawal of treatments for critically ill patients. Across such practices, we can see that while there is a legal and moral presumption in favour of preserving life, avoiding death should not always be the pre-eminent goal.[66]

Withholding or withdrawal of life-sustaining therapies such as ventilator support, inotropic support, or antibiotics occurs in the knowledge that the patient will most probably die from their underlying disease.[67] This is considered ethically acceptable and clinically desirable if it reduces unnecessary patient suffering in those whose prognosis is considered hopeless (i.e. 'futile'). While there is some acceptance of the concepts of withdrawing and withholding of treatment, there is less agreement as to how such practices can be operationalised in critical care. Country-specific strategies have been used to address this, for example, Australia's consensus statement on agreed practice for recognising and responding to people in need of end-of-life care in acute hospitals.[68] Similarly, in the UK, care pathways have been used with some success,[69] although now personalised plans of care are more favoured.[70]

However, there are marked differences in the foregoing of life-sustaining treatments between countries, and even within states. What may be adopted legally and ethically in one country may not be acceptable in another. For example, a recent publication highlights current challenges experienced by clinicians in Japan where, despite clear support from end-of-life guidelines, the practice of treatment withdrawal is limited.[71] Further, complexities in care arise due to the differing views held internationally on whether withdrawal of treatment and withholding of treatment are ethically the same.[72] In Australasia, whether active treatment is withdrawn or withheld, the same legal and ethical principles apply. The Australian and New Zealand Intensive Care Society (ANZICS) and College of Intensive Care Medicine of Australia and New Zealand (CICM) recommend that, when treatment withdrawal or withholding has been discussed and agreed with the family, an 'alternative care plan' with a focus on dignity and patient comfort be implemented. It is suggested that such discussions are recorded in the patient notes including the basis for the decision, those involved in the discussions and the specifics of treatment(s) being withheld or withdrawn.[73]

Although doctors and nurses appear clear in their support for treatment withdrawal in cases of futility, the public at large hold different perceptions about this aspect of care. This is demonstrated in results from the Ethicatt study[74] where an end-of-life decision-making questionnaire was administered to doctors, nurses, patients and family members across ICUs in six European countries. Less than 10% of doctors and nurses wanted their life prolonged by all available means, compared with 40% of patients and 32% of families. When asked where they would prefer to be cared for if they had a terminal illness with a short time to live, more doctors and nurses preferred care at home or in a hospice and more patients and families preferred care in intensive care. Differences in responses were based on the respondent's country.[74] A similar spread of views across healthcare staff and the general public was demonstrated when consulted about physician-assisted suicide in the USA.[75] It is therefore interesting that North American observational studies demonstrate healthcare staff consult families more often than European healthcare staff[74,76] with some seriously ill patients indicating a willingness to participate in end-of-life decisions, while others did not.[77]

It is clear that having in-depth knowledge of the critical care environment and of clinical treatments influences clinicians' views on the practice of treatment withdrawal or limitation. Cultural, religious, philosophical and professional attitudes also influence views held in this area. In a UK study[78] reviewing the use of treatment withdrawal guidelines, staff reported concern over the legal, moral, ethical and professional accountability issues involved in this area. The study demonstrated that medical decisions to withdraw treatment were inconsistent within medical teams and in similar patients. With such a range of factors influencing decision making about withdrawal and withholding of treatment, it is not surprising that gaining consensus on complex clinical situations, such as withdrawal of treatment, can be difficult. In cases where there is uncertainty about the efficacy or appropriateness of a life-sustaining treatment, it may be considered preferable to commence treatment, with an option to withdraw treatment after broad consultation has occurred. However, managing such situations can be challenging as conflicts can occur about when and how to withdraw life-sustaining treatment;[13] this is an area that critical care nurses can actively contribute to in supporting the processes of decision making at end of life.[65]

Although it is essential that all members of the critical care team contribute to such discussions, legal responsibility and accountability for the decision lies with the senior treating doctor. Where conflict arises with family members, especially if a family member has medical power of attorney (or equivalent), the doctor must take this into consideration and respect the rights of any patient legal representative. It is unlikely that withdrawal of treatment will occur until a consensus decision is reached. This is a different situation to that of a person who is legally declared brain dead[73] where different ethical challenges are posed[79] (see Chapter 29).

Once a decision to limit or withdraw treatment has been agreed, a plan is made as to how this will occur, which treatments will be withdrawn/withheld, when and by whom. It is at this stage that critical care nurses play an important role in managing end-of-life care.[80] Concepts of caring for the dying patient in a critical care unit are no different to those in a hospital ward or hospice. The principles of care encompass privacy, dignity, relief of pain, provision of comfort and support for patient and relatives. Recognising and being respectful of the religious, spiritual and cultural needs of the patient and family are also important. Care given at this time continues beyond the moment of the patient's death with particular attention placed on how the death of the person is pronounced, how the family is notified of this death and the immediate bereavement support offered to the family, including discussions about possible autopsy. Compassionate care to the family at this time is essential.

Decision-making principles

Despite significant advances in critical care medicine, approximately 20% of patients admitted to ICUs do not survive.[81] The majority of patients who die in critical care do so after planned withdrawal of life-prolonging therapies, as opposed to dying after unexpected and unsuccessful cardiopulmonary resuscitation.[82] Given the complex nature of the decisions made at end of life, it is unsurprising that key ethical challenges arise. These mainly focus on arguments about quality of life, best interest, and whether treatment is futile.

Although debate about quality of life is often engaged with when justifying the continuation or discontinuation of life-sustaining treatment in critical care,[9] there is no single agreed definition of quality of life. When making decisions about medical treatments based on quality of life arguments, it is important therefore that consideration is given to the personal preferences and wellbeing of the individual together with review of the person's independent health and welfare status.[13]

Best interest is a further guiding principle for making decisions in, and about, healthcare. It is defined as acting in a way that optimally promotes good for the individual and is referred to when one person makes a decision on behalf of another, as when a doctor makes a decision to cease life-sustaining treatment for a particular patient. The best interest principle is often invoked in situations where the patient may be assessed as unable to participate in the decision-making process. The best interest principle relies on decision makers holding an understanding of, and knowing the views held by, the person in question (e.g. critically ill patient). The best interest principle poses particular challenges including how assumptions are made about what quality of life means for individuals, and whether those views are current i.e. have been recently communicated to a significant other, and therefore not been changed over time.[83]

The third ethical position often explored at end of life is whether ongoing medical treatment is futile. In other words, whether the treatment has no apparent physical benefit to the patient (physiological futility) or where the benefit of recovery of the patient is outweighed by the burden of survival, that is the person survives but with potential of physical or mental incapacity.[7] Treatment is considered futile if the medical therapy will never enable the person to achieve a state beyond permanent unconsciousness or that it is unlikely that the person will ever be discharged alive from intensive care.[84] This acknowledges that physiological decay of the body due to old age and/or illness will exceed the body's response to medical treatments.[85] Futility is a concept in widespread use in healthcare ethics and poses clinical challenges and international debate.[86] Futility is often used by critical care doctors and nurses as a rationale for why lifesaving or life-sustaining medical treatments are considered not in the patient's best interest. While this is logical, the concept of futility should not be used unethically, for example to coerce relatives into agreeing to cease treatment in a patient.[87]

Clinicians usually reflect on past clinical experiences, experiential knowledge gained from colleagues, and reported empirical data to conclude that treatments are futile.[88] Although there is no international definition of futility, some country-specific and profession-specific guidance exist to inform care.[17] Futile interventions are seen to cause pain and discomfort at end of life, give false hope to patients and family, delay palliative care and expend limited medical resources. While the ethical requirement to respect patient autonomy entitles a patient to choose or reject the medically acceptable treatment options, it does not entitle patients to receive whatever treatments they want, including futile treatments. Clinicians are only required to offer treatments consistent with professional standards and that give benefit to the patient. With respect to the law governing withholding and withdrawing treatment, there have been few cases internationally where courts have been consistent in concluding that there is no duty to provide life-sustaining treatment that is futile.[89] Fig. 4.1 outlines factors influencing ethical decision-making processes in healthcare delivery.

Understanding patient preferences at end of life: advance directives

Advance directives can be completed for individuals wanting to document future healthcare preferences for when they are no longer able to make decisions for themselves. With the increasing availability of medical technology, use of advance directives has improved.[90,91] An advance directive, also known as a living will, a personal directive or an advance care directive, sets out instructions by a competent individual specifying what actions should be taken for their health in the event that they are no longer able to make decisions due to illness or incapacity. The five wishes advance directive created by 'Ageing with Dignity', a non-profit organisation in the USA, is one example of an advance directive.[92] There are also national frameworks for advanced care directives[93] and specialty specific exemplars, e.g. the Western Australian Cancer and Palliative Care Network Advance Health Directive.[94] Some people are hesitant to document their end-of-life care plan so there is legal provision for the appointment of a person holding enduring power of attorney for matters of health[76] (see below). When it comes to addressing end-of-life care in the paediatric ICU (PICU) or the neonatal ICU

FIGURE 4.1 Factors influencing decision-making processes in healthcare ethics.

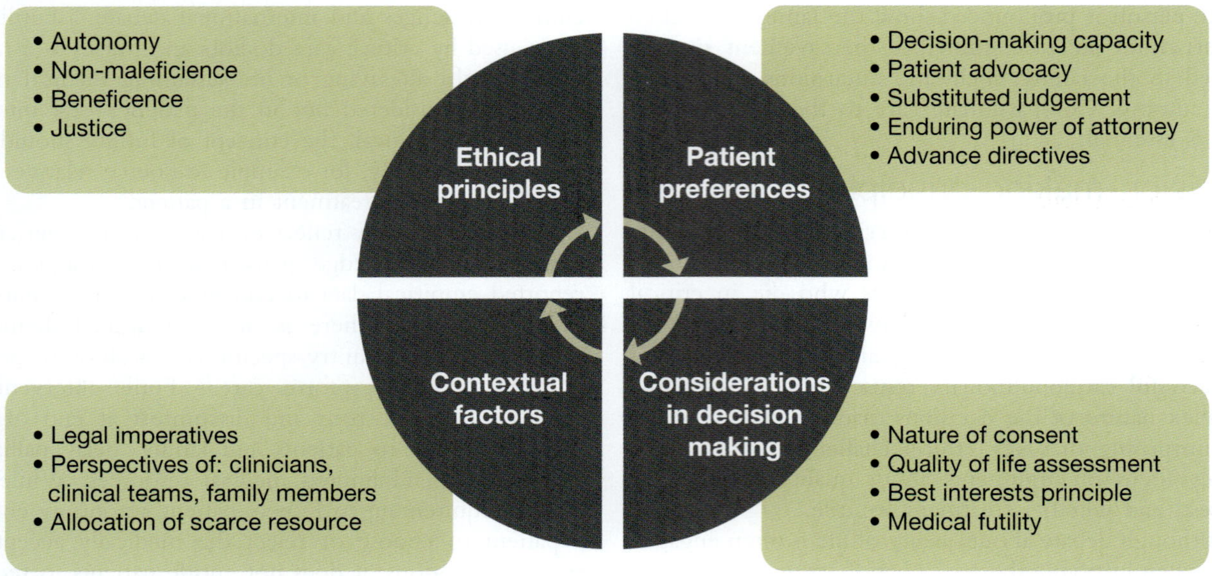

Source: Adapted from Rischbieth & Benbenishty, ACCCN's Critical Care Nursing 2nd ed., Elsevier, 2012.

(NICU) there are a number of ethical complexities that are outside the scope of this chapter to address comprehensively. An increasing number of resources, however, are available to nurses working in PICU and NICU to support their understanding of best practice end-of-life care in these settings.[95,96]

Regarding preference for treatment, cardiopulmonary resuscitation (CPR) remains the only intervention that patients explicitly state that they do, or do not want.[97] If patients have acute, reversible illness conditions, they should have the right to CPR. However, discussions may occur regarding the withholding of CPR in patients with irreversible or terminal illnesses. This is an important point to consider as every patient will have CPR, unless documented otherwise. The decision to withhold CPR may be termed a 'do not resuscitate' (DNR), 'do not attempt resuscitation' (DNAR) or 'not for resuscitation' (NFR) order. While such 'orders' reflect a decision against any resuscitation treatment, there are other types of resuscitation orders seen written in patient notes that use limited treatment, including 'for defibrillation only' or 'for one round of advanced life support only'. These can be confusing for staff and families who may perceive such orders to be half-hearted attempts at resuscitation or, indeed, that no care is meant to be given.[97] As each patient case is considered on its own merit, it is important that any medical orders or directives are well-documented in the patient's notes or on the appropriate forms so that misinterpretations do not occur. It is important that clear discussion and broad consultation across the clinical team(s) and patient/family occurs. A management plan that incorporates assessment of patient and family understanding, disclosure of the patient's situation, and discussion and consensus gaining with the patient and family can be particularly useful.[98]

Understanding patient preferences: surrogate decision makers and patient advocates

Patient advocacy has, at its heart, a focus on patient rights, values and interests. It seeks to promote autonomy when patients are unable or incapable of participating in making decisions about their healthcare. If a person does not have the mental capacity to make medical decisions, a surrogate decision maker should be identified. Substituted judgement is where an appropriate surrogate attempts to determine what the patient would have wanted in his/her present circumstances[84] by utilising the values and preferences of the patient. Making a substituted judgement is a relatively informal process, in the sense that the patient has not formally appointed the proxy decision maker. Rather, the role of proxy tends to be assumed on the basis of an existing relationship between the proxy and the patient, for example, next of kin or family member. However, this informal arrangement means that making an accurate substituted judgement can be difficult[99] and that the proxy might not be the most appropriate person for this role.

There are more formally recognised patient advocate roles and internationally 'medical or healthcare agent', 'medical power of attorney' and 'enduring guardian' are terms and roles related to this concept of patient advocacy. A patient advocate for healthcare is usually someone chosen by an individual (e.g. a partner, child, good friend over 18 years of age) to make medical decisions on their behalf should a situation arise where they lack decisional capacity. Most patient advocates are known to, and appointed by the person, or are representatives of recognised bodies to safeguard vulnerable persons (e.g. guardianship boards, Office of the Public Advocate). Each country has legislation in place to protect the patient, patient advocate and healthcare team and therefore legal consultation should occur to fully understand the conditions and safeguards in place.

Euthanasia and physician-assisted suicide in critical care

Euthanasia is a subject currently undergoing much international debate. Euthanasia is generally understood as the termination of a person's life in order to relieve suffering. It is carried out because it is requested by the person. Although the concept of euthanasia is supported in some places, it remains illegal across most of the world. With confusion occurring about the difference between treatment withdrawal and euthanasia, the primary distinction between the two acts relates to the issue of 'intent'.[100] If the primary intention of the intervention (e.g. a lethal injection) is to cause death, this is regarded as euthanasia. If the primary intention of the intervention is to reduce pain and suffering, this may not be regarded as euthanasia but this may still be tested legally in a court of law. It is this complexity that causes the vigorous 'for' and 'against' debates about euthanasia. Those opposing euthanasia do so in the belief of the sanctity of life, that life is God-given, and that effective symptom control should be able to keep individuals comfortable. Other opponents raise the concern that, if euthanasia were made legal, the laws regulating it could be abused and this would lead to euthanasia being used with people not expressing a wish to die. Those in support of euthanasia argue that a civilised society should support a person's autonomy and self-determinism and that people should die in dignity and without pain. If people are not able to terminate their own life, others should be allowed to help them to do so.

Several countries have considered the physician's role in euthanasia (termed physician-assisted suicide) including the USA and the Netherlands. Many other countries, including the UK, NZ and Australia, have ongoing public, professional and legal debate on this matter. Oregon was the first state in the USA to legalise physician-assisted suicide when it passed the *Death with Dignity Act* in 1997.[101] The *Death with Dignity Act* outlines a rigorous process for assisted dying with strict criteria requiring details pertaining to: the patient's request; the patient's suffering; information provided to the patient; the presence of reasonable alternatives; consultation with another physician; and the applied method of ending life. Under the *Death with Dignity Act*, physicians may not administer the medication; patients must ingest it independently. This is a constantly changing landscape in healthcare, for example, we are yet to understand the impact of the recent change as the Australian state of Victoria became the country's first to legalise assisted dying.[102]

This is clearly a contentious area with continuing evidence of conflicting views[103] about physician-assisted suicide in critical care, and lack of understanding among critical care staff as to terminology in this area.[104] It is important to note that there are also cultural and geographical variations that influence attitudes to euthanasia with some societies (e.g. China) presenting different cultural traditions, customs, religious beliefs that impact on professional ethics.[105] Therefore, country-specific best practice must be sought; many of which will often include ongoing exploration of treatment options to support symptom relief, and use of other specialist teams and professionals leading to an agreed future treatment plan.[98]

Making decisions with others: patient, family and clinical team perspectives

Critical care nurses aim to bring the ethical principles of patient autonomy, beneficence and non-maleficence to their daily bedside practices. Discussions can be held direct with patients to determine their treatment wishes. However, there are times in critical care, where it can be difficult to uphold patient autonomy, for example when patients are unconscious or sedated with no advance directives. For many patients, family members then become surrogate decision makers, and the patient's wishes are known through them.

However, communication can be a complicated process especially when difficult and challenging information is exchanged over a short timeframe. Communication can become even more complex if doctors and nurses lack communication skills,[106] or are fearful of holding discussions with family members because of concerns about litigation.[107] Collectively, these factors can lead to misunderstandings and confusion about what the patient wants, what the family wish for, and what critical care staff feel is achievable. Indeed, upholding patient autonomy and working with surrogate decision makers have been identified as frequent ethical situations challenging nurses on a daily basis.[108] This is despite the fact that nurses at the bedside are well-placed to support the patient/family make choices congruent with their values and wishes.[109]

Critical care doctors (and nurses) often receive requests for potentially inappropriate treatment for their family member.[110] Such situations need careful management to ensure that open communication channels are maintained between healthcare staff and family members. Asking questions to understand whose perspectives and whose ethical principles are being used to inform the requests can be helpful. Fear of loss can make distressed families focus on what is best for them as a family, rather than what may be best for the patient. Careful use of appropriate language can help families understand the gravity of situations, especially at end of life.[111] Talking about withdrawal of treatment, rather than withdrawal of care can ensure that family members are clear about what is, and what is not being offered for their family member; and this may ease ethical and moral distress.

Some situations in critical care can be ambiguous for families, for example a patient who is brain dead, but who looks to be pink and 'breathing'. Nursing staff may continue to talk to the patient while providing care, despite the family being informed that the patient is brain dead with no possibility of recovery. This may be confusing for some family members, whilst others may be comforted by staff talking to their family member. There is no right and wrong here, rather that such situations reinforce the need for all staff to be sensitive to how their words and actions may be perceived, and be clear with families as to what is informing these. Cultural sensitivity also needs to be demonstrated given that some families (e.g. traditional Chinese) prefer to keep information about death and dying away from patients in order to protect their loved one from any distress during end of life.[112] What is important is that doctors and nurses have a heightened awareness as to the emotional distress that families may be under at this time, and to ensure that communication with families is sensitive, timely, clear and compassionate.

Critical care is delivered by a team, and yet team members may have different perspectives on what 'good' critical care looks like; this is informed by different professional ethical decision-making frameworks. While the values of patients' rights, justice and quality of life are central to medicine's ethical framework, empirical work demonstrates that patient dignity, comfort and respect for patients' wishes are central to nurses' ethical framework.[113] At end of life, medical staff focus on making difficult decisions whereas nurses focus on supporting patients and families in crisis,[114] and enabling them to be involved in end-of-life decisions so that decisions match with stated care preferences, expectations and values.[115] Despite the contribution that nurses can make to decision making in critical care, the nursing voice can be silent. Several studies demonstrate the lack of engagement by nurses during decision making,[116,117] especially in countries such as Brazil and Japan. While this highlights specific cultural challenges, in sensitive areas such as end of life, it is generally recommended that open communication occurs with all doctors and nurses involved.[118]

Practice is made more challenging for doctors and nurses when further ethical conflicts result from organisational ethical issues, e.g. allocation of funding and resources, and administration support – or lack of it.[119] In situations where complex ethical dilemmas are faced, access to debriefing, interdisciplinary education, or a clinical ethicist/clinical ethics committee[120] may help in bringing together those involved, and offer an ethical review to mediate the problem.

Developing moral resilience to maintain ethical competence

In reading through the preceding sections, the many aspects of critical care nursing that hold moral and ethical challenge are clearly visible. Ethical issues in practice range from the 'big' subjects, such as assisted dying or when treatment should, or should not, be offered through to the 'everyday' ethical challenges of nursing practice, such as the use of chemical versus physical restraints for patients.[121] While professional codes of conduct exist to highlight ethical values that should inform the actions of nurses, the reality of upholding these values in practice, is more challenging.

If decisions are made where nurses' professional or personal ethical views have not been considered, this can result in a perception that unsatisfactory decisions have been made[122] with nurses experiencing the despair and hopelessness associated with moral distress. Moral distress occurs when nurses face ethical conflicts but are unable to respond to them in a way that maintains their personal or professional integrity.[122] The impact of this is felt by the individual nurse (e.g. burnout) and by organisations (e.g. increased turnover, shortage of workforce, staff becoming increasingly disengaged).[122]

The development of moral resilience is one way to mitigate moral distress. Moral resilience is described as an ability to choose how one responds to ethical challenges in ways that preserves integrity and minimises one's own suffering. As individuals, nurses can foster greater self-awareness to become more familiar with their moral values and their own strengths and limitations. They can develop self-regulatory capacities so that they are able to uphold their moral position in the face of external approval,[123] and develop ethical competence in developing a moral vocabulary and an openness to understanding the values of others.[122]

Healthcare organisations also need to develop fair and transparent ethical decision-making processes, at every level.[124] Traditionally strategies to address moral distress have focused on improving understanding, awareness and communication between individuals and included education to build skills in ethical decision making, conflict resolution, and interdisciplinary collaboration.[125] To address moral distress and build moral resilience requires an organisational and professional commitment to develop practice areas as moral communities[126] where ethically-driven practice is central. This will be essential to address the moral and ethical challenges that critical care nurses face in the future.

Ethics in research

When conducting research studies involving humans, all researchers must meet ethical codes of conduct that ensure valid consent and mitigation of harm to participants. There are various ethical guidelines for the conduct of research globally, for example the Declaration of Helsinki is regarded as an authoritative source.[127] In the UK, the General Medical Council provides guidance to researchers in the form of its Good Medical Practice Statement.[128] Healthcare research in Australia is performed in accordance with guidelines issued by the National Health and Medical Research Council (NHMRC), while in NZ the guidelines are issued by the Health Research Council (HRC).

Most countries now have national guidelines in place that are used to inform researchers conducting research with human participants; members of an ethics review committee reviewing/approving research; those involved in research governance; and, potential research participants. Such guidelines will also set up the expected composition of local level (site specific) research and ethics bodies.[12,129] In Australa and NZ the NHMRC and HRC respectiviely hold statutory authority, and health service and university human research ethics committees (HRECs) are required to consider research proposals in accordance with the relevant recommended processes and procedures outlined by these councils (see *Online resources* for a list of relevant resources provided by the NHMRC and HRC).

Application of ethical principles

When considering human clinical research in the context of critical care, the concept of *respect for persons* is linked to the ethical principle of autonomy.[12] In human research, respect for persons demands that participants receive adequate information and choose to participate voluntarily in the research without coercion. Similar criteria as for consent to treatment should be applied by researchers seeking to recruit participants into their study. Although there may be some variation between organisations and jurisdictions, Box 4.4 provides the type of information that potential participants should be provided with to meet ethical requirements for consent in medical research.[29] When research studies are being considered in critical care areas, surrogate consent may be applicable.[130]

Other important and relevant ethical principles for consideration in human research are beneficence and non-maleficence. *Beneficence* in the research context is expressed by the researcher's responsibility to minimise the risk of harm or discomfort to research participants.[12] Research protocols should be designed to ensure that respect for dignity and wellbeing takes precedence over any expected knowledge benefits from the research. With regard to *justice* in research, this requires that within a population there is a fair distribution of 'benefits and burdens' for research participation. In using this concept it is the scientific objective, as opposed to membership of either a privileged or vulnerable population, that should determine the participants for a study, and the sample population should be selected to most equitably share the risks and benefits of the research.

BOX 4.4

Information requirements for participant consent in medical research

Consent to medical research documentation should include the following:[23]

- A statement that the study involves research
- An explanation of the purposes of the research
- The expected duration of the subject's participation
- A description of the procedures to be followed
- Identification of any procedures that are experimental
- A description of any reasonably foreseeable risks or discomforts to the subject
- A description of any benefits to the subject or to others that may reasonably be expected from the research
- A disclosure of appropriate alternative procedures or courses of treatment, if any, that might be advantageous to the subject
- A statement describing the extent, if any, to which confidentiality of records identifying the subject will be maintained
- For research involving more than minimal risk, an explanation as to whether any compensation, and an explanation as to whether any medical treatments are available, if injury occurs and, if so, what they consist of, or where further information may be obtained
- An explanation of whom to contact for answers to pertinent questions about the research and research subjects' rights, and whom to contact in the event of a research-related injury to the subject
- A statement that participation is voluntary, refusal to participate will involve no penalty or loss of benefits to which the subject is otherwise entitled, and the subject may discontinue participation at any time without penalty or loss of benefits, to which the subject is otherwise entitled

When recruiting research participants, it is important to ensure that any initial approach is made appropriately. When the study involves recruitment of hospital inpatients, this approach should be made by someone directly involved in their care, with the aim of seeking permission to then be approached by the investigators specifically about the research. If the study involves recruitment of individuals from the community, this can be done by public display (e.g. flyers, published advertisements) that provides the contact details of the researcher. Control for involvement in the research is then with the participant to make contact with the researcher. While these processes may be interpreted as putting an extra barrier to recruitment, the principles of respect and autonomy for persons are upheld as the potential for coercive recruitment is reduced. Another guiding value in ethical research is that of *integrity*. This requires that the researcher be committed to the search for knowledge and to the principles of ethical research, conduct and results dissemination.[12]

Human research ethics committees

HRECs play a central role in the ethical supervision of research involving humans. Individual research institutes/centres, universities, regional/local health authorities and hospitals will have an HREC (or equivalent body) and articulate requirements for research to be conducted in their institution. The HREC will review proposals for research involving humans to ensure that the research is soundly designed, and conducted according to high ethical standards such as those articulated in Australia in the *National Statement on Ethical Conduct in Human Research 2007* (known as the National Statement) which incorporates updates as of May 2015.[12] Individual HRECs have protocols for submission of ethics applications, compliance, monitoring and complaints-handling processes. Importantly, no research study involving humans can be commenced until ethical clearance has been formally given by the relevant HREC(s).

The role of an HREC should not be confused with another form of clinical ethics committee that has been established in some hospitals and health services to provide closed forums for clinicians to raise ethical and legal concerns associated with particular clinical treatments or decisions. These are advisory committees that can also take into account patients' and or their families' wishes when this raises complex decision making with clinicians. In addition to providing clinicians with advice on particular cases these committees may also assist with the development of organisational policies on patient care and facilitate staff and patient education about ethical issues.

Research involving unconscious persons

The question of whether it is justifiable to include an unconscious patient in a research project without his or her consent is a problematic issue that most critical care researchers and HRECs have to attend to.[12,131] Paramount in these considerations is the careful weighing up of potential risks and benefits by a competent individual. However, analysis of these risks and benefits by a surrogate on behalf of an incompetent individual poses a range of ethical difficulties. Most national and international guidelines concur that such research is justified as long as safeguards are in place. Both the National Statement[12] and the Operational Standards[132] outline categories of vulnerable persons and the relevant ethical considerations that apply to these groups. The governing bodies recommend careful consideration of these highly vulnerable groups. Of note, the New Zealand Operational Standards[132] recognise that research on unconscious patients is appropriate, but emphasise the need for communication with the family or other legal representatives wherever possible. These Standards do note that in emergency situations consultation with the family/legal representatives may not be possible, but that the 'healthcare practitioner must always act in the best interests of the consumer.'[132]

Clinical trials

Clinical trials are a specific type of research study that explores whether a medical treatment, drug or device is safe and effective for humans. As these trials use people/patients as subjects in the study, these studies must follow strict scientific standards that are set within each country. The Therapeutic Goods Administration (TGA) in Australia has adopted the *Note for Guidance on Good Clinical Practice* to replace the *Guidelines for Good Clinical Research Practice*,[133] but at the same time note there is some overlap with The National Statement, which prevails. The TGA has published an annotated version for the Australian regulatory context. The *Note for Guidance on Good Clinical Practice*[133] is an internationally accepted standard for the designing, conducting, recording and reporting of clinical trials.

The Australian government, through the NHMRC, has funded and established the Australian Clinical Trial Registry (ACTR) at the NHMRC Trials Centre in Sydney, which complies with these requirements. Clinical trials must be registered online prior to subject recruitment, as there are important implications for future research publication in journals. The World Health Organization (WHO) has developed the International Clinical Trial Registry Platform (ICTRP)[134] as a global project to facilitate access to information about controlled trials and their results. The Clinical Trials Search Portal provides access to a central database containing the trial registration data sets provided by the registries listed. It also provides links to the full original records. To facilitate the unique identification of trials, the Search Portal bridges (groups together) multiple records about the same trial.[134]

Ethics in publication

One of the key ways in which research findings are disseminated is through publication in peer-reviewed journals. Many international high quality journals, including *Australian Critical Care*, support the implementation of the *Committee of Publication Ethics (COPE) Code of Conduct and Best Practice Guidelines*[135] for journal editors and publishers. These guidelines recognise the important roles of editors, editorial boards and publishers in promoting and supporting ethical practices in reporting research. Therefore, journal editors are increasingly requiring that researchers demonstrate evidence of their ethics review process before a manuscript/study is considered for publication.

In Australia the NHMRC *Australian Code for the Responsible Conduct of Research (2007)*[136] provides guidance on the minimum requirements for authorship of research. Authorship is defined as substantial participation, where all the following conditions are met:

- conception and design, or data collection or analysis/interpretation of data
- drafting the article, or revising it critically for important intellectual content
- final approval of the version to be published.[136]

Authors must also ensure that all those who have contributed to the work are recognised and acknowledged. Acquisition of research funding or general supervision of a research group is not considered sufficient for authorship. Intellectual honesty should be paramount and used to inform publication ethics and to prevent misconduct.[136] Furthermore, under best practice guidelines, journals should ensure processes whereby researchers are obliged to disclose any potential competing interests before a manuscript is published and ensure all published reports and reviews of research papers have been peer reviewed by suitably qualified persons and, where needed, publish corrections, clarifications, retractions and apologies.[135]

Summary

Managing ethical issues in any healthcare setting can be complex and, at times, contentious. As has been explored in this chapter, the critical care environment provides some unique challenges where the patient is particularly vulnerable; decision-making potentially complex; and resource utilisation challenging. Critical care nurses therefore need to use ethical principles to guide care of the critically ill and inform the conduct of clinical human research. As nurses provide a continuous presence at the bedside and a key voice heard in clinical management and leadership discussions across critical care, it is important that nurses develop and maintain a strong ethical and moral compass to guide care delivered.

Case study

Peter, a 67-year-old male, was brought into the emergency department (ED) after taking 40 × 500 mg of paracetamol. He refused treatment on arrival, was coherent and not showing signs of mental incapacity. His wife, Lucy, had died 2 years prior of a brain tumour. Recently, Peter had been diagnosed with metastatic bowel cancer which had spread to the liver. He had previously refused further investigation into the disease and any treatment. In the ED he was assessed and passed the Mental State Examination and apart from suicidal ideation was not displaying any symptoms of major depression. His cognitive function was not impaired. ED staff informed him of the outcome if he continued to refuse treatment, which he understood. He gave a document that was typed up and in a plastic sleeve to the ED staff which declared his wishes to die now and to avoid a long and painful death from cancer. He was well aware of the consequences of taking the paracetamol overdose and wished to be cared for in hospital until he died, but to not receive any lifesaving treatment. He asked that his daughter not be told until he had passed away.

A treatment option considered by staff was to physically restrain Peter (due to his physical resistance of medical intervention), insert a nasogastric tube, administer charcoal and n-acetylcysteine and transfer him to the ICU.

An alternate option was to consult with the full clinical team and the medical director and seek legal advice, given Peter was assessed as having mental capacity and therefore had the right to refuse treatment.

CASE STUDY QUESTIONS

1 Consider the issues of mental capacity raised by the *Case study* and answer the following question parts:
   a How are assessments about someone's mental capacity made in your clinical area?
   b What legal, professional and organisational processes and guidance are in place to assist this?
   c What actions would you take if your assessment of a patient's mental capacity were not reflective of others in your team?

2 If a similar case presented to your hospital, how would it be managed and what factors would guide the approach to be taken?

3 In your practice, are there decisions made by adult patients with capacity that challenge you in thinking there are limits to someone's autonomy? What are those circumstances and how are these managed in practice?

4 Ethically, is there a difference between a competent person making a well-thought-through request as opposed to an irrational person?

RESEARCH VIGNETTE

Brooks LA, Manias E. Barriers, enablers and challenges to initiating end-of-life care in an Australian intensive care unit context. Aust Crit Care 2017;30(3):161-166

Abstract

Background: Patients admitted to Australian intensive care units are often critically unwell, and present the challenge of increasing mortality due to an ageing population. Several of these patients have terminal conditions, requiring withdrawal of active treatment and commencement of end-of-life (EoL) care.

Objectives: The aim of the study was to explore the perspectives and experiences of physicians and nurses providing EoL care in the ICU. In particular, perceived barriers, enablers and challenges to providing EoL care were examined.

Methods: An interpretative, qualitative inquiry was selected as the methodological approach, with focus groups as the method for data collection. The study was conducted in Melbourne, Australia in a 24-bed ICU. Following ethics approval intensive care physicians and nurses were recruited to participate. Focus group discussions were discipline specific. All focus groups were audio-recorded then transcribed for thematic data analysis.

Results: Five focus groups were conducted with 11 physicians and 17 nurses participating. The themes identified are presented as barriers, enablers and challenges. Barriers include conflict between the ICU physicians and external medical teams, the availability of education and training, and environmental limitations. Enablers include collaboration and leadership during transitions of care. Challenges include communication and decision making, and expectations of the family.

Conclusions: This study emphasised that positive communication, collaboration and culture are vital to achieving safe, high quality care at EoL. Greater use of collaborative discussions between ICU clinicians is important to facilitate improved decisions about EoL care. Such collaborative discussions can assist in preparing patients and their families when transitioning from active treatment to initiation of EoL care. Another major recommendation was to implement EoL care leaders from nursing and medical disciplinary backgrounds, and patient support coordinators, to encourage clinicians to communicate with other clinicians and with family members about plans for EoL care.

Critique

This interpretive qualitative Australian study explores how doctors and nurses experience and perceive barriers, enablers and challenges to providing EoL care in the ICU. The paper begins with a succinct outline of the study's context. Current state of knowledge with regards to the provision at EoL is highlighted including the importance of open communication with family members, the need for collaborative interdisciplinary team working, and organisational support for staff (education and emotional support). The aim of the study is clearly stated and the underpinning research questions described. A particular strength of this section is the provision of definitions for 'barriers', 'enablers' and 'challenges' so that readers understand how the authors are using these terms. These details, which researchers often assume a shared understanding of, enhances the integrity of the research.

This qualitative study undertook focus groups with doctors and nurses in a single intensive care site in order to gain in-depth understanding about provision of EoL. As exploratory, guided, interactive conversations, focus groups are a suitable data collection method to uncover beliefs held about a particular issue. It is stated that ethics approval was given by the participating health service although no further details are provided. It is usual for ethical approval to be granted by a recognised HREC, for example a university-based or health agency HREC at local, state or national jurisdictional level. For this study, it would appear that local arrangements were in place for review of the research proposal to ensure that the study met the requirements for ethical conduct and participants were protected. The setting is described with detail of the type and size of unit and workforce numbers. Given the focus of the study, it would have been helpful to provide information regarding EoL care, for example mortality data, EoL education, EoL case conferences.

The sampling strategy is well described outlining purposeful sampling and the criteria for selection. Recruitment details are given (email sent to eligible staff), although it is unclear who sent the email and how any potential for coercion was avoided, noting this omission may have been due to word constraints set by the journal.

The focus group is explored in good detail and provision of the focus group template is helpful. The focus groups were discipline-specific, that is, with either doctors or nurses. It is worth noting that there are benefits to this approach, in that it may be more practical to organise and offer opportunity for participants to speak more freely. However, data collected from interdisciplinary focus groups are helpful in explicitly revealing points of similarity and tensions across cultures and groups. There is no detail of an observer being used during data collection. Observers can be helpful in focus groups to take notes of what is said and document non-verbal signs and body language that can enrich data through collection of subtle nuances that transcription of the narrative text alone can miss. This data can bring further understanding about group interaction. Data management and the thematic data analysis are well described.

There is rigorous detail given about the participants. Clear tabulated information is provided summarising demographic and qualification characteristics, and explanatory notes made about codes used to indicate quotes taken from physician and nursing groups. The findings are presented under three concepts used in the research aim: barriers, enablers and challenges. While these help provide structure to the paper, it is noted that these areas were used in the original study research question. It is therefore not clear whether or how these were thematically developed from the data. More detail about this process would have been helpful. That being said, the themes are well-supported by data extracts. The discussion section of the paper explores all key points raised by the data, with a particular focus on the need for improved communication and decision-making skills. Study limitations are stated.

The paper concludes by recommending more structured EoL education for physicians and nurses and improved collaboration among clinical teams, both clearly derived from study findings. The study was published in a peer-reviewed, clinical journal and adds to the body of knowledge about EoL in the ICU.

Learning activities

1 Consider the decision-making and communication challenges reported in the *Research vignette* paper by Brooks et al (2017). Reflect on your experiences in this area of EoL. What are some of the actions that you could take to improve collaboration in care?

2 You are on duty when a patient who has ingested a poisonous substance is admitted. The patient does not want medical intervention, and only wants pain relief. What ethical and legal issues need consideration for this person? How can these be managed?

3 There is a colleague at work who frequently refuses to care for long-term patients and who appears to be getting more stressed and anxious at work. Think about the section on moral distress in this chapter. What could you do to offer support?

4 What are the ethical principles involved in clinical research? How can you safeguard the rights of patients who are involved in clinical trials?

Online resources

AUSTRALIA

Australian state and territory privacy law, www.oaic.gov.au/privacy/other-privacy-jurisdictions/state-and-territory-privacy-law

National Health and Medical Research Council (NHMRC), An ethical framework for integrating palliative care principles into the management of advanced chronic or terminal conditions, www.nhmrc.gov.au/_files_nhmrc/publications/attachments/rec31_ethical_framework_palliative_care_terminal_110908.pdf

National Health and Medical Research Council (NHMRC), Challenging ethical issues in contemporary research on human beings, 2007, current, www.nhmrc.gov.au/_files_nhmrc/publications/attachments/e73.pdf

National Health and Medical Research Council (NHMRC), Health ethics, research integrity, 2016, https://www.nhmrc.gov.au/research/responsible-conduct-research-0

National Health and Medical Research Council (NHMRC), National Statement on Ethical Conduct in Human Research 2007, updated 2015

NEW ZEALAND

Health Act 1956 (NZ), www.legislation.govt.nz/act/public/1956/0065/latest/DLM305840.html

Health Research Council of New Zealand (HRCNZ), Ethics overview, www.hrc.govt.nz/ethics-and-regulatory/nz-ethics-overview and www.hrc.govt.nz/ethics-and-regulatory/

Health Research Council of New Zealand (HRCNZ), Guidelines for researchers on health research involving Maori, revised 2010, www.hrc.govt.nz/news-and-publications/publications/guidelines-researchers-health-research-involving-m%C4%81ori/

National Ethics Advisory Committee NZ, http://neac.health.govt.nz/home/

New Zealand multi-region ethics committees, http://ethics.health.govt.nz/about-committees/archived-minutes-and-reports-pre-2012/multi-region-committee/

New Zealand Privacy Commissioner website, www.privacy.org.nz

Public Health and Disability Act 2000 (NZ), Amended as NZ Public Health and Disability Amendment Bill 2010, www.parliament.nz/en-nz/pb/legislation/bills/digests/49PLLawBD17731/new-zealand-public-health-and-disability-amendment-bill

EUROPE & UK

Council for International Organisations of Medical Sciences (CIOMS), International Ethical Guidelines for Health-related Research Involving Humans, 2002, Fourth Edition, https://cioms.ch/shop/product/international-ethical-guidelines-for-biomedical-research-involving-human-subjects-2/

European Network of Research Ethics Committees – EUREC, http://www.eurecnet.org/index.html

World Health Organization, List of Ethics Committees, 2015, http://apps.who.int/ethics/nationalcommittees/NEC_full_web.pdf

World Health Organization, Operational Guidelines for Ethics Committees that Review Biomedical Research, 2000, www.who.int/tdr/publications/training-guideline-publications/operational-guidelines-ethics-biomedical-research/en

World Medical Association, Declaration of Helsinki, updated 2013

http://irb.sinica.edu.tw/doc/regulation/DECLARATION%20OF%20HELSINKI%20(2013).pdf *or*

European Commission – Public Health, https://ec.europa.eu/health/home_en

NORTH AMERICA

National Institutes of Health, Research Involving Human Subjects, https://humansubjects.nih.gov/

Office for Human Research Protections, https://www.hhs.gov/ohrp/

Panel on Research Ethics, Navigating the Ethics of Human Research, http://www.pre.ethics.gc.ca/eng/index/

Tri Council Policy Statement, Ethical Conduct for Research Involving Humans, 2010, http://www.pre.ethics.gc.ca/pdf/eng/tcps2/TCPS_2_FINAL_Web.pdf

US Department of Health and Human Services, Federal Policy for the Protection of Human Subjects ('Common Rule') https://www.hhs.gov/ohrp/regulations-and-policy/regulations/common-rule/index.html

ASIA

Ethical Guidelines for Biomedical Research on Human Participants, http://icmr.nic.in/ethical_guidelines.pdf

Ethics in Human Experimentation, Bio-medical Ethics, http://icmr.nic.in/human_ethics.htm

Medical Research Ethics Committee, Kuala Lumpur, http://nih.gov.my/web/mrec/

AFRICA

Egyptian Network of Research Ethics Committees, http://www.enrec.org/

Health Professions Council of South Africa Guidelines for Good Practice in the Health Care Professions General Ethical Guidelines for Health Researchers, http://www.hpcsa.co.za/Uploads/editor/UserFiles/downloads/conduct_ethics/rules/generic_ethical_rules/booklet_6_gen_ethical_guidelines_for_researchers.pdf

South African Medical Research Council Ethics Committee, Standard, http://www.mrc.ac.za/ethics/StandardOperatingProcedures.pdf

OTHERS

International Committee of Medical Journal Editors (ICMJE) Recommendations (The Uniform Requirements), www.icmje.org.

Medical Research Council of Canada (MRC), National Science and Engineering Research Council of Canada (NSERC) and the Social Science and Humanities Research Council of Canada (SSHRC), Tri-Council Policy Statement: Ethical conduct for research involving humans, Ottawa, MRC, NSERC & SSHRC, 1998

Further reading

Benatar S. Reflections and recommendations on research ethics in developing countries. Soc Sci Med 2002;54(7):1131–41.

DeAngelis CD, Drazen JM, Frizelle FA, et al. Clinical trial registration: a statement from the International Committee of Medical Journal Editors. JAMA 2004;292:1363–4.

Hurley C. A model to support the ethical elements of decisions made by advanced level practitioners. Nurs Crit Care 2011;16:53–4.

Kim Y-S, Kang SW, Ahn JA. Moral sensitivity relating to the application of the code of ethics. Nurs Ethics 2013;20(4):470–8.

McGowan CM. Legal issues. Legal aspects of end-of-life care. Crit Care Nurse 2011;31(5):64–9.

Settle PD. Nurse activism in the newborn intensive care unit: actions in response to an ethical dilemma. Nurs Ethics 2014;21(2):198–209.

Woods M. Beyond moral distress: preserving the ethical integrity of nurses. Nurs Ethics 2014;21:127–8.

References

1. International Council of Nurses (ICN). Code of Ethics. 2012. Available from: http://www.icn.ch/publications/position-statements. [Accessed 26 May 2018].
2. NMBA Professional Codes and Guidelines. 2018. Available from: http://www.nursingmidwiferyboard.gov.au/Codes-Guidelines-Statements/Professional-standards.aspx. [Accessed 26 May 2018].
3. Tschudin V. The words private and costly certainly figure large in nurses work. Nurs Ethics 2002;9(2):119.
4. Department of Health. Report of the Mid Staffordshire NHS Foundation Trust Public Inquiry. London: The Stationary Office; 2013.
5. Commonwealth of Australia. Public Interest Disclosure Bill 2013 [Provisions]. 2013. Available from: https://www.aph.gov.au/Parliamentary_Business/Committees/Senate/Legal_and_Constitutional_Affairs/Completed_inquiries/2010-13/publicinterestdisclosure/report/inde. [Accessed 26 May 2018].
6. McIlwraith J, Madden B. Health care and the law. 6th ed. Sydney: Thomson Reuters (Professional) Australia; 2014.
7. Beauchamp TL, Childress JF. Principles of biomedical ethics. 5th ed. New York: Oxford University Press; 2001.
8. McPherson P, Stakenberg S. Values, ethics and advocacy. In: Berman A, Snyder S, Levett-Jones T, et al, editors. Kozier and Erb's fundamentals of nursing, vol. 1. 2nd Australian ed. Frenchs Forest: Pearson; 2010.

9. Johnstone M-J. Bioethics: a nursing perspective. 5th ed. Sydney: Elsevier; 2009.
10. Nursing and Midwifery Board of Australia (NMBA). Code of Ethics for Nurses and Midwives in Australia. May 2018. Available from: http://www.nursingmidwiferyboard.gov.au/Codes-Guidelines-Statements/Professional-standards.aspx. [Accessed 26 May 2018].
11. The National Commission for the Protection of Human Subjects of Biomedical & Behavioral Research. The Belmont Report: Ethical principles and guidelines for the protection of human subjects of research. 1979; (78-0014). Available from: http://videocast.nih.gov/pdf/ohrp_appendix_belmont_report_vol_2.pdf. [Accessed 26 May 2018].
12. National Health and Medical Research Council (NHMRC). National Statement on Ethical Conduct in Human Research 2007 (updated May 2015). 2007. Available from: http://www.nhmrc.gov.au/guidelines/publications/e72. [Accessed 26 May 2018].
13. Bailey S. Ethically defensible decision-making in health care: challenges to traditional practice. Aust Health Rev 2002;25(2):27–31.
14. Nelson JE, Puntillo KA, Pronovost PJ, et al. In their own words: patients and families define high-quality palliative care in the intensive care unit. Crit Care Med 2010;38(3):808–18.
15. Angelucci P, Carefoot S. Working through moral anguish. Nurs Manage 2007;38(9):10–12.
16. Staunton P, Chiarella M. Law for nurses and midwives. 8th ed. Sydney: Elsevier; 2017.
17. South Australian Government. Consent to Medical Treatment and Palliative Care Act 1995. 2015. Available from: https://www.legislation.sa.gov.au/LZ/C/A/CONSENT%20TO%20MEDICAL%20TREATMENT%20AND%20PALLIATIVE%20CARE%20ACT%201995/CURRENT/1995.26.AUTH.PDF. [Accessed 26 May 2018].
18. New Zealand Government. Privacy Act 1993: Reprint 2017. Available from: http://www.legislation.govt.nz/act/public/1993/0028/latest/DLM296639.html. [Accessed 26 May 2018].
19. Commonwealth of Australia. Privacy Act 1988 – C2014C00669. 2014. Available from: https://www.oaic.gov.au/privacy-law/privacy-act/. [Accessed 26 May 2018].
20. Australian state and territory privacy law. Available from: http://www.oaic.gov.au/privacy/other-privacy-jurisdictions/state-and-territory-privacy-law. [Accessed 26 May 2018].
21. United Nations. The Universal Declaration of Human Rights 1948, 2014. Available from: http://www.un.org/en/universal-declaration-human-rights/index.html. [Accessed 26 May 2018].
22. Grech C. Factors affecting the provision of culturally congruent care to Arab Muslims by critical care nurses. Aust Crit Care 2008;21(3):167–71.
23. Bloomer MJ, Al-Mutair A. Ensuring cultural sensitivity for Muslim patients in the Australian ICU: considerations for care. Aust Crit Care 2013;26(4):193–6.
24. Nursing and Midwifery Board of Australia. Registered nurse standards for practice. 2016. Available from: http://www.nursingmidwiferyboard.gov.au/Codes-Guidelines-Statements/Professional-standards/registered-nurse-standards-for-practice.aspx. [Accessed 26 May 2018].
25. National Health and Medical Research Council (NHMRC). Cultural competency in health: a guide for policy, partnerships and participation. Canberra: Australian Government; 2006. Available from: https://www.nhmrc.gov.au/guidelines/publications/hp19-hp26. [Accessed 26 May 2018].
26. Commonwealth of Australia Department of Health. Aboriginal and Torres Strait Islander Health Curriculum Framework. Canberra. 2014. Available from: http://www.health.gov.au/internet/main/publishing.nsf/Content/72C7E23E1BD5E9CFCA257F640082CD48/$File/Health%20Curriculum%20Framework.pdf. [Accessed 26 May 2018].
27. Queensland Health. Delegated consent position statement. Brisbane: Queensland Government; 2013. Available from: https://www.health.qld.gov.au/__data/assets/pdf_file/0022/156082/delegated_consent_pos_sta.pdf. [Accessed 26 May 2018].
28. Rogers vs Whitaker (1992). 175 CLR 479. McIlwraith J, Madden B, editors. In: Health care and the law. Sydney: Thomson Reuters; 2014.
29. Rischbieth A, Blythe D. Ethics handbook for researchers, Australian and New Zealand Intensive Care Society (ANZICS) Clinical Trials Group (CTG). Melbourne: Wakefield Press; 2005.
30. Health and Disability Commissioner. Annual report of the Health and Disability Commissioner for the year ended 30 June 2002. Auckland: New Zealand Government; 2002.
31. Government of the United Kingdom. Human Rights Act. London. 1998. Available from: http://www.legislation.gov.uk/ukpga/1998/42. [Accessed 26 May 2018].
32. O'Neill O. Some limits of informed consent. J Med Ethics 2003;29(1):4–7.
33. Kon AA, Davidson JE, Morrison W, et al; American College of Critical Care Medicine & American Thoracic Society. Shared decision making in ICUs: an American College of Critical Care Medicine and American Thoracic Society policy statement. Crit Care Med 2016;44(1):188–201.
34. Aveyard H. Implied consent prior to nursing care procedures. J Adv Nurs 2002;39(2):201–7.
35. McConnell T. Inalienable rights: the limits to informed consent in medicine and the law. New York: Oxford University Press; 2000.
36. Nursing and Midwifery Council. The Code: professional standards of practice and behaviour for nurses and midwives. London.: NMC; 2015. Available from: https://www.nmc.org.uk/standards/code/. [Accessed 26 May 2018].
37. Office of the Queensland Parliamentary Council. Health Practitioner Regulation National Law Act 2009. Reprint 2018. Available from: https://www.legislation.qld.gov.au/view/html/inforce/current/act-2009-045. [Accessed 26 May 2018].
38. Ministry of Health. The Health Practitioners Competence Assurance Act 2003 (New Zealand). 2003 2018. Available from: http://www.legislation.govt.nz/act/public/2003/0048/latest/whole.html. [Accessed 26 May 2018].

39. Department of Health. Australian National Guidelines for the Management of Health Care Workers known to be infected with Blood Borne Viruses, Australian Government. 2012. Available from: http://www.health.gov.au/internet/main/publishing.nsf/Content/cda-cdna-bloodborne.htm. [Accessed 26 May 2018].
40. Hurley C. A model to support the ethical elements of decisions made by advanced level practitioners. Nurs Crit Care 2011;16:53–4.
41. Weng L, Joynt G, Lee A, et al. Attitudes towards ethical problems in critical care medicine: the Chinese perspective. Intensive Care Med 2011;37(4):655–64.
42. Fernandes MIIM. Ethical issues experienced by intensive care unit nurses in everyday practice. Nurs Ethics 2013;20(1):72–82.
43. Langeland K, Sørlie V. Ethical challenges in nursing emergency practice. J Clin Nurs 2011;20(13–14):2064–70.
44. Pauly BM, Varcoe C, Storch J. Framing the issues: moral distress in healthcare. HEC Forum 2012;24:1–11.
45. Edbrooke D, Corcoran M, Dean J, et al The cost of intensive care. CMIC 2000. 2000. Available from: https://www.uninet.edu/cimc2000/conferencia/conf47/Edbrooke.htm. [Accessed 26 May 2018].
46. Persad G, Wertheimer A, Emanuel EJ. Principles for allocation of scarce medical interventions. Lancet 2009;373(9661):423–31.
47. Eastman N, Philips B, Rhodes A. Triaging for adult critical care in the event of overwhelming need. Intensive Care Med 2010;36(6):1076–82.
48. Liu J, Chen XX, Wang XLJ. Ethical issues in neonatal intensive care units. J Matern Fetal Neonatal Med 2016;29(14):2322–6.
49. Nguyen Y-L, Angus DC, Boumendil A, et al. The challenge of admitting the very elderly to intensive care. Ann Intensive Care 2011;1(29):1–7.
50. Nates JL, Nunnally M, Kleinpell R, et al. ICU admission, discharge, and triage guidelines: a framework to enhance clinical operations, development of institutional policies, and further research. Crit Care Med 2016;44(8):1553–602.
51. Stelfox HT, Lane D, Boyd JM, et al. A scoping review of patient discharge from intensive care: opportunities and tools to improve care. Chest 2015;147(2):317–27.
52. Oerlemans AJM, van Sluisveld N, van Leeuwen ESJ, et al. Ethical problems in intensive care unit admission and discharge decisions: a qualitative study among physicians and nurses in the Netherlands. BMC Med Ethics 2015;16(9):1–10.
53. Kraus CK, Levy F, Kelen GD. Lifeboat ethics: considerations in the discharge of inpatients for the creation of hospital surge capacity. Disaster Med Public Health Prep 2007;1(1):51–6.
54. Nates JL, Nunnally M, Kleinpell R, et al. ICU admission, discharge, and triage guidelines: a framework to enhance clinical operations, development of institutional policies, and further research. Crit Care Med 2016;44(8):1553–602.
55. Hall K. Intensive care ethics in evolution. Bioethics 1997;11(3–4):241–5.
56. Oberle K, Hughes D. Doctors' and nurses' perceptions of ethical problems in end-of-life decisions. J Adv Nurs 2001;33(6):707.
57. George NR, Kryworuchko J, Hunold KM, et al. Shared decision making to support the provision of palliative and end-of-life care in the emergency department: a consensus statement and research agenda. Acad Emerg Med 2016;23(12):1394–402.
58. Downar J. Rapid response teams and end-of-life care. Can Respir J 2014;21(5):268.
59. Solverson KJ, Roze des Ordons AL, Doig CJ. Withholding and withdrawing life support: difficult decisions around care at the end of life. Can J Anaesth 2018;65(1):9–13.
60. Skjaker SA, Hoel H, Dahl V, et al. Factors associated with life-sustaining treatment restriction in a general intensive care unit. PLoS ONE 2017;12(7):1–5.
61. Manalo MF, Fidelis C. End-of-life decisions about withholding or withdrawing therapy: medical, ethical, and religio-cultural considerations. Palliat Care 2013;7:1–5.
62. Society of Critical Care Medicine Ethics Committee. Attitudes of critical care professionals concerning forgoing life-sustaining treatments. Crit Care Med 1992;20:320–6.
63. Chung GS, Yoon JD, Rasinski KA, et al. US physicians' opinions about distinctions between withdrawing and withholding life-sustaining treatment. J Relig Health 2016;55(5):1596–606.
64. Sprung CL, Cohen SL, Sjokvist P, et al; Ethicus Study Group. End-of-life practices in European intensive care units: the Ethicus Study. JAMA 2003;290(6):790–7.
65. Latour JM, Fulbrook P, Albarran JW. EfCCNa survey: European intensive care nurses' attitudes and beliefs towards end-of-life care. Nurs Crit Care 2009;14(3):110–21.
66. Orlowski J. Ethics in critical care medicine. Baltimore: University Publishing Group; 1999.
67. Luce JM, White DB. The pressure to withhold or withdraw life-sustaining therapy from critically ill patients in the United States. Am J Respir Crit Care Med 2007;175(11):1104–8.
68. Australian Commission on Safety and Quality in Health Care (ACSQHC). National consensus statement: essential elements for safe and high-quality end-of-life care in acute hospitals. Sydney: ACSQHC; 2015. Available from: https://www.safetyandquality.gov.au/wp-content/uploads/2015/05/National-Consensus-Statement-Essential-Elements-forsafe-high-quality-end-of-life-care.pdf. [Accessed 26 May 2018].
69. Walker R, Read S. The Liverpool care pathway in intensive care: an exploratory study of doctor and nurse perceptions. Int J Palliat Nurs 2010;16(6):267–73.
70. Chan RJ, Webster J, Bowers A. End-of-life care pathways for improving outcomes in caring for the dying. Cochrane Database Syst Rev 2016;(2):CD008006.
71. Makino J, Fujitani S, Twohig B, et al. End-of-life considerations in the ICU in Japan: ethical and legal perspectives. J Intensive Care 2014;2(1):1–7.

72. Wilkinson D, Savulescu J. A costly separation between withdrawing and withholding treatment in intensive care. Bioethics 2014;28(3):127–37.
73. Australian and New Zealand Intensive Care Society (ANZICS), College of Intensive Care Medicine of Australia and New Zealand. The ANZICS statement on withholding and withdrawing treatment. 2013. Available from: https://cicm.org.au/CICM_Media/CICMSite/CICM-Website/Resources/Professional%20Documents/IC-14-Statement-on-Withholding-and-Withdrawing-Treatment.pdf. [Accessed 26 May 2018].
74. Sprung CL, Carmel S, Sjokvist P, et al; ETHICATT Study Group. Attitudes of European physicians, nurses, patients, and families regarding end-of-life decisions: the ETHICATT study. Intensive Care Med 2007;33(1):104–10.
75. Bachman JG, Alcser KH, Doukas DJ, et al. Attitudes of Michigan physicians and the public toward legalizing physician-assisted suicide and voluntary euthanasia. N Engl J Med 1996;334(5):303–9.
76. Sjokvist P, Cook D, Berggren L, et al. A cross-cultural comparison of attitudes towards life support limitation in Sweden and Canada. Clin Intensive Care 1998;9(2):81–5.
77. Uhlmann RF, Pearlman RA, Cain KC. Physician' and spouses' predictions of elderly patients' resuscitation preferences. J Gerontol 1988;43(5):M115–21.
78. Ravenscroft AJ, Bell M. 'End-of-life' decision making within intensive care – objective, consistent, defensible? J Med Ethics 2000;26(6):435.
79. National Health and Medical Research Council (NHMRC). Organ and tissue donation after death, for transplantation: guidelines for ethical practice for health professionals. 2007. Available from: https://www.nhmrc.gov.au/guidelines-publications/e75. [Accessed 26 May 2018].
80. Long-Sutehall T, Willis H, Palmer R, et al. Negotiated dying: a grounded theory of how nurses shape withdrawal of treatment in hospital critical care units. Int J Nurs Stud 2011;48(12):1466–74.
81. Barber K, Falvey S, Hamilton C, et al. Potential for organ donation in the United Kingdom: audit of intensive care records. BMJ 2006;332(1124):1–4.
82. Connolly C, Miskolci O, Phelan D, et al. End-of-life in the ICU: moving from 'withdrawal of care' to a palliative care, patient-centred approach. Br J Anaesth 2016;117(2):143–5.
83. Chaet D. The AMA Code of Medical Ethics' opinions relevant to patient- and family- centered care. AMA J Ethics 2016;18(1):45–8.
84. Loretta MK. The best interests standard for incompetent or incapacitated persons of all ages. J Law Med Ethics 2007;35(1):187–96.
85. Morgan J. End-of-life care in UK critical care units – a literature review. Nurs Crit Care 2008;13(3):152–61.
86. Coombs M, Long-Sutehall T, Shannon S. International dialogue on end of life: challenges in the UK and USA. Nurs Crit Care 2010;15(5):234–40.
87. Haynes LI. Palliative care: attitudes and practices of trauma care providers. Arizona: The University of Arizona; 2017.
88. Aghabarary M, Dehghan Nayeri N. Medical futility and its challenges: a review study. J Med Ethics Hist Med 2016;9(11):1–13.
89. Willmott L, White B, Downie J. Withholding and withdrawal of 'futile' life-sustaining treatment: unilateral medical decision-making in Australia and New Zealand. J Law Med 2013;20(4):907–24.
90. Chiarchiaro J, Arnold RM, White DB. Reengineering advance care planning to create scalable, patient- and family-centered interventions. JAMA 2015;313(11):1103–4.
91. Caring info. Advanced care planning ahead. 2016. Available from: http://www.caringinfo.org/i4a/pages/index.cfm?pageid=3289. [Accessed 26 May 2018].
92. Wynn F. Reflecting on the ongoing aftermath of heart transplantation: Jean-Luc Nancy's L'intrus. Nurs Inq 2009;16(1):3–9.
93. Australian Government Department of Health and Ageing. A national framework for advance care directives. 2011. Available from: https://www.dementia.org.au/files/start2talk/5.0.4.1%20AHMAC%20framework.pdf. [Accessed 26 May 2018].
94. Government of Western Australia. WA Cancer and Palliative Care Network. Advance care planning. Available from: http://www.healthnetworks.health.wa.gov.au/cancer/palliative/. [Accessed 26 May 2018].
95. Michelson KN, Siegel LB. Palliative care in the PICU. In: Wheeler D, Wong H, Shanley T, editors. Pediatric critical care medicine. London: Springer; 2014. p. 141–8.
96. Mullen JE, Reynolds MR, Larson JS. Caring for pediatric patients' families at the child's end of life. Crit Care Nurse 2015;35(66):46–55.
97. Lackman V. Do-not-resuscitate orders: nurse's role requires moral courage. Medsurg Nurs 2010;19(4):249–52.
98. New South Wales Government. Advanced Care Directives (NSW) – Using. Sydney: NSW Government. 2005. Available from: http://www1.health.nsw.gov.au/pds/ActivePDSDocuments/GL2005_056.pdf. [Accessed 26 May 2018].
99. Phillips J. Clarifying substitute judgement: the endorsed life approach. J Med Ethics 2015;41(9):723–30.
100. Sanchini V, Nardini C, Boniolo G. The withholding/withdrawing distinction in the end-of-life debate. Multidiscip Respir Med 2014;9(13):1–3.
101. Ganzini L, Nelson H, Schmidt T, et al. Physicians' experiences with the Oregon Death with Dignity Act. N Engl J Med 2000;342:557–63.
102. Hutchinson S, Brown G Euthanasia bill passes Victorian parliament. The Australian. 20 October 2017. Available from: http://www.theaustralian.com.au/national-affairs/state-politics/euthanasia-bill-passes-victorian-parliament/news-story/ec70c5edbdb24c721aa82889d7540456. [Accessed 26 May 2018].
103. Goligher EC, Ely EW, Sulmasy DP, et al. Physician-assisted suicide and euthanasia in the ICU: a dialogue on core ethical issues. Crit Care Med 2017;45(2):149–55.
104. Kranidiotis G, Ropa J, Mprianas J, et al. Attitudes towards euthanasia among Greek intensive care unit physicians and nurses. Heart Lung 2015;44(3):260–3.

105. Lin LB. Clinical review: ethics and end-of-life care for critically ill patients in China. Crit Care 2013;17(6):1–5.
106. Brighton LJ, Koffman J, Hawkins A, et al. A systematic review of end-of-life care communication skills training for generalist palliative care providers: research quality and reporting guidance. J Pain Symptom Manage 2017;54(3):417–25.
107. Ha JF, Longnecker N. Doctor patient communication: a review. Ochnsner J 2010;10(1):38–43.
108. Ulrich CM, Taylor C, Soeken K, et al. Everyday ethics: ethical issues and stress in nursing practice. J Adv Nurs 2010;66(11):2510–19.
109. Price D, Knotts S. Communication, comfort, and closure for the patient with cystic fibrosis at the end of life: the role of the bedside nurse. J Hosp Palliat Nurs 2017;19(4):303–4.
110. Bosslet GT, Kesecioglu J, White DB. How should clinicians respond to requests for potentially inappropriate treatment? J Intensive Care Med 2016;42:422–5.
111. Curtis JR, Sprung CL, Azoulay E. The importance of word choice in care of critically ill patients and their families. J Intensive Care Med 2014;40:606–8.
112. Cheng F, Ip M, Wong KK, et al. Critical care ethics in Hong Kong: cross-cultural conflicts as East meets West. J Med Philos 1998;23(6):616–27.
113. Flannery L, Ramjan LM, Peters K. End-of-life decisions in the Intensive Care Unit 9 (ICU) – Exploring the experiences of ICU nurses and doctors – a critical literature review. Aust Crit Care 2016;29(2):97–103.
114. Epstein EG. Moral obligations of nurses and physicians in neonatal end-of-life care. Nurs Ethics 2010;17(5):577–89.
115. Murray MA, Miller T, Fiset V, et al. Decision support: helping patients and families to find a balance at the end of life. Int J Palliat Nurs 2004;10(6):270–7.
116. Ferrand E, Lemaire F, Regnier B, et al; French RESSENTI Group. Discrepancies between perceptions by physicians and nursing staff of intensive care unit end-of-life decisions. Am J Respir Crit Care Med 2003;167:1310–15.
117. Yaguchi A, Truog RD, Curtis JR, et al. International differences in end-of-life attitudes in intensive care unit: results of a survey. Arch Intern Med 2005;165:1970–5.
118. Joynt GM, Lipman J, Hartog C, et al. The Durban World Congress Ethics Round Table IV: health care professional end-of-life decision making. J Crit Care 2015;30(2):224–30.
119. Gaudine A, LeFort SM, Lamb M, et al. Ethical conflicts with hospitals: the perspective of nurses and physicians. Nurs Ethics 2011;18(6):756–66.
120. Hall RM. Ethical consultations in the ICU: by whom and when? Crit Care Med 2014;42(4):983–4.
121. Holt J, Convey H. Ethical practice in nursing care. Nurs Stand 2012;27(13):51–6.
122. Rushton CH. Moral resilience: a capacity for navigating moral distress in Critical Care. AACN Adv Crit Care 2016;27(1):111–19.
123. O'Connell C. Gender and the experience of moral distress in critical care nurses. Nurs Ethics 2015;22(1):32–42.
124. Rushton CH, Schoonover-Shoffner K, Kennedy MS. A collaborative state of the science initiative: transforming moral distress into moral resilience in nursing experts recommend strategies to develop moral resilience and support ethical practice. Am J Nurs 2017;117(2):S2–6.
125. Grace P, Robinson E, Jurchak M, et al. Clinical ethics residency for nurses: an education model to decrease moral distress and strengthen nurse retention in acute care. J Nurs Adm 2014;44(12):640–6.
126. Austin W. The ethics of everyday practice: healthcare environments as moral communities. ANS Adv Nurs Sci 2007;30(1):81–8.
127. World Medical Association (WMA). The WMA Declaration of Helsinki – Ethical principles for medical research involving human subjects. 2013. Available from: https://www.wma.net/policies-post/wma-declaration-of-helsinki-ethical-principles-for-medical-research-involving-human-subjects/. [Accessed 26 May 2018].
128. General Medical Council. Consent: patients and doctors making decisions together. London: GMC; 2008. Available from: https://www.gmc-uk.org/-/media/documents/consent—english-0617_pdf-48903482.pdf. [Accessed 26 May 2018].
129. Research and Ethical Boards USA. Policy and procedures manual: Research ethics board 2014. Available from: https://www.psi.org/wp-content/uploads/2014/10/REB_Policy_Procedures_Manual.pdf. [Accessed 26 May 2018].
130. The SAFE Study Investigators. A comparison of albumin and saline for fluid resuscitation in the intensive care unit. N Engl J Med 2004;350(22):2247.
131. Council for International Organizations of Medical Sciences (CIOMS). International ethical guidelines for biomedical research involving humans. Fourth edition, Geneva. 2016. Available from: https://cioms.ch/wp-content/uploads/2017/01/WEB-CIOMS-EthicalGuidelines.pdf. [Accessed 26 May 2018].
132. New Zealand Ministry of Health. Operational standard for ethics committees: updated edition. Wellington: Ministry of Health.; 2006. Available from: https://www.parliament.nz/resource/0000162273. [Accessed 26 May 2018].
133. Australian Therapeutic Goods Administration (TGA). Note for Guidance on Good Clinical Practice (CPMP/ICH/135/95) Annotated with TGA comments. 2018. Available from: https://www.tga.gov.au/publication/note-guidance-good-clinical-practice. [Accessed 26 May 2018].
134. World Health Organization (WHO). International Clinical Trials Registry Platform (ICTRP). 2018. Available from: http://www.who.int/ictrp/en/. [Accessed 26 May 2018].
135. Committee on Publication Ethics (COPE). Code of Conduct and Best Practice Guidelines. 2018. Available from: https://publicationethics.org/resources/code-conduct. [Accessed 26 May 2018].
136. National Health and Medical Research Council (NHMRC). Australian Code for the Responsible Conduct of Research. 2007. Available from: https://www.nhmrc.gov.au/guidelines-publications/r39. [Accessed 26 May 2018].

Section 2

Principles and practice of critical care

Chapter 5

Essential nursing care of the critically ill patient

Bernadette Grealy, Lotta Johansson, Fiona Coyer

KEY WORDS

bowel management
eye care
infection control
intra-hospital transport
oral care
patient positioning and mobility
personal hygiene
pressure injury
urinary catheter care

Learning objectives

After reading this chapter, you should be able to:

- identify risks posed to critically ill patients relating to inadequate physical care and hygiene
- describe eye- and oral-related risks associated with critical illness and mechanical ventilation
- describe best practice in the provision of physical care and hygiene
- describe factors of importance in the care of critically ill patients with special needs such as older adults and overweight patients
- describe preventive nursing care measures necessary for critically ill patients
- understand the key elements of safe transfer of critically ill patients within the hospital setting
- understand the principles of infection-control risk identification and management for critically ill patients.

Introduction

This chapter is about essential nursing care. Because it is often referred to as basic nursing, nurses may not prioritise it. Yet, how well patients are cared for has a direct effect on their sense of wellbeing and their recovery. 'Interventional patient hygiene' is a systematic, evidence-based approach to nursing actions designed to improve patient outcomes using a framework of hygiene, catheter care, skin care, mobility and oral care.[1] This chapter focuses on physical care, infection control, preventive therapies and transport of critically ill patients. The first two areas are closely linked: poor-quality physical care increases the risk of infection. The final areas are essential features of critical care nursing.

Comfort is a paramount concern in intensive care. Two key areas of care – reducing risk and providing quality care – are closely related and served by a series of principles (Table 5.1). Implementing evidence-based essential nursing care is a key strategy to reduce avoidable errors and improve patient outcomes.[1] If patients are assessed thoroughly and on a regular basis, problems may be detected and treated early, preventing the development of

TABLE 5.1
Principles of practice

REDUCING RISKS TO PATIENTS	PROVISION OF QUALITY CARE
• Recognition of the specific needs of critically ill patients, particularly those who are unconscious, sedated or immobile • Recognition of specific complications that may require special observation or treatment • Vigilant monitoring and early recognition of signs of deterioration • Selection, implementation and evaluation of specific preventive measures • Management of potentially detrimental environmental factors that may affect the patient	• Development of knowledge and skills for practice • Evidence-based practice • Optimal use of protocol-driven therapy • Competent, efficient and safe practice • Selection and application of appropriate nursing interventions • Monitoring the consequences of nursing interventions • Review and evaluation of nursing practices • Continuity of care • Effective critical care team functioning

unnecessary complications. Although this chapter focuses on the physical dimension of nursing care, patients' psychosocial care should not be ignored (see Chapters 6 and 7). Further, while this chapter describes essential nursing care, care bundles, which encompasses groups of activities, are described in Chapter 3.

Practice tip

Introducing yourself to patients and their family members or support persons is professionally appropriate and reassuring to them.

Ensure patients and their support persons know your name when you are caring for them; introducing yourself is professionally appropriate and reassuring to patients and their support persons.

Skin integrity

One of the most basic needs of patients is to maintain intact, healthy, moisturised skin. Intact skin is the body's first line of defence against the invasion of microorganisms, provides a protective barrier from numerous environmental threats, and facilitates retention of moisture. Maintaining the critically ill patient's skin integrity is one of the most fundamental yet critical goals of nursing practice.

Personal hygiene

It is important to provide the critically ill patient with effective personal hygiene as poor hygiene may increase the risk of bacterial colonisation and subsequent infection.[2] Daily bed baths are usually provided for most critically ill patients, although their effectiveness at reducing bacterial colonisation is questionable.[2] However, bed baths provide an opportunity to achieve other clinical goals such as skin examination, comfort and stimulating circulation.[3] Personal hygiene is closely related to an individual's esteem and sense of wellbeing. It may also influence family members' perception of the quality of care the patient is receiving and the confidence they have in the staff. Family members may want to help with the provision of essential care and help monitor the patient and be an adjunct to the nurse. This is an individually based approach with the family as a partner with the registered nurse (see Chapter 8). Daily bathing with 2% chlorhexidine gluconate-impregnated washcloths are used in some intensive care units (ICU). While international guidelines do not recommend the use of antiseptic-impregnated wash clothes, a recent meta-analysis suggests they may have some benefits to reduce bloodstream infections.[4]

Assessment of personal hygiene

Assessment of critical care patients' personal hygiene should be undertaken on two levels: first, determining what patients are able, and want, to do for themselves and second, the nurse's assessment of what is required. As with all aspects of care, the patient has the right to refuse personal hygiene measures. Many critical care patients are unable to participate in decision making; in these cases it is the nurse's responsibility to determine what level of care is necessary.[3] Consideration of the patient's specific condition may influence when and how personal hygiene is performed. For example, the patient may have to be moved slowly when changing bed linen because of their cardiovascular instability, or they may require a blanket while bathing if they are hypothermic. Finally, providing essential care should be timed to promote optimal rest. There are a number of areas to consider when assessing the skin (Table 5.2).

Essential hygiene care

A daily bed bath with intermittent washes of the face and hands is standard care; however, the following key points should be considered:

- patients who are sweating, incontinent, bleeding or with leaking wounds should be promptly washed and their linen changed as often as necessary.
- it may be appropriate to give prophylactic pain relief before commencing a bed bath.
- timing should be based on patient preference, clinical stability and to avoid disruption to patients' sleep.[3]

TABLE 5.2
Skin and tissue assessment

FACTOR	OBSERVATIONS
Colour of the skin	• Jaundice, erythema, pallor, cyanosis
Condition of the skin	• Skin turgor (elasticity): evidence of oedema (taut skin), dehydration (dryness, tenting of the skin), age-related or steroid-related damage (thin, papery, easily torn skin), skin tears • Presence of: rash, cellulitis, irritation, bruising, swelling
Tissue perfusion	• Hypoperfusion: capillary refill time, cool extremities, pulse strength and volume, blanching of the skin • Hyperaemia: very warm, red areas of skin • Thrombus formation: warm, red, swollen areas (especially calves)
Moisture	• Excessive sweating • Skin damage caused by moisture, especially in skinfolds: under the breasts, in the groin, between the buttocks
Wounds, drains, cannulae, catheters	• Evidence of inflammation, infection, pressure damage, skin excoriation caused by leaking exudates, correct positioning of drains, need to redress wounds

- planning ahead to coordinate patient repositioning helps avoid unnecessary delays and interruptions that affect the dignity of the patient.
- privacy for the patient should be of paramount concern.
- perform the bed bath promptly to prevent patient shivering.
- use of a low pH skin cleanser is recommended and no-rinse pH balanced cleansers is preferred to alkaline soaps where washing and then rinsing is required.[5]
- normal shampoo can be used to wash the patient's hair; however, hair caps and washing products are available that are easier to use for bedridden patients.
- male facial hair should be managed as per the patient's normal routine, such as maintaining a beard or shaving.
- ears should be gently inspected for debris or injury.
- clean nails should be maintained. Care should be taken if nails require trimming, especially if the patient has brittle nails or is diabetic.

Practice tip 2

Although personal grooming is not vital from a health perspective, it is a factor in how we see ourselves and how others identify with us. With the many changes that come with illness and therapies applied in critical care, it is important to keep the patient's 'look' as normal as possible – simple things such as styling hair or trimming beards – if not for the patients themselves, who might be unaware, then for their families.

Impaired skin integrity

Impaired skin integrity in the critically patient encompasses a number of conditions; pressure injuries, moisture-associate skin damage (MASD), medical adhesive-related skin injuries (MARSI) and skin tears. Information about each of these conditions are provided.

Pressure injury

The term 'pressure injury' rather than 'pressure ulcer' is used in Australasia and North America.[6] Other terms used include bed sore and decubitus ulcer. The majority of pressure injuries are considered preventable adverse events.[6] The risk of developing a pressure injury is 3.8 times more likely in intensive care patients compared to non-intensive care hospitalised patients.[7] Pressure injury risk for critically ill patients can be attributed to their immobility, lack of sensory protective mechanisms, sub-optimal tissue perfusion and environmental factors that cause pressure and friction.[8] Significant risk factors include age, number of days since admission, malnutrition and delays in the use of pressure-relieving mattresses.[8] The commonest locations for pressure injuries are the sacrum, the heels and the head.[7]

Pressure injury risk assessment tools can help nurses identify at-risk patients.[8] Risk assessment should be undertaken as soon as possible after the patient's admission and within 8 hours of admission.[8] There are several pressure injury risk assessment tools available such as the Braden score, the revised Jackson/Cubbin pressure risk calculator,[9] and the Conscious level-Mobility-Haemodynamics-Oxygenation-Nutrition (COMHON) index. The latter was designed specifically for use in ICU and identifies many factors that need to be considered and monitored prior to and during procedures for pressure injury prevention[10] (Table 5.3). A

TABLE 5.3
Components of the revised Jackson/Cubbin pressure area risk calculator[61]

RISK ASSESSMENT CATEGORIES	SCORING
• Age • Weight/tissue viability • Past medical history affecting condition • General skin condition • Mental status • Mobility • Haemodynamics • Respiration • Oxygen requirements • Nutrition • Incontinence • Hygiene	• Score range = 12–48 • One point is deducted for each of the following: ○ The patient has spent time in surgery/scan in the past 48 h ○ The patient has received blood products ○ The patient is hypothermic • A lower score indicates higher risk • A score of <29 indicates high risk

comprehensive head-to-toe skin assessment for pressure should be completed at least daily, including a review of pressure-relieving devices. Skin should be inspected at each episode of patient repositioning. Skin assessment should include testing for blanching response and checking for areas of oedema, induration, redness or localised heat.[8] Pressure injury prevention practices include alternating the use of pressure-relief mattresses, low-pressure mattresses and air-flow mattresses. For bariatric patients (usually those heavier than 150 kg), specialist beds and mattresses are required.[8]

Intensive care patients are at risk of pressure injuries and injury from a number of devices in everyday use, such as endotracheal tubes and nasogastric tubes (Table 5.4).[11] Close attention to detail with frequent observation of the patient, the patient's position and the presence and location of equipment is required to prevent skin damage.[12] It is imperative to choose the correct size of the device for the patient, cushion and protect the skin with dressings where appropriate, inspect the skin in contact with the device regularly, and be aware of the presence of oedema under devices and the potential for skin injury. It is also important to remove aids such as compression stockings and cervical collars to assess the skin. Vulnerable patients, such as those with poor

TABLE 5.4
Risk of pressure injuries from commonly used equipment

RISK FACTOR	COMMENTS
Endotracheal tubes (ETTs)	The ETT should be repositioned from one corner of the mouth to the other on a daily basis to prevent pressure on the same area of oral mucosa and lips. Care should also be taken when positioning and tying ETT tapes: friction burns may be caused if they are not secure; pressure sores may be caused if they are too tight (particularly above the ears and in the nape of the neck). Moist tapes exacerbate problems and harbour bacteria
Oxygen saturation probes	Repositioning of oxygen saturation probes 1–2-hourly prevents pressure on potentially poorly perfused skin. If using ear probes, these must be positioned on the lobe of the ear and not on the cartilage, as this area is very vulnerable to pressure and heat injury
Blood pressure cuffs	Non-invasive blood pressure cuffs should be regularly reattached and repositioned. If left in position without reattachment for long periods of time they can cause friction and pressure damage to skin. Care should be taken to ensure that tubing is not caught under the patient, especially after repositioning
Urinary catheters, central lines and wound drainage	The patient should be checked often to ensure that invasive lines are not trapped under the patient. In addition to causing skin injury, they may function ineffectively
Bed rails	Limbs should not press against bed rails; pillows should be used if the patient's position or size makes this likely
Oxygen masks	Use correct-size mask and hydrocolloid protective dressing on the bridge of the nose to assist with prevention of pressure from non-invasive or CPAP masks, especially when these are in constant or frequent use
Splints, traction and cervical collars	Devices such as leg/foot splints, traction and cervical collars can all cause direct pressure when in constant use and friction injury if they are not fitted properly. ICU patients often have rapid body mass loss (especially muscle) following admission, so daily assessment is required

TABLE 5.5
Monitoring pressure injuries (PIs)

FACTOR	ACTIONS
Size	• Objectively assess length, width and depth
Stage/grading	• Use a standardised measure to grade the injury (e.g. International NPUAP and EPUAP Pressure Ulcer Classification System)
Documentation	• Note the absence/presence/location of PIs on admission and discharge • Keep a record of nursing interventions and treatments used to treat PIs
Treatment	• Monitor response to therapy by assessing the size and stage/grade of the PI on a daily basis
Observing other sites	• Dependent areas of the body are susceptible: sacrum, heels, back of the head, hips, shoulders, elbows, knees • Areas of the body where equipment is causing pressure are susceptible: nose, ears, corners of the mouth, fingertips • Areas of the body where tissue perfusion is poor are susceptible: extremities

tissue perfusion, anaemia, oedema, diaphoresis and poor sensory perception, can develop pressure injuries relatively quickly. Pressure injuries caused by equipment are entirely avoidable.

All pressure points and any pressure injuries should be monitored closely. The key areas of monitoring are identified in Table 5.5. It is important to use standardised methods to objectively assess pressure injuries and their response to therapy. If a patient develops one pressure injury, there is a good chance another could develop. Nursing intervention includes the placing of patients in positions that avoid pressure on the affected area(s), employing measures such as good fluid management to improve tissue perfusion, reducing the risk of infection and promoting tissue granulation with the use of appropriate dressings. The application of layered silicone foam dressings has been shown to have a positive impact in reducing sacral pressure injury incidence in critically ill patients.[13]

The International NPUAP–EPUAP-PPPIA Pressure Ulcer Classification System[8] categorises pressure injuries as follows:

- Stage I: non-blanchable redness of intact skin
- Stage II: partial thickness skin loss or blister
- Stage III: full thickness skin loss (fat visible)
- Stage IV: full thickness tissue loss (muscle/bone visible)
- Unstageable pressure injury: depth unknown
- Suspected deep tissue injury: depth unknown
- Mucosal injury.[12]

Skin injuries are now differentiated from mucosal injuries. Mucosal pressure injuries are defined as injuries found on mucous membranes with a history of a medical device in use at the location of the injury. These injuries cannot be staged.[14]

Practice tip 3

It is worthwhile knowing the key features of the beds and mattresses commonly used in your area so that you can use them effectively to match patient requirements for bed functions, bed type (e.g. bariatric suitability) and pressure prevention (e.g. high-, medium- or low-risk mattress systems).

Moisture-associated skin damage

MASD is an umbrella term for skin damage due to excess moisture or prolonged exposure to moisture. This includes: peri-stomal dermatitis where healthy skin around the stoma is exposed to stomal effluent; peri-wound dermatitis where healthy skin surrounding a wound is exposed to wound exudate; intertriginous dermatitis where sweat trapped in skin folds, for example under the breasts, in the armpits or under the abdominal pannus, causes skin inflammation; and incontinence-associated dermatitis (IAD) where the skin has prolonged exposure to urine, stool or both urine and stool.

Incontinence-associated dermatitis

IAD, a type of MASD, is a preventable skin condition that occurs when the skin has prolonged or repeated exposure to urine, stool or both. It is characterised by patchy or consolidated inflammation of the epidermis and, potentially, the dermis.[14] The inflammation is observed as erythema, with repeated exposure to the irritants resulting in denudation of the skin's superficial layers, which may present as erosion, with vesicles or bullae, and clear exudates. The patient may experience itching or burning sensations and often severe pain.[15] Complications of IAD include increased risk of

TABLE 5.6
Treatment of skin tears

FACTOR	INTERVENTIONS
Cleansing	• Gently clean skin with saline or non-toxic wound cleaner • Allow to dry or pat dry carefully
Skin flap	• Approximate the skin tear flap/tissue, if present, as closely as possible
Dressing	• Provide appropriate topical wound care, such as a moist wound dressing • Remove any product with an adhesive backing with utmost care to avoid further trauma • Secure non-adherent dressing with a gauze or tubular non-adhesive wrap • Change dressings according to the manufacturer's recommendations
Documentation	• Record details of skin tear, describe or photograph wound, record details of dressings and implementation of measures to reduce the risk of further occurrences

developing a pressure injury or a perineal skin infection.[15] It is recognised that IAD development is influenced by the type of incontinence, with the presence of frequent liquid faeces placing a patient at the highest risk.[15] The prevalence of faecal incontinence in the ICU has been reported to be as high as 78%, with the prevalence of diarrhoea reported to be 13%.[16] Prevention and treatment of IAD involves removing or reducing skin exposure to urine and faeces or both.[15] Prevention and management of IAD should include a skin protection product designed to form a barrier between the skin and the irritant. While prevention and treatment regimens include cleansing and protection, treatment may also require the management of a possible skin infection.[17]

Medical adhesive-related skin injuries

Medical adhesives are used commonly in the intensive care setting, yet patient skin injuries caused by medical adhesive remain an under-reported complication. Skin injury occurs when skin to adhesive attachment is stronger than the skin cell to skin cell attachment, causing the epidermal layers to separate or complete separation of the epidermis from the dermis.[18] This may be seen as skin stripping, tension injuries or blisters, skin tears, irritant contact or allergic dermatitis, maceration or folliculitis. A history of patient allergies and sensitivities should be obtained and documented. The skin underneath adhesives should be assessed at least daily for evidence of damage, and a comprehensive assessment performed to determine injury severity. Prevention of MARSI includes identification of at-risk patients, for example older adult critically ill patients, patients with dermatological conditions, gross oedema, malnutrition or dehydration. Care of these patients includes the use of gentler adhesives, barrier products and medical adhesive removers.[18]

Skin tears

Skin tears result from routine activities such as dressing, positioning and transferring.[19] Dependent patients who require total care, older adults, those with fragile skin (particularly those with a history of previous skin tears), those who require the use of devices to assist lifting, those who are cognitively or sensorially impaired and those who have skin problems such as oedema, purpura or ecchymosis are at greatest risk. Most skin tears occur on the arms and the back of the hands. The International Skin Tear Advisory Panel classification system[19] uses three categories to describe skin tears: skin tears without tissue loss; skin tears with partial tissue (flap) loss; and skin tears with complete tissue (flap) loss.

Skin tears can be prevented by careful handling of patients to reduce skin friction and shear during repositioning and transfers. Padded bed rails, pillows and blankets can be used to protect and support arms and legs. Paper-type or non-adherent dressings should be used on frail skin, and should be removed gently and slowly. Wraps or nets can be used instead of surgical tape to secure dressings and drains in place. Application of a moisturising lotion to dry skin helps to keep it adequately hydrated. Treatment of skin tears[19] is outlined in Table 5.6. The focus of nursing care should be on careful cleansing and protection of the skin tear to prevent further damage and documentation of interventions and healing progress.

Practice tip 4

Monitor any bruising regularly, as these areas may be at risk of developing skin tears.

Eye care

The eyes are one of the most sensitive parts of the human body. Simple bedside procedures such as turning on lights at night or assessing pupil reactions can be uncomfortable. There are a number of physiological processes that protect the eye. For example, the eye is protected from dryness by frequent lubrication facilitated by blinking. Antimicrobial substances in tears help prevent infection, and the tear ducts provide drainage. When the eye is unable to close properly, the tear film evaporates more quickly.[20] If any of these defence mechanisms are compromised the eyes are at greater risk of injury.[21]

There is considerable risk to patients' eyes while they are in the ICU.[22] The blink response may be slowed or absent in some patients, such as individuals receiving sedatives and muscle relaxants, or those with Guillain–Barré syndrome. A number of complications can result, such as keratopathy, corneal ulceration and viral or bacterial conjunctivitis.[21] Corneal abrasions may occur within 48 hours of ICU admission and in up to 40–60% of critically ill patients.[21,23] When the eyes are exposed they are at greater risk of injury and infection, and conjunctival oedema (see more information below) can lead to sub-conjunctival haemorrhage. For the intensive care patient, who often has multiple intravenous lines, nasogastric tubes, ventilation tubes and their various connections, there is potential to unintentionally damage one of the eyes with one of these devices during position changes.

Eye assessment

Eye assessment should be undertaken and findings documented as soon as possible after admission and thereafter at least every 12 hours, even for conscious patients who are able to blink spontaneously. Do not forget to check if the patient wears contact lenses and, if they are in situ, take them out to reduce risk of corneal surface infection. Document if the patient normally uses glasses or contact lenses. If the glasses are present but not used, they should be labelled and stored safely.

The general principles of eye assessment are shown in Table 5.7, including a full examination of the eye's external structure, colour and response. Various assessment tools have been developed for this purpose; however, a universally accepted protocol for the protection of eyes in the ICU does not exist.[24] Thorough eye assessment should assess appearance (which may provide indications of disease or trauma) and physical and neurological functions. If there is concern about any aspect of a patient's eyes, a referral for assessment should be made to an ophthalmologist.

The risk of corneal abrasion or iatrogenic trauma is greatest when patients are unable to close their eyes spontaneously.[25] The second at-risk group is those patients receiving positive pressure ventilation, who may develop conjunctival oedema (chemosis), sometimes referred to as 'ventilator eye'.[21] Thirdly, patients who are exposed to high flows of air/oxygen, such as that with continuous positive airway pressure (CPAP) systems, may be vulnerable to its drying effects. Finally, all patients are at risk of eye inflammation and infection. Serious infections with bacteria such as pseudomonas can progress rapidly, resulting in blindness if not treated promptly.

Essential eye care

The goals of eye care are to provide comfort and protect the eyes from injury and infection. Eye care and the administration of artificial tears should be provided as required, if the patient complains of sore or dry eyes or if there is visible evidence of encrustation. If a patient is receiving high-flow oxygen therapy via a mask, they may benefit from regular 4-hourly administration of artificial tears to lubricate the eyes,[25] although this may be unnecessary while they are sleeping. An evidence-based eye care guideline for critically ill patients is outlined in Table 5.8.[26] Further recommendations relate to regular monitoring, reporting and timely referral of ophthalmologic complications.

For at-risk patients, the general consensus is that eye care should be performed using a sterile technique, cleansing the eye from the outside towards the nose usually with saline and gauze; however, eye care regimens have not been rigorously researched. Cotton wool is not recommended because of the presence of particulates that may cause corneal abrasions. Eyedrops should be administered gently, inserting the drop in the uppermost part of the opened eye and as close to the eye as possible without touching it. Sometimes eyedrops can sting, so it is advisable to warn the patient of this possibility. Regular scheduled eye care with an ocular lubricant plus eye closure with tape or wrap is used to

TABLE 5.7
Assessment of the eyes

EXTERNAL STRUCTURE	COLOUR	REACTION
• Is it bulging or misshapen? • Is the pupil circular? • What size are the pupils? • Are both pupils the same size? • Is the pupil clear? • Is there any visible trauma? • Is it weeping? • Does it look dry or moist?	• Is the sclera its normal off-white colour or is there evidence of jaundice or haemorrhage? • Does it look red and inflamed?	• Is the blink reflex present? • Do both pupils react to light with equal speed? • Is there a composite reaction to light in the opposite eye?

TABLE 5.8
Eyecare in the critically ill

Assessment	Patients must be assessed for risk factors for iatrogenic eye complications
	Daily assessment of the ability of the patient to maintain eyelid closure
	Weekly assessment of iatrogenic eye complication (at the microepithelial level) using instillation or fluorescein or a cobalt blue pen torch
Management	Eyelid closure should be maintained either passively or mechanically
	All patients who cannot achieve eyelid closure should receive 2-hourly eye care
	Eye care should be cleaning with saline-soaked gauze and administration of an eye-specific lubricant

Adapted from Marshall A, Elliott R, Rolls K, et al. Eye care in the critically ill: clinical practice guideline. Aust Crit Care 2008;21(2);97–109, with permission.

reduce the potential for corneal abrasions or subsequent corneal ulceration or infection in patients who are either paralysed or heavily sedated.[22]

Practice tip 5

Another source of irritant to the eyes can be the constant air flow from air-conditioning vents or fans, so check that your patient at risk is not positioned directly in line with these vents or poorly positioned fans.

Conjunctival oedema (chemosis)

Conjunctival oedema (chemosis) or 'ventilator eye', is a common problem associated with positive pressure ventilation, positive end-expiratory pressure (PEEP) above 5 cmH_2O and prone positioning.[20] Although the oedema itself usually resolves without treatment when ventilation is discontinued, it may be advisable to seek an ophthalmic opinion if there is concern. Evidence is inconclusive concerning the best method of treatment for conjunctival oedema, but evidence supports the use of artificial tear ointment and maintaining eye closure as effective measures to reduce corneal abrasions.[20]

Severe oedema often results in the patient's inability to maintain eye closure. Under these circumstances, the majority opinion is that eye closure may be maintained by applying a wide piece of adhesive tape horizontally to the upper part of the eyelid.[19] This usually anchors the lid in the closed position, while allowing the eyelid to be opened for pupil assessment and access for eye care. It is not necessary to change the tape at each pupil assessment using this method. However, the use of tape may be inappropriate for patients whose skin is very friable. Furthermore, if the eyelid becomes sore and inflamed, taping should be discontinued and an alternative method employed to close the eyes, e.g. cover the eye with polyethylene film, which has been shown to reduce the incidence of corneal abrasion.[25] This should be changed 4-hourly with eye care and assessment. Commercially available eye-closing tape products are also available along with gel eye dressings, which may be used instead of polyethylene film.[27,28] Current evidence indicates that polyethylene film is the superior and most cost-effective product for maintaining the ocular surface.[28] When it is not possible to close the eyes, artificial tear ointment has been shown to reduce the incidence of corneal abrasion.

Oral hygiene

Poor oral hygiene is unpleasant, causing halitosis and discomfort. Mouth care is one of the most basic nursing activities; neglecting it can lead to serious complications or increase risk, such as ventilator-associated pneumonia in the ventilated patient.[29] Attendance to oral hygiene including the removal of dental plaque that harbours pathogens is an important component of nursing care.[30] Using a well-developed oral protocol can improve the oral health of ICU patients. However, the practice of mouth care is not always evidence based.[31] Factors associated with poor quality of oral care include lack of education, insufficient time, non-prioritising of oral care and the perception that it is unpleasant.[32] Saliva produces protective enzymes, but absence of mastication, for example due to the presence of an endotracheal tube (ETT) or deep sedation, leads to a reduction in saliva production. An ETT can cause pressure areas in the mouth (which may be exacerbated if the patient is oedematous) and may thus need to be relocated regularly to a different position in the patient's mouth.

Oral assessment

Mouth care should be reviewed regularly, based on a thorough assessment of the oral cavity. Oral assessment tools have been designed specifically for intubated patients.[33] Essentially, a healthy mouth is characterised by several factors, as identified in Box 5.1; all of which should be assessed as a basis for good oral care.

BOX 5.1

Characteristics of a healthy mouth

- Pink moist oral mucosa and gums. Absence of coating, redness, ulceration or bleeding
- Pink, moist tongue. No coating, cracking, blisters or areas of redness
- Clean teeth/dentures; free of debris, plaque and dental caries
- Well-fitting dentures
- Adequate salivation
- Smooth and moist lips. No cracking, bleeding or ulceration
- No difficulties eating or swallowing

Essential oral care

Oral care aims to ensure healthy oral mucosa, prevent halitosis, maintain a clean and moist oral cavity, prevent pressure sores from devices such as ETTs, prevent trauma caused by grinding of teeth or biting of the tongue and reduce bacterial activity that leads to local and systemic infection.[29] Keeping the mucosa moist is the basic rule for oral care. Oral care for a non-intubated conscious patient with a healthy mouth generally involves daily observation of the mucosa and twice-daily tooth brushing with a non-irritant fluoride toothpaste. Oral care should generally be performed 2-hourly for unconscious patients, although the evidence is inconclusive and frequency ranges from 2- to 12-hourly.[34] If the mouth is unhealthy, it may be necessary to provide oral hygiene even more frequently.

The basic method for oral care is to use a soft toothbrush and toothpaste (even for intubated patients), which will assist with gum care as well as cleaning teeth.[31] Toothpaste loosens debris[31] and fluoride helps to prevent dental caries.[35] Brush teeth, tongue, and ETT if present. If the patient has a bone-anchored bridge, brush extra carefully in the gap between the jawbone and the tooth to prevent infection up in the jawbone. Lately, it has been debated but not yet fully explored if and in what degree the surfactant sodium lauryl sulfate (SLS) (found in many toothpastes) interfere with chlorhexidine.[36] Choose a toothpaste without SLS to prevent reduced effect of chlorhexidine. Be aware that some toothpastes contain small amounts of milk proteins and eggs, important if the patient is allergic. Rinse away the toothpaste properly, as toothpaste dries the oral mucosa. Using mouth swabs only for oral hygiene is ineffective, and toothbrushes perform substantially better than foam swabs in removing plaque.[35] Thirst is one of the most distressing symptoms critically ill patients suffer;[37] therefore, regular sips of fluid or mouth washing with water is recommended. Immunosuppressed patients or those on high-dose antibiotics may also require antifungal treatment to treat oral thrush.

There are many oral hygiene products and solutions available to suit the needs of all patients. Commercial mouthwashes should be used as a comfort measure to supplement toothbrushing.[30] A range of other products is available to treat oral problems, for example benzydamine hydrochloride (anti-inflammatory), aqueous lignocaine (anaesthetic) and nystatin (antifungal). Chlorhexidine gluconate mouthwash has long been – and is still – used as a part of the oral hygiene care to prevent ventilator-associated pneumonia (VAP) of adult critically ill patients receiving mechanically ventilation. However, the extent to which chlorhexidine is beneficial for patient outcomes is not clear and requires further investigation as a recently published review found only moderate evidence of significant effects.[30] Chlorhexidine gluconate mouthwash has the disadvantage of an unpleasant taste and can discolour teeth.

Practice tip 6

If patients object to the taste of the chlorhexidine gluconate mouthwash, consider a follow-up rinse of water.

Practice tip 7

Performing oral hygiene with toothbrush and toothpaste in an intubated patient and ensuring the mouth is rinsed well may be assisted by the use of a dental sucker, which is flexible. This disposable device attached to a continuous suction system can be positioned in the mouth to aid in the continual removal of fluids while brushing and rinsing is performed.

Patient positioning and mobilisation

Positioning patients correctly is important for their comfort and the reduction of complications associated with pressure areas[7] and joint immobility. Lying in bed for long periods can be a painful experience. Neuromyopathy from critical illness and disuse atrophy from prolonged immobility is described as contributing to intensive care-acquired weakness.[38] This weakness may contribute to prolonged ventilation and intensive care length of stay as well as delayed return to physical normality.[39] Cardiovascular stability, respiratory function and cerebral or spinal function are all factors that influence the positioning of patients in critical care areas.

The primary goals of essential nursing care for patient positioning are:

- to position the patient comfortably
- to enhance therapeutic benefits

- to prevent pressure injuries, venous thromboembolism and pulmonary dysfunction
- to ensure the limbs are supported appropriately and to maintain flexible joints
- to facilitate patient activity to minimise muscle atrophy
- to implement early mobilisation as the patient's condition allows.

Practice tip 8

Movement of the lower legs, ankles and feet can be achieved in conjunction with a gentle massage or application of moisturiser. Family members may wish to undertake this, giving them an opportunity to provide the patient with care and touch.

Assessment of body positioning

Patients at highest risk of complications related to their position are those who are unable to move for long periods. For example, unstable patients whose status is compromised when they are moved, patients who are in critical care for a long time, older adult and frail or malnourished patients and patients who are unable to move themselves (e.g. due to sedation, trauma, surgery or obesity) are all at risk. Other risk factors exist such as age, length of intensive care stay, use of adrenaline and/or noradrenaline infusions; patients with comorbidities such as cardiovascular disease and diabetes and unstable patients.[40] However, even previously fit patients who experience a critical illness can develop severe limitations in their mobility. Regular musculoskeletal assessment should be made, focusing on the patient's major muscles and joints and the degree of mobility. Table 5.9 offers a simple guide to assessment, which includes visual and physical assessment of all limbs and joints. Provided there are no contraindications, function should be stimulated by regular passive then active movements of all limbs and joints to maintain both flexibility and comfort.

TABLE 5.9
Musculoskeletal assessment

MUSCLES AND JOINTS	MOBILITY
• Power/strength • Range of movement • Symmetry • Tenderness and pain • Inflammation, swelling, wasting	• Degree of independence • Need for assistance • Adherence/compliance with physiotherapy/ mobility regimen • Need for planned rest periods • Use of splints or collar

Positioning and mobilising patients

Positioning the patient to achieve maximum comfort, therapeutic benefit and pressure area relief and employing active and passive exercises to maintain muscle and joint integrity and progress to regaining mobility are important nursing activities. Provided there are no specific contraindications, the immobile patient should be positioned with the head raised by 30° or more, as research has demonstrated that it improves mortality and helps reduce VAP.[40] When combined with thromboembolic prophylaxis, gastric ulcer prophylaxis and daily sedation assessment, VAP may be reduced by around 45%.[41]

The routine standard for immobilised patients in ICU is 2-hourly body repositioning, although the optimal interval for turning critically ill patients is unknown.[7] Repositioning promotes comfort, relaxation and rest; helps inflate both lungs, improves oxygenation and helps mobilise airway secretions; to orient the patient to the surroundings and for a change of view; and to improve circulation to limbs through movement.[42]

Good body alignment helps prevent pressure points, contractures and unnecessary pain or discomfort for the patient.[42] Here, careful consideration should be given to factors (outlined in Table 5.10) such as haemodynamic and cardiopulmonary responses of the patient, the timing and method of positioning patients and whether there are any restrictions on movement. For example, for patients with spinal injuries, log-rolling may be required (see Chapter 17).

Mobilisation for the critically ill patient can be described as a graduated increase in range of activity from positioning, passive movement, sitting upright in bed, sitting in a chair to actually ambulating.[40] Two groups of safety factors need to be considered prior to mobilising the critically ill patient: those specific to the patient and their physical and physiological condition and those extrinsic to the patient such as the environment, staffing and devices. Creating an individualised mobility plan that can be adapted according to patient assessment and general health progress will optimise early movement and mobilisation. Early mobilisation improves patient outcomes. It is best achieved through a multidisciplinary team approach.[43]

Practice tip 9

Even small readjustments in positioning may improve patient comfort and often can be made without much effort by the nurse or disturbance to the resting patient. Most electric beds provide for adjustments to the backrest angle, knee bend and bed tilt, and adjustments can be easily made. In addition to comfort, these adjustments will aid in pressure changes between repositioning of the patient.

TABLE 5.10
Factors to consider when positioning patients

FACTORS	COMMENTS
Haemodynamic and cardiopulmonary responses	• Placing patients in the left lateral position can cause a (usually harmless) fall in oxygenation for a few minutes
Timing	• Position the patient to avoid clashes with treatment/investigations such as chest physiotherapy or chest X-ray • Consider the need for the patient to rest
Method	• The need to use lifting devices • The availability of staff to perform a safe manoeuvre • The placement of pillows to support limbs, to facilitate both comfort and respiratory efficiency • Use of bed adjustments to create 'chair' positions to prepare patients to sit out of bed
Restrictions on positioning	• The need for spinal alignment • Cerebral injury • Haemodynamic instability • Respiratory compromise • Access to devices for therapies • Body size

Practice tip 10

When planning repositioning, ensure there are enough staff to give the patient a sense of security, which also ensures the patient's devices (e.g. IV lines) are managed. Check that all devices are placed to accommodate the repositioning before you begin to move the patient.

Active and passive exercises

Physical activity is essential to healthy functioning and beneficial for the cardiovascular system,[40] yet spontaneous physical activity decreases by as much as 50% in hospitalised patients.[44] Inactivity, age and the inflammatory process that occurs during critical illness combine to progress muscle breakdown and loss of physical function in older hospitalised patients with muscle mass reduction, which occurs as early as several hours from the onset of immobility.[44] Active exercises are those that can be performed by the patient with no, or minimal, assistance. Passive exercises are performed when patients are either too weak or incapable of active exercise. Exercises can be employed to help patients develop power and regain function, and assist in venous return and maintenance of normal sensations of movement.[44] They should be performed at least daily. Passive exercises put the main joints through their range of movement, which helps reduce joint stiffness and maintain muscle integrity, preventing contractures. Shoulders, hands, hips and ankles are particularly at risk of stiffness and muscle contracture. It is important, however, to ensure that joints and muscles are not overstretched, as this is painful for patients and can cause permanent injury. Splints may be used when the patient is resting, to maintain joints in a neutral position.[44] The physiotherapist's advice should be sought regarding the correct range of movement and the frequency of passive exercises; particularly important for burn-injured patients.

Concern has been expressed about the effects of limb movements on head-injured patients; however, two early seminal studies detected no significant cardiovascular or neurological changes during passive exercises in neurosurgical patients,[45] and found no detrimental effects on cerebral perfusion or intracranial pressure (ICP), whether ICP was raised or not.[46]

Rotational therapy

Continuous lateral rotation therapy or kinetic bed therapy is an intervention in which the patient is rotated continually, on a specialised bed, through a set number of degrees; it helps to relieve pressure areas and can significantly improve oxygenation. Continuous lateral rotation therapy may reduce the prevalence of VAP in patients requiring long-term ventilation.[47] Appropriate evaluation of the benefits and suitability of the patient for continuous lateral rotation therapy should be undertaken by the team and the therapy implemented according to local protocols. In implementing this therapy, the goal is to achieve continuous rotation through the maximum angle that the patient tolerates for 18 hours per day.[47]

Venous thromboembolism (VTE) prophylaxis

Deep vein thrombosis (DVT) and pulmonary embolism (PE) are separate conditions collectively referred to as venous thromboembolism (VTE).[48] Blood clots form in major veins of the lower body due to poor venous flow, endothelial injury to the vein, trauma, venous stasis or coagulation disorders.[49] Pulmonary emboli occur when a part of a thrombosis moves through the circulation and lodges in the pulmonary circulation. VTE is a major risk factor for hospitalised patients in general and critically ill patients in particular, due to blood vessel damage, coagulation disorders and limited mobility leading to venous stasis.[48] Further, around 50% of patients with DVT will also suffer a PE, which can be fatal.[48] Patients with VTE may also develop post-thrombotic syndrome where tissue injury occurs leading to pain, paraesthesia, pruritus, oedema, venous dilatation and venous ulcers.[49]

It is important to consider the individual patient (age, body mass index) and their history (previous VTE, coagulation disorders) along with their current condition, whether it be surgical or medical, and features of their treatment (immobilisation) when determining risks for VTE.[50] Both the risk assessment and the patient's current condition will determine the most appropriate VTE prophylaxis strategy.[51] Prophylaxis consists of a combination of pharmacological and mechanical interventions that may be used together or separately according to the degree of risk for VTE and/or contraindications to particular therapies. The use of combined therapies is supported by reviews and guidelines.[49,51] The National Health and Medical Research Council clinical practice guideline for the prevention of venous thromboembolism (DVT and PE) in patients admitted to Australian hospitals[48] provides a comprehensive guide to risks and management relating to VTE for critical care in Australia.

Low-molecular-weight heparin or unfractionated heparin is the most common pharmacological therapy prescribed, while other medications will be prescribed for patients according to individual factors.[48,52] In principle, it is advised that graduated compression stockings are used for all general, cardiac, thoracic and vascular surgical patients until full mobility is achieved irrespective of pharmacological prophylaxis.[48,51] Mechanical prophylaxis is provided through a range of graduated compression stockings and various pneumatic venous pump or sequential compression devices.[53,54] It is important to make sure that the relevant devices are fitted correctly and monitored closely.

Along with pharmacological and mechanical venous thromboembolism prophylaxis, maintaining patients' hydration and implementing early mobilisation are key components of care in preventing VTE.[48,50] Rauen et al[55] describe the most common reasons cited for lack of proper VTE prophylaxis as being lack of knowledge among healthcare providers and underestimation of the risk of VTE along with overestimation of the potential risk of bleeding from prophylaxis. Given the risks of VTE for critically ill patients, it is clearly important that nurses contribute to lowering risks for their patients by knowing the range of risk factors for their patients, along with the appropriate pharmacological prophylaxis that may be prescribed. It is also important to know how to appropriately implement and manage the mechanical prophylactic devices and, most importantly, facilitate the early mobilisation of the patient.

Bowel management

Although bowel care is an essential nursing care, there is limited research on the topic specific to ICU patients. Good bowel care promotes patient comfort and reduces the risks of associated problems such as nausea, vomiting and abdominal/pelvic discomfort. Maintaining good bowel care in the critically ill patient can have changing foci from promoting defecation to containing diarrhoea, as throughout critical illness, gut function is influenced by changing therapies, medications, nutrition, hydration and mobility of the patient. Enteral feeding is often cited in the literature as a cause of diarrhoea,[56] but poor gastric fluid intake causes constipation, and improved gut motility decreases the risk of aspiration and subsequent pneumonia. Additional to the need to manage faecal incontinence, the two spectrums of constipation and diarrhoea are particular challenges for nurses to provide patient-specific, effective management in a sensitive and dignified way for their critically ill patient.

Bowel care can be one of the most distressing aspects of nursing care, from a patient's perspective. Often patients find bowel care to be awkward and embarrassing, and the routines that individuals may have developed, especially the older adult, to sustain effective bowel function in their daily lives are then interrupted by their illness, and their loss of control over their body for this function can be particularly distressing. Sensitive nursing care that respects the dignity of the patient is paramount.

Bowel assessment

Initial bowel assessment should be undertaken to determine the patient's usual bowel habits, as a daily bowel action is not common for most of the population. In general, older patients are more susceptible to constipation. Gut function should be assessed at the start of each nursing shift[56] (Box 5.2). Studies suggest that use of a protocol improves bowel care in critically ill patients.[57,58] Protocols may include rectal examination undertaken if the patient has not had their bowels open for 3

BOX 5.2

Assessment of gut function

- Observation of nasogastric aspirate volume
- Visual inspection and palpation of abdomen, noting any tenderness, pain or distension
- Recording the frequency, nature and quantity of bowel actions
- The presence or absence of bowels sounds

TABLE 5.11
Bristol stool form scale

GRADE	DESCRIPTION
0	No bowel movement
1	Separate hard lumps; like nuts; hard to pass
2	Sausage-shaped but lumpy
3	Like a sausage but with cracks on the surface
4	Like a sausage or snake but smooth and soft
5	Soft blobs with clear-cut edges; easily passed
6	Fluffy pieces with ragged edges; a mushy stool
7	Watery; no solid pieces; entirely liquid

Lewis SJ, Heaton KW. Stool form scale as a useful guide to intestinal transit time. Scand J Gastroenterol. 1997;32 (9):920–4. Reprinted by permission of the publisher, Taylor & Francis Ltd., http://www.tandfonline.com.

consecutive days,[58] and alternative therapies as determined from the examination results. For some patients in whom defecation is problematic, it may be appropriate to objectively assess the quality of faecal stools using a tool such as the Bristol stool form scale, which uses a 7-point grading system to assess stool consistency (Table 5.11).[58] Establishing the cause of faecal incontinence is important as this will direct the treatment and management plan. Faecal incontinence may occur in conditions such as neurological and spinal conditions, intestinal diseases such as Crohn's, cognitive impairment such as dementia or may be the result of anal sphincter or rectal injury or dysfunction, medications or intestinal impaction and overflow.[59]

Practice tip 11

When undertaking bowel assessment consider the patient's normal diet and any laxatives routinely taken, as this information may influence any bowel regimen developed for the patient.

Essential bowel care

Nursing care is based on providing privacy and managing patient embarrassment, increasing exercise where possible, ensuring adequate fibre and fluid in the diet, reducing unnecessary use of drugs that cause constipation and appropriate use of laxative agents. Where bowel care is concerned, it is always appropriate to first explain to patients what is to be done, and to gain their consent if they are conscious. Constant reassurance is important so that patients feel safe and secure in the knowledge that their privacy will be maintained to the greatest degree possible.

Peristaltic movement of the gut is stimulated by exercise. Although difficult in the intensive care setting, many patients are awake, and even those who require sedation should be sedated with the minimal amount necessary for their safety, as this will enable some degree of movement. Promoting patient mobility, especially voluntary movement, helps to improve gut motility.

Ensuring the appropriate administration of fluid and an adequate dietary fibre intake[60] helps to prevent constipation and maintain normal bowel function. Although enteral feeding increases faecal bulk and provides gastric fluid, which helps to maintain gut motility, Bishop et al[61] found a higher rate of enteral nutrition was strongly associated with a looser type of stool. Choice of enteral formula is important, and Chapter 19 contains an in-depth discussion on the principles of enteral feeding.

The use of sedatives is often an ascribed cause of constipation in critically ill patients. This is not due to their direct effect, but due to the subsequent immobility of patients when sedatives are used. Opiates, which are often used to control pain, slow propulsive gut contraction. In a small cohort study, Sawh et al[62] reported the successful resumption of target enteral feeding after treating opioid-induced constipation with subcutaneous methylnaltrexone. The main drugs that cause constipation in critical care settings are analgesics, anaesthetic agents, anticonvulsants, diuretics and calcium channel blockers. Although it is difficult to avoid giving these drugs, their judicious use in tandem with other preventive measures will help avoid constipation. Antiemetic and prokinetic agents can also be used in critical care patients and Bishop et al[61] found the administration of ondansetron was a significant predictor of defecation on that day in their critical care patient cohort.

Constipation

Constipation is common in critically ill patients; its incidence varies from 5–83%.[63] Variations in incidence may be attributed to the lack of a consistent definition for constipation. Constipation is described as fewer than three bowel movements per week, incomplete evacuation, hard or difficult to pass stools or the requirement of manual faecal removal, according to the American Gastroenterological Association.[64]

Causes of constipation in critically ill patients range from shock and reduced gut motility to changes in nutrition and lack of mobility. The consequences of constipation are not well defined but can include increased abdominal distension and resulting impedance of lung function, inability to establish adequate enteral nutrition and increased acquired bacterial infections.[65] The prevention of constipation is particularly important for patients with high cervical spinal injuries, as if left untreated it may cause potentially fatal autonomic dys-reflexia.[65] De Azevedo et al[60] discussed the need to determine whether constipation is a marker of severity and poor prognosis in critically ill patients or if it is a dysfunction contributing to a worsening clinical condition. However, the need for effective prevention and management of constipation in critically ill patients is clear.

Non-pharmacological methods to reduce constipation include exercise or moving, increasing fluid intake and adding dietary fibre.[56] These means should be implemented routinely before the need to use laxatives arises. There are many types of laxatives available, which can be given to prevent or treat constipation. Bulk-forming agents work by increasing faecal size; stimulants, such as senna, increase peristalsis; and osmotic agents draw fluid into the gut. Faecal impaction should be treated with enemas, not stimulant laxatives. In general, existing protocols advise that treatment of constipation should commence with senna administration and, if ineffective after 2–3 days, lactulose should be commenced.[57]

Diarrhoea

Diarrhoea can be a major problem for intensive care patients, and in severe cases may lead to electrolyte imbalances, dehydration, malnutrition (see also Chapter 19) and skin breakdown. Furthermore, it can be very distressing for the patient, who may also suffer from abdominal distension, nausea and cramp-like pain. Investigations should be implemented to determine the cause of the diarrhoea and the patient should be managed with appropriate precautions to prevent cross-contamination if the cause is infectious. If laxatives are being given they should be stopped, and a stool specimen should be obtained for microbiological examination. Anti-motility drugs may be used, except with bloody diarrhoea or proven infection with *E. coli*.[57] Appropriate rehydration should be implemented. If patients are being fed enterally there may be a reduction in episodes of diarrhoea if fibre-enriched feed is used.[56]

Faecal containment devices should be used in severe cases of diarrhoea in conjunction with all other measures to support the patient's comfort.[66] Broadly, indications for use of a faecal containment device are persistent diarrhoea, diagnosis of *C. difficile* infection, peri-anal wound or skin breakdown in the presence of incontinence, plus the patient must have anal sphincter tone to enable securement of the device balloon.[66,67] Firstly the patient should be assessed for their suitability for using the incontinence system against the manufacturer's guidelines. And then whether there are any conditions or factors to prevent safe use of the device for individual patients, such as allergy to the materials in the product, risk of autonomic dysreflexia in spinal cord injury patients, or rectal and anal conditions.[66,67] It is imperative that both medical and nursing consultation occurs, along with patient consent before use of such devices as the potential for complications ranges from discomfort and failure of the device through to infection and rectal and bowel injuries. Faecal management devices and associated rectal haemorrhage, or development of recto-urethral and ano-vaginal fistulas have been reported.[68-70] An appropriate bowel therapy regimen and close monitoring of these systems should be implemented to optimise functioning and reduce risk.

Practice tip 12

Monitoring the security and position of a faecal management system is necessary for effective functioning of the system as well as the prevention of pressure-related injury and potential rectal bleeding.

Urinary catheter care

Urinary catheters are inserted into many critically ill patients. Catheter-associated urinary tract infections (CAUTI) are a common cause of infection in this group and are associated with increased mortality and length of stay in the ICU.[71] Monitoring the incidence of CAUTI is a requirement in many jurisdictions. In principle, urinary catheters should be inserted only when deemed clinically necessary, and they should be removed as soon as they are no longer required clinically. Alternatives to urinary catheterisation should be considered; however, most critically ill patients require accurate monitoring of their urinary output and fluid balance, and a catheter is required for this reason.[72] CAUTI are primarily caused by contamination from the healthcare worker or from the patient's own flora during catheter insertion or management of the urinary drainage system or via reflux of contaminated urine.[73] While routine screening for urinary tract infection is not required,[73] critical care nurses should be mindful of the risk factors for CAUTI such as prolonged catheterisation, older patients, impaired immunity and any breaches in good practices related to the insertion and maintenance of urinary catheters and drainage.[73] The consequences of poor urinary catheter care and management are not only distressing to the patient but detrimental to their health.

Urinary catheterisation assessment

The rationale for urinary catheter insertion outlined in Table 5.12 should be carefully considered and a portable ultrasound to evaluate the volume of bladder urine may help with the assessment.[72] Once it is established that a urinary catheter is necessary, the type of catheter should be determined. While the primary purpose of urinary catheters is management of urine drainage, the choice of catheter type may be influenced by the concurrent need for urinary temperature monitoring. The smallest size catheter possible is used to reduce bladder neck and urethral damage[73] although narrow-bore tubes flex easily, which can be problematic in male catheterisation. Larger-diameter catheters may be required to drain haematuria and clots. The routine use of antibiotic-impregnated catheters or silver alloy catheters is not currently recommended.[73]

Urinary catheterisation essential care

Catheter insertion and maintenance should be according to facility policies and undertaken by people appropriately trained in the procedures.[73] Aseptic techniques

TABLE 5.12
Urinary catheter quick reference

COMPONENT OF CARE	CONSIDERATIONS
Rationale for insertion and/or continuing use *Reevaluate continuing use daily against rationale and remove catheter as soon as possible when no longer required*	Acute urinary retention or bladder obstruction Need for accurate measurement of urinary output in critically ill patients Perioperative use for selected surgical procedures Assist in healing of open sacral or perineal wounds in incontinent patients Patient requiring prolonged immobilisation, e.g. spinal injury Patient admitted with chronic indwelling catheter Exceptional circumstances such as to improve end-of-life care
Insertion *Use principles of aseptic non-touch technique*	Follow documented facility policy on urinary catheter insertion Staff performing procedure follow policy and are trained in technique Use sterile equipment, including sterile drape Use aseptic technique when inserting catheter and connecting to sterile drainage system Clean meatus with sterile normal saline before catheter insertion Use appropriate sterile, single-use lubricant or anaesthetic gel Secure catheter after insertion to prevent movement and urethral traction Document insertion information in patient record
Maintenance *Consider each shift:* • *How long has the catheter been in situ?* • *Is the catheter still required?* • *Are there any indications of infection or complications?* • *Is the drainage system being managed appropriately?*	Maintain aseptic continuously closed system drainage Perform hand hygiene and use non-sterile gloves prior to any manipulation of the drainage system Position drainage bag to prevent backflow or contact with floor Empty drainage bag frequently to maintain urine flow and prevent reflux and empty before patient transport Use separate urine collection container for each patient, avoiding contact between drainage bag and container. This collection container should be discarded if single use or cleaned and sterilised if reusable Change drainage bags only according to manufacturers' guidelines or patients clinical need, without clamping as it is unnecessary Daily meatal hygiene via routine hygiene Avoid use of bladder irrigation, instillation or washouts as routine measures to prevent catheter-associated infections Document all related assessment and procedures for the catheter and drainage system

Adapted from NHMRC Australian guidelines for the prevention and control of infection in healthcare, http://www.nhmrc.gov.au; 2010 [accessed December 2017].

should be adhered to during catheter insertion, and hand hygiene should be performed before and after and gloves used during any manipulation of the catheter or drainage system.[73]

The urine drainage system should be sterile and continuously closed with an outlet designed to avoid contamination.[72] It should have a sample port for taking urine samples. Where appropriate, patients should be given a choice of system suited to their needs. For example, a shorter drainage tube with a leg-bag may be more comfortable for a patient who is mobile. All procedures involving the catheter and drainage system should be documented in the clinical notes, including size and type of catheter, balloon size and the date of insertion. If an anticipated date of removal is also documented at the time of insertion and subsequent assessments, it may trigger staff to remove the catheter as soon as possible.

Catheter maintenance

The ongoing need for a urinary catheter should be assessed on a daily basis. The introduction of criteria that enable registered nurses to remove catheters without a medical review may result in a reduction in catheter-related infections. Routine hygiene at appropriate intervals for patient comfort is adequate for urethral meatal care.[73]

Urinary catheters should be changed according to clinical need and with regard to the manufacturer's guidelines, and the closed drainage system should be broken only for limited, clearly defined clinical reasons. Bladder washout or irrigation should be avoided and only performed for a specific clinical reason, such as intermittent irrigation for clots or debris. If obstruction is likely, a closed continuous irrigation system may be utilised. Contamination of the drainage system outlet must be avoided during emptying. An aseptic technique and sterile equipment must be used when taking a urine sample via the sample port.

The whole drainage system should be maintained with patient comfort in mind, and care should be taken to ensure that the patient is not lying on the drainage tube, which can cause pressure sores and blockage. Furthermore, the catheter itself should be positioned and then secured so that it is not pulling on the urethra or kinked. The drainage bag should be kept below the level of the bladder at all times to maintain an unobstructed flow of urine,[73] and it should be emptied into a disinfected or single-use container. The drainage bag should be changed according to the manufacturer's instructions, which is usually in the range of 5–7 days. In addition, it should be replaced if it is leaking, if there has been a break in the closed system or whenever the catheter is changed.

Practice tip 13

Use a catheter support device or bandage on the leg to secure the urinary catheter. It lessens tension and irritation from catheter movement, patient comfort is improved, and it also promotes effective drainage and, in restless patients, may prevent accidental catheter removal as well.

Care of the older adult

Older adults are being admitted to the ICU in greater numbers as this section of the population continues to grow. There are no absolute definitions of older persons, but the United Nations describes 60 plus years as older, while many developed countries use 65 plus years as older.[74]

There are a multitude of physiological changes that result from ageing. Common causes of anaemia in older persons are iron deficiency and the presence of chronic disease or inflammation followed by chronic kidney dysfunction. When critically ill, anaemia may contribute to the older patient's fatigue, so careful consideration should always be given to planning activities such as hygiene and mobilisation. Some older patients are quite fragile, because of anorexia of ageing,[75,76] and, after 65 years of age, a person may have less body fat and lower weight as a consequence of reduced food intake. Acute illness or injury risks increasing the extent of malnutrition.[77] Other consequences include impaired muscle function and decreased bone mass, which impair mobility and lead to increased falls. Mobility problems are exacerbated by both loss of muscle mass and function and degenerative joint disease.[78] However, early mobilisation is as important for older adults as it is for younger persons with critical illness to prevent ICU-acquired weakness and reduce duration of mechanical ventilation.[79] Older adults' functional and cognitive status should be assessed and documented as soon as possible after admission, either through an evaluation tool or from the patient's family to identify patients at high risk of cognitive disabilities. In addition, daily monitoring should be performed to pay attention to potential changes. In ventilated patients, it is important to optimise sedation and pain management strategies to reduce the incidence of intensive care-associated delirium.[80,81]

Loss of muscle mass and then muscle activity reduces metabolic function and subsequently causes loss of body heat, so care should be taken to ensure the older adult is well covered at all times with additional lightweight warming devices available to be used as required.[82]

Skin, the biggest organ, is often the most visible sign of age in the older patient. The epidermis atrophies, especially in exposed areas of the body, and once over 65 years, blistered skin takes longer to repair than in a young adult. From fragile to easily bruised skin or moist skin folds in those who are overweight, careful hygiene care is required and consideration should be given to the use of specific products for these patients.

Practice tip 14

Pay extra attention to the positioning of devices when used with older adult patients and check them more frequently than normal, as the patient may not have full sensation in the affected area or the physical ability to adjust the device themselves, or the confidence to tell you that the device is causing pressure or discomfort. Examples may be non-invasive blood pressure cuffs that are left on too long or sequential compression device leggings that have slipped.

Persistent abdominal discomfort and pain should be triggers for considering bowel obstruction in older adults, as with age the colon is hypotonic resulting in slower stool transit and subsequent increased hardening of the stool from dehydration.[78] Faecal incontinence in older adults can be due to loss of anal sphincter tone and, therefore, planning for toileting is a practical way of managing continence and eliminating the distress caused by this problem. Symptoms of urinary tract infection, such as dysuria and frequency, are less likely to be as obvious in the older adult as in the young, as the capacity of the bladder decreases with age and especially if the patient suffers from stress incontinence already. As with other functions, ageing blunts the immune system response, which results in increased susceptibility of the older adult to infection. This, along with the additional deterioration in skin integrity and likely increased exposure to antibiotics over time, means that this group of patients may be at greater risk of hospital-acquired infections and multi-resistant organisms.[83]

Consideration should be given to a suitable environment for the older patients, such as increased soundproofing, more comfortable and supportive chairs, cutlery, and utensils that are easy to grip to enable meals that are more comfortable. Above all, nurses should adjust some of their behaviours with the older person, such as speaking clearly, listening carefully without interruption, anticipating frequent personal care needs and allowing time to enable mobilisation without haste, all of which may help to facilitate feelings of independence and control of their circumstances for these patients.[84]

Bariatric considerations

Obesity continues to be a major health issue around the world; an even a higher proportion of obese patients in the ICU exists compared to normal population.[85] Total body weight (TBW) in kg and body mass index (BMI) (weight (kg)/lengths (m^2)) are two common methods to classify under-, overweight and obesity in adults. While BMI is widely used, it has limitations as age and muscle mass are not included in the calculation. Lean body weight, a descriptor of weight devoid of all adipose tissue, and predicted normal body weight that takes into account gender, height and weight to estimate the fractional fat mass, are two other measures used. What applies to all bariatric care is that each patient is unique and all measures and treatments must be decided in relation to the individual patient's conditions and needs.

People who are obese contend with a negative bias[86] but this same negative bias from health professionals including nurses may then interfere with their ability to obtain quality healthcare.[87] The key to providing quality, patient-centred, sensitive care to the bariatric patient is R-E-S-P-E-C-T: **r**apport, **e**nvironment/**e**quipment, **s**afety, **p**rivacy, **e**ncouragement, **c**aring/**c**ompassion and **t**act.[87] Simple things such as an appropriately-sized gown and suitable bed linen that provide the patient with adequate covering are often not well-organised for this patient group, unless the nurse takes the time to arrange specific supplies if they are not routinely available.[88]

Respiratory considerations

Obese patients may have increased intraabdominal pressure and decreased chest wall compliance resulting in a decrease in low functional residual capacity and expiratory reserve volume. Obstructive sleep apnoea is common in the obese population. It is a state characterised by short episodes of apnoea (breathing cessation), accompanied by nocturnal oxygen desaturation and fragmented sleep[89] and results in impaired pulmonary gas exchange both at rest and with exercise.[90,91] These significant changes in static and dynamic respiratory mechanics adversely affect the patient in the form of changes in breathing such as increased respiratory rate, increased oxygen consumption, increased work of breathing and decreased tidal volumes. As a result, more oxygen is required and time to desaturation is decreased.[92] Lowered functional residual capacity increases the risk of atelectasis and therefore non-invasive ventilation and CPAP are tools necessary to help derecruitment (alveolar closing). To help obese patients in their work of breathing, positioning is important and a continuous active mobilisation regime may be necessary. When the airway is secured, the patient should sit in a reversed Trendelenburg position (head up, feet down), sometimes called 'beach chair position'. This position should decrease pressure on the diaphragm and therefore decrease intrathoracic pressure and as a result improve respiratory compliance and gas exchange.[93] If possible, the patient should be mobilised to bedside and standing as early as possible. Only a few studies have investigated prone position in severe hypoxemic obese patients with acute respiratory distress syndrome (ARDS). De Jong[94] found that the prone position was a safe method that may improve oxygenation more than in non-obese patients; however, another study found that abdominally obese patients cared for in the prone position developed renal failure and hypoxic hepatitis more frequently than non-obese patients.[95] More research in this area is needed.

Ventilation mode should be oriented on ideal bodyweight tidal volume 6–8 mL/kg. An individually adapted PEEP level is important. PEEP levels that are too low may result in atelectasis while excessive tidal volumes and high PEEP may generate higher autoPEEP and shear force and thus lung damage. Unfortunately, optimal PEEP level in obese critically ill patients is still unknown. As weaning often takes a longer time in bariatric patients, post-extubation non-invasive ventilation should be considered. Although there are risks with tracheostomy, this should be discussed early as well as a no-sedation strategy. Ensure there is a secure fit of tracheostomy support device – adjustment for increased neck circumference may be needed.

Circulation

Obesity affects the circulatory system in various ways through increased blood volume, decreased fibrinolysis, and increased blood viscosity. Polycythemia and increased activity of the renin–angiotensin system cause an increase in total blood volume and cardiac output.[91,96] Close glucose monitoring regimens should be implemented and appropriately calculated dosages for medications prescribed. As obese persons often have venous stasis disease, VTE prophylaxis is recommended with weight-adjusted dosing of medications.[49,97] Combining pharmacological and mechanical prophylaxis is recommended for this high-risk group. Care must be taken with measuring the limb to obtain the correct size legging or stocking. Early mobilisation is important. Extra consideration must be given to the patient's skin. Observe the entire skin costume several times daily. Be extra observant for exposed places like breast and lumps and keep the skin dry and clean.

Drugs and diets

There are many factors affecting the distribution, binding and elimination of drugs in obesity (Box 5.3). Therefore, drug doses must be individually adjusted to provide

BOX 5.3

Pharmacologic concerns in obesity

- Greater than normal amount adipose tissue
- Increased lean body mass
- Increased blood volume
- Smaller than normal fraction total body water
- Increased cardiac output
- Decreased pulmonary function
- Increased proteins, free fatty acids
- Increased renal blood flow
- Increased glomerular filtration rate
- Abnormal liver function

effects based on the patient's characteristics, thereby minimising side effects.[98] Drug doses are not necessarily administered according to the actual body weight, but more often are based on other dosing approaches. Sedation in the bariatric patient needs to be carefully managed to avoid the resultant risk of respiratory failure and need for ventilation. Reducing narcotic usage through use of combinations of other analgesia along with sedatives will also reduce the risk of respiratory failure.[99]

Equipment

Adapted techniques to enhance patient assessment may be required, such as auscultating over the left lateral chest wall to hear heart sounds while the patient is positioned towards their left side or using a thigh or regular blood pressure cuff on the patient's forearm. The use of arterial monitoring rather than non-invasive blood pressure measurements for patients receiving titrated vasoactive infusions should be considered, because of the difficulty in obtaining accurate readings if the cuff is not sized or positioned correctly. Use specific bariatric equipment and techniques to move patients safely for both the patient and the staff involved. It is important to be aware of the weight capacities of various facilities, such as lifts and equipment, which may be required in the care of the bariatric patient. Overweight patients can be challenging in any setting, and it is important to consider the health and safety of the staff involved in lifting and moving patients. Equally important is maintaining the patient's dignity and feeling of safety and minimising their self-consciousness during repositioning, irrespective of the method required. Lifts and hoists and other equipment that are designed for heavier people should be used.[100] A well-thought-out strategy by an interdisciplinary group can work through the local issues within a hospital or unit and produce a bariatric kit, containing a range of equipment appropriate to the needs of the bariatric patients in various settings including the ICU.

Practice tip 15

Ensure adequate equipment for obese patients is available including beds and wheelchairs. Identify and document weight capacity of equipment, such as how much weight beds and lifts can handle to ensure safe care.

General principles of infection control in critical care

Effective infection control is vital in the critical care setting to prevent further health risks to critically ill patients already compromised by their disease or trauma. Critically ill patients often require multiple invasive devices and therapies to manage their illness and, while vital to patient management, they are not without risks, such as the increased potential for infection. VAP, CAUTIs and central line-associated bloodstream infection (CLABSI) are all aligned with invasive device use and form a significant source of healthcare-acquired infections (HAIs) within critical care.[101] Critical care staff themselves need to protect against contracting infections while providing care for their patients.

When patients are admitted to critical care it is impossible to identify whether or not they are newly colonised with bacteria, or are carrying an infection, without further investigation.

'Standard Precautions' are applied in the management of all patients regardless of the reason for their admission. Standard precautions include: hand hygiene, respiratory hygiene and cough etiquette; the use of appropriate personal protective equipment; safe handling of sharps, waste and used linen; appropriate cleaning and environmental controls; appropriate reprocessing of reusable equipment; and the use of aseptic non-touch techniques during procedures.[101]

Continuing emphasis on respiratory hygiene, cough etiquette and effective hand hygiene to limit influenza and other respiratory illnesses is vital.[101] Further 'Transmission-based Precautions' are implemented as required in response to suspicion (while awaiting confirmation from tests) or diagnosis of a condition in which standard precautions may not be sufficient to control the transmission of microorganisms.[101] Transmission-based precautions appropriately applied to specific microorganisms disrupt their method of transmission to other patients, visitors and healthcare workers. Transmission-based precautions include continuation of standard precautions, the use of personal protective equipment specific to the risk of transmission, individual patient equipment where possible and specific cleaning protocols for shared equipment, placement of patients in single rooms (or cohorted if appropriate) and specific air filtration or circulation and environmental cleaning protocols.[101]

TABLE 5.13
Transmission-based precautions and infectious conditions

TRANSMISSION-BASED PRECAUTIONS	EXAMPLES OF INFECTIOUS CONDITIONS
Contact	MROs: MRSA, MRGN, VRE, ESBL, CRE Gastrointestinal pathogens: *C. difficile*, Norovirus Highly contagious skin infections
Droplet	Influenza RSV Meningococcal
Airborne	Pulmonary TB Chickenpox (varicella), measles (rubella) SARS, MERS

CRE = carbapenem resistant Enterobacteriaceae; ESBL = extended-spectrum beta-lactamase-producing (Enterobacteriaceae); MERS = Middle East respiratory syndrome coronavirus; MRGN = Multi-resistant Gram-negative bacilli; MRO = multi-resistant organism; MRSA = methicillin-resistant *Staphylococcus aureus*; RSV = pertussis; SARS = severe acute respiratory syndrome; TB = tuberculosis; VRE = vancomycin-resistant enterococcus.
Adapted from NHMRC Australian guidelines for the prevention and control of infection in healthcare, <http://www.nhmrc.gov.au>; 2010 [accessed 12.17].

There are three types of transmission-based precautions recommended to counteract the various infectious agents: 'Contact Precautions', 'Droplet Precautions' and 'Airborne Precautions'[101] (Table 5.13). These types of precautions are applied with refinement to the use of personal protective equipment, room requirements and recommendations for visitors specific to the mode of transmission of the organism. Critical care nurses should be knowledgeable about both local and national guidelines and protocols for infection control in order to provide safe care to all their patients. Failure to consistently apply standard precautions and, when implemented, transmission-based precautions, adds to the patient's risk of healthcare-associated infections, especially in those who are critically ill.

Although good hand hygiene is the single most effective tool in infection control,[102,103] the key components of effective infection control are surveillance, prevention and control, which are described in more detail.

Surveillance

ICU patients may be colonised or infected with a multi-resistant organism (MRO) prior to admission,[104] so routine screening should be undertaken to detect the presence of bacteria.[105] Local conditions, risk factors and protocols will provide guidance, but commonly critically ill patients will be screened for multi-resistant *Staphylococcus aureus* (MRSA) and vancomycin-resistant *Enterococcus* (VRE) on admission.[104-106] In the 1980s, a landmark study established that hospital-acquired infection may be reduced by around one-third if surveillance and prevention programs are implemented.[106] Reporting surveillance data to the clinical team regularly can aid with infection control strategy compliance.

Prevention

Core components and principles in the management of infection control within healthcare facilities set by the World Health Organization (WHO) and outlined by organisations like the Centers for Disease Control and Prevention (CDC) USA and the International Federation of Infection Control and International Society for Infectious Diseases are adopted as practice guidelines in local jurisdictional publications.[101] Health services should apply designated guidelines and operate within clearly defined infection-control procedures, which are based on standard precautions for all patients and situations with transmission-based precautions applied in response to patient condition and infection risk.[101] Critical care nurses should refer to their specific hospital infection-control policies regarding details of procedures that must be followed.

Control

Once an organism has been identified, the goal is to limit its spread. Colonisation refers to the presence of microorganisms in any amount, whereas infection means that pathological tissue injury or disease has occurred due to the invasion and multiplication of the microorganism.[106] Typically, surveillance measures identify many patients who are colonised with MRSA or VRE and, although they themselves are not infected, it is important to stop the spread of bacteria to patients more vulnerable and thus more susceptible to opportunistic infection, by implementing transmission-based precautions.[101,107] Key measures demonstrated to be effective in managing multi-resistant bacterial infections in ICUs include early identification of infected patient and use of contact precautions, along with containment of equipment such as stethoscopes and thermometers for exclusive use of a single patient.

Due to the vulnerable nature of critically ill patients, specific issues are described in more detail including: hand hygiene, personal protective equipment (PPE), MROs, HAIs, VAP and CLABSI. Management of environmental cleanliness is a key factor in infection control. This extends to cleaning standards and frequency, waste management, water quality, air quality and circulation, the changing of bed linen and its handling for disposal or removal for cleaning.

Practice tip 16

When using open tracheal suctioning techniques, ensure that the ventilator connection is not contaminated during the procedure while disconnected from the tracheal tube.

Hand hygiene

At the core of standard precautions is effective hand hygiene, which reduces the spread of bacteria and is the most effective and least expensive method of preventing healthcare-associated or nosocomial infection.[102,103] Constant diligence is required to ensure good hand hygiene, as compliance can be variable;[101,102] however, regular education programs, feedback and reminders are known to support improvement.[102,103] The five moments for hand hygiene created by the WHO in 2009[102] can be adopted for local implementation, such as by Hand Hygiene Australia.[101] Evidence led to the use an alcohol-based hand rub for hand hygiene unless the hands are soiled but regular soap and water is still recommended and particularly in the presence of *C. difficile* or Norovirus and outbreaks.[101,107] Given the frequency of hand hygiene while caring for patients, clinicians should monitor their hand skin integrity and be alert to any product irritation. The use of alcohol hand rubs is associated with higher rates of hand hygiene compliance although effectiveness is dependent on technique.[101,102]

Practice tip 17

Good hand hygiene is vital before and after all interventions with patients. There are multiple objects in a single ward or unit, such as computer keyboards and door handles, that are touched by many people within a day. Movement of contaminants from inanimate objects to patients and the reverse is possible if adherence to good hand hygiene is not upheld. Remember the five moments for hand hygiene.

Practice tip 18

Compliance with local protocols for surveillance, isolation and use of PPE for MROs and infectious conditions is vital to the management of all patients, and the safety of personnel and visitors in critical care units.

Personal protective equipment

PPE may include any and all of the following: plastic aprons, gowns (single use or sterile), gloves (single use or sterile), masks ranging from surgical to particulate filter N95 mask or P2 respirators and eye protection such as goggles or face shields that also protect mucous membranes of the mouth and nose.[101] Specific sequences for putting on and taking off PPE that minimise the risk of contamination should be taught to all key personal.[101]

Epidemic outbreaks of severe acute respiratory syndrome (SARS) coronavirus occurred in Canada, China, Hong Kong, Singapore and Vietnam[108] in 2003 and cases were reported in over 25 countries.[108] SARS was transmitted between patients, healthcare workers and hospital visitors, and large within-hospital outbreaks were associated with aerosol-generating procedures such as bronchoscopy, endotracheal intubation and the use of aerosol therapy,[102] which are commonplace in critical care areas. In Hong Kong, more than 20% of cases were healthcare workers.[108,109] Because of the high level of morbidity and mortality associated with SARS,[108,110] the risk to healthcare staff is considerable and, during the Hong Kong SARS outbreak, healthcare workers wore full head covers with a visor.[111]

Previous research has demonstrated relatively low rates of compliance with standard precautions, ranging from 16% to 44%.[106] The SARS outbreaks emphasised the need for effective infection-control procedures, especially for airborne pathogens. With airborne pathogens such as pulmonary tuberculosis or the Middle East respiratory syndrome coronavirus (MERS-CoV),[112,113] airborne precautions[101] using properly fitted N95 masks (face mask with 95% or greater filter efficiency), gowns and gloves are implemented to reduce the spread of the organism, plus the use of airborne infection isolation rooms or negative air pressure rooms with room exhaust via high-efficiency particulate air (HEPA) filtration and strict control of family visiting.[108] Additional measures may include the use of high-efficiency bacterial filters to filter patients' expired air, closed suction systems and ventilator scavenging systems.[111]

MERS-CoV was first reported in 2012 in Saudi Arabia and most cases have been in countries near to the Arabian Peninsula and from travellers returning home from the area to over 17 countries to date.[112] A large outbreak in North Korea was reported in 2015 where 186 persons were affected linked to a single traveller back from the Middle East.[112] The severity of respiratory infection symptoms varies, with mortality highest in those requiring ventilation for confirmed MERS-CoV infections, i.e. MERS.[113]

The influenza H1N1 pandemic alerted everyone to the need for vigilance in infection control. The use of 'droplet precautions' is the main feature of infection control for influenza, along with early testing.[114] The influenza outbreak also drew attention to the need for vaccinations. Influenza vaccines are developed as the influenza A virus changes. All healthcare workers and especially those in critical care should be knowledgeable of the vaccinations that may be available to them through their employers and those that are recommended by local jurisdictions. A variation of the avian influenza A (H7N9) virus was first reported in China in 2013[114] and most recently again in July 2017.[115]

Practice tip 19

Remember, hand hygiene is performed before putting on PPE and after removing PPE. Hand hygiene is also performed after removal of gloves.

Multi-resistant organisms

MROs, or multi-drug-resistant organisms, are collective terms for a number of infections with antimicrobial resistance (AMR). While the early diagnosis of an MRO and immediate implementation of organism-specific 'transmission-based precautions' is key to management, it is true that MRSA and extended-spectrum beta-lactamase-producing Enterobacteriaceae (ESBL-E) have reached epidemic proportions. Multiple strains of MRSA have been identified, and in many studies ICUs have the highest incidence.[116] In the past decade VRE has become a serious health issue and more recently, carbapenem-resistant Enterobacteriaceae (CRE).[116] Other multi-resistant organisms include multi-drug resistant *Pseudomonas aeruginosa* and *Acinetobacter* spp.[101] As with MRSA, transmission of the MROs above is associated with contact. However, there is also a multi-drug-resistant TB and according to the WHO promoting World TB day on 2nd February 2018, there were 490,000 persons who developed this condition in 2016.[117]

MRO management includes routine screening on and during ICU admission and using key methods for reducing their spread. Combating growing AMR is a WHO global health priority and this can be aided with effective infection prevention and control and only prescribing antibiotics when required.

Healthcare-acquired infections

Nosocomial, or hospital- or healthcare-acquired, infection (HAI) is a major problem in critical care that may affect up to 20% of patients, with a mortality of around 30%.[101] Critically ill patients are 5–10 times more likely to become infected than hospital ward patients.[101] Multi-drug-resistant bacteria are a worldwide problem; their acquisition by patients can lead to infection with the same bacteria, and multiple antibiotic therapy encourages the proliferation of resistant organisms.[118] The diligent focus on antibiotic stewardship assists in the optimal use of antibiotics.[118] Antibiotic or antimicrobial stewardship facilitates a factual review of prescribing, provision of guidance and education to support best practice among other activities. Countries may have a national body to provide governance or reports for healthcare providers on this important topic, such as the Australian report AURA,[118] which provides factual updates on the national surveillance data and trends for AMR and use and prescribing appropriateness of antibiotics.[118]

Medical devices or therapies may expose patients to the potential risk of acquiring an HAI. This risk may occur during the insertion procedure or subsequent maintenance care of the medical device, unless appropriate techniques are used. The use of an aseptic technique during insertion of a device is a feature of infection control, asepsis being the elimination of pathogens. Aseptic non-touch technique is a format for guiding practice in the application.[101] Standard aseptic non-touch technique involves standard hand hygiene, a general aseptic field and non-sterile or sterile gloves and is used for minor procedures that are simple and of short duration, that is, less than 20 min. Examples of procedures include simple wound dressings and intravenous cannulation or urinary catheterisation by proficient practitioners. Surgical aseptic non-touch technique is used for complex or lengthy procedures such as insertion of a central venous catheter and involves the use of full barrier precautions (sterile gown and gloves, face mask), extensive drapes and critical aseptic field.[101] Box 5.4 provides some basic points to guide management of the use of medical devices in critical care.

BOX 5.4

Invasive device management

- Does the patient need the invasive device for effective management of their condition?
- Is the chosen device the most suitable for the individual patient, e.g. size and type of device?
- Are the healthcare professional/s trained to safely insert and manage the device?
- Use the appropriate aseptic procedure for device insertion.
- Follow management protocols to minimise the risk of infection while the device is in situ.
- Monitor the patient for signs and symptoms of infection.
- Review the need for the device in the management of the patient daily and remove as early as possible.

Adapted from NHMRC. Australian guidelines for the prevention and control of infection in healthcare, <http://www.nhmrc.gov.au>; 2010 [accessed 12.17].

The commonest HAIs occur at surgical sites, the urinary tract, lower respiratory tract and bloodstream. For the critically ill patient intravascular cannulas including central venous catheters, urinary catheters, enteral or nasogastric tubes and artificial airways and ventilation are some of the healthcare devices associated with risk. See the section on urinary catheters for information regarding CAUTI.

Ventilator-associated pneumonia

VAP is common in intensive care and usually occurs within 48 hours of initiating ventilation.[119] Changing

TABLE 5.14
Strategies to prevent VAP

MEASURE	INTERVENTIONS
Infection control measures	• Hand hygiene • Active surveillance • Appropriate PPE when managing ventilation-related devices, e.g. ETT, ventilator circuits, tracheal suctioning
Gastrointestinal tract	• 2-hourly oral hygiene • Stress ulcer prophylaxis • Avoid gastric over-distention • Enteral nutrition
Patient position	• Semi-recumbent with head raised to >30° • Rotational bed therapy
Artificial airway	• Respiratory airway care • Avoid unplanned extubations • Secure tracheal airway cuff • Inline or intermittent subglottic secretion removal
Mechanical ventilation	• Maintenance of ventilation equipment, heat and moisture exchangers, safe removal of condensate from circuits • Minimisation of ventilation time • Daily interruption to sedation and/or assessment for readiness to wean therapy and/or extubate • Non-invasive mechanical ventilation

ETT = endotracheal tube; PPE = personal protective equipment; VAP = ventilator-associated pneumonia.
Adapted from NHMRC. Australian guidelines for the prevention and control of infection in healthcare. http://www.nhmrc.gov.au; 2010 [accessed December 2017].

entire team practices and behaviours is critical to successful reduction of VAP within an ICU.[119] A number of strategies that are effective in helping to prevent infection[117] are identified in Table 5.14; two of the simplest and most effective are raising the head of the bed and frequent effective oral hygiene.[33] Good analgesia and minimising sedation plus avoidance of muscle-relaxant medications along with early mobilisation are some of the other strategies that may contribute to the reduction of VAP. Using a heat and moisture exchanger limits the need to change ventilator circuits, while maintaining a closed ventilator circuit and the use of closed suction systems for endotracheal suction assist with prevention strategies.

Selective digestive decontamination continues to be studied extensively. In theory, the use of antimicrobial agents to reduce gut flora in intubated intensive care patients reduces the risk of pneumonia due to micro aspiration (see Chapter 19). Although most studies have demonstrated a reduction in the incidence of VAP, the use of chlorhexidine was reported to be less successful,[120] with an inconsistent reduction in ICU mortality, and continuing concerns about the promotion of AMR with its prolonged use.[119] Related information on respiratory failure, VAP and ventilation can be found in Chapters 14 and 15.

Central line-associated bloodstream infection

The use of central lines is common in critical care areas. The definition by the International Sepsis Forum of catheter-related sepsis is at least one peripheral positive blood culture plus at least one of the following: a positive catheter tip culture; a positive hub or exit-site culture; or a positive paired central and peripheral blood culture where the central culture is positive 2 hours earlier than the peripheral culture or has five times the growth.[121] CLABSI is one of the most important and severe infections that can occur in ICU. Renal failure may significantly increase the risk of infection.[121] Implementing quality improvement measures to ensure adherence to evidence-based infection control guidelines results in a significant reduction of catheter-related bloodstream infection.[122]

After implementing strategies to reduce CLABSI, staff engagement in constant vigilance is required to maintain success.[123] Use of antibiotic-impregnated catheters reduce bacteraemia,[124] which can be used safely for up to 7 days[125] unless restricted by manufacturer guidelines. Current practice supports the use of maximal barriers (head cap, face mask, sterile body gown, sterile gloves and full-size body drape) during routine insertion of central venous catheters along with antiseptic solutions to prepare the skin, and catheter insertion by appropriately trained personnel.[101] Chapter 3 contains information on central line care bundles and checklists. Although chlorhexidine solutions are recommended, their effectiveness depends upon the strength of the solution. In Australia and in Sweden decontamination of the insertion site is with 0.5% chlorhexidine gluconate in 70% isopropyl alcohol.[101] Nurses are responsible for the maintenance of central venous catheters once inserted, including care of the insertion site dressing and infusion line management. Dressings should be replaced whenever their seal is broken or every 7 days.[126] Catheter hubs are another site of colonisation for microorganisms such as *Staphylococcus epidermidis*, and effective hand hygiene combined with non-touch aseptic techniques when accessing the catheter hub should be implemented. Intravenous administration sets containing blood products or lipids or parenteral nutrition infusions are changed when the infusion completes or daily, while others are changed according to local protocols. Infusions such as propofol or nitroglycerine may have additional manufacturer guidelines regarding administration set changes.[127]

After removal of the catheter, and once homeostasis has been established, the site should be covered with an occlusive dressing, which should be left in place for 48 hours to minimise the risk of infection. The catheter should be examined after removal and any damage reported. It may be hospital or unit policy to send the catheter tip for culture and sensitivity; however, a recent single-centre study has shown that colonisation is heaviest at the intravascular proximal segment compared to the distal tip of the catheter.[128]

> **Practice tip 20**
>
> Unless contraindicated in a specific patient, a central venous catheter dressing should be changed whenever there is evidence of fluid accumulation or loss of the dressing's occlusive seal.

Transport of critically ill patients: general principles

The transport of critically ill patients may occur for several reasons, such as from an accident site, categorised as pre-hospital transport, or to move a patient to another facility for treatment, which is known as inter-hospital transport, or within a hospital from one department to another, this being intra-hospital transport.[129] This section will focus on intra-hospital transport, while inter-hospital transport is described in Chapter 23. There are three major groups of critically ill patients undergoing intra-hospital transport. First, there are those unstable patients transported from the emergency department (ED)[130] to the ICU or radiology, Cardiac Intervention Unit or the operating theatres. Another significant group are those deteriorating patients within a hospital ward or persons attended to by a Medical Emergency Response team, who require emergency transfer to the ICU. Finally, patients within the ICU often require transport to imaging departments for scans or operating theatres for procedures or cardiac catheterisation laboratory for angiography.

Guidelines for the transport of critically ill patients are available in many countries including Australia and New Zealand, France, USA and UK[129,130-132] with the principles applying to intra-hospital and other transport.[129,133] Specific guidelines may need to be observed for certain groups of patients, for example those with head injury. While the patients from the ED or from Medical Emergency Calls are generally being moved to facilities where more treatment or care can be provided, the decision to transport an intensive care patient for diagnostic tests or interventions not possible within the ICU is given careful consideration as to the benefits to be gained, as transporting such patients is not without risk and the goal should be no reduction in care during transport.[129,133-136] To reduce the risk of adverse events during transport, various diagnostic tests or surgical procedures should be evaluated in terms of their potential to be undertaken in the critical care unit.[131]

Considerations

Fanara et al[136] outlined a diversity of adverse events during intra-hospital transport. In one study 16.8% of intra-hospital transport adverse events were considered serious.[137] Bergman et al identified categories of hazards pre-, during and post intra-hospital transport as: team, tasks, tools and technologies, environment and organisation.[134] Recognition of the risk of adverse events during intra-hospital transports has long been a concern in critical care and remains so today.[135-137] The primary focus of assessment should be on patient safety and the prevention of adverse events. A transport 'event' can be any event that has an adverse impact and can be patient-, staff- or equipment-related.[135,137] The patient may be adversely affected during transport, ranging from anxiety or pain to respiratory or cardiovascular compromise.[135] Staff may have difficulty with managing the patient's needs during transport and equipment-related problems during transport of critically ill patients are a major consideration along with device dislodgement.[136,137] Risk–benefit assessment is helpful to identify patients with a high risk of complications.[134] For example, the potential risk of moving a severely head-injured patient with unstable ICP may outweigh the potential benefit of a CT scan. Parmentier-Decrucq et al[137] found sedation of the patient before transport, PEEP >6 cmH_2O and the need for fluid infusion for transport to be risk factors for any adverse event during intra-hospital transport. Meticulous planning for all aspects of the transport, based on a thorough assessment of the patient's anticipated needs, is the key to safe intra-hospital transport.[129,133] Consideration of specific patient needs such as the availability of lifting devices for transferring bariatric patients from bed to CT table or appropriate warming devices for the use of older adult patients during lengthy interventional radiological procedures need to be communicated to the procedural areas prior to transport commencing so that no delays occur. A comprehensive guide of information addressing key components of intra-hospital transport of critically ill patients should be available to personnel at every hospital.[129,131]

Safe transport requires accurate assessment and stabilisation of the patient before transport.[129] Key elements[130] are identified in Box 5.5. Securing vascular accesses should be a primary concern, while some consideration may be given to having two intravenous accesses in situ. All equipment should be checked for functionality prior to transport and, while it is vital to ensure that sufficient equipment is taken to maintain the patient, unnecessary equipment complicates the logistics of managing the transport smoothly. Specifically-constructed transport beds or attachments such as equipment tables designed

BOX 5.5

Key elements of safe transfer

- Experienced staff
- Appropriate equipment
- Full assessment and investigation
- Extensive monitoring
- Careful stabilisation of patient
- Reassessment
- Continuing care during transfer
- Direct handover
- Documentation and audit

Reproduced from Wallace PGM, Ridley SA. ABC of intensive care: transport of critically ill patients. Br Med J 1999;319(7206):368–71, with permission.

to support and secure equipment safely during transfer are useful and protect the patient from equipment misplacement injuries.[129,134] The period of transport should ideally be as short as possible, although safety should not be sacrificed for speed. Pre-planning the route of transport and good dialogue between department staff can help to maximise the efficiency of transport and reduce unnecessary delays.[131,135] At all times, the team must be confident that all safety considerations have been made. Both 'haste' and 'pressure to proceed' with transport are contributing factors in adverse events.[134] Adverse events are described in various studies relating to poor preparation and decisions, lack of situational awareness, deficits in skill and ad-hoc work-arounds or non-compliance with designated procedures or practices.[134]

Practice tip 21

Transport preparation should include: 1) establishing the need and purpose of transport; 2) time duration relating to the route to be taken, length of procedure and return journey; 3) necessary equipment; 4) patient preparation; 5) appropriately skilled and numbers of staff; 6) supplies required to continue therapies during transport event; and 7) consideration of emergency and contingency plans.

Essential nursing care during transport

Essential care during transport involves major components: the patient, the team, the monitoring and therapy equipment, and the preparation. Importantly, the patient and their family should be given an explanation of why the transport is necessary, how long the procedure is expected to take and that the transport process includes a team accompanying the patient to continue monitoring and provide required treatment.

The level of experience and specialty of personnel involved in the transport of critically ill patients are factors influencing safe transport.[129,131] Staff should be trained in the various aspects of patient transport,[129,138] including competent management and troubleshooting of all equipment required for particular patient needs, e.g. intra-aortic balloon pump. Team members should be aware of their specific roles, the expected standards to be maintained and ensure excellent communication both within the team and with associated department personnel throughout the transport procedure. Nursing responsibilities during transport of the patient include all aspects of patient and therapy monitoring, comfort and maintaining appropriate documentation. Continuous or frequent monitoring of the patient's vital signs and physiological parameters and equipment alarms and parameters should be undertaken throughout the transport event, and all equipment should be checked regularly to ensure correct functioning. Gas reserves of oxygen cylinders and battery time of all devices require pre-transport calculation before being used and vigilant attention during transport. Patient safety is paramount and close attention to detail is required. Throughout the transport, patients should be reassured regarding their condition and the progress of the purpose of the transport.

Practice tip 22

Staff involved in patient transports should be knowledgeable about the most efficient route to take as well as the facilities at their destination such as power and gas supplies.

Equipment

Equipment used during patient transport must be robust, lightweight and battery-powered,[134] and must adhere to relevant national manufacturing and safety standards. Equipment-related complications occur in around a third of transports.[138] All equipment must be adequately secured during transport, and must be available continuously to the operator.[129] Oxygen requirements should be calculated in advance (or it should be established that piped oxygen is available at the destination department) to ensure an adequate supply, both for the journey and for the duration of the investigation/procedure. Staff responsibility for the safe management of the patient during transport extends to competence with troubleshooting equipment and responsiveness to unexpected equipment, environmental or logistical situations of varying degrees of seriousness.[139] Standard equipment for inter-hospital transport is identified in Table 5.15[129] and, while some items may be unnecessary for all intra-hospital transport, this Table provides

TABLE 5.15
Monitoring during transport

CLINICAL PATIENT MONITORING	EQUIPMENT MONITORING
• Circulation • Respiration • Oxygenation • Neurological • Pain score • Patient comfort	• Pulse oximeter, and capnography • Breathing system alarms • Electrocardiograph • Physiological pressures • Other clinically indicated equipment • Audible and visual equipment alarms

Adapted from College of Intensive Care Medicine Australia and New Zealand (CICM). Guidelines for transport of critically ill patients. http://www.cicm.org.au; 2015 [accessed December 2017].

a useful checklist so that all necessary equipment is taken. Development of institutional checklist to aid the safe transport of critically ill patients may be common; however, not all may contain all the relevant aspects of the transport such as pre- (preparation) during and post-transport with each component informed by analysis of local events and factors such as transport routes and logistical challenges.[135,140] Additional specialist equipment may be required for certain patients, such as spare tracheostomy tubes in case of accidental extubation.

Practice tip 23

To ensure safe equipment preparation, especially during emergency transport events, have two nurses perform independent checks against a transport checklist that includes battery life and gas cylinder data for equipment in your unit as a standard transport preparation practice. Consider additional length infusion lines and ventilation circuits if the destination requires, such as magnetic resonance imaging (MRI) scans.

Before transport, all equipment should be prepared and checked, including the function of visible and audible alarms. All non-essential therapy should be discontinued temporarily during the transport, such as enteral nutrition. Where possible, therapies should be simplified, such as exchanging chest drainage systems for one-way valves, or disconnecting completed infusion administration sets from intravenous lines. The patient's physical safety should be maintained, and care should be taken to ensure that bed rails are used and the patient's limbs are secure and not likely to be injured by equipment. All vital monitoring and therapy equipment should be transferred to portable equipment, and the patient should be stabilised before being moved. Some transport equipment ventilators may not provide identical parameters or functioning to a ventilator the patient is already using, so time must be taken to adjust the transport ventilator to effective ventilation for the patient. If the patient is being transported for MRI, it is important to ensure that all equipment is compatible.

Practice tip 24

If ceasing nutrition during patient transport, make sure that the patient is not at risk of hypoglycaemia from concurrent insulin therapy.

Monitoring

The need for monitoring relates to both the patient and equipment, as identified in Table 5.16.[129] Some monitoring should be continuous, such as cardiac, oxygen saturation, capnography if the patient is intubated and arterial, pulmonary artery and intracranial monitoring if the respective devices are in situ. Recent articles describe the particular complexities of transport for patients with traumatic brain injuries, from the clamping of external ventricular drains during transport and potential intracranial haemodynamic complications[140] to the potential for secondary insults due to instability,[141] to the rise in ICP observed in one series of patients during vertical movement in an elevator.[142] Intermittent monitoring of central venous pressure (CVP), non-invasive blood pressure and respiratory rate should be undertaken as indicated by the patient's condition.[129]

A complete record should be made on one of either the ICU chart, specific transport form or electronic record of all details of the patient's condition, personnel involved, clinical events, observations and therapy given during transport. Pre-determining minimum documentation and observation standards during transport will enhance patient safety and ongoing management. The transporting team should hand over directly to the receiving team providing continuing care for the patient[134,136] or should remain during the intervention/procedure to manage the patient's care.

TABLE 5.16
Standard equipment for intra-hospital transport

RESPIRATORY SUPPORT EQUIPMENT	CIRCULATORY SUPPORT EQUIPMENT	OTHER EQUIPMENT	PHARMACOLOGICAL AGENTS
• Airway management equipment, including intubation set, range of ETTs and laryngeal mask airways, hand ventilation set with PEEP valve and emergency surgical airway set • Oxygen, masks, nebuliser • Pulse oximeter and capnography • Sufficient oxygen supply • Suction equipment • Portable ventilator with disconnect and high-pressure alarms • Pleural drainage equipment	• Monitor/defibrillator/external pacer combined unit • Non-invasive blood pressure device • IV cannula, IV fluids, pressure infusion set, infusion pumps • Arterial cannulae and arterial monitoring device • Syringes and needles, sharps' disposal container • Pericardiocentesis equipment	• Nasogastric tube and bag • Dressings, antiseptic lotions, bandages, tape, • Torch • Thermal insulation and temperature monitor • PPE for transport team	• Checked and clearly labelled drugs: standard resuscitation drugs and those specific to the patient's condition

ETT = endotracheal tube; IV = intravenous; PPE = personal protective equipment.
Adapted from College of Intensive Care Medicine Australia and New Zealand (CICM). Guidelines for transport of critically ill patients. http://www.cicm.org.au; 2013 [accessed April 2014].

Summary

In the management of critically ill patients there is always an initial focus on assessing and treating the patient's most life-threatening and immediate problems. Early attention should then be given to the implementation of preventive therapies such as VTE prophylaxis and pressure injury prevention, along with a thorough assessment of physical care needs and a subsequent plan of management. Recovery for patients to normal functioning after a critical illness is dependent upon a multitude of factors and is a dynamic process over time; however, much of the essential nursing care given to critically ill patients assists in both reducing deficits associated with their episode of illness and reducing the time taken to achieve normal functioning.

Good personal hygiene is at the heart of essential nursing care, and many other aspects of essential care (e.g. eye care and oral care) are closely related. Personal hygiene is often attended to when patients are repositioned, and whenever they are moved the nurse has an opportunity to assess patients, particularly their dependent pressure areas. Bowel and urinary catheter care are vital but often neglected areas of care. When patients are critically ill, the development of preventable complications such as constipation and urinary tract infection may have significant consequences for them. All critically ill patients are at risk of infection, and essential nursing care requires effective application of surveillance, prevention and control measures that should be applied equally to all patients. This principle is embedded in the recommended use of standard precautions.

Critically ill patients are often transferred to other departments for further investigation or specific interventions. All transports pose a potential risk to patients, particularly if they are unstable. Essential nursing care of patients during transfer is based on thorough assessment and preparation in an attempt to anticipate their every need so that adverse events do not occur. This chapter has provided a comprehensive overview of the general but essential nursing care of critically ill patients. It offers a guideline for nurses that is relevant for most patients, most of the time. As with all other aspects of nursing practice, nursing care and intervention should be based on a thorough assessment of each individual patient and tailored to their needs and preferences.

Case study

Mr Y is a 54-year-old male living independently at home. He travels frequently on regional planes between home in the city and the rural centre where he works in the mines. He has had ear discomfort and earaches in the past associated with pressure from the flights. He was brought to the local hospital ED by family following nearly 4 days of otalgia, headaches and the onset of confusion. Mr Y had symptoms of fever, tachycardia, hypotension and lethargy indicating sepsis. Examination of Mr Y's right eardrum showed local inflammation with a discharge, right otitis media. Microbiological swabs of the ear discharge were taken along with blood for cultures. An intravenous cannula was inserted and intravenous fluids given to rehydrate Mr Y and broad-spectrum antibiotics were commenced intravenously. Neurological observations were initiated and performed hourly. The family confirmed that Mr Y's confusion was unusual and new. Mr Y's headache was persisting and while his Glasgow Coma Score was 14, given the onset and increasing confusion, a CT scan was arranged.

Nursing care for Mr Y was primarily directed at keeping him comfortable and quiet as he was disturbed by his headache and initially aware of and worried about his confusion. He also has some dizziness, so movements were conducted slowly. Preparation of Mr Y for transport to the imaging department for the CT was organised and included provision of oxygen and suction and cardiac, non-invasive blood pressure and SpO_2 monitoring. During CT with Mr Y lying supine, his confusion increased. The CT showed right mastoiditis and pneumocephalus with otitis media as the source. Mr Y was referred and then transported to another hospital with neurosurgical services. On arrival at the hospital he was reviewed by the neurosurgeon and subsequently prepped for the operating theatre. Mr Y underwent drainage of his ear and left frontoparietotemporal craniotomy with evacuation of subdural empyema and insertion of intracranial pressure monitoring (ICP).

Mr Y was admitted to the ICU postoperatively intubated and ventilated, with arterial pressure monitoring, central venous catheter and urinary catheter in situ. Mr Y remained sedated with propofol infusion. He was positioned supine with head slightly raised (less than 30°) with close monitoring of ICP and cerebral perfusion pressure (CPP) at 70 mmHg on arrival. Initial observations showed raised temperature monitored via urinary catheter and sinus tachycardia of 124 and large volume of urine in the drainage bag. The urinary catheter had been inserted intra-operatively. His bed was fitted with a pressure-relieving mattress and his initial skin assessment was limited due to the reluctance to move Mr Y until his neurological status could be better evaluated, and it was noted that a sacral silicone dressing had been applied pre-operatively. Mr Y's visible skin was intact and perfusion good.

The next 48 h were focused on close monitoring of Mr Y's ICP and CPP, observing for any polyuria, monitoring blood sodium levels and ongoing neurological assessments. Mr Y remained sedated and ventilated and nursing care was clustered to minimise any adverse impact on ICP, when care such as endotracheal and oral suctioning, oral hygiene and eye care and personal hygiene were performed, while recognising that Mr Y was at risk of developing VAP if diligent care was not taken. Significant repositioning of Mr Y was limited, but careful attention to small adjustments to the angles of the bed enabled some pressure prevention strategies to be implemented frequently.

Results from microbiology testing of the ear discharge swab and blood cultures showed *Streptococcus pneumoniae* in both samples. The infectious diseases team was consulted and the initial broad-spectrum antibiotic of vancomycin was continued for 7 days with ceftriaxone intravenous added for longer administration. Antibiotics for cerebral abscess can be required for up to 8 weeks.

Mr Y was prepared and transported with full monitoring, on a portable ventilator to imaging for a repeat CT. During the transport and CT, the RN's responsibility was to ensure the security of the intraventricular drain and prevent any inadvertent drainage of cerebral spinal fluid (CSF) through poor positioning of the ICP system or inadvertent adjustment of the drainage controls. Spare propofol medication was taken during the transport.

Over the following days Mr Y's management and care was focused on neurological and cerebral pressure monitoring and treatment with antibiotics and the introduction of Levetiracetam for the management of seizures. In addition, close attention was given to the prevention of complications such as pressure injury due to the limitations in patient repositioning, further infections due to invasive devices, VAP prevented by raised head of bed and attentive oral hygiene. Because of the risks of raised ICP, the environment was kept quiet and stimuli of Mr Y limited. However, the nurses provide continual quiet explanations of care and provision of reassurance, both to Mr Y and his family.

On day 8 Mr Y's Glasgow Coma Scale (GCS) score was eyes 4, verbal 1 and motor 6 and he was extubated and ICP drain removed. On day 10 M. Y was discharged to the ward with an ongoing left-sided weakness and expressive aphasia.

CASE STUDY QUESTIONS

1 What are the options for pressure injury prevention when movement is limited?
2 What is the significance of obtaining microbiology specimens prior to antibiotic administration?

RESEARCH VIGNETTE

Santamaria N, Gerdtz M, Sage S, et al. A randomised controlled trial of the effectiveness of soft silicone multi-layered foam dressings in the prevention of sacral and heel pressure ulcers in trauma and critically ill patients: the border trial. Int Wound J 2015; 12:302–308

Abstract

The prevention of hospital-acquired pressure ulcers in critically ill patients remains a significant clinical challenge. The aim of this trial was to investigate the effectiveness of multilayered soft silicone foam dressings in preventing intensive care unit (ICU) pressure ulcers when applied in the emergency department to 440 trauma and critically ill patients. Intervention group patients (n=219) had Mepilex® Border Sacrum and Mepilex® Heel dressings applied in the emergency department and maintained throughout their ICU stay. Results revealed that there were significantly fewer patients with pressure ulcers in the intervention group compared to the control group (5 versus 20, P=0.001). This represented a 10% difference in incidence between the groups (3.1% versus 13.1%) and a number needed to treat ten patients to prevent one pressure ulcer. Overall there were fewer sacral (2 versus 8, P=0.05) and heel pressure ulcers (5 versus 19, P=0.002) and pressure injuries overall (7 versus 27, P=0.002) in interventions than in controls. The time to injury survival analysis indicated that intervention group patients had a hazard ratio of 0.19 (P=0.002) compared to control group patients. We conclude that multilayered soft silicone foam dressings are effective in preventing pressure ulcers in critically ill patients when applied in the emergency department prior to ICU transfer.

Critique

This study investigated a novel single intervention, the application of multilayered soft silicone foam dressings, to prevent hospital-acquired pressure injuries in the ICU. Prevention of hospital-acquired pressure injuries is, as the authors argue, a persistent and significant clinical challenge. The study used an open-label randomised controlled trial design to determine the effectiveness of multilayered soft silicone foam dressings in preventing sacral and heel pressure injury development in trauma or critically ill patients who were admitted to the ICU via the ED. The study was conducted in a single metropolitan tertiary hospital with a mixed medical and surgical 24-bed ICU. At the time of the study, the ICU admitted approximately 2000 patients per annum.

Patients were included in the study if they were over 18 years of age and had an ED and subsequent ICU admission for trauma and /or critical illness. Excluded patients were those with suspected or actual spinal injury preventing the patient being repositioned, a sacral or heel pressure injury on admission to the ED, and trauma to the sacrum or heels. Eligible patients were randomised in the ED to receive either the intervention or the control study procedures. Randomisation was undertaken in the ED by an ED research nurse who retrieved the next envelope in a pre-prepared series of envelopes determining group allocation. The control group received standard care measures that included ongoing pressure injury risk assessment, use of a standard support surface during their ICU admission and stated standard ICU pressure injury prevention practices (e.g. regular repositioning and skin care). The intervention group received the standard care measures plus the application of a multilayered soft silicone foam dressing to the sacrum and both heels. The heel dressings were secured with elastic tubular bandages. All dressing were changed every 3 days unless soiled or dislodged.

The study end-point was the pressure injury incidence rate in both groups. Study measures included patient demographic and clinical characteristics, severity of illness as determined by the Australasian Triage Score (ED) and the Acute Physiology and Chronic Health Evaluation (APACHE) II score (ICU). Pressure injury risk was determined by the Braden Scale score. All patients had data collected daily and a daily visual inspection of the skin underneath the dressings where the dressing was partially peeled back so the skin could be observed and assessed for the presence of a pressure injury. Pressure injuries were staged according to national guidelines current at the time of the study.

This study used an appropriate design, a randomised control design, to test the effectiveness of a single novel intervention. Patient enrolment, group allocation, follow-up and analysis was according to the international Consolidated Standards of Reporting Trials (CONSORT) protocol. The CONSORT statement provides a standard way for authors to report trial findings, facilitating complete and transparent reporting, and aiding critical appraisal and interpretation. Because patients were recruited on certain days only and it is not clear if all potential patients were screened for inclusion, it is possible selection bias, where the patients included in the study differ in some systematic way from the general population, may have occurred.

Randomising patients increases the likelihood that both the control and treatment/intervention group are similar in relation to a variety of both known and unknown characteristics, and thus makes it more likely that any differences in outcomes between groups is due to the treatment/intervention. To limit the potential for bias, outcome assessors should be independent of the recruiters and those delivering the intervention, and when possible, they should be blinded to group allocation. The authors do not identify if the outcome assessors were independent and they were not blinded. While the latter seems difficult to achieve, use of photographs could have been used. The fact that the outcome assessors were not being blinded to either the study hypotheses or the intervention allocation. This was noted as a study limitation by the authors.

The application of dressings, as a prophylactic intervention to prevent pressure injury development, warrants further investigation. Many different dressing are available and the properties or composition of each dressing varies from multilayered soft silicone foam to silicone adhesive composite hydrocellular foam and polyurethane film. A consensus document published in 2016 outlines the rationale for, and role of, dressing use in the prevention of pressure injuries.[143] However, further research in the form of a comparison trial is required to determine the most effective dressing type in terms of patient outcomes and cost effectiveness.

Learning activities

1 List the benefits and risks of faecal containment devices.
2 Outline ICU patient preparation for transfer to the operating theatre.
3 What criteria do you use to evaluate the positioning in bed of your patients?
4 Name some of the significant infection risks for patients in ICU.
5 Summarise circulatory and respiratory challenges in the care of obese patients.
6 Describe how patients in intensive care are at risk of eye damage.

Online resources

Australian Department of Health, www.health.gov.au

Australian Wound Management Association, www.awma.com.au

Cochrane Collaboration, www.cochrane.org

College of Intensive Care Medicine of Australia and New Zealand (CICM), www.cicm.org.au

Communicable Diseases Network Australia (CDNA), www.health.gov.au/cdna

European Pressure Ulcer Advisory Panel, www.epuap.org

Hand Hygiene Australia, www.hha.org.au

National Health and Medical Research Council, www.nhmrc.gov.au

National Institute of Clinical Studies (NICS), www.nhmrc.gov.au/nics/index.htm

Skin Tear Advisory Panel, www.skintears.org/pdf/Skin-Tear-Resource-Kit.pdf

Therapeutic Goods Australia, www.tga.gov.au/index.htm

US Centers for Disease Control and Prevention, www.cdc.gov

World Health Organization, www.who.int/en

Further reading

Coyer F, Stotts NA, Blackman VS. A prospective window into medical device-related pressure ulcers in intensive care. Int Wound J 2013;doi:10.1111/iwj.12026.

Brummel NE, et al. Understanding and reducing disability in older adults following critical illness. Crit Care Med 2015;43(6): 1265–75.

Bergman LM, Pettersson ME, Chaboyer WP, et al. Safety hazards during intrahospital transport: a prospective observational study. Crit Care Med 2017;45:e1043–9.

References

1. Vollman KM. Interventional patient hygiene: discussion of the issues and a proposed model for implementation of nursing care basics. Intensive Crit Care Nurs 2013;29:250–5.
2. Powers J, Peed J, Burns L, et al. Chlorhexidine bathing and microbial contamination in patients' bath basins. Am J Crit Care 2012;21(5):338–43.
3. El-Soussi AH, Asfour HI. Examining bed-bath practices of critically ill patients. J Nurs Ed Prac 2016;6(12):1–10.
4. Afonso E, Blot K, Blot S. Prevention of hospital-acquired bloodstream infections through chlorhexidine gluconate-impregnated washcloth bathing in intensive care units: a systematic review and meta-analysis of randomised crossover trials. Eurosurveillance 2016;21(46):27–37.
5. Martin ET. Bathing hospitalized dependent patients with pre-packaged disposable washcloths instead of traditional basins: a case-crossover study. Am J Infect Control 2017;45(9):90.
6. National Pressure Ulcer Advisory Panel (NPUAP). National Pressure Ulcer Advisory Panel (NPUAP) announces a change in terminology from pressure ulcer to pressure injury and updates the-stages of pressure injury; 2016. Online. Available from: http://www.npuap.org/national-pressure-ulcer-advisory-panel-npuap-announces-a-change-in-terminology-from-pressure-ulcer-to-pressure-injury-and-updates-the-stages-of-pressure-injury/. [Accessed January 2018].
7. Coyer F, Miles S, Gosley S, et al. Pressure injury prevalence in intensive care versus non-intensive care patients: a state-wide comparison. Aust Crit Care 2017;30:244–50.
8. National Pressure Ulcer Advisory Panel, European Pressure Ulcer Advisory Panel and Pan Pacific Pressure Injury Alliance. In: Haesler Emily, editor. Prevention and treatment of pressure ulcers: clinical practice guideline. Cambridge Media: Osborne Park; 2014.
9. Garcia-Fernandez FP, Pancorbo-Hidalgo PL, Agreda Soldevilla JJ. Predictive capacity of risk assessment scales and clinical judgement for pressure ulcers: a meta-analysis. J Wound Ostomy Continence Nurs 2014;41(1):24–34.
10. Fulbrook P, Anderson A. Pressure inury risk assessment in intensive care: comparison of inter-rater reliability of the COMHON (Conscious level, Mobility, Haemodynamics, Oxygenation, Nutrition) index with three scales. J Adv Nurs 2016;72(3):680–92.
11. Coyer F, Stotts NA, Blackman VS. A prospective window into medical device-related pressure ulcers in intensive care. Int Wound J 2014;11(6):656–64.
12. National Pressure Ulcer Advisory Panel. Mucosal pressure ulcers: an NPUAP position statement. Washington DC: National Ulcer Advisory Panel; 2009.
13. Tayyib N, Coyer F. Effectiveness of pressure ulcer prevention strategies for adult patients in intensive care units: a systematic review. Worldview Evid Based Nurs 2016;13(6):432–44.
14. Coyer F, Campbell J. Incontinence-associated dermatitis in the critically ill patient: an intensive care perspective. Nurs Crit Care 2017;doi:10.1111/nicc.12331.
15. Beeckman D, Campbell J, Campbell K, et al. Proceedings of the Global IAD Expert Panel. Incontinence-associated dermatitis: moving prevention forward. Wounds International; 2015. Online. Available from: www.woundsinternational.com. [Accessed January 2018].

16. Garcia CB, Binks R, De Luca E, et al. Prevalence, management and clinical challenges associated with acute faecal incontinence in the ICU and critical care settings: the FIRST™ cross-sectional descriptive survey. Int Crit Care Nurs 2012;28(4):242–50.
17. Coyer F, Gardner A, Doubrovsky A. An interventional skin care protocol (InSPiRE) to reduce incontinence-associated dermatitis in critically ill patients in the intensive care unit: a before and after study. Int Crit Care Nurs 2017;40:1–10.
18. McNichol L, Lund C, Rosen T, et al. Medical adhesives and patient safety: state of the science: consensus statements for the assessment, prevention, and treatment of adhesive-related skin injuries. J Wound Ostomy Continence Nurs 2013;40(4):E1–2.
19. LeBlanc K, Baranoski S, the International Skin Tear Advisory Panel 2013. Skin tears: the state of the science: consensus statements for the prevention, prediction, assessment and treatment of skin tears. Adv Skin Wound Care 2011;24(9 Suppl.):2–15.
20. Nair PN, White E. Care of the eye during anaesthesia and intensive care. Int Care Med 2014;15(1):40–3.
21. Grixti A, Sadri M, Edgar J, et al. Common ocular surface disorders in patients in intensive care units. Ocul Surf 2012;10(1):26–42.
22. Alansari MA, Hijazi MH, Maghrabi KA. Making a difference in eye care of the critically ill patients. J Intensive Care Med 2015;30(6):311–17.
23. Kuruvilla S, Jayanthi P, Sarada D, et al. Incidence and risk factor evaluation of exposure keratopathy in critically ill patients: a cohort study. J Crit Care 2015;30(2):400–4.
24. Kam KY, Haldar RS, Papamichael E, et al. Eye care in the critically ill: A National Survey and Protocol. J Intensive Care Soc 2013;14(2):150–4.
25. Dawson D. Development of a new eye care guideline for critically ill patients. Intensive Crit Care Nurs 2005;21(2):119–22.
26. Marshall AP, Elliott R, Rolls K, et al. Eye care in the critically ill: clinical practice guidelines. Aust Critical Care 2008;21(2):97–109.
27. Ezra DG, Chan M, Solebo L, et al. Randomised trial comparing ocular lubricants and polyacrylamide hydrogel dressings in the prevention of exposure keratopathy in the critically ill. Intensive Care Med 2009;35(3):455–61.
28. So HM, Lee CCH, Leung AKH, et al. Comparing the effectiveness of polyethylene covers (Gladwrap) with lanolin (Duratears) eye ointment to prevent corneal abrasions in critically ill patients: a randomized controlled study. Int J Nurs Stud 2008;45(11):1565–71.
29. Micik S, Besic N, Johnson N, et al. Reducing risk for ventilator associated pneumonia through nursing sensitive interventions. Int Crit Care Nurs 2013;29(5):261–5.
30. Hua F, Xie H, Worthington HV, et al. Oral hygiene care for critically ill patients to prevent ventilator-associated pneumonia. Cochrane Database Syst Rev 2016;(10):CD008367.
31. Dale C, Angus JE, Sinuff T, et al. Mouth care for orally intubated patients: a critical ethnographic review of the nursing literature. Intensive Crit Care Nursing 2013;29(5):266–74.
32. Allen Furr L, Binkley CJ, McCurren C, et al. Factors affecting quality of oral care in intensive care units. J Adv Nurs 2004;48(5):454–62.
33. Prendergast V, Kleiman C, King M. The bedside oral exam and the Barrow oral care protocol: translating evidence-based oral care into practice. Intensive Crit Care Nurs 2013;29(5):282–90.
34. Binkley C, Furr LA, Carrico R, et al. Survey of oral care practices in US intensive care units. Am J Infect Control 2004;32(3):161–9.
35. Pearson LS, Hutton JL. A controlled trial to compare the ability of foam swabs and toothbrushes to remove dental plaque. J Adv Nurs 2002;39(5):480–9.
36. Elkerbout TA, De Slot EB, Van der Weijden G. Chlorhexidine mouthwash and sodium lauryl sulphate dentifrice: do they mix effectively or interfere? Int J Dental Hygiene 2016;14(1):42–52.
37. Puntillo K, Nelson J, Weissman D, et al. Palliative care in the ICU: relief of pain, dyspnea, and thirst – A report from the IPAL-ICU Advisory Board. Intensive Care Med 2014;40(2):235–48.
38. Kress JP, Hall JB. ICU-acquired weakness and recovery from critical illness. N Engl J Med 2014;370:1626–35.
39. Vanpee G, Hermans G, Segers J, et al. Assessment of limb muscle strength in critically ill patients: a systematic review. Crit Care Med 2014;42(3):701–11.
40. Hodgson CL, Stiller K, Needham DM, et al. Expert consensus and recommendations on safety criteria for active mobilization of mechanically ventilated critically ill adults. Crit Care 2014;18:658. https://doi.org/10.1186/s13054-014-0658-y.
41. Resar R, Pronovost P, Haraden C, et al. Using a bundle approach to improve ventilator care processes and reduce ventilator-associated pneumonia. Jt Comm J Qual Patient Saf 2005;31(5):243–8.
42. Gosselink R, Roeseler J. Physiotherapy in critically ill patients. In: Tubaro M, Vranckx P, Price S, et al, editors. The ESC textbook of intensive and acute cardiovascular care. Oxford: Oxford University Press; 2015.
43. Phelan S, Lin F, Mitchell M, et al. Implementing early mobilisation in the intensive care unit: an integrative review. Int J Nurs Stud 2018;77:91–105. doi:10.1016/j.ijnurstu.2017.09.019.
44. Casey CM. The study of activity: an integrative review. J Gerontol Nurs 2013;39(8):12–25.
45. Koch SM, Fogarty S, Signorino C, et al. Effect of passive range of motion on intracranial pressure in neurosurgical patients. J Crit Care 1996;11(4):176–9.
46. Brimioulle S, Moraine JJ, Norrenberg D, et al. Effects of positioning and exercise on intracranial pressure in a neurosurgical intensive care unit. Phys Ther 1997;77(12):1682–9.
47. Schieren M, Piekarski F, Dusse F, et al. Continuous lateral rotational therapy in trauma – A systematic review and meta-analysis. J Trauma Acute Care Surg 2017;83(5):926–33.
48. NHMRC. Clinical practice guideline for the prevention of venous thromboembolism (deep vein thrombosis and pulmonary embolism) in patients admitted to Australian hospitals. Melbourne: National Health and Medical Research Council; 2009.

49. Kakkos SK, Caprini JA, Geroulakos G, et al. Combined intermittent pneumatic leg compression and medication for prevention of deep vein thrombosis and pulmonary embolism in high-risk patients. Coch Database Syst Rev 2011;(4):CD005258.pub2, doi:10.1002/14651858.
50. Geerts WH, Bergqvist D, Pineo GF, et al. Prevention of venous thromboembolism: American College of Chest Physicians evidence-based clinical practice guidelines. Chest 2008;133:S381–453.
51. Sachdeva A, Dalton M, Amaragiri SV, et al. Elastic compression stockings for prevention of deep vein thrombosis. Coch Database Syst Rev 2010;(7):CD001484, doi:10.1002/14651858.
52. Douketis J, Cook D, Meade M, et al. Prophylaxis against deep vein thrombosis in critically ill patients with severe renal insufficiency with the low-molecular-weight heparin dalteparin: an assessment of safety and pharmacodynamics: the DIRECT study. Arch Intern Med 2008;168:1805–12.
53. Griffen M, Kakkos SK, Geroulakos G, et al. Comparison of three intermittent pneumatic compression systems in patients with varicose veins: a hemodynamic study. Int Angiol 2007;26(2):158–64.
54. Lachiewicz PF, Kelley SS, Haden LR. Two mechanical devices for prophylaxis of thromoboembolism after total knee arthroplasty. A prospective, randomised study. J Bone Joint Surg 2004;86(8):1137–41.
55. Rauen CA, Flynn-Makic MB, Bridges E. Evidence-based practice habits: transforming research into bedside practice. Crit Care Nurse 2009;29(2):46–59.
56. Rushdi TA, Pichard C, Khater YH. Control of diarrhea by fiber-enriched diet in ICU patients on enteral nutrition: a prospective randomized controlled trial. Clin Nutr 2004;23(6):1344–52.
57. McPeake J, Gilmore H, MacIntosh G. The implementation of a bowel management protocol in an adult intensive care unit. Nurs Crit Care 2011;16(5):235–42.
58. Riegler G, Esposito I. Bristol scale stool form. A still valid help in medical practice and clinical research. Tech Coloproctol 2001;5(3):163–4.
59. Bianchi J, Segovia-Gomez T. The dangers of faecal incontinence in the at-risk patient. Wound Int 2012;3(3):15–21. Available: http://www.woundsinternational.com.
60. de Azevedo RP, Machado FR. Constipation in critically ill patients: much more than we imagine. Rev Bra Ter Intensiva 2013;25(2):73–4.
61. Bishop S, Young H, Goldsmith D, et al. Bowel motions in critically ill patients: a pilot observational study. Crit Care Resusc 2010;12(3):182–5.
62. Sawh SB, Selvaraj IP, Danga A, et al. Use of methylnaltrexone for the treatment of opioid-induced constipation in critical care patients. Mayo Clin Proc 2012;87(3):255–9.
63. Mostafa SM, Bhandari S, Ritchie G, et al. Constipation and its implications in the critically ill patient. Br J Anaesth 2003;91(6):815–19.
64. Locke GR, Pemberton JH, Phillips SF. American Gastroenterological Association Medical Position Statement: guidelines on constipation. Gastroenterology 2000;119(6):1761–6.
65. Gacouin A, Camus C, Gros A, et al. Constipation in long-term ventilated patients; associated factors and impact on intensive care outcomes. Crit Care Med 2010;38(10):1933–8.
66. All Wales Guidelines for Faecal Management Systems; 2010. Online. Available from: http://welshwoundnetwork.org/dmdocuments/all_wales_faecal_systems.pdf. [Accessed December 2017].
67. Yates A. Faecal incontinence: a joint approach to guideline development. Nurs Times 2011;107(12):12. Online. Available from: http://www.nursingtimes.net/continence. [Accessed June 2014].
68. Bright E, Fishwick G, Berry D, et al. Indwelling bowel management system as a cause of life-threatening rectal bleeding. Case Rep Gastroenterol 2008;2(3):341–55.
69. A'Court J, Yiannoullou P, Pearce L, et al. Rectourethral fistula secondary to a bowel management system. Intensive Crit Care Nurs 2014;30:226–30.
70. Massey J, Gatt M, Tolan DJ, et al. An ano-vaginal fistula associated with the use of a faecal management system: a case report. Colorectal Dis 2010;12(7):e173–4.
71. Chant C, Smith OM, Marshall JC, et al. Relationship of catheter associated urinary tract infection to mortality and length of stay in critically ill patients: a systematic review and meta-analysis of observational studies. Crit Care Med 2011;39(5):1167–73.
72. Gould CV, Umscheid CA, Agarwal RK, et al; the Healthcare Infection Control Practices Advisory Committee (HICPAC). Guideline for prevention of catheter-associated urinary tract infections 2009. Online. Available from: https://www.cdc.gov/infectioncontrol/guidelines/cauti/. [Accessed March 2018].
73. Mitchell B, Ware C, McGregor A, et al. ASID (HICSIG)/AICA Position Statement: preventing catheter-associated urinary tract infections in patients. Healthcare Infect 2011;16:45–52. Online. Available from: http://www.publish.csiro.au/journals/hi. [Accessed December 2017].
74. Bagshaw SM, Webb SAR, Delaney A, et al. Very old patients admitted to intensive care in Australia and New Zealand: a multi-centre cohort analysis. Crit Care 2009;13(2):R45.
75. de Boer A, Ter Horst GJ, Lorist MM. Physiological and psychosocial age-related changes associated with reduced food intake in older persons. Ageing Res Rev 2013;12(1):316–28.
76. Atalayer D, Astbury NM. Anorexia of aging and gut hormones. Aging Dis 2013;4(5):264–75.
77. Finocchiaro D, Hook J. Enteral nutritional support of the critically ill older adult. Crit Care Nurs Q 2015;38(3):253–8.
78. Pisani MA. Considerations in caring for the critically ill older patient. J Intensive Care Med 2009;24(2):83–95.
79. Brummel NE, et al. Understanding and reducing disability in older adults following critical illness. Crit Care Med 2015;43(6):1265–75.

80. Chen L, Lim FA. Stuck inside a cloud: optimizing sedation to reduce ICU-associated delirium in geriatric patients. Crit Care Nurs Q 2015;38(3):245–52.
81. Kirksey KM, McGlory G, Sefcik E. Pain assessment and management in critically ill older adults. Crit Care Nurs Q 2015;38(3):237–44.
82. Strøm C, Rasmussen L, Steinmetz J. Practical management of anaesthesia in the elderly. Drugs Aging 2016;33(11):765–77.
83. Chernecky C, Macklin D, Blackburn P. Catheter-related bloodstream infections (CR-BSI) in geriatric patients in intensive care units. Crit Care Nurs Q 2015;38(3):280–92.
84. Chang CW, Chen YM, Su CC. Care needs of older patients in the intensive care units. J Clin Nurs 2012;21(5–6):825–32.
85. Dennis DM, Bharat C, Paterson T. Prevalence of obesity and the effect on length of mechanical ventilation and length of stay in intensive care patients: a single site observational study. Aust Crit Care 2017;30(3):145–50.
86. Puhl RM, Brownell KD. Confronting and coping with weight stigma: an investigation of overweight and obese adults. Obesity (Silver Spring) 2006;14(10):1802–15.
87. Bejciy-Spring SM. R-E-S-P-E-C-T: a model for the sensitive treatment of the bariatric patient. Bariatr Nurs Surg Patient Care 2008;3(1):47–56.
88. Hales C, Coombs M, de Vries K. The challenges in caring for morbidly obese patients in Intensive Care: a focused ethnographic study. Aust Crit Care 2018;31(1):37–41.
89. Pedoto A. Lung physiology and obesity: anesthetic implications for thoracic procedures. Anesthesiol Res Pract 2012;154208.
90. Parameswaran K, Todd DC, Soth M. Altered respiratory physiology in obesity. Can Respir J 2006;13(4):203–10.
91. Lotia S, Bellamy MC. Anaesthesia and morbid obesity. Cont Edu Anaesth Crit Care Pain 2008;8(5):151–6.
92. De Jong A, Chanques G, Jaber S. Mechanical ventilation in obese ICU patients: from intubation to extubation. Crit Care 2017;21(1):63.
93. Fischer AJ, Kaese S, Lebiedz P. Management of obese patients with respiratory failure – A practical approach to a health care issue of increasing significance. Respir Med 2016;117:174–8.
94. De Jong A, Molinari N, Sebbane M, et al. Feasibility and effectiveness of prone position in morbidly obese patients with ARDS: a case-control clinical study. Chest 2013;143(6):1554–61.
95. Weig T, Janitza S, Zoller M, et al. Influence of abdominal obesity on multiorgan dysfunction and mortality in acute respiratory distress syndrome patients treated with prone positioning. J Crit Care 2014;29(4):557–61.
96. Oppenheimer BW, Berger KI, Rennert DA, et al. Effect of circulatory congestion on the components of pulmonary diffusing capacity in morbid obesity. Obesity (Silver Spring) 2006;14(7):1172–80.
97. Berrios LA. The ABCDs of managing morbidly obese patients in intensive care units. Crit Care Nurse 2016;36(5):17–26.
98. Leykin Y, Miotto L, Pellis T. Pharmacokinetic considerations in the obese. Best Pract Res Clin Anaesthesiol 2011;25(1):27–36.
99. King DR, Velmahos GC. Difficulties in managing the surgical patient who is morbidly obese. Crit Care Med 2010;38(9 Suppl.):S478–82.
100. Hignett S, Griffiths P. Risk factors for moving and handling bariatric patients. Nurs Stand 2009;24(11):40–8.
101. NHMRC. Australian guidelines for the prevention and control of infection in healthcare; 2010. Online. Available from: http://www.nhmrc.gov.au. [Accessed December 2017].
102. WHO Guidelines on hand hygiene in healthcare; 2009. Online. Available from: http://www.who.int/gpsc/5may/tools. [Accessed December 2017].
103. Grayson L, Russo P, Ryan K. Hand hygiene. Australia manual. Australian Commission for Safety and Quality in Healthcare; 2009. Online. Available from: http://www.hha.org.au/. [Accessed December 2017].
104. Orsi GB, Raponi M, Franchi C, et al. Surveillance and infection control in an intensive care unit. Infect Control Hosp Epidemiol 2005;26(3):321–5.
105. Haley RW, Culver DH, White JW, et al. The efficacy of infection surveillance and control programs in preventing nosocomial infections in US hospitals. Am J Epidemiol 1985;121(2):182–205.
106. Lim S-M, Webb SAR. Nosocomial bacterial infections in intensive care units. Organisms and mechanisms of antibiotic resistance. Anaesthesia 2005;60(9):887–902.
107. Hardy KJ, Hawkey PM, Gao F, et al. Methicillin resistant Staphylococcus aureus in the critically ill. Br J Anaesth 2004;92(1):121–30.
108. Johnson PDR, Martin R, Burrell LJ, et al. Efficacy of an alcohol/chlorhexidine hand hygiene program in a hospital with high rates of nosocomial methicillin-resistant staphylococcus aureus (MRSA) infection. Med J Aust 2005;183(10):509–14.
109. Gamage B, Moore D, Copes R, et al. Protecting health care workers from SARS and other respiratory pathogens: a review of the infection control literature. Am J Infect Control 2005;33(2):114–21.
110. Ho W, Hong Kong Hospital Authority Working Group on SARS Central Committee of Infection Control. Guideline on management of severe acute respiratory syndrome (SARS). Lancet 2003;361(9366):1313–15.
111. Chan D. Clinical management of SARS patients in ICU. Connect 2003;2(3):76–9.
112. WHO. Middle East respiratory syndrome coronavirus [MERS-CoV] summary and literature update – as of 11 June 2014. Online. Available from: http://www.who.int/crs/disease/coronavirus_infections/archive_updates/en/. [Accessed December 2017].
113. CDC. Middle East Respiratory Syndrome (MERS). Online. Available from: http://www.cdc.gov/coronavirus/MERS/index.html. [Accessed February 2018].
114. Webb SA, Seppelt IM, ANZIC Influenza Investigators. Pandemic (H1N1) 2009 influenza ('swine flu') in Australia and New Zealand intensive care. Crit Care Resus 2009;11(3):170–2.

115. WHO Human Infection with Avian Influenza A(H7N9) virus. Online. Available from: www.who.int. [Accessed February 2018].
116. WHO Guidelines on Core Components of Infection Prevention and Control Programmes at the Nataional and Acute Health Care Facility Level. Online. Available from: http://www.who.int/infection-prevention/. [Accessed February 2018].
117. WHO Multi Drug Resistant TB (MDRTB) Fact Sheet. Online. Available from: www.who.int. [Accessed December 2017].
118. AURA 2016 Summary report. Online. Available from: www.safetyandquality.gov.au. [Sourced January 2018].
119. Sedwick MB, Lance-Smith M, Reeder SJ, et al. Using evidence-based practice to prevent ventilator-associated pneumonia. Crit Care Nurs 2012;32(4):41–50.
120. Price R, MacLennan G, Glen J, SuDDICU collaboration. Selective digestive or oropharyngeal decontamination and topical oropharyngeal chlorhexidine for prevention of death in general intensive care: systematic review and network meta-analysis. BMJ 2014;348:g2197.
121. Hosoglu S, Akalin S, Kidir V, et al. Prospective surveillance study for risk factors of central venous catheter-related bloodstream infections. Am J Infect Control 2004;32(3):131–4.
122. Berenholtz S, Pronovost P, Lipsett P, et al. Eliminating catheter-related bloodstream infections in the intensive care unit. Crit Care Med 2004;32(10):2014–20.
123. Southworth SL, Henman LJ, Kinder LA, et al. The journey to zero central catheter-associated bloodstream infections: culture change in an intensive care unit. Crit Care Nurs 2012;32(2):49–54.
124. Rowley S, Clare S. Improving standards of aseptic practice through an ANTT trust-wide implementation process: a matter of prioritisation and care. Br J Infect Prevention 2009;10(1):S18–23.
125. Hanna HA, Raad II, Hackett B, et al. Antibiotic-impregnated catheters associated with significant decrease in nosocomial and multidrug-resistant bacteremias in critically ill patients. Chest 2003;124(3):1030–8.
126. Moureau NL, Deschneau M, Pyrek J. Evaluation of the clinical performance of a chlorhexidine gluconate antimicrobial transparent dressing. J Infect Prevention 2009;10:S13–17.
127. Rickard C, Lipman J, Courtney M, et al. Routine changing of intravenous administration sets does not reduce colonization or infection in central venous catheters. Infect Control Hosp Epidemiol 2004;25(8):650–5.
128. Koh DBC, Robertson IK, Watts M, et al. Density of microbial colonization on external and internal surfaces of concurrently placed intravascular devices. Am J Crit Care 2012;21(3):162–71.
129. Australasian College for Emergency Medicine and Australian and New Zealand College of Anaesthetists and College of Intensive Care Medicine Australia and New Zealand (CICM). Guidelines for transport of critically ill patients; 2015. Online. Available from: http://www.cicm.org.au/. [Accessed January 2018].
130. Intrahospital transport of critically ill patients (excluding newborns) recommendation of the Société Française d'Anesthésie et de Réanimation (SSFAR) and the Société Française de Medicine d'Urgence (SFMU). Ann Intensive Care 2012;2:1.
131. Warren J, Fromm RE, Orr RA, et al; ACoCCM. Guidelines for the inter- and intrahospital transport of critically ill patients. Crit Care Med 2004;32(1):256–62.
132. Intensive Care Society. Guidelines for transport of the critically ill adult. 3rd ed. London: Intensive Care Society; 2011.
133. Wallace PGM, Ridley SA. ABC of intensive care: transport of critically ill patients. Br Med J 1999;319(7206):368–71.
134. Bergman LM, Pettersson ME, Chaboyer WP, et al. Safety hazards during intrahospital transport: a prospective observational study. Crit Care Med 2017;45:1043–9.
135. Schwebei C, Clec'h C, Magne C, et al; OUTCOMEREA Study Group. Safety of intrahospital transport in ventilated critically ill patients: a multicenter cohort study. Crit Care Med 2013;41(8):1919–28.
136. Fanara B, Mazon C, Barbot O, et al. Recommendations for the intra-hospital transport of critically ill patients. Crit Care 2010;14:R87.
137. Parmentier-Decrucq E, Poissy J, Favory R, et al. Adverse events during intrahospital transport of critically ill patients: incidence and risk factors. Ann Intensive Care 2013;3:10.
138. Jia L, Wan H, Gao Y, et al. High incidence of adverse events during intra-hospital transport of critically Ill patients and new related risk factors: a prospective, multicenter study in China. Crit Care 2016;20:12.
139. Brunsveld-Reinders AH, Arbous MS, Kuiper SG, et al. A comprehensive method to develop a checklist to increase safety of intrahospital transport of critically ill patients. Crit Care 2015;19:214.
140. Chaikittisilpa N, Lele AV, Lyons VH, et al. Risks of routinely clamping external ventricular drains for intrahospital transport in neurocritically ill cerebrovascular patients. Neurocrit Care 2017;28(2):196–204.
141. Martin M, Cook F, Lobo D, et al. Secondary insults and adverse events during intrahospital transport of severe traumatic brain injured patients. Neurocrit Care 2017;26(1):87–95.
142. Trofimov A, Kalentiev G, Yunev M, et al. Intrahospital transfer of patients with traumatic brain injury: increase in intracranial pressure. Acta Neurochir Suppl 2016;122:125–7.
143. World Union of Wound Healing Societies (WUWHS) Consensus Document. Role of dressings in pressure ulcer prevention. Wounds International, 2016. Online. Available from: www.woundsinternational.com. [Accessed 28 February 2018].

Chapter 6

Patient comfort and psychological care

Rosalind Elliott, Leanne Aitken

KEY WORDS

anxiety
agitation
alcohol withdrawal
delirium
pain assessment and pain management
sedation assessment and management
sedation protocols
sleep promotion

Learning objectives

After reading this chapter, you should be able to:

- implement appropriate evidence-based strategies to reduce patient anxiety
- describe the subtypes of delirium
- discuss strategies to potentially prevent, or reduce the duration and severity of, delirium in the critically ill patient
- implement and evaluate delirium assessment screening instruments for the critically ill
- implement screening strategies to identify patients at risk of substance dependence
- implement alcohol withdrawal assessment monitoring instruments
- integrate best practice into pain assessment and management
- describe the different instruments available to assess sedation needs in critically ill patients and discuss the benefits and limitations of each
- determine methods to promote rest and sleep for critically ill patients.

Introduction

Promotion of comfort, psychological health and wellbeing of patients is an essential aspect of care for critically ill patients. Patients experience significant discomfort and ongoing compromise of their psychological health both while in the critical care environment and beyond. Effective management of both patient comfort and psychological health also influences patients' physical health. Aspects of patient comfort and psychological health that are most relevant in the care of the critically ill include the recognition and management of anxiety, delirium, withdrawal from alcohol or other substances, pain, sedation and sleep and inclusion of the patient's family in promoting comfort and psychological health. Despite widespread recognition of the need for regular assessment using validated instruments and targeted management to achieve patient comfort, there are repeated reports indicating absent or infrequent and incomplete assessment, with a lack of subsequent care, internationally.[1-3]

Although each of the concepts of anxiety, delirium, pain, sedation and sleep are reviewed sequentially through this chapter, in reality it is often difficult to separate them as their effects are additive or synergistic. While it is important to ensure that assessment incorporates each of the individual concepts, management may often target multiple aspects concurrently.

Anxiety

Patients may experience anxiety both during and following a period of critical illness. Anxiety has been defined as an unpleasant emotional arousal or condition caused by a perceived threat or stressor.[4] Within that broad definition there are two related, but conceptually different constructs, specifically state and trait anxiety.[5] Trait anxiety, a personality characteristic, refers to the tendency of people to perceive situations as stressful or anxiety-provoking. In contrast, and of more immediate concern during the care of critically ill patients, is state anxiety, an emotional state that exists at a given moment in time and is characterised by 'subjective feelings of tension, apprehension, nervousness, and worry'[5] and is associated with activation of the autonomic nervous system.

Factors contributing to anxiety include:[6-10]

- preexisting high trait anxiety
- current or previous dependence on alcohol or illicit substance/opioids
- previous mental illness
- unwanted symptoms such as pain, sleeplessness, thirst, and discomfort and immobility
- interventions including mechanical ventilation, invasive devices, repositioning and suctioning
- increased severity of illness
- unwanted side effects of medications
- adverse and unfamiliar environmental conditions such as noise and light
- extended ICU length of stay
- concerns about current illness together with underlying chronic disease and the ongoing impact of illness on recovery.

Anxiety has been identified in approximately half of critically ill patients, with the majority of patients reporting moderate-to-severe anxiety.[6,11-13] Patterns of anxiety vary widely; high levels of anxiety early or later in the ICU stay are frequent.[11] The prevalence of anxiety in critically ill patients appears to be similar across countries and cultures.[9,13,14]

Physiological and psychological responses to anxiety reflect a stress response and incorporate avoidance behaviour, increased vigilance and arousal, activation of the sympathetic nervous system and release of cortisol from the adrenal glands.[15] The humoral response, mediated by the hypothalamic–pituitary–adrenal (HPA) axis, regulates this activity. Physiological changes occur to multiple body systems, with the most relevant including constriction of blood vessels, increased heart rate, relaxation of airways, increased secretion of epinephrine and norepinephrine as well as increased glucose production,[15] and result in behavioural, psychological/cognitive and social manifestations (Table 6.1).[16-18] Anxiety can lead to negative outcomes for critical care patients.

Anxiety assessment

The importance of anxiety assessment, with the aim of ameliorating the adverse effects of anxiety, is widely accepted. However, recognition and interpretation of anxiety is complex, particularly when signs and symptoms are masked by critical illness and its treatment. History and previous experience are vital adjuncts to

TABLE 6.1
Clinical indicators of anxiety

PHYSIOLOGICAL	BEHAVIOURAL	PSYCHOLOGICAL/COGNITIVE	SOCIAL
Heart rate	Restlessness	Confusion	Seeking reassurance
Blood pressure	Agitation	Anger	Need for attention/companionship
Chest pain	Sleeplessness	Negative thinking	Limiting interaction
Respiratory rate	Hypervigilance	Verbal expression of stress/ anxiety	
Shortness of breath	Fighting ventilator	Crying	
Altered O_2 saturation	Facial grimacing/tension	Inability to retain and process information	
Coughing/choking feeling	Uncooperative		
Diaphoresis	Rapid speech		
Pallor	Difficulty verbalising		
Cold and clammy	Distrustful/suspicious		
Dry mouth	Avoidance/ desire to leave stressful area		
Pain			
Headache			
Nausea and vomiting			
Swallowing difficulty			

TABLE 6.2
Anxiety self-report assessment scales

SCALE	NUMBER OF ITEMS	COMMENTS
Hospital Anxiety and Depression Scale (HADS)[22]	14 (including 7 anxiety items)	Easy and fast to complete
		Extensively used and therefore international comparisons are available
		Demonstrated validity[25]
Depression Anxiety and Stress Scale 21 (DASS 21)[23]	21 (including 7 anxiety items)	Items measured on scale of 0 (did not apply to me at all) to 3 (applied to me very much or most of the time)
		Demonstrated validity in clinical populations[26]
Spielberger State Anxiety Inventory (SAI)[24]	20 items	Items measured on a scale of 1 (not at all) to 4 (very much so)
		Validity demonstrated in various populations[5]
		Too long for routine clinical use, but may be useful in associated research; attempts to shorten the SAI have provided inconsistent results[5,27]
Visual Analogue Scale – Anxiety (VAS-A)[21]	1 item	10 cm/100 mm line from 'not at all anxious' to 'very anxious'
		Demonstrated validity[21]
Faces Anxiety Scale[18]	1 item	5 possible responses or 'faces' to reflect anxiety
		Fast and easy to use
		Validity has been demonstrated in a small number of ICU cohorts[18,28-30]

patient assessment and diagnosis and often provide information that is vital to effective care and treatment.[19] Alterations in levels of biochemical markers, such as cortisol and catecholamines, that are frequently associated with anxiety may also be attributed to physiological stress.[16] Thus, anxiety rating scales are advocated and may offer benefits not found with unstructured clinical assessment.[20]

Practice tip

Remember a patient's history and previous experiences are vital to 'knowing the person' so if a patient is unable to communicate ask their family and friends about past experiences of illnesses, hospitalisations, phobias, likes and dislikes and usual coping strategies.

A structured approach to assessment is needed to accurately and consistently understand patients' anxiety. A number of self-report scales are available to assess anxiety (Table 6.2). These scales require a degree of cognitive acumen and an ability to communicate responses; a challenge for many critically ill patients. In addition, some scales have up to 21 items, making them both time-consuming and unmanageable for routine use. Patients with visual and auditory impairments may require additional assistance, such as larger print, hearing aids or glasses in order to complete the forms.

The visual analogue scale for anxiety (VAS-A) is a single-item measure which is fast and simple to complete, and has been shown to have good reliability and validity.[21] The VAS-A comprises a 100-millimetre vertical line, with the bottom marker labelled 'not anxious at all' and the top marker labelled 'the most anxious I have ever been'.

Similarly, the Faces Anxiety Scale, another single-item self-reporting scale which was developed by Australian researchers, accurately detects anxiety in critically ill patients.[18] There are five possible responses to assess anxiety (Fig. 6.1).

Anxiety management

The detrimental short- and long-term effects of high anxiety levels and importance of ameliorating or managing this unpleasant psycho-physiological state are widely accepted.[31,32] Although pharmacological interventions such as anxiolytic medications and analgesia are well-recognised and frequently used, non-pharmacological treatments i.e. environmental and nurse-initiated interventions are also useful.

Non-pharmacological treatments

An advantage of non-pharmacological treatments is that they can be nurse-initiated. They may be implemented when units are designed or refurbished (Table 6.3). Although the benefits of some complementary therapies may be widely accepted in the community, use of

FIGURE 6.1 Faces Anxiety Scale

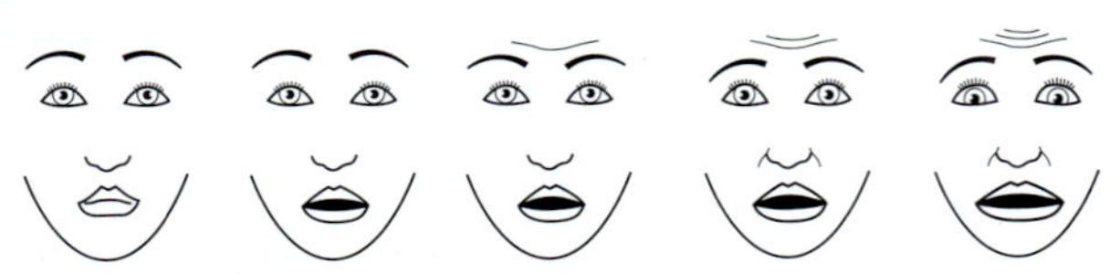

Adapted from McKinley S, Coote K, Stein-Parbury J. Development and testing of a Faces Scale for the assessment of anxiety in critically ill patients. J Adv Nurs 2003;41(1):73–9, with permission.

TABLE 6.3
Non-pharmacological measures to reduce anxiety

NURSE-INITIATED TREATMENTS	ENVIRONMENTAL FACTORS
Patient massage[35]	Provision of natural light[37]
Aromatherapy[38,39]	Calming wall colours such as blue, green and violet
Music therapy[33,41]	Noise reduction with consideration of alarms, paging systems, talking etc[40]

them in critical care is dependent on their acceptance, safety, efficacy and patient consent. While the level of evidence is low, beneficial effects for some complementary therapies such as music therapy and massage have been reported and include lowered blood pressure, heart rate and respiratory rate; improved sleep; and reduced stress (and concomitant sedative medication requirements), anxiety and pain.[33-37] As with any therapy, each non-pharmacological treatment may have different effects on individual patients; consequently, ongoing assessment is essential. In addition, the safety of these therapies during critical illness has not been well demonstrated, necessitating thorough monitoring and caution throughout administration.

Practice tip

Consider using music as an adjunct for patient care. If the patient likes music, ask about their music likes and dislikes (styles, instruments, artists) and when they like to listen to music. Document this information, then request the family to bring a music player with a selection of their preferred music and headphones. Then, prepare the patient for a rest period. Ensure that analgesia is sufficient, there are no planned interventions, and the patient is comfortable, then commence at least 30 minutes of uninterrupted music. See Chlan et al.[42] for more information about providing music as an adjunct to care.

Practice tip

Prioritise the assessment and treatment of discomfort and anxiety. This will greatly reduce sedative medication requirements.

Other strategies to reduce anxiety include communication and information sharing by the healthcare team and inclusion of family members in care processes. The presence of a family member can provide additional reassurance and inner strength (see Chapter 7). In addition, the very presence of the nurse has been reported to be a great source of security, reducing feelings of vulnerability.[43]

Pharmacological treatment for anxiety

Treatment for pain and other reversible physiological causes of anxiety and agitation should be a priority. If anxiety and agitation continue, despite the incorporation of non-pharmacological interventions, pharmacological treatment with relevant medications may be initiated. A brief overview of these medications in the treatment of unrelieved anxiety is provided in Table 6.4. Generally, non-benzodiazepine sedative medications such as propofol are recommended in preference to benzodiazepines.[44]

Delirium

Delirium is a significant concern for critically ill patients and clinicians. It is a central nervous dysfunction in which behaviours and physiological responses are not conducive to healing and recovery. Arguably, the condition has been under-recognised and under-treated[46] and is only recently receiving the attention it deserves. Early detection and treatment of delirium is vital, as it is associated with adverse clinical outcomes such as prolonged duration of ventilation and hospitalisation and higher rates of morbidity and mortality.[47-50] Furthermore, long periods of delirium have been associated with long-term cognitive impairment[51] and an increase in delusional memories.[52,53]

There are three subtypes of delirium: hypoactive, hyperactive and combined (a combination of both).[54] Disturbances in attention (e.g. reduced ability to direct, focus, sustain and shift attention) and awareness (e.g. reduced orientation to the environment) that develop over a short period of time (e.g. hours to a few days) are characteristic of all subtypes of delirium.[54] This contrasts with dementia in which cognitive decline occurs over months and years. Cognitive and perceptive ability often fluctuates through the day worsening at night. A change in an additional cognitive domain such as memory deficit, disorientation or language disturbance that is not better accounted for by a preexisting, established or evolving other neurocognitive disorder and does not occur in the context of a severely reduced level of arousal such as coma is diagnostic of delirium. There should also be evidence from the patient's history, physical examination

TABLE 6.4
Pharmacological treatment for anxiety[44,45]

DRUG GROUP	DRUG/DOSE RANGE	ACTION	SIDE EFFECTS	COMMENT
Sedative hypnotic agent	Propofol 10–100 mcg/kg/min (infusion)	General anaesthetic agent	Hypotension Respiratory depression Myocardial depression when given as bolus Reported to affect memory May cause dreams	Dedicated intravenous line Infusions recommended High metabolic clearance Patient's conscious level increases more quickly once drug is ceased Expensive
Non-benzodiazepine sedative	Dexmedetomidine 0.2–0.7 mcg/kg/h (infusion)	Highly selective alpha-2-adrenoceptor agonist	Initial hypertension may be experienced Hypotension Bradycardia may persist Hyperglycaemia	Minimal respiratory depression No amnesic effect Rapid onset Infusions preferred Role as first line agent not yet demonstrated
Benzodiazepine sedative	Diazepam 5–10 mg bolus	Block encoding on GABA receptors	Long-acting metabolites Hypotension Respiratory depression	No analgesia properties
	Midazolam 0.5–10 mg/h (infusion) 1–2 mg (bolus)		Less likely to have above side effects, but they may still occur	Useful as continuous infusion Rapid onset No analgesia properties Amnesic effect
	Lorazepam 0.01–0.1 mg/kg/h (≤10 mg/h)		Less likely to have above side effects, but they may still occur	Not licensed for use in some countries Strong anxiolytic

Source: Barr et al., 2013 & Reardon et al., 2013.

or laboratory findings that the disturbance is a direct physiological consequence of another medical condition or substance intoxication or withdrawal.[55] Alcohol, nicotine or illicit substance/opioid dependence is more common than many clinicians suspect and this is often a result of history-taking that lacks detail.[56] This topic is explored more thoroughly in the next section.

Lethargy, slow quiet speech and reduced alertness are typical behaviours of hypoactive delirium.[55] Given that many patients with hypoactive delirium appear 'quietly' confused, delirium may not be recognised and treated.[46] Behaviours evident in hyperactive delirium such as hyperactivity and agitation cannot go unnoticed by clinicians and present overt risks of self-injury such as unintentional extubation/decannulation and intravenous/arterial device removal. Combined delirium is characterised by fluctuations in activity and attention levels including the behaviours of both hyperactive and hypoactive subtypes.

Reports in the healthcare literature about the prevalence of delirium in ICU vary widely from 10% to 80%,[1,57] an unsurprising finding given that it is notoriously difficult to diagnose in patients who are unable to communicate verbally. The prevalence in other critical care areas such as emergency departments is generally reported to be lower,[58] likely because the patients' severity of illness varies.

The exact pathophysiology of delirium is not yet fully understood; however, imbalances in brain cholinergic and dopaminergic neurotransmitter systems are thought to be responsible.[59] Many predisposing and precipitating risk factors have been identified[59-61] (Table 6.5) and current opinion suggests that there is an additive effect: patients with more than one predisposing factor will require less noxious precipitating factors to develop delirium than patients who have none.[61] Predisposing risk factors are those that exist prior to the occurrence of critical illness, while precipitating risk factors occur during the course of critical illness and may be disease-related or iatrogenic. Prevention and therapeutic management of risk factors is the mainstay delirium treatment.

Practice tip

Perform a patient assessment to identify predisposing and contributing risk factors for delirium (Table 6.5). Interview the family if the patient is unable to provide a history. Discuss your findings with the multidisciplinary health care team and develop a plan for prevention (using the strategies suggested in this chapter). Document and evaluate.

TABLE 6.5
Risk factors for delirium

PREDISPOSING RISK FACTORS	PRECIPITATING RISK FACTORS[57,62-65]
Advanced age	Increased severity of illness
Dementia	Metabolic, fluid and electrolyte disturbance (particularly uraemia)
Illicit substance use	Systemic inflammatory response (particularly infection)
Excessive intake of alcohol	Hypoxia
Smoking	Acute injury affecting the CNS
Sensory deficits	Medications that affect acetylcholine transmission, e.g. atropine, fentanyl
Renal insufficiency	Psychoactive medications, e.g. benzodiazepines, opioids
Previous cerebral damage	Prolonged pain
Hypertension	Excessive noise
Congestive heart failure	Sleep deprivation
History of depression	Immobility
Genetic propensity	
Functional dependence and frailty	

Assessment of delirium

The increased morbidity and mortality associated with delirium make it imperative to incorporate reliable and valid assessment in routine care.[66] A practical delirium assessment screening instrument for the critically ill cannot be reliant on patient–assessor verbal communication. Both the Intensive Care Delirium Screening Checklist (ICDSC)[66] (Fig. 6.2) and the Confusion Assessment Method for the Intensive Care Unit (CAM-ICU)[67] (Fig. 6.3) have been shown to fulfil these requirements, although clinical judgement should also be retained in the screening process.[68,69]

The ICDSC contains eight items based on the *Diagnostic and Statistical Manual of Mental Disorders* (DSM-IV) criteria for delirium and was validated in a study conducted within ICU.[66] It is also simple to use and easily integrated into patient documentation. All features of delirium are incorporated such as sleep pattern disturbances and hypo- or hyperactivity. The first step in using the ICDSC is an assessment of conscious level using a five-point scale (A–E). Only patients whose conscious level is sufficient for them to respond to moderate physical stimuli (C–E on the scale) are able to be assessed. The eight items of the ICDSC are rated present (1) or absent (0). A score of four or higher is considered to be indicative of delirium.[66]

The CAM-ICU was also validated for screening delirium in the ICU population (see *Further reading* for more information).[67] Acute onset of mental status changes or fluctuating course is assessed using neurological observations conducted over the previous 24 hours. Inattention is tested in patients who are unable to communicate verbally by using either picture recognition or a random letter test. Disorganised thinking is assessed by listening to the patient's speech and, for patients who are unable to verbally communicate, a simple command is provided such as 'hold up the same number of fingers as me' (while the assessor holds up their fingers). Any conscious level other than 'alert' is considered 'altered'. An overall score is not derived from the CAM-ICU; delirium is either present or absent.[67]

Prevention and treatment of delirium

Although the causes of delirium are thought not to be strictly 'psychological' in nature, many interventions and preventative strategies focus on reducing anxiety, maintaining safety and providing a calming and low stimulus environment together with ameliorating or eliminating risk factors. Individual patient risk factors should be identified and where possible modified (even in the absence of delirium). Potential preventative measures include:

- adequate pain relief
- reassurance to reduce anxiety
- judicious use of sedative medications, particularly benzodiazepine medications (avoidance of continuous infusions)
- correction of the physiological effects of critical illness (e.g. hypoxia, hypotension, infection and fluid and electrolyte imbalance)
- optimisation of the sleep cycle
- early mobilisation
- treatment of the underlying illness.

Research investigating the prevention and management of delirium in ICU is growing; however, evidence for the majority of interventions is low. There is emerging evidence that intervention bundles directed towards preventing delirium among other aspects of care in ICU patients may be beneficial.[40,71,72] Given the hypothesised underlying pathophysiology of delirium, it is not surprising that strategies to promote and maintain good quality sleep and avoidance of benzodiazepines are emphasised in these 'bundles'. Regardless of the efficacy of the interventions[73] to date, the creation of environmental conditions that are conducive to rest and sleep, in particular sound reduction and adjusting light levels appropriate for the time of day, as well as sedation minimisation, delirium monitoring and early mobilisation, have not been shown to cause harm and therefore represent good practice.

In cases where non-pharmacological strategies are not successful antipsychotic medications (e.g. olanzapine) or the selective alpha-2-adrenoceptor agonist, dexmedetomidine may be considered.[44] Although frequently used, there is little evidence showing the efficacy of haloperidol and atypical antipsychotics in reducing the duration of delirium in adult ICU patients (and humans generally).[74,75] Evidence is inconsistent[76] but dexmedetomidine has shown promise in both reducing the duration and incidence of delirium in critically ill patients.[77,78] It

FIGURE 6.2 Intensive care delirium screening checklist (ICDSC).

PATIENT EVALUATION	DAY 1	DAY 2	DAY 3	DAY 4	DAY 5
Altered level of consciousness* (A-E)					
	If A or B do not complete patient evaluation for the period				
Inattention					
Disorientation					
Hallucination – delusion – psychosis					
Psychomotor agitation or retardation					
Inappropriate speech or mood					
Sleep/wake cycle disturbance					
Symptom fluctuation					
TOTAL SCORE (0-8)					

Level of consciousness*:		Score
	A: no response	none
	B: response to intense and repeated stimulation (loud voice and pain)	none
	C: response to mild or moderate stimulation	1
	D: normal wakefulness	0
	E: exaggerated response to normal stimulation	1

SCORING SYSTEM:
The scale is completed based on information collected from each entire 8-hour shift or from the previous 24 hours.
Obvious manifestation of an item = 1 point. No manifestation of an item or no assessment possible = 0 point.
The score of each item is entered in the corresponding empty box and is 0 or 1.

1. Altered level of consciousness:
A) No response or B) the need for vigorous stimulation in order to obtain any response signified a severe alteration in the level of consciousness precluding evaluation. If there is coma (A) or stupor (B) most of the time period then a dash (-) is entered and there is no further evaluation during that period.
C) Drowsiness or requirement of a mild to moderate stimulation for a response implies an altered level of consciousness and scores 1 point.
D) Wakefulness or sleeping state that could easily be aroused is considered normal and scores no point.
E) Hypervigilance is rated as an abnormal level of consciousness and scores 1 point.

2. Inattention: Difficulty in following a conversation or instructions. Easily distracted by external stimuli Difficulty in shifting focuses. Any of these scores 1 point.

3. Disorientation: Any obvious mistake in time, place or person scores 1 point.

4. Hallucination, delusion or psychosis: The unequivocal clinical manifestation of hallucination or of behaviour probably due to hallucination (e.g, trying to catch a non-existent object) or delusion. Gross impairment in reality testing. Any of these scores 1 point.

5. Psychomotor agitation or retardation: Hyperactivity requiring the use of additional sedative drugs or restraints in order to control potential dangerousness (e.g. pulling out IV lines, hitting staff), hyperactivity or clinically noticeable psychomotor slowing. Any of these scores 1 point.

6. Inappropriate speech or mood: Inappropriate, disorganised or incoherent speech. Inappropriate display of emotion related to events or situation. Any of these scores 1 point.

7. Sleep/wake cycle disturbance: Sleeping less than 4 hours or waking frequently at night (do not consider wakefulness initiated by medical staff or loud environment). Sleeping during most of the day. Any of these scores 1 point.

8. Symptom fluctuation: Fluctuation of the manifestation of any item or symptom over 24 hours (e.g. from one shift to another) scores 1 point.

Adapted from Bergeron N, Dubois MJ, Dumont M, et al. Intensive care delirium screening checklist: evaluation of a new screening tool. Intensive Care Med 2001;27(5):859–64.

should also be noted that any medication designed to enhance cognition has the potential to make delirium worse and there are many potential unwanted side effects (e.g. Q-T interval prolongation for some antipsychotics[79] and bradycardia and hypotension for alpha-2-adrenoceptor agonists[77]); therefore these medications should be used judiciously in the critically ill.

Alcohol, benzodiazepine, nicotine and opioid withdrawal

Patients who are dependent on alcohol (ethanol), benzodiazepines, nicotine or opioids are at risk of developing a withdrawal syndrome in the initial stages of treatment in ICU. Withdrawal from opioids may also occur later

FIGURE 6.3 Confusion Assessment Method – Intensive Care Unit (CAM-ICU).[70]

CAM-ICU Worksheet

Feature 1: Acute Onset or Fluctuating Course Positive if you answer 'yes' to either 1A or 1B.	Positive	Negative
1A: Is the patient different than his/her baseline mental status? Or 1B: Has the patient had any fluctuation in mental status in the past 24 hours as evidenced by fluctuation on a sedation scale (e.g. RASS), GCS, or previous delirium assessment?	Yes	No
Feature 2: Inattention Positive if either score for 2A <u>or</u> 2B is less than 8. Attempt the ASE letters first. If patient is able to perform this test and the score is clear, record this score and move to Feature 3. If patient is unable to perform this test <u>or</u> the score is unclear, then perform the ASE Pictures. If you perform both tests, use the ASE Pictures' results to score the Feature.	Positive	Negative
2A: ASE Letters: record score (enter NT for not tested) <u>Directions</u>: Say to the patient, "*I am going to read you a series of 10 letters. Whenever you hear the letter 'A', indicate by squeezing my hand.*" Read letters from the following letter list in a normal tone. SAVEAHAART Scoring: Errors are counted when patient fails to squeeze on the letter "A" and when the patient squeezes on any letter other than "A".	Score (out of 10):_____	
2B: ASE Pictures: record score (enter NT for not tested) Directions are included on the picture packets.	Score (out of 10):_____	
Feature 3: Disorganised Thinking Positive if the combined score is less than 4	Positive	Negative
<u>3A: Yes/No Questions</u> (Use either Set A or Set B, alternate on consecutive days if necessary): Set A 1. Will a stone float on water? 2. Are there fish in the sea? 3. Does one pound weigh more than two pounds? 4. Can you use a hammer to pound a nail? Set B 1. Will a leaf float on water? 2. Are there elephants in the sea? 3. Do two pounds weigh more than one pound? 4. Can you use a hammer to cut wood? Score___(Patient earns 1 point for each correct answer out of 4) <u>3B: Command</u> Say to patient: "Hold up this many fingers" (Examiner holds two fingers in front of patient) "Now do the same thing with the other hand" (Not repeating the number of fingers). (If pt is unable to move both arms, for the second part of the command ask patient "Add one more finger") Score___(Patient earns 1 point if able to successfully complete the entire command)	Combined Score (3A + 3B): _____ (out of 5)	
Feature 4: Altered Level of Consciousness Positive if the Actual RASS score is anything other than "0" (zero)	Positive	Negative
Overall CAM-ICU (Features 1 and 2 and either Feature 3 or 4):	Positive	Negative

Source: © E. Wesley Ely, MD, MPH. Pulmonary and Critical Care and Health Services Research. Vanderbilt University and VA-GRECC. www.icudelirium.org.

in the illness trajectory for patients who receive large doses of analgesics for painful injuries and conditions ('iatrogenic dependency'). Unrecognised and therefore untreated withdrawal from any substance may lead to prolonged length of stay and duration of mechanical ventilation and increased risk of infection and delirium and even mortality.[80] Opioid and nicotine withdrawal is unpleasant but rarely physiologically dangerous. However, sudden cessation of ethanol or benzodiazepines in the setting of prolonged use and neurobiological adaptation may lead to alcohol withdrawal syndrome (AWS) or benzodiazepine withdrawal and serious complications.[81] Therefore early identification of the possibility of withdrawal (within 24 hours for alcohol) is essential to ensure timely treatment.

As ethanol mimics γ-aminobutyric acid (GABA) in the brain, regular and excessive intake of ethanol leads to changes in the inhibitory GABA and excitatory glutamate systems, decreased endogenous GABA levels, fewer and less sensitive GABA receptors and glutamate system activation.[81] Postsynaptic *N*-methyl-D-aspartate (NMDA) receptors are more reactive and glutamate concentration increases. Therefore, cessation of ethanol may lead to unopposed neuronal excitation and resulting autonomic hyperactivity.

Criteria for classifying withdrawal are based on history of heavy alcohol use, symptoms and effect of symptoms on physical and mental functioning which cannot be accounted for by another mental disorder.[55] Frequency and quantity of alcohol consumption together with other factors including previous detoxification episodes and withdrawal seizures and structural brain lesions are thought to be predictive of AWS symptom severity.[82] Withdrawal may occur 6–24 hours after cessation or significant reduction in intake. The physiological basis of benzodiazepine withdrawal is similar resulting in autonomic hyperactivity. The severity is in part dependent on the half-life of the type of benzodiazepine. The most severe form of AWS, delirium tremens, occurs from 12 to 72 hours after cessation and is characterised by fluctuating conscious level, including attention and cognitive deficits (hallucinations, confusion and delirium), and severe hyperthermia and hypertension. The result of untreated delirium tremens may be withdrawal seizures, cardiovascular and respiratory failure, multiorgan dysfunction and death.[81]

The international estimation of opioid use disorder (OUD) in the population is approximately 5%.[83-85] Given the concomitant adverse health effects of OUD, a significant number of people with OUD who are at risk of opioid withdrawal are treated in ICU. Data for nicotine withdrawal in critical care are also likely to reflect population rates for daily tobacco smoking which range from 14% in Australia, North America and parts of Europe[86,87] to over 30% in parts of Asia.[88] The underlying physiology of withdrawal symptoms is similar for these chemicals. Opioids act on the dopaminergic mesolimbic system. Dependency results in lower levels of endogenous opioids and down regulation of the dopaminergic system[89] so withdrawal produces unpleasant symptoms such as dysphoria, anxiety, joint pain, diarrhoea and vomiting.[90] Similarly nicotine dependency results in neurological adaptation that is desensitisation to nicotine which causes up-regulation of nicotinic acetylcholine receptors (nAchRs). The nAchRs modulate many mood enhancing neurotransmitters, dopamine, and acetylcholine causing a physiological 'need' and nicotine-seeking behaviour. Withdrawal symptoms related to reduced levels of neurotransmitters are unpleasant. Neither opioid nor nicotine withdrawal is life-threatening but may result in delirium or agitation which increases the risk of self-injury.

It is estimated that up to 33% of patients treated in ICU with continuous infusions for an extended time experience iatrogenic opioid withdrawal.[91,92] The incidence of iatrogenic benzodiazepine withdrawal is estimated to be lower (8%)[87] although opioid and benzodiazepine withdrawal often occurs simultaneously and the signs are non-specific so the exact incidence for either iatrogenic withdrawal is unclear. The risk of withdrawal can be reduced by using all opioids and sedative medications judiciously based on individual patient needs (to maintain comfort and a calm and cooperative patient).[5,44] It is also recommended that medications are tapered for patients who require continuous opioid and sedative infusions for several days or a program of methadone replacement is instituted to facilitate a gradual reduction (5–10% per day) of the infusion doses.[92]

Screening for and assessment of withdrawal symptoms

Identification of withdrawal is challenging because symptoms may be the same for the underlying illness unless the reason for treatment in ICU is related to alcohol, benzodiazepine or opioid consumption (in which case the likelihood of withdrawal is high).[80] Thus no screening or assessment scales have been specifically validated for use in ICU and history-taking is a vital adjunct to assessment and diagnosis. As highlighted earlier, history-taking with regard to alcohol and substance use often lacks detail. A brief interview schedule such as the 4-item CAGE questionnaire[93] (administered to the patient's proxy if the patient is unable to participate taking care to maintain confidentiality) is a recommended approach to guide history taking. Screening questions pertain to previous intentions to '**C**ut down' drinking, **A**nnoyance about being criticised for drinking, previous **G**uilty feelings about drinking and need to drink first thing in the morning ('**E**ye opener'). The presence of two or more of these features indicates that alcohol dependency is likely and requires further investigation. An alternative is the Prediction of Alcohol Withdrawal Severity Scale (PAWSS).[82] Although the frequency and amount of a substance consumed is important it should also be noted that the definition of 'excessive intake' of any substance varies and is dependent on factors such as gender, body size and fat composition, liver function and genetic composition.

In cases in which alcohol withdrawal is suspected it is recommended that withdrawal assessment scales (Table 6.6) are used to guide treatment and monitor progress particularly in the first 24–48 hours.[80] Although not necessarily tested in ICU, both the Clinical Institute Withdrawal Assessment of Alcohol Scale, revised (CIWA-Ar), and AWS Scale have been shown to perform well in clinical practice[94] so the context and patient specifics should dictate choice of scale. To overcome the limitations of using the CIWA-Ar with non-verbal patients (e.g. mechanically ventilated)[80,95] clinicians recommend using it with a sedation or agitation scale. The AWS[96] scale overcomes the difficulty of requiring a verbal response and may be more appropriate for the ICU population.

The Fagerström Test for Nicotine Dependence (FTND) is a commonly used validated tool to assess

TABLE 6.6
Widely used alcohol withdrawal assessment scales

SCALE	DESCRIPTION	COMMENT
The Clinical Institute Withdrawal Assessment for Alcohol (CIWA-Ar) scale[97]	10-item scale Maximum score 67; higher scores indicate more severe withdrawal; <8 = mild withdrawal; 8–15 = moderate withdrawal; >20 = severe withdrawal Administer a minimum of every hour until symptoms subside	Widely used in ICU setting Patient must be able to verbally communicate to complete 4 items (7–10) Best used together with the sedation-agitation scale to guide treatment Scores <8–10 indicate that pharmacological treatment probably not necessary
Alcohol Withdrawal Syndrome (AWS) Scale[97]	Consists of two subscales; somatic symptoms = s and mental symptoms = m S subscale: pulse rate, diastolic blood pressure, temperature, breathing rate, sweating, tremor M subscale: agitation, contact, orientation, hallucination, anxiety Maximum score: 55; higher scores indicate more severe withdrawal; 5 = mild; 6–9 = moderate; and ≥10 = severe Administer every hour until symptoms subside	Allows separate assessment of somatic and mental withdrawal symptoms. Developed specifically for patients with severe withdrawal or delirium (but not for ICU patients); does not need verbal response from patient

likelihood of nicotine withdrawal.[98] The score ranges from 0 to 10; higher scores indicate higher dependency. The FTND relies on self-report so has some limitations for use in ICU. Recent pack-year history (packs per day × number of years smoking) may also provide the clinician with useful information about the likelihood of withdrawal.

Withdrawal screening and assessment tools specifically designed for other substances such as opioids have poor validity and reliability.[99] Clinical judgement is primarily used to monitor and guide treatment.

Practice tip

The CAGE ('**C**ut down' drinking, **A**nnoyance about being criticised for drinking, previous **G**uilty feelings and need to drink first thing in the morning ['**E**ye opener']) screening approach can be adapted for use for detecting dependence to other substances such as benzodiazepines. Practice using the adapted screening approach next time you care for a patient who is suspected to be dependent on benzodiazepines and opioids.

Management of withdrawal

Comprehensive supportive care underpins the management of any withdrawal syndrome. Withdrawal from many substances does not necessarily require pharmacological treatment and depends on the substance and the severity of withdrawal. Supportive care (e.g. maintenance of fluid and electrolyte balance and serum thiamine levels) may be all that is required for minor alcohol withdrawal. Clinicians should be aware that the psychological 'need' for alcohol or any other substance may continue beyond the period of physiological withdrawal. People with a preexisting substance dependency may require ongoing psychological support and understanding; the involvement of specialist 'drug and alcohol' health care teams is advised.

Treatment for alcohol withdrawal comprises pharmacological agents guided by symptom severity. A loading dose of benzodiazepine followed by tapering doses should be used. Diazepam is the conventional approach, however; other medications such as barbiturates, dexmedetomidine, clonidine, ketamine and propofol (often in combination with benzodiazepines) have been explored.[100] Barbiturates are indicated in the setting of severe withdrawal requiring escalating benzodiazepine doses.[101] Further research is required before recommendations for treatment of AWS with other pharmacological agents can be made. Wernicke's encephalopathy is a potential catastrophic consequence of AWS caused by overwhelming metabolic demands on brain cells that have depleted intracellular thiamine. Thiamine and B vitamin complex supplementation is an essential component of treatment reducing mortality and morbidity.[102]

As the underlying pathophysiology of benzodiazepine withdrawal is the same as AWS, a similar treatment regimen of a tapering dose of a long-acting benzodiazepine is advised together with supportive therapy. 'Benzodiazepine sparing' treatment regimens incorporating dexmedetomidine are also recommended.[44] It should be noted that continuous infusion of dexmedetomidine over several days may result in dependency. Low dose flumazenil is a novel approach provided as multiple bolus intravenous doses together with or without benzodiazepine tapering to reduce withdrawal symptoms.[103] Efficacy and safety has largely been tested in ambulatory care settings; guidelines for use during critical illness are not available.

Mild opioid withdrawal may be treated with supportive therapy alone, but moderate-to-severe withdrawal is treated with tapering doses of methadone.[104] More recently buprenorphine has been found to control withdrawal symptoms better than methadone and may reduce long-term dependence.[105] The first dose of buprenorphine is administered when withdrawal symptoms are moderate reducing the risk of precipitated withdrawal.[104] Other anxiolytic medications such as clonidine, dexmedetomidine and benzodiazepines may also play a role in reducing somatic withdrawal symptoms.[104]

Nicotine replacement therapy (NRT) has been associated with adverse outcomes, consequently universal use of NRT is not recommended for the critically ill.[106,107] It should be reserved for patients for whom the risk of not providing NRT (e.g. severe agitation attributable to nicotine withdrawal) outweighs potential harms.[108] The usual regimen for NRT comprises transdermal administration of tapering doses of 24-hour release nicotine impregnated patches.

Comprehensive guidance for all substance withdrawal syndromes is beyond the scope of this textbook. The reader is advised to consult papers published in journals such as *Alcohol and Alcoholism* and *Journal of Chemical Dependency* and relevant textbooks[109,110] (see *Further reading*) as well as local practice guidelines.

Practice tip

Next time you care for a patient who has experienced alcohol withdrawal ask them about the symptoms and strategies other than medications that helped reduce their discomfort.

Pain

Pain is an unobservable, inherently subjective, experience. The nebulous multifaceted nature of pain has led to significant difficulties in not only understanding the mechanisms underlying the experience but also assessing and managing the phenomenon.

Pain is a sensation widely experienced by critical care patients and is one of the stressors most commonly reported by former and current ICU patients.[53,111] In particular, apparently innocuous procedures such as turning or positioning may cause mild or moderate pain while invasive procedures (e.g. chest drain removal) are often severely painful.[112] Arguably, pain management is not always afforded the same emphasis as more 'life-threatening' conditions such as haemodynamic instability. However, its alleviation is an essential element of critical care nursing and should be emphasised in order to reduce potential suffering and the need for sedative medication. Myths such as the possibility that patients may become dependent on analgesics, that the very young and elderly have higher tolerance for pain, and our cultural tendency to reward high pain tolerance may lead to inadequate pain management. In critical care, nurses assume a fairly autonomous role in titrating analgesic medication. With this increased autonomy comes a responsibility to be knowledgeable and aware of effective pain management and assessment of the 'fifth vital sign'.

Pathophysiology of pain

Pain is transmitted to the central nervous system via one of two pathways. The fast pain pathway occurs when the stimuli are carried by small myelinated A-delta fibres, producing a sharp, prickling sensation that is easily localised. The slow pathway acts in response to polymodal nociceptors, is carried by small unmyelinated C fibres and produces a dull, aching or burning sensation. It is difficult to locate, acts after fast pain, and is considered to be more unpleasant than fast pain.[113]

Perceptions of pain are thought to occur in the thalamus, whereas behavioural and emotional responses occur in the hypothalamus and limbic system.[113] Perceptions of pain are influenced by prior experience, and by cultural and normative practices, which helps to explain individual reactions to pain.[113]

There are negative physiological effects of pain that include a sympathetic response with increased cardiac work, thus potentially compromising cardiac stability.[114] Respiratory function may be impaired in the critically ill undergoing surgical procedures when deep-breathing and coughing is limited by increased pain, thus reducing airway movement and increasing the retention of secretions and possibility of nosocomial pneumonia.

Adverse psychological sequelae of poorly-treated pain include diminished feelings of control and self-efficacy and increased fear and anxiety. An inability to engage in rehabilitation and health-promoting activities may transpire. The long-term effects of undertreated pain are not clearly understood but almost certainly impact on recovery and may even lead to worsening chronic pain.[115] When these unwanted outcomes are considered alongside the physiological effects of poorly-treated pain, the vital importance of pain management is evident.

Pain assessment

Pain is whatever the experiencing person says it is, existing whenever he [sic] *says it does.*[116]

The nebulous quality and subjective nature of the pain experience lead to considerable problems in its assessment. Compounding this is the challenge of assessment for the critically ill who often have insufficient cognitive acumen to articulate their needs and an inability to communicate verbally. A common language and process in which to assess pain is essential in ameliorating some of these challenges. Furthermore, accurate assessment and consistent recording are fundamental aspects of pain management. Without these vital components, it is impossible to evaluate interventions designed to reduce pain. Despite the importance of assessing pain there is evidence to suggest that formal assessment (or at least documentation of that assessment) only occurs about 50% of the time.[1]

Since the pain experience is subjective, all attempts should be made to facilitate patient communication of the nature, intensity, body part affected and characteristics of their pain. The patient's usual communication aids, such as glasses and hearing aid, should be used. Whenever patients cannot verbally communicate other strategies must be established and used consistently. For example, strategies involving nodding, hand movements, facial expressions, eye blinks, mouthing answers and writing can be highly effective, not only for pain assessment but also to express other feelings and concerns. In cases when there is limited motor function but the patient is cognitively able, the speech pathologist may be able to advise on alternative communication strategies.

When possible, a patient's health history (from the family if the patient is unable), including any existing painful conditions, should be taken. Quite apart from the presenting condition, which may be painful, critical care patients may have significant comorbidities such as rheumatoid/osteoarthritis and chronic back pain. It is imperative that the patient's usual pain management strategies are identified and implemented if possible. For example, factors that relieve the pain or increase its intensity should be recorded, along with its relationship to daily activities such as sleep, appetite and physical ability.

Regardless of the patient's communication capability, strategies to ensure consistent objective assessment and management should be implemented. Laminated cards displaying body diagrams, words to describe pain and pain intensity measures (including visual analogues and numerical scales) are useful instruments in meeting these requirements. Verbal numerical reporting scales and visual analogue scales (VAS) are commonly used. These are outlined in Table 6.7. VAS can be difficult to administer to critically ill patients; however, a combined

TABLE 6.7
Pain scales

SCALE	DESCRIPTION	COMMENTS
Verbal numeric reporting scale	Self-rating scale Single-item scale Scale from 0 (no pain) to 10 (worst pain ever)	Patient must be able to communicate verbally Needs to understand concept of rating pain Dependent on prior pain experiences Simple, easy to use
Visual analogue scale	Self-rating scale Single-item A horizontal line with equal divisions is used for the patient to rate current pain level (no pain is on far left and worst pain is far right)	Patient can communicate by pointing Needs to understand concept of rating pain Dependent on patient's prior pain experiences Simple, easy to use
McGill Short Pain Questionnaire[121]	Measures quality of pain Uses 15 descriptor words to measure sensory effect of pain Can be used in conjunction with a pain intensity scale	Gives more information about the patient's pain[112] Takes longer to administer
Behavioural Pain Scale (Fig. 6.4)[118]	Based on pain-related behaviours: the sum of three items Higher scores indicate higher pain intensity (range: 3–12)	Patient does not have to communicate Simple, easy to use Includes 'ventilator compliance' (may no longer be relevant for pain assessment when using modern ventilators)
Checklist of Nonverbal Pain Indicators (CNPI)[119]	Developed for cognitively impaired adults Based on the presence/absence of 5 non-verbal pain behaviours (one is non-verbal vocalisation, e.g. groaning) and verbal complaints Score 0–6 (score of 1 allocated for the presence of a pain behaviour/verbal complaint), higher scores indicate more pain	Patient does not have to communicate Simple, easy to use No patient report at all Not as reliable for immobile patients[149]
Critical Care Pain Observation Tool (CPOT)[120]	Based on previously developed instruments using pain-related behaviour to assess pain, e.g. BPS 4 items: facial expression, body movements, muscle tension and compliance with ventilator or vocalisation Higher scores indicate more pain (range: 0–8)	Patient does not have to communicate Simple, easy to use Includes 'ventilator compliance' (may no longer be relevant for pain assessment when using modern ventilators) or vocalisation in extubated patients

FIGURE 6.4 Behavioural Pain Scale.

Item	Description	Score
Facial expression	Relaxed	1
	Partially tightened (e.g. brow lowering)	2
	Fully tightened (e.g. eyelid closing)	3
	Grimacing	4
Upper limbs	No movement	1
	Partially bent	2
	Fully bent with finger flexion	3
	Permanently retracted	4
Compliance with ventilation	Tolerating movement	1
	Coughing but tolerating ventilation for most of the time	2
	Fighting ventilator	3
	Unable to control ventilation	4

Source: Payen JF, Bru O, Bosson JL, et al. Assessing pain in critically ill sedated patients by using a behavioral pain scale. Crit Care Med 2001;29(12):2258–63.

VAS and numerical reporting scale includes the benefit of a visual cue with the ability to quantify pain intensity.

Other physiological and behavioural pain indicators may be used to assess pain in less responsive or unconscious patients.[117] Several instruments have been developed and validated for use in the critically ill adult patient including the Behavioural Pain Scale (BPS) (Fig. 6.4),[118] Checklist of Non-verbal Pain Indicators (CNPI)[119] and the Critical Care Pain Observation Tool (CPOT)[120] (http://ajcc.aacnjournals.org/content/15/4/420/T1.expansion.html). Briefly, scores are assigned to categories such as altered body movements, restlessness and synchronisation with the ventilator, providing a global score for comparison after pain relief interventions. The BPS and the CPOT are considered to be the most valid and reliable behavioural pain assessment instruments for patients who are unable to communicate verbally.[44] The CPOT offers several benefits over the BPS including use of an indicator assessing muscle tension where resistance to passive movement is assessed as 0 = relaxed; 1 = tense or rigid; 2 = very tense or rigid; and an alternative indicator to compliance with ventilation that can be used in extubated patients – assessments include whether the patient is talking in normal tone or no sound = 0; sighing, moaning = 1; crying out, sobbing = 2.

Nurses should not rely solely on changes in physiological parameters, including cardiovascular (elevated blood pressure and heart rate) and respiratory recordings to assess pain intensity, as other pathophysiological or treatment-related factors may be responsible.[122] Classic reactions to stressors (e.g. pain), such as increased heart rate and blood pressure, do not always occur in critically ill patients and are therefore unreliable pain assessment methods.[122] A potential explanation is that autonomic tone may be dysfunctional in a large proportion of ICU patients.[123] In haemodynamically-stable long-term critical patients, vital signs may be useful if used in conjunction with other forms of assessment.[44]

In addition, it is particularly important to regularly consider and search for potential sources of pain in unresponsive patients and those who are unable to communicate. Nurses should assume pain is present if there is a reason to suspect pain; an analgesic trial may assist in identifying this. As a general rule, analgesia medication should be administered to patients who are heavily sedated or receiving muscle relaxants as a precaution.

Pain management

Although pain management is discussed here independently, in practice it is often combined with sedative administration to reduce anxiety. However, pain management should always be the first goal for achieving overall patient comfort (the so called analgosedation approach[124]). Efforts to improve patient comfort for intubated patients often favour the concurrent use of both sedative and analgesic medications.[44] This practice therefore makes it difficult to assess the single effect of each medication on the patient's pain and highlights its multidimensional properties. In addition to pharmacological treatment of pain, non-pharmacological strategies can be effective as an adjunct to drug therapy or as an alternative.

Pain relief may be required for preexisting injuries or prior to specific procedures to prevent pain. Being turned is often cited as a painful procedure; however, wounds, drain removal, tracheal suction, femoral catheter removal, placement of a central venous catheter and wound dressings and coughing may also cause considerable discomfort.[111] Guidelines and written protocols for procedures such as femoral sheath removal and insertion of a central venous catheter can significantly reduce pain intensity as they often contain reminders to provide analgesia. Some procedures, such as insertion of invasive devices, require additional pain management such as local anaesthetics. This highlights the potential need for additional pain protocols linked to key standard procedures (e.g. patient turning) to reduce patients' pain experience.

Pain-relieving medication can be administered via a number of routes, including oral, enteral feeding tube, intravenous, rectal, topical, subcutaneous, intramuscular, epidural and intrathecal. For all routes of administration, assessment of the patient's suitability and contraindications for use are an essential part of the decision-making process. Patient-controlled analgesia for intravenous and, more recently, epidural analgesia is commonly part of critical care nursing.

Epidural pain management requires additional evaluation, including sensory and functional assessment, because both local anaesthetic opioid medications are used. Sensory function should be regularly checked using a dermatome chart to gauge segments that are blocked by the local anaesthetic agent. In addition to sensory blockade, regular assessment for lower limb motor deficit is required to detect changes in motor response, which may impair the ability to mobilise safely. Sudden or subtle changes may also indicate a complication such as epidural haematoma. The Bromage Assessment Scale is often used to assess motor response. The catheter site must be regularly checked to identify complications such as bleeding, haematoma and infection early and to ensure catheter patency. Intrathecal administration of analgesic medications has similar contraindications and complications to epidural analgesia and requires similar precautions. It is important to note that intrathecal (as compared to intravenous) administration does not eliminate all opioid side effects (see *Further reading*).

Practice tip

Epidural administration of medication does not preclude mobilisation. However, certain safety measures should be taken. Ensure that the epidural catheter is well secured: view the site before mobilising and apply extra tape. Monitor blood pressure and heart rate before and during the initial stages of mobilising. Two healthcare personnel should assist during the first attempt to mobilise.

Non-pharmacological treatment for pain

Non-pharmacological strategies to reduce pain are linked to some key strategies to reduce stress. Excessive pain may lead to stress as the body attempts to maintain homeostasis and stress may exacerbate pain. Strategies to reduce stress and pain include both comfort measures and diversional interventions, which require the nurse to individualise and adapt strategies to match the patient's needs and preferences. Diversional methods may include distraction strategies, and aim to refocus the patient's thinking away from the pain and on to other more pleasant thoughts or activities. Research has highlighted the importance patients place on the presence of family members in the facilitation of emotional and physical strategies of pain management.[125,126] Some interventions that may be effective are listed in Table 6.8.

TABLE 6.8
Non-pharmacological treatment for pain

COMFORT MEASURES	DIVERSIONAL MEASURES
Repositioning[44]	Relaxation
Oral and endotracheal suctioning	Breathing exercises
Mouth, oral and/or wound care	Visual imagery
Reassurance and information	Music therapy[41]
Massage	Family presence[126]

Non-pharmacological interventions have the benefit of being nurse-initiated, non-invasive and able to be personalised. These strategies may not reduce pain intensity significantly on their own but have the capacity to enhance the effects of analgesic medication and humanise the critically ill patient's experience, particularly when family members are included.[125]

Pharmacological treatment for pain

Pharmacological treatment for pain in critically ill patients centres on opioid medications, which act as opioid agonists binding to the μ-receptors in the brain, central nervous system and other tissues.[44] Opioid medications have a rapid action and are readily titrated, and their metabolites, if present, are less likely to accumulate. Morphine sulfate and fentanyl are routinely used in critical care, and their properties, side effects and nursing implications are outlined in Table 6.9. (For ischaemic chest pain management, see Chapter 10.)

Other medications such as non-steroidal anti-inflammatory drugs (NSAIDs) act by inhibition of an enzyme within the inflammatory cascade, and may produce analgesia (especially when combined with opioids) for bone and soft tissue injuries. As with all medication, side effects and contraindications can be serious and, in the case of NSAIDs, include gastrointestinal bleeding, renal insufficiency and exacerbation of asthma. Paracetamol is another medication that may be highly effective for mild pain and, when combined with opioid medications, provides analgesia for bone and soft tissue injuries.

An alternative to opioid medication for procedural pain is ketamine.[127,128] Single doses of the medication are effective in achieving analgesia during severely painful interventions such as deep wound care (e.g. burn injury). Ketamine is usually administered in conjunction with midazolam to reduce any potential emergent effects.

Pain relief is a primary goal for critical care nursing and requires regular assessment of pain intensity. No single medication is ideal for all patients, and clinicians

TABLE 6.9
Analgesics

DRUG/DRUG DOSE	PROPERTIES	SIDE EFFECTS	NURSING IMPLICATIONS
Morphine sulfate 1–10 mg/h (IV infusion), 1–4 mg (IV bolus)	Water-soluble Peak effect 30 min Half-life: 3–7 h Sedative effect and release of histamines[44]	Vasodilatory effect Decreased gastric motility Respiratory depression Nausea and vomiting[113]	Intermittent doses, rather the need for continuous infusions[44]
Fentanyl 25–200 mcg/h (IV infusion), 25–100 mcg/h (IV bolus)	Lipid-soluble Synthetic opioid 80–100 times more potent than morphine Peak effect in 4 min Half-life: 1.5–6 h[44]	Respiratory depression Bradycardia Muscular rigidity	Useful where: Hypotension or tachycardia needs to be avoided Gastric and/or histamine side effects occur with morphine
Tramadol hydrochloride 100 mg (IV bolus), then 50–100 mg 4–6/24 h	Soluble in water and ethanol Synthetic Centrally acting opioid-like analgesic	Nausea, vomiting Dizziness, dry mouth Headache Sweating	Intermittent doses only
NSAIDs	Analgesia and antipyretic	Gastrointestinal Some have anticoagulant side effects	Oral or rectal Renal clearance
Ketamine 20 mg (IV bolus), then 10–20 mg every 5–10 min[113]	Analgesic and dissociative anaesthetic for painful procedures Onset of action 1–2 min Analgesic/anaesthetic effects last 5–15 min Half-life 3 h	Hypertension and respiratory depression (administer slowly) Increased intracranial pressure Hallucinations	Use for painful procedures e.g. wound dressings Administer 2 mg of midazolam at the start of the procedure or continue midazolam infusion to minimise the dysphoric and hallucinogenic side effects

NSAIDs = non-steroidal anti-inflammatory drugs.

need to carefully select, monitor and titrate the doses of any agent. In the case of major thoracic or abdominal surgery patient-controlled analgesia may provide the most effective pain management strategy (see Chapter 12). Non-pharmacological strategies add to the relief of pain and come under the domain of nursing care. Without adequate pain management, patients will be unable to achieve adequate rest and sleep, both essential for healing and wellbeing.

Sedation

Maintaining adequate levels of sedation is a core component of care during critical illness, when patients are treated with invasive and difficult-to-tolerate procedures and interventions. A primary aim of nursing critically ill patients is to provide comfort, and adequate sedation is fundamental to this. Individualising sedation management is crucial to effective treatment, with accurate assessment a core requirement. An appropriate level of sedation is essential for all patients – this may require no sedation for some patients while others may require a significant level. Adequate sedation is paramount for those patients receiving muscle relaxants. In association with sedation management, it is essential that adequate pain relief and anxiolysis are provided to all critically ill patients.

There is growing evidence of the detrimental effects of sedation on outcomes in critically ill patients. A light, rather than deep, level of sedation is associated with shorter duration of mechanical ventilation and shorter length of ICU stay.[44,129] There is also beginning, although sometimes conflicting, evidence to suggest that lighter levels of sedation are beneficial for improved psychological recovery, particularly in relation to delusional memories.[130,131] Strategies to achieve light sedation are now the mainstay of sedation assessment and management for the critically ill.

Assessment of sedation

Assessment of the effect of all sedative treatments is essential. When pharmacological agents are used there is always a risk of over- or under-sedation, and both can have significant negative effects on patients.[132] Over-sedation may lead to detrimental physiological effects including cardiac, renal and respiratory depression and can result in longer duration of mechanical ventilation, associated complications and recovery.

FIGURE 6.5 Richmond Agitation–Sedation Scale (RASS)[135]

Richmond Agitation Sedation Scale (RASS)

Sore	Term	Description	
+4	Combative	Overtly combative, violent, immediate danger to staff	
+3	Very agitated	Pulls or removes tube(s) or catheter(s); aggressive	
+2	Agitated	Frequent non-purposeful movement, fights ventilator	
+1	Restless	Anxious but movements not aggressive vigorous	
0	Alert and calm		
−1	Drowsy	Not fully alert, but has sustained awakening (eye-opening/eye contact) to *voice* (≥10 seconds)	Verbal Stimulation
−2	Light sedation	Briefly awakens with eye contact to *voice* (<10 seconds)	Verbal Stimulation
−3	Moderate sedation	Movement or eye opening to *voice* (but not eye contact)	Verbal Stimulation
−4	Deep sedation	No response to voice, but movement or eye opening to *physical* stimulation	Physical Stimulation
−5	Unarousable	No response to *voice* or *physical* stimulation	Physical Stimulation

Procedure for RASS Assessment

1. Observe patient
   a. Patient is alert, restless, or agitated. (score 0 to +4)
2. If not alert, state patient's name and *say* to open eyes and look at speaker.
   b. Patient awakens with sustained eye opening and eye contact. (score −1)
   c. Patient awakens with eye opening and eye contact, but not sustained. (score −2)
   d. Patient has any movement in response to voice but no eye contact. (score −3)
3. When no response to verbal stimulation, physically stimulate patient by shaking shoulder and/or rubbing sternum.
   e. Patient has any movement to physical stimulation. (score −4)
   f. Patient has no response to any stimulation. (score −5)

Source: Reprinted with permission of the American Thoracic Society. Copyright © 2019 American Thoracic Society. Sessler CN, Gosnell M, Grap MJ, et al. The Richmond Agitation–Sedation Scale: validity and reliability in adult intensive care patients. Am J Respir Crit Care Med 2002;166:1338–44. The "American Journal of Respiratory and Critical Care Medicine" is an official journal of the American Thoracic Society.

Under-sedation has the opposite effect on the cardiac system, with hypertension, tachycardia, arrhythmias, ventilator dyssynchrony, agitation and distress, with the potential for accidental self-harm.

Objective sedation scales provide an effective method of assessing and monitoring consciousness or arousal level, as well as evaluating parameters such as cognition, agitation and patient–ventilator synchrony (Figs 6.5 and 6.6). A number of sedation scales have been developed for use in intensive care (Table 6.10), with variable strengths and weaknesses.[133] Even though clinicians are frequently concerned about the reliability of sedation assessment in patients with neurological compromise, there is evidence that the Richmond Agitation–Sedation Scale (RASS) is reliable.[134]

Bispectral index monitoring provides an objective measurement of sedation level. A self-adhesive electrode pad is secured to the patient's forehead to continuously record cortical activity which is scored on a scale from 0 (absence of brain activity) to 100 (completely aware). There is not yet consensus on the most appropriate brain activity level for intensive care patients or what role bispectral index can offer in their care.[142,143] More studies to evaluate the efficacy of bispectral index are required.

Sedation protocols

Patients' sedation needs are complex. There is growing awareness of the need to ensure optimal pain management prior to considering sedation, with the knowledge that sedation will not always be required once adequate pain management has been implemented (see *Pain* above).

In situations where sedation is required, one of the strategies used is a sedation protocol. The aim of sedation protocols is to improve sedation management by encouraging regular discussion of sedation goals among the healthcare team, while enabling nurses to manage ongoing sedative needs. Not all patients' sedative needs will be met within the sedation protocol; in these instances, specific care should be planned and implemented by the multidisciplinary healthcare team.

Sedation protocols offer a framework, or algorithm, within which clinicians can manage specific patient care with prearranged outcomes. Aspects of sedation management that should be incorporated into sedation protocols include:

- the sedation scale to be used, as well as frequency of assessment

FIGURE 6.6 Riker Sedation-Agitation Scale (SAS)[141]

Riker Sedation-Agitation Scale (SAS)

Score	Term	Description
7	Dangerous agitation	Pulling at ET tube, trying to remove catheters, climbing over bedrail, striking at staff, thrashing side-to-side
6	Very agitated	Requiring restraint and frequent verbal reminding of limits, biting ETT
5	Agitated	Anxious or physically agitated, calms to verbal instructions
4	Calm and cooperative	Calm, easily arousable, follows commands
3	Sedated	Difficult to arouse but awakens to verbal stimuli or gentle shaking, follows simple commands but drifts off again
2	Very sedated	Arouses to physical stimuli but does not communicate or follow commands, may move spontaneously
1	Unarousable	Minimal or no response to noxious stimuli, does not communicate or follow commands

Guidelines for SAS Assessment

1. Agitated patients are scored by their most severe degree of agitation as described.
2. If patient is awake or awakens easily to voice ('awaken' means responds with voice or head shaking to a question or follows commands), that's a SAS 4 (same as calm and appropriate – might even be napping).
3. If more stimuli such as shaking is required but patient eventually does awaken, that's SAS 3.
4. If patient arouses to stronger physical stimuli (may be noxious) but never awakens to the point of responding yes/no or following commands, that's a SAS 2.
5. Little or no response to noxious physical stimuli represents a SAS1.

Source: Riker RR, Picard JT, Fraser GL. Prospective evaluation of the Sedation-Agitation Scale for adult critically ill patients. Crit Care Med 1999;27(7):1325–9.

- an algorithm-based process for selecting the most appropriate sedative agent
- the range of sedative agents that might be considered and associated administration guidelines
- a target sedation score
- when to commence, increase, decrease or cease sedative agents
- when to seek review by a medical officer.

Sedation protocols usually also incorporate an analgesia component, frequently with an emphasis on pain assessment and management as the first step to achieve patient comfort.

Although sedation protocols have widespread support, there is mixed evidence regarding the benefits of their implementation. It is likely that sedation protocols provide most benefit in settings where ratios of critical care nurses and medical officers to patients are low (that is, are not available or limited in numbers).

Practice tip

Assessing and managing pain first, prior to providing any sedation, will improve comfort and reduce the need for sedation in many patients.

Nurse-led sedation protocols

Nurse-led sedation protocols are usually ordered by a doctor or advanced practice nurse with prescribing rights, contain guidance regarding sedation management and are usually used by nurses although they may have input from pharmacists or other members of the healthcare team. While some studies show benefits associated with nurse-led sedation protocols, particularly in relation to hospital length of stay, others do not.[144] Until further research is undertaken, sedation protocols should be considered on a local basis where current practice conditions indicate potential benefit from care standardisation. Appropriate evaluation of the impact of protocol implementation should be undertaken.

Practice tip

Patients should be kept 'calm and cooperative' unless there is a reason for deeper sedation. Strategies to minimise sedation include discussion and agreement of a target sedation score and regular assessment of pain, agitation and delirium.

TABLE 6.10
Sedation scales

SCALE	DESCRIPTION	COMMENT
Richmond Agitation–Sedation Scale (RASS)[135]	Scores from −5 (unarousable) to +4 (combative) 4 levels of agitation, 1 level for 'calm and alert', 5 levels of sedation	Assesses patient's responses in relation to the type of stimulus given (i.e. verbal or physical), plus consideration of cognition and sustainability Thorough testing of psychometric properties with positive results including good inter-rater reliability
Riker Sedation-Agitation Scale (SAS)[141]	Scored from 1 (unarousable) to 7 (dangerous agitation) 3 levels of agitation, 1 level of 'calm and cooperative', 3 levels of sedation	Multiple criteria for each level which, although increase complexity, result in better discrimination between scores Thorough testing of psychometric properties with positive results including good inter-rater reliability
Ramsay sedation scale[136]	Scores from 1 (agitated/restless) to 6 (no response) 4 levels of sedation, 1 level of 'cooperative, oriented and tranquil' and 1 level of 'anxious, agitated or restless'	Easy to administer No differentiation between different levels of anxiety, restlessness and agitation Unable to distinguish between a light plane of unconsciousness and a deep coma Lack of clarity between each score Limited testing of psychometric properties
Motor activity Assessment Scale (MAAS)[137]	Scored from 0 (unresponsive) to 6 (dangerously agitated) 3 levels of agitation, 1 level of 'calm and cooperative', 3 levels of sedation	Very similar to SAS Multiple criteria for each level which, although increase complexity, result in better discrimination between scores Limited psychometric testing
Vancouver Interactive and Calmness Scale (VICS)[138]	Two domains (interaction and calmness) each containing 5 questions Each question is scored on a 6-point scale from 'strongly agree' to 'strongly disagree', resulting in a potential total score of 30 for each domain	Thorough assessment of calmness (in contrast to agitation) with multiple levels of scoring available Differentiation between each of the points on the 6-point scale difficult Moderate psychometric testing completed, with positive results
Adaptation to the Intensive Care Environment (ATICE)[139]	Designed to measure the level of adaptation of mechanically ventilated patients to the ICU environment Two domains – consciousness (awakeness and comprehension items) and tolerances (calmness, ventilator synchrony and face relaxation items)	Different scales for assessment of each item Moderate psychometric testing completed, with positive results
Minnesota Sedation Assessment Tool (MSAT)[140]	Two domains – motor activity (assessed on 4-point scale) and arousal (assessed on 6-point scale) Assessed over previous 10 min	Good descriptive differentiation of points on scales Moderate psychometric testing completed, with positive results

Sedation minimisation protocols

A range of multidimensional protocols developed for use by all the multidisciplinary team for the purpose of minimising the amount of sedation delivered and minimising the patients' sedation level have been developed. Some of these have been incorporated into bundles such as the Wake Up and Breathe Program[177] or the expanded ABCDEF bundle.[178] Like nurse-led sedation protocols, benefits have been demonstrated in some settings[179,180] but not in all,[181] therefore any plans to implement such a protocol should take into account local practice and ensure continuous evaluation of the benefits as well as adverse events.

Daily interruption of sedation

A specific form of sedation protocol is the daily interruption of sedation. Although the initial study in this area found benefits in reduced duration of mechanical ventilation and ICU length of stay,[145,146] these benefits have not been demonstrated subsequently. In both a meta-analysis of data from nine studies including 1282 patients and a multicentre study of 423 patients in 16 centres across Canada and the USA, no improvement in duration of mechanical ventilation, ICU or hospital length of stay or rates of delirium was seen.[147,148] Further, in the multicentre study, patients who received daily interruption of sedation required higher daily doses of some sedative and analgesic agents and greater nurse workload was required for patients in this group.[148] From a practical perspective, there are growing reports of clinicians' concerns regarding patient comfort such as agitation and pain, as well as adverse events such as device removal during sedation interruption.[149,150] Given this evidence, daily interruption of sedation cannot be recommended. Instead, the mainstay of achieving good practice in this setting is maintaining appropriate targets for sedation levels that are as light as possible and based on individual patient needs.

Sleep

The function of sleep is not yet fully understood; however, it is considered to be required for many bodily functions.[151] It is vital for wellbeing and sleep disruption or deprivation leads to psychological and physical ill health, as well as death.[152] Sleep is considered to be physically and psychologically restorative and essential for healing and recovery from illness. Arguably, critically ill people are in greater need of undisrupted sleep given their need for healing and recovery, but are more likely to experience poor quality sleep.[153,154]

Sleep in the healthy adult comprises one consolidated period of 6–8 hours (mean 7.5 hours) in each 24-hour period occurring at night according to natural circadian rhythms.[155] There are two main sleep states: rapid eye movement sleep (REM) (approximately 25% of total sleep time [TST]) and non-rapid eye movement sleep (non-REM) (approximately 75% of TST). Non-REM sleep is composed of four stages: stages 1 and 2 or light sleep and stages 3 and 4 or slow wave sleep (SWS) or deep sleep, which must be completed in sequence in order to enter REM sleep. The consolidated sleep period consists of four to six sleep cycles: stages 1–4 followed by REM sleep, which lasts 60–90 minutes. (More recent sleep staging guidelines have combined stages 3 and 4 so that there are now only three stages of non-REM sleep;[156] however, the foremost sleep medicine textbook continues to use the conventional 1–4 staging nomenclature.[155]) All sleep stages are important to health and, unfortunately, critically ill patients commonly experience little deep or REM sleep.

Evidence suggests that, although critically ill patients may experience normal sleep quantities, the quality is poor with very few experiencing SW or REM sleep.[157,158] Sleep is highly disrupted and distributed across 24 hours with roughly equal amounts occurring in the day and at night.[159,160] These findings, obtained using polysomnography (PSG), have been corroborated by patients' self-reports of their sleep in critical care.[151,162] Patients consistently rate their overall sleep quality as poor and, more specifically, they report light sleep with frequent awakenings and considerable difficulty falling asleep and returning to sleep.[163] Many factors are thought to affect the patient's ability to sleep, including those intrinsic to the patient such as abnormal temperature and pain, others that are environmental such as noise and light, and those that are treatment related such as medications, tubes and mechanical ventilation.[161,164]

There are changes in sleep architecture over the adult lifespan that require consideration in the context of critical care nursing. TST and the percentage of SWS decline (TST by 10 minutes and SWS by 2% per decade) and light sleep increases slightly (by 5% between 20 and 70 years) with age.[165] REM sleep remains fairly constant with an approximate 0.6% decline per decade until age 70 when REM increases with a simultaneous decrease in TST.[166] Time spent awake after sleep onset increases with age by 10 minutes per decade after age 30.[165]

Sleep assessment/monitoring

The patient's sleep history should be taken as soon as possible after admission. The person closest to the patient (ideally living in the same home) may be willing to provide a sleep history if the patient is unable to communicate verbally. The requirement for nocturnal non-invasive ventilation or sleep medication should be considered with the multidisciplinary team. Particular attention should be paid to reports of daytime sleepiness, dissatisfaction with sleep and bed partner reports of excessive snoring as these may indicate an undiagnosed sleep disorder. Usual sleep habits such as 'going to bed', 'getting up' and shower times should be accommodated while the patient is treated in critical care whenever possible.

Unfortunately, few objective methods of assessing sleep reliably in critically ill patients are available. PSG, a method of recording electroencephalography, electrooculography and electromyography, is the 'gold standard' for assessing sleep. PSG data are analysed according to Rechtschaffen and Kales' (R & K)[167] criteria to provide TST and sleep stage times. Difficulties applying standard R & K sleep criteria to critically ill patients' sleep data and the need for a trained operator to undertake analysis preclude its routine clinical use in critical care. Actigraphy is another method of recording sleep that has been attempted in the critically ill. Modern actigraphs are small wristwatch devices (they may also be located on the ankle) containing accelerometers that detect motion in a single axis or multiple axes.[168] Although actigraphy has been shown to be feasible in the critically ill population[168,169] there is some evidence that actigraphy provides an overestimation of sleep time given critically ill patients are typically immobile for long periods regardless of sleep state. The other objective method that has been attempted in critical care is bispectral index

TABLE 6.11
Sleep assessment instruments

INSTRUMENT	DESCRIPTION	COMMENTS
Richards-Campbell Sleep Questionnaire[172]	Five VAS (0–100 mm) Total score derived from average of the 5 scales (high scores indicate good sleep)	Patient does not need to be able to write (nurse can mark the line as instructed by patient) Patient requires sufficient level of cognitive function to use it
Sleep in Intensive Care Questionnaire[173]	Seven questions (some have more than one item) Likert scales 1–10 No global score Good for organisational changes in practice	Patient does not need to be able to write (nurse can circle the response as instructed by patient) Patient requires sufficient level of cognitive function to use it Not yet validated
Nurses' observation checklist[174]	Tick box table Assignment of a category: 'awake', 'asleep', 'could not tell' and 'no time to observe' every 15 min	No training required Typically, nurses tend to overestimate sleep Better for trend over several nights

monitoring.[170] At present, considerable algorithm development using comparisons with PSG data are required before it is a viable option to measure sleep accurately in any setting, although there is some early evidence of feasibility.[171]

The most reliable option for the critical care clinician to assess sleep is a patient self-report (in any case, the patient is best placed to judge the adequacy of their sleep if they are able). Two instruments have been specifically developed for use in critical care: the Richards-Campbell Sleep Questionnaire (RCSQ)[172] and the Sleep in Intensive Care Questionnaire (SICQ) (Table 6.11).[173] The RCSQ comprises five 100-mm VAS: sleep depth, latency, awakenings, time awake and quality of sleep. It was validated in 70 male patients where there was a moderate correlation between total RCSQ score and PSG sleep efficiency index, $r = 0.58$, ($p < 0.001$).[172] The SICQ is better suited for use when assessing a unit/organisation-wide change in practice rather than for individual patient's sleep (Table 6.11).

Up to 50% of patients treated in critical care may be unable to complete a sleep self-assessment, in which case the only remaining option is nurse assessment. The Nurses' Observation Checklist (NOC)[174] can be used to obtain the bedside nurses' assessments of the patient's sleep quantity. It is a relatively simple instrument to use. However, evidence from many studies suggests that nurses tend to overestimate sleep time, so sleep time derived from the NOC may be better used as a trend rather than a definitive report for an individual night's sleep.[175,176]

Sleep promotion and maintenance

There is a growing, although still small and often low-quality, body of evidence of interventions that are effective in promoting sleep for patients in ICU. These interventions can be grouped into two categories including optimising patient comfort and adapting the environment to be more conducive to normal sleep routines. Multidimensional interventions that incorporate a number of strategies have been found to be beneficial.[40] Individualised approaches to all aspects of care are best and this is particularly important when promoting and maintaining sleep in the critically ill. The following information, based on research and expert opinion, provides some general advice that may promote and maintain sleep and, at the very least, create conditions conducive to rest.

Comfort measures

- Ensure pain relief is offered and administered if pain is suspected
- Reduce anxiety by providing information and the opportunity to have questions answered. Anxiolytics such as benzodiazepines may also be required
- Provide night-time sedation as required (remember sedation is not natural sleep and patients may only appear to be asleep; however, it is possible to be sedated and asleep)
- Consider providing a light massage or music therapy unless contraindicated to help patients relax[25]
- Provide an extra cover for warmth (metabolic rate typically drops during sleep)
- Request the patient's family to provide some of the patient's own personal belongings such as pillows and toiletries
- Ear plugs and eye covers may assist some patients,[25,177] and have been shown to reduce the risk of delirium although patients provided with ear plugs and eye covers should have the ability to remove them without assistance if they wish.

Care activities

- Attend to nursing care at the beginning of the night to reduce the likelihood of disturbing sleep during the night, for example:
  - redress wounds and empty drainage bags
  - wash, clean teeth and change gown and sheets
  - reposition with suitable pressure support measures
  - level the transducer at the phlebostatic axis to ensure accurate haemodynamic monitoring so you do not need to disturb the patient again later
  - ensure intravenous lines and drains are accessible.
- Plan care activities to allow the patient 1.5–2-hour periods of undisturbed time during the night. Negotiate with other healthcare personnel to allow these uninterrupted periods at night and during daytime rest times. 'Cluster care', for example, time medication administration, planned ETT suctioning and pressure area care to coincide.
- Provide the daily bath to suit patient needs rather than organisational needs (either before settling for the night or during normal waking hours).

Practice tip

Enabling the patient to experience good quality and quantities of sleep should be a major priority for critical care nursing. Demonstrate your commitment to improving rest and sleep for intensive care patients by incorporating sleep into the treatment reminder system used in the unit you work in (e.g. FASTHUG becomes FASSTHUG).

Environmental

- Reduce noise levels especially during rest times and at night, which may require a unit-wide change in practice as several critical care studies highlight the association between noise levels and sleep disruption.[189,179] Noise levels in adult critical care areas consistently exceed hospital noise standards; for example, the World Health Organisation guidelines that recommend noise during the night inside a hospital should not exceed 40 dB, with particular attention given to sound levels in the ICU.[180]
- Ensure lights are sufficiently dimmed and window blinds drawn during rest times and at night and that lighting is bright and blinds opened at all other times. It is known that critically ill patients' melatonin metabolism is non-circadian so it is particularly important to attempt to use lighting that encourages normal circadian rhythm.[181,182] Generally, critical care areas contain fluorescent lights that may emit up to 600 lux. Light levels between 50 and 100 lux at night, even for relatively brief periods, are known to suppress melatonin production, a vital hormone in the promotion of sleep and maintenance of circadian rhythm.[155,183] It is well known that artificial lights emit light with sufficient short wave content to affect melatonin secretion.

Practice tip

Ask your patient (or their relatives) about their usual night-time 'settling routine' for sleep. Try to emulate the routine as closely as possible. Then check if this improved their sleep.

Treatments

- Discuss the need for alternative mechanical ventilation settings at night with the medical team. Hyperventilation caused by inappropriately high inspiratory pressure can cause hypocapnia, which may lead to central apnoeas and sleep disturbance.[184]
- Many medications administered in critical care affect sleep architecture. Even vasoactive medications such as adrenaline have the capacity to affect the quality of sleep. Sedatives, especially benzodiazepines and opioids, reduce time in stages 3 and 4 and REM, thus reducing the amount and quality of sleep.[185-187] However, pain relief and anxiolysis may be essential for sleep to occur, but an awareness of potential adverse medication reactions is important in the prevention of escalating sleep disturbances.
- Specific sleep-promoting medications may be administered once non-pharmacological interventions have been attempted. Table 6.12 contains a summary of the commonly used medications for the general management of insomnia. It should be noted that investigations of the effectiveness of these medications have not been undertaken in the critically ill.

Practice tip

Next time you are at work in ICU take the time to consider the sound level. At an appropriate time and position in the ICU, close your eyes for 1 minute and consider whether you would be able to rest. In addition, find a patient who is well enough to be discharged to the hospital ward and ask them about the factors that they found most disruptive to rest and sleep while they were being treated in ICU.

Melatonin

Melatonin is used for the short-term alleviation of insomnia. This naturally-occurring hormone is both sleep-promoting and sleep-maintaining. Despite its use

TABLE 6.12

Summary of commonly used medications used for sedation and sleep promotion

MEDICATION	MEDICATION CLASS	TYPICAL HYPNOTIC DOSE RANGE (ADULT)	ADDITIONAL INFORMATON
Temazepam	Benzodiazepine	Oral/enteral: 10–20 mg once per night (30 min before settling)	May help sleep onset and sleep maintenance but tends to reduce duration of slow wave sleep (some patients may report lack of restorative sleep)[185] Adverse effects may outweigh benefits for some patients High likelihood of dependency if used long-term Reduce dose in liver failure Check liver function[188]
Propofol	Intravenous sedative/ anaesthetic agent	Intravenous: mechanical ventilation: 1.0–3.0 mg/kg/h Self-ventilating: no greater than 0.5 mg/kg/h	May help sleep onset and maintenance but little evidence of improving sleep quality (self-report)[189] Short-term use only Continuous respiratory monitoring Check liver function
Zolpidem	Non-benzodiazepine hypnotic	Oral/enteral: 5–10 mg once per night (immediately before settling)	Improves sleep onset and maintenance for slow release preparation[190] Short-term use only (2–4 weeks) Associated with hallucinations Extended half-life in liver impairment
Zopiclone	Non-benzodiazepine hypnotic	Oral/enteral: 3.75–7.5 mg once per night (immediately before settling)	Improves sleep onset and maintenance Short-term use only (2–4 weeks) Associated with hallucinations Extended half-life in liver impairment
Haloperidol	Typical antipsychotic	Provide maintenance doses used for treatment of delirium for night-time settling Intravenous (slow): 2–10 mg which can be repeated Oral/enteral: 5–15 mg per day	Monitor QT interval and liver function Observe for extrapyramidal symptoms No more than 100 mg/day
Olanzapine	Atypical antipsychotic	Oral/enteral: 2.5–20 mg once per night several hours before settling	Evidence for the effectiveness for sleep is weak[188] Short-term use only May cause hypotension
Quetiapine	Atypical antipsychotic	Oral/enteral: 25–200 mg once per night 1 h before settling	Evidence for the effectiveness for sleep is weak[188] Short-term use only May cause hypotension Monitor QT interval
Amitriptyline	Tricyclic antidepressant	Oral/enteral: 25–150 mg once per night 1–2 h before settling	Use only if also required for pain relief or as antidepressant[188] Monitor QT interval and for anticholinergic effects Increased seizure risk
Doxepin	Tricyclic antidepressant	Oral/enteral: 25–150 mg once per night 1– 2 h before settling	Improves sleep maintenance[189] Monitor QT interval and for anticholinergic effects Increased seizure risk
Mirtazapine	Noradrenergic and specific serotonergic antidepressant	Oral/enteral: 15–60 mg once per night 1–2 h before settling	Little evidence of effectiveness for sleep Use only if also required as antidepressant[190] Higher doses may have a stimulatory effect

TABLE 6.12
Summary of commonly used medications used for sedation and sleep promotion—cont'd

MEDICATION	MEDICATION CLASS	TYPICAL HYPNOTIC DOSE RANGE (ADULT)	ADDITIONAL INFORMATON
Ramelteon	Melatonin agonist	Oral/enteral: 8 mg once per night 1–2 h before settling	Modest evidence for improving sleep onset[190] Relatively safe with little of dependency
Melatonin	Melatonin (exogenous)	Oral/enteral: 0.2–5 mg (depending age and weight) taken 30–60 minutes before settling Slow release oral: 1 mg	Limited evidence of effectiveness for sleep in ICU patients[192] (or healthy individuals) More research is required Relatively safe
Suvorexant	Orexin receptor antagonist	Oral/enteral: 10 mg 1 hour before settling	Some effectiveness to improve sleep onset and maintenance but not recommended[188] Moderate potential for dependency
Dexmedetomidine	Alpha-agonist	Intravenous: loading dose 1 mcg/kg over 10–20 min followed by maintenance infusion 0.2–1 mcg/kg/h titrated to effect	EEG evidence of substitute for sleep[194] but further research is required to confirm this subjectively Not to be used as a continuous infusion for more than 24 h Continuous respiratory monitoring

Practice tip

If after interviewing the patient or their family about their usual sleep and assessing their sleep in ICU you suspect they might have an existing untreated sleep disorder, request the treating medical team to make a sleep medicine referral. Untreated sleep problems long-term may be associated with increased risk of cardiovascular disease and cancer.

as a treatment for primary insomnia, e.g. jet lag and shift work, the effectiveness of exogenous melatonin for most sleep disorders has not been established.[191,192] Several small scale studies have been undertaken to examine whether melatonin improves either sleep or delirium in the critically ill, and although there are some promising signs, evidence remains limited, conflicting and inconclusive.[193] Difficulties occur in emulating the typical endogenous pulsatile secretion of the hormone and, together with its short half-life, these probably explain why many study results are inconclusive. The high doses required to achieve an adequate plasma level overnight when administered once at the beginning of the night are likely to persist in the body and may upset normal circadian rhythm. The typical dose is 3–5 mg once or twice a day.

The current advice of the authors based on evidence available to date is that it is better to provide conditions that encourage the normal circadian secretion of endogenous melatonin (i.e. provide lighting and activity levels appropriate for the time of day) than to administer exogenous melatonin.

Summary

Meeting the psychological needs of patients is essential in the care of critically ill patients. In this chapter the various methods that are available to assess and then effectively manage aspects of patient care related to anxiety, delirium, pain, sedation and sleep are outlined. Assessment of these aspects of the patient's condition require thorough clinical assessment, with a range of validated instruments available to help improve consistency over time and between clinicians, as well as to inform decisions regarding the most appropriate interventions. Although these aspects of care have been reviewed sequentially in this chapter, in reality they are closely interrelated and should be considered concurrently.

Case study

A 58-year-old woman, Rebecca, was found unconscious by her husband in their home at 18:00 hours (he last saw her at 08:30 hours). A strong smell of alcohol was noted and an empty box of paracetamol (24 tablets of 500 mg) was found near her (it was unclear how many she had ingested). She was intubated by paramedics and brought to hospital. On arrival Rebecca was unresponsive (Glasgow Coma Scale (GCS): 3), her serum alcohol concentration was 3.0% and paracetamol level 150 mg/L.

Rebecca was known to be alcohol dependent. Her husband revealed that this began after their only child died from leukaemia aged 10 years (10 years ago). After one session of grief counselling she declined further assistance. He reported that she had been 'dry' on and off over the last 5 years but for the last few months he had noticed her breath smelled of alcohol. He was reluctant to address this as she was low in mood and confidence. She was undernourished (weight: 45 kg; height: 165 cm) but had no other health problems, rarely saw a GP, was a 'non-smoker' and did not take drugs.

An infusion of acetylcysteine was started and a computerised tomography (CT) of her head and neck was performed (findings were unremarkable). On arrival in ICU her neurological status improved but she was agitated and uncooperative (Richmond Agitation–Sedation Scale (RASS) score: +3). A low dose propofol infusion was started and as alcohol withdrawal was likely (all components of the CAGE screening interview with her husband were positive), the AWS Scale was used to monitor her symptoms. Her AWS score was 15; she was sweating and experiencing intermittent visual hallucinations. Small doses of IV diazepam were given. Subsequently RASS scores were 0 to +1 and AWS scores were 5–6 after diazepam.

Twenty-four hours after ICU admission Rebecca was extubated but her serum liver function tests were 'trending up' and she had right upper quadrant abdominal pain. Rebecca's liver function tests deteriorated (a regimen of lactulose was started), her renal function was poor, she became drowsy (GCS: 9) and was hypertensive. A CT scan of her head revealed loss of sulci and other features consistent with cerebral oedema. She was reintubated. Intermittent analgesia (IV opioids) and sedation (low dose propofol) were provided when necessary. She became anuric and required continuous renal replacement therapy (CRRT).

Rebecca's liver function tests improved 5 days after admission but her renal function remained poor so CRRT continued. On day 9 she was extubated. She was 'positive' for delirium when screened with the Confusion Assessment Method-ICU (CAM-ICU). During periods of delirium she was distressed and agitated but cooperative. She was low in mood and withdrawn but denied suicidal ideation (when not delirious Rebecca explained that she wanted the 'pain to go away'). She was tearful and expressed shame about her alcohol dependence and continuously apologised for circumstances that had brought her to hospital. By day 15 she was no longer delirious but continued to experience difficulty sleeping.

TREATMENT

A small team of nurses was allocated to improve continuity of care and communication with input from the entire multidisciplinary team including physiotherapy, dietician, social work and occupational therapy. Rehabilitation started with an emphasis on developing function to address Rebecca's own goals, which were specifically to walk her dog and return to work as an academic. She agreed to talk to the drug and alcohol team about her future plans.

- Rebecca was encouraged to express her feelings and talk about her child if she wished
- After the period of alcohol withdrawal, non-pharmacological interventions were used to manage delirium; benzodiazepines were avoided
- Rebeccca was reassured that it was immaterial how and why she required treatment in ICU – nobody was judging her and that she would be provided with the treatment and care she required
- Rebecca was visited by her husband whenever she wished (the ICU had an open visiting policy)
- She was given an appetite stimulant 30 minutes before meals and her husband was asked to bring in her favourite foods
- Her husband was provided with support, details of grief counsellors and advice about carer support
- Antidepressant medication was prescribed by the mental health team

- The drug and alcohol team visited her to discuss future plans and her alcohol abstinence strategies
- A summary of her day's achievements, however small, were written on a whiteboard in her room
- A sleep enhancing routine was instigated, which involved settling early with a warm wash, teeth brushing, playing relaxing music, face mask and ear plugs (when delirium was no longer a problem) and access to her own audio player through the night to listen to a relaxation exercise. All care at night was clustered so that she had consolidated 2-hour rest periods.

Rebecca was treated in ICU for 3 weeks (and went home after 6 weeks in hospital). Her renal function improved. Generalised deconditioning (frailty) and a chest infection requiring high flow oxygen delayed her ICU discharge.

RECOVERY

Rebecca's physical recovery was uneventful; however, she continued to experience severe low mood even with treatment from the drug and alcohol team and mental health team. Three months after she had returned home her husband visited the ICU and expressed his gratitude for his wife's treatment. He reported that she had almost walked to the park, was abstinent from alcohol and was planning to return to work. At that time Rebecca stated that she did not feel ready to visit ICU.

DISCUSSION

Rebecca's recovery was complicated by significant psychosocial challenges on a background of alcohol dependence. Depression was ever present so at times Rebecca's psychological care needs were greater than her physical needs. Rebecca's husband was her main support and with her agreement his involvement was welcomed by the entire team.

Her husband stated that a coordinated patient goal-directed approach to her early rehabilitation was instrumental in her recovery. Input from the mental health and drug and alcohol teams was essential for rehabilitation to reduce the risk of relapse and depression.

CASE STUDY QUESTIONS

1. After the period of alcohol withdrawal Rebecca continued to experience delirium. List Rebecca's risk factors for developing delirium and the non-pharmacological nursing interventions that were used in caring for her, as well as any additional strategies that might have been used.
2. One of the interventions used to assist Rebecca to sleep was 'music of her choice'. Explain the underlying rationale for choosing this intervention.

RESEARCH VIGNETTE

Flannery AH, Oyler DR, Weinhouse GL. The impact of interventions to improve sleep on delirium in the ICU: a systematic review and research framework. Crit Care Med 2016; 44: 2231–2240

Abstract

Objective: This study aimed to assess whether interventions targeted at improving sleep in the ICU were associated with reductions in ICU delirium. Secondary outcomes include duration of delirium and ICU length of stay.

Data sources: MEDLINE, CINAHL, Web of Science, Scopus, WorldCat, and International Pharmaceutical Abstracts were searched from inception to January 2016.

Study selection: Studies investigating any type of sleep intervention (non-pharmacologic or pharmacologic) and assessing the impact on ICU delirium were included. Any type of study design was permitted so long as the delirium assessment was made at least daily with a validated delirium assessment tool.

Data extraction: The following data were extracted: first author, year of publication, study design, ICU type, components of sleep intervention, use of sleep assessment tool, patient age, sex, severity of illness, sleep measures, delirium assessment tool, incidence of delirium, duration of delirium, and ICU length of stay. The incidence of delirium was used to compare rates of ICU delirium across studies. Methodologic quality of included studies was evaluated using the Effective Public Health Practice Project quality assessment tool.

Data synthesis: Of 488 citations screened, 10 studies were identified for inclusion in the final review, six of which demonstrated a statistically significant reduction in the incidence of ICU delirium associated with sleep intervention. Four studies assessed duration of delirium, of which, three reported a shorter duration of delirium with sleep intervention. Two studies associated sleep intervention with a reduced ICU length of stay. In regard to quality assessment and risk of bias, only one study was assessed as strong. Multiple identified confounders and the significant qualitative assessment of heterogeneity limit both the conclusions that can be drawn from these findings and the quantitative pooling of data.

Conclusions: Although sleep interventions seem to be a promising approach for improving delirium-related outcomes, studies are limited by bias issues, varying methodologies, and multiple confounders, making the evidence base for this conclusion limited at best. Future studies would benefit from a systematic approach to studying the link between sleep intervention and delirium-related outcomes, which is outlined in the context of reviewing the existing literature.

Critique

The role of sleep in affecting delirium, as well as influencing other aspects of long-term recovery has been noted. The search in this review was extensive and generally appropriate, although it would have been advantageous to see it extended to databases such as Embase that has better coverage of some European journals and PsycINFO with an increased emphasis on behavioural interventions, as well as languages beyond English. The review process was rigorously conducted, with two people independently undertaking screening and identifying relevant literature, extracting the data and assessing the study quality.

The prevailing theme of the results is that there is a likelihood that sleep interventions have a positive benefit in regard to delirium, with six of the 10 studies reporting a statistically significant reduction in the incidence of delirium and a further three of the four studies that reported duration of delirium reporting a reduction. Further, two of the five studies that reported ICU length of stay reported a statistically significant reduction.

The limitations of the body of evidence are recognised by the authors, with only one of the 10 included studies being rated as having strong methodology, with a further six rated as moderate and three as week. Unfortunately, the body of evidence as a whole suffers from issues of bias, heterogeneity, varying methodologies, and multiple confounders that influence the relationship between the interventions that were implemented, patients' sleep and the delirium experienced.

While the link between sleep and delirium has not been definitively demonstrated, this review provides further evidence of the likely relationship between sleep and delirium. Further challenges exist in accurately and reliably measuring sleep. Various concerns have been raised about the appropriateness of using objective measures such as PSG, and practical considerations such as resourcing usually preclude this as a routine feature of ICU practice. Consequently, use of self-report measures such as the RCSQ appear the most ideal and various studies have demonstrated feasibility for many ICU patients, including those who are awake while still being intubated and ventilated. Increasing awareness of the importance of monitoring sleep, both to guide interventions designed to help patients achieve better sleep, and also to influence other outcomes including delirium, is essential. Consider implementing a process of routine sleep assessment as one of the essential elements of critical care patient monitoring.

Learning activities

1 The assessment of anxiety and pain is integral to critical care nursing:
   - discuss the assessment strategies you would use to differentiate between anxiety and pain
   - list any special considerations associated with your choices.

2 Outline some non-pharmacological strategies that could be employed to reduce pain.

3 Discuss how family could help with the management of the patient's anxiety.

4 Critically ill patients who experience delirium require highly skilled and informed nursing. The following exercises may enhance your ability to manage patients with delirium:
   - identify risk factors for the patient and think of ways to ameliorate them (in practice always discuss with the multidisciplinary team)
   - highlight nursing interventions that may reduce the potential for delirium. Describe the rationale for your selection of nursing interventions using current research.

5 Outline the differences between delirium and dementia.

6 Effective treatment for alcohol and substance withdrawal is dependent on identifying symptoms early. Outline the strategies to identify patients at risk of alcohol withdrawal in critical care.

7 Why is thiamine and complex B vitamin supplementation considered a vital component of treatment for alcohol dependence?

8 Compare and contrast the various pain assessment instruments and discuss the relative merits and disadvantages of using each of these instruments. Now repeat the exercise for each of the instruments for sedation assessment instruments and the delirium assessment instruments.

9 Using the references provided in this chapter:
   - highlight the importance of good quality sleep in health and illness
   - identify theories that explain the function of sleep.

10 Think about the last time you experienced fragmented sleep or insufficient sleep and describe how you felt in terms of your:
   - mood
   - cognitive function
   - physical function
   - appetite
   - motivation.

Online resources

Australasian Sleep Association, www.sleep.org.au

ICU Delirium and Cognitive Impairment Study Group, www.icudelirium.org

Healthtalk.org (Former patients talk about their experience): http://www.healthtalk.org/peoples-experiences/intensive-care/intensive-care-patients-experiences/topics

Further reading

Devlin JW, Skrobik Y, Gelinas C, et al. Clinical practice guidelines for the prevention and management of pain, agitation/sedation, delirium, immobility, and sleep disruption in adult patients in the ICU. Crit Care Med 2018;46:e825–e873.

Bergeron N, Dubois MJ, Dumont M, et al. Intensive Care Delirium Screening Checklist: evaluation of a new screening tool. Intensive Care Med 2001;27:859–64.

DAS Taskforce, Baron R, Binder A, et al. Evidence and consensus based guideline for the management of delirium, analgesia, and sedation in intensive care medicine. Revision 2015 (DAS-Guideline 2015) – short version. Ger Med Sci 2015;13:Doc19. http://www.egms.de/static/en/journals/gms/2015-13/000223.shtml. [Accessed 21 March 2018].

Ely EW, Inouye SK, Bernard GR, et al. Delirium in mechanically ventilated patients: validity and reliability of the confusion assessment method for the intensive care unit (CAM-ICU). JAMA 2001;286:2703–10.

Erickson CK. Addiction essentials: the go-to guide for clinicians and patients. New York: WW Norton; 2011.

Fishman S, Ballantyne J, Rathmell JP. Bonica's Management of pain. 4th ed. Philadelphia: Lippincott Williams & Wilkins; 2009.

Hardin KA. Sleep in the ICU: potential mechanisms and clinical implications. Chest 2009;136:284–94.

Kampman K, Jarvis M. American Society of Addiction Medicine (ASAM) national practice guideline for the use of medications in the treatment of addiction involving opioid use. J Addict Med 2015;9:358–67.

Kyranou M, Puntillo K. The transition from acute to chronic pain: might intensive care unit patients be at risk? Ann Intensive Care 2012;2:36.

References

1. Elliott D, Aitken LM, Bucknall TK, et al. Patient comfort in the intensive care unit: a multicentre, binational point prevalence study of analgesia, sedation and delirium management. Crit Care Resusc 2013;15(3):213–19.
2. Richards-Belle A, Canter RR, Power GS, et al. National survey and point prevalence study of sedation practice in UK critical care. Crit Care 2016;20(1):355.
3. Kotfis K, Zegan-Baranska M, Zukowski M, et al. Multicenter assessment of sedation and delirium practices in the intensive care units in Poland – is this common practice in Eastern Europe? BMC Anesthesiol 2017;17(1):120.
4. Spielberger CD. Anxiety: current trends in theory and research: I. New York: Academic Press; 1972.
5. Abed MA, Hall LA, Moser DK. Spielberger's state anxiety inventory: development of a shortened version for critically ill patients. Issues Ment Health Nurs 2011;32(4):220–7.
6. Castillo MI, Cooke M, Macfarlane B, et al. Factors associated with anxiety in critically ill patients: a prospective observational cohort study. Int J Nurs Stud 2016;60:225–33.
7. Tate JA, Devito Dabbs A, Hoffman LA, et al. Anxiety and agitation in mechanically ventilated patients. Qual Health Res 2012;22(2):157–73.
8. Lamas DJ, Owens RL, Nace RN, et al. Opening the door: the experience of chronic critical illness in a long-term acute care hospital. Crit Care Med 2017;45(4):e357–62.
9. Oh J, Sohn JH, Shin CS, et al. Mutual relationship between anxiety and pain in the intensive care unit and its effect on medications. J Crit Care 2015;30(5):1043–8.
10. Vesz PS, Costanzi M, Stolnik D, et al. Functional and psychological features immediately after discharge from an intensive care unit: prospective cohort study. Rev Bras Ter Intensiva 2013;25(3):218–24.
11. Chlan L, Savik K. Patterns of anxiety in critically ill patients receiving mechanical ventilatory support. Nurs Res 2011;60(3 Suppl.):S50–7.
12. Chung CR, Yoo HJ, Park J, et al. Cognitive impairment and psychological distress at discharge from intensive care unit. Psychiatry Investig 2017;14(3):376–9.
13. Fink RM, Makic MB, Poteet AW, et al. The ventilated patient's experience. Dimens Crit Care Nurs 2015;34(5):301–8.
14. De Jong MJ, Chung ML, Roser LP, et al. A five-country comparison of anxiety early after acute myocardial infarction. Eur J Cardiovasc Nurs 2004;3(2):129–34.
15. Bear MF, Connors BW, Paradiso MA. Neuroscience exploring the brain. Philadelphia: Lippincott Williams & Wilkins; 2007.
16. Porth C. Essentials of pathophysiology: concepts of altered health states. Philadelphia: Lippincott Williams & Wilkins; 2011.
17. Frazier SK, Moser DK, Riegel B, et al. Critical care nurses' assessment of patients' anxiety: reliance on physiological and behavioral parameters. Am J Crit Care 2002;11(1):57–64.
18. McKinley S, Coote K, Stein-Parbury J. Development and testing of a Faces Scale for the assessment of anxiety in critically ill patients. J Adv Nurs 2003;41(1):73–9.
19. Jackson JC, Santoro MJ, Ely TM, et al. Improving patient care through the prism of psychology: application of Maslow's hierarchy to sedation, delirium, and early mobility in the intensive care unit. J Crit Care 2014.
20. DAS Taskforce, Baron R, Binder A, et al. Evidence and consensus based guideline for the management of delirium, analgesia, and sedation in intensive care medicine. Revision 2015 (DAS-Guideline 2015) – short version. Ger Med Sci 2015;13:Doc19.
21. Hornblow AR, Kidson MA. The visual analogue scale for anxiety: a validation study. Aust N Z J Psychiatry 1976;10(4):339–41.
22. Zigmond A, Snaith R. The Hospital Anxiety and Depression Scale. Acta Psychiatr Scand 1983;67(6):361–70.
23. Lovibond S, Lovibond P. Manual for the depression anxiety stress scales, 2nd ed. Sydney Psychology Foundation; 1995.
24. Spielberger C, Gorsuch R, Lushene R. Manual for the state-trait anxiety inventory. Palo Alto: Consulting Psychologist Press; 1983.
25. Hu RF, Jiang XY, Chen J, et al. Non-pharmacological interventions for sleep promotion in the intensive care unit. Cochrane Database Syst Rev 2015;(10):Cd008808.
26. Ng F, Trauer T, Dodd S, et al. The validity of the 21-item version of the Depression Anxiety Stress Scales as a routine clinical outcome measure. Acta Neuropsychiatr 2007;19:304–10.
27. Chlan L, Savik K, Weinert C. Development of a shortened state anxiety scale from the Spielberger State-Trait anxiety Inventory (STAI) for patients receiving mechanical ventilatory support. J Nurs Meas 2003;11(3):283–93.
28. McKinley S, Madronio C. Validity of the Faces Anxiety Scale for the assessment of state anxiety in intensive care patients not receiving mechanical ventilation. J Psychosom Res 2008;64(5):503–7.

29. McKinley S, Stein-Parbury J, Chehelnabi A, et al. Assessment of anxiety in intensive care patients by using the Faces Anxiety Scale. Am J Crit Care 2004;13(2):146–52.
30. Gustad LT, Chaboyer W, Wallis M. Performance of the Faces Anxiety Scale in patients transferred from the ICU. Intensive Crit Care Nurs 2005;21(6):355–60.
31. Milton A, Bruck E, Schandl A, et al. Early psychological screening of intensive care unit survivors: a prospective cohort study. Crit Care 2017;21(1):273.
32. Nikayin S, Rabiee A, Hashem MD, et al. Anxiety symptoms in survivors of critical illness: a systematic review and meta-analysis. Gen Hosp Psychiatry 2016;43:23–9.
33. Chlan LL, Weinert CR, Heiderscheit A, et al. Effects of patient-directed music intervention on anxiety and sedative exposure in critically ill patients receiving mechanical ventilatory support: a randomized clinical trial. JAMA 2013;309(22):2335–44.
34. Davis T, Jones P. Music therapy: decreasing anxiety in the ventilated patient: a review of the literature. Dimens Crit Care Nurs 2012;31(3):159–66.
35. Alves da Silva T, Stripari Schujmann D, Yamada da Silveíra LT, et al. Effect of therapeutic Swedish massage on anxiety level and vital signs of Intensive Care Unit patients. J Bodyw Mov Ther 2017;21(3):565–8.
36. Boitor M, Gelinas C, Richard-Lalonde M, et al. The effect of massage on acute postoperative pain in critically and acutely ill adults post-thoracic surgery: systematic review and meta-analysis of randomized controlled trials. Heart Lung 2017;46(5):339–46.
37. Rashid M. Two decades (1993-2012) of adult intensive care unit design: a comparative study of the physical design features of the best practice examples. Crit Care Nurs Q 2014;37(1):3–32.
38. Halm MA. Essential oils for management of symptoms in critically ill patients. Am J Crit Care 2008;17(2):160–3.
39. Lytle J, Mwatha C, Davis KK. Effect of lavender aromatherapy on vital signs and perceived quality of sleep in the intermediate care unit: a pilot study. Am J Crit Care 2014;23(1):24–9.
40. Patel J, Baldwin J, Bunting P, et al. The effect of a multicomponent multidisciplinary bundle of interventions on sleep and delirium in medical and surgical intensive care patients. Anaesthesia 2014;69(6):540–9.
41. Mofredj A, Alaya S, Tassaioust K, et al. Music therapy, a review of the potential therapeutic benefits for the critically ill. J Crit Care 2016;35:195–9.
42. Chlan L, Heiderscheit A. A tool for music preference assessment in critically ill patients receiving mechanical ventilatory support. Music Ther Perspect 2009;27(1):42–7.
43. McKinley S, Nagy S, Stein-Parbury J, et al. Vulnerability and security in seriously ill patients in intensive care. Intensive Crit Care Nurs 2002;18(1):27–36.
44. Barr J, Fraser GL, Puntillo K, et al. Clinical practice guidelines for the management of pain, agitation, and delirium in adult patients in the intensive care unit. Crit Care Med 2013;41(1):263–306.
45. Reardon DP, Anger KE, Adams CD, et al. Role of dexmedetomidine in adults in the intensive care unit: an update. Am J Health Syst Pharm 2013;70(9):767–77.
46. Spronk PE, Riekerk B, Hofhuis J, et al. Occurrence of delirium is severely underestimated in the ICU during daily care. Intensive Care Med 2009;35(7):1276–80.
47. Karnatovskaia LV, Johnson MM, Benzo RP, et al. The spectrum of psychocognitive morbidity in the critically ill: a review of the literature and call for improvement. J Crit Care 2015;30(1):130–7.
48. Ouimet S, Kavanagh BP, Gottfried SB, et al. Incidence, risk factors and consequences of ICU delirium. Intensive Care Med 2007;33(1):66–73.
49. Han JH, Shintani A, Eden S, et al. Delirium in the emergency department: an independent predictor of death within 6 months. Ann Emerg Med 2010;56(3):244–52 e1.
50. Salluh JI, Wang H, Schneider EB, et al. Outcome of delirium in critically ill patients: systematic review and meta-analysis. BMJ 2015;350:h2538.
51. Wilcox ME, Brummel NE, Archer K, et al. Cognitive dysfunction in ICU patients: risk factors, predictors, and rehabilitation interventions. Crit Care Med 2013;41(9 Suppl. 1):S81–98.
52. Svenningsen H, Tonnesen EK, Videbech P, et al. Intensive care delirium - effect on memories and health-related quality of life - a follow-up study. J Clin Nurs 2014;23(5–6):634–44.
53. Roberts BL, Rickard CM, Rajbhandari D, et al. Factual memories of ICU: recall at two years post-discharge and comparison with delirium status during ICU admission – a multicentre cohort study. J Clin Nurs 2007;16(9):1669–77.
54. Meagher DJ, Leonard M, Donnelly S, et al. A longitudinal study of motor subtypes in delirium: relationship with other phenomenology, etiology, medication exposure and prognosis. J Psychosom Res 2011;71(6):395–403.
55. American Psychiatric Association. Diagnostic and statistical manual of mental disorders (DSM-5®): American Psychiatric Pub; 2013.
56. Broyles LM, Colbert AM, Tate JA, et al. Clinicians' evaluation and management of mental health, substance abuse, and chronic pain conditions in the intensive care unit. Crit Care Med 2008;36(1):87–93.
57. van den Boogaard M, Schoonhoven L, van der Hoeven JG, et al. Incidence and short-term consequences of delirium in critically ill patients: a prospective observational cohort study. Int J Nurs Stud 2011.

58. Mariz J, Santos NC, Afonso H, et al. Risk and clinical-outcome indicators of delirium in an emergency department intermediate care unit (EDIMCU): an observational prospective study. BMC Emerg Med 2013;13(1):2.
59. Maldonado JR. Acute brain failure: pathophysiology, diagnosis, management, and sequelae of delirium. Crit Care Clin 2017;33(3):461–519.
60. Zaal IJ, Devlin JW, Peelen LM, et al. A systematic review of risk factors for delirium in the ICU. Crit Care Med 2015;43(1):40–7.
61. Boogaard Mvd, Pickkers P, Slooter AJC, et al. Development and validation of PRE-DELIRIC (PREdiction of DELIRium in ICu patients) delirium prediction model for intensive care patients: observational multicentre study. BMJ 2012;344.
62. Aldemir M, Ozen S, Kara IH, et al. Predisposing factors for delirium in the surgical intensive care unit. Crit Care 2001;5(5):265–70.
63. Girard TD, Ely EW. Delirium in the critically ill patient. Handb Clin Neurol 2008;90:39–56.
64. McPherson JA, Wagner CE, Boehm LM, et al. Delirium in the cardiovascular ICU: exploring modifiable risk factors. Crit Care Med 2013;41(2):405–13.
65. Girard TD, Pandharipande PP, Ely EW. Delirium in the intensive care unit. Crit Care 2008;12(Suppl. 3):S3.
66. Bergeron N, Dubois MJ, Dumont M, et al. Intensive care delirium screening checklist: evaluation of a new screening tool. Intensive Care Med 2001;27(5):859–64.
67. Ely EW, Inouye SK, Bernard GR, et al. Delirium in mechanically ventilated patients: validity and reliability of the Confusion Assessment Method for the Intensive Care Unit (CAM-ICU). JAMA 2001;286(21):2703–10.
68. Neto AS, Nassar AP Jr, Cardoso SO, et al. Delirium screening in critically ill patients: a systematic review and meta-analysis. Crit Care Med 2012;40(6):1946–51.
69. Shi Q, Warren L, Saposnik G, et al. Confusion assessment method: a systematic review and meta-analysis of diagnostic accuracy. Neuropsychiatr Dis Treat 2013;9:1359–70.
70. Ely EW, Margolin R, Francis J, et al. Evaluation of delirium in critically ill patients: validation of the confusion assessment method for the intensive care unit (CAM-ICU). Crit Care Med 2001;29(7):1370–9.
71. Kamdar BB, King LM, Collop NA, et al. The effect of a quality improvement intervention on perceived sleep quality and cognition in a medical ICU. Crit Care Med 2013;41(3):800–9.
72. Smith CD, Grami P. Feasibility and effectiveness of a delirium prevention bundle in critically ill patients. Am J Crit Care 2016;26(1):19–27.
73. Flannery AH, Oyler DR, Weinhouse GL. The impact of interventions to improve sleep on delirium in the ICU: a systematic review and research framework. Crit Care Med 2016;44(12):2231–40.
74. Neufeld KJ, Yue J, Robinson TN, et al. Antipsychotics for prevention and treatment of delirium in hospitalized adults: a systematic review and meta-analysis. J Am Geriatr Soc 2016;64(4):705–14.
75. Weaver CB, Kane-Gill SL, Gunn SR, et al. A retrospective analysis of the effectiveness of antipsychotics in the treatment of ICU delirium. J Crit Care 2017;41:234–9.
76. Kawazoe Y, Miyamoto K, Morimoto T, et al. Effect of dexmedetomidine on mortality and ventilator-free days in patients requiring mechanical ventilation with sepsis: a randomized clinical trial. JAMA 2017;317(13):1321–8.
77. Cruickshank M, Henderson L, MacLennan G, et al. Alpha-2 agonists for sedation of mechanically ventilated adults in intensive care units: a systematic review. Health Technol Assess 2016;20(25):1–118.
78. Reade MC, Eastwood GM, Bellomo R, et al. Effect of dexmedetomidine added to standard care on ventilator-free time in patients with agitated delirium: a randomized clinical trial. JAMA 2016;315(14):1460–8.
79. Hale GM, Kane-Gill SL, Groetzinger L, et al. An evaluation of adverse drug reactions associated with antipsychotic use for the treatment of delirium in the intensive care unit. J Pharm Pract 2016;29(4):355–60.
80. Awissi DK, Lebrun G, Coursin DB, et al. Alcohol withdrawal and delirium tremens in the critically ill: a systematic review and commentary. Intensive Care Med 2013;39(1):16–30.
81. Schuckit MA. Recognition and management of withdrawal delirium (delirium tremens). N Engl J Med 2014;371(22):2109–13.
82. Maldonado JR, Sher Y, Ashouri JF, et al. The 'Prediction of Alcohol Withdrawal Severity Scale' (PAWSS): systematic literature review and pilot study of a new scale for the prediction of complicated alcohol withdrawal syndrome. Alcohol 2014;48(4):375–90.
83. Australian Institute of Health and Welfare. Non-medical use of pharmaceuticals: trends, harms and treatment, 2006-07 to 2015-16. Canberra: AIHW; 2017.
84. US Department of Health and Human Services (HHS). Facing addiction in America: the surgeon general's report on alcohol, drugs, and health. Washington, DC: HHS; 2016.
85. United Nations Office on Drugs and Crime. World Drug Report 2017. United Nations, 2017.
86. Banks E, Joshy G, Weber MF, et al. Tobacco smoking and all-cause mortality in a large Australian cohort study: findings from a mature epidemic with current low smoking prevalence. BMC Med 2015;13(1):38.
87. Greenhalgh EM, Bayly M, Winstanley MH. 1.2 Overview of major Australian data sets. In: Scollo MM, Winstanley MH, editors. Tobacco in Australia: facts and issues. Melbourne: Cancer Council Victoria; 2015.
88. Ng M, Freeman MK, Fleming TD, et al. Smoking prevalence and cigarette consumption in 187 countries, 1980-2012. JAMA 2014;311(2):183–92.
89. Koob GF, Volkow ND. Neurobiology of addiction: a neurocircuitry analysis. Lancet Psychiatry 2016;3(8):760–73.
90. Donroe JH, Tetrault JM. Substance use, intoxication, and withdrawal in the critical care setting. Crit Care Clin 2017;33(3):543–58.

91. Wang PP, Huang E, Feng X, et al. Opioid-associated iatrogenic withdrawal in critically ill adult patients: a multicenter prospective observational study. Ann Intensive Care 2017;7(1):88.
92. Awissi DK, Lebrun G, Fagnan M, et al. Alcohol, nicotine, and iatrogenic withdrawals in the ICU. Crit Care Med 2013;41(9 Suppl. 1):S57–68.
93. Ewing JA. Detecting alcoholism. The CAGE questionnaire. JAMA 1984;252(14):1905–7.
94. Mirijello A, D'Angelo C, Ferrulli A, et al. Identification and management of alcohol withdrawal syndrome. Drugs 2015;75(4):353–65.
95. Sutton LJ, Jutel A. Alcohol Withdrawal syndrome in critically ill patients: identification, assessment, and management. Crit Care Nurse 2016;36(1):28–38.
96. Wetterling T, Kanitz RD, Besters B, et al. A new rating scale for the assessment of the alcohol-withdrawal syndrome (AWS scale). Alcohol Alcohol 1997;32(6):753–60.
97. Sullivan JT, Sykora K, Schneiderman J, et al. Assessment of alcohol withdrawal: the revised clinical institute withdrawal assessment for alcohol scale (CIWA-Ar). Br J Addict 1989;84(11):1353–7.
98. Heatherton TF, Kozlowski LT, Frecker RC, et al. The Fagerstrom test for Nicotine Dependence: a revision of the Fagerstrom Tolerance Questionnaire. Br J Addict 1991;86(9):1119–27.
99. Chiu AW, Contreras S, Mehta S, et al. Iatrogenic Opioid withdrawal in critically ill patients: a review of assessment tools and management. Ann Pharmacother 2017;51(12):1099–111.
100. Dixit D, Endicott J, Burry L, et al. Management of acute alcohol withdrawal syndrome in critically ill patients. Pharmacotherapy 2016;36(7):797–822.
101. Perry EC. Inpatient management of acute alcohol withdrawal syndrome. CNS Drugs 2014;28(5):401–10.
102. Thomson AD, Cook CC. Parenteral thiamine and Wernicke's encephalopathy: the balance of risks and perception of concern. Alcohol Alcohol 1997;32(3):207–9.
103. Hood SD, Norman A, Hince DA, et al. Benzodiazepine dependence and its treatment with low dose flumazenil. Br J Clin Pharmacol 2014;77(2):285–94.
104. Kampman K, Jarvis M. American Society of Addiction Medicine (ASAM) national practice guideline for the use of medications in the treatment of addiction involving opioid use. J Addict Med 2015;9(5):358–67.
105. Gowing L, Ali R, White JM, et al. Buprenorphine for managing opioid withdrawal. Cochrane Database Syst Rev 2017;(2):CD002025.
106. Ng K, Gillies M, Griffith D. Effect of nicotine replacement therapy on mortality, delirium, and duration of therapy in critically ill smokers: a systematic review and meta-analysis. Anaesth Intensive Care 2017;45(5):556–61.
107. Kowalski M, Udy AA, McRobbie HJ, et al. Nicotine replacement therapy for agitation and delirium management in the intensive care unit: a systematic review of the literature. J Intensive Care 2016;4(1):69.
108. Wilby KJ, Harder CK. Nicotine replacement therapy in the intensive care unit: a systematic review. J Intensive Care Med 2014;29(1):22–30.
109. Erickson CK. Addiction essentials: the go-to guide for clinicians and patients. New York: WW Norton & Co; 2011.
110. Mack AH. Clinical textbook of addictive disorders. New York: The Guilford Press; 2016.
111. Puntillo KA, Max A, Chaize M, et al. Patient recollection of ICU procedural pain and post ICU burden: the memory study. Crit Care Med 2016;44(11):1988–95.
112. Puntillo KA, Max A, Timsit JF, et al. Determinants of procedural pain intensity in the intensive care unit. The Europain(R) study. Am J Respir Crit Care Med 2014;189(1):39–47.
113. Fishman S, Ballantyne J, Rathmell JP. In: Fishman SM, Ballantyne JC, Rathmell JP, editors. Bonica's Management of pain. 4th ed. Philadelphia: Lippincott Williams & Wilkins; 2009.
114. Milgrom LB, Brooks JA, Qi R, et al. Pain levels experienced with activities after cardiac surgery. Am J Crit Care 2004;13(2):116–25.
115. Dunwoody CJ, Krenzischek DA, Pasero C, et al. Assessment, physiological monitoring, and consequences of inadequately treated acute pain. J Perianesth Nurs 2008;23(1 Suppl.):S15–27.
116. McCaffery M. Understanding your patient's pain. Nursing (Lond) 1980;10(9):26–31.
117. Herr K, Coyne PJ, Key T, et al. Pain assessment in the nonverbal patient: position statement with clinical practice recommendations. Pain Manag Nurs 2006;7(2):44–52.
118. Payen JF, Bru O, Bosson JL, et al. Assessing pain in critically ill sedated patients by using a behavioral pain scale. Crit Care Med 2001;29(12):2258–63.
119. Feldt KS. The checklist of nonverbal pain indicators (CNPI). Pain Manag Nurs 2000;1(1):13–21.
120. Gélinas C, Fillion L, Puntillo KA, et al. Validation of the critical-care pain observation tool in adult patients. Am J Crit Care 2006;15(4): 420–7.
121. Melzack R. The short-form McGill Pain Questionnaire. Pain 1987;30(2):191–7.
122. Arbour C, Gelinas C. Are vital signs valid indicators for the assessment of pain in postoperative cardiac surgery ICU adults? Intensive Crit Care Nurs 2010;26(2):83–90.
123. Frazier SK, Moser DK, Schlanger R, et al. Autonomic tone in medical intensive care patients receiving mechanical ventilation and during a CPAP weaning trial. Biol Res Nurs 2008;9(4):301–10.
124. Wiatrowski R, Norton C, Giffen D. Analgosedation: improving patient outcomes in ICU sedation and pain management. Pain Manag Nurs 2016;17(3):204–17.

125. Fredriksen ST, Svensson T. The bodily presence of significant others: intensive care patients' experiences in a situation of critical illness. Int J Qual Stud Health Well-being 2010;5(4).
126. Gelinas C, Arbour C, Michaud C, et al. Patients and ICU nurses' perspectives of non-pharmacological interventions for pain management. Nurs Crit Care 2013;18(6):307–18.
127. MacPherson RD, Woods D, Penfold J. Ketamine and midazolam delivered by patient-controlled analgesia in relieving pain associated with burns dressings. Clin J Pain 2008;24(7):568–71.
128. Zor F, Ozturk S, Bilgin F, et al. Pain relief during dressing changes of major adult burns: ideal analgesic combination with ketamine. Burns 2010;36(4):501–5.
129. Balzer F, Weiss B, Kumpf O, et al. Early deep sedation is associated with decreased in-hospital and two-year follow-up survival. Crit Care 2015;19:197.
130. Samuelson KA, Lundberg D, Fridlund B. Light vs heavy sedation during mechanical ventilation after Oesophagectomy – a pilot experimental study focusing on memory. Acta Anaesthesiol Scand 2008;52(8):1116–23.
131. Treggiari MM, Romand JA, Yanez ND, et al. Randomized trial of light versus deep sedation on mental health after critical illness. Crit Care Med 2009;37(9):2527–34.
132. Jackson DL, Proudfoot CW, Cann KF, et al. A systematic review of the impact of sedation practice in the ICU on resource use, costs and patient safety. Crit Care 2010;14(2):R59.
133. Robinson BR, Berube M, Barr J, et al. Psychometric analysis of subjective sedation scales in critically ill adults. Crit Care Med 2013;41(9 Suppl. 1):S16–29.
134. Yu A, Teitelbaum J, Scott J, et al. Evaluating pain, sedation, and delirium in the neurologically critically ill-feasibility and reliability of standardized tools: a multi-institutional study. Crit Care Med 2013;41(8):2002–7.
135. Sessler CN, Gosnell M, Grap MJ, et al. The Richmond Agitation–Sedation Scale: validity and reliability in adult intensive care patients. Am J Respir Crit Care Med 2002;166:1338–44.
136. Ramsay MA, Savege TM, Simpson BR, et al. Controlled sedation with alphaxalone-alphadolone. Br Med J 1974;2(5920):656–9.
137. Devlin JW, Boleski G, Mlynarek M, et al. Motor Activity Assessment Scale: a valid and reliable sedation scale for use with mechanically ventilated patients in an adult surgical intensive care unit. Crit Care Med 1999;27(7):1271–5.
138. de Lemos J, Tweeddale M, Chittock D. Measuring quality of sedation in adult mechanically ventilated critically ill patients. The Vancouver Interaction and Calmness Scale. Sedation Focus Group. J Clin Epidemiol 2000;53(9):908–19.
139. De Jonghe B, Cook D, Griffith L, et al. Adaptation to the Intensive Care Environment (ATICE): development and validation of a new sedation assessment instrument. Crit Care Med 2003;31(9):2344–54.
140. Weinert C, McFarland L. The state of intubated ICU patients: development of a two-dimensional sedation rating scale for critically ill adults. Chest 2004;126(6):1883–90.
141. Riker RR, Picard JT, Fraser GL. Prospective evaluation of the Sedation-Agitation Scale for adult critically ill patients. Crit Care Med 1999;27(7):1325–9.
142. Anderson J, Henry L, Hunt S, et al. Bispectral index monitoring to facilitate early extubation following cardiovascular surgery. Clin Nurse Spec 2010;24(3):140–8.
143. Weatherburn C, Endacott R, Tynan P, et al. The impact of bispectral index monitoring on sedation administration in mechanically ventilated patients. Anaesth Intensive Care 2007;35(2):204–8.
144. Aitken LM, Bucknall T, Kent B, et al. Protocol-directed sedation versus non-protocol-directed sedation to reduce duration of mechanical ventilation in mechanically ventilated intensive care patients. Cochrane Database Syst Rev 2015;(1):Cd009771.
145. Kress JP, Gehlbach B, Lacy M, et al. The long-term psychological effects of daily sedative interruption on critically ill patients. Am J Respir Crit Care Med 2003;168(12):1457–61.
146. Kress JP, Pohlman AS, O'Connor MF, et al. Daily interruption of sedative infusions in critically ill patients undergoing mechanical ventilation. N Engl J Med 2000;342(20):1471–7.
147. Burry L, Rose L, McCullagh IJ, et al. Daily sedation interruption versus no daily sedation interruption for critically ill adult patients requiring invasive mechanical ventilation. Cochrane Database Syst Rev 2014;(7):Cd009176.
148. Mehta S, Burry L, Cook D, et al. Daily sedation interruption in mechanically ventilated critically ill patients cared for with a sedation protocol: a randomized controlled trial. JAMA 2012;308(19):1985–92.
149. Rose L, Fitzgerald E, Cook D, et al. Clinician perspectives on protocols designed to minimize sedation. J Crit Care 2015;30(2):348–52.
150. Sneyers B, Laterre PF, Bricq E, et al. What stops us from following sedation recommendations in intensive care units? A multicentric qualitative study. J Crit Care 2014;29(2):291–7.
151. Siegel JM. Why we sleep. Sci Am 2003;289(5):92–7.
152. Gallicchio L, Kalesan B. Sleep duration and mortality: a systematic review and meta-analysis. J Sleep Res 2009;18(2):148–58.
153. Kamdar BB, Needham DM, Collop NA. Sleep deprivation in critical illness: its role in physical and psychological recovery. J Intensive Care Med 2012;27(2):97–111.
154. Pisani MA, Friese RS, Gehlbach BK, et al. Sleep in the intensive care unit. Am J Respir Crit Care Med 2015;191(7):731–8.
155. Kryger MH, Roth T, Dement WC. Elsevier Freedom Collection EBA. Principles and practice of sleep medicine. 6th ed. Philadelphia: Elsevier; 2017.

156. Iber C, Ancoli-Israel S, Chesson A, et al, editors. AASM Manual for the scoring of sleep and associated events: rules, terminology and technical specification. 1st ed. Westchester. American Academy of Sleep Medicine; 2007.
157. Friese RS, Diaz-Arrastia R, McBride D, et al. Quantity and quality of sleep in the surgical intensive care unit: are our patients sleeping? J Trauma 2007;63(6):1210–14.
158. Hardin KA, Seyal M, Stewart T, et al. Sleep in critically ill chemically paralyzed patients requiring mechanical ventilation. Chest 2006;129(6):1468–77.
159. Elliott R, McKinley S, Cistulli P, et al. Characterisation of sleep in intensive care using 24-hour polysomnography: an observational study. Crit Care 2013;17(2):R46.
160. Drouot X, Cabello B, d'Ortho M-P, et al. Sleep in the intensive care unit. Sleep Medicine Reviews [Internet] 2008 070808; doi:10.1016/j.smrv.2007.11.004.
161. Aitken LM, Elliott R, Mitchell M, et al. Sleep assessment by patients and nurses in the intensive care: an exploratory descriptive study. Aust Crit Care 2017;30(2):59–66.
162. Ritmala-Castren M, Axelin A, Kiljunen K, et al. Sleep in the intensive care unit – nurses' documentation and patients' perspectives. Nurs Crit Care 2017;22(4):238–46.
163. Nicolás A, Aizpitarte E, Iruarrizaga A, et al. Perception of night-time sleep by surgical patients in an intensive care unit. Nurs Crit Care 2008;13(1):25–33.
164. Beltrami FG, Nguyen XL, Pichereau C, et al. Sleep in the intensive care unit. J Bras Pneumol 2015;41(6):539–46.
165. Ohayon MM, Carskadon MA, Guilleminault C, et al. Meta-analysis of quantitative sleep parameters from childhood to old age in healthy individuals: developing normative sleep values across the human lifespan. Sleep 2004;27(7):1255–73.
166. Floyd JA, Janisse JJ, Jenuwine ES, et al. Changes in REM-sleep in percentage over the adult lifespan. Sleep 2007;30(7):829–36.
167. Rechtschaffen A, Kales A. A manual of standardized terminology: techniques and scoring system for sleep stages of human subjects. Los Angeles: UCLA Brain Information Service/Brain Research Institute; 1968.
168. Kamdar BB, Kadden DJ, Vangala S, et al. Feasibility of continuous actigraphy in patients in a medical intensive care unit. Am J Crit Care 2017;26(4):329–35.
169. Raj R, Ussavarungsi K, Nugent K. Accelerometer-based devices can be used to monitor sedation/agitation in the intensive care unit. J Crit Care 2014;29(5):748–52.
170. Nieuwenhuijs D, Coleman EL, Douglas NJ, et al. Bispectral index values and spectral edge frequency at different stages of physiologic sleep. Anesth Analg 2002;94(1):125–9.
171. Giménez S, Romero S, Alonso JF, et al. Monitoring sleep depth: analysis of bispectral index (BIS) based on polysomnographic recordings and sleep deprivation. J Clin Monit Comput 2017;31(1):103–10.
172. Richards KC, O'Sullivan PS, Phillips RL. Measurement of sleep in critically ill patients. J Nurs Meas 2000;8(2):131–44.
173. Freedman NS, Kotzer N, Schwab RJ. Patient perception of sleep quality and etiology of sleep disruption in the intensive care unit. Am J Respir Crit Care Med 1999;159(4 Pt 1):1155–62.
174. Edwards GB, Schuring LM. Pilot study: validating staff nurses' observations of sleep and wake states among critically ill patients, using polysomnography. Am J Crit Care 1993;2(2):125–31.
175. Beecroft JM, Ward M, Younes M, et al. Sleep monitoring in the intensive care unit: comparison of nurse assessment, actigraphy and polysomnography. Intensive Care Med 2008;34(11):2076–83.
176. Richardson A, Crow W, Coghill E, et al. A comparison of sleep assessment tools by nurses and patients in critical care. J Clin Nurs 2007;16(9):1660–16668.
177. Hu RF, Jiang XY, Hegadoren KM, et al. Effects of earplugs and eye masks combined with relaxing music on sleep, melatonin and cortisol levels in ICU patients: a randomized controlled trial. Crit Care 2015;19:115.
178. Tainter CR, Levine AR, Quraishi SA, et al. Noise levels in surgical ICUs are consistently above recommended standards. Crit Care Med 2016;44(1):147–52.
179. Darbyshire JL, Young JD. An investigation of sound levels on intensive care units with reference to the WHO guidelines. Crit Care 2013;17(5):R187.
180. Berglund B, Lindvall T, Schwela DH. Guidelines for Community Noise Geneva World Health Organisation; 1999.
181. Korompeli A, Muurlink O, Kavrochorianou N, et al. Circadian disruption of ICU patients: a review of pathways, expression, and interventions. J Crit Care 2017;38:269–77.
182. Engwall M, Fridh I, Johansson L, et al. Lighting, sleep and circadian rhythm: an intervention study in the intensive care unit. Intensive Crit Care Nurs 2015;31(6):325–35.
183. Chan MC, Spieth PM, Quinn K, et al. Circadian rhythms: from basic mechanisms to the intensive care unit. Crit Care Med 2012;40(1):246–53.
184. Cabello B, Thille AW, Drouot X, et al. Sleep quality in mechanically ventilated patients: comparison of three ventilatory modes. Crit Care Med 2008;36(6):1749–55.
185. Bourne RS, Mills GH. Sleep disruption in critically ill patients - pharmacological considerations. Anaesthesia 2004;59(4):374–84.
186. Hardin KA. Sleep in the ICU: potential mechanisms and clinical implications. Chest 2009;136(1):284–94.

187. Roehrs T, Roth T. Drug-related sleep stage changes: functional significance and clinical relevance. Sleep Med Clin 2010;5(4):559–70.
188. Matheson E, Hainer BL. Insomnia: pharmacologic therapy. Am Fam Physician 2017;96(1):29–35.
189. Lewis SR, Schofield-Robinson OJ, Alderson P, et al. Propofol for the promotion of sleep in adults in the intensive care unit. Cochrane Database Syst Rev 2018;(1):Cd012454.
190. Wilt TJ, MacDonald R, Brasure M, et al. Pharmacologic treatment of insomnia disorder: an evidence report for a clinical practice guideline by the American College of Physicians. Ann Intern Med 2016;165(2):103–12.
191. Buscemi N, Vandermeer B, Hooton N, et al. Efficacy and safety of exogenous melatonin for secondary sleep disorders and sleep disorders accompanying sleep restriction: meta-analysis. BMJ 2006;332(7538):385–93.
192. Mo Y, Scheer CE, Abdallah GT. Emerging role of melatonin and melatonin receptor agonists in sleep and delirium in intensive care unit patients. J Intensive Care Med 2016;31(7):451–5.
193. Lewis SR, Pritchard MW, Schofield-Robinson OJ, et al. Melatonin for the promotion of sleep in adults in the intensive care unit. Cochrane Database Syst Rev 2018;(5):Cd012455.
194. Huupponen E, Maksimow A, Lapinlampi P, et al. Electroencephalogram spindle activity during dexmedetomidine sedation and physiological sleep. Acta Anaesthesiol Scand 2008;52(2):289–94.

Chapter 7

Family and cultural care of the critically ill patient

Marion Mitchell, Denise Wilson

KEY WORDS

bereavement
communication
continuity of care
cultural care
cultural humility
cultural safety
cultural responsiveness
end-of-life
family care
minority or marginalised groups
models of care
patient, family-centred care
spiritual care

Learning objectives

After reading this chapter, you should be able to:

- describe models of care and evaluate how they meet patient and family needs
- recognise appropriate resources to enhance communication
- develop an understanding of the needs of families and patients who die in the ICU
- evaluate and implement appropriate strategies for working with families from a diversity of cultures
- recognise and implement the needs of the critically ill and/or dying patient who is from a different culture.
- recognise the various spiritual considerations for families and their patients who are dying or who have died.

Introduction

Care of critically ill patients is complex and multifactorial. Although management of the haemodynamic parameters and healthcare interventions is an essential component of effective care of the critically ill, the psychosocial health and wellbeing of patients are intimately related to their wellness and eventual illness outcome. There is a tendency, due to the technologically complex nature of nursing in critical care areas, for novice critical care nurses to focus their attention on the management of medical treatment regimens. This is an important part of their learning trajectory. However, nurses need to be guided to see beyond the waveforms and physical parameters to see the patient in the bed as an individual with unique needs. The previous chapter examined specific aspects of the psychological wellbeing of the critically ill with strategies to improve patient outcomes. This chapter extends the focus to incorporate the family into the caring paradigm and introduces the concept of person-centred, patient-centred, and patient, family-centred care. The word family in this chapter is defined as whomever the patient considers to be their family and will generally incorporate those who have a lasting relationship with the patient irrespective of any legal or blood ties.

Nursing practices that incorporate the patient's family into the care of the critically ill acknowledge, support and promote the vital part families play in the illness continuum.

The assessment, understanding and incorporation of the patient's and family's cultural needs are essential elements of nursing the critically ill, and involve the entire interdisciplinary team. These elements are important for both the recipients of the care (the patient and family) and the critical care nurse, as the practice of nursing all aspects of the patient's wellbeing brings humanity into critical care nursing. Cultural factors include social factors and human behaviours associated with emotional and spiritual needs.[1] In this chapter, models of nursing are examined with particular reference to the philosophy of patient, family-centred care, which may be an appropriate nursing model for use within critical care settings. The specific needs of the families of critically ill patients, as well as the implications for critical care nursing, are discussed. The differing world views on health and illness are highlighted for consideration of appropriate care. Many of the populations for whom we provide care exhibit diversity of gender and sexual identity, sexuality, ethnicity, country of origin and cultural practices. Effective communication is crucial to meet both patient and their families' needs. The complexity of patient communication together with the addition of linguistically diverse patients is outlined and suggestions for clinical practice provided. End-of-life care is discussed in general terms and specific cultural considerations are highlighted with particular reference to racial or ethnic minority groups and other marginalised groups (such as, transgendered youth).

Overview of models of care

Nurses manage their daily activities and patient care in response to both the critical care unit's model of care delivery and the individual nurse's personal philosophy of what and how nursing is constructed. These are both influenced by broader hospital, national and international priorities together with guidance from professional organisations.[2-4] Alternative models of care are examined in this section and their use in critical care areas discussed. Nursing models define shared values and beliefs that guide practice. Various philosophies and models of nursing care delivery have evolved over the decades and contrast with the 'medical model', which focuses on the diagnosis and treatment of disease.[5] Models such as primary nursing and team nursing as seen in various health care facilities have organisational and management properties, whereas patient-centred practice is another model where a partnership is developed between health professionals and the patient and their family.[5-7]

Patient-centred care

Patient-centred care shifts control in health-related decisions from the healthcare professional to the patient – the recipient of care, thus challenging some existing paradigms.[8] This model has patient empowerment as the core element. To facilitate empowerment, patients need to be well informed in such a way that they can understand the information to help with their decisions.[9] It is incumbent upon critical care nurses to have a conversation with patients about their illness perceptions, priorities and future plans. Having a clear understanding of patients' concepts of illness, their cultural beliefs and intent is vital.[9] Treating patients with respect and providing care that is responsive to individual patient preferences, needs and values is fundamental to acknowledging patient identity and empowerment.[7]

Implementation of patient-centred care requires a culture change and therefore needs support at an individual, professional level and at an organisational level.[10,11] A study in the USA examined how critical care nurses communicate with patients and families within a patient-centred care framework that was operating within their unit. They found that nurses predominantly communicated information related to the patient's acute biophysical status. Although the nurses in the study supported the importance of shared power and responsibility, they exhibited few examples in practice. They reflected that they felt sharing power fell within the domain of intensivists' discussions with patients and families rather than theirs.[12] Nurses deferring responsibility for communication in such a way highlights the importance of a whole-of-team approach to patient-centred care where healthcare professionals share the responsibility of meaningfully involving patients and their families in decisions and care options. Nurses need to have adequate support to meet the intense demands that come with caring for the critically ill for them to overcome the barriers to achieving optimum patient-centred care.[6,10]

Person-centred care

Person-centred care is another term used. The *Oxford English Dictionary* defines 'patient' in passive terms as the receiver of care whereas a 'person' is acknowledged as being an individual in their own right.[13] Those who read about patient-centred care (as outlined above) will understand that the word 'patient' in the context of patient-centred care is far from the passive role in this dictionary definition. However, if consumers are to understand healthcare organisations' working paradigms, semantics and first impressions are important. The term 'person-centred care' emphasises the individual nature of the person with the illness. It promotes the perception of equal power and a shared partnership between the person and healthcare provider/s. Here, the person is an acknowledged expert for their own health values and goals. The partnership is both collaborative and respectful and highlights the importance of knowing the person behind the patient and understanding that the patient is more than their illness.[14]

There is a scarcity of evaluations of person-centred care in critical care areas.[15] However, some evidence, outside the critical care environment, is coming out of the Centre for Person-Centred Care in the University of Gothenburg in Sweden where improved patient outcomes have been reported.[15] In one in-hospital study of chronic heart failure patients, length of stay was reduced by a third with no compromise in their perceived quality of care when person-centred care was compared to usual care. The individualised care plan based on understanding each patient's needs was seen to be a major contributing factor in reducing hospital stay.[16] In another study of patients with chronic heart failure in the USA, person-centred care was explored in five wards in a single hospital that implemented a person-centred care approach.[12] Person-centred care was evaluated in relation to how it reduced patients' uncertainty about their illness. The differing organisational and operational features of the ward were examined. In wards where goal setting, planning, control and stability were evident, patients' uncertainty in illness was reduced, which the authors linked to a person-centred approach to care.[12] Within an intensive care unit (ICU) environment, however, a truly shared partnership with the patient may be problematic, where critical illness restricts patient involvement in decision making and care planning. In reality, it is generally family members who provide the link between the patient and healthcare team.

During the 1980s, the role of the family was one focus of nursing debate and discussion. Friedman believed families were the greatest social institution influencing individuals' health in our society.[17] A worldwide trend is for health professionals to value the role of family members in providing ongoing, post-acute care,[18] with the reality being that families provide considerable support during rehabilitation phases of critical illnesses. The family is strongly incorporated within these philosophies and whichever model is selected, it must be practical and understood in the clinical setting for which it is intended. There are entire organisations, such as Plaintree, that provide resources for patients, families and organisations on how to implement strategies to enhance the philosophy of person-centred care.[19]

Patient, family-centred care

Patient, family-centred care is a third term you may see used. This is intended to describe sharing of responsibility of patient care decisions with the family, where appropriate, and thus highlights the importance of family in critical care areas. This developed during the early 1990s, primarily in North America in the area of children's nursing, where incorporating the family was considered fundamental to the care of the patient.[20] Over the past decades, the scope and extent of family-centred care has broadened and the Institute for Family-Centered Care now defines family-centred care more broadly to patient, family-centred care which it describes as 'an innovative approach to the planning, delivery, and evaluation of healthcare that is governed by mutually beneficial partnerships among healthcare providers, patients and families'.[21] Patient, family-centred care applies to patients of all ages, and it may be practised in any healthcare setting.[22]

Patient, family-centred care is founded on mutual respect and partnership among patients, families and healthcare providers. It incorporates all aspects of physical and psychosocial care, from assessment to care delivery and evaluation.[21] Five elements of patient and family participation include 1) a physical presence 2) having needs met 3) effective communication 4) decision making 5) contributing to care.[23] Healthcare providers that value the family/patient partnership during a critical illness strive to facilitate relationship building and provide amenities and services that facilitate families being connected and physically near their hospitalised relative.[18] Parent and nurse perceptions on the quality of patient, family-centre care have been examined in a study of 11 neonatal ICUs in Europe where innovative text-messaging data collection methods were used. Although parents perceived high levels of patient and family-centred care, there were areas for improvement such as providing emotional support to parents, including parents in decision making and encouraging fathers to participate in their infant's care.[24]

Many nurses also value family involvement in the care of their own sick relative.[25,26] Other strategies to improve patient, family-centred care within adult critical care areas include involving family members in partnering with the nursing staff to consider the involvement they, and the patient, would like them to have, which may include providing fundamental care to their sick relative.[27] Family members can decide in consultation and negotiation with the direct care nurse the care that they want, and are able to provide that aligns with the patient's preferences. This care may vary from moisturising their relative's skin to a full sponge and will require negotiation. Such acts of caring allow family members to connect in what they see as a meaningful way with their sick relative. In addition, it can also improve communication with critical care nurses and facilitate close physical and emotional contact with their relative.[28] An independent nursing intervention such as partnering with family to provide care constitutes an example of how to operationalise a patient, family-centred care model in the clinical setting and assists in the evaluation of other future interventions directed to improve patient, family-centred approaches.

To date, there have been limited quality evaluation studies assessing the efficacy of patient, family-centred interventions. However, some have shown a reduction in length of ICU stay, improved patient and family satisfaction scores and psychological symptoms.[29] Patient and family experience would likely benefit from a whole-of-unit approach where there is a cultural shift to a patient, family-centred care philosophy rather than the current research that predominantly focuses on single elements of patient, family-centred care in isolation.[9,29,30] It is acknowledged that taking care of critically ill patients requires considerable knowledge and skill. When family members are incorporated into the caring paradigm, as advocated within patient, family-centred care, health professionals equally need specific knowledge and skills. This information should be initiated in foundation degrees, continued within postgraduate studies and via ongoing professional development opportunities.[12,31] Internationally it is recognised that the benefits of involving families extends to the promotion of safe practice.[10,32,33]

Professional critical care associations in both USA and Australia have shown leadership and have provided direction by way of guidelines with multiple recommendations for practice[9] and a position statement on partnering with families in critical care.[4] These documents are based on low levels of evidence highlighting the need for future evaluation research. The family knows the patient best, has their best interest foremost and is the one constant throughout the illness. Importantly, family members frequently provide ongoing care beyond the ICU, and involving them during the critical illness phase supports their ability to provide immediate feedback and prolonged care to their relative. Partnering with families is not necessarily time-consuming but, to be able to do this, an understanding of their needs is required.[17,34]

Needs of family during critical illness

Family members of critically ill patients have little time to prepare or adapt to the demands of an ICU admission resulting in anxiety, worry and stress. Critical care nurses have a responsibility to support family members through this confronting period of their lives.[35] Understanding their needs is fundamental to being able to provide appropriate support measures. Consistently, family needs include the need for assurance, information, proximity, comfort and support and although there will always be the need to individualise care, assurance and information needs are paramount.[36] Assurance needs are closely related to information needs where family members want to know the diagnosis, treatment options, plan of care and short and longer term goals.[35] The manner in which family needs are met is directly related to family members' satisfaction with the care their relative receives and is considered a legitimate quality indicator in many hospitals.[37,38]

On a very practical level family members are often the decision makers on treatment options due to the impaired cognitive state of the patient. Their contribution to healthcare decisions is sought in both acute and ongoing care situations as they have insight and knowledge of the patient on an entirely different level to that of health professionals.[39] Importantly, family members provide not only support in the critical illness situation, but also continuity of care through rehabilitation. This responsibility together with the often sudden critical illness may create stress, anxiety, depression and/or posttraumatic stress disorder (PTSD) for family members.[40,41] A primary outcome of patient, family-centred care is to reduce the risk of stress-related reactions to the ICU experience, which is often traumatic for family members.[42,43]

> **Practice tip**
>
> Suggest to a family member that they might like to provide some care to their relative with your help. This will need some discussion as you will want to gain an understanding of their relationship with the patient and what they feel the patient might want and what is possible in the situation. They might want to comb their hair or massage their hands. Alternatively, they might like to read something to them that they know will be of interest. By giving the family member permission to do these things, you will be making them feel involved, helpful and contributing to the patient's care. It will also give you insight into the person your patient really is – their likes and dislikes.

Stress and anxiety associated with having a critically ill relative can hinder a family's coping ability, adaptation, decision making[44] and long-term health with the possibility that posttraumatic stress disorder (PTSD) may develop in family members of ICU patients.[45-48] Families that experience stress before the critical illness do not cope as well, and may need additional assistance.[49] As many as half of family members report symptoms of anxiety and depression, indicating it is a very real problem.[47,50] These figures are concerning, particularly when symptoms continue beyond 6 months post ICU.[45,51] Early identification and prevention strategies are an important area for further research. Meeting the needs of families during this stressful and demanding time has the capacity to reduce their stress and promote positive coping strategies.[47]

A combined healthcare team approach is needed to meet the family's needs, as differing perceptions among the healthcare team can result in non-unified approaches that are potentially confusing. The needs of families with critically ill relatives are complex and multifactorial, reinforcing the need for an all-of-team approach.[52] Family members' needs were recognised in Molter's influential study in 1979 in which she researched the specific needs of ICU patients' family members. Although Molter's sample was small ($n = 40$), 45 potential needs of family members were identified and ranked in order of importance.[53] Family needs continue to be researched[40,48,54,55] and can be generally grouped into the need for: 1) information, 2) reassurance, 3) proximity, 4) support and 5) comfort.[44] More specifically, families' needs include the following:[44]

- to know their relative's progress and prognosis
- to have their questions answered honestly
- to speak to a doctor at least once a day
- to be given consistent information by staff

- to feel their relative is looked after by competent and caring people
- to feel confident that staff will call them at home if changes occur in their relative's condition
- to be given a sense of hope
- to know about transfer plans as they are being made.

Meeting information needs

Families' needs for information and reassurance are paramount during a critical illness, which is often unexpected or unexplained. Seven out of the top 10 requirements of families are related to information needs.[56] When information is provided, it is important to spend sufficient time with family members to ascertain understanding. A self-designated family member can act as the primary receiver of information and take the responsibility of relaying the information to others. It is not sufficient to think, 'But I told them all that yesterday'. Communication is a two-way process and as such needs to be received in a meaningful way as well as given appropriately. Repeating information in different ways, multiple times may be necessary. In a case study report of a mother and her adult war-injured son, the mother tells how she tried to remember things the staff told her. She said, 'I loved how my questions would be answered when we asked (except for the daily one about his brain damage) and how most people did not take offense at me writing down everything. I know that I was scared to death most of the entire time'.[40 p.18]

Strategies to improve communication with family members can include conversations around their current concerns and needs.[35] Once the needs have been identified, specific strategies can be developed to meet those needs. Some critical care areas may choose to have an additional strategy of a designated nursing position that focuses on family advocacy within a patient, family-centred care philosophy.[57]

Interdisciplinary patient rounds that meaningfully include the family demonstrate an inclusive and open communication process that values all contributors as they collectively make an individual plan of care for the patient.[9,40] Our paediatric critical care colleagues lead the way and are trialling ways to not just introduce but also to improve patient rounds that routinely include the family. Beck and colleagues trialled a revised process that focused the objectives of the round to one of advancing the care of the patient in a time-efficient manner. They successfully implemented a standard plan of day template that included a checklist for review of quality and safety indicators. They reported a culture of improvement together with halving of the rounding time from 4 to 2 hours.[58]

New ways to practice can be daunting and we know that our attitudes and perceptions are one of the greatest influences of our behaviour. Canadian researchers surveyed their medical and nursing staff on their perceptions of family-centred rounds to gain an understanding of their staff's views.[59] Just one-third of the nurses and two-thirds of the medical staff felt comfortable with the idea or thought that family should be given an option to attend family rounds. Experienced nurses held greater reservations and less comfort with the thought than did less experienced nurses (58% versus 26%).[59] The promotion of patient, family-centred care has led to family presence at rounds as not being discretionary but rather recognised as gold standard.[60] Understanding unit culture and individual clinicians' perceptions provide foundation for future strategies to progress achieving this standard of care.

In addition, routine family meetings may be a useful way to improve communication and understanding.[54] Frequently, however, family meetings are called when the family is needed to make critical decisions about the ongoing care of their relative rather than as a proactive and positive strategy that allows for patient and family preferences to be integrated into patient care.[54] Family conferences with the interdisciplinary team should be organised in a staged and planned manner, with the first occurring within the first 48 hours of admission, the second after around 3 days and a third when there is a significant change in treatment goals.[56,61] Fundamental topics for the interdisciplinary meetings with the family could include the patient's condition and prognosis together with short- and long-term treatment goals.[37,61,62] Family conferences provide time for discussion among family members with the healthcare team as a resource and also for the team to make an assessment of the family's understanding of the situation. Importantly, they provide an opportunity to develop an awareness of specific family needs that the team can endeavour to meet.[37] Unhurried family conferencing allows opportunities for families to pose questions and longer family conferences can result in families feeling greater support and significantly reduced PTSD symptoms.[63] Providing family members, prior to the meeting, with an outline of the purpose of the meeting and points for discussion can be helpful. This meeting guide prompts family members to jot down their questions beforehand and ensures their questions are discussed,[64] as it is well recognised that families forget, or are hesitant to ask their questions. Although family conferencing has been found beneficial, it is advocated that multiple modes of communication and information sharing are required. Individualised and/or general information via leaflets, brochures and internet-based information and support strategies are also helpful.[37,63,65]

To promote communication, nurses can discuss with the family whether they would like a phone call or text message at night updating them on their relative's condition. It is important to follow through on prearranged strategies. Alternatively, nurses can give them a time to phone before change of shift. This will help to allay their anxiety and promotes positive communication and trust. When patients are transferred from critical care, families and patients may become anxious or concerned by the reduced level of care in the new ward area. This can be alleviated by providing families with verbal and individualised written transfer information as a means to help prepare them for transfer.[66] In addition, a structured transferring plan helps critical care nurses feel better equipped to ensure they give families the information they need at this important time of transfer.[66]

Family presence

Patients find that family provides a link to whom they were before their illness and that they provide support and comfort.[67] This, together with the families' need to be physically close to their critically ill relative, support the concept of unrestrictive family presence. Central to family presence is the need for due consideration of patient confidentiality and privacy.[9,68,69]

Family-friendly policies with few restrictions that centre on genuine patient care issues require the support of critical care nurses, medical officers and others.[9] Flexibility is particularly relevant for families who live long distances from the hospital and have to travel for many hours in order to be with there for their relative. Unrestrictive family presence is not common. In the UK, around 80% of 206 surveyed ICUs restricted both the duration and number of visitors.[70] A similar situation was found to be the case in USA where from 606 hospitals, 90% restricted family presence.[71] Sweden reports the least restrictive policies with only 30% of surveyed units having some restrictions.[71] The disparity has been assisted by clear practice guidelines from critical care associations in the USA and Australia that guide clinicians to support family members and patients by recommending open or flexible family presence at the bedside.[4,9]

Family-friendly policies have been found to have an unintended but positive outcome in that they improve quality indicators with higher patient satisfaction levels.[58] Once introduced, an Australian study found that ICU staff report satisfaction with the policy change. Interestingly, the vast majority of families chose to be with their relative between 11 o'clock in the morning and 8 o'clock at night.[30] Family members are not just 'visitors': they have an intimate relationship with the patient which helps to form crucial components of the patient's identity.[72,73] Remember that there are often different meanings or interpretations of 'family', with family often meaning more than just the immediate nuclear family but rather inclusive of wider family networks (aunties, uncles, cousins, for instance). Examples of people whose families are a wider collective group are Gypsy Roma Travellers, people from European countries (such as Italy and Greece), and indigenous peoples (such as New Zealand Māori and Australian First People). The notable difference from these family constellations in comparison to nuclear families is that each of its members have responsibilities and obligations not only to the other members but also to the family as a collective group. Negotiation of family presence processes that consider these cultural understandings is imperative and it is discussed later in this chapter why it is important that families are included in nursing care in critical care contexts.

Practice tip

Sometimes the number of 'close' family members can be overwhelming for critical care nurses. Remember that for those families comprising extended family networks, identifying each family's needs in terms of providing the patient support and negotiating a system of communication through one or two spokespersons is helpful.

There is a genuine concern by some parents or carers that children should not come to see family members who are critically ill as they may find the ICU environment and presence traumatic. However, this needs to be balanced against a child who experiences separation anxiety, which can be intense and have a negative impact on their adaptive functioning. In addition, when children are appropriately supported, they are more likely to not be frightened but rather curious about their surroundings.[74] Children may have questions and it is recommended that they be prepared well with adequate information before, during and after their time with their relative in the critical care area.

Patients, however, may want visiting restricted as some patients find them stressful or tiring. Contrary to popular belief, unrestricted visiting hours are not associated with long visits. In three separate studies where unrestricted family presence was introduced, the number of hours that family members spent with the patient varied and usually family came during the day. This suggests that when family members have free access to their sick relative they do not perceive a sense of duty to be there all day and night.[16,75,76] Participating in patient care is one way for family members to feel closer to their critically ill family member and at the same time promotes family integrity.[77,78] Most family members, however, will not ask if they can help with care[26] as this is seen as the nurses' domain in adult critical care areas.[9] Nurses, therefore, should invite family members to be part of the patient's care, with massaging and helping to wash the patient being popular activities.[27] Providing care allows the family members to feel connected emotionally with their relative and provides a means to get to know and communicate with the nurses, which families consider important. Family members appreciate invitations from nurses as this allows them to feel more in control[24] in a situation where family members do not often experience this.[79,80] For family participation to work effectively and safely, a number of guiding principles should be incorporated, as outlined in Table 7.1. It is useful for critical care nurses to explore their beliefs and practices concerning family participation, as

TABLE 7.1
Family participation in patient care

PRINCIPLE	PROCEDURE
Consent	Gain patient consent beforehand where possible For some cultures belief about illness mean families take on the decision making to relieve patients of this burden. Thus, consent may be devolved to a family member
Building of trust	Relationships are important for building trust Introduce the concept of family members' involvement in care after a period during which a rapport is developed, which includes agreeing on roles and expectations
Individualise for patient and family	Offer suitable options from which family members can choose: for example, massaging feet and hands, cleaning teeth and feeding may be appropriate options for short-term patients, whereas additional options may exist for long-term patients
Safety	The registered nurse should remain physically close by at all times
Promote achievement of goals	Provide sufficient information to the family member to support successful completion of the care
Reflect on outcomes	Provide feedback to family members on how they performed the task
Continuity of care	Document the care the family members participated in and any relevant information, especially information shared by family members

many support family participation but do not always implement these beliefs in their practice.

Communication

The ability to communicate effectively is an underlying tenet of nursing practice and a fundamental need for people. As mentioned previously in the context of caring for family members, for communication to occur, there needs to be a two-way passage of ideas, thoughts and messages. It is a basic requirement to be able to comprehend what is being conveyed before one can interpret, internalise and respond. This is referred to as health literacy and is defined by the Institute of Medicine as 'the degree to which individuals have the capacity to obtain, process, and understand basic health information and services needed to make appropriate health decisions.'[81] Families with deficient health literacy will misunderstand medical terminology around their relative's care or illness and this is problematic.[82] In addition to health literacy issues, patients have physical impediments to communication that cause, or adds to, anxiety, frustration, stress and depression as they lose control over their life and healthcare decisions.[83]

It is therefore imperative for healthcare professionals to find ways to communicate with patients in simple non-technical everyday language that is understandable and is targeted at their health literacy level. Critically ill patients commonly have communication difficulties due to either mechanical devices (e.g. endotracheal tubes), cognitive impairment from the disease and/or pharmacological medications or language difficulties. Therefore, effective communication is challenging, and critical care nurses and other staff need additional knowledge and understanding of these complex situations to assist in meeting the key communication needs of patients and families. With the objective for minimal levels of patient sedation in mechanically-ventilated patients, the need to find effective communications strategies is more relevant than ever.[83] It is equally important to continue speaking to critically ill patients who are unconscious as it has been known for decades that sedated and unconscious patients can hear and recall some verbal communication once they regain consciousness.[84,85]

It is important to focus communication with critically ill patients on what is important to them as they fatigue easily and have difficulty maintaining concentration. Asking them for their needs and assessment of pain and comfort is critical. Providing reassurance, with both speech and touch contributes to a sense of empathy and feelings of safety for the patient within an environment that takes into consideration the cultural perspective.[86] Communicating empathy is further supported by family members' presence and their interaction with their relative. In addition, constructive strategies should be identified to overcome difficulties with patient communication. Augmentative and alternative communication methods are advocated where different ways to communicate can be tried for individual patients to convey their ideas/thoughts.[87]

The following methods may be used individually or together to enhance communication, and many can readily be initiated by nurses:[87,88]

- body language
- lip reading
- writing

- alphabet boards
- communication boards
- pictures
- gestures, including nodding and blinking of the eyes
- tablets, e.g. iPads and smartphones
- speaking tracheostomy tube with inflated cuff
- electrolarynx

Practice tip

When you are meeting your patient's relatives for the first time that day, ask them about how they think their relative is progressing. You will get a better understanding of their comprehension of the illness situation and health literacy than if you provide information to them. This understanding will enable you to structure the way you communicate for the rest of your shift. Check with them when they last spoke to the doctor and see if that is a priority for them that day. If they want to speak with the doctor, try to plan ahead so this can be achieved during their time in the unit.

An effective strategy to promote good communication is for health professionals to seek and maintain eye contact (if culturally appropriate). This may mean the nurse or doctor sitting down on a chair beside the bed to facilitate face-to-face communication. This act also conveys a sense of the importance the health professional is placing on the interaction by taking time to ensure they understand each other. Associated with this is the need to use commonly understood language. One method of checking patients' responses is to repeat these back to them. A quiet environment reduces extraneous noise and potential interruptions, and may promote communication and concentration. When communication seems unsuccessful, talking loudly will not improve the interaction; one good strategy is for the nurse and patient to agree to try again later. Communication methods that are found to be effective, such as facial expression, head nods and eye blinks used to respond to questions, should be passed on to the next nurse and recorded in the patient's notes to promote continuity of care.

Practice tip

Check with the patient's family if they wear glasses or hearing aids. Ask them to bring them in next time they come ensuring the cases are clearly named with the patient's identification label. Ask for extra batteries for the hearing aids. These will assist communication.

Language barriers may necessitate the assistance of an interpreter as miscommunication is detrimental to the development of trust and impacts on decision making. Interpreters require some knowledge of healthcare terminology to ensure the content is adequately translated. An independent person ensures that the patient receives the message in its entirety from the health professional but in practice, interpreters are not always available.[89-92]

It is widely acknowledged that communicating with critically ill and/or mechanically-ventilated patients is challenging for the healthcare professional, the patient and their family. Specific communication skills workshops for ICU nurses have been advocated.[93,94] In addition, skill acquisition on different ways to communicate needs to be a feature of postgraduate and unit level education programs to support critical care nurses in their ability to successfully use appropriate communication strategies, mechanical devices and technology to connect meaningfully with our patients.[93] Effective communication with the patient or their family is vital in order to determine their cultural beliefs and practices to further enhance appropriate communication and promote understanding.

Cultural care

The challenge for critical care nurses is to establish positive working relationships with the patient (when possible) and family so their important values, beliefs and practices can be shared and incorporated into plans of intervention and treatment. It is not always possible to 'know' another person's culture in any great depth, or 'know' all cultural beliefs and practices of the patients and families a critical care nurse will encounter. Therefore, establishing relationships with the patient and the family during their critical care experience is crucial. It also demonstrates both respect for, and the value of, patients and their families and the cultural beliefs and practices they hold. This enables critical care teams to better meet their needs.

Although people's ethnicities or nationalities may provide a clue to their culture, it is not a reliable indicator and ignores the multiple cultural groups people belong to that extend beyond ethnicity, such as age and gender. Furthermore, with increasing migration globally and inter-ethnic marriages, some people identify with more than one ethnic group. Making assumptions about a person's culture and reliance on universal approaches to direct nursing practice engenders risks to nursing practice and potentially compromises the outcomes of interactions and interventions. Even within cultural groups (e.g. indigenous, racial or ethnic minority groups, immigrant groups, and other marginalised cultural groups), variations and sharing in beliefs and practices can exist. Such differences result from the interactions with the various groups a person belongs to, responses to societal changes and the socialisation of immigrants into a new country or those countries where colonisation has occurred.

Acculturation (whereby people acquire aspects of the dominant culture such as food or dress) and assimilation (the integration and adoption of dominant cultural practices by people from ethnic minority groups) are two concepts that are associated with cultural diversity.[95] People are also influenced by the other 'cultural' groups they belong to (e.g. women's or men's groups, belonging to the disabled community, older people's groups), which all have their own particular views of the world, values, beliefs, and practices. Thus, person-centred care of patients and their families is imperative to incorporating specific cultural needs in the planning and delivery of interventions. This section outlines important strategies critical care nurses can develop for working with patients and their families to identify the essential beliefs and practices they need to have incorporated into treatment and intervention plans during a stressful time in an unfamiliar environment. Such actions can optimise their spiritual wellbeing and lessen some of the stress they feel.

Defining culture

Wepa describes culture: 'Our way of living is our culture. It is our taken-for-grantedness that determines and defines our culture. The way we brush our teeth, the way we bury people, the way we express ourselves through art, religion, eating habits, rituals, humour, science, law and sport; the way we celebrate occasions is our culture. All these actions we carry out consciously and unconsciously'.[96 p.31] Reid and colleagues[97] describe culture as:

- intergenerational transmission of patterns of meaning using a variety of modes such as stories, song, cultural symbols
- a social construction that shapes our sense of being and social expectations of behaviour and communication
- a sense of belonging through a system of meaningful actions and behaviours so that we know who we are and how we belong.

Simply, culture refers to the values, beliefs and practices that patients, family members and nurses undertake in their daily lives. It determines how they view the world, and their orientation to health, illness, life and death.[98,99]

Culture involves a shared set of rules and perspectives acquired through the processes of socialisation and internalisation. These provide a frame of reference to guide how members interpret such phenomena as health and illness and death and dying. This, in turn, influences their actions and interactions.[99] Culture is a more specific way of describing how groups of people function on a daily basis, influenced by their beliefs, relationships and the activities they engage in.

Understanding that culture, ethnicity and race are not the same thing is crucial to meeting the cultural needs of patients and their families. Race is generally determined on the basis of physical characteristics and is often used to socially classify people broadly as Caucasians, Europeans, Polynesians or Asians, for example.[100] However, assigning people to a homogeneous group is problematic, and is the antithesis of cultural diversity,[101] particularly as globally countries are becoming increasingly ethnically diverse. Furthermore, homogenisation does not account for the diversity that exists within many groups in contemporary society, which is increasing with globalisation, marriage between people from different ethnic groups, and the subsequent acculturation and assimilation that occurs. For example, new immigrants may adhere more strongly to traditional cultural values, beliefs and practices than those who have been in a country for two or more generations. Ethnicity extends beyond the physical characteristics associated with race to include such factors as common origins, language, history and dress – it is usually associated with nations,[101] although a number of ethnic groups may exist within a nation.

Culture is internalised and embodied, therefore, it is important for critical care nurses to understand that it is something that is not always visible or identifiable by people's everyday behaviours, especially for those who belong to the dominant culture. It is often implicit, such as our values and beliefs that guide what is important in our lives, and is not something people have had to share until such a time that their cultural values, beliefs and practices become challenged.[87] For instance, when a person and their family are in the foreign environment of a critical care unit, or they are facing the end of life of one of their family members. At this time, what is important for many patients and their families seems to become secondary to the illness or trauma that led to their being in a critical care setting and can cause distress and conflict if left unresolved.

Differing world views

Culture influences how people view the world, what they believe in and how they do things, particularly with regard to practices around health, dying and death. The critical care environment is unfamiliar for patients and families, especially as health professionals' beliefs, practices and world views may not align with their own. What is important for critical care nurses may not be important for the patient or the family, and may lead to tension and dissatisfaction when patients' and families' views are at variance. This does not mean that one world view is necessarily more right or wrong – they are different.

The biomedical model influences the way healthcare services are structured and delivered.[102] As a dominant model it heavily influences the necessary focus on the physical wellbeing of patients within critical care environments. Focusing on the management of disease and illness, and using processes that lead to health issues being fragmented and reduced to presenting signs and symptoms and diagnoses, risks excluding what is important for the patient and family.[103] This contrasts with indigenous and minority group cultures, for example, which tend to have a holistic eco-spiritual world view, with a strong spiritual dimension that extends beyond a disease and illness focus.[104] As will be discussed later in this chapter, spiritual wellbeing has greater value and importance for some people – it can be just as significant, and for some, more important than their physical wellbeing. The world view of critical care nurses is influenced by the cultural beliefs, practices and life circumstances of each nurse, and the 'world view' of the critical care service that drives its service delivery. The result is that, consequently, patients and their families become sandwiched between differing world views. Culturally responsive practice is contingent on nurses having respectful relationships and being willing to let the person and family lead in terms of what they need (all the while balancing the critically ill patient's physical needs).[105,106]

Research highlights the lack of alignment that can occur between the needs of consumers of health services and the intentions of healthcare providers such as nurses.[104] It is the potential for the non-alignment between patients and families and healthcare providers that critical care nurses need to be aware of, as dissatisfaction with the care being delivered can arise when the patient's and family's needs are not recognised or attended to,[107] leading to unnecessary tensions and conflicts between patients, families and nurses. A nurse's willingness to acknowledge and respect patients' world views and the things that are important to them minimises the likelihood of any dissatisfaction occurring,[104] as it values their specific needs during their critical care experience.

Practice tip

Being able to deliver culturally responsive nursing care requires the nurse to undergo a process of education and critical self-reflection of culture, own cultural beliefs and practices, and the possible influences these may have on practice.[108]

Where the worldviews of patients and families are considerably different from that of the nurse, nurses should identify the beliefs they hold about the patient and family, the impact of these interactions on the patient and family and the power the nurse can utilise during such interactions.[101] Sometimes a nurse's personal beliefs will be in conflict with professional nursing beliefs, which necessitates choosing between personal and professional beliefs in the practice setting. For example, a nurse's personal beliefs about life, death and body tissues may be compromised by the duty to care for a patient with brain death awaiting the removal of organs for transplant. This may also be compounded by nursing staff shortages, less-than-desirable skill mixes and the acuity and complexity that critical care nurses are faced with daily. Therefore, it is vital, not only for the individual nurse, but also for the team of critical care nurses to develop strategies, such as processes and procedures, that can optimise the development of working relationships with patients from different cultural backgrounds.[109]

Cultural responsiveness

Cultural responsiveness refers to strategies for responding to a patient's and their family's cultural backgrounds, and depends on the cultural competence of nurses so that they feel culturally safe.[103] An important factor to consider regarding culturally responsive care is recognising the individualistic culture on which many health services are based. That is, the focus is only on patients and their presenting illness or trauma. This is mostly because health systems and services are designed on western biomedical approaches to health care. However, for many people belonging to minority cultural groups their focus is on the collective family – that is, all members and the family as a whole. This collective concept is similar to the notion of holism whereby the whole is greater than the sum of its parts. From a cultural perspective, embedded in families that function collectively is the notion that the family is an integral part of a person and likewise each of its members are critical to the family as whole. Therefore, the focus of the family is on the responsibilities and obligations that each of its members have to other members as well as to the family as a whole. These families have extended family networks that extend in composition beyond that of nuclear family constructions, which are more constrained in size and make-up.

Different models exist to assist in the integration of the cultural beliefs and practices of patients and their family in critical care nursing practice. For example, Leininger's cultural care diversity and universality theory[110] requires nurses to deliver culturally congruent nursing care for people of varying or similar cultures. Ramsden's work on cultural safety[111,112] focuses on the delivery of nursing care to patients (whose cultural beliefs and practices differ from that of the nurse) that is determined appropriate and effective by the patients and families who are the recipients of that care. These models have been used to guide nursing practice in Australia, New Zealand and North America. Such models require that critical care nurses recognise patients' and families' views of their health experience and any that subsequently have discordant priorities.

Practice tip

Culturally responsive care leading to a patient and their family feeling culturally safe is not a destination or an endpoint. It is a career-long endeavour aided by being humble and critically self-reflective, and drawing on past experiences that were both optimal and less than optimal – the outcome should be on improving the quality of care for future patients and families.[113]

TABLE 7.2
Levels of cultural practice

LEVEL OF CULTURAL PRACTICE	INDICATORS
1 Awareness	Recognition that differences between groups of people extend beyond socioeconomic differences
2 Sensitivity	Recognition that difference is valid, which initiates a critical exploration of personal cultural beliefs and practices as a 'bearer' of culture that may affect others
3 Safety	Delivery of a safe service as a result of undergoing education about culture and nursing practice, and reflecting on their own and others' practice

Adapted from Wood PJ, Schwass M. Cultural safety: a framework for changing attitudes. Nurs Prax NZ 1993;8(1): 4–15.

Wood and Schwass have described three levels at which a nurse may practise with respect to cultural issues (Table 7.2).[114] These levels, ranging from cultural awareness to cultural safety, describe the differing characteristics of nurses' cultural care. For example, a nurse practising in an organisation where cultural safety is required would need not only to recognise differences between groups of people, but also to deliver differing cultural care to patients and their families after undergoing appropriate education. It is insufficient for nurses to be simply culturally aware or culturally sensitive because, to a large extent, these are relatively passive activities. Critical care nurses need to demonstrate to patients and their families that they have a genuine desire to incorporate important cultural practices into the patient and family care. Therefore, this requires critical care nurses to demonstrate actions and undertake practices so that patients and their families feel culturally safe.

From a transcultural nursing perspective, culturally responsive nursing care requires the nurse to incorporate cultural knowledge, the nurse's own cultural perspective and the patient's cultural perspective into intervention plans.[103] However, it is not possible to collate cultural knowledge specific to various groups owing to the diversity that exists both among and within groups.[115] This difficulty in 'knowing' a culture relates to the diversity not only between different groups of people, but also the differences that exist within their 'group', and despite education in cultural competence inequities in quality of care continue to exist.[107] Moreover, the reliance on 'evidence' without inclusion of people's sociocultural contexts can result in an incongruence in the health beliefs systems of patients and their family and nurses.[113] Therefore, critical care nurses are advised to critically examine theories and models to guide their practice, to ensure they deliver appropriate and effective care for the patients and families they work with.

Practice tip

It is important to be mindful of the diversity that exists within 'cultural' groups, and therefore, avoid acting on stereotypes and assumptions.

Competence is an important dimension of nursing practice, as it provides users of nursing services with confidence in nurses' knowledge, skills and attitudes necessary to undertake their practice. Given the importance of culture in the delivery of nursing care, the measurement of cultural competence is also important. There is evidence of numerous variations on the concept of cultural competence.[115-118] The attributes of cultural competence include cultural awareness, cultural knowledge, cultural understanding, cultural sensitivity, cultural interaction and cultural skill.[116-118] However, the inherent need for the acquisition and use of culturally-specific information limits the application of these attributes; the collation of culturally-specific information is increasingly problematic, particularly as our communities become more diverse in their composition. Therefore, the acquisition of specific knowledge based on a person's racial, ethnic or cultural background is inadequate with increasing cultural diversity. Cultural competence has evolved to be more grounded in person-centred care, aided by a range of skills including compassion, empathy, active listening, and attending to the patient's and the family's needs.[119]

Practice tip

The ability to deliver culturally responsive nursing practice involves critical self-reflection to became self-aware, culminating in nurses taking action to improve the patient's and family's health experience and integrating their important beliefs and practices into treatment and intervention plans.

Fundamental to providing culturally responsive nursing care is cultural humility. Minkler[120 p.256] maintains '… cultural humility is the notion that while we can't be competent in another's culture, we can engage in self-reflection, learning our own biases, being open to other's cultures, and committing ourselves to authentic partnership and redressing power imbalances.' Cultural responsiveness is about aiming to practice in a sound manner rather than merely behaving correctly.[103] Durie encouraged the development of cultural safety (which focuses on the patient's and their family's experience and determination of the appropriateness of care received), to a construct that can measure the capability of the health worker, such as the critical care nurse.[121] Culturally competent nursing practice is about:

- the nurses' knowledge about their own cultural beliefs and practices and the impact these may have on others
- the actions and capability of the nurse to improve the patient's health experience, and the integration of culture in clinical practice
- delivering culturally competent and safe care.[103]

Cultural competence provides a framework to objectively measure the nurse's performance, although there is variation in frameworks.[109] Fundamental for the critical care nurse to deliver culturally responsive care, which is competent and safe, is determining the cultural needs of patients and families, and the provision of patient-centred care that focuses on their individual needs and expectations.

Working with culturally and linguistically diverse patients and families

Globalisation has resulted in increasing immigration and migration among countries, thus populations are increasing in their cultural and linguistic diversity. Thirty-five percent of Australians,[122] 25% of New Zealanders,[123] 20.6% of Canadians,[124] 13% of Americans,[125] and 13% of those from UK and Wales[126] were born overseas. Immigrants arrive from various countries globally, but especially the European, Asian and African continents. Labels assigned to groups of 'immigrants', such as Asians or Indians, are misleading and far from the homogeneity they infer. Added to the complexity of trying to determine ways of working with culturally and linguistically diverse patients and families is the variation in their degree of acculturation – for example, some may be second- or third-generation born into another country and highly acculturated into the respective culture of their country of current residence, or they may be new immigrants with traditional cultural beliefs and practices. Therefore, given the diversity that exists it is difficult to provide specific guidelines on working with culturally and linguistically diverse patients and their families, although some common principles can apply. Ruston and Smith[127] argue that we categorise people according to what we know. When we encounter groups of people that are seen as different or 'outsiders' who disrupt this categorisation we then tend to classify people using a non-rational approach that lends itself to negative stereotyping, discrimination and stigmatisation. Such approaches are generally based on misinformation that is reinforced by negative societal and media portrayal of such groups.[128]

A fundamental starting point for working with culturally and linguistically diverse patients is to establish their capacity to communicate in the dominant cultural language, for example English. Determining the language a patient uses on a daily basis, and whether they can speak and write in dominant language, will indicate whether an interpreter is needed. Family members or friends can be used as interpreters when care is being undertaken on a daily basis, although a professional or accredited interpreter should be used when important information is to be shared or when decisions need to be made. This avoids the potential for family members or friends 'censoring' the information conveyed during discussions. How the patient wishes to be addressed, cultural values and beliefs related to communication (e.g. eye contact, personal space or social taboos), preferences related to healthcare providers (that is culture, gender or age), the nature of family support, and usual food and nutrition are other areas that should be explored with the patient or family, whichever is appropriate (Table 7.3).

Campinha-Bacote's[129] mnemonic, ASKED, provides a process for self-reflection to make explicit your knowledge and skills and desires to work with people who are culturally and linguistically diverse. The following questions can be asked:

- Awareness: what awareness do you have of the stereotypes, prejudices and racism that you hold about those in cultural groups that are different from your own?
- Skill: what skills do you have to undertake a cultural assessment in an appropriate and safe manner?
- Knowledge: how knowledgeable are you about the world views of the various cultural and ethnic groups within your community?
- Encounters: what face-to-face interactions have you initiated with people from different cultural groups than yourself?
- Desire: what is the extent of your desire to be culturally safe or competent in your nursing practice?

When critical care nurses understand their position on nursing people from other cultures, strategies can be adopted to improve their responsiveness and the quality of care delivered. Working with culturally and linguistically diverse people should be based on the following framework:

1. Partnership: aim to work in partnership with the patient and family. Prior negative experiences may influence the development of a productive relationship. A respectful, genuine, non-judgemental attitude is necessary to develop a productive relationship with the patient and family, and providing time for responses is important.
2. Participation: where possible involve the patient and family in their care, if this is appropriate. This will involve the critical care nurse explaining the treatment and intervention routines.

TABLE 7.3
Considerations for working with those from other cultures

ISSUE	CONSIDERATIONS
Holistic, spiritual world view	For some people, health and wellbeing is not just physical wellbeing but the social, spiritual, emotional and cultural wellbeing of the whole family and community The family and extended family may be more important than individuals on their own
Beliefs around hospitalisation and places to die	Identify previous health care experiences and talk to the family about concerns they may have about the care they will be receiving and the cultural practices they would like observed Be clear, consistent and honest in responses to questions about a patient's condition – avoid communication that expects people to 'read between the lines' Avoid doing things that are culturally offensive, so enquire respectfully about what is needed to avoid this
Traditional healing	Explore traditional healing remedies and 'medicines' that can complement western medicine Facilitate access for traditional healers when requested
Connections	In many minority cultural groups, extended families are important and these members should be included Connections to the environment are important – this means enquiring whether there are cultural processes that need to be undertaken with regard to body tissues/fluids/parts
Elders	In many minority cultural groups, elders are respected members and hold an important status. Thus, an unwell elder may have a lot of visitors because of his/her respected status Elders may be a spokesperson for the family, making identification of a spokesperson important
Establishing relationships	Showing attitudes and actions that are genuine, and a willingness to listen and to share where you have come from and who you are, are helpful in establishing relationships Establish and maintain a positive partnership relationship that promotes participation and that protects people's values and beliefs Community health workers may provide vital links with cultural minority communities
Diversity	Often people belonging to minority groups are grouped under one label but are diverse in their values, beliefs and practices Have conversations with the family and community elders about important cultural information
Language	Facilitate use of interpreters Always check out understanding of the information shared Avoid using health care jargon when explaining things Have culturally appropriate resources developed

Adapted from Eckermann A-K, Dowd T, Chong E, et al. Binan Goonj: bridging cultures in Aboriginal health. 3rd ed. Sydney: Churchill Livingstone; 2010, with permission.

3 Protection: determine specific cultural and spiritual values, beliefs and practices, and enable these to be practised during the patient's time in the critical care unit. Where possible these should be accommodated, although there may be instances when this is not possible. In such situations, the patient and family should be fully informed of the rationale for this.

Determining the cultural needs of patient and family

Given the great diversity that occurs within contemporary cultural groups, it is crucial to develop a relationship so important cultural values, beliefs and practices can be identified and incorporated into the patient's plan of care. Critical care nurses can then better understand a patient's or family's behaviours when the patient is critically unwell. Discovering the values and beliefs a patient and their family have about health, illness, death and dying, and what they believe may make their health worse, is a good starting point and will provide insight into the type of support and caring behaviours that may be observed. In addition to this, identifying how health and illnesses are managed in the person's daily life will provide an indication of whether traditional healers are used, along with healing remedies such as herbs and prayer, for example. Understanding the patient's locus of control can also provide an indication of whether they will play an active role in the outcome of an illness, or whether there is a fundamental belief that illnesses are caused by some external force.

Promoting a genuine, welcoming atmosphere and the use of effective communication (that is, compassionate and consistent) invite the family to be involved early in the patient's critical care experience, and are essential to determine the cultural needs of the patient and family (Table 7.4).[130] While communication has been mentioned earlier, interpreting cultural needs requires the critical care nurse to be attentive to communication. Nurses are advised to talk less, attend to details that may arise and simply listen. The need to intervene and to dominate discussions and 'interviews' with the family[130] from the nurse's perspective needs to be curbed, so time is made available for cultural beliefs and practices to be shared.[106,131] Understanding and supporting the patient and family can be improved by the nurse's empowering them through the processes of listening carefully, use of silence (to provide space to process information and questions), and validating what they have to say. The process of involving patients and their family in assessment, decision making and care planning enabling a greater 'client orientation' (versus management orientation) is more likely to be nurses who engage in and facilitate patient/family-centred care that focuses on the individual needs of patients and their family.[106] Research has found a transformational patient care style that actively involves patients and their family predicts greater satisfaction and more likely to result in their expectations and needs being met.[132]

Working in partnership with a family can bridge the cultural 'gap', and give families the opportunity to be well informed, which can assist with their stress and coping.[133] However, this is not always easy to achieve in challenging situations, such as when various members of a large family come and go, compounded by changing nurses with shift changes. Receiving clear and consistent information about the patient, including his/her progress, from all members of the healthcare team can reduce cross-cultural confusion and misunderstanding, especially as messages are prone to distortion and change when many are involved. A strategy to manage this may involve discussing the management of information dissemination with the family, and the identification of one or two family members who become the point of contact through which staff discuss and communicate information about the patient.[104,134] Often, apparent 'cultural conflicts' will arise as a result of communication problems with the family; communicating information in a clear and understandable manner helps prevent these problems from occurring.

For many cultural groups the presence of family is vital to both the patient's and family's spiritual wellbeing. Therefore, facilitating a family presence at the patient's bedside and possibly including them in the care of the patient is important. For some cultures there is a belief that family members should shoulder the burden of information and decision making so the patient can expend their energy and focus on getting better. In some cases to burden the patient with information about their condition, especially its gravity, or having to make decisions, is believed to contribute to a negative outcome. Thus, positively engaging families and, where practical, patients in collaborative relationships, involving them in the care and decision making and ensuring their cultural values, beliefs and practices are protected are ways critical care nurses can respect the cultural traditions of those patients who are from different cultural and linguistic backgrounds.

> **Practice tip**
>
> The EPICS Bundle[133] is a mnemonic that helps to plan and provide family-centred care:
>
> - Evaluate the patient's and family's cultural beliefs, and their needs and expectations and decide what adaptations are needed to their plan of care
> - Plan care with the patient and family and validating this with the patient
> - Involve the family in nursing care decisions
> - Communicate compassionately and consistently the patient's progress and rationale for any changes in care
> - Support families with compassion and empathy

A culturally diverse health workforce

Increasing the representation of people belonging to minority group cultures or marginalised groups within the health workforce has been recognised internationally as an important mechanism for improving cultural safety within healthcare facilities.[135,136] Research has demonstrated that indigenous people, for instance, are more likely to access mainstream health services if there is an indigenous workforce.[137]

Key to culturally responsive care in the critical care setting is a culturally diverse nursing workforce that is reflective of the population the health service serves. Increasing the ethnic and racial diversity among the health workforce is seen as a way to advance the health care workforce that is culturally competent and improving the quality of care people receive.[138,139] The under-representation of cultural minority and marginalised groups is associated with the lack of culturally competent evidence-based nursing care.[140] Cohen and others maintain, '… health care providers must have a firm understanding of how and why different belief systems, cultural biases, ethnic origins, family structures, and a host of other culturally determined factors influence the manner in which people experience illness, adhere to medical advice, and respond to treatment. Such differences are real and translate into real differences in the outcomes of care.'[138 p.92] Furthermore, they contend that cultural competence cannot be simply learned from textbooks and didactic learning, but instead needs to have

TABLE 7.4
Communication cues and principles

PRINCIPLE	CONSIDERATIONS
Establish a relationship	The first few minutes of your initial interaction with a person from another culture are critical for effective communication Avoid perpetuating people's experiences with western systems where language has reinforced dominant and submissive power relationships Obtaining information from patients and family members is regarded as a privilege, not a right To prove they are worthy and can be trusted with the receipt of knowledge a nurse may have to spend time building rapport and establishing common ground before exploring the 'business at hand' Be prepared to share information about yourself. As family and where people are geographically from can be important to people, positioning yourself within your family context and your 'place' is important. For example, sharing where you are from, relationships you are comfortable talking about (children, brothers, sisters, grandparents), the sports team you support and food you like is culturally appropriate
Consider kinship relationships	Certain people will have rights to access particular knowledge and make specific decisions within family and community The passing of information often depends on a person's position in the family/community or relationship with the holder of information Identify the relationships between the patient, and his/her attending family and friends and the relationships between family and friends Establish spokespersons – remembering that there might be different spokespersons for different elements of the person's life Identify who can make decisions on behalf of the patient (e.g. in the capacity of next of kin) Consider what might constitute gendered or generational considerations in conversations
Body language	Become familiar with non-verbal forms of communication where possible, e.g. hand signs and facial gestures Do not assume people from other cultures make direct eye contact. If the person is avoiding eye contact he/she will be listening and is not being rude Body language may also extend into close proximity within the client's personal space, this is particularly evident when the opposite sex is conducting the consultation; ask for permission to conduct any physical examinations
Use of silence	Use of silence is a key feature of communication with and between people belonging to some cultures. Pauses or silence during an interaction may mean that a person is thinking carefully before speaking or divulging information. The use of silence may also be a time for translation between languages. Pauses may be quite pronounced and time should be allowed for responses before seeking to fill in the silence by repeating the question. Active listening requires that you consider the importance of the use of silence, especially when people are from a different culture, in considering the information shared in the conversation Cultural protocols may also mean there are times when it is culturally inappropriate to respond Try reframing the question in a different way, or ask if the person may like someone else to respond
Shame	Shame is a term often used in some cultures, and will be named accordingly. 'Shame' describes a person's feeling of utmost embarrassment about something. It can be used in both serious and humorous terms
Providing information and asking questions	'Reading between the lines' is a concept that is difficult to understand if English is not your first language and western culture is unfamiliar Be direct in your communication – carefully consider how to describe clinical progression, while at the same time not diminishing the severity of a situation because family may need to be informed and travel long distances to join the patient Do not assume nodding or saying yes means that a message is understood – it is often easier to say yes – this is known as gratuitous concurrence. Perceived/actual power relationships between the health professional and the person and their family may prompt the person not to contradict or disappoint and may lead to the person providing what they think is an agreeable response
Improve communication outcomes	Provide opportunities for more than one person to ask questions Follow up on individual messages in different ways to ensure full understanding has been gained Use open rather than closed questions Avoid using compound questions (e.g. 'Is it this way, that way or the other way?') Avoid asking questions in a way that is framed in expectation of a positive response Ask only one question at a time, and give the person time to consider the question and formulate a response

people who have 'insider' insights into the way cultural beliefs impact outcomes, and the contribution these can make to the access and quality of care delivered by relatively monocultural health care services.

Cultural responsiveness and patient-centred, individualised care

'Individualised care requires the patient and nurse to work together to identify a path towards health that maintains the integrity of the patient's sense of self and is compatible with their personal circumstances'.[141] This means the critical care nurse ideally working in collaboration with the family to identify important cultural needs and the inclusion of beliefs and practices that need to be observed during the patient's critical care experience; in other words, eliciting a patient's view to ensure person-centred care.[142] It is recognised that 'the work' of the nurse involves responding, anticipating, interpreting and enabling, all of which are crucial for individualised care.[143] Indeed, partnership requires the nurse not only to work with the patient and family but also to identify the power that the nurse possesses and the potential for its inadvertent misuse.[134] Patient- and family-centred care requires critical care nurses to observe each of the following:

- interacting respectfully with the patient and their family, and treating them with dignity
- communicating clearly, without jargon
- sharing information fully and honestly
- using the strengths of the family to enhance their sense of control and independence
- working with patients and their family collaboratively.[144]

Facilitating the inclusion of cultural beliefs and practices requires identification and then incorporation in the patient's plan of care. However, given the resource constraints and the culture of some health services, universal approaches to planning care may be adopted for convenience. The critical care nurse is discouraged from adopting a 'one-size-fits-all' approach to nursing practice, as this disregards the cultural systems of the patient and family.[104] Patient-centred care is optimised by nurses having sufficient information about the patient and family in order to identify their needs and plan interventions. Incorporating each family's cultural beliefs and practices provides a 'bigger picture' of the patient[104] than would have been gained by simply focusing on the presenting disease or illness and its management. Such an approach to patient-centred care enables the critical care nurse to become familiar with the context of the patient's life circumstances and how they interpret illness, and also improves the quality of care and interactions they have with patients and families.[144,145]

Critical care nurses are potentially influential and can advocate for family-centred care,[146] although sometimes the nurse will want to have a full understanding of a cultural belief or practice before being willing to incorporate it. This is an example of where the identification and acceptance of cultural beliefs and practices of the family (to the extent that they will not deliberately harm the patient), and working with the family on how these are incorporated in an intervention plan, can be beneficial to all parties. Once this has occurred, it is crucial this information is documented, thereby making visible the patient's individualised care.[147]

Practice tip

Determining cultural needs means the critical care nurse must:

- identify a spokesperson to communicate information to so the messages the family receives are consistent
- engage in genuine communication and partnership with the patient and family
- be willing to listen, understand and validate information received

Practice tip

To optimise interactions with people from a culture different from yours as a critical care nurse:

- avoid making assumptions
- avoid culturally offensive practices that are known and learned
- remember that actions speak louder than words
- be willing to ask the patient or family for clarification or validation.

Closely related to cultural aspects of care is spirituality, which for some people is based in religion. Aspects to consider when patients have religious needs are reviewed next.

Spiritual and religious considerations

Spiritual care and being with a patient and family are important in providing quality care, especially nearing the end of a person's life.[148,149] Despite spirituality being viewed as an important component of holistic nursing care, it is an area that is not always well attended to within the critical care environment.[1,150,151] While for some people spirituality is embedded within religion, for others it is a metaphysical or existential experience.[1] Therefore, it is important for critical care nurses to avoid assuming that spirituality and religion are the same entity. Spirituality is grounded with a person's culture, the two aligning with their fundamental values and beliefs. It is highly subjective, unique and person or family-centred, transcending scientific and objective explanations. When not attended to it can be the source of spiritual distress.[148]

> **Practice tip**
>
> Critical care nurses can be supported in providing spiritual care by seeking the assistance from chaplains in the first instance.

> **Practice tip**
>
> At the time of identifying the cultural needs of a patient and family, also identify their spiritual care needs. Asking and having a conversation is a good place to begin.

Spiritual and religious beliefs and practices contribute to a person's spiritual wellness,[1,148] on one hand, while on the other a critical care nurse's religion may influence how care is delivered.[152] Spiritual and religious beliefs can be closely aligned with a person's culture and vary in how life, dying and death are viewed, and may dictate how life is conducted.[1,153-155] Any breaches can have profound effects on a patient's wellbeing and, in some cases, how a family member may consequently interact with the patient. This has important implications for critical care nurses undertaking everyday practices and common procedures where religious beliefs dictate a different approach. A common example is blood transfusions for those belonging to the Jehovah's Witness religion. Having a standardised list of religions and procedural considerations is flawed due to the variations that exist, and in some instances the variations are great. Thus, as part of the initial assessment the critical care nurse should determine whether the patient has religious beliefs and practices that must be observed or not, and incorporate these into the care plan.

When a family member becomes critically ill, spiritual and religious beliefs and practices become an important coping mechanism in terms of making sense of the experience, as well as being a source of faith and hope. While it can be helpful to the critical care nurse to have an overview of the main religious beliefs and practices (Table 7.5), caution must be used and should not preclude working with the patient's family to ascertain exactly what their beliefs and preferences are. Having said this, a patient may have adopted a religion that is separate from their family. In such circumstances, family cannot be relied upon as informants and, in some situations, there may be a conflict between the religious values and practices of the patient and those of the family. Religious beliefs and practices, like cultural beliefs and practices, will vary between orthodox or traditional and contemporary interpretations.

Patients generally fall into three groups with regard to their religious practices.[153] There are those who:

1. practise their religious beliefs regularly
2. practise their religious beliefs on an irregular basis, often in times of need and stress
3. have no religious interests.

All patients should have access to religious support where they indicate a need. Therefore, it is beneficial for critical care nurses to have knowledge of how to access the relevant religious resources if needed. The focus of the critical care setting often involves going to extreme lengths to keep patients alive, which may well be in direct opposition to some religious beliefs. Spiritual and religious beliefs can either facilitate or disrupt the process of living or dying.[156-158] There are several useful principles underpinning practice when nursing patients with specific religious needs (Table 7.6).

In addition to these principles, contact and communication between the patient, family and the critical care nurse are important,[1] and can enable a person's spiritual or religious needs to be determined. The critical care nurse should ascertain whether the patient and family have any spiritual or religious beliefs and practices to be observed during their time in the critical care setting.[1,153] Once the spiritual or religious beliefs and practices have been determined, the critical care nurse can facilitate opportunities for the patient and/or family to carry out their beliefs and practices, and avoid any insensitive actions and pay attention to any spiritual distress evident in the patient and family members.[153]

> **Practice tip**
>
> Spiritual intelligence enables nurses to be more resilient and adaptable when faced with challenges and stresses often arising within critical care contexts, and is essential for quality of care that includes spiritual care.[159]

A person's spirituality, whether informed by religion or some other basis, manifests in a variety of relationships with self, others, nature and 'divine' beings. It is the essence of who a person is, or who groups of people are. While assessing spiritual or religious needs is one aspect, presence and being with, empathetic listening, reality orientation of the family and enabling visiting and contact are all important nursing activities that can support the spiritual and religious needs of patients and their families.[152,160,161] When families are confronted with the possibility of death, the documentation of a death plan that outlines the preferred care during the process of dying and death is recommended.[153] Death plans are about what a patient and family want and empowerment, differing from advance directives, which outline what is not wanted (e.g. cardiopulmonary resuscitation). Through formal discussion with the patient

TABLE 7.5
Overview of key religious beliefs and practices

RELIGION	PRACTICES TO BE AWARE OF	BELIEFS ABOUT ILLNESS, LIFE AND DEATH
Protestantism	Prayer and the Bible are important for support. Minister, vicar or pastor may visit the sick person and the family	Illness is an accepted part of life, although euthanasia is not allowed. There is a belief in the afterlife, with the dead being buried or cremated
Roman Catholicism	Prayer and the Bible are important. Some may have restrictions on eating meat on Fridays of Lent, Ash Wednesday and Good Friday. Priest may undertake communion with and anoint the sick person	Illness is an accepted part of life, although euthanasia is forbidden. There is a belief in the afterlife, with the dead being buried or cremated
Judaism	There are orthodox and non-orthodox forms of Judaism. Procedures should be avoided on the Sabbath (from sundown on Friday to sundown on Saturday). Dietary restrictions around pork, shellfish and the combination of meat and dairy products extend to the use of dishes and utensils. Gelatin is a product that is used for medication capsules, for example. Frequent praying, especially for the sick person who should not be left alone. The Rabbi will attend the sick person	Illness is an accepted part of life, with euthanasia being forbidden, thus saving or prolonging life is important and those on life support stay on it until death. The Sabbath is a time that is considered sacred and when restrictions on activities are observed. There is a belief that the human spirit is immortal. There are special processes for managing the dead person, who should be buried as soon as possible after death. Thus, consultation with the Rabbi is important. Postmortem examination is allowed only if necessary
Buddhism	Prayer and meditation are important, using prayer books and scriptures, supported by teacher and Buddhist monks. The Buddhist is generally vegetarian. Patients may refuse treatments (e.g. narcotic medications) that alter consciousness	Illness originates from a sin in a previous life. There is a belief in afterlife, and the dead are buried or cremated. Living things should not be killed; this belief extends to euthanasia
Hinduism	Prayer and meditation are important, and are supported by a Guru. Some Hindus are vegetarian. The dying patient may have threads tied around the neck or wrist and be sprinkled with water; these threads are sacred and are not removed after death. The body is not washed after death	Illness is usually a punishment and must be endured. Some Hindus have healing practices based on their faith. There is a belief that the dead are reincarnated; they are usually cremated
Sikhism	Morning and evening prayer are important and should not be interrupted for routine care. Some Sikh have undergone initiation and carry on their bodies the 5 Ks (kesh (uncut hair), kengha (wooden comb), kach/kachera (cotton shorts), kara (steel bracelet) and kirpan (strapped sword) at all times. Hair should not be cut unless urgent for lifesaving treatment. Some Sikhs may or may not be vegetarians – those who eat meat only eat meat that is not ritually prepared. Gelatin capsules or fish oil may be unacceptable	Illness and death are believed to be the will of God, and the artificial extension of life over extended periods of time may not be encouraged. Sikhs believe in life after death and in rebirth, and therefore, that the soul's existence is eternal.
Islam (Muslims)	Private prayer, facing Mecca several times a day, requires a private space. The patient may like to be positioned towards Mecca. Guided by the Qur'an (Koran), which outlines the will of Allah (the creator of all) as given through Muhammad (the prophet). Muslims fast during Ramadan, and eating pork and drinking alcohol are forbidden. Stopping treatment goes against Allah. Talking about death should be avoided; designated male relatives will decide what information patient and family should receive	Life and death are predetermined by Allah, and any suffering must be endured in order to be rewarded in death. It is believed that dying the death of a martyr will be rewarded in death by going to paradise. Thus, staying true to the Qur'an is crucial. There is a belief in the afterlife, and the dead are buried as soon as possible after death, on the side facing Mecca

Adapted from Blockley C. Meeting patients' religious needs. Kai Tiaki Nurs NZ 2001/2002;7(11):15–7. Other sources: Hoffman L. A focus on: Judaism. Community Practitioner 2018;91(2):31–3. And Nesbitt E. A focus on: Sikhism. Community Practitioner 2018;91(3):33–6.

TABLE 7.6
Principles for recognising religious needs

PRINCIPLE	AREAS FOR CONSIDERATION
Diversity exists between and within the various religions	Determine values and beliefs related to health, illness, dying, death and any specific requirements for undertaking everyday nursing cares and procedures
Spirituality is an essential part of care planning and the delivery of quality care	Spiritual and religious needs should be documented in the care plan to ensure continuity and quality of care
Interpersonal skills and therapeutic use of self are essential to engaging and being present with the patient and family	Approach the patient with a genuine, non-judgemental attitude Avoid imposing own religious or spiritual beliefs on the patient and family
Being knowledgeable about a patient's religious values about life, health, illness, death and dying enables the critical care nurse to be respectful and accommodating n their care	Consult family, if they share same religion, and/or consult appropriate representative of the patient's religion. Areas to explore should include the following to determine: • religious values regarding life, health, illness, dying and death • nature of the ideal environment • processes surrounding dying, if appropriate to the patient • beliefs regarding nutrition and hydration • use of touch • gender-specific care • family presence, involvement and support • care after death
Philosophies and policies should be cognisant of the cultural and religious diversity within the critical care patient population	Policies should be cognisant of cultural and religious diversity, and include management of the following: • visiting • modesty • gender-specific care • communication • language and the use of interpreters

and/or family, religious and end-of-life needs can be determined, and a management plan developed for implementation.

Practice tip

Research shows that many critical care nurses feel unprepared and unsupported to deliver spiritual care, making this challenging for them psychologically and emotionally. Make developing spiritual care as part of critical care nursing practice an ongoing professional development activity.

End-of-life care and bereavement

Internationally, mortality rates in ICUs vary considerably and are a feature of the models of care including admission criteria and discharge destinations.[162] Specifically, within Australia and New Zealand the Intensive Care Society Centre for Resource and Evaluation reported on data from 165 Australasian ICUs about discharge of 172,167 patients. The ICU mortality rates from New Zealand and Australia across tertiary, metropolitan, rural, paediatric and private ICUs ranged from 7.8% to 5.2% respectively. The impact is that somewhere around 13,000 families in these two countries alone were bereaved during the reporting year of 2014/2015.[163] End-of-life and bereavement care therefore constitutes a core component of the comprehensive care we provide to patients, families and staff. Death can occur as a result of sudden decline in the patient's condition, or as a result of ceasing active treatment to palliation. Patient death in critical care areas is found to have a significantly different effect on family members from a death in another in-hospital area as the critical illness is often sudden and unexpected. Family may be unprepared for their relative's death in the highly medicalised critical care environment. Where possible, patient, family-centred decision making, together with effective communication and attention to symptom management, is optimal. Practical and emotional support for family and patients is important and scrutiny of the way we manage these important areas provides quality indicators for critical care areas.[37,164] Nurses have crucial influence at end of life. As essential advocates, educators and facilitators, they can initiate conversations and bring patient wishes to the forefront of care ensuring every effort is made to guide care that is patient, family-centred.[158]

Patient comfort and palliative care

Maintaining patient comfort and support for families and staff are primary requirements of nursing patients during the end stages of life. Avoiding distress and suffering for patients and their families are fundamental components to providing a 'good death' together with individualising care by enacting the patient and family's wishes.[165] Advanced directives and 'not for resuscitation' orders should be in place to prevent mismanagement and misunderstanding of patient wishes (see Chapter 4).[37] Key elements of palliative care incorporate management of physical, psychological and spiritual symptoms which is a shared responsibility of the health care team. Maintenance of patient comfort through protocols or guidelines to reduce symptom distress with non-pharmacological strategies, analgesics and sedatives is extremely important from the patient, family and nurses' perspective.[82,166-168] Although this may seem fundamental there is evidence to suggest that this is still not achieved. Major recommendations from a USA study of 322 critical care nurses indicated end-of-life care needed to be improved in a number of ways including: the provision of a private, peaceful environment; timely, truthful communication with patient and family members; the need for 1:1 nurse to patient ratio; and early recognition of futile treatments.[167]

Collaboration and early involvement by palliative care teams is one way to integrate end-of-life care for patients who either remain in critical care areas or are transferred from the unit to other areas. Withholding or withdrawing treatment requires careful consideration and preparation for symptom management for the patient, their family and staff. Choices of bolus or infusion administration of medications need to be based on patient comfort issues. Oxygen therapy is continued in the most appropriate form, and an oral airway may improve patient comfort and aid secretion clearance. Medications may be administered to reduce copious oral secretions and enhance comfort.

The attainment of humane nursing care must include heightened efforts in achieving quality indicators, such as mentioned above – adequate management of pain and nausea, agitation and restlessness. Both critical care staff and families should continue to communicate with the patient by speaking and touching as this can have a calming influence. Comfort measures to enhance holistic care delivery should continue together with emotional support and environmental modifications promoting a quiet, private and respectful setting.[169]

Patient dignity should be a priority, with gowns, or personal attire essential elements of care. The management of symptoms further allows patients to maintain their dignity. Privacy for patients and their families allows an opportunity for them to communicate as they so wish. As indicated in previous sections of this chapter, patient and family culture, beliefs and spiritual values are important considerations that underpin care.[168,170] Caring for patients and their families can be quite challenging and supporting each other in these situations will share the burden and provide direction to novice critical care nurses on ways to alleviate suffering and care for oneself.

> **Practice tip**
>
> Discuss with a colleague end-of-life care processes in your unit. Do you have a current guideline or policy document to provide direction? Are family conferences held regularly to ensure family are kept well informed or do you use a different method of communicating updates? What would you like to see implemented in your unit to improve end-of-life care?

Family care

Care of the family is supported by proactive palliative care interventions that include empathic, informative communication with interdisciplinary team meetings and family conferences that are not rushed where families are integral to decision making and goal planning.[37,65,171] The desire to participate in decision making varies from family to family, and families' choices cannot be assumed. Decision-making support for family members is complex and to date there is little evidence of effective support mechanisms; however, those that have a patient, family-centred focus are more likely to meet the unique needs of the families.[172] An example of how we should not assume we know best and how to individualise care was reported in a study from The Netherlands where family members were interviewed 2 months following the death of their relative in ICU. Some families wanted the monitoring systems turned off whereas others wanted to be able to see the patient's decline visually.[173] Something that was universal to all family members was the need to have their questions answered and recognition that nurses did this very well.

Structured communication between the healthcare team and families can assist with timely decisions, goal formation about care and preparation for the process of palliation. Although there are a number of family meeting tools available, they predominantly focus on supporting staff in the process.[174] Ideally, such tools should also support family participation with the preparation of questions, identification of topics for discussion or clarification and sharing concerns and fears, together with overall goals for the meeting. Emotional and practical support can be given to families by providing written material about the critical care area, local facilities and specific information on bereavement.[65] Privacy is not always possible in the busy, sometimes open-plan critical care environment, but maximising efforts in this regard for dying patients and their families provides a more conducive environment for strengthening patient–family relationships, communication and dignity. Communication is enhanced with family conferences, which provide a structured process where family members and patients' healthcare teams can share goals and understanding of end-of-life care.

Family conferences are a way to meet family needs, and enhance communication and understanding of the patient situation. These become an essential element of care when end-of-life discussions are needed. Privacy, away from the direct clinical environment, is important to allow uninterrupted time for families to meet with their relative's healthcare team.[175] When family conferences have been instituted early in the admission, a family/staff relationship will be established that supports ongoing communicating about end-of-life care.[61,176]

It is important to have the interprofessional team (for example: intensivist, social worker, case manager, direct care nurse, chaplain) meeting with the patient's family at this time to ensure a comprehensive approach to the coordination of patient care and family support.[62] This approach helps in both the understanding and provision of consistent information. Where possible, involving all significant family members in the family conference allows them to hear the same information, ask individual questions and discuss options. These collectively reduce family and/or family/staff conflict[80] and support those families that prefer to make decisions as a collective.

Family members of ICU patients are at a high risk of anxiety and depression. In a large ICU multicentre French study, 73% of family members experienced anxiety and 35% were diagnosed with depression around the time of discharge or death of their relative.[177] This mental health morbidity is likely related to the burden of the critical illness and potential or imminent demise of a loved one. Family member's depression, grief and anxiety can be manifested by physiological, behavioural, psychological/cognitive and social indicators. The physiological stress response with increased cortisol excretion and poor sleep patterns[43] can affect family interactions with each other and with staff. At times of end-of-life discussions, family members may exhibit confusion, anger and/or threatening behaviour, making it difficult for everyone involved. Importantly, these emotions make it challenging for family to grasp and understand the often complex patient situation. Strategies such as family conferences are important as they potentially improve communication channels and promote understanding, thereby reducing conflict situations.

Planning for the family conference around end-of-life issues involves ensuring a common time for significant family members and the critical care team to meet. If a key family member is away or overseas, a conversation over the internet may be the best option as video facilities will allow better communication than with a telephone call. Where there are complex family situations with extended families or previous partners, care must be taken to try to avoid a poorly functioning group. There may also be an estranged partner who wants to be included, which may add to the dynamics of the situation. The critical care team will need to exhibit great diplomacy in such complex situations to keep the group and meeting meaningful and productive. There is no rule as how to manage these situations but the foremost consideration is how to serve the best interests of the patient. Family members unable to attend the family conferences should be relayed information in a timely way by a self-designated family spokesperson. This person is generally one who is more resilient and coping better than others with the end-of-life discussions who can take the responsibility for communicating the situation to other family members. Reassurance that the patient will not be abandoned and care will remain of the highest quality is important to families and fundamental to the care we provide.

A well-organised critical care team will meet prior to the family conference and ensure all relevant information is gathered and that there is a shared understanding. Curtis and colleagues[178] suggest the use of a five-point approach during the family conference, which may be useful around end-of-life meetings. This approach is termed 'VALUE': 1) valuing family statements; 2) acknowledging emotion; 3) listening; 4) understanding the patient as a person; and 5) eliciting questions. The critical care team's ability to listen to the family is a key element and has been found to significantly increase a family's satisfaction with end-of-life care.[171]

The healthcare team that provides information and discusses palliation and end-of-life care needs to clearly indicate to families that, although they are involved in much of the decision making,[61] the decision to withdraw treatment is a medical one in Australia but may be quite different elsewhere. This notwithstanding, consensus and shared decision making remains the aim as careful consideration of the patient's wishes, the family perspective and the futility or otherwise of further treatment are considered within an ethical framework.[61,175] Importantly, the differences between withdrawal of life-sustaining treatment and the provision of end-of-life care processes need to be distinguished for families.[179] How best to meet the needs of families at these times is not well understood, partly due to the sensitive nature of researching this area of care as we strive to do no harm, and partly due to individual responses to the circumstances that restrict generalisability of findings. Maintaining a patient, family-centred approach seeking feedback on their needs helps us to individualise the care we provide and remains the best available approach in these circumstances where one-size-does not fit all.

While the family grapple with the process of grieving,[180] we do know that nurses need to provide physical and psychological care for patients and families. This can be achieved when there is patient, family-centred decision making, good communication, continuity of care and emotional and practical support; and spiritual support can assist with this.[181] Individualising the care to the family is essential, and support measures should be instituted based on their needs which can change rapidly as the situation changes. Importantly, grief manifests in different ways, and grieving is a complex process. Bereaved families in intensive care demonstrate complex bereavement processes and, without support, prolonged grief reactions can occur. In a longitudinal study nearly half (46%) of bereaved family members had complicated grief 1 year later when measured by the Inventory of Complicated Grief Scale.[182] Complicated grief patterns are detrimental as they decrease the family's ability to cope with everyday needs, increase the need for health services and may progress to unresolved grief.[183]

The detrimental effects of long-term unresolved grief after the death of a loved one are well documented.[183] The preferred term is 'prolonged grief disorder' (previously called complicated grief), which has clinically disabling grief symptoms including, amongst others, a preoccupation with thoughts of the loss, avoidance of reminders of the loss, disbelief over the person's death, feeling lonely since the loss, feeling that the future holds no purpose and feeling stunned or shocked by the loss.[184] These symptoms can result in elevated morbidity and mortality levels associated with depression, cardiac events (including a higher risk of sudden cardiac death), hypertension, neoplasms, ulcerative colitis, suicidal tendencies and social dysfunction (including alcohol abuse and violence).[43,183] These potentially harmful outcomes provide strong motivation for critical care clinicians to initiate family support mechanisms such as bereavement services.[185] Bereavement care aims to reduce the immediate physical and emotional distress for those grieving, while improving the long-term morbidity associated with unresolved grief.

Although critical care clinicians in the UK,[186] USA,[185] Europe and Canada[187] are developing guidelines for bereavement care in critical care, little evidence-based research has been conducted on bereavement care strategies.[185] One study, however, conducted a broader evaluation of 113 ICUs in the UK and summarised bereavement care from the perspective of senior nursing clinicians. The senior nurses considered that they were proficient in providing written information to families but lacking in their provision of a respectful and quiet physical environment.[155] Others suggest that our care needs to incorporate key elements including physical and psychosocial comfort and culturally sensitive communication and family care.[188] Bereavement services in 153 Australasian ICUs were reported to also incorporate distribution of information to families in the majority of ICUs; fewer, however, had bereavement follow-up services (50% of ICUs in New Zealand and 23% in Australia).[30] Follow-up services were more common in Denmark where 72% of the reporting 46 ICUs offering these services to ICU families following the death of a relative in ICU.[189] It is imperative to rigorously assess new and existing bereavement interventions as to how well they meet the needs of families. Legitimising research on this vulnerable group is required to improve end-of-life care for families and patients.

Care of the critical care nurse

The two previous sections have focused on care for the dying patient and their family. Critical care nurses who care for both patients and families also require care in end-of-life situations.[146,190] Caring for dying patients is emotionally draining and highly demanding of the critical care nurse, who may not have the knowledge and understanding of palliative care and death in the critical care environment. Peer support and unit guidelines on palliative care may provide support and reduce caregiver burden.[168,185,191,192]

Dealing with the death of patients may be exacerbated in some critical care environments, particularly in the rural setting, where the nurse may know the patient outside the work environment. Effective palliation is more likely to occur when the interdisciplinary team collectively develops their unit's palliative care and bereavement services with care and attention to staff's needs together with those of patients and their families.[181,185]

In the main, nurses depend on colleagues and friends for support when patients die, and they may value the opportunity to discuss the patient and family situation by way of debriefing sessions. 'Debriefing' sessions can have a number of interpretations. For example, debriefing in critical care often takes the form of an opportunity to share feelings. Alternatively, it may involve a procedural clinical review of events where the objective is to understand and learn from the situation.[193] Both forms of debriefing are important, together with the opportunity for peer discussion to provide mutual support within the interdisciplinary team.[194] Accessing experts from outside the unit's usual resources may also be helpful in particularly challenging situations.[193]

Dealing with death is never easy; however, an awareness of colleagues' needs is a key to providing support as mental and physical exhaustion can develop.[195] The term compassion fatigue is defined 'as a state of tension and preoccupation with the traumatised patients by re-experiencing the traumatic event … associated with the patient'.[196 p.1435] Nurses' experiences of caring for critically ill or dying patients and their families have the potential to gradually lead to compassion fatigue.[195] This is detrimental; not only to the nurse, but also to patients and families as the nurse endeavours to protect and distance themselves from further emotional situations. A workplace culture that includes positive inter- and intra-disciplinary relationship influences the ability of nurses to provide compassionate care. Shared understanding of the plan of care for the patient is an important factor as is having your experiences validated by your team. Influences from outside the workplace also impact on our ability to provide compassionate care. Our values about patient care and lifestyle factors including family demands influence our caring capacity.[197]

One way to explore compassion amongst critical care nurses is to structure 'Compassion cafes' into regular education sessions.[198] Compassion cafes are described as a way to provide a safe, supportive space away from the ICU where nurses can share their experiences within a collegial environment. Importantly, they focus on recognition of compassion fatigue and strategies to reduce its occurrence.[199] Sharing experiences and knowledge around end-of-life care[189] helps protect against compassion fatigue[197] and not unexpectedly, compassion fatigue has been linked to reduced job satisfaction and an intention to leave the profession.[200] A number of strategies are important to enhance the care we are able to provide during end-of-life care. Caring for ourselves and our colleagues are fundamental to being able to care for patients and their families.

Practice tip

Think back to the last time you were involved with a patient who was being palliated. What were the things that worked well for you? Did you feel supported, or provide support to your colleagues? Were you able to care for the patient and their family as you would have liked? Did you have the resources to be able to provide a peaceful and dignified place to be? Having read this chapter, is there feedback you can provide to your colleagues and leadership team on ways to improve palliative care in your unit?

Summary

The psychosocial, cultural and religious needs of critically ill patients and their families are just as important as their physical needs, and care needs to be taken not to overlook these. In this chapter a holistic and patient, family-centred approach to practice is presented, which enables individualised plans of care that include specific psychosocial, cultural and religious needs of critically ill patients and their families. Health, illness, death and dying are sociocultural constructions, and can have different meanings for critically ill patients and their families. Cultural and spiritual care are an important aspect of people's wellbeing, and essential for critical nurses to be mindful of. Thus, culturally and linguistically diverse patients and families have specific cultural values, beliefs and practices that critical care nurses need to determine, which may involve the assistance of an interpreter. These patients require the critical care nurse to interact with them in a manner that facilitates the identification of their needs on an individual basis. The old adage 'actions speak louder than words' is worthy of consideration when working with these patients in the critical care setting. It is important that individual patient and family plans of care are developed that include their participation and reflect their important beliefs and practices that need to be included in their critical care experience. In order to meet the needs of the critically ill patient and family, the critical care nurse is advised to identify personal beliefs, practices and expectations that may influence professional decision making and interactions with the patient and family.

Case study

Johnny, is a 36-year-old man admitted to the critical care unit with a severe head injury after being hit by a speeding car at the roadside where the family were currently living. He has been stabilised on life support to manage his cerebral oedema but his condition is listed as critical. He is married to Keiza and they have five young children, aged 18 months old to 12 years. Johnny is self-employed and is the family's sole source of income. The information the admitting nurse has received indicates that Johnny and Keiza identify as Gypsy Roma Travellers (GRTs). Given Johnny's status, the family have indicated the need for wider family members to be present and that this is very important for them, especially at this time when Johnny's life is under threat. At the bedside the critical care nurse is challenged by several concerned family members, including Johnny's partner, children, siblings, cousins, aunties and uncles, who all want to be present. Keiza and other family members are showing signs of distrust, and when spoken to appear to be defensive, responding with somewhat hostile attitudes. The critical care nurse is somewhat concerned and wanting to restrict visitors to Johnny's partner and children – as per the critical care visitation policy. However, the critical care nurse:

- is aware that for the family such an action is totally unacceptable – they need to be with the patient
- is vaguely aware that GRTs do not have positive experiences with health services

- is unaware of their cultural and spiritual needs, and the importance of family, particularly with the potential for death and dying.

The critical care nurse has just received a handover from the nurse involved in stabilising Johnny, and explains she knows little about his family. While being somewhat overwhelmed, the nurse decides to draw upon what she knows about being culturally responsive and practising with cultural humility. Thus, she recognises prejudices she holds about Gypsy Roma Travellers, mainly derived from interactions with her own family and friends, which is not going to help her. The nurse first introduces herself to the family, telling them her name, where she was from, and what her role is in caring for Johnny. She then politely asked who the family members were and how they were connected to Johnny. She then tells the family that she needs to talk with them after she has done her initial checking of Johnny's condition. The nurse indicated that she was aware that often Gypsy Roma Traveller communities did not have positive experiences when accessing health services; however, she wanted to understand what important needs the critical care people should know when caring for Johnny and the family. She then asked them to select a spokesperson who the staff could communicate with about important information about Johnny and his progress while she was doing Johnny's checks. She intended to document this information in Johnny's plan of care to assist other nurses caring for Johnny and interacting with the family.

CASE STUDY QUESTIONS

1. Generally, Gypsy Roma Travellers have negative experiences and discrimination with health professionals. In what ways could having an analysis of Gypsy Roma Travellers' histories, contemporary socioeconomic deprivation, and the family's past experiences help shape critical nurses' practice?
2. When confronted by large family groups, reflect on your thoughts, the actions you undertake, and how you evaluate whether your actions are driven by your personal and/or professional values and beliefs, and if you are being culturally responsive in these situations.
3. In what ways do you think the family's trust is important for identifying their needs that should be integrated into Johnny's plan of care, and communicated to other critical care nurses and other staff?

RESEARCH VIGNETTE

Beckstrand RL, Lamoreaux N, Luthy KE, Macintosh JLB. Critical care nurses' perceptions of end-of-life care obstacles: comparative 17-year data. Dimens Crit Care Nurs 2017; 36(2):94-105

Abstract

Background: Nurses working in intensive care units (ICUs) frequently care for patients and their families at the end of life (EOL). Providing high-quality EOL care is important for both patients and families, yet ICU nurses face many obstacles that hinder EOL care. Researchers have identified various ICU nurse-perceived obstacles, but no studies have been found addressing the progress that has been made for the last 17 years.

Objective: The aims of this study were to determine the most common and current obstacles in EOL care as perceived by ICU nurses and then to evaluate whether meaningful changes have occurred since data were first gathered in 1998.

Methods: A quantitative-qualitative mixed methods design was used. A random, geographically dispersed sample of 2000 members of the American Association of Critical-Care Nurses was surveyed.

Results: Five obstacle items increased in mean score and rank as compared with 1999 data including 1) family not understanding what the phrase 'lifesaving measures' really means, 2) providing lifesaving measures at families' requests despite patient's advance directive listing no such care, 3) family not accepting patient's poor prognosis, 4) family members fighting about the use of life support, and 5) not enough time to provide EOL care because the nurse is consumed with lifesaving measures attempting to save the patient's life. Five obstacle items decreased in mean score and rank compared with 1999 data including 1) physicians differing in opinion about care of the patient, 2) family and friends who continually call the nurse rather than calling the designated family member, 3) physicians who are evasive and avoid families, 4) nurses having to deal with angry families, and 5) nurses not knowing their patient's wishes regarding continuing with tests and treatments.

Conclusions: Obstacles in EOL care, as perceived by critical care nurses, still exist. Family-related obstacles have increased over time. Obstacles related to families may not be easily overcome as each family, dealing with a dying family member in an ICU, likely has not previously experienced a similar situation. On the basis of the current top five obstacles, recommendations for possible areas of focus include 1) improved health literacy assessment of families followed by earlier directed, appropriate, and specific EOL information; 2) improved physician/team communication; and 3) ensuring patients' wishes are followed as written. In general, patient- and family-centered care using clear and open EOL communication regarding wishes and desires between patients and families, their physicians, and nurses will help decrease common obstacles, thus improving the quality of EOL care provided to dying patients and families.

Critique

These researchers examined critical care nurses' views on end-of-life care within ICUs. They highlight that caring for patients who will die in ICU, and their families, is both a complex and yet relatively common occurrence. The rationale for their study was that when we understand the issues, we are better able to remediate to overcome them in order to improve the care we provide. The purpose was to uncover the most common obstacles experienced by critical care nurses delivering end-of-life care. The authors were also interested in mapping changes in nurses' perception over time as they compared their results with similar studies conducted in 1998 and 1999. The research questions clearly aligned with their purpose.

This study used a mixed methods design; however, quantitative data from a 72-item survey are reported in this manuscript and a later publication provides data from open-ended survey responses on suggestions on ways to overcome the obstacles.[167] It is unfortunate that the entire results could not be reported in the one publication as the purpose of a mixed methods design is to combine or merge the two forms of data in such a manner as to answer the research questions persuasively.[211]

A random sample of 2000 was drawn from members of the professional critical care nurses association in the USA which has just over 100,000 members. To be eligible to participate, nurses had to reside in the USA and have minimal experience of providing end-of-life care for an ICU patient. They were recruited via mail and a follow-up reminder was sent 3 months later. The accuracy of the mailing address was dependent on the currency of the association's database and may have been a reason for the reduced response rate. The self-administered survey had 72 items including demographic details and the National Survey of Critical Care Nurses Perceptions of End-of-life Care which the lead author had used in the previous studies in 1998 and 1999. High internal consistency was reported at 0.89 for the reliability of the obstacle items.

Data from 509 critical care nurses were analysed (response rate of 26.7%). In spite of the relatively lengthy survey, missing data constituted less than 2% for most variables. Respondents were experienced critical care nurses: they had a mean age of 45 years with over 15 years' experience in critical care nursing and over 65% had provided end-of-life care to 30 or more ICU patients. Participants were asked to rate a set of 29 obstacle items from 0 [not an obstacle] to 5 [an extremely large obstacle]. The top three rated obstacles included: 1) family members not understanding what 'lifesaving measures' really means (mean [SD], 4.05 [0.97]), 2) multiple doctors for the one patient differed in opinion regarding the direction of care (mean [SD], 3.94 [1.13]), and 3) using life-sustaining measures, at the families' request, although the patient signed advanced directives requesting no such treatments (mean [SD], 3.92 [1.23]). When the obstacles were compared with the 1999 results, three obstacles, all relating to family members, significantly increased in severity: 1) family not accepting what the doctors tell them about prognosis, 2) visiting hours are too liberal, and 3) family not understanding what 'lifesaving' measures mean. These obstacles to providing end-of-life care require addressing as they all are connected with the manner in which nurses or doctors communicate with family. The researchers discuss the need for an assessment of family members' health literacy levels before communication of patient-related information occurs but they fail to provide further direction on how this could be managed. As communication is a primary need for families, it is imperative that nurses and doctors understand how to assess understanding at this crucial time where end-of-life decision making and care occurs. Quality communication with family could alleviate many of the listed obstacles – in fact seven out of the top 10 obstacles from the current study involve family. The need for improved communication is endorsed in the authors' paper reporting qualitative findings where the nurses considered that earlier, honest communication with family that is realistic would improve end-of-life care.[165]

Nine obstacles improved significantly over the time period with the greatest improvements in the ICU layout allowing for privacy; visiting hours less restrictive and patients' pain better controlled. It is welcoming that the nurses' considered that they were better able to manage patients' pain – a fundamental provision of care and patient–family-centred need. Similarly, having more support from social workers and religious leaders indicates progress in how ICUs have access and involve allied health and ancillary services that improve the care we provide. Conversely, it is somewhat of concern that doctors are still avoiding family members at a time when they need to be informed and frequently see the doctor as the authoritative and best informed professional.

In the second paper by the authors who report thematic analysis from the open-ended items, the three top themes included ensuring a 'good death'; early, honest and more realistic communication and appropriate 1:1 nurse: patient staffing ratios.[167] When patient–family-centred care is practised, symptom control will be paramount together with striving for a quiet, respectful private space for families and their dying relatives. Nurse: patient ratios that are 1:1 are commonplace in some countries including Australia, New Zealand and the UK; however, in countries where this is not the case, a strong argument supported by critical care and local guidelines needs to be developed to enable quality care.

A significant limitation of this study is that there is a predominance of responses from highly experienced critical care nurses. Perceptions of issues related to end-of-life care may have been quite different from the perspective of less experienced nurses whom, it could be argued, need more support. A future study could target students enrolled in critical care programs as they are more likely to be less experienced in the speciality. The size or type of ICU is not reported, which may have impacted on the resources available to them. A brief description of the model of nursing care would have made it clearer for the international readership.

In summary, the authors provide an informative overview of obstacles to the provision of end-of-life care in ICU that have changed over time from the perspective of critical care nurses. Addressing the needs of family remain paramount and a particular focus on their understanding and health literacy is recommended. Patient–family-centred care will provide support for improved communication between the interdisciplinary team, patient and family members.

Learning activities

1 In the critical care setting, the focus is on individuals and the physical health status. In this chapter the importance of patient- and family-centred nursing care is discussed, which requires critical care nurses to not only focus on a very unwell patient's physical status but also on their wider health and wellbeing needs and those of their family. This requires not only consideration of the people before you but also an understanding of the contextual factors that can enhance or impede patient- and family-centred nursing care. Identify the contextual factors in your critical care setting that might influence your practice by completing the following activities:

   a List those organisational policies and practices you can identify in the clinical practice setting that might influence nursing practice.

   b Identify the characteristics of a clinician who practices patient- and family-centred nursing practice and how these promote exemplary nursing care.

   c Imagine you were a patient in the critical care unit in which you work, what would be important to you about the nursing care you received?

   d Imagine you had a family member in a critical care unit, write down those things you consider most important about the care that you and your family member receive. Compare this with the list provided earlier in the chapter in the section *Needs of family during critical illness*.

   e Reflecting on the four activities above, write down how you can improve your patient- and family-centred care practice and identify those factors that would impede this practice and what strategies you could undertake to minimise their effects.

2 When considering culturally responsive care as a career-long endeavour, it is useful for critical care nurses to identify where on that journey they may be and what the need to undertake to progress further. Think about two situations involving patients and their families from another culture than your own – one where the interactions went well, the patient's and family's needs were respected and met, and the outcomes were positive, and the other where the situation was challenging and marred by conflict and family disatisfaction. How might you need to develop your knowledge, skills and strategies to optimise your cultural responsiveness? To assist you answering this question, consider the following:
   a Identify the factors that facitilitated a positive outcome, and then the challenges and barriers that made reaching a positive outcome problematic.
   b Identify the cultural factors related to your personal and professional expectations, and those of the patient and family. How might these be sources of potential conflict?
   c What knowledge, skills and strategies might be needed for working in a culturally responsive way with patients and families from different cultures?

3 Spiritual intelligence, according to Moradnezhad et al (2017),[159] involves the following activities: creating existential thinking, creating personal meaning, transcendental awareness, and consciousness state expansion. In what ways would these activities assist critical care nurses to develop their ability to respond better to patients' and their families' spiritual needs? To help you assist with this activity, the following questions can guide self-reflection and/or discussion with your peers:
   a Why would critical care nurses need to develop their spiritual intelligence?
   b What benefits would emerge from having a higher level of spiritual intelligence derived from the activities that Moradnezhad et al[159] suggest within the critical care setting?
   c How would critical care nurses having a higher level of spiritual intelligence assist them to respond better to patients' and their families' spiritual needs?

4 You are to attend a family conference for the patient you are caring for. In preparation for this family conference, consider the following:
   a What approach you would adopt if this is the first time participating in a family conference
   b The information you would need to gather to prepare in readiness for the family conference
   c The key people you would approach to get additional information, if today is the first time you have cared for the patient
   d What considerations will be needed if children are going to be present
   e The documentation required in the patient's clinical file following the family conference.

Online resources

Arctic University of Norway's Centre for Sami Studies, https://en.uit.no/om/enhet/forsiden?p_dimension_id=88182

Australian Indigenous Health InfoNet, www.healthinfonet.ecu.edu.au

Cooperative Research Centre for Aboriginal Health, www.crcah.org.au/index.cfm

eMedical Journal of Australia articles on Aboriginal health, www.mja.com.au/Topics/Aboriginal%20health.htm

Hauora: Māori standards of health IV: A study of the years 2000–2005, https://www.otago.ac.nz/wellington/departments/publichealth/research/erupomare/research/otago019494.html

Māori, www.Maori.org.nz/tikanga/?d=page&pid=sp44&parent=42

Information about Māori protocol and beliefs, www.Maori.org.nz/tikanga/?d=page&pid=sp44&parent=42)

New Zealand Ministry of Health website (access to Māori health-related publications and resources), www.moh.govt.nz

Office of Aboriginal Health–WA, http://www.aboriginal.health.wa.gov.au/home

Patient-centred care: Improving quality and safety by focusing care on patients and consumers, www.safetyandquality.gov.au/wp-content/uploads/2012/01/PCCC-DiscussPaper.pdf

YouTube: Discrimination of Romani, https://www.youtube.com/watch?v=N8MZz3Ehuil

Further reading

Abrahamsson A, Lindmark U, Gerdner A. Sense of coherence of reindeer herders and other Samis in comparison to other Swedish citizens. Int J Circumpolar Health 2013;72(1):20633.

Best O, Fredericks B, editors. Yatdjuligin: Aboriginal and Torres Strait Islander nursing and midwifery care. 2nd ed. Melbourne, VIC: Cambridge University Press; 2018.

Carson B, Dunbar T, Chenhall RD, et al, editors. Social determinants of Indigenous health. Crows Nest: Allen and Unwin; 2007.

Cormack D, Stanley J, Harris R. Multiple forms of discrimination and relationships with health and wellbeing: findings from national cross-sectional surveys in Aotearoa/New Zealand. Int J Equity Health 2018;17:26.

Creswell JW, Plano Clark VL. Designing and conducting mixed methods research. 3rd ed. Thousand Oaks, California: SAGE; 2018.

Durie M. Whaiora. Auckland: Oxford University Press; 1998.

Eckermann A-K, Dowd T, Chong E, et al. Bridging cultures in Aboriginal health. 3rd ed. Sydney: Churchill Livingstone; 2010.

Gjernes T. Perceptions of risk and uncertainty among Sámi women involved in reindeer herding in Northern Norway. Health, Risk & Society 2008;10(5):505–16.

Isaacs AN, Pyett P, Oakley-Browne MA, et al. Barriers and facilitators to the utilization of adult mental health services by Australia's Indigenous people: seeking a way forward. Int J Ment Health Nurs 2010;19(2):75–82.

Lally S. Gypsies and Travellers: their history, culture and traditions. Community Pract 2015;88(1):30–3.

McFadden A, Siebelt L, Gavine A, et al. Gypsy, Roma and Traveller access to and engagement with health services: a systematic review. Eur J Pub Health 2018;28(1):74–81.

Parekh N, Rose T. Health inequalities of the Roma in Europe: a literature review. Cent Eur J Public Health 2011;19(3):139–42.

Reeskens T, Hooghe M. Cross-cultural measurement equivalence of generalized trust. Evidence from the European Social Survey (2002 and 2004). Soc Indic Res 2008;85(3):515–32.

Stojanovski K, Holla A, Hoxha I, et al. The influence of ethnicity and displacement on quality of antenatal care: the case of Roma, Ashkali, and Balkan Egyptian communities in Kosovo. Health Hum Rights 2017;19(2):35–48.

Tipa Z, Wilson D, Neville S, et al. Cultural responsiveness and the family partnership model. Nurs Prax N Z 2015;31(2):35–49.

Wallace M, Sarles S. EB49 Changing culture to cultivate patient- and family-centered care. Crit Care Nurs 2012;32(2):e30.

Wepa D. Cultural safety in Aotearoa New Zealand. Melbourne: Cambridge University Press; 2015.

Wright LM, Leahey M. Nurses and families: a guide to family assessment and intervention. 6th ed. Philadelphia: FA Davis; 2013.

References

1. Canfield C, Taylor D, Nagy K, et al. Critical care nurses' perceived need for guidance in addressing spirituality in critically ill patients. Am J Crit Care 2016;25(3):206–11.
2. National Safety and Quality Health Services Standards. Australian Commission on Safety and Quality in Health Care, 2017. Available from: https://www.safetyandquality.gov.au/wp-content/uploads/2017/12/National-Safety-and-Quali-ty-Health-Service-Standards-second-edition.pdf. [Accessed 5 April 2018].

3. World Health Organisation. WHO patients for patient safety programme, 2013. Available from: http://www.who.int/gpsc/5may/5may2013_patient-participation/en/. [Accessed 5 April 2018].
4. Mitchell ML, Gill F, Grealy B, et al ACCCN Position Statement - Partnering with Families in Critical Care, 2015. Available from: https://www.acccn.com.au/documents/item/289. [Accessed 5 April 2018].
5. Jost SG, Bonnell M, Chacko SJ, et al. Integrated primary nursing: a care delivery model for the 21st-century knowledge worker. Nurs Adm Q 2010;34(3):208–16.
6. Jakimowicz S, Perry L, Lewis J. An integrative review of supports, facilitators and barriers to patient-centred nursing in the intensive care unit. J Clin Nurs 2017;26(23–24):4153–71.
7. Jakimowicz S, Perry L. A concept analysis of patient-centred nursing in the intensive care unit. J Adv Nurs 2015;71(7):1499–517.
8. Delaney LJ. Patient-centred care as an approach to improving health care in Australia. Collegian 2018;25(1):119–23.
9. Davidson JE, Aslakson RA, Long AC, et al. Guidelines for family-centered care in the neonatal, pediatric, and adult ICU. Crit Care Med 2017;45(1):103–28.
10. Australian Commission on Safety and Quality in Health Care (ACSQHC). Discussion paper: Patient-centred care: Improving quality and safety by focusing care on patients and consumers, 2010. Available from: https://www.safetyandquality.gov.au/wp-content/uploads/2012/01/PCCC-DiscussPaper.pdf. [Accessed 5 April 2018].
11. Epstein RM, Fiscella K, Lesser CS, et al. Why the nation needs a policy push on patient-centered health care. Health Aff 2010;29(8):1489–95.
12. Slatore CG, Hansen L, Ganzini L, et al. Communication by nurses in the intensive care unit: qualitative analysis of domains of patient-centered care. Am J Crit Care 2012;21(6):410–18.
13. Oxford Dictionary. 2014. Available from: www.oxforddictionaries.com/definitions/english/. [Accessed 5 April 2018].
14. Ekman I, Swedberg K, Taft C, et al. Person-centered care – ready for prime time. Eur J Cardiovasc Nurs 2011;10(4):248–51.
15. Centre for Person-Centred Care University of Gothenburg S. Research. Available from: https://gpcc.gu.se/english/research. [Accessed 5 April 2018].
16. Fumagalli S. Reduced cardiocirculatory complications with unrestrictive visiting policy in an intensive care unit: results from a pilot, randomized trial. Circulation 2006;113(7):946–52.
17. Friedman M. Family nursing: research, theory and practice. 5th ed. Stamford: Appleton & Lange; 2003.
18. Wright LM. Nurses and families: a guide to family assessment and intervention. 6th ed. Philadelphia: F A Davis & Company; 2013.
19. Plaintree Organisation. Resources, 2018. Available from: https://planetree.org/resources/ [Accessed 5 April 2018].
20. Espezel HJE, Canam CJ. Parent-nurse interactions: care of hospitalized children. J Adv Nurs 2003;44(1):34–41.
21. Institute for Patient- and Family-Centered Care. Patient- and Family-Centered Care, 2012. Available from: http://www.ipfcc.org/about/pfcc.html. [Accessed 5 April 2018].
22. de Beer J, Brysiewicz P. The conceptualization of family care during critical illness in KwaZulu-Natal, South Africa. Health SA Gesondheid 2017;22:20–7.
23. Olding M, McMillan SE, Reeves S, et al. Patient and family involvement in adult critical and intensive care settings: a scoping review. Health Expectations 2016;19(6):1183–202.
24. Raiskila S, Lehtonen L, Tandberg BS, et al. Parent and nurse perceptions on the quality of family-centred care in 11 European NICUs. Aust Crit Care 2016;29(4):201–9.
25. Engström B, Uusitalo A, Engströmemail Å. Relatives' involvement in nursing care: a qualitative study describing critical care nurses' experiences. Intensiv Crit Care Nurs 2011;27(1):1–9.
26. Garrouste-Orgeas M, Willems V, Timsit J-F, et al. Opinions of families, staff, and patients about family participation in care in intensive care units. J Crit Care 2010;25(4):634–40.
27. Mitchell M, Chaboyer W, Burmeister E, et al. Positive effects of a nursing intervention on family-centered care in adult critical care. Am J Crit Care 2009;18(6):543–52.
28. Mitchell M. Family-centred care - are we ready for it? An Australian perspective. Nurs Crit Care 2005;10(2):54–5.
29. Goldfarb MJ, Bibas L, Bartlett V, et al. Outcomes of patient- and family-centered care interventions in the ICU: a systematic review and meta-analysis. Crit Care Med 2017;45(10):1751–61.
30. Mitchell ML, Coyer F, Kean S, et al. Patient, family-centred care interventions within the adult ICU setting: an integrative review. Aust Crit Care 2016;29(4):179–93.
31. Eggenberger SK, Sanders M. A family nursing educational intervention supports nurses and families in an adult intensive care unit. Aust Crit Care 2016;29(4):217–23.
32. de Silva D. Helping measure person-centred care. London: The Health Foundation; 2014. Available from: https://www.health.org.uk/sites/health/files/HelpingMeasurePersonCentredCare.pdf. [Accessed 6 April 2018].
33. Scottish Government. The healthcare quality strategy for NHS Scotland. Edinburgh: The Scottish Government; 2010. Available from: http://www.scottishneurological.org.uk/content/res/quality_strategy.pdf. [Accessed June 2018].
34. Kean S, Mitchell M. How do intensive care nurses perceive families in intensive care? Insights from the United Kingdom and Australia. J Clin Nurs 2014;23(5–6):663–72.

35. Wilson MEMD, Kaur SMD, Gallo De Moraes AMD, et al. Important clinician information needs about family members in the intensive care unit. J Crit Care 2015;30(6):1317–23.
36. Al-Mutair AS, Plummer V, O'Brien A, et al. Family needs and involvement in the intensive care unit: a literature review. J Clin Nurs 2013;22(13–14):1805–17.
37. Nelson JE. Improving comfort and communication in the ICU: a practical new tool for palliative care performance measurement and feedback. Qual Saf Health Care 2006;15(4):264–71.
38. Ekwall A, Gerdtz M, Manias E. The influence of patient acuity on satisfaction with emergency care: perspectives of family, friends and carers. J Clin Nurs 2008;17(6):800–9.
39. Szalados JE. Legal issues in the practice of critical care medicine: a practical approach. Crit Care Med 2007;35(Suppl.):S44–58.
40. Aiken LJ, Bibeau PD, Cilento BJ, et al. A personal reflection: a case study in family-centered care at the national naval medical center in Bethesda, Maryland. Dimens Crit Care Nurs 2010;29(1):13–19.
41. Hwang DY, Yagoda D, Perrey HM, et al. Anxiety and depression symptoms among families of adult intensive care unit survivors immediately following brief length of stay. J Crit Care 2014;29(2):278–82.
42. Bandari R, Heravi-Karimooi M, Rejeh N, et al. Information and support needs of adult family members of patients in intensive care units: an Iranian perspective. J Res Nurs 2015;20(5):401–22.
43. Buckley T, Sunari D, Marshall A, et al. Physiological correlates of bereavement and the impact of bereavement interventions. Dialogues Clin Neurosci 2012;14(2):129–39.
44. Lee LYK, Lau YL. Immediate needs of adult family members of adult intensive care patients in Hong Kong. J Clin Nurs 2003;12(4):490–500.
45. Azoulay E, Pochard F, Kentish-Barnes N, et al. Risk of post-traumatic stress symptoms in family members of intensive care unit patients. Am J Respir Crit Care Med 2005;171(9):987–94.
46. McAdam JL, Fontaine DK, White DB, et al. Psychological symptoms of family members of high-risk intensive care unit patients. Am J Crit Care 2012;21(6):386–94.
47. Petrinec AB, Mazanec PM, Burant CJ, et al. Coping strategies and posttraumatic stress symptoms in post-ICU family decision makers. Crit Care Med 2015;43(6):1205–12.
48. de Beer J, Brysiewicz P. The needs of family members of intensive care unit patients: a grounded theory study. S Afr Med J 2017;32(2):44–9.
49. Leske J. Protocols for practice: applying research at the bedside, interventions to decrease family anxiety. Crit Care Nurs 2002;22(6):61–5.
50. Jones C, Backman C, Griffiths RD. Intensive care diaries and relatives' symptoms of posttraumatic stress disorder after critical illness: a pilot study. Am J Crit Care 2012;21(3):172–6.
51. Jones C, Skirrow P, Griffiths RD, et al. Post-traumatic stress disorder-related symptoms in relatives of patients following intensive care. Intensive Care Med 2004;30(3):456–60.
52. Kinrade TJA, Tomnay JE. The psychosocial needs of families during critical illness comparison of nurses' and family members' perspectives. Aust J Adv Nurs 2009;27(1):82–8.
53. Molter NC. Needs of relatives of critically ill patients: a descriptive study. Heart Lung 1979;8(2):332–9.
54. Hickman RL, Douglas SL. Impact of chronic critical illness on the psychological outcomes of family members. AACN Advanced Critical Care 2010;21(1):80–91.
55. Kentish-Barnes N, Lemiale V, Chaize M, et al. Assessing burden in families of critical care patients. Crit Care Med 2009;37:S448–56.
56. Mitchell ML, Courtney M, Coyer F. Understanding uncertainty and minimizing families' anxiety at the time of transfer from intensive care. Nurs Health Sci 2003;5(3):207–17.
57. Nelson DP, Polst G. An interdisciplinary team approach to evidence-based improvement in family-centered care. Crit Care Nurs Q 2008;31(2):110–18.
58. Beck K, Albert E, Johnsen A, et al. Pediatric Intensive Care Unit rounding improvements. BMJ Qual Improv Rep 2016;5(1):u208902.w3600.
59. Santiago C, Lazar L, Jiang D, et al. A survey of the attitudes and perceptions of multidisciplinary team members towards family presence at bedside rounds in the intensive care unit. Intensive Crit Care Nurs 2014;30(1):13–21.
60. Abraham M, Moretz JG. Implementing patient- and family-centered care: part I understanding the challenges. Pediatr Nurs 2012;38(1):44–7.
61. Cypress BS. Family conference in the Intensive Care Unit: a systematic review. Dimens Crit Care Nurs 2011;30(5):246–55.
62. Moore CD, Bernardini GL, Hinerman R, et al. The effect of a family support intervention on physician, nurse, and family perceptions of care in the surgical, neurological, and medical intensive care units. Crit Care Nurs Q 2012;35(4):378–87.
63. Soltner C, Lassalle V, Galienne-Bouygues S, et al. Written information that relatives of adult intensive care unit patients would like to receive – A comparison to published recommendations and opinion of staff members. Crit Care Med 2009;37(7):2197–202.
64. Nelson JE, Walker AS, Luhrs CA, et al. Family meetings made simpler: a toolkit for the intensive care unit. J Crit Care 2009;24(4):626.e7–14.
65. Lautrette A, Darmon M, Megarbane B, et al. A communication strategy and brochure for relatives of patients dying in the ICU. N Engl J Med 2007;356(5):469–78.
66. Mitchell M, Courtney M. An intervention study to improve the transfer of ICU patients to the ward - evaluation by ICU nurses. Aust Crit Care 2005;18(3):123–8.

67. Mitchell ML, Coyer F, Kean S, et al. Patient, family-centred care interventions within the adult ICU setting: an integrative review. Aust Crit Care 2016;29(4):179–93.
68. Schwarzkopf D, Behrend S, Skupin H, et al. Family satisfaction in the intensive care unit: a quantitative and qualitative analysis. Intensive Care Med 2013;39(6):1071–9.
69. McGowan C. Patients' confidentiality. Crit Care Nurs 2012;32(5):61–4.
70. Hunter JD, Goddard C, Rothwell M, et al. A survey of intensive care unit visiting policies in the United Kingdom. Anaesthesia 2010;65(11):1101–5.
71. Liu V, Read J, Scruth E, et al. Visitation policies and practices in US ICUs. Crit Care 2013;17(2):R71.
72. Molter NC. Families are not visitors in the critical care unit. Dimens Crit Care Nurs 1994;13(1):2–3.
73. Mitchell ML, Chaboyer W. Family centred care – a way to connect patients, families and nurses in critical care: a qualitative study using telephone interviews. Intensive Crit Care Nurs 2010;26(3):154–60.
74. Kean S. Children and young people visiting an adult intensive care unit. J Adv Nurs 2010;66(4):868–77.
75. Garrouste-Orgeas M, Philippart F, Timsit JF, et al. Perceptions of a 24-hour visiting policy in the intensive care unit. Crit Care Med 2008;36(1):30–5.
76. Mitchell ML, Aitken LM. Flexible visiting positively impacted on patients, families and staff in an Australian intensive care unit: a before-after mixed method study. Aust Crit Care 2017;30(2):91–7.
77. Van Horn ER, Kautz D. Promotion of family integrity in the acute care setting: a review of the literature. Dimens Crit Care Nurs 2007;26(3):101–7.
78. Maxwell KE, Stuenkel D, Saylor C. Needs of family members of critically ill patients: a comparison of nurse and family perceptions. Heart Lung 2007;36(5):367–76.
79. Arockiasamy V, Holsti L, Albersheim S. Fathers' experiences in the neonatal intensive care unit: a search for control. Pediatrics 2008;121(2):e215–22.
80. Davidson JE. Family-centered care: meeting the needs of patients' families and helping families adapt to critical illness. Crit Care Nurs 2009;29(3):28–34, quiz 5.
81. National Institutes of Health. Health Literacy, Maryland: National Institutes of Health; Available from: https://nnlm.gov/initiatives/topics/health-literacy. [Accessed 20 April 2018].
82. Beckstrand RL, Lamoreaux N, Luthy KE, et al. Critical care nurses' perceptions of end-of-life care obstacles: comparative 17-year data. Dimens Crit Care Nurs 2017;36(2):94–105.
83. Baumgarten M, Poulsen I. Patients' experiences of being mechanically ventilated in an ICU: a qualitative metasynthesis. Scand J Caring Sci 2015;29(2):205–14.
84. Green A. An exploratory study of patients' memory recall of their stay in an adult intensive therapy unit. Intensive Crit Care Nurs 1996;12(3):131–7.
85. Lawrence M. The unconscious experience. Am J Crit Care 1995;4(3):227–32.
86. Lorie A, Reinero DA, Phillips M, et al. Culture and nonverbal expressions of empathy in clinical settings: a systematic review. Patient Educ Couns 2017;100(3):411–24.
87. Ten Hoorn S, Elbers PW, Girbes AR, et al. Communicating with conscious and mechanically ventilated critically ill patients: a systematic review. Crit Care 2016;20(1):333.
88. McNaughton D, Light J. The iPad and mobile technology revolution: benefits and challenges for individuals who require augmentative and alternative communication. Augment Altern Commun 2013;29.
89. Ahmed S, Lee S, Shommu N, et al. Experiences of communication barriers between physicians and immigrant patients: a systematic review and thematic synthesis. Patient Exp J 2017;4(1):122–40.
90. Travaline J. Communication in the ICU: an essential component of patient care. J Crit Illn 2002;14:451–6.
91. Hupcey JE. Feeling safe: the psychosocial needs of ICU patients. J Nurs Scholarsh 2000;32(4):361–7.
92. Misak CJ. The critical care experience: a patient's view. Am J Respir Crit Care Med 2004;170(4):357–9.
93. Dithole K, Sibanda S, Moleki MM, et al. Exploring communication challenges between nurses and mechanically ventilated patients in the intensive care unit: a structured review. Worldviews 2016;13(3):197–206.
94. Dithole KS, Thupayagale-Tshweneagae G, Akpor OA, et al. Communication skills intervention: promoting effective communication between nurses and mechanically ventilated patients. BMC Nurs 2017;16:74.
95. Lara M, Gamboa C, Kahramanian MI, et al. Acculturation and Latino health in the United States. In: LaVeist TA, Isaac LA, editors. Race, ethnicity and health: a public health reader. 2nd ed. San Francisco: Jossey-Bass; 2013. p. 215–52.
96. Wepa D. Culture and ethnicity: what is the question? In: Wepa D, editor. Cultural safety in Aotearoa New Zealand. Auckland: Pearson Prentice Hall Health; 2005. p. 30–8.
97. Reid J, Varona G, Fisher M, et al. Understanding Māori 'lived' culture to determine cultural connectedness and wellbeing. J Popul Res 2016;33(1):31–49.
98. Dempsey J, Hillege S, Hill R, editors. Fundamentals of nursing and midwifery: a person-centred approach to care. 2nd ed. Australia, New Zealand. Sydney: Lippincott, Williams & Wilkins; 2013.

99. Charon JM. Symbolic interactionism: an introduction, an interpretation, an integration. 10th ed. Upper Saddle River: Prentice-Hall; 2009.
100. Gushue GV, Mejia-Smith BX, Fisher LD, et al. Differentiation of self and racial identity. Couns Psychol Q 2013;26(3–4):343–61.
101. Wepa D. Cultural safety in Aotearoa New Zealand. 2nd ed. Melbourne: Cambridge University Press; 2015.
102. Davidson JE, Daly BJ, Agan D, et al. Facilitated sensemaking: a feasibility study for the provision of a family support program in the intensive care unit. Crit Care Nurs Q 2010;33(2):177–89.
103. Wilson D, Hickey H. Māori health: Māori- and whānau-centred practice. In: Wepa D, editor. Cultural safety in Aotearoa New Zealand. Melbourne, Australia: Cambridge University Press; 2015. p. 235–51.
104. Wilson D, Heaslip V, Jackson D. Improving equity and cultural responsiveness with marginalised communities: understanding competing worldviews. J Clin Nurs 2018;00:1–10.
105. Heyland DK, Davidson J, Skrobik Y, et al. Improving partnerships with family members of ICU patients: study protocol for a randomized controlled trial. Trials 2018;19:1–11.
106. Mol MMC, Boeter TGW, Verharen L, et al. Patient- and family-centred care in the intensive care unit: a challenge in the daily practice of healthcare professionals. J Clin Nurs 2017;26(19–20):3212–23.
107. McKinnon J. The case for concordance: value and application in nursing practice. Br J Nurs 2013;22(13):766–71.
108. Almutairi AF, Adlan AA, Nasim M. Perceptions of the critical cultural competence of registered nurses in Canada. BMC Nurs 2017;16:1–9.
109. Gill GK, Babacan H. Developing a cultural responsiveness framework in healthcare systems: an Australian example. Divers Equal Health Care 2012;9(1):45–55.
110. Leininger MM. Cultural care diversity and universality: a theory of nursing. New York: National League for Nursing Press; 2001.
111. Ramsden IM. Cultural safety and nursing education in Aotearoa and Te Waipounamu. Wellington: Victoria University of Wellington; 2002.
112. Ramsden I. Kawa Whakaruruhau: cultural safety in nursing education in Aotearoa. Wellington, New Zealand. Nursing Council of New Zealand 1991.
113. Lee H, Fitzpatrick JJ, Baik S-Y. Why isn't evidence based practice improving health care for minorities in the United States? Appl Nurs Res 2013;26(4):263–8.
114. Wood PJ, Schwass M. Cultural safety: a framework for changing attitudes. Nursing Praxis in New Zealand 1993;8(1):4–15.
115. McDonough S, Chopra P, Tuncer C, et al. Enhancing cultural responsiveness: the development of a pilot transcultural secondary consultation program. Australas Psychiatry 2013;21(5):494–8.
116. Dudas KI. Cultural competence: an evolutionary concept analysis. Nursing Educ Perspect 2012;33(5):317–21.
117. Perng S-J, Watson R. Construct validation of the Nurse Cultural Competence Scale: a hierarchy of abilities. J Clin Nurs 2012;21(11/12):1678–84.
118. Ingram RR. Using Campinha-Bacote's process of cultural competence model to examine the relationship between health literacy and cultural competence: health literacy and cultural competence. J Adv Nurs 2012;68(3):695–704.
119. Betancourt JR, Green AR. Linking cultural competence training to improved health outcomes. In: Laveist TA, Isaac LA, editors. Race, ethnicity and health: a public health reader. San Francisco: Jossey-Bass; 2013.
120. Minkler M. Community organizing and community building for health and welfare. 3rd ed. New Brunswick: Rutgers University Press; 2012.
121. Durie M Cultural competence and medical practice in New Zealand. Australian and New Zealand Boards and Council Conference; November 21; Wellington, New Zealand 2001.
122. Australian Bureau of Statistics. 6250.0 - Characteristics of recent migrants, Australia, November 2016. Canberra, ACT: Australian Bureau of Statistics; 2017. Available from: https://secure.abs.gov.au/ausstats/abs@.nsf/0/E92EA270A32AF8F1CA256953007D9AFA?Opendocument.
123. Statistics New Zealand. Quick stats: About culture and identity 2014. Available from: http://archive.stats.govt.nz/Census/2013-census/profile-and-summary-reports/quickstats-culture-identity/birthplace.aspx.
124. Statistics Canada. Immigration and ethnocultural diversity in Canada 2015. Available from: https://www12.statcan.gc.ca/nhs-enm/2011/as-sa/99-010-x/99-010-x2011001-eng.cfm.
125. United States Census Bureau. Quick facts United States 2017. Available from: https://www.census.gov/quickfacts/fact/table/US/PST045217.
126. UK Office for National Statistics. Health and social care, 2016. Available from: https://www.ons.gov.uk/peoplepopulationandcommunity/healthandsocialcare.
127. Ruston A, Smith D. Gypsies/travellers and health: risk categorisation versus being 'at risk'. Health Risk Soc 2013;15(2):176–93.
128. Smith D, Ruston A. 'If you feel that nobody wants you you'll withdraw into your own': Gypsies/Travellers, networks and healthcare utilisation. Soc Health Ill 2013;35(8):1196–210.
129. Campinha-Bacote J. The process of cultural competence in the delivery of healthcare services: a model of care. J Transcult Nurs 2002;13(3):181–4.
130. Ellis L, Gergen J, Wohlgemuth L, et al. Empowering the 'cheerers': role of surgical intensive care unit nurses in enhancing family resilience. Am J Crit Care 2016;25(1):39–45.
131. Boles J. Bearing bad news: supporting patients and families through difficult conversations. Pediatr Nurs 2015;41(6):306–8.
132. Huynh HP, Sweeny K, Miller T. Transformational leadership in primary care: Clinicians' patterned approaches to care predict patient satisfaction and health expectations. J Health Psychol 2018;23(5):743–53.
133. Knapp SJ, Sole ML, Byers JF. The EPICS Family Bundle and its effects on stress and coping of families of critically Ill trauma patients. Appl Nurs Res 2013;26(2):51–7.

134. Wilson D, Barton P. Indigenous hospital experiences: a New Zealand case study. J Clin Nurs 2012;21(15–16):2316–26.
135. Boucher NA. Direct engagement with communities and interprofessional learning to factor culture into end-of-life health care delivery. Am J Public Healt 2016;106(6):996–1001.
136. Cometto G, Witter S, Boerma T, et al. Tackling health workforce challenges to universal health coverage: setting targets and measuring progress. Bull World Health Organ 2013;91(11):881–9.
137. Mbuzi V, Fulbrook P, Jessup M. Indigenous peoples experiences and perceptions of hospitalisation for acute care: a metasynthesis of qualitative studies. Int J Nurs Stud 2017;71:39–49.
138. Cohen JJ, Gabriel BA, Terrell C. The case for diversity in the health care workforce. Health Affairs (Millwood) 2002;21(5):90–102.
139. American Association of Colleges of Nursing. Diversity, inclusion, & equity in academic nursing: AACN position statement 2017. Available from: http://www.aacnnursing.org/Portals/42/News/Position-Statements/Diversity-Inclusion.pdf.
140. Doolen J, York NL. Cultural differences with end-of-life care in the critical care unit. Dimens Crit Care Nurs 2007;26(5):194–8.
141. Procter S. Whose evidence? Agenda setting in multi-professional research: observations from a case study. Health, Risk & Society 2002;4(1):45–59.
142. Petroz U, Kennedy D, Webster F, et al. Patients' perceptions of individualized care: evaluating psychometric properties and results of the individualized care scale. Can J Nurs Res 2011;43(2):80–100.
143. Shaw J, Pemberton S, Pratt C, et al. Shadowing: a central component of patient and family-centred care. Nursing Management - UK 2014;21(3):20–3.
144. Bredemeyer S, Reid S, Polverino J, et al. Implementation and evaluation of an individualized developmental care program in a neonatal intensive care unit. J Spec Pediatr Nurs 2008;13(4):281–91.
145. Suhonen R, Valimaki M, Leino-Kilpi H. Individualized care, quality of life and satisfaction with nursing care. J Adv Nurs 2005;50(3): 283–92.
146. Coombs M, Mitchell M, James S, et al. Intensive care bereavement practices across New Zealand and Australian intensive care units: a qualitative content analysis. J Clin Nurs 2017;26(19–20):2944–52.
147. Jansson I, Pilhamar E, Forsberg A. Factors and conditions that have an impact in relation to the successful implementation and maintenance of individual care plans. Worldviews Evid Based Nurs 2011;8(2):66–75.
148. Bone N, Swinton M, Hoad N. Critical care nurses' experiences with spiritual care: the spirit study. Am J Crit Care 2018;27(3):212–19.
149. Coombs M. A scoping review of family experience and need during end of life care in intensive care. Nursing Open 2015;2(1):24–35.
150. Abu-El-Noor N. ICU nurses' perceptions and practice of spiritual care at the end of life: implications for policy change. Online J Issue Nurs 2016;21(1):6.
151. Ramezani M, Ahmadi F, Mohammadi E, et al. Spiritual care in nursing: a concept analysis. Int Nurs Rev 2014;61(2):211–19.
152. Kisorio LC, Langley GC. Intensive care nurses' experiences of end-of-life care. Intensive Crit Care Nurs 2016;33:30–8.
153. Blockley C. Meeting patients' religious needs. Kai Tiaki Nursing New Zealand 2001;7(11):15–17.
154. Cook D, Rocker G. Dying with dignity in the Intensive Care Unit. New Engl J Med 2014;370(26):2506–14.
155. Berry M, Brink E, Metaxa V. Time for change? A national audit on bereavement care in intensive care units. J Intensive Care Soc 2017;18(1):11–16.
156. Halligan P. Caring for patients of Islamic denomination: critical care nurses' experiences in Saudi Arabia. J Clin Nurs 2006;15(12): 1565–73.
157. Kongsuwan W, Locsin RC. Promoting peaceful death in the intensive care unit in Thailand. Int Nurs Rev 2009;56(1):116–22.
158. Banjar AK. Till death do us part: the evolution of end-of-life and death attitudes. Can J Crit Care Nurs 2017;28(3):34–40.
159. Moradnezhad M, Seylani K, Navab E, et al. Spiritual intelligence of nurses working at the intensive care units of hospitals affiliated with Tehran University of Medical Sciences. Nursing Practice Today 2017;4(4):170–9.
160. Kisorio LC, Langley GC. End-of-life care in intensive care unit: family experiences. Intensiv Crit Care Nurs 2016;35:57–65.
161. Sprung CL, Maia P, Bulow H-H, et al. The importance of religious affiliation and culture on end-of-life decisions in European intensive care units. Intens Care Med 2007;33(10):1732–9.
162. Murthy S, Wunsch H. Clinical review: international comparisons in critical care - lessons learned. Crit Care 2012;16(2):218.
163. Australia and New Zealand Intensive Care Society. Intensive care: Centre for Outcome and Resource evaluation. Resource and activity report 2014-2015: ANZICS Centre for Outcome and Resource Evaluation (CORE); 2016. Available from: http://www.anzics.com.au/Downloads/ANZICS%20CORE%20Annual%20Report%202015.pdfCarlton. [Accessed 12 April 2018].
164. Gries CJ, Curtis JR, Wall RJ, et al. Family member satisfaction with end-of-life decision making in the ICU. Chest 2008;133(3):704–12.
165. Kehl KA. Moving toward peace: an analysis of the concept of a good death. Am J Hosp Palliat Care 2006;23(4):277–86.
166. Edwards J, Voigt L, Nelson J, et al. Ten key points about ICU palliative care. Intensive Care Med 2017;43(1):83–5.
167. Beckstrand RL, Hadley KH, Luthy KE, et al. Critical care nurses' suggestions to improve end-of-life care obstacles: minimal change over 17 years. Dimens Crit Care Nurs 2017;36(4):264–70.
168. Gaeta S, Price KJ. End-of-life issues in critically ill cancer patients. Crit Care Clin 2010;26(1):219–27.
169. Ranse K, Yates P, Coyer F. End-of-life care practices of critical care nurses: a national cross-sectional survey. Aust Crit Care 2016;29(2):83–9.

170. Myburgh J, Abillama F, Chiumello D, et al. End-of-life care in the intensive care unit: Report From the Task Force of World Federation of Societies of Intensive and Critical Care Medicine. J Crit Care 2016;34:125–30.
171. Schaefer KG, Block SD. Physician communication with families in the ICU: evidence-based strategies for improvement. Curr Opin Crit Care 2009;15(6):569–77.
172. Pignatiello G, Hickman RL Jr, Hetland B. End-of-life decision support in the ICU: where are we now? West J Nurs Res 2018;40(1):84–120.
173. Noome M, Dijkstra BM, van Leeuwen E, et al. Exploring family experiences of nursing aspects of end-of-life care in the ICU: a qualitative study. Intensiv Crit Care Nurs 2016;33:56–64.
174. Singer AE, Ash T, Ochotorena C, et al. A systematic review of family meeting tools in palliative and intensive care settings. Am J Hosp Palliat Care 2016;33(8):797–806.
175. Siegel MD. End-of-life decision making in the ICU. Clin Chest Med 2009;30(1):181–94.
176. Seaman JB. Improving care at end of life in the ICU: a proposal for early discussion of goals of care. J Gerontol Nurs 2013;39(8):52–8.
177. Pochard F, Darmon M, Fassier T, et al. Symptoms of anxiety and depression in family members of intensive care unit patients before discharge or death. A prospective multicenter study. J Crit Care 2005;20(1):90–6.
178. Curtis JR, Ciechanowski PS, Downey L, et al. Development and evaluation of an interprofessional communication intervention to improve family outcomes in the ICU. Contemp Clin Trials 2012;33(6):1245–54.
179. Coombs MA, Parker R, Ranse K, et al. An integrative review of how families are prepared for, and supported during withdrawal of life-sustaining treatment in intensive care. J Adv Nurs 2017;73(1):39–55.
180. Krueger G. Meaning-making in the aftermath of sudden infant death syndrome. Nurs Inq 2006;13(3):163–71.
181. Nelson JE, Angus DC, Weissfeld LA, et al. End-of-life care for the critically ill: a national intensive care unit survey. Crit Care Med 2006;34(10):2547–53.
182. Anderson WG, Arnold RM, Angus DC, et al. Posttraumatic stress and complicated grief in family members of patients in the Intensive Care Unit. J Gen Intern Med 2008;23(11):1871–6.
183. Stroebe M, Schut H, Stroebe W. Health outcomes of bereavement. Lancet 2007;370(9603):1960–73.
184. Golden A-MJ, Dalgleish T. Is prolonged grief distinct from bereavement-related posttraumatic stress? Psychiatry Res 2010;178(2):336–41.
185. Kuschner WG, Gruenewald DA, Clum N, et al. Implementation of ICU palliative care guidelines and procedures. Chest 2009;135(1):26–32.
186. Department of Health. Bereavement care services: a synthesis of the literature. London: Department of Health; 2011.
187. Cook D, Rocker G, Heyland D. Dying in the ICU: strategies that may improve end-of-life care. Can J Anaesth 2004;51(3):266–72.
188. Preciado A, Vachhani A, Gilbert A, et al. Innovative solutions: the C.O.R.E. to sociocultural care in nursing. Dimens Crit Care Nur 2012;31(5):283–6.
189. Egerod I, Kaldan G, Coombs M, et al. Family-centered bereavement practices in Danish intensive care units: a cross-sectional national survey. Intensive Crit Care Nurs 2018;45:52–7.
190. Mitchell M, Coombs M, Wetzig K. The provision of family-centred intensive care bereavement support in Australia and New Zealand: results of a cross sectional explorative descriptive survey. Aust Crit Care 2017;30(3):139–44.
191. Quenot JP, Rigaud JP, Prin S, et al. Suffering among carers working in critical care can be reduced by an intensive communication strategy on end-of-life practices. Intensive Care Med 2012;38(1):55–61.
192. Shaw DJ, Davidson JE, Smilde RI, et al. Multidisciplinary team training to enhance family communication in the ICU. Crit Care Med 2014;42(2):265–71.
193. Rogers S, Babgi A, Gomez C. Educational interventions in end-of-life care: part I. Adv Neonatal Care 2008;8(1):56–65.
194. Simpson N, Knott CI. Stress and burnout in intensive care medicine: an Australian perspective. Med J Aust 2017;206(3):107–8.
195. Sacco TL, Ciurzynski SM, Harvey ME, et al. Compassion satisfaction and compassion fatigue among critical care nurses. Crit Care Nurs 2015;35(4):32–43. quiz.
196. Figley CR. Compassion fatigue: Psychotherapists' chronic lack of self care. J Clin Psychol 2002;58(11):1433–41.
197. Jones J, Winch S, Strube P, et al. Delivering compassionate care in intensive care units: nurses' perceptions of enablers and barriers. J Adv Nurs 2016;72(12):3137–46.
198. Strube P, Henderson A, Mitchell ML, et al. The role of the nurse educator in sustaining compassion in the workplace: a case study from an intensive care unit. J Contin Educ Nurs 2018;49(5):221–4.
199. Winch S, Henderson AJ, Kay M, et al. Understanding compassion literacy in nursing through a clinical compassion cafe. J Contin Educ Nurs 2014;45(11):484–6.
200. Jakimowicz S, Perry L, Lewis J. Compassion satisfaction and fatigue: a cross-sectional survey of Australian intensive care nurses. Aust Crit Care 2017.

Chapter 8

Recovery and rehabilitation

Janice Rattray, Leanne Aitken

KEY WORDS

cognitive dysfunction

health-related quality of life

intensive care unit-acquired weakness

post-intensive care syndrome

posttraumatic stress symptoms

psychological sequelae

Learning objectives

After reading this chapter, you should be able to:

- discuss the physical, psychological and cognitive sequelae some survivors experience after critical illness
- identify the risk factors associated with poor physical, psychological and cognitive sequelae
- outline the common functional, psychological, cognitive and health-related quality of life (HRQOL) instruments used to assess patient outcomes after a critical illness
- identify a range of potential interventions that may prevent or reduce the short- and long-term consequences of critical illness.
- examine the benefits and challenges for implementing interventions in intensive care unit (ICU), in hospital after ICU discharge and after hospital discharge to improve recovery and rehabilitation.

Introduction

Millions of people each year experience a critical illness requiring admission to an intensive care unit (ICU). Although overall survival rates are generally above 80% at hospital discharge, recovery for individuals is often delayed beyond 6 months postdischarge.[1] Physical de-conditioning and neuromuscular dysfunction[2] as well as psychological[3-5] and cognitive sequelae[6] are common, adding to the burden of illness for survivors, carers, the healthcare system and broader society.

Although ICU clinicians have traditionally focused on survival as the principal indicator of patient outcome and unit performance, physical, psychological and cognitive functioning and health-related quality of life (HRQOL) have now emerged as legitimate patient outcomes from both practice and research perspectives.[1,7] With this shifting focus towards long-term health and wellbeing has also come a reconsideration and re-conceptualisation of critical care as only one component in the continuum of care for a critically ill patient. An episode of critical illness is now viewed as a continuum that begins with the onset of acute clinical deterioration, includes the ICU admission and continues until the patient's risk of late sequelae has returned

FIGURE 8.1 The continuum of critical illness.

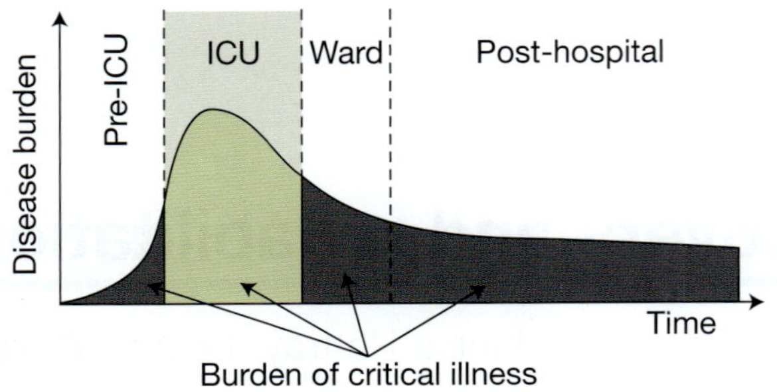

Source: Angus DC, Carlet J. Surviving intensive care: a report from the 2002 Brussels Roundtable. Intensive Care Med 2003;29(3):368-77.

to the baseline risk of a similar individual who has not incurred a critical illness[1,8] (Fig. 8.1). Timing of this recovery trajectory is variable, and related to a number of individual, illness and treatment factors. Interventions need to be delivered in a manner that takes into account this trajectory and related factors and incorporates the expertise of all members of the multidisciplinary team.

Reviews of numerous observational studies confirm delayed recovery in HRQOL[9] with physical, psychological and cognitive symptoms prevalent:

- weakness: approximately 40%[2,10,11]
- delirium: up to 81% with average of 32%[12]
- anxiety: up to 45%[3,13]
- depression: approximately 30%[4]
- posttraumatic stress symptoms: approximately 20%[5]
- cognitive dysfunction: 36–62%.[6]

Recognition of the frequency, and co-occurrence, of these elements of compromise has led to the development of the term 'post-intensive care syndrome' (PICS) to 'describe new or worsening impairments in physical, cognitive, or mental health status arising after critical illness and persisting beyond acute care hospitalisation'.[1] While significant sequelae therefore exist for a substantial proportion of critical illness survivors, limited evidence is currently available to support specific interventions for improving their recovery.

In further chapters of this book patient comfort and psychological issues including comfort and sedation management and delirium monitoring while in ICU (Chapter 6) and breathing trials and weaning from mechanical ventilation (Chapter 15) are discussed. Common physical and psychological sequelae associated with a critical illness, and how this impacts on a survivor's HRQOL, are discussed in this chapter. Common instruments measuring physical, psychological, cognitive and HRQOL are described. Rehabilitation strategies, commencing in-ICU and extending both post-ICU and post-hospital that can be delivered by the multidisciplinary team are also discussed.

Compromise following a critical illness

Examination of patient outcomes beyond survival is an important contemporary topic for critical care practice and research. Patient outcomes after a critical illness or injury were traditionally measured using a number of objective parameters (e.g. number of organ failure-free days, 28-day status, or 1-year mortality). Other measures that examined patient-centred concepts such as functional status, HRQOL, psychological health and cognitive function have become more prevalent in the past 10 years.[1] The notion of 'survivorship' in this patient group is receiving increasing interest [14,15] recognising that the recovery trajectory from a critical illness may be long and incomplete, mapping this path is a complex process.

Health-related quality of life

Survivors of critical illness or trauma experience compromised HRQOL for varying periods of time after leaving ICU. HRQOL covers a number of physical, psychological, emotional and social domains of life and is now generally accepted as an important outcome measure. Within this chapter, we guide the reader to the commonly used measures but present the physical and psychological issues separately. Ongoing physical and psychological problems tend to impact negatively on social, environmental and economic elements in life,[16] and many patients and families experience a significant economic challenge during the recovery process. Although some patients recover quickly and do not report ongoing issues, others report significant and protracted compromise in their quality of life.[17] It is clear that survivors of critical illness have markedly lower HRQOL than other members in the community when matched for age and gender. Although there is convincing evidence of this widespread compromise, we also know that recovery patterns vary for individual patients, with some recovering rapidly. Factors that have been shown to influence components of quality of life include age, comorbidities[18] lower socioeconomic status, social integration,[19] gender, severity of illness, primary diagnosis,[9] frailty[20] and length of ICU stay, although few of these factors appear to affect people in a consistent manner. Individual characteristics will also influence recovery although this is an area where there is limited research. For example, those with an emotion-focused coping style may have better mental health-related quality of life.[21]

ICU-acquired weakness

Critical illness myopathy (CIM), polyneuropathy (CIP) and neuromyopathy (CINM) syndromes occur in

50–100% of ICU survivors.[2,11] ICU-acquired weakness (ICU-AW) has come into use as a term that encompasses these syndromes of muscle wasting and functional weakness in patients with a critical illness who have no other plausible aetiology.[22,23] The three syndromes above form the sub-categories of ICU-AW, with CINM used when both myopathy and axonal polyneuropathy are evident. Development of ICU-AW is associated with a number of risk factors that occur during intensive care treatment:[24,25]

- critical illness: sepsis, systemic inflammatory response syndrome (SIRS), multi-organ system failure, catabolic state
- treatments: mechanical ventilation, hyperglycaemia, hypoalbuminaemia, parenteral nutrition, glucocorticoids, sedatives, neuromuscular blocking agents, immobility.

Local and systemic inflammation acts synergistically with bed rest and immobility to alter metabolic and structural function of muscles,[26] resulting in muscle atrophy and contractile dysfunction, loss of flexibility, CIP, heterotopic ossification and entrapment neuropathy.[22] Muscle wasting can occur rapidly, with patients losing up to 30% of their muscle mass within 10 days of being admitted to the ICU.[27] This muscle loss contributes to weakness and disability and a prolonged recovery period. These neuromuscular dysfunctions are diagnosed by clinical assessment, diagnostic studies (electrophysiology, ultrasound) or histology of muscle or nerve tissue.

The syndrome of ICU-AW manifests as prolonged weaning time, inability to mobilise and reduced functional capacity. Patients with ICU-AW also experience increased mortality.[28] ICU-AW has also been linked with reductions in both functional ability and HRQOL that may persist for months or years after discharge, although effects appear to be inconsistent across different groups of critical illness survivors.[29-31]

Clinical assessment

Clinical assessment includes identification of generalised weakness following the onset of a critical illness, exclusion of other diagnoses (e.g. Guillain–Barré syndrome) and measurement of muscle strength. Instruments are available to assess both volitional and non-volitional muscle strength.[32] Manual muscle testing is commonly assessed using the Medical Research Council (MRC) Scale,[33] a 0–5-point ordinal scale:

0 = no contraction
1 = flicker or trace of muscle contraction
2 = full range of active movement with gravity eliminated
3 = reduced power but active movement against gravity
4 = reduced power but active movement against gravity and resistance
5 = normal power against gravity and full resistance.

For patients who are awake and cooperative, each muscle group is assessed sequentially for strength and symmetry:

- upper limb: deltoid, biceps, wrist extensors
- lower limb: quadriceps, gluteus maximus, ankle dorsiflexion.

Weakness is evident in patients with an MRC sum score of <48 (<4 in all testable muscle groups); this should be re-tested after 24 hours. Weakness (<4 MRC Scale) is associated with worse survival up to 5 years after critical illness.[34]

Hand-held dynamometry and handgrip dynamometry can also be used to measure volitional muscle strength using a calibrated device for patients who are conscious and cooperative. The benefit of these measures is increased objectivity to obtain continuous data.[32] All volitional strength measurements may be affected by the level of awareness and cooperation of patients, as well as their motivation, although inter-rater reliability of the MRC sum score as well as hand-held dynamometry and handgrip dynamometry has been shown to be good to very good.[32,33]

Diagnostic testing

Electrophysiological testing (nerve conduction studies, needle electromyography) may be useful to differentiate between CIM and CIP, although this distinction is difficult and often not required in the clinical setting.[24,33] Histology for CIP is primarily noted as distal axonal degeneration in both sensory and motor fibres, while the characteristic findings in CIM are patchy loss of myosin (thick filaments), necrosis and fast twitch fibre atrophy.[22]

Practice tip

Current clinical recommendations to limit muscle wasting in ICU include:

- minimising patient exposure to corticosteroids and neuromuscular blocking agents
- limiting depth of sedation
- moderate glycaemic control
- early mobilisation

Psychological health

Psychological responses to a critical illness and patients' memories of experiences during an ICU admission have been explored using quantitative[35,36] and/or qualitative approaches.[37-39] Some survivors reported increased anxiety, including transfer anxiety (discharge from ICU);[3] depression[4]; posttraumatic stress;[5,40] hallucinations;[35] and continuing cognitive dysfunction.[6,41]

For some patients, recovery from a critical illness results in short- and long-term psychological dysfunction (e.g. anxiety, depression and posttraumatic stress symptoms), which potentially result in additional health problems, reduced HRQOL,[9,42] reduction in social activities and functioning and failure to engage with rehabilitation programs.[43] Our understanding of these sequelae and their consequences has improved over the past decade in part due to increased research activity. The introduction of follow-up services within the UK has also contributed significantly to this increased understanding through the regular collection of a range of measures that assess physical and psychological symptoms. Many of these services are nurse-led, multidisciplinary services (discussed later in the chapter), and we must not underestimate the contribution of their routine clinical observations. Risk factors have been identified and a range of interventions tested. These will be discussed later in the chapter.

Anxiety and depression

The most commonly used measure to assess anxiety and depression in this patient population is the Hospital Anxiety and Depression Scale (HADS)[3] and this will be discussed later in the chapter. This measure has two 'cut-off' scores to indicate possible (8–10) or probable (>11) presence of either an anxiety or depressive disorder. In a number of recent systematic reviews prevalence rates of anxiety and depression have been reported. Nikayin et al.[3] reported anxiety pooled prevalence rates with 20% of patients demonstrating probable (>11) anxiety disorder at 6 months, reducing to 17% at 12-14 months, and Rabiee et al.,[4] reported probable depressive disorder around 17% at six months reducing to 13% at 12–14 months. These figures are higher when the lower 'cut-off' score is used with 34% reporting significant anxiety symptoms at 12–14 months and 29% symptoms of depression, and although these latter figures do not represent a clinical disorder, it is clear that for many patients they have ongoing, enduring issues.

Patients often exhibit high levels of distress at the time of hospital discharge and these tend to reduce during the first year after discharge.[13,44] However, the episodic timing of assessments may not fully capture the potentially varied trajectory of anxiety and depression symptoms, and establish whether full resolution is achieved, or identify a later onset problem. For example, in patients with acute respiratory distress syndrome (ARDS), levels of depression increased from 16% at 1 year after discharge to 23% at 2 years,[45] while patients with ongoing physical care needs were more likely to exhibit depressive symptoms.[46] This may reflect prolonged recovery in general. A rise in depression scores may therefore be a reflection of that prolonged physical recovery. Our lack of understanding of symptom trajectory has implications for both symptom monitoring and care delivery after ICU discharge.

Anxiety and depression are also associated with other aspects of recovery and, in particular, HRQOL. Depressed and/or anxious patients tend to rate their HRQOL as poorer than those who are not.[45,47] However, what is less clear is the direction of this relationship; it could be that patients with a poorer HRQOL tend to be depressed or anxious rather than depression or anxiety leading to perceptions of poorer HRQOL.

Patients who have or have had psychological problems prior to intensive care are likely to continue to have or will develop these again after discharge,[3,43] and this is true for both anxiety and depression. Individuals who demonstrate trait anxiety are more likely to be anxious after critical illness.[13]

Few risk factors for anxiety and depressive symptoms have been consistently identified. In a general population, depression is more commonly associated with being female and middle-aged, yet this is not so in intensive care survivors.[4] Length of stay, admission diagnosis, illness severity, sedation regimens including daily sedation withdrawal and light sedation, sleep problems after discharge have been associated with either anxiety or depressive symptoms in univariate analyses, but not consistently in multivariate analyses.[3,48] Rather it is a preexisting psychological or psychiatric problem, distress at time of hospital discharge, and memories of the critical illness experience that appear to be related to subsequent symptoms.[13,43] The latter has consistently been identified as a predictor of subsequent psychological recovery, and those patients who experience distressing memories that are often described as nightmares or hallucinations or extreme fear are more likely to have ongoing psychological problems.[3,13,43]

Although assessment of pre-ICU status is difficult, in some cases this information can be obtained from relatives or caregivers e.g. if a patient is receiving antidepressant or anxiolytic medication or has seen a psychiatrist or psychologist. It is becoming increasingly clear that anxiety, depression and posttraumatic stress tend to co-exist.[43,49] While these may be related, they have important distinct differences and treatments.

Posttraumatic stress

In recent years there has been increasing interest in the development of posttraumatic stress reactions such as posttraumatic symptomatology (PTSS) or posttraumatic stress disorder (PTSD) as a response to critical illness,[40] and there is increasing recognition of these symptoms as a significant problem for some intensive care survivors.[50] What has been difficult to establish is whether it is being critically ill per se or the environment and treatments within critical care that predispose survivors to develop posttraumatic stress symptoms.[40] Individuals are required to meet a number of criteria before a diagnosis of PTSD is considered, and in 2013 the American Psychiatric Association presented the DSM-V criteria for PTSD (see Box 8.1 for these criteria).[51]

Many symptoms of posttraumatic stress that patients experience in the initial days after intensive care discharge may be considered a normal reaction, and it is important that practitioners clearly separate the normal from the abnormal response. This is achieved by assessing

BOX 8.1

Posttraumatic stress disorder diagnostic criteria[51]

Criterion A: Stressor – The person was exposed to: death, threatened death, actual or threatened serious injury or actual or threatened sexual violence, as follows (one required):

1 Direct exposure
2 Witnessing, in person
3 Indirectly, by learning that a close relative or close friend was exposed to trauma. If the event involved actual or threatened death, it must have been violent or accidental
4 Repeated or extreme indirect exposure to aversive details of the event(s) usually in the course of professional duties. This does not include indirect non-professional exposure through electronic media, television, movies or pictures

Criterion B: Intrusion symptoms – The traumatic event is persistently re-experienced in the following way (one required):

1 Recurrent, involuntary and intrusive memories
2 Traumatic nightmares
3 Dissociative reactions (e.g. flashbacks), which may occur on a continuum from brief episodes to complete loss of consciousness
4 Intensive or prolonged distress after exposure to traumatic reminders
5 Marked physiological reactivity after exposure to trauma-related stimuli

Criterion C: Avoidance – Persistent effortful avoidance of distressing trauma-related stimuli after the event (one required):

1 Trauma-related thoughts or feelings
2 Trauma-related external reminders

Criterion D: Negative alterations in cognitions and mood – Negative alterations in cognitions and mood that began or worsened after the traumatic event (two required):

1 Inability to recall key features of the traumatic event (usually dissociative amnesia: not due to head injury, alcohol or drugs)
2 Persistent (and often distorted) negative beliefs and expectations about one's self or the world (e.g. I am bad, the world is completely dangerous)
3 Persistent distorted blame of self or others for causing the traumatic event or for resulting consequences
4 Persistent negative trauma-related emotions (e.g. fear, horror, anger, guilt or shame)
5 Markedly diminished interest in (pre-traumatic) significant activities
6 Feeling alienated from others (e.g. detachment or estrangement)
7 Constricted affect: persistent inability to experience positive emotions

Criterion E: Alterations in arousal and reactivity – Trauma-related alterations in arousal and reactivity that began or worsened after the traumatic event (two required):

1 Irritable or aggressive behaviour
2 Self-destructive or reckless behaviour
3 Hypervigilance
4 Exaggerated startle response
5 Problems in concentration
6 Sleep disturbance

Criterion F: Duration
Persistence of symptoms (in Criteria B, C, D and E) for more than 1 month

Criterion G: Functional significance
Significant symptom-related distress or functional impairment (e.g. social, occupational)

Criterion H: Exclusion
Disturbance is not due to medication, substance use, or other illness

Source: US Department of Veterans Affairs. PTSD: National Center for PTSD Washington, DC: US Department of Veterans Affairs; 2014 [cited 2018 23/03/2018]. http://www.ptsd.va.gov.

the severity and duration of symptoms, and their effect on an individual's life. PTSD should not be diagnosed until at least 1 month after the event, and until the symptoms have been present for 1 month. Symptoms commonly cause problems in relation to work, social or other important activities.[52]

Signs of posttraumatic stress include four main symptom areas: intrusive thoughts, avoidance behaviours, negative alterations in cognitions and mood and hyper-arousal symptoms.[52] Individuals can re-experience a traumatic event through involuntary unwanted thoughts, often in the form of 'flashbacks' and/or 'nightmares'. Individuals experiencing these thoughts often develop avoidant behaviours in the belief this action will reduce the intrusive thoughts. Avoidant behaviours for intensive care patients can range from simply avoiding television programs about hospitals, not talking about their ICU experience or, more seriously, non-attendance at a follow-up clinic or other hospital outpatient appointments. The latter also compounds the issue of accurate prevalence. It is these two symptom clusters (avoidant behaviours and intrusive thoughts) that appear more prevalent in

ICU survivors.[53] Negative alterations in cognitions and mood may include continuing self-blame or blaming others about the cause or consequences of the critical illness.[52] Hyper-arousal behaviours include difficulties in concentrating or falling asleep. ICU survivors may be preoccupied with these intrusive thoughts, concerns about future health issues, and may engage in negative health behaviours.[53]

Current research has concentrated on prevalence of symptoms at one point in time or group changes over time. Few have considered different trajectories. A number of these have been proposed within the wider PTSS/PTSD literature and include resilient, recovery, delayed reaction and chronic.[54,55] The first trajectory, as the name suggests, consists of those with few symptoms at any time point; a recovery trajectory represents those patients who may exhibit initial distress but this reduces over time; a delayed reaction will result in symptoms worsening over time and those with chronic distress will have consistently high levels of symptoms.[54] In a study of trauma survivors over a period of 6 years, Bryant and colleagues[54] described these four trajectories but include a fifth – worsening/recovery where symptoms worsened over time and then recovered. The majority of patients were in the resilient group (73%) with 10% worsening, 8% worsening/recovery, 6% recovery and 5% chronic. An independent predictor of a poorer trajectory was admission to an ICU.[54] We do not know whether ICU patients experience similar trajectories and this is an important gap. Recognising such trajectories has implications for what and how we deliver short and long-term psychological therapies.

As with other psychological symptoms such as anxiety and depression, it has been difficult to establish the prevalence of PTSD after intensive care because of the use of self-report measures, different research designs, varied patient case-mix and international variations in the delivery of intensive care. These variations have resulted in over-estimation of the prevalence of PTSD and PTSS.[56] Patients may have significant PTSS without developing PTSD and it is mainly these symptoms that are assessed using the self-report measures. Reported prevalence of significant PTSS or PTSD ranges from 5% to 64%, with an average of around 20% experiencing significant issues[53] during the first year after discharge.[57,58] What is important is that once PTSS or PTSD is established, it is enduring and without treatment may last for several years.

There are certain risk factors that predict posttraumatic stress symptoms, although also not consistently.[5,40] Those more consistently associated include: previous psychiatric history,[43] previous stressful events,[49] frightening intensive care experience, use of restraints,[59] and benzodiazepine use.[5,40] The literature is more equivocal in relation to age, gender, admission diagnosis, length of ICU stay, and mechanical ventilation and although these have been cited previously as risk factors, results from a recent systematic review are less compelling.[5,40]

Interestingly, individual characteristics such as employment and level of education also appear to predict those most at risk.[60,61] Early signs of acute stress or depression are a strong predictor of ongoing problems.[62] Ongoing sleep problems which can be prevalent after intensive care have been associated with PTSS in one study;[62] however, it is unclear whether poor sleep quality mediates PTSS or PTSS causes sleep problems. This is an area for further study.

We have limited understanding of factors that protect against the development of psychological problems. There is little research in this patient group exploring the role of an individual's coping strategies, social support and resilience.[40] Understanding these will assist us to better predict those at risk.

What is evident in the emerging literature is the effect of patients' subjective intensive care experiences.[5,62-64] These experiences, reported as unpleasant memories of being in ICU consistently predict subsequent poorer psychological outcomes.[37,39,65] They are discussed later in this chapter. While this evidence appears strong, that related to delirium is contradictory. In a systematic review no consistent relationship between delirium and subsequent emotional outcome was identified.[66]

Memories and perceptions

Interestingly, illness severity does not consistently predict a PTSS reaction,[40] but such a reaction is more likely to be influenced by patients' perceptions of their intensive care experience. This is one of the unique features of being in intensive care: patients have limited recall for factual events and often report large gaps where they remember very little about their critical illness. Some patients will report upsetting or unpleasant factual memories such as pain, oxygen masks on a patient's face and difficulty breathing.[50] However, frequently, patients' accounts include disturbing recollections with memories of 'odd perceptual experiences',[38,67] 'nightmares' or 'hallucinations'.[50] While not all patients experience these, those who do so tend to report memories that are persecutory in nature,[50] are often associated with feelings of being elsewhere,[68] or fighting for survival. These memories often seemed 'real' and were distressing to patients at the time, and may be recalled with the same detail years afterwards.[69] For some time, it was thought that having factual memories was a protective mechanism [47,70] to reduce negative psychological outcomes and early work was promising. However, findings have not been replicated consistently,[40] and further work is needed to understand the consequences of these experiences.

Cognitive dysfunction

Cognitive impairment in survivors of critical illness has only been recognised and measured in the past decade. Although there is some variation in prevalence and severity, in general more than 50% of survivors report cognitive impairment at the time of hospital discharge and approximately one-quarter continue to have problems

TABLE 8.1
Summary of reviews of cognitive impairment

AUTHORS	NUMBER OF STUDIES	DURATION OF FOLLOW-UP	INCIDENCE OF COGNITIVE IMPAIRMENT	OTHER FINDINGS OF NOTE
Wilcox et al 2013[6]	31 studies: ARDS pts – 11 studies Mixed ICU pts – 20 studies	ARDS pts: 1– 241 months Mixed pts: 2 weeks – 8.3 years	ARDS pts hosp discharge: 70–100% 1 yr: 46–78% 2 yrs: 25–47% Mixed pts hosp discharge: 39– 51% 3–6 mths: 13–79% 12 mths: 10–71%	Mixed findings in relation to the potential predictors of CI including hypoxaemia, preexisting depression, Some evidence that CI may be more severe or more frequent following sepsis, hypoglycaemia and longer duration of delirium
Wolters et al 2013[71]	19 studies: ARDS pts – 7 studies mixed ICU pts – 12 studies	2–156 months	ARDS pts: 4–56% Mixed pts: 4–62%	Studies that used only screening test data reported lower rates of CI than studies using neuropsychological testing No identified higher risk of CI in studies of elderly patients

NB: 15 of the studies reviewed by Wolters et al (2013)[71] are also covered in the review by Wilcox et al (2013).[6]

12 months later (Tables 8.1 and 8.2).[6,71] Cognitive problems include memory, attention and executive function, which in turn includes reasoning and decision making. These can have significant impact upon the daily life of not just patients but families and have been linked to other aspects of recovery such as psychological health,[72] as well as longer term dementia.

Various factors have been linked to cognitive impairment including delirium, hypoxaemia, hypotension, glucose dysregulation, use of sedatives, sepsis and inflammation and sleep efficiency.[6,41] Although many of these relationships appear inconsistent, and may be more problematic in specific sub-groups of the critical care population, delirium has repeatedly been shown to be highly predictive of cognitive impairment, particularly in regard to duration of delirium. Characteristics such as age and previous health have not been found to be related to the development of cognitive impairment, with young, previously healthy patients just as likely as older patients to develop problems.

Practice tip

When conducting discharge education for patients and their families, don't forget to tell them that problems with memory, decision making and reasoning are common after critical illness.

These will resolve over time for many but, because they persist for some, you may want to suggest where patients and carers may access information about seeking help.

Measuring patient outcomes following a critical illness

The measurement of health outcomes after critical illness is vital – both to determine patient recovery and inform decisions about ongoing care. Measures related to HRQOL and physical, psychological and cognitive function are discussed.

It is unclear how long patient outcomes following critical illness should be measured, but given that ongoing compromise exists for months to years post-hospital discharge, such measurement should continue for a similar time, for example 6–12 months. In the research setting there is a need to extend follow-up of patients beyond 2 years to determine the long-term morbidities associated with critical illness and care.[1]

Measures of HRQOL after a critical illness

The range of HRQOL instruments available is large but can be divided into two groups: generic to all illnesses or specific to a particular disease state. One limitation of generic instruments is that, while they can be applied to a broad spectrum of populations, they may not be responsive to specific disease characteristics, and this is problematic in the usually heterogeneous critical care population. A generic instrument that measures baseline HRQOL and exhibits responsiveness in a recovering critically ill patient with demonstrated reliability and validity has been elusive, although recent outcomes from stakeholder consultations, including agreed core outcome sets have provided some consensus[1,73] (Table 8.3).

TABLE 8.2
Summary of studies examining cognitive function after critical illness (published since the reviews summarised in Table 8.1)

AUTHOR / COUNTRY	DESIGN	N / % MALES	COHORT	ACUITY / ICU LOS	AGE	INSTRUMENT	MAIN FINDINGS
Pandharipande 2013[41]/ USA	Prospective cohort study with 3-and 12- month follow-up	In-hospital cohort: 420/821 (51%); follow-up cohort: 234/467 (50%)	Medical and surgical ICU patients with respiratory failure, cardiogenic shock or septic shock	APACHE II: median 25 (IQR: 19–31); duration of MV: median 3 (IQR: 1–8)	Median 61 (IQR: 51–71) years	RBANS Trail Making Test B	Median RBANS cognition scores at 3 and 12 months were 79 (IQR 70–86) and 80 (IQR 71– 87) respectively; these scores were 1.5 SD below age-adjusted population mean and were similar to scores for patients with mild cognitive impairment 40% of patients at 3 months and 34% of patients at 12 months had scores similar to those for patients with moderate traumatic brain injury
Baumbach 2016/Germany	Prospective cohort study with 3- and 6- month follow-up	Not reported	Surgical and medical ICU patients	APACHE II: median 16 (IQR: 12–23) ICU LOS: median 2.2 (IQR 1.8–4.0) days	Not reported	Functional Assessment of Cancer Therapy – Cognitive Function (FACT-Cog)	Patients were significantly more cognitively impaired than family member controls at 3 and 6 months after ICU discharge
de Azevedo 2017/Brazil	Prospective cohort study with >3- month follow-up	In-hospital cohort 374/724 (52%); Follow-up cohort 206/413 (50%)	Medical and surgical ICU patients	APACHE IV: median 35 (IQR: 23–53) ICU LOS: median 11 (IQR: 6–23) days	In-hospital cohort median 59 (IQR: 47–73); Follow-up cohort median 57 (IQR 46–72)	Forward and backward digit span to assess attention and memory; Rey Auditory Verbal Learning Test to assess verbal memory; clock-drawing test to evaluate executive function; verbal fluency test to assess language; Mini-Mental State Examination to assess global mental state	Cognitive impairment identified in 206 (50%) of patients – 120 (29%) had mild or moderate cognitive impairment, 86 (21%) had severe cognitive impairment

TABLE 8.3
HRQOL instruments used for patients following a critical illness

INSTRUMENT	ITEMS	CONCEPTS/DOMAINS
Medical outcomes study (SF-36)[74,75]	36	Physical: functioning, role limitations, pain, general health Mental: vitality, social, role limitations, mental health; health transition; variable response levels (2–5)
Euro–Qol-5 dimensions (EQ-5D)[76,77]	5	Mobility, self-care, usual activities, pain/discomfort, anxiety/depression; 3 response levels; cost-utility index
15D[76,78]	15	Mobility, vision, hearing, breathing, sleeping, eating, speech, elimination, usual activities, mental function, discomfort, distress, depression, vitality and sexual activity; 5-point ordinal scale (1 = full function; 5 = minimal/no function)
Quality of life–Italian (QOL–IT)[79]	5	Physical activity; social life; perceived quality of life; oral communication; functional limitation; varied response levels (4–7)
Assessment of Quality of Life (AQOL)[80]	15	Illness (3 items); independent living (3 items); physical senses (3 items); social relationships (3 items); psychological wellbeing (3 items); 4 response levels; enables cost-utility analysis
Quality of life–Spanish (QOL–SP)[81]	15	Basic physiological activities (4 items); normal daily activities (8 items); emotional state (3 items)
Sickness impact profile (SIP)[82]	68	Physical: somatic autonomy; mobility control; mobility range Psychosocial: psychic autonomy and communication; social behaviour; emotional stability; developed from original 136-item
Nottingham Health Profile (NHP)[83]	45	Experience: energy, pain, emotional reactions, sleep, social isolation, physical mobility Daily life: employment, household work, relationships, home life, sex, hobbies, holidays
Perceived quality of life (PQOL)[84]	11	Satisfaction with: bodily health; ability to think/remember; happiness; contact with family and friends; contribution to the community; activities outside work; whether income meets needs; respect from others; meaning and purpose of life; working/not working/retirement; each scored on 0–100 scale

SF-36 is the most commonly used and validated instrument in the literature, including with a variety of critically ill patient groups (e.g. general ICU, ARDS, trauma and septic shock).

Measures of physical function following a critical illness

Numerous instruments have been developed to examine the physical capacity of individuals, usually focusing on functional status ranging from independent to dependent.[85,86] The range of instruments available to measure various aspects of physical function has evolved in the past decade, particularly in regard to the availability of measures useful within the intensive care environment.

Previously available measures such as the Six Minute Walk Test (6MWT), Barthel Index and Functional Independence Measure (FIM) are valuable to assess patients after critical illness. In addition, physical activity associated with cardiac or pulmonary dysfunction may be assessed using perceived breathlessness (dyspnoea) during exercise by the modified Borg scale,[87] ranging from 0 (no dyspnoea) to 10+ (maximal). The Borg scale is commonly used with other physical activity instruments, e.g. the 6MWT.[88]

The limitation of many of these measures is that they require alert, cooperative patients able to participate in functional activities, whereas critically ill patients are not always able to participate to this level. In response, a range of new instruments have been developed including the Chelsea critical care physical assessment tool (CPAx),[89] the Physical Function ICU Test (PFIT-s),[90] the ICU Mobility Scale (IMS)[91] and the Functional Status Score – ICU (FSS-ICU).[92] Each of these measures has been designed to measure a slightly different aspect of function and have different benefits and limitations that mean they should be used for different purposes as outlined in Fig. 8.2.

Measures of psychological function after a critical illness

The psychological recovery process and trajectory for survivors of a critical illness remains an important but relatively under-researched area.[94] Exploration of the impact

FIGURE 8.2 Outcome measures used to assess physical function in patients during and after critical illness[93]

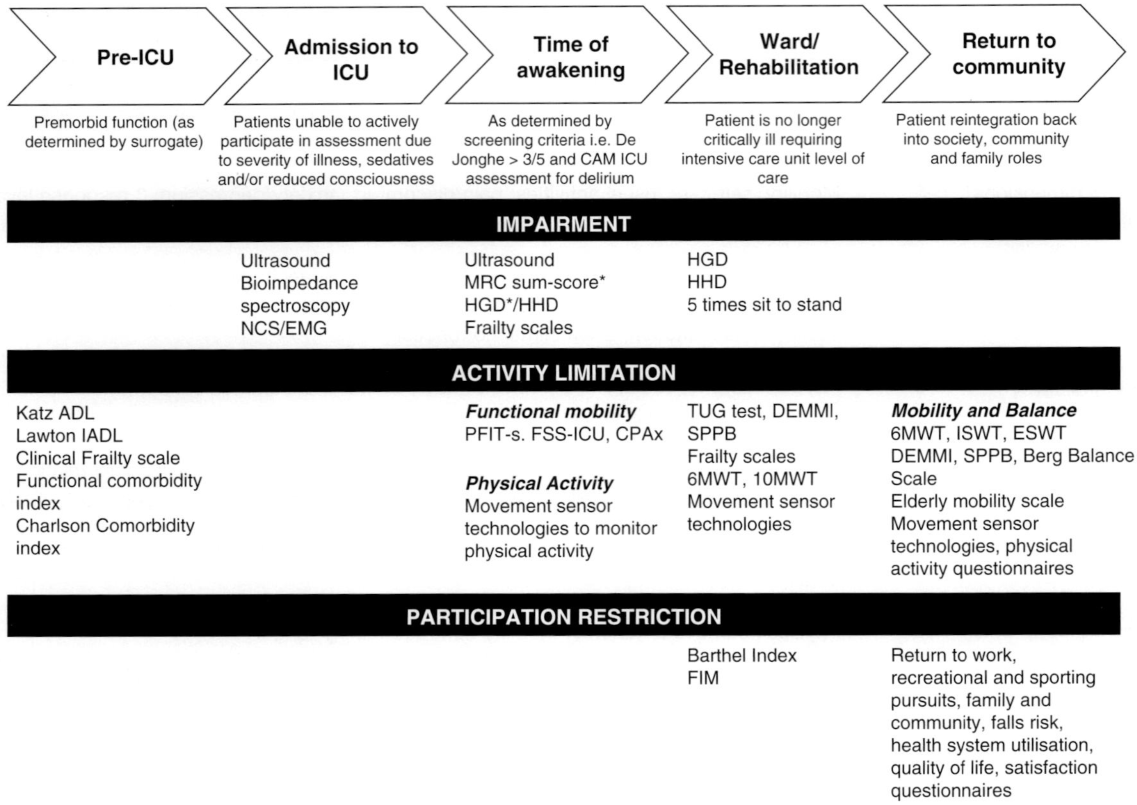

Source: Reprinted with permission from Springer Nature. Parry SM, Granger CL, Berney S, Jones J, et al. Assessment of impairment and activity limitations in the critically ill: a systematic review of measurement instruments and their clinimetric properties. Intensive Care Med 2015;41(5):744–62.

of the intensive care experience, including ongoing stress and distress[95,96] and memories for the patient,[97,98] has now emerged in the literature as an important area of research and practice. Instruments that assess mood and mental wellbeing after a critical illness focus on psychological constructs, including anxiety, depression, fear and post-traumatic stress symptoms[99] (Table 8.4). Constructs that relate to an individual during a critical illness episode also include agitation and confusion/delirium[100] (discussed further in Chapter 6).

Assessment of psychological outcomes has relied mainly on self-report questionnaires administered via either a postal survey or a structured interview format. Few studies have included clinical assessments such as the Clinical Administered PTSD Scale, the 'gold standard' for diagnosing PTSD.[108] This means, therefore, that such questionnaires are screening tools that can be used to identify individuals at risk of developing a significant clinical problem. They are not diagnostic and this is an important point when considering designing, implementing and evaluating any intervention. A number of standardised questionnaires have demonstrated reliability and validity in this patient group, but the use of different questionnaires makes it difficult to generalise findings. The recently developed Intensive Care Psychological Assessment Tool (IPAT)[109] is slightly different in that it has been designed specifically for the purpose of identifying which ICU patients are at risk of subsequent distress.

These instruments often include 'cut-off' or 'threshold' scores that enable screening for the presence or severity of a disorder. For example, a score of 8–10 on either subscale of the HADS indicates the possible presence of a disorder, while a score of 11 or above indicates probable presence of such a condition.[103] One limitation of these self-report measures is that while sensitivity (ability to correctly identify all patients with the condition) can be high, specificity (ability to correctly identify all patients without the condition) is less easy to determine, and therefore the incidence of psychological distress may be overstated. This makes estimation difficult and is one of the challenges in establishing the actual magnitude of psychological distress after a critical illness. Other challenges include the recruitment of different cohorts or sub-groups of patients (e.g. patients with adult respiratory distress syndrome or acute lung injury). Variations in the international provision of ICU services also mean that differences may exist in case-mix in the areas of illness severity, planned or unplanned admissions, ages and reasons for admission.

TABLE 8.4
Examples of common measures of psychological function after critical illness

INSTRUMENT	MEASUREMENT	SCORE RANGE
Impact of Event Scale (IES);[101] IES-R[102]	15-item; assesses levels of posttraumatic distress; two subscales: intrusive thoughts, avoidance behaviours; revised form (IES-R) adds hyper-arousal subscale (7 items)	Frequency of thoughts over past 7 days; 0 = no thoughts; 5 = often; higher scores indicate greater distress: scores ≥11 on either subscale indicates a clinical disorder
Hospital Anxiety and Depression Scale (HADS)[103]	14-item (4-point scale); measures mood disorders in non-psychiatric patients; focuses on psychological rather than physical symptoms of anxiety and depression	Score ≥11 on either subscale indicates a clinical disorder
Center for Epidemiologic Studies – Depression Scale (CES–D)[104]	20-item self-report scale assesses frequency and severity of depressive symptoms experienced in the previous week	Score range 0–60; higher scores reflect increased symptoms and severity
Kessler 10 (K-10)[105]	10-item (5-point scale) self-report measure of non-specific psychological distress over the past 4 weeks	Score range 10–50; higher scores reflect greater distress
Posttraumatic stress disorder (PTSD) checklist (PCL)[106]	20-item (5-point scale) self-report assessment of symptoms of PTSD corresponding to DSM-V criteria	Score range 20–100; higher scores reflect increased symptoms of PTSD
Posttraumatic Stress Symptoms 14 (PTSS 14)[107]	14-item extended version of the PTSS 10 to cover all aspects of PTSD consistent with Diagnostic and Statistical Manual of Mental Disorders (DSM-IV) symptom categories	2 parts: Part A – Assessment of traumatic memories from ICU; Part B – Posttraumatic stress disorder symptoms; score range 14–98
Intensive Care Psychological Assessment Tool (IPAT) (Wade et al, 2014[109])	14-item scale covering hopelessness, tension, panic, delusions, intrusive memories, sadness, sleeplessness, communication difficulties, hallucinations and disorientation	Non-parametric factor analysis reduces this scale to 10 and awaiting further psychometric testing. 3 response formats: no; yes a bit; yes a lot Trigger scores still require to be confirmed

Measures of cognitive function after a critical illness

Cognitive or neuropsychological assessment of critical illness survivors has only become more common in the past 10 years. Comprehensive and lengthy testing batteries exist, although those used in studies examining recovery after critical illness have tended to favour the slightly shorter testing (Table 8.5). Most of these tests require more than 30 minutes for this assessment, which may tire some people, particularly early in their recovery phase after critical illness. In addition, some of the tests need to be administered by qualified psychology or psychiatry personnel, although some instruments that can be administered by research personnel, both in person and over the telephone, have recently been developed. Neuropsychological instruments are non-invasive. Repeated testing with the same instrument on multiple occasions may lead to practice effects; in other words, the critical illness survivor learns how to perform better on the test. Hence, instruments with multiple versions prove beneficial in some circumstances. Where neuropsychological testing can be carried out, it enables assessment of the nature, severity, prevalence and incidence of cognitive impairment.[110] Cross-cultural differences do exist in some of the domains measured in neuropsychological assessment so where comparison to normative data is required for analysis and interpretation, for example in the Repeatable Battery for the Assessment of Neuropsychological Status (RBANS), country-specific data are required.[111]

In the past the most commonly used brief measure was the Mini-Mental State Examination (MMSE);[112] however, criticisms of insensitivity, susceptibility to ceiling effects and limited capacity to differentiate between cognitive domains are often levelled at brief measures. In contrast, more lengthy measures such as the RBANS,[113] Trail Making Test,[114] the Wechsler Memory Scale – revised[115] and the Wechsler Adult Intelligence Scale – revised[116] provide more detail and better differentiation of memory problems but often tire those being tested, particularly older people and those who are still recovering from critical illness. Scales such as the Montreal Cognitive Assessment[117] or The Telephone Interview

TABLE 8.5
Neuropsychological instruments to assess cognitive function in patients following a critical illness

INSTRUMENT	MEASUREMENT	SCORE RANGE / COMMENTS
Mini-Mental State Examination (MMSE)[112]	11 items in 5 domains including orientation, memory, attention and concentration, delayed recall, language	Score of ≤23, or 2 points below maximum in any domain, indicates the presence of moderate-to-severe cognitive impairment; 5–10 minutes to administer
Montreal Cognitive Assessment (MoCA)[117]	Eight cognitive domains including attention and concentration, executive functions, memory, language, visuoconstructional skills, conceptual thinking, calculations, orientation	Requires 10 minutes to administer; total possible score is 30 with scores ≥26 indicating normal cognition; a version that can be conducted over the phone (referred to as MoCA – Blind) is available
Repeatable Battery for the Assessment of Neuropsychological Status (RBANS)[113]	Measurement of multiple areas of cognitive functioning across 5 indices covering the domains of immediate memory, visuospatial/constructional, language, attention, delayed memory	RBANS must be administered by a qualified psychologist; designed as a paper-and-pencil screening battery; has multiple versions to allow for multiple testing without problems of practice effect
The Telephone Interview of Cognitive Status – Modified (TICS-M)[118,119]	Abbreviated 13 item measure that includes four domains: orientation; registration, recent memory and delayed recall (memory); attention/calculation; semantic memory, comprehension and repetition (language).	Maximum score of 39; requires approximately 10 minutes to administer
Trail Making Test[114]	Part A requires the rapid connection of 25 sequential numbers; Part B measures visual scanning, visuospatial sequencing and cognitive set shifting by requiring connection of 25 alternate numbers and letters in ascending sequence	Score is obtained as the number of seconds required to complete each part (the examiner points out errors as they occur, so correction time is included); this is then converted to a 10-point scale with 10 as the best possible score in each part; Total score ≤12 indicates impairment
Wechsler Memory Scale – Revised (WMS-R)[115]	Measures different memory functions in adults; 7 sub-tests including spatial addition, symbol span, design memory, general cognitive screener, logical memory, verbal paired associates, visual reproducing	Performance reported as 5 index scores including auditory memory, visual memory, visual working memory, immediate memory and delayed memory
Wechsler Adult Intelligence Scale – Revised (WAIS-R)[116]	Measures intelligence in adults and older adolescents; although it is used to measure intelligence rather than cognition, it is often used in combination with WMS-R	10 core sub-tests and 5 supplemental sub-tests; 4 index scores (verbal comprehension and working memory that combine to provide Verbal IQ Index; perceptual organisation and processing speed that combine to provide Performance IQ Index) as well as the overall full-scale IQ

of Cognitive Status – Modified version (TICS-M)[118] are now frequently used, given they provide a balance between length and detail, and can be administered over the telephone.

Improving recovery following a critical illness

Survivors of critical illness experience multidimensional and protracted compromise over weeks to months and often extending to years. Interventions to improve recovery following critical illness can be delivered at multiple time points in the critical illness continuum. Some of these interventions are the primary responsibility of the multidisciplinary critical care team, are delivered while the patient remains in ICU and are directed towards limiting the detrimental effects of intensive care or promoting recovery as early as possible. Other interventions to improve recovery may be delivered after the patient has left the ICU but remains in the hospital or after discharge from hospital. These later strategies are often delivered in collaboration with other members of the healthcare team. Although there is only limited evidence of specific strategies that are effective in improving recovery, the body of evidence unpinning these strategies is starting to build.

Interventions delivered in ICU

Interventions to improve long-term recovery that are delivered in the ICU focus on strategies to minimise the detrimental effects of critical illness and the associated care. These interventions might focus on one aspect of care, for example sedation minimisation or early mobilisation, or might be multidimensional, for example targeting sedation minimisation, optimisation of sleep and limitation of the use of restraints as a combined intervention. The majority of interventions delivered within the ICU are targeted at improving physical function.

Interventions to minimise ICU-AW, particularly in relation to muscle deconditioning from disuse (e.g. sedation; bed rest) have recently focused on active exercises and mobility, including while patients are intubated and ventilated.[120] Multiple studies and quality improvement projects have demonstrated the safety and feasibility of ICU-based early mobilisation interventions, often with short-term benefits for patients when interventions are delivered early in ICU,[121] although few interventions have had sufficient testing yet to show sustained improvement in patient outcomes. As identified in a systematic review, where interventions have shown benefit, they have sometimes been in isolated areas of function, for example ability to walk without assistance, rather than widespread across all aspects of patients' function and quality of life.[122] Interventions that have shown initial benefit in small studies include in-bed cycling using an ergometer,[123] a combination of functional electrical stimulation and cycling[124] early exercise and mobilisation,[125] and studies that focus on multidisciplinary or team-based activities to promote mobilisation[126] (Table 8.6). This is an area where there is increased interest and research activity, with the potential to be an improved evidence base in the near future.

In addition, strategies primarily directed towards minimising sedation, and therefore facilitating more patient movement, have demonstrated effectiveness (see Chapter 6 for further details).

Effective implementation of any of these interventions requires a change in how critical care clinicians care for their patients and this requires a cultural shift with a multidisciplinary team approach and changes in care processes.[131–134] Strong leadership in the process, beliefs about capability and the benefits of the activity, as well as a culture of safety and improvement within the ICU are perceived as important factors to aid implementation of interventions such as early mobilisation. Involving the family in interventions to support recovery, including early mobilisation, has also been proposed,[135] and although this has not yet been confirmed in research as an effective strategy, it has great potential and few disadvantages if appropriate preparation is provided.

Implementation of 'early' activity for ICU patients relates to after clinical stabilisation is evident, and includes those still intubated. Factors to ensure patient safety

TABLE 8.6
Studies of in-ICU mobility over the past 10 years

FIRST AUTHOR/ COUNTRY	DESIGN	N/AGE	COHORT	INTERVENTION	MAIN FINDINGS
Burtin 2009[123]/ Belgium	Randomised controlled trial	90/57	Prolonged ICU (expected 12-day LOS)	Daily exercise; 20 mins with bedside cycle ergometer[a] from day 5, 5 days/week	6MWD (hospital discharge): 196 vs 143 m (<0.05) Isometric quadriceps: 2.37 vs 2.03 Newton (n.s.) SF-36 PF: 21 vs 15 (p < 0.01) ICU LOS: 25 vs 24 days (n.s.) Hospital LOS: 36 vs 40 days (n.s.)
Schweickert 2009[125]/USA	2-site randomised controlled trial	104/56	ICU patients with <72 hours MV	Exercise and mobilisation (PT and OT)[b] for stable and awake patients; activity based on patient stability and tolerance	Independent function (hospital discharge): 59% vs 35% (p = 0.02) Ventilator free days: 23.5 vs 21.1 (n.s.) ICU LOS: 5.9 vs 7.9 days (n.s.) Hospital LOS: 13.5 vs 12.9 days (n.s.) Barthel Index (hospital discharge): 75 vs 55 (n.s.) 1 serious adverse event in 498 therapy sessions (desaturation <80%) and 4% sessions discontinued due to patient instability

Continued

TABLE 8.6
Studies of in-ICU mobility over the past 10 years—cont'd

FIRST AUTHOR/ COUNTRY	DESIGN	N/AGE	COHORT	INTERVENTION	MAIN FINDINGS
Bourdin 2010[127]/ France	Cohort	20/68	≥7 days ICU ≥2 days MV	Protocol of chair sitting, tilt-table, walking activities; 33% during MV	Contraindication to mobility intervention on 230/524 (43%) patient days 425 mobility interventions performed, complete data on 275 (65%) 91 (33%) interventions during MV Common interventions were sitting in chair (55%), tilt-up ± arm support (33%), walking 11% Adverse event occurred in 3% interventions (no harm)
Needham 2010[128]/USA	Before/ after Quality Improvement (QI) project	57/52	≥2 days MV	Structured QI model, multidisciplinary team, new PT and OT referral and sedation reduction guidelines	Reduced benzodiazepine dose (pre: 50%, post: 25%, p = 0.02) Increased number of functional mobility treatments (pre: 56%, post: 78%, p = 0.03)
Pohlman 2010[129]/ USA	Intervention arm of randomised controlled trial	49/58	<3 days MV with expected further MV	Sedation interruption, PT/OT rehabilitation protocol,[c] sessions 25–30 minutes	Intubated participants sat at edge of bed in 60%, stood in 33% and ambulated in 15% of sessions
Denehy 2013[130]/ Australia	Randomised controlled trial	150/61	>5 days in ICU	Exercise rehabilitation in ICU, ward and outpatients	No major adverse events No significant differences at hospital discharge, 3, 6 or 12 months in 6MWD, TUG, AQOL, SF-36
Parry 2014[124]/ Australia	Observational	16/63	Septic ICU patients, >48 hours MV, in ICU >4 days	FES-cycling intervention 20–60 minutes daily, 5 times/week[d]	Number of cycling sessions – 8/patient Total cycling sessions provided 69 (73%) out of possible 95 1 minor adverse event (SPO2 86% requiring FiO2 increase)
Schaller et al 2016[126] / Multinational	RCT	200/65	Surgical ICU patients, MV <48 hours and expected to require at least another 24 hours MV	Goal-directed mobilisation using interprofessional approach[e]	Improved level of mobilisation Reduced SICU LOS in intervention group (7 [5-12] vs 10 [6-15] days, p=0.0054) Increased functional mobility at hospital discharge More adverse events in intervention group compared with control group (25 [2.8%] vs 10 [0.8%]) but no serious adverse event

6MWD = 6-minute walk distance; AQOL = Assessment of Quality of Life instrument; FES = Functional Electrical Stimulation; MV = mechanical ventilation; n.s. = not significant; OT = occupational therapy; PT = physiotherapy; SF-36 = Short Form 36 Health Survey; TUG = Timed Up and Go test.

[a]Passive or active cycling, 6 levels of increasing resistance; sedated patients received passive cycling at 20 cycles/minute.

[b]Daily passive ROM for unresponsive; after daily interruption of sedation, assisted and independent active ROM supine, bed mobility (transferring to upright sitting and balance) and activities of daily living (ADLs), transfer training (sit-to-stand from bed to chair), pre-gait exercises, walking.

[c]Passive ROM for unresponsive; assisted and independent active ROM supine, bed mobility (lateral rolling, transferring to upright sitting), balance, ADLs, transfer training, walking.

[d]Supine motorised cycle ergometer attached to a current-controlled stimulator, muscles were stimulated at specific stages throughout cycling phase based on normal muscular activation patterns regulated by the bicycle software.

[e]Goal-directed mobilisation using interprofessional approach incorporating closed-loop communication and an algorithm to drive mobilisation

during mobilisation have been identified, including confirming that a patient has sufficient cardiovascular and respiratory reserve and cognitive function.[136,137] Potential barriers to mobilisation during mechanical ventilation (e.g. acute lung injury, vasoactive infusions) have also been examined and include clinical instability, excessive staff turnover, morale issues and a lack of respect among disciplines.[131,132] Physiotherapy recommendations for physical deconditioning include development of 'exercise prescriptions' and 'mobilising plans'.[138] Activities range from passive stretching and range of motion exercises for limbs and joints to positioning, resistive muscle training to electrical stimulation, aerobic training and muscle strengthening and ambulation.[139] Specific mobility activities include:

- in-bed (range of motion, roll, bridge, sitting on the edge of the bed)
- standing at the side of the bed
- standing on the tilt-table
- transfer to and from bed to chair
- marching on the spot
- walking
- neuromuscular electrical stimulation
- bedside cycle ergometry.

Patient support for each activity ranges from assistance with 1–2 staff through to independence under supervision. Inspiratory muscle training has been used for weakness associated with prolonged mechanical ventilation, using resistance and threshold-training devices. While there is evidence that inspiratory muscle training is effective,[140-142] this evidence is not consistent[143] and some risks including mortality have been identified.[144]

Mobilisation practices have been explored in multicentre point prevalence and observational assessments in various countries, with widespread reports of limited mobilisation despite widespread recognition of the benefits of such mobilisation.[145-148] As noted earlier, a culture of patient wakefulness and early in-ICU activity and mobility is advocated but challenged by the status quo of work practices and health professional role delineations.[131,149] A re-engineering of work processes and practices to promote patient activity is therefore required to ensure optimal outcomes for survivors of a critical illness. Few reports of achieving this change are available, but initial evidence in single centres suggests it is possible to change practice in the local environment using various interventions such as those based on effective teamwork to increase the number of patients mobilising.[150-152]

Interventions to improve psychological recovery

Although there is now strong empirical evidence that some patients experience significant psychological dysfunctions after a critical illness, it is less clear how and when to treat these symptoms.[153] Traditional therapies for posttraumatic stress include cognitive behaviour therapy[154] and eye movement desensitising and reprocessing.[155] The latter approach was tested in a small pilot study (n=10), and produced some positive results with all participants demonstrating significant symptom reduction.[155]

However, there may be scope for some specific interventions to be administered when the patient is in intensive care, prior to hospital discharge or when they are at home. There is some evidence to support the minimisation of sedation, particularly with benzodiazepines, while the patient is in ICU, and strategies to achieve this that are relevant to each ICU context should be implemented (see Chapter 6 for more details).[59,156]

Early detection and identification of patients at risk are important, and are included as a quality standard in recent UK National Institute for Clinical Excellence (NICE) guidelines.[157] The NICE guidelines[157] emphasised regular assessment of patient recovery including psychological recovery. Assessment periods include during intensive care, ward-based care, before discharge home or community care and 2–3 months after ICU discharge, with the use of existing referral pathways and stepped care models to treat identified psychological dysfunctions. These services are usually well established and allow patients to be treated by appropriately qualified practitioners. The role of critical care practitioners may therefore be to establish the causes of psychological disturbances associated with critical illness, identifying at-risk patients through systematic and standardised screening activities, closely monitoring identified patients and referring to appropriate specialties where appropriate, to optimise their recovery trajectory while not introducing any further harm. Once a patient has a diagnosis of anxiety, depression or posttraumatic stress, treatment should follow national guidelines, for example NICE guidelines for the management of adult patients with depression (see the NICE website, http://www.nice.org.uk/Guidance/CG90).

Early evidence of the benefits of in-ICU psychological care delivered by clinical psychologists as a way of reducing anxiety, depression and posttraumatic stress symptoms is promising.[158] However, this was a single centre study in a sub-group of trauma patients using historical controls; therefore, further work is necessary before considering wider implementation. Interestingly the intervention included stress management techniques and cognitive and emotional restructuring. A more recent large multicentre study is being undertaken currently within the UK. A large multicenter study has recently been completed in which a nurse-led preventative psychological intervention delivered in intensive care was evaluated; however, improved psychological health for patients was not demonstrated.[159]

Systematic follow-up services may offer appropriate assessment and support during recovery for individuals identified with psychological disturbances. Intensive care follow-up clinics where patients have the opportunity to discuss their intensive care experiences and receive information about what had happened to them could be a useful intervention, although there are currently no empirical data to support this,[95] and further research work is required. In a recent quasi-experimental study evaluating a nurse-led follow-up program, more severe PTSS symptoms in the experimental group receiving the follow-up were reported.[64] This is both an interesting and concerning finding. Differences between groups go some way in explaining this finding with the experimental group being younger and having a shorter stay in intensive care, but the authors themselves highlight the need to be cautious about timing interventions and the importance of 'watchful waiting'. We must be mindful also of the premise of 'doing no harm' when developing, delivering and evaluating interventions.

Interventions that include provision of information

Giving information is thought to be important in 'bridging' a perceived memory gap that might help a patient make sense of their critical illness experience, and thus improve psychological outcome. This may involve a more structured discharge planning process or the use of diaries for intensive care patients. A diary approach has been adopted in a number of European ICUs;[160-162] however, there has been a great deal of variation in how the diaries are compiled and viewed by a patient, as well as how much support is offered to them to explain diary content.[163] To this point in time the use of such diaries tends to be atheoretical,[164] with limited long-term exploration of the effect of the diary intervention on patient outcomes. While there is a small amount of evidence that supports their use,[165] further empirical work is necessary to ensure their effectiveness.

The provision of a personalised discharge summary as a component of discharge planning is another approach. This has been shown to be both desired by some survivors[166] and feasible to produce with an average time to completion of 15 minutes.[167] However the effectiveness of this as an intervention to reduce negative psychological outcomes has not yet been tested and further research is required.

One further study focusing on psychological rehabilitation after discharge home was conducted to examine the effect of consultations that focused on provision of information and constructing an illness narrative.[168] In this multicentre, non-blinded, randomised controlled trial (RCT), patients received a nurse-led intervention delivered at the ICU follow-up clinic about 3 months after hospital discharge, with further telephone-based consultations 5 and 10 months after discharge. No differences in quality of life were identified in the two groups of patients, although when anxiety was categorised as low or high, there were fewer anxious patients in the intervention group suggesting there may be some benefit in some patients.[168]

It is important to note, however, that not all patients wish to be reminded of their ICU experience; this is especially the case for patients who demonstrate avoidant behaviours. Two studies have reported that approximately 50% of patients do not wish to know what has happened to them during intensive care.[47,169] Others may wish not to be reminded of being critically ill but wish to concentrate on recovery.[95] A recent systematic review suggested that giving information via some type of consultation did not demonstrate better psychological outcomes.[170] We have to be mindful of not doing harm and that interventions may not be appropriate for all patients at the same point in time.

Ward-based post-ICU recovery

Follow-up services for survivors of a critical illness have occurred sporadically in individual units with interested clinician teams, but there is currently no widespread systematic approach to recovery and rehabilitation and the management of physical, psychological or cognitive dysfunctions.[1]

Commencement or continuation of rehabilitation activities in the general wards after discharge from ICU highlights a potentially different set of challenges, particularly in terms of physiotherapy resources, involvement of other medical teams and compliance to a prescribed plan. Although some cohorts of critically ill patients (e.g. pulmonary, cardiac, stroke, brain injury) have defined rehabilitation pathways, patients with other clinical presentations may not be routinely prescribed a rehabilitation plan or be able to access relevant services.

For patients who survive to ICU discharge, up to 10% will die prior to hospital discharge.[171,172] Some work in Europe on prognosis post-ICU discharge using the 4-point Sabadell Score (0 = good prognosis; 1 = long-term poor prognosis; 2 = short-term poor prognosis; 3 = expected hospital death) demonstrated that subjective intensivist assessment was able to predict the risk of patient mortality and conversely those patients potentially suitable for rehabilitation.[173]

Specific ward-based rehabilitation interventions following ICU discharge are beginning to be investigated. Designing and implementing such an intervention is challenging because of the heterogeneous nature of intensive care patients who have increasing complexity and ill-defined recovery trajectories. Furthermore, these patients tend to be 'scattered' throughout the hospital making coordination of care post-ICU difficult. Some exploratory work in the UK implemented a generic rehabilitation assistant to support enhanced physiotherapy and nutritional rehabilitation in collaboration with ward-based staff.[174,175] Following the MRC framework for complex interventions, the intervention focused primarily on physical recovery from ICU discharge to 3 months. The generic rehabilitation assistant was able to provide information and explanation of the patient's time in intensive care, facilitate discussions with the multidisciplinary team, assist in goal setting and provide enhanced ward-based rehabilitation.[176] Results demonstrated no significant improvement in primary outcomes (Rivermead Mobility Index) but patients were significantly more satisfied with physiotherapy, nutritional support, coordination of care and information provision.[177] In contrast, in one small Austrian study a ward-based early rehabilitation study was effective in reducing hospital length of stay and improving functional recovery, while also being safe and cost-effective.[178] Given the dearth of evidence, and inconsistent results, in this area further research is required to test specific interventions during the post-ICU hospital period aimed at improving the recovery trajectory and health outcomes for patients with limited physical function. As noted with in-ICU rehabilitation, the optimal duration, intensity and frequency of interventions is not yet clear.

Recovery after hospital discharge

Of patients who survive their critical illness to hospital discharge, up to 20% will die within 12 months, and their risk of death is three times higher than for the general population.[172,179] Functional recovery can be delayed in some individuals for 6–12 months or longer. In a Norwegian study, only half of 194 patients had returned to work or study 1 year after surviving their critical illness.[180]

There is, however, only limited research and mixed study findings identifying specific interventions during the post-hospital period that may improve a patient's recovery trajectory and health outcomes. Most work has involved practice evaluations or studies of outpatient 'ICU follow-up' clinics, while there is some work exploring home-based programs that predominantly focus on physical recovery.

ICU follow-up clinics

Systematic follow-up for survivors of a critical illness after hospital discharge emerged in the UK in the early 1990s, after a number of government reviews on the cost and effectiveness of critical care services highlighted the need to evaluate longer term patient outcomes, in particular quality of life,[181] and recognised that patients had sequelae that were best understood and managed by ICU clinicians. There has, however, been limited evidence of the benefits of an ICU follow-up clinic although these have been implemented widely in the UK. While there are clear recommendations about follow-up that includes a comprehensive review of patient progress, recent guidelines fall short of specifically recommending this is through clinic provision.[182]

The first intensive care follow-up clinics were established in the UK in the early 1990s,[183] driven by a few interested and committed intensive care clinicians. A recent UK survey indicated that approximately 27% of UK ICUs offered a follow-up service.[184] Although there are few reports of clinics operating outside the UK, occasional clinics do exist.[185,186] Different clinic models have evolved as nurse-led, doctor-led or a combination of multidisciplinary team members with more than half in the UK nurse-led. Many clinics restrict patients invited to return to those with an ICU length of stay of at least 3 or 4 days. This decision is often based upon resources rather than evidence, as patients who have a shorter stay may also have subsequent physical and psychological problems.[187]

Common practice is to invite patients to attend a first clinic appointment approximately 2–3 months after discharge from intensive care or hospital, although timing has to be flexible given the length of hospital stay for some patients. For many, one appointment is sufficient,[188] but others have continuing problems and may need to return on a number of occasions. Some clinics routinely offer return appointments up to 1 year after discharge, determined on an individual patient basis. Attendance can be problematic; only 70–90% in some studies with non-attendance occurring because a patient has no identified problems (shorter ICU length of stay, less ill) or, more importantly, because of individual limitations (limited mobility, living a distance away from the clinic or significant posttraumatic stress symptoms including avoidant behaviours).[187,189]

While these services developed in a relatively ad hoc manner, tended to be underfunded and used a variety of models in their delivery, the purposes for such a service are similar (Box 8.2). Patient who attend clinical appointments tend to report high levels of satisfaction,[188] and a recent Australian study reported that many patients who had received prolonged ventilation indicated that a follow-up clinic would have been beneficial.[190] It is undeniable though that much of our understanding of the longer term consequences of critical illness has emerged as a consequence of patients attending follow-up clinics.

BOX 8.2

Purpose of an intensive care follow-up service

- Review and assess patient progress
- Facilitate early identification of problems and refer to appropriate specialties where necessary
- Coordinate care
- Support a rehabilitation program
- Discuss the intensive care experience and offer patient the opportunity to comment on care
- Offer patient the opportunity to visit the ICU
- Provide a forum for relatives to ask questions
- Use information to inform delivery of intensive care

TABLE 8.7
Sample clinic assessment tool

SUBJECT AREA	RATIONALE
General health	Assessed on a linear analogue or forced choice response to elicit a patient's subjective account of how they view their general health and how it has changed since critical illness
Medications	Review of medications commenced during the critical illness and continued postdischarge, with advice provided to the patient's GP[187]
Movement and mobility, household management and joints	Assess mobility problems, often due to continuing fatigue and weakness, but also perhaps joint problems;[191] identify impact on daily activities[157]
Breathing and tracheostomy	Breathlessness is common after critical illness and there are a number of potential difficulties post-tracheostomy; these can be identified and the patient referred to the appropriate specialist
Sleep and eating	Sleep and concentration disturbances are common, and muscle loss and weakness are important contributors to delayed recovery[157]
Urology/reproduction, skin and senses	Patients may have sexual problems[192] and skin and nail problems
Recreation, work and lifestyle change	Patients may experience difficulties reintegrating into society and in particular returning to work
Memory, concentration, decision making	This will provide an indication of ongoing cognitive problems that may influence ongoing recovery[6]
Intensive care experience	Patients rarely remember factual events of their time in ICU, but their memories are often of unpleasant and disturbing events;[50] offering an opportunity to discuss actual events and sometimes distressing memories can be beneficial[188]
Quality of life	The ultimate aim of treatment and care is to return a patient to an acceptable and optimal quality of life; it is important to gauge how patients perceive their life quality, and may identify areas for practice improvement

Clinic activities

Patient progress is reviewed for identification of subsequent problems and timely referral to appropriate services for further treatment. A major advantage of follow-up clinics is the increased understanding of patient recovery, as a range of physical and psychological assessments can be conducted (see an example in Table 8.7). Content of assessment is informed by the understanding and knowledge of the problems patients commonly face during their recovery period. Critical care and rehabilitation staff, however, need to ensure that issues are not 'problematising' for aspects of recovery that are not of concern to the patient.

Content of an assessment tool structures the clinic visit and identifies any patient problems. These assessments can include the use of standardised questionnaires of HRQOL, physical function, psychological status and cognitive function and other free-text responses that incorporate patient comments and other issues. Use of standardised questionnaires is, however, inconsistent,[183,184] which limits evaluation and comparisons of clinic outcomes. Common examples of questionnaires and tests are listed in Tables 8.3–8.5 and Fig. 8.2. The issue of respondent burden must be considered and questionnaire fatigue recognised. This can be managed in part by asking patients to bring completed questionnaires with them to the clinic appointment. Administration, scoring and interpretation of questionnaires must also be managed in accordance with instrument guidelines.

Referral to appropriate specialists using a systematic approach and timely response times are necessary, as other healthcare professionals will not usually be present when patients attend the clinic. Delays in treatment following identification of significant posttraumatic symptomatology can result in PTSD that is enduring and lasts for several years.[193] Implementing defined referral criteria and pathways can, however, be challenging particularly when a clinic is nurse-led.[187] While identification of referrals during a follow-up clinic reflects a potential unmet need for these patients, one survey reported that 51% of clinics had no formal referral mechanisms.[183] This referral activity also reflects an additional function of the clinic in coordinating patient care after hospital discharge.

Coordination of care for these patients with complex needs often includes multiple outpatient appointments and investigations at a time when they are least able to cope with this complexity. An additional patient benefit of returning to a follow-up clinic is in supporting them to negotiate their way through this complex care, coordinate outpatient appointments and to have someone whom they know help them understand and interpret the entire critical illness and recovery experience.[187] The follow-up clinic can also be a vehicle for supporting and evaluating a rehabilitation program. Rehabilitation in the form of a 6-week supported self-help manual with weekly telephone calls and completion of a diary demonstrated an improvement in physical recovery at 8 weeks and 6 months after intensive care discharge.[194]

As noted earlier, a unique element of a patient's intensive care experience is their limited recall of factual events but a common experience of 'nightmares' and 'hallucinations' that can be distressing both at the time and during recovery. The benefits of having an opportunity to discuss their experiences with intensive care staff should not be underestimated, and as such effective communication skills are vital for those delivering ICU clinic services.[195] Patients value being able to speak to 'experts' about their experience, being given information about what happened to them in ICU and also receiving reassurances about the length of time that recovery will take and that their distressing memories are common. Clinics also offer patients the opportunity to comment on their care both during and after intensive care.[188] This is important not just for the patient but to inform care delivery. For ICUs that complete patient diaries, the follow-up clinic is often the place where these are introduced and discussed with the patient.[162,165,196]

Offering the patient an opportunity to visit the ICU is possible during the follow-up clinic appointment. As noted earlier, the lack of factual memory of intensive care often leaves patients with gaps that may be distressing. Visiting the ICU may therefore be beneficial for some patients, particularly when they report odd perceptual experiences, and enable them to make sense of some of these experiences. However, care should be taken, as some patients may find this experience distressing and appropriate explanation and support is essential.

A follow-up clinic also provides an important forum for relatives. Relatives may have different needs to a patient, and it is common to encourage relatives to attend with the patient. Relatives may not only have short- and long-term consequences for their emotional wellbeing and physical health,[197] but also be faced with supporting a patient who has unrealistic expectations about their recovery. Clinic attendance by relatives varies[187] and may be related to them having no identified problems or unanswered questions about the patient's recovery, or being unable to attend because of work commitments. Some relatives, however, may not attend because of also adopting avoidant strategies if they are experiencing posttraumatic stress symptomatology,[198] depression[199] or other health problems.

Clinic evaluation

Given the development of follow-up clinics and the nature of implementation, formal evaluation is difficult and this is reflected in the paucity of empirical evidence. Anecdotally, nurses who deliver these clinics consider them beneficial and patients seem to value them. Intuitively, it is a good idea for intensive care practitioners who have unique insights into patient experiences to follow their patients after discharge. Three approaches to follow-up clinic evaluation are evident: a service evaluation,[189] a qualitative study[188] and a pragmatic, randomised controlled trial;[187] each provides different insights.

Twenty-five interviews were performed to evaluate one service, with a number of important themes evident: patients valued easy access to the clinic, being well-treated by staff and not having to wait long to be seen. Some patients attended because they simply received the appointment, while others identified the need to have questions answered, and wanted to discuss their distressing dreams and hallucinations.[189] Although there was an insightful account of the development and initial evaluation, no demonstrable patient benefits were evident.

Four main themes emerged from another study of 34 patients: continuity of care; receiving information; importance of expert reassurance; and giving feedback to intensive care staff.[188] Continuity of care enabled reassurance to patients that their progress was being monitored and any problems dealt with if referral to other specialties was needed. Opinions varied about the number of clinic appointments and this reflects individual perceptions and needs. Receiving information was invaluable because of the poor memory for factual events. General information about what had happened to them in ICU was also important for gauging the length of time needed for recovery. Patients also found specific information about tracheostomy scars and other specific areas beneficial. While much of this information could be delivered by non-ICU staff, it was noted patients and relatives were specifically reassured by experts familiar with their ICU experiences.[188] Being informed that other patients had similar experiences, particularly with problems sleeping or the nightmares and hallucinations, was also comforting to patients. Clinics also offered the patient the opportunity to give feedback to ICU staff, and allowed patients and relatives to thank staff for the care received.

The PRaCTICaL study randomised eligible patients to a control group of usual care (in-hospital review by a liaison nurse) or intervention group (a physical rehabilitation handbook and a nurse-led intensive care follow-up clinic 2–3 months after discharge and 6 months later).[187] Referral pathways were developed with 'fast-track' access to psychiatric or psychological services. There were no demonstrated differences between groups for the primary (HRQOL: SF-36) or secondary outcome measures (anxiety and depression: HADS; posttraumatic stress: Davidson Trauma Scale). There were also no differences between patients who had a short intensive care stay and those with longer stays.[187]

Despite the lack of evidence to support any improvement in outcome, there is little doubt that patients value intensive care follow-up.[200] There are a number of reasons for the lack of empirical evidence. Our contemporary understanding of patient recovery is evolving constantly. The clinics tend to see all patients at the same time in the recovery process and this may not be appropriate, and perhaps the timing of the clinic is either too late or too early for some patients. It may be that studies have been based on an outdated intervention that did not recognise other challenges such as the effects of delirium or cognitive compromise. Sample sizes tend to be relatively small and often fail to identify what can be small sub-groups of patients who might benefit from a specific intervention.

Other models that incorporate a more person-centred approach and allow more flexibility should therefore be considered. Telephone contact in the initial weeks after discharge can offer some reassurance to patients and also identify early problems. Patients could then be referred to other specialties, have their outpatient appointments coordinated or be invited to return to a follow-up clinic if they experience identified difficulties. Home visits could also be an option for those who are physically or practically unable to return to a clinic or for those with avoidant behaviours. There may be opportunity to incorporate technological solutions such as web-based resources which can provide information about the recovery process and incorporate feedback. One such site is http://edinburghroyalinfirmary.criticalcarerecovery.com/ where patients can access a range of information about the recovery process, be directed to other sites, and importantly how to access help.

Other considerations

It is important to consider that while interventions may not always benefit patients, it also has to be demonstrated that they cause no harm and, therefore, initiating a new service has governance issues. There are also knowledge and skill-set development issues. Intensive care nurses tend not to have training in managing patients on an outpatient basis and new skills have to be learned. They may also not have knowledge and experience in managing many of the patient problems evident at follow-up, in particular the psychological and cognitive issues. Other considerations include accommodation, documentation, communication with other healthcare professionals and evaluation processes. Table 8.8 provides an example of how these issues were addressed when setting up a follow-up service in a Scottish teaching hospital.

Home-based care

Although there are home-based programs to manage ongoing care for some clinical cohorts (e.g. patients with heart failure), no specific follow-up programs currently exist to support survivors of a critical illness. Initial studies in this setting are also yet to identify an optimal intervention to improve recovery. A small number of studies that have predominantly focused on physical rehabilitation have been undertaken where various interventions lasting from 6 to 12 weeks after hospital discharge have been examined; inconsistent results have been identified.

Four studies have been conducted in the UK. In the first study of 126 patients who were provided with a self-help manual that included instructions for exercise as well as two phone calls in the 6-week period improved physical function as measured on the SF-36 was reported.[194] In contrast, a self-help manual was used by Cuthbertson and colleagues over a 3-month period after hospital discharge and no difference in either physical function or mental health on the SF-36 was reported by the 192 participants.[187] Similarly, in an RCT of 60 patients who were in ICU >96 hours, an individually tailored (personalised) exercise program did not improve the primary outcome of physical functioning although there were some short-term improvements in some other aspects of quality of life.[201] Some improvements were identified in the UK where a 5-week multidisciplinary peer-supported rehabilitation program (InS:PIRE) was tested in a quality improvement study (with historical controls).[202] A small improvement in QOL for study patients was identified in comparison to controls. In addition, self-efficacy scores increased during the 5-week program – this was sustained to 12 months. Importantly, there was also a trend towards more InS:PIRE patients returning to employment/volunteering than historical controls. In Australia two studies have also been undertaken. In the first, 195 patients received a graded, individualised endurance and strength training intervention at home that incorporated a printed manual, three home visits and four follow-up phone calls over 8 weeks post-hospital discharge.[203] No difference in physical function on the SF-36 or 6-minute walk test was reported. More recently, Denehy and colleagues provided 150 patients with an exercise program that commenced in ICU and continued through their ward stay and first 8 weeks post-hospital discharge; patients attended outpatients clinics for exercise twice a week for 60 minutes in this post-hospital phase.[130] No difference in physical function was identified. One home-based study has been conducted in the USA where 21 patients received a multi-component intervention incorporating physical, functional and cognitive training.[204] Despite the small patient numbers, improved physical and cognitive functions were identified in patients who received the intervention.

Further research is therefore required to determine what elements of interventions are effective, and at what

TABLE 8.8
Examples of considerations in setting up a nurse-led follow-up service

CONSIDERATION	ACTION
Staff preparation and training	Attend at least one established clinic • Arrange to access educational preparation in relation to psychiatric problems • Discussion and frequent contact with relevant healthcare practitioner, e.g. consultant psychiatrist, psychologist • Observe or 'shadow' a community psychiatric nurse
Accommodation	• Arrange outpatient accommodation with an area close to but separate from the ICU
In-hospital follow-up	• Introduce patients to the presence of the follow-up clinic prior to hospital discharge • Identify how best to communicate with the patient after discharge, i.e. telephone consultation, home visit or clinic appointment
Timing of clinic and number of appointments	• Initial appointment 2–3 months after ICU discharge • Further appointments determined by patient need or request • All patients can contact the follow-up nurse without formal appointments
Structure of clinic	• Patient's case notes reviewed prior to the clinic appointment and discussed between nurse and intensivist • General assessment questionnaire forms the basis of the discussion between the nurse and patient • Standardised measures include for example Short Form 36, HADS and Intensive Care Experience Questionnaire and the Mini-Mental State Examination • Consider offering patients a visit to the ICU but ensure they are ready for this, e.g. if they do not 'trigger' referral on the HADS
Documentation	• General assessment questionnaire will form the basis of the record of appointment; the nurse records any additional information on this form
Referral criteria	• Develop and negotiate clear referral criteria for the relevant specialties, in collaboration with intensivists, other medical specialties and allied health professionals
Letter to GP	• A letter summarising the appointment and any recommendations is sent to the patient's GP

time points these interventions should be delivered; a number of these are currently underway. It must be noted that much of the evidence fails to address specific problems or issues with minority, often indigenous populations or people who live remotely. This criticism can be applied to the international literature and indicates an area worthy of further exploration. With further study, future continuity of care and follow-up services after hospital discharge should enable the development of a series of seamless services that start recovery and rehabilitation activities for a patient while in ICU, are carried through to hospital discharge and continue into the community setting.

Summary

In summary we now have increasing evidence of the significant burden of health issues faced by critical illness survivors. We know many face a prolonged and difficult recovery period that will include physical and psychological problems and that these affect not just the patient themselves but family members and other carers. Patients' lives may be significantly altered after critical illness, placing a social and economic burden on the patient and family but also on the healthcare system. Quality of life is often viewed as diminished and we now need to look to focusing on two main areas by identifying a) effective interventions that can be delivered by the multidisciplinary team that will reduce these burdens and improve overall life quality and b) the patients most likely to benefit from these interventions. Currently health systems are not organised in such a way as to recognise these problems and, therefore, care after ICU discharge tends to be ad hoc and does not follow a recognised rehabilitation pathway. There is a need to look at and learn from other long-term conditions and to adopt approaches that recognise the concept of survivorship after critical illness[15,205] and develop the appropriate systems and processes that will improve life after critical care.

Case study

Mr Paterson was a 45-year-old man admitted to ICU with abdominal sepsis secondary to a ruptured diverticulum. He required 10 days of mechanical ventilation, 5 days renal support, and was in ICU for a total of 15 days. He was sedated through much of this time, though in keeping with local policy his sedation was light and titrated according to his RASS score. Mr Paterson's wife and young children visited him each day while he was in the ICU. He appeared to recognise them but they were unsure. Mr Paterson was then discharged to the high dependency unit for 3 days and then to a surgical ward for a further 10 days. An ICU liaison nurse saw him on one occasion prior to discharge from the ward where he initially had some confusion, appeared fatigued, and was suffering from hallucinations. He was sent an outpatient appointment to attend the nurse-led ICU follow-up clinic around 3 months after hospital discharge.

Mr Paterson and his wife both attended the clinic. He was progressing slowly and struggling with every day activities. He was easily tired, still having some hallucinations from his time in ICU although he was not distressed with these. He indicated to the clinic nurse that he could not understand why he was so tired and unable to return to his work as a storekeeper at a local DIY store. This was causing him and his wife some financial worries, concerns about his progress, and making Mr Paterson irritable and short-tempered with his children. Mrs Paterson was tearful and appeared to be struggling to cope. Mr Paterson had visited his general practitioner (GP) and described these problems, but was told it was quite common to experience these after a lengthy hospitalisation and time in the ICU.

CASE STUDY QUESTIONS

1. How and when should Mr Paterson have been screened or assessed specifically for physical problems and how could his discharge planning have better prepared him for going home from hospital?
2. What strategies might have been commenced in ICU, particularly in collaboration with Mrs Paterson, that might have helped with Mr Paterson's initial time at home. Discuss the evidence underpinning the strategies you suggest.

RESEARCH VIGNETTE

Hickmann CE, Castanares-Zapatero D, Bialais EJ et al. Teamwork enables high level of early mobilization in critically ill patients. Ann Intensive Care 2016;6(1):80. CC BY 4.0.

Abstract

Background: Early mobilisation in critically ill patients has been shown to prevent bed-rest-associated morbidity. Reported reasons for not mobilising patients, thereby excluding or delaying such intervention, are diverse and comprise safety considerations for high-risk critically ill patients with multiple organ support systems. This study sought to demonstrate that early mobilisation performed within the first 24 h of ICU admission proves to be feasible and well tolerated in the vast majority of critically ill patients.

Results: General practice data were collected for 171 consecutive admissions to our ICU over a 2-month period according to a local, standardised, early mobilisation protocol. The total period covered 731 patient-days, 22 (3 %) of which met our local exclusion criteria for mobilisation. Of the remaining 709 patient-days, early mobilisation was achieved on 86 % of them, bed-to-chair transfer on 74%, and at least one physical therapy session on 59 %. Median time interval from ICU admission to the first early mobilisation activity was 19 h (IQR = 15–23). In patients on mechanical ventilation (51%), accounting for 46 % of patient-days, 35% were administered vasopressors and 11% continuous renal replacement therapy. Within this group, bed-to-chair transfer was achieved on 68% of patient-days and at least one early mobilisation activity on 80%. Limiting factors to start early mobilisation included restricted staffing capacities, diagnostic or surgical procedures, patients' refusal, as well as severe hemodynamic instability. Hemodynamic parameters were rarely affected during mobilisation, causing interruption in only 0.8% of all activities, primarily due to reversible hypotension or arrhythmia. In general, all activities were well tolerated, while patients were able to self-regulate their active early mobilisation. Patients' subjective perception of physical therapy was reported to be enjoyable.

Conclusions: Mobilisation within the first 24 h of ICU admission is achievable in the majority of critical ill patients, in spite of mechanical ventilation, vasopressor administration, or renal replacement therapy.

Critique

This observational study provides a description of frequency and characteristics of early mobilisation in a single ICU in Belgium. Early mobilisation (within 24 h) is considered the standard of care and incorporates a progressive range of physical activities from passive to active including transfers in chair, cycle ergometer, verticalisation, standing, leg press and assisted walking. To achieve this mobilisation there is a multidisciplinary(physical therapists, nurses, physicians) review of all patients each morning, with a plan for the day developed. Senior physical therapist to patient ratio is 1:14 from 7.30 a.m. to 5.00 p.m. Monday – Friday; additionally, senior physical therapist to physical therapy students is 1:2. In addition, the nurse patient ratio is 1:1.6 from 7.30 a.m. to 4.00 p.m. No information about staffing levels outside these times are provided.

Over a 2-month period 171 patients were either admitted or already a patient in ICU. This group of patients had a mean APACHE II score of 18±7 and half of the patients were mechanically ventilated. Just over 80% (n = 139) of the patients were mobilised during the first 24 hours of their admission – with seating in a chair being the first activity for 79% of patients.

Eight patients requested their mobilisation activity be discontinued, while a further 11 activities were discontinued due to medical/nursing procedures. Adverse events occurred in 10 mobilisation activities, representing 0.8% of all activities. These adverse events included hypotension, hypertension, tachycardia, faintness, seizures and wound ooze. Importantly, all adverse events were reversible following interruption of the activity and were assessed to have no adverse impact on clinical outcome.

Although this paper summarises activity in a single centre, where only approximately half the patient population is mechanically ventilated it does provide evidence that, with team commitment to early mobilisation, it is possible to achieve such activity in the majority of patients. The authors perceive teamwork to be essential to carrying out early mobilisation, although unfortunately no evaluation of whether that team consultation actually occurred, and what was included in that consultation, has been included in the study. Other contextual elements of this particular setting may be important in achieving mobilisation, although these are not able to be identified with the limited description of setting and without comparison to other ICUs. Resourcing in regard to numbers of physical therapists and nurses has been provided to assist with planning in other settings.

Single centre observational studies such as this are an essential component of building an evidence base, although they should be used to inform the development of larger, multisite studies conducted across many different settings to determine facilitators, barriers, positive outcomes and adverse events or complications in various settings.

Learning activities

1. Identify the changes in patient care in your ICU that could be introduced to facilitate improved long-term recovery and rehabilitation of your patients. Discuss the potential barriers and facilitators to implementing these changes.
2. Develop an educational plan for delivery in your ICU to help staff understand the physical, psychological and cognitive challenges that patients experience after critical illness.
3. Patients transferred from ICU to the ward may have complex care needs. In your hospital, if a follow-up service was planned, how do you think this should be developed?
4. Review the evidence for psychological assessment and management of patients after a critical illness and intensive care admission.

Online resources

ICU Steps, www.icusteps.com

Johns Hopkins Outcomes After Critical Illness and Surgery, https://www.hopkinsmedicine.org/pulmonary/research/outcomes_after_critical_illness_surgery/index.html

Patient-reported Outcome and Quality of Life Instruments Database (PROQOLID), https://eprovide.mapi-trust.org/about/about-proqolid

Patient-Centered Outcomes Research Institute, www.pcori.org

PTSD NICE Guidelines, www.nice.org.uk/CG26

Rehabilitation after critical illness in adults, https://www.nice.org.uk/Guidance/CG83

Mobilisation-network.org, http://www.mobilization-network.org/Network/Welcome.html

Further reading

Azoulay E, Vincent JL, Angus DC, et al. Recovery after critical illness: putting the puzzle together-a consensus of 29. Crit Care 2017;21(1):296. Available from: https://ccforum.biomedcentral.com/articles/10.1186/s13054-017-1887-7

Berry A, Beattie K, Bennett J, et al. Physical activity and movement: a guideline for critically ill adults. Agency for Clinical Innovation, NSW Government, ISBN 978-1-74187-976-6, 2017. Available from: https://www.aci.health.nsw.gov.au/__data/assets/pdf_file/0005/239783/ACI17131_PAM_Guideline.pdf.

National Institute for Health and Clinical Excellence. Rehabilitation after critical illness. NICE clinical guideline 83. 2009 March: 1–91. Available from: http://www.nice.org.uk/CG83; 2009 [accessed 14.03.2018].

References

1. Needham DM, Davidson J, Cohen H, et al. Improving long-term outcomes after discharge from intensive care unit: report from a stakeholders' conference. Crit Care Med 2012;40(2):502–9.
2. Jolley SE, Bunnell AE, Hough CL. ICU-acquired weakness. Chest 2016;150(5):1129–40.
3. Nikayin S, Rabiee A, Hashem MD, et al. Anxiety symptoms in survivors of critical illness: a systematic review and meta-analysis. Gen Hosp Psychiatry 2016;43:23–9.
4. Rabiee A, Nikayin S, Hashem MD, et al. Depressive symptoms after critical illness: a systematic review and meta-analysis. Crit Care Med 2016;44(9):1744–53.
5. Parker AM, Sricharoenchai T, Raparla S, et al. Posttraumatic stress disorder in critical illness survivors: a metaanalysis. Crit Care Med 2015;43(5):1121–9.
6. Wilcox ME, Brummel NE, Archer K, et al. Cognitive dysfunction in ICU patients: risk factors, predictors, and rehabilitation interventions. Crit Care Med 2013;41(9 Suppl. 1):S81–98.
7. Reay H, Arulkumaran N, Brett SJ. Priorities for future intensive care research in the UK: results of a James Lind Alliance Priority Setting Partnership. J Intensive Care Soc 2014;15(4):288–96.
8. Angus DC, Carlet J. Surviving intensive care: a report from the 2002 Brussels Roundtable. Intensive Care Med 2003;29(3):368–77.
9. Oeyen SG, Vandijck DM, Benoit DD, et al. Quality of life after intensive care: a systematic review of the literature. Crit Care Med 2010;38(12):2386–400.
10. Fan E, Dowdy DW, Colantuoni E, et al. Physical complications in acute lung injury survivors: a two-year longitudinal prospective study. Crit Care Med 2014;42(4):849–59.
11. Appleton RT, Kinsella J, Quasim T. The incidence of intensive care unit-acquired weakness syndromes: a systematic review. J Intensive Care Soc 2015;16(2):126–36.
12. Salluh JI, Wang H, Schneider EB, et al. Outcome of delirium in critically ill patients: systematic review and meta-analysis. BMJ 2015;350:h2538.
13. Castillo MI, Cooke M, Macfarlane B, et al. Factors associated with anxiety in critically ill patients: a prospective observational cohort study. Int J Nurs Stud 2016;60:225–33.
14. Iwashyna TJ, Netzer G, Langa KM, et al. Spurious inferences about long-term outcomes: the case of severe sepsis and geriatric conditions. Am J Respir Crit Care Med 2012;185(8):835–41.
15. Kean S, Salisbury LG, Rattray J, et al. 'Intensive care unit survivorship' - a constructivist grounded theory of surviving critical illness. J Clin Nurs 2017;26(19–20):3111–24.
16. Griffiths J, Hatch RA, Bishop J, et al. An exploration of social and economic outcome and associated health-related quality of life after critical illness in general intensive care unit survivors: a 12-month follow-up study. Crit Care 2013;17(3):R100.

17. Dowdy DW, Eid MP, Sedrakyan A, et al. Quality of life in adult survivors of critical illness: a systematic review of the literature. Intensive Care Med 2005;31:611–20.
18. Orwelius L, Nordlund A, Nordlund P, et al. Pre-existing disease: the most important factor for health related quality of life long-term after critical illness: a prospective, longitudinal, multicentre trial. Crit Care 2010;14(2):R67.
19. Orwelius L, Backman C, Fredrikson M, et al. Social integration: an important factor for health-related quality of life after critical illness. Intensive Care Med 2011;37(5):831–8.
20. Bagshaw SM, Stelfox HT, Johnson JA, et al. Long-term association between frailty and health-related quality of life among survivors of critical illness: a prospective multicenter cohort study. Crit Care Med 2015;43(5):973–82.
21. Dettling-Ihnenfeldt DS, de Graaff AE, Beelen A, et al. Coping style and quality of life in Dutch intensive care unit survivors. Rehabil Psychol 2016;61(2):165–72.
22. Stevens RD, Marshall SA, Cornblath DR, et al. A framework for diagnosing and classifying intensive care unit-acquired weakness. Crit Care Med 2009;37(10 Suppl.):S299–308.
23. Barreiro E. Models of disuse muscle atrophy: therapeutic implications in critically ill patients. Ann Transl Med 2018;6(2):29.
24. Parry SM, Puthucheary ZA. The impact of extended bed rest on the musculoskeletal system in the critical care environment. Extrem Physiol Med 2015;4:16.
25. de Jonghe B, Lacherade JC, Sharshar T, et al. Intensive care unit-acquired weakness: risk factors and prevention. Crit Care Med 2009;37(10 Suppl.):S309–15.
26. Winkelman C. Mechanisms for muscle health in the critically ill patient. Crit Care Nurs Q 2013;36(1):5–16.
27. Puthucheary ZA, Rawal J, McPhail M, et al. Acute skeletal muscle wasting in critical illness. JAMA 2013;310(15):1591–600.
28. Hermans G, Van Mechelen H, Clerckx B, et al. Acute outcomes and 1-year mortality of intensive care unit-acquired weakness. a cohort study and propensity-matched analysis. Am J Respir Crit Care Med 2014;190(4):410–20.
29. Villeneuve PM, Clark EG, Sikora L, et al. Health-related quality-of-life among survivors of acute kidney injury in the intensive care unit: a systematic review. Intensive Care Med 2016;42(2):137–46.
30. Bein T, Weber-Carstens S, Apfelbacher C. Long-term outcome after the acute respiratory distress syndrome: different from general critical illness? Curr Opin Crit Care 2018;24(1):35–40.
31. Dettling-Ihnenfeldt DS, Wieske L, Horn J, et al. Functional recovery in patients with and without intensive care unit-acquired weakness. Am J Phys Med Rehabil 2017;96(4):236–42.
32. Vanpee G, Hermans G, Segers J, et al. Assessment of limb muscle strength in critically ill patients: a systematic review. Crit Care Med 2014;42(3):701–11.
33. Fan E, Cheek F, Chlan L, et al. An official American Thoracic Society Clinical Practice guideline: the diagnosis of intensive care unit-acquired weakness in adults. Am J Respir Crit Care Med 2014;190(12):1437–46.
34. Dinglas VD, Aronson Friedman L, Colantuoni E, et al. Muscle weakness and 5-year survival in acute respiratory distress syndrome survivors. Crit Care Med 2017;45(3):446–53.
35. McKinley S, Fien M, Elliott R, et al. Health-related quality of life and associated factors in intensive care unit survivors 6 months after discharge. Am J Crit Care 2016;25(1):52–8.
36. Hweidi IM, Nizamli FM. Stressors in intensive care units in Syria: patients' perceptions. J Res Nurs 2015;20(2):114–26.
37. Guttormson JL. 'Releasing a lot of poisons from my mind': patients' delusional memories of intensive care. Heart Lung 2014;43(5): 427–31.
38. Engstrom A, Nystrom N, Sundelin G, et al. People's experiences of being mechanically ventilated in an ICU: a qualitative study. Intensive Crit Care Nurs 2013;29(2):88–95.
39. Cutler LR, Hayter M, Ryan T. A critical review and synthesis of qualitative research on patient experiences of critical illness. Intensive Crit Care Nurs 2013;29(3):147–57.
40. McGiffin JN, Galatzer-Levy IR, Bonanno GA. Is the intensive care unit traumatic? What we know and don't know about the intensive care unit and posttraumatic stress responses. Rehabil Psychol 2016;61(2):120–31.
41. Pandharipande PP, Girard TD, Jackson JC, et al. Long-term cognitive impairment after critical illness. N Engl J Med 2013;369(14): 1306–16.
42. de Miranda S, Pochard F, Chaize M, et al. Postintensive care unit psychological burden in patients with chronic obstructive pulmonary disease and informal caregivers: a multicenter study. Crit Care Med 2011;39(1):112–18.
43. Davydow DS, Zatzick D, Hough CL, et al. A longitudinal investigation of posttraumatic stress and depressive symptoms over the course of the year following medical-surgical intensive care unit admission. Gen Hosp Psychiatry 2013;35(3):226–32.
44. Chan KS, Aronson Friedman L, Bienvenu OJ, et al. Distribution-based estimates of minimal important difference for hospital anxiety and depression scale and impact of event scale-revised in survivors of acute respiratory failure. Gen Hosp Psychiatry 2016;42:32–5.
45. Hopkins RO, Weaver LK, Collingridge D, et al. Two-year cognitive, emotional, and quality-of-life outcomes in acute respiratory distress syndrome. Am J Respir Crit Care Med 2005;171(4):340–7.
46. Choi J, Tate JA, Rogers MA, et al. Depressive symptoms and anxiety in intensive care unit (ICU) survivors after ICU discharge. Heart Lung 2016;45(2):140–6.
47. Rattray JE, Johnston M, Wildsmith JA. Predictors of emotional outcomes of intensive care. Anaesthesia 2005;60(11):1085–92.

48. McKinley S, Aitken LM, Alison JA, et al. Sleep and other factors associated with mental health and psychological distress after intensive care for critical illness. Intensive Care Med 2012;38(4):627–33.
49. Paparrigopoulos T, Melissaki A, Tzavellas E, et al. Increased co-morbidity of depression and post-traumatic stress disorder symptoms and common risk factors in intensive care unit survivors: a two-year follow-up study. Int J Psychiatry Clin Pract 2014;18(1):25–31.
50. Wade DM, Brewin CR, Howell DC, et al. Intrusive memories of hallucinations and delusions in traumatized intensive care patients: an interview study. Br J Health Psychol 2014.
51. US Department of Veterans Affairs. PTSD: National Center for PTSD. Washington, DC: US Department of Veterans Affairs; 2014. [cited 23 Mar 2018].
52. American Psychiatric Association. Diagnostic and statistical manual of mental disorders (DSM-5®): American Psychiatric Pub, 2013.
53. Jackson JC, Jutte JE, Hunter CH, et al. Posttraumatic stress disorder (PTSD) after critical illness: a conceptual review of distinct clinical issues and their implications. Rehabil Psychol 2016;61(2):132–40.
54. Bryant RA, Nickerson A, Creamer M, et al. Trajectory of post-traumatic stress following traumatic injury: 6-year follow-up. Br J Psychiatry 2015;206(5):417–23.
55. Pietrzak RH, Van Ness PH, Fried TR, et al. Trajectories of posttraumatic stress symptomatology in older persons affected by a large-magnitude disaster. J Psychiatr Res 2013;47(4):520–6.
56. Jackson JC, Hart RP, Gordon SM, et al. Post-traumatic stress disorder and post-traumatic stress symptoms following critical illness in medical intensive care unit patients: assessing the magnitude of the problem. Crit Care 2007;11:1–11.
57. Wade DM, Howell DC, Weinman JA, et al. Investigating risk factors for psychological morbidity three months after intensive care: a prospective cohort study. Crit Care 2012;16(5):R192.
58. Jones C, Bäckman C, Capuzzo M, et al. Precipitants of post-traumatic stress disorder following intensive care: a hypothesis generating study of diversity in care. Intensive Care Med 2007;33(6):978–85.
59. Wade D, Hardy R, Howell D, et al. Identifying clinical and acute psychological risk factors for PTSD after critical care: a systematic review. Minerva Anestesiol 2013;79(8):944–63.
60. Davydow DS, Gifford JM, Desai SV, et al. Depression in general intensive care unit survivors: a systematic review. Intensive Care Med 2009.
61. Schandl A, Bottai M, Hellgren E, et al. Developing an early screening instrument for predicting psychological morbidity after critical illness. Crit Care 2013;17(5):R210.
62. Elliott R, McKinley S, Fien M, et al. Posttraumatic stress symptoms in intensive care patients: an exploration of associated factors. Rehabil Psychol 2016;61(2):141–50.
63. Castillo MI, Cooke ML, Macfarlane B, et al. Trait anxiety but not state anxiety during critical illness was associated with anxiety and depression over 6 months after ICU. Crit Care Med 2016;44(1):100–10.
64. Jonasdottir RJ, Jonsdottir H, Gudmundsdottir B, et al. Psychological recovery after intensive care: outcomes of a long-term quasi-experimental study of structured nurse-led follow-up. Intensive Crit Care Nurs 2018;44:59–66.
65. Chahraoui K, Laurent A, Bioy A, et al. Psychological experience of patients 3 months after a stay in the intensive care unit: a descriptive and qualitative study. J Crit Care 2015;30(3):599–605.
66. Nouwen MJ, Klijn FA, van den Broek BT, et al. Emotional consequences of intensive care unit delirium and delusional memories after intensive care unit admission: a systematic review. J Crit Care 2012;27(2):199–211.
67. Egerod I, Bergbom I, Lindahl B, et al. The patient experience of intensive care: a meta-synthesis of Nordic studies. Int J Nurs Stud 2015;52(8):1354–61.
68. Meriläinen M, Kyngäs H, Ala-Kokko T. Patients' interactions in an intensive care unit and their memories of intensive care: a mixed method study. Intensive Crit Care Nurs 2013;18(6):320–31. 29(2):78-87.
69. Zetterlund P, Plos K, Bergbom I, et al. Memories from intensive care unit persist for several years–a longitudinal prospective multi-centre study. Intensive Crit Care Nurs 2012;28(3):159–67.
70. Weinert C, Sprenkle M. Post-ICU consequences of patient wakefulness and sedative exposure during mechanical ventilation. Intensive Care Med 2008;34(1):82–90.
71. Wolters AE, Slooter AJ, van der Kooi AW, et al. Cognitive impairment after intensive care unit admission: a systematic review. Intensive Care Med 2013;39(3):376–86.
72. Duggan MC, Wang L, Wilson JE, et al. The relationship between executive dysfunction, depression, and mental health-related quality of life in survivors of critical illness: results from the BRAIN-ICU investigation. J Crit Care 2017;37:72–9.
73. Needham DM, Sepulveda KA, Dinglas VD, et al. Core outcome measures for clinical research in acute respiratory failure survivors. An international modified Delphi consensus study. Am J Respir Crit Care Med 2017;196(9):1122–30.
74. Ware JE Jr. SF-36 health survey update. Spine 2000;25(24):3130–9.
75. Ware JE, Snow KK, Kosinski M. SF-36 health survey: manual and interpretation guide. Lincoln: Quality Metric Incorporated; 2000.
76. Vainiola T, Pettila V, Roine RP, et al. Comparison of two utility instruments, the EQ-5D and the 15D, in the critical care setting. Intensive Care Med 2010;36(12):2090–3.
77. Brooks R. EuroQol: the current state of play. Health Policy (New York) 1996;37(1):53–72.
78. Sintonen H. The 15D instrument of health-related quality of life: properties and applications. Ann Med 2001;33:328–36.

79. Capuzzo M, Grasselli C, Carrer S, et al. Validation of two quality of life questionnaires suitable for intensive care patients. Intensive Care Med 2000;26(9):1296–303.

80. Hawthorne G, Richardson J, Osborne R. The Assessment of Quality of Life (AQoL) instrument: a psychometric measure of health-related quality of life. Qual Life Res 1999;8(3):209–24.

81. Rivera Fernandez R, Sanchez Cruz JJ, Vazquez Mata G. Validation of a quality of life questionnaire for critically ill patients. Intensive Care Med 1996;22(10):1034–42.

82. de Bruin AF, Diederiks JP, de Witte LP, et al. The development of a short generic version of the Sickness Impact Profile. J Clin Epidemiol 1994;47(4):407–18.

83. Hunt S, McKenna S, McEwan J, et al. Measuring health status: a new tool for clinicians and epidemiologists. J R Coll Gen Pract 1985;35:185–8.

84. Patrick DL, Danis M, Southerland LI, et al. Quality of life following intensive care. J Gen Intern Med 1988;3:218–23.

85. Elliott D, Denehy L, Berney S, et al. Assessing physical function and activity for survivors of a critical illness: a review of instruments. Aust Crit Care 2011;24(3):155–66.

86. Tipping CJ, Young PJ, Romero L, et al. A systematic review of measurements of physical function in critically ill adults. Crit Care Resusc 2012;14(4):302–11.

87. Borg GA. Psychophysical bases of perceived exertion. Med Sci Sports Exerc 1982;14:377–81.

88. American Thoracic Society. Guidelines for the six-minute walk test. Am J Respir Crit Care Med 2002;166:111–17.

89. Corner EJ, Soni N, Handy JM, et al. Construct validity of the Chelsea critical care physical assessment tool: an observational study of recovery from critical illness. Crit Care 2014;18(2):R55.

90. Skinner EH, Berney S, Warrillow S, et al. Development of a physical function outcome measure (PFIT) and a pilot exercise training protocol for use in intensive care. Crit Care Resusc 2009;11(2):110–15.

91. Hodgson C, Needham D, Haines K, et al. Feasibility and inter-rater reliability of the ICU Mobility Scale. Heart Lung 2014;43(1):19–24.

92. Thrush A, Rozek M, Dekerlegand JL. The clinical utility of the functional status score for the intensive care unit (FSS-ICU) at a long-term acute care hospital: a prospective cohort study. Phys Ther 2012;92(12):1536–45.

93. Parry SM, Granger CL, Berney S, et al. Assessment of impairment and activity limitations in the critically ill: a systematic review of measurement instruments and their clinimetric properties. Intensive Care Med 2015;41(5):744–62.

94. Jackson JC, Mitchell N, Hopkins RO. Cognitive functioning, mental health, and quality of life in ICU survivors: an overview. Crit Care Clin 2009;25(3):615–28, x.

95. Rattray J, Hull A. Emotional outcome after intensive care: literature review. J Adv Nurs 2008;64(1):2–13.

96. Jones C. Aftermath of intensive care: the scale of the problem. Br J Hosp Med (Lond) 2007;68(9):464–6.

97. Hopkins RO. Haunted by delusions: trauma, delusional memories, and intensive care unit morbidity. Crit Care Med 2010;38(1):300–1.

98. Ringdal M, Plos K, Ortenwall P, et al. Memories and health-related quality of life after intensive care: a follow-up study. Crit Care Med 2010;38(1):38–44.

99. Brewin CR. Systematic review of screening instruments for adults at risk of PTSD. J Trauma Stress 2005;18(1):53–62.

100. Griffiths J, Fortune G, Barber V, et al. The prevalence of post traumatic stress disorder in survivors of ICU treatment: a systematic review. Intensive Care Med 2007;33(9):1506–18.

101. Horowitz MJ, Wilner N, Alvarez W. Impact of Event Scale: a measure of subjective stress. Psychosom Med 1979;41(3):209–18.

102. Weiss DS. The impact of event scale - revised. In: Wilson JP, Keane TM, editors. Assessing psychological trauma and PTSD. 2nd ed. New York: The Guilford Press; 2004.

103. Zigmond A, Snaith R. The Hospital anxiety and depression scale. Acta Psychiatr Scand 1983;67(6):361–70.

104. Radloff LS. The CES-D Scale: a self-report depression scale for research in the general population. Applied Psychological Measurement 1977;1(3):385–401.

105. Kessler RC, Barker PR, Colpe LJ, et al. Screening for serious mental illness in the general population. Arch Gen Psychiatry 2003;60(2):184–9.

106. Weathers FW, Litz BT, Keane TM, et al The PTSD Checklist for DSM-5 (PCL-5). National Center for PTSD. Available from: www.ptsd.va.gov, 2013.

107. Stoll C, Kapfhammer HP, Rothenhausler HB, et al. Sensitivity and specificity of a screening test to document traumatic experiences and to diagnose post-traumatic stress disorder in ARDS patients after intensive care treatment. Intensive Care Med 1999;25(7):697–704.

108. Hull AM, Rattray J. Competing interests declared: early interventions and long-term psychological outcomes. Crit Care 2013;17(1):111.

109. Wade DM, Hankins M, Smyth DA, et al. Detecting acute distress and risk of future psychological morbidity in critically ill patients: validation of the intensive care psychological assessment tool. Crit Care 2014;18(5):519.

110. Wergin R, Modrykamien A. Cognitive impairment in ICU survivors: assessment and therapy. Cleve Clin J Med 2012;79(10):705–12.

111. Green A, Garrick T, Sheedy D, et al. Repeatable Battery for the Assessment of Neuropsychological Status (RBANS): preliminary Australian normative data. Aust J Psychol 2008;60(2):72–9.

112. Folstein MF, Folstein SE, McHugh PR. Mini-mental state. A practical method for grading the cognitive state of patients for the clinician. J Psychiatr Res 1975;12(3):189–98.

113. Randolph C, Tierney MC, Mohr E. The Repeatable Battery for the Assessment of Neuropsychological Status (RBANS): preliminary clinical validity. J Clin Exp Neuropsychol 1998;20(3):310–19.
114. Reitan RM. The relation of the trail making test to organic brain damage. J Consult Psychol 1955;19(5):393–4.
115. Wechsler D. Wechsler memory scale - Revised. San Antonio, TX: Psychological Corporation; 1997.
116. Wechsler D. Wechsler adult intelligence scale - Revised. San Antonio, TX: Psychological Corporation; 1997.
117. Nasreddine ZS, Phillips NA, Bedirian V, et al. The Montreal Cognitive Assessment, MoCA: a brief screening tool for mild cognitive impairment. J Am Geriatr Soc 2005;53(4):695–9.
118. de Jager CA, Budge MM, Clarke R. Utility of TICS-M for the assessment of cognitive function in older adults. Int J Geriatr Psychiatry 2003;18(4):318–24.
119. Cook SE, Marsiske M, McCoy KJM. The use of the Modified Telephone Interview for Cognitive Status (TICS-M) in the detection of amnestic mild cognitive impairment. J Geriatr Psychiatry Neurol 2009;22(2):103–9.
120. Calvo-Ayala E, Khan BA, Farber MO, et al. Interventions to improve the physical function of ICU survivors: a systematic review. Chest 2013;144(5):1469–80.
121. Connolly B, O'Neill B, Salisbury L, et al. Physical rehabilitation interventions for adult patients during critical illness: an overview of systematic reviews. Thorax 2016;71(10):881–90.
122. Castro-Avila AC, Seron P, Fan E, et al. Effect of early rehabilitation during Intensive Care Unit stay on functional status: systematic review and meta-analysis. PLoS ONE 2015;10(7):e0130722.
123. Burtin C, Clerckx B, Robbeets C, et al. Early exercise in critically ill patients enhances short-term functional recovery. Crit Care Med 2009;37(9):2499–505.
124. Parry SM, Berney S, Warrillow S, et al. Functional electrical stimulation with cycling in the critically ill: a pilot case-matched control study. J Crit Care 2014;29(4):695, e1–7.
125. Schweickert WD, Pohlman MC, Pohlman AS, et al. Early physical and occupational therapy in mechanically ventilated, critically ill patients: a randomised controlled trial. Lancet 2009;373(9678):1874–82.
126. Schaller SJ, Anstey M, Blobner M, et al. Early, goal-directed mobilisation in the surgical intensive care unit: a randomised controlled trial. Lancet 2016;388(10052):1377–88.
127. Bourdin G, Barbier J, Burle JF, et al. The feasibility of early physical activity in intensive care unit patients: a prospective observational one-center study. Respir Care 2010;55(4):400–7.
128. Needham DM, Korupolu R, Zanni JM, et al. Early physical medicine and rehabilitation for patients with acute respiratory failure: a quality improvement project. Arch Phys Med Rehabil 2010;91(4):536–42.
129. Pohlman MC, Schweickert WD, Pohlman AS, et al. Feasibility of physical and occupational therapy beginning from initiation of mechanical ventilation. Crit Care Med 2010;38(11):2089–94.
130. Denehy L, Skinner EH, Edbrooke L, et al. Exercise rehabilitation for patients with critical illness: a randomized controlled trial with 12 months of follow-up. Crit Care 2013;17(4):R156.
131. Carrothers KM, Barr J, Spurlock B, et al. Contextual issues influencing implementation and outcomes associated with an integrated approach to managing pain, agitation, and delirium in adult ICUs. Crit Care Med 2013;41(9 Suppl. 1):S128–35.
132. Barber EA, Everard T, Holland AE, et al. Barriers and facilitators to early mobilisation in Intensive Care: a qualitative study. Aust Crit Care 2015;28(4):177–82, quiz 83.
133. Nickels M, Aitken LM, Walsham J, et al. Clinicians' perceptions of rationales for rehabilitative exercise in a critical care setting: a cross-sectional study. Aust Crit Care 2016.
134. Goddard SL, Lorencatto F, Koo E, et al. Barriers and facilitators to early rehabilitation in mechanically ventilated patients-a theory-driven interview study. J Intensive Care 2018;6:4.
135. Rukstele CD, Gagnon MM. Making strides in preventing ICU-acquired weakness: involving family in early progressive mobility. Crit Care Nurs Q 2013;36(1):141–7.
136. Hodgson CL, Stiller K, Needham DM, et al. Expert consensus and recommendations on safety criteria for active mobilization of mechanically ventilated critically ill adults. Crit Care 2014;18(6):658.
137. Conceicao T, Gonzales AI, Figueiredo F, et al. Safety criteria to start early mobilization in intensive care units. Systematic review. Rev Bras Ter Intensiva 2017;29(4):509–19.
138. Gosselink R, Bott J, Johnson M, et al. Physiotherapy for adult patients with critical illness: recommendations of the European Respiratory Society and European Society of Intensive Care Medicine Task Force on Physiotherapy for Critically Ill Patients. Intensive Care Med 2008;34(7):1188–99.
139. Kayambu G, Boots R, Paratz J. Physical therapy for the critically ill in the ICU: a systematic review and meta-analysis. Crit Care Med 2013;41(6):1543–54.
140. Moodie L, Reeve J, Elkins M. Inspiratory muscle training increases inspiratory muscle strength in patients weaning from mechanical ventilation: a systematic review. J Physiother 2011;57(4):213–21.
141. Tonella RM, Ratti L, Delazari LEB, et al. Inspiratory muscle training in the Intensive Care Unit: a new perspective. J Clin Med Res 2017;9(11):929–34.

142. Nepomuceno BRV Jr, Barreto MS, Almeida NC, et al. Safety and efficacy of inspiratory muscle training for preventing adverse outcomes in patients at risk of prolonged hospitalisation. Trials 2017;18(1):626.
143. Condessa RL, Brauner JS, Saul AL, et al. Inspiratory muscle training did not accelerate weaning from mechanical ventilation but did improve tidal volume and maximal respiratory pressures: a randomised trial. J Physiother 2013;59(2):101–7.
144. Bissett BM, Leditschke IA, Neeman T, et al. Inspiratory muscle training to enhance recovery from mechanical ventilation: a randomised trial. Thorax 2016;71(9):812–19.
145. Jolley SE, Dale CR, Hough CL. Hospital-level factors associated with report of physical activity in patients on mechanical ventilation across Washington State. Ann Am Thorac Soc 2015;12(2):209–15.
146. Hodgson C, Bellomo R, Berney S, et al. Early mobilization and recovery in mechanically ventilated patients in the ICU: a bi-national, multi-centre, prospective cohort study. Crit Care 2015;19:81.
147. Nydahl P, Ruhl AP, Bartoszek G, et al. Early mobilization of mechanically ventilated patients: a 1-day point-prevalence study in Germany. Crit Care Med 2014;42(5):1178–86.
148. Berney SC, Harrold M, Webb SA, et al. Intensive care unit mobility practices in Australia and New Zealand: a point prevalence study. Crit Care Resusc 2013;15(4):260–5.
149. Bailey PP, Miller RR 3rd, Clemmer TP. Culture of early mobility in mechanically ventilated patients. Crit Care Me 2009;37(10 Suppl.):S429–35.
150. Hickmann CE, Castanares-Zapatero D, Bialais E, et al. Teamwork enables high level of early mobilization in critically ill patients. Ann Intensive Care 2016;6(1):80.
151. Drolet A, DeJuilio P, Harkless S, et al. Move to improve: the feasibility of using an early mobility protocol to increase ambulation in the intensive and intermediate care settings. Phys Ther 2013;93(2):197–207.
152. Dinglas VD, Parker AM, Reddy DR, et al. A quality improvement project sustainably decreased time to onset of active physical therapy intervention in patients with acute lung injury. Ann Am Thorac Soc 2014;11(8):1230–8.
153. Mehlhorn J, Freytag A, Schmidt K, et al. Rehabilitation interventions for postintensive care syndrome: a systematic review. Crit Care Med 2014;42(5):1263–71.
154. Ehlers A, Hackmann A, Grey N, et al. A randomized controlled trial of 7-day intensive and standard weekly cognitive therapy for PTSD and emotion-focused supportive therapy. Am J Psychiatry 2014;171(3):294–304.
155. Hulme T. Using eye movement therapy to reduce trauma after intensive care. Nursing Times (online) 2018;114(3):18–21.
156. Long AC, Kross EK, Davydow DS, et al. Posttraumatic stress disorder among survivors of critical illness: creation of a conceptual model addressing identification, prevention, and management. Intensive Care Med 2014;40(6):820–9.
157. National Institute for Health and Clinical Excellence. Rehabilitation after critical illness. NICE clinical guideline 83. 2009. Available from: http://www.nice.org.uk/CG83.
158. Perris A, Bonizzoli M, Iozzelli D, et al. Early intra-intensive care unit psychological intervention promotes recovery from post traumatic stress disorders, anxiety and depression symptoms in critically ill patients. Crit Care 2011;15:R41.
159. Wade DM, Mouncey PR, Richards-Belle A, et al. Effect of a nurse-led preventive psychological intervention on symptoms of posttraumatic stress disorder among critically ill patients: a randomized clinical trial. JAMA 2019;321(7):665–75.
160. Nydahl P, Knuck D, Egerod I. The extent and application of patient diaries in German intensive care units. Connect: the world of critical care nursing. 2010;7(2):122–6.
161. Egerod I, Schwartz-Nielsen K, Hansen G, Laerkner E. The extent and application of patient diaries in Danish ICUs in. Nurs Crit Care 2006;12(3):159–67.
162. Egerod I, Storli SL, Akerman E. Intensive care patient diaries in Scandinavia: a comparative study of emergence and evolution. Nurs Inq 2011;18(3):235–46.
163. Aitken LM, Rattray J, Hull A, et al. The use of diaries in psychological recovery from intensive care. Crit Care 2013;17(6):253.
164. Ullman AJ, Aitken LM, Rattray J, et al. Intensive care diaries to promote recovery for patients and families after critical illness: a Cochrane systematic review. Int J Nurs Stud 2015;52(7):1243–53.
165. Jones C, Backman CG, Capuzzo M, et al. Intensive care diaries reduce new onset post traumatic stress disorder following critical illness: a randomised, controlled trial. Crit Care 2010;14(5):168–78.
166. Bench SD, Day T, Griffiths P. Involving users in the development of effective critical care discharge information: a focus group study. Am J Crit Care 2011;20(6):443–52.
167. Bench SD, Heelas K, White C, et al. Providing critical care patients with a personalised discharge summary: a questionnaire survey and retrospective analysis exploring feasibility and effectiveness. Intensive Crit Care Nurs 2014;30(2):69–76.
168. Jensen JF, Egerod I, Bestle MH, et al. A recovery program to improve quality of life, sense of coherence and psychological health in ICU survivors: a multicenter randomized controlled trial, the RAPIT study. Intensive Care Med 2016;42(11):1733–43.
169. Rattray J, Crocker C, Jones M, et al. Patients' perception of and emotional outcome after intensive care: results from a multicentre study. Nurs Crit Care 2010;15(2):86–93.
170. Jensen JF, Thomsen T, Overgaard D, et al. Impact of follow-up consultations for ICU survivors on post-ICU syndrome: a systematic review and meta-analysis. Intensive Care Med 2015;41(5):763–75.

171. Moran JL, Solomon PJ. Fixed effects modelling for provider mortality outcomes: analysis of the Australia and New Zealand Intensive Care Society (ANZICS) Adult Patient Data-base. PLoS ONE 2014;9(7):e102297.
172. Gayat E, Cariou A, Deye N, et al. Determinants of long-term outcome in ICU survivors: results from the FROG-ICU study. Crit Care 2018;22(1):8.
173. Fernandez R, Serrano JM, Umaran I, et al. Ward mortality after ICU discharge: a multicenter validation of the Sabadell score. Intensive Care Med 2010;36(7):1196–201.
174. Salisbury LG, Merriweather JL, Walsh TS. Rehabilitation after critical illness: could a ward-based generic rehabilitation assistant promote recovery? Nurs Crit Care 2010;15(2):57–65.
175. Salisbury LG, Merriweather JL, Walsh TS. The development and feasibility of a ward-based physiotherapy and nutritional rehabilitation package for people experiencing critical illness. Clin Rehabil 2010;24(6):489–500.
176. Ramsay P, Salisbury LG, Merriweather JL, et al. A rehabilitation intervention to promote physical recovery following intensive care: a detailed description of construct development, rationale and content together with proposed taxonomy to capture processes in a randomised controlled trial. Trials 2014;15:38.
177. Walsh TS, Salisbury LG, Merriweather JL, et al. Increased hospital-based physical rehabilitation and information provision after Intensive Care Unit discharge: the RECOVER randomized clinical trial. JAMA Intern Med 2015;175(6):901–10.
178. Gruther W, Pieber K, Steiner I, et al. Can early rehabilitation on the general ward after an Intensive Care Unit stay reduce hospital length of stay in survivors of critical illness?: a randomized controlled trial. Am J Phys Med Rehabil 2017;96(9):607–15.
179. Williams TA, Dobb GJ, Finn JC, et al. Determinants of long-term survival after intensive care. Crit Care Med 2008;36(5):1523–30.
180. Myhren H, Ekeberg O, Stokland O. Health-related quality of life and return to work after critical illness in general intensive care unit patients: a 1-year follow-up study. Crit Care Med 2010;38(7):1554–61.
181. UK NHS Audit Commission. Critical to Success. The place of efficient and effective critical care services within the acute hospital. London: Audit Commission for Local Authorities and the National Health Service in England and Wales; 1999.
182. National Institute for Clinical Excellence (NICE). Rehabilitation after critical illness in adults: Quality standard. Available from: nice.org.uk/guidance/qs158 2017.
183. Griffiths JA, Barber VS, Cuthbertson BH, et al. A national survey of intensive care follow-up clinics. Anaesthesia 2006;61(10):950–5.
184. Connolly B, Douiri A, Steier J, et al. A UK survey of rehabilitation following critical illness: implementation of NICE Clinical Guidance 83 (CG83) following hospital discharge. BMJ Open 2014;4(5):e004963.
185. Modrykamien AM. The ICU follow-up clinic: a new paradigm for intensivists. Respir Care 2012;57(5):764–72.
186. Duarte PAD, Costa JB, Duarte ST, et al. Characteristics and outcomes of Intensive Care Unit survivors: experience of a multidisciplinary outpatient clinic in a teaching hospital. Clinics 2017;72(12):764–72.
187. Cuthbertson BH, Rattray J, Campbell MK, et al. The PRaCTICaL study of nurse led, intensive care follow-up programs for improving long term outcomes from critical illness: a pragmatic randomised controlled trial. BMJ 2009;339:b3723.
188. Prinjha S, Field K, Rowan K. What patients think about ICU follow-up services: a qualitative study. Crit Care 2009;13(2):R46.
189. Cutler L, Brightmore K, Colqhoun V, et al. Developing and evaluating critical care follow-up. Nurs Crit Care 2003;8:116–25.
190. Farley KJ, Eastwood GM, Bellomo R. A feasibility study of functional status and follow-up clinic preferences of patients at high risk of post intensive care syndrome. Anaesth Intensive Care 2016;44(3):413–19.
191. Griffiths RD, Jones C. Seven lessons from 20 years of follow-up of intensive care unit survivors. Curr Opin Crit Care 2007;13(5):508–13.
192. Griffiths J, Gager M, Alder N, et al. A self-report-based study of the incidence and associations of sexual dysfunction in survivors of intensive care treatment. Intensive Care Med 2006;32(3):445–51.
193. Kapfhammer HP, Rothenhausler HB, Krauseneck T, et al. Posttraumatic stress disorder and health-related quality of life in long-term survivors of acute respiratory distress syndrome. Am J Psychiatry 2004;161(1):45–52.
194. Jones CP, Skirrow PM, Griffiths RDMDF, et al. Rehabilitation after critical illness: a randomized, controlled trial. Crit Care Med 2003;31(10):2456–61.
195. Hazzard A, Harris W, Howell D. Taking care: practice and philosophy of communication in a critical care follow-up clinic. Intensive Crit Care Nurs 2013;29(3):158–65.
196. Akerman E, Granberg-Axell A, Ersson A, et al. Use and practice of patient diaries in Swedish intensive care units: a national survey. Nurs Crit Care 2010;15(1):26–33.
197. Paul F, Rattray J. Short- and long-term impact of critical illness on relatives: literature review. J Adv Nurs 2008;62(3):276–92.
198. Paul F, Hendry C, Cabrelli L. Meeting patient and relatives' information needs upon transfer from an intensive care unit: the development and evaluation of an information booklet. J Clin Nurs 2004;13(3):396–405.
199. Choi J, Sherwood PR, Schulz R, et al. Patterns of depressive symptoms in caregivers of mechanically ventilated critically ill adults from intensive care unit admission to 2 months postintensive care unit discharge: a pilot study. Crit Care Med 2012;40(5):1546–53.
200. Williams TA, Leslie GD. Beyond the walls: a review of ICU clinics and their impact on patient outcomes after leaving hospital. Aust Crit Care 2008;21(1):6–17.
201. McDowell K, O'Neill B, Blackwood B, et al. Effectiveness of an exercise program on physical function in patients discharged from hospital following critical illness: a randomised controlled trial (the REVIVE trial). Thorax 2017;72(7):594–5.

202. McPeake J, Shaw M, Iwashyna TJ, et al. Intensive Care Syndrome: Promoting Independence and Return to Employment (InS:PIRE). Early evaluation of a complex intervention. PLoS ONE 2017;12(11):e0188028.
203. Elliott D, McKinley S, Alison J, et al. Health-related quality of life and physical recovery after a critical illness: a multi-centre randomised controlled trial of a home-based physical rehabilitation program. Crit Care 2011;15(3):R142.
204. Jackson JC, Ely EW, Morey MC, et al. Cognitive and physical rehabilitation of intensive care unit survivors: results of the RETURN randomized controlled pilot investigation. Crit Care Med 2012;40(4):1088–97.
205. Iwashyna TJ. Survivorship will be the defining challenge of critical care in the 21st century. Ann Intern Med 2010;153(3):204–5.

Chapter 9

Cardiovascular assessment and monitoring

Frances Lin, Thomas Buckley

Learning objectives

After reading this chapter, you should be able to:

- describe the normal blood flow through the cardiovascular system
- define each stage of the cardiac action potential and its application to electrocardiography
- describe the determinants of cardiac output and their interpretation in cardiovascular assessment and monitoring
- describe the reasons for the assessment and monitoring of critically ill patients
- summarise the key principles underpinning cardiac assessment and monitoring
- identify the recommended anatomical landmarks for cardiac auscultation and identify normal and common abnormal heart sounds
- describe the physiological bases and reasons for different types of haemodynamic monitoring
- critique and evaluate current clinical practice on haemodynamic monitoring and integrate best evidence in clinical practice.

KEY WORDS

cardiovascular assessment
cardiovascular electrophysiology
cardiovascular macrostructure
chest X-ray
coronary perfusion
diagnostic imaging
electrocardiography
haemodynamic monitoring
heart sounds

Introduction

This chapter reviews the support of cardiovascular function in the face of many compromises to the system. It is essential for the reader to have a thorough knowledge of both electrical and mechanical functions of the cardiac system. Methods for assessment of cardiovascular elements are discussed, along with best practice ideas and diagnostic techniques.

Related anatomy and physiology

The cardiovascular system is essentially a transport system for distributing metabolic requirements to, and collecting byproducts from, cells throughout the body. The heart pumps blood continuously through two separate circulatory systems: to the lungs and to all other parts of the body (Fig. 9.1). Structures on the right side of the heart pump blood through the lungs (the pulmonary circulation) to be oxygenated. The left side of the heart pumps oxygenated

FIGURE 9.1 The systemic and pulmonic circulations.

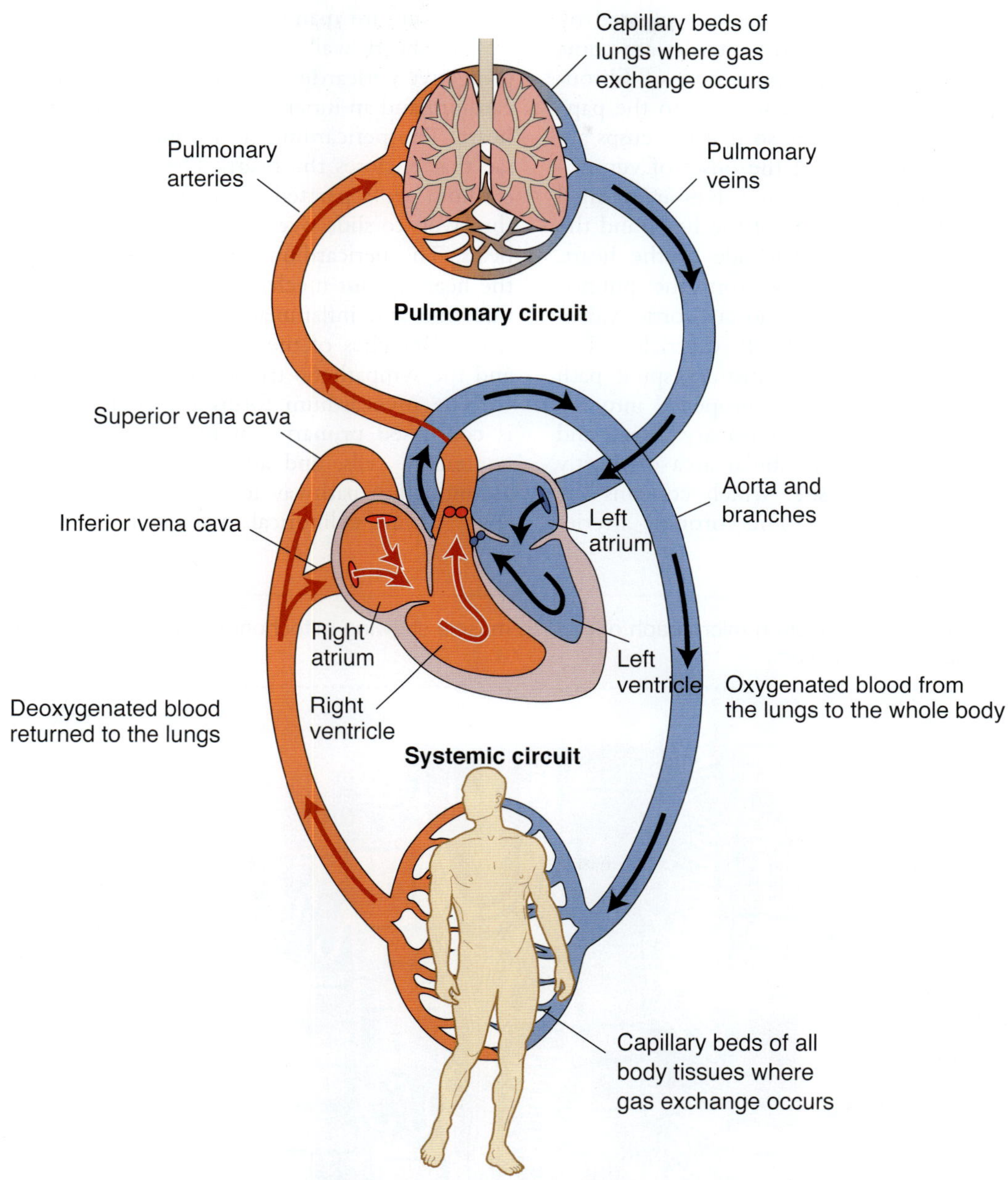

Adapted from Novak B, Filer L, Latchett R. The applied anatomy and physiology of the cardiovascular system. In: Hatchett R, Thompson D, editors. Cardiac nursing: a comprehensive guide. Philadelphia: Churchill Livingstone Elsevier; 2002, with permission.

blood throughout the remainder of the body (the systemic circulation). The two systems are connected, so the output of one becomes the input of the other.

Cardiac macrostructure

The heart is cone-shaped and lies diagonally in the mediastinum towards the left side of the chest. The point of the cone is called the apex and rests just above the diaphragm; the base of the cone lies just behind the mediastinum. The adult heart is about the size of that individual's fist, weighs approximately 300 g and is composed of chambers and valves that form the two separate pumps. The upper chambers, the atria, collect blood and act as a primer to the main pumping chambers, the ventricles. As the atria are low-pressure chambers, they have relatively thin walls and are relatively compliant. As the ventricles propel blood against either pulmonary or systemic pressure, they have much thicker and more muscular walls than the atria. As pressure is higher in the systemic circulation, the left ventricle is much thicker than the right ventricle. Dense fibrous connective tissue rings provide a firm anchorage for attachments of atrial and ventricular muscle and valvular tissue.[1]

One-way blood flow in the system is facilitated by valves. Valves between the atria and ventricles are composed of cusps or leaflets sitting in a ring of fibrous tissue and collagen. The cusps are anchored to the papillary muscles by chordae tendineae so that the cusps are pulled together and downwards at the onset of ventricular contraction. The atrioventricular valves are termed the tricuspid valve in the right side of the heart and the mitral or bicuspid valve in the left side of the heart. Semilunar valves prevent backflow from the pulmonary artery (pulmonic valve) and aorta (aortic valve) into the corresponding right and left ventricles. The muscles in the ventricles follow a distinct spiral path so that, during contraction, blood is propelled into the respective outflow tracts of the pulmonary artery and aorta. The aortic valve sits in a tubular area of mostly non-contractile collagenous tissue, which contains the opening of the coronary arteries. The coronary arteries run through deep grooves that separate the atria and ventricles. The two sides of the heart are divided by a septum, which ensures that two separate but integrated circulations are maintained.[2]

The heart wall has three distinct layers: the outer protective pericardium, a medial muscular layer or myocardium and an inner layer or endocardium that lines the heart. The pericardium is a double-walled, firm fibrous sac that encloses the heart. The two layers of the pericardium are separated by a fluid-filled cavity, enabling the layers to slide over each other smoothly as the heart beats. The pericardium provides physical protection for the heart against mechanical force and forms a barrier to infection and inflammation from the lungs and pleural space. Branches of the vagus nerve, the phrenic nerves and the sympathetic trunk enervate the pericardium.

The myocardium forms the bulk of the heart and is composed primarily of myocytes. Myocytes are the contractile cells, and autorhythmic cells, which create a conduction pathway for electrical impulses. Myocytes (Fig. 9.2) are cylindrical in shape and able to branch to

FIGURE 9.2 Diagram of an electron micrograph of cardiac muscle showing mitochondria, intercalculated discs, tubules and sarcoplasmic reticulum.

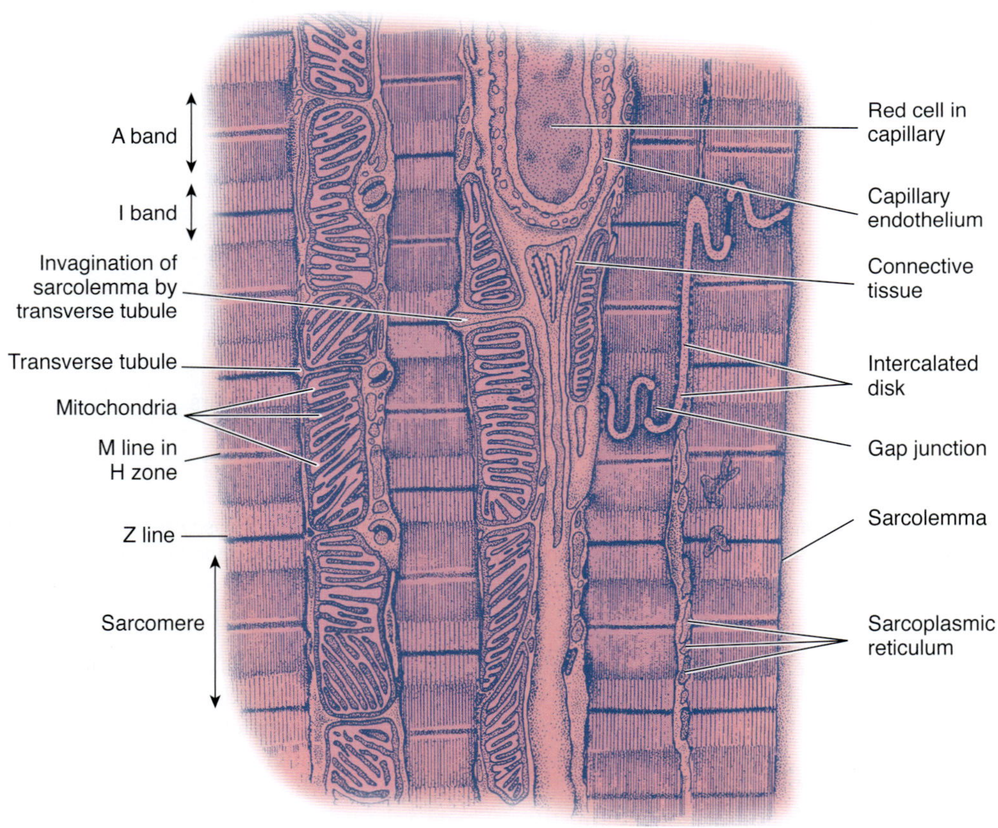

Adapted from Urden L, Stacy KL, Lough ME, editors. Thelan's critical care nursing: diagnosis and management. 6th ed. St Louis: Elsevier; 2010, with permission.

interconnect with each other. The junctions between myocytes are termed intercalated discs and contain desmosomes and gap junctions. Desmosomes act as anchors to prevent the myocytes from separating during contraction. Gap junctions contain connexons, which allow ions to move from one myocyte to the next. The movement of ions from cell to cell ensures that the whole myocardium acts as one unit, termed a functional syncytium. When ischaemia occurs, the gap junctions may uncouple, so ions do not move as freely. Uncoupling may also contribute to the poor conduction evidenced on ECG during ischaemia.[3]

The endocardium is composed primarily of squamous epithelium, which forms a continuous sheet with the endothelium that lines all arteries, veins and capillaries. The vascular endothelium is the source of many chemical mediators, including nitric oxide and the endothelin involved in vessel regulation. It has been theorised that the endocardium may also have this function.[1]

Coronary perfusion

The heart is perfused by the right and left coronary arteries that arise from openings in the aorta called the coronary ostia (Fig. 9.3). The right coronary artery (RCA) branches supply the atrioventricular node, right atrium and right ventricle, and the posterior descending branch supplies the lower aspect of the left ventricle. The left coronary artery divides into the left anterior descending artery (LAD) and the circumflex artery (CX) shortly after its origin. The LAD supplies the interventricular septum and anterior surface of the left ventricle. The CX supplies the lateral and posterior aspects of the left ventricle. This is the most common distribution of the coronary arteries, but it is not uncommon for the RCA to be small and the CX to supply the inferior wall of the left ventricle. The coronary arteries ultimately branch into a dense network of capillaries to support cardiac myocytes.[1] Anastomoses between branches of the coronary arteries often occur in mature individuals when myocardial hypoxia has been present. These anastomoses are termed collateral arteries, but the contribution to normal cardiac perfusion during occlusion of coronary arteries is unclear.[4]

The cardiac veins collect venous blood from the heart. Cardiac venous flow is collected into the great coronary vein and coronary sinus and ultimately flows into the right atrium. Lymph drainage of the heart follows the conduction tissue and flows into nodes and into the superior vena cava.[5]

Physiological principles

An understanding of the principles of cardiac physiology is essential for safe management of the critically ill patient. While the primary role of the circulatory system is to provide sufficient blood flow to meet metabolic demands, this requires adequate myocardial contraction, coordinated electrical conduction and adequate intravascular volume.

Mechanical events of contraction

Energy is produced in the myocytes by a large number of mitochondria contained within the cell. The mitochondria produce adenosine triphosphate (ATP), a molecule that is able to store and release chemical energy. Other

FIGURE 9.3 Location of the coronary arteries.

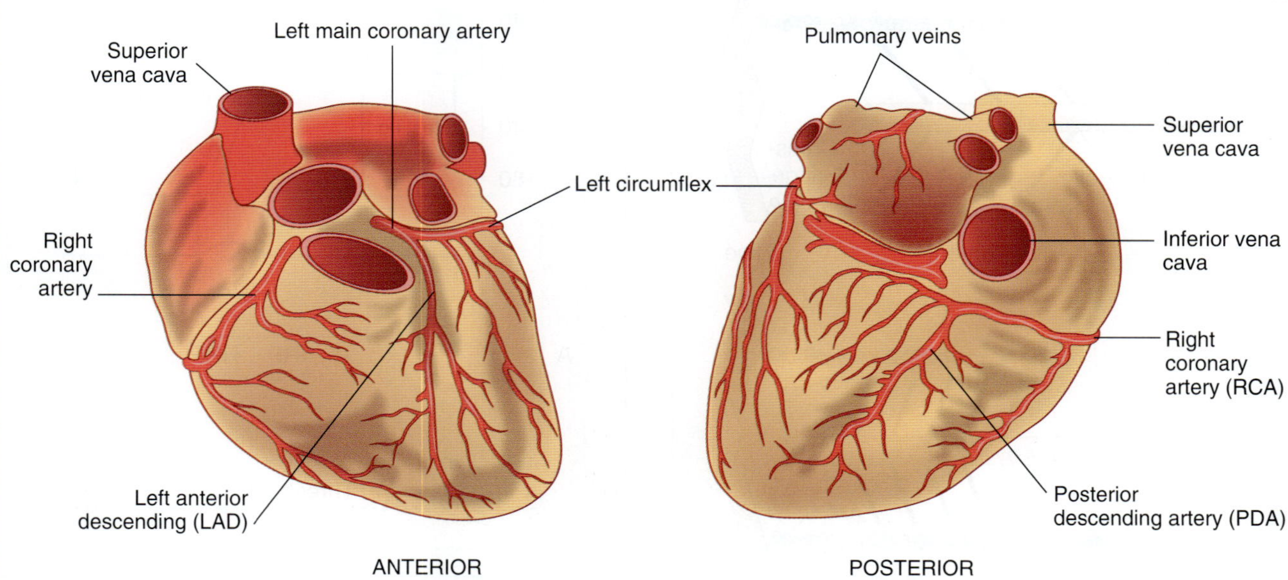

Adapted from Urden L, Stacy KL, Lough ME, editors. Thelan's critical care nursing: diagnosis and management. 6th ed. St Louis: Elsevier; 2010, with permission.

organelles in the myocyte, called sarcoplasmic reticulum, are used to store calcium ions. The myocyte cell membrane (sarcolemma) extends down into the cell to form a set of transverse tubules (T tubules), which rapidly transmit external electrical stimuli into the cell. Cross-striated muscle fibrils, which contain contractile units, fill up the myocyte. These fibrils are termed sarcomeres.

The sarcomere contains two types of protein myofilaments, one thick (myosin) and one thin (actin, tropomyosin and troponin) (Fig. 9.4). The myosin molecules of the thick filaments contain active sites that form bridges with sites of the actin molecules on the thin filaments. These filaments are arranged so that during contraction, bridges form and the thin filaments are pulled into the lattice of the thick filaments. As the filaments are pulled towards the centre of the sarcomere, the degree of contraction is limited by the length of the sarcomere. Starling's law states that, within physiological limits, the greater the degree of stretch, the greater the force of contraction. The length of the sarcomere is the physiological limit because too great a stretch may disconnect the myosin–actin bridges.[2]

Electrical events of depolarisation, resting potential and action potential

Automaticity and rhythmicity are intrinsic properties of all myocardial cells. However, specialised autorhythmic cells in the myocardium generate and conduct impulses in a specific order to create a conduction pathway. This pathway ensures that contraction is coordinated and rhythmical, so that the heart pumps efficiently and continuously. Electrical impulses termed action potentials are transmitted along this pathway and trigger contraction in myocytes. Action potentials represent the inward and outward flow of negative and positive charged ions across the cell membrane (Fig. 9.5).

Cell membrane pumps create concentration gradients across the cell membrane during diastole to create a resting electrical potential of −80 mV. Individual fibres are separated by membranes but depolarisation spreads rapidly because of the presence of gap junctions. There are five key phases to the cardiac action potential:

0 depolarisation
1 early rapid repolarisation
2 plateau phase
3 final rapid repolarisation
4 resting membrane phase.[6]

The contractile response begins just after the start of depolarisation and lasts about 1.5 times as long as the depolarisation and repolarisation (Fig. 9.6).

The action potential is created by ion exchange triggered by an intracellular and extracellular fluid

FIGURE 9.4 Actin and myosin filaments and other cross-bridges responsible for cell contraction.

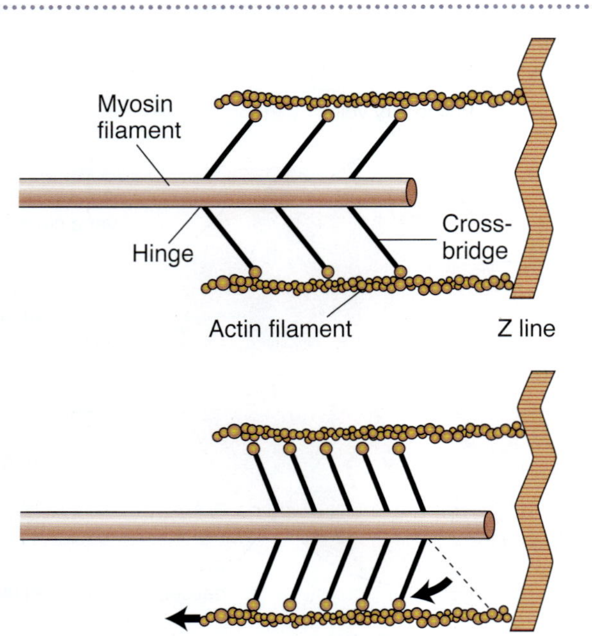

Adapted from Urden L, Stacy KL, Lough ME, editors. Thelan's critical care nursing: diagnosis and management. 6th ed. St Louis: Elsevier; 2010, with permission.

FIGURE 9.5 (A) Action potential in a 'fast-response', non-pacemaker myocyte: phases 0–4, resting membrane potential –80 mV, absolute refractory period (ARP) and relative refractory period (RRP). (B) Action potential in a 'slow response', pacemaker myocyte. The upward slope of phase 4, on reaching threshold potential, results in an action potential.

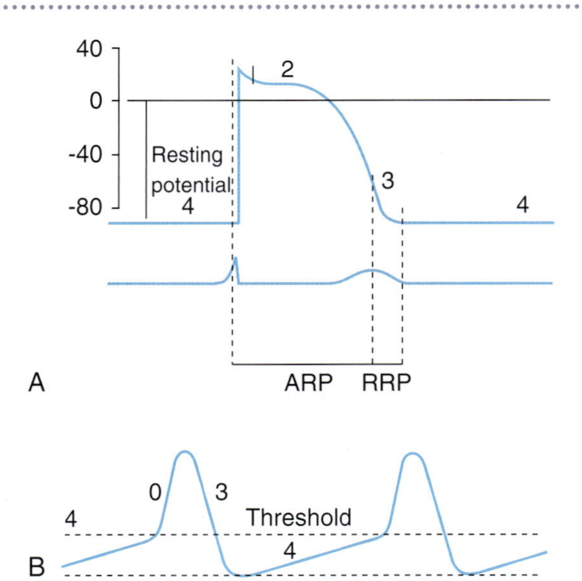

Adapted from Bersten AD, Soni N, Oh TE. Oh's intensive care manual. 7th ed. Oxford: Butterworth-Heinemann; 2013, with permission.

FIGURE 9.6 Action potential.

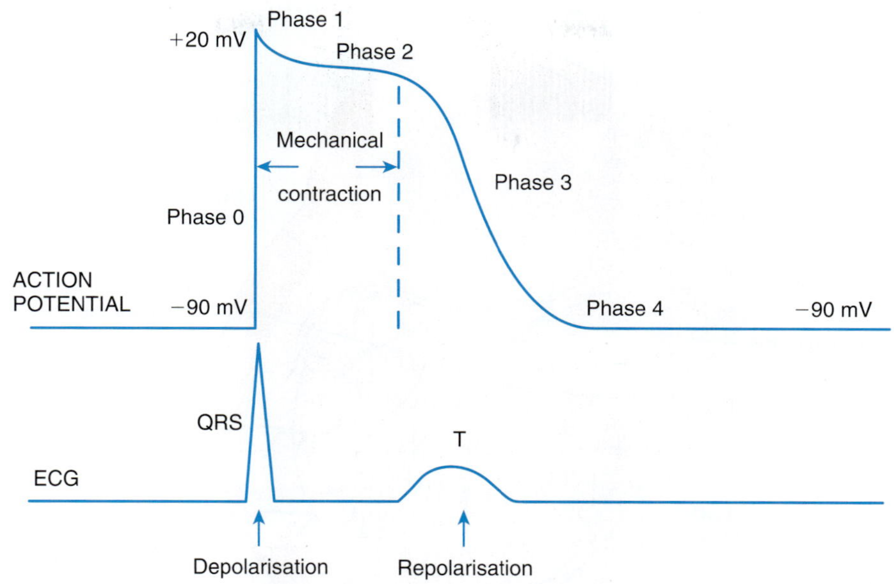

Adapted from Urden L, Stacy KL, Lough ME, editors. Thelan's critical care nursing: diagnosis and management. 6th ed. St Louis: Elsevier; 2010, with permission.

trans-membrane imbalance. There are three ions involved: sodium, potassium and calcium. Normally, extracellular fluid contains approximately 140 mmol/L sodium and 4 mmol/L potassium. In intracellular fluid these concentrations are reversed.[6] The following is a summary of physiological events during a normal action potential:

- At rest cell membranes are more permeable to potassium and, consequently, potassium moves slowly and passively from intracellular to extracellular fluid. At this time fast sodium and slow calcium channels are closed and the resting membrane potential is very negative (–90 mV).
- During depolarisation (phase 0), rapid ion movement caused by sodium flowing into the cell alters the electrical potential from –90 mV to +30 mV. At this time potassium channels close.
- In phase 1 the sodium channels close and potassium begins to leave the cell. This is followed by a brief influx of calcium via the fast channel and then more via the slower channel to create a plateau (phase 2), the duration of which determines stroke volume due to its influence on the contractile strength of the muscle fibres.
- The third phase occurs when the calcium channels are inactivated allowing potassium to leave the cell more rapidly, restoring the negative charge and causing rapid depolarisation.
- The final resting phase occurs when slow potassium leakage allows the cell to increase its negative potential or charge (phase 4) to ensure that it is more negative than surrounding fluid, before the next depolarisation occurs and the cycle repeats.[6]

Cardiac muscle is generally slow to respond to stimuli and has relatively low ATPase activity. Its fibres are dependent on oxidative metabolism and require a continuous supply of oxygen. The lengths of fibres and the strength of contraction are determined by the degree of diastolic filling in the heart. The force of contraction is enhanced by catecholamines.

Depolarisation is initiated in the sinoatrial (SA) node and spreads rapidly through the atria, then converges on the atrioventricular (AV) node; atrial depolarisation normally takes 0.1 second. There is a short delay at the AV node (0.1 s) before excitation spreads to the ventricles. This delay is shortened by sympathetic activity and lengthened by vagal stimulation. Ventricular depolarisation takes 0.08–0.1 s, and the last parts of the heart to be depolarised are the posteriobasal portion of the left ventricle, the pulmonary conus and the upper septum.

The electrical activity of the heart can be detected on the body surface because body fluids are good conductors; the fluctuations in potential that represent the algebraic sum of the action potentials of myocardial fibres can be recorded on an electrocardiogram (see later in this chapter).

Cardiac macrostructure and conduction

The electrical and mechanical processes of the heart differ but are connected. The autorhythmic cells of the

FIGURE 9.7 Cardiac conduction system. AV = atrioventricular; LBB = left bundle branch; RBB = right bundle branch.

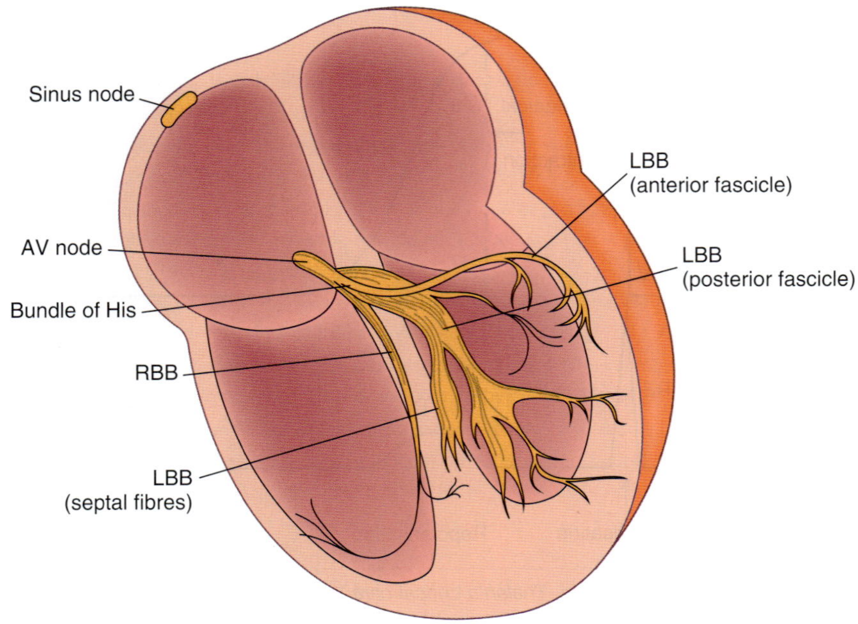

Adapted from Urden L, Stacy KL, Lough ME, editors. Thelan's critical care nursing: diagnosis and management. 6th ed. St Louis: Elsevier; 2010, with permission.

cardiac conduction pathway ensure that large portions of the heart receive an action potential rapidly and simultaneously. This ensures that the pumping action of the heart is maximised. The conduction pathway is composed of the sinoatrial (SA) node, the atrioventricular (AV) node, the bundle of His, right and left bundle branches and Purkinje fibres (Fig. 9.7). The cells contained in the pathway conduct action potentials extremely rapidly, 3–7 times faster than general myocardial tissue. Pacemaker cells of the sinus and atrioventricular nodes differ, in that they are more permeable to potassium, so that potassium easily 'leaks' back out of the cells triggering influx of sodium and calcium back into cells. This permits the spontaneous automaticity of pacemaker cells.[7]

At the myocyte, the action potential is transmitted to the myofibrils by calcium from the interstitial fluid via channels. During repolarisation (after contraction), the calcium ions are pumped out of the cell into the interstitial space and into the sarcoplasmic reticulum and stored. Troponin releases its bound calcium, enabling the tropomyosin complex to block the active sites on actin, and the muscle relaxes.

The cardiac conduction system and the mechanical efficiency of the heart as a pump are directly connected. Disruption to conduction may not prevent myocardial contraction but may result in poor coordination and lower pump efficiency. Interruption to flow through the coronary arteries may alter depolarisation. Disrupted conduction from the SA to the AV node may allow another area in the conduction system to become the new dominant pacemaker and alter cardiac output. Although the autonomic nervous system influences cardiac function, the heart is able to function without neural control. Rhythmical myocardial contraction will continue because automaticity and rhythmicity are intrinsic to the myocardium.[1,7]

Cardiac output

Cardiac performance is altered by numerous homeostatic mechanisms. Cardiac output is regulated in response to stress or disease, and changes in any of the factors that determine cardiac output will result in changes to cardiac output (Fig. 9.8). Cardiac output is the product of heart rate and stroke volume; alteration in either of these will increase or decrease cardiac output, as will alteration in pre-load, afterload or contractility.[1]

Determinants of cardiac output

In the healthy individual, the most immediate change in cardiac output is seen when heart rate rises. However, in the critically ill, the ability to raise the heart rate in response to changing circumstances may be limited, and a rising heart rate may have negative effects on homeostasis, due to decreased diastolic filling and increased myocardial oxygen demand.[8]

FIGURE 9.8 Determinants of cardiac function and oxygen delivery.

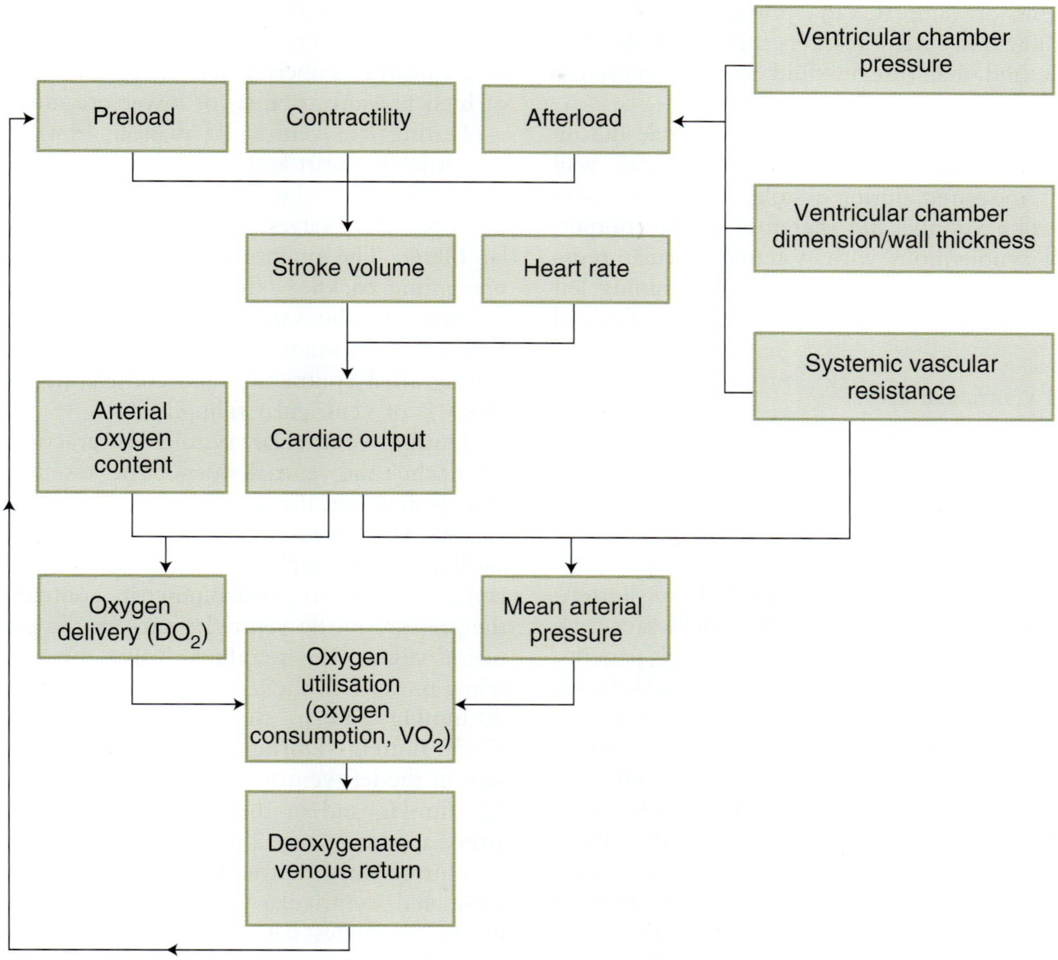

Adapted from Elliott D. Shock. In: Romanini J, Daly J, editors. Critical care nursing: Australian perspectives. Sydney: Harcourt Brace; 1994, with permission.

Preload is the load imposed by the initial fibre length of the cardiac muscle before contraction (i.e. at the end of diastole). The primary determinant of preload is the amount of blood filling the ventricle during diastole and, as indicated in Fig. 9.8, it is important in determining stroke volume. Preload influences the contractility of the ventricles (the strength of contraction) because of the relationship between myocardial fibre length and stretch. However, a threshold is reached when fibres become overstretched, and force of contraction and resultant stroke volume will fall.

Preload reduces as a result of large-volume loss (e.g. haemorrhage), venous dilation (e.g. due to hyperthermia or drugs), tachycardias (e.g. rapid atrial fibrillation or supraventricular tachycardias), raised intrathoracic pressures (a complication of intermittent positive pressure ventilation [IPPV]), and raised intracardiac pressures (e.g. cardiac tamponade). Some drugs such as vasodilators can cause a decrease in venous tone and a resulting decrease in preload. Preload increases with fluid overload, hypothermia or other causes of venous constriction, and ventricular failure. Body position will also affect preload, through its effect on venous return.

The volume of blood filling the ventricles is also affected by atrial contraction: a reduction in atrial contraction ability, as can occur during atrial fibrillation, will result in a reduction in ventricular volume, and a corresponding fall in stroke volume and cardiac output.[9]

Preload of the left side of the heart, assessed at the end of filling of the left ventricle from the left atrium using the pulmonary capillary wedge pressure (PCWP), is assumed for clinical purposes to reflect left ventricular end-diastolic volume (LVEDV). Due to the non-linear relationship between volume and pressure, caution must, however, be taken when interpreting these values, as rises in LVEDP may indicate pathology other than increased preload.[10] Traditionally, preload of the right side of the heart has been indirectly assessed at the end of filling of the right ventricle from the right atrium through central venous pressure (CVP) monitoring, although CVP, as well as other static markers such as PCWP can be unreliable and their use in fluid responsiveness has been challenged.[11]

Afterload is the load imposed on the muscle during contraction, and translates to systolic myocardial wall tension. It is measured during systole, and is inversely related to stroke volume and therefore cardiac output, but it is not synonymous with systemic vascular resistance (SVR), as this is just one factor determining left ventricular afterload.[12] Factors that increase afterload include:

- increased ventricular radius
- raised intracavity pressure
- increased aortic impedance
- negative intrathoracic pressure
- increased SVR.

As afterload rises, the speed of muscle fibre shortening and external work performed falls, which can cause a decrease in cardiac output in critically ill patients. Afterload of the right side of the heart is assessed during the ejection of blood from the right ventricle into the pulmonary artery. This volume is indirectly assessed by calculating pulmonary vascular resistance. Ventricular afterload can be altered to clinically affect cardiac performance. Reducing afterload will increase the stroke volume and cardiac output, while also reducing myocardial oxygen demand. However, reductions in afterload are associated with lower blood pressure, and this limits the extent to which afterload can be manipulated.[12]

Contractility is the force of ventricular ejection, or the inherent ability of the ventricle to perform external work, independent of afterload or preload. It is difficult to measure clinically. It is increased by catecholamines, calcium, relief of ischaemia and digoxin. It is decreased by hypoxia, ischaemia and certain drugs such as thiopentone, beta-adrenergic blockers, calcium channel blockers or sedatives. Such changes affect cardiac performance, with increases in contractility causing increased stroke volume and cardiac output. Increasing contractility will increase myocardial oxygen demand, which could have a detrimental effect on patients with limited perfusion. Stroke volume is the amount of blood ejected from each ventricle with each heartbeat. For an adult, the volume is normally 50–100 mL/beat, and equal amounts are ejected from the right and left ventricle.

Cardiac output is dependent on a series of mechanical events in the cardiac cycle (Fig. 9.9). As normal average heart rate is maintained at approximately 70 beats per minute (bpm), the average phases of the cardiac cycle are completed in less than a second (0.8 s). Electrical stimulation of myocardial contraction ensures that the four chambers of the heart contract in sequence. This allows the atria to act as primer pumps for the ventricles, while the ventricles are the major pumps that provide the impetus for blood to flow through the pulmonary and systemic vascular systems. The phases of the cardiac cycle are characterised by pressure changes within each of the heart chambers, resulting in blood flow from areas of high pressure to areas of lower pressure.[1]

During late ventricular diastole (rest), pressures are lowest in the heart and blood returns passively to fill the atria. This flow also moves into the ventricle through the open AV valves, producing 70–80% of ventricular filling. The pulmonic and aortic valves are closed, preventing backflow from the pulmonary and systemic systems into the ventricles. Depolarisation of the atria then occurs, sometimes referred to as atrial kick, stimulating atrial contraction and completing the remaining 20–30% of ventricular filling.[1,2]

During ventricular systole (contraction), the atria relax while the ventricles depolarise, resulting in ventricular contraction. Pressure rises in the ventricles, resulting in the AV valves closing. When this occurs, all four cardiac valves are closed, blood volume is constant and contraction occurs (isovolumetric contraction). When the pressure in the ventricles exceeds the pressure in the major vessels, the semilunar valves open. This occurs when pressure in the left ventricle reaches approximately 80 mmHg and in the right ventricle approximately 27–30 mmHg. During the peak ejection phase, pressure in the left ventricle and aorta reaches approximately 120 mmHg and in the right ventricle and pulmonary artery approximately 25–28 mmHg.

During early ventricular diastole, the ventricles repolarise and ventricular relaxation occurs. The pressure in the ventricles falls until the pressures in the aorta and pulmonary artery are higher and blood pushes back against the semilunar valves. Shutting of these valves prevents backflow into the ventricles, and pressure in the ventricles declines further. During ventricular contraction, the atria have been filling passively, so the pressure in the atria rises to higher than that in the ventricles and the AV valves open, allowing blood flow to the ventricles. Any rise in heart rate will shorten the resting period, which may impair filling time and coronary artery flow as these arteries fill during diastole.[2]

Regulation of cardiac output

The heart is a very effective pump and is able to adapt to meet the metabolic needs of the body. The activities of the heart are regulated by two responsive systems: intrinsic regulation of contraction and the autonomic nervous system.

Intrinsic regulation of contraction responds to the rate of blood flow into the chambers. Blood flow into the heart depends on venous return from systemic and pulmonic veins and varies according to tissue metabolism, total blood volume and vasodilation. Venous return contributes to end-diastolic volume (preload) and pressure, which are both directly related to the

FIGURE 9.9 The cardiac cycle.

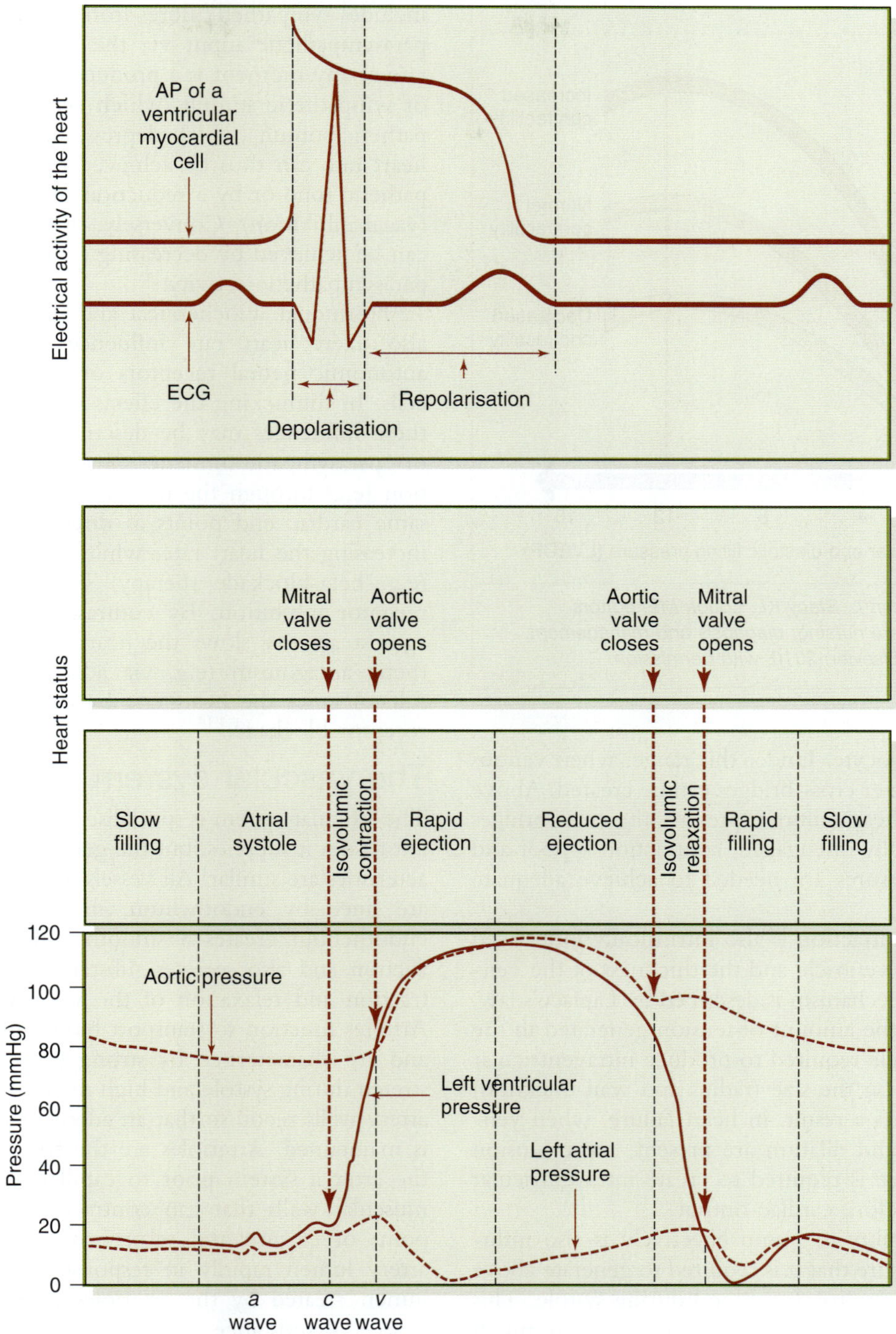

Adapted from Urden L, Stacy KL, Lough ME, editors. Thelan's critical care nursing: diagnosis and management. 6th ed. St Louis: Elsevier; 2010, with permission.

force of contraction in the next ventricular systole. The intrinsic capacity of the heart to respond to changes in end-diastolic pressure can be represented by a number of length–tension curves and the Frank–Starling mechanism (Fig. 9.10). According to this mechanism, within limits, the greater the stretch of the cardiac muscle fibre before contraction, the greater the strength of contraction. The ability to increase strength of contraction in response to increased stretch exists because there is an optimal range of cross-bridges that can be created between actin and

FIGURE 9.10 The Frank–Starling curve. As left ventricular end-diastolic pressure increases, so does ventricular stroke work.

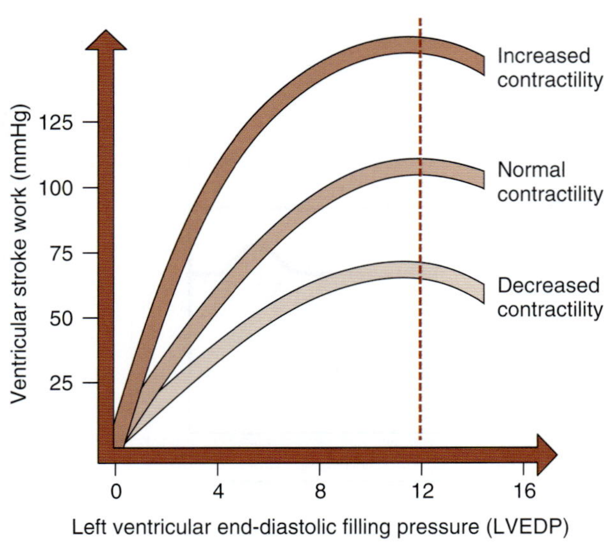

Adapted from Urden L, Stacy KL, Lough ME, editors. Thelan's critical care nursing: diagnosis and management. 6th ed. St Louis: Elsevier; 2010, with permission.

myosin in the myocyte. Under this range, when venous return is poor, fewer cross-bridges can be created. Above this range, when heart failure is present, the cross-bridges can become partially disengaged, contraction is poor and higher filling pressures are needed to achieve adequate contractile force.[1]

Ventricular contraction is also intrinsically influenced by the size of the ventricle and the thickness of the ventricle wall. This mechanism is described by Laplace's law, which states that the amount of tension generated in the wall of the ventricle required to produce intraventricular pressure depends on the size (radius and wall thickness) of the ventricle. As a result, in heart failure, when ventricular thinning and dilation are present, more tension or contractile force is required to create intraventricular pressure and therefore cardiac output.

The heart's ability to pump effectively is also influenced by the pressure that it is required to generate above end-diastolic pressure to eject blood during systole. This additional pressure is usually determined by how much resistance is present in the pulmonary artery and aorta, and is in turn influenced by the peripheral vasculature. This SVR, known and measured as afterload, causes resistance to flow in relation to the left ventricle and is influenced by vascular tone and disease.[13]

Autonomic nervous system control and regulation of heart rate

Although the pacemaker cells of the heart are capable of intrinsic rhythm generation (automaticity), inputs from the autonomic nervous system regulate heart rate changes in accordance with body needs by stimulating or depressing these pacemaker cells. Cardiac innervation includes sympathetic fibres from branches of T1–T5 and parasympathetic input via the vagus nerve. The heart rate at any moment is a product of the respective inputs of sympathetic stimuli (which accelerate) and parasympathetic stimuli (which depress) on heart rate. Rises in heart rate can thus be achieved by an increase in sympathetic tone or by a reduction in parasympathetic tone (vagal inhibition). Conversely, slowing of the heart rate can be achieved by decreasing sympathetic or increasing parasympathetic activity.[14]

Hormonal, biochemical and pharmacological inputs also exert heart rate influences by their effects on autonomic neural receptors or directly on pacemaker cells. In mimicking the effects of direct nervous inputs, these influences may be described as sympathomimetic or parasympathomimetic. Sympathomimetic stimulation (e.g. through the use of isoprenaline) achieves the same cardiac end points as direct sympathetic activity, increasing the heart rate, while sympathetic antagonism (e.g. beta-blockade therapy) slows the heart through receptor inhibition. By contrast, parasympathomimetic agonist activity slows the heart rate, while parasympathetic antagonism (e.g. via administration of atropine sulfate) raises the heart rate by causing parasympathetic receptor blockade.[1,14]

The vascular system

The vascular system is specialised according to the different tissues it supplies, but the general functions and characteristics are similar. All vessels in the circulatory system are lined by endothelium, including the heart. The endothelium creates a smooth surface, which reduces friction and also secretes substances that promote contraction and relaxation of the vascular smooth muscle. Arteries function to transport blood under high pressure and are characterised by strong elastic walls that allow stretch during systole and high flow. During diastole, the artery walls recoil so that an adequate perfusion pressure is maintained. Arterioles are the final small branches of the arterial system prior to capillaries, and have strong muscular walls that can contract (vasoconstrict) to the point of closure and relax (vasodilate) to change the artery lumen rapidly in response to tissue needs. The lumen created by the arterioles is the most important source of resistance to blood flow in the systemic circulation (just under 50%).

Capillaries function to allow exchange of fluid, nutrients, electrolytes, hormones and other substances through highly permeable walls between the blood plasma and interstitial fluid (Fig. 9.11). Just before the capillary beds are precapillary sphincters, bands of smooth muscle that adjust flow in the capillaries. Venules collect blood from the capillaries to veins. Excess tissue fluid is collected by the lymphatic system. Lymphatic veins have a similar structure to the cardiovascular system veins described

FIGURE 9.11 The structure of arteries, veins and capillaries.

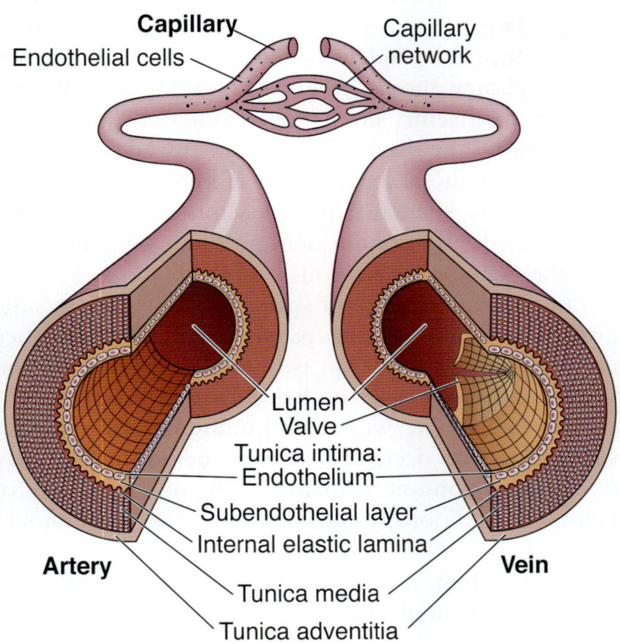

Adapted from Novak B, Filer L, Latchett R. The applied anatomy and physiology of the cardiovascular system. In: Hatchett R, Thompson D, editors. Cardiac nursing: a comprehensive guide. Philadelphia: Churchill Livingstone Elsevier; 2002, with permission.

below, with lymph returning to this system at the right side of the heart.

Veins collect and transport blood back to the heart at low pressure and serve as a reservoir for blood, with ability to dilate and constrict as required. Therefore, veins are numerous and have thinner, less muscular walls, which can dilate to store extra blood (up to 64% of total blood volume at any time). Some veins, particularly in the lower limbs, contain valves to prevent backflow and ensure one-way flow to the heart. In addition to intravascular pressure changes, venous return is promoted during standing and moving by the muscles of the legs compressing the deep veins, promoting blood flow towards the heart.

Blood pressure

Blood flow is maintained by pulsatile ejection of blood from the heart and pressure differences between the blood vessels. Traditionally, blood pressure is measured from the arteries in the general circulation at the maximum value during systole and the minimum value occurring during diastole. The cardiovascular system must supply blood according to varying demands and in a range of circumstances, with at least a minimal blood flow to be maintained to all organs. At a local level this is achieved by autoregulation of individual arteries, such as the coronary arteries, in response to the metabolic needs of the specific tissue or organ. The exact mechanism is unknown, but it has been proposed that increased vascular muscle stretch and/or metabolites and decreased oxygen levels are detected and cells release substances such as adenosine.[1] These substances result in rapid vasodilation and increased perfusion. The vascular endothelium actively secretes prostacyclin and endothelial-derived relaxing factor (nitric oxide), both vasoactive agents.[15]

There are three main regulatory mechanisms of blood pressure control: a) short-term autonomic control, b) medium-term hormonal control and c) long-term renal system control.

Autonomic control

The cardiovascular control centre connects with the hypothalamus to control temperature, the cerebral cortex and the autonomic system to control cardiac activity and peripheral vascular tone. Information about blood pressure and resistance is sensed by neural receptors (baroreceptors) in the aortic arch and the carotid sinuses, which detect changes in blood supply to the body and the brain. Impulses from these receptors initiate a blood-pressure regulating reflex in the cardiovascular centre, which activates the parasympathetic system and sympathetic system to alter cardiac activity and dilation or constriction of arterioles and veins to lower or raise blood pressure. The cardiovascular system also maintains a constant resting tone of intermediate tension in the arteries.[1]

Hormonal control

Changes in blood pressure are also detected by the adrenal medulla, which secretes catecholamines as cardiac output declines. The two main catecholamines, adrenaline (epinephrine) and noradrenaline (norepinephrine), mimic the action of the sympathetic system by binding to and stimulating adrenergic receptors. Adrenergic receptors are located in smooth muscle cells of vascular beds including the peripheral veins and arterioles supplying the skin, kidneys, skeletal muscles and mucosa.[1]

The main action of adrenaline occurs by binding to the beta-1 adrenoreceptors (located mainly in the heart but also found in platelets and the non-sphincter part of the gastrointestinal tract), causing an increase in the rate and contraction of the heart, aggregation of platelets and relaxation of the non-sphincter part of the gastrointestinal tract. Adrenaline also binds to beta-2 receptors, located on blood vessels, the bronchi, gastrointestinal tract, skeletal muscle, liver and mast cells (inflammatory cells). Activation results in vasodilatation of small coronary arteries, bronchodilation, relaxation of the gastrointestinal tract, glycogenolysis (breakdown of glycogen to glucose) in the liver, tremor in skeletal muscle and inhibition of histamine (an inflammatory amine responsible for increased permeability of capillaries).

Noradrenaline binds to both beta and alpha receptors. Alpha-1 and alpha-2 adrenoreceptors are found in the central and peripheral nervous system and are located on vascular and non-vascular smooth muscle. Alpha-1 adrenergic stimulation causes vasoconstriction and is the main mechanism of the vasopressor action of noradrenaline. Presynaptic alpha-2 receptors inhibit the release of noradrenaline and thus serve as an important receptor in the negative feedback control of noradrenaline release.[16] Postsynaptic alpha-2 receptors are located on liver cells, platelets and the smooth muscle of blood vessels and, when activated, cause platelet aggregation and blood vessel constriction.[17] Noradrenaline results in very little beta-2 activity. Clinically, the positive inotropic and chronotropic effects of noradrenaline, from beta-1 simulation, are counterbalanced by the increased afterload from elevated SVR (alpha-1 adrenergic agonist effect).

Renal control

Renal control of blood pressure in the long term occurs via control of blood volume. Generally, as blood pressure or volume rises, the kidneys produce more urine; conversely, as blood pressure or volume falls, the kidneys produce less urine.

In addition to longer term fluid regulation, during acute illness or time of acute hypotension, the renin–angiotensin–aldosterone system (RAAS) plays an important role in maintaining blood pressure. This negative feedback system both reabsorbs intravascular fluid and increases peripheral resistance, in an effort to increase blood pressure.[1] Further details on the RAAS system can be found in Chapter 18.

Assessment

It is essential that the critical care nurse conducts a comprehensive cardiac assessment on a critically ill patient. The nursing assessment aims to define patient cardiovascular status as well as inform implementation of an appropriate clinical management plan. The focus of the cardiovascular assessment varies according to the setting, clinical presentation and treatments commenced, if any. However, the main priority should be to determine whether the patient is haemodynamically stable or requiring initiation or adjustment of supportive treatments.

A thorough cardiac assessment requires the critical care nurse to be competent in a wide range of interpersonal, observational and technical skills. A cardiac assessment should be performed as part of a comprehensive patient assessment and should consider the following elements.

It is important to create a health history, if not already obtained. This history should aim to elicit a description from the patient or their family of the present illness and chief complaint. A useful guide in taking a specific cardiac history is to use direct questions to seek information regarding symptom onset, course, duration, location and precipitating and alleviating factors. Some common cardiovascular disease-related symptoms to be observed for include: chest discomfort or pain, palpitations, syncope, generalised fatigue, dyspnoea, cough, weight gain or dependent oedema. Chest pain, discomfort or tightness should be initially considered indicative of cardiac ischaemia until proven otherwise by further examination and diagnostic assessment. Additionally, a health history should be inclusive of known cardiovascular risk factors, such as hyperlipidaemia or hypertension, and any medications the patient may be taking including over-the-counter medications.

Prior to inspecting or palpating the patient, the nurse should observe the patient's general appearance noting whether the patient is restless, able to lie flat, in pain or distress, is pale or has decreased level of consciousness. Patients with compromised cardiac output will likely have decreased cerebral perfusion and may have mental confusion, memory loss or slowed verbal responses. Additionally, assessment of any pain should be noted.

Specific physical assessment in relation to cardiovascular function should be inclusive of:

- vital signs
- respiratory assessment for signs of pulmonary oedema (shortness of breath or basal crepitations)
- assessment of neck vein distension for signs of right-sided venous congestion
- assessment for signs of peripheral oedema
- capillary refill time with >3 seconds return indicative of sluggish capillary return; indicative of reduced effective circulating volume
- 12-lead ECG for signs of ischaemia or cardiac pathology
- appearance and temperature of the skin for signs of peripheral constriction or dehydration
- core body temperature measurement
- urine output with < 0.5 mL/kg/h a potential indicator of decreased renal perfusion.

Assessment of pulse

In the critical care environment, the heart rate can be observed from a cardiac monitor; however, this does not give qualitative information about the arterial pulse. Routinely performed as part of most patient assessments, information gathered from pulse assessment can give useful cues and direct further assessments. Although the radial pulse is distant from the central arteries, it is useful for gathering information on rate, rhythm and strength. Heart rate below 60 bpm is defined as 'bradycardia' (*brady* is Greek for slow, and *kardia* means heart). A heart rate greater than 100 bpm per minute is called 'tachycardia' (*tachy* is Greek meaning swift). An important aspect of pulse assessment involves assessment for regularity. Detection of an irregular pulse should trigger further investigation and prompt ECG assessment for atrial fibrillation, a condition in which atrial contraction becomes lost due to chaotic electrical activity with variable ventricular response. In addition to rate and rhythm, assessment of pulse, especially if palpated in the carotid or femoral artery, can reveal a bounding pulse that may be indicative of hyperdynamic state or aortic regurgitation. An alternating strong and weak pulse, known as *pulsus alternans*, may be observed in advanced heart failure.

Auscultation of heart sounds

Auscultation of the heart involves listening to heart sounds over the pericardial area using a stethoscope.[18] While challenging to achieve competence in, cardiac auscultation is an important part of cardiac physical examination and relies on a sound understanding of cardiac anatomy, cardiac cycle and physiologically associated sounds. For accurate auscultation, experience in assessment of normal sounds is critical and can only be obtained through constant practice. When auscultating heart sounds, normally two sounds are readily audible and they are known as the first (S1) and second (S2) sounds. A useful technique when listening to heart sounds is to feel the carotid pulse at the same time as auscultation, which will help identify the heart sound that corresponds with ventricular systole.

Practice tip

When learning to interpret heart sounds, feel the carotid pulse at the same time as auscultation of the heart, which will help identify the heart sound that corresponds with ventricular systole (S1 will be heard simultaneously with the pulse).

The first heart sound (S1) occurs at the beginning of ventricular systole, following closure of the intracardiac valves (mitral and tricuspid valves). This heart sound is best heard with the diaphragm of the stethoscope and loudest directly over the corresponding valves (4th intercostal space (ICS) left of the sternum for the tricuspid and 5th ICS left of the mid-clavicular line for the mitral valve). Following closure of these two valves, ventricular contraction and ejection occurs and a carotid pulse may be palpated at the same time that S1 is audible.[19]

The second heart sound (S2) occurs at the beginning of diastole, following closure of the aortic and pulmonary valves and can be best heard over these valves (2nd ICS to the right and left of the sternum, respectively). It is important to remember that both S1 and S2 result from events occurring in *both* left and right sides of the heart. As left-sided heart sounds are normally loudest and occur slightly before right-sided events, careful listening during inspiration and expiration may result in left and right events being heard separately. This is known as physiological splitting of heart sounds, a normal physiological event. A guide to placement of the stethoscope when listening to heart sounds is presented in Table 9.1.

TABLE 9.1
Guide to placement of the stethoscope when listening to heart sounds

STETHOSCOPE PLACEMENT		AUDITABLE REGION OF HEART
2nd intercostal space	Right of sternum	Aortic valve
2nd intercostal space	Left of sternum	Pulmonary valve
4th intercostal space	Left side of sternum	Tricuspid valve
5th intercostal space	Mid-clavicular line	Mitral valve

In assessment of the critically ill patient extra heart sounds, labelled S3 and S4, may be heard during times of extra ventricular filling or fluid overload. Often referred to as 'gallops', these extra heart sounds are accentuated during episodes of tachycardia. S3, ventricular gallop, occurs during diastole in the presence of fluid overload. Considered physiological in children or young people, due to rapid diastolic filling, S3 may be considered pathological when due to reduced ventricular compliance and associated increased atrial pressures. As S3 occurs early in diastole, it will be heard and associated more closely with S2.[19]

S4 is a late diastolic sound and may be heard shortly before S1. S4 occurs when ventricular compliance is reduced secondary to aortic or pulmonary stenosis, mitral regurgitation, systemic hypertension, advanced age or ischaemic heart disease. In patients with severe ventricular dysfunction, both S3 and S4 may be audible although, when coupled with tachycardia, these may be difficult to differentiate and will require specialist assessment.

The critical care nurse auscultating the heart should also listen for a potential pericardial rub. This 'rubbing' or 'scratching' sound is secondary to pericardial inflammation and/or fluid accumulation in the pericardial space. To differentiate pericardial rub from pulmonary rub, if possible the patient should be instructed to hold their breath for a short duration as pericardial rub will continue to be audible in the absence of breathing, heard over the 3rd ICS to the left of the mid-sternum. Detection of pericardial rub warrants further investigation by ultrasound.

TABLE 9.2
Classification of heart murmurs using the Levine scale

Grade 1	Low intensity and difficult to hear
Grade 2	Low intensity, but audible with a stethoscope but no palpable thrill
Grade 3	Medium intensity and easily heard with a stethoscope
Grade 4	Loud and audible and with palpable thrill
Grade 5	Very loud but cannot be heard outside the praecordium and with palpable thrill
Grade 6	Audible with the stethoscope away from the chest

Adapted from Johnson K, Rawlings-Anderson K. Oxford handbook of cardiac nursing. 2nd ed. New York: Oxford University Press.

Practice tip

To differentiate pericardial rub from pulmonary rub, ask the patient to hold their breath for a short duration, as pericardial rub will continue to be audible in the absence of breathing and pleural rub will not be audible while the patient is not breathing.

In addition to pericardial rub, murmurs may also be audible. Murmurs are generally classified and characterised by location with the most common murmurs associated with the mitral or aortic valves, due to either stenosis or regurgitation at these locations. Murmurs are best thought of as turbulent flow or vibrations associated with the corresponding valve and can be of variable pitch. Specialist cardiac referral is indicated upon detection of cardiac murmurs to differentiate pathological murmurs, as seen during valvular dysfunction or myocardial infarction, from innocent systolic 'high flow' murmurs detected in children or adolescents as a result of vigorous ventricular contraction. Murmurs may be classified using the Levine scale,[20] shown in Table 9.2.

Continuous cardiac monitoring

In the case of the critically ill patient, there are two main forms of cardiac monitoring, both of which are used to generate essential data: continuous cardiac monitoring and the 12-lead ECG. Internationally, a minimum standard for an ICU requires availability of facilities for cardiovascular monitoring.[21-23] Continuous cardiac monitoring allows for rapid assessment and constant evaluation with, when required, the instantaneous production of paper recordings for more detailed assessment or documentation into patient records. In addition, practice standards for electrocardiographic monitoring in hospital settings have been established.[24]

It is common practice for five leads to be used for continuous cardiac monitoring, as this allows a choice of seven views. The five electrodes are placed as follows:

- right and left arm electrodes: placed on each shoulder
- right and left leg electrodes: placed on the hips or level with the lowest ribs on the chest
- V-lead views can be monitored: for V1 place the electrode at the 4th ICS, right of the sternum; for V6 place the electrode at the 5th ICS, left mid-axillary line.

The monitoring lead of choice is determined by the patient's clinical situation. Generally, two views are better than one. V1 lead is best to view ventricular activity and differentiate right and left bundle branch blocks; therefore, one of the channels on the bedside monitor should display a V lead, preferably V1, and the other display lead II or III for optimal detection of arrhythmias. When the primary purpose of monitoring is to detect ischaemic changes, leads III and V3 usually present the optimal combination.[24]

The skin must be carefully prepared before electrodes are attached, as contact is required with the body surface and poor contact will lead to inaccurate or unreadable recordings, causing interference or noise. Patients who are sweaty need particular attention, and it may be necessary to shave the areas where the electrodes are to be placed in very hairy people.

12-lead ECG

The Dutch physiologist Einthoven was one of the first to represent heart electrical conduction as two charged electrodes, one positive and one negative. The body can be likened to a triangle, with the heart at its centre, and this has been called Einthoven's triangle. Cardiac electrical activity can be captured by placing electrodes on both arms and on the left leg. When these electrodes are connected to a common terminal with an indifferent electrode that remains near zero, an electrical potential is obtained. Depolarisation moving towards an active electrode produces positive deflection.

The 12-lead ECG consists of six limb leads and six chest leads. The limb leads examine electrical activity along a vertical plane. The standard bipolar limb leads (I, II, III) record differences in potential between the two limbs by using two limb electrodes as positive and negative poles (Fig. 9.12): leads I, II, and III all produce positive deflections on the ECG because the electrical current flows from left to the right and from upwards to downwards. Placement should be:

- I = negative electrode in right arm and positive electrode in left arm

FIGURE 9.12 Einthoven's triangle formed by standard limb leads.

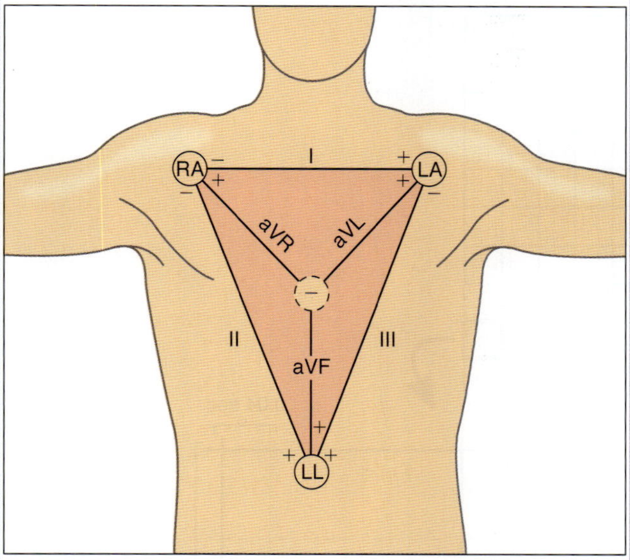

Adapted from Urden L, Stacy KL, Lough ME, editors. Thelan's critical care nursing: diagnosis and management. 6th ed. St Louis: Elsevier; 2010, with permission.

FIGURE 9.13 Position of chest leads.

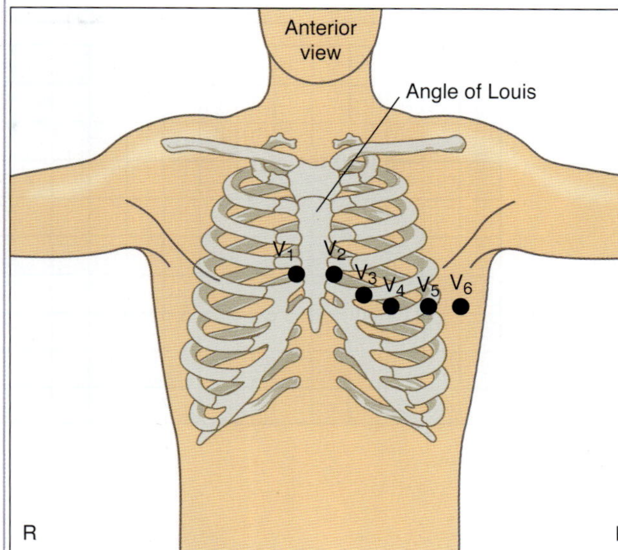

Adapted from Urden L, Stacy KL, Lough ME, editors. Thelan's critical care nursing: diagnosis and management. 6th ed. St Louis: Elsevier; 2010, with permission.

- II = negative electrode in right arm and positive electrode in left leg
- III = negative electrode in left arm and positive electrodes in left leg.

The three unipolar limb leads (aVR, aVL, aVF) record activity of the heart's frontal plane. Each of these unipolar leads has only one positive electrode (the limb electrode such as left arm, right arm or left leg), with the centre of Einthoven's triangle acting as the negative electrode. The waveforms of these leads are usually very small; therefore, they are augmented by the ECG machine to increase the size of the potentials on the ECG strip. These three leads view the heart at different angles:

- Lead aVR produces a negative reflection because the electrical activity moves away from the lead. Lead aVR does not provide a specific view of the heart.
- Lead aVL produces a positive deflection because the electrical activity moves towards the lead. Lead aVL views the electrical activity from the lateral wall.
- Lead aVF also produces a positive deflection on the ECG because the electrical activity flows towards this lead. It views the electrical activity from the inferior wall.

The six unipolar chest leads (precordial leads) are designated V1–6 and examine electrical activity along a horizontal plane from the right ventricle, septum, left ventricle and the left atrium. They are positioned in the following way (Fig. 9.13):

- V1 = 4th ICS, to the right of the patient's sternum
- V2 = 4th ICS, to the left of the patient's sternum
- V3 = equidistant between V2 and V4
- V4 = 5th ICS on the mid-clavicular line
- V5 = 5th ICS, anterior axillary line
- V6 = 5th ICS on the mid-axilla line

Amplitude (voltage) in the ECG is measured by a series of horizontal lines on the ECG trace (Fig. 9.14). Lines are 1 mm apart and represent increments of 0.1 mV. Amplitude reflects the wave's electrical force and has no relation to the muscle strength of ventricular contraction. Duration of activity within the ECG is measured by a series of vertical lines also 1 mm apart (Fig. 9.14). The time interval between each line is 0.04 s. Every 5th line is printed in bold, producing large squares. Each represents 0.5 mV (vertically) and 0.2 s (horizontally).[6]

Key components of the ECG

Key components of the cardiac electrical activity are termed PQRST (Fig. 9.15):

- The P wave represents electrical activity caused by spread of impulses from the SA node across the atria and appears upright in lead II. Inverted P waves indicate atrial depolarisation from a site other

FIGURE 9.14 ECG graph paper.

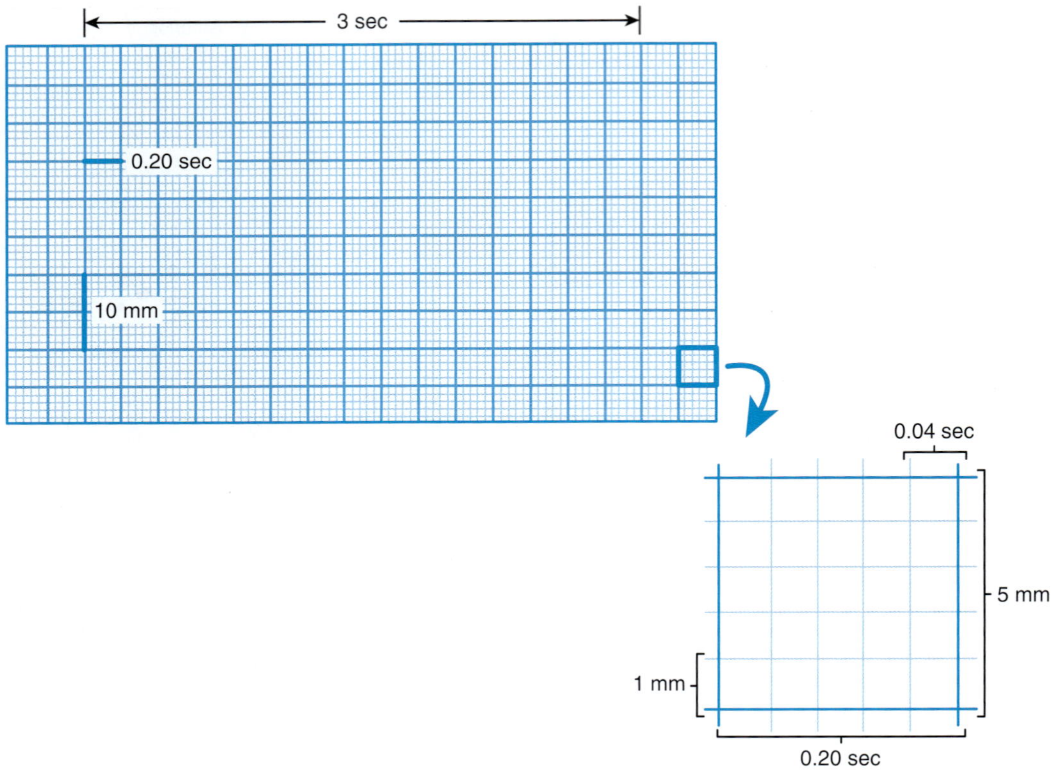

Adapted from Urden L, Stacy KL, Lough ME, editors. Thelan's critical care nursing: diagnosis and management. 6th ed. St Louis: Elsevier; 2010, with permission.

FIGURE 9.15 Normal ECG.

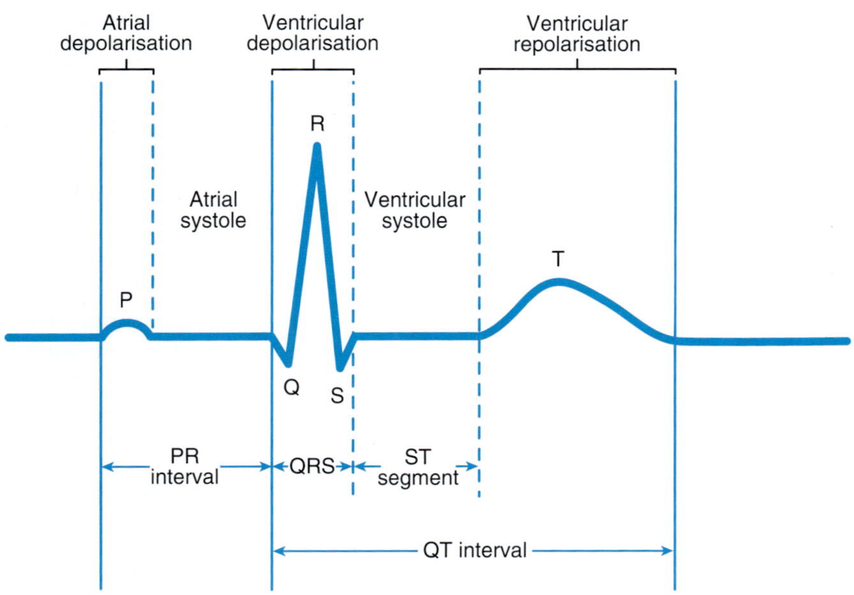

Adapted from Urden L, Stacy KL, Lough ME, editors. Thelan's critical care nursing: diagnosis and management. 6th ed. St Louis: Elsevier; 2010, with permission.

than the SA node. Normal P wave duration is considered to be less than 0.12 s.

- The P–R interval reflects the total time taken for the atrial impulse to travel through the atria and AV node. It is measured from the start of the P wave to the beginning of the QRS complex, but is lengthened by AV block or some drugs. Normal P–R interval is 0.12–0.2 s.
- The QRS complex is measured from the start of the Q wave to the end of the S wave and represents the time taken for ventricular depolarisation. Normal QRS duration is 0.08–0.12 s. Anything longer than 0.12 s is abnormal and may indicate conduction disorders such as bundle branch block. The deflections seen in relation to this complex will vary in size, depending on the lead being viewed. However, small QRS complexes occur when the heart is insulated, as in the presence of pericardial effusion. Conversely, an exaggerated QRS complex is suggestive of ventricular hypertrophy. Normal, non-pathological Q waves are often seen in leads I, aVL, V5, V6 from septal depolarisation, which are less than 25% of the R height and 0.04 s. A 'pathological' Q wave (>0.04 s plus >25% of R wave height) may indicate a previous myocardial infarction; however, not every myocardial infarction will result in a pathological Q wave and some abnormal Q waves, in combination with other ECG changes and patient symptoms, may indicate a current myocardial infarction. Pathological Q waves may also be seen in non-ischaemic conditions such as Wolff–Parkinson–White syndrome (WPW).
- The Q–T interval is the time taken from ventricular stimulation to recovery. It is measured from the beginning of the QRS to the end of the T wave. Normally, this ranges from 0.35 to 0.45 s, but shortens as heart rate increases. It should be less than 50% of the preceding cycle length.
- The T wave reflects repolarisation of the ventricles. A peaked T wave indicates hyperkalaemia, myocardial infarction (MI) or ischaemia, while a flattened T wave usually indicates hypokalaemia. An inverted T wave occurs following an MI, or ventricular hypertrophy. A normal T wave is 0.16 s. The height of the T wave should be less than 5 mm in all limb leads, and less than 10 mm in the precordial leads.
- The ST segment is measured from the J point (junction of the S wave and ST segment) to the start of the T wave. It is usually isoelectric in nature, and elevation or depression indicates some abnormality in the onset of recovery of the ventricular muscle, usually due to myocardial injury.
- The U wave is a small positive wave sometimes seen following the T wave. Its cause is still unknown but it is exaggerated in hypokalaemia. Inverted U waves may be seen and are often associated with coronary heart disease (CHD), and these may appear transiently during exercise testing.

Practice tip

The 6-second measurement for heart rate calculation is particularly useful when the patient's heart rate is irregular. Count the R waves on a 6-s strip and multiply by 10 to calculate the rate for 1 minute.

ECG interpretation

Interpretation of a 12-lead ECG is an experiential skill, requiring consistent exposure and practice. Some steps to aid interpretation are noted below:

- Calculate heart rate
  - There are many ways to calculate the heart rate. One way is to count the R waves on a 6-second strip and multiply by 10 to calculate the rate (the top of the ECG paper is usually marked at 3-second intervals)
  - Use an ECG ruler if one is available
- Check R–R intervals (rhythm)
  - Is the rhythm regular?
  - To assess regularity, mark the duration of two neighbouring R waves (R–R interval) on a plain piece of paper and move this paper to check other R–R intervals on the ECG strip. R–R intervals should be uniform in a normal ECG, which indicates that the patient has a regular ECG rhythm
- Locate P waves (check atrial activity)
  - Observe for the presence or absence of P waves
  - Check regularity and shape
  - Is the P wave positive?
  - The relationship between P waves and QRS complexes: is there a P wave preceding every QRS complex?
  - What is the duration of the P wave?
- Measure P–R interval (check AV node activity)
  - What is the duration of the P–R interval?
- Measure QRS duration (check ventricular activity)
  - Is the ventricular electrical activity normal?
  - Is the QRS complex too wide or narrow?
  - Check the presence of a Q wave. If present, is it normal or pathological?
- Note other clues
  - Observe whether the isoelectric line is present between the S and T waves.
  - Examine the T wave to see whether it is positive, negative or flat: is it less than 0.16 s?

- Examine the duration of the Q–T interval: is it too long?
- Observe for any extra complexes and note their rate and shape, and whether they have the same or different morphology.

> **Practice tip**
>
> The presence of Q waves does not always indicate past MI. Q waves may be secondary to:
>
> - physiological and positional effects
> - myocardial injury or replacement
> - ventricular enlargement
> - altered ventricular conduction.
>
> Other patient clinical information is needed to interpret the significance of Q waves. ECG interpretation should always take a patient's clinical information (patient symptoms, complaints, other haemodynamic information) into account.

> **Practice tip**
>
> Think of the leads I, II, III, aVR, aVL, aVF, V1–V6 as the 'eyes' that are looking at the heart's electrical activity from different angles and view the heart's different areas.

Haemodynamic monitoring

The dynamic movement of the blood in the cardiovascular system is referred to as haemodynamics. Haemodynamic monitoring is performed to provide the clinician with a greater understanding of the pathophysiology of the problem being treated than would be possible with clinical assessment alone. Knowledge of the evidence that underpins the technology and the processes for interpretation is therefore essential to facilitate optimal usage and evidence-based decisions.[25]

This section explores the principles related to haemodynamic monitoring and the different types of monitoring available, and introduces the most recent and appropriate evidence related to haemodynamic monitoring. The reasons for haemodynamic monitoring are generally threefold:

1. to establish a precise health-related diagnosis
2. to determine appropriate therapy
3. to monitor the response to that therapy.

Haemodynamic monitoring can be non-invasive or invasive, and may be required on a continuous or intermittent basis depending on the needs of the patient. In both cases, signals are processed from a variety of physiological variables, and these are then clinically interpreted within the individual patient's context.[25]

Non-invasive monitoring does not require any device to be inserted into the body and therefore does not breach the skin. Directly measured non-invasive variables include body temperature, heart rate, blood pressure, respiratory rate and urine output, while other processed forms can be generated by the ECG, arterial and venous Dopplers, transcutaneous pulse oximetry (using an external probe on a digit such as the finger or on the ear) and expired carbon monoxide monitors.

Invasive monitoring requires the vascular system to be cannulated and pressure or flow within the circulation interpreted. Invasive haemodynamic monitoring technology includes:

- systemic arterial pressure monitoring
- CVP
- pulmonary artery pressure
- cardiac output.

Invasive monitoring has also facilitated greater use of blood component analyses, such as arterial and venous blood gases.

The invasive nature of this monitoring allows the pressures that are sensed at the distal ends of the catheters to be transduced, and to continuously display and monitor the corresponding waveforms. The extent of monitoring should reflect how much information is required to optimise the patient's condition, and how precisely the data are to be recorded. As Muller argues, a great deal of information is generated by this form of monitoring, and the clinical value of this is questionable. It is important to note that these invasive monitoring strategies are not substitutes for careful examination and do not replace the clinicians' clinical decision making. The accuracy of the values obtained and the critical care professionals' ability to interpret the data and choose an appropriate intervention directly affect the patient's condition and outcome.[26]

Principles of haemodynamic monitoring

A number of key principles need to be understood in relation to invasive haemodynamic monitoring of critically ill patients. These include haemodynamic accuracy, the ability to trend data and the maintenance of minimum standards. These are reviewed below.

Haemodynamic accuracy

Accuracy of the value obtained from haemodynamic monitoring is essential as this information is used to guide patient care. Electronic equipment for this purpose has four components (Fig. 9.16):

1. an invasive catheter attached to high-pressure tubing
2. a transducer to detect physiological activity
3. a flush system
4. a recording device, incorporating an amplifier to increase the size of the signal, to display information.

FIGURE 9.16 Haemodynamic monitoring system.

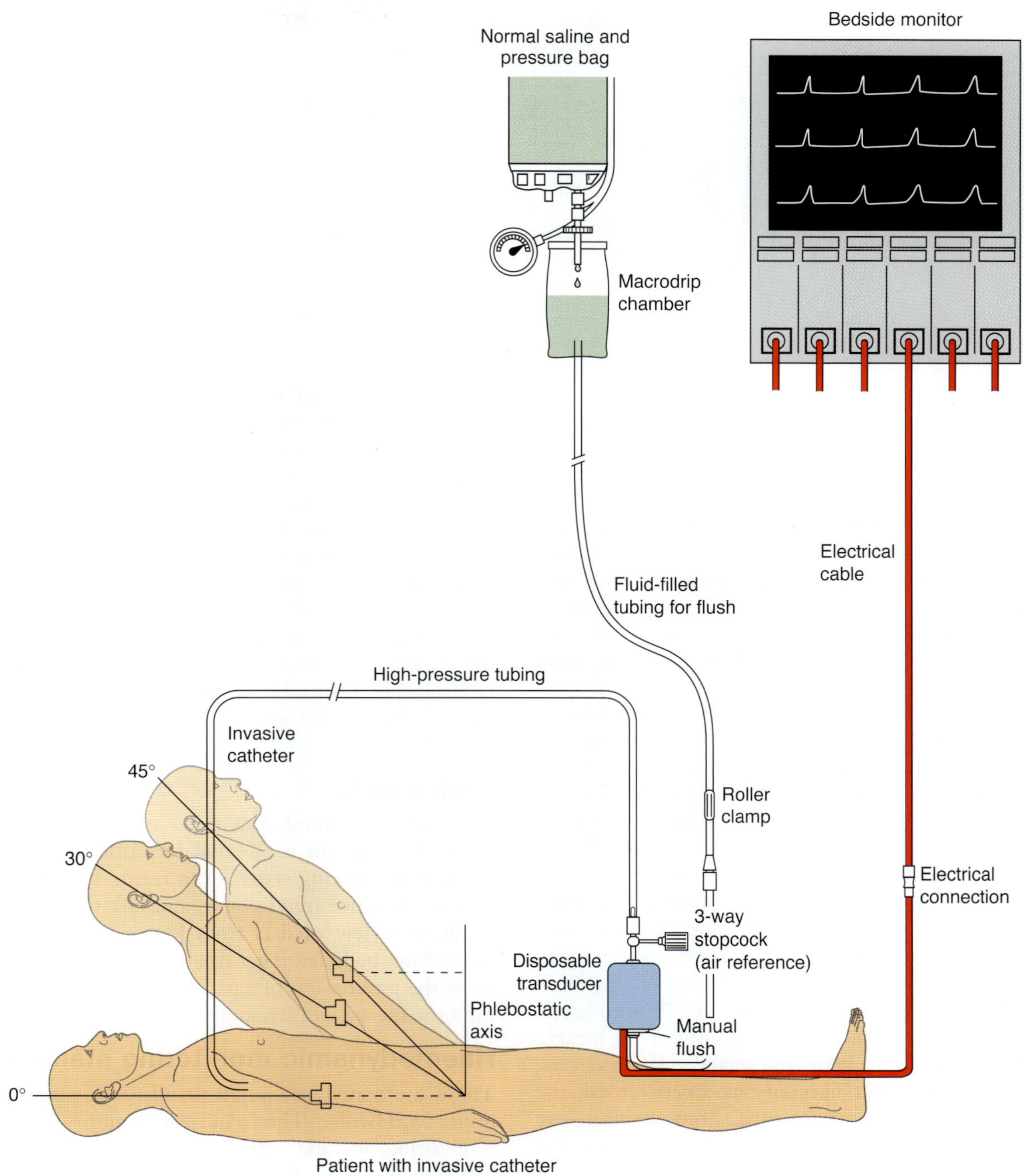

Adapted from Urden L, Stacy KL, Lough ME, editors. Thelan's critical care nursing: diagnosis and management. 6th ed. St Louis: Elsevier; 2010, with permission.

High-pressure (non-distensible) tubing reduces distortion of the signal produced between the intravascular device and the transducer; the pressure is then converted into electrical energy (a waveform). Fluid (0.9% sodium chloride) is routinely used to maintain line patency using a continuous pressure system. No difference in adding heparin in the flush system or using 0.9% sodium chloride alone has been found in maintaining the potency of the pressure system.[27,28] The pressure of the flush system fluid bag should be maintained at 300 mmHg, which normally delivers a continual flow of 3 mL/hour.

FIGURE 9.17 Normal dynamic response test.

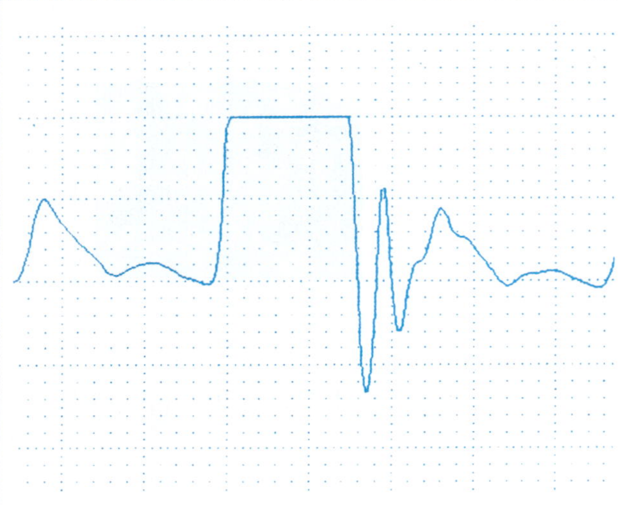

FIGURE 9.18 Overdamped dynamic response test.

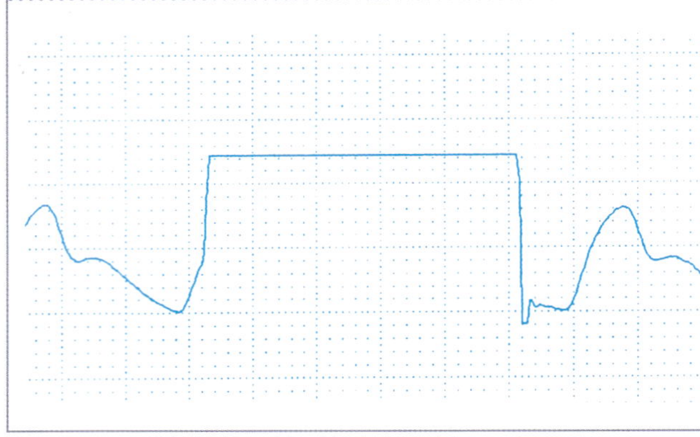

Accuracy is dependent on levelling the transducer to the appropriate level (and altering this level with changes in patient position as appropriate), then zeroing the transducer in the pressure monitoring system to atmospheric pressure (called calibration) as well as evaluating the response of the system by fast-flush wave testing. The transducer must be levelled to the reference point of the phlebostatic axis, at the intersection of the 4th intercostal space and the mid-thoracic anterior–posterior diameter (not the mid-axillary line). Error in measurement can occur if the transducer is placed above or below the phlebostatic axis. Thus, when the patient's position changes, the transducer must be re-levelled to maintain the accuracy of the measurement.

Zeroing the transducer system to atmospheric pressure (calibration of the system) is achieved by turning the three-way stopcock nearest to the transducer open to the air, and closing it to the patient and the flush system. The monitor should display zero (0 mmHg), as this equates to current atmospheric pressure (760 mmHg at sea level). With the improved quality of transducers, repeated zeroing is not necessary as, once zeroed, the drift from the baseline is minimal. Some critical care units, however, continue to recalibrate transducer(s) at the beginning of each clinical shift.

Fast-flush square wave testing, or dynamic response measurement, is a way of checking the dynamic response of the monitor to signals from the blood vessel. It is also a check on the accuracy of the subsequent haemodynamic pressure values. The fast-flush device within the system, when triggered and released, exposes the transducer to the amount of pressure in the flush solution bag (usually 300 mmHg). The pressure waveform on the monitor will show a rapid rise in pressure, which then squares off before the pressure drops back to the baseline (Fig. 9.17).

Interpretation of the square wave testing is essential; the clinician must observe the speed with which the wave returns to the baseline as well as the pattern produced. One to three rapid oscillations should occur immediately after the square wave, before the monitored waveform resumes. The distance between these rapid oscillations should not exceed 1 mm or 0.04 s. Absence, or a reduction, of these rapid oscillations, or a 'square wave' with rounded corners, indicates that the pressure monitoring system is overdamped; in other words, its responsiveness to monitored pressures and waveforms is reduced (Fig. 9.18). An underdamped monitoring system will produce more rapid oscillations after the square wave than usual.

Data trends

The ability to trend data via a monitor or a clinical information system is essential for critical care practice. Current monitoring systems can retain data for a period of time, produce trend graphs and link to other devices to allow review of data from locations other than the immediate bedside. The data trends can be used to assess the progression of a patient's clinical condition and monitor the patient's response to treatment.

Haemodynamic monitoring standards

There are stated minimum standards for critical care units worldwide. The standards require that patient monitoring include circulation, respiration and oxygenation, with the following essential equipment available for every patient: an ECG that facilitates continual cardiac monitoring; a mechanical ventilator, pulse oximeter; and other equipment available where necessary to measure intra-arterial and pulmonary pressures, cardiac output, inspiratory pressure and airway flow, intracranial pressures and expired carbon dioxide.[27]

Blood pressure monitoring

Indirect and direct means of monitoring blood pressure are widely used in critical care units. These are outlined in more detail below.

Non-invasive blood pressure monitoring

Non-invasive blood pressure monitoring requires the use of a manual or electronic sphygmomanometer. Oscillation in the pressure generated by alterations in arterial flow is captured either through auscultation or automatic sensing. On auscultation, a number of Korotkoff sounds can be heard as the cuff pressure is released:[29]

- a sharp thud that is heard when the patient's systolic pressure is reached
- a soft tapping, intermittent in nature
- a loud tapping, intermittent in nature
- a low, muffled noise that is continuous in nature and is heard when the diastolic pressure is reached; as the cuff pressure diminishes further, the sound disappears.

For critically ill patients, this method of blood pressure monitoring has limitations and is often used when invasive methods cannot be utilised. It is a less accurate alternative, as results vary with the size of cuff used, equipment malfunction and incorrect placement of the sphygmomanometer (this must be placed at heart level).[30] In addition, the pressures generated by the inflating cuff, particularly those generated by automatic machines, can be high, and frequent measurements of blood pressure by this method may become uncomfortable for the patient. It is therefore important that skin integrity be checked regularly to prevent ischaemia and that the frequency of automated inflations be minimised.

Invasive intra-arterial pressure monitoring

Arterial pressure recording is indicated when precise and continuous monitoring is required, especially in periods of fluid volume, cardiac output and blood pressure instability.[30,31] An arterial catheter is commonly placed in the radial artery, although other sites can be accessed, including the brachial, femoral, dorsalis pedis and axillary arteries. Arterial catheter insertion is performed aseptically, and it is important that collateral circulation, patient comfort and risk of infection be assessed before insertion is attempted. The radial artery is the most common site, as the ulnar artery provides additional supply to extremities if the radial artery becomes compromised.

Complications of arterial pressure monitoring include:

- infection
- arterial thrombosis
- distal ischaemia
- air embolism
- accidental disconnection (the insertion sites should be always visible)
- accidental drug administration through the arterial catheter; all arterial lines and connections should be clearly identified as such (e.g. marked with red stickers or have red bungs).

Blood pressure is the same at all sites along a vertical level but when the vertical level is varied, pressure will change. To prevent ventilator-associated pneumonia, ventilated patients are often sat up to 45°. It is important to remember that blood pressures can be measured and recorded at different positions. Consequently, referencing is required to correct for changes in hydrostatic pressure in vessels above and below the heart; if not, the blood pressure will appear to rise when this is not really the case. It is important to zero the monitoring system at the left atrial level.[31]

Arterial waveform

A steep upstroke (corresponding to ventricular systole) is followed by brief, sustained pressure (anacrotic shoulder). At the end of systole pressure falls in the aorta and left ventricle, causing a downward deflection (Fig. 9.19). A dicrotic notch can be seen in the downward deflection which represents the closure of the aortic valve. The systolic pressure corresponds to the peak of the waveform. The arterial pressure waveform changes its contours when recorded at different sites. It can become sharper in distal locations.

Disease process has an effect on waveforms: for example, atherosclerosis causes an increase in systolic waveform, as well as a decrease in the size of the diastolic wave and dicrotic notch due to changes in elasticity. Cardiomyopathy causes reduced stroke volume and mean arterial pressure, and there is a late secondary systolic peak seen on the waveform.

Invasive arterial pressure versus cuff pressure

At times, the accuracy of the invasive arterial pressure reading may be checked by comparing the reading against that generated by a non-invasive device using an inflating cuff. However, there is no basis for comparing these values. Invasive blood pressure values are a measure of the actual pressure within the artery whereas those

FIGURE 9.19 Arterial pressure waveform.

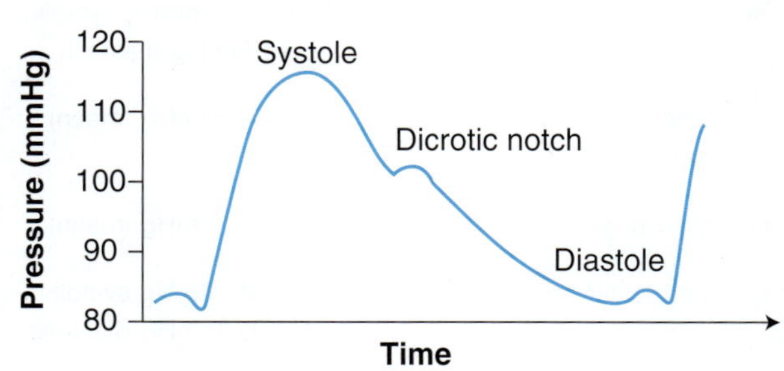

Adapted from Urden L, Stacy KL, Lough ME, editors. Thelan's critical care nursing: diagnosis and management. 6th ed. St Louis: Elsevier; 2010, with permission.

from the cuff depend on flow-induced oscillations in the arterial wall. Pressure does not equal flow, as resistance does not remain constant. Studies found that the non-invasive cuff blood pressure method can be unreliable in measuring systolic blood pressure when the blood pressure is low, for example, when a patient is in shock. In addition, radial arterial pressure is normally higher than that obtained by brachial non-invasive pressure monitoring because the smaller vessel size exerts greater resistance to flow, and therefore generates a higher pressure reading.[30,31]

Invasive cardiovascular monitoring

For many critically ill patients, haemodynamic instability is a potentially life-threatening condition that necessitates urgent action. Accurate assessment of the patient's intracardiac status is therefore essential. A number of values can be calculated; the measurements commonly made are listed in Tables 9.3 and 9.4.

Preload

As noted earlier, preload is the filling pressure in the ventricles at the end of diastole. CVP is used clinically as a surrogate estimate of preload in the right ventricle, although this may be an unreliable predictor because CVP is affected by intrathoracic pressure, vascular tone and obstruction.[29] PCWP, obtained using a pulmonary artery catheter, is frequently used as a surrogate estimate of left ventricular preload but again, due to unreliability, this parameter provides only an estimate rather than a true reflection of volume.[30,31] In view of this, other modalities are now being explored, including right ventricular end-diastolic volume evaluation via fast-response pulmonary artery catheters, left ventricular end-diastolic area measured by echocardiography and intrathoracic blood volume measured by transpulmonary thermodilution.[25]

TABLE 9.3
Haemodynamic pressures

PARAMETER	RESTING VALUES
Central venous pressure	0 to +8 mmHg (mean)
Right ventricular pressure	+15 to +30 mmHg systolic; 0 to +8 mmHg diastolic
Pulmonary artery wedge pressure	+5 to +15 mmHg (mean)
Left atrial pressure	+4 to +12 mmHg (mean)
Left ventricular pressure	90 to 140 mmHg systolic; +4 to +12 mmHg diastolic
Aortic pressure	90 to 140 mmHg systolic; 60 to 90 mmHg diastolic; 70 to 105 mmHg (mean)

Central venous pressure monitoring

Central venous catheters are inserted to facilitate the monitoring of CVP; facilitate the administration of large amounts of IV fluid or blood; provide long-term access for fluids, drugs, specimen collection and/or parenteral feeding. CVP monitoring has been used for many years to evaluate circulating blood volume, despite discussion as to its validity to do so.[25] However, it is a common monitoring practice and continues to be used. Therefore, clinicians need to be aware of possible limitations to this form of measurement and interpret the data accordingly. CVP monitoring can produce erroneous results: a low CVP does not always mean low volume and it may reflect other pathology, including peripheral dilation due to sepsis. Hypovolaemic patients may have normal CVP due to sympathetic nervous system activity increasing vascular tone. An increase in CVP can also be seen in patients on mechanical ventilation with application of PEEP.[32]

Central venous catheters used for haemodynamic monitoring are classed as short-term percutaneous (non-tunnelled) devices. Short-term percutaneous catheters are inserted through the skin, directly into a central vein, and usually remain in situ for only a few days or for a maximum of 2–3 weeks. They are easily removed and changed, and are manufactured as single- or multi-lumen types. However, they can be easily dislodged, are thrombogenic due to their material and are associated with a high risk of infection.[33]

A number of locations can be used for central venous catheter insertion. The two commonly used sites in critically ill patients are the subclavian and the internal jugular veins. Other less common sites are the antecubital fossa (generally avoided but may be used when the patient cannot be positioned supine), the femoral vein (associated with high infection risk and the external jugular vein although the high incidence of anomalous anatomy and the severe angle with the subclavian vein make this an unpopular choice).[34,35]

Internal jugular cannulation has a high success rate for insertion; however, complications related to insertion via this route include carotid artery puncture and laceration of local neck structures arising from needle probing. There are a number of key structures adjacent to the vein, including the vagus nerve (located posteriorly to the internal jugular vein), the sympathetic trunk (located behind the vagus nerve) and the phrenic nerve (located laterally to the internal jugular). Damage can also occur to the sympathetic chain, which leads to Horner's syndrome (constricted pupil, ptosis and absence of sweat gland activity on that side of the face). Central venous catheters inserted in the internal jugular vein pose a number of nursing challenges that can cause fixation problems and the need for repeated dressing

TABLE 9.4
Normal haemodynamic values

PARAMETER	DESCRIPTION	NORMAL VALUES
Stroke volume (SV)	Volume of blood ejected from left ventricle/beat SV = CO/HR	50–100 mL/beat
Stroke volume index (SVI)	Volume of blood ejected/beat indexed to BSA	25–45 mL/beat
Cardiac output (CO)	Volume of blood ejected from left ventricle/min CO = HR × SV	4–8 L/min
Cardiac index (CI)	A derived value reflecting the volume of blood ejected from left ventricle/min indexed to BSA CI = CO/BSA	2.5–4.2 L/min/m^2 (normal assumes an average weight of 70 kg)
Mean arterial pressure (MAP)	[(2 × diastolic) + systolic] /3	70–105 mmHg
Flow time corrected (FTc)	Systolic flow time corrected for heart rate	330–360 ms
Systemic vascular resistance (SVR)	Resistance left heart pumps against SVR = [(MAP – RAP) × 79.9]/CO	900–1300 dyn•s/cm^5
Systemic vascular resistance index (SVRI)	Resistance left heart pumps against indexed to body surface area SVRI = [(MAP – RAP) × 79.9]/CI	1700–2400 dyn•s/cm^5/m^2
Pulmonary vascular resistance (PVR)	Resistance right heart pumps against PVR = [(mPAP – LVEDP) × 79.9]/CO	20–120 dyn•s/cm^5
Pulmonary vascular resistance index (PVRI)	Resistance right heart pumps against indexed to body surface area PVRI = [(mPAP – LVEDP) × 79.9]/CI	255–285 dyn•s/cm^5/m^2
Mixed venous saturation (SvO_2)	Shows the balance between arterial O_2 supply and oxygen demand at the tissue level	70%
Left ventricular stroke work index (LVSWI)	Amount of work performed by LV with each heartbeat (MAP – LVEDP) × SVI × 0.0136	50–62 g-m/m^2
Right ventricular stroke work index (RVSWI)	Amount of work performed by RV with each heartbeat (mPAP – RAP) × SVI × 0.0136	7.9–9.7 g-m/m^2
Right ventricular end-systolic volume (RVESV)	The volume of blood remaining in the ventricle at the end of the ejection phase of the heartbeat	50–100 mL/beat
Right ventricular end-systolic volume index (RVESVI)		30–60 mL/m^2
Right ventricular end-diastolic volume (RVEDV)	The amount of blood in the ventricle immediately before a cardiac contraction begins	100–160 mL/beat
Right ventricular end-diastolic volume index (RVEDVI)		60–100 mL/m^2

BSA = body surface area; HR = heart rate; RAP = right atrial pressure.
Adapted from:
Leeper B. Monitoring right ventricular volumes: a paradigm shift. AACN Clinical Issues 2003;14(2):201–19.
Schummer W. Central venous pressure. Validity, informative value and correct measurement. Anaesthetist 2009;58(5):499–505.

changes. These include beard growth, diaphoresis and poor control of oral secretions.

The subclavian approach is used often, perhaps because of a reported lower risk of catheter-related bloodstream infection.[34] Coagulopathy is a significant contraindication for this approach, as puncture of the subclavian artery is a known complication. There is also a risk of pneumothorax, which rises if the patient is receiving IPPV.[36] Complications of any central venous access catheter include air embolism, pneumothorax, hydrothorax and haemorrhage.

Pulmonary artery pressure monitoring

Pulmonary artery pressure (PAP) monitoring began in the 1970s, led by Drs Swan, Ganz and colleagues,[36] and was subsequently adopted in ICUs worldwide. Pulmonary artery catheterisation facilitates assessment of filling pressure of the left ventricle through the pulmonary artery wedge (occlusion) pressure (Fig. 9.20). By using a thermodilution pulmonary artery catheter (PAC), cardiac output and other haemodynamic measurements can also be calculated. PAP monitoring is a diagnostic tool that can assist in determination of the nature of a haemodynamic problem and improve diagnostic accuracy. In addition to measuring postero-anterior (PA) pressures, PAC may also be used for accessing blood for assessment of mixed-venous oxygenation levels (see Chapter 13).

The benefits of PAP monitoring have been scrutinised in recent years. A Cochrane systematic review on PAC use by Rajaram et al[37] suggests that there was no difference in mortality rates, hospital length of stay and ICU length of stay in patients with or without PACs, and there was no difference in clinical benefit or harm in either group of patients. The PAC insertion is invasive, and increases the cost of patients' hospitalisation. Consequently, the use of PAC in clinical practice has dropped 50–65% in recent years, although the PAC is still considered a useful monitoring tool that helps with diagnosis in clinical practice.[37]

Thus, the indications of PAP monitoring are largely based on health professionals' clinical experience and expertise. It has been suggested that PAP monitoring may be indicated for adults in severe hypovolaemic or cardiogenic shock, where there may be diagnostic uncertainty, or where the patient is unresponsive to initial therapy. The PAP is used to guide administration of fluids, inotropes and vasopressors. PAP monitoring may also be utilised in other cases of haemodynamic instability when the diagnosis is unclear. It may be helpful when clinicians want to differentiate hypovolaemia from cardiogenic shock or, in cases of pulmonary oedema, to differentiate cardiogenic from non-cardiogenic origins. However, in their Cochrane review, Rajaram et al concluded that more studies are needed to investigate the benefit of PAC use in subgroup patients including reversing shock states and improving organ function.[37] Complications do arise from PACs, as these catheters share all the complications of central lines and are additionally associated with a higher incidence of arrhythmia, valve damage, pulmonary vascular occlusion, emboli/infarction (reported incidence of 0.1–5.6%) and, very rarely, knotting of the catheter.[37]

A number of measurements can be taken via the PAC, either by direct measurement, for example using PCWP, which is used as a surrogate estimate of left ventricular preload (LVEDV), or through calculation of derived parameters such as cardiac output (CO) and cardiac index (CI) (see Table 9.4 for descriptors and normal values).

PCWP monitoring

PCWP, or pulmonary artery occlusion pressure (PAOP), is measured when the PAC balloon is inflated with no more than 1–1.5 mL air. The inflated balloon isolates the distal measuring lumen from the pulmonary arterial pressures, and measures pressures in the capillaries of the pulmonary venous system, and indirectly the left atrial pressure. The PAP waveform looks similar to that of the arterial waveform, with the tracing showing a systolic peak, dicrotic notch and a diastolic dip (Fig. 9.21). When the balloon is inflated, the waveform changes shape and becomes much flatter in appearance, providing a similar waveform to the CVP. There are two positive waves on the tracing: the first reflects atrial contraction and the second reflects pressure changes from blood flow when the mitral valve closes and the ventricles contract. The PCWP should be read once the 'wedge' trace stops falling at the end-expiratory phase of the respiratory cycle (Fig. 9.21).

If balloon occlusion occurs with <1 mL of air, the balloon is wedged in a small capillary and consequently will not accurately reflect LA pressure. Conversely, if 1.5 mL air does not cause occlusion, the balloon may have burst (which can result in an air embolus) or it may be floating in a larger vessel. If balloon rupture is suspected, no further attempts to inflate the balloon should be made, and interventions to minimise the risk of air embolism should be initiated.

Note: it is essential that the balloon be deflated as soon as the wedge has been recorded, as continued occlusion will cause distal pulmonary vasculature ischaemia and infarction.

Left atrial pressure monitoring

Left atrial pressure (LAP) monitoring directly estimates left heart preload. It used to require an open thorax to enable direct cannulation of the atrium. It was used only in the postoperative cardiac surgical setting, although such use has been infrequent since the widespread use of PAC. Recent advancement in cardiac implantable devices development enables the patients to self-monitor LAP under their doctors' guidance, which was found to be a valuable tool to improve the management of patients with advanced heart failure. Other modes of monitoring can also be used to achieve comprehensive left atrial assessment, such as Doppler echocardiography.[38]

FIGURE 9.20 Pulmonary artery catheter.

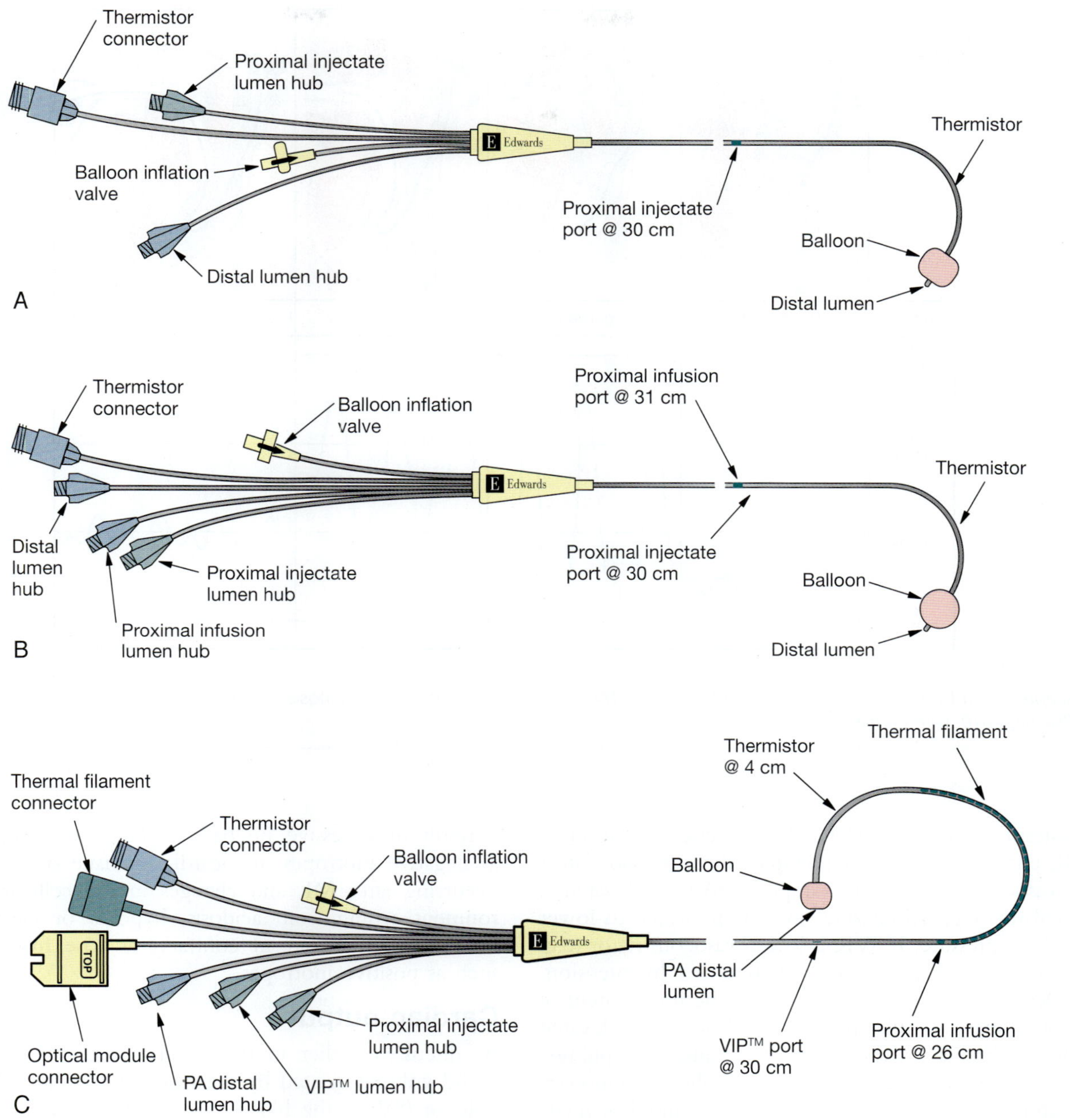

Adapted from Urden L, Stacy KL, Lough ME, editors. Thelan's critical care nursing: diagnosis and management. 6th ed. St Louis: Elsevier; 2010, with permission.

Afterload

As previously noted, afterload is the pressure that the ventricle produces to overcome the resistance to ejection generated in the systemic or pulmonary circulation by the arteries and arterioles. It is calculated by CO studies: left heart afterload is reflected as SVR, and right heart afterload is reflected as pulmonary vascular resistance (PVR) (see Table 9.4).

Systemic and pulmonary vascular resistance

SVR is a measure of resistance or impediment of the systemic vascular bed to blood flow. An elevated SVR can be caused by vasoconstrictors, hypovolaemia or late septic shock. A lowered SVR can be caused by early septic shock, vasodilators, morphine, nitrates or hypercarbia. Afterload is a major determinant of blood pressure, and gross vasodilation causes peripheral pooling and

FIGURE 9.21 Pulmonary artery pressure and wedge waveforms.

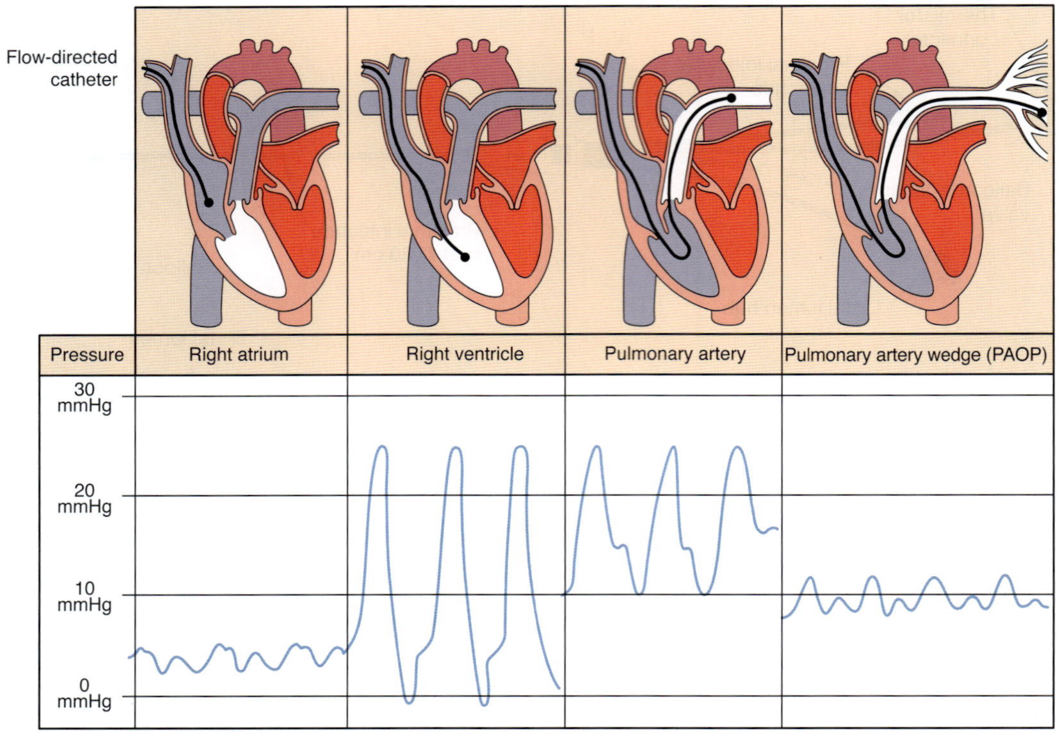

Adapted from Urden L, Stacy KL, Lough ME, editors. Thelan's critical care nursing: diagnosis and management. 6th ed. St Louis: Elsevier; 2010, with permission.

hypotension, reducing SVR. The precise estimation of SVR enables safer use of therapies such as vasodilators and vasoconstrictors. For example, if SVR is elevated, a vasodilator (e.g. hydralazine) may be indicated to lower the blood pressure. If SVR is low, a vasoconstrictor (e.g. noradrenaline) should be considered to treat hypotension.

PVR is a measure of resistance or the impediment of the pulmonary vascular bed to blood flow. An elevated PVR ('pulmonary hypertension') is caused by pulmonary vascular disease, pulmonary embolism, pulmonary vasculitis or hypoxia. A lowered PVR is caused by medications such as calcium channel blockers, aminophylline or isoprenaline, or by the delivery of O_2.

Contractility

Contractility reflects the force of myocardial contraction, and is related to the extent of myocardial fibre stretch (preload, see above) and wall tension (afterload, see above). It is important because it influences myocardial oxygen consumption. Contractility of the left side of the heart is measured by calculating the left ventricular stroke work index (LVSWI), although the clinical use of this value is not widespread.

Right ventricular stroke work index (RVSWI) can be similarly calculated. Contractility can decrease as a result of excessive preload or afterload, drugs such as negative inotropes, myocardial damage such as that occurring after MI, and changes in the cellular environment arising from acidosis, hypoxia or electrolyte imbalances. Increases in contractility arise from drugs such as positive inotropes.

Cardiac output

As discussed earlier in the chapter, CO refers to the blood volume ejected by the heart in 1 minute. Stroke volume (SV) is the blood ejected by the heart in one beat. Therefore, CO can be calculated as the heart rate multiplied by SV. The SV is determined by the heart's preload, afterload and the contractility.

The variety of CO measurement techniques has grown over the past decade since the development of thermodilution PACs, pulse-induced contour devices, less invasive techniques such as Doppler, and non-invasive continuous haemodynamic monitoring methods. Vincent et al[39] provides an overview of advantages and disadvantages of these different measurement methods.

As many critically ill patients require mechanical ventilation support, the associated rises in intrathoracic pressure, as well as changing ventricular compliance, make accurate haemodynamic assessment difficult with the older technologies. Therefore, volumetric measurements of preload, such as right ventricular end-systolic volume (RVESV), right ventricular end-diastolic volume (RVEDV) and index (RVESVI/RVEDVI) as well as measurements of right ventricular ejection fraction (RVEF) may be used to more accurately determine CO. The parameters RVEF, CO and/or CI and SV are generated using thermodilution technology, and from these the parameters of RVEDV/RVEDVI and RVESV/RVESVI can be calculated (see Table 9.4 for normal values). The availability of continuous modes of assessment has further improved a clinician's ability to accurately assess, and then effectively treat, these patients.

The Fick principle

Several CO measurement methods use the Fick principle. In 1870, Fick proposed that 'in an organ, the uptake or release of an indicator substance is the product of the arterial-venous concentration of this substance and the blood flow to the organ'.[40] Using oxygen as the indicator substance, the calculation of CO is as follows:

$$CO = VO_2/(CaO_2 - CvO_2)$$

where VO_2 is oxygen consumption, CaO_2 is arterial oxygen concentration, and CvO_2 is venous oxygen concentration.

Thermodilution methods

Thermodilution methods calculate CO by using temperature change as the indicator in Fick's method. CO and associated pressures such as global end-diastolic volume can be calculated using a thermodilution PAC. CO can be monitored intermittently or continuously using the PA catheter. Intermittent measurements obtained every few hours produce a snapshot of the cardiovascular state over that time. By injecting a bolus of 5–10 mL of crystalloid solution, and measuring the resulting temperature changes, an estimation of SV is calculated. Cold injectate (run through ice) was initially recommended, but studies now support the use of room temperature injectate, providing there is a difference of 12°C between injectate and blood temperature. Three readings are taken at the same part of the respiratory cycle (normally end expiration), and any measurements that differ by more than 10% should be disregarded (see Table 9.4 for normal values). Since the 1990s, the value of having continuous measurement of CO has been recognised and this has led to the development of devices that permit the transference of pulses of thermal energy to pulmonary artery blood – the pulse-induced contour method.[41]

Pulse-induced contour CO

Pulse-induced contour cardiac output (PiCCO) provides both intermittent and continuous assessment of CO, and requires a central venous line and an arterial line with a thermistor (not a PAC).[41] A known volume of thermal indicator (usually room temperature saline) is injected into the central vein. The injectate disperses both volumetrically and thermally within the cardiac and pulmonary blood. When the thermal signal is detected by the arterial thermistor, the temperature difference is calculated and a dissipation curve generated. From these data, the CO can be calculated. These continuous CO measurements have been well researched and appear to be equal in accuracy to those produced by intermittent injections required for the earlier catheters.[42] The parameters measured by PiCCO include the following:

- PiCCO: derived normal value for CI, 2.5–4.2 L/min/m^2.
- Global end-diastolic volume (GEDV): the volume of blood contained in the four chambers of the heart; assists in the calculation of intrathoracic blood volume. Derived normal value for global end-diastolic blood volume index, 680–800 mL/m^2.
- Intrathoracic blood volume (ITBV): the volume of the four chambers of the heart plus the blood volume in the pulmonary vessels; more accurately reflects circulating blood volumes, particularly when a patient is artificially ventilated. Derived normal value for ITBV index, 850–1000 mL/m^2.
- Extravascular lung water (EVLW): the amount of water content in the lungs; allows quantification of the degree of pulmonary oedema (not evident with X-ray or blood gases). Derived normal value for extravascular lung water index is 3–7 mL/kg. EVLW has been shown to be useful as a guide for fluid management in critically ill patients. An elevated EVLW may be an effective indicator of severity of illness, particularly after acute lung injury or in acute respiratory distress syndrome (ARDS), when EVLW is elevated due to alterations in hydrostatic pressures. Other patients at risk of high EVLW are those with left heart failure, severe pneumonia and burns. There may be an association between high EVLW and increased mortality, the need for mechanical ventilation and a higher risk of nosocomial infection. A decision tree outlining processes of care guided by information provided by PiCCO is provided in Fig. 9.22.

PiCCO removes the impact of factors that can cause variability in the standard approach of CO measurement, such as injectate volume and temperature, and timing of the injection within the respiratory cycle.[42] The additional fluid volume injected with the standard technique is significant in some patients; with the continuous technology, this is eliminated. A further advantage is that virtually real-time responses to treatment can be obtained, removing the time delay that was a potential problem with standard thermodilution techniques.[42]

An arterial catheter is widely used in critical care to enable frequent blood sampling and blood pressure monitoring, and is used to measure beat-by-beat CO, obtained from the shape of the arterial pressure wave. The area under the systolic portion of the arterial pulse

FIGURE 9.22 PiCCO decision tree.

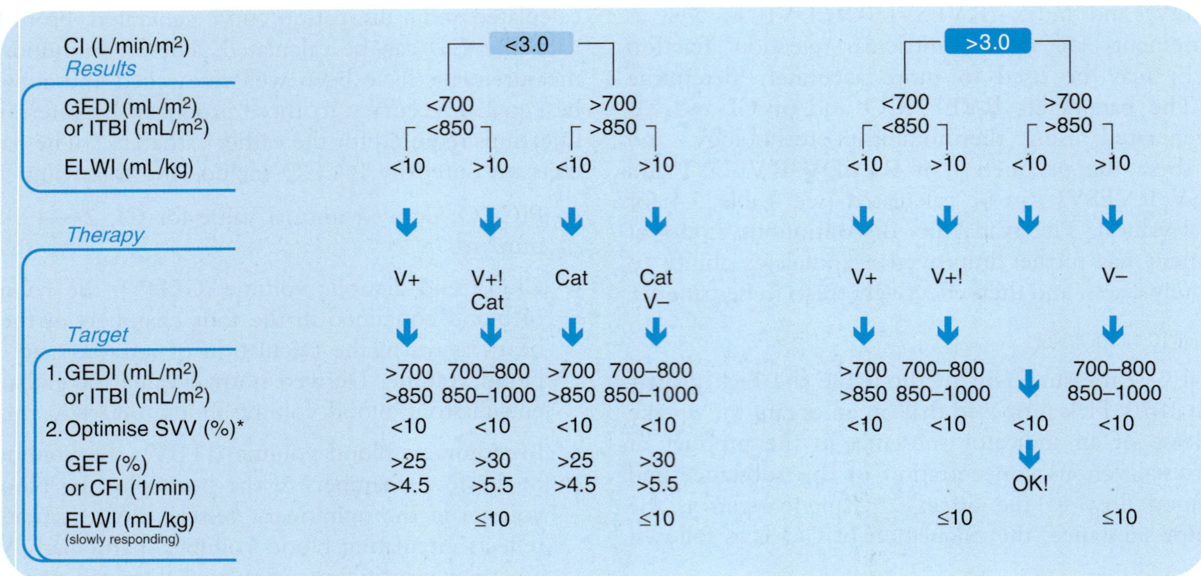

V+ = volume loading (! = cautiously) V- = volume contraction Cat = catecholamine / cardiovascular agents
*SVV only applicable in ventilated patients without cardiac arrhythmia

Without guarantee

wave from the end of diastole to the end of the ejection phase is measured and combined with an individual calibration factor. The algorithm is capable of computing each single SV after being calibrated by an initial transpulmonary thermodilution.

PiCCO preload indicators of ITBV and GEDV are more sensitive and specific to cardiac preload than the standard cardiac filling pressures of CVP and PCWP, as well as RVEDV. One advantage of ITBV and GEDV is that they are not affected by mechanical ventilation and therefore give correct information on the preload status under almost any condition. Extravascular lung water (EVLW) correlates moderately well with severity of ARDS, length of ventilation days, ICU stay and mortality,[43] and appears to be of greater accuracy than the traditional assessment of lung oedema by chest X-ray. Disadvantages of PiCCO include its potential unreliability when heart rate, blood pressure and total vascular resistance change substantially.[41]

Lithium dilution cardiac output (LiDCO)

Lithium can be used as an alternative indicator to estimate CO, which is a method that has been used since its introduction in the 1990s. The LiDCO is calculated using lithium dilution. Isotonic lithium chloride is injected as a bolus (0.002–0.004 mmol/kg) via either central or peripheral venous route, then a concentration-time curve is generated by an ex vivo ion-selective electrode attached to the arterial pressure line. The CO is calculated from the lithium dose and the area under the concentration-time curve.[44] It is considered to be a simpler method as it only requires an arterial line. The LiDCO measurement method has been found to be as accurate as the PAC thermodilution technique.[45]

Doppler ultrasound methods

Oesophageal Doppler monitoring enables calculation of CO from assessment of SV and heart rate, but uses a less invasive technique than those outlined previously.[45] SV is assessed by measuring the flow velocity and the area through which the forward flow travels. Flow velocity is the distance one red blood cell travels forward in one cardiac cycle, and the measurement provides a time velocity interval. The area of flow is calculated by measuring the cross-sectional area of the blood vessel or heart chamber at the site of the flow velocity measurement.[37] Oesophageal Doppler monitoring can be performed at the level of the pulmonary artery, mitral valve or aortic valve.

According to Doppler principles, the movement of blood produces a waveform that reflects blood flow velocity, in this case in the descending thoracic aorta (Fig. 9.23), that is captured by the change in frequency of an ultrasound beam as it reflects off a moving object.[23] This measurement is combined with an estimate of the cross-sectional area of the aorta so that the SV, CO and CI can be calculated, using the patient's age, height and weight.[37]

FIGURE 9.23 Oesophageal Doppler waveforms.

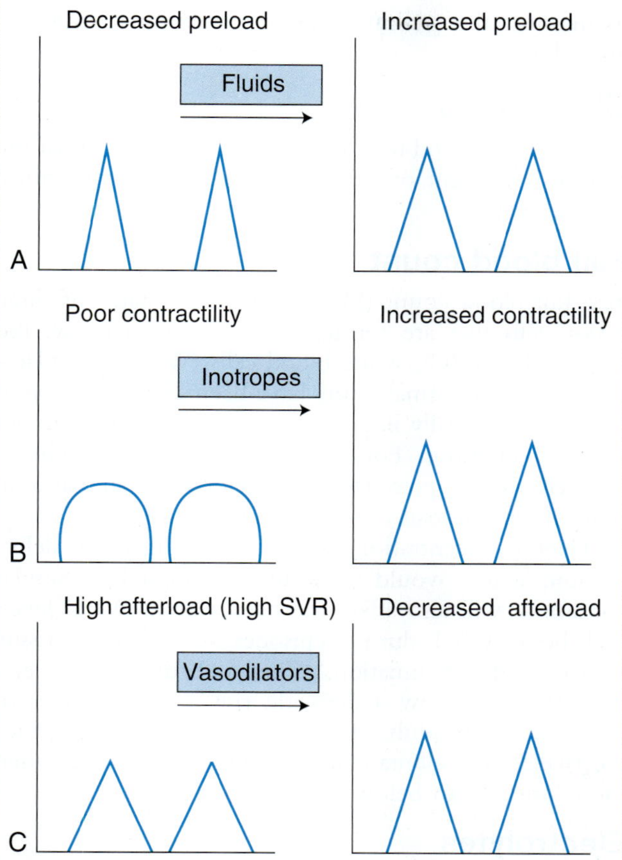

Oesophageal Doppler monitoring provides an alternative for patients who would not benefit from PAC insertion,[46] and can be used to provide continuous measurements under certain conditions: the estimate of cross-sectional area must be accurate; the ultrasound beam must be directed parallel to the flow of blood; and there should be minimal variation in movement of the beam between measurements. There is some debate at present among clinicians about the accuracy of oesophageal Doppler monitoring for calculating CO.[47] This form of monitoring can be used perioperatively and in the critical care unit, on a wide variety of patients.[46] It should not, however, be used in patients with aortic coarctation or dissection, oesophageal malignancy or perforation, severe bleeding problems or with patients on an intra-aortic balloon pump.[47]

The Doppler probe that sits in the oesophagus is approximately the size of a nasogastric tube, is semi-rigid and is inserted using a similar technique. The patient is usually sedated but the method has been used in awake patients. In such cases, however, the limitation is that the probe is more likely to require more frequent repositioning.

The waveform that is displayed on the monitor is triangular in shape (Fig. 9.23) and captures the systolic portion of the cardiac cycle – an upstroke at the beginning of systole, the peak reflecting maximum systole and the downward slope of the ending of systole. The waveform captures real-time changes in blood flow and can therefore be seen as an indirect reflection of left ventricular function. Changes to haemodynamic status will be reflected in alterations in the triangular shape (Fig. 9.23).

Ultrasonic CO monitor

The ultrasonic cardiac output monitor (USCOM) monitors CO non-invasively using continuous Doppler ultrasound waves by placing an ultrasound transducer probe supra- or parasternally. The principles of CO calculation in this method are the same as for oesophageal Doppler monitoring. The use of non-invasive USCOM has been found to provide adequate clinical data in patients in different shock categories, and to be safe and cost-effective; however, CO can be difficult to measure in some patients.[39]

Impedance cardiography

Transthoracic bioimpedance (impedance cardiography) is another form of non-invasive monitoring used to estimate CO. It measures the amount of electrical resistance generated by the thorax to high-frequency, low magnitude currents. This measure is inversely proportional to the content of fluid in the thorax: if the amount of thoracic fluid increases, then transthoracic bioimpedance falls. Changes in CO can be reflected as a change in overall bioimpedance. The technique requires six electrodes to be positioned on the patient: two in the upper thorax/neck area and four in the lower thorax. These electrodes also monitor electrical signals from the heart.

Overall, transthoracic bioimpedance is determined by: 1) changes in tissue fluid volume; 2) volumetric changes in pulmonary and venous blood caused by respiration; and 3) volumetric changes in aortic blood flow produced by myocardial contractility. Accurate measurements of changes in aortic blood flow are dependent on the ability to measure the third determinant, while filtering out any interference produced by the first two determinants. Any changes to position or to electrode contact will cause alterations to the measurements obtained, and recordings should therefore be undertaken with the electrodes positioned in the same location as previous readings. Caution is required for patients with high levels of perspiration (which reduces electrode contact), atrial fibrillation (irregular R–R intervals make estimation of the ventricular ejection time difficult) or pulmonary oedema, pleural effusions or chest wall oedema (which alter bioimpedance readings irrespective of any changes in CO). The use of transthoracic bioimpedance in critically ill patients is less reliable, due in part to limitations of its usefulness in patients who have pulmonary oedema, and not applicable in cardiothoracic surgery.[39]

Practice tip

Current evidence-based literature suggests that haemodynamic measurements such as CVP, PAWP and PAP can be accurately measured with a patient position of supine to head – up to 60°.

Diagnostics

Apart from the haemodynamic monitoring methods to facilitate cardiac assessment of a patient's clinical condition, various diagnostic tests are often used. Echocardiography and blood tests are the most commonly used in critical care. Other tests such as computerised tomography (CT) and nuclear medicine cardiac examination are also used when indicated. Exercise stress tests and cardiac angiography are also used and are reviewed in Chapter 10.

Echocardiography

Echocardiography (frequently shortened to ECHO) is often used in critical care to assess cardiovascular conditions such as heart failure, hypertensive heart disease, valve disease and pericardial disease in critically ill patients. It adopts a technique of detecting the echoes produced by a heart from a beam of very high frequency sound – ultrasound. Two-dimensional, three-dimensional and contrast ECHO images can be obtained using the non-invasive transthoracic technique or the invasive transoesophageal technique (TOE). The transthoracic ECHO uses a transducer probe externally to the heart to obtain images (same as a normal ultrasound technique). This method is painless and does not require sedation. The TOE technique involves placing a transducer probe into the oesophageal cavity to assess the function and structure of the heart. This method produces better images of the heart than the normal transthoracic ECHO. However, this method requires sedation during the procedure and the patient needs to fast for a few hours prior to the examination.

Two-dimensional ECHO images are valuable resources for assessment of the function and structure of the heart. Three-dimensional images offer more realistic visualisation of its structure and function. Contrast ECHO provides enhanced images of left and right ventricular definition to facilitate the diagnosis of complex cardiac conditions such as congenital heart defects, valve stenosis and regurgitation. The contrast ECHO technique uses gas air microbubbles, produced by hand-agitating a syringe containing 10 mL of normal saline with a small amount of air, injected into the peripheral vein to produce images of the heart functions.

In the critical care setting, the preparation of critically ill patients for this examination is important. The nurse needs to help the sonographer to position the patient to achieve the best results. For TOE preparation, fasting time must be followed to avoid complications such as respiratory aspiration. The nurse will also need to assist the anaesthetist and the TOE operator, and continue to monitor the patient's clinical conditions during the procedure.

Blood tests

A number of blood tests are often conducted to assist the clinical assessment of critically ill patients in the critical care setting.

Full blood count

The full blood count (FBC) assesses the status of three major cells that are formed in the bone marrow: red blood cells (RBC), white blood cells (WBC) and platelets. Although normal values have been given (see *Appendix B*), for critically ill patients changes will occur under certain conditions. For example, haemoglobin (Hb) is reduced in the presence of haemorrhage and also in acute fluid overload causing haemodilution.

Haemoconcentration can occur during acute dehydration, which would show up as a high Hb. Similar conditions will also affect the haematocrit. WBC levels will be elevated during episodes of infection, tissue damage and inflammation. When infections are severe, the FBC will show a dramatic rise in the number of immature neutrophils. Platelets are easily lost during haemorrhage, and spontaneous bleeding is a danger when the count falls to below 20 3 10^9/L.[48]

Electrolytes

The assessment of electrolyte levels in critically ill patients is important in diagnosing the patient's condition. Electrolyte imbalances, such as potassium and calcium level changes, can cause cardiovascular abnormalities such as arrhythmias. Electrolyte levels are often checked regularly in critically ill patients.

The functions of electrolytes and their cardiac implications are listed in Table 9.5.

Cardiac enzymes

Cardiac biochemical markers, such as troponin, are proteins that are released from damaged myocardial cells that are detectable by performing blood tests. Troponin elevation is considered a significant biomarker for patients with MI; however, it can also be elevated in non-MI patients.[48] Thus, diagnosis for critically ill patients with elevated cardiac troponin levels should be made with support from other data. See Table 9.6 for cardiac enzyme parameters and normal values. For abnormal cardiac enzymes in MI, please refer to Chapter 10.

Chest X-ray

Chest X-ray is the oldest non-invasive way to visualise the heart and blood vessels, and is one of the most commonly taken diagnostic procedures in critical care. To interpret a chest X-ray for cardiac diagnosis, basic knowledge of the normal anatomical cardiac structure

TABLE 9.5
Electrolyte functions and pathophysiology

ELECTROLYTE	FUNCTIONS	COMMON IMBALANCES AND CAUSES	SIGNS AND SYMPTOMS
Potassium	Maintains normal functions of nerve and muscle cells Acid–base balance	*Hyperkalaemia* Renal failure, dehydration, diabetes, diuretic medications	Muscle weakness, ECG changes in cardiac toxicity, severe hyperkalaemia (serum K between 6 and 6.5 mEq/L) needs prompt attention because it can cause life-threatening arrhythmia
		Hypokalaemia Kidney disease, diarrhoea, vomiting, diuretic medications	Muscle weakness, respiratory failure, ECG changes
Sodium	Regulates body fluid movement Maintains cell functions Acid–base balance	*Hypernatraemia* Renal failure, dehydration, diarrhoea, vomiting	Thirst, confusion, hyperreflexia, seizures
		Hyponatraemia Acute renal failure, heart failure, pancreatitis, peritonitis, burns	Altered personality, confusion, seizures, coma, death
Calcium	Bone metabolism Blood coagulation Muscle contraction Nerve conduction	*Hypercalcaemia* Hyperparathyroidism, vitamin D toxicity, cancer	Polyuria, constipation, nausea, vomiting, muscle weakness, confusion, coma, ECG changes (shortened QT intervals)
		Hypocalcaemia Hypoparathyroidism, vitamin D deficiency, renal disease	Paraesthesias, tetany. In severe cases, seizures, encephalopathy, ECG changes (prolonged ST and QT intervals), heart failure
Magnesium	Activates sodium–potassium pumps Inactivates calcium channels Neuromuscular transmission	*Hypermagnesaemia* Renal failure	Hypotension, respiratory depression, AV conduction disturbances, which can lead to cardiac arrest (often in renal failure patients)
		Hypomagnesaemia Inadequate intake and absorption, or increased excretion, due to hypercalcaemia or diuretics	Anorexia, nausea, vomiting, lethargy. It may contribute to hypokalaemia development therefore cardiac arrhythmias may be present *Note*: associated hypocalcaemia is common in hypomagnesaemia
Phosphorus	Intracellular energy production (ATP) and enzyme regulation Tissue oxygen delivery Bone metabolism	*Hyperphosphataemia* Kidney failure, metabolic and respiratory acidosis	Usually asymptomatic. However, when concurrent hypocalcaemia, symptoms of hypocalcaemia may be present
		Hypophosphataemia Burns, diuretic medications, respiratory alkalosis, acute alcoholism	Usually asymptomatic. Severe cases may have muscle weakness, heart failure, coma

For cardiac implications of electrolytes imbalances, see Chapter 10 and Chapter 11.
Adapted from:
Urden LD, Stacey KM, Lough ME, editors. Critical care nursing: diagnosis and management. St Louis: Elsevier; 2014, with permission.
Moser DK, Reigel B. Cardiac nursing: a companion to Brauwald's heart disease. St Louis: Elsevier; 2008, with permission.

TABLE 9.6
Cardiac biochemical markers: description and normal values

ENZYME	DESCRIPTION	NORMAL VALUE
Troponin T (cTnT)	Detected within 2–3 h after infarction, and may remain elevated for 7–10 d	<0.1 ng/mL
Troponin I (cTnI)	Detected within 2–3 h of infarction, and may remain elevated for up to 14 d	<0.03 ng/mL
Creatine kinase (CK)	Serum CK are elevated following muscle or neurological injury. Creatine kinase myocardial bound (CK–MB) is useful in quantifying the degree of infarction and timing of onset. Levels rise 3–6 h and peak 12–24 h after infarction	Adult female: 30–135 units U/L; Adult male: 55–170 units U/L CK–MB: 0–5% of total CK
Aspartate aminotransferase (AST)	Detection and monitoring of liver cell damage. No cardiac-specific isoenzymes; today rarely used because it is released after renal, cerebral and hepatic damage	<40 U/L
Lactate dehydrogenase (LDH)	Of no value in the diagnosis of myocardial infarction. Occasionally useful in the assessment of patients with liver disease or malignancy (especially lymphoma, seminoma, hepatic metastases); anaemia when haemolysis or ineffective erythropoiesis suspected. Although it may be elevated in patients with skeletal muscle damage, it is not useful in this situation. Post-AMI, cardiac-specific isoenzyme LDH^1 peaks between 48 and 72 h	110–230 U/L
D-Dimer	Presence indicates deep vein thrombosis, myocardial infarction, DIC	<0.25 ng/L

DIC = disseminated intravascular coagulation.
Please note different laboratories may use slightly different reference values. Please always check with the values provided by your laboratory.
Adapted from Pragana KD, Pragana TJ. Mosby's diagnostic and laboratory test reference. 13th ed. St Louis: Elsevier; 2016.

is important to identify abnormality, and a basic understanding of the chest X-ray is essential. Please review the basic concepts, such as what water, air and bone show on X-ray, and the concepts of anteroposterior (AP) and PA films, in Chapter 13 before you move on to the next section.

Cardiac chest X-ray interpretation

To interpret the chest X-ray for cardiac assessment, the following steps should be followed to ensure a thorough diagnosis:[49]

1. The heart size needs to be checked first to see if the size of the heart is appropriate. The cardiac silhouette should be no more than 50% of the diameter of the thorax; this is called the cardiothoracic ratio. The position of the heart should be ⅓ of the heart shadow to the right of the vertebrae and ⅔ of the shadow to the left of the vertebrae. The size of the heart can be determined in a matter of seconds, even by the novice clinician, since this can be simply determined by visualising the cardiothoracic ratio.
2. The shape of the heart should be inspected next. The border of the heart on the X-ray film is determined by the heart anatomy. The border is formed by: the right atrial shadow as the right convex cardiac border, the superior vena cava as the superior border and the left ventricle as the left heart border and cardiac apex. In the frontal chest X-ray, the right ventricle is not a border-forming structure because it is directly superimposed on the cardiac silhouette. Similarly, the normal left atrium should not be visible on a posteroanterior (PA) film. The border of the heart should be sharp. If the left atrium is enlarged, a convex superior left heart border is seen.
3. On the superior border the aortic arch and the pulmonary arteries should be identified next. The aortic arch is called the knob. The pulmonary arteries and their branches radiate outward from the hila (Fig. 9.24). The hilum in the mediastinal region is formed by the pulmonary arteries and the main stem bronchi shadows on the film. The focus of this step is to check for prominence of vessels in this region, as this suggests vascular abnormalities.

Chest X-ray in diagnosing cardiac conditions

For CHD assessment, an initial chest X-ray film is useful to exclude other causes of chest pain, such as pneumonia, pneumothorax and aortic aneurysm, and to assess whether heart failure and/or pulmonary congestion are

FIGURE 9.24 Chest PA radiograph. The convex right cardiac border is formed by the right atrium (thin arrows), and the heavy arrows indicate the location of the superior vena cava.

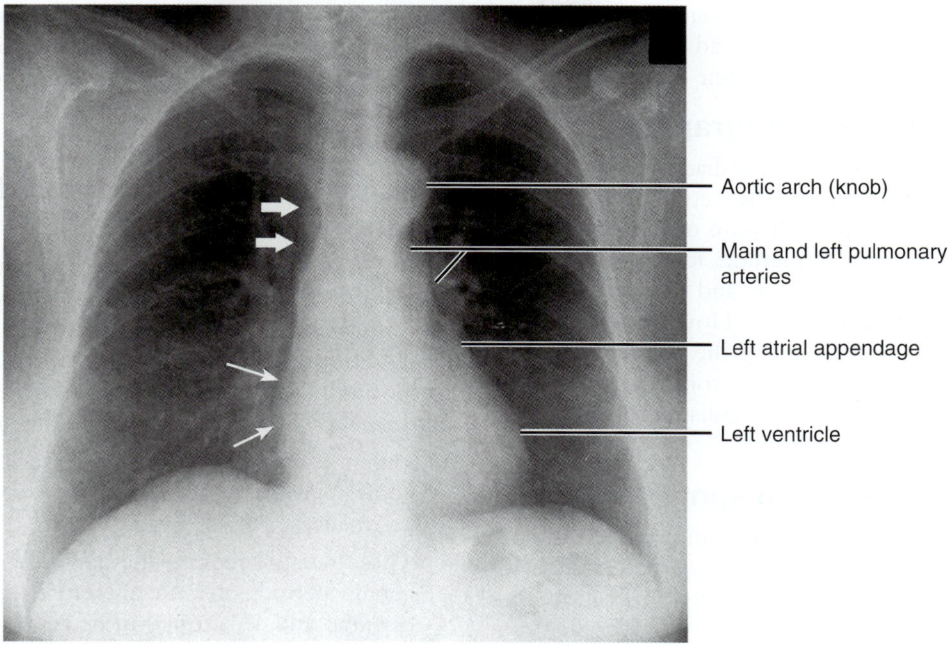

Source: Erkonen WE, Wilbur LS. Radiology 101: the basics and fundamentals of imaging. 3rd ed. Philadelphia, PA: Lippincott Williams and Wilkins; 2009, with permission.

present. Patients with chronic heart failure show cardiomegaly, Kerley B lines or pulmonary oedema. Cardiomegaly is seen as an enlarged heart on the X-ray film. Kerley B lines on the X-ray film are the result of pulmonary congestion and fluid accumulation in the interstitium. Although cardiomegaly and pulmonary oedema indicate heart failure, the chest X-ray alone cannot diagnose the condition. Other tests are needed to thoroughly assess patients for accurate diagnosis.

Practice tip

Critical care nurses should take a systematic approach to interpreting chest X-rays. The respiratory and cardiac structures, tubes, wires and other devices should all be identified in the chest X-ray film.

A widened mediastinum and abnormal aortic contour may indicate aortic dissection. Similar to heart failure, further tests such as TOE, magnetic resonance imaging (MRI) or angiography are needed to confirm the diagnosis. Subtle abnormalities in the hilar region may indicate pulmonary hypertension (PAH). A decrease in pulmonary vascular markings and prominent main and hilar pulmonary arterial shadows in the lung fields on the chest film are classic signs of pulmonary hypertension. However, the sensitivity of this for excluding PAH is lacking. In pericardial disease, the chest X-ray often appears normal unless the accumulated fluid in the pericardial space is over 250 mL. Note that accumulation of fluid is indicated in many cardiac conditions; therefore, other tests need to be carried out to confirm the diagnosis.[48]

The positions of a PAC, a central venous catheter and pacing wires can be identified on the chest X-ray. The positions of these catheters need to be checked regularly to ensure the catheters and wires are in appropriate places. More details on how to identify the catheters and pacing wires are given in Chapter 13.

Due to individual variations in shape, size and rotation of the heart, and the complexity of cardiac signs, chest X-rays often play a minor role in cardiac diagnosis. A patient's clinical condition and other diagnostic test results must be taken into account when diagnosing a cardiac condition.[48]

Practice tip

Comparison of earlier chest X-ray film(s) with the current film is important to diagnose a patient's clinical progress, response to treatment and any movements of catheter positions.

Other diagnostic tests of cardiac function

Since 2000, more non-invasive diagnostic imaging techniques are used to aid cardiac assessment. Some of these techniques have shown significant advantages, such as lowered cost, but they also have their limitations.

Cardiac computed tomography

Cardiac computed tomography (cardiac CT) is a recent development in diagnosing cardiac conditions such as suspected CHD and in the evaluation of coronary artery bypass grafts. It provides a method for visualising the anatomical structures of the heart and coronary arteries reliably and accurately in patients.[50] However, limitations remain with this method including the inability to assess the haemodynamic relevance of a coronary artery lesion. In addition, the most appropriate radiation and contrast doses have not been determined.[51]

Magnetic resonance imaging

MRI is a non-invasive method that can provide cardiac-specific biochemical information about factors such as tissue integrity, cardiac aneurysms, ejection fraction and CO. These techniques are sometimes considered superior to radiography and ultrasound examination methods because the MRI is not affected by bone structure. The techniques include perfusion imaging, atherosclerosis imaging and coronary artery imaging.[43] MRI is considered an accurate method for predicting the presence of significant coronary artery disease. However, MRI use in critically ill patients has its limitations. Because of the magnetic field required for this method, the patient cannot be fitted with any pumps or machines that have metal parts in them. Organising appropriate equipment for critically ill patients who are undergoing this test can be a challenge.

Nuclear medicine cardiac studies

There are several types of radionuclide imaging methods available to assess a patient's cardiac status, including radionuclide isotopes, thallium scan and stress test radionuclide scan. The purpose of radionuclide imaging is to assess the perfusion status of cardiac muscle. When lowered perfusion in cardiac muscle is identified this may indicate heart muscle damage. Radionuclide imaging is often used in patients who have been diagnosed with a MI when further investigation is required to determine if interventions such as cardiac stent or coronary artery bypass surgery are likely to benefit the patient.

Nursing care of patients undergoing diagnostic tests

All of the above methods have advantages and benefits in assessing the cardiac condition of a patient. For the critical care nurse, preparation of patients for these examinations is important because patients often need to be transported to the radiology or nuclear medicine departments. Important considerations include:

- Patient's allergy profile in relation to imaging contrast needs to be evaluated before the requests are made.
- These tests all require the patient to lie still for certain periods of time; therefore, explanation is essential and sedation may be required during the procedure.
- Appropriate equipment, such as non-metal equipment, needs to be organised beforehand if the patient is having an MRI study.

Practice tip

Hearing aids and partial dental plates with metal parts must be removed prior to MRI. Additionally, patients with implantable devices such as permanent pacemakers cannot have an MRI. Critical care patients are at increased risk of adverse events during intra-hospital transport; therefore, close monitoring and documenting the patient's clinical condition during transport are imperative.

Summary

The cardiovascular system is essentially a transport system for distributing metabolic requirements to, and collecting byproducts from, cells throughout the body. A thorough understanding of anatomical structures and physiological events is critical to inform a comprehensive assessment of the critically ill patient. Findings from assessment should define patient cardiovascular status as well as inform the implementation of a timely clinical management plan. A thorough cardiac assessment requires the critical care nurse to be competent in a wide range of interpersonal, observational and technical skills.

Current minimum standards for critical care units in many parts of the world require that patient monitoring include circulation, respiration and oxygenation. For many critically ill patients, haemodynamic instability is a potentially life-threatening condition that necessitates urgent action. In the critical care environment two main forms of cardiac monitoring are commonly employed: continuous cardiac monitoring and the 12-lead ECG. Accurate assessment of the patient's intracardiac status is frequently employed and often considered essential to guide management. Strong research evidence has shown that there is no increased harm or benefit in using pulmonary artery monitoring in critically ill patients; therefore, the decision to use pulmonary artery monitoring as a diagnostic tool depends on the clinical need and clinician expertise. In day-to-day management of critically ill patients, critical care nurses must ensure they are skilled and educated in the techniques of non-invasive and invasive cardiovascular monitoring techniques and technologies, and be able to synthesise all data gathered and base their practice on the best available evidence to date.

Case study

Mr Garry Jones is an 81-year-old man presented to the emergency department (ED) with acute abdominal pain. On arrival to the ED, his heart rate (HR) was 130 bpm, blood pressure (BP) was 85/55 mmHg, and temperature was 38°C. His oxygen saturation (SaO^2) was 93% on 6 L/min oxygen. He has not passed any urine for the past 4 hours according to his family. He was given 1 L of intravenous normal saline as soon as he was admitted. An urgent CT scan of his abdomen showed extra luminal gases with suspected faeces, which indicated possible perforated bowel. He was given broad spectrum antibiotics then underwent urgent surgery. Surgery confirmed the diagnosis of perforated bowel and faecal peritonitis. A bowel resection with extensive peritoneal washout was performed.

He was admitted to ICU following the surgery ventilated and sedated. He had a central venous catheter (CVC) and an arterial line in situ on arrival to ICU. He was ventilated on SIMV with a pressure support of 10 cmH^2O, PEEP of 5 cmH^2O, FiO^2 0.40, and respiratory rate of 10/min. His blood gas results were pH 7.30, PaO^2 88, PCO^2 25, lactate: 2.9. He had 5 L of fluid resuscitation during surgery; however, he remained hypotensive. On arrival to ICU, his observations were: HR 120 bpm, BP 90/55 mmHg, temperature 35.9° C. He was on noradrenaline infusion at 0.1 mcg/kg/min.

GENERAL INFORMATION

Past history of hypertension. Height 175 cm, weight 140 kg. He is an ex-smoker but has not smoked for 2 years. Drinks an average 1–2 glasses of wine per night but he used to be a heavy drinker (amount unknown). He has recently been diagnosed with early stage dementia. He was on propranolol (80 mg sustained-release once a day).

DISCUSSION

This patient was in septic shock from perforated bowel. He showed signs of sepsis with multi-organ involvement including hemodynamic instability, respiratory dysfunction, and renal dysfunction. The diagnosis and subsequent treatment were consistent with best available evidence (antibiotic treatment, identify and treat the underlying cause, fluid resuscitation, and hemodynamic management as indicated).

CASE STUDY QUESTIONS

1 On admission to ICU, what cardiac and hemodynamic monitoring should be commenced and why?
2 Is CO monitoring needed for Mr Jones? If yes, what monitoring option is appropriate and why?

RESEARCH VIGNETTE

Toscani L, Aya HD, Antonakaki D, et al. What is the impact of the fluid challenge technique on diagnosis of fluid responsiveness? A systematic review and meta-analysis. Crit Care 2017;21(1):207

Abstract

Background: The fluid challenge is considered the gold standard for diagnosis of fluid responsiveness. The objective of this study was to describe the fluid challenge techniques reported in fluid responsiveness studies and to assess the difference in the proportion of 'responders' (PR), depending on the type of fluid, volume, duration of infusion and timing of assessment.

Methods: Searches of MEDLINE and Embase were performed for studies using the fluid challenge as a test of cardiac preload with a description of the technique, a reported definition of fluid responsiveness and PR. The primary outcome was the mean PR, depending on volume of fluid, type of fluids, rate of infusion and time of assessment.

Results: A total of 85 studies (3601 patients) were included in the analysis. The PR were 54.4% (95% CI 46.9–62.7) where <500 mL was administered, 57.2% (95% CI 52.9–61.0) where 500 mL was administered and 60.5% (95% CI 35.9–79.2) where >500 mL was administered (p = 0.71). The PR was not affected by type of fluid. The PR was similar among patients administered a fluid challenge for <15 minutes (59.2%, 95% CI 54.2–64.1) and for 15–30 minutes (57.7%, 95% CI 52.4–62.4, p = 1). Where the infusion time was ≥30 minutes, there was a lower PR of 49.9% (95% CI 45.6–54, p = 0.04). Response was assessed at the end of fluid challenge, between 1 and 10 min, and >10 min after the fluid challenge. The proportions of responders were 53.9%, 57.7% and 52.3%, respectively (p = 0.47).

Conclusions: The PR decreases with a long infusion time. A standard technique for fluid challenge is desirable.

Critique

This systematic review and meta-analysis evaluates studies related to intravenous fluid challenges, an area of practice that is the cornerstone of haemodynamic management of critically ill patients. A strength of this systematic review was the use of a predefined protocol and well-defined inclusion criteria to ensure studies are related to the review objective and question. Another strength of the review was the conduct of a meta-analysis on several primary variables. An advantage of conducting a meta-analysis is that it provides a powerful method of combining analysis for extracted data, giving weighted values for each variables effect size. This review included studies that were conducted in ICU or operating theatres with adult patients, where fluid challenge was used as preload or part of the treatment algorithm.

This review informs clinical practice with the following key findings of note. The study highlights that there are different ways to define clinical fluid responsiveness from the studies reviewed including changes to CI, CO, SV and SV index. Another finding of clinical interest was the lack of difference in the proportion of responders between those receiving <500 mL (n=8, 12.7%) in comparison to those receiving > 500 mL (n=5, 7.9%), although the numbers in both groups were very small. In addition, it should be noted that the most common volume infused in studies was 500 mL (n=50, 79.4%). Another clinically informative finding was that when fluid was administered within 30 min, this was more effective in detecting responders than >30 min, supporting the theory that rapid fluid administration rapidly increases venous return and RVEDV. Therefore, administering fluids at a slower rate of infusion is likely to be less effective. The finding from the meta-analysis that timing of assessment of patient response did not impact on detection of response is somewhat surprising and the authors suggest that this may have resulted from the high proportion of studies that used PACs to measure CO, a method they propose does not accurately detect immediate changes in SV.

In summary, this is an informative systematic review that highlights the variance in practice in relation to fluid challenges in critically ill patients and the variance in monitoring effectiveness. Findings suggest that the proportion of patients who respond to fluid challenge infusions is dependent on the technique used with a rapid infusion more likely to result in a positive response. The study also highlights the need for standardisation of practice in this complex clinical practice.

Learning activities

1 Briefly discuss the main ion movement at each of the following phases of the cardiac action potential:
   a depolarisation
   b early rapid repolarisation
   c plateau phase
   d final rapid repolarisation
   e resting membrane phase.
2 Describe the correct placement of the precordial leads when doing a 12-lead ECG.
3 Describe what PQRST represents on an ECG and identify the normal duration for each segment.

4 Describe what systemic vascular resistance (SVR) is and what clinical condition can cause an elevated or lowered SVR.

5 Describe the main determinants of CO.

6 Describe the limitations of CVP monitoring and why.

Online resources

American Heart Association, www.americanheart.org

European Society of Cardiology, https://www.escardio.org/

Australian and New Zealand Intensive Care Society, www.anzics.com.au

United Kingdom Intensive Care Society, https://www.ics.ac.uk/

Australian College of Critical Care Nurses, www.acccn.com.au

British Association of Critical Care Nurses, www.baccn.org.uk

Critical Care Forum, www.ccforum.com/home

National Heart Foundation of Australia, www.heartfoundation.org.au

World Federation of Critical Care Nurses, www.wfccn.org

Further reading

Chung F-T, Lin S-M, Lin S-Y, et al. Impact of extravascular lung water index on outcomes of severe sepsis patients in a medical intensive care unit. Resp Med 2008;102(7):956–61.

Erkonen WE, Wilbur LS. Radiology 101: the basics and fundamentals of imaging. 3rd ed. Philadelphia: Lippincott Williams & Wilkins; 2009.

Patil H, Vaidya O, Bogart D. A review of causes and systemic approach to cardiac troponin elevation. Clin Cardiol 2011;34(12):723–8.

Rajaram SS, Desai NK, Kalra A, et al. Pulmonary artery catheters for adult patients in intensive care. Cochrane Database Syst Rev 2013;(2):CD003408.

Asgar Pour H, Yavuz M. Effects of fever on haemodynamic parameters in neurosurgical intensive care unit patients. Intensive Crit Care Nurs 2014;30(6):325–32.

Preau S, Dewavrin F, Demaeght V, et al. The use of static and dynamic haemodynamic parameters before volume expansion: a prospective observational study in six French intensive care units. Anaesth Crit Care Pain Med 2016;35(2): 93–102.

Khunti K. Accurate interpretation of the 12-lead ECG electrode placement: a systematic review. Health Educ J 2014;73(5):610–23.

Siegenthaler N, Giraud R, Saxer T, et al. Haemodynamic monitoring in the intensive care unit: results from a web-based Swiss survey. Biomed Res Int 2014;2014:129593.

Vincent J-L, et al. Clinical review: update on hemodynamic monitoring – a consensus of 16. Crit Care 2011;15(4):229.

References

1. Hall E, Guyton A. Textbook of medical physiology. 13th ed. Philadelphia: Elsiever; 2016.
2. Costanzo L. Physiology. 6th ed. Philadelphia: Elseiver; 2017.
3. Ozcan C, Palmeri M, Horvath TL, et al. Role of uncoupling protein 3 in ischemia-reperfusion injury, arrhythmias, and preconditioning. Am J Physiol Heart Circ Physiol 2013;304(9):H1192–200.
4. eMedMD.com. Anatomy of the coronary arteries 2018. Available from: http://www.emedmd.com/content/anatomy-coronary-arteries.
5. McCance K, Huether S, editors. Pathophysiology: the biologic basis for disease in adults and children. St Louis: Mosby; 2014.
6. Conover MB. Understanding electrocardiography. St. Louis: Mosby; 2003.

7. Burkhard S, van Eif V, Garric L, et al. On the evolution of the cardiac pacemaker. J Cardiovasc Dev Dis 2017;4(2).
8. Modell H, Cliff W, Michael J, et al. A physiologist's view of homeostasis. Adv Physiol Educ 2015;39(4):259–66.
9. Heijman J, Algalarrondo V, Voigt N, et al. The value of basic research insights into atrial fibrillation mechanisms as a guide to therapeutic innovation: a critical analysis. Cardiovasc Res 2016;109(4):467–79.
10. Reddy YNV, El-Sabbagh A, Nishimura RA. Comparing pulmonary arterial wedge pressure and left ventricular end diastolic pressure for assessment of left-sided filling pressures. JAMA Cardiol 2018;3(6):453–4.
11. Monnet X, Marik PE, Teboul J-L. Prediction of fluid responsiveness: an update. Ann Intensive Care 2016;6:111. http://doi.org/10.1186/s13613-016-0216-7.
12. Vincent JL. Understanding cardiac output. Crit Care 2008;12(4):174.
13. Sloop GD, Weidman JJ, St Cyr JA. The systemic vascular resistance response: a cardiovascular response modulating blood viscosity with implications for primary hypertension and certain anemias. Ther Adv Cardiovasc Dis 2015;9(6):403–11.
14. Gordan R, Gwathmey JK, Xie LH. Autonomic and endocrine control of cardiovascular function. World J Cardiol 2015;7(4):204–14.
15. Rajendran P, Rengarajan T, Thangavel J, et al. The vascular endothelium and human diseases. Int J Biol Sci 2013;9(10):1057–69.
16. Russell JA. Presynaptic alpha-2 receptors inhibit norepinephrine release in tracheal smooth muscle. Respir Physiol 1987;70(1):25–35.
17. Gavras I, Gavras H. Role of alpha2-adrenergic receptors in hypertension. Am J Hypertens 2001;14(6 Pt 2):171S–177S.
18. Chizner MA. Cardiac auscultation: rediscovering the lost art. Curr Probl Cardiol 2008;33(7):326–408.
19. Redlarski G, Gradolewski D, Palkowski A. A system for heart sounds classification. PLoS ONE 2014;9(11):e112673.
20. Silverman ME, Wooley CF, Samuel A. Levine and the history of grading systolic murmurs. Am J Cardiol 2008;102(8):1107–10.
21. Australian and New Zealand College of Intensive Care Medicine (CICM). Minimum standards for intensive care units 2011. Available from: https://www.cicm.org.au/CICM_Media/CICMSite/CICM-Website/Resources/Professional%20Documents/IC-1-Minimum-Standards-for-Intensive-Care-Units.pdf.
22. Valentin A, Ferdinande P, Esicm Working Group on Quality Improvement. Recommendations on basic requirements for intensive care units: structural and organizational aspects. Intensive Care Med 2011;37(10):1575–87.
23. Professional Standards Committee of the Faculty of Intensive Care Medicine and the Standards SaQCotICS. Core Standards for Intensive Care Units 2013. Available from: https://www.ficm.ac.uk/sites/default/files/Core%20Standards%20for%20ICUs%20Ed.1%20(2013).pdf.
24. Sandau KE, Funk M, Auerbach A, et al. Update to practice standards for electrocardiographic monitoring in hospital settings: a scientific statement from the American Heart Association. Circulation 2017;136(19):e273–344.
25. Tsang R. Hemodynamic monitoring in the cardiac intensive care unit. Congenit Heart Dis 2013;8(6):568–75.
26. Sakka SG. Hemodynamic monitoring in the critically ill patient – current status and perspective. Front Med (Lausanne) 2015;2:44.
27. Zhong L, Wang H-L, Xu B, et al. Normal saline versus heparin for patency of central venous catheters in adult patients – a systematic review and meta-analysis. Crit Care 2017;21:5.
28. Robertson-Malt S, Malt G, Farquhar V, et al. Heparin versus normal saline for patency of arterial lines (Review). Cochrane Database Syst Rev 2014;(5):CD007364.
29. Pickering TG, Hall JE, Appel LJ, et al. Recommendations for blood pressure measurement in humans and experimental animals: part 1: blood pressure measurement in humans: a statement for professionals from the Subcommittee of Professional and Public Education of the American Heart Association Council on High Blood Pressure Research. Circulation 2005;111(5):697–716.
30. Ribezzo S, Spina E, Di Bartolomeo S, et al. Noninvasive techniques for blood pressure measurement are not a reliable alternative to direct measurement: a randomized crossover trial in ICU. Scientific World Journal 2014;2014:353628.
31. Saugel B, Dueck R, Wagner JY. Measurement of blood pressure. Best Pract Res Clin Anaesthesiol 2014;28(4):309–22.
32. Shojaee M, Sabzghabaei A, Alimohammadi H, et al. Effect of positive end-expiratory pressure on central venous pressure in patients under mechanical ventilation. Emergency 2017;5(1):e1.
33. Spelman T, Pilcher DV, Cheng AC, et al. Central line-associated bloodstream infections in Australian ICUs: evaluating modifiable and non-modifiable risks in Victorian healthcare facilities. Epidemiol Infect 2017;145(14):3047–55.
34. Loveday HP, Wilson JA, Pratt RJ, et al. epic3: National evidence-based guidelines for preventing healthcare-associated infections in NHS hospitals in England. J Hosp Infect 2014;86:S1–70.
35. World Health Organization. Preventing bloodstream infections from central line venous catheters. Available from: URL: http://www.who.int/patientsafety/implementation/bsi/en/index html. 2012.
36. Swan HJC, Ganz W, Forrester J, et al. Catheterization of the heart in man with use of a flow-directed balloon-tipped catheter. New Engl J Med 1970;283(9):447–51.
37. Rajaram SS, Desai NK, Kalra A, et al. Pulmonary artery catheters for adult patients in intensive care [Internet]. Cochrane Database Syst Rev 2013;(2):CD003408.
38. Roşca M, Lancellotti P, Popescu BA, et al. Left atrial function: pathophysiology, echocardiographic assessment, and clinical applications. Heart 2011;97(23):1982–9.
39. Vincent J-L, Rhodes A, Perel A, et al. Clinical review: update on hemodynamic monitoring – a consensus of 16. Crit Care 2011;15(4):229.
40. Lough ME. Cardiovascular diagnostic procedures. In: Urden LD, Stacey KM, Lough ME, editors. Critical care nursing. Maryland Heights: Elsevier; 2018. p. 199–275.

41. Huygh J, Peeters Y, Bernards J, et al. Hemodynamic monitoring in the critically ill: an overview of current cardiac output monitoring methods. F1000Res 2016;5:F1000. Faculty Rev-2855.
42. Litton E, Morgan M. The PiCCO monitor: a review. Anaesth Intensive Care 2012;40:393–409.
43. Ripley DP, Musa TA, Dobson LE, et al. Cardiovascular magnetic resonance imaging: what the general cardiologist should know. Heart 2016;102(19):1589–603.
44. LiDCO. Cardiac output 2018. Available from: http://www.lidco.com/education/cardiac-output/.
45. Drummond KE, Murphy E. Minimally invasive cardiac output monitors. Continuing Edu Anaesth Crit Care Pain 2012;12(1):5–10.
46. Singer M. Oesophageal Doppler. Curr Opin Crit Care 2009;15:244–8.
47. Wilson RJT. Oesophageal Doppler monitoring – the emperor's new clothes? Anaesthesia 2013;68(10):1072–3.
48. Pagana K, Pagana T, Pagana T. Mosby's diagnostic and laboratory test reference. 13th ed. St Louis: Elsevier; 2016. p. 1088.
49. Erkonen WE, Smith WL. Radiology 101: the basics and fundamentals of imaging. 3rd ed. Philadelphia: Lippincott William & Wilkins; 2009. p. 384.
50. Wijesekera NT, Duncan MK, Padley SPG. X-ray computed tomography of the heart. Br Med Bull 2010;93(1):49–67.
51. Ropers D. Multislice computer tomography for detection of coronary artery disease. J Interv Cardiol 2006;19(6):574–82.

Chapter 10

Cardiovascular alterations and management

Andrea Driscoll, Karen Smith

Learning objectives

After reading this chapter, you should be able to:

- explain the pathophysiology of coronary artery disease, clinical manifestations of acute coronary syndromes and management of events
- discuss the care for a patient with chest pain
- list the diagnostic tests used to assess myocardial ischaemia
- discuss the pathways for reperfusion therapies in STEMI
- outline the clinical manifestations of right and left ventricular failure
- discuss the goals of heart failure treatment
- discuss the pathophysiologies of the four different types of cardiomyopathy and how they affect cardiac function
- outline the actions of angiotensin-converting enzyme inhibitors, angiotensin neprilysin receptor inhibitors, beta-blockers, loop diuretics and spironolactone and how they relate to the pathophysiology of heart failure.

Introduction

The support of cardiovascular function in the face of many compromises is reviewed in this chapter. It focuses on two of the most prevalent and fatal cardiovascular diseases: coronary heart disease and heart failure. These diseases are also a common comorbidity in elderly patients admitted to critical care units. The first section on coronary heart disease reviews the pathophysiological concepts of acute coronary syndromes (ACS), associated myocardial ischaemia and complications, with detailed consideration of the clinical implications, assessment and associated management. Heart failure is discussed in terms of the body's compensatory mechanisms and the clinical sequelae and associated clinical features of heart failure. Nursing and medical management is outlined including the management of acute exacerbations of heart failure. Finally, other cardiovascular disorders commonly managed in critical care units are reviewed, ranging from other forms of heart failure to hypertensive emergencies and aortic aneurysms. The case study presented at the end of the chapter highlights the key aspects of the management of heart failure in patients admitted to critical care units.

KEY WORDS

acute coronary syndrome
acute heart failure
aortic aneurysm
arrhythmia
cardiomyopathy
endocarditis
hypertensive emergencies
left ventricular failure
myocardial infarction
percutaneous coronary intervention
right ventricular failure
ventricular aneurysm

Cardiovascular disease

Cardiovascular disease (CVD), encompassing diseases of the heart and circulation, retains a key influence on morbidity, mortality and health care expenditure.[1] CVD has been reported to be responsible for an estimated 17.7 million deaths worldwide in 2015 reflecting 31% of all global deaths.[2] Of these approximately 7.4 million have been associated with coronary heart disease (CHD),[2-4] a condition resulting from a reduction or complete obstruction of blood flow through the coronary arteries due to narrowing from atherosclerosis and/or thrombus formation. Death rates over the last three decades have fallen by about 75%, primarily due to improvements in risk factors and healthcare for those at risk. However, in the most recent decade there has been a plateau in this mortality decline in the 55–69 year olds.[4] Despite improvements, the burden of CHD remains high, with 16% of males and 13% of females being affected by the disease in Australia.[4] It was responsible for 31% of all hospitalisation for CVD, in all age groups with the exception of those over 85 where hospitalisation for heart failure and cardiomyopathy were more common.

Although some patients may be asymptomatic, the most common manifestations of CHD are chest pain due to angina, ACS which includes acute myocardial infarction [AMI] and unstable angina and sudden death due to cardiac arrest. CHD may also cause arrhythmias and heart failure.[5]

Myocardial ischaemia

When coronary blood supply is insufficient to meet myocardial tissue demand for oxygen, myocardial ischaemia occurs. Critical restriction to blood flow occurs when the diameter of the lumen of the blood vessel is reduced by more than half either as a result of coronary artery narrowing through the build-up of fatty deposits and the development of plaque (atherosclerosis) or the formation of a thrombus or blood clot causing occlusion. Coronary blood flow is also determined by perfusion pressure, which can be adversely affected by abnormalities in blood flow (valvular disease), vessel wall (coronary spasm) and the blood (anaemia, polycythaemia).[5] Myocardial oxygen demand is influenced by heart rate, strength of myocardial contraction and left ventricular wall tension. The myocardium receives most of its blood supply during diastole; hence a rise in heart rate that decreases the duration of diastole will also decrease coronary perfusion. Sympathetic stimulation increases the force of contraction and therefore oxygen demand. Left ventricular wall tension increases with the changes in preload associated with filling and afterload associated with systemic vascular resistance. During activity, pyrexia and arrhythmias, these effects may compound due to sympathetic stimulation, causing increased oxygen demand and reduced coronary perfusion resulting in symptoms of angina.

Angina

Angina (angina pectoris) is the most common manifestation of CHD and is the term used to describe the symptoms of discomfort that occur during myocardial ischaemia. The classic angina pattern consists of retrosternal constricting chest pain/discomfort, which may radiate to the arms, throat, jaw, teeth, back or epigastrium.[6] Associated symptoms often include shortness of breath, nausea, vomiting, sweating, palpitations and weakness.

A fixed coronary artery lesion, causing limitation of oxygen supply at times of increased demand, results in stable angina. Therefore, symptoms arise during periods of physical and emotional stress and resolve within 2–10 min of rest. Symptoms tend to be worse in the morning (coinciding with a peak in blood pressure), after heavy meals and in cold weather. The severity of symptoms has little correlation with the progress of the disease. However, a patient with a typical history of angina has a high probability of CHD and a higher risk of AMI and coronary death during the next 5 years.[7]

Acute coronary syndromes

ACS include unstable angina, often related to transient ischaemia, and AMI associated with myocardial necrosis.[6-9] According to electrocardiographic changes AMI is further classified into ST elevation myocardial infarction (STEMI) and non-ST elevation MI (NSTEMI). ACS are associated with the underlying disease process of arthrosclerosis and the development of atheromatous plaque consisting of lipids, cells fibrin and cell debris which form over time causing narrowing of the vessel lumen. ACS develops due to the fissuring or rupture of the plaque leading to release of vasoconstrictor substances and potentially triggering coagulation activity (Fig. 10.1) causing a reduction in coronary blood flow and subsequent damage to myocardial cells.[8,10] The diagnosis of ACS will be made based on the combination of clinical history, the presence or absence of ST elevation on a 12-lead electrocardiograph (ECG) and alterations in cardiac biomarkers (commonly troponin), as defined in the third universal definition of AMI.[8,10] The presence of ST elevation in the 12 lead ECG will activate well-defined critically time-dependent care pathways to achieve rapid opening of the affected coronary artery and reperfusion by primary percutaneous coronary intervention (PCI) or thrombolysis. ACS typically presents as a recent history of angina (within the past 4–6 weeks); a change in symptoms including increased frequency, more easily provoked or occurring in the absence of physical or emotional stress, more severe or prolonged and/or less responsive to nitrate therapy. ACS is a medical emergency, with approximately one-fifth of ACS patients at risk of AMI and death within 30 days.[8]

Myocardial infarction (MI) occurs when blood flow to the myocardium is severely impaired for more than 20 min as myocardial cell necrosis begins. A coronary artery thrombus arising from an atherosclerotic plaque is

FIGURE 10.1 (**A**) Plaque rupture exposes thrombogenic lipid. A white thrombus is formed by activated platelets adhering. This lesion is unstable and may lead to thrombin activation. (**B**) Thrombin activation leads to a mesh of fibrin and red blood cells, leading to a 'red thrombus'.

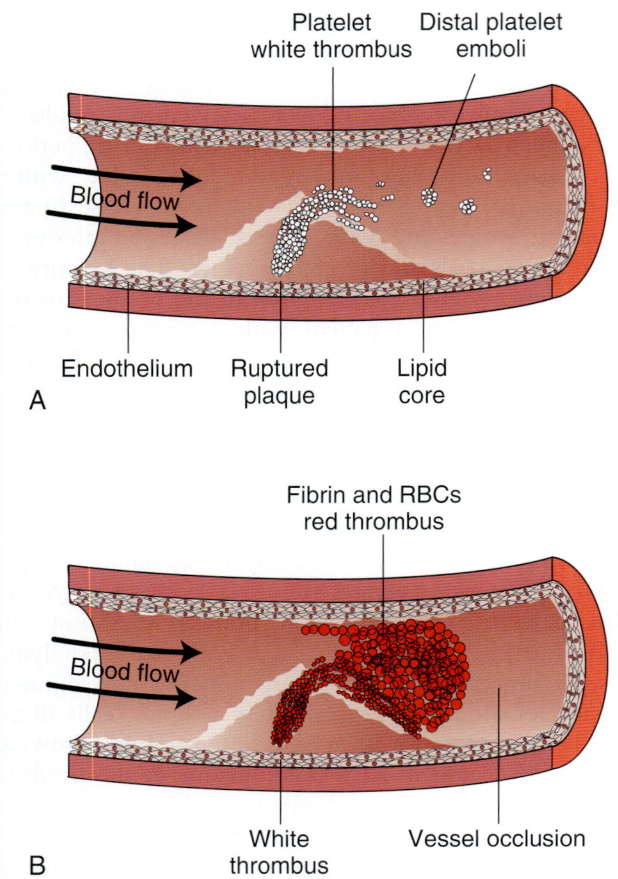

Adapted from Bersten AD, Soni N, Oh TE. Oh's intensive care manual. 5th ed. Oxford: Butterworth-Heineman; 2003 with permission.

found in the majority of patients dying of AMI.[10] Cellular death begins in the subendocardial layer and progresses through the full muscle thickness, so that by 2–4 hours with total occlusion a full 'transmural' infarction will result. However, the full extent of tissue death may occur as a single incident or evolve over several days, depending on the degree of obstruction to blood flow. The size and location of the infarction will influence the clinical manifestations and risk of death and determine treatment. The size of the infarction is determined by the extent, severity and duration of the ischaemic event, the amount of collateral circulation and the metabolic demands placed on the myocardium. Usually the ventricle wall is affected, with a small infarction often resulting in a dyskinetic wall (altered movement), whereas a large infarction may result in akinesis (no movement).

The location and impact of the infarction will depend on which coronary artery has been obstructed:

- Left anterior descending (LAD) affects the function of the left ventricle and interventricular septum, including ventricular conduction tissue. Patients with anteroseptal MI are at high risk of heart failure, cardiogenic shock and mortality due to pump deficits.
- Circumflex (CX) affects the left ventricle lateral and posterior walls and the sinoatrial (SA) node in 40% of people.[5,11] The impact on pump efficiency of lateral and posterior wall necrosis is not as severe as anteroseptal infarctions, although patients are at more risk of arrhythmias.
- Right coronary artery (RCA) affects the inferior wall of the left ventricle and the right ventricle, as well as the AV node in most patients (90%) and the SA node in 60% of people. There is potentially severe impact on ventricular function if both the inferior wall and the right ventricle are affected, as well as a high risk of arrhythmias due to SA and AV node involvement.

Clinical features

Patients with AMI most often present with chest pain. This pain is described as central crushing retrosternal pain, which lasts longer than 20 min and is not relieved by nitrate therapy. The pain may radiate to the neck, jaw, back and shoulders and is often accompanied by 'feelings of impending doom', sweating and pallor. Nausea is often associated with the pain, due to vagal nerve stimulation. Depending on the size and location of the AMI, patients may also present with sudden death or with varying degrees of syncope and heart failure. Women may present with different symptoms.[6,12]

Patient assessment and diagnostic features

A key feature of assessment of the patient with chest pain is the use of protocols and guidelines to promote rapid implementation of revascularisation procedures such as primary PCI and thrombolysis when no contraindications to treatment exist. This process begins at the point of contact, often in the community with 12-lead ECG transmission to the hospital where rapid, early triage models of care are in place.[13] Clinical assessment methods used will depend on the condition of the patient but should occur within 10 min of arrival.[9,10,12] This initial history will focus on the nature of presenting symptoms such as pain and symptoms assessment can be aided by the use of an acronym such as PQRST or OLDCARTs (Tables 10.1 and 10.2) to incorporate precipitating and palliative factors, qualitative descriptors, onset, location, radiation, severity and duration.[14] Intensity can be rated on a pain scale.[14] Asking patients for descriptive words is useful in assessment as many patients will deny pain and instead use words such as pressure, tightness or constriction. It is essential not to ignore other presentations,

TABLE 10.1
The PQRST criteria for assessing chest pain

P	Precipitating	Exercise and activity Stress and anxiety Cold weather
	Palliating	Stop activity Rest Nitroglycerine
Q	Quality	Heavy, tight, choking, vice-like, constricting
R	Region, Radiation	Left side of chest, shoulder, arm and jaw Retrosternal and radiating to the neck
S	Severity	Rate pain on scale of 1 (no pain) to 10 (worst pain possible)
T	Time	Pain lasts longer than 10 min despite nitroglycerine Pain comes and goes but lasts longer than 20 min

Adapted from Hudak CM, Gallo BM, Morton PG. Critical care nursing, a holistic approach. 7th ed. Philadelphia: Lippincott; 1998.

as patients with atypical symptoms, such as women, diabetics and the elderly often have a delayed diagnosis and treatment and a higher mortality.[7,12,13] Differentiating current pain from any previous pain is also useful in differential diagnosis. Pain relief should be a priority not only for comfort but to reduce associated physiological responses including sympathetic stimulation and vasoconstriction which are detrimental to an already compromised coronary circulation. Recurrent chest discomfort requires urgent reassessment, including immediate ECG.

The brief history should also include a short cardiovascular risk profile: 1) previous cardiac history such as angina, MI, revascularisation and 2) family history, smoking, hypertension, diabetes. A more complete history, which includes detailed information about risk factors, can be acquired when the patient is stabilised. This information will be essential to guide patient education and rehabilitation and to plan discharge.

Practice tip

Because of changes in neuroreceptors, older patients and diabetic patients may not describe the typical anginal pain. Women also may not describe classic angina symptoms and may use different descriptors from men.[6] Be alert for prodromal symptoms, such as increased shortness of breath, weakness and fainting.

Timmis A. Acute coronary syndromes. BMJ 2015;351:h5849.

TABLE 10.2
OLDCARTS framework for assessing chest pain

DESCRIPTION	QUESTIONS TO ASK TO YIELD THE INFORMATION
Onset	When did the pain begin?
Location	Where is the pain? Can the patient point to the location of the pain?
Duration	How long does the pain last? Is it persistent or intermittent?
Characteristics	Describe the pain: is it crushing, stabbing, indigestion-like, dull, or ache, for example?
Associating factors	What other symptoms are associated with the pain, such as nausea and/or vomiting, weakness, fatigue, breathlessness, syncope, feeling cold and clammy?
Relieving factors/radiation	Does the pain radiate, such as down the arm or up into the neck, for example? Does the pain stop when activity ceases, or is it relieved by sitting forward or resting?
Treatment/temporal factors	Is pain relieved by rest or a decrease in physical activity? Is it relieved by the use of glyceryl trinitrate? Is pain comparable to previous ischaemic chest pain?
Severity (intensity)	A numerical scale (1 no pain to 10 worse pain experienced) is used to gauge pain severity

Source: Seidel HM, Ball JW, Dains JE, Benedict GW. Mosby's Guide to physical examination. 6th ed. Mosby, 2003.

Physical examination

Physical manifestations vary and depend on the impact of pain, size and location of the infarction in the individual. Heart rate and blood pressure may be raised due to anxiety. Impaired left ventricular function may result in dyspnoea, tachycardia, hypotension, pallor, sweating, nausea and vomiting. Impaired right ventricular function may be indicated by jugular vein distension and peripheral oedema. Abnormalities in heart sounds may be present, including a muffled and diminished first heart sound due to decreased contractility. A fourth heart sound is common, whereas a third heart sound is uncommon. Many patients develop a pericardial rub after about 48–72 hours due to an inflammatory response to the damaged myocardium. Additional findings occur with complications, and these are discussed in the related specific sections below.

Electrocardiographic examination

Patients with chest discomfort should be assessed by an appropriately qualified person and have a 12-lead ECG recorded within 10 min of first acute clinical contact to determine the presence and extent of myocardial ischaemia, the risk of adverse events and to provide a baseline for subsequent changes.[15,16] Most importantly, the ECG is essential to determine whether emergency reperfusion is required, and is recommended as the sole test for selecting patients for PCI or thrombolysis. Where ST-segment monitoring is available, this should be continuous. Alternatively, if chest discomfort persists, ECGs should be repeated every 15 min. Even when chest pain resolves it is important to record a series of 12-lead ECGs during admission to determine changes over time. (The normal ECG is covered in Chapter 9, whereas this section addresses ischaemic changes in the ECG.)

Myocardial ischaemia, injury or infarction causes cellular alterations and affects depolarisation and repolarisation[17] resulting in T wave inversion or ST-segment depression in the leads facing the ischaemic area.[13,17] Ischaemic T waves are usually symmetrical, narrower and more pointed. ST-segment depression of 1 mm for 0.08 seconds is indicative of ischaemia, especially when forming a sharp angle with an upright T wave.[18] These changes are reversible with reduction in demand (e.g. by rest, nitrates).

MI is associated with a typical pattern of ECG changes over time including evolution of the ST segments, Q-wave development and T wave inversion as described below, but these changes too are not universal. The distinction between the various ACS, including ST-elevation acute coronary syndrome (STEACS), ST-elevation MI (STEMI) and non-ST-elevation MI (non-STEMI), is important for ensuring appropriate assessment and protocol-based treatment.[9,10,12,15,16]

The location and extent of ischaemia or infarction may be evident on the ECG leads overlying the affected area, as follows:

- anteroseptal wall of left ventricle, V1–V4
- anterior wall of the left ventricle, V1–V6, I and aVL
- lateral wall of left ventricle, I, aVL,V5 and V6
- inferior wall of left ventricle, II, III and aVF.

Additional electrodes can be placed on the right chest wall using the same landmarks as the left chest to view the right ventricle (see Chapter 9). Further posterior electrodes, V7–V9, may be placed over the posterior left chest to view the posterior wall. Other indicative signs of posterior wall damage are a dominant r wave in V1 and/or ST depression in V3 and V4, as these may be reciprocal changes. If these signs are present a left-sided ECG, V7–V9, should be done to confirm or rule out a posterior infarction.

Continuous ECG monitoring is essential for the early detection of arrhythmias, which often accompany AMI and may be life-threatening. The arrhythmia may be due to poor perfusion of the conduction tissue. More often, arrhythmias occur because ischaemic tissue has a lower fibrillatory threshold and ischaemia is not being managed. Arrhythmias also result from left ventricular failure.

Typical ECG evolution pattern

The initial ECG features of MI are ST-segment elevation with tall T waves recorded in leads overlying the area of damaged myocardium. These changes gradually change, or evolve, over time, with ST segments returning to baseline (within hours), while Q waves develop (hours to days) and T waves become inverted (days to weeks). The time course for the evolutionary changes is accelerated by reperfusion, e.g. PCI, thrombolysis or surgery. Thus, an almost fully-evolved pattern may be seen within hours if successful reperfusion has been undertaken (see Figs 10.2–10.4 for examples). Given the expected time course for evolution, it is possible to approximate how recently infarction has occurred, which is essential in determining management:

- Acute (or hyperacute): there is ST elevation but Q waves or T inversion have not yet developed (Fig. 10.5).
- Recent: Q waves have developed. ST-segment elevation may still be present. Evolution is underway. The infarction is more than 24 hours old.
- Old (fully evolved): Q waves and T inversion are present. ST segments are no longer elevated. Infarction occurred anything from a few days to years ago.

Biomarkers

Cardiac troponins T and I are structural proteins, which now are the preferred biomarkers for identification of myocardial necrosis given their sensitivity and specificity. Furthermore, high sensitivity troponin assays can detect

FIGURE 10.2 Acute inferoposterior infarction: ST elevation in indicative leads II, III and aVF. The ST-segment depression in I and aVL is reciprocal to the inferior infarction. Also, ST depression in anterior leads (V1–V3) is reciprocal to posterior wall infarction. Posterior leads (not shown here) were recorded and revealed ST elevation in V7, V8 and V9. This patient had acute (100%) obstruction at the ostium of the RCA.

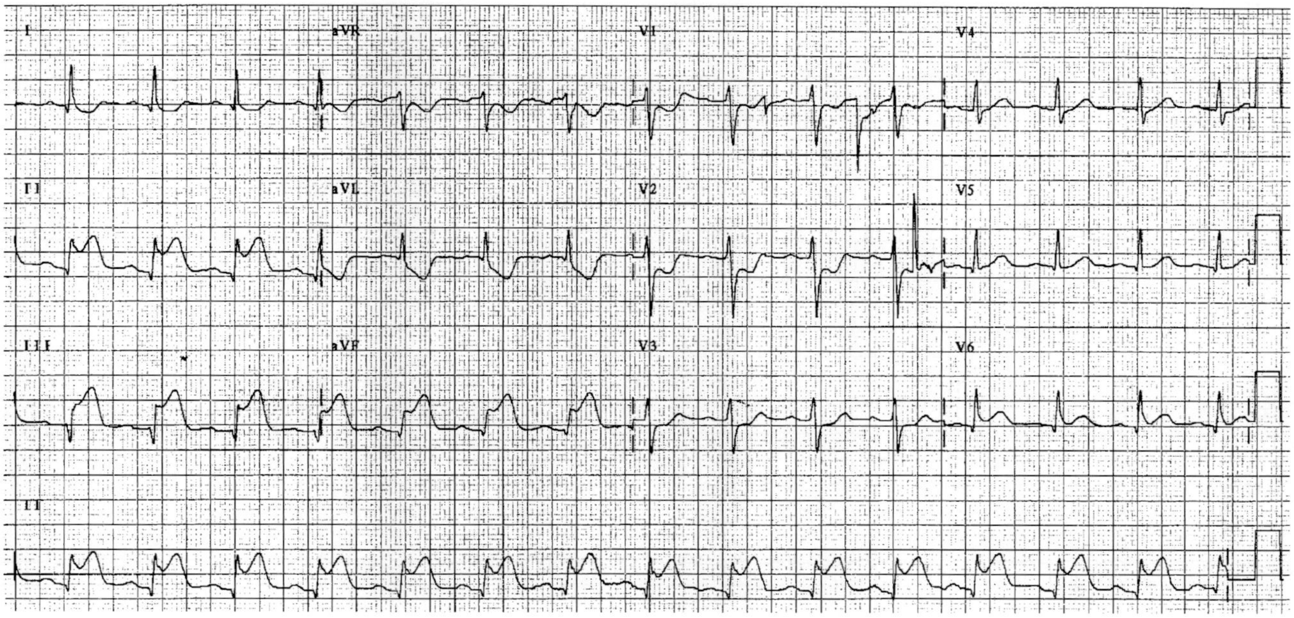

FIGURE 10.3 The same patient as in Fig. 10.2, recorded only 1 h later, after stenting of the RCA with an evolving inferoposterior infarction. Note the ST segments in II, III and aVF are still elevated but returning to baseline. The reciprocal ST depression is likewise diminishing and can now be seen only in aVL, V1 and V2. Q waves have already developed in inferior leads.

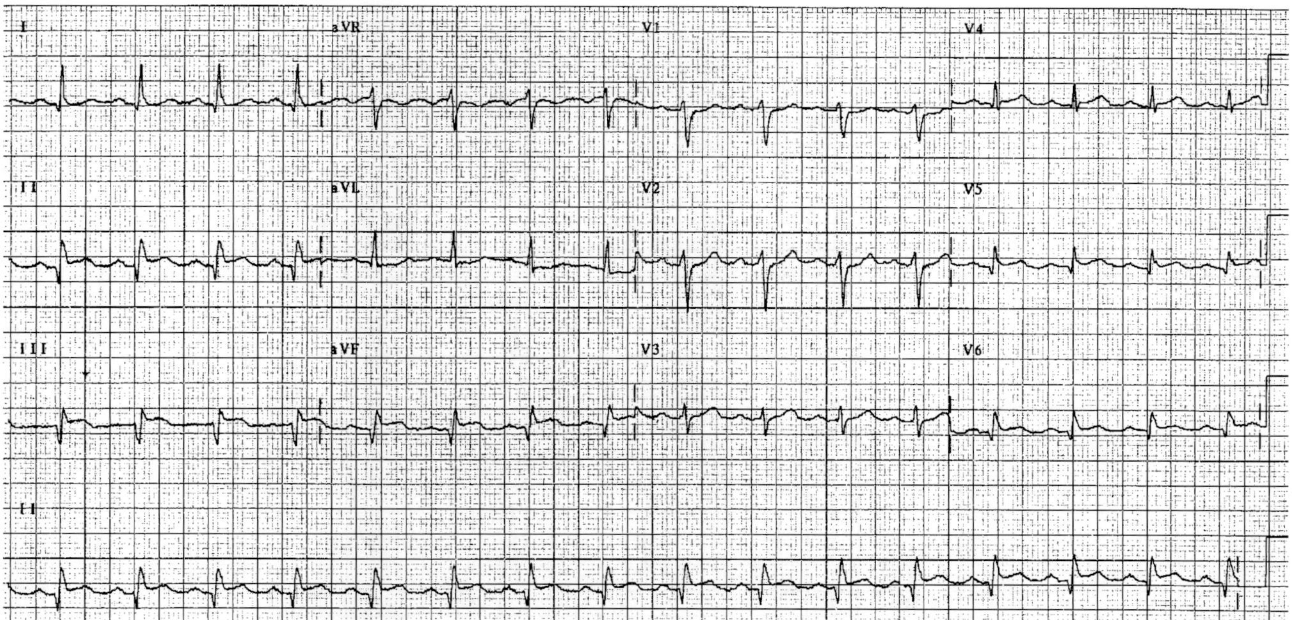

FIGURE 10.4 The same patient again, recorded a further 21 h later. An almost fully evolved pattern is now present. Note the ST segments inferiorly have almost completely returned to baseline (as have the reciprocal changes). The Q waves remain, and T waves have now inverted inferiorly.

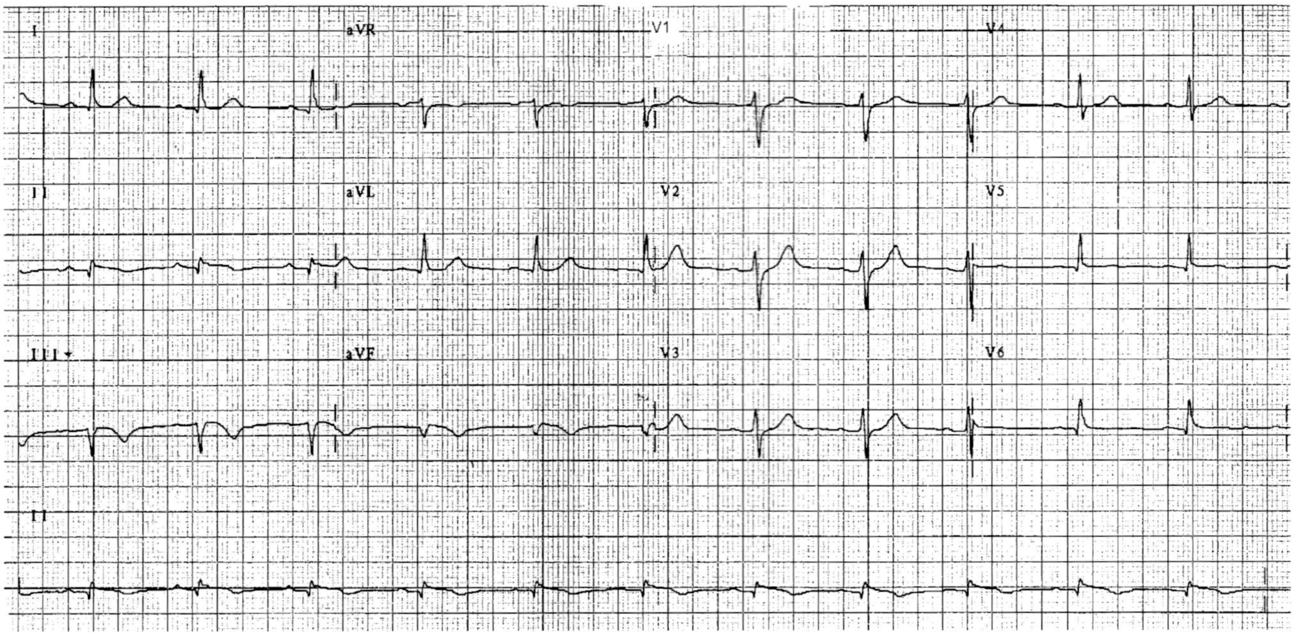

FIGURE 10.5 Acute anterolateral infarction in a patient with anterior descending coronary artery obstruction. Note the ST elevation and tall (hyperacute) T waves across the chest leads V1–V6 recorded on admission.

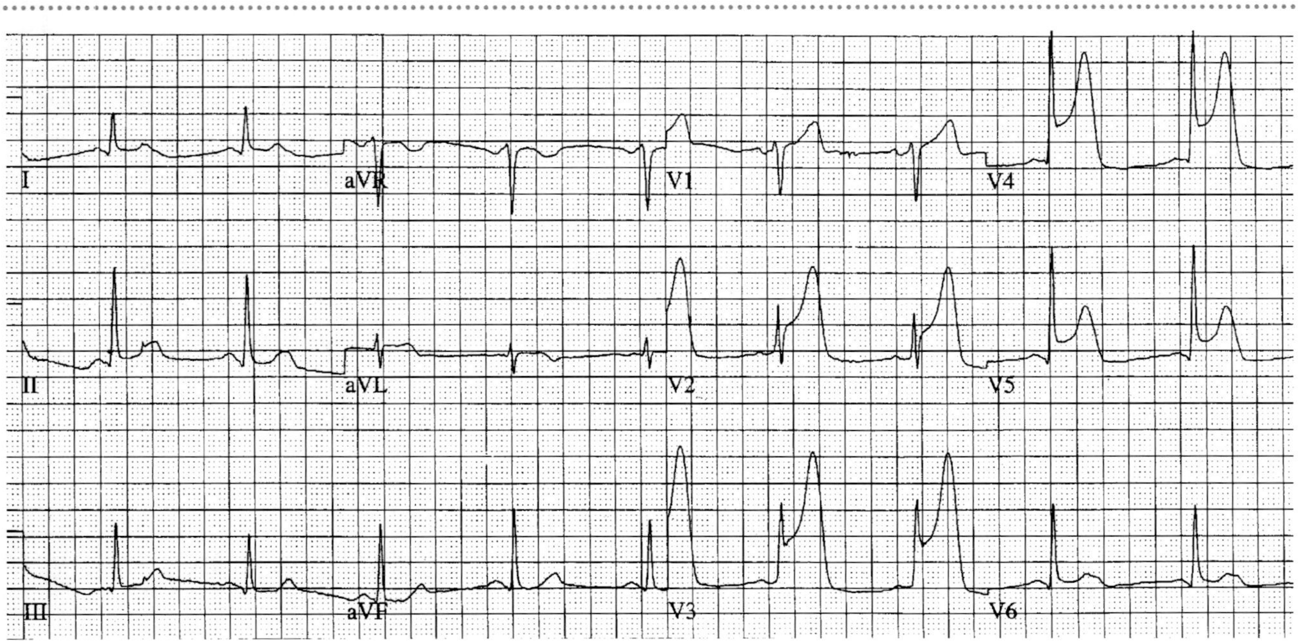

plasma elevation, within 1–3 hours, supporting early diagnosis and subsequent risk stratification of patients with suspected ACS.[19,20] Troponin elevation is defined as at least one value exceeding the 99th percentile of the assays upper reference limit and detection of a rise and/or fall of the measurements is essential to support the diagnosis of acute MI.[10] Measurement of troponin should occur at hospital presentation and predefined time periods according to unit protocols alongside thorough clinical assessment to allow accurate differential diagnosis of AMI from other medical conditions associated with elevations in cardiac troponin levels e.g. including myocarditis, heart failure and renal disease.

Coronary angiography and left heart catheterisation

Coronary angiography gives a detailed picture of coronary artery disease. Specially designed catheters are advanced with the assistance of a guidewire into the ascending aorta via the radial[12] or less frequently the femoral arteries and manoeuvred into the ostium of each coronary artery. Contrast media is then injected and images are taken from several views to provide detailed information on the extent, site and severity of coronary artery lesions and the blood flow into each artery. This flow is graded using the Thrombolysis in Myocardial Infarction (TIMI) studies system (Table 10.3). Typically, a left ventricular angiogram is performed during the same procedure to assess the appearance and function of the left ventricle, mitral and aortic valves. If CHD is present, treatment is determined as appropriate according to the severity (PCI, coronary artery bypass grafting or medical therapy). The nursing care for coronary angiography is similar to PCI and is covered under that section.

Given that conventional angiography only provides information related to the lumen of the artery, the use of alternative imaging techniques is increasing e.g. coronary computed tomography angiography (CTA) or magnetic resonance imaging (MRI) angiography to visualise the coronary anatomy and provide additional information about the atherosclerotic plaques within the vessel wall.

Non-invasive investigations

A number of investigations may aid the clinical diagnosis for patients with a suspected diagnosis of angina. These investigations which may be either anatomical (e.g. computerised tomography-coronary angiography [CT-CA]) or functional (e.g. exercise tolerance testing [ETT] or cardiac imaging) can help confirm the presence of underlying atherosclerotic disease and guide risk stratification related to severity of ischaemia.[21] A baseline 12-lead electrocardiogram (ECG) should be performed in every patient with suspected angina. While an abnormal resting ECG increases the probability that a patient has coronary artery disease (CAD) and may highlight the presence of other conditions such as atrial fibrillation or left ventricular hypertrophy, it is important to remember that a normal 12-lead ECG does not exclude a diagnosis of CAD and further investigation may be required.[21]

Recent guidelines have reduced the emphasis of ETT within the diagnostic screening process; however, practice may be influenced by the availability of local investigative resources.[20] For some time it has been recognised that false-positive ETTs are more common in populations with a lower incidence of CHD, including women.[21,22] The main diagnostic ECG abnormality during ECG exercise testing consists of a horizontal or down-sloping ST-segment depression >0.1 mV, persisting for at least 0.06–0.08 seconds after the J-point, in one or more ECG leads. Stress imaging techniques i.e. echocardiography performed in the presence of physical (treadmill of bike) or pharmacological (e.g. dobutamine) stressors, myocardial perfusion scintigraphy (SPECT/PET), or Stress MRI may also detect ischæmic change and wall motion abnormalities. Comparisons of the diagnostic accuracy of various non-invasive tests used in patients with suspected stable angina favour CT-CA due to its high sensitivity and specificity (0.96 and 0.79, respectively) in detecting obstructive CAD.[21] Given the high negative predictive value of CT-CA in the absence of stenosis, patients and referring physicians can be reassured that initiating medical therapy is sufficient without the need for further testing or invasive therapies.[22]

TABLE 10.3
Thrombolysis in myocardial infarction (TIMI) flow grades in coronary arteries

TIMI 0	No perfusion and no antegrade flow beyond the occlusion
TIMI 1	Penetration with minimal perfusion, and contrast does not opacify the entire bed distal to the stenosis during the picture run
TIMI 2	Partial perfusion and contrast opacifies the entire coronary bed distal to the stenosis, although entry to this area is slower than with unaffected coronary beds
TIMI 3	Complete perfusion and filling and clearance of contrast is rapid and comparable to other coronary beds

Adapted from Belenkie I, Knudtson ML, Roth DL, et al. Relation between flow grade after thrombolytic therapy and the effect of angioplasty on left ventricular function: a prospective randomized trial. Am Heart J 1991;121(2 Pt 1):407–16113.

Furthermore initial trial data suggest that the inclusion of CTA can clarify diagnosis, and aid the implementation of more appropriate treatment plans with the potential of preventing future AMI.[22]

Chest radiography

An initial chest X-ray film is useful to exclude other causes of chest pain, such as pneumonia, pneumothorax and aortic aneurysm, and to assess whether heart failure and/or pulmonary congestion are present. If the diagnosis is clearly ACS or AMI, this step can wait until after thrombolysis or PCI.

Patient management

The management of stable angina patients is aimed at: 1) secondary prevention of cardiac events, 2) symptom control with medication, 3) revascularisation and 4) rehabilitation (Fig. 10.6).[9] (Revascularisation by coronary artery bypass graft is reviewed in Chapter 12; revascularisation by percutaneous coronary angioplasty is reviewed in the next section.)

Treatment of patients with ACS aims at rapid diagnosis, identification of the presence or absence of ST elevation and risk stratification. When ST elevation is present optimal reperfusion strategies are immediately implemented to re-establish flow through the occluded coronary artery, ensure myocardial perfusion and minimise the area of myocardial ischaemia/infarction. In those without ST elevation, the priority is risk stratification using a validated tool such as Global Registry of Acute Events (GRACE) or Thrombolysis in Myocardial Infarction (TIMI)[16] to allow early implementation of evidence-based therapies and interventions.

The optimal place to manage ACS or MI patients is in the coronary or cardiac care unit, where continuous, specialised nursing care is available and there is rapid access to treatments.[23-27] Secondary prevention of cardiac events includes the provision of medications, such as antiplatelet therapy and lipid-lowering therapy.[6,8,12,18]

In addition, treatment aims to:

- stablise the patient's condition
- decrease myocardial workload
- maximise oxygen delivery to tissues
- control pain and sympathetic stimulation
- prevent and detect complications
- preserve ventricular function
- reduce morbidity and mortality.

Reperfusion therapy

Reperfusion therapy includes coronary angioplasty, ideally with a stent, or thrombolytic therapy (also termed fibrinolysis). Patients fast-tracked for reperfusion therapy have one or more of the following indications: 1) ischaemic or infarction symptoms for longer than 20 min; 2) onset of symptoms within 12 hours; 3) ECG changes (ST elevation of 1 mm in contiguous limb leads, ST elevation of 2 mm in contiguous chest leads; left bundle branch block). Systematic reviews have highlighted the superiority of primary PCI over thrombolysis in relation to short and long-term mortality, stroke, re-infarction, recurrent ischaemia and need for coronary artery bypass grafting for STEMI patients. The greatest benefits were noted within the first 12 h of symptom onset. As such STEMI guidelines recommend immediate treatment with primary PCI when this can be delivered within 90–120 min of first medical contact.[2,15,16] However, when primary PCI is not available many will still benefit from immediate thrombolysis and transfer to a facility providing PCI.

Thrombolytic therapy

Thrombolytic therapy has been demonstrated to produce a significant reduction in mortality in the high-risk group described above.[28] The greatest reduction in mortality occurs, therefore, if the reperfusion occurs within the first 'golden' hour of presentation.[28] Thrombolysis can be delivered effectively in many settings where other methods of reperfusion are not available. Clots formed in response to injury normally dissolve using the body's fibrinolytic processes as tissue repair takes place. This requires the presence of the proenzyme plasminogen, which is converted into the enzyme plasmin when activated by macrophages and degrades the clot. Thrombolytic agents, including tissue-type plasminogen activator (tPA), have been developed that trigger conversion of plasminogen to plasmin and therefore break down clots. It is essential to screen patients for contraindications to thrombolysis quickly but thoroughly so that therapy can be commenced as soon as possible. Contraindications are given in the National Health Foundation of Australia (NHFA) Guidelines (Fig. 10.6).[9]

Tenecteplase is one of the most commonly prescribed thrombolytic agents and is a drug tissue-type plasminogen activator (tPA) that is available as alteplase, tenecteplase and reteplase. These agents are of human origin, made by recombinant DNA techniques.[29] The drug activates only plasminogen present in blood clots, so the risk of haemorrhage is decreased. Unlike streptokinase, tPA can be given repeatedly without risk of anaphylactic reaction. Often patients with anterior ischaemic changes are treated with tPA (alteplase) based on the GUSTO-1 trial that showed improved outcomes in terms of reduction of ischaemia.[30] Alteplase is usually given by infusion, whereas reteplase, which has a longer half-life, can be given in two bolus injections. In the pre-hospital setting, weight-adjusted tenecteplase is the preferred agent for ease of administration through an IV bolus in a pre-hospital setting.[6,9,29]

Nursing management of patients post-thrombolysis focuses on monitoring and detection of bleeding complications and/or return of ischaemia. Care is as follows:

- continuous observations to assess changes in neurological state including orientation, any IV sites and urinalysis for the presence of bleeding. Along

FIGURE 10.6 Management of acute coronary syndromes.[9]

Heart Foundation®

Assessment protocol for suspected ACS using point-of-care assays

IMPORTANT NOTICE: Management protocols never replace clinical judgement. The care outlined in this protocol must be altered if it is not clinically appropriate for the individual patient.

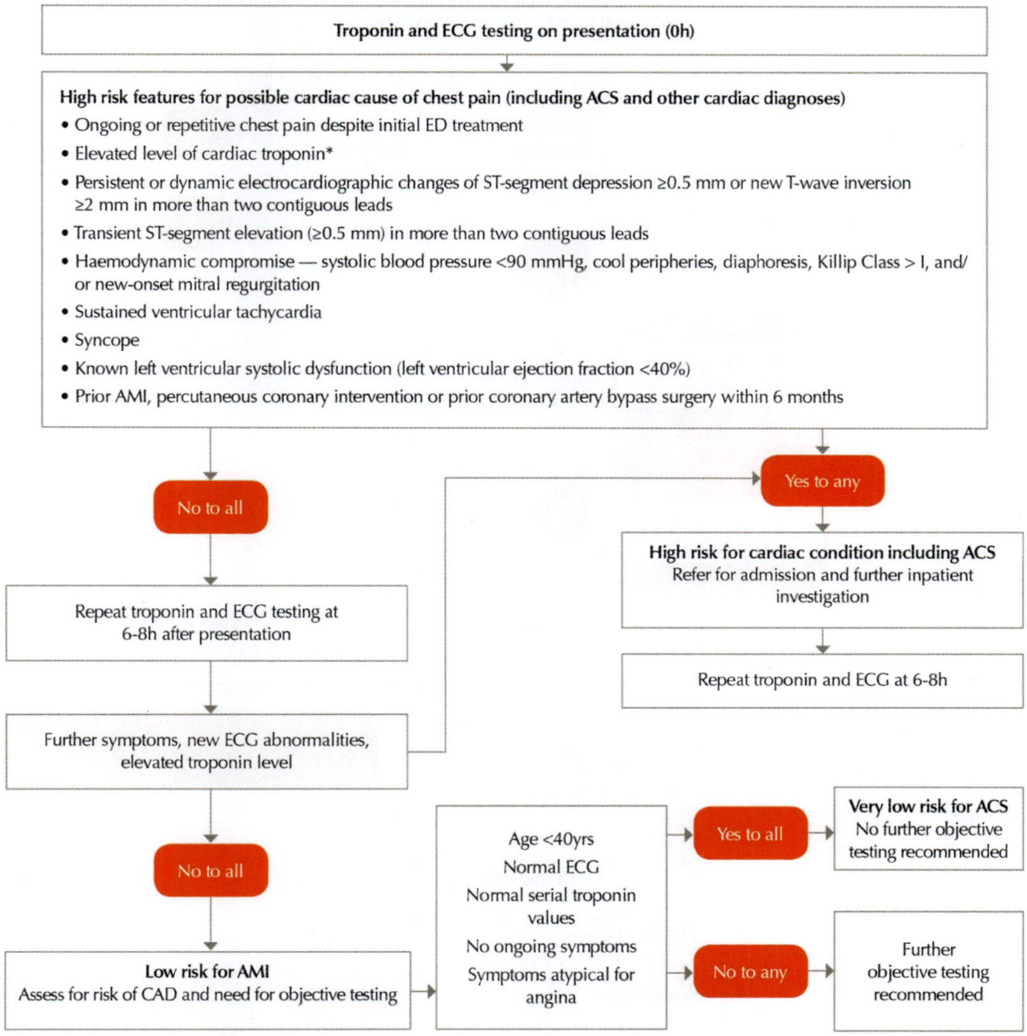

Note: It is important to validate the local Suspected ACS assessment protocol (Suspected ACS-AP). We recommend evaluating three components: Routinely monitor and assess patients receiving the local Suspected ACS-AP; continuously evaluate adherence to the Suspected ACS-AP; conduct ongoing assessment of the 30-day outcome associated with the application of the Suspected ACS-AP. *Elevated troponin defined as >99th percentile of a normal reference population. AMI, acute myocardial infarction; CAD, coronary artery disease; ECG, electrocardiogram; ED, emergency department

This figure has been reproduced from National Heart Foundation of Australia and Cardiac Society of Australia and New Zealand (NHFA and CSANZ); Chew DP, Scott IA, Cullen L et al. NHFA and CSANZ: Australian clinical guidelines for the management of acute coronary syndromes 2016. Heart Lung Circ 2016; 25:895–951.

Source: Reproduced with permission by National Heart Foundation of Australia. This figure has been reproduced from National Heart Foundation of Australia and Cardiac Society of Australia and New Zealand (NHFA and CSANZ); Chew DP, Scott IA, Cullen L, et al. NHFA and CSANZ: Australian clinical guidelines for the management of acute coronary syndromes 2016. Heart Lung Circ 2016;25:895–951. © 2016 National Heart Foundation of Australia, ABN 98 008 419 761.

Continued

FIGURE 10.6—cont'd

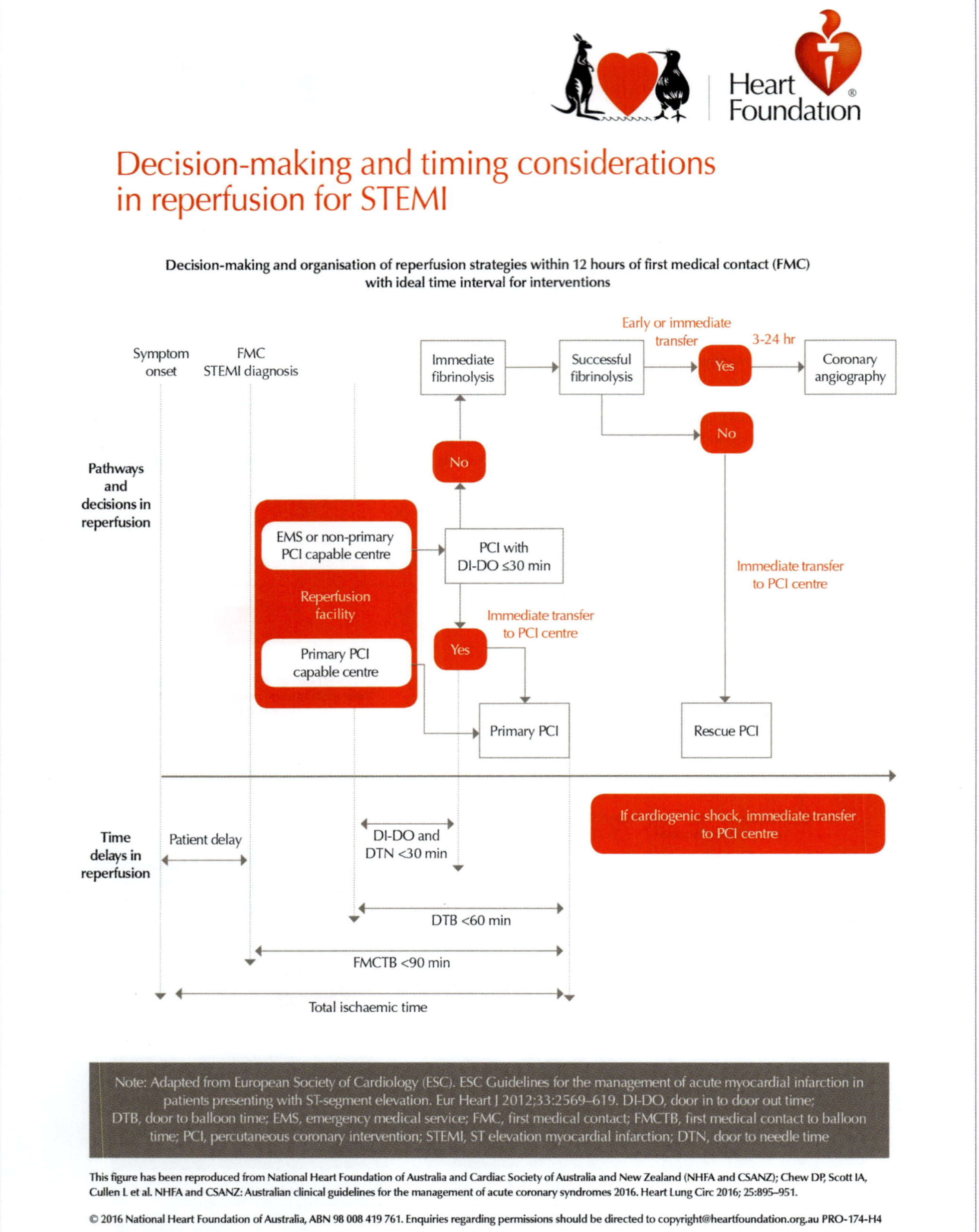

Source: Reproduced with permission by National Heart Foundation of Australia. This figure has been reproduced from National Heart Foundation of Australia and Cardiac Society of Australia and New Zealand (NHFA and CSANZ); Chew DP, Scott IA, Cullen L, et al. NHFA and CSANZ: Australian clinical guidelines for the management of acute coronary syndromes 2016. Heart Lung Circ 2016;25:895–951. © 2016 National Heart Foundation of Australia, ABN 98 008 419 761.

with vital signs, these are attended every 15 min for the first hour, half-hourly for an hour and then hourly according to the patient's condition; however, patients are advised to report any bleeding post-discharge as well.

- ECG monitoring: includes 12-lead ECG on return and continuous ECG monitoring and chest pain assessment to detect reocclusion and arrhythmias. Some arrhythmias, particularly idioventricular arrhythmias, are associated with reperfusion and tend to be benign. ST-segment monitoring and assessment of pain help evaluate the effectiveness of the thrombolysis. Patients need to be requested to inform nursing staff of any chest pain or discomfort. Should this be present a repeat 12-lead ECG should be completed.
- IV anticoagulants such as heparin and/or oral antiplatelet drugs, such as ticagrelor or clopidogrel: may be given following thrombolysis to prevent reocclusion in the stent.

Thrombolysis is considered to have failed if the patient is still in pain and the ST segment has not resolved within 60–90 min.[16] If thrombolysis fails, patients are at high risk for other interventions, so repeat thrombolysis is often the only treatment option. Salvage or rescue angioplasty may be undertaken if available at the site.

FIGURE 10.7 PTCA procedure.[74]

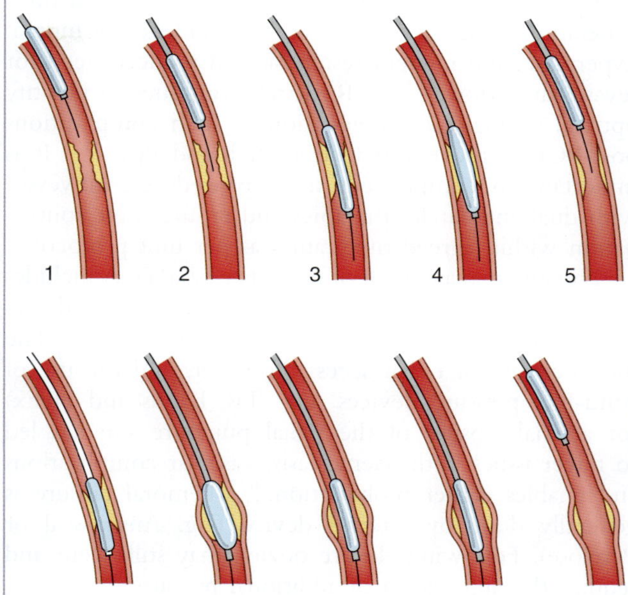

Source: Urden L, Stacy K, Logh M, Thelan's Critical care nursing: Diagnosis and management. 5th ed. St Louis: Mosby, 2006.

Coronary angioplasty

Following an identified need for coronary revascularisation, clinicians need to decide whether this should be undertaken by PCI or surgery. Coronary artery bypass grafting was traditionally the first-line option but with the evolution of PCI technology, the introduction of drug eluting stents (DES), and comparable clinical outcomes in specific populations, the role of surgery has been challenged.[21,31] PCIs include percutaneous transluminal coronary angioplasty (PTCA) procedures which are used more commonly than coronary artery bypass grafts (CABG) for revascularisation even in the older population. During PTCA a catheter is introduced, commonly through the radial artery, and advanced to the area of occlusion or stenosis within the coronary arteries into under the guidance of imagery. The artery is then dilated by inflating a fine balloon to widen the lumen of the artery, and then a coronary artery stent (a fine lattice scaffold) is inserted to prevent the artery from recoiling (Fig. 10.7). Over 90% of PCI procedures now involve implantation of one or more coronary stents.[21,31] Rapid advances in stent technology and the use of second and third generation DES has helped to prevent or slow down endothelialisation and reduce but not entirely eliminate stent restenosis, including in small calibre vessels.[21,31-33]

The choice of revascularisation technique is often complex and will require careful consideration of the individual's medical and surgical suitability for the procedure as well as the patient's individual preferences based on an informed choice associated with risks and benefits. Factors influencing the revascularisation decision may include the extent and severity of underlying CAD, for example single versus multivessel disease or the presence of left main-stem disease. Associated comorbidities e.g. diabetes mellitus and renal impairment as well as the patient's age and quality of life may also influence the final decision.[21] Long-term outcomes with PTCA for silent ischaemia following AMI have demonstrated a significant reduction in cardiac death, recurrent MI, or the needs for revascularisation, with less evidence of ischaemia on exercise testing at 4 years despite the PTCA patients being on less beta-blockers.[32] PCI and CABG now offer comparable outcomes in patients with left main-stem disease in the short to medium term; however, current evidence supports the benefit of CABG over PCI in patients with a greater disease burden and more complex CHD in terms of improved mortality and less need for revascularisation in the longer term.[21]

Primary angioplasty is the recommended first-line therapy for patients with STEMI as it results in a higher rate of patency of the affected artery (>90%), lower rates of cerebrovascular accident (CVA) and re-infarction and higher short-term survival than thrombolysis.[9,16] PTCA is recommended in all patients presenting with chest pain who meet the indications for reperfusion when: 1) facilities are available and it can be achieved within recommended guideline times (90–120 min); 2) there are contraindications to fibrinolytic therapy described above; 3) ischaemia would result in large anterior AMI within

4 hours; or 4) haemodynamic instability or cardiogenic shock is present.

Following primary PCI, the use of second and third generation stents has minimised the incidence of intimal hyperplasia and in-stent restenosis and reduced need for revascularisatrion.[21,31,32,33] Research continues to identify optimal strategies for prevention of such complications post-PCI to prevent reduction of blood flow.[33,34] It is important to complement these procedures, however, with dual antiplatelet therapies and ensure their continuation within agreed timeframes as per unit protocols.

Nursing management of patients post-PTCA includes care of the puncture site to prevent bleeding and detect arterial changes (including clot and aneurysm).[35-37] The increased use of radial access, however, and the use of band-like pressure devices (e.g. TR Bands and Helix) for arterial closure of the radial puncture site has led to fewer issues with haemostasis, vascular complications and enables earlier mobilisation.[36,37] Femoral closure is generally done by internal device (e.g. Angio-seal or Perclose). Following closure oozing may still occur and require the application of additional pressure.

Following PCI, specific care will be determined by access site:

- Observations: observe access site for haemorrhage and haematoma; assess perfusion to the lower limb, including colour, warmth and pulses. This monitoring is needed frequently in the first few hours, when complications are most likely to occur.
- ECG monitoring: includes 12-lead ECG following completion of the procedure, ongoing ECG monitoring and chest pain assessment to detect reocclusion. Patients need to be requested to inform nursing staff of any chest pain or discomfort.
- Vital signs: may be recorded every 15 min for the first hour, half-hourly for 1 h and then hourly according to the patient's condition.
- Removal of sheath: is usually performed by medical or specially trained nursing staff.
- Achievement of haemostasis: use either application of pressure for at least 5 min or vascular sealing.[36]
  - Pressure application can be by a manual-compression device (such as Femostop, RADI Medical Systems, Uppsala, Sweden) and less often digital, to maintain a pressure of about 20 mmHg.
  - Vascular sealing uses a device such as the Angio-seal vascular closure device (St Jude Medical Inc., St Paul, MN). This includes a collagen plug and a small biodegradable plate inside the artery, which is held in place by a small suture, tamping tube and small spring on the exterior. The tension spring is removed and the suture trimmed half an hour after application. This enables the patient to mobilise and reduces nursing time.[35]
- Assess: international normalised ratio (INR), prothrombin (PT) and partial thromboplastin time (PTT), as bleeding is more likely to occur if anticoagulants are above the therapeutic range. Weight-adjusted heparin (100 units/kg) is usually used during PTCA to prevent thrombus formation, and glycoprotein IIb/IIIa inhibitors may be used to prevent platelet aggregation and thrombus formation for patients at high risk of adverse events.[16]
- Bed rest (2–6 h): is used to discourage the patient from moving the joint of the insertion site to prevent clot displacement and haematoma formation. Initially, the patient should lie relatively flat if femoral artery access has been used, then progress to sitting. The period of rest has been demonstrated to be safely reduced to 1 h in low-risk patients (normotensive and normal platelet count).[35]
- Pain relief: is used primarily to promote comfort for patients who find bed rest causes pain and discomfort.
- Urine output: adequate urine output is essential as radiographic IV contrast is cleared by the kidneys, so it is vital that nurses ensure good hydration and monitor initial urine output.
- Oral antiplatelet drugs, such as ticagrelor, clopidogrel or ticlopidine in addition to aspirin: may be given prior to the procedure to prevent later reocclusion in the stent. Dual antiplatelet therapy should continue for 6 months; however, longer treatment durations may be used where the risks of atherothrombotic events outweigh the risk of bleeding.[16]

Many patients find the PTCA procedure and confirmation of CHD diagnosis stressful.[38] It is an important nursing role to provide patients with preparatory information about the procedure and care required during recovery. As family members provide valuable support and reminders about recovery, these people should be included in any information sessions. The patient and family need to be provided with information about the possibility of restenosis, mobility restrictions at home and the lifestyle changes needed to reduce the risk of worsening CHD.

Practice tip

Increased hydration can aggravate problems with urination when on bed rest, particularly in older men with prostate enlargement. If a femoral access site is used in these patients, it is easier for the patient to urinate while turned on their side, using pillow support to maintain the position.

Practice tip

If a femoral access site has been used, bleeding may track between the patient's legs and pool, and this will be invisible to a cursory inspection, particularly if the patient is obese. Always move the patient's thigh during regular inspections.

Nursing management of ACS and MI patients

The nursing role in patients with ACS includes reducing myocardial workload and maximising cardiac output, provision of treatments, careful monitoring to determine the effects of treatment and detect complications, rapid treatment of complications, comfort and pain control, psychosocial support and teaching and discharge planning. Suffering an acute cardiac event results in loss of control over life, the constant presence of nurses and their open and honest communication provides the security and reassurance patients require.[38,39] A calm, caring manner during nursing care is essential to establish rapport and lower patient and family anxiety. Patients should be given sufficient information to understand their condition and immediate treatment plan but not overloaded with unnecessary facts.[38,39] Individual evaluation of the patient and the family is necessary to determine the most appropriate management of visiting.

Reduction of myocardial workload includes ensuring the patient has bed rest, providing support with activities and limiting stress. Continuous cardiac monitoring (preferably including ST monitoring) and evaluation of heart rate and rhythm, shortness of breath, chest discomfort and blood pressure are essential to determine ischaemia, treatment effects, myocardial workload and complications. This monitoring should occur within the acute phase, reducing as the patient recovers. Oxygen saturation levels should be routinely assessed and provision of oxygen by mask or nasal cannulae provided only if levels are reduced.[12] A systematic review found no conclusive evidence to support routine supplementary oxygen therapy in AMI.[40] Symptom relief should be provided, including analgesia for pain. Analgesia management should be conducted by nurses because of their continued contact and thus more accurate assessment and treatment of pain.[41,42] It is essential to treat pain, not only for the distress it causes patients but also because pain causes stimulation of the sympathetic nervous system (SNS). SNS responses include elevated heart rate and potential for arrhythmias, peripheral vasoconstriction and increased myocardial contractility and, therefore, an overall increase in myocardial oxygen demand. Effective treatments for pain include IV morphine and nitrates. The IV route is preferable, as absorption is predictable and additional punctures in thrombolysed/anticoagulated patients are not required. Morphine has the additional benefit of reducing anxiety in a distressing situation and should be initially provided at a dose of 2.5–5 mg at 1 mg/min, followed by 2.5-mg doses as indicated. While there is little randomised controlled trial evidence to support this particular practice, it is generally accepted to be appropriate. A standardised method of pain evaluation and charting should be used to ensure consistent assessment and treatment. An antiemetic such as metoclopramide should be given concurrently to lessen and prevent nausea. Other drugs, such as beta-blockers and nitrates, decrease myocardial workload, contributing to pain reduction.

Medications

Provision of medications and assessment of the effectiveness of treatment is a major component of the nurse's role in caring for the cardiac patient. Many of the medications are accompanied by side effects and interactions with other drugs, which the nurse must monitor. An array of medications is used to treat ACS patients, including aspirin, lipid-lowering agents, beta-blockers, ace inhibitors and organic nitrates (Table 10.4).

TABLE 10.4
Medications used in the treatment of ACS

AGENT	ACTION	SIDE EFFECTS/CAUTION	COMMENTS
	ANTIPLATELET AGENTS		
Aspirin	Inhibits cyclooxygenase (COX-1) and prevents platelet synthesis of thromboxane A2, a vasoconstrictor and stimulant of platelet aggregation May provide benefits from anti-inflammatory properties in reducing plaque rupture[16]	Gastrointestinal (GI) irritation and bleeding; use enteric-coated tablets to minimise gastric irritation	Noted to reduce the risk of vascular events (cardiovascular death, AMI and non-fatal stroke) by 50%.[16] Lifelong use is recommended for secondary prevention

Continued

TABLE 10.4
Medications used in the treatment of ACS—cont'd

AGENT	ACTION	SIDE EFFECTS/CAUTION	COMMENTS
		ANTIPLATELET AGENTS	
Ticagrelor	Reversibly and noncompetitively binds the adenosine diphosphate (ADP) $P2Y_{12}$ receptor on the platelet surface which prevents ADP-mediated activation of the GPIIb/IIIa receptor complex thereby reducing platelet aggregation[43]	Adverse side effects reported for P2Y12-receptor antagonists are bleeding, transient bradycardia and dyspnea[16] Ticagrelor should be administered with caution or avoided in patients with advanced sinoatrial disease. Caution is advised in patients at risk of increased bleeding due to trauma, surgery, or other pathological conditions and in those with asthma or COPD Care is required when delivering with other drugs and other anticoagulants[16]	Reversible, direct-acting inhibitor of the adenosine diphosphate receptor $P2Y_{12}$ that has a more rapid onset and more pronounced platelet inhibition than clopidogrel RCTs have demonstrated reductions in atherothrombotic events (MI or CVA) with no increase in overall rate of major bleeding but had an increase in rate of non-procedural bleeding
Clopidogrel	Adenosine diphosphate (ADP) receptor agonist; prevents the binding of ADP to its platelet receptor, thus inhibiting platelet aggregation[43]	Inhibits P450 liver enzyme; care is required when delivering with other drugs and other anticoagulants	Clopidogrel produces fewer GI effects than aspirin and is more effective in patients with recent stroke, MI and peripheral vascular disease
Ticlopidine	As for clopidogrel	Severe side effects including neutropenia and liver abnormalities	Used less frequently due to its adverse side effect profile
Tirofiban, eptifibatide, lamifiban, abciximab	Glycoprotein IIb/IIIa receptor antagonists prevent the final step of platelet aggregation and fibrinogen cross linking[16] Used most commonly to inhibit thrombus formation in ACS	Bleeding, thrombocytopenia, nausea, fever and headache; doses need to be reduced in renal failure	Although much of the evidence for their use precedes the use of the current $P2Y_{12}$ blockers, they are still considered for use in ACS patients at high risk of adverse cardiovascular events or those undergoing complex interventional procedures
Anticoagulant therapy Unfractionated heparin Low molecular weight heparin (LMWH) Direct thrombin inhibitors e.g. hirudin bivalirudin, Synthetic penta-saccharides e.g. fondaparinux	Limit further formation of thrombus in the acute phase The main effect of unfractionated heparin (UH) is on the inhibition of thrombin induced platelet aggregation[43] LMWH has been shown to have even greater benefit then UH in reducing subsequent MI, and need for revascularisation with treatment effects enduring for up to 12 months in NSTEMI[16] Bind directly to thrombin(factor IIa) and inhibits the conversion of fibrinogen to fibrin.[43] Blocks platelet activation and aggregation Selectively activated factor X inhibitor[87]	Need for aPTT monitoring Convenience in administration, no need for aPTT monitoring Eliminated even in patients with moderate-to-severe renal function. Require only once a day administration due to long half-life. Caution in impaired liver or renal function where risk of haemorrhage increases. Dose adjustment required for low body weight[43]	Reduces death and re-infarction In contrast to UH in STEMI, LMWH prevented 21 deaths or MIs per 1000 patients at the expense of four non-fatal bleeds Evidence favours progressively LMWHs and treatment durations >48 h Pentasaccharides appear to have the best safety and efficacy profiles: less adverse bleeding events combined with a reduction in short to medium-term mortality[43]

TABLE 10.4
Medications used in the treatment of ACS—cont'd

AGENT	ACTION	SIDE EFFECTS/CAUTION	COMMENTS
	ANTIPLATELET AGENTS		
BETA-BLOCKERS	Reduce cardiac workload (heart rate and force of contraction) and myocardial oxygen demand by blocking beta-adrenergic receptors, preventing sympathetic stimulation of the heart[43]	Contraindications include significant AV block, bradycardia, hypotension, history of asthma or uncontrolled heart failure	In the absence of bradycardia or hypotension, immediate IV and oral beta-blockade should be considered in ACS patients[16]
ACE INHIBITORS e.g. Ramipril	Cause dilation of arteries and veins by competitively inhibiting the conversion of angiotensin I to angiotensin II (a potent endogenous vasoconstrictor) and by inhibiting bradykinin metabolism; these actions result in preload and afterload reductions on the heart. ACE inhibitors also promote sodium and water excretion by inhibiting angiotensin II induced aldosterone secretion; elevation in potassium may also be observed. Can reduce cardiac and vascular remodelling[43]	Common side effects dry cough and hypotension Uncommon but life-threatening effect may be angioedema Can cause renal impairment – requires monitoring of urea and electrolytes. Exert caution in times of dehydration	Recommended in high-risk patients with vascular disease (unstable angina) in the absence of documented heart failure. All-cause mortality, MI, and stroke were reduced. Observed benefits appear independent of the associated BP reductions particularly marked in patients with diabetes mellitus Major mortality and morbidity benefits have been reported in patients with HF or LVSD post AMI. Treatment should be initiated within 36 h of the acute event[16]
NITRATES Glyceryl trinitrate (IV, sublingual and spray) Isosorbide mononitrate	Potent peripheral vasodilators, particularly in venous capacitance vessels, thereby reducing preload and to a lesser extent afterload, to reduce myocardial workload Dilate normal and atherosclerotic coronary blood vessels to increase myocardial oxygen supply Used to manage unstable angina and reduce blood pressure in the critical care setting, where there is some evidence for symptomatic relief	Reflex tachycardia, hypotension, syncope and migraine-like headache; generally occur in first few days of treatment, then subside. Blood pressure should be monitored	Tolerance to the vasodilator effect occurs, so intermittent treatment is most effective. In the case of transdermal delivery, if treatment is withheld for 8–12 h in every 24 h, therapeutic activity is restored
	LIPID-LOWERING STATINS		
Atorvastatin, simvastatin, fluvastatin, pravastatin	Inhibit 3-hydroxy-3-methylglutaryl-coenzyme-A (HMG-CoA) reductase, the enzyme that limits the rate of cholesterol synthesis in the liver, thereby reducing plasma cholesterol	Headache, gastrointestinal upset, inflammation of voluntary muscles and altered liver function; taking statins with food may reduce GI symptoms	There is strong evidence supporting the secondary prevention benefits of statins therefore they should be commenced for long-term maintenance before discharge[16]

ACS: acute coronary syndrome; CVA: cerebrovascular accident; LMWH: low molecular weight heparin; LVSD: left ventricular septal defect.
Adapted from SIGN Acute Coronary Syndrome Guideline 148[16] *and Opie LH, Gersh BJ. Drugs for the heart. 7th ed. Philadelphia: Saunders; 2009.*

Symptom control

Control of anginal symptoms with medication usually includes sublingual glyceryl trinitrate (GTN) for immediate symptom control and one or more antianginal medications for sustained symptom management.[44] These medications are described in the next section. The choice of medication may depend on how acceptable the patient finds the reduction in symptoms and the presence of side effects. Patients need to take antianginal agents continuously, regardless of symptoms. Patients should also be encouraged to take sublingual GTN prophylactically.

Angina may also be managed by treating associated conditions that precipitate angina e.g. anaemia, thyrotoxicosis and avoiding situations that trigger angina. Education needs to be directed at awareness of symptoms and management of unstable angina and AMI symptoms, and the need for emergency care. Although these patients are at low risk of further cardiovascular events in the short term, in the medium to long term, risk may accumulate. Patients with angina may also benefit from comprehensive rehabilitation interventions.[45] While some national guidelines recommend cardiac rehabilitation (CR) for patients with stable angina, a recent Cochrane review focusing on exercise-based interventions highlighted the need for more research in this area.[46]

Angiotensin-converting enzyme (ACE) inhibitors have been recommended for all post-AMI patients while in hospital, with review of prescription at 4–6 weeks post-discharge. Patients with left ventricular failure should be maintained on ACE inhibitors. Similarly, diuretics provide the mainstay of the management of left ventricular failure if it is present. Diabetic patients have a higher mortality after AMI in both acute and long-term phases. Guidance supporting the use of insulin for targeted glucose control has become more flexible but still aims to maintain glucose levels below 180 mg/dL or 11 mmol while avoiding hypoglycaemia in ACS patients.[47]

Transfer to a step-down unit or general ward usually occurs when the patient is pain-free and is haemodynamically stable. Stability means that patients are not dependent on IV inotropic or vasoactive support and have no arrhythmias. Discharge home after AMI varies, but usually occurs at day 2 or 3 for low-risk patients.[44]

Emotional responses and patient and family support

ACS or AMI is usually accompanied by feelings of acute anxiety and fear, as most patients are aware of the significant threat posed to their health.[25,48] For many patients it may also be the first experience of acute illness and associated aspects such as ambulance transport, emergency care and hospitalisation, so they may experience shock and disbelief as well. Fast-track processes such as pre-hospital triage require patients and their families to process a large amount of information and make decisions quickly, and this, added to an alien environment, full of unfamiliar technology and personnel, can be quite distressing. However, the environment can also promote a feeling of security for patients and their families.[25]

Anxiety is a common response to the stress of an acute cardiac event and leads to important physiological and psychological changes.[49] The SNS is stimulated, resulting in increased heart rate, respiration and blood pressure. These responses increase the workload of the heart and therefore myocardial oxygen demand. In an acute cardiac event, these demands occur when perfusion is already poor and may lead to worse outcomes, including ventricular arrhythmias and increased myocardial ischaemia. Therefore, staff working in emergency and coronary care should employ strategies to reduce a patient's anxiety. Chapter 6 provides a more detailed description of psychological care.

Increasing a patient's sense of control, calm and confidence in care reduces the patient's sense of vulnerability, whether it is realistic or not.[25] This can be achieved by:

- providing order and predictability in routines, allowing the patient to make choices, providing information and explanations and including the patient in decision making using a calm, confident approach
- open and honest communication with patients and families
- restricting the number and type of visitors in the acute phase is customary, but many patients may feel safer if a family member is present
- provision of comprehensive information to families, with more concise information in understandable language for patients.

Nurses need to monitor patients for signs of excessive anxiety, including facial expressions and behavioural changes. However, overt behaviours may be controlled by the patient, so careful conversation and/or use of specific assessments may be necessary to detect anxiety. The move to the step-down or general ward may also be stressful to the patient and family. This move needs to be planned and discussed, and promoted as a sign of recovery.

Cardiac rehabilitation

CR has been defined as 'the coordinated sum of activities required to influence favourably the underlying cause of cardiovascular disease, as well as to provide the best possible physical, mental and social conditions, so that the patients may, by their own efforts, preserve or resume optimal functioning in their community and through improved health behaviour, slow or reverse progression of disease'.[50] CR is recommended as an integral part of comprehensive care of CHD patients.[45,46,50] Although exercise therapy has consistently been identified as a central element of CR, The British Association for Cardiovascular Prevention and Rehabilitation (BACPR) describe six core components of CR which include: health behaviour change and education; lifestyle risk factor management (including physical activity and exercise, healthy eating and body composition, tobacco cessation and relapse prevention), psychosocial health; medical risk management; long-term strategies; and audit and evaluation (Fig. 10.8).[50]

It is important to identify and address misconceptions and provide information regarding the disease process, prognosis, and an optimal approach to recovery. Early mobilisation is encouraged and discharge planning remains a very important element to streamline

FIGURE 10.8 BACPR Core components[50]

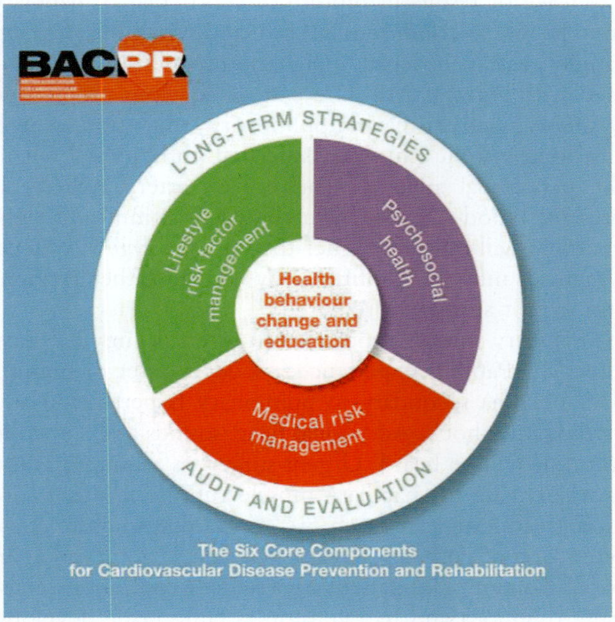

Source: The British Association for Cardiovascular Prevention and Rehabilitation. 3rd ed. British Cardiovascular Society. London (available online http://www.bacpr.com).

the transition between hospital and community care. Since discharge may be within 48–72 hours even from the acute phase, it is important to provide psychological support.[44-46, 48-50] Input focusing on health and lifestyle behaviour change, risk factor modification, and psychosocial wellbeing can also support self-management of their long-term cardiac condtion.[44-50] There is a strong evidence base supporting the benefits for CR in cardiac conditions yet many people do not participate in CR following acute events.[51,52] An updated Cochrane review confirmed that exercise-based CR reduces cardiovascular mortality, hospital admissions and improves quality of life.[53] Additional benefits have been shown for improvements in exercise tolerance, symptoms, serum lipids, psychological wellbeing and cessation of smoking.[53] CR provision centres around adequate and timely assessment of the patients' needs and the provision of a tailored and individualised program to provide support throughout the inpatient, immediate discharge period, and outpatient stages of the patient's recovery. The focus will eventually be on chronic disease management and maintaining risk modification behaviour. Within CR provision incorporation of the principles of adult learning may optimise learning and behaviour change. These principles include recognition of 'readiness to learn and change behaviour. Adults are ready to learn most effectively when they are physically and emotionally stable and are aware of the problem or need to learn. Nurses, because of their expertise and continual presence, are best placed to assess and provide education at optimal times.

Complications of myocardial infarction

Despite declines in death rates from MI, many patients will experience complications, most of which occur within the first 24 hours.[54,55]

Cardiogenic shock

Cardiogenic shock occurs as a complication of MI and although advances in reperfusion therapy have been associated with improvements in survival, in-hospital mortality remains high (27%–51%).[54,55] Evidence supports the mortality benefit of early PCI; however, what is not clear is whether, as the majority of patients with cardiogenic shock have multivessel disease, revascularisation via PCI should be performed in the culprit artery alone.[55] The recent results of the CULPRIT-SHOCK trial confirmed that the 30-day risk of a composite of death or severe renal failure leading to renal-replacement therapy was lower among those who initially underwent PCI of the culprit lesion only than among those who underwent immediate multivessel PCI. There were no significant differences in bleeding complications between the two groups.[55]

In addition to revascularisation procedures, efforts to reduce mortality associated with cardiogenic shock have been directed towards improvements in mechanical circulatory support (MCS) therapies. Intra-aortic balloon pumps (IABP) were commonly used to support patients in cardiogenic shock. However, the results of the IABP-SHOCK II trial following acute MI showed no benefit with routine IABP placement in addition to revascularisation.[56] This has resulted in decreased use of IABPs in clinical practice and less prominence of this therapy in guideline recommendations.[7,12] Although other devices and advanced therapies have shown promise in the treatment of cardiogenic shock, more data from randomised clinical trials are needed.[56] Cardiogenic shock and the related management are described in more detail in Chapter 21.

Arrhythmias

Arrhythmias often occur in ACS and are often the cause of death in the pre-hospital phase. Management of the pre-hospital phase focuses on community education and an effective, rapidly responsive ambulance service, as exemplified in Seattle in the USA.[51] Similarly within Europe survival benefits have been significantly associated with increases in bystander CPR.[57] Arrhythmias may be generated by poorly perfused tissue and electrolyte alterations, and increased sympathetic tone during infarction, but are more often due to a failing left ventricle. Arrhythmias may also be related to revascularisation procedures, although debate exists as to whether this indicates evidence of reperfusion or ongoing ischaemia.[58,59] It is essential to rapidly and effectively treat arrhythmias in the ACS context. The goal of treatment is to maintain hemodynamic stability and cardiac output while reducing workload. Management of arrhythmias is described in Chapter 11.

Pericarditis and pericardial effusion

Pericarditis is inflammation of the visceral and parietal layers of the pericardium that cover the heart. Although perhaps less common in this era of early and aggressive revascularisation, a recent study demonstrated that 31 (4%) of 743 patients undergoing primary PCI for acute STEMI developed early post-MI pericarditis (PMIP), most with pericardial effusion within 4 days of MI.[60] Another retrospective analysis of 13,387 ACS patients (2000–2013) identified only 90 patients (0.67%) with PMIP, 84.4 % of whom had suffered a STEMI. This reflected a 35% reduction in PMIP prevalence since 2000.[61]

As pericarditis is associated with chest pain, this is often confused with ischaemic pain, particularly due to the presence of ST-segment elevation on the ECG. However, pericardial pain increases with deep inspiration and a pericardial rub is often present. Electrocardiographically, the elevated ST segments of pericarditis are typically concave upwards (saddle-shaped) and often widespread, contrasting with convex ST-segment elevation limited to the distribution of a single coronary artery in infarction. In addition, depression of the PR segment is commonly present.[62] Pericarditis normally responds to anti-inflammatory treatment by aspirin, indomethacin and/or corticosteroids. Approximately 1–5% of AMI patients develop pericarditis as a late complication, 2 weeks to a few months post-AMI.[63] Usually, this late-onset pericarditis is associated with Dressler's syndrome and may be an autoimmune response to myocardial injury. This is a chronic condition requiring systemic corticosteroid treatment.

Due to the accumulation of excessive pericardial fluid a pericardial effusion may develop most commonly in anterior STEMI, with large infarcts, and when heart failure is present. A recent French study of 908 participants identified pericardial effusion in 6.6% of the patients.[64] Such patients have the potential for rapid deterioration, the development of cardiac tamponade and cardiac arrest associated with pulseless electrical activity (PEA), which developed in 0.8% of these patients due to left ventricular free wall rupture.[65] The detection of a moderate-to-severe pericardial effusion (≥10 mm) early after STEMI should raise the concern of potential sudden cardiac death through cardiac tamponade given its association with a 5-fold increase in mortality.[65] Although it is often associated with left ventricular free wall rupture (FWR), in 80% of cases, it can also be produced by heart failure and myocardial haemorrhage may result from anticoagulant or antiaggregant therapies. Pericardiocentesis and blood pressure control may also be life-saving; however, emergency surgical intervention for tamponade may be required particularly when associated with EMD.[65]

Structural defects

Myocardial tissue death may be catastrophic if it is extensive or results in rupture of ventricular or papillary muscle. These conditions are rare and symptoms develop rapidly. Intraventricular septal rupture is usually associated with anterior MI. The patient develops progressive dyspnoea, tachycardia and pulmonary congestion, as well as a loud systolic murmur associated with a thrill felt in the parasternal area. If a pulmonary artery catheter is present, blood samples from the right atrium and right ventricle will reveal a higher than usual oxygen content. Diagnosis must be confirmed by cardiac catheterisation, and urgent surgery is required.

Papillary muscle rupture most often occurs 2–7 days after MI. Patients experience a sudden onset of pulmonary oedema secondary to pulmonary hypertension and cardiogenic shock. Additional heart sounds and a systolic murmur will be heard. Urgent surgery is required, as the mortality rate for papillary muscle rupture without surgical treatment, can reach 80%.[61] Cardiac rupture most often occurs within 5 days of MI and is commonest in older women. The patient experiences continuous chest pain, dyspnoea and hypotension as tamponade develops. Symptoms may worsen rapidly and result in PEA unless surgery is undertaken immediately. Fortunately, with the increasing use of early and effective revasculation therapies, these complications have become less common affecting approximately 2.3% of AMIs. Clinicians should, however, remain alert to these serious and potentially lethal complications following ACSs.[61]

Heart failure

In normal circumstances, the heart is a very effective, efficient pump with reserve mechanisms available to allow output to meet changing demands. These mechanisms include: 1) increasing heart rate to increase total cardiac output; 2) dilation to create muscle stretch and more effective contraction; 3) hypertrophy of myocytes over time to generate more force; and 4) increasing stroke volume by increasing venous return and increased contractility. Heart failure is a complex clinical condition that is characterised by an underlying structural abnormality or dysfunction that results in the inability of the ventricle to fill with or eject blood. The condition is also known as congestive cardiac failure, a term commonly used in the USA but not in Australia. Chronic heart failure (CHF) describes the long-term inability of the heart to meet metabolic demands.

The burden of disease associated with heart failure is on the rise due to our ageing population, the prevalence of CHD and hypertension, the decrease in fatality from ACS and improved methods of diagnosis. Survival rates and prognosis for heart failure patients are extremely poor. Approximately 30% of patients diagnosed with heart failure will die within 1 year of discharge[66,67] and the majority will die within 5 years.[67] The outcomes associated with heart failure are worse than most common forms of cancer.[68] Heart failure continues to be the most common cause of hospitalisation in the elderly. Over 50% of patients newly diagnosed with heart failure have concurrent ischaemic heart disease, hypertension, diabetes mellitus.[1] The causes of heart failure can be categorised according to: 1) myocardial disease, 2) arrhythmias, 3) valve disease, 4) pericardial disease and 5) congenital heart disease.[69] Myocardial disease may be caused by MI and fibrosis from prolonged ischaemic heart disease, which accounts for approximately two-thirds of systolic heart failure causing systolic dysfunction and a reduced ejection fraction.

Arrhythmias, including both brady- and tachyarrhythmias, may cause heart failure due to changes in filling time affecting preload and resultant cardiac output. Myocardial oxygen demand is increased and, if the heart is poorly perfused, muscle contraction will be affected. Frequent premature contractions and atrial fibrillation disturb mechanical coordination so that the ventricles may not be adequately filled for efficient contraction. Heart failure patients are also at high risk of sudden cardiac death due to ventricular fibrillation or tachycardia. Valvular disease-causing heart failure usually involves valves on the left side of the heart (mitral and/or aortic valves). Aortic stenosis results in an increase in afterload and ventricular hypertrophy develops with reduced diastolic compliance resulting in a reduced ejection fraction. Mitral stenosis is usually due to rheumatic heart disease. Valvular incompetence results in a dilated ventricle to accommodate the regurgitant volume. Stroke volume increases in an attempt to empty its contents and ventricular muscle mass increases. However, over time the ventricle is unable to maintain the increased workload and heart failure develops. Valvular heart disease and treatment are described in more detail in Chapter 12.

There are several terms used to describe the pathology and signs and symptoms of heart failure. These include:

- Backward failure: refers to the systemic and pulmonary congestion that occurs as a result of failure of the ventricle to expel its volume.
- Forward failure: is due to an inadequate cardiac output and leads to decrease in vital organ perfusion.
- Acute heart failure: includes the initial hospitalisation for the diagnosis of heart failure and exacerbations of CHF.
- CHF: develops over time as a result of the inability of compensatory mechanisms to maintain an adequate cardiac output to meet metabolic demands. It refers to a long-term diagnosis of heart failure.
- Heart failure with reduced ejection fraction (HF*r*EF) or systolic heart failure: refers to the inability of the ventricle to contract adequately during systole resulting in a reduced ejection fraction of <50%[69,70] and an increased end-diastolic volume. This is the most common form of heart failure.
- Heart failure with preserved ejection fraction (HF*p*EF) or diastolic heart failure: indicates normal systolic function with a normal ejection fraction (EF≥50%)[70,71] but impaired relaxation so there is a resistance to filling with increased filling pressures. Diastolic dysfunction usually occurs in conjunction with systolic dysfunction and is more common in the elderly.
- Low cardiac output syndrome: this occurs in response to hypovolaemia and/or hypertension. Severe vasoconstriction further reduces the cardiac output.
- High cardiac output syndrome: is the result of an increase in metabolic demands causing a decrease in systemic venous return leading to an increase in stroke volume and cardiac output. Burns and sepsis are the main causes.
- Left-sided heart failure: occurs when there is a reduced left ventricular stroke volume resulting in accumulation of blood in the pulmonary system.
- Right-sided heart failure: is the congestion of blood in the systemic system due to the inability of the right ventricle to expel its blood volume.

Responses to heart failure

When heart failure occurs, several adaptive responses are initiated by the body in an attempt to maintain normal perfusion (Fig. 10.9). These mechanisms are successful in the normal heart but contribute to decreased effectiveness in the failing heart. The compensatory mechanisms include:

- SNS response
- renin–angiotensin–aldosterone system (RAAS)
- Frank–Starling response
- neurohormonal response.

The SNS is the first response to be stimulated in heart failure. It occurs within seconds of a reduction in cardiac output and the parasympathetic system becomes inhibited. The baroreceptor reflexes are activated in response to a reduced arterial pressure. The beta-adrenergic receptors located in the heart are activated, resulting in an increase in heart rate and contractility to increase stroke volume and cardiac output. SNS response in the peripheral vascular system results in vasoconstriction, which increases systemic venous return and mean systemic filling pressures. This results in an increase in venous return, preload and afterload (Fig. 10.9). The consequence of this activation is increased myocardial oxygen demand. Although blood flow to essential organs is maintained, perfusion to the kidneys, gastrointestinal system and skin is reduced and peripheral resistance increased. Chronic activation of vasoconstrictors contributes to the progression of cardiac

FIGURE 10.9 Flowchart of the pathophysiology of heart failure.[113]

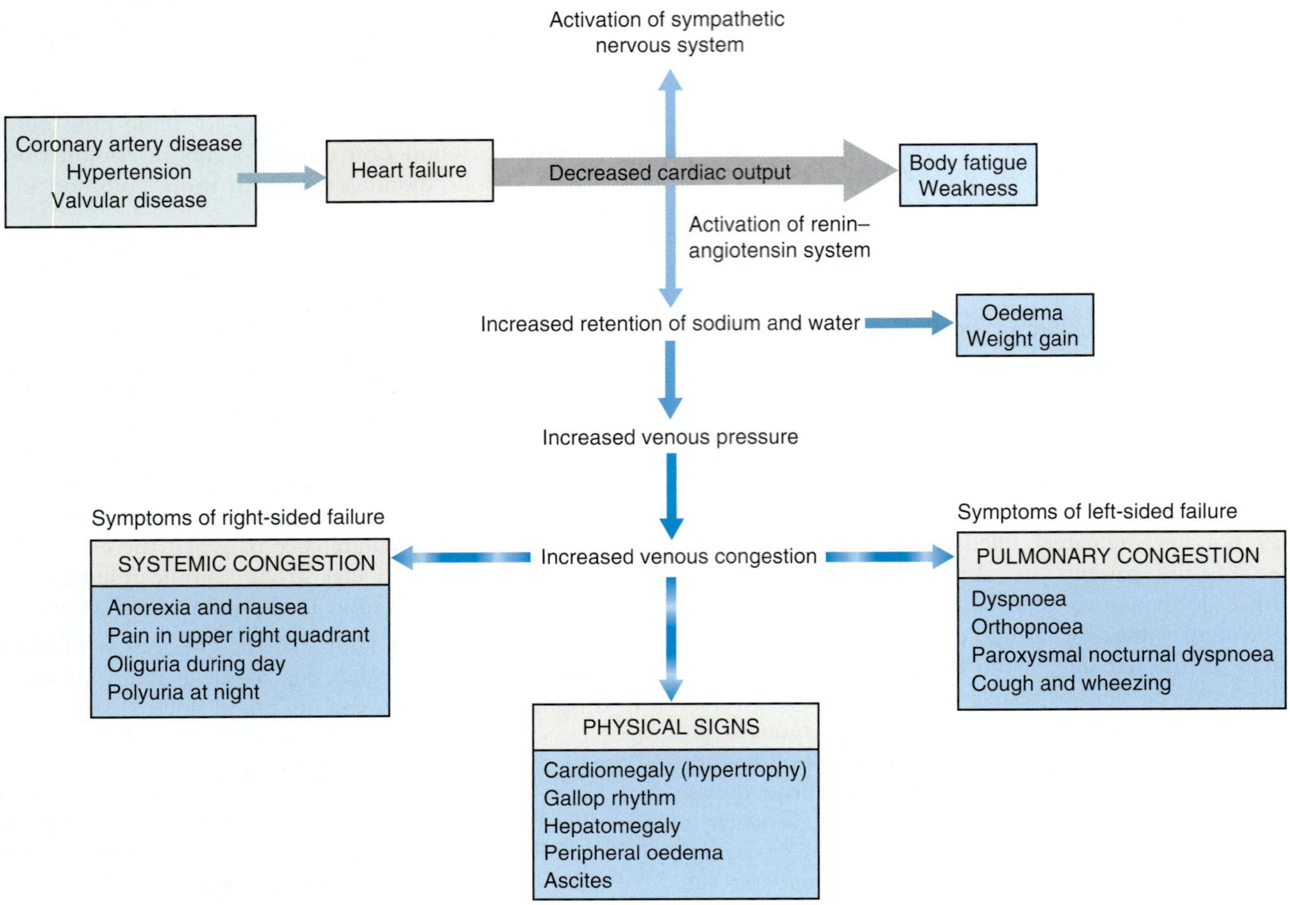

Source: Bryant B, Knights K, Saterno E. Pharmacology for health professionals. 2nd ed. Sydney: Mosby, 2007.

failure through increased resistance and effects on cardiac structure, causing hypertrophy and fibrosis and down-regulation of beta-adrenergic receptors and endothelial dysfunction. Chronic poor perfusion to skeletal muscles may contribute to changes in muscle metabolism, resulting in further reductions in exercise tolerance.

The next compensatory mechanism to be activated is the RAAS. This is stimulated within minutes, in response to a decrease in kidney perfusion resulting in a decrease in glomerular filtration rate. Activation of this response results in an increase in systemic venous return and sodium and water reabsorption, which then increases the circulating blood volume, systemic filling pressures and venous return enhancing preload and afterload (see Chapter 9). The Frank–Starling response is also activated. As the end-diastolic volume increases (preload) in response to SNS stimulation, ventricular dilation occurs stimulating the Frank–Starling response. As the myocardial fibres are stretched during diastole the force of contractility also increases to expel the increasing preload. This is a major mechanism of the heart to maintain a normal cardiac output. Optimal contractility occurs when the diastolic volume is 12–18 mmHg.[72] However, when the ventricle is damaged, such as in MI, the SNS increases heart rate and contractility, further increasing cardiac workload and exacerbating myocardial dysfunction, which increases end-diastolic volume (preload) and ventricular dilation further, and heart failure progresses. As ventricular dilation continues, ventricular hypertrophy results. The myocardium also increases its muscle mass in an attempt to increase contractility, called ventricular remodelling. However, over time ventricular hypertrophy results in changes to end-diastolic compliance and contractility due to the thickened ventricular wall, impaired muscle function and growth of collagen. These result in further impairment of ventricular function (Fig. 10.10). Ventricular hypertrophy also has a depressant effect on ventricular compliance, heart rate and contractility resulting in an increase in end-diastolic pressure with no associated increase in contractility. As the pulmonary artery pressures increase, pulmonary oedema and cardiogenic shock develop.

The final compensatory mechanism to be activated is the neurohormonal response, which takes days to be activated. This response involves the activation of vasopressin and atrial natriuretic peptide (ANP). Vasopressin is a potent vasoconstrictor and also an antidiuretic hormone. ANP is important in the regulation of cardiovascular volume homeostasis. It is released from the atria in response to atrial stretching due to an increased circulating blood volume. ANP blocks the effect of the SNS, RAAS and vasopressin. It reduces tachycardia via the baroreceptors and reduces circulating blood volume by increasing salt and water excretion in the kidneys. Plasma ANP is increased in acute heart failure but depleted in CHF.

While in the healthy heart these compensatory mechanisms would result in an adequate cardiac output, in heart failure they do not, depending on the aetiology. In ischaemic heart failure the damaged myocardium is unable to respond adequately to the Frank–Starling response and ventricular remodelling develops. Heart failure caused by hypertension or valvular heart disease results in persistent pressure or volume overload, which is exacerbated by the Frank–Starling response and SNS compensatory mechanisms. This causes ventricular remodelling and depletion of noradrenaline and a reduction of inotropic response to the cardiac SNS. These all exacerbate the reduction in circulating blood volume and kidney perfusion. Many patients with heart failure often have a high plasma renin activity due to the continual activation of the RAAS compensatory mechanism.

FIGURE 10.10 Function curves of left ventricular pressure during various stages of heart failure.[73]

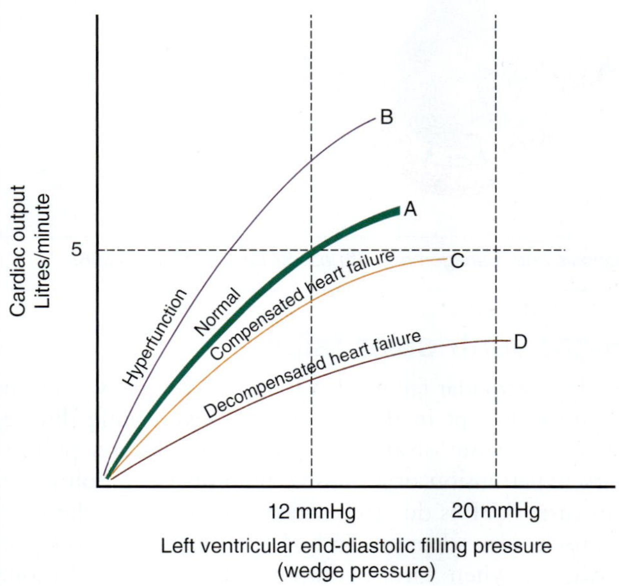

Source: Michaelson CR. Congestive heart failure. St Louis: Mosby, 1983.

In heart failure patients the inadequate cardiac output results in signs and symptoms of hypoperfusion (oliguria, cognitive impairment and cold peripheries) and congestion of the venous and pulmonary systems (acute pulmonary oedema, dyspnoea, hypoxaemia, peripheral oedema and liver congestion). Classification of signs and symptoms is usually considered in the context of left or right ventricular failure.

Left ventricular failure

Left ventricular failure (LVF), compared with other forms of heart failure, is characterised by breathlessness, orthopnoea and paroxysmal nocturnal dyspnoea, irritating cough and fatigue (Table 10.5). LVF or HF*r*EF exists when the ventricle has an ejection fraction of less than 50%,[70,71] resulting in increased end-diastolic volume and increased intraventricular pressure. The left atrium is unable to empty into the left ventricle adequately and pressure in the left atrium rises. This pressure is reflected in the pulmonary veins and causes pulmonary congestion. When pulmonary venous congestion exceeds 20 mmHg, fluid moves into the pulmonary interstitium. Raised pulmonary interstitial pressure reduces pulmonary compliance, increases the work of breathing and is experienced by the patient as shortness of breath. Increased blood volume in the lung also

TABLE 10.5
Clinical manifestations of failure of right and left sides of the heart

LEFT VENTRICULAR FAILURE		RIGHT VENTRICULAR FAILURE	
SIGNS	**SYMPTOMS**	**SIGNS**	**SYMPTOMS**
Tachypnoea	Dyspnoea	Peripheral oedema	Fatigue
Tachycardia	Orthopnoea	Raised JVP	Weight gain
Bibasal crackles	PND	Raised central venous pressure	Anorexia
Haemoptysis	Fatigue	Ascites	
Cough	Nocturia	Hepatomegaly	
Pulmonary oedema			
Raised pulmonary artery pressure			
S3 heart sound			

JVP: jugular venous pressure.

FIGURE 10.11 Pathophysiology of pulmonary oedema. As pulmonary oedema progresses, it inhibits oxygen and carbon dioxide exchange at the alveolar–capillary interface. (**A**) Normal relationship. (**B**) Increased pulmonary capillary hydrostatic pressure causes fluid to move from the vascular space into the pulmonary interstitial space. (**C**) Lymphatic flow increases and pulls fluid back into the vascular or lymphatic space. (**D**) Failure of lymphatic flow and worsening of left-sided heart failure causes further movement of fluid into the interstitial space and then into the alveoli.[74]

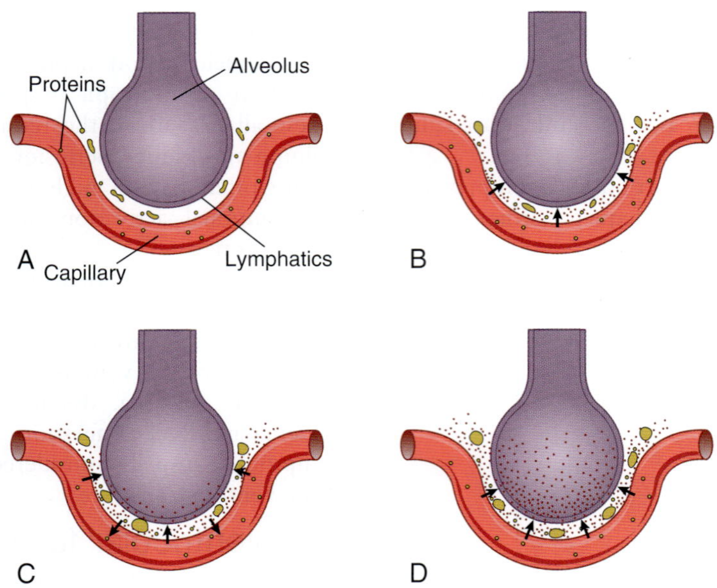

Source: Urden L, Stacy K, Logh M, Thelan's Critical care nursing: Diagnosis and management. 5th ed. St Louis: Mosby, 2006.

initiates shallow, rapid breathing and the sensation of breathlessness. Patients also experience orthopnoea (dyspnoea while lying flat) and paroxysmal nocturnal dyspnoea because, when lying down, blood is redistributed from gravity-dependent areas of the body to the lung. Sitting upright or standing, and sleeping with additional pillows, relieves breathlessness at night.

Acute pulmonary oedema results when pulmonary capillary pressure exceeds approximately 30 mmHg, and then fluid from the vessels begins to leak into the alveoli (Fig. 10.11). This fluid leak decreases the area available for normal gas exchange and severe shortness of breath results, often accompanied by pink, frothy sputum and noisy respirations. This causes patients to experience severe anxiety and decreased oxygen levels. Pulmonary oedema is a medical emergency and requires urgent treatment.

In addition to pulmonary symptoms, patients with LVF experience signs and symptoms related to decreased left ventricular output, including weakness, fatigue, difficulty in concentrating and decreased exercise tolerance. These symptoms may be present for some time before an accurate diagnosis of heart failure is made, because they are non-specific and are consistent with other diagnoses such as depression. Other signs that are useful in diagnosis include the presence of S3 (ventricular gallop), crackles over lung fields that do not clear with a cough, cardiomegaly and the presence of pulmonary vessels on chest X-ray.

Right ventricular failure

Right ventricular failure (RVF) does not usually occur in isolation, except in the presence of severe lung disease, such as chronic obstructive pulmonary disease, pulmonary hypertension or a massive pulmonary embolus.[74] In this case, RVF is due to resistance to outflow. The right ventricle can adapt to fairly large changes in volume; however, when cardiac output decreases, end-diastolic volume increases, and the right atrium is unable to empty adequately. Right atrial pressure rises and is reflected into the venous system. Jugular vein distension occurs, and the veins are usually visible above the clavicle. Symptoms of right heart failure are not as specific as LVF and are mostly related to low cardiac output and raised venous pressure (see Table 10.5). Ascites and oedema tend to progress insidiously, and dependent oedema in the feet and ankles is often most prominent. Weight gain is an important sign as 1 kg of weight gain equals 1 litre of excess fluid. Liver congestion may result in tenderness, ascites and jaundice. Nausea and anorexia may be present and are a result of an increased intraabdominal pressure. Many signs are not readily distinguishable from LVF, including extra heart sounds.

Patient assessment, diagnostic procedures and classification

Assessment and diagnosis are summarised in a diagnostic algorithm (Fig. 10.12). A full assessment and history are

FIGURE 10.12 Diagnostic algorithm for a patient with suspected heart failure.[70]

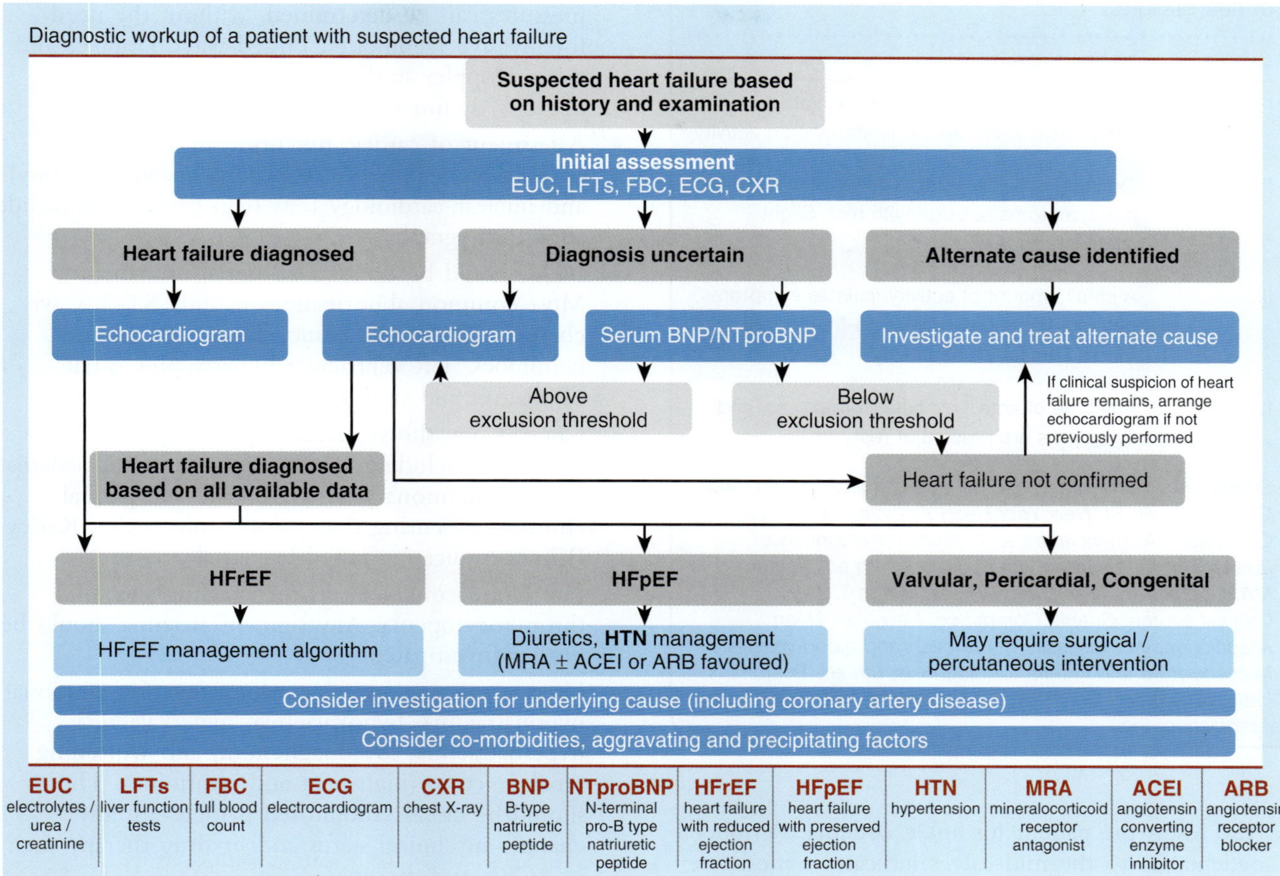

Atherton JJ, Sindone A, De Pasquale CG, et al. National Heart Foundation of Australia and Cardiac Society of Australia and New Zealand: Guidelines for the Prevention, Detection, and Management of Heart Failure in Australia. Heart, Lung and Circulation 2018; 27(10):1123-208, with permission.

essential to determine the cause(s) of CHF and to assess the severity of the disease. A careful physical assessment is important for initial diagnosis and to evaluate the effectiveness of treatments and progress of the disease. The depth and time taken to conduct the assessment depend on the severity of symptoms. The physical examination of the patient focuses on cardiovascular and pulmonary assessment.

Cardiovascular assessment includes:

- Pulse rate and rhythm: the pulse rate is generally elevated due to a low cardiac output. However, if the patient is prescribed beta-adrenergic blocking agents and/or angiotensin-converting enzyme inhibitors (ACEIs), the pulse rate may be low.
- Palpation of the precordium and apical impulse: may be displaced laterally and downward to the left due to an increased heart size.
- Auscultation of a third heart sound (S3 gallop): occurs due to a low ejection fraction and diastolic dysfunction. A fourth heart sound may also be present due to a decrease in ventricular compliance.
- Assessment of jugular venous pressure (JVP): is performed to estimate the degree of venous volume. If raised it reflects hypervolaemia, RVF and reduced right ventricular compliance. It can also be raised in the presence of tricuspid valve disease. The hepatojugular reflex is also assessed by pressing on the liver and observing an increase in JVP. This results in an increase in blood flow to the right atrium.
- Blood pressure: lying and standing blood pressure are measured to assess postural hypotension due to a low cardiac output and also the prescribing of beta-adrenergic blocking agents and ACEIs.
- Peripheries: look for the presence of cyanosis that may be due to vasoconstriction. Assess the fingers for clubbing, which indicates long-term cyanosis usually as a consequence of congenital heart disease.

TABLE 10.6
New York Heart Association functional classification of heart failure

CLASS	DEFINITION
I	Normal daily activity does not initiate symptoms. There are no limitations on activity
II	Ordinary activities initiate onset of symptoms, but symptoms subside with rest. Slight limitation of daily activities
III	A small amount of activity initiates symptoms; patients are usually symptom-free at rest. Marked limitation of activity
IV	Any type of activity initiates symptoms, and symptoms are present at rest

Source: Adapted from Dolgin M, Association NYH, Fox AC, Gorlin R, Levin RI, New York Heart Association. Criteria Committee. Nomenclature and criteria for diagnosis of diseases of the heart and great vessels. 9th ed. Boston, MA: Lippincott Williams and Wilkins; March 1, 1994. Original source: Criteria Committee, New York Heart Association, Inc. Diseases of the heart and blood vessels. Nomenclature and criteria for diagnosis, 6th ed. Boston: Little, Brown and Co. 1964, p 114. ©1964 American Heart Association, Inc.

Also assess the patient for ankle oedema. Peripheral oedema up to the mid-calves indicates a moderate amount of excess fluid and the patient may require a bolus dose of diuretic medication.

Pulmonary assessment includes chest auscultation for inspiratory crepitations that do not clear with coughing. They are initially heard in the bases but as congestion increases, they become diffuse. General assessment of the patient includes daily weighing and looking for signs of cachexia (usually associated with severe CHF), anaemia and dizziness.

Heart failure is usually classified according to the severity of symptoms. In CHF, the New York Heart Association (NYHA) Functional Classification is commonly used to classify patients based on the activity level that initiates symptoms (Table 10.6).

Diagnostic tests

Tests used to diagnose heart failure include the following:

- Transthoracic echocardiography is the most useful investigation to confirm diagnosis. This is the gold standard diagnostic test for heart failure and should always be undertaken when possible.[70,71] This test is vital, as it can distinguish systolic dysfunction (left ventricular ejection fraction [LVEF] <50%) from diastolic dysfunction, and therefore help determine treatment. Information on left and right ventricular sizes, volumes, left ventricular thrombus and ventricular wall thickness and motion can be provided. Assessment of valve structure and function as well as intracardiac and pulmonary pressures can be determined, without the need for invasive techniques. Pulsed-wave Doppler and tissue Doppler studies can be used to determine diastolic dysfunction.
- Assessment of cardiac function can also be done by invasive techniques (e.g. coronary angiography) and nuclear cardiology tests (e.g. gated radionuclide angiocardiography).
- ECG should be done as an initial investigation. Most common abnormalities include ST-T wave changes, left bundle branch block, left anterior hemiblock, left ventricular hypertrophy, atrial fibrillation and sinus tachycardia.
- Chest X-ray shows cardiomegaly and pulmonary markings, including evidence of interstitial oedema: perihilar pulmonary vessels, small basal pleural effusions obscuring the costophrenic angles, Kerley B lines (indicating raised left atrial pressure).
- Full blood count checks for anaemia and mild thrombocytopenia. Any signs of anaemia should be further investigated.
- Urea, creatinine and electrolytes tests for dilutional hyponatraemia, hypokalaemia, hyperkalaemia, hypernatraemia, low magnesium, and worsening renal function (high urea and creatinine). These should be closely monitored if there are any changes in clinical status and/or drug therapy such as ACEIs and diuretics.
- Liver function tests check for elevated levels of AST, ALT, lactate dehydrogenase (LDH) and serum bilirubin.
- Thyroid function tests are performed particularly in patients with no history of coronary artery disease and who develop atrial fibrillation.
- Urinalysis is conducted to measure specific gravity and proteinuria.
- Myocardial ischaemia and viability need to be assessed in patients with heart failure and coronary artery disease. These can be assessed by a stress ECG, stress echocardiography or a myocardial perfusion study. Coronary angiography is useful to determine the contribution of coronary artery disease in these patients.
- Natriuretic peptides include plasma ANP and B-type natriuretic peptide (BNP). BNP or N-terminal proBNP (NTproBNP) is not recommended to be used as the only test to diagnose CHF as an elevated or reduced BNP or NTproBNP may be due to other causes, such as atrial fibrillation, in the elderly or the prescribing of an angiotensin receptor neprilysin inhibitor (ARNI) will artificially increase BNP levels so NTproBNP should be done on these patients.

FIGURE 10.13 Management of HF*r*EF.[70]

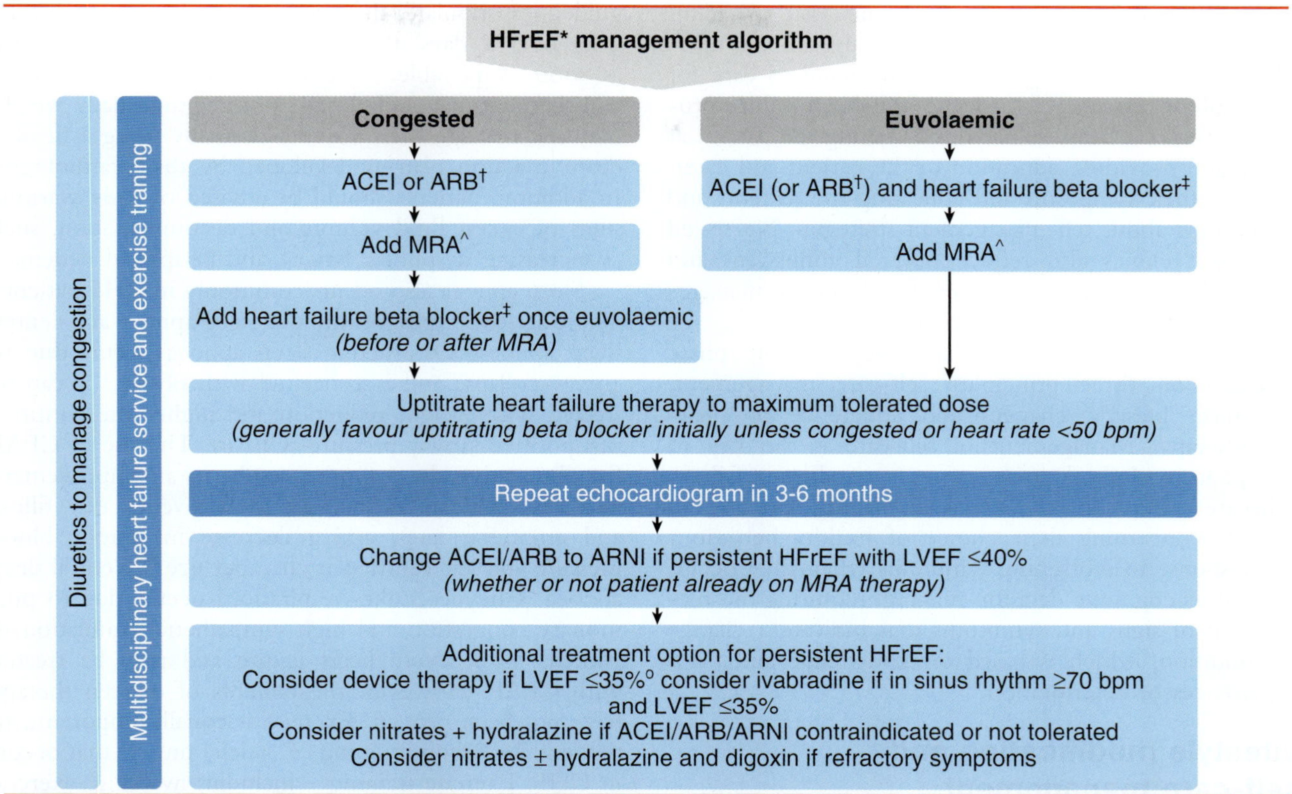

HFrEF	ACEI	ARB	MRA	ARNI	LVEF	ICD	CRT
heart failure with reduced ejection fraction	angiotensin converting enzyme inhibitor	angiotensin receptor blocker	mineralocorticoid receptor antagonist	angiotensin receptor neprilysin inhibitor	left ventricular ejection fraction	implantable cardioverter defibrillator	cardiac resynchronisation therapy

* HFrEF refers to patients with symptoms ± signs of heart failure associated with an LVEF less than 50% (unless otherwise specified)
† ARB should only be used if ACEI is contraindicated or not tolerated
‡ Carvedilol, bisoprolol, metoprolol succinate, nebivolol
^ Commencing MRA usually avoided if serum K >5 mmol/L or CrCl <30 mL/minute
° ICD and/or CRT

Source: Atherton JJ, Sindone A, De Pasquale CG, et al. National Heart Foundation of Australia and Cardiac Society of Australia and New Zealand: Guidelines for the prevention, detection, and management of heart failure in Australia. Heart, Lung and Circulation 2018;27(10):1123–208.

However, it is useful to use BNP/NTproBNP in conjunction with other diagnostic tests, particularly to differentiate between dyspnoea due to heart failure and dyspnoea due to chronic obstructive pulmonary disease.

- Endomyocardial biopsy should be conducted if there is a suspicion of cardiomyopathy.

Patient management

Treatment of CHF is lifelong and multifactorial, requiring a well-coordinated, multidisciplinary approach. The goals of heart failure treatment are to identify and eliminate the precipitating cause, promote optimal cardiac function, enhance patient comfort by relieving signs and symptoms and help the patient and family cope with any lifestyle changes. Clinical practice guidelines have been developed to guide the treatment of heart failure on the basis of ventricular dysfunction and grade of symptoms (Figs 10.12 and 10.13).[70,71,75]

Planning for hospital discharge begins early in the admission and aims to promote quality of life for the patient and prevent unnecessary admissions. Several healthcare services have been implemented to support the transition from hospital to home as it is during the first 30 days post-discharge that nearly 25% of heart failure patients are readmitted to hospital.[76] There are currently over 80 outreach heart failure programs throughout Australia that support heart failure patients post-discharge.[77] The main goals of these programs are to reduce symptom burden, improve functional capacity and minimise hospital readmissions. These programs range from in-hospital visits to facilitate discharge planning to nurse-led heart failure outpatient clinics, home visit programs and heart failure-specific exercise programs. Several meta-analyses of home visit programs have shown a reduction in hospital admissions and mortality[78,79] and these programs are now standard care for heart failure patients.[70,71,75] Home visit heart failure programs involve a heart failure nurse visiting the patient at home and providing education to the patient and carer, assessing their symptoms and educating the patients and their carers about self-management strategies. Nurse-led outpatient clinics also reduce hospital admissions and mortality[80,81] and play an important role in the management of heart failure patients post-discharge.

Management of heart failure post the acute phase is based on three principles: self-care management, long-term lifestyle changes and adherence to pharmacotherapy. Management of self-care is the key to non-pharmacological management of heart failure. Self-care refers to the decision-making process of patients concerning their choice of healthy behaviour and response to worsening symptoms when they occur. It involves cognitive decision making, requiring the recognition of signs and symptoms that indicate a change in condition, which is based on knowledge and prior experiences of deterioration.[82,83]

Lifestyle modification and self-care management

Patient education is the key to self-management and must include family members to be effective. Patient education should include information on the following:

- the disease process – this involves discussing what heart failure is, signs and symptoms and why they occur, and strategies to improve their symptoms
- lifestyle changes
- medications and side effects
- self-monitoring and acute symptoms
- importance of adherence to the medications and management plan.

There are numerous resources available for patient and carer education. The Heart Foundation has an excellent resource titled 'Living well with CHF' and other resources (https://www.heartfoundation.org.au/your-heart/heart-conditions/heart-failure-the-facts). Also 'heart online' (http://www.heartonline.org.au) and 'Heart failure matters' (https://www.heartfailurematters.org/en_GB) are excellent resources for health professionals providing information for patients and carers. Both of these websites also provide resources for health professionals regarding heart failure management and tools such as surveys.

Restriction of fluid to 1.5L/day is one of the most important strategies that patients can adhere to in order to improve their symptoms. However, it is only recommended in patients with signs and symptoms of fluid overload.[70,71,75] Patients are encouraged to weigh themselves daily and to identify any increase in weight as an increase of 1 kg equals 1 litre of excess fluid. National guidelines stipulate that, if their weight increases by 2 kg over 2 days, they need to see their local doctor as soon as possible.[70,75] Patients who adhere to their management plan and closely monitor their daily weight may self-manage their volume status by using a flexible diuretic action plan as developed by their cardiologist. In addition, patients should be advised of early warning signs of excess fluid volume and decompensation, such as increasing dyspnoea, fatigue and peripheral oedema.

Sleep apnoea also occurs commonly in CHF patients. There are two types: obstructive sleep apnoea and central sleep apnoea. Obstructive sleep apnoea occurs due to airway collapse and is associated with obesity. It can be treated with weight reduction and night-time continuous positive airway pressure (CPAP). The use of CPAP for obstructive sleep apnoea results in an improvement in LVEF due to an increase in left ventricular filling and emptying rates, and a decrease in systolic blood pressure and left ventricular chamber size.[84] Central sleep apnoea (Cheyne–Stokes respiration) occurs due to pulmonary congestion and high sympathetic stimulation in patients with severe heart failure and may be treated with CPAP. However, the benefits of oxygen therapy have not been proven. Exercise is equally important, to prevent the deconditioning of skeletal muscle that occurs in CHF. Exercise training – including walking, exercise bicycle and light resistance – has been shown to improve functional capacity, symptoms, neurohormonal abnormalities, quality of life and mood in CHF.[85] National clinical heart failure guidelines all recommend that stable CHF patients, regardless of age, should be considered for referral to a tailored exercise program (preferably a heart failure-specific exercise program) or modified CR program.[70,71,75] Heart failure exercise programs comprise resistance training and have been shown to improve functional capacity, heart failure symptoms and survival and reduce hospitalisations.[85] In patients with symptomatic heart failure physical activity should be undertaken under the supervision of trained heart failure specialists, e.g. a physiotherapist or exercise physiologist, who can tailor the level of exercise to the degree of severity of symptoms. Many CHF patients have comorbidities such as arthritis, which make exercise programs difficult, but maintaining general activity should be encouraged.

Dietary sodium intake should be reduced to 2 g/day for patients with moderate-to-severe heart failure and patients to eat a healthy diet and maintain a healthy weight.[70,71,75] Reduction in sodium intake helps reduce fluid retention, diuretic requirements and potassium excretion. A large proportion of an individual's sodium intake can come from processed foods, so patients are encouraged to read nutrition labels and reduce the intake of these foods. Salt intake can also be reduced by avoiding adding salt in cooking or to meals. As CHF patients who are overweight have an increased demand on their heart, weight loss by lowering dietary fat intake may improve symptoms and quality of life. In patients with moderate-to-severe heart failure, cardiac cachexia and anaemia are common, which further exacerbate weakness and fatigue. These patients will require a referral to a dietician for nutritional support. Other lifestyle changes are: cease smoking, ideally cease alcohol intake or otherwise limit alcohol to less than two standard drinks/day (alcohol is a myocardial toxin and reduces contractility), limit caffeinated drinks to 1–2 drinks/day (to decrease the risk of arrhythmias), control diabetes and have annual vaccinations for influenza and regular pneumococcal disease vaccinations.[70,71,75]

Palliative care may be appropriate for patients with end-stage heart failure who are experiencing significant symptoms, prescribed maximal pharmacotherapy, and have poor response to treatment. It is important that all patients have an advanced care plan in place and that this has been discussed with family members. Advanced care plans should be discussed soon after the patient's first hospital admission for treatment of decompensated heart failure.

Pharmacotherapy in patients with heart failure is vital and includes an array of drugs that require careful management. Nurse practitioners are authorised to titrate some heart failure medications, including diuretics, beta-adrenergic blocking agents, ACEIs, angiotension receptor blocking agents (ARBs) and ARNIs. Pharmacists also provide essential patient education and support the optimisation of medication treatments and management of complex medication schedules. Some major hospitals have a pharmacist outreach program where a pharmacist visits the patient at home.

Practice tip

When considering if a patient is suitable for palliation, discussion also needs to include deactivation of their pacemaker or implantable cardioverter defibrillator (ICD).

Medications

Pharmacological management relies on the following categories of drugs: ACEIs, ARNI, beta-adrenergic blocking agents, ARBs, diuretics, ivabradine, inotropes, and antiarrhythmic drugs. Antiarrhythmic drugs are reviewed in Chapter 11. The main actions and adverse effects of these drugs in heart failure are summarised in Table 10.7.

Angiotensin-converting enzyme inhibitors

ACEIs are the cornerstone of CHF treatment, as they have been demonstrated to prolong survival, improve patient symptoms and exercise tolerance, prevent hospitalisation and improve ejection fraction in CHF patients.[86,87] All patients with symptomatic systolic left ventricle (LV) dysfunction should be prescribed either an ACEI, ARNI or ARB.[70,71,75] ACEIs (such as captopril, enalapril, lisinopril) act on the renin–angiotensin system by specifically preventing the conversion of angiotensin I to angiotensin II.[43] As a result, systemic vascular resistance (afterload) is decreased. This is particularly important in preventing the progression of CHF, because blockade of the renin–angiotensin system prevents further development of systolic dysfunction. In addition, because angiotensin II also stimulates the release of aldosterone, sodium and water retention are decreased (preload). This may also be beneficial when ACEIs are prescribed with diuretics, as potassium loss is limited. Further, ACEIs inhibit the breakdown of bradykinin (a vasodilator), which also contributes to decreasing vascular resistance. The total reduction of systemic vascular resistance reduces the workload of the heart without affecting heart rate or cardiac output.

Common adverse effects of ACEIs primarily result from hypotension, including dizziness and headache. Other side effects include hyperkalaemia, deterioration of renal function and an unproductive cough, which may respond to asthma prophylactic medications. Initial doses of ACEIs should be low, as severe – though transient – symptomatic hypotension can occur, worsening of renal function and hyperkalaemia. The dose of ACEIs needs to be gradually increased to maximum dose over two months to optimise the survival and functional capacity benefits. This group of drugs is contraindicated in patients with bilateral renal artery stenosis due to the danger of developing renal failure. One important adverse effect of ACEIs is that they cannot be taken in conjunction with non-steroidal anti-inflammatory drugs (NSAIDs) as NSAIDs reduce the action of ACEIs.[88]

Practice tip

A dry, non-productive cough is often associated with the introduction of ACEI medication, but is often mistaken for a symptom of other conditions, so patients may not report the symptom as new. The cough usually begins within 1–2 days of commencing therapy and uptitration of dose.

Practice tip

Heart failure is a disease of the elderly. Many elderly patients have arthritis. However, elderly patients with heart failure must avoid taking NSAID medications, especially when taking ACEIs, as NSAIDs counter the action of ACEIs. In such cases we usually recommend taking long-acting paracetamol or glucosamine for relief from arthritis pain.

TABLE 10.7
Common medications for the treatment of heart failure

DRUG/EXAMPLE	ACTION	MAJOR ADVERSE EFFECTS
ACE inhibitor Captopril Enalapril	Decrease systemic vascular resistance by stopping angiotensin I conversion to II; decreased sodium and water retention	Symptomatic hypotension Hyperkalaemia Unproductive cough Renal failure Rash
Beta-adrenergic blockers Bisoprolol Carvedilol Metoprolol CR/XL	Reduce systemic vascular resistance and heart rate by blocking adrenoreceptors in arteries and heart	Hypotension Bronchoconstriction
ARNI Entresto	Blocks selective AT1 receptor causing a reduction in vasoconstriction, sodium and water retention	Symptomatic hypotension Hyperkalaemia Risk of angioedema
Potassium-sparing diuretics Spironolactone	Increase urine volume by aldosterone blocking and sodium retention	Hyperkalaemia Rash Gynaecomastia
ARB Candesartan Irbesartan	Block the angiotensin II receptor that responds to angiotensin II stimulation; decreased sodium and water retention. Alternative to ACEI	Symptomatic hypotension Hyperkalaemia Renal failure
Ivabradine	Reduces heart rate through inhibition of the sinoatrial node	Bradycardia Dizziness Ventricular arrhythmias AF
Loop diuretics Frusemide	Increase urine volume by decreasing reabsorption of chloride and sodium	Hypokalaemia Ototoxicity Rash
Thiazide diuretics Chlorothiazide Hydrochlorothiazide	Increase urine volume by decreasing reabsorption of sodium	Hypokalaemia Hyperglycaemia Sensitivity: rash
Cardiac glycosides Digitalis	Increase myocardial contractility and decrease heart rate by inhibiting sodium pump in myocytes	Tachycardia AV block Nausea and vomiting Disorientation Visual disturbances

ARNI: angiotensin receptor neprilysin inhibitor

ARNI

ARNIs are a new class of drugs that act on the RAAS and the neprilysin peptide system. The neprilysin peptide system increases the circulating natriuretic peptides which reduce the symptoms and progression of heart failure. The first drug in this new class is called LCZ696, which is a combination of valsartan and sacubitril (neprilysin inhibitor). The valsartan component blocks the AT1 receptor and sacubitril inhibits neprilysin promoting a higher concentration of circulating natriuretic peptides. In symptomatic patients diagnosed with HF*r*EF it is now recommended that patients are prescribed an ARNI to replace ACEI and ARBs.[70,71,75] ARNIs have demonstrated they reduce hospital readmissions and improve survival.[89,90] To minimise the risk of angioedema, it is recommended that ACEIs are ceased for at least 36 hours prior to the initiation of an ARNI. There is a contraindication with the combined use of ACEI or ARB and an ARNI. Current clinical guidelines recommend that patients who are eligible to be prescribed an ARNI commence low dose of ACEI or ARB prior and then switch over to an ARNI.[70,71,75] The dose of ARNI should also be gradually increased 2–4 weekly until optimal dose is reached. More clinical trials are being conducted on the safety of prescribing an ARNI without commencing an ACEI or ARB prior and also its efficacy in HFpEF.

Common adverse effects of ARNIs include: increased risk of angioedema, symptomatic hypotension, hyperkalaemia, renal impairment, and a cough.[70,71,89,90]

Beta-adrenergic blocking agents

All patients with symptomatic systolic left ventricular dysfunction should be prescribed a beta-adrenergic blocking agent. Beta-adrenergic blocking agents (carvedilol, metoprolol CR/XL, bisoprolol, nebivolol) are used in CHF to inhibit the adverse effects of chronic activation of the SNS and improve ventricular function. In heart failure $beta_2$ receptors predominate with $beta_1$ receptors being downregulated. In heart failure beta-adrenergic blocking agents reduce this neurohormonal activity. The addition of a beta-adrenergic blocker has been demonstrated to reduce symptoms, reduce hospitalisations and prolong survival in patients.[91] Similar to ACEIs, the dose of beta-adrenergic blocking agents needs to be gradually increased. Once the patient is euvolaemic they should be commenced on low dose and gradually increased to maximal dose over several months.

In patients with chronic obstructive pulmonary disease (COPD), selective $beta_1$ blockers are prescribed. Patients will require close monitoring for signs of deterioration of their COPD. Other adverse events are: symptomatic hypotension, bradycardia and worsening heart failure. Also, during the uptitration of beta-adrenergic blocking agents, many patients complain of feeling slightly confused in the morning; this usually disappears after 2–3 weeks.

Angiotensin receptor blocking agents

The primary use of ARBs is in patients who are intolerant of an ACEI such as ACEI cough. They have a similar action as ACEIs; however, ARBs block the angiotensin II receptor that responds to angiotensin II stimulation. ACEIs, on the other hand, act on the enzyme that produces angiotensin II.[87] They have similar benefits as ACEIs, such as improving survival, LVEF and heart failure symptoms and reducing hospitalisations.[92] Similar to ACEIs, ARBs are commenced on a low dose and gradually uptitrated to optimal dose over two months. Adverse effects are: deterioration in renal function, hyperkalaemia and symptomatic hypotension.[43]

Diuretics

Diuretics are one of the mainstays of management of heart failure, primarily to decrease the sodium and water retention response to the low cardiac output state. A combination of diuretics may be used if oedema persists on one diuretic. Most often, diuretics will be used in combination with ACEIs.

- Loop diuretics: (frusemide, ethacrynic acid and bumetanide) act on the ascending limb of the loop of Henle of the nephron. They prevent the reabsorption of chloride and sodium ions from the loop, so that increased concentrations are present in the loop, attracting more water and increasing urine volume. Intravenous administration of frusemide is often used to manage preload in acute exacerbations. In fluid-overloaded patients, the aim is to achieve increased urine output and a weight reduction of 0.5–1 kg daily, until clinical euvolaemia is achieved. Hypokalaemia is a common adverse effect, and patients on long-term diuretics need regular monitoring and may require potassium supplements. Hyponatraemia may also occur at high doses, and needs careful management in heart failure patients. Ototoxicity, presenting as tinnitus, vertigo and deafness, can occur at high doses, so IV delivery of frusemide should be no faster than 4 mg/min.
- Thiazide and thiazide-like diuretics: (chlorothiazide, hydrochlorothiazide, chlorthalidone) act on the ascending loop of the nephron and decrease sodium reabsorption. As a result, the fluid in the collecting ducts is more concentrated and attracts more water. Thiazides also cause peripheral arteriole vasodilation, which may be beneficial in hypertensive patients. Adverse effects are similar to loop diuretics due to potassium and sodium loss, and supplementation may be necessary. When ACEIs are prescribed concurrently, there is less potassium loss (details below). Hyperglycaemia can occur, so diabetics need monitoring. Impotence may also occur, as well as sensitivity due to the presence of sulfonamide in the drug structure.
- Aldosterone antagonists: are potassium-sparing diuretics and include spironolactone. Aldosterone acts on the distal convoluted tubule of the nephron to cause sodium retention and thus water retention, although potassium is lost. Antagonists stop this action, so potassium is not lost and not as much sodium retained, thus there is minor diuresis. Spironolactone is particularly useful in CHF because there is excessive aldosterone production, causing oedema. There is the potential that spironolactone, by blocking aldosterone systemically, may prevent the negative effects of aldosterone on the heart, such as fibrosis, hypertrophy and arrhythmogenesis. Adverse effects include hyperkalaemia, which may occur more readily in CHF patients because of renal failure, and, because of its potentially lethal effects, spironolactone requires regular monitoring. Other effects include hyponatraemia and feminisation effects such as gynaecomastia. In patients with HF*p*EF, spironolactone has been shown to reduce heart failure-related hospitalisations; however, there was no reduction in all-cause hospitalisations.[93] Spironolactone is recommended for use in patients with symptomatic (NYHA class II–IV) HF*r*EF in addition to other pharmacotherapy such as ACEIs. Aldosterone antagonists have additional survival benefits and reduce hospital readmission.[93-95]

Ivabradine

Ivabradine is a sinoatrial node inhibitor resulting in heart rate reduction which reduces cardiac workload and myocardial oxygen demand. It is recommended for use in patients with HF*r*EF with EF≤35%, sinus rhythm >70 beats per min and prescribed optimal dose of medical therapy including beta-adrenergic blocker and ACEI, ARNI or ARB.[70,71,75] Adverse effects include: bradycardia, dizziness, ventricular arrhythmias, and atrial fibrillation (AF). Initially, patients should be prescribed low dose ivabradine of 2.5–5 mg BD which is then uptitrated every 2 weeks to a target dose of 7.5 mg BD.

Inotropic agents

This category of drugs increases cardiac contractility. The group includes cardiac glycosides (digoxin) and dopamine agonists (dopamine, dobutamine), sympathomimetics (adrenaline, noradrenaline) and calcium sensitising agents (levosimendan). Inotropes are used as IV infusions in severe heart failure, acute exacerbations of CHF and for palliative care or bridging to transplant in very severe CHF. These drugs have both inotropic and chronotropic actions, so that cardiac contractility and heart rate are both increased to improve cardiac output. Continuous ambulatory infusions of inotropic agents such as dobutamine are administered to patients with severe heart failure as a bridge to transplantation, which allows these patients to be discharged home with support from a home visit nurse. A more detailed overview of these medications is in Chapter 21.

Cardiac glycosides

Cardiac glycosides such as digitalis inhibit the sodium pump such that the exchange between sodium and calcium is impaired. This results in calcium stores being released and intracellular calcium levels rising. As more calcium is available for contraction, contractility and cardiac output increase. These changes in ion movement and additional effects, which enhance parasympathetic stimulation, result in decreased impulse generation by the sinoatrial (SA) node. This is known as a negative chronotropic effect. Conduction is also slowed through the atrioventricular (AV) node and ventricles, allowing more filling time, and therefore having a positive effect on cardiac output. The negative chronotropic effects are particularly beneficial in patients with the atrial fibrillation that is so common in CHF. Digitalis may also affect cardiopulmonary baroreceptors to reduce sympathetic tone, which may be a valuable offset to excessive sympathetic stimulation in CHF.

The most important adverse effects of digoxin are caused by changes in conduction: tachycardia, fibrillation and AV block. Digoxin may also cause nausea and vomiting due to direct brain effects and gastrointestinal irritation. Digitalis has a narrow margin of safety, a long half-life and side effects that can be fatal, so assay of plasma drug levels must be conducted regularly and at initiation and change of treatment. Excessive digoxin causes disorientation, hallucinations and visual disturbances. Potassium levels directly alter the effect of digoxin, so that low levels enhance effects and high levels reduce effects.

Arrhythmias are common in heart failure and need to be treated. The agent must be carefully selected, as CHF patients often have complex medication regimens and interactions may occur. Also, some ventricular anti-arrhythmics, such as class 1 agents (e.g. flecainide), are associated with sudden death in CHF. ICD therapy is also effective in treating ventricular arrhythmias. ICDs reduce mortality by 20–30%[96] and are first-line therapy in patients with a history of ventricular fibrillation (VF) or sustained VT, LVEF ≤30% with NYHA class II–III, at least 40 days post-MI, and prescribed optimal pharmacotherapy or NYHA class I with LVEF ≤35% and prescribed optimal pharmacotherapy.[70,71,75] Cardiac resynchronisation therapy (CRT) (also known as biventricular pacing) is also indicated in patients with symptomatic heart failure to reduce asynchronous pacing of the left ventricle (QRS duration >150 ms).[70,71,75] Systolic function is improved when the left and right ventricles are paced simultaneously. Often patients with a prolonged QRS will have a combination of an ICD with CRT therapy. ICDs and CRT are discussed in more detail in Chapter 11.

In severe heart failure, when patients do not respond to pharmacological treatment, mechanical measures such as cardiopulmonary bypass and left ventricular assist devices may be used. In appropriate candidates, cardiac transplant may also be an option. These procedures are covered under cardiac surgery.

Acute exacerbations of heart failure

Acute exacerbations of heart failure usually occur as episodes of decompensation due to progression of the disease, exacerbation of their comorbidities or non-adherence to their management plan.[97] Acute episodes usually present as congestive heart failure with associated pulmonary oedema, cardiogenic shock (see Chapter 21) or respiratory failure.[70] Patients with severe dyspnoea due to pulmonary congestion with an oxygen saturation of less than 94% should be administered oxygen therapy.[70] If their hypoxaemia does not improve, they may benefit from bilevel positive airway pressure (BiPAP) to support ventilation and gas exchange. The use of continuous positive airway pressure ventilation (CPAP) or BiPAP in acute pulmonary oedema will reduce the need for intubation and mechanical ventilation. If their oxygen saturation is greater than 94% then oxygen therapy should not be used as it causes vasoconstriction and reduces cardiac output.[70]

Once the patient has been stabilised in ICU/CCU it is important to confirm a diagnosis of acute heart failure and to identify and treat potential precipitants of their exacerbation. Some of the most common precipitants include: ACS, tachyarrhythmias, sepsis, non-adherence to their heart failure management plan and/or medications, anaemia, hypoxia, acute renal failure, and/or metabolic/hormonal imbalances such as thyroid dysfunction or diabetic ketoacidosis. In addition to a thorough clinical examination, diagnostic tests on admission in the emergency department include: chest X-ray, 12-lead ECG, echocardiography within 48 hours if haemodynamically unstable or suspected cardiac structure dysfunction, natriuretic peptides to exclude acute heart failure, cardiac troponins if there is a history of CHD, and other biochemistry and haematology investigations as indicated by their clinical condition.

The mainstay of treatment of an acute exacerbation is pharmacological, so a combination of medications is given, usually comprising diuretics and vasodilators such as nitrates. Opiates are only to be considered to relieve anxiety in patients with severe dyspnoea.[70] Opiates are to be used with caution as they reduce the respiratory drive and respiratory workload. Nitrates cause vasodilatation and epicardial artery dilatation and reduce preload, which also helps to relieve symptoms of pulmonary congestion particularly at night when filling pressures are increased due to the recumbent position of sleeping. Diuretics should be administered intravenously to optimise the excretion of intra- and extravascular cellular fluid to reduce circulating blood volume to reduce cardiac workload. Fluid restriction, usually to 1.5 L in 24 hours, is commenced. Various positive inotropes may be administered at low dose (e.g. IV dobutamine causes vasodilatation; IV dopamine improves renal function) to improve contractility and reduce systemic venous return. A higher dose of inotropes should only be used if the patient has symptomatic hypotension or hypoperfusion to increase cardiac output and blood pressure. Levosimendan or phosphodiesterase III inhibitors may be used for hypotension or hypoperfusion to reverse the effect of beta-blockade to increase cardiac output and blood pressure and improve peripheral perfusion.[72] Vasopressors may also be used in cardiogenic shock (see Chapter 21). Vasopressors should only be used short-term as they increase afterload which may further reduce perfusion. If the patient is in rapid atrial fibrillation, digoxin, beta-blockers or amiodarone may be used to control their ventricular rate. A more detailed discussion of these medications is in Chapter 11.

Various mechanical devices are also available, e.g. intra-aortic balloon pump, LVAD (discussed in Chapter 12). CRT with or without an ICD may be implanted. CRT is recommended in NYHA class II–III or ambulatory class IV patients on optimal pharmacological therapy, LVEF ≤35%, left bundle branch block with a QRS duration >150 ms, and sinus rhythm.[71,75] All of these criteria must be fulfilled. Criteria for implantation of an ICD include: symptomatic patients (NYHA class II–IV) and LVEF ≤35%, LVEF <30% at least 40 days post AMI.[71,75] If a patient is to have an ICD implanted, extensive counselling pre- and post-implantation must be undertaken with the patient and carer to ensure they are aware of the painful and unexpected shocks that may be delivered. Some patients may also progress to a heart transplant which is discussed further in Chapter 12.

Most patients in acute heart failure have poor perfusion of the gastrointestinal system and, combined with dyspnoea, a resultant limited appetite. Small, easily ingested meals are best. While the patient is on bed rest, nursing care to prevent problems related to immobility is important. Skin care is particularly important, as poor skin perfusion and oedema place the CHF patient at higher risk of skin breakdown.

Selected cases

Cardiomyopathy

As the term implies, the cardiomyopathies are primary disorders of the myocardium in which there are systolic, diastolic or combined abnormalities. Classification of the most common forms of cardiomyopathy is made on the basis of the dominant abnormality, which may be dilation, hypertrophy or restricted filling. However, each has different haemodynamic effects and therefore requires different treatment.

Dilated cardiomyopathy

Dilated cardiomyopathy (DCM) is the most common form of cardiomyopathy and is characterised by ventricular and atrial dilation and systolic dysfunction.[98] All four chambers become enlarged, which is not in proportion to the degree of hypertrophy. It presents as heart failure of variable severity, sometimes complicated by thromboembolism, at least partly due to atrial fibrillation, which is common. Conduction abnormalities are common in DCM further exacerbating AV dyssynchrony and left ventricular dysfunction. DCM is the most common cause of sudden cardiac death due to ventricular arrhythmias. Annual mortality from DCM ranges from 10% to 50%.[98] Idiopathic DCM is the most common cause of heart failure in young people. Aetiology of DCM includes CHD, myocarditis, cardiotoxins, genetics and alcohol misuse.

Diagnosis

Many of the features of DCM are non-specific. Heart failure, as mentioned, is present with typical symptoms of dyspnoea, fatigue, peripheral oedema and cardiomegaly. S3 and S4 heart sounds may be present on auscultation. Atrial and ventricular arrhythmias are common, particularly atrial fibrillation, ventricular tachycardia, ventricular fibrillation and torsades de pointes. Left bundle branch block (LBBB) is often present, which worsens systolic performance and shortens survival, especially when the QRS interval is markedly prolonged.[98] Echocardiography demonstrates the defining abnormalities and may be useful in revealing atrial thrombus. Occasionally, endocardial biopsy is undertaken to differentiate from myocarditis or rarer causes of cardiomyopathy.

Patient management

Treatment for DCM is similar to that of heart failure and includes beta-adrenergic blocker therapy, ACEIs/ARBs, ARNIs, diuretics and antiarrhythmic therapy where indicated or, if necessary, an ICD for recurrent haemodynamically significant ventricular arrhythmias.[98] The use of CRT has produced significant clinical improvements and is recommended for DCM patients with NYHA functional class II–III or ambulatory class IV, optimal medical therapy, LVEF <35% and sinus rhythm with LBBB with a QRS >150 ms.[70] Cardiac transplantation is considered when standard therapies fail to influence clinical progression and left ventricular assist devices and ICDs may be used as a bridge to transplantation.

Hypertrophic cardiomyopathy

Hypertrophic cardiomyopathy (HCM) is a genetic abnormality that gives rise to inappropriate hypertrophy especially in the intraventricular septum with preserved or hyperdynamic systolic function. The main abnormality with HCM is diastolic rather than systolic as in DCM. The hypertrophy is not a compensatory response to excessive load, such as in aortic stenosis or hypertension. Left ventricular hypertrophy of variable patterns is seen, occasionally with disproportionate septal hypertrophy, which causes left ventricular outflow tract obstruction in which HCM progresses to hypertrophic obstructive cardiomyopathy (HOCM). In HCM the muscle mass is large and hypercontractile, but the left ventricular cavity is small. The increase in left ventricular systolic pressure and the altered relaxation cause diastolic dysfunction and impaired ventricular filling. Mitral regurgitation is common. These abnormalities combine to produce pulmonary congestion and dyspnoea due to raised end-diastolic pressure. Sudden cardiac death, often after exertion or other increases in contractility, is sometimes seen in HCM and is thought to be partly attributable to outflow obstruction.[71] It is the most common cause of death in athletes.[71]

Diagnosis

Echocardiography will confirm the presence and pattern of hypertrophy and the presence (or absence) of an outflow tract gradient. Examination findings include cardiomegaly and pulmonary congestion. An S4 heart sound is common, and the ECG shows left ventricular hypertrophy and often ventricular arrhythmias. When the obstructive form hypertrophic obstructive cardiomyopathy (HOCM) is present, a systolic murmur, mitral regurgitation murmur and deep narrow Q waves on ECG may be present.[98] The majority of patients are asymptomatic and, when they present to hospital, it will be with severe symptoms of dyspnoea, angina and syncope. Angina is the result of an imbalance between oxygen supply and demand due to the increased myocardial mass and not due to atherosclerosis.

Patient management

Treatment for HCM is aimed at the prevention of sudden cardiac death and pharmacotherapy to increase diastolic filling and to reduce the left ventricular outflow tract obstruction. Pharmacotherapy includes beta-adrenergic blocker or calcium channel blocker therapy, as these decrease contractility and lessen outflow tract obstruction. Care is necessary with medication selection, as vasodilation may worsen obstruction, causing haemodynamics to suffer.[98] The impact of atrial fibrillation, by worsening the ventricular filling defect, can be dramatic in HCM patients and will require antiarrhythmics and anticoagulation. If ventricular arrhythmias are present, or there is a family history of sudden cardiac death, treatment with an ICD should be considered.[98] For severely symptomatic patients or those worsening despite maximal drug treatment, surgical myectomy to reduce the size of the septum and lessen obstruction may be necessary and can result in a marked improvement of symptoms.[99] Septal ablation with alcohol injected into the first septal branch of the LAD artery is a less invasive alternative, a procedure that is usually undertaken with pacemaker insertion as AV block is produced. Although surgical myectomy remains the gold standard, both treatments provide effective symptom relief and improvement in heart failure severity.[99] If the patient with HCM deteriorates and is hospitalised, positive inotropes, chronotropes and nitrates worsen left ventricular outflow tract obstruction and should be avoided. However, beta-adrenergic blockers, amiodarone and calcium antagonists such as verapamil are indicated.[98] Due to the familial nature of HCM, relatives aged 12–18 years also need to be screened for HCM.

Restrictive cardiomyopathy

Restrictive cardiomyopathies (RCMs) limit diastolic distensibility or compliance of the ventricles. The stiff ventricular walls produce diastolic dysfunction and there is impaired ventricular filling. Infiltrates into the interstitium and the replacement of normal myocardium with abnormal tissue hamper this relaxation.[98] Initially, systolic function and wall thickness are normal. However, as the disease progresses systolic dysfunction occurs. RCM is commonly caused by myocardial infiltration, as in amyloidosis, sarcoidosis, fibrosis or cardiac metastases, or may be idiopathic. Endomyocardial disease is more common in tropical countries, but in the Western world, RCMs are the least common form of cardiomyopathy.[98]

Diagnosis

Clinically, heart failure (increase in JVP, dyspnoea, S3 and S4 heart sounds and oedema), particularly right ventricular, and infiltration of the conduction system may cause conduction defects and heart block. Low-voltage ECGs are commonly seen. Patients commonly present with decreased exercise tolerance due to the impaired ability to increase heart rate and cardiac output because of reduced ventricular filling. RCM must be distinguished from constrictive pericarditis (which it may closely resemble), as pericarditis may be easily managed. If echocardiography demonstrates a restrictive pattern, a myocardial biopsy may be undertaken to determine its aetiology, especially in the case of systemic infiltrative disease.

Patient management

There is no treatment for RCM so the aim of therapy is to relieve symptoms. This includes diuretics, corticosteroids and pacing. The use of nitrates should be initiated with caution as the filling defect can be worsened by decreased venous return or hypovolaemia. Generally, prognosis is poor with many dying within 1–2 years of diagnosis.[98]

Hypertensive emergencies

Acute, uncontrolled hypertension is often divided into two categories: hypertensive emergencies and hypertensive urgencies. In hypertensive emergencies blood pressure needs to be reduced within 1 hour to prevent end-organ damage, such as hypertensive encephalopathy, papilloedema or aortic dissection.[100] Immediate blood pressure reduction with IV agents under critical care monitoring is needed. By contrast, hypertensive urgencies are those in which end-organ damage is not occurring and, although prompt management is required, this can be approached more gradually with oral antihypertensive agents under close supervision, without necessarily requiring admission to a critical care unit. Previous hypertension is not always present, but because of chronic adaptive vascular changes may provide some level of protection against acute tissue injury. Symptoms may not develop until the blood pressure exceeds 220/110 mmHg, whereas in patients without previous hypertension, hypertensive emergencies may occur at levels of even 160/100 mmHg.[101] When the diastolic pressure is persistently above 130 mmHg, there is risk of vascular damage and it must be treated.

Diagnosis

A thorough history is taken, including any hypertension management, known renal or cerebrovascular disease, eclampsia in previous pregnancies if gravid or use of stimulants or illicit drugs such as cocaine. Patient assessment should include evidence of: end-organ damage, such as back pain (aortic dissection); neurological damage, such as headache, altered consciousness, confusion, visual loss, stupor or seizure activity (encephalopathy); cardiac damage, such as chest pain, ST-segment changes, cardiac enlargement or the development of heart failure or pulmonary oedema; and renal damage, such as oliguria and azotaemia.[101] Serum urea, creatinine, electrolytes, urinalysis, ECG and chest X-ray should be performed.

Patient management

More severe, or malignant, hypertension may cause retinal haemorrhage or papilloedema, and emergency treatment should immediately be instituted. Other contexts in which there is a need for rapid treatment of severe hypertension include intracranial bleeding, AMI, phaeochromocytoma, recovery from cardiac surgery and bleeding from vascular procedure sites. Hypertensive emergencies in pregnancy threaten both the mother and the fetus.[102]

The aim of treatment is to acutely lower the blood pressure, but neither too quickly nor too dramatically. Recommendations vary, but an initial aim of 150/110–160/100 mmHg within 2–6 hours, or a 25% reduction in mean arterial pressure within 2 hours, has been described.[103,104] Continuous direct arterial pressure monitoring should be in place during treatment. Intravenous sodium nitroprusside, a rapidly acting arterial and venous dilator, is most frequently used, at doses of 0.25–10 mcg/kg/min.[104] Weaning of nitroprusside is undertaken after the later introduction of oral antihypertensives. Care is required to avoid hypotension during treatment, as well as rebound hypertension as nitroprusside is withdrawn. Rapidly acting beta-adrenergic blocking agents with short half-lives, such as IV esmolol, may be used at doses of 50–100 mcg/kg/min (or higher) in patients without standard contraindications to beta-adrenergic blockers (asthma, heart failure).[104] Glyceryl trinitrate infusions at 10–100 mcg/min or higher are used for combined venous and arterial dilation, especially if there is angina.[104] Intravenous frusemide may be introduced during the acute phase. After intravenous therapies have been established and progress towards target pressures is made, oral agents are introduced. These include oral beta-adrenergic blockers, calcium channel blockers, ACEIs and diuretics.

Infective endocarditis

Infective endocarditis (IE) remains a potentially life-threatening disorder. Despite improvements in the management of IE it is still associated with high mortality and severe complications.[105] Infective endocarditis is no longer isolated to the native valve and may include an infection of any structure within the heart e.g. prosthetic valves, implanted devices and chordae tendineae.[106] The development of endocarditis has been observed, with factors such as longer life, IV drug use, prosthetic valves, greater rates of cannulation during hospitalisation, cardiac surgery, resistant organisms and increased numbers of immunocompromised patients from immunosuppressant drugs and human immunodeficiency virus/acquired immune deficiency syndrome HIV/AIDS.[106,107]

Infection of the endocardium, often with involvement of the cardiac valves, occurs most commonly due to staphylococcal, streptococcal, enterococcal and HAECK (*Haemophilus parainfluenzae*, *H. aphrophilus*, *H. paraphrophilus*, *H. influenzae*, *Actinobacillus actinomycetemcomitans*, *Cardiobacterium hominis*, *Eikenella corrodens*, *Kingella kingae* and *K. denitrificans*) organisms.[107,108] IE can be acute or subacute. Acute IE progresses over days to weeks with destruction of valves and metastatic infection. Subacute

IE occurs over weeks to months and is milder than acute IE. Endothelial damage occurs in the endocardium. Platelet-fibrin deposits form and a lesion develops. Bacterial colonisation then occurs and vegetation adheres to the endocardial lesion. Many of the signs and symptoms of IE are due to the immune response to the microorganism. The patient presents with fever, and general features of febrile illness, which may include septic shock. Joint pain is common and septic arthritis is sometimes seen. Cardiac symptoms develop when there is valvular involvement, which may manifest as erosion through valve leaflets producing regurgitation, fusing of valve leaflets or vegetations (outgrowths from valve structures), producing valvular stenosis or regurgitation.[109]The mitral valve is more commonly affected, but aortic valve involvement carries a worse prognosis.[105,107] Conduction system involvement manifests as arrhythmias and conduction defects. Embolic complications are relatively common and multifactorial. Septic emboli, embolisation of atrial thrombi when atrial fibrillation is present and fragmentation of vegetations may all give rise to pulmonary and systemic emboli. These most often present as splenic infarction, stroke, peripheral vascular occlusion and renal failure.[105]

Diagnosis

Diagnosis of IE is based on the modified Duke criteria, echocardiography (transthoracic or transoesophageal) alongside clinical judgement.[105,106] These are based on the presence of microorganisms (identified in blood cultures), pathological lesions (vegetation or abscess present) and clinical criteria. The clinical criteria are based on two major criteria, or one major and three minor criteria, or five minor criteria. Major clinical criteria are:

- positive blood culture
- evidence of endocardial involvement (positive echocardiography, abscess, partial dehiscence of a prosthetic valve or new valvular vegetation).

Minor clinical criteria include:

- fever with body temperature >38°C
- predisposing heart condition or intravenous drug use
- vascular signs: arterial emboli, intracranial haemorrhage, Janeway lesions (erythematous spots on the palms and feet) or conjunctival haemorrhages
- immunological signs: Osler nodes (painful, reddened nodules on the fingers and the feet) or glomerulonephritis.[107]

Echocardiography may reveal vegetations, abscess and valvular abnormalities, but endocarditis is more a clinical diagnosis based on the appearance of febrile illness, positive blood cultures with organisms known to cause endocarditis, new murmur and vascular features. Positive blood cultures remain central to the diagnosis. At least three sets are taken at 30-min intervals, each containing 10 mL of blood which should be obtained from a peripheral vein rather than from a central venous catheter (because of the risk of contamination and misleading interpretation), using a meticulous sterile technique. Once the causative microorganism has been identified, blood cultures should be repeated after 48–72 hours to check the effectiveness of treatment.[105]

Patient management

Prosthetic valve endocarditis must be aggressively managed, as mortality may be high.[105] Current guidelines recommend a multidisciplinary team-based approach to improve outcomes.[110] This use of this team-based approach, which included standardised medical therapy, recommended surgical interventions and close follow-up for 1 year significantly reduced the 1-year mortality, from 18.5% to 8.2%.[111] Approximately 40–50% of patients undergo cardiac surgery during hospitalisation.[111]

During their hospitalisation close observation is required to identify and manage any infection-related complications (e.g. perivalvular abscesses, progressive HF, septic emboli and stroke). HF is the most frequent complication of IE (42–60% of cases) and one of the most frequent reasons for surgery. It is associated with new or worsening regurgitation, more often in the aortic rather than the mitral valve, and less commonly due to intracardiac fistulae. Valve obstruction, although more rare, may also lead to HF (see section, Acute exacerbations of heart failure). Due to the febrile illness it is important not to overlook hydration and dietary status. Uncontrolled infection as the second commonest indication for surgical intervention although optimal timing for this remains unclear. Due to the observation that persistently positive blood cultures 48–72 hours after initiation of antibiotics are an independent risk factor for hospital mortality suggests that surgery should be considered at this time after the exclusion of other causes of persistent positive blood cultures.[105] The aim of surgery is the total removal of infected tissues and repair or replacement of the affected valve(s).

Antibiotic therapy is provided empirically until blood culture and sensitivities are established after which specific therapy will be delivered. The first 2 weeks of inpatient therapy is often considered as the critical phase with the option to consider outpatient antibiotic therapy beyond this point.

Prophylactic antibiotic coverage should be undertaken for at-risk patients 1 hour before dental procedures are to be performed, in particular for those with previous rheumatic fever or endocarditis, or prosthetic valves.[105] Antibiotic prophylaxis for genitourinary and gastrointestinal procedures is no longer recommended.[105]

Patients who have suffered from IE remain at high risk of relapse and reoccurrence risk (2–6%) and therefore they and their families need to be aware of the importance of obtaining blood cultures (× 3) if they develop a fever before taking any antibiotics. If blood stream infection is confirmed as the cause, then re-evaluation for possible IE is required. Regular clinic review within the first year is recommended with blood sampling where infection may be suspected and reinforcement of the principles of IE prevention at each follow-up visit. Echocardiography should be performed at the completion of antimicrobial therapy and repeated at intervals, particularly during the first year of follow-up to monitor the development of secondary HF. Good oral health maintenance, preventive dentistry and advice about skin hygiene, including tattoos and skin piercing, are mandatory.

Aortic aneurysm

The aorta is the major blood vessel leaving the heart. An aneurysm is a local dilation or outpouching of a vessel wall and comes in several forms (Fig. 10.14).[28] Most aortic aneurysms are fusiform and saccular, and occur in the abdominal aorta creating an increase in aortic diameter to 3 cm or more. A fusiform aneurysm is uniform in shape with symmetrical dilation that involves the whole circumference of the aorta.[111] A saccular aneurysm has dilation of part of the aortic wall so the dilation is very localised.[111] A dissecting aneurysm occurs when the layers of the wall of the aorta continue to separate and fill with blood, resulting in obstructed blood flow. The aorta is particularly susceptible to aneurysm formation because of constant stress on the vessel wall and the absence of penetrating vasa vasorum that normally provide perfusion to the adventitia. As the blood flows through the aneurysm it becomes turbulent and some blood may stagnate along the walls, allowing a thrombus to form. This thrombus in addition to atherosclerotic debris may embolise into the distal arteries compromising their circulation. Atherosclerosis is the most common cause of aneurysm, because plaque formation erodes the vessel wall.[112] Other causes include syphilis, infection, inflammatory diseases and trauma. Aneurysms occur most often in men and in people with the risk factors of hypertension or smoking. Approximately 80% of aortic aneurysms rupture into the left retroperitoneum, which may contain the rupture. However, the other 20% rupture into the peritoneal cavity and uncontrolled haemorrhage results.[112]

Patients often experience no symptoms until the aneurysm is extensive or ruptures. Clinical presentation varies and depends on the location and expansion rate. Aneurysms of the ascending aorta tend to affect the aortic root and cause valve regurgitation. Expansion of the aneurysm may also compress the vena cavae, leading to engorged neck and superficial veins, or compress the large airways, causing respiratory distress. The first symptom most patients experience is pain, which may be steady and continuous from local compression or sudden and severe in the case of dissection or rupture, usually in the lower back. In this case, the pain is usually associated with syncope and is an acute emergency. Depending on the site of the aneurysm, there is usually an absence or decrease in the pulses below the site of the aneurysm, most commonly in the limbs. The renal arteries may be affected, resulting in decreased urine output and renal failure. The spinal blood flow may also be affected, resulting in paraplegia and, if the carotid arteries are affected, there may be altered consciousness. Infrarenal aneurysms are the most common form of aortic aneurysm and are located below the renal arteries. Bruits can also be heard over the aneurysm.

FIGURE 10.14 Aneurysm. Major types of aneurysm: (**A**) fusiform aneurysm has an entire section of an artery dilated, occurring most often in the abdominal aorta due to atherosclerosis; (**B**) sacculated aneurysm affects one side of an artery, usually in the ascending aorta; (**C**) dissecting aneurysm results from a tear in the intima, causing blood to shunt between the intima and media; (**D**) pseudoaneurysm usually results from arterial trauma, such as intra-aortic balloon pump catheter or an arterial introducer; the opening does not heal properly and is covered by a clot that can burst at any time.[28]

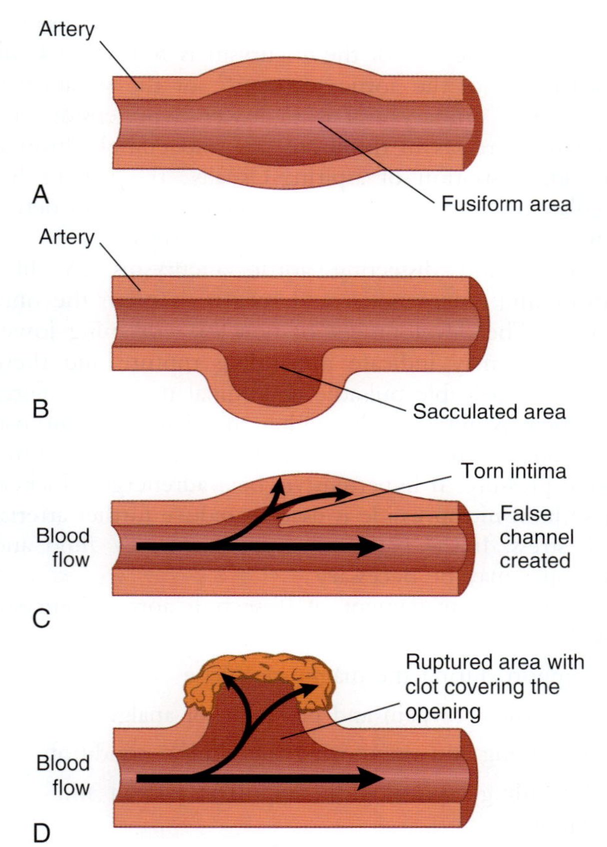

Source: Fibrinolytic Therapy Trialists' Collaborative Group. Indications for fibrinolytic therapy in suspected acute myocardial infarction: collaborative overview of early mortality and major morbidity results from all randomised trials of more than 1000 patients. The Lancet 1994;343(8893):311–22.

Diagnosis

A chest X-ray is usually the first investigation and may reveal a widened mediastinum or enlarged aortic knob.

Some aneurysms will be hidden, so normal chest X-ray does not exclude the diagnosis. If available, a CT scan using contrast dye provides accurate information on the location and size of the aneurysm. Transoesophageal echocardiography (TOE) provides an accurate diagnosis and is the preferred investigation in dissecting aneurysms. TOE can clearly identify the tear/flap, to enable classification of the aneurysm. There are some limitations in viewing the ascending aorta, and patients with respiratory dysfunction may have difficulty with lying flat for the procedure and having a light anaesthetic.

Patient management

Management of asymptomatic aneurysms is conservative, unless the size of the aneurysm is > 1.5 times the normal size of the aortic segment[103] or the situation is acute. The primary aim is to lower hypertension and prevent increases in thrombus size and emboli through the administration of aspirin. Usually, the patient has regular monitoring to assess the aneurysm and to determine the timing and need for surgical repair.

Acute and dissecting aortic aneurysms are life-threatening emergencies, and surgery is often the only option. The development of new or worsening lower back pain may indicate impending rupture and there may be a palpable pulsatile abdominal mass. The faster treatment is initiated, the higher the chances of survival with optimal recovery. The primary goal is to control blood pressure. If hypertensive, beta-adrenergic blockers or sodium nitroprusside is used to reduce further arterial wall stress. If the patient is hypotensive, IV fluid and inotropes may be necessary.

Nursing management of dissecting aortic aneurysm involves the following:

- support during the diagnostic phase
- assessment of pain and provision of analgesia
- stabilising and monitoring the clinical condition
- providing psychological support to patient and family
- preparation for surgery and long-term care.

Assessment of the patient's symptoms and effects of the aneurysm is essential. This includes careful assessment and recording of symptoms, including pain level and intensity, peripheral pulses, oxygen saturation levels, blood pressure in both arms and neurological symptoms to assist with diagnosis and detect progression. Intravenous analgesia is essential to control the severe pain, and an antiemetic is useful to prevent opiate side effects. Opiates may also contribute to a sedative effect and slight vasodilation, which are both beneficial. Oxygen therapy via mask should be administered as indicated by oxygen saturation levels. Blood pressure control is vital, and usually IV medications are titrated to a narrow mean arterial pressure (MAP) range of 60–75 mmHg. Close observation of fluid balance to detect changes in renal perfusion and maintain appropriate blood volume is also essential. Finally, preparation for surgery is necessary, and must include the patient and family.

Ventricular aneurysm

Less than 5% of patients post-STEMI, particularly a transmural anterior infarction, develop a left ventricular aneurysm.[109] Post-STEMI, dyskinetic or akinetic areas of the left ventricle are common and known as regional wall motion abnormalities. It is in these areas that there is a risk of an aneurysm developing. Ventricular aneurysms are more likely to develop post-anterior STEMI with a totally occluded LAD with poor collateral circulation.

Aneurysms form when the intraventricular tension stretches the dyskinetic area and a thin, weak layer of necrotic muscle and fibrous tissue develops and bulges with each contraction of the ventricle resulting in a reduction in stroke volume. Aneurysms range from 1–8 cm in diameter and are four times more likely to occur at the apex and anterior wall rather than the inferoposterior wall.[109] Large ventricular aneurysms may result in a reduction in stroke volume causing an increase in myocardial oxygen demand resulting in angina and heart failure. The mortality rate in people with ventricular aneurysms is four times higher than those with no aneurysm due to a higher risk of tachyarrhythmias and sudden cardiac death. Unlike aortic aneurysms these aneurysms rarely rupture so their management is usually conservative.

Diagnosis

Diagnosis of a ventricular aneurysm is by echocardiography. Ventricular aneurysm should be considered when ST-segment elevation persists beyond 1 week after MI.

Patient management

Management of a left ventricular aneurysm consists of aggressive management of STEMI and reperfusion therapy. Long-term anticoagulation therapy with warfarin is required. A complication of a ventricular aneurysm includes the development of an intraventricular thrombus within the aneurysmal pocket which, if mobilised, becomes arterial emboli. Also due to the high risk of tachyarrhythmias, antiarrhythmic therapy is indicated. An ICD may also be necessary if antiarrhythmic therapy is unsuccessful in suppressing tachyarrhythmias. Surgical aneurysmectomy may also be required, if heart failure and angina become severe, and is usually successful.

Summary

Compromise of the cardiovascular system, as either a primary or secondary condition, is a common problem that necessitates admission of patients to a critical care area. Prompt and appropriate assessment and treatment are required to ensure adequate oxygen supply to the tissues throughout the body. The most common cardiovascular problems experienced by patients include CHD, arrhythmias and cardiogenic shock; however, heart failure and selected conditions such as cardiomyopathies, hypertensive emergencies, endocarditis and aortic aneurysm also occur. Appropriate assessment and management are essential to prevent secondary complications arising. Important principles covered in this chapter are summarised below.

- CHD:
  - Incorporates myocardial ischaemia, angina and ACS.
  - Early patient assessment and diagnosis are essential to facilitate prompt intervention.
  - Initial diagnosis is based on history, clinical assessment, electrocardiographic and biochemical examination, with coronary angiography, exercise testing and chest radiography available to provide later detail.
  - Early restoration of blood flow – including reperfusion therapy and coronary angioplasty – to reduce myocardial damage is a core component of treatment.
  - Other goals of care include reducing plaque and clot formation in coronary arteries, reducing the workload of the heart, controlling symptoms, providing psychosocial support to the patient and family and educating the patient about the disease process, lifestyle and future responses to illness.
- Heart failure:
  - May affect either the left, right or both ventricles, resulting in different signs and symptoms.
  - Diagnosis is usually made on the basis of echocardiography, ECG, and chest X-ray.
  - In acute heart failure, CPAP or BiPAP may be necessary to improve hypoxaemia.
  - Pharmacological therapy of acute heart failure consists of beta-adrenergic blockers, ACEIs/ARNIs/ARBs, MRAs and diuretics. Inotropes may also be used, such as low dose dopamine and dobutamine, to improve renal perfusion and contractility.
  - Many patients with heart failure will also have a pacemaker with CRT and/or a defibrillator to improve cardiac function and reduce the incidence of sudden death.
  - Patient care must be lifelong and coordinated between all members of the healthcare team. Broad interventions, including medications, diet and lifestyle modification, may be appropriate for some patients, while palliative care might be more appropriate for other patients.

Case study

Mr Aran Blackmore, a 52-year-old man presented to the emergency department (ED) with a 2-month history of a dry cough, 2 weeks of increasing shortness of breath on exertion (SOBOE), orthopnoea and paroxysmal nocturnal dyspnoea (PND) and a 1-week history of increasing abdominal pain/discomfort. For the past 2 weeks he has had to sleep sitting up, which is unusual for him. During the past week Mr Blackmore has been experiencing difficulty in carrying out tasks at work. He works full-time as a furniture removalist. He has not experienced any chest pain or peripheral oedema. Due to his abdominal pain, he has had a decreased appetite and lost 10 kg over the past few weeks. He has a long history as a heavy smoker but no COPD. He has no medical comorbidities and is usually very fit, not overweight and takes no medications.

A CXR was done in ED which showed cardiomegaly and congestion. He underwent testing for pulmonary embolism (PE): D-dimer was 557. CTPA showed bilateral pleural effusions suggestive of acute heart failure (AHF). He was afebrile, pulse 113 beats/min and regular, respiratory rate of 22 beats/min, blood pressure 106/75 and oxygen saturation was 96% on room air. NYHA functional class was IV (shortness of breath [SOB] at rest). His JVP was +2 and he had no peripheral oedema. He had dual heart sounds (S1, S2) and a third heart sound (S3). U&E blood test results included: Na 140 mmol/L; K 5.1 mmol/L; urea 5.4 mmol/L; creatinine 72 umol/L; eGFR>90; and albumin 33 g/L. LFTs were abnormal: ALP 97 U/L; ALT 77 U/L; GGT 70 U/L; AST 47 ng/L, which was due to hepatic congestion. Other pathology included: CRP 10.4 mg/L; NTproBNP 9,981 ng/L; and hsTroponinT 20 ng/L. An ECG was taken in the ED (Fig. 10.15).

FIGURE 10.15 Case study – Mr AB's ECG on presentation to ED.

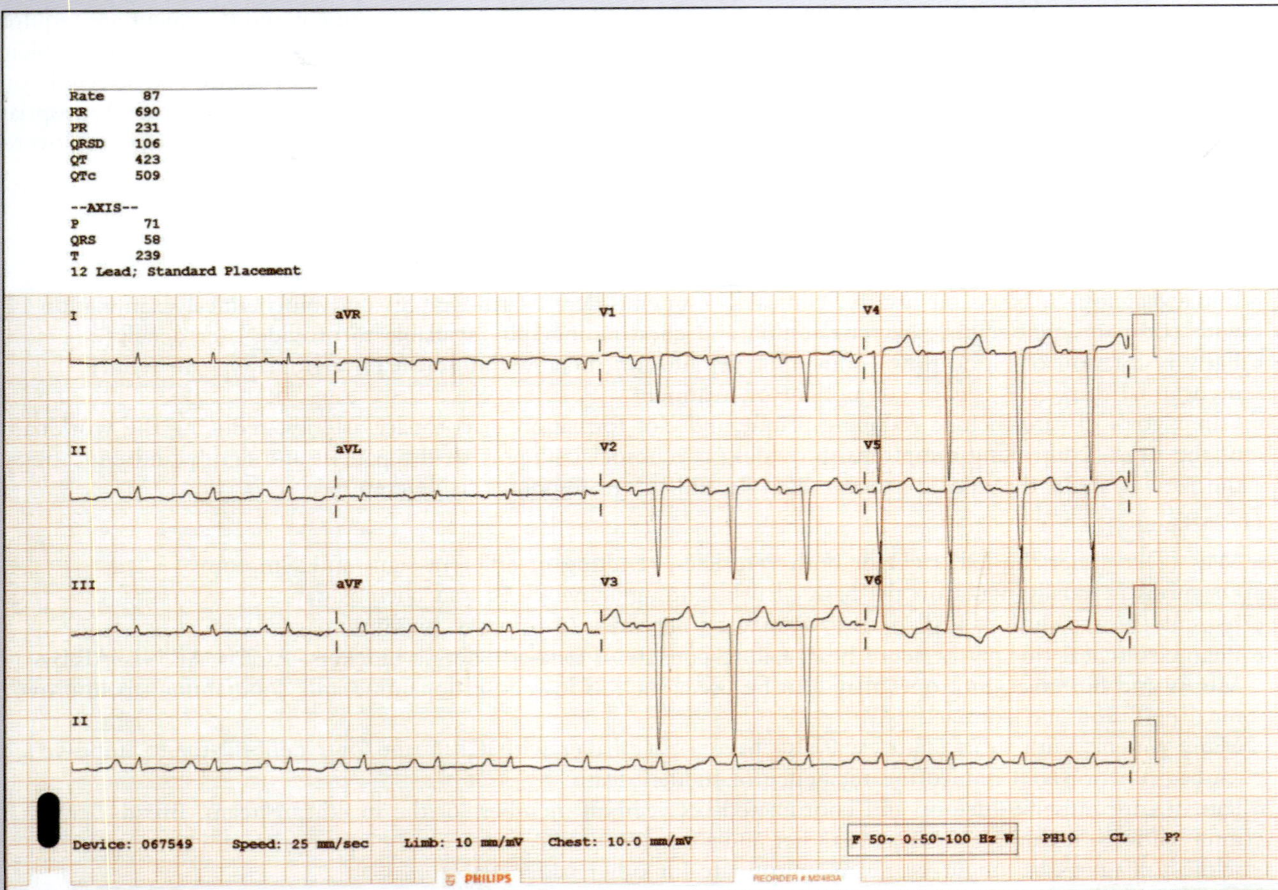

In ED Mr Blackmore was prescribed frusemide 80 mg IV and transferred to ward for further diuresis. During his inpatient stay, Mr Blackmore had an echocardiography which showed severely dilated left ventricle with severe left ventricular and moderate right ventricular systolic dysfunction with a LVEF of 9% and e/e ratio of 21%. An e/e >15% is indicative diastolic dysfunction. Moderately enlarged left atrium, mildly enlarged right atrium and mild to moderate mitral regurgitation were identified. He underwent investigation for the primary cause of his dilated cardiomyopathy but these did not reveal a cause. Coronary angiogram showed only minor diffuse coronary disease. The primary cause was thought to be viral cardiomyopathy.

During his hospital stay Mr Blackmore was gradually commenced on the gold standard pharmacotherapy for heart failure: beta-adrenergic blocker, ACEI, loop diuretic and aldosterone antagonist. IV frusemide was switched to oral; however, he subsequently developed fluid overload. Due to difficulties with ongoing fluid management, he was commenced on a frusemide IV infusion at 18 mg/h and transferred to CCU for ongoing monitoring. A good diuresis was achieved with weight loss. During his hospital stay Mr Blackmore lost a total of 10 kg of weight. This equates to 10 L of additional fluid in his body, most likely around his abdomen.

During his stay in CCU, Mr Blackmore's dose of beta-adrenergic blocker was increased. However, he showed further signs of decompensated heart failure – blood pressure fell to 85/50 with symptoms of dizziness and pulse of 52 beats/min. His beta-adrenergic blocker was ceased and he was closely monitored for further signs of decompensation which may have necessitated IV inotropes and/or temporary pacing. Due to his persistent fluid overload, IV fluid boluses were unable to be given to increase his blood pressure. Several attempts were made to increase the dose of Mr Blackmore's carvedilol during his hospitalisation. However, they were unsuccessful due to his decompensation of low blood pressure, difficulties in achieving euvolaemia and poor tolerance of beta-adrenergic blockers. The plan was to increase the dose of his beta-adrenergic blocker in outpatients once he was euvolaemic.

Mr Blackmore's remaining hospitalisation was uneventful. He was transferred to the ward and then a few days later discharged home. His fluids were restricted to 1.5 L/day, and he was weighed daily. Education was provided to him and his family about the diagnosis of heart failure, prognosis and management of his heart failure at home. Mr Blackmore was also informed that he was unable to drive his furniture removalist truck due to his LVEF being less than 40%. This is based on the Australian Traffic Authority Commission heavy vehicle driving conditions. Mr Blackmore's LVEF was 9%. On discharge his medications were: carvedilol 3.25 mg BD, ramipril 2.5 mg daily, spironolactone 12.5 mg daily, and frusemide 40 mg mane. Once he has recovered from his hospitalisation and his ramipril is at 5 mg mane, he will be changed over to Entresto 24/26 mg BD. He was also referred to a heart failure management program and to be seen in heart failure clinic within 2 weeks of discharge.

CASE STUDY QUESTIONS

1 What are the signs and symptoms related to right ventricular failure?
2 What is your interpretation of the 12-lead ECG in Figure 10.15?
3 Why was it important to determine the aetiology of Mr Blackmore's heart failure?
4 What is the significance of an S3 heart sound in the clinical setting of heart failure?
5 During Mr Blackmore's early stay in hospital, why was oral frusemide unsuccessful in maintaining a diuresis?
6 When Mr Blackmore was discharged from hospital, why was he prescribed carvedilol, ramipril, spironolactone and frusemide? Include in your answer the reason for prescribing these medications and their actions and major side effects.

RESEARCH VIGNETTE

Ayton DR, Barker AL, Peeters GME, et al. Exploring patient-reported outcomes following percutaneous coronary intervention: a qualitative study. Health Expectations 2018;21(2):457–65.

Abstract

Background: Percutaneous coronary intervention (PCI) is a common cardiac procedure used to treat obstructive coronary artery disease. Patient-centred care is a priority in cardiovascular health having been shown to increase patient satisfaction, engagement with rehabilitation activities and reduce anxiety. Evidence indicates that patient-centred care is best achieved by routine collection of patient-reported outcomes (PROs). However, existing patient-reported outcome measures (PROMs) have limited the patient involvement in their development.

Aims: To identify and explore outcomes, patients perceive as important following PCI.

Methods: A qualitative design was adopted. Eight focus groups and five semi-structured interviews were conducted with 32 patients who had undergone PCI in the previous 6 months. Outcomes were identified and mapped under the US Food and Drug Administration (FDA) PROs domains of feeling (physical and psychological outcomes), function and evaluation. Inductive and deductive analysis methods were used with open, axial and thematic coding.

Results: Consistent with prior studies, patients identified feeling and function outcomes such as reductions in physical and psychological symptoms and the ability to perform usual activities as important. Participants also identified a range of new outcomes, including confidence to return to usual activities and evaluation domain such as adverse effects of medications and the importance of patient communication.

Conclusion: The findings of this research should be considered in the design of a cardiac PROM for PCI patients. A PROM which adequately assesses these outcomes can provide clinicians and hospital staff with a foundation in which to address these concerns or symptoms.

Critique

The aim of this qualitative study was to explore the outcomes that patients perceived as important following PCI, a common procedure in the treatment of cardiac patients with stable angina and also with ACS. Within this study, however, it is not known whether the participants received PCI as an elective (for stable angina) or emergency (acute coronary syndrome) procedure, which may have influenced their experiences and subsequent recovery. The chosen qualitative methodology is appropriate to meet the aim of exploring the subjective experiences of cardiac patients. In conducting the study, data were collected from 32 participants across four hospital sites; five of these were through individual interviews and 27 took part in one of eight focus groups. There is limited information on the recruitment process with no detail of sample stratification criteria (e.g. age gender, education level, PCI centre etc.) to ensure diversity of participants, nor how individuals were selected or allocated to either the focus group or individual interview. Details of the number of participants within each focus group was also absent; however, since eight groups were completed this suggests suboptimal numbers to gain the intended benefits of focus group discussion and interaction. It is not clear whether ethical approval was obtained nor how and when informed consent was obtained. Although information is provided about the time period of recruitment, the time period and duration of the focus groups and interviews is absent.

Interviews were audio recorded, transcribed verbatim and analysed using inductive and deductive coding methods. Emergent themes were mapped against 3 FDA PROs domains of: 1) feeling (physical and psychological outcomes); 2) function which often related to their ability to fulfil their normal supportive roles in within their family unit; and 3) evaluation which related to their perceived success of the procedure and engagement in rehabilitation and recovery strategies. Analysis of data by two independent researchers and presentation of themes to all authors for feedback enhances rigour; however, they do not elaborate on whether the transcripts or interpretation were returned to participants to verify accuracy of transcriptions and analysis.

The authors acknowledge a number of limitations in their study including the potential differences in recovery associated with different clinical presentations, the need to consider further the experience of emergency versus elective PCI. The low response rate of 8% was also acknowledged; there was little discussion of strategies to mitigate against this poor response such as reminders, or the influence of those actually approaching participants for consent (e.g. insurers). Similarly, there is an absence of details related to the distribution of participants across the four hospital sites, nor any information on any similarities or differences in these centres. Although the authors report that 34 patients were ineligible to take part due to the timing of their PCI, the rationale for this is unclear, particularly given that they met the original eligibility criteria. Mapping the emergent data against the FDA PRO domains is a strength of this work. While sample bias has been acknowledged, the authors could also have commented on the high number of participants in rehabilitation, which may reflect a sample bias with those already motivated to positively change their lifestyle. A particular strength of this work has been their ability to develop, refine and validate a 5-item PROM to assess these issues that matter to patients in their recovery after PCI thus supporting person-centred care delivery. This paper provides an interesting insight into issues that are relevant and important to patients through their recovery following PCI.

Learning activities

1 Follow two ACS patient journeys, one each for patient presenting with either a STEMI or NSTEMI, consider their immediate management and longer term care needs. Compare and contrast the patient experiences from the two pathways.

2 Examine the 12-lead ECG of a patient with ACS, and identify the key features of this ECG in relation to STEMI or non-STEMI. Compare this to the features of a normal ECG.

3 Discuss the compensatory mechanisms that are activated in heart failure and their effects on the cardiovascular system.

4 Discuss the gold standard pharmacotherapy for patients with HF*r*EF. Relate the action of each group to their effect on the pathophysiological compensatory mechanisms.

5 Analyse the ECG of a patient with heart failure. What are the electrocardiographcal features of left and/or right ventricular hypertrophy? Why do these changes occur in terms of the electrophysiological pathway?

6 Observe an echocardiograph and ask the sonographer to explain what is visualised on the screen, particularly in Doppler mode. Ask them to identify areas of valvular dysfunction and any evidence of dyssynchrony between the ventricles.

Online resources

American Heart Association, www.heart.org/HEARTORG/

Australian Institute of Health and Welfare, www.aihw.gov.au

British Heart Foundation, www.bhf.org.uk

Cardiac Society of Australia and New Zealand, www.csanz.edu.au

European Society of Cardiology, www.escardio.org

Heart Education Assessment and Rehabilitation Toolkit (HEART), www.heartonline.org.au

HEARTe. Chest Heart and Stroke Scotland (CHSS) educational resource, www.heartelearning.org

Heart failure matters, www.heartfailurematters.org

National Heart Foundation of Australia, www.heartfoundation.com.au

National Heart Foundation of New Zealand, www.heartfoundation.org.nz

Patient information on living with heart failure, www.heartfoundation.org.au/SiteCollectionDocuments/Living well with chronic heart failure.pdf

Further reading

Woods SL, Froelicher ESS, Motzer SU, et al, editors. Cardiac nursing. 6th ed. Baltimore: Lippincott, Williams & Wilkins; 2010.

Zipes DP, Libby P, Bonow RO, et al, editors. Braunwald's heart disease: a textbook of cardiovascular medicine. 10th ed. Philadelphia: Elsevier Saunders; 2014.

References

1. Benjamin EJ, Virani SS, Callaway CW, et al. Heart disease and stroke statistics – 2018 update: a report from the American Heart Association. Circulation 2018;137:e67–492.
2. World Health Organisation Cardiovascular disease fact sheet; Deaths from coronary heart disease. Online. Available from: http://www.who.int.
3. Lozano R, Naghavi M, Foreman K, et al. Global and regional mortality from 235 causes of death for 20 age groups in 1990 and 2010: a systematic analysis for the Global Burden of Disease Study 2010. Lancet 2012;380(9859):2095–128.
4. Australian Institute of Health and Welfare 2016. Australia's Health, Canberra.
5. Hall J. Guyton and Hall textbook of medical physiology. 13th ed. Philadelphia: Elsevier; 2016.
6. Timmis A. Acute coronary syndromes. BMJ 2015;351:h5849.
7. Rapsomaniki E, Shah A, Perel P, et al. Prognostic models for stable coronary artery disease based on electronic health record cohort of 102 023 patients. Eur Heart J 2014;35(13):844–52.
8. Thygesen K, Alpert JS, Jaffe AS, et al. Third universal definition of myocardial infarction. Eur Heart J 2012;33(20):2551–67.
9. Chew DP, Scott IA, Cullen L, et al. National Heart Foundation of Australia and Cardiac Society of Australia and New Zealand Australian clinical guidelines for the management of acute coronary syndromes. Med J Aust 2016;2016:128–33.
10. Chew D, Aroney C, Aylward P, et al. 2011 addendum to the Guidelines for the Management of Acute Coronary Syndromes 2006. Heart Lung Circ 2011;20:S111–12.

11. Noble A, Johnson R, Thomas A, et al. The cardiovascular system. Basic science and clinical conditions. 2nd ed. Edinburgh: Churchill Livingston; 2010.
12. Ibanez B, James S, Agewall S, et al. 2017 ESC guidelines for the management of acute myocardial infarction in patients presenting with ST-segment elevation. The Task Force for the Management of Acute Myocardial Infarction in Patients Presenting with ST-segment Elevation of the European Society of Cardiology (ESC). Eur Heart J 2018;39(2):119–77.
13. Nam J, Caners K, Bowen JM, et al. Systematic review and meta-analysis of the benefits of out-of-hospital 12-lead ECG and advance notification in ST-segment elevation myocardial infarction patients. Ann Emerg Med 2014;64(2):176–86, e9.
14. O'Donovan K. Nursing assessment of the causes of chest pain. Br J Cardiac Nurs 2013;8(10):483–8.
15. Chew DP, Scott IA, Cullen L, et al. National Heart Foundation of Australia & Cardiac Society of Australia and New Zealand: Australian clinical guidelines for the management of acute coronary syndromes. Heart Lung Circ 2016;25(9):895–951.
16. Scottish Intercollegiate Guidelines Network (SIGN). Acute coronary syndrome. Edinburgh: SIGN; 2016. Online. Available from: http://www.sign.ac.uk. April 2016 (SIGN publication no. 148).
17. McCance K. Structure and function of the cardiovascular and lymphatic systems, understanding pathophysiology. St Louis: Mosby; 2010.
18. Moliterno DJ, Sgarbossa EB, Armstrong PW, et al. A major dichotomy in unstable angina outcome: st depression versus t-wave inversion: GUST0-II Results. J Am Coll Cardiol 1996;27:(2 Suppl 1; Suppl A).
19. Reichlin T, Hochholzer W, Bassetti S, et al. Early diagnosis of myocardial infarction with sensitive cardiac troponin assays. N Engl J Med 2009;361(9):858–67.
20. Hamon M, Pristipino C, Di Mario C, et al. Consensus document on the radial approach in percutaneous cardiovascular interventions: position paper by the European Association of Percutaneous Cardiovascular Interventions and Working Groups on Acute Cardiac Care and Thrombosis of the European Society of Cardiology. EuroIntervention 2013;8(11):1242–51.
21. Scottish Intercollegiate Guidelines Network (SIGN). Management of stable angina. Edinburgh: SIGN; 2018. Online. Available from: http://www.sign.ac.uk. April 2018 (SIGN publication no. 151).
22. Williams MC, Hunter A, Shah ASV, et al. Use of coronary computed tomographic angiography to guide management of patients with coronary disease. J Am Coll Cardiol 2016;67(15):1759–68.
23. Cross E, Goodacre S. Patient satisfaction with chest pain unit care: findings from the Effectiveness and Safety of Chest Pain Assessment to Prevent Emergency Admissions (ESCAPE) cluster randomised trial. Emerg Med J 2010;27(10):774–8.
24. Tierney S, Cook G, Mamas M, et al. Nurses' role in the acute management of patients with non-ST-segment elevation acute coronary syndromes: an integrative review. Eur J Cardiovasc Nurs 2012;12(3):293–301.
25. Nakano A, Mainz J, Lomborg K. Patient perception and assessment of admission to acute cardiac care unit. Eur J Cardiovasc Nurs 2008;7(1):10–15.
26. Macdonald N, Jones J, Leslie SJ. Acute coronary syndromes – the role of the CCU nurse. Part I: initial management. Br J Cardiac Nurs 2016;11(9):453–8.
27. De Luca G, Biondi-Zoccai G, Marino P. Transferring patients with ST-segment elevation myocardial infarction for mechanical reperfusion: a meta-regression analysis of randomized trials. Ann Emerg Med 2008;52(6):665–76.
28. Fibrinolytic Therapy Trialists' Collaborative Group. Indications for fibrinolytic therapy in suspected acute myocardial infarction: collaborative overview of early mortality and major morbidity results from all randomised trials of more than 1000 patients. Lancet 1994;343(8893):311–22.
29. Guillermin A, Yan DJ, Perrier A, et al. Safety and efficacy of tenecteplase versus alteplase in acute coronary syndrome: a systematic review and meta-analysis of randomized trials. Arch Med Sci 2016;12(6):1181–7.
30. Investigators GUSTO. An international randomized trial comparing four thrombolytic strategies for acute myocardial infarction. N Engl J Med 1993;329(10):673–82.
31. Maron DJ, Spertus JA, Mancini GBJ, et al. Impact of an initial strategy of medical therapy without percutaneous coronary intervention in high-risk patients from the Clinical Outcomes Utilizing Revascularization and Aggressive DruG Evaluation (COURAGE) Trial. Am J Cardiol 2009;104(8):1055–62.
32. Siontis GCM, Stefanini GG, Mavridis D, et al. Percutaneous coronary interventional strategies for treatment of in-stent restenosis: a network meta-analysis. Lancet 2015;386(9994):655–64.
33. Zheng F, Xing S, Gong Z, et al. Five-year outcomes for first generation drug-eluting stents versus bare-metal stents in patients with st-segment elevation myocardial infarction: a meta-analysis of randomised controlled trials. Heart Lung Circ 2014;23(6):542–8.
34. Chevalier B. In-stent restenosis treatment: quest for the best device. Lancet 2015;386(9994):627–8.
35. Shoulders-Odom B. Management of patients after percutaneous coronary interventions. Crit Care Nurse 2008;28(5):26–41.
36. Schiks IEJM, Schoonhoven L, Aengevaeren WRM, et al. Ambulation after femoral sheath removal in percutaneous coronary intervention: a prospective comparison of early vs. late ambulation. J Clin Nurs 2009;8(13):1862–70.
37. Ferrante G, Rao SV, Jüni P, et al. Radial versus femoral access for coronary interventions across the entire spectrum of patients with coronary artery disease. JACC Cardiovasc Interv 2016;9(14):1419–34.
38. Trotter R, Gallagher R, Donoghue J. Anxiety in patients undergoing percutaneous coronary interventions. Heart Lung 2011;40(3):185–92.
39. Liljeroos M, Snellman IM, Ekstedt MH. A qualitative study on the role of patient-nurse communication in acute cardiac care. J Nurs Educ Pract 2011;1(1):17–24.

40. Cabello JB, Burls A, Emparanza JI, et al. Oxygen therapy for acute myocardial infarction. Cochrane Database Syst Rev 2013;(8): CD007160.
41. Jarvis S. Diagnosis, management and nursing care in acute coronary syndrome. Nurs Times 2017;113(3):31–5.
42. Task Force M, Montalescot G, Sechtem U, et al. 2013 ESC guidelines on the management of stable coronary artery disease. The Task Force on the Management of Stable Coronary Artery Disease of the European Society of Cardiology. Eur Heart J 2013;34(38):2949–3003.
43. Opie LH, Pfeffer MA. Inhibitors of angiotensin-converting enzyme, angiotesin II receptor, aldosterone and renin. In: Opie LH, Gersh BJ, editors. Drugs for the heart. 7th ed. Philadelphia: Saunders; 2009.
44. Jones DA, Rathod KS, Howard JP, et al. Safety and feasibility of hospital discharge 2 days following primary percutaneous intervention for ST-segment elevation myocardial infarction. Heart 2012;98:1722–7.
45. Furze G. Angina rehabilitation: exercise is not enough. Procedia-Social and Behavioral Sciences 2010;5:1545–9.
46. Long L, Anderson L, Dewhirst AM, et al. Exercise-based cardiac rehabilitation for adults with stable angina. Cochrane Database Syst Rev 2018;(2):CD012786.
47. McGuire DK. Diabetes and the Cardiovascular system. In: Mann DL, Zipes DP, Libby P, et al, editors. Braunwald's Heart disease: a textbook of cardiovascular medicine, vol. 2. Philadelphia: Elsevier Saunders; 2015. p. 1392.
48. Blumenthal JA, Feger BJ, Smith PJ, et al. Treatment of anxiety in patients with coronary heart disease: rationale and design of the UNderstanding the benefits of exercise and escitalopram in anxious patients WIth coroNary heart Disease (UNWIND) randomized clinical trial. Am Heart J 2016;176:53–62.
49. De Jong M. Impact of anxiety on cardiac disease. In: Moser DRB, editor. Cardiac nursing: a companion to Braunwald's heart disease. St Louis: Saunders Elsevier; 2008.
50. The British Association for Cardiovascular Prevention and Rehabilitation. 3rd ed. British Cardiovascular Society, London. Online. Available from: http://www.bacpr.com.
51. Dalal HM, Doherty P, Taylor RS. Cardiac rehabilitation. BMJ 2015;351:h5000. Available from: https://www.bacpr.com/pages/page_box_contents.asp?pageID=791.
52. Herber OR, Smith K, White M, et al. 'Just not for me' – contributing factors to nonattendance/noncompletion at phase III cardiac rehabilitation in acute coronary syndrome patients: a qualitative enquiry. J Clin Nurs 2017;26(21–22):3529–42.
53. Anderson L, Thompson DR, Oldridge N, et al. Exercise-based cardiac rehabilitation for coronary heart disease. Cochrane Database Syst Rev 2016;(1):CD001800.
54. Van Diepen S, Katz JN, Albert NM, et al. Contemporary management of cardiogenic shock: a scientific statement from the American Heart Association. Circulation 2017;136(16):E232–68.
55. Thiele H, Akin I, Sandri M, et al. PCI strategies in patients with acute myocardial infarction and cardiogenic shock. N Engl J Med 2017;377(25):2419–32.
56. Thiele H, Zeymer U, Neumann F-J, et al. Intraaortic balloon support for myocardial infarction with cardiogenic shock. N Engl J Med 2012;367(14):1287–96.
57. Møller Nielsen A, Lou Isbye D, Knudsen Lippert F, et al. Engaging a whole community in resuscitation. Resuscitation 2012;83(9):1067–71.
58. Tatli E, Alicik G, Buturak A, et al. Arrhythmias following revascularization procedures in the course of acute myocardial infarction: are they indicators of reperfusion or ongoing ischemia? ScientificWorldJournal 2013;7 pages.
59. Bonnemeier H, Ortak J, Wiegand UKH, et al. Accelerated idioventricular rhythm in the post-thrombolytic era: incidence, prognostic implications, and modulating mechanisms after direct percutaneous coronary intervention. Ann Noninvasive Electrocardiol 2005;10(2): 179–87.
60. Imazio M, Negro A, Belli R, et al. Frequency and prognostic significance of pericarditis following acute myocardial infarction treated by primary percutaneous coronary intervention. Am J Cardiol 2009;103(11):1525–9.
61. Lador A, Hasdai D, Porter A, et al. Trends in frequency and prognosis of post myocardial infarction pericarditis: ACSIS 2000–2013. Eur Heart J 2017;38(Suppl. 1):ehx504.P3646.
62. Wagner GS, Strauss DG. Marriott's practical electrocardiography. 12th ed. Philadelphia: Lippincott, Williams Williams & Wilkins; 2014.
63. M. M. Pericardial, myocardial and endocardial disease in cardiac nursing. 6th ed. Baltimore: Wolters Kluwere Health / Lippincott Williams and Wilkins; 2010.
64. Gueret P, Khalife K, Jobic Y, et al. Echocardiographic assessment of the incidence of mechanical complications during the early phase of myocardial infarction in the reperfusion era: a French multicentre prospective registry. Arch Cardiovasc Dis 2008;101(1):41–7.
65. Figueras J, Barrabés JA, Serra V, et al. Hospital outcome of moderate to severe pericardial effusion complicating ST-elevation acute myocardial infarction. Circulation 2010;122(19):1902–9.
66. Chen J, Normand ST, Wang Y, et al. National and regional trends in heart failure hospitalization and mortality rates for medicare beneficiaries, 1998-2008. JAMA 2011;306(15):1669–78.
67. Joffe SW, Webster K, McManus DD, et al. Improved survival after heart failure: a community-based perspective. J Am Heart Assoc 2013;2(3):e000053.
68. Australian Bureau of Statistics. 3303.0 - Causes of Death Australia 2017. Online. Available from: http://www.abs.gov.au/Ausstats/abs@.nsf/0/B482831519147814CA257B2E000D8171.
69. Abraham WT, Krum H. Heart failure: a practical approach to treatment. New York: McGraw Hill Medical; 2007.

70. Atherton JJ, Sindone A, De Pasquale CG, et al. National Heart Foundation of Australia and Cardiac Society of Australia and New Zealand: guidelines for the prevention, detection, and management of heart failure in Australia. Heart Lung Circ 2018;27(10):1123–208.
71. Yancy CW, Jessup M, Bozkurt B. 2013 ACCF/AHA guideline for the management of heart failure: a report of the American College of Cardiology Foundation/American Heart Association Task Force on practice guidelines. Circulation 2013;128:1810–52.
72. Soine L. Heart failure and cardiogenic shock. In: Woods SLFE, Motzer SU, Bridges EJ, editors. Cardiac nursing. 6th ed. Baltimore: Lippincott, Williams & Wilkins; 2010.
73. Michaelson CR. Congestive heart failure. St Louis: Mosby; 1983.
74. Urden L, Stacy K, Logh M. Thelan's Critical care nursing: diagnosis and management. 5th ed. St Louis: Mosby; 2006.
75. Ponikowski P, Voors AA, Anker SD, et al. 2016 ESC Guidelines for the diagnosis and treatment of acute and chronic heart failure The Task Force for the diagnosis and treatment of acute and chronic heart failure of the European Society of Cardiology (ESC). Developed with the special contribution of the Heart Failure Association (HFA) of the ESC. Eur Heart J 2016;37(27):2129–200.
76. Dharmarajan K, Hsieh AF, Lin Z, et al. Diagnoses and timing of 30-day readmissions after hospitalization for heart failure, acute myocardial infarction, or pneumonia. JAMA 2013;309(4):355–63.
77. Driscoll A, Worrall-Carter L, Hare DL, et al. Evidence-based chronic heart failure management programs: reality or myth? Qual Saf Health Care 2009;18(6):450–5.
78. McAlister FA, Stewart S, Ferrua S, et al. Multidisciplinary strategies for the management of heart failure patients at high risk for admission. J Am Coll Cardiol 2004;44(4):810–19.
79. Whellan DJ, Hasselblad V, Peterson E, et al. Meta-analysis and review of heart failure disease management randomized controlled clinical trials. Am Heart J 2005;149(4):722–9.
80. Phillips CO, Singa RM, Rubin HR, et al. Complexity of program and clinical outcomes of heart failure disease management incorporating specialist nurse-led heart failure clinics. A meta-regression analysis. Eur J Heart Fail 2005;7(3):333–41.
81. Driscoll A, Currey J, Tonkin A, et al. Nurse-led titration of angiotensin converting enzyme inhibitors, beta-adrenergic blocking agents, and angiotensin receptor blockers for people with heart failure with reduced ejection fraction. Cochrane Database Syst Rev 2015;(12):CD009889.
82. Driscoll A, Davidson P, Clark R, et al. Tailoring consumer resources to enhance self-care in chronic heart failure. Aust Crit Care 2009;22(3):133–40.
83. Riegel B, Dickson VV. A Situation-specific theory of heart failure self-care. J Cardiovasc Nurs 2008;23(3):190–6.
84. Kaneko Y, Floras JS, Usui K, et al. Cardiovascular effects of continuous positive airway pressure in patients with heart failure and obstructive sleep apnea. N Engl J Med 2003;348(13):1233–41.
85. Piepoli MF, Corrà U, Benzer W, et al. Secondary prevention through cardiac rehabilitation: from knowledge to implementation. A position paper from the Cardiac Rehabilitation Section of the European Association of Cardiovascular Prevention and Rehabilitation. Eur J Cardiovasc Prev Rehabil 2010;17(1):1–17.
86. Group CTS. Effects of enalapril on mortality in severe congestive heart failure. N Engl J Med 1987;316(23):1429–35.
87. Investigators SOLVD. Effect of enalapril on survival in patients with reduced left ventricular ejection fractions and congestive heart failure. N Engl J Med 1991;325(5):293–302.
88. Ailabouni W, Eknoyan G. Nonsteroidal anti-inflammatory drugs and acute renal failure in the elderly. Drugs Aging 1996;9(5):341–51.
89. McMurray JJV, Packer M, Desai AS, et al. Angiotensin-neprilysin inhibition versus enalapril in heart failure. N Engl J Med 2014;371(11): 993–1004.
90. Packer MMJ, Desai AS, et al; on behalf of the PARADIGM-HF Investigators and Committees. Angiotensin receptor neprilysin inhibition compared with enalapril on the risk of clinical progression in surviving patients with heart failure. Circulation 2015;131(1):54–61.
91. Hjalmarson Å, Goldstein S, Fagerberg B, et al. Effects of controlled-release metoprolol on total mortality, hospitalizations, and well-being in patients with heart failure: the metoprolol cr/xl randomized intervention trial in congestive heart failure (merit-hf). JAMA 2000;283(10):1295–302.
92. McMurray JJV, Östergren J, Swedberg K, et al. Effects of candesartan in patients with chronic heart failure and reduced left-ventricular systolic function taking angiotensin-converting-enzyme inhibitors: the CHARM-Added trial. Lancet 2003;362(9386):767–71.
93. Pitt B, Remme W, Zannad F, et al. Eplerenone, a selective aldosterone blocker, in patients with left ventricular dysfunction after myocardial infarction. N Engl J Med 2003;348(14):1309–21.
94. Pitt B, Pfeffer MA, Assmann SF, et al. Spironolactone for heart failure with preserved ejection fraction. N Engl J Med 2014;370(15):1383–92.
95. Pitt B, Zannad F, Remme WJ, et al. The effect of spironolactone on morbidity and mortality in patients with severe heart failure. N Engl J Med 1999;341(10):709–17.
96. Bokhari F, Newman D, Greene M, et al. Long-term comparison of the implantable cardioverter defibrillator versus amiodarone. Eleven-year follow-up of a subset of patients in the Canadian Implantable Defibrillator Study (CIDS). Circulation 2004;110:112–16.
97. Fitzgerald AA, Powers JD, Ho PM, et al. Impact of medication nonadherence on hospitalizations and mortality in heart failure. J Card Fail 2011;17(8):664–9.
98. Wynne JA, Braunwald E. The cardiomyopathies and myocarditis. In: Zipes DP, Libby P, Bonow RO, et al, editors. Braunwald's Heart disease: a textbook of cardiovascular medicine. 7th ed. Philadelphia: Elsevier Saunders; 2008. p. 1404.

99. Ralph-Edwards A, Woo A, McCrindle BW, et al. Hypertrophic obstructive cardiomyopathy: comparison of outcomes after myectomy or alcohol ablation adjusted by propensity score. J Thorac Cardiovasc Surg 2005;129(2):351–8.
100. Kaplan NM. Systemic hypertension: mechanisms and diagnosis. In: Zipes DP, Libby P, Bonow RO, et al, editors. Braunwald's Heart disease: a textbook of cardiovascular medicine. 7th ed. Philadelphia: Elsevier Saunders; 2008. p. 807.
101. Pacheco HG, Victorino NM, Urquiza JPN, et al. Patients with hypertensive crises who are admitted to a coronary care unit: clinical characteristics and outcomes. J Clin Hypertens (Greenwich) 2013;15(3):210–14.
102. Vidaeff A, Carroll MA, Ramin S. Acute hypertensive emergencies in pregnancy. Crit Care Med 2005;33(10):S307–12.
103. Shapiro S. Cardiac problems in critical care. In: Bongard FS, Sue DY, editors. Current critical care: diagnosis and treatment. 2nd ed. New York: Lange Medical Books/McGraw-Hill; 2002.
104. Baas LS. Hypertensive emergencies. In: Baird MSKJ, Swearingen PL, editors. Manual of critical care nursing: nursing interventions and collaborative management. 5th ed. St Louis: Elsevier Mosby; 2005.
105. Habib G, Lancellotti P, Antunes MJ, et al. 2015 ESC guidelines for the management of infective endocarditis. The Task Force for the Management of Infective Endocarditis of the European Society of Cardiology (ESC) endorsed by: European Association for Cardio-Thoracic Surgery (EACTS), the European Association of Nuclear Medicine (EANM). Eur Heart J 2015;36(44):3075–128.
106. Nakagawa T, Wada H, Sakakura K, et al. Clinical features of infective endocarditis: comparison between the 1990s and 2000s. J Cardiol 2014;63(2):145–8.
107. Baddour LMFW, Suri RM, Wilson WR, et al. Cardiovascular infections. In: Mann D, Zipes D, Libby P, editors. Braunwald's Heart disease: a textbook of cardiovascular medicine. 10th ed. Philadelphia: Elsevier Saunders; 2015. p. 1524.
108. Baas LS. Acute infective endocarditis. In: Baird MSKJ, Swearingen PL, editors. Manual of critical care nursing: nursing interventions and collaborative management. 5th ed. St Louis: Elsevier Mosby; 2005.
109. Mega JL, Morrow DA, et al. ST-elevation myocardial infarction management. In: Mann D, Zipes D, Libby P, editors. Braunwald's Heart disease: a textbook of cardiovascular medicine. 10th ed. Philadelphia: Elsevier Saunders; 2015. p. 1136.
110. Nishimura RA, Otto CM, Bonow RO, et al. 2014 AHA/ACC guideline for the management of patients with valvular heart disease: executive summary: a report of the American College of Cardiology/American Heart Association Task Force on Practice Guidelines. J Am Coll Cardiol 2014;63(22):2438–88.
111. Braverman AC, et al. Diseases of the aorta. In: Mann D, Zipes D, Libby P, editors. Braunwald's heart disease: a textbook of cardiovascular medicine. 10th ed. Philadelphia: Elsevier Saunders; 2015. p. 1278.
112. Noble AJR, Thomas A, Bass P. The cardiovascular system. Basic science and clinical conditions. 2nd ed. Philadelphia: Elsevier Saunders; 2010.
113. Bryant B, Knights K, Saterno E. Pharmacology for health professionals. 2nd ed. Sydney: Mosby; 2007.

Chapter 11

Cardiac rhythm assessment and management

Malcolm Dennis, Michael Sampson

Learning objectives

After reading this chapter, you should be able to:

- describe the mechanisms implicated in the development and propagation of cardiac arrhythmias
- recognise commonly observed arrhythmias, and discuss the factors that lead to their development
- evaluate the haemodynamic consequences of each arrhythmia, and its prognostic implications
- identify assessment and treatment strategies that ensure that specific arrhythmias are managed safely and effectively
- discuss the principles and indications for pacemaker therapy
- recognise abnormal pacemaker activity on the ECG and discuss the causes and corrective actions for complications during temporary pacing
- describe the principles and benefits of cardiac resynchronisation therapy (CRT), including the factors that limit the effectiveness of the therapy
- discuss the principles and indications for treatment of arrhythmias including ablation therapies, permanent pacing, cardioverter defibrillators, cardioversion and defibrillation.

KEY WORDS

ablation
arrhythmia
atrial
bradycardia
cardiac resynchronisation therapy
cardioversion
implantable cardioverter defibrillator
pacemaker
tachycardia
ventricular

Introduction

The coordination of normal cardiac function relies on intrinsic electrical activity.[1] This activity initiates the heartbeat and coordinates effective contraction. Cardiac arrhythmias are disturbances in this normal electrical activity, with varying impact on cardiac performance. They may be asysmptomatic, have only mild impact, or may be accompanied by a rapid decline in cardiac output. When severe and sustained, the patient becomes shocked, and organ dysfunction develops unless rapid action is taken. In the worst-case scenario, arrhythmias present as, or lead to, cardiac arrest.

How patients respond to arrhythmias depends on current state of health, existing left ventricular function, comorbidity and the nature of the arrhythmia.[2] The likelihood of severe compromise is greater in arrhythmias developing during critical illness. Arrhythmia management therefore encompasses an understanding of the causes and effects of arrhythmias, an appreciation of how they are likely to affect the individual, and a systematic assessment of the patient. Such understandings are important, given the higher incidence of arrhythmias in the critically ill population. Atrial fibrillation (AF), for example, affects at least 2% of the general population; this increases dramatically in acute care environments.[3,4] Half of patients with septic shock will develop AF, and a third of those undergoing cardiac surgery.[5,6]

This chapter covers the mechanisms of arrhythmia formation, their causes and prognostic features, ECG recognition, and treatment in the acute setting. Cardiac rhythm management devices (pacemakers and defibrillators) are covered later in the chapter.

The cardiac conduction system

The heart is an electromechanical organ; the contraction of cardiac myocytes is initiated and coordinated by electrical activity created by the depolarisation and repolarisation of the cardiac cell membrane.[7] This is discussed in more detail in Chapter 9; recall that the movement of ions across the cell membrane creates cardiac electrical activity, with sodium and calcium entry largely responsible for depolarisation, and potassium egress causing repolarisation. Ions move through channels in the cell membrane that open and close in response to various stimuli, including the voltage across the cell membrane.

In normal health, depolarisation commences in the sinus node and spreads across both atria, creating the P wave on the ECG.[8] The wave of depolarisation from the sinus node reaches the ventricles via the atrioventricular (AV) node, before conducting to the bundle of His, right and left bundle branches, and Purkinje fibres (Fig. 9.7). In the normal heart, the AV node is the only electrical connection between the atria and the ventricles. A small delay in conduction through the AV node permits complete atrial emptying before ventricular excitation. This slow AV nodal conduction also limits conduction to the ventricles during atrial tachyarrhythmias, protecting against excessively rapid ventricular rates. Thus, the atrial rates of 300/min during atrial flutter, or 400 or more during AF usually result in ventricular rates less than 170 beats/min.

Practice tip

During atrial arrhythmias, drugs are often used to further slow AV node conduction and reduce the ventricular rate. This is referred to as rate control. Rate control drugs include beta-blockers, diltiazem, verapamil and digoxin. These drugs also slow the heart rate during sinus rhythm.

Sinus rhythm

The normal rhythm of the heart originates in the sinus node and is referred to as sinus rhythm. Sinus rhythm is defined by rates of 60–100 per minute.[9] Sinus rates less than 60 are termed sinus bradycardia, and greater than 100 as sinus tachycardia.[9,10] An example of normal sinus rhythm can be found in Fig. 11.1.

The key features of this rhythm are:

- Regular P waves with a normal and consistent morphology. P waves upright in the inferior ECG leads
- One P wave in front of every QRS complex
- A normal and consistent PR interval (0.12–0.20 seconds)
- A heart rate between 60 and 100 beats/min.

The QRS complex is usually narrow during sinus rhythm (not more than 0.11 seconds); however, it will be broad if there is bundle branch block. A number of variations of sinus rhythm occur, and these are discussed below. The ECG criteria for rhythms arising in the sinus node are summarised in Table 11.1.

Sinus bradycardia

The sinus node is heavily innervated by both sympathetic and parasympathetic fibres. During sleep, parasympathetic tone predominates, and the heart rate falls. Sinus bradycardia (< 60/min) is normal during sleep and is common during rest in athletes.[1] In the non-athlete, heart rates below 50 beats/min are less common. Possible causes include drugs that slow the sinus node, myocardial ischaemia (especially when due to right coronary artery disease), hypoxia and vagal stimulation

FIGURE 11.1 Sinus rhythm with a heart rate of 78 beats/min. Every P wave is identical, and is followed by a narrow QRS. The PR interval is normal.

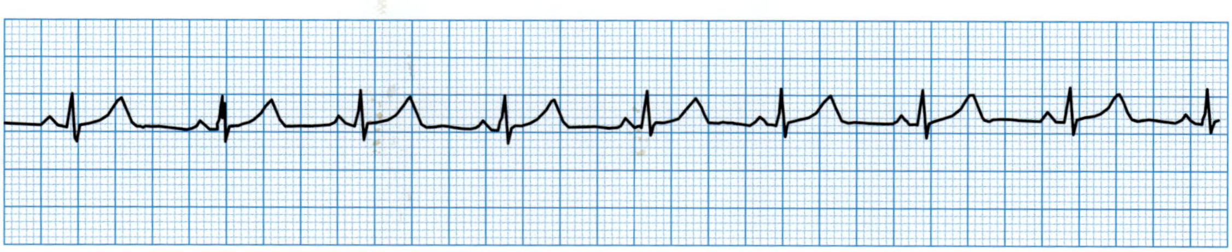

(e.g. nausea, vomiting or painful procedures).[1] In older people, sick sinus syndrome, a degenerative disease of the sinus node, is another common cause.[11] The ECG shows the same features as sinus rhythm, though with a rate less than 60/min (Fig. 11.2).

Symptoms are generally proportional to the degree of sinus slowing but will also be more marked during critical illness due to higher oxygen demands.[7] If compromised, negative chronotropic (heart rate slowing) drugs should be discontinued if possible, and positive chronotropes given to increase the heart rate. Intravenous atropine blocks parasympathetic activity, increasing the heart rate. The drug is given in increments of 500 mcg, up to a maximum of 3 mg.[2] Alternative drugs include glycopyrrolate, adrenaline, isoprenaline and dopamine, while glucagon can be useful in beta-blockers or calcium channel blockers overdose.[12] If drug treatment is ineffective the patient may need transvenous or transcutaneous pacing.[13] Epicardial pacing wires are commonly in place for bradycardia management following cardiac surgery.

TABLE 11.1
ECG criteria for rhythms arising in the sinus node

RHYTHM	ECG CRITERIA
Sinus rhythm (SR)	Regular rhythm Heart rate between 60 and 100 beats/min QRS complex usually narrow Upright P waves precede the QRS complex (commonly inverted in III, aVR, V1) PR interval is consistent, and between 120 and 200 ms (3–5 small squares)
Sinus bradycardia (SB)	As SR, but heart rate less than 60 beats/min
Sinus tachycardia (ST)	As SR, but heart rate greater than 100 beats/min
Sinus arrhythmia	As SR, but P-P interval increases with inspiration and decreases with expiration
Sinus exit block	SR with a sudden missed beat. Pause is a multiple of the usual P-P interval
Sinus arrest	SR with a sudden missed beat. Pause is not a multiple of the usual P-P interval

Sinus tachycardia

In adults, a sinus rate above 100 beats/min is termed sinus tachycardia (Fig. 11.3).[10] This is a normal response to exercise but is abnormal at rest. Possible causes include physical or psychological stress, pain, bleeding, anaemia, hypoxaemia and hypoglycaemia.[8] In these contexts, sinus tachycardia is physiologically appropriate and a useful pointer to underlying abnormalities. Inotropes and sympathomimetics also accelerate the sinus rate. Some causes may be covert, for example internal bleeding or pulmonary embolus, so thorough assessment is required.

Treatment of sinus tachycardia should aim to correct the underlying abnormality, for example controlling bleeding or relieving pain. Slowing sinus tachycardia with drugs such as beta-blockers is generally not indicated and may worsen any haemodynamic compromise. A rare exception to this is 'inappropriate sinus tachycardia', a condition in which unexplained sinus tachycardia is seen at rest.[14] Slowing the heart rate during normal sinus rhythm also has therapeutic benefit in the long-term management of coronary heart disease and

FIGURE 11.2 Sinus bradycardia. The heart rate is 50 beats/min.

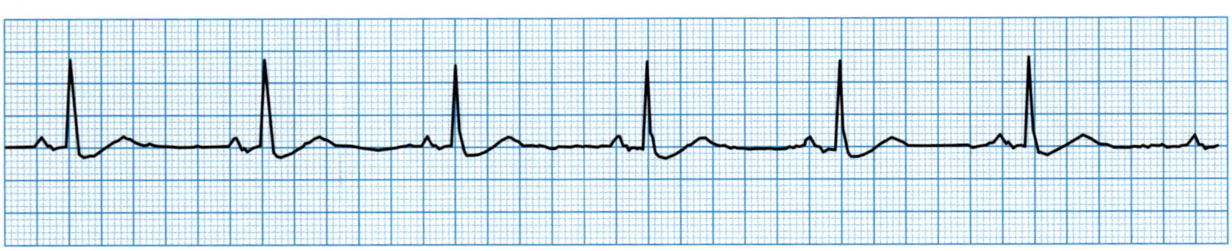

FIGURE 11.3 Sinus tachycardia. The heart rate is 114 beats/min.

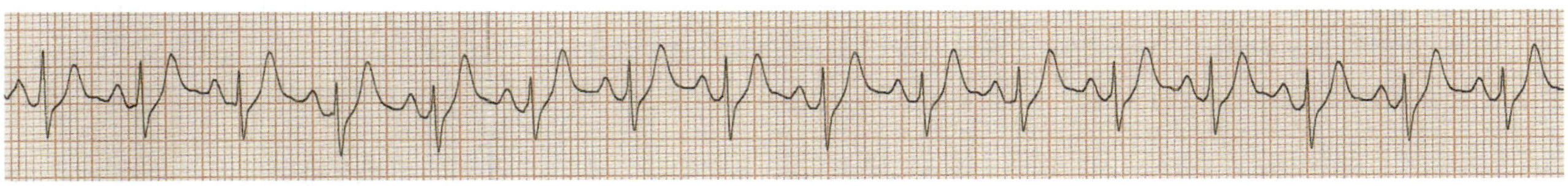

chronic heart failure.[15,16] Drugs used to slow sinus node discharge include beta-blockers, calcium channel blockers, and the selective sinus node inhibitor ivabradine.[17]

Sinus arrhythmia

In young, healthy people a beat-to-beat variation in heart rate can often be seen, resulting in a slightly irregular rhythm. This is referred to as sinus arrhythmia.[1] Sinus arrhythmia is caused by variations in vagal tone during breathing. During inspiration, vagal tone declines and heart rate increases. During expiration, the opposite occurs, and heart rate slows. Sinus arrhythmia therefore sometimes shows a cyclical pattern of mild acceleration and deceleration of the heart rate that can be matched with respiration (Fig. 11.4). As with normal sinus rhythm, every P wave is identical in morphology, and the PR interval is constant. If this is not the case, then the rhythm may not be sinus arrhythmia; sinus pauses or atrial ectopic beats can produce a similar variation in sinus rate, but will be characterised by sudden changes in rate, in other words very early or very late beats. Sinus arrhythmia by itself does not require treatment.

Sinus pause, arrest and exit block

Sinus pause and exit block describe sudden interruptions in sinus rhythm, resulting in longer than expected intervals between beats. In sinus arrest the sinus node fails to depolarise.[1] Alternatively, sinus impulses may fail to conduct out of the sinus node because of fibrosis or ischaemic tissue surrounding it; this is termed sinus exit block.[18] On the ECG, both sinus arrest and sinus exit block are characterised by an interval between beats that is much longer than the baseline rhythm. No P wave or QRS complex can be seen during this pause in the rhythm. If the cause is sinus exit block, the pause will be a multiple of the length of the previous P-P interval, because the sinus node is still firing but the beat has not conducted out of the node (Fig. 11.5). If the cause is sinus arrest, there is no relationship between the length of the pause and the underlying sinus rate (Fig. 11.6).

Occasional short pauses are relatively common, especially in people taking rate-limiting medications. In most cases, there is a degree of underlying sinus node dysfunction or sick sinus syndrome.[11] The mechanism of the pause (i.e. sinus arrest or sinus exit block) is not

FIGURE 11.4 Sinus arrhythmia. Note the cyclical rise and fall of the heart rate, which accelerates at each end of the strip, and slows in the middle.

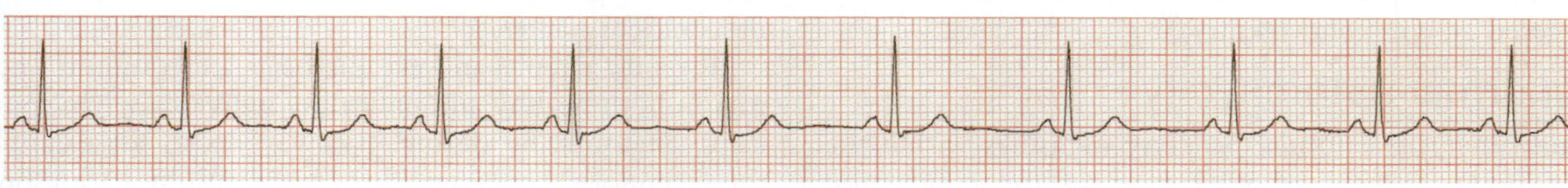

FIGURE 11.5 Sinus exit block. An abrupt rate drop follows the first three sinus beats. As the P–P interval spanning the pause is exactly twice the P–P interval of the preceding beats, the pause could be due to sinus exit block.

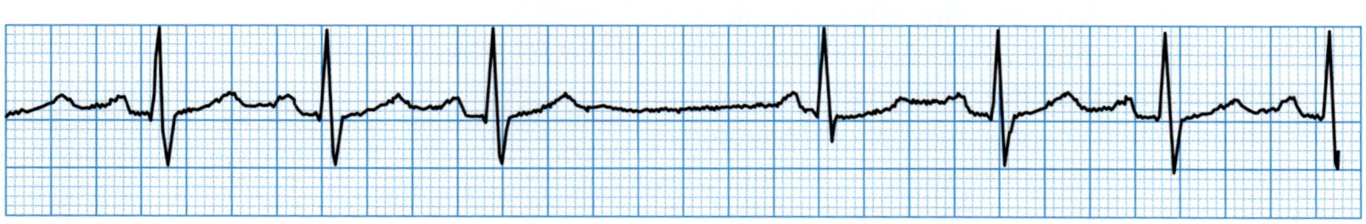

FIGURE 11.6 Sinus arrest. Two beats of sinus rhythm at 60/min are followed by two sinus pauses, the first at 2 s, and the second at 3.2 s.

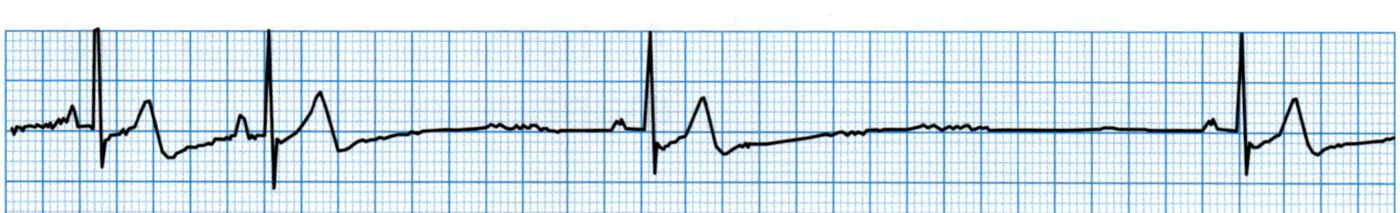

important in practice, as treatment is based on the length of the pauses recorded, and the symptoms reported by the patient. Short pauses (<3 seconds) are often asymptomatic; however, longer pauses can cause dizziness or syncope. Longer pauses are often termed sinus arrest. When significant pauses are recorded in the absence of rate-limiting medications, and the patient is symptomatic, a permanent pacemaker is usually implanted.[1]

Practice tip

Very early atrial ectopic beats which are blocked by the AV node are a common cause of apparent pauses. Non-conducted P waves may be partially concealed in the T wave of the preceding beat. When evaluating a pause on the ECG, always examine the previous T wave and consider whether it has a normal shape; if it is distorted it may contain a non-conducted P wave.

Arrhythmias mechanisms

Arrhythmias occur when electrical impulse generation or conduction is abnormal.[1] In other words, depolarisation commences somewhere outside of the sinus node, or an impulse arising normally fails to conduct through the heart in the usual manner. Mechanisms to explain arrhythmia formation include abnormal automaticity, triggered activity, and reentry.[19]

Abnormal automaticity

Automaticity is a normal property of tissues within the sinus node, as well as other parts of the conduction system, and allows these areas to initiate cardiac rhythms spontaneously.[10] Under normal circumstances, the SA node has the highest rate of depolarisation, and therefore acts as the primary pacemaker. Under abnormal conditions such as ischaemia or autonomic dysfunction, sinus automaticity may become depressed, or the automaticity of subsidiary pacemakers enhanced. This allows a subsidiary pacemaker to take control of the heart, resulting in abnormal rhythms arising in the atria, AV junction or ventricles. Non-pacemaker cells may also develop automaticity when conditions are abnormal, for example during physiologic stress, hypokalaemia, acidaemia, and hypoxemia.[20,21] These are conditions frequently encountered in critically ill individuals, and for this reason abnormal automaticity is more common in this group than in the general population.

Triggered activity

Triggered activity describes abnormal electrical impulses arising during the repolarisation phase of the action potential. During the return towards the resting membrane potential, membrane voltages can be disturbed.[21] These voltage changes may be sufficient for cells to prematurely reach the threshold potential for re-excitation, giving rise to ectopic beats and sustained ventricular arrhythmias. When occurring during phase 2 or 3 of the action potential, these voltage changes are termed 'early depolarisations', and when in phase 4, 'late after depolarisations'.

Increased intracellular calcium (such as during ischaemia, or digoxin or sympathomimetic administration), and prolonged repolarisation are the major causes of triggered arrhythmias. A number of inherited long QT syndromes exist, and there are many drugs which prolong the QT interval.[22] Amiodarone, erythromycin and propofol are among those seen commonly in critical care.[23] Triggered activity, especially torsade de pointes, occurs more readily when there is bradycardia, electrolyte disturbance or ischaemia.

Reentry

Reentry is the most common mechanism underlying tachyarrhythmias. The major requirements for reentry are an area of conduction block and an area of slow conduction. If a wave of depolarisation reaches an area of block (e.g. an area of scar tissue), conduction may continue to spread if a route (or circuit) around the block is available. If conduction is slow enough, the wave of depolarisation may spread around the circuit with enough time having elapsed for tissues to have repolarised. If so, then conduction may continue to endlessly circulate around the circuit, with each 'lap' of the circuit giving rise to another QRS and rapid atrial or ventricular rates.[19]

Reentry circuits and ectopic beats are common findings in both healthy and unhealthy individuals.[21] In some cases, anatomically distinct pathways exist, for example the accessory pathways that cause Wolff–Parkinson–White syndrome (see later in the chapter). More commonly, reentry circuits develop through pathological processes such as ischaemia, infarction and fibrosis. These conditions create areas of block, slowed conduction, and multiple potential reentry circuits.[21]

Practice tip

Antiarrhythmic drugs such as flecainide, sotalol and amiodarone alter the electrical properties of cardiac cells, changing the action potential, helping to prevent or terminate reentry arrhythmias. These changes may alter conduction or refractoriness so as to cause other arrhythmias. This potential for antiarrhythmic drugs to trigger arrhythmias is referred to as proarrhythmia, limiting the usefulness of these drugs.[21]

Arrhythmias and arrhythmia management

Arrhythmia differentiation requires knowledge of ECG criteria and a systematic approach to interpretation. The flow diagram in Fig. 11.7 gives an overview of this

FIGURE 11.7 Stepwise approach to arrhythmia identification.

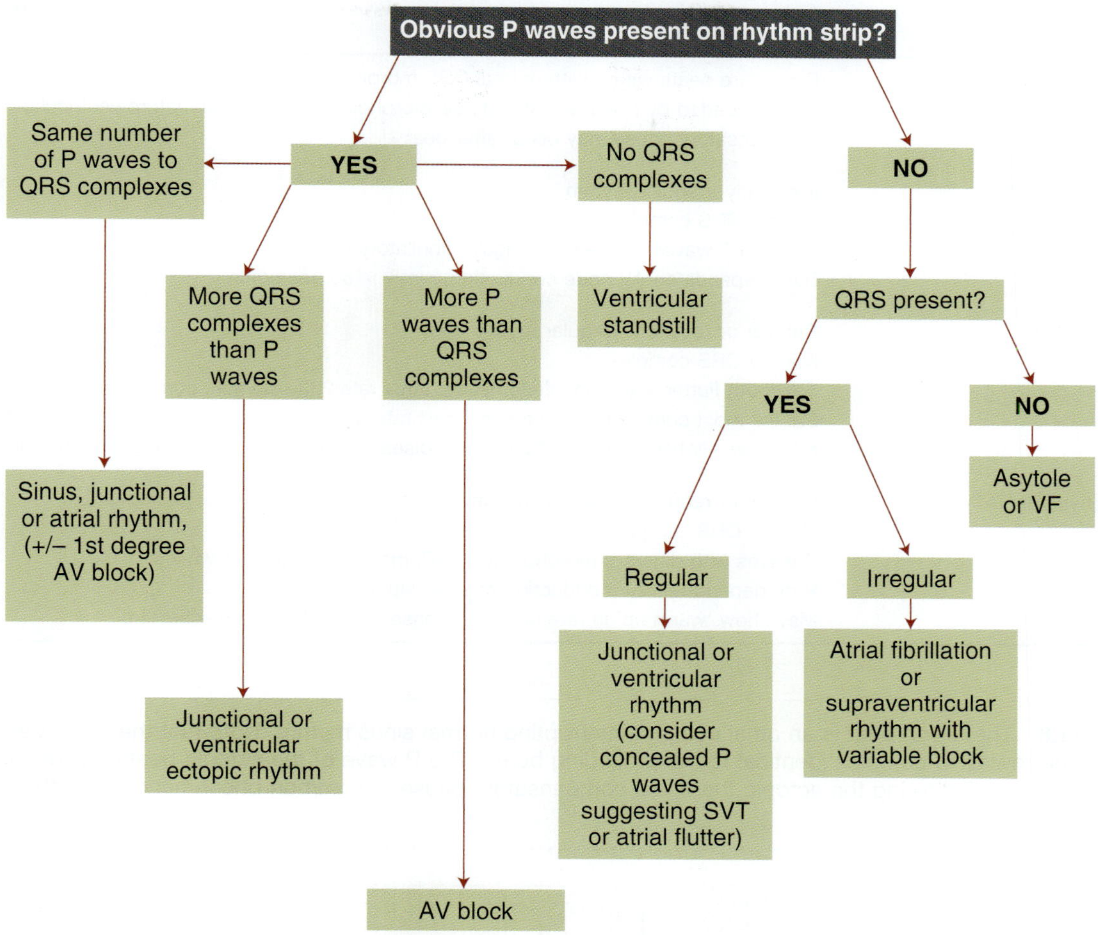

process, while a more detailed consideration of rhythm recognition and management can be found below under the heading for each arrhythmia.

Atrial arrhythmias

Atrial arrhythmias are commonly encountered in clinical practice.[1] While they rarely result in death, they frequently cause symptoms including palpitations, shortness of breath, fatigue, dizziness, and syncope. They also increase the risk of thromboembolic events such as stroke. Atrial arrhythmias may present as persistent rhythms, or in paroxysmal episodes that may terminate spontaneously within a few hours or days. In critically ill people, they may cause haemodynamic instability, prolong hospital stay, and increase mortality.[24] Atrial arrhythmias include ectopic beats, AF, atrial flutter, and atrial tachycardia. The ECG rhythm criteria for these arrhythmias are summarised in Table 11.2.

Atrial ectopic beats

Atrial ectopics are single beats arising outside of the sinus node due to abnormal automaticity, reentry, or triggered activity.[10] On the ECG, atrial ectopics appear as early beats with the same QRS morphology as preceding sinus beats (Fig. 11.8). The P wave is usually a different shape to the sinus P wave, because the depolarising wavefront through the atria is altered. Atrial ectopics may arise in either atrium and are a common and relatively benign occurrence. They do not generally need treatment, unless they trigger sustained atrial arrhythmias.[21] As described earlier, very premature atrial ectopics may fail to conduct through the AV node, resulting in dropped beats.

Atrial fibrillation

AF is the most common arrhythmia, affecting at least 2% of the population of developed countries.[3] This rises significantly in critically ill populations. Incidence also increases with age; by age 85, at least 10% of people have developed AF.[25] The arrhythmia occurs most frequently in people with hypertension or structural heart disease and is also common in chronic diseases of the lung. Acute triggers include heart failure, systemic infection, hyperthyroidism, and alcohol abuse. In a significant

TABLE 11.2
ECG criteria for rhythms arising in the atria

RHYTHM	ECG CRITERIA
Atrial ectopics (AE) Also premature atrial contraction (PAC)	Premature beats with a with normal QRS morphology QRS preceded by P waves with altered morphology precede premature ventricular Compensatory pause may occur after beat
Atrial fibrillation (AF)	Irregularly-irregular rhythm Narrow QRS complex Discrete P waves not seen – irregular fibrillatory baseline Rate depends on AV node conduction, rarely >180 beats/min
Atrial flutter (AFl)	Regular or regularly-irregular rhythm Narrow QRS complex Sawtooth flutter waves in inferior leads, atrial rate 200–430/min, commonly around 300/min 2:1 the most common presentation (heart rate around 150 beats/min), 1:1 rare unless atrial rate slow. Higher degree of AV block in diseased AV nodes, or when rate control drugs given
Atrial tachycardia (AT)	Regular or regularly-irregular rhythm Narrow QRS complex P waves with different morphology to SR, may be hidden in T waves Rate depends on AV conduction may be rapid if 1:1, 2:1 May show 'warm up' in rate or sudden onset, depending on mechanism

FIGURE 11.8 The fourth beat is an atrial ectopic, interrupting normal sinus rhythm. Note that the beat is early and has a narrow QRS complex identical to the preceding beats. The P wave of the ectopic beat is hidden in the preceding T wave. Following the ectopic there is a compensatory pause, a common phenomenon after this type of beat.

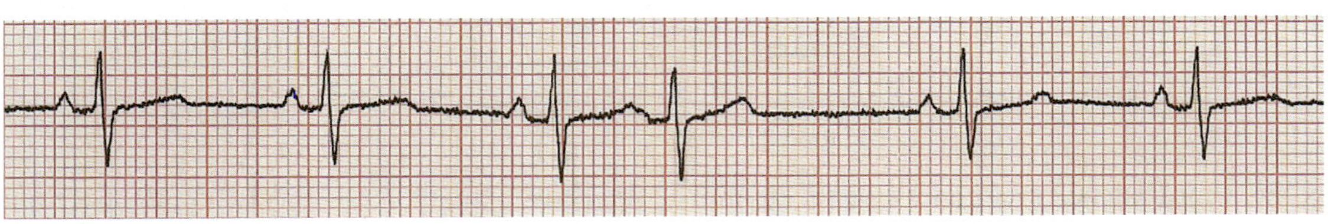

minority of individuals, no underlying cause is found. In these cases, a genetic predisposition is likely; studies have identified multiple genetic variations that increase the risk of AF.[26]

Commonly, the trigger for AF initiation is rapid ectopy arising from the pulmonary veins.[27] This rapid electrical activity produces multiple reentry circuits which collide, extinguish and reform, leading to uncoordinated atrial depolarisation. The atria fibrillate, or quiver, and effective contraction is lost. Fibrillatory waves at 400–600/min are seen, though the AV node blocks most of these, producing a maximal ventricular rate of 180 per min. Those that do pass through conduct at irregular intervals, leading to an irregularly-irregular rhythm on the ECG (Fig. 11.9).[10] The QRS is narrow, unless there is intraventricular conduction delay, and the P wave is replaced by rapid and irregular undulations of the fibrillatory waves. If AV node conduction is normal, the heart rate may be rapid. If there is AV node disease, or the patient is taking rate slowing drugs, the heart rate will be slower; bradycardia is possible.[25]

Acute management

Loss of effective atrial contraction during AF has two important consequences. First, cardiac output falls due to reduced preload.[8] This may result in significant hypotension, especially in patients with limited cardiovascular reserve. Second, there is pooling and stasis of blood within the left atrium, leading to clot formation. These may embolise into the arterial system, causing stroke, limb ischaemia or bowel infarction.[28] The treatment of AF aims to slow the heart rate (rate control), restore sinus rhythm (rhythm control), and to reduce stroke risk.[29]

Rate control may be sufficient to control symptoms and stabilise cardiovascular function,[29] though rhythm

FIGURE 11.9 Atrial fibrillation with a rapid (uncontrolled) ventricular response. The rate is around 170/min and the rhythm irregularly-irregular.

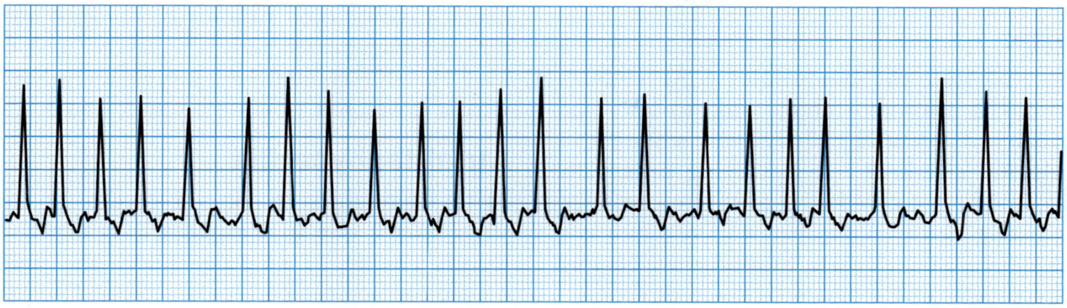

control reduces haemodynamic instability in cardiac surgical AF populations.[30]

Acute rhythm control is achieved using antiarrhythmic drugs or direct current (DC) cardioversion.[2] Amiodarone is a common choice and is often given as an intravenous loading dose of 300 mg over 1 hour, followed by an infusion of 900 mg over the following 24 hours. Although effective, its use may also be limited by hypotension. It causes phlebitis, so administration via a central venous catheter is recommended.[31] DC cardioversion is preferred if the patient is showing signs of shock, heart failure, myocardial ischaemia or syncope.[2] Although DC cardioversion has a high success rate, recurrence of AF is common and chronic drug therapy may be necessary.

Stroke risk reduction is based on assessment of risk, as well as planned treatment strategy. The risk of stroke is increased when AF has been persistent for 48 hours or more, and is higher for several weeks after cardioversion, regardless of whether this achieved using drugs or cardioversion.[29] Ideally, anticoagulation is given for at least 3 weeks before cardioversion, and for 4 weeks afterwards. Pre-procedural echocardiography has become routine to rule out atrial thrombus. Post-procedure anticoagulation should be commenced as soon as practical if urgent (non-anticoagulated) cardioversion has been necessary.[29]

Ongoing need for anticoagulation should be assessed using the CHA_2DS_2-VASC score, which allocates points according to age, gender and comorbidity (Table 11.3).[32] A score of two or more is an indication for long-term anticoagulation with warfarin or a direct oral anticoagulant (DOAC). Unfractionated heparin can be used instead in patients who are unconscious or nil by mouth. The decision to anticoagulate can be difficult in critically ill patients, as bleeding risk may outweigh the benefits of stroke risk reduction.

TABLE 11.3
CHA_2DS_2-VASC score. Anticoagulation is mandated if the individual scores ≥2

RISK FACTORS	POINTS
Congestive heart failure/left ventricular dysfunction	1
Hypertension	1
Age 75 or more	2
Diabetes mellitus	1
Stroke/transient ischaemic attack/ thromboembolic event	2
Vascular disease (coronary heart disease, peripheral vascular disease, aortic plaque)	1
Age 65–74	1
Female gender	2
Maximum score	9

Long-term management

In the longer term, some individuals with AF will benefit from catheter ablation.[33] In this procedure, electrode catheters are inserted via the femoral veins and advanced to the right atrium. The left atrium is entered via transeptal puncture. Energy sources including radiofrequency (heat) or cryo (freezing) are used to create encircling lesions arounds the pulmonary veins, referred to as pulmonary vein isolation (PVI), or within atrial muscle.[33] AF ablation carries a small risk of complication including stroke, cardiac tamponade, and vascular injury, but offers a better chance of long-term rhythm control than drugs or cardioversion.[29] Success rate may be as high as 80–90% in patients with paroxysmal AF and normal hearts, although it declines with increasing cardiovascular comorbidity and duration of the arrhythmia.[33]

In cases where all other treatments have failed, or are undesirable, an 'ablate and pace' strategy may be implemented.[29] This involves ablating the AV node so that (uncorrectable) AF can no longer conduct. As complete heart block results, permanent pacemaker implantation is also necessary. Ongoing fibrillation of the atria may result in imperfect symptom control.[34]

Atrial flutter

Atrial flutter arises from the same causes as AF (above). It carries a similar thromboembolic risk to AF, and acute management is identical.[29] However, while AF is caused by chaotic electrical activity arising principally from the left atrium, typical atrial flutter is an organised rhythm originating in the right atrium. The cause is a single reentry circuit that sweeps around the tricuspid valve annulus, usually in a counterclockwise direction.[21] This results in characteristic 'sawtooth' flutter waves in the inferior ECG leads, often at rates around 300 beats/min (Fig. 11.10). Most commonly there is 2:1, 3:1 or 4:1 AV block, resulting in regular, narrow complex ventricular rates around 150, 100, and 75 respectively.[35] Variable AV conduction results in a regularly-irregular rhythm.

Although the acute management of atrial flutter mirrors that of AF, long-term management usually involves catheter ablation because this is simple and effective in this arrhythmia.[21] As with AF, catheters are introduced via the femoral veins; however, transseptal puncture is not required. A lesion is created across the narrowest part of the reentry circuit, which is found between the inferior vena cava and the tricuspid valve annulus. This location gives the procedure its technical name; cavotricuspid isthmus (CTI) ablation. CTI ablation is often carried out as a daycase procedure under local anaesthesia, and has a success rate of 90% or more, with a lower risk of complication than AF ablation.[36]

Atrial tachycardia

Atrial tachycardia describes a rhythm arising in either atria, usually due to a rapidly firing ectopic focus or a reentry circuit.[21] Like atrial flutter, the rhythm can be regular or regularly-irregular, depending on the ratio of conducted to non-conducted beats through the AV node. Unlike flutter, regular P waves appear, although some may be concealed in the T wave (Fig. 11.11). P wave morphology is usually unlike that of sinus rhythm, unless the abnormal focus is close to the sinus node. At rates less than 200/min, 1:1 conduction may occur, and differentiation from sinus tachycardia may be difficult.

Atrial tachycardia is less common than AF or flutter, and much more variable in its presentation. In younger patients with normal hearts, it often arises from abnormal automaticity in the right atrium and has a benign prognosis with no increase in stroke risk.[1] In older patients,

FIGURE 11.10 Atrial flutter with variable block. Note the sawtooth baseline, which is characteristic of typical atrial flutter. The atrial rate is regular and is a little faster than 300/min, while the ventricular rate is irregular because of the variable block. At times the ventricular rate is close to 150/min (when there is 2:1 block) and at other times close to 100/min (when there is 3:1 block).

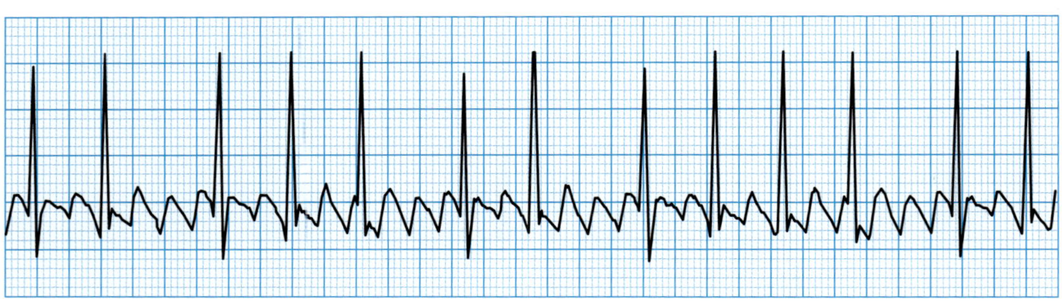

FIGURE 11.11 Atrial tachycardia. In this narrow complex tachycardia, the rhythm is very regular and the rate close to 210/min. It is not possible to clearly identify P waves within the T waves.

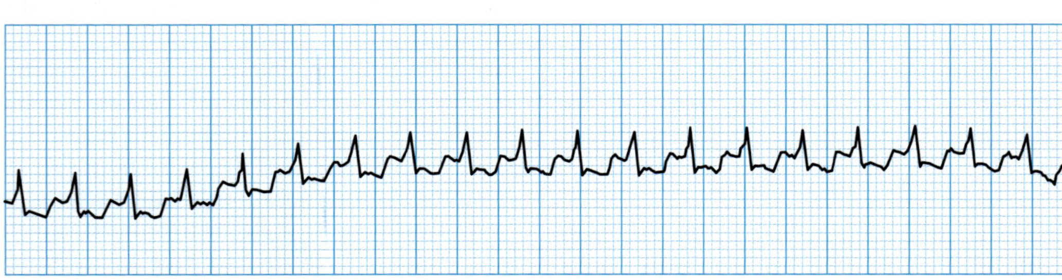

and those with structural heart disease, it more commonly arises from the left atrium or pulmonary veins, in which case it has the same prognostic features as AF. Left atrial tachycardia is a common complication following pulmonary vein isolation, and often involves a macro-reentrant circuit around the mitral valve annulus or roof of the left atrium.[37] Atrial tachycardias are treated in the same way as AF and flutter; catheter ablation is often used outside of the acute setting.

Multifocal atrial tachycardia

Atrial tachycardia may arise from more than one focus, in which case the term multifocal atrial tachycardia is used. There are multiple P wave morphologies (typically three or more), and the rhythm is usually irregular (Fig. 11.12). Multifocal atrial tachycardia is most commonly seen in chronic obstructive pulmonary disease and other chronic lung diseases.

Supraventricular tachycardia

The term supraventricular tachycardia (SVT) can be used in several ways. In its broadest sense, it refers to any rhythm originating above the ventricles, and therefore includes AF, atrial flutter and atrial tachycardia. In rhythm recognition, however, SVT often has a much more specific meaning, and refers to a regular, narrow complex tachycardia with no visible atrial activity (Fig. 11.13).[38] Although this ECG appearance can be due to atrial tachycardia, in more than 90% of cases it is due to a reentrant circuit that includes the AV node.[21] These arrhythmias are caused by minor congenital abnormalities in the conduction system, and are seen in people of all ages, including children. Unlike the atrial arrhythmias, there is no increase in the incidence of underlying heart disease compared to the general population.[21]

SVT is usually paroxysmal in nature, although persistent forms do occur. Typically, episodes last minutes rather than hours, and terminate spontaneously. The most common symptom is palpitation, although breathlessness, chest pain, dizziness and syncope are also possible.[39] Reentrant SVT falls into two distinct types; atrioventricular nodal reentrant tachycardia (AVNRT), and atrioventricular reentrant tachycardia (AVRT).[38]

Atrioventricular nodal reentrant tachycardia

AVNRT accounts for 60% of SVT and is slightly more prevalent in women.[40] The arrhythmia is caused by functional differences in the conduction pathways into the AV node, referred to as dual AV node physiology.[21] Atrial impulses conduct into the AV node via both a fast and a slow pathway, which have different conduction speeds and refractory periods. The fast pathway is responsible for the normal PR interval (<0.20 seconds). If blocked, conduction via only the slow pathway produces PR intervals >0.30 seconds). AVNRT occurs when an ectopic beat is blocked in the fast pathway, but still reaches the AV node through the slow pathway with a PR interval >0.30 seconds. The impulse then conducts back into the atria in a retrograde manner via the fast pathway, only to conduct again along the slow pathway-fast pathway circuit. With each circuit, a wave of depolarisation spreads through the atria and ventricles almost simultaneously, creating a rapid regular rhythm in which the P wave is hidden by the QRS complex. The QRS complex is narrow, because conduction to

FIGURE 11.12 Multifocal atrial tachycardia. After three beats of sinus rhythm, the rate abruptly rises during a paroxysm of multifocal atrial tachycardia, which spontaneously reverts. The resultant tachycardia is irregular, and P waves of varying shapes can sometimes be clearly seen while others can be gleaned only by the deformity of T waves.

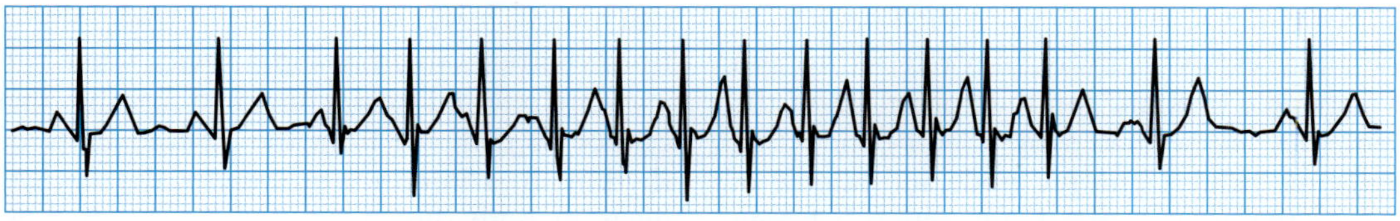

FIGURE 11.13 Supraventricular tachycardia. There are regular, narrow QRS complexes at a rate of 180 beats/min. No atrial activity can be seen (the biphasic waveform between the QRS complexes is the T wave).

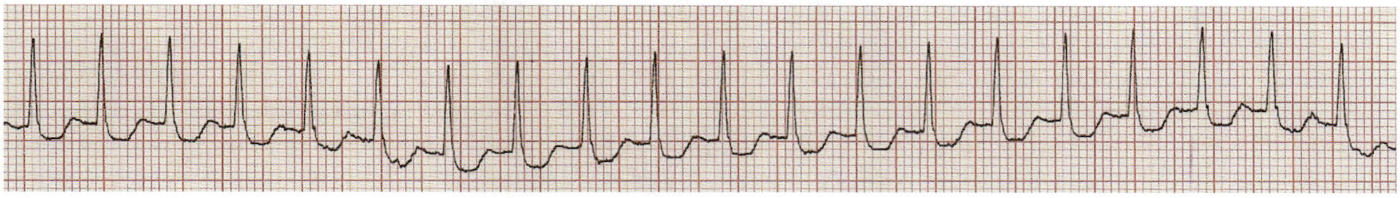

FIGURE 11.14 Atrioventricular nodal reentry tachycardia (AVNRT). Lead V1. There is sinus rhythm initially. A premature atrial ectopic conducts with a long P–R interval (0.36 s), initiating onset of AVNRT at a rate of 140/min. Note the P waves during the tachycardia can be seen distorting the end of the QRS (the 'pseudo R wave in V1' of AVNRT), which is not present before the tachycardia.

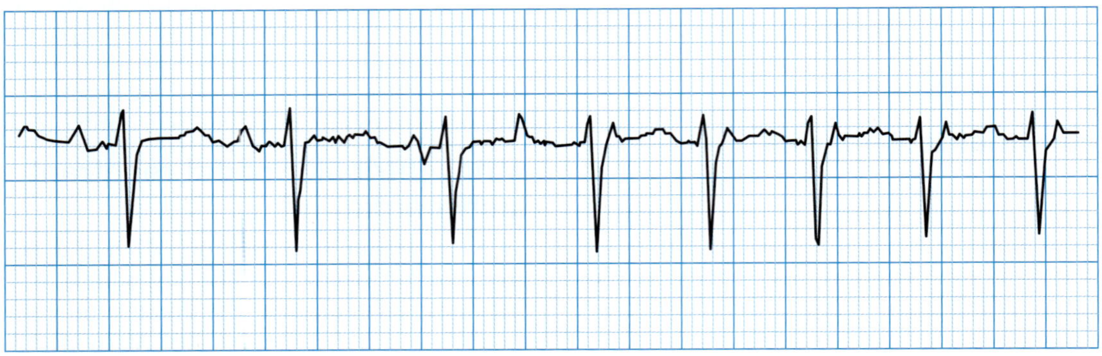

FIGURE 11.15 Antidromic AVRT, recorded using an ambulatory monitor. The patient was a fit young man, who complained of palpitation during exercise. Antidromic AVRT was reproduced during an EP study, and a left-sided accessory pathway found and ablated. Note the wide QRS which can be indistinguishable from ventricular tachycardia.

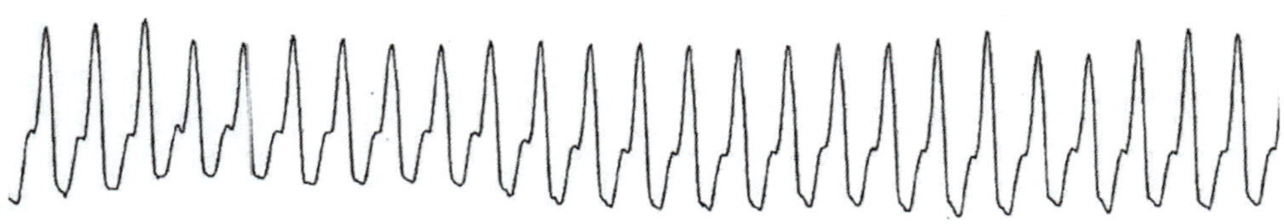

the ventricles occurs normally via the bundle of His and bundle branches. Sometimes, the P wave can be seen just after the QRS complex, distorting its shape or appearing in the sinus tachycardia (ST) segment.[40] This is usually most obvious in lead V1 (Fig. 11.14).

Atrioventricular reentrant tachycardia

Atrioventricular reentrant tachycardia (AVRT) occurs in patients with an accessory pathway, also referred to as a bypass tract or bundle of Kent.[41] In the normal heart, the atria and ventricles are separated by a non-conducting layer of connective tissue.[8] The AV node and bundle of His are therefore the only electrical connection between the atria and ventricles. An accessory pathway is a minor congenital abnormality in which one or more strands of myocardium cross this fibrous barrier, creating an alternative pathway for electrical conduction.[21] Orthodromic AVRT occurs when an atrial ectopic beat travels down through the AV node, and returns to the atria via the accessory pathway. Conduction may then cycle continuously via this reentry circuit of the AV node and accessory pathway giving rise to tachycardia. The retrograde P waves occur later than in AVNRT, and may be seen in the ST segment or T wave.[40] A reverse circuit is possible, though uncommon, in which the impulse travels down the accessory pathway, and back up through the AV node. This is referred to as antidromic (as opposed to orthodromic) AVRT and has an appearance very similar to monomorphic ventricular tachycardia (VT); the rhythm is regular and fast, with a broad QRS complex and no obvious P waves (Fig. 11.15).[41]

One reason that antidromic AVRT is uncommon is that most accessory pathways are only able to conduct from ventricles to atria, and not vice versa.[42] These pathways are referred to as 'concealed' because their presence cannot be deduced from the 12-lead ECG during sinus rhythm. In a minority of individuals, the pathway conducts in both directions, and is described as 'manifest' because it causes a change to the resting 12-lead ECG referred to as pre-excitation (excitation of the ventricles earlier via the accessory pathway than can be achieved via the AV node). The ECG signs of pre-excitation are a shortening of the PR interval and a slurring of the first part of the QRS complex referred to as a delta wave (Fig. 11.16).[41] Features of pre-excitation coupled with arrhythmias involving the accessory pathway comprise the Wolff–Parkinson–White syndrome, which is associated with a small increase in the risk of sudden cardiac death.[43] This occurs if AF is rapidly conducted down the accessory pathway, causing degeneration to ventricular

FIGURE 11.16 Pre-excitation during sinus rhythm. Note the short PR interval (<120 ms) and slurred upstroke of the QRS complex (delta wave).

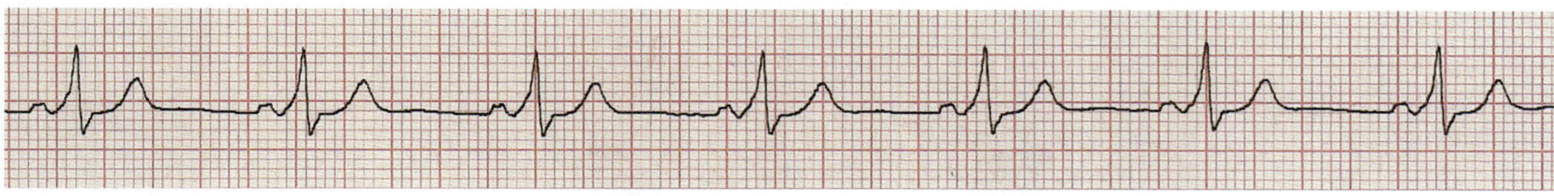

FIGURE 11.17 Pre-excited AF in a young woman. Note the irregular rhythm. Most of the QRS complexes are wide, as the impulses from the atria have conducted down the accessory pathway. Conduction via the AV node rather than the accessory pathway is seen in the middle four beats, the first of which is probably fusion with accessory pathway conduction. The pathway was successfully ablated.

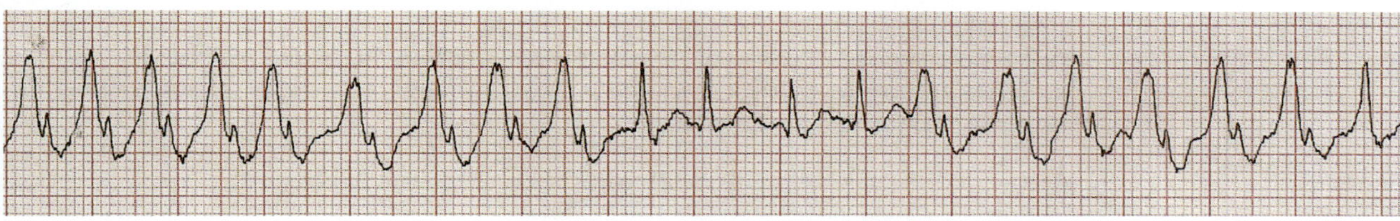

fibrillation. Pre-excited AF can be recognised by an irregular rhythm with a broad QRS complex that is not typical of either left or right bundle branch block (Fig. 11.17), often at rates approaching 300/min.[42] Antiarrhythmic drugs or DC cardioversion are recommended.[2]

Treatment of SVT due to AVNRT and AVRT

In both AVNRT and AVRT, the AV node is part of the reentry circuit. Slowing AV node conduction therefore terminates these rhythms and is the primary approach in acute management.[2] Simple methods include carotid sinus massage and the Valsalva manoeuvre, and are effective in 25% of cases.[38] If these fail, incremental adenosine doses (6 mg, 12 mg) may be used to abruptly block AV conduction. While effective, adenosine-induced AV block is usually very unpleasant and sedation is often co-administered.[39] Verapamil 2.5 mg–5 mg IV is a good alternative, and unlike adenosine can be used in asthmatic patients.[2] SVT rarely causes serious haemodynamic compromise; if this occurs DC cardioversion should be performed.

Practice tip

Failure to terminate SVT with adenosine suggests that either the drug has been given too slowly (it has a very short half-life) or that the rhythm is not SVT. Adenosine should be given as a rapid bolus in a large, proximal vein followed by an immediate flush. Always record a rhythm strip during drug administration; if the rhythm is not SVT, the underlying P waves or flutter waves will be apparent during the pause in ventricular activity.

Beyond the acute setting, ablation success rates exceed 90% for SVT.[40] The aim of ablation is to prevent symptomatic episodes and to reduce the risk of sudden cardiac death in patients with Wolff–Parkinson–White syndrome. AVNRT ablation is relatively simple as the reentry circuit is in the right atrium and involves ablation of just the slow pathway. Complications are uncommon, although there is a small risk (1 in 200) of damage to the AV node requiring permanent pacing.[40] AVRT can be more challenging. Sixty percent of pathways are found on the left side of the heart, necessitating transseptal puncture and introducing a small risk of thromboembolic complication.[44] More than one pathway may exist and reaching some pathways with a catheter can be difficult. Nonetheless, success rates are high and complications relatively uncommon, occurring in 2–4% of cases.[40]

Ventricular arrhythmias

Ventricular arrhythmias may occur as single beats (ectopics), couplets, non-sustained runs (more than three ectopic beats), or in sustained rhythms. Self-limiting runs of ventricular arrhythmia are sometimes asymptomatic, but more frequently cause palpitation, dizziness or loss of consciousness. Sustained arrhythmias more commonly produce hypotension of varying severity, and can cause cardiac arrest. They are therefore a more alarming finding than atrial arrhythmias and warrant urgent assessment and treatment. The ECG rhythm criteria for ventricular arrhythmias are summarised in Table 11.4.

Ventricular ectopic beats

Ventricular ectopic beats are also known as premature ventricular contractions (PVCs). On the ECG, they can

TABLE 11.4
ECG rhythm criteria for ventricular and cardiac arrest arrhythmias

RHYTHM	ECG CRITERIA
Ventricular ectopics Also premature ventricular contraction (PVC)	Premature beats with a broad QRS complex (≥0.12 s) Discordant T wave No preceding P wave Compensatory pause may occur after beat
Ventricular tachycardia (VT)	Three or more consecutive wide QRS beats (≥0.12 s), at rate >100/min Rate range 100–240/min P waves may be absent, dissociated or retrogradely conducted after each QRS Usually regular, sometimes irregular at onset of rhythm and prior to reversion
Ventricular fibrillation (VF)	No recognisable/organised QRS. Irregular baseline deflections of variable amplitude at 300–500/min. P waves not discernible
Torsades de pointes (TdP)	Broad complex tachycardia. Some irregularity. Rate 220–330/min Obvious polymorphism of QRS with 'sinusoidal twisting' around the baseline and transitions between polarity of QRS complexes – first positive then negative. Baseline ECG shows QT prolongation May appear monomorphic in some leads
Asystole	Absence of QRS complexes. ECG baseline may show some slow undulation
Ventricular standstill	Regular P waves but no QRS complexes or T waves
Agonal rhythm	Extremely slow ventricular rate (<20 beats/min). Usually with markedly wide QRS complexes The wide QRS and T wave amalgam often referred to as a 'sine wave' rhythm. Commonly a terminal rhythm

FIGURE 11.18 Ventricular ectopics. The second and fifth beats are PVCs. Note the broad QRS complex, discordant T wave, and lack of preceding P wave. These PVCs are monomorphic; they have the same shape, and therefore originate from the same part of the ventricle.

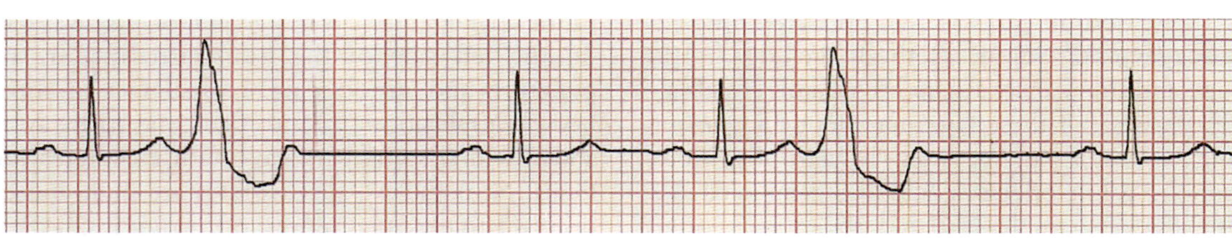

be recognised as single, early beats with a broad QRS complex (Fig. 11.18). There is no preceding P wave, and T waves are inscribed in opposite direction to the QRS deflection. In addition to being wide (≥0.12 s), the QRS complex often large and bizarre in appearance, and may be notched.[35]

Single PVCs are common and relatively benign, especially in structurally normal hearts.[1] They frequently arise from a single focus within the heart (unifocal) producing a single, uniform QRS shape (monomorphic). Increasing frequency of PVCs may precede more sustained arrhythmias, especially if they are polymorphic or occur in couplets or triplets (two or three consecutive PVCs). An increasing frequency of ventricular ectopy in the critically ill individual suggests an increased risk of sustained ventricular arrhythmia and should prompt patient assessment and optimisation. Electrolytes should be checked and replaced if necessary, especially potassium and magnesium, and efforts made to optimise myocardial oxygenation and acid-base balance.[21] When ventricular ectopics occur with every other beat, the resulting rhythm is referred to as ventricular bigeminy (Fig. 11.19), and if every third beat, ventricular trigeminy. Box 11.1 lists patterns of ectopy suggesting a greater risk of sustained arrhythmia.

Monomorphic ventricular tachycardia

VT is described as a 'run' of three or more consecutive ventricular ectopic beats, at a rate greater than 100/min.[1] Most VT is monomorphic; on the ECG, it appears as a

FIGURE 11.19 Ventricular bigeminy. Every other beat is a ventricular ectopic.

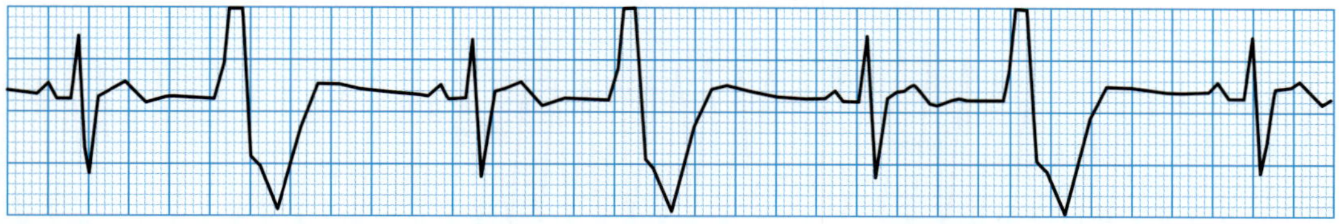

FIGURE 11.20 The onset of ventricular tachycardia. There are three sinus beats, followed by a ventricular ectopic which emerges from the T wave of the final sinus beat, triggering VT. The resulting rhythm is fast and regular, with a wide QRS, discordant T waves, and no obvious P waves.

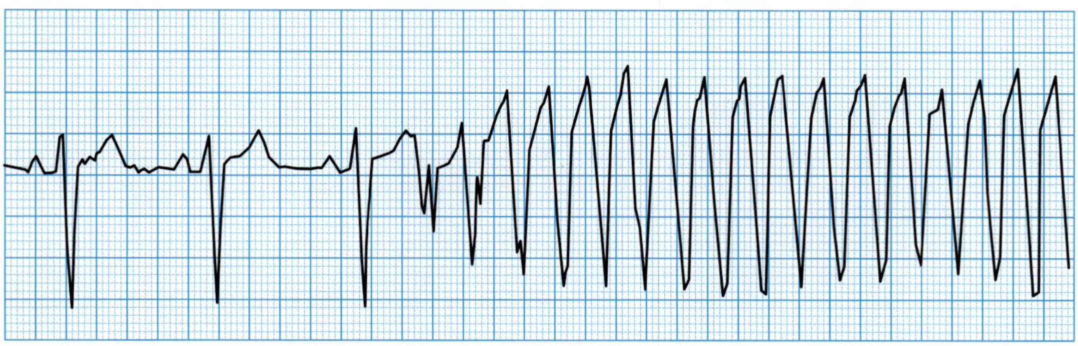

BOX 11.1

Patterns of ventricular ectopy suggestive of a higher risk of arrhythmia

- Increasing frequency of ectopy
- Polymorphic ectopics
- Couplets or triplets
- Bigeminy or trigeminy
- Three or more ectopics in a row (non-sustained ventricular tachycardia)
- R-on-T ectopics
- Bradycardia-dependent ectopics when the Q-T interval is long

rapid, regular rhythm with broad QRS complexes that are often bizarre and notched (Fig. 11.20).[35] P waves do not precede the QRS complex, although dissociated (slower) P waves may distort the T waves. When present, these dissociated P waves are a useful diagnostic feature as they do not occur during aberrant conduction of SVT or antidromic AVRT. Other features that are diagnostic of monomorphic VT include capture and fusion beats. These are beats in which an occasional sinus impulse manages to conduct as far as the ventricles, and either captures them for a single beat, or fuses with a ventricular impulse. Very fast VT is sometimes described as ventricular flutter (Fig. 11.21).

The most common cause of monomorphic VT is structural heart disease, especially coronary artery disease.[1] The rhythm is common during acute myocardial ischaemia and is a common cause of death in this setting.[45] The usual mechanism is reentry.[21] In critically ill people, the rhythm may also arise due to abnormal automaticity, or triggered activity, secondary to metabolic derangement, increased sympathetic drive, and medication use. In 10% of patients evaluated in the outpatient setting, monomorphic VT occurs in the context of a normal heart and has a relatively benign prognosis.[46]

In critically ill people, monomorphic VT frequently causes haemodynamic compromise, and may result in cardiac arrest. Immediate assessment is necessary. If the patient is pulseless, immediate defibrillation and cardiopulmonary resuscitation (CPR) are indicated.[47] If cardiac output is present, the patient should be assessed for haemodynamic instability, shock, myocardial ischaemia, heart failure and syncope.[2] If any of these are present, DC cardioversion should be performed as soon as possible. An infusion of amiodarone is often started post-cardioversion to prevent further episodes of VT. In the stable patient who has no adverse features, drug therapy alone is sufficient, although careful monitoring for clinical deterioration is necessary. As with ventricular

FIGURE 11.21 Ventricular flutter in a 16-year old female recovering from tricyclic overdose. The heart rate is 300 beats/min.

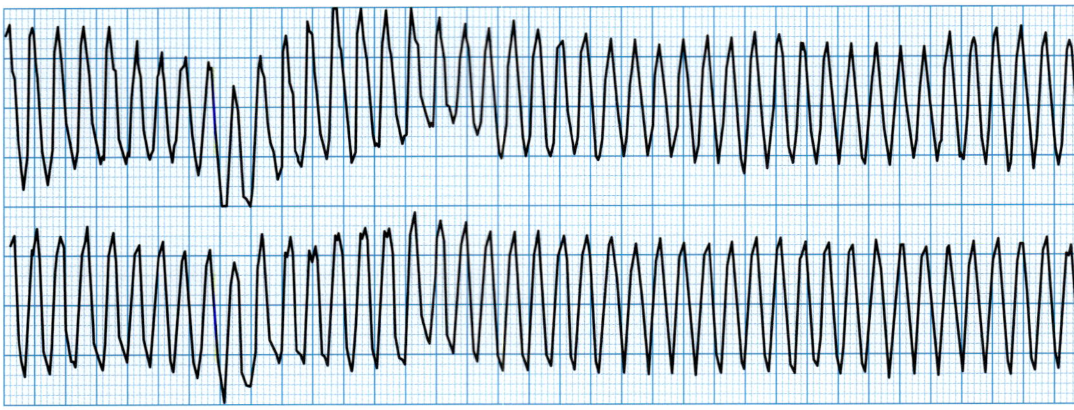

FIGURE 11.22 Torsades de pointes (TdP) tachycardia. After three beats of sinus rhythm, a ventricular ectopic beat emerging from the T wave triggers the onset of TdP. Note the characteristic sinusoidal twisting around the baseline, changing direction of the QRS, and rapid rate (300/min).

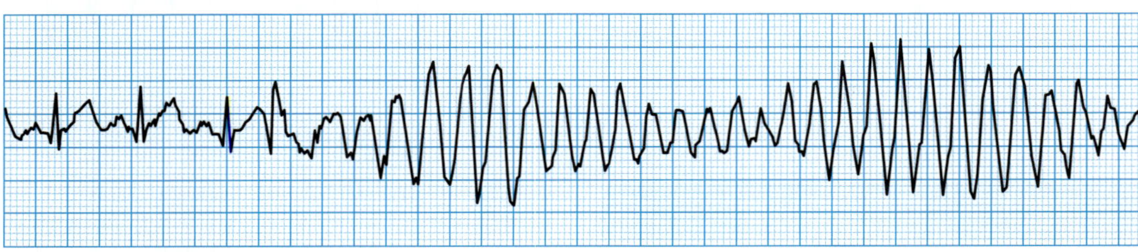

ectopics, patient optimisation is essential. Overdrive pacing may terminate VT if available. The ventricles are briefly paced at a higher rate than the VT, and then the pacing abruptly terminated, hopefully interrupting the reentrant circuit and allowing sinus rhythm to resume. There is a small risk of converting the rhythm to ventricular fibrillation (VF), so this treatment is usually reserved for situations where drugs are ineffective.[1] Cardioversion equipment should be on hand.

> **Practice tip**
>
> Although amiodarone is currently the drug of choice for ventricular arrhythmias, lignocaine was widely used in the past and remains an effective alternative, especially in the context of acute coronary syndromes. Unlike amiodarone, it causes little or haemodynamic disturbance; however, overdose can cause central nervous dysfunction including slurred speech, dizziness, numbness and seizures.

Polymorphic ventricular tachycardia

In polymorphic VT, the shape and orientation of the QRS complex is variable. The QRS may alternate between two discrete morphologies on a beat-to-beat basis (seen most commonly in digitalis intoxication) or switch between groups of beats, with first one morphology and then another (bidirectional VT).[35] Torsades de pointes (TdP) is the commonest polymorphic VT. In this arrhythmia, the QRS undergoes a gradual transition from a negative QRS complex, to a positive one, and then back again. There is usually an ill-defined transition between the two, and the amplitude of the QRS complex tends to rise and fall, producing an overall appearance that is sometimes described as a 'sinusoidal twisting'.[48] The key ECG features are a rapid, broad complex tachycardia with a varying QRS morphology (Fig. 11.22). The rate is often around 300 beats/min, and the rhythm is generally regular, although it appears less so when there is a change in QRS direction. No atrial activity can be seen.

TdP is caused by triggered activity and is associated with delayed repolarisation, seen as QT interval prolongation on the ECG during sinus rhythm (a corrected QTc of more than 450 ms in men, or 460 ms in women).[49] Bradycardia or pause increase the likelihood of TdP in susceptible patients, as does electrolyte depletion.[50] The rhythm often occurs in short, self-terminating bursts, but may be highly recurrent. Syncope is likely if sustained. Electrolyte replacement, especially magnesium, and isoprenaline or pacing to increase the heart rate and shorten the QT interval, are the cornerstones of treatment.[50] Drugs that prolong the QT interval (including amiodarone and sotalol) should be avoided or withdrawn. If TdP is sustained, cardiac arrest occurs, and immediate CPR and defibrillation should be performed.[47] Although increasing the sinus, or pacing, rate will often prevent further episodes of TdP, overdrive pacing is not effective in terminating the rhythm.

Practice tip

Risk factors for QT prolongation and TdP include congenital long QT syndrome, older age, female gender, renal or hepatic impairment, and the use of drugs that prolong the QT interval. Measurement of the QT interval is an important part of care for these patients and should be performed at least 8-hourly.[51]

Update to practice standards for electrocardiographic monitoring in hospital settings: a scientific statement from the American Heart Association. Circulation 2017;136:e273–e344.

Ventricular fibrillation

During VF there are no recognisable QRS complexes, and the rhythm is fast, chaotic and disorganised (Fig. 11.23).[48] The ventricles fibrillate (quiver), and effective ventricular contraction ceases, with complete loss of cardiac output. Immediate defibrillation and CPR are required; amiodarone may be given if defibrillation is unsuccessful, or recurrence occurs.[47] The arrhythmia is a common cause of death during acute myocardial ischaemia, although like VT it also occurs in the context of critical illness. VF is the mechanism of sudden death in some inherited syndromes, for example the Brugada syndrome.[52]

Long-term management of ventricular arrhythmias

Any patient surviving a cardiac arrest due to VT or VF should be offered an implantable cardioverter defibrillator (ICD), unless occurring during the acute phase of myocardial infarction (MI).[53] ICD implantation may also be advised in patients with sustained VT without cardiac arrest, and in individuals with significant left ventricular systolic dysfunction.[53] Other approaches to management include long-term antiarrhythmic drug use, often beta-blockers and amiodarone, or the use of catheter ablation. This is a developing field of practice; however, success rates of around 80% have been demonstrated in individuals with ischaemic VT.[54] In normal heart VT, success rates are higher.[46] Although VF is not generally amenable to catheter ablation, recent work in Brugada patients has shown that modification of arrhythmogenic substrate can prevent further VF in these individuals.[55,56]

Asystole, ventricular standstill and agonal rhythm

In a significant proportion of cardiac arrests asystole, ventricular standstill or agonal rhythm may be the first rhythm encountered or may develop during attempted resuscitation of other arrhythmias as cells exhaust their energy substrates.[47] Ischaemia, hyperkalaemia and acidosis should be considered when asystole, ventricular standstill or agonal rhythms occur unexpectedly. The ECG rhythm criteria for these arrhythmias are summarised in Table 11.4.

FIGURE 11.23 Ventricular fibrillation. The rhythm is rapid, irregular and wholly disorganised. Here the fibrillatory waves are large, or coarse. In many instances fibrillatory waves are of lower amplitude.

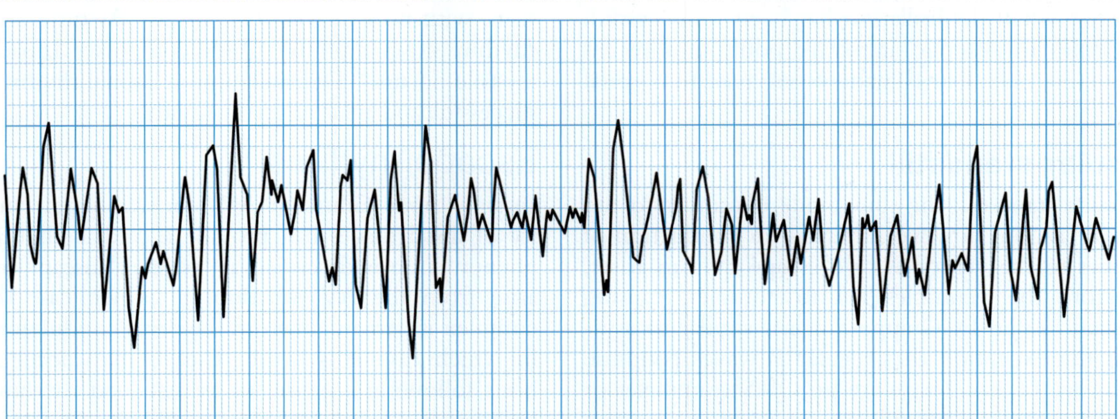

FIGURE 11.24 Asystole. No electrical activity can be seen. Note the characteristic fluctuation of the baseline.

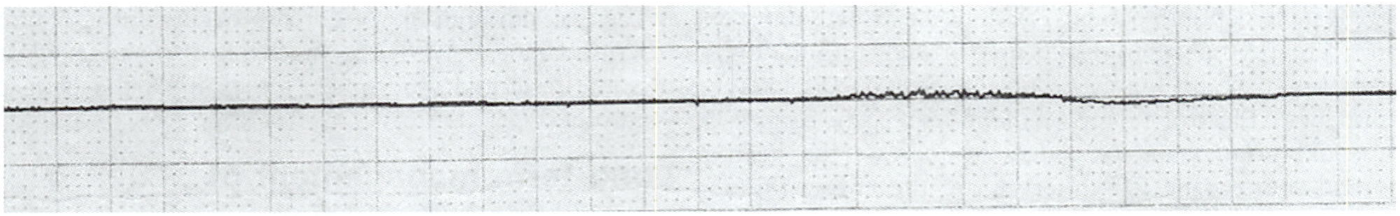

FIGURE 11.25 Ventricular standstill. P waves at a rate of 80 per min can be seen, but there are no QRS complexes. The patient may respond to emergency pacing.

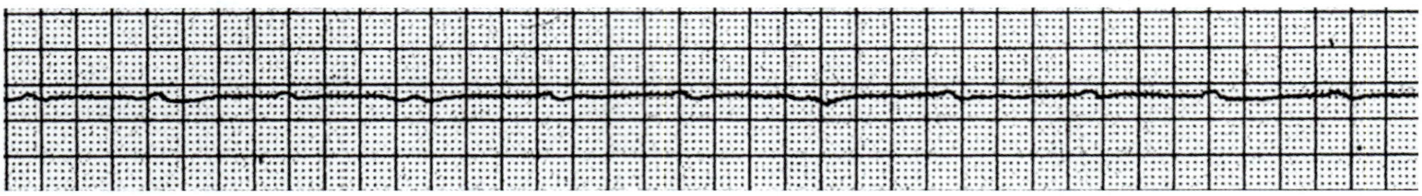

FIGURE 11.26 Agonal rhythm. Note the extremely wide QRS complexes. This is usually a terminal rhythm.

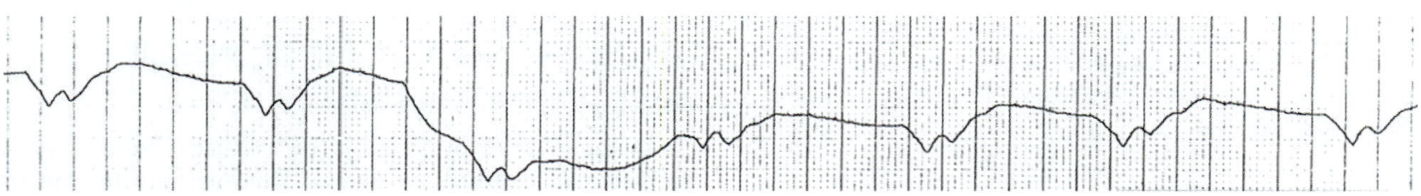

Asystole

Asystole is the complete absence of cardiac electrical activity (Fig. 11.24).[35] The heart does not contract, and cardiac arrest occurs. Commonly, the baseline has a slight wander; if it is completely flat, ECG lead disconnection should be considered. The treatment of asystole is CPR, intravenous adrenaline, and reversal of underlying causes.[47] Major haemorrhage is a common cause of asystole, although the rhythm is also seen late in cardiac arrest when defibrillation has been unsuccessful. The outcomes in asystolic arrest are poor; in a recent national survey, only 1 in 10 patients survived to hospital discharge.[57]

Ventricular standstill

In ventricular standstill, the sinus node continues to fire in a normal fashion; however, there is no conduction of the impulses to the ventricles. No escape rhythm arises, and therefore the ventricles fail to contract, causing cardiac arrest.[47] The ECG appearance is similar to asystole, with the exception that regular P waves continue to appear (Fig. 11.25). There are no QRS complexes or T waves. Ventricular standstill may occur in the context of existing complete heart block, which is discussed below.[2] Emergency pacing is the first-line treatment.[47] If this is unsuccessful, CPR, adrenaline, and a search for reversible causes must be commenced.

Agonal rhythm

Agonal rhythm is seen in dying patients, and in the late stages of unsuccessful resuscitation attempts.[47] It rarely produces a palpable pulse. On the ECG, slow, irregular and wide QRS complexes of varying amplitude are seen, with no P waves (Fig. 11.26). As time elapses, the rhythm slows and the QRS complexes broaden until asystole occurs.[48] Defibrillation of agonal rhythm is rarely successful and may result in asystole.

Escape rhythms

In sinus node failure or AV block, inherent automaticity of distal tissues can provide a cardiac rhythm.[8] This phenomenon is described as 'escape'.[1] Escape beats may arise from the AV junction, in which case the QRS complex is narrow, or from the distal conduction system, in which case it is broad. Escape may occur as single beats following a pause, or as sustained rhythms during bradycardia. Table 11.5 summarises the ECG features of the escape rhythms.

Junctional rhythm

Junctional rhythm is an escape rhythm arising from the AV node or bundle of His.[21] The rhythm is regular, with a narrow QRS complex and a rate typically between 40 and 60 beats/min.[35] Depending on where the escape arises within the AV junction, inverted P waves are seen before the QRS (with a short PR interval), after the QRS, or are hidden by the QRS complex (Fig. 11.27).[1] If there is abnormal enhancement of automaticity, an accelerated junctional rhythm may be seen; this has the same features, but the heart rate is between 60 and 100 beats/min. Junctional rhythm is often well tolerated, but the slow heart rate and loss of atrial kick can compromise patients who are acutely unwell or who have limited haemodynamic reserve. If treatment is necessary, it follows the same format as sinus bradycardia.

TABLE 11.5
ECG rhythm criteria for escape rhythms

RHYTHM	ECG CRITERIA
Junctional escape beat	Beat following a pause in SR, escape rate 40–60 beats/min Narrow QRS complex Inverted P waves may precede the QRS with short PR interval, or may be concealed within the QRS or ST segment
Junctional rhythm	Regular rhythm with a heart rate of 40–60 beats/min Narrow QRS complex P waves inverted inferiorly and may precede QRS with short P–R interval or may be concealed within the QRS or ST segment
Accelerated junctional rhythm	As per junctional rhythm, but heart rate 60–100 beats/min.
Junctional tachycardia	As per junctional rhythm, but rate >100 beats/min
Idioventricular rhythm	Regular rhythm with a rate between 20-40 beats/min Broad QRS complex P waves may be absent, retrogradely conducted, or dissociated from ventricular rhythm.
Accelerated idioventricular rhythm (AIVR)	As idioventricular rhythm, but heart rate >60 beats/min

Idioventricular rhythm

If both the sinus and AV nodes fail, an idioventricular (escape) rhythm may arise from the distal conduction system. These distal pacemakers are slow (20–40/min) and less reliable; there is a small risk of asystole or ventricular standstill.[1] The heart rate may be too slow to generate an adequate cardiac output, so acute rate restoration is often necessary. Positive chronotropes and/or pacing may be necessary.[2] On the ECG, the QRS complex is wide and bizarre, with discordant T waves. If P waves are present, they are dissociated from the QRS complex.

Accelerated idioventricular rhythm

Accelerated idioventricular rhythm (AIVR) is commonly seen after percutaneous coronary intervention or thrombolytic therapy, in which case it generally implies treatment success (Fig. 11.28).[58] The arrhythmia is caused by increased automaticity and like other automatic rhythms may display 'warm-up' behaviour, i.e. it may gradually accelerate rather than displaying the sudden jump in heart rate typical of reentrant arrhythmias.[21] When AIVR occurs in the context of reperfusion, it usually produces a stable cardiac output and requires no treatment; termination usually occurs spontaneously.

Atrioventricular blocks

Atrioventricular (AV) blocks occur when conduction of atrial depolarisation is slowed or fails to conduct to the ventricles.[1] Conduction failure may be intermittent or persistent, and may occur at the level of the AV node or within the distal conduction system. Its clinical significance depends on its degree, resulting heart rate, width of the QRS complex, and effect upon the patient.

FIGURE 11.27 Sinus bradycardia followed by onset of junctional escape rhythm. The sinus rate is initially 37 beats/min, but then slows further, allowing the junctional escape to emerge at 35/min. The junctional beats are not preceded by P waves, instead P waves can be seen distorting the ST segment of these last 2 beats.

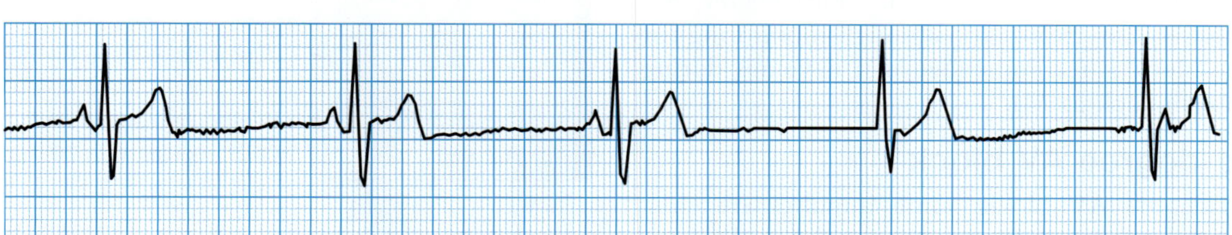

FIGURE 11.28 Accelerated idioventricular rhythm (AIVR) following reperfusion in myocardial infarction. An accelerated ventricular focus emerges at 65/min, taking over from the slower sinus rate of 60/min. It then accelerates gradually until settling at a rate of 85/min by the end of the second strip. This display of rate 'warm up' at onset is a characteristic of arrhythmias due to increased automaticity. The distortion of the ST segment from the third beat of AIVR onwards is due to retrograde conduction to the atria, creating an inverted P wave.

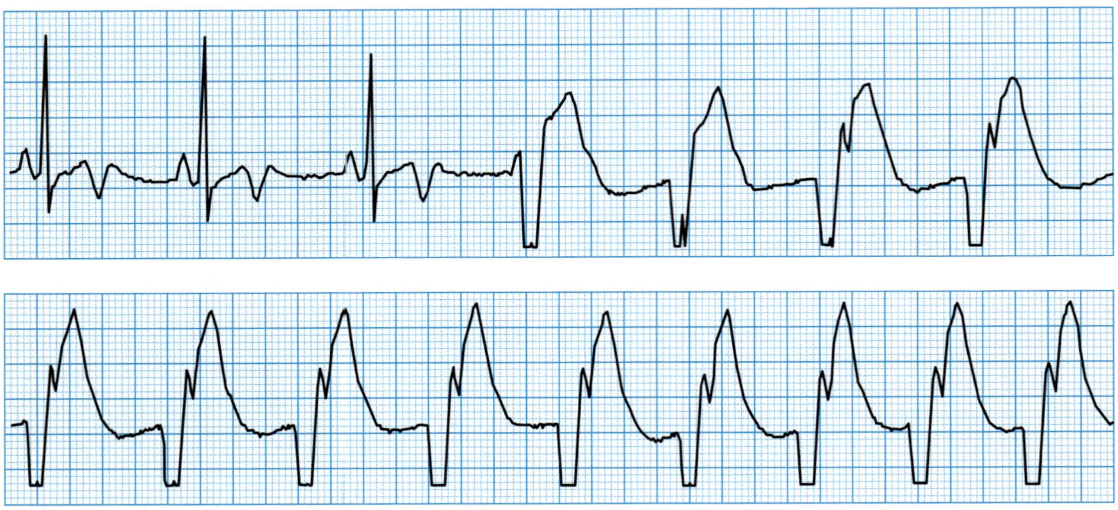

Slow conduction through the AV node may occur quite occasionally during sleep, or as a consequence of athletic training.[1] It may also result from the use of rate slowing or antiarrhythmic drugs, which may also slow the distal conduction system. More severe AV block is often the consequence of acute or chronic damage to the heart; AV blocks can therefore complicate acute coronary syndromes and myocarditis, as well as non-cardiac conditions such as Lyme disease.[35] Approximately 50% of AV blocks are due to progressive degenerative disease of the conduction tissues.[59] The ECG rhythm criteria for atrioventricular block are summarised in Table 11.6.

TABLE 11.6
ECG rhythm criteria for atrioventricular (AV) block

RHYTHM	ECG CRITERIA
First-degree AV block (1° AVB)	Regular rhythm. Every P wave followed by a QRS complex. PR interval >0.20 s
Second-degree AV block Mobitz type I (Wenckebach)	Regularly-irregular rhythm. Intermittent non-conducted P waves PR intervals show progressive PR interval prolongation until 'dropped' beat
Second-degree AV block Mobitz type II	Regularly-irregular, or regular rhythm Intermittent non-conducted P waves PR intervals of conducted beats is consistent
Third-degree AV block (3° AVB) Also: complete heart block (CHB)	No P waves conduct. No uniform PR intervals or PR relationships P waves may be buried in QRS complex and T wave bradycardia, appearing as: • Junctional escape rhythm – normal QRS, regular, rate 40–60/min • Ventricular escape rhythm – wide QRS, regular, rate 20–40/min

First-degree AV block

In first-degree AV block, conduction is slowed, but every impulse from the sinus node is conducted to the ventricles.[48] On the ECG, the PR interval is greater than 0.20 seconds, but every P wave is followed by a QRS (Fig. 11.29). Conduction delay is usually within the AV node, and is a common and benign finding in athletes, and during sleep.[1] Acute progression to higher levels of block may occur, although an increase in the frequency of AF and need for permanent pacing in the longer term has been demonstrated.[60] First-degree AV block rarely requires treatment, although monitoring for progressive block is recommended if it develops during an acute event such as MI.[59]

Second-degree AV block

In second-degree AV block, some impulses are conducted from the atria to the ventricles, while others are blocked. It can therefore be described as an intermittent

FIGURE 11.29 First-degree AV block. The PR interval is extended at 250 ms, but every P wave is followed by a QRS complex.

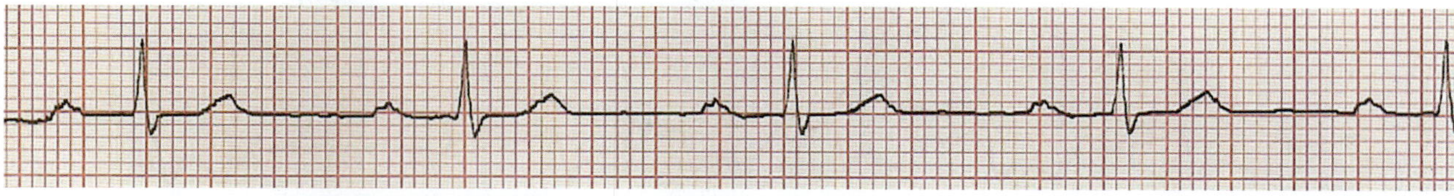

FIGURE 11.30 Second-degree AV block, Mobitz type I. Every third P wave is not conducted (3:2 conduction). The PR interval can be seen to lengthen before the dropped beats (*). After the dropped beats the cycle starts with a PR interval of 0.18 s. It then extends to 0.25 s before again dropping a beat.

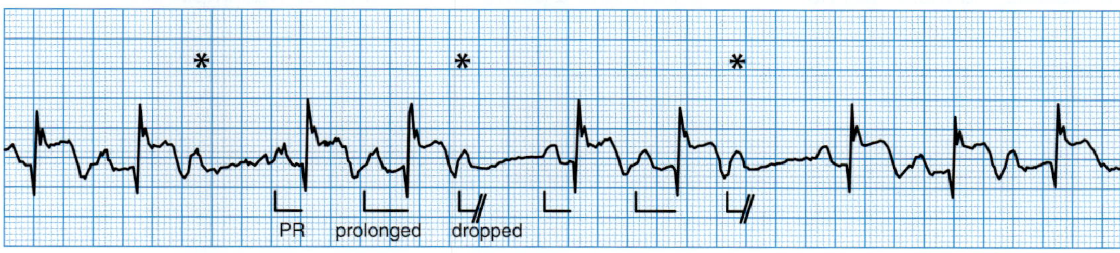

block. It can be further divided into several categories according to ECG appearance:

- Mobitz type I, also referred to as Wenckebach
- Mobitz type II
- 2:1 AV block.

Mobitz type I (Wenckebach)

Mobitz type I block is caused by conduction delay within the AV node, and is a normal finding during sleep and in athletes, in which case it reflects high vagal tone.[61] Like first-degree heart block, it may complicate acute MI in which case vigilance for clinical deterioration is necessary. Often, the heart rate is preserved, and no treatment is required.

On the ECG, the key feature of Mobitz type I is a lengthening of the PR interval over several beats, followed by conduction failure.[35] The PR interval lengthens with each beat, until a P wave is not followed by a QRS complex (Fig. 11.30). After the dropped beat, the PR interval returns to baseline and the cycle resumes. This produces a rhythm that is regularly-irregular; there are periods of regular rhythm (when each P wave is conducted) interspersed with pauses (caused by the dropped beats). Symptoms are generally proportional to the frequency of dropped beats and the absolute ventricular rate.

Mobitz type II

Mobitz type II is generally more serious. The block may be within the AV node or the distal conduction system, and commonly reflects myocardial disease.[59] There is a greater risk of progression to complete heart block so careful assessment and observation are required.[1] If the heart rate is slow, significant haemodynamic impairment may occur, necessitating drug treatment or pacing.[47]

On the ECG, some P waves will be followed by QRS complexes, while others will not.[35] Unlike Mobitz type I, the PR interval of the conducted beats is uniform (Fig. 11.31). The rhythm may be regular-irregular, or regular if there is a consistent ratio of conducted to blocked beats. The QRS is often wide, reflecting distal conduction system disease.

2:1 AV block

Second-degree AV block sometimes occurs in a pattern where every other beat is blocked, resulting in 2:1 conduction to the ventricles (Fig. 11.32).[59] Using normal ECG criteria it is impossible to classify this as either Mobitz I or Mobitz II, because only one PR interval is seen before each dropped beat. Bennett suggests that 2:1 AV block with a broad QRS complex is likely to be due to distal conduction disease and should therefore be treated as Mobitz type II.[1]

Third-degree (complete) AV block

In complete AV block, there is no conduction between the atria and the ventricles. An escape rhythm usually arises below the level of the block; however, if this fails ventricular standstill or asystole will occur. Urgent intervention and continuous monitoring are therefore essential.[47] If the block is in the AV node or bundle of

FIGURE 11.31 Second-degree AV block, Mobitz type II. A non-conducted beat confirms the second-degree block. There is no progressive prolongation of the P–R interval before the dropped beat (*).

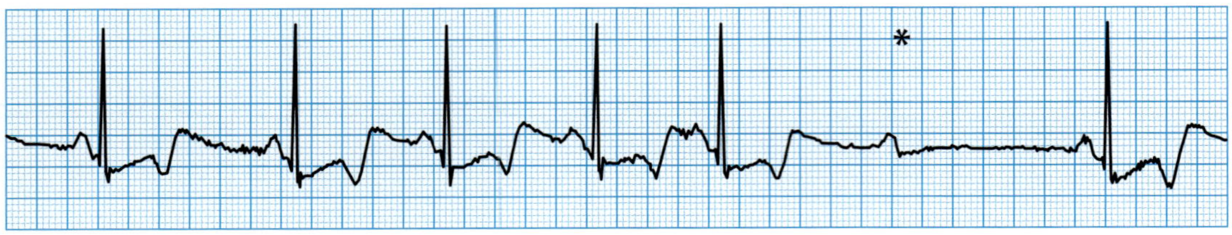

FIGURE 11.32 2:1 AV block. There is a non-conducted P wave just after the T wave of each beat. The 12-lead ECG of this elderly patient demonstrated right bundle branch block, and left-axis deviation, signifying severe distal conduction disease. As there was no obvious precipitant, a permanent pacemaker was implanted immediately.

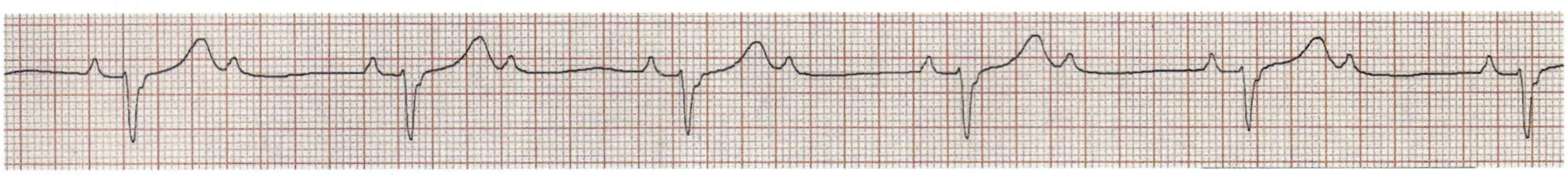

FIGURE 11.33 Complete heart block. Note the P waves (*) at a rate of 90–100/min and the ventricular rate of 40/min. The P waves bear no relationship to the QRS complexes – they are dissociated. The 7th P wave is premature and different in morphology, suggesting an atrial ectopic beat.

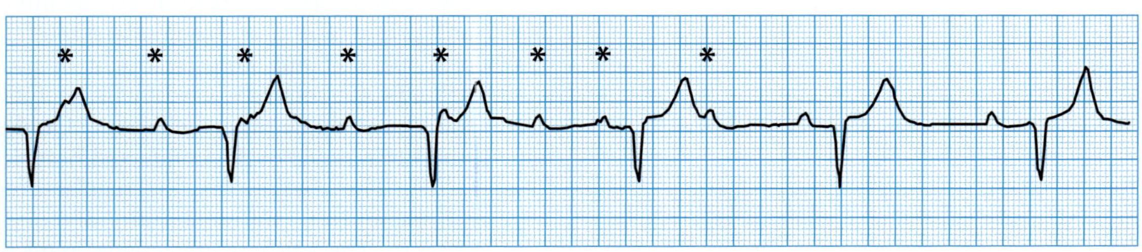

His, a narrow complex escape rhythm may arise. This often produces a stable rhythm with an adequate heart rate. Block in the distal conduction system results in a wide complex escape rhythm, which will be slower and less stable. Urgent treatment, including pacing, is usually required for complete heart block with a broad QRS.[47]

On the ECG, complete heart block appears as a regular rhythm. Both QRS complexes and P waves appear at regular intervals; however, there is no association between them.[35] Some P waves will be buried in the T waves or hidden by the QRS complexes; mapping out both the QRS and P wave rhythm can be helpful in determining the rhythm (Fig. 11.33).

Management of AV blocks

As with all arrhythmias, assessment of ventricular rate and patient condition are as important as rhythm recognition. If there is bradycardia and the patient demonstrates shock, syncope, myocardial ischaemia, or heart failure, urgent action should be taken to increase the rate.[2] Atropine may have less effect in AV blocks with broad QRS complexes but is still attempted; pacing is generally required. The management of bradycardia is discussed more fully in the section on sinus bradycardia.

In the longer term, patients with Mobitz II or complete AV block should be assessed for a permanent pacemaker, unless there are reversible causes.[62] In the context of acute MI, AV blocks are often transient and reversible during inferior infarction, but permanent and irreversible in anterior infarction.[45] When recovery is not expected, a permanent pacemaker should be implanted as soon as possible as temporary systems are unreliable and more prone to complications.[13] In all forms of AV block, the 12-lead ECG should be carefully evaluated for evidence of underlying conduction system disease, in particular bundle branch blocks and axis deviation.[62]

Antiarrhythmic drugs

Antiarrhythmic drugs have a range of properties, based on their effect on cardiac ion channels or receptors for the autonomic nervous system. Some drugs influence the automaticity and conduction speed of the sinus and AV nodes, while others affect the depolarisation and/or repolarisation of myocardial cells.[21] The Vaughan Williams classification organises these drugs into four groups (I–IV) based on the principal effect of the drug at the cell membrane. Later, class I was subdivided into three, and an additional class, V, was added to accommodate drugs that did not fit into the original system. The system is imperfect; many drugs have effects from several classes, and classification does not necessarily predict clinical utility (Table 11.7).[63]

The drugs most commonly used in critical care, including notes on their uses and limitations in the acute setting, are listed in Table 11.8. The most common problems that these drugs share is a negative inotropic effect, hypotension, a slowing of SA and AV node function, and a risk of proarrhythmia.[64] During IV drug administration, the ECG should be continuously monitored for the development of new arrhythmias, bradycardia or AV block, and resuscitation facilities should be immediately available.[47] Of all the drugs, amiodarone is probably the safest in the acute setting, and the most effective.[65] The drug is associated with an impressive range of adverse effects; however, these are dose dependent and more problematic with chronic rather than acute use.[2]

TABLE 11.7
Vaughan Williams classification system[21,63]

CLASS	ACTION	DRUGS
IA	Block sodium channels Prolong the action potential and decrease conduction velocity, increase refractory period. Work in both atria and ventricles	Ajmaline Cibenzoline Disopyramide Pilsicainide Procainamide Quinidine
IB	Block sodium channels Shorten action potential duration and decrease refractory period Ventricular site of action	Lignocaine (lidocaine) Mexiletine Phenytoin
IC	Block sodium channels Marked slowing of conduction velocity with little effect on duration of action potential or refractory period. Work in both atria and ventricles	Flecainide Propafenone
II	Block beta-adrenoceptors on the heart (and elsewhere) Decrease sympathetic tone to the heart Decrease SA and AV node automaticity and conduction velocity	Atenolol Carvedilol Esmolol Metoprolol Nadolol Propranolol
III	Block potassium channels Increase duration of action potential by prolonging repolarisation	Amiodarone Dronedarone Dofetilide Ibutilide Sotalol
IV	Block calcium channels Decrease SA and AV node automaticity and conduction velocity	Diltiazem Verapamil
V	Other: various mechanisms that do not fit into original classification	Adenosine Atropine Digoxin Ivabradine Ranolazine Vernakalant

Cardiac pacing

Artificial cardiac pacing is most commonly used to provide protection against bradycardia and/or AV block. Slow heart rates can be sustained by repetitive electrical stimulation at a programmed rate. Temporary pacing may be provided in an emergency, providing rhythm protection while reversible factors are overcome (biochemical or drug influence, myocardial ischaemia) or as a bridge to permanent pacemaker implantation.[66] Separate from such bradycardia protection, pacing may be undertaken to treat or suppress arrhythmias,[67] or to improve contractile performance.

Principles of pacing

A paced rhythm can be achieved by delivering electrical stimuli through pacing leads connected to the myocardium. Pacing lead systems require two electrodes, a negative electrode via which impulses are delivered to the myocardium, and a positive electrode via which the electrical circuit is completed. These two electrodes may exist as two separate leads or may be incorporated into a single lead with the two electrodes incorporated into them. Electrical impulses of sufficient strength stimulate the myocardium surrounding the electrode to depolarise and then propagate through the entire myocardium to initiate contraction.[64,68,69]

Pacing leads (electrodes) may be positioned in contact with the endocardium via transvenous access, or attached to the epicardium at the time of cardiac surgery.[70] For epicardial pacing, two separate leads are usually attached to each chamber paced (atrial/ventricular), with one wire connected to each of the negative and positive terminals of the pacemaker (pulse generator).[69] For transvenous pacing, a single lead is advanced to the apex of the right ventricle. These leads have a pacing electrode (negative pole) at their tip and a circumferential (or

TABLE 11.8
Antiarrhythmic drugs commonly used in critical care[2,21,47,63-65]

DRUG	INTRAVENOUS DOSE	INDICATION	CONSIDERATIONS	POSSIBLE ADVERSE EFFECTS
Adenosine	6 mg by rapid bolus into central or large peripheral vein. If first dose ineffective, double to 12 mg and repeat after 1–2 min	Termination of AVNRT or AVRT Diagnostic application to induce AV block and reveal atrial activity	Avoid in asthma, heart failure or second-/third-degree AV block unless pacemaker fitted. Warn patient of unpleasant but transient effects (e.g. chest pain)	AVB/ventricular standstill; transient chest pain/ nausea/dizziness/ breathlessness
Amiodarone	Loading dose of 300 mg over 20–60 mins, followed by maintenance infusion of 900 mg over 23 h	Atrial and ventricular arrhythmias	Potentiates digoxin and warfarin. Causes phlebitis so CVC administration recommended Hypotension linked to speed of administration. Little negative inotropy	Hypotension; bradycardia; AVB; QT prolongation; with long-term use – thyroid and hepatic dysfunction, pulmonary fibrosis, photosensitivity
Atropine	500 mcg, repeated every 3–5 min to a max of 3 mg	Bradycardia	Blocks vagal tone and therefore less effective in ventricular escape rhythms	Tachycardia, blurred vision; dry mouth; urinary retention; confusion
Digoxin	0.75–1 mg IV over at least 2 h then oral/NGT if necessary (usual daily dose 125–250 mcg)	Rate control of narrow complex arrhythmias, especially AF and flutter	Narrow therapeutic index and renal excretion – toxicity more likely in renal impairment, hypokalaemia, and elderly. Mild positive inotropic effect	Bradycardia; AVB; nausea/vomiting; dizziness; blurred or yellow vision (suggests toxicity). At toxic levels, causes atrial or ventricular arrhythmia
Flecainide	2 mg/kg over 10–30 min (150 mg max), followed if necessary by infusion of 1.5 mg/kg/h for 1 h, then 100–250 mcg/kg/h for up to 24 h. Max dose in 24 h 600 mg	Supraventricular and ventricular arrhythmias, pre-excited AF	Avoid in structural heart disease (increased risk of proarrhythmia). Negative inotrope	Hypotension; bradycardia; AVB; proarrhythmia; QRS prolongation
Lignocaine	Loading bolus of 50–100 mg over a few minutes, immediately followed by a reducing infusion of 4 mg/min for 30 min, 2 mg/min for 2 h, then 1 mg/min	Ventricular tachycardia, especially after acute MI	If hepatic/renal dysfunction: dose modification necessary to avert toxicity. Avoid hypokalaemia	Dizziness, paraesthesia or drowsiness; confusion; respiratory depression; convulsions; hypotension; bradycardia; AVB
Metoprolol	Up to 5 mg at 1–2 mg/ min. Repeat after 5 min if necessary, max dose 10–15 mg	Rate control of narrow complex arrhythmias. Termination of SVT	Contraindicated in asthma, high grade AV block. Negative inotrope	Hypotension; bradycardia; AVB; symptom provocation in asthma, COPD, diabetes, and peripheral vascular disease
Sotalol	75–150 mg over 5h. Usual maintenance dose 75–150 mg once or twice daily (equivalent to 80–160 mg oral)	Supraventricular and ventricular arrhythmias	Highest risk drug for QT prolongation and torsades de pointes – QTc monitoring recommended. Negative inotrope. Avoid in significant renal impairment	As for metoprolol; QT prolongation

TABLE 11.8
Antiarrhythmic drugs commonly used in critical care—cont'd

DRUG	INTRAVENOUS DOSE	INDICATION	CONSIDERATIONS	POSSIBLE ADVERSE EFFECTS
Verapamil	5–10 mg over 2–3 min, a further 5 mg after 5 min if required	Rate control of narrow complex arrhythmias. Termination of SVT and some normal heart VT	Potentiates digoxin, negative inotrope	Hypotension; bradycardia; AVB; constipation; flushing/ headache

AVB = atrioventricular block; COPD = chronic obstructive pulmonary disease; CVC = central venous catheter; GI = gastrointestinal; NGT = nasogastric tube.

'ring') electrode slightly proximal to this (the positive electrode). In an emergency, these transvenous ventricular pacing wires can be inserted promptly and establish a supportive ventricular rate.[69,71,72] Temporary transvenous pacing is almost always undertaken as ventricular pacing only. By contrast, in the cardiac surgical patient, where direct lead attachment to the epicardium is straightforward, pacing may be undertaken as single chamber (atrial or ventricular) or dual chamber (atrial and ventricular).

Temporary transvenous wires are vulnerable to movement.[71] Unlike permanent pacing leads, which are 'fixed' in some manner to the myocardium,[73] temporary leads are simply blunt-ended leads that rely on lodging in muscular folds (trabeculae) near the apex of the right ventricle to hold the lead in position. Activity limitation and strict rest in bed are therefore recommended for the patient with temporary transvenous pacing who is pacemaker-dependent.[74]

The details and descriptions of pacing in this section apply equally to temporary and permanent pacing. However, strategies for the correction of problems are oriented more towards temporary pacing, where clinicians can perform corrective actions.

Bipolar vs unipolar pacing: achieving capture and sensing

In the examples above, both negative and positive electrodes are positioned on or within the chamber being paced, a configuration labelled bipolar pacing, which predominates in pacing practice. Alternatively, unipolar pacing is sometimes necessary, in which only one (the negative) electrode is in contact with the heart, while the positive pole is positioned elsewhere on the body. Both pacing and sensing of the intrinsic rhythm require continued function of both electrodes and leads. Interrupting the integrity or the connections of either the positive or negative lead will interrupt both sensing and pacing as neither is possible without a complete electrical circuit.[69]

To capture the myocardium, the current must travel via the negative electrode to the heart and return to the pulse generator via the positive terminal.[69,74] Most commonly, the stimulus excites the myocardial cluster immediately surrounding the negative electrode and a wave of depolarisation advances throughout the atria or ventricles from that point. The resultant pattern of depolarisation through the chamber is different from normal conduction and so P waves and QRS complexes bear a different morphology to intrinsic rhythms. In ventricular pacing the QRS morphology closely resembles a left bundle branch block (LBBB) pattern, with a wide, sometimes notched, QRS and with ST and T wave changes similar to LBBB.[69,75]

Myocardial disease may decrease the responsiveness (threshold) of the tissue surrounding the electrode and interfere with successful capture.[76] This may be overcome by increasing the pacemaker output, but may require repositioning of the lead to contact more responsive tissue. Where repositioning of the lead is not practical, a unipolar configuration may be successful to restore capture.[76] An ECG dot or 'skin suture' placed on the body (usually anterior torso), and connected to the positive pacemaker terminal can act as the positive limb of the circuit. This alters the current path of the pacemaker stimulus and the new current path may encounter responsive tissue, restoring capture.

Major pacemaker controls

All temporary pacemakers give the operator control over the pacing mode, rate, output (strength of the applied stimulus), sensitivity (to intrinsic rhythm) and (in dual-chamber modes) the AV interval. Additional controls such as output pulse width, upper tracking rate and the post-ventricular atrial refractory period (for DDD mode) are available on some temporary and all permanent devices. Table 11.9 describes the major parameters that can be directly controlled on temporary devices.

Pacing terminology

To aid in communication when discussing pacing functions, international agreement on terminology has been reached (Table 11.10). A 5-letter code[77] describes the pacing (and/or defibrillation) capabilities of any given device in terms of chambers involved in pacing, sensing or other functions such as rate-responsive

TABLE 11.9
Pacemaker controls and settings

CONTROL	FUNCTION
Base rate	Sets the rate at which the pacemaker will discharge: pacing occurs at this rate unless the patient's own rate is faster and is sensed by the pacemaker. Typically set at 60–100/min
Maximum tracking rate (also upper tracking rate)	Sets the upper limit for which atrial tracking will be permitted – i.e., the fastest rate which ventricular pacing will occur in response to atrial rhythms. Usually 130–140 per min. Provides protection against tracking atrial tachyarrhythmias
Ventricular output	The size, or strength, of the stimulus delivered to the ventricles. In temporary devices this is an adjustable current (measured in milliamperes [mA]). Output is increased until capture (successful stimulation) is achieved. The minimum current required to achieve capture is termed the output threshold. Impulses delivered below the threshold value will not capture the myocardium. Temporary pacemakers have an adjustable output range of 0.1–25 mA
Atrial output	The size or strength of the stimulus delivered to the atria. Range 0.1–20 mA
Atrial and ventricular pulse width	Only adjustable on some devices. Allows adjustment of the duration for which the pacemaker output is applied to the myocardium. Selectable range typically 1.0–2.0 ms in 0.25-ms increments. Increasing the pulse width enhances ability to gain capture
Atrioventricular delay	The interval between the delivery of the atrial and ventricular pacing stimuli. Normally this is set in the same range as normal P–R intervals (between 0.12 and 0.20 s)
Sensitivity	Affects the ability of the pacemaker to detect the presence of spontaneous cardiac activity. Sensitivity settings can be adjusted between 1.0 and 20 millivolts (mV). Set at 1.0 mV the device is very sensitive (able to sense small electrical signals from the heart). Set at higher values, the device becomes less sensitive (higher voltage signals required to be detected), with the risk that QRS complexes or P waves will not be sensed

TABLE 11.10
Pacemaker terminology[56]

CHAMBER PACED	CHAMBER SENSED	RESPONSE TO SENSING	PROGRAMMABLE FUNCTIONS	ANTITACHYARRHYTHMIA FUNCTIONS
O, none	O, none	O, none	O, none	O, none
A, atrium	A, atrium	T, triggered	P, simple programmable	P, pacing
V, ventricle	V, ventricle	I, inhibited	M, multi-programmable	S, shock
D, dual (A & V)	D, dual (A & V)	D, dual (T & I)	C, communicating	D, dual (P & S)
			R, rate responsive	

pacing capabilities. A pacemaker designated as VVIR, for example, is capable of **V**entricular pacing, sensing of **V**entricular activity, **I**nhibiting pacing in response to sensing of ventricular activity, as well as possessing **R**ate responsiveness. While the first three positions in the terminology relate to all types of pacing, the fourth and fifth letters relate only to permanent pacing and have not been used in this chapter.

Mode selection

The ease of inserting a temporary transvenous pacing lead in the right ventricle makes it the first choice for acute pacing in any form of bradycardia. Most commonly this will be in VVI (demand) mode. In the post-cardiac surgical patient where atrial and ventricular leads can readily be positioned, DDD is the preferred mode. This is true for permanent pacing also. The exception to this is where AF is present. Even though dual-chamber leads may be placed in case of future reversion of AF, while in AF VVI pacing should be used.[75] It is not possible to achieve capture of a fibrillating chamber, rendering atrial pacing unproductive. In addition, to remain in DDD while AF is present may also produce undesirable rapid ventricular pacing, and may be proarrhythmic.

Capture

A pacing stimulus which successfully generates a P wave or QRS complex is said to have 'captured' the atria or

FIGURE 11.34 Ventricular pacing at 86/min. There is capture on the first five beats but none of the remaining pacing spikes are followed by the expected wide QRS of capture. Note that, while there is capture, the patient's own rhythm is suppressed. When capture is lost, the patient's slower rate emerges. Consistent capture needs to be re-established, by either increasing the pacemaker output or correcting factors that depress myocardial responsiveness.

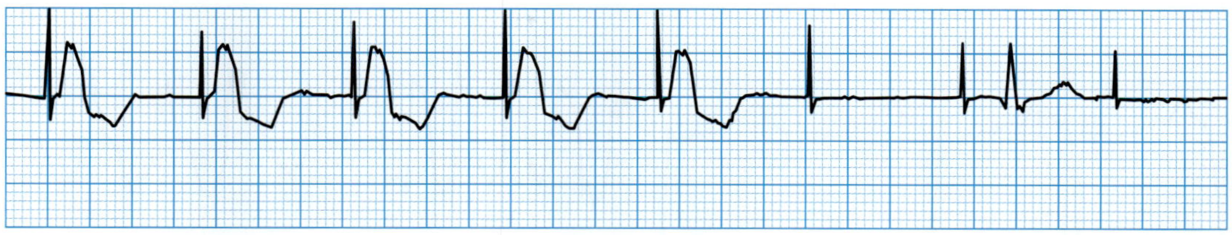

FIGURE 11.35 Demand ventricular pacing at a rate of 60/min. The patient's rate increases after the first two paced beats and inhibits the pacemaker. It then slows to below 60/min and the pacemaker recommences 'on demand'.

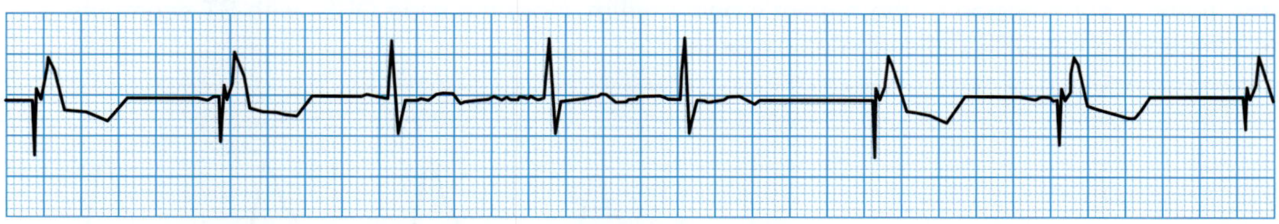

ventricles respectively. If pacing stimuli are not followed by a P wave or a QRS complex, 'failure to capture' is said to be occurring and requires immediate corrective action (Fig. 11.34).

Output and threshold

The strength of the pacing stimulus applied is termed the pacing 'output', and is adjustable by the operator. For temporary pacing this is more often an adjustable current, and with permanent pacing an adjustable voltage. When first establishing pacing, the output is increased gradually until 100% capture is achieved. The minimum output required to achieve capture is termed the output threshold. This pacing threshold may vary significantly with changes in biochemistry, arterial pH, myocardial perfusion, drugs and other factors.[71,78–80] To accommodate potential threshold changes, output settings on the pulse generator are set with a 'safety margin', i.e. the pulse generator is set to deliver outputs that are at least double the threshold value.[79]

In addition to the strength of the applied stimulus, some temporary pacemakers feature an adjustable pulse width. This is the duration over which the stimulus is applied and typical ranges are 0.1–2.0 milliseconds. Capture is a product of pulse amplitude and pulse duration,[76] and so increasing pulse width, if available, may restore capture even when maximum output has been unable to capture.

Practice tip

Thresholds for stimulation are more volatile in the temporary pacemaker patient in whom ischaemia or postoperative biochemical, pH and haemodynamic changes are common. Monitoring should be focused on confirming capture and low heart rate limits should be set to 5 or 10 beats below the base pacing rate.

Demand versus asynchronous pacing

Demand pacing

The so-called 'demand' modes predominate in pacing. In these modes, pacing is provided only on demand; that is, when the heart rate falls below a nominated level (demand rate) (Fig. 11.35). Demand pacing requires pacemaker detection of the patient's intrinsic cardiac rhythm. If an intrinsic rhythm is sensed, it 'inhibits' the pacemaker from delivering a pacing stimulus (pacing is not delivered and timing cycles recommence). The demand modes ensure that pacing is provided only when needed, and also protect against pacing during arrhythmically vulnerable moments in the cardiac cycle. Ventricular pacing delivered at the time of the T wave may induce ventricular tachyarrhythmias[81] (Fig. 11.36), while atrial pacing during atrial repolarisation (shortly after the P wave) may precipitate atrial tachyarrhythmias.

FIGURE 11.36 Intermittent asynchronous pacing due to incomplete sensing. Set pacing rate 66/min. The 1st, 3rd and 4th beats are sensed and appropriately inhibit pacing. However, a pacing spike can be seen at the apex of the T wave of the 2nd beat, which does not cause arrhythmia. The next pacing spike, just after the apex of the T wave of the 5th beat, arrives during the period of increased excitability in the action potential and precipitates ventricular tachycardia.

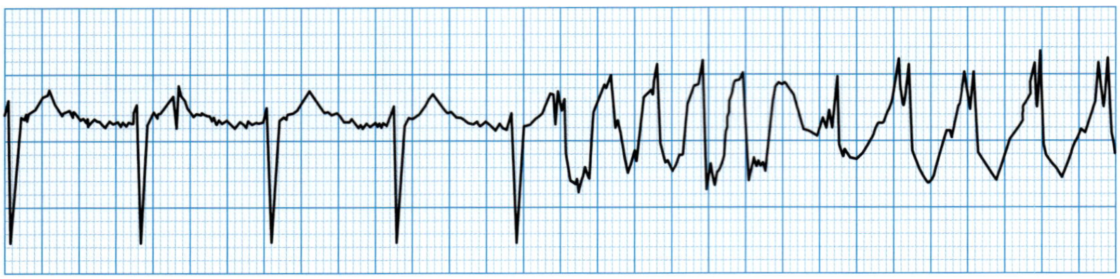

FIGURE 11.37 Onset of ventricular pacing. At the start of the strip the patient's heart rate is around 70/min. The pacemaker is then turned on with the rate set at 80/min. Capture is achieved immediately and, because the pacing rate is faster, there is suppression of the patient's own rhythm. Note the wide QRS, with ST segments and T waves in opposite direction to the QRS deflection as expected.

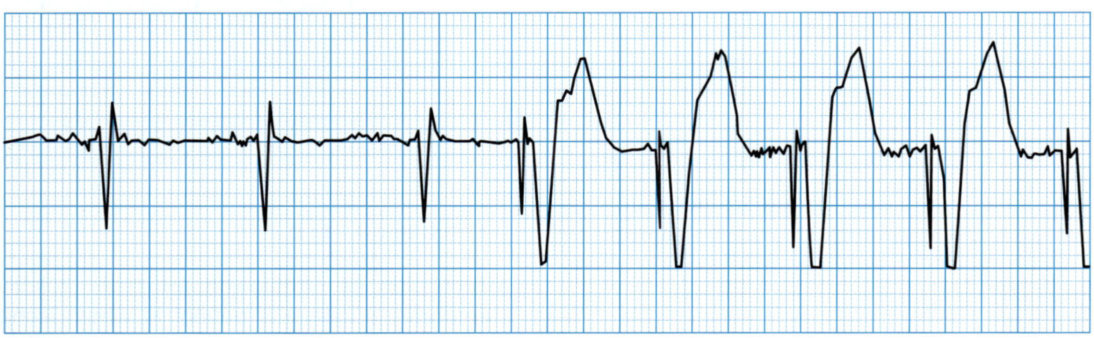

Asynchronous pacing

Pacing may be delivered in an asynchronous mode, that is, without the capability of sensing the heart's inherent rhythm. When in an asynchronous mode, the pulse generator will pace perpetually at the set rate, irrespective of whether the patient is generating their own rhythm. The main applications of non-sensing modes are: 1) when there is oversensing, or risk of oversensing, such as in environments with strong electromagnetic fields and 2) when patients would otherwise be asystolic or critically bradycardic if pacing were interrupted (pacemaker-dependent).[68,82,83] In demand modes of pacing, false sensing of electromagnetic interference is able to inappropriately inhibit pacing, returning patients to their own unreliable rhythm.[82] Temporary reprogramming to non-sensing modes (AOO, VOO, DOO) is commonly undertaken during surgery to prevent false pacemaker inhibition by electrocautery.[76] The appropriateness of continuing in an asynchronous mode should always be reconsidered if the patient's rate re-emerges in competition with the pacing due to the risk of precipitating arrhythmias.

Single chamber pacing: ventricular pacing

Stimulation of just the ventricles results in the generation of a ventricular ectopic rhythm. Functionally this will be no different from an intrinsic ventricular rhythm. There will be loss of atrioventricular synchrony, and the loss of atrial kick may cause low cardiac output and hypotension.[84] To offset the loss of atrial kick, ventricular pacing is sometimes undertaken at slightly higher rates than normally seen in the resting patient (e.g. 70–80/min, rather than 50–60/min).

The paced QRS complex will be wide (>0.12 seconds) and often notched, resembling a ventricular ectopic rhythm. Pacing from near the right ventricular apex will produce an ECG that closely resembles LBBB morphology, with left-axis deviation. ST segments and T waves will appear in the opposite direction to the major QRS direction in all leads.[78]

Ventricular pacing protects against bradycardia or AV block by stimulating the ventricles at a set rate (Fig. 11.37). Temporary ventricular pacing may also be undertaken to prevent bradycardia-dependent tachyarrhythmias such as torsade de pointes.[85] In this context, pacing at faster rates provides protection by reducing the QT interval, as well as preventing pauses which commonly give rise to ectopy and onset of torsade de pointes.[86]

Practice tip

If haemodynamic status is suboptimal during ventricular pacing (low blood pressure and/or cardiac output), consider changing the pacing rate. A faster pacing rate may offset the loss of atrial kick and so restore cardiac output despite low stroke volume. Alternatively, turning down the pacing rate may reveal an underlying (slower) sinus rhythm that produces improved cardiac output due to the inclusion of atrial kick.

Single chamber pacing: atrial pacing

Atrial pacing alone is indicated when there is sinus node dysfunction in the presence of reliable AV conduction.[66,83] The characteristic arrhythmias of such patients are symptomatic sinus bradycardia and/or sinus pause/arrest that may be syncopal. For atrial-only pacing to be undertaken, there needs to be confidence that AV conduction is intact, and that it will remain intact in the future[87] as the annual incidence of progression to AV block is 1% in these patients.[88] If there is AV block, atrial pacing alone is unsuitable, and dual-chamber pacing should be considered.[66,83,87] Atrial-only pacing is uncommon.

Atrial pacing tends to produce low-amplitude P waves, which vary from the typical P waves of sinus rhythm (Fig. 11.38). They may at times be difficult to identify on the ECG. Appropriate lead selection is important to reveal the atrial depolarisation and confirm atrial capture. It is common for the AV interval (P–R interval) to extend slightly (e.g. to 0.20–0.22 seconds) during atrial pacing compared with sinus rhythm, as the time taken for atrial impulses to traverse the atria from the pacing focus is longer than the sinus-to-AV node conduction interval.

Atrial pacing and AV block

Any degree of AV block is possible during atrial pacing and it must be remembered that AV block is rate-dependent.[87,88] Thus, the severity of AV block may be worsened not only by AV node deterioration but also by changes in the atrial pacing rate. Thus, a patient with first-degree block may develop second-degree block if the atrial pacing rate is increased, without this implying worsening AV node function. Conversely, AV block developing during atrial pacing may be lessened or overcome by reducing the atrial pacing rate. An example of such rate-dependent AV block behaviour is demonstrated in Figs 11.39–11.41.

Practice tip

If AV block is encountered during atrial pacing and is causing significant bradycardia, consideration should be given to reducing the atrial pacing rate to see whether the severity of the AV block can be reduced.

Dual-chamber pacing

Pacing of both the atria and ventricles offers the benefit of atrial kick as well as a guarantee of a ventricular rhythm. Thus, it provides protection against bradycardia and AV block. As with either atrial or ventricular pacing, demand modes have been preferred in dual-chamber pacing, unless oversensing and pacemaker dependence warrant asynchronous pacing. Particular features of the DDD pacing mode have made it the predominant mode in both permanent and postsurgical temporary pacing.

Pacing stimuli are delivered to the atria and ventricles at a selected rate. After delivery of the atrial stimulus there is a programmed delay of usually 0.16–0.24 seconds (equivalent to a P–R interval) before delivery of the ventricular pacing stimulus (Fig. 11.42). If the patient is able to conduct the atrial depolarisation to the ventricles themselves before the ventricular pacing is

FIGURE 11.38 Commencement of atrial pacing. The patient's own sinus rhythm is around 65/min at the start of the strip. Pacing is turned on at a rate of around 70/min, and causes suppression of the slower sinus rhythm. Note that the commonly seen changes during pacing compared with sinus rhythm are present here – paced P waves are lower in amplitude than the sinus beats, and the P–R interval prolongs slightly during pacing.

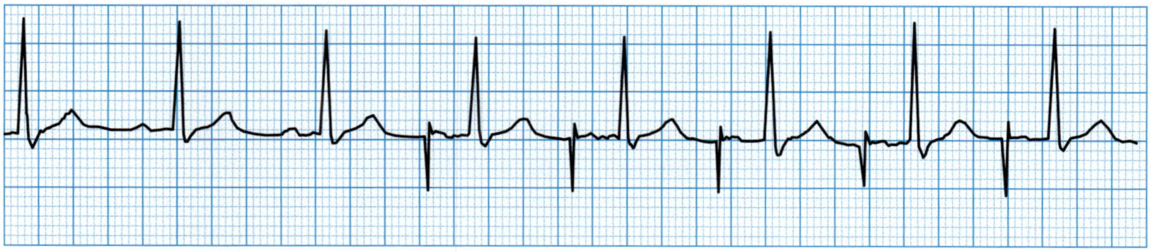

FIGURE 11.39 Atrial pacing at 70/min with first-degree AV block. Note the long P–R interval, at almost 0.4 s; particular caution is warranted in increasing the rate as, although AV conduction is 1:1, it is already very slow. See Figs 11.40 and 11.41 for worsening of AV block as the atrial rate is increased.

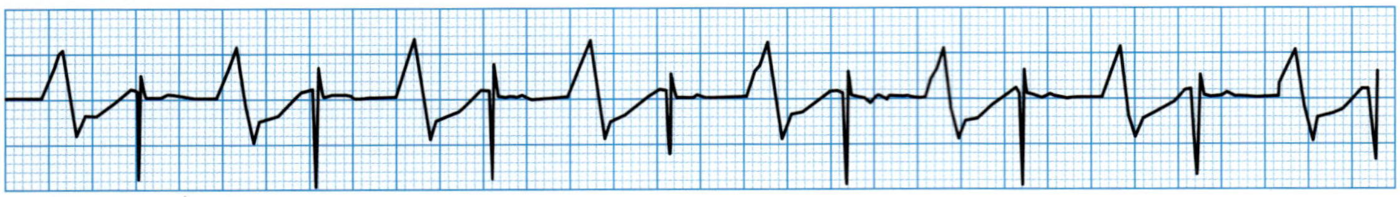

FIGURE 11.40 Second-degree AV block type I with 3:2 conduction. The same patient as above, with worsening AV block after increasing the atrial pacing rate to 80/min. Note the 1:1 conduction has been lost and there are dropped beats. After each of the dropped beats the P–R is 0.30 s, which extends to 0.46 s on the next beat, before dropping of the third beat of each cycle.

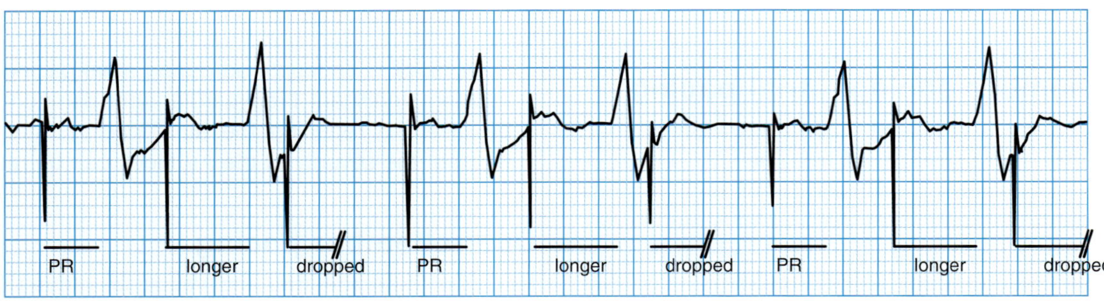

FIGURE 11.41 The same patient again, now with the atrial pacing at 86/min. At the faster atrial rate, AV conduction has worsened further. There is now a 2:1 block yielding a ventricular rate of 43/min.

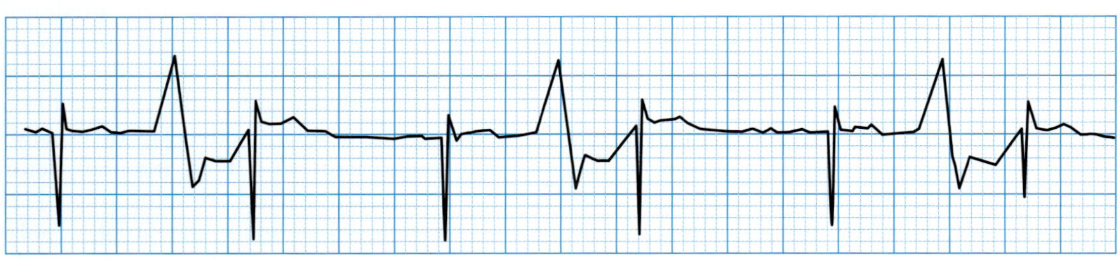

due, then the pacemaker senses the resultant QRS and inhibits ventricular pacing.

A dual-chamber pacemaker may demonstrate atrial and ventricular pacing at the set rate and at the set AV delay as described above, or may operate as simply atrial pacing if normal AV node conduction occurs before the programmed AV delay has elapsed. Deliberately prolonging the programmed AV delay provides greater opportunity for patients to conduct to the ventricles by themselves. In permanent pacing, there is emphasis on promoting intrinsic ventricular conduction by programming longer AV delays, or other measures. This is because of evidence from the DAVID trial which revealed increased heart failure and dilated cardiomyopathy secondary to chronic pacing from the apex of the right ventricle.[89] Short-term (temporary) pacing does not carry this same risk, and increasing the AV delay beyond the range of a normal PR interval carries a small arrhythmic risk[90] (Fig. 11.43).

DDD pacing: the 'universal' pacing mode

The introduction of the DDD mode (dual-chamber pacing, dual-chamber sensing and dual responses [inhibition and triggered ventricular pacing]) added an important dimension to dual-chamber pacing: the ability to synchronise ventricular pacing to spontaneous atrial

FIGURE 11.42 Dual-chamber pacing at a rate of 72/min. Note the atrial spikes are followed by P waves (atrial capture), then after an AV interval of 0.20 s there is a ventricular spike, followed by a QRS complex (ventricular capture).

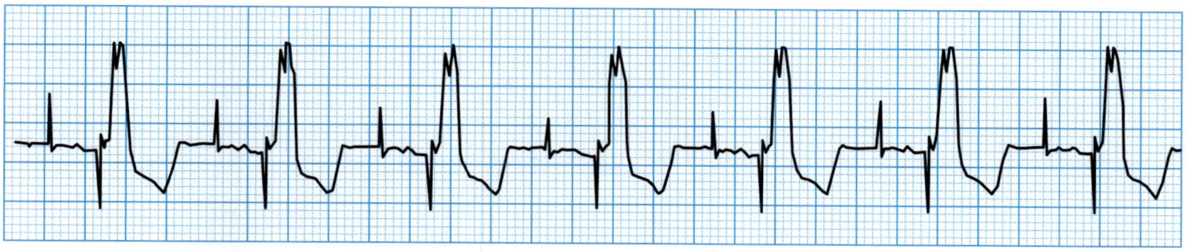

FIGURE 11.43 AV pacing to promote intrinsic conduction. There is initially AV pacing at a rate of 75/min, with an AV delay of 0.16 s. The AV delay is then increased to 0.30 s, during which the patient can be seen to conduct spontaneously through to the ventricles to produce a spontaneous narrow QRS. These are sensed by the pacemaker and inhibit the ventricular pacing.

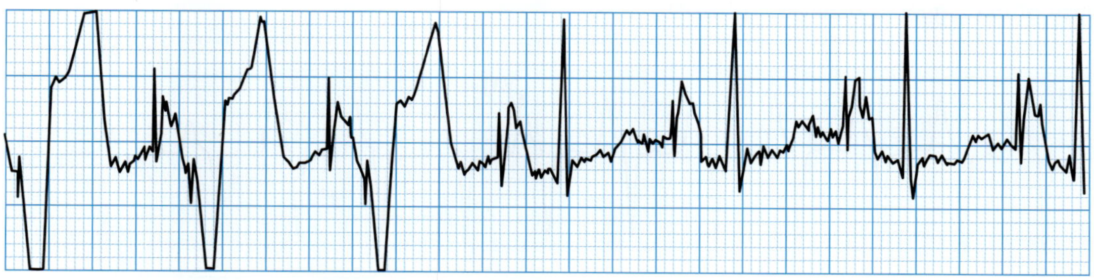

activity in patients with AV block.[83] In addition to the normal bradycardia and AV block protection, the DDD mode features a 'triggered' function. If the pacemaker detects a P wave but a QRS does not follow within the preset AV interval (AV block), the pacemaker will be triggered to provide ventricular pacing at the end of the programmed AV interval.[76] In short, the pacemaker paces the ventricles after any P wave. This means that the ventricular rate can be brought back under control of the sinus node, even though there is AV block. Consequently, in a DDD pacemaker it is common to see ventricular pacing at a range of different rates as it responds to sinus activity. This triggered behaviour of the DDD device is sometimes called 'P-synchronous ventricular pacing',[76] although 'atrial tracking' is a more practical term as the ventricular pacing 'tracks' the atrial rate (Figs 11.44 and 11.45).

Atrial tracking allows the pacemaker to pace the ventricles in response to the atrial rate sensed by the pacemaker. This is desirable when the atrial rate is controlled by the sinus node, but is inappropriate during atrial arrhythmias. For example, in the patient with AV block it is beneficial to pace the ventricles after each sinus P wave. In contrast, atrial tracking at a 1:1 rate during atrial flutter would produce an intolerable ventricular rate, and during AF the tracking rate could be even higher. For this reason, an 'upper rate' for atrial tracking is programmed in the DDD pacemaker. The upper rate controls the maximal rate at which ventricular pacing can be provided (how fast it may track the atria at a 1:1 ratio). This is typically set to around 120–130 per min. In younger patients it may be set higher, e.g. 140–170/min. If the atrial rate exceeds the upper rate for tracking, then it is no longer possible for all of the atrial beats to be tracked. DDD pacemakers will start 'dropping' beats when the atrial rate exceeds the upper tracking rate, analogous to the behaviour of the AV node.

Documentation of paced rhythm

It will be apparent from descriptions above that at different times the DDD pacemaker may be pacing either the atria *or* the ventricles, pacing both the atria *and* the ventricles, or pacing neither, depending on the patient's sinus and AV node capabilities. Merely documenting 'DDD' does not convey anything about pacemaker dependence or reveal recovery of sinus or AV nodal capabilities. A representation which conveys atrial and ventricular activity is more useful, and is shown below in Table 11.11. Note the information contained may be obtained from either cardiac monitoring or from the pace indicators on the pacemaker.

FIGURE 11.44 ECG excerpt from a patient with sinus rhythm and 2:1 AV block. The non-conducted P waves are partially concealed but can be seen distorting the T waves (arrows). Although the sinus node can generate a rate of 75/min, the patient is rendered bradycardic by the AV block.

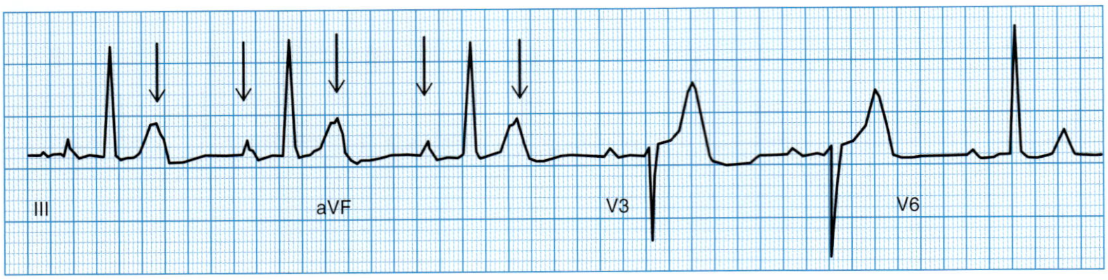

FIGURE 11.45 The same patient as above, 2 h later. A DDD pacemaker has been inserted and, although some of the pacing spikes are difficult to see, all QRSs are paced beats. The sinus rate is again close to 75/min, and atrial tracking ensures that a paced QRS follows each P wave. The ventricular rate has been brought back under control of the sinus node. Note that, although set to a back-up rate of 60/min, the pacemaker is pacing much faster than this because of the triggered behaviour of DDD.

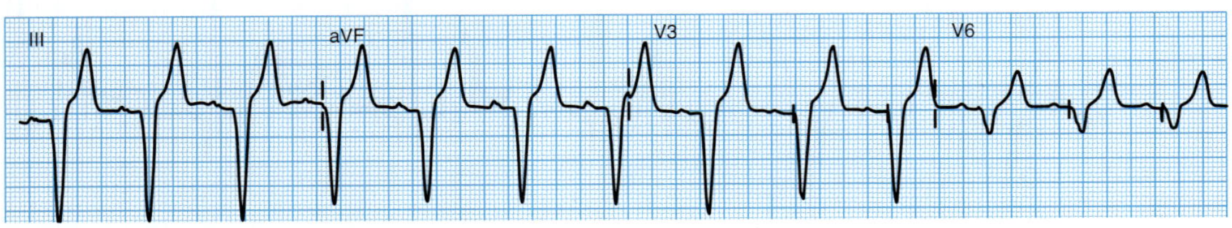

TABLE 11.11
Representative documentation of current rhythm during dual-chamber pacing

SUGGESTED DOCUMENTATION	INFORMATION CONVEYED
AP-VP Atrial paced, ventricular paced	Sinus rate is less than base rate. AV block is at least first degree
AP-VS Atrial paced, ventricular sensed	Sinus rate is less than base rate AV conduction is occurring normally (recovered)
AS-VP Atrial sensed, ventricular paced	Sinus rate has recovered and is greater than base rate. AV block is first degree or worse.
AS-VS Atrial sensed, Ventricular sensed	Sinus rate has recovered. Normal AV conduction has recovered

External ('transthoracic') pacing

Emergency pacing may be undertaken noninvasively via external pacing electrodes, and is termed 'external' or 'transthoracic' pacing. Adhesive defibrillation pads are applied in either the anteroposterior (preferred) or standard apico-basal positions as per defibrillation. These are connected to a defibrillator with additional pacing capability. Pacing stimuli of large current (10–200 mA) are necessary to achieve myocardial capture, and frequently also cause uncomfortable or painful skeletal muscle stimulation. Its use is therefore usually reserved for highly symptomatic/life-threatening bradyarrhythmias, and only as a short-term bridge to invasive pacing. Sedation is usually required.

External/transthoracic cardiac pacing provides ventricular pacing only, and the patient should be assessed not only for reliable capture, but also for an adequate pulse and blood pressure during pacing. Pacing may be in either demand or asynchronous mode, usually at rates of 40–80 beats/min.

Practice tip

The high current pacing spikes of transthoracic pacing may conceal the resultant QRS on bedside monitors. Filters on the monitors of the pacer/defibrillator unit make them a more reliable source of capture confirmation.

FIGURE 11.46 Intermittent failure to capture. The 1st, 2nd, 6th and 7th spikes gain ventricular capture but the rest do not. Note the significant pause during failure to capture, in which there is atrial but not ventricular activity. Symptoms during failure to capture depend on the rate of any underlying rhythm.

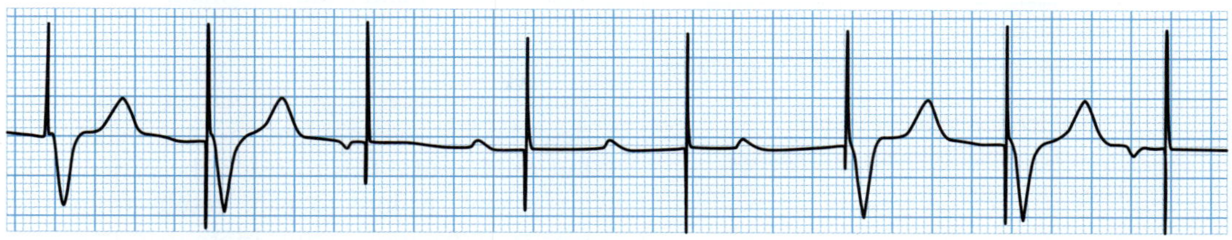

FIGURE 11.47 Atrial pacing with intermittent failure to capture (output set at 14 mA). Note that capture is evident following the 1st, 3rd, 5th, 7th and 8th pacing spikes, but not the others. Fortunately, here the patient has an underlying sinus rhythm, so that the impact of failure to capture is of no great consequence.

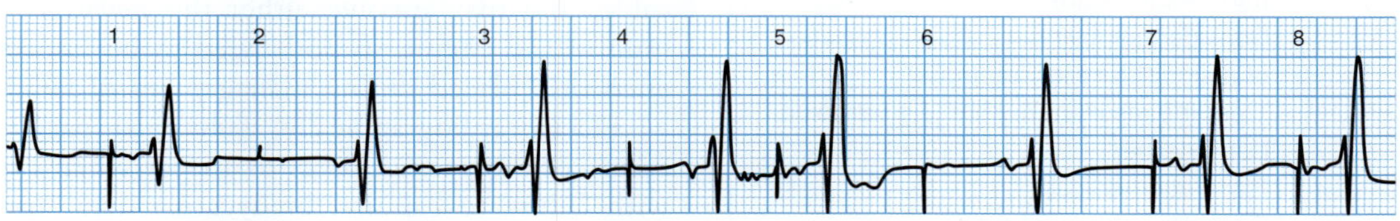

Complications of pacing

Effective pacing may be disturbed by problems related to pacing leads, myocardial responsiveness, programmed values, the pulse generator itself (including power sources), and interactions between these factors.[68–72] Four major disturbances to pacing are described below. These provide the bulk of pacing problems encountered and, because they may either interrupt pacing or precipitate serious arrhythmias, critical care nurses need to be competent in their recognition and management.

Failure to capture

When pacing spikes do not successfully stimulate the heart this is termed 'failure to capture'. Pacing spikes are evident on the ECG but are not followed by either QRS complexes (in ventricular pacing) or P waves (in atrial) (Figs 11.46 and 11.47). Failure to capture may occur when the myocardial responsiveness (threshold) worsens, or when impulses do not reach responsive myocardium. Note that dislodgement of a lead from the myocardium will still show pacing spikes on the ECG as long as the lead is in contact with body fluids or tissue. This is a critical distinction when troubleshooting failure to capture (spikes are present) from failure to pace (no spikes are present) as management of the two is distinctly different. Repositioning of leads must therefore be included in considerations during management of failure to capture.

Failure to capture may present as a clinical emergency and requires immediate attention. With failure to capture, patients are left to generate their own rhythm, which may be unacceptably slow. Failure to capture may be complete (no spikes capturing) or intermittent (with only some spikes achieving capture). Even occasional spikes with failure to capture require immediate attention, as complete failure to capture may ensue. Causes and management of failure to capture[76,79,80,91,92] are listed in Table 11.12. Patient factors which cause failure to capture are the same as causes of bradycardia and/or AV block, and are essentially causes of conduction system depression. This is useful in guiding investigation of clinical reasons for failure to capture. Likewise, treatment includes the same measures used to treat bradycardia and AV block. Positive chronotropes are useful both for managing the resultant bradycardia, and for potentially restoring capture.

Failure to sense

Sensing of the intrinsic cardiac rhythm is necessary to achieve demand pacing.[93] If rhythms are not sensed, pacing will proceed at a fixed rate and in competition with the native rhythm (Figs 11.48 and 11.49). By definition, pacing continues to occur despite the intrinsic rhythm being faster than the set pacing rate. Pacing spikes may thus be delivered during the excitable period of the action potential and trigger tachyarrhythmias[94] (Fig. 11.36). The risk of arrhythmias is greatest when ventricular pacing spikes are delivered just after the peak of the T wave, especially when there is myocardial ischaemia or infarction, or hypokalaemia. Immediate restoration of appropriate sensing needs to be undertaken. Causes and management of failure to sense[81,91,93] are

TABLE 11.12
Failure to capture: causes and management

CAUSES	MANAGEMENT
Output too low	Increase output Increase pulse width if feature is available
Changing capture threshold	Check for and treat ischaemia, hyperkalaemia, acidosis or alkalosis Lead maturation
Antiarrhythmic drugs	Consider cessation or dose reduction
Lead migration/ dislodgement	Reposition lead if able Reverse polarity of leads (for epicardial wires) Position patient on left side (if transvenous lead) Consider unipolar pacing via application of a skin suture (or electrode) Treat the resultant rhythm (e.g. atropine, isoprenaline) Place another lead Consider external pacing

detailed in Box 11.2. Remember, however, that sensing controls are inverse: lowering numerical settings (e.g. from 5 to 2 mV) increases the sensitivity (as does unipolar configuration[95]), while increasing the value (from 1 to 4 mV) makes the pacemaker less sensitive.

Failure to pace

Failure to pace is an imperfect term that is used to describe the event when the pacemaker does discharge but the impulse fails to reach the patient.[76] Pacing spikes are absent. Failure to pace results from a break in the electrical (pacing) circuit. Note that if either the negative or positive leads are disconnected from the pacemaker then the result will be failure to pace. The flashing pace indicators on temporary pacemakers confirm that pacing is occurring, but the spikes fail to appear on the ECG. Most commonly, failure to pace is due to a loose connection in the lead system or a fractured lead or bridging cable, and may involve either the negative or positive limb of the circuit, so both need to be inspected, tightened or replaced during management of failure to pace.

Electrocardiographically, failure to pace appears as failure of the pacing spikes to appear when expected. As with failure to capture, bradycardia may ensue. Failure to pace may present as complete loss of pacing, or just

FIGURE 11.48 Ventricular pacing with failure to sense. At the start of the strip there is ventricular pacing. A junctional rhythm appears at a slightly faster rate than the ventricular pacing, but despite this the pacemaker continues to fire, delivering the spikes into the ST segment and T wave. Appropriate sensing of the last three beats of the strip would have caused inhibition of these pacing spikes. Note also the pacing spikes delivered inappropriately into the QRS and ST segment do not capture as the ventricles are refractory.

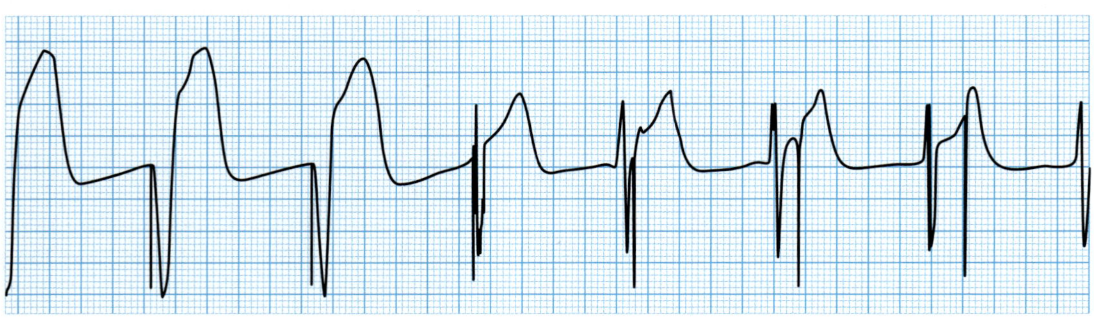

FIGURE 11.49 Atrial failure to sense. The first three beats show atrial pacing. Then there are two spontaneous P waves (4th and 5th beats). These P waves should have inhibited the atrial pacing, but pacing spikes can be seen at the start of the QRS of the 4th beat and in the ST segment of the 5th beat. (Note also, the 3rd pacing spike is strictly a fusion beat as the intrinsic P wave and the pacing spike have occurred simultaneously.)

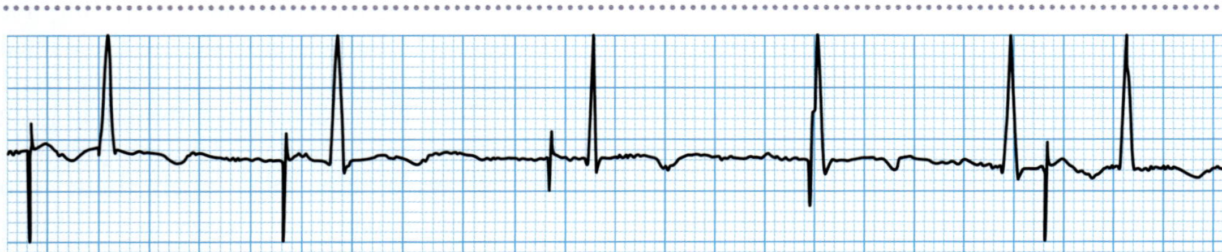

BOX 11.2

Failure to sense: causes and management

Causes:

- Sensitivity set too low (too high a number)
- Programmed to asynchronous mode (AOO, VOO or DOO)
- Altered sensing threshold (lead maturation)
- Decreased myocardial voltages
- Lead movement/dislodgement

Management:

- Increase sensitivity (to a lower number)
- Check/tighten connections
- If epicardial leads, reverse the polarity of the electrodes (reverse connections of positive and negative electrodes)
- Increase the pacing rate to overdrive the competing rhythm
- If underlying rhythm satisfactory, consider turning pacemaker off
- Consider placement of an alternative sensing electrode (skin suture) to create unipolar pacing

pacing at a slower rate than set (Figs 11.50 and 11.51). If the patient's rhythm is very slow, failure to pace can be a clinical emergency. Even if there is an adequate rhythm, the situation requires immediate attention. Causes and management of failure to pace[68,76,93] are detailed in Box 11.3.

Practice tip

The ECG usually does not help to distinguish between oversensing and failure to pace, and instead – at least with temporary pacing – the distinction is made by inspecting the flashing pacing indicators. If the *pacing* indicator continues to flash during periods where the spikes do not appear, then the problem is failure to pace (an interrupted electrical circuit). Alternatively, if the *sense* indicator is flashing during a period where the spikes do not appear, then the problem is oversensing.

Oversensing

As in failure to pace, pacing spikes fail to appear when oversensing occurs.[68,95] Rather than sensing only intrinsic cardiac activity, the pacemaker may sense electrical signals (electromagnetic interference) from other sources. The

FIGURE 11.50 At the start of the strip there is ventricular pacing at a rate of around 85/min. However, the pacing spikes abruptly cease and the patient is left to generate his/her own slower rate. Spikes do reappear but these are slower than the programmed rate. This could be either failure to pace or oversensing during ventricular pacing, and differentiation cannot be made absolutely from this strip. Rather, pacing indicators need to be examined to aid this differentiation. This was a case of ventricular failure to pace due to a poor connection of the pacing leads to the bridging cable.

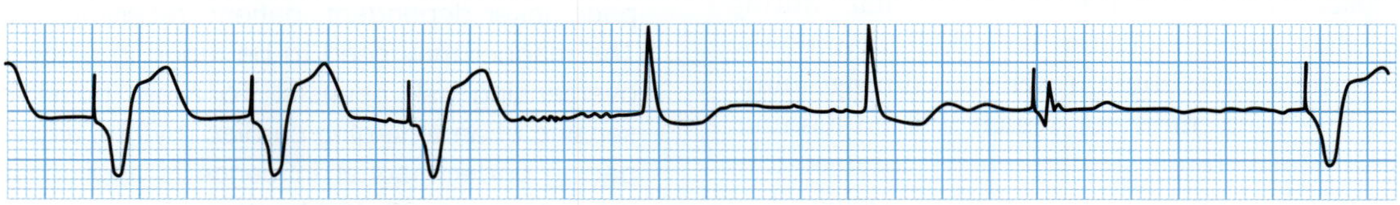

FIGURE 11.51 Atrial pacing with failure to pace. There is sudden disappearance of the pacing spikes after the first three beats. From this strip alone, the distinction between failure to pace and oversensing cannot be made. However, the pacing indicator was flashing through such pauses, rather than the sensitivity indicator, confirming failure to pace. The connection between the pacing wires and the bridging cable needed tightening and immediately corrected the problem.

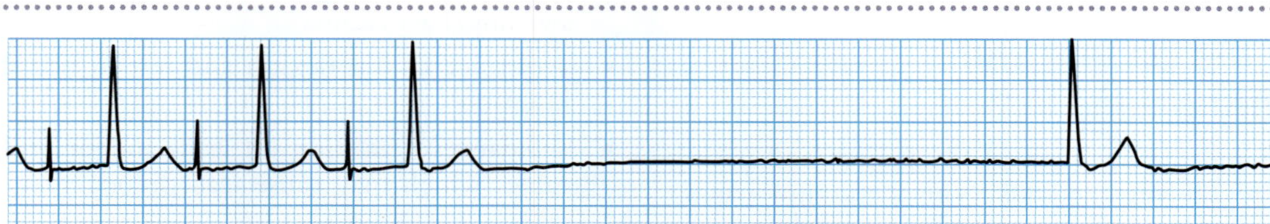

BOX 11.3

Failure to pace: causes and management

Causes:

- Disconnected lead/loose connections – commonest cause
- Pacemaker turned off or dysfunctional
- Output turned off
- Battery depleted
- Fractured lead (may be internally fractured but outwardly intact)

Management:

- Check that pacemaker is turned on
- Check all connections and leads, and tighten/replace if necessary
- Change battery
- Replace the bridging cable between the pacemaker and the pacing leads
- Ensure output is turned on
- Complete circuit with skin suture to positive terminal of the pacemaker, and try each of the existing wires in the negative terminal
- Differentiate from oversensing
- Assess and support rhythm and haemodynamics

device will respond as if these were genuine signals and inhibit pacing. Oversensing is a common event during temporary pacing and electrocardiographically may be indistinguishable from failure to pace, as both appear as missing pacing spikes. Pacing indicators displayed on temporary pacemakers therefore become vital: during oversensing the 'sense' indicator will flash despite the absence of a true cardiac rhythm, whereas during failure to pace it is the 'pace' indicator which will be flashing.

Oversensing may result in momentary interruptions to pacing (pauses) or complete cessation of pacing. The clinical impact depends on the duration of oversensing, and on the patient's ability to generate an underlying rhythm. Electromagnetic interference resulting in oversensing may arise from a variety of causes, originating from the patient (muscle movement) or external sources (devices). The sources of oversensing[68,95] may be difficult to establish clinically but should be sought and corrected where possible. Causes and management of oversensing are detailed in Box 11.4.

Care of the patient with temporary pacing

Monitoring and management of the patient and pacing largely fall to the nursing staff. Nurses monitor pacing performance and the detection of pacing abnormalities, the integrity of the pacing system, the avoidance of clinical situations or physical changes that may alter pacing effectiveness, patient safety and the prevention of complications.

Nursing responsibilities in the care of the patient with a pacemaker include:

- pacemaker site inspection for inflammation/swelling/haematoma
- avoidance of hip flexion and rest in bed if femoral insertion
- avoidance of traction on leads and/or bridging cables which may cause lead dislodgement
- vital signs, circulatory observations etc, at intervals appropriate to the overall patient context

BOX 11.4

Oversensing: causes and management

Causes:

- Muscle potentials other than QRS complexes:
  - Cardiac: T waves, U waves, P waves
  - Non-cardiac: shivering, fasciculations, seizure activity, any skeletal muscle movement
- External electrical interference:
  - Electrocautery, TENS machines
  - Electrical devices (rare)
  - Movement of the connecting pins at the connection to the pulse generator (common)
- Management:
  - Reduce sensitivity (turn sensitivity to higher number)
  - Consider disabling the sensitivity altogether (i.e. asynchronous, VOO, AOO, DOO mode)
  - Consider reversing the polarity of the wires (positive to negative)
  - Remove the source of interference where it can be identified

Practice tip

A ring magnet placed over a permanent pacemaker causes a permanent pacemaker to revert to an asynchronous mode (VOO or DOO). It is thus a management strategy for symptomatic oversensing or for contexts where there is risk of oversensing (e.g. the pacemaker-dependent patient receiving diathermy). The magnet may need to be taped in place while the oversensing risk persists. To avoid possible undersensing of an emerging cardiac rhythm, asynchronous pacing under magnet influence is applied at an elevated rate (e.g. 90–100 beats/min).

- rhythm monitoring:
  - return of intrinsic rhythm or progression to pacemaker dependence
  - detection of pacing associated arrhythmias
- confirmation of capture and sensing
- assessment of haemodynamic adequacy during both paced and spontaneous rhythms (BP, CO, perfusion, symptoms)
- strip documentation of rhythm 6-hourly and daily 12-lead ECG
- chest X-ray to confirm the position of the wire/ absence of complications
- checking and tightening of all connections (leads to bridging cable, bridging cable to pulse generator) at commencement of the shift and during all pacing adverse events
- confirmation of battery status each shift
- performance of pacemaker threshold assessment each shift or daily.

Protection against microshock

Normally, small electrical stimuli (even static electricity applied to the body) dissipate through body tissues and never reach sufficient current density at the heart to produce arrhythmias. However, pacing wires provide a direct route to the heart, so that even minor electrical sources may achieve sufficient current density at the heart to precipitate arrhythmias.[96] Protection strategies include nursing patients in cardiac-protected areas, insulating lead connector pins when pacing is not in use and using rubber gloves at all times when handling pacing wires.[96]

Battery depletion in a temporary pacemaker

A standard 9V battery powers a temporary pacemaker for up to a week. It is prudent to commence treatment with a new battery to avoid unexpected power failure during use.

Indicators of declining battery status are usually displayed when less than 24 hours of battery life remains: flashing battery icons appear on the digital screens of newer generation devices while on both new and older non-digital screen devices, pacemakers will stop supplying power to the flashing sense/pace LEDs while pacing continues. Battery replacement should be undertaken as soon as reasonably possible as these indicators are not obvious until looked for, so some time may have elapsed before detection by staff.

Changing the battery on a temporary device carries the risk of interrupting pacing, which may be disastrous in the pacemaker-dependent patient. It is worth noting, however, that temporary pacemakers carry a small stored charge which is enough to sustain pacing for about 10 seconds. If a well-rehearsed procedure is undertaken, battery change can be performed without interrupting pacing for even a single beat. An understanding of the behaviour of the device in use should be established before undertaking battery replacement, along with a clear understanding of prompt power restoration if powering down occurs.

Pacemaker function testing

Routine pacemaker checks should be undertaken regularly in the patient with a temporary pacemaker. Temporary pacing leads and wires are prone to movement and other causes of sensing and capture threshold variation. Variations may also be marked when there is myocardial, biochemical and haemodynamic volatility as often seen in critically ill patients. Pacemaker tests are performed to reveal the return of underlying rhythm, which may be being concealed by pacing, and to measure thresholds for capture and sensing as these values may change with time and in response to changing myocardial responsiveness[72,79,83,94] Regular checking allows detection of threshold changes, and setting of sensing and output safety margins, in order to avert unexpected failure to capture or sense.

Practices employed to test temporary pacemakers vary widely, as do attitudes to whether this may or may not be undertaken by nurses. The sample protocol shown in Box 11.5 provides an organised approach to testing during which safety has been emphasised. Because of the varying attitudes to nursing responsibilities, the use of this approach should be ratified at individual institutions before use. Many departments stipulate competency certification, and may further stipulate that these procedures apply to routine testing in patients without haemodynamic compromise. An alternative approach to the unstable patient is also provided below.

Testing pacemaker thresholds is performed daily or on each shift, but not if the patient is unstable, using the steps described in Box 11.5. The test should be carried out promptly, with attention to avoiding undue bradycardia or periods of asynchronous pacing. The patient should be advised that pacemaker assessment is being undertaken and to report any sensations/symptoms during testing.

Pacemaker testing in the unstable pacemaker-dependent patient

Greater caution must be applied in the testing of pacemaker functions if the patient has marked haemodynamic instability or has little or no underlying rhythm. It is common for pacemaker testing to be avoided altogether in such circumstances although this may be misguided. Routine testing of pacemaker function as described in Box 11.5 may not be suitable, but testing for underlying rhythm and some level of testing of capture threshold, so as to be confident of safety margins, are beneficial. Testing allows early identification of any emerging influences on pacing efficacy, and may avert their progression to an acute disruption to pacing. Planning and measured responses to identified abnormalities are thus possible.

BOX 11.5

Routine temporary pacemaker testing protocol: underlying rhythm, output and sensitivity threshold test

1. Store current values in memory (for devices with memory). If rhythm difficulty is encountered during testing, these original settings can be immediately re-established by depressing the stored values mode selector.
2. Test for underlying rhythm. Gradually decrease rate in 10 beat/min steps until evidence of underlying rhythm (ULR) emerges:
   (a) If ULR present, observe whether sensing is now occurring.
   (b) If still pacing at 50/min (no emergence of ULR), return to initial settings; do not continue to test sensitivity or output thresholds.
   (c) Document attempt and ULR less than 50/min.
   If ULR is haemodynamically acceptable, continue.
3. Test sensitivity threshold. Having confirmed haemodynamically adequate ULR:
   (a) Turn pacing rate to half the patient's rate.
   (b) Turn output to minimum (not off).
   (NB: Sensitivity testing requires that failure to sense is created for a brief period, so steps 3a and 3b are designed to minimise danger of arrhythmias.)
   While observing the sense indicator on the pacemaker:
   - decrease sensitivity (increasing the number) until failure to sense (the sense indicator stops flashing – pacing indicator will now be flashing);
   - increase sensitivity (decreasing the number) until sensing resumes;
   - note the value at which sensing returns – this is the threshold value for sensing; and
   - set sensitivity to half this value.
4. Test output threshold (continuing from step 3 above the pacing will now be set at a low rate, and at minimum output):
   - Increase the pacing rate to 10 greater than ULR.
   While watching the monitor:
   - gradually increase the output until capture is achieved;
   - note the value at which capture occurs – this is the threshold value; and
   - set output to double this value as a safety margin (minimum 5 mA).
5. Store new values in memory and document settings.

For the patient with haemodynamic instability and/or inotrope use, testing for underlying rhythm becomes of even greater importance as pacing may either prevent or conceal the return of sinus rhythm capability, and cardiac output may be as much as 50% greater with the atrial kick of sinus rhythm than during pacing (Fig. 11.52). In searching for underlying rhythm it may take several seconds for the sinus node to 'warm up' and express itself, so the rate should be reduced gradually and only to reasonable levels (sinus rates of less than 50 are unlikely to be beneficial). It is advisable to have additional cardiology or intensive care personnel present during such non-routine testing.

Threshold testing in the pacemaker-dependent patient is also contentious as loss of capture during testing may be poorly tolerated. If the capture threshold is not measured; however, a rising threshold and loss of safety margins cannot be identified, and may only become apparent upon development of acute failure to capture, possibly with outputs already set to maximum and, therefore, no scope for recovering capture. An alternative approach to testing thresholds in this context is useful. Rather than formally measuring threshold by creating loss of capture, the output may be decreased to a value that confirms safety margins are still possible, but without having lost capture at any point, e.g. where thresholds have previously been modest, decreasing output to 10 mA on a device with an output capability of 20 mA. If there is still capture at 10 mA, further reductions can be avoided because a 10-mA safety margin has been demonstrated.

Permanent pacing

For bradyarrhythmias that are not due to temporary reversible factors or that are likely to be sustained or recurrent, permanent pacemaker implantation may be undertaken, usually in DDD mode.[84,97] Atrial capture cannot be achieved in AF[97] so, if chronic, rate-responsive ventricular pacing is used.[97,98] A dual-chamber device is still used for when atrial fibrillation is intermittent, with automatic mode switching by the device between DDD (during sinus rhythm) and VVI (during AF).

Patients with sinus node dysfunction are more likely to have rate-responsive pacing enabled so that the pacemaker can adjust pacing rates to activity and exercise. Typical pacemaker longevity is 8–12 years.

Positioning of the ventricular lead in the right ventricular outflow tract has largely supplanted the historically routine placement at the right ventricular apex.[99]

Leads are steroid-tipped to limit any lead contact-induced inflammatory changes, and consequent threshold increases.[73] Changes are most evident in the first month, so discharge pacing outputs are set high, and chronic output settings determined at the first postoperative review in 6–8 weeks.

FIGURE 11.52 Unveiling haemodynamically superior underlying rhythm (strips are continuous). Initially there is ventricular pacing at a rate of 68/min. No atrial activity can be seen and the blood pressure is 85/50 mmHg with noradrenaline support at 8 mcg/min. Across the top strip the paced rate is reduced, allowing P waves to emerge at a rate of 60/min (arrow) and then accelerate to around 70/min across the lower strip. Note the impressive BP increase to 125/65 mmHg allowing discontinuation of noradrenaline infusion. (Note also: cardiac index recorded during V pace 1.7 L/min/m^2, during sinus rhythm 2.3 L/min/m^2.) Importantly, there was no suggestion of sinus capability until the pacing rate was reduced.

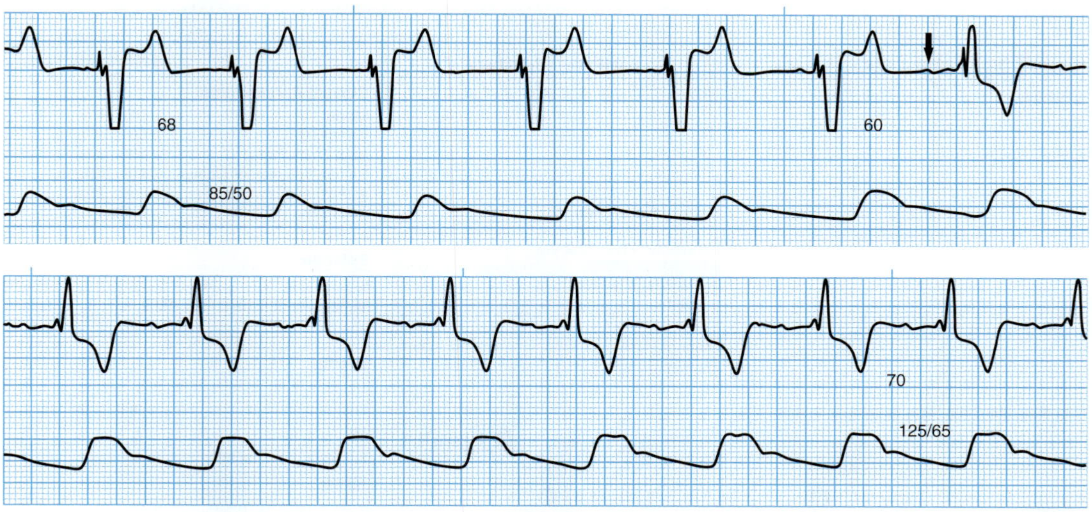

Pacemaker parameters: programming and status reports

Knowledge of current pacemaker programming is crucial to interpreting pacemaker behaviour to enable determination of whether a change in behaviour represents a pacing problem or is simply an automated behaviour. Device printouts should be available whenever a device is interrogated or reprogrammed. The summary pages outline the operating parameters, active automated features, results from recent tests and battery status (see Fig. 11.53 for an example). Important elements include:

- Patient/device details: patient name, type of device, date and time of the printout
- Predicted battery longevity (assuming 100% pacing), and magnet rate (the asynchronous rate which will apply upon magnet placement)
- Current parameters: base rate, maximum atrial tracking rate, AV delay, output settings and pulse widths for both chambers
- Episodes: summary of any arrhythmia episodes that have been recorded since the last interrogation and any automatic mode switching events that have occurred
- Test results: the results of device and lead testing performed during the current interrogation, including graphic trends of all test results over time
- Sense results: the results of the sensing tests carried out in the current interrogation, the last session's values and sensing trends
- Lead impedance: rising impedance accompanies progressive lead fracture and falling impedance suggests degradation of lead insulation.

Cardiac resynchronisation therapy

Cardiac resynchronisation therapy (CRT) involves the use of pacing to improve the performance of the left ventricle in heart failure patients. Initially, CRT was undertaken only in patients with severe heart failure (New York Heart Association Class III–IV with ejection fraction <30%) due to dilated cardiomyopathy and with wide LBBB,[100,101] but its proven efficacy in all major randomised controlled studies[102-106] has seen the range of indications expand to include patients with less severe heart failure (New York Heart Association Class I and II).[107] Ischaemic cardiomyopathies with LBBB are also amenable to CRT. CRT is typically only undertaken after demonstrating failure to respond to optimal medical therapy.

Optimum systolic performance requires all segments of the ventricles to contract more or less synchronously. However, in LBBB septal depolarisation occurs well in advance of the delayed conduction to the posterolateral left ventricular wall, creating ventricular dyssynchrony, with the septum contracting before the lateral wall,[108] resulting in reduced ejection fraction and cardiac output.

FIGURE 11.53 FastPath Summary from a St Jude Medical Accent™ dual-chamber pacemaker (St Jude Medical Sylmar CA), highlighting basic parameters, events and test results recorded during pacemaker interrogation. Any test results or settings followed by an 'A' in a circle denote automated features. Thus, this device will automatically test capture thresholds and set outputs according to these tests every 8 h or if ever there is non-capture. Similarly, sensing is automatically tested and automatic sensitivity algorithms allow for changing myocardial voltages. Lead impedance measurements are automatically tested daily, and the pacemaker can automatically switch from bipolar to unipolar to maintain normal capture and sensing if impedance measurements violate alarm limits. See text for additional details.

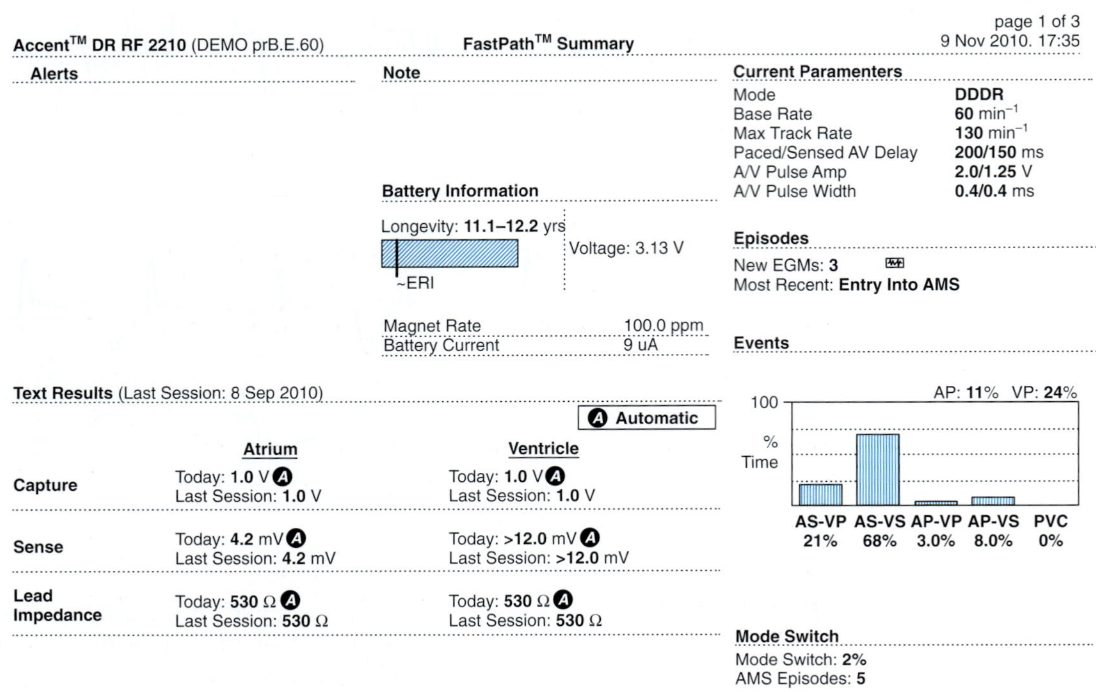

Similarly, ventricular relaxation becomes dyssynchronous, which may lessen myocardial perfusion and limit ventricular filling, both of which contribute to heart failure severity.[108] The majority of patients with LBBB have dyssynchrony and systolic dysfunction, and the impact of this becomes more pronounced when there is existing myocardial disease and/or heart failure. With very wide LBBB (e.g. >0.14 seconds) the impact is greater, as the dyssynchrony between the septal and free wall contraction is exaggerated.[101,108–110]

In CRT, pacing leads on both the right ventricular (RV) septum and the left ventricular (LV) posterolateral wall are used to stimulate both muscle masses at the same time, with the aim of restoring synchronous contraction and improving heart failure.[111] LV and RV pacing stimuli may be delivered simultaneously, although programming of LV stimulation prior to RV pacing by 10–60 milliseconds is more common. The major determinant of CRT success is the degree of QRS duration reduction.[112,113] Expected clinical outcomes of CRT include:[102–112]

- arrest or limit the progression of heart failure
- improvement in New York Heart Association functional class
- improvement in quality of life
- improvement in physical function
- improvement in ejection fraction and reduction in ventricular size
- reduced hospitalisations for heart failure
- cardiovascular mortality reduction.

The right ventricular lead is implanted in standard fashion, positioned either at the RV apex or outflow tract. Most commonly, the left ventricular lead is also positioned transvenously, with the lead advanced via the coronary sinus into a coronary vein on the lateral or posterolateral LV wall. In a minority of cases when access is poor a separate mini-thoracotomy may be necessary for positioning of an epicardial LV lead.

Two types of devices currently exist: CRT-P (pacemaker), which is a pacemaker achieving resynchronisation, and CRT-D (defibrillator), which adds resynchronisation to an ICD. The latter devices are more commonly implanted as the combination of severe heart failure and ventricular tachyarrhythmias is frequently present.[114,115]

Practice tip

For the patient with a CRT device whose heart failure is worsening, investigate whether there are device-related factors that may be correctable:

- Is the patient being ventricularly paced >95% of the time? If not, they will be losing the potential benefit of resynchronisation.
- Can you determine whether there is capture from both the LV and RV leads? Compare with old ECGs where available.

Responders and non-responders to CRT

An improvement in symptoms of heart failure may develop immediately, with restored LV synchrony impacting on dyspnoea even as early as the first post-operative night. It is important to stress to patients that they should not be discouraged by absence of obvious early improvement. A significant additional benefit can be anticipated for most patients as they undergo ventricular alterations to the new pattern of LV contraction under biventricular pacing.[116,117] This 'reverse remodelling' takes time (up to 6–12 months). Patients who show symptom, functional class, and LV measurement improvement are termed responders. Response rates have improved with device capabilities and better understanding of techniques for optimising programming.

Failure to respond to CRT (non-responders)[104,106,116] may be due to device- or lead-related factors, or because of cardiac factors which contribute to worsening heart failure, especially myocardial ischaemia, atrial fibrillation[115] and diminishing responses to adjunctive pharmacological therapy.

It should be noted that the preference in CRT is to see *paced* ventricular rhythms rather than the patient's own QRS complexes as pacing produces a synchronised contraction of the LV compared to the patient's native, dyssynchronous contraction. The aim is for >95% of ventricular beats to be paced to achieve the desired benefit from CRT. While failure to improve is termed non-response, patients in whom their heart failure progression is halted are still deriving significant benefit from device implantation.

Among correctible factors are loss of capture by either the LV or RV lead, resulting in loss of resynchronisation and likely return of heart failure symptoms. With a standard pacemaker, loss of capture is quickly obvious as pacing spikes fail to produce QRS complexes. With two leads, however, loss of capture by only one of the ventricular leads will still appear as capture from the remaining ventricular lead. Additional indications for loss of capture by only one lead are therefore necessary. See below.

AF is particularly problematic for CRT patients as they are generally more dependent on atrial kick and the faster rates also reduce ventricular filling times.[115] Additionally, because they conduct with their own LBBB rather than receiving biventricular pacing they lose the benefit of resynchronisation.

Optimisation of device programming

Optimum device programming can have a significant impact on the benefit conferred by CRT.[101] It is not practical for all patients to undergo regular echocardiography for optimisation of programming and so alternative approaches to optimisation have been developed. The critical timing factors that should be optimised are the atrioventricular (AV) delay and the delay between stimulation of the left and right ventricles (V–V delay).[118] Electrocardiographic optimisation has largely supplanted echocardiography and can be performed quickly and without need for specialist equipment and personnel.[112] Automated optimisation algorithms are also becoming increasingly available.[119,120] The impact of effective optimisation may be sufficient to convert non-responders to responders.

ECG markers of optimum CRT performance

Assessment of CRT systems is most easily made via the ECG; changes may alert clinicians to the need for reprogramming, such as during readmissions for heart failure.[121,122] The markers are simple and can best be identified from V1 on the ECG.

In LBBB, lead V1 features a wide, negative QRS complex resulting in ventricular dyssynchrony.[123] When the heart is paced from the right ventricle, the QRS is wide and resembles LBBB. Lead V1 will have a wide, negative QRS. Pacing from the left ventricle produces a wide QRS, but conduction, spreading from left to right, produces an upright QRS in V1. When pacing from both ventricles, the resultant ECG becomes narrower, and V1 shows either a normalised pattern (narrow, with negative QRS), or more commonly, a hybrid QRS somewhere in between RV pacing and LV pacing, with a narrower QRS results. The narrower the QRS the greater the likelihood of clinical response.[112,122]

The hybrid pattern sought in V1 is a QRS which becomes more upright. Usually this is as a biphasic QRS with an R wave followed by an S wave (an rS or Rs pattern),and the taller the R wave, the greater the likelihood of clinical response to CRT.[122,124,125] In the patient representing with worsening heart failure, ECG changes from these expected patterns should be identified as reprogramming may return optimum device performance.

Recognising failure to capture in a CRT device

Recognising failure to capture in CRT is made difficult by the fact that both ventricles are paced. Failure of pacing to produce QRS complexes will only occur if

FIGURE 11.54 Comparative appearance of lead during biventricular pacing, and alternately with loss of capture by the left ventricular, then right ventricular lead. In the top strip there is Bi-V pacing with a narrow QRS, which is negative in V1. In the same strip, loss of LV capture results in RV-only pacing. The QRS widens to beyond 0.12 s and becomes more deeply negative in V1. In the second strip RV-only becomes Bi-V pacing after re-establishing LV capture. The QRS returns to its initial morphology as in strip 1. In the third strip Bi-V pacing is present initially followed by loss of RV capture, resulting in LV-only pacing. Note that the QRS becomes upright in V1 and again widens to well beyond 0.12 s. In the lower strip LV-only pacing precedes the return to the previous Bi-V morphology as RV capture is restored.

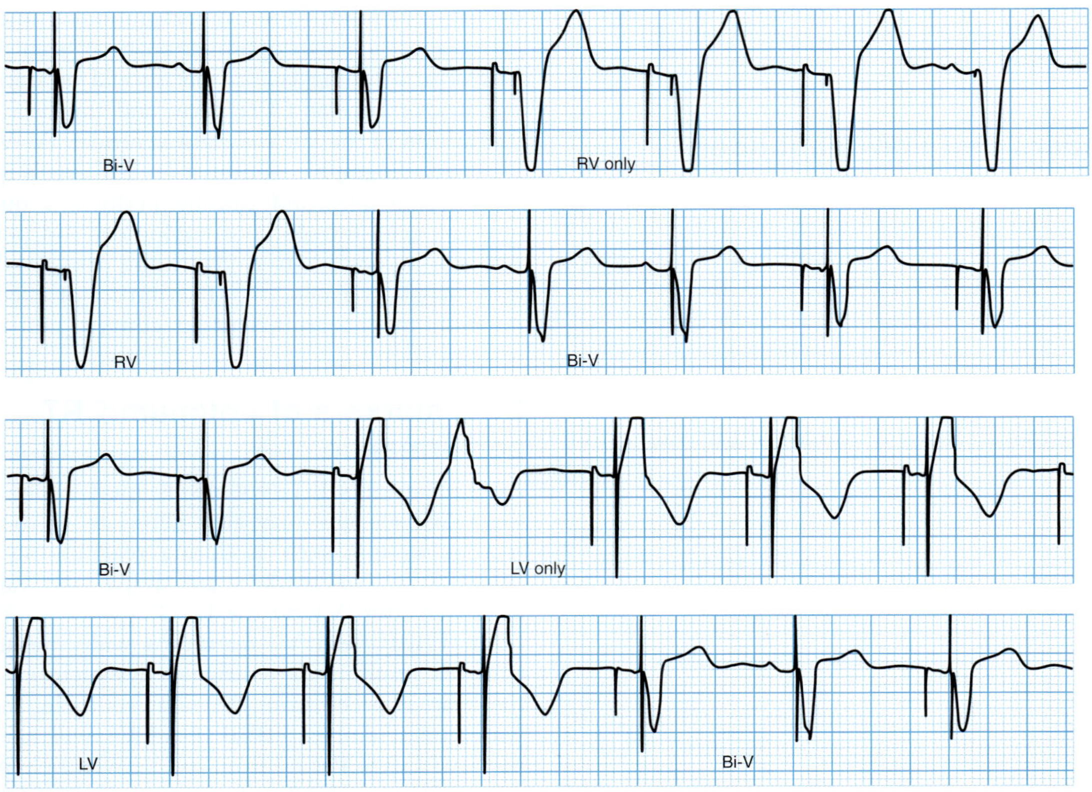

there is failure to capture from *both* LV and RV leads.[120] The ECG, during failure to capture by just the LV lead, will still show capture from the RV lead, and vice versa. Instead of loss of the QRS, to identify loss of capture it is necessary to look more closely at QRS morphology and vectors to confirm capture or loss of capture from either the left or right ventricular lead.[120,122] Lead V1 (or MCL1) and lead I are the most helpful in confirming RV, LV or biventricular (Bi-V) capture. Specific changes include:

- RV capture only (loss of LV capture): the QRS will be wide (>0.12 seconds) with left-axis deviation; lead V1 (or MCL1) will be a negative complex, most commonly as a QS complex. QRS in lead I will be upright, as an R wave or sometimes rSR[104] (Fig. 11.54).
- LV capture only (loss of RV capture): the QRS will be wide (>0.12 s) with right-axis deviation; lead V1 (or MCL1) will be an upright complex, either as an R wave, or less commonly as an rSR. QRS in lead I will be a negative complex, either as a QS or rS complex[104] (Fig. 11.54).
- Biventricular capture: the QRS may be negative (and narrow), or more commonly overall upright (RS or rS pattern)[113,121,124] with the axis deviated most commonly to the right.[121,122,125]

Phrenic nerve stimulation in CRT patients

On occasion LV pacing may stimulate the phrenic nerve producing repetitive diaphragmatic contraction of varying intensities. These may be continuous and uncomfortable or painful, disturb sleep, and are usually visible on inspection. Programming may overcome the problem but, if unsuccessful, reoperation to reposition the LV lead may be necessary, or resynchronisation therapy may need to be abandoned altogether. Advances in lead design have delivered greater options for programming to overcome phrenic nerve stimulation.

Cardioversion and defibrillation

Electrical cardioversion can be applied as an adjunct to pharmacological therapy in the management of tachyarrhythmias. The aim of cardioversion is to excite all myocardial cells at the same time with the result that all of the heart will also be refractory at the same time. If this is achieved, the circulating stimulus of reentry dies out for lack of non-refractory tissue to conduct through. If the applied shock does not depolarise the greater bulk of myocardium, then non-depolarised cells are still available for conduction and the arrhythmia may persist. External shocks of 100–200 joules (biphasic) are required for sufficient current density to reach the myocardium and depolarise the greater bulk of cells, thus extinguishing available pathways.[126] Drugs or biochemical correction may be necessary to prevent recurrence. Success rates from cardioversion range from 70% to 95% depending on the rhythm.[126] Arrhythmias due to increased automaticity are less amenable to cardioversion, as there is a higher chance of early arrhythmia recurrence; and for arrhythmias occurring as a complication of digitalis toxicity, cardioversion (but not defibrillation) is contraindicated.

Early defibrillation increases survival from VF. The success of public-access defibrillator schemes has warranted their increased availability.[127,128] Automatic external defibrillators (AEDs) in the home or community simplify the task of applying defibrillation by non-healthcare responders and increase access to definitive electrical management for patients suffering ventricular arrhythmias. For patients at increased risk for arrhythmia development, or for those who have survived previous arrhythmic cardiac arrest, an ICD may be necessary. Emergency defibrillation is discussed more completely in Chapter 25

Elective cardioversion

Elective direct current reversion (DCR, or cardioversion) applied under short-acting sedation or anaesthesia is undertaken for non-cardiac arrest arrhythmias.[128] These include AF, tachycardia or flutter, conscious VT, AV nodal reentry tachycardia, and conscious tachyarrhythmias complicating Wolff–Parkinson–White syndrome. The time available for preparation is variable and depends on the haemodynamic impact of the arrhythmia. Patients admitted for reversion of AF or flutter may be stable throughout their hospitalisation, whereas patients with conscious VT may initially demonstrate stability, only to decompensate later without warning.

Unlike emergency defibrillation, cardioversion shocks are synchronised to the cardiac cycle so that they are delivered into the QRS complex. Unsynchronised shocks, if delivered into the T wave, may precipitate VF. With successful synchronisation, a marker is inscribed over each ECG on the monitor.

When time permits the patient should be thoroughly investigated, including physical examination, neurological assessment, palpation of peripheral pulses, electrocardiograph, biochemistry, and serum drug levels where necessary.[129] Fasting should be ensured. If AF or flutter are present echocardiography is undertaken to rule out atrial thrombus, as restoration of atrial contraction may cause pulmonary or systemic arterial embolisation. The patient should be fully informed of the rationale for and nature of the procedure and have all necessary preparatory tasks explained to them.

The cardioversion team should include a minimum of one medical officer, skilled in emergency rhythm management and airway management including intubation, and two critical care nurses, who prepare the patient and equipment, assist in sedation, perform the cardioversion, document events and manage aftercare. Usually there is a cardiologist and anaesthetist present for the separate roles. All team members should confirm readiness, confirm synchronisation, and correct defibrillator energy settings (in joules). The patient is sedated (e.g. midazolam) or anaesthetised (e.g. propofol), pre-oxygenated, and cardioverted under ECG and oximetry monitoring. Electrical safety, and ensuring that all personnel are clear of the bed, is the responsibility of the nurse delivering cardioversion, whether via paddles or hands-free electrodes.

After the procedure the patient should be closely monitored for return to wakefulness, airway protection capability, effective respiration and gas exchange, rhythm stability, blood pressure, and for any changes in neurological status or peripheral pulses. Pain and inflammation at cardioversion discharge sites may be lessened by application of topical ibuprofen 5% cream 2 hours before elective DCR, where this is feasible.[130] Energy requirements for reversion of atrial tachycardia or flutter may be as little as to 50 joules (J).[130,131] The 2010 recommendations of the European Resuscitation Council[128] are for initial shocks at 70–120 J (biphasic) for atrial flutter, and 120–150 J for cardioversion of AF and VT. If initial shocks are unsuccessful, repeat attempts at higher energy settings (up to 360 J) may be undertaken.

Implantable cardioverter defibrillators

Implantable cardioverter defibrillators (ICDs) may be implanted for survivors of sudden cardiac death (SCD) or haemodynamically significant, potentially lethal, ventricular arrhythmias.[132] They have been repeatedly demonstrated in large clinical trials to provide significantly improved survival compared with pharmacological treatment.[133-136] This 'secondary prevention' application of ICDs dominated the early indications for devices, with trial meta-analysis demonstrating a mean 27% mortality reduction compared with antiarrhythmics.[133] More recently indications have expanded to 'primary prevention' in patients without prior cardiac arrest, as it has become clear that heart failure patients with ejection fractions <30% (including both ischaemic

FIGURE 11.55 Successful antitachycardia pacing delivered by an implantable cardioverter defibrillator. Three simultaneous strips show the presence of sustained ventricular tachycardia (VT). After the first eight beats, pacing is applied at a rate slightly faster than the tachycardia. Entrainment, or capture, by the pacemaker is best seen in lead II, where the QRS morphology clearly changes. After 11 paced beats, ATP is ceased, revealing interruption of the VT.

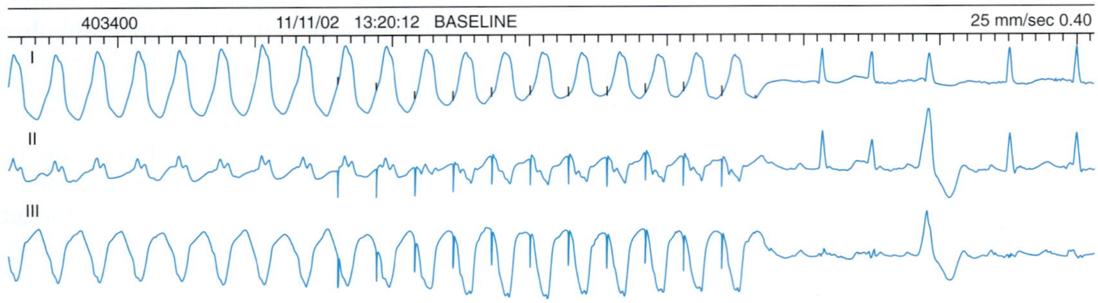

and non-ischaemic cardiomyopathies) have a high risk of sudden cardiac death due to ventricular arrhythmias.[136,137]

The modern ICD features both antibradycardia and antitachycardia capabilities. As antibradycardia devices they possess all the capabilities of standard pacemakers, increasingly in the DDD mode. However, if there is no history of bradycardia, they may be programmed at low base pacing rates (e.g. 40/min). If there is significant heart failure the antibradycardia arm may be provided as biventricular pacing (to achieve cardiac resynchronisation). Antitachycardia features are those therapies provided to treat ventricular tachyarrhythmias and include antitachycardia pacing (ATP), also termed overdrive pacing, as well as cardioversion (for VT) and defibrillation (for very fast VT or VF). Refer to Fig. 11.55 for an example of antitachycardia pacing.

ICDs are most commonly positioned in the left pectoral region, leaving the right side of the chest available for conventional placement of external defibrillator paddles should they ever become necessary. Atrial leads are normal atrial pacing leads, but the ventricular ICD leads are slightly larger than pacing leads and carry the normal ventricular pacing circuitry, as well as coils encircling the lead that emit the high-energy shock discharges. Single coil systems have one coil positioned on the lead at the level of the RV cavity, and shocks travel from this coil to the metal casing of the ICD. Dual coil leads feature this same RV coil as well as a second coil in the superior vena cava. In these systems, shocks can be configured to travel from the RV coil to the superior vena cava coil, from the RV coil to the ICD, or from the RV coil to both the superior vena cava coil and the ICD. Configurations can impact significantly on the defibrillation threshold, and changes to the shock vector may be undertaken for patients with high defibrillation thresholds.

All modern ICDs provide biphasic shock waveforms only. Arrhythmia detection and classification usually require only a few seconds, and charging to maximum joules in a new device takes up to 10 seconds. As the battery declines charge time may increase to 15–20 seconds or longer. Maximum energy delivery capabilities vary between manufacturers but are all in the range of 30–40 J.

Typically, shocks for VF and very fast VT are provided at the maximum available capability of the device, but for less fast ventricular tachycardia, lower 'cardioversion' shocks may be attempted first (e.g. 15–25 J). If initial shocks are unsuccessful, progressive shock strength escalation occurs.[132]

Defibrillation thresholds may be measured at the time of implantation of the ICD; however, this practice has decreased significantly because of inherent risks in inducing VF, and because it is recognised that clinical VF may behave differently to induced VF.[138,139]

ICDs are usually programmed to deliver up to six 'therapies' during a tachyarrhythmia episode. For VF, this usually means six attempts at defibrillation at maximum joules after which further antitachycardia therapies are aborted. No more shocks will be delivered. Antibradycardia pacing operation will continue. If the tachyarrhythmia is interrupted at any point and then recurs, the six-therapy counter will recommence. For VT, attempts may first be made to overdrive pace. So-called ATP aims to interrupt VT by pacing the ventricles slightly faster than the VT rate so as to interrupt reentry, the major cause of VT (see Fig. 11.55 for example of reversion). A number of attempts at ATP may be programmed, often with slightly faster rates at each successive attempt. This is especially true if the patient is known to tolerate their VT reasonably well. If ATP is unsuccessful, devices progress to shocks of increasing strength.

Tachyarrhythmia detection and classification

ICDs are configured to classify and treat arrhythmias first on the basis of rate. Defibrillation algorithms using high-energy settings (30–40 J) are followed when the rate is very fast (e.g. >200/min), as syncope is likely even if the rhythm is not VF (e.g. very fast VT). At slower rates, other antitachycardia options may first be attempted. Additionally, at rates where the rhythm could be ventricular or supraventricular, attempts are made to discriminate between ventricular and supraventricular tachycardias (SVTs) using a variety of criteria. SVT discrimination by a device uses similar criteria to those by which a clinician would differentiate between VT and SVT and includes regularity or irregularity of the rhythm, sudden or gradual onset, similar or different morphology to the previous sinus rhythm, and atrioventricular relationships. If these discriminators indicate that a tachyarrhythmia is supraventricular, therapy can be withheld, avoiding inappropriate therapy. The major device capabilities and programming options of an ICD are shown in Fig. 11.56.

Patients receiving ICDs require particular education and support, as the experience of shocks can be painful and disturbing. Anticipation of shocks can cause anxiety and/or depression,[140] especially in patients who have experienced shocks while conscious. Inappropriate therapy delivery remains a significant problem, and as many as 25% of ICD therapies were reported as inappropriate shocks during early experience, delivered due either to supraventricular arrhythmias or oversensing of electromagnetic interference.[140,141] Refinement of rhythm discrimination has seen the incidence of inappropriate shocks reduced significantly with time. The avoidance of strong electrical fields (welding, generators) should be stressed, as well as direct contact with devices such as transcutaneous electrical nerve stimulation (TENS) machines or electrocautery devices.[73] If surgery requiring diathermy becomes necessary, antitachycardia therapies are usually programmed to 'OFF' to avoid inappropriate detection and treatment. The ability to undergo magnetic resonance imaging (MRI) should be determined on an individual basis, as some, but not all ICDs, are approved for use in the MRI environment.

Patients should be encouraged to rest after any therapy delivery and, where multiple discharges occur, they should report to a healthcare facility for assessment.[142] If inappropriate shocks are being delivered (shocks delivered despite the patient not being in VT or VF), further shocks may be suspended by the placement of a ring magnet over the device.[143] This suspends the antitachycardia features of the device while the magnet is in place – no therapy will be delivered by the device. Cardiac monitoring is imperative while a magnet is in place to detect any development of genuine ventricular arrhythmias as these would not be treated by the device. Removal of the magnet will immediately reactivate antitachycardia therapies. Back-up (antibradycardia) pacing functions remain active and unaffected during magnet application.

In the event of unsuccessful reversion of a ventricular arrhythmia by ICD therapy, standard advanced life support protocols should be applied. External defibrillation can be undertaken with paddles in normal apicobasal or anteroposterior positions, taking care to avoid positioning paddles over the ICD.[142] External chest compressions can safely be undertaken by rescuers, including during device therapy.[144]

Practice tip

If cardiac arrest occurs in a patient with an ICD in place, all standard therapies should be undertaken, including CPR, drug administration, and immediate preparation for external defibrillation. If device shocks are unsuccessful, proceed to external defibrillation.

End-of-life care in the patient with an ICD

ICDs often create uncertainty among healthcare workers as to how death may occur. In the palliative patient, where active resuscitation is not to be pursued, the decision to disable antitachycardia therapies is often taken. This can be achieved by reprogramming the ICD, and there is often sufficient time to incorporate this step into palliative planning. If time does not permit this, tachyarrhythmia treatment can be suspended by securing a ring magnet over the ICD (tape it in place). Thus, if the terminal rhythm is VT or VF, therapies will not be delivered.

Other than by disabling therapy, cardiac death may occur by normal mechanisms. However, cardiac depressive factors will not cause bradycardia or asystole because of the pacemaker function. What would otherwise be a bradyarrhythmic death will instead become eventual failure to capture by the pacemaker. Similarly, if the cardiac impact of acute or terminal illness produces tachyarrhythmias, these same influences will increase the defibrillation threshold and antitachycardia therapies will become unsuccessful. Devices offer no protection against pulseless electrical activity.

FIGURE 11.56 Implantable cardioverter defibrillator (ICD) programmed parameter summary report from St Jude Medical ICD Ellipse™ dual chamber ICD model 2277-36 (St Jude Medical, Sylmar CA). Similar to the report shown earlier for a pacemaker, the report includes battery status and test results for lead impedances, sensing and capture thresholds for the atrial and ventricular lead. The battery status section also displays the most recent time (in seconds) taken for the device to charge to a maximum joule shock and the date. In the parameters section are the programmed settings for pacing and defibrillation behaviours. The tachyarrhythmia treatments are shown at the right of the parameters section and show the device behaviour for tachycardias occurring at different rates. In the so-called 'VF zone', the ICD will respond to any arrhythmia faster than 214 beats/min (whether it is VF or fast VT). As rhythms at this rate are likely to be syncopal, ICDs are usually programmed to proceed directly to delivering shocks rather than spending time delivering ATP unless, as here, a single attempt at ATP is selected to be delivered while the device is charging (and therefore not delaying the time to first shock delivery). Shocks in the VF zone are more commonly at maximum joules although first shocks may be of lesser strength with subsequent escalation. In the VT-2 zone, a different strategy has been programmed for VT between 181 and 214/min. Three attempts at delivering ATP have been programmed and, if unsuccessful, the ICD will progress to increasing energy levels (20, 30, 36 J) if reversion is not achieved. An additional strategy has been included for slower forms of VT (150–181/min) (VT-1 zone). As VT at these rates is more likely to be tolerated greater use of ATP is often programmed so as to avoid shocks if possible. Two different ATP regimes have been set, with the second set of six pacing attempts more aggressive than the first set of six. If ATP is unsuccessful, the device progresses to escalating shocks. Details of how the device is set to discriminate between VT and SVT, as well as the set-up of the pacing strategies, are given in separate sections of these reports. Also shown on the summary are any VT/VF episodes since the last device check. In this case there had been two episodes of VT and two of VF. Recordings of these arrhythmias and treatments are recorded elsewhere in the report.

15 Mar 2019
6:48 am
In-Clinic

FastPath™ Summary — ⚠ 7 Alerts — Page 1 of 2

Battery
Longevity: 5.4-5.8 yrs
~ERI — > 6 yrs

Implant Date:	21 Sep 2017
Last Max Charge	10.0 sec (8 Jan 2019)
Battery Current	14 uA
Remaining Capacity to ERI	83%

Test Results 15 Mar 2019 — Ⓐ Automatic

	Capture	Sense	Lead Impedance
A	**1.0V @ 0.5ms** (Bi) Ⓐ 0.875V @ 0.5ms (Bi) 14 Jan 2019	**4.0mV** (Bi) Ⓐ 4.0mV (Bi) 14 Jan 2019	**600 Ω** (Bi) Ⓐ 580 Ω (Bi) 13 Feb 2019
V	**1.0V @ 0.5ms** (Bi) Ⓐ 1.0V @ 0.5ms (Bi) 14 Jan 2019	**>12.0mV** (Bi) Ⓐ >12.0mV (Bi) 14 Jan 2019	**580 Ω** (Bi) Ⓐ 580 Ω (Bi) 13 Feb 2019
HV			**42 Ω** (RV to SVC & Can) Ⓐ 41 Ω (RV to SVC & Can) 13 Feb 2019

Parameters

Mode	DDDR	Zone Configuration	VT-1	VT-2	VF
Base Rate	65 min-1	Detection Criteria	150 min-1	181 min-1	214 min-1
Max Track Rate	110 min-1	Therapy **(ENABLED)**	▸**ATP x6**	▸**ATP x3**	ATP x1
Paced AV Delay	200 ms		▸**ATP x6**	▸**20.0 J**	▸**30.0 J**
Sensed AV Delay	150 ms		▸**30.0 J**	30.0 J	▸**36.0 J**
			▸**36.0 J x2**	36.0 J x2	36.0 J x4

Capture & Sense

	A	V
ACap™ Confirm/V. AutoCapture	On	On
Pulse Amplitude	2.0 V Ⓐ	1.25 V Ⓐ
Pulse Width	0.5 ms	0.5 ms
AutoSense	On	On
Sensitivity	Auto Ⓐ	Auto Ⓐ

Diagnostics Summary Since 20 Mar 2018

AP	3.5 %
VP	14 %
AMS Episodes	6
Mode Switch	<1%
AT/AF Burden	<1%

VT/VF Episodes: 4 Since 14 Jan 2019

	VT-1	VT-2	VF
Episodes	0	2	2
ATP Delivered		0	0
Shocks Delivered		2	0

SVT Episodes: 0
Non-sustained Episodes: 0

Summary

Alteration to the electrophysiological function of the heart is very common in patients admitted to critical care settings. Arrhythmia detection is largely the responsibility of the critical care nurse, who must maintain accurate monitoring, constantly observe for the development of arrhythmias, assess their clinical impact and assist in identifying causative factors. The critical care nurse must also deliver the care and management of arrhythmias, including pharmacological and electrical therapies, being aware of complications and management of complications of these treatments.

Case study

Three days following coronary artery bypass graft surgery, Mr Schmidt, a 78-year-old male, remained in cardiogenic shock requiring high dose adrenaline and noradrenaline infusions, and intra-aortic balloon pump support. He remained sedated, intubated and ventilated.

Rhythm: the underlying rhythm was unknown as pacemaker testing had not been undertaken due to his severe shock state. VVI pacing (two standard ventricular epicardial wires), output 13 mA. Atrial wires present but had been described as 'non-functional'

Cardiac index 1.4 L/min/m^2, right atrial pressure 23 mmHg, mean pulmonary artery pressure 27 mmHg.

A monitor alarm highlighted abrupt onset of asystole and complete loss of pacing spikes. No underlying escape rate rhythm emerged and asystole persisted (Fig. 11.57).

Before progressing, make your own judgements about the initial rhythm shown in Fig. 11.57 and how it should be treated. Additionally, what can be said about the function of the pacemaker and how should it be managed?

CPR and standard ALS practices were commenced with no immediate impact on the rhythm, and the question of resuscitative futility was raised.

The digital display of the pacemaker was still active, ruling out battery depletion. The 'emergency pacing mode' was selected. Not available on all pacemakers, this mode delivers asynchronous pacing at 80 beats/min at maximum output and is a useful first step whenever asystole or severe bradycardia develops while pacing is on. Asynchronous pacing will immediately correct the situation if the absence of spikes is due to oversensing. If, however, the problem persists after selecting asynchronous pacing then the problem is failure to pace, and every effort should be directed to re-establishing an intact pacing circuit.

Inspection of pacing leads and bridging cables for integrity and security of connections revealed the cause – the connector pin at the end of the positive pacing lead had been snapped off at the connection to the bridging cable. Without the positive electrode, pacing spikes could not be delivered.

With persistent asystole despite full resuscitative efforts, and a non-functioning pacing system, futility was agreed upon and the decision was made to withdraw treatments. An attempt to restore pacing via conversion to unipolar pacing was made as a final effort.

FIGURE 11.57 Ventricular pacing at 80 beats/min followed by abrupt, complete interruption to pacing and asystole. Atrial activity cannot be seen and no ventricular rhythm emerges.

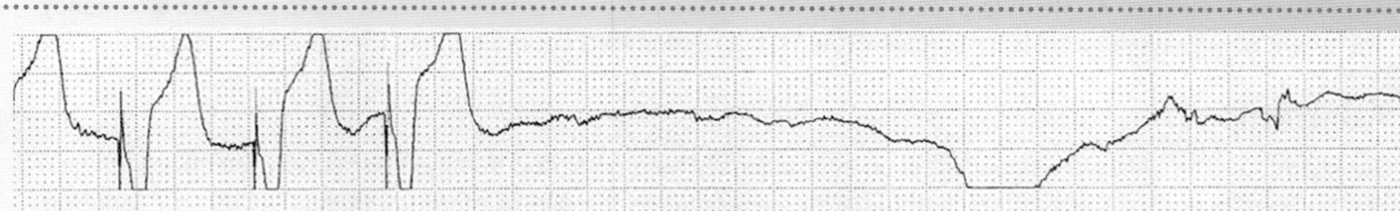

FIGURE 11.58 Restoration of ventricular pacing at 80 beats/min upon conversion to unipolar pacing. 100% capture is evident.

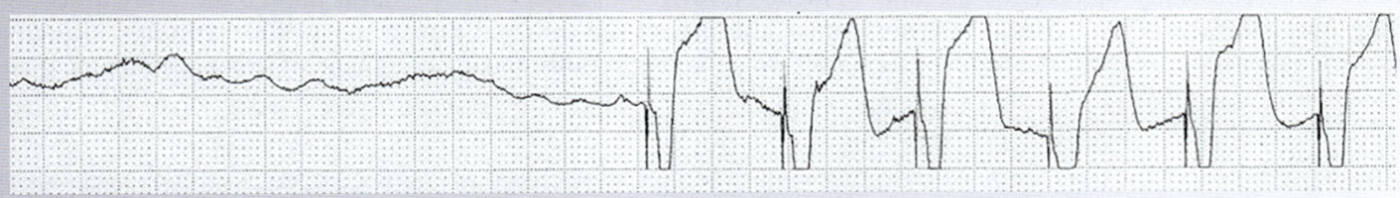

Unipolar pacing was achieved using an ECG dot on the anterior chest and the use of a modified ECG cable, connected to the ECG dot at one end and to the positive connection of the bridging cable at the other (this cable lead had previously been modified for this purpose, with a connector pin meeting connection dimensions. If it had not been available, a commercial pacing skin suture could be used).

The strip in Fig. 11.58 shows the response upon plugging the cable into the positive terminal. Ventricular pacing spikes resume immediately, with 100% capture. Note the very large spikes which are typically seen during unipolar pacing. Of additional note, atrial pacing spikes had not appeared despite the selection of the emergency (DOO) pacing mode. Subsequent investigation of the status of the atrial pacing wires revealed a loose connection of the negative pin at the bridging cable. Thus, there was also atrial failure to pace. Simply tightening this connection restored atrial pacing and atrial capture. Capture via both leads remained reliable and intrinsic conduction eventually re-emerged. Circulatory support was weaned and the patient discharged home alive.

Of note, the need for unipolar pacing was obvious in this case as the positive connector pin had been snapped off. Even if this had not been the case conversion to unipolar pacing was still indicated by failure to pace. If the first step of tightening all connections does not correct failure to pace, then components (even if outwardly intact) need to be replaced – first the bridging cable and then the positive electrode via the skin suture or ECG dot connection. If unsuccessful a new pacing lead would be necessary.

CASE STUDY QUESTIONS

1 Had the steps above not been effective for failure to pace, what additional tactics are available to manage this complication?

2 Atrial pacing wires were available in this patient but had been described as not working:

   a During the ventricular standstill would it have been worth trying to restore the function of the atrial pacing?

   b What would be the advantages (if any) of restoring atrial lead function after the patient's rhythm had been restored?

3 What tools do you have in your unit or hospital for converting temporary pacing systems from bipolar to unipolar? Review the particulars of your equipment and how they are used.

RESEARCH VIGNETTE

Appelboam A, Reuben A, Mann C et al. Postural modification to the standard Valsalva manoeuvre for emergency treatment of supraventricular tachycardias (REVERT): a randomised controlled trial. Lancet 2015; 386:1747-1753

Abstract

Background: The Valsalva manoeuvre is an internationally recommended treatment for supraventricular tachycardia, but cardioversion is rare in practice (5–20%), necessitating the use of other treatments including adenosine, which patients often find unpleasant. We assessed whether a postural modification to the Valsalva manoeuvre could improve its effectiveness.

Methods: We did a randomised controlled, parallel-group trial at emergency departments in England. We randomly allocated adults presenting with supraventricular tachycardia (excluding AF and flutter) in a 1:1 ratio to undergo a modified Valsalva manoeuvre (done semi-recumbent with supine repositioning and passive leg raise immediately after the Valsalva strain), or a standard semi-recumbent Valsalva manoeuvre. A 40-mmHg pressure, 15 s standardised strain was used in both groups. Randomisation, stratified by centre, was done centrally and independently, with allocation with serially numbered, opaque, sealed, tamper-evident envelopes. Patients and treating clinicians were not masked to allocation. The primary outcome was return to sinus rhythm at 1 min after intervention, determined by the treating clinician and electrocardiogram and confirmed by an investigator masked to treatment allocation.

Findings: We enrolled 433 participants between Jan 11, 2013, and Dec 29, 2014. Excluding second attendance by five participants, 214 participants in each group were included in the intention-to-treat analysis. 37 (17%) of 214 participants assigned to standard Valsalva manoeuvre achieved sinus rhythm compared with 93 (43%) of 214 in the modified Valsalva manoeuvre group (adjusted odds ratio 3·7 (95% CI 2·3–5·8; $p<0.0001$). We recorded no serious adverse events.

Interpretation: In patients with supraventricular tachycardia, a modified Valsalva manoeuvre with leg elevation and supine positioning at the end of the strain should be considered as a routine first treatment, and can be taught to patients.

Critique

The Valsalva manoeuvre is the first-line treatment for supraventricular tachycardia (SVT) in current practice guidelines.[2] The technique is simple, non-invasive, and can be taught to patients for use in the home, potentially avoiding the need for Emergency Department attendance. Its main limitation is low success; in this paper a success rate between 5 and 20% is suggested for a standard Valsalva. This is usually achieved by asking the patient to blow into a 10 mL syringe to try and blow the plunger out. This causes expiration against a closed glottis, and an increase in intrathoracic pressure which reduces preload and cardiac output.[8] This leads to a compensatory increase in heart rate and vasoconstriction, mediated by increased sympathetic tone. When the manoeuvre is terminated, intrathoracic pressure falls, and preload and cardiac output rise, causing a reflex surge in parasympathetic (vagal) tone that slows heart rate and AV node conduction speed. The transient drop in conduction speed through the AV node is sufficient to interrupt reentry and terminate SVT in some people.

In this study, the authors postulated that laying patients flat and raising their legs to 45° for 15 seconds immediately after the Valsalva manoeuvre would further augment preload, and result in a stronger vagal response that would be more effective in terminating SVT. This hypothesis was supported; of 214 people performing a standard Valsalva, only 17% reverted to sinus rhythm. This increased to 43% in the modified Valsalva group. Adenosine was subsequently required by 69% of patients in the standard Valsalva group, but only 50% in the modified group. The study was well conducted, with rigorous randomisation, multiple centres, and a standardised approach to both the interventions and the measurement of outcome. Baseline demographics, medical history and physiological data were similar in the two groups. There was no loss to follow up, and no cross-over between the two groups. Although it was impossible to blind the researchers or participants, a source of potential bias, data analysis was blinded. It should be pointed out, however, that while the study was conducted in multiple hospitals, these were all located in a single country. Some caution should therefore be used when extrapolating these findings to other countries or healthcare settings.

This is a thought-provoking study for several reasons. First, the intervention was highly effective, as well as safe, with no serious adverse events recorded in either group. This is unusual in healthcare interventions. Second, the improved outcome was achieved at zero cost, using simple and readily available materials. There is a potential cost saving in drugs and intravenous lines. This is increasingly important in all healthcare systems, where cost containment, and value for money, are important drivers of policy. Finally, there is a real benefit for patients. Receiving adenosine is a highly unpleasant experience; the drug induces transient, complete heart block, and produces symptoms including chest pain, breathlessness and a sensation of impending doom. A more effective Valsalva allows more patient to avoid this unpleasant treatment, or even to avoid hospital attendance altogether.

Learning activities

1 Practice using a systematic approach to rhythm interpretation by collecting rhythms from your department and applying the criteria in Tables 11.1–11.6.

2 Review the contents of emergency pacing systems located in your unit. Familiarise yourself with use of bridging cables, pulse generators and equipment for converting bipolar to unipolar pacing. If uncertain with any equipment, utilise your education staff or contact equipment company representatives to review with you.

3 Perform supervised pacemaker testing according the guidelines in Box 11.5. The aim of practice should be to perform testing with minimum interruptions to pacing and sensing in the various steps of the procedure.

4 Draw a series of simple diagrams of the heart's conducting system, then sketch and label the differing sequences of sinoatrial, AV junctional and ventricular conduction events that occur with second-degree AV block types I and II and third-degree AV block. Compare and contrast the relative conduction events occurring with each AV block type and their relationship to the surface ECG rhythm patterns that are typically observed in each.

5 A patient with dilated cardiomyopathy is admitted with worsening heart failure. He has had a biventricular pacemaker implanted previously. What cardiac rhythm or ECG changes may be present which may contribute to his heart failure?

6 You are caring for a 68-year-old gentleman with chronic AF who develops intermittent non-sustained runs of VT. The man has been admitted to critical care for the management of acute renal failure and has a history of coronary artery disease and chronic obstructive pulmonary disease. With reference to antiarrhythmic classifications (Table 11.7) and with further reading, consider the relative benefits and risks of administering flecainide, sotalol or amiodarone for the treatment of this man's VT.

Online resources

'Life in the Fast Lane' is as an excellent online resource for concise information on arrhythmias and 12-lead ECG abnormalities. It is to the point, up to date, and discusses features, clinical considerations and management, http://lifeinthefastlane.com

'ECG Corner' is an open learning platform for the medical community working in cardiology. It has a high-quality lecture series, especially for progressing beyond the basics of electrocardiography and arrhythmias. The site is sponsored by Abbott, and the courses are designed and delivered by Hein Wellens and Geronimo Farre, www.ecgcorner.org:

ECG quizzes and teaching materials: http://library.med.utah.edu/kw/ecg/, http://ekgreview.com/, http://biotel.ws/quizzes/ekgs/ekgs.htm, www.ecglibrary.com/ecghome.html, http://en.ecgpedia.org, www.learntheheart.com/ecg-review/ecg-quiz

ECRI Institute Alarm Safety Resource site, www.ecri.org/forms/pages/Alarm_Safety_Resource.aspx

European Heart Rhythm Association (EHRA), www.escardio.org/communities/EHRA/Pages/welcome.aspx

European Resuscitation Council, www.erc.edu/index.php/mainpage/en/ECG

Pacing resources, www.sjmprofessional.com, www.medtronic.com/for-healthcare-professionals/education-training

Further reading

Conover MB. Understanding electrocardiography. 8th ed. St Louis: Mosby; 2002.

For reasonably down to earth discussion of pacemakers and ICDs, the 3-part series by Tom Kenny is valuable, the new editions are imminent:

- The nuts and bolts of cardiac pacing. 2nd edn. Wiley-Blackwell, 2008.
- The nuts and bolts of ICD therapy. Blackwell-Futura, 2005.
- The nuts and bolts of cardiac resynchronization therapy, 2007. Blackwell-Futura.

Brignole M, Auricchio A, Baron-Esquivias G, et al. 2013 ESC Guidelines on cardiac pacing and cardiac resynchronization therapy: the Task Force on cardiac pacing and resynchronization therapy of the European Society of Cardiology

(ESC). Developed in collaboration with the European HeartRhythm Association (EHRA). Eur Heart J 2013;34(29):2281–329. doi:10.1093/eurheartj/eht150. [Epub 2013 Jun 24]; PubMed PMID: 23801822.

Drew B, Ackerman M, Funk M, et al. Prevention of torsades de pointes in hospital settings: a scientific statement from The American Heart Association and The American College of Cardiology Foundation. J Am Coll Cardiol 2010;55(9):934–47.

Epstein A, DiMarco J, Ellenbogen K, et al. American College of Cardiology Foundation; American Heart Association Task Force on Practice Guidelines; Heart Rhythm Society. 2012 ACCF/AHA/HRS focused update incorporated into the ACCF/AHA/HRS 2008 guidelines for device-based therapy of cardiac rhythm abnormalities: a report of the American College of Cardiology Foundation/American Heart Association Task Force on Practice Guidelines and the Heart Rhythm Society. J Am Coll Cardiol 2013;61(3):e6–75. doi:10.1016/j.jacc.2012.11.007.

References

1. Bennett DH. Bennett's Cardiac arrhythmias: practical notes on interpretation and treatment. 8th ed. London: Hodder Arnold; 2013.
2. Pitcher D, Nolan J. Peri-arrest arrhythmias. Resuscitation Council UK, London; 2015.
3. Colilla S, Crow A, Petkun W, et al. Estimates of current and future incidence and prevalence of atrial fibrillation in the U.S. adult population. Am J Cardiol 2013;112(8):1142–7.
4. Arrigo M, Bettex D, Rudiger A. Management of atrial fibrillation in critically ill patients. Crit Care Res Pract [Internet] 2014;2014:840615.
5. Walkley AJ, Wiener JM, Ghorbrial LH, et al. Incident stroke and mortality associated with new-onset atrial fibrillation in patients with severe sepsis. JAMA 2011;306(20):2248–55.
6. Filardo G, Damiano RJ, Ailawadi G, et al. Epidemiology of new-onset atrial fibrillation following coronary artery bypass graft surgery. Heart 2018;0:1–8. doi:10.1136/heartjnl-2017-312150.
7. Pappano AJ, Wier WJ. Cardiovascular physiology. 10th ed. Philadelphia: Elsevier/Mosby.; 2013.
8. Klabunde RE. Cardiovascular physiology concepts. 2nd ed. Philadelphia: Lippincott, Williams & Wilkins; 2012.
9. Bonnemeier H, Richardt G, Potratz J, et al. Circadian profile of cardiac autonomic nervous modulation in healthy subjects: differing effects of aging and gender on heart rate variability. J Cardiovasc Electrophysiol 2003;14:791–9.
10. Hampton JR. The ECG made easy. 8th ed. London: Churchill Livingstone; 2013.
11. Ewy GA. Sick sinus syndrome: synopsis. J Am Coll Cardiol 2014;64:539–40.
12. Graudins A, Lee HM, Druda D. Calcium channel antagonist and beta-blocker overdose: antidotes and adjunct therapies. Br J Clin Pharmacol 2016;81(3):453–61.
13. Poulidakis E. Transvenous temporary cardiac pacing. Hospital Chronicles 2014;9(3):190–8.
14. Olshansky B, Sullivan RM. Inappropriate sinus tachycardia. J Am Coll Cardiol 2013;61(8):793–801.
15. Fox K, Ford I, Steg PG, et al. Ivabradine in stable coronary artery disease without clinical heart failure. N Engl J Med 2014;371(12):1091–9.
16. Ponikowski P, Voors AA, Anker SD, et al. 2016 ESC Guidelines for the diagnosis and treatment of acute and chronic heart failure: the Task Force for the diagnosis and treatment of acute and chronic heart failure of the European Society of Cardiology (ESC) Developed with the special contribution of the Heart Failure Association (HFA) of the ESC. Eur Heart J 2016;37(27):2129–200.
17. Scheinman M, Vedantham V. Ivabradine. A ray of hope for inappropriate sinus tachycardia. J Am Coll Cardiol 2012;60(15):1330–2.
18. Monfredi O, Dobrzynski H, Mondal T, et al. The anatomy and physiology of the sinoatrial node – a contemporary review. PACE. 2010;33:1392–406.
19. Antzelevitch C, Burashnikov A. Overview of basic mechanisms of cardiac arrhythmia. Card Electrophysiol Clin 2011;3(1):23–45.
20. Grandi E, Sanguinetti MC, Bartos DC, et al. Potassium channels in the heart: structure, function and regulation. J Physiol 2017;595(7): 2209–28.
21. Fogoros RN, Mandrola JM. Fogoros' electrophysiologic testing. 6th ed. Oxford: Wiley Blackwell; 2018.
22. Abrams DJ, MacRae CA. Long QT syndrome. Circulation 2014;129(14):1524–9.
23. Konstantopoulou A, Tsikrikas S, Asvestas D, et al. Mechanisms of drug-induced proarrhythmia in clinical practice. World J Cardiol 2013;5(6):175.
24. Shaver CM, Chen W, Janz DR, et al. Atrial fibrillation is an independent predictor of mortality in critically ill patients. Crit Care Med 2015;43(10):2104.
25. Andrade J, Khairy P, Dobrev D, et al. The clinical profile and pathophysiology of atrial fibrillation: relationships among clinical features, epidemiology, and mechanisms. Circ Res 2014;114(9):1453–68.
26. Christophersen IE, Ellinor PT. Genetics of atrial fibrillation: from families to genomes. J Hum Genet 2016;61(1):61.
27. Haisseguerre M, Jais P, Shah DC, et al. Spontaneous initiation of atrial fibrillation by ectopic beats originating in the pulmonary veins. N Engl J Med 1998;339:659–66.
28. Lip GY, Lane DA. Stroke prevention in atrial fibrillation: a systematic review. JAMA 2015;313(19):1950–62.
29. January CT, Wann LS, Alpert JS, et al. 2014 AHA/ACC/HRS guideline for the management of patients with atrial fibrillation: a report of the American College of Cardiology/American Heart Association Task Force on Practice Guidelines and the Heart Rhythm Society. J Am Coll Cardiol 2014;64(21):e1–76.

30. Gillinov AM, Bagiella E, Moskowitz AJ, et al. Rate control versus rhythm control for atrial fibrillation after cardiac surgery. N Engl J Med 2016;374(20):1911–21.
31. Hannibal GB. Peripheral phlebitis related to amiodarone infusion. AACN Adv Crit Care 2016;27(4):465–71.
32. Lip GY, Nieuwlaat R, Pisters R, et al. Refining clinical risk stratification for predicting stroke and thromboembolism in atrial fibrillation using a novel risk factor-based approach: the Euro Heart Survey on atrial fibrillation. Chest 2010;137:263–72.
33. Calkins H, Hindricks G, Cappato R, et al. 2017 HRS/EHRA/ECAS/APHRS/SOLAECE expert consensus statement on catheter and surgical ablation of atrial fibrillation. Heart Rhythm 2017;14(10):e275–444.
34. Brignole M, Botto GL, Mont L, et al. Predictors of clinical efficacy of 'Ablate and Pace' therapy in patients with permanent atrial fibrillation. Heart 2012;98(4):297–302.
35. Houghton AR, Gray D. Making sense of the ECG: a hands-on guide. 4th ed. Boca Raton: CRC Press; 2014.
36. Perez FJ, Schubert CM, Parvez B, et al. Long-term outcomes after catheter ablation of cavo-tricuspid isthmus dependant atrial flutter: a meta-analysis. Circ Arrhythm Electrophysiol 2009;2:393–401.
37. Wasmer K, Mönnig G, Bittner A, et al. Incidence, characteristics, and outcome of left atrial tachycardias after circumferential antral ablation of atrial fibrillation. Heart Rhythm 2012;9(10):1660–6.
38. Whinnett ZI, Sohaib SA, Davies DW. Diagnosis and management of supraventricular tachycardia. BMJ 2012;345:e7769.
39. Appelboam A, Reuben A, Mann C, et al. Postural modification to the standard Valsalva manoeuvre for emergency treatment of supraventricular tachycardias (REVERT): a randomised controlled trial. Lancet 2015;386(10005):1747–53.
40. Page RL, Joglar JA, Caldwell MA, et al. 2015 ACC/AHA/HRS guideline for the management of adult patients with supraventricular tachycardia: a report of the American College of Cardiology/American Heart Association Task Force on Clinical Practice Guidelines and the Heart Rhythm Society. Heart Rhythm 2016;13(4):e136–221.
41. Mark DG, Brady WJ, Pines JM. Pre-excitation syndromes: diagnostic consideration in the ED. Am J Emerg Med 2009;27:878–88.
42. Thanavaro JL, Thanavaro S. Clinical presentation and treatment of atrial fibrillation in Wolff-Parkinson-White syndrome. Heart Lung 2010;39:131–6.
43. Obeyesekere M, Gula LJ, Skanes AC, et al. Risk of sudden death in Wolff-Parkinson-White syndrome: how high is the risk? Circulation 2012;125:659–60.
44. Chugh A, Bogun F, Morady F. Catheter ablation of accessory pathways. In: Wilber DJ, Packer DL, Stevenson WG, editors. Catheter ablation of cardiac arrhythmias: basic concepts and clinical applications. 3rd ed. Oxford: Blackwell Publishing.; 2008.
45. Hreybe H, Saba S. Location of acute myocardial infarction and associated arrhythmias and outcome. Clin Cardiol 2009;32(5):274–7.
46. Prystowsky EN, Padanilam BJ, Joshi S, et al. Ventricular arrhythmias in the absence of structural heart disease. J Am Coll Cardiol 2012;59(20):1733–44.
47. Resuscitation Council (UK). Advanced life support. 7th ed. London: RCUK; 2016.
48. Wagner GS, Strauss DG. Marriott's practical electrocardiography. 12th ed. Baltimore: Lippincott, Williams & Wilkins; 2013.
49. Rautaharju PM, Surawicz B, Gettes LS. AHA/ACCF/HRS recommendations for the standardization and interpretation of the electrocardiogram. Part IV: the ST segment, T and U waves, and the QT interval. A scientific statement from the American Heart Association Electrocardiography and Arrhythmias Committee, Council on Clinical Cardiology; the American College of Cardiology Foundation; and the Heart Rhythm Society. Circulation 2009;119:e241–50.
50. Drew BJ, Ackerman MJ, Funk M, et al; on behalf of the American Heart Association Acute Cardiac Care Committee of the Council on Clinical Cardiology; Council on Cardiovascular Nursing; American College of Cardiology Foundation. Prevention of torsade de pointes in hospital settings: a scientific statement from the American Heart Association and the American College of Cardiology Foundation. Circulation 2010;121:1047–60.
51. Sandau KE, Funk M, Auerbach A, et al. Update to practice standards for electrocardiographic monitoring in hospital settings: a scientific statement from the American Heart Association. Circulation 2017;136:e273–344.
52. John RM, Tedrow UB, Koplan BA, et al. Ventricular arrhythmias and sudden cardiac death. Lancet 2012;380:1520–9.
53. Al-Khatib SM, Stevenson WG, Ackerman MJ, et al. 2017 AHA/ACC/HRS guideline for management of patients with ventricular arrhythmias and the prevention of sudden cardiac death: a report of the American College of Cardiology/American Heart Association Task Force on Clinical Practice Guidelines and the Heart Rhythm Society. J Am Coll Cardiol 2017;24390.
54. Ling Z, Hari A, Tandri H. VT ablation: new developments and approaches. Curr Treat Options Cardiovasc Med 2014;16(4):297–310.
55. Nademanee K, Veerakul G, Chandanamattha P, et al. Prevention of ventricular fibrillation episodes in Brugada syndrome by catheter ablation over the anterior right ventricular outflow tract epicardium. Circulation 2011;123:1270–9.
56. Brugada J, Pappone C, Berruezo A, et al. Brugada syndrome phenotype elimination by epicardial substrate ablation. Circ Arrhythm Electrophysiol 2015;8(6):1373–81.
57. Nolan JP, Soar J, Smith GB, et al. Incidence and outcome of in-hospital cardiac arrest in the United Kingdom National Cardiac Arrest Audit. Resuscitation 2014;85(8):987–92.
58. Bonnemeier H, Ortak J, Wiegand UK, et al. Accelerated idioventricular rhythm in the post-thrombolytic era: incidence, prognostic implications, and modulating mechanisms after direct percutaneous coronary intervention. Ann Noninvasive Electrocardiol 2005;10(2):179–87.
59. Vogler J, Breithardt G, Eckardt L. Bradyarrhythmias and conduction blocks. Rev Esp Cardiol 2012;65:656–67.

60. Cheng S, Keyes MJ, Larson MG, et al. Long-term outcomes in individuals with prolonged PR interval or first-degree atrioventricular block. JAMA 2009;301(24):2571–7.
61. Sharma S, Drezner JA, Baggish A, et al. International recommendations for electrocardiographic interpretation in athletes. Eur Heart J 2017;ehw631.
62. Brignole M, Auricchio A, Baron-Esquivias G, et al. 2013 ESC Guidelines on cardiac pacing and cardiac resynchronization therapy: the Task Force on cardiac pacing and resynchronization therapy of the European Society of Cardiology (ESC). Developed in collaboration with the European Heart Rhythm Association (EHRA). Eur Heart J 2013;34(29):2281–329.
63. Dan GA, Martinez-Rubio A, Agewall S, et al Antiarrhythmic drugs – clinical use and clinical decision making: a consensus document from the European Heart Rhythm Association (EHRA) and European Society of Cardiology (ESC) Working Group on Cardiovascular Pharmacology, endorsed by the Heart Rhythm Society (HRS), Asia-Pacific Heart Rhythm Society (APHRS) and International Society of Cardiovascular Pharmacotherapy (ISCP). Europace 2018; Feb 9.
64. Joint Formulary Committee. British national formulary. 75th ed. London: BMJ Group and Pharmaceutical Press; 2018.
65. Opie LH, Gersh BJ. Drugs for the heart. 8th ed. Philadelphia: Elsevier Saunders; 2013.
66. Carlson MD, Wilkoff BL, Maisel WH, et al. Recommendations from the Heart Rhythm Society Task Force on Device Performance Policies and Guidelines endorsed by the American College of Cardiology Foundation and the American Heart Association (AHA) and the International Coalition of Pacing and Electrophysiology Organizations (COPE). Heart Rhythm 2006;3(10):1250–73. https://doi.org/10.1016/j.hrthm.2006.08.029.
67. Viskin S, Glikson M, Fish R, et al. Rate smoothing with cardiac pacing for preventing torsade de pointes. Am J Cardiol 2000;86(9).
68. Mattingly E. AANA Journal course: update for nurse anesthetists – arrhythmia management devices and electromagnetic interference. AANA J 2005;73(2):129–36.
69. Overbay D, Criddle L. Mastering temporary invasive cardiac pacing. Crit Care Nurse 2004;24(3):25–32.
70. Swerdlow CD, Gillberg JM, Olson WH. Sensing and detection. In: Ellenbogen KA, Kay GN, Lau CP, et al, editors. Clinical cardiac pacing, defibrillation, and resynchronization therapy. 3rd ed. Philadelphia: Elsevier Saunders; 2007.
71. Hayes DL, Friedman PA. Cardiac pacing, defibrillation and resynchronization. 2nd ed. Singapore: Wiley-Blackwell; 2008.
72. Laczika K, Thalhammer F, Locker G, et al. Safe and efficient emergency transvenous ventricular pacing via the right supraclavicular route. Anesth Analg 2000;90(4):784–9.
73. Kay GN, Shepard RB. Cardiac electrical stimulation. In: Ellenbogen KA, Kay GN, Lau CP, et al, editors. Clinical cardiac pacing, defibrillation, and resynchronization therapy. 3rd ed. Philadelphia: Elsevier Saunders; 2007.
74. Drew BJ, Califf RM, Funk M, et al. Practice standards for electrocardiographic monitoring in hospital settings: an American Heart Association scientific statement from the Councils on Cardiovascular Nursing, Clinical Cardiology, and Cardiovascular Disease in the Young: endorsed by the International Society of Computerized Electrocardiology and the American Association of Critical-Care Nurses. Circulation 2004;110:2721–46.
75. Kusumoto FM, Goldschlager N. Cardiac pacing. N Engl J Med 1996;334:89–99.
76. Chan T, Brady W, Harrigan R. Diagnosis: pacemaker failure to capture. Emergency Medicine News 2007;29(1):11.
77. Bernstein AD, Camm AJ, Fletcher RD, et al. The NASPE/BPEG generic pacemaker code for antibradyarrhythmic and adaptive rate pacing and antitachyarrhythmic devices. PACE 1987;10:794–9.
78. Sgarbossa EB, Pinski SL, Gates KB, et al. Early diagnosis of acute myocardial infarction in the presence of ventricular paced rhythm. Am J Cardiol 1996;77(5):423–44.
79. Schuchert A, Frese J, Stammwitz E, et al. Low settings of the ventricular pacing output in patients dependent on a pacemaker: are they really safe? Am Heart J 2002;143(6):1009–11.
80. Ellenbogen KA, Wood MA. Cardiac pacing and ICDs. 4th ed. Oxford: Blackwell Publishing; 2005.
81. Tommaso C, Belic N, Brandfonbrener M. Asynchronous ventricular pacing: a rare cause of ventricular tachycardia. PACE 1982;5(4): 561–3.
82. Ahmed FZ, Morris GM, Allen S, et al. Not all pacemakers are created equal: MRI conditional pacemaker and lead technology. J Cardiovasc Electrophysiol 2013;24(9):1059–65.
83. Hayes DL, Zipes DP. Cardiac pacemakers and cardioverter-defibrillators. In: Braunwald E, Dipes DP, Libby P, editors. Heart disease: a textbook of cardiovascular medicine. 6th ed. Philadelphia: WB Saunders; 2001.
84. Slink M, Hellkamp A, Estes M, et al. High incidence of pacemaker syndrome in patients with sinus node dysfunction treated with ventricular-based pacing in the Mode Selection Trial (MOST). J Am Coll Cardiol 2004;43(11):2066–71.
85. Sweeney MO, Ruetz LL, Belk P, et al. Bradycardia pacing-induced short-long-short sequences at the onset of ventricular tachyarrhythmias. A possible mechanism of proarrhythmia? J Am Coll Cardiol 2007;50(7):614–22.
86. Fisher JD, Teichman SL, Eerrick A, et al. Antiarrhythmic effects of VVI pacing at physiologic rates: a crossover controlled evaluation. PACE 1987;10:822–30.
87. Kristensen L, Nielsen JC, Pedersen AK, et al. AV block and changes in pacing mode during long-term follow-up of 399 consecutive patients with sick sinus syndrome treated with an AAI/AAIR pacemaker. Pacing Clin Electrophysiol 2001;24(3):358–65.
88. Brandt J, Anderson H, Fahraeus T, et al. Natural history of sinus node disease treated with atrial pacing in 213 patients: implications for selection of stimulation mode. J Am Coll Cardiol 1992;20(3):633–9.

89. Wilkoff BL, Cook JR, Epstein AE, et al. Dual chamber pacing or ventricular backup pacing in patients with an implantable defibrillator: the Dual Chamber and VVI Implantable Defibrillator (DAVID) trial. JAMA 2002;288:3115–23.
90. Dennis MJ, Sparks PB. Pacemaker mediated tachycardia as a complication of the autointrinsic conduction search function. Pacing Clin Electrophysiol 2004;27(6Pt1):824–6.
91. Safavi-Naeini P, Saeed M. Pacemaker troubleshooting. common clinical scenarios. Tex Heart Inst J 2016;43(5):413–18.
92. Kahloon MU, Aslam AK, Aslam AF, et al. Hyperkalaemia induced failure of atrial and ventricular pacemaker capture. Int J Cardiol 2005;105(2):224–6.
93. Elmi F, Tullo N, Khalighi K. Natural history and predictors of temporary epicardial pacemaker wire function in patients after open heart surgery. Cardiology 2002;98(4):175–80.
94. Sachin S, Rajesh S, Rajeev M, et al. Temporary pacemaker induced ventricular fibrillations in Cath Lab due to R on T phenomenon. Int J Case Rep Short Rev 2018;4(1):6–8.
95. Mond HG. Unipolar versus bipolar pacing – poles apart. Pacing Clin Electrophysiol 1991;14(9):1411–24.
96. Boumphrey S, Langton JA. Electrical safety in the operating theatre. Br J Anaesth 2003;3(1):10–14.
97. Connolly SJ, Kerr CR, Gent M, et al. Effects of physiologic pacing versus ventricular pacing on the risk of stroke and death due to cardiovascular causes. N Engl J Med 2000;342(19):1385–91.
98. Lamas GA, Lee KL, Sweeney MO, et al. For the mode selection trial in sinus-node dysfunction. Ventricular pacing or dual-chamber pacing for sinus node dysfunction. N Engl J Med 2002;346(2):1854–62.
99. Mond HG, Hikkock RJ, Stevenson IH, et al. The right ventricular outflow tract: the road to septal pacing. Pacing Clin Electrophysiol 2007;30:482–91.
100. Bakker P, Meijburg H, De Vries JW, et al. Biventricular pacing in end-stage heart failure improves functional capacity and left ventricular function. J Interv Card Electrophysiol 2000;4(2):395–404.
101. Hawkins NM, Petrie MC, MacDonald MR, et al. Selecting patients for cardiac resynchronization therapy: electrical or mechanical dyssynchrony? Eur Heart J 2006;27:1270–81.
102. Linde C, Leclerq C, Rex S, et al. Long-term benefits of biventricular pacing in congestive heart failure: results from the MUSTIC study. J Am Coll Cardiol 2002;40:433–40.
103. Cleland JGF, Subert JC, Erdmann E, et al. Longer-term effects of cardiac resynchronization therapy on mortality in heart failure [The Cardiac Resynchronisation-Heart Failure (CARE-HF) trial extension phase]. Eur Heart J 2006;27:1928–32.
104. Auricchio A, Stellbrink C, Sack S, et al. Pacing Therapies in Congestive Heart Failure (PATH-CHF) Study Group. Long-term clinical effect of hemodynamically optimized cardiac resynchronisation therapy in patients with heart failure and ventricular conduction delay. J Am Coll Cardiol 2002;39:2026–33.
105. Young JB, Abraham WT, Smithe AL, et al. Combined cardiac resynchronization and implantable cardioverter defibrillation in advanced chronic heart failure: the MIRACLE ICD trial. JAMA 2003;289:2685–94.
106. Bristow MR, Saxon LA, Boehmer J, et al. Comparison of Medical Therapy, Pacing, Defibrillation in Heart Failure (COMPANION) Investigators. Cardiac resynchronization therapy with or without an implantable defibrillator in advanced chronic heart failure. N Engl J Med 2004;350:2140–50.
107. Ghi S, Constantin C, Klersy C, et al. Interventricular and intraventricular dyssynchrony are common in heart failure patients, regardless of QRS duration. Eur Heart J 2004;25:571–8.
108. Littmann L, Symanski JD. Hemodynamic implications of left bundle branch block. J Electrocardiol 2000;33(Suppl1):115–21.
109. Verrnooy K, Verbeek XA, Peschar M, et al. Left bundle branch block induces ventricular remodelling and functional septal hypoperfusion. Eur Heart J 2005;26:91–8.
110. Sundell J, Engblom E, Koistinen J, et al. The effects of cardiac resynchronization therapy on left ventricular function, myocardial energetics and metabolic reserve in patients with dilated cardiomyopathy and heart failure. J Am Coll Cardiol 2004;43:1027–33.
111. Peichl P, Kautzner J, Cihak R, et al. The spectrum of inter- and intraventricular conduction abnormalities in patients eligible for cardiac resynchronization therapy. Pacing Clin Electrophysiol 2004;27(8):1105–12.
112. Varma N, O'Donnell D, Bassiouny M, et al. Programming cardiac resynchronization therapy for electrical synchrony: reaching beyond left bundle branch block and left ventricular activation delay. J Am Heart Assoc 2018;7:e007489:1–12. doi:10.1161/JAHA. 117.007489.
113. Alonso C, Leclercq C, Victor F, et al. Electrocardiographic predictive factors of long-term clinical improvement with multisite biventricular pacing in advanced heart failure. Am J Cardiol 1998;84:1417–21.
114. Abraham WT, Fisher WG, Smith AL, et al; MIRACLE Study Group. Multicenter InSync Randomized Clinical Evaluation: cardiac resynchronization in chronic heart failure. N Engl J Med 2002;13(346):1845–53.
115. Daubert JC. Atrial fibrillation and heart failure: a mutually noxious association. Europace 2004;5:S1–4.
116. Pappone C, Ćalović Ž, Vicedomini G, et al. Multipoint left ventricular pacing improves acute hemodynamic response assessed with pressure-volume loops in cardiac resynchronization therapy patients. Heart Rhythm 2013;11(3):394–401.
117. Thibault B, Dubuc M, Khairy P, et al. Acute haemodynamic comparison of multisite and biventricular pacing with a quadripolar left ventricular lead. Europace 2013;15(7):984–91.
118. Brabham WW, Gold MR. The role of AV and VV optimization for CRT. J Arrhythm 2013;29(3):153–61.

119. Meine TJ. An intracardiac EGM method for VV optimization during cardiac resynchronization therapy. Heart Rhythm J 2006;3:AB30–5.
120. Kenny T. The nuts and bolts of cardiac resynchronization therapy. Massachusetts: Blackwell Futura; 2007.
121. Barold SS, Herweg B. Usefulness of the 12-lead electrocardiogram in the follow-up of patients with cardiac resynchronization devices. Part I. Cardiol J 2011;18(5):476–86.
122. Sweeney MO, Hellkamp AS, van Bommel RJ, et al. QRS fusion complex analysis using wave interference to predict reverse remodelling during cardiac resynchronization therapy. Heart Rhythm 2014;11:806–13.
123. Jackson T, Sohal M, Chen Z, et al. A U-shaped type II contraction pattern in patients with strict left bundle branch block predicts super-response to cardiac resynchronization therapy. Heart Rhythm 2014;11:1790–7.
124. Van Deursen CJM, Blaauw Y, Withens MI, et al. The value of the 12-lead ECG for evaluation and optimization of cardiac resynchronization therapy in daily clinical practice. J Electrocardiol 2014;47:202–11.
125. Bode WD, Bode MF, Gettes L, et al. Prominent R wave in ECG lead V1 predicts improvement of left ventricular ejection fraction after cardiac resynchronization therapy in patients with or without left bundle branch block. Heart Rhythm 2015;12:2141–7.
126. Miller JM, Zipes DP. Management of the patient with cardiac arrhythmias. In: Braunwald E, Zipes DP, Libby P, editors. Heart disease: a textbook of cardiovascular medicine. 6th ed. Philadelphia: WB Saunders; 2001.
127. The Public Access Defibrillation Trial Investigators. Public-access defibrillation and survival after out-of-hospital cardiac arrest. N Engl J Med 2004;351:637–46.
128. Deakin C, Nolan J, Sunde K, et al. European Resuscitation Council Guidelines for Resuscitation 2010 Section 3. Electrical therapies: automated external defibrillators, defibrillation, cardioversion and pacing. Resuscitation 2010;81:1293–304.
129. Valenzuela TD, Bjerke HS, Clark LL, et al. Rapid defibrillation by nontraditional responders: the Casino Project. Acad Emerg Med 1998;5:414–15.
130. Ambler JJ, Zideman DA, Deakin CD. The effect of topical non-steroidal anti-inflammatory cream on the incidence and severity of cutaneous burns following external DC cardioversion. Resuscitation 2005;65(2):173–8.
131. Pinski SL, Sgarbossa EB, Ching E, et al. A comparison of 50-J versus 100-J shock for direct current cardioversion of atrial flutter. Am Heart J 1999;137:439–42.
132. Pinski KL, Fahy GJ. Implantable cardioverter defibrillators. Am J Med 1999;106:446–58.
133. The Antiarrhythmics versus Implantable Defibrillators (AVID) Investigators. A comparison of antiarrhythmic-drug therapy with implantable defibrillators in patients resuscitated from near-fatal ventricular arrhythmias. N Engl J Med 1997;337:1576–83.
134. Conolly SJ, Gent M, Roberts RS, et al. Canadian Implantable Defibrillator Study (CIDS): a randomized trial of the implantable cardioverter defibrillator against amiodarone. Circulation 2000;101:1297–302.
135. Kuck KH, Cappato R, Siebels J, et al. Randomized comparison of antiarrhythmic drug therapy with implantable defibrillators in patients resuscitated from cardiac arrest. The Cardiac Arrest Study Hamburg (CASH). Circulation 2000;102:748–54.
136. Moss AJ, Hall WJ, Cannom D, et al. Multicentre Automatic Defibrillator Implantation Trial Investigators. Improved survival with an implanted defibrillator in patients with coronary artery disease at high risk for ventricular arrhythmias. N Engl J Med 1996;335(26):1933–40.
137. Mark DB, Nelson CL, Anstrom KJ, et al. Cost-effectiveness of ICD therapy in the sudden cardiac death in heart failure trial (SCD-HeFT). Circulation 2006;114(2):135–42.
138. Swerdlow C, Shivkumar K, Zhang J. Determination of the upper limit of vulnerability using implantable cardioverter defibrillator electrograms. Circulation 2003;107:3028–33.
139. Viskin S, Rosso R. The top 10 reasons to avoid defibrillation threshold testing during ICD implantation. Heart Rhythm 2008;5(3):391–3.
140. Sola CL, Bostwick JM. Implantable cardioverter-defibrillators, induced anxiety, and quality of life. Mayo Clinic Proc 2005;80(2):232–7.
141. Daubert JP, Zareba W, Cannom DS, et al. (MADIT II Investigatores). Inappropriate implantable cardioverter-defibrillator shocks in MADIT II: frequency, mechanisms, predictors and survival impact. J Am Coll Cardiol 2008;51(14):1357–65.
142. Kruse J, Finkelmeier B. Permanent pacemakers and implantable cardioverter-defibrillators. In: Finkelmeier BA, editor. Cardiothoracic surgical nursing. 2nd ed. Philadelphia: Lippincott, Williams & Wilkins; 2000.
143. Jacob S, Panaich SS, Maheshwari R, et al. Clinical application of magnets on cardiac rhythm management devices. Europace 2011;13(9):1222–30.
144. Jacobson C, Gerity D. Pacemakers and implantable defibrillators. In: Woods S, Froelicher E, Underhill Motzer S, editors. Cardiac nursing. 5th ed. Philadelphia: Lippincott, Williams & Wilkins; 2005.

Chapter 12

Cardiac surgery and transplantation

Sher Michael Graan, Jayne Bancroft

Learning objectives

After reading this chapter, you should be able to:

- outline cardiac surgical procedures including coronary artery bypass graft surgery and valve repair and replacement
- describe the indications, advantages and disadvantages of using cardiopulmonary bypass
- outline methods of myocardial preservation during cardiac surgery
- outline immediate postoperative management of cardiac surgical patients
- outline the principles of counterpulsation in intra-aortic balloon pumping (IABP)
- outline the benefits and timing methods of balloon inflation and deflation, including assessment of timing and timing errors
- describe the nursing management of IABP complications, including limb perfusion, bleeding and immobility-related complications
- discuss methods of weaning IABP and management of intra-aortic balloon catheter removal
- discuss the immediate postoperative care of heart transplant recipients
- describe the clinical manifestations of postoperative complications in heart transplant recipients
- identify signs and symptoms of rejection in heart transplant recipients
- evaluate the effectiveness of nursing interventions in the postoperative management of heart transplant recipients.

KEY WORDS

arrhythmia
cardiac surgery
cardiopulmonary bypass
counterpulsation
denervation
heart transplant
intra-aortic balloon pump
ischaemic reperfusion injury
valve replacement, repair

Introduction

Many critically ill patients experience compromised cardiac function, as either a primary or secondary condition. This chapter follows on from those situations examined in Chapter 10, and reviews care of patients with conditions that lead to admission to specialised critical care units. The burden of cardiovascular disease (CVD) is the highest globally, the World Health Organization reported that CVD was the number one cause of death in 2015 with 17.7 million deaths, which is 31% of all global deaths (7.4 million were due to coronary heart diseases (CHD) alone) and 37% of death caused by CVD were premature deaths (under the age of 70).[1] In Europe, cardiovascular diseases accounted for 45% (3.9 million) of all deaths; just less than half of mortality was due to coronary heart diseases and in 2015, 85 million people were living in Europe with CVD.[2] Cardiovascular diseases in Australia affect one in six Australians and accounted for 31% of all deaths in 2011,[3] with acute coronary syndrome affecting 69,500 Australians and contributing to 13% of all deaths in 2013.[3] Currently, cardiovascular diseases are the second most common health issue, with the level of burden in Australia slightly lower than other developed nations (25.8% versus 33.7%).[4] In 2013–14 there were 149,000 hospitalisations (1.5% of all hospitalisation) due to CHD and caused 13% of all deaths.[3]

In this chapter, three topics will be discussed. First, the management of a patient who requires cardiac surgery for coronary artery disease or valvular disease including the use of cardiopulmonary bypass, will be described. Second, the use and management of intra-aortic balloon counterpulsation in cardiac surgical and medical patients will be reviewed. Finally, the management of patients following heart transplantation, including the prevention and management of immediate postoperative complications, will be reviewed.

Cardiac surgery

The focus of this section is on cardiac surgery for repair of structural abnormalities and repair or replacement of stenotic or regurgitant valves, as well as bypass grafting of coronary artery lesions. The structural abnormalities resulting from myocardial infarction have been described in Chapter 10. In this chapter, structural and functional abnormalities that are causing valvular disease (mitral, aortic, tricuspid or pulmonic valves) and ventricular defects will be discussed.

Valvular disease

The incidence and types of valvular disease have changed over the past 50 years.[4] Valvular disorders, such as mitral stenosis and aortic regurgitation, often arise from infectious diseases such as rheumatic fever (β-haemolytic streptococcal pharyngitis) and syphilis, which are much less common today. Conversely, there has been a rise in the rate of valvular diseases due to degenerative changes including leaflet degeneration and/or annulus calcification, which are common in ageing. In contrast to these trends, the prevalence of rheumatic fever and rheumatic valvular disorders among Aboriginal people (one of the highest in the world) and Pacific Islanders living in New Zealand is six times higher than the general population.[5] Globally, rheumatic heart diseases are the most common cause of acquired cardiac disease affecting 32 million people mainly in developing countries and causing 275,000 deaths per year.[1] Other causes of valvular diseases are congenital valve diseases (common in the younger population, with respect to e.g. bicuspid valves) and endocarditis.

Two valvular abnormalities that alter the blood flow across the valve are common. Stenotic valves have a tightened, restricted orifice causing the valve to not fully open. There is a restriction to forward flow of blood, which must be forced through the valve at higher pressure (Fig. 12.1). The high pressure combined with incomplete emptying of the chamber may increase the end-systolic volume, which will result in hypertrophy and dilation of the affected chamber(s) as a compensatory mechanism. The second valvular abnormality is valve regurgitation, which is also called incompetence or insufficiency. In this condition the incomplete closure of the valve leaflets results in backflow of blood into the chamber increasing its end diastolic volume, which may cause chamber hypertrophy and dilation.

In both of these conditions heart failure may result as the pressure in the ventricles and atria grows and this pressure is reflected back into the pulmonary or venous system. Although the heart contains four valves, the majority of disorders affect the mitral and aortic valves in the left side of the heart.

Aortic valve disease

The aortic valve is located between the left ventricle and the aorta with a normal surface area of 2–3 cm.[2] Mild aortic stenosis is a narrowing of the opening of the valve area to less than 1.5 cm^2 and a pressure gradient between the left ventricle and aorta of more than 25 mmHg; severe aortic stenosis is defined as a valve area of less than 1.0 cm^2 and a pressure gradient of more than 55 mmHg (Fig. 12.1). Aortic stenosis often results from degenerative changes or congenital abnormalities such as a bicuspid aortic valve (with a prevalence of 0.5% in the general population), which may also cause regurgitation. Aortic stenosis increases left ventricle afterload, causing impedance to left ventricle ejection. This increases left ventricle end-systolic volume and left ventricle systolic pressure, resulting in left ventricle hypertrophy and dilation. Increased myocardial oxygen demands from the hypertrophied muscle also mean that angina is common.

Clinical manifestations of aortic stenosis include low cardiac output, increased left ventricle workload, angina, dyspnoea, syncope and fatigue. On auscultation, additional heart sounds are heard as a systolic ejection murmur and a loud S4. Left heart failure with pulmonary congestion is usually a late sign. The ECG may show left ventricular hypertrophy with strain patterns.

Aortic regurgitation may occur acutely when the aortic valve is damaged by endocarditis, trauma or aortic dissection, and presents as a life-threatening emergency. Chronic aortic regurgitation usually results from

FIGURE 12.1 Valvular stenosis and regurgitation: (**A**) normal position of valve leaflets (cusps) when the valve is open and closed; (**B**) open position of a stenosed valve (left) and closed position of a regurgitant valve (right); (**C**) haemodynamic effect of mitral stenosis shows the mitral valve is unable to open completely during left atrial systole, limiting left ventricular filling; (**D**) haemodynamic effect of mitral regurgitation shows the mitral valve does not close completely during left ventricular systole, allowing blood to re-enter the left atrium.

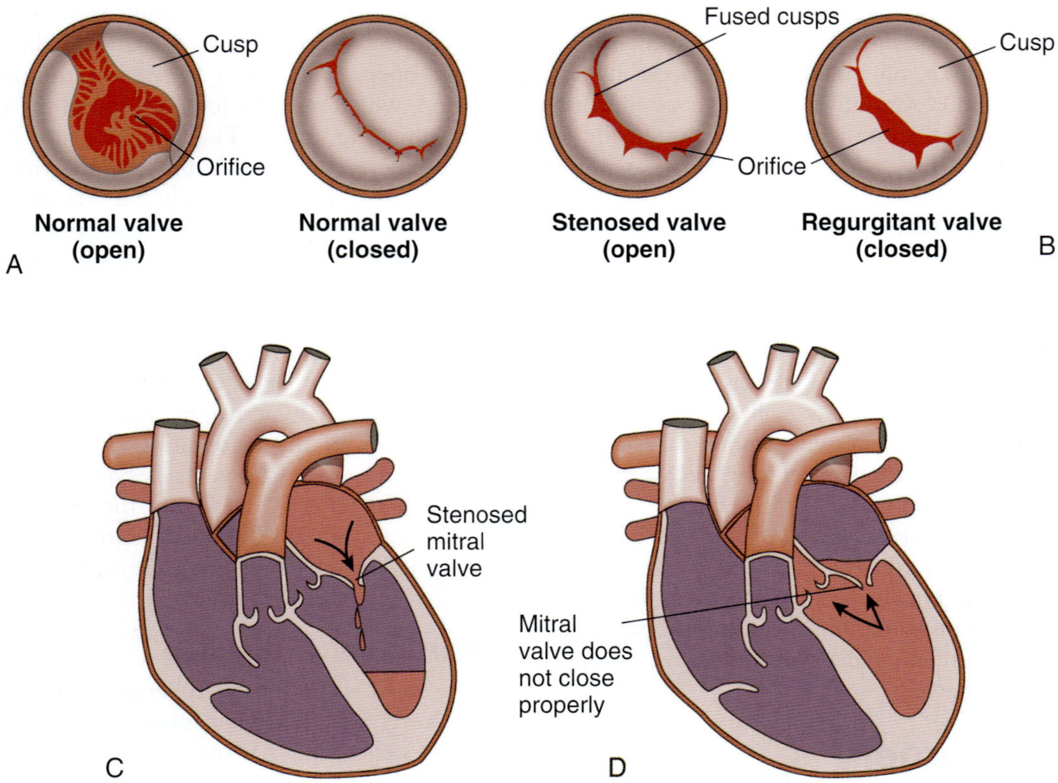

Adapted from Badhwar V, Esper S, Brooks M, et al. Extubating in the operating room following adult cardiac surgery safely improves outcomes and lowers costs. J Thorac Cardiovasc Surg 2014;148(6):3101-9, e1, with permission.

rheumatic heart disease, syphilis or congenital conditions. In aortic regurgitation reflux of blood to the left ventricle during diastole, due to incomplete closure of the valve, increases left ventricle end diastolic pressure and volume. This results in left ventricle dilation and hypertrophy and left heart failure. When left heart failure occurs, left atrial pressure rises and may cause pulmonary congestion and pulmonary hypertension.

In acute aortic regurgitation, the patient presents with signs and symptoms of acute left ventricle failure, cardiogenic shock and acute pulmonary oedema.[6] Patients with chronic aortic regurgitation may remain asymptomatic for years, finally presenting with signs of left heart failure including fatigue, palpitation, syncope, angina and dyspnoea. On auscultation, a diastolic murmur can be heard. The ECG may show left ventricular hypertrophy due to volume overload and a chest X-ray may reveal cardiomegaly and features of acute pulmonary oedema.

Mitral valve disease

Mitral stenosis is a chronic and progressive narrowing of the mitral valve orifice (normally 4–6 cm^2), restricting blood flow from the left atrium to the left ventricle. Patients may exhibit symptoms when the valve area is <2 cm^2 and they will have symptoms at rest when the valve area is <1 cm^2.

Mitral valve stenosis often occurs as a result of rheumatic heart disease, degenerative valve diseases and, less often, from systemic lupus erythematosus. These diseases cause damage to the leaflets and chordae tendineae, so that during healing the scars contract and seal, restricting the aperture. The incomplete emptying of the left atrium causes increased left atrial pressure and left atrial enlargement, and results in pulmonary congestion and pulmonary hypertension. In chronic conditions, this pressure may also affect the right ventricle, causing right ventricular failure, but left ventricular function is usually intact.[5] Lung compliance is reduced, causing dyspnoea, orthopnoea and nocturnal paroxysmal dyspnoea. Patients may complain of fatigue, low exercise tolerance, cough and haemoptysis. On auscultation a low-pitched diastolic murmur and an opening snap can be heard. The ECG may show left atrial enlargement and possibly atrial fibrillation (AF), and a chest X-ray may reveal right ventricular hypertrophy, left atrium enlargement and features of pulmonary oedema.

In mitral valve regurgitation, the mitral valve is not closing during left ventricular systole, causing backflow of blood into the left atrium, which creates elevated atrial and pulmonary pressures, and possibly pulmonary oedema.[5] Acute mitral regurgitation is often caused by acute myocardial infarction (AMI) resulting in papillary muscle rupture, trauma or infectious endocarditis, and patients may present with signs and symptoms of acute left ventricular failure, acute pulmonary oedema and cardiogenic shock. The causes of chronic mitral regurgitation are rheumatic diseases, congenital mitral valve prolapse or degenerative changes. The patient may complain of weakness, fatigue, exertional dyspnoea, palpitation and symptoms of pulmonary congestion and right ventricular failure such as cough, dyspnoea, orthopnoea and lower extremity oedema. On auscultation, a third heart sound and a pansystolic murmur can be heard. ECG may show left atrial enlargement, left ventricular hypertrophy, P mitrale and possibly AF, and a chest X-ray may reveal left ventricular hypertrophy, left atrium enlargement and features of pulmonary oedema.

Tricuspid valve disease

Tricuspid stenosis (normal area is 7 cm^2) is often seen with aortic or mitral valve diseases, and rarely in isolation. The restriction of blood flow from the right atrium to the right ventricle causes systemic venous congestion. On auscultation, a diastolic murmur can be heard. Tricuspid regurgitation is most commonly a functional disorder due to annulus dilation as a result of increased right ventricle pressure and hypertrophy, mitral stenosis, pulmonary embolism, cor pulmonale or right ventricle AMI. The backflow of blood from the right ventricle to the right atrium causes systemic venous congestion. On auscultation, a pansystolic murmur can be heard. In both stenosis and regurgitation of the tricuspid valve patients present with a high central venous pressure (CVP) and jugular venous pressure (JVP), hepatomegaly, ascites and peripheral oedema, and their ECG may show P pulmonale and possibly AF, and a chest X-ray may reveal prominent right heart border.

Pulmonic valve disease

Pulmonic valve stenosis is rare in isolation and is often due to a congenital defect. The restriction to blood flow from the right ventricle to the pulmonary arteries causes right ventricular hypertrophy and dilation, and the patient presents with exertional dyspnoea, syncope, cyanosis and a systolic murmur, and a split S2 heart sound. The ECG may show right ventricular hypertrophy.

Pulmonic valve regurgitation is also a rare condition that is usually caused by a congenital defect or pulmonary hypertension or is iatrogenic (e.g. post-balloon valvuloplasty). Patients might be asymptomatic, but in severe cases they present with signs and symptoms of right ventricular failure.

Cardiac surgical interventions

The most common cardiac surgical procedures include coronary artery bypass graft (CABG) surgery, to bypass lesions within the coronary arteries, and repair or replacement of stenotic or regurgitant valves. During these procedures preservation of systemic circulation, ventilation and perfusion of the myocardium is required and is often achieved with the aid of cardiopulmonary bypass (CPB).

Coronary artery bypass graft surgery

The pathophysiology and implications of ischaemic heart disease are explained in detail in Chapter 10. Single lesions can be treated by angioplasty and stent; however, patients with a left main coronary artery lesion, multiple (double- or triple-vessel) disease, longer lesions and failed angioplasty may need CABG surgery.[6]

In CABG a section of vein or artery is used to bypass a blockage in the patient's coronary artery. The vessels used for grafting arise from arteries (internal mammary artery or radial artery and, less commonly, gastro-epiploic artery) or veins (saphenous vein). Saphenous veins are harvested from the legs, and the radial artery from the forearm, and each is used as a free graft with anastomoses at the ascending aorta and distal to lesions to one or more coronary arteries. When saphenous veins are used as grafts (SVG), they often develop diffuse intimal hyperplasia, which ultimately contributes to re-stenosis. Patency rates are lowest in saphenous vein grafts attached to small coronary arteries or coronary arteries supplying myocardial scars. Consequently, arterial grafts are used more often, as they are more resistant to intimal hyperplasia. Internal mammary arteries (IMAs) and radial artery grafts may be used.[7] The IMA remains attached to the subclavian artery and is mobilised from the chest wall and anastomosed to the coronary artery distal to the occlusion (Fig. 12.2). If the radial artery is being harvested for grafting, the collateral circulation in the forearm is assessed. Echo colour Doppler provides the best accuracy in assessing forearm circulation, although the clinical Allen test is quite commonly used. The disadvantage of the Allen test is that it gives false patency results around 5% of the time.[8] A selection of IMA, SVG and radial artery grafts may be necessary over time as repeat procedures are needed or in patients with extensive disease requiring multiple grafts.

For single-vessel disease, particularly of the left anterior descending (LAD) artery, a new approach to CABG – minimally invasive direct coronary artery bypass grafting (MIDCABG) – has been used. This procedure uses intercostal incisions and a thoracoscope instead of

FIGURE 12.2 Coronary artery bypass grafts. CX = circumflex artery; LAD = left anterior descending; LIMA = left internal mammary artery; LM = left main; RCA = right coronary artery; SVG = saphenous vein graft.

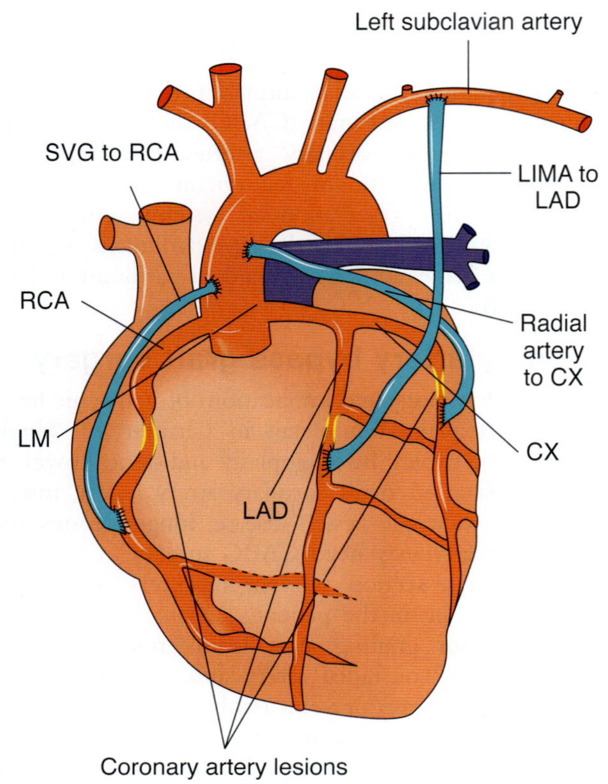

Source: Courtesy Tahiba Pirzada.

a sternotomy to access the heart and coronary arteries. MIDCABG is also often performed without CPB (off-pump coronary artery bypass, OPCAB); instead, the heart is slowed with beta-blockers to allow the surgery to be performed on a beating heart.[9–11] OPCAB procedures may also be performed using full or partial sternotomy to provide access for multiple vessel grafting. Both procedures have been successful responses to the drive to reduce the need for transfusion, recovery times, patient stays in hospital and costs.[9–11]

In the last decade robotically-assisted cardiac surgery has evolved in America and Europe and has been introduced at a small number of Australian hospitals for CABG and mitral valve surgery. This technique has further reduced the invasiveness of cardiac surgery, as little more than stab wounds are required in the right chest for thoracoscopy and the robotic instruments. Avoiding true thoracotomy or sternotomy improves postoperative pain experience, is associated with quicker recovery and shortens length of stay.[12–14]

Although CABG is the most common cardiac surgical procedure undertaken in Australia, the incidence of hospitalisation for CABG has declined since 2004/05 from 0.7 to 0.5 procedures/1,000 population in 2013–14,[3,4] but the rate of CABG has not changed in major European countries from 2006 to 2014.[2] The decline in surgery rates is due to changes in the treatment of CHD, including the advent of percutaneous coronary intervention (PCI). More procedures are now being performed in older patients, with 73% of current patients aged over 60 years.[3] CABG is used to relieve the symptoms of angina by increasing coronary blood flow distal to occlusive coronary lesions. It is a palliative, not curative, treatment as the underlying disease process continues. CABG is more effective than percutaneous transluminal coronary angioplasty (PTCA) in patients with extensive, multivessel disease with improved survival over a 3–5-year period by 5%, and a 4–7-fold reduction in the need for reintervention.[15] CABG is also used in left main vessel lesions due to the high risk of extensive infarction associated with PTCA in this area. CABG surgery is commonplace, and many cardiothoracic centres have highly efficient, effective systems in place with mortality rates as low as 2%.

Valve repair and replacement

Valve surgery is usually undertaken to repair the patient's valve or, more often, to replace the valve with a mechanical or tissue prosthesis. The clinical decision for valve surgery is primarily based on the clinical state of the patient using the New York Heart Association (NYHA) classification system and echocardiographic findings.[6] The type of surgery used will depend on the valves involved, the valvular pathology, the severity of the condition and the patient's clinical condition. Often valve surgery is not a single procedure, and it may involve multiple valves, CABG, pacemaker and an implantable cardioverter defibrillator (ICD). Valve surgery is palliative, not curative, and patients will require lifelong health care.

Valve repair may involve resecting and/or suturing prolapsed or torn leaflets (valvuloplasty) and repairing the ring of collagen the valve sits in (annuloplasty) and is commonly used for mitral and tricuspid regurgitation. Commissurotomy (incising valve leaflets and debriding calcification) is the treatment of choice for mitral stenosis. Both repair processes have demonstrated lower operative mortality than replacement, although complete valve competence may not be achievable. Open procedures are preferred because thrombi and calcification can thereby be removed.

Valve replacement may be necessary, but could be associated with higher risks due to the long-term disease process and poor underlying left ventricular function. The most common indication for valve replacement is aortic stenosis, which accounts for around 60% of valve surgery.[6,16] Prosthetic valves may be mechanical or biological. Mechanical valves are made of metal alloys, pyrolite carbon and Dacron (Fig. 12.3). Biological valves are constructed from porcine, bovine or human cardiac tissue. Mechanical valves are more durable but have an increased risk of thromboembolism, so lifelong

FIGURE 12.3 Prosthetic valves: (**A**) the Bjork-Shiley valve, with a pyrolyte-carbon disc that opens to 60°; (**B**) the Starr-Edwards caged-ball valve model 6320, with satellite ball; (**C**) the St Jude Medical mechanical heart valve, with a mechano-central flow disc; (**D**) the Hancock II porcine aortic valve, with stent and sewing ring covered in Dacron cloth 5.

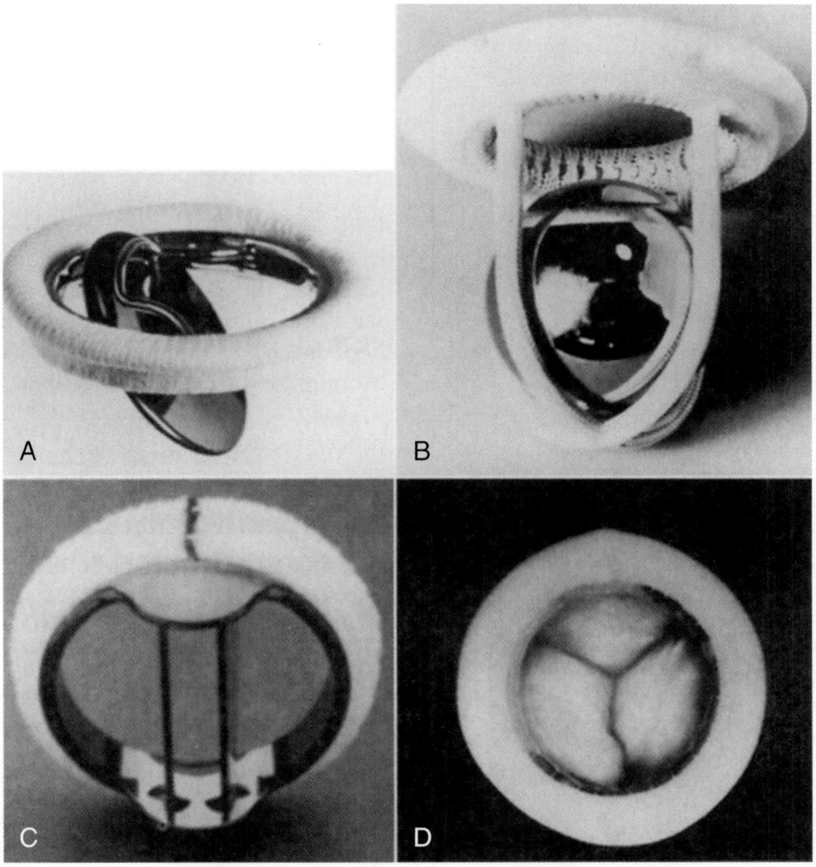

Source: Urden LD, Satcy KM, Lough ME. Thelan's Critical Care Nursing Diagnosis and Management. 5th ed. 2006, St Louise: Mosby.

anticoagulation is required. Biological valves suffer from the same problems as the patient's valve (i.e. calcification and degeneration). The choice of valve depends on the age of the patient and potential difficulties with taking anticoagulants.

For elderly patients with high risk of open heart surgery and higher comorbidity, trans-catheter aortic valve implantation (TAVI) of commercial artificial valves (for example Medtronic CORE Valve or Edwards Sapien) has been used. This procedure is usually performed in a catheter laboratory, via femoral artery approach, similar to angiography procedure and light anaesthesia. This procedure carries higher risks of all-cause 1-year mortality of 13.9–16.3%, major vascular complications of 9.3–12.3% and 2.6% incidence of stroke.[17,18]

Mortality is higher for valvular surgery than for CABG, reflecting the underlying loss of ventricular function and additional procedures that are common. Risk stratification models have been developed to help determine the patients that are most likely to have poor recovery and outcomes.[19] The major factors that contribute to poor outcomes are worse left ventricular function and age over 70 years.[15]

Cardiopulmonary bypass

CPB was developed to enable surgery to be performed on a still, relatively bloodless heart, while preserving the patient's circulation. CPB temporarily performs the functions of the heart in circulating blood and of the lungs by enabling gas exchange with the blood. Silicone cannulae are inserted into the venae cavae or right atrium, and venous blood is circulated through a circuit outside the body. In this circuit the blood is oxygenated, carbon dioxide removed and blood temperature controlled. Drugs and anaesthetics may be added. A roller pump is generally used to provide the pressure to create blood flow in the circuit and back to the patient's aorta.

Adverse effects of CPB are diverse, and include the following (Table 12.1):[6,11,20,21]

- haematological effects due to exposure of the blood to tubing and gas exchange surfaces, which initiates surface activation of the clotting cascade;

TABLE 12.1
Summary of the impact and side effects of CPB

BODY SYSTEM	CPB IMPACT	SIDE EFFECTS
Haematology	Surface activation of clotting cascade	↓ WBC, ↓ HcT, ↓ platelets Thromboembolism formation
Pulmonary	SIRS activation (CPB circuit) Lung deflation (during surgery)	↑ Capillary permeability and leakage Pulmonary congestion ↓ Surfactant production Atelectasis Impaired gas exchange
Cardiovascular	Volume changes SIRS activation	Fluid shift ↓ Myocardial contractility and CO Vasodilation and ↓ SVR
Neurological	Poor cerebral perfusion Thromboembolism Post-pump delirium or psychosis	↑ Risk of CVA Short-term memory deficit ↓ Attention Sensory deficit
Renal	↓ CO and renal perfusion	↓ Urine output, and ↑ risk of ARF

ARF = acute renal failure; CO = cardiac output; CPB = cardiopulmonary bypass; CVA = cardiovascular accident; HcT = haematocrit; SIRS = systemic inflammatory response syndrome; SVR = systemic vascular resistance; WBC = white blood cells.

also blood component damage due to shear stress from the roller action of the pump, which reduces haematocrit, leucocyte and platelet count

- pulmonary effects due to activation of systemic inflammatory response syndrome (SIRS), which increases capillary leakage, and lung deflation during surgery leading to postoperative atelectasis
- cardiovascular effects due to volume changes, fluid shifts and decreased myocardial contractility, which decreases cardiac output; this is most severe during the first 6 hours, but usually resolves within 48–72 hours
- neurological effects due to poor cerebral perfusion and generation of thromboemboli from aortic cannulation, which can lead to cerebrovascular accidents
- renal effects due to decreases in cardiac output during initiation of CPB, which decreases renal perfusion
- post-pump delirium or psychosis, which occurs in 32% of CPB patients, although the cause has not been identified; symptoms include short-term memory deficit, decreased attention and inability to respond to and integrate sensory information
- activation of a systemic inflammatory response, which may cause vasodilation and increased cardiac output.

These effects are well documented, and routine CPB management and postoperative care are designed to minimise and treat the complications. Heparin is added at the commencement of CPB and is reversed with protamine (1 mg of protamine for every 100 U of heparin) when CPB ceases; activated clotting times are monitored throughout and after CPB. Blood returning to the circulation is filtered, and surgical procedures proceed carefully to reduce microemboli. Monitoring and maintenance of adequate arterial flow rates are used to prevent low perfusion. Temperature gradients and a rewarming process are instituted slowly so that cardiac output can meet metabolic demands.

Myocardial preservation

One of the processes involved in CPB is that the aorta is clamped where a cannula is inserted to return blood to the circulation. This clamp prevents blood flow into the coronary arteries; therefore, the myocardium must be protected from ischaemia during the cardiac surgical procedure. This protection is achieved through several mechanisms directed towards reducing oxygen demand: first, oxygen demand is reduced by mild-to-moderate hypothermia (28–32°C); second, myocardial temperature is reduced (0–4°C) by infusing cold fluids directly into the coronary arteries; and third, normal conduction is prevented by arresting the heart during diastole, by infusing a concentrated potassium solution into the coronary arteries. Return to normal rhythm is usually achieved by circulation of warm blood, though defibrillation may be necessary.

Sternal closing options

The traditional wire closure of the sternum has been used for decades, but due to high risk of infection and postoperative sternal wound dehiscence, other techniques have developed. One method is the use of a biological bone adhesive, such as Kryptonite, when combined with a standard sternal wire has shown enhancement of mechanical strength, prevention of sternal dehiscence, reduction in postoperative pain and improvement in quality of life, but further research is needed.[22] Other techniques such as the use of sternal clips or rigid fixation (e.g. using SternaLock® system) have been developed, although they still require further evaluation to determine effectiveness and confirm the

FIGURE 12.4 Sternal closing options: **(A)** use of sternal wire; **(B)** use of sternal clip; and **(C)** use of sternal wires 'figure of 8' method.

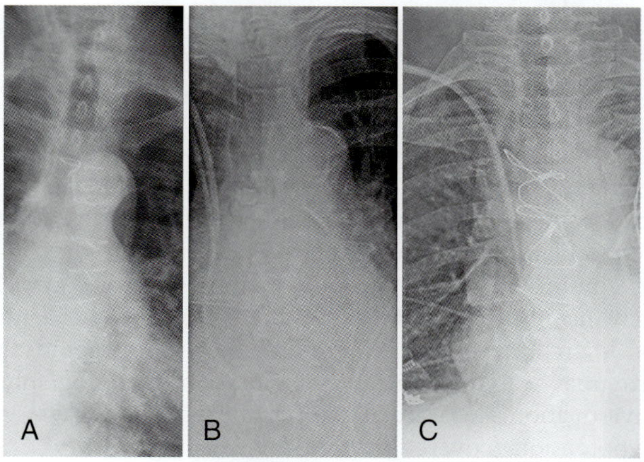

lack of complications.[23,24] Use of these methods of sternal closure necessitates having the correct equipment available to enable rapid re-opening of the sternum in case of emergency (Fig. 12.4).

Patient management

The often-rapid turnaround from complete dependence in intensive care to discharge in post-cardiothoracic surgery patients can provide particularly rewarding nursing experiences. However, this rapid progression is also often marked by haemodynamic instability, arrhythmias and biochemical and haematological changes. The increased emphasis on rapid weaning and extubation, often occurring during turbulent anaesthetic recovery, presents one of the more volatile periods in ventilatory support, requiring knowledgeable and skilled nursing and medical management. In addition to the management of ventilation, temporary pacemaker therapies and mechanical circulatory assist devices (IABP and ventricular assist), effective pain management and rapid mobilisation provide opportunity for the development of broad and detailed expertise.

Patients are usually admitted to the intensive care unit for 1–2 days although, when early extubation is undertaken, they may spend only hours in a recovery unit before progressing to a cardiothoracic high-dependency area, where nurse-to-patient ratios may be 1:2 to 1:3.

The immediate postoperative period

Patients should be transported to intensive care accompanied by at least an anaesthetist, an appropriately qualified nurse and transport personnel under continuous cardiac monitoring and assisted ventilation. It is a requirement to include capnography during patient transport to detect ventilator disconnection, dysfunction or endotracheal tube migration. Intensive care or theatre nursing staff may be a component of the transport team. The admission to intensive care requires a team approach, with the participation of intensive care nursing and medical staff and/or technician input. The immediate postoperative decision making on patient management is influenced by handover from anaesthetists and the surgical team, settling in procedures and collegial assistance.[25–27] Admission activities are commonly divided between nurses, with one nurse taking responsibility for the patient and establishing monitoring and haemodynamic assessment and management, and a second nurse managing ventilation and endotracheal tube security, as well as managing chest drains, gastric tube and urinary catheter. If staffing permits, additional nurses may take responsibility for documentation, performing arterial blood gases, 12-lead ECG and providing assistance as required.

The objectives of immediate postoperative management of cardiac surgical patients may include:

- optimisation of cardiovascular performance
- reestablishment and/or maintenance of normothermia
- promotion of haemostasis
- ventilatory support and management
- prevention and management of arrhythmias
- optimisation of organ perfusion.

Haemodynamic monitoring and support

Typical haemodynamic monitoring includes an intraarterial catheter for continuous blood pressure monitoring and arterial blood sampling. Cardiac output and preload measurement are achieved most commonly with either a pulmonary artery or central venous catheter configured for pulse contour cardiac output (PiCCO) monitoring (see Chapter 9).

Preload measures provided by the pulmonary artery catheter include right atrial pressure (RAP) to approximate right ventricular filling and pulmonary artery pressure (PAP) to approximate right ventricular systole and provide insight into pulmonary vascular resistance and left heart function. The pulmonary capillary wedge pressure (PCWP) is available to approximate left ventricular filling and left heart function. Alternatively, the PiCCO monitoring system represents preload by intrathoracic blood volume index (ITBVI) and global end-diastolic volume index (GEDVI). In addition, the extravascular lung water index (EVLWI) can demonstrate the accumulation of interstitial lung water.[28]

Cardiac output is measured by either intermittent or continuous thermodilution via pulmonary artery catheters, or measured intermittently and then approximated continuously on a beat-to-beat interpretation of pulse contour by the PiCCO monitoring system. Cardiac output measurement can be combined with other pressure variables to calculate systemic and pulmonary vascular resistance, stroke volume and measures of ventricular work.

Certain common haemodynamic patterns are seen in the early postoperative phase. These must be detected through thorough monitoring and interpretation of variables, and managed according to specific needs. During the initial 2 hours of recovery period, 95% of patients will experience haemodynamic instability.[29–31]

> **Practice tip**
>
> The choice of inotropes and vasoactive drugs should be based on the haemodynamic findings, for example: a patient with low systemic vascular resistance (SVR) and low contractility (low CO and BP) will need an ino-constrictor such as adrenaline or dopamine; a patient with high SVR and low contractility will need an ino-dilator such as milrinone or dobutamine.

Hypertension

Hypertension is present in up to 30% of patients initially,[32,33] as hypothermia, stress responses, pain and hypovolaemia contribute to vasoconstriction.[26,34] When the SVR is excessive, the high afterload may contribute to low cardiac output.[34] Rewarming to normothermia with space blankets or heated air blankets, fluid administration, administration of sedation or analgesics and infusion of IV vasodilators (glyceryl trinitrate or sodium nitroprusside) are all commonly used to overcome vasoconstriction when contributing to hypertension.[26,33,34] Occasionally, beta-blockers are used. Hypertension increases myocardial workload and contributes to bleeding.

Hypotension

Transient hypotension requiring treatment is common at some stage during the postoperative period. Contributing factors to hypotension include hypovolaemia and decreased venous return (from polyuria, bleeding, ventilation and positive end-expiratory pressure and excess vasodilation), contractile impairment (from ischaemia or infarction, hypothermia and negative inotropic influences), pericardial tamponade and vasodilation (from excess vasodilator therapy, or as part of an inflammatory response to CPB).[32,33]

Hypotension may present with reduced or elevated preload, reduced or elevated cardiac output and reduced or elevated SVR. When hypovolaemia is present, cardiac output will be low and SVR usually high. Hypovolaemia is diagnosed by measuring preload indicators, as pressure (RAP, PAP, PCWP) or volume (ITBVI, GEDVI).[35] Choice of colloids or crystalloid fluids for volume restoration in the postoperative period has no effect on mortality,[27] but colloids affect clot formation and strength and also produce greater haemodilution, which is associated with more blood product transfusion.[30,36] Blood returned from the CPB circuit ('pump blood') usually accompanies the patient to ICU, and this should be readministered at a rate suitable to filling indices and blood pressure.

Hypotension accompanied by elevated preload and low cardiac output usually represents cardiac dysfunction or pericardial tamponade, and the distinction should be quickly sought.[37–39] When such left ventricular dysfunction is present, there is usually compensatory vasoconstriction and tachycardia, although heart rate responses may be unreliable due to cardioplegia, cold, conduction disease[26] and preoperative beta-blocking agents. Inotropic agents, including milrinone hydrochloride, adrenaline, dopamine or dobutamine, may become necessary (these are covered more completely in Table 21.7 and its accompanying text). When the profile of severe left ventricular dysfunction is persistent (either at the time of coming off bypass or later in intensive care), IABP may be instituted. ECG assessment for new ischaemia or infarction should be made, which if of significant size, may warrant surgical re-exploration or angiographic investigation. Pericardial tamponade is also a cause of hypotension (covered later in this chapter).

A fourth common postoperative profile is hypotension with normal or elevated cardiac output in the presence of low SVR. This may occur with excess vasodilator administration, the use of postoperative epidural infusions and vasodilation from a systemic inflammatory response to CPB and other factors such as reinfusion of collected operative site blood.[31] The inotrope milrinone hydrochloride is popular in the postoperative phase because of its dilating effect on radial artery grafts,[32] but often contributes to hypotension through its systemic vasodilator properties. When hypotension is attributable to vasodilation, metaraminol or noradrenaline may be used.[35] Arginine vasopressin, by infusion, could be used as an effective alternative vasoconstrictor for cardiac surgical patients, but early introduction of vasopressin demonstrated improved haemodynamic response.[40]

A mean arterial pressure of 70–80 mmHg is generally targeted in the postoperative period.[26,32] This can sometimes be reduced if there has been ventriculotomy or if there is concern about the status of the aorta. The cardiac index should be maintained above 2.2 L/min/m^2, as hypoperfusion develops below these values. When at these levels, additional assessments are often undertaken, such as mixed venous oxygen saturation measurement (to assess oxygen delivery deficits) and arterial pH and lactate measurements (to detect metabolic acidosis from anaerobic metabolism).

In addition to assessment of preload, contractility and afterload, heart rate and rhythm should be assessed for their input to cardiac output and blood pressure. Extremes of rate and arrhythmias alter ventricular filling and may need correction. If temporary pacing wires are present, pacing strategies for haemodynamic improvement include rate rises (even if already in the normal range)[21] and the provision of dual-chamber or atrial pacing as alternatives to ventricular pacing only in order to maximise atrioventricular synchrony and the contribution of atrial kick to blood pressure. Alternatively, if ventricular pacing is present, reducing the rate to permit expression of a slower sinus rhythm may, with the provision of atrial kick, improve cardiac output and blood pressure (refer to Chapter 11 for more information on pacing).

Practice tip

Be aware of an apparent paradox: hypertension may occur even if there is hypovolaemia. The intense vasoconstriction often seen postoperatively not only raises blood pressure but aids venous return so that RAP is normal. It may not be until the patient has warmed and dilated that the true filling status is revealed. When the patient is cold and has normal filling pressures, be prepared for possible hypotension, and the need for significant fluid resuscitation, on rewarming.

Rhythm monitoring and postoperative arrhythmias

Continuous rhythm monitoring is necessary while the patient is in intensive care, and telemetry monitoring is usually continued until discharge from hospital. Lead selection is often haphazard, but a chest lead in the V1 position (or lead MCL1) generally provides the best information on atrial and ventricular activity.[41] Unlike many leads, these two leads reliably demonstrate normal rhythms, bundle branch block and ventricular rhythms,[41] and may be useful in confirming pulmonary artery catheter irritation as the cause of ventricular arrhythmias.[42]

A 12-lead ECG is performed on admission to the ICU and should be compared with the preoperative ECG. It should be assessed for signs of new ischaemia or infarction, new bundle branch block and arrhythmias or conduction disturbances. Pericarditis, a frequent complication of surgery, appears as ST-segment elevation (often, but not always, in many leads), and may mask or mimic myocardial infarction. The nurse should look for the classic concave upward, or 'saddle-shaped' ST segment, to distinguish pericardial changes from the more convex upward ST segment of infarction. Worsening of pain on inspiration and a pericardial rub help to confirm pericarditis.[41]

AF is the most common postoperative arrhythmia and contributes significantly to postoperative morbidity and hospital length of stay.[43] It occurs in up to 30–50% of patients, most often on days 2–3 postoperatively.[37] Many patients revert without treatment, but when treatment becomes necessary, beta-blockers and amiodarone appear to be the most successful agents for correction.[44] Digitalis is effective for rate control and IV magnesium is often used, although further evidence for its use is needed. Atrial pacing to prevent AF is being increasingly explored but a clear recommendation on pacing sites and protocols has yet to emerge. In contrast, atrial overdrive pacing can be an effective means to immediately and safely interrupt atrial flutter.[43,44]

Ventricular ectopic beats are common and by themselves do not require treatment unless they accompany ischaemia or biochemical disturbance,[45] in which case they may progress to more complex arrhythmias. Consideration should always be given to the pulmonary artery catheter as the cause (including both correctly and incorrectly positioned catheters),[42] as this is an easily corrected influence. Ventricular tachycardia and fibrillation are uncommon and usually denote myocardial disturbance such as ischaemia or infarction, shock, electrolyte disturbance, hypoxia or increased excitation due to high circulating catecholamine levels.[45] Standard approaches to resuscitation according to protocols in Chapter 24 apply, including standard cardiopulmonary resuscitation (CPR) over the recent sternotomy. When ventricular fibrillation cannot be corrected, consideration is often given to re-exploration of the chest to examine graft patency and/or provide internal cardiac massage. The cardiac surgical intensive care unit should be equipped to enable emergency re-exploration for such purposes.

Practice tip

Appropriate patient management should be based on frequent assessment and evaluation of their condition, especially during the immediate postoperative period, to achieve:

- optimal preload
- optimal contractility
- optimal afterload.

Ventilatory support

Ventilation should be approached according to the general principles described in Chapter 15. As anaesthesia is not typically reversed at the end of the operation, patients are generally admitted apnoeic, and within 1–3 hours return to wakefulness and spontaneous breathing.

Ensuring a secure airway is an initial priority; the following should be undertaken:

- Confirmation of endotracheal tube (ETT) position and its security immediately on admission:
  - auscultation for equal bilateral air entry to rule out right main bronchus intubation
  - recording of the ETT insertion length to detect ETT migration
  - postoperative chest X-ray, taken within 30 minutes, should also be examined for ETT positioning
- Initial ETT care:
  - assessment for air leak around the cuff (via performance of minimal occlusive volume or pressure tests) and auscultation of the neck
  - ensure ETT is adequately secured and positioned so as not to apply undue pressure against soft tissues of the mouth and lips.

TABLE 12.2
Postoperative ventilation settings

NOMINAL OR GENERALLY ACCEPTABLE SETTINGS	ALTERNATIVES TO NOMINAL SETTINGS AND REASONS FOR VARIATION
SIMV with volume control ventilation	Pressure control suitable. Generally used only if there is significant hypoxaemia or the need to exert greater control on pulmonary pressure. Hybrid modes such as Autoflow, pressure-regulated volume control or volume control plus (VC+) are also suitable, generally for the same indications as pressure control
Tidal volume 8–10 mL/kg	Lower tidal volumes (6–8 mL/kg) when there is known compliance disorder (atelectasis, pulmonary oedema, fibrosis) or unexplained high plateau pressures
Mandatory rate 10 L/min	Faster rates may be necessary if low tidal volume strategies become necessary. Lower rates if gas-trapping risk due to airways disease. Adjust according to $PaCO_2$ level
Inspiratory flow 30–50 L/min to provide I: E ratio of 1:2 to 1:4 acceptable	Slower flows to prolong the inspiratory time may be necessary if there is atelectasis and hypoxaemia, or if there is a desire to lessen inspiratory pressures. Faster flows to enhance expiratory time necessary only if gas-trapping risk
PEEP minimum levels of 5 cmH_2O	Higher levels of PEEP according to severity of hypoxaemia
Pressure support 5–10 cmH_2O	Automated pressure support modes such as automatic tube compensation (autoadjusted pressure support to overcome flow resistance of tracheal tubes) or volume support (autoadjusted pressure support to achieve target tidal volume on spontaneous breaths) exist. There is no pressing indication for their use in uncomplicated cardiac surgical patients
Permissive hypercapnoea rarely necessary	Particularly important to avoid if existing pulmonary hypertension, as may worsen acutely with respiratory acidosis
FiO_2 initially 0.8–1.0 then wean down according to PaO_2/SaO_2	According to PaO_2/SaO_2

FiO_2 = fraction of inspired oxygen; PEEP = positive end expiratory pressure; SIMV = synchronised intermittent mandatory ventilation mode.

There has been a general trend to more rapid ventilatory weaning in recent years, and in some centres 'fast-track' cardiac surgical recovery includes extubation at the end of the operation before transfer to a recovery unit for suitable patients. Indices of respiration show no improvement when intubation is maintained for longer compared with early extubation,[46] and pooled results from randomised early extubation trials show earlier ICU discharge and shorter lengths of stay (by 1 day) when early extubation is undertaken.[46,47]

Apart from these fast-track approaches, ventilation is commonly employed for 2–6 hours in the uncomplicated patient. Reasons for continuing ventilation beyond this time frame may include:

- intraoperative neurological event
- gas exchange deficit with unresolved hypoxaemia
- ventilatory inadequacy
- significant haemodynamic insufficiency or instability
- patients returning from theatre late in the evening may sometimes continue ventilation overnight to optimise postextubation breathing ability.

For many patients, ventilation is provided purely for initial airway and apnoea protection rather than for treatment of pulmonary deficits. In the absence of pulmonary disease, many centres provide fairly uniform approaches to parameter settings that aim at sustaining ventilation and oxygenation, while limiting traumatic risk to the lungs (Table 12.2). However, approaches to ventilation will need to be tailored in the presence of operative complications or coexisting lung disease.

Ventilation challenges specific to the postoperative cardiac setting include:

- atelectasis due to operative access
- pneumothorax (pleural opening for grafts, or ventilation-induced trauma)
- pulmonary hypertension from cardiac failure or valve disease
- cardiogenic shock/post-pump failure
- SIRS due to CPB
- early or rapid weaning that is undertaken before complete readiness, leading to failure at weaning attempt

- surgical pain limiting spontaneous effort and potentially leading to atelectasis or sputum retention.

Approaches to weaning

As patients often have no underlying pulmonary pathology, and have been ventilated for brief periods only, rapid weaning phases have become the norm in most centres. In many instances, as soon as the patient wakes and begins spontaneous breathing activity, he/she may be suitable for at least a trial of spontaneous breathing in continuous positive airway pressure (CPAP) mode, usually with some modest level of pressure support (e.g. 5–10 cmH_2O). If tolerated and the patient maintains an adequate minute volume, SpO_2 and $PaCO_2$, extubation may be considered within as little as another 30 min. Normal demonstrations of airway protection capability (e.g. neuromuscular control, gag, swallow, cough and patient strength) should be sought before extubation (see Chapter 15 for details).

These short ventilation times and rapid weaning carry a greater risk of weaning failure. Patients may initially wake and appear to sustain spontaneous ventilation well for some time, only to lapse back under anaesthetic influence. A return to greater ventilatory support may be necessary. Failure to wean carries greater significance in the cardiac surgical patient with existing pulmonary hypertension, as respiratory acidosis causes pulmonary vasoconstriction, abruptly worsening pulmonary hypertension and the risk of pulmonary oedema and/or right ventricular failure.

When ventilation has been more prolonged due to postoperative pulmonary problems, weaning may be approached more cautiously, as might be applied to the general longer-term ventilated patient. Gradual mandatory rate reduction or increasing periods of spontaneous ventilation interspersed with periods of greater assistance have been employed.[46,48]

Postoperative bleeding

The harvest sites for radial arteries or saphenous veins are uncommon sources of significant blood loss and are generally easily managed with dressings or compression. Intrathoracic bleeding, however, may be torrential and threaten life. Occasionally, surgical bleeding from the aorta, arterial grafts or myomectomy sites may exceed replacement capabilities, and at times patients succumb to overwhelming haemorrhage. Maintenance of drain patency and strict recording of losses and total fluid balance are paramount, and fluid balance assessments over shorter intervals, even every 5–10 min, become necessary during active bleeding. Because of the potential rates of bleeding, the cardiac surgical unit must be equipped to institute rapid volume replacement, and have access to adequate blood and blood product stores, blood warmers and all necessary procoagulant therapies. In addition, dedicated equipment should be available to facilitate emergency resternotomy to control haemorrhage.

One or more chest drains are inserted to remove and monitor blood loss, but the positioning of drains is variable, depending in part on the procedure performed, the surgical route taken and surgeon preference. Regardless of these considerations there will always be a retrosternal/anterior mediastinal drain, as the sternum is generally the major source of bleeding in the absence of complications. Additional drains may be inserted in the pericardial or pleural spaces. Pericardial drains are more likely to be inserted following aortic valve surgery, whereas pleural drains become necessary following mammary artery harvesting or when the pleura is opened for any other reason. Pleural drains may be anterior, posterior or 'wrap-around' configurations in which they project over the anterior lung, following the pleural space first from midline to lateral and then, finally, the posterior pleural space.

Reportable postoperative blood losses vary, but greater than 100 mL/h, or greater than 400 mL in the first 4 hours, would generally be regarded as excessive and worthy of surgeon notification. Importantly, excessive bleeding does not always represent a surgical defect that reoperation might correct, as there are many contributors to impaired haemostatic capability in the cardiac surgical patient (see below).

Chest drainage should be monitored closely and, while bleeding is active, volumes should be assessed every 5 min and patency of drains ensured to avert tamponade. Sudden cessation of drainage should always raise the possibility of the loss of tube patency and risk of tamponade, but tamponade may also occur while drainage continues, as collections and compressions may occur at sites isolated from drains, or losses may simply be occurring faster than that able to be removed by patent drains.

Chest drains should also be observed for bubbling, to assess for air leaks originating from either system faults or patient leaks. When bubbling can be attributed to the patient, the patency of tubes becomes additionally important to avert tension pneumothorax, which may accumulate rapidly, even over the course of a few breaths in the ventilated patient.

Blood transfusions are not aimed at restoring haemoglobin to normal levels and, despite variations in acceptable levels, relative anaemia is almost universally tolerated. Haemoglobin levels are thus not routinely treated unless below 80 g/L, except in the elderly or when there are significant comorbidities.[49–52] From these levels patients return to normal haemoglobin status within 1 month postoperatively.

Contributors to impaired haemostatic capability

Many factors may contribute to postoperative bleeding by their influence on coagulation and haemostatic ability. CPB is used in the majority of cardiac surgical cases and exerts many influences on coagulation, as do additional factors such as preoperative medications, anaemia or coagulopathies. Contributing factors include:

- CPB influences:
  - o heparinisation, haemodilution, platelet damage and altered function
  - o disseminated intravascular coagulation (DIC) following activation of the SIRS post-CPB
- preoperative anticoagulant/antiplatelet medications commonly encountered
- aspirin, warfarin, clopidogrel
- preoperative anaemia due to aortic valve disease, autologous blood donation or the various chronic anaemias
- clotting factor deficiency
- hypothermia
- coexisting coagulopathies
- increased fibrinolytic activity
- surgical defects such as failure of access site closure, or vascular anastomosis defects.

Bedside assessment of bleeding

The activated clotting time (ACT) is the most commonly used assessment of coagulation and heparin activity during cardiac surgery and subsequently in intensive care. It measures the time to onset of fibrin formation (initial clot development). The ACT has been valuable because it can be inexpensively and efficiently performed at the bedside, providing prompt results and requiring only modest personnel training. Bleeding patients with a prolonged ACT come under consideration for administration of protamine or other agents.[53] Treatable levels vary from greater than 120 seconds to greater than 150 seconds among different centres.

A limitation of ACT measurements is that they provide no information about clotting processes beyond initial fibrin formation, so clotting deficits such as impaired clot strength or the presence of significant fibrinolysis as contributors to bleeding are not revealed by this test.[54,55] By contrast, the thromboelastograph (TEG) measures the clotting process as it proceeds over time.[54,55] TEG monitoring not only reveals abnormalities early in the clot process (time to fibrin formation, as would be demonstrated by the ACT) but also the subsequent development of clot strength, clot retraction and, finally, fibrinolytic activity for each of their contributions in the bleeding patient.[54,55] TEG monitoring, although considerably more expensive than the ACT, is now available as a bedside or operating room technology and offers better insight into bleeding causes. In addition, because TEG monitoring identifies deficiencies at the various stages of clot formation, development of clot strength and the presence of undue fibrinolytic activity, it may permit better matching of procoagulant, blood product or antifibrinolytic therapy to needs.[53–55]

No matter which of the above technologies is used at the bedside, the patient with significant bleeding should be evaluated more fully as soon as bleeding develops. Blood should be drawn and sent for laboratory assessment, including full blood examination, clotting profile and measures of fibrinolytic activity.

Heparin reversal

CPB requires full heparinisation (initially 300 IU/kg), which is reversed at end-operation.[56,57] The specific antidote, protamine sulfate, is administered as bypass is ceased, at a dose of 1 mg per 100 IU heparin used (i.e. 3 mg/kg).[58] If reversal is less than complete, as evidenced by a prolonged ACT, further protamine sulfate (at doses of 25–50 mg over 5–10 min) may be necessary.

Management of bleeding

Treatment approaches to bleeding once the patient is in intensive care include further protamine administration if the ACT remains prolonged, blood and blood product administration (platelets, clotting factors, fresh frozen plasma), procoagulants (desmopressin acetate [DDAVP]) and anti-fibrinolytic agents (see Table 12.3 for more details). Other general measures such as rewarming the patient and preventing or treating hypertension should be undertaken.

Autotransfusion

Chest drain systems used in cardiothoracic surgery can be configured for retransfusion of collected blood during rapid blood loss. If losses are fresh, and are collected with reliable sterility, they can be transfused back into the patient. Blood that has been collected and left standing in the drain receptacle rapidly becomes unsuitable for retransfusion, and so autotransfusion is generally limited to blood that has collected over 1–2 hours, rarely longer. Blood filters should always be used for protection against clots that may have developed in the drain receptacle. A small proportion of centres are using Intraoperative Cell Salvage (e.g. Cell Saver autologous blood recovery system) to recover blood loss from the chest drain system, wash the red blood cells and re-infused to the patient in case of postoperative massive bleeding.[59]

Pericardial tamponade

Postoperative pericardial tamponade results from the accumulation of blood or effusion fluid within the pericardium. An increasing volume within the pericardial space eventually compresses cardiac chambers, impeding venous return and therefore causing low cardiac output and hypotension. Pericardial tamponade is an emergency and varies in severity from shock to pulseless electrical activity.[38,39,60] Described as one of the extra-cardiac obstructive shocks, pericardial tamponade often resembles cardiogenic shock. The low cardiac output and hypotension result in oliguria, altered mentation, peripheral hypoperfusion and development of lactic acidosis. Compensation includes tachycardia and marked vasoconstriction, elevating the SVR. As in cardiogenic shock, there is usually elevation of the filling pressures (right atrial, pulmonary artery and PCWPs), sometimes with a particularly suggestive merging of the pulmonary

TABLE 12.3
Management of the bleeding patient post-cardiac surgery[26,54-58]

THERAPY	DOSE	COMMENTS / ISSUES
Protamine sulfate	25–50 mg slow IV (<10 mg/min); may be repeated if ACT prolonged	Specific antidote to heparin. May cause hypotension. Contraindicated in patient with seafood allergy
Aprotinin (Trasylol)	Continuous infusion of 2 million units over 30 min, then 500,000 units per hour	Antifibrinolytic. Proteinaceous. Anaphylaxis risk on re-exposure. Alert should be posted on history
Desmopressin acetate (DDAVP)	0.4 mcg/kg IV	Promotes factor VIII release; limited evidence for use
'Pump blood' (blood retrieved from bypass circuit at end-operation)	Often 400–800 mL	This is the remaining blood in bypass circuit; usually centrifuged before returning to patient. Note: this blood contains heparin from CPB
Whole blood/packed cells	As necessary to achieve Hb >80 g/L or more, according to needs	Autologous blood sometimes available when patients have donated blood preoperatively
Fresh frozen plasma	As necessary	'Broad-spectrum' factor replacement; contains most factors. Useful adjunct to massive blood transfusion
Platelet concentrates	As necessary	Generally ABO and Rh compatible preferred
Epsilon-aminocaproic acid (Amicar)	100 mg/kg IV followed by 1–2 g/h	Antifibrinolytic. Inhibits plasminogen activation
Cryoprecipitate	10 units IV	Contains factor VIII and fibrinogen (factor I)
Calcium chloride or gluconate	10 mL 10% solution	Used to offset citrate binding of calcium in stored blood
Prothrombinex	20–50 IU/kg IV	Contains factors II, IX and X

ACT = activated clotting time; CPB = cardiopulmonary bypass.

artery diastolic, right atrial and pulmonary artery wedge pressures.[38,39,60] Additional features that may be present include muffled heart sounds, decreased QRS voltage, electrical alternans, narrowing pulse pressure and pulsus paradoxus, along with features of increasing anxiety and/or dyspnoea in the awake patient.

Echocardiography is the definitive assessment tool to reveal the presence of pericardial collections as well as identifying the impact on relaxation, filling and contraction of each cardiac chamber. The chest X-ray is of limited use and may show little, even with significant pericardial collections.

Importantly, the 'classic' or typical haemodynamic profile described above is not uniformly seen in tamponade, and tamponade should never be excluded because the haemodynamic status does not match this profile. This may be because classic tamponade implies uniform compression of the entire heart, which may not be the case with haemorrhagic tamponade. A clot may develop over just one chamber rather than occupying the entire pericardium, and so there may be compromise to only a single chamber rather than the whole heart.[38,39,60]

Management of pericardial tamponade

The management of pericardial tamponade includes limiting further losses into the pericardium, relief of pericardial pressure through evacuation of blood or clots and management of the haemodynamic impact of tamponade.

Steps to control bleeding and blood pressure as described above may limit further losses into the pericardium. All steps should be taken to maintain or re-establish chest tube patency (crushing clots within tubing – often referred to as 'milking' the tubes – is not recommended but continues to be used as a last resort) and to ensure free flow of blood from the chest by avoiding dependent tubing loops or by instigating side-to-side rolling of the patient to possibly bring collections into proximity of drain tubes. When tube patency is in doubt, the surgeon may even pass a suction catheter or a balloon-tipped catheter (such as Fogarty catheter) through the chest drain under aseptic conditions in an attempt to remove clots at the drain tip.[38,39,60] If the above measures do not relieve tamponade, consideration is given to re-exploring the pericardium, either by returning to the operating theatre or, in an emergency, to the intensive care unit, although this is less preferable.

Emergency opening of the sternotomy and mediastinal re-exploration requires a coordinated team response and, where possible, operating room staff should be included to manage the sterile field and assist the surgeon. Equipment and disposable materials should be counted and documented in the manner normally applied in theatre. When the situation has been stabilised, consideration should be given to returning to theatre for final assessment and chest closure.[38,39,60]

Practice tip

Given the variability of presentation of cardiogenic shock, and the importance of accurate identification, clinicians should search for tamponade whenever there is haemodynamic instability postoperatively, especially when the haemodynamic status does not match classic patterns for the major shock states. The management of postoperative cardiac arrest accompanying any arrhythmia, as well as pulseless electrical activity, should include consideration of tamponade.

Assessment and management of postoperative pain

As much an art as a science, pain control in the cardiac surgical patient remains a major challenge and continues to provide uncertainty and opportunities for nursing clinicians and researchers. Principles are similar to those outlined in Chapter 6. Surgical pain is often complicated by pericardial inflammation and pain management must be balanced against the promotion of spontaneous breathing, chest physiotherapy, mobilisation and participation in education and lifestyle modification programs.

Analgesic options for pain control include intravenous, oral or rectal analgesics, non-steroidal anti-inflammatory medications and, less commonly, epidural therapies and nerve blocks. Intravenous opiates and codeine/paracetamol preparations provide the mainstay of postoperative analgesia. When insufficient, or when clinical and electrocardiographic features suggest pericarditis, non-steroidal anti-inflammatory drugs such as rectal indomethacin are appropriate, except in patients with renal impairment due to their renal side effects of reducing glomerular filtration rate and acute deterioration of renal function.[61] The place of IV COX-2 inhibitors such as parecoxib appears uncertain, as analgesic efficacy now must be weighed against emerging data suggesting increased thrombotic complications.[62] Chronic post-surgical pain could persist in up to 10% of patients especially female gender, younger ages and in overweight patients. Although the main mechanism of this chronic pain is not established yet, well-controlled perioperative pain management regardless of the methods has shown to be a convincing preventative strategy.[63,64]

Fluid and electrolyte management

Fluid therapy in the postoperative period is aimed at maintaining blood volume, replacing recorded and insensible losses and providing adequate preload to sustain haemodynamic status. Isotonic dextrose solutions (5%) or dextrose 4% + saline 0.18% are commonly used at approximately 1.5 L/day as maintenance fluids.[26,30]

Potassium replenishment is generally necessary according to measured serum potassium. Polyuria is usually evident in the early postoperative period due to deliberate haemodilution while on CPB. With polyuria comes potassium loss, which must be treated to avert atrial or ventricular ectopy and tachyarrhythmias. Because of these predictable potassium losses, protocols for potassium replacement may be instituted, with standing orders for potassium replacement (e.g. 10 mmol over 1 hour if the serum potassium is <4.5 mmol/L, or 20 mmol over 2 hours if <4.0 mmol/L). Main line hydration infusions may also have added potassium to avoid hypokalaemia. Hypomagnesaemia may also develop due to polyuria, and is likewise proarrhythmic. Supplementation (magnesium chloride) is often used for arrhythmia management postoperatively, but its effectiveness has been questioned in many trials.[65,66]

Hyperkalaemia occurs less often but is seen particularly when there is impaired renal function. Additional contributors to a rising potassium level include acidosis, administration of stored blood, haemolysis, inotrope use and any postoperative use of depolarising muscle relaxants such as suxamethonium.

Emotional responses and family support

The experience of being diagnosed with a cardiac disorder, waiting for surgery, the surgical experience and recovery is an emotional journey for patients and their families. Regardless of low mortality rates, the possibility of death and painful wounds can concern patients. Consequently, patients undergoing cardiac surgery often experience anxiety and depression,[67] and women appear to be more vulnerable to these emotions in relation to cardiac surgery than men.[68] In addition, the same levels of anxiety, depression and stress have been experienced by patients' spouses but significantly reduce over time in both patients and their families. It has been suggested that providing appropriate information about the procedures to both patients and their spouses will assist them to deal better with their psychological state in the recovery period.[69] The use of a 30-min preoperative education session on psychosocial wellbeing has been shown to significantly reduce the rate of pre- and postoperative anxiety in cardiac surgical patients; therefore, training provided to nurses and physicians on emotional support of these patients is essential.[70]

Similarly, adequate preparation of the patient and their family in the preoperative period will assist them with their stress and anxiety coping strategies as well as reduce their work stress after their return to work.[69,71] The preoperative preparation is usually provided by nurses and should incorporate information and support about the procedures and recovery period, so that patients and their families are better equipped during their recovery. Emphasis should be on identifying the intrapersonal stressors, such as pain and discomfort, invasive lines and surgical procedures, for individual patients to assist them coping with their perioperative and rehabilitation period.[69,72] However, patients who have had their surgery postponed or who have been operated on in an emergency setting may need additional support. Also, critical pathways for cardiac surgery do not include assessing the patient's psychological state, so nurses must take care to consider this aspect. Printed information regarding the surgery, recovery and emotions will be useful for the patient and family (for further information refer to Chapter 6, *Patient comfort and psychological care*, and Chapter 7, *Family and cultural care of the critically ill patient*).

Intra-aortic balloon pumping

Intra-aortic balloon pumping (IABP) is a widely-used circulatory assist therapy that has become straightforward in application and relatively free of complications.[73–75] The primary aim of IABP is to assist repairing an existing imbalance between myocardial oxygen supply and demand. The main indications are for cardiogenic shock, myocardial infarction or ischaemia, haemodynamic support for PCI and weaning from CPB. The combined effects of increasing cardiac output and mean arterial pressure (increasing oxygen supply) and decreasing myocardial workload (reducing oxygen demand) make IABP therapy ideal for the management of infarct-related cardiogenic shock,[73–75] for which it should be regarded as standard management.

IABP therapy involves placement of a balloon catheter in the descending thoracic aorta. This catheter is most commonly advanced from a percutaneous femoral artery access until the tip of the catheter is situated just below the left subclavian artery (Fig. 12.5). A chest X-ray or fluoroscopy should reveal the catheter tip just below the aortic arch, or at the level of the second anterior intercostal space or fifth posterior intercostal space (Fig. 12.6). The conventional catheter has two lumens: a monitoring lumen, which opens at the catheter tip from which the aortic pressure waveform is monitored; and a helium drive lumen, through which the helium

FIGURE 12.5 Intra-aortic balloon catheter. On the left the inflated catheter can be seen behind the heart, with its tip below the arch of the aorta and the left subclavian artery. The balloon cycles between inflated (during diastole) and deflated (during systole), as on the right. Blood fills the aorta while the balloon is deflated, and with inflation the balloon almost fills the descending aorta, displacing 40 mL blood from the aorta to the coronary and systemic circulation.

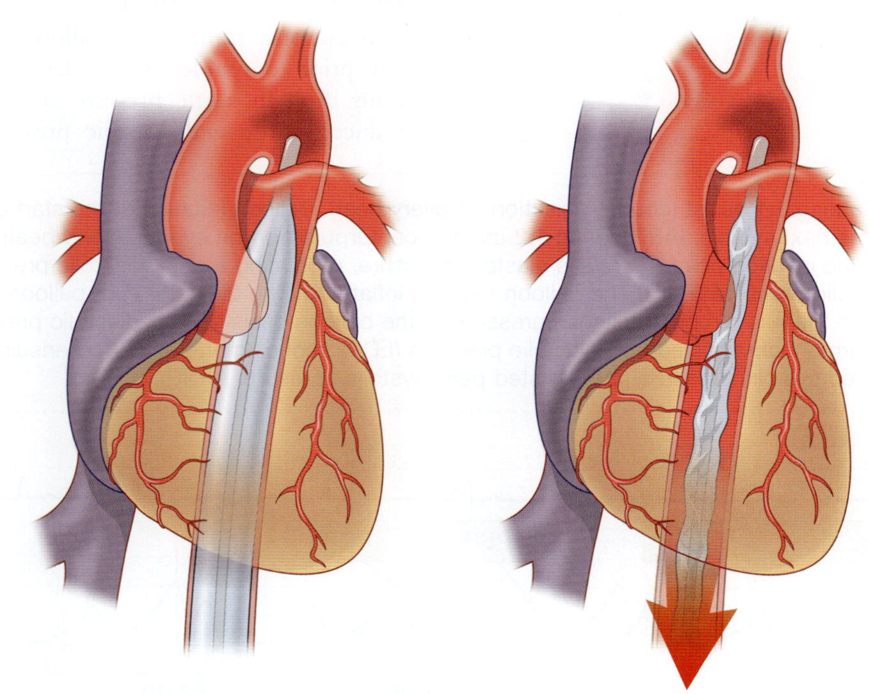

is shuttled from the pumping console to the catheter balloon. The newer fibreoptic catheter has an additional lumen for electrical signal acquisition and transmission from the tip of catheter; together with the automation mode this has improved IABP timing through enabling faster adjustment to patient rate and rhythm changes. Balloon volumes range from 25 mL (paediatric use) to 34–50 mL in adults (most commonly used is a 40 mL balloon) and are selected according to patient height (e.g. a 40 mL balloon is used for a patient height of 162–183 cm).

FIGURE 12.6 IABP catheter position in CXR; the tip is located in the second intercostal space anterior ribs or fifth intercostal space posterior ribs.

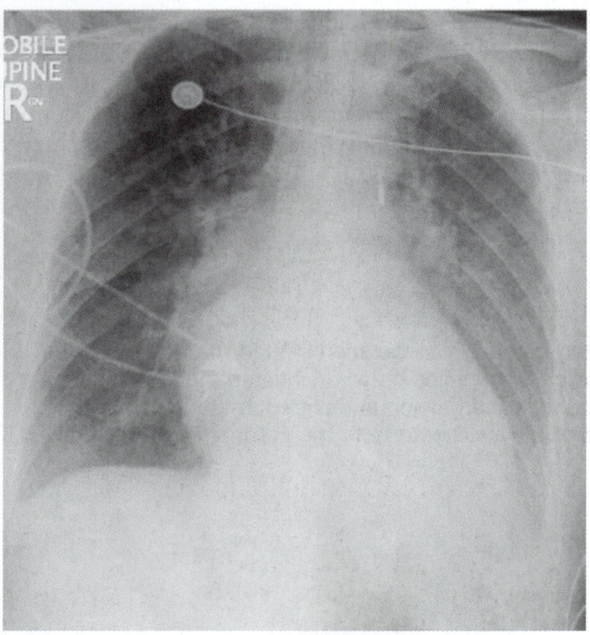

Principles of counterpulsation

When IABP is initiated, the balloon will be inflated rapidly at the onset of diastole of each cardiac cycle and then deflated immediately just before the onset of the next systole; this sequence is referred to as counterpulsation.

Balloon inflation

At the onset of diastole, the balloon is rapidly inflated with (most commonly) 40 mL of helium. This inflation causes a sudden rise in pressure in the aortic root during diastole, raising mean arterial pressure and, importantly, coronary perfusion pressure. The blood displaced by the balloon expansion improves blood flow into the coronary circulation (which fills largely during diastole), as well as to the brain and systemic circulation. Thus, there is improved myocardial oxygen supply and increased mean arterial pressure, as well as improved systemic perfusion.[6,64] The balloon remains inflated for the duration of diastole. The arterial pressure wave should reveal a sharp rise in pressure at the dicrotic notch, with a second pressure peak now appearing on the waveform, described as the ‘augmented diastolic’ or ‘balloon-assisted peak diastolic’ pressure. This peak is usually at least 10 mmHg higher than the systolic pressure (Fig. 12.7).

Balloon deflation

As the inflated balloon largely obstructs the aorta, it must be deflated to permit systolic emptying of the left ventricle. Two separate approaches to the timing of balloon deflation have emerged: ‘conventional timing’ and ‘real timing’.

Conventional timing

In conventional timing, the balloon is deflated immediately prior to systole. Rapid deflation induces a precipitous drop in aortic pressure at the end of diastole (a reduced aortic end-diastolic pressure). This reduces

FIGURE 12.7 IABP during 1:1 assist (counterpulsation on every beat). Balloon inflation at the start of diastole and deflation just before the next systole. IABP during 1:2 assist (counterpulsation on every second beat). Inflation of the balloon rapidly at the inflation point (IP) raises diastolic pressure, producing a peak diastolic pressure (PDP) that exceeds the peak systolic pressure (PSP). The balloon remains inflated during diastole. With balloon deflation just prior to the next systole there is a rapid decline in pressure to the balloon-assisted end-diastolic pressure (BAEDP), which is lower than normal non-assisted end-diastolic pressure (EDP), reducing afterload. The ensuing systole is achieved with a reduced systolic pressure (the assisted peak systolic pressure, APSP).

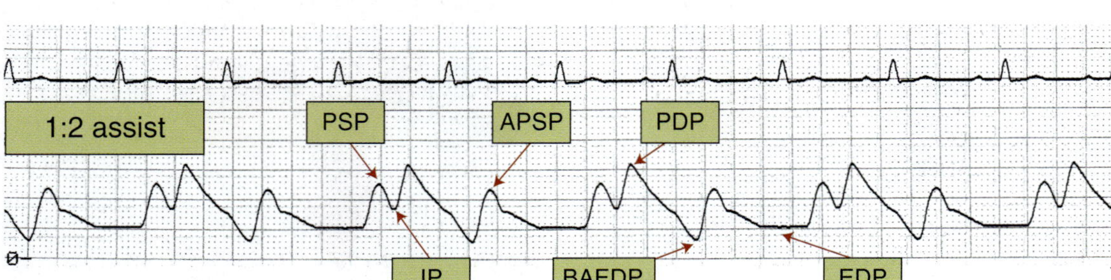

the duration of the left ventricle isovolumetric contraction phase of the cardiac cycle (most oxygen-consuming phase of the cardiac cycle), reduces the left ventricular afterload and improves left ventricular emptying, improving stroke volume and cardiac output.[6,73,76] In addition, less pressure is required for left ventricular emptying, so systolic work and oxygen demands on the myocardium are reduced.[6,73,76] Thus, deflation during conventional timing should see the aortic pressure drop to below normal at end-diastole, just in advance of the subsequent systole. Systolic pressure should also be lower than during a non-assisted beat.

Real timing

In contrast to conventional timing, during real timing (also referred to as R wave deflate) the balloon remains inflated for slightly longer, and is deflated not before but at the same time as systole. The reduction in aortic end-diastolic pressure is therefore not seen, but deflating simultaneously with left ventricular contraction still favourably affects left ventricular emptying.[6,77] Thus, there is improved stroke volume, systolic pressure reduction and decreased ventricular work and oxygen demand as seen during conventional timing.[6,77] Box 12.1 summarises the impact of balloon inflation and deflation on haemodynamic status and the oxygen supply/demand balance.

The arterial pressure wave reveals the impact of IABP therapy on haemodynamic status. Placing the pump into 1:2 assist (balloon pumping on only every second beat) is useful to highlight balloon pump impact and how assisted beats vary from the normal pressure cycle during systole and diastole. Fig. 12.7 depicts the impact of IABP on haemodynamic status and the arterial pressure waveform.

BOX 12.1

Effects of intra-aortic balloon counterpulsation

- Balloon inflation:
  - increased aortic diastolic pressure (augmented, or balloon-assisted peak diastolic pressure, balloon aortic end-diastolic pressure [BAEDP])
  - increased mean arterial pressure
  - increased myocardial perfusion and oxygen supply
  - increased cerebral and systemic perfusion
- Balloon deflation:
  - decreased afterload
  - increased stroke volume and cardiac output
  - decreased LV congestion, decreased PCWP, decreased pulmonary congestion
  - decreased left ventricular workload
  - decreased systolic pressure
  - decreased myocardial oxygen demand
  - decreased duration of isovolumetric contraction

Complications of intra-aortic balloon pumping

Serious complications are uncommon during IABP treatment and have continued to decrease in frequency during the past decade with advances in pump technology and the advent of smaller catheter sizes.[78,79] Limb ischaemia remains the most common serious complication, especially in patients with existing vasculopathy,[78,79] providing impetus to the development of smaller catheters, which have now reached 7.5 French gauge. Additional complications, such as bleeding, catheter migration, thromboembolism, insertion-site vascular damage, thrombocytopenia and device-related problems such as timing inaccuracy, device failure and gas leaks, also occur but are less common. These are described below.

Patient management

Prevention of complications, as well as optimisation of the impact of counterpulsation, form the major components of nursing care of a patient being treated with IABP. Thorough understanding of the impact of the presence of the balloon, as well as the beneficial and detrimental effects of counterpulsation, is essential.

Maintenance of limb perfusion

The use of smaller-gauge catheters has reduced the potential for obstruction of arterial flow past the catheter to the lower limbs, as has the trend to sheath-less insertion. Nevertheless, the threat of limb ischaemia remains an important issue in patient care, as IABP is most commonly undertaken in patients with atherosclerosis, potentially involving the lower limbs, even in the absence of overt peripheral vascular deficits. Identification of patients at risk (known claudication, chronically cold feet and peripheral vascular diseases) may be useful to ensure appropriate vigilance and prompt intervention where necessary. Peripheral perfusion may also be compromised by arterial embolisation should thrombi develop on the catheter. Although catheter materials are non-thrombogenic, the risk of thrombi formation remains and is heightened if periods of catheter stasis (interrupted pumping) are encountered. Systemic heparinisation is not recommended routinely for thromboembolic prevention as it increases the risk of bleeding except for specific indications.[80]

Hourly assessments of peripheral perfusion (colour, warmth, movement, sensation) should be performed to identify potential deficits. Dorsalis pedis and posterior tibialis pulses should be palpated and may sometimes require examination with a Doppler probe. Deficits should be promptly reported and consideration given to catheter removal or reinsertion on the contralateral limb. When pulses cannot be demonstrated, the limb should be assessed for the development of compartment syndrome. At times, the viability of a limb must be weighed against the potential survival benefit of IABP to the patient.

Prevention and treatment of bleeding

Significant bleeding is uncommon,[79] but blood loss may occur from the femoral arterial access site. In addition to physical factors at the insertion site, contributors to bleeding include heparinisation, thrombocytopenia from the physical effect of the pump on platelets and/or other anticoagulants or antiplatelet agents used for the primary disease. Regular observation should be made of the insertion site for bruising or external bleeding, as well as other possible sites of bleeding due to heparinisation. Treatment includes manual pressure at the insertion site or use of compression devices such as FemoStop®, reinforcement of dressings and/or topical procoagulant agents. Monitoring of coagulation status and haemoglobin should be undertaken and blood or blood products may (uncommonly) be required.

Prevention of immobility-related complications

The need for immobilisation of the patient, and in particular the leg, is often over-emphasised, and may heighten the risk of atelectasis, pressure area development and venous stasis and thrombosis. Sensible limitation of leg movement is advised, but patients can generally still move in bed, and should still be turned 2-hourly for pressure relief as long as the insertion site is adequately protected and supported. The femoral access limits flexion at the hip beyond 30°, which may also hamper effective chest physiotherapy and increase the risk of atelectasis and pneumonia.

Migration of the balloon catheter towards the aortic arch or towards the abdominal aorta may cause compromised perfusion to the left arm (occlusion of left subclavian artery), kidneys (renal arteries) or abdominal viscera (superior mesenteric artery). Therefore, neurovascular observation of the upper limbs, urine output and bowel sounds are part of nursing management of the patient with IABP in situ.

Weaning of IABP

Weaning of IABP therapy is generally undertaken once the patient has stabilised, is free of ischaemic signs and symptoms and is on minimum or no inotropic support. Algorithms have been offered for approaches to weaning therapy, with no haemodynamic or mortality benefit.[81,82] Weaning is carried out by either gradual reductions in balloon inflation volume (volume weaning) or gradual reductions in assist frequency from 1:1 through 1:2 and 1:4 (ratio weaning). Hybrids of the two approaches are sometimes used. Support is reduced at intervals while the patient is observed for haemodynamic deterioration, pulmonary congestion and the return of ischaemic signs and symptoms.

Assessment of timing and timing errors

Accurate timing of inflation and deflation in relation to the cardiac cycle is required to maximise IABP benefit. Errors in timing may lessen the potential benefit, or in some cases may worsen cardiac performance and increase demands on the myocardium. Nurses are required to continually assess the haemodynamic impact of balloon pumping and the accuracy of timing via inspection of the arterial pressure waveform, and to adjust timing to optimise the impact of balloon pumping. The development of automated IABP counterpulsation has reduced timing errors by automatic trigger signal recognition and selection, accuracy of automatic setting for optimal inflation and deflation timing and automatic adjustment to changing patient conditions. Therefore, the automated mode of counterpulsation is recommended.[83]

Early inflation

Early inflation will at times be difficult to differentiate from correct inflation timing but is recognised by the onset of inflation soon after the peak systolic pressure, before the pressure has declined to the level of the dicrotic notch (Fig. 12.8). Early inflation may limit the stroke volume and cardiac output, as terminal systole is impeded, and may result in increased myocardial oxygen demands, increased left ventricle workload and premature valve closure. The inflation point should be adjusted (to later) until the inflation upstroke emerges smoothly out of the dicrotic notch.

Late inflation

The arterial pressure waveform reveals the onset of diastole (the dicrotic notch) before balloon inflation commences (Fig. 12.9). This generally results in a lower augmented diastolic pressure than could otherwise be achieved. As the duration of balloon inflation is lessened, the desired rise in mean arterial pressure and coronary perfusion will not be achieved. The inflation marker should be set to 'earlier' until the inflation upstroke emerges smoothly out of the dicrotic notch.

Early deflation

Deflating the balloon earlier than necessary shortens the duration for which the balloon remains inflated and therefore limits the benefit of IABP. When deflation is very early, it may cause harm. Deflation sees the aortic pressure drop markedly but there is now time for blood to fill the space left by the balloon before systole commences. Aortic end-diastolic pressure increases and may even exceed the normal end-diastolic pressure, increasing the duration of the isovolumetric phase, worsening left ventricular afterload and increasing myocardial oxygen demand (Fig. 12.10). Correction is achieved by setting deflation to later until the pressure drop of deflation occurs just in advance of the succeeding systole.

FIGURE 12.8 IABP during 1:2 assist. Early inflation. The inflation point (IP) can be seen high in the downstroke of systole, in this case well before the dicrotic notch (DN).

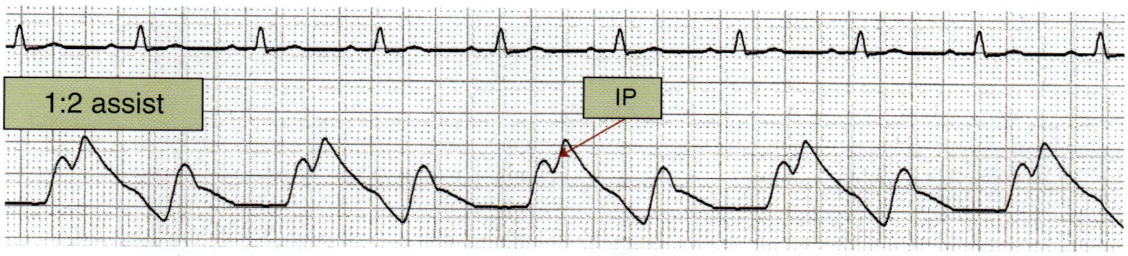

FIGURE 12.9 IABP during 1:2 assist. Late inflation. Note that the inflation point (IP) occurs well after the dicrotic notch (DN). Late inflation is also obvious in 1:1 assist with balloon inflation well after the dicrotic notch.

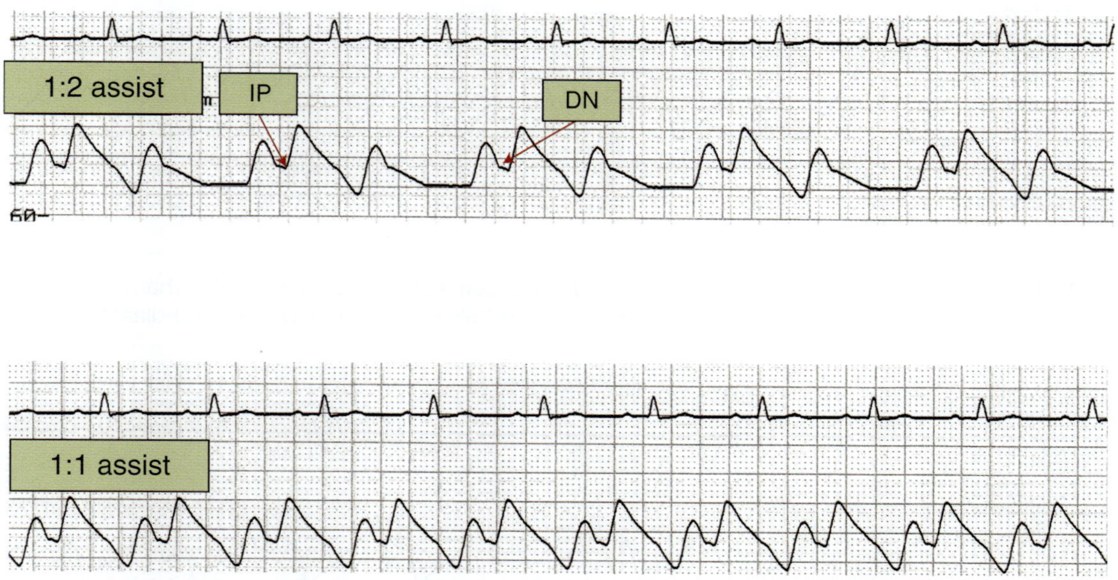

Late deflation

When deflation begins too late, systole commences before complete emptying of the intra-aortic balloon. The typical reduction of aortic end-diastolic pressure is not seen. When significantly late, the end-diastolic pressure may even be increased, prolonging the duration of the isovolumetric contraction phase and worsening afterload. As systole occurs against an incompletely deflated balloon, the stroke volume and cardiac output suffer and ventricular work and oxygen demand increase (Fig. 12.11). Deflation should be set to earlier until the systolic upstroke emerges out of the reduced end-diastolic pressure dip.

Alarm states

Alarm functions vary according to manufacturer and model. The main alarm states common to most devices, and their causes and significance, are shown in Table 12.4.

Importantly, in most alarm states the pump consoles will revert to standby, suspending pumping. The balloon is at risk of developing thrombi within the folds of the balloon while deflated, and these can be liberated as arterial emboli on recommencement of pumping. Therefore, it is important to treat alarm states promptly, to limit the duration of balloon stasis. If interruption to pumping is prolonged, intermittent manual inflation of the balloon with a syringe is recommended (e.g. once every 5–10 min).

Gas loss alarms

Most devices will determine the severity of gas losses and classify them as slow, rapid or disconnect. In all gas loss states it is imperative that assessments be made to exclude balloon rupture and helium leak into the arterial circulation. Small gas losses of helium may or may not be of clinical significance, but the delivery of

FIGURE 12.10 IABP during 1:2 assist. Early deflation. The balloon has been deflated well in advance of the subsequent systole. The aortic pressure does drop off (not much from non-assisted diastole) but then begins to rise again before the next systole gets underway, and may even exceed the normal end-diastolic pressure. Early deflation is also obvious in 1:1 assist.

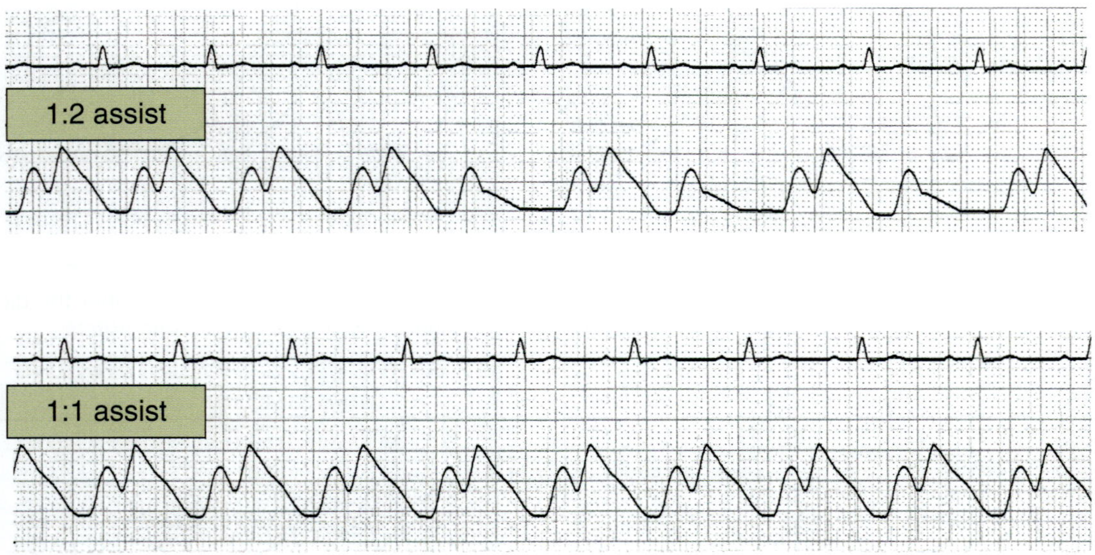

FIGURE 12.11 IABP during 1:2 assist. Late deflation. The late deflation is seen here as the sharp drop-off before systole and a balloon-assisted end-diastole that does not fall to below the normal patient end-diastolic pressure.

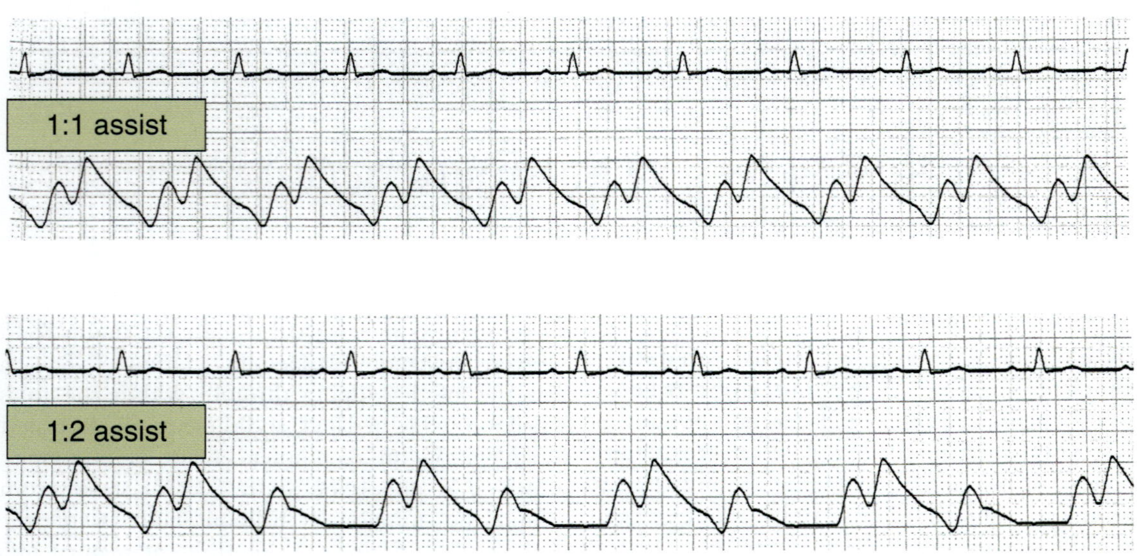

sizeable helium volumes may behave as gas emboli and, if delivered into the coronary circulation, may result in lethal arrhythmias or neurological complications if delivered into the cerebral circulation.[84] In all gas loss alarm states, the helium drive line should be inspected for the presence of blood to indicate loss of integrity of the balloon. If blood is present in the drive line (Fig. 12.12), pumping should be suspended and no attempts at recommencing balloon pumping should be made. Prompt removal and/or replacement, along with thorough patient assessment, is essential.

Heart transplantation

The ultimate goal of organ transplantation is to provide an improved quality of life and long-term survival for

TABLE 12.4
Intra-aortic balloon pump alarm states

ALARM STATE	CAUSES / SIGNIFICANCE
Catheter alarm	Obstruction (complete or subtotal) of the catheter, drive line or balloon Device reverts to standby (non-assist); commonly due to catheter flexion at insertion site due to limb position or excessive surface-to-vessel depth
Loss of trigger	ECG trigger: signal disrupted or low in amplitude, or asystole Pressure trigger: pulse pressure below threshold for detection Pacer trigger: pacing spikes not detected or absent (including demand pacing) Device reverts to standby until restoration of trigger; alternative trigger selection may be necessary
Gas loss alarms	Leak in circuit/drive line or balloon; gas leak may be to the environment or into the patient as a helium embolus Pump reverts to standby; refilling of circuit may be necessary
Low augmentation	Augmented diastolic pressure is lower than operator-selected alarm level; pumping is not interrupted
Pneumatic drive	Functional problem with the pump inflation/deflation pneumatic system Device reverts to standby; alarm may sometimes be activated during tachycardia; 1:2 assist or assist at reduced augmentation may be possible until a replacement device is accessed
Autofill failure	Routine 2-hourly refilling of the system with helium may fail if gas tank is incompletely open or if circuit leaks cause volume loss during the filling attempt Device reverts to standby
System failure	Console self-testing has identified component malfunction Device reverts to standby; restarting may be possible but a replacement device should be accessed
Low helium supply	Helium tank empty or incompletely opened
Low battery	Reconnect to power and recharge

FIGURE 12.12 Intra-aortic balloon rupture and presence of blood in the helium drive line.

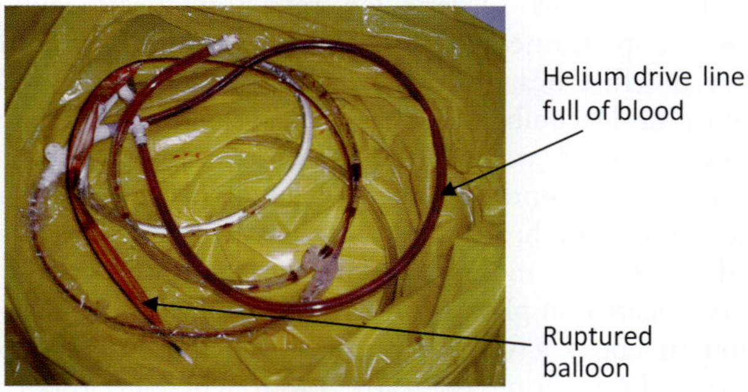

patients with end-stage heart disease. To optimise patient outcomes, the early postoperative management of these patients requires critical care clinicians with specific expertise to collaborate with a multidisciplinary team of health professionals. In the following sections, the important management issues in the early postoperative period for heart transplant recipients are discussed. The major long-term complications of heart transplantation are also discussed briefly as survivors may be readmitted to critical care with life-threatening complications years after their transplant.

Patients with certain chronic heart, respiratory and lung diseases may be referred for organ transplantation assessment when their disease state is such that their life expectancy is less than 2 years and quality of life intolerable. Patients who receive organ transplants are commonly debilitated and may have an acute on chronic presentation at the time of surgery. The surgical procedure is lengthy, up to 12 hours, and involves CPB. The duration and nature of the surgery in patients with severely compromised health status serve to compound the often critical condition of such patients in the early postoperative period.

The immediate period following surgery is commonly the first contact that critical care clinicians have with transplant recipients and their families. The exception may be patients awaiting heart transplantation who are supported by an intra-aortic balloon pump or mechanical circulatory support, also known as a ventricular assist device (VAD), as a 'bridge to transplantation' (Fig. 12.13). Ideally, patients with mechanical circulatory support are returned to a sound physical, mental and nutritional state prior to receiving a transplant and, as

FIGURE 12.13 Pump, monitor and controller. (**A**) HeartWare implanted HVAD® pump. (**B**) HeartWare® monitor with HeartWare® controller and HeartWare® batteries. (**C**) HeartMate 3.

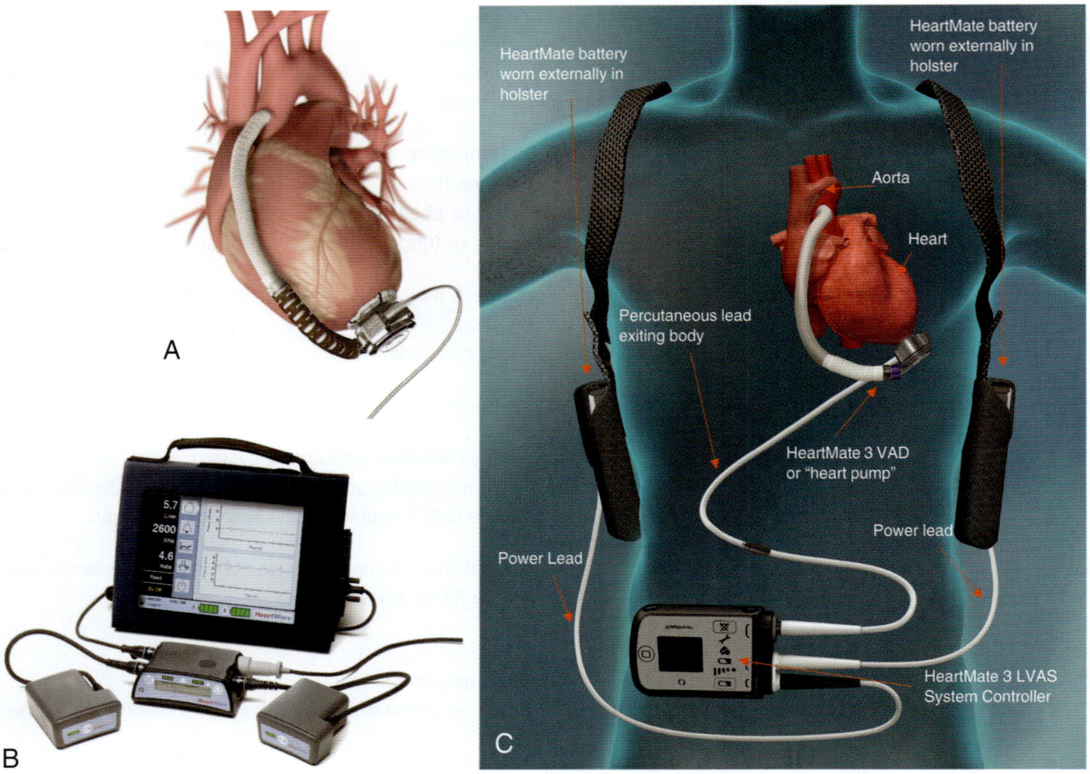

part of their recovery, await transplantation in the ward or home setting. For specific management of patients on mechanical circulatory support, readers are referred to specific resources (e.g. websites and operating manuals for individual mechanical circulatory support devices: Medtronic (HeartWare®), Abbott (Thoratec®) and SynCardia).

Heart transplantation is a life-saving and cost-effective form of treatment that enhances the quality of life for many people with chronic heart failure. Legislation that defined brain death and enabled beating-heart retrieval was enacted in Australia from 1982. This legislation heralded the establishment of formal transplant programs. In Australia, the first heart program commenced in 1983.[85,86] With worsening shortage of donor hearts, the growing interest of using DCD (donation after cardiac death) hearts has emerged, especially as the use of DCD livers, kidneys and lungs have significantly contributed to transplant numbers. St Vincent's in Sydney performed the world's first DCD heart using the TransMedics Organ Care System (OCS) in 2014. Early outcomes have been very encouraging and experience to date suggests that DCD donors can contribute significantly to transplant.[87,88] The success of transplantation in the current era as a viable option for end-stage organ failure is primarily due to the discovery of the immunosuppressive agent cyclosporin A. In this section, heart transplantation as a component of critical care nursing is discussed, with reference to evidence-based practices.

History

Heart transplant surgery for refractory heart failure was first performed in Australia in 1968, only months after the first heart transplant was performed in South Africa in December 1967.[89] However, high mortality rates associated with severe acute rejection and infection within months of surgery led to a reduction in the number of heart transplants performed worldwide, and in effect a moratorium occurred with the procedure. Heart transplantation was finally established in the modern era as a viable treatment option for end-stage heart failure during the early 1980s when cyclosporin A, a then-novel immunosuppressive agent, dramatically improved patients' survival rates by reducing episodes of acute rejection and lowering attendant infectious complications.[90]

Incidence

Heart transplants in the modern era have been performed in Australia since 1986 and in New Zealand since 1987. In 2016, 136 heart transplants were performed in Australia and New Zealand.[91,92] In Europe, 587 heart transplants were performed,[93] an annual figure that has been relatively static for the past 5 years. As the annual number of transplants globally is likely to remain relatively stable because of limited organ availability, future management of end-stage heart failure may involve the insertion of a left ventricular assist device (LVAD) designed for long-term permanent mechanical circulatory support, so-called 'destination therapy'. In the early years, the VADs available were primarily used as 'bridge to transplantation' therapy (i.e. support for a failing native heart until a suitable heart became available), not 'destination therapy', although both purposes were shown to be viable options in the REMATCH study.[94] While this is still the case in Australia and New Zealand, recent global reports show about 46% of VADs are now used as 'destination therapy'.[95] This change has been facilitated by improvements in device technologies and the experiences of clinicians in managing this unique cohort. Survival with continuous flow VADs is now at 80% to the first year and 70% at 2 years.[95] The notion of patients with VADs permanently due to advances in device design and capability (e.g. fully implantable with internal batteries) may not be as futuristic as once thought.

Outcomes from heart transplantation

Currently, the centres around the world that submit data to the International Society of Heart and Lung Transplantation (ISHLT) indicates a 1-year survival at 84.5% and a 5-year survival at 72.5% with a 21% survival at 20 years.[96] In Australia and New Zealand, approximately 88% of heart transplant patients survive to 1 year, and 83% survive to 5 years.[97]

Indications

The vast majority of patients referred for heart transplantation have persistent NYHA functional class IV symptoms (see Chapter 10), secondary to ischaemic heart disease or some form of dilated cardiomyopathy.[98] In ICUs and cardiac units, patients with cardiogenic shock requiring either continuous intravenous inotropic support or cardiovascular support with an intra-aortic balloon pump or VAD are referred for transplant consideration.[98] Commonly, patients listed for transplantation have a life expectancy of less than 2 years without transplantation. Accepted contraindications for heart transplantation include active malignancy, complicated diabetes, morbid obesity, uncontrolled infection, active substance abuse and an inability to comply with complex medical regimens.[99] Currently, 50% of transplanted patients globally are between 50 and 64 years of age.[98] Age has become a relative contraindication, with 16 days old being the youngest and 71 years of age being the oldest to have received a transplant to date.[97] However, the presence of multiple comorbidities in patients over 70 years of age would be expected to exclude the majority of such patients from consideration.[100,101] Other relative contraindications include renal failure and an irreversible high transpulmonary gradient (mean PAP minus pulmonary artery wedge pressure) of greater than 15 mmHg[98,102] (see section on *Early allograft dysfunction and failure* below). In the context of a rigorous postoperative regimen of polypharmacy, frequent follow-up medical appointments and routine cardiac biopsies, a strong social support network, absence of psychiatric illnesses and a willingness to participate actively in the recovery process are highly desirable characteristics of prospective recipients.[103]

Patients referred for heart transplant assessment must have exhausted all other accepted pharmacological and surgical treatment options for end-stage heart failure, such as optimal therapeutic doses of common heart failure medications; revascularisation via CABG surgery or PTCA; continuous IV infusions of dobutamine in the community/home setting; IV levosimendan (a calcium sensitiser); antiarrhythmic drugs to suppress, or an internal cardiac defibrillator to treat potentially lethal arrhythmias; and insertion of a biventricular pacemaker (i.e. chronic resynchronisation therapy) to re-establish atrioventricular synchrony (see Chapter 11).

The average costs associated with heart transplantation are high, at approximately AUD$35,000 for the first year and approximately AUD$15,000 for each ongoing year, depending on the drug regimen and episodes of rejection or infection. As some immunosuppressant drugs have come off patent, these costs have been reduced. However, the high incidence of chronic heart failure and associated hospitalisation costs are also considerable. The number of Australians aged >45 years developing any form of heart failure with clinical overt signs and symptoms is estimated to be more than 60,000 per annum. Based on conservative high mortality rates (≈50% at 5 years and ≈75% at 10 years) these data would suggest a minimum prevalence of 350,000 to 400,000 Australians with clinically overt heart failure.[104] The number of de novo hospitalisations for heart failure per annum is estimated to be 27,468 (45% from 61,444 incident cases) associated with 226,000 days of hospital stay. The annual direct cost of managing heart failure in the community is close to $900 million and as part of an acute hospitalisation $1.8 billion (total direct cost =$2.7 billion). Transplantation for end-stage heart failure is actually a viable and economical treatment option for individuals and society; it is, however, a limited resource available to only a few recipients.[102]

Forms of heart transplant surgery

The most common heart transplant surgery is orthotopic transplantation, with two surgical techniques used: the standard or bicaval approaches. The standard technique has been used since the 1960s and involves anastomoses of the donor and native atria.[105] Complications associated with the standard technique can include abnormal atrial contribution to ventricular filling and tricuspid and mitral valve insufficiency.[106,107] Since the mid-1990s, the bicaval technique as described by Dreyfus et al[108] has gained favour. The main advantage of the bicaval approach is the maintenance of atrial-conducting pathways and the

FIGURE 12.14 **Left**: Completion of bicaval transplant technique, showing the inferior vena caval, superior vena caval, aortic and pulmonary artery anastomoses. **Right**: Commencement of the left atrial anastomosis.

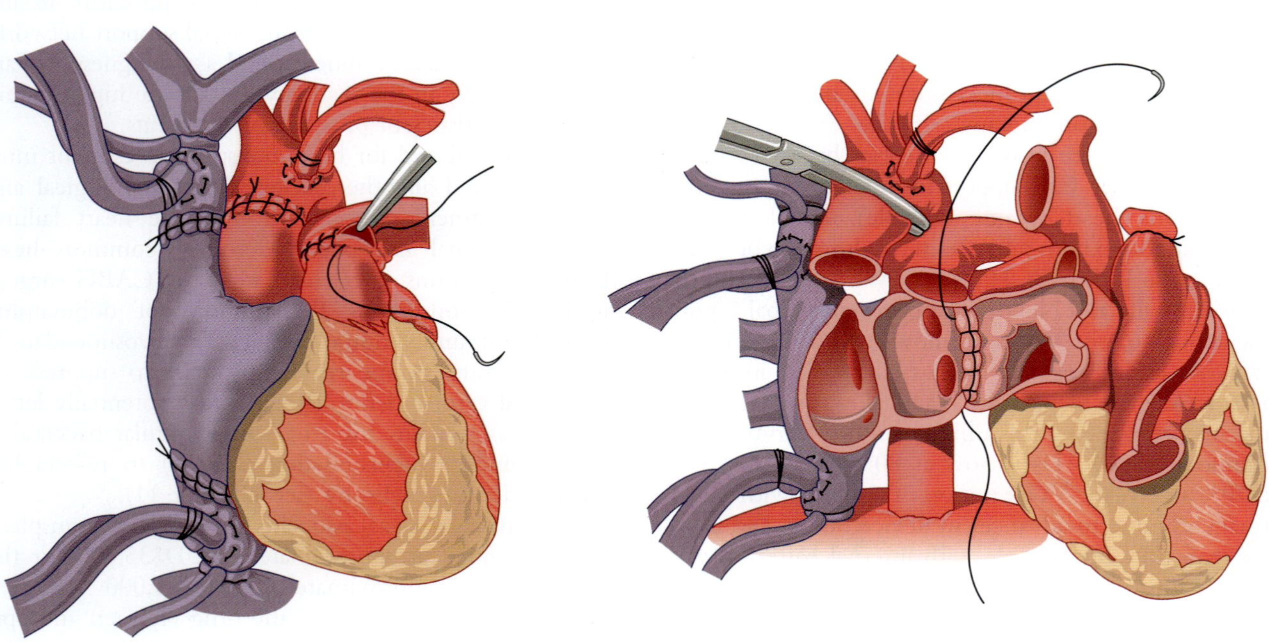

Adapted from Kirklin JK, Young JB, McGiffin DC. Heart transplantation. Philadelphia: Churchill Livingstone; 2002, with permission.

likelihood of promoting sinus rhythm and its associated superior atrial haemodynamics[108] (Fig. 12.14). Reported potential disadvantages include stenoses in the inferior and superior vena cava at the anastomosis sites.[108]

The second form of heart transplant surgery is heterotopic transplantation, although these account for only a handful of heart transplants globally. In this procedure, the donor heart is implanted in the right side of the chest next to the native heart[109] to augment native systolic function. Heterotopic heart transplantation is primarily indicated in patients with pulmonary hypertension refractory to pulmonary vasodilator therapies. It may also be considered in patients with a large body surface area who are unlikely to receive a suitably large-sized donor heart to enable an orthotopic procedure to take place,[105,110] or when the donated organ is unsuitable as an orthotopic graft.[9] Heterotopic transplantation is usually performed to support the left ventricle (LVAD configuration), but can be configured to support biventricular function (biventricular ventricular assisted device configuration). Fig. 12.15 shows a chest X-ray of the donor heart next to the native heart and the LVAD configuration for heterotopic heart transplantation is illustrated in Fig. 12.16.

Patient management

Postoperative nursing and collaborative management of orthotopic heart transplant recipients involve full haemodynamic monitoring with a pulmonary artery catheter

FIGURE 12.15 Chest X-ray showing heterotopic heart transplant.

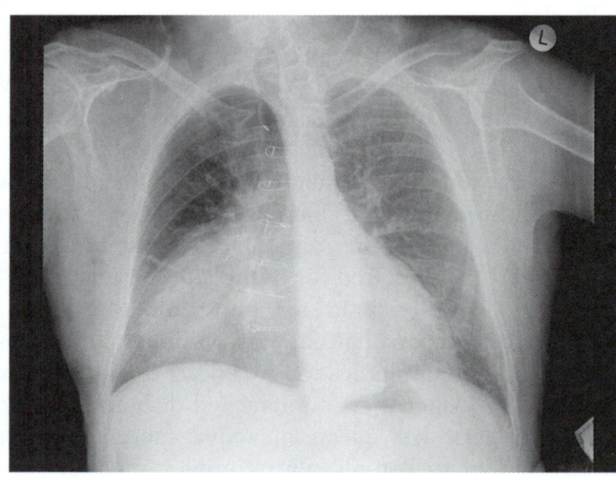

(PAC), a triple- or quad-lumen central venous catheter (CVC), arterial line, indwelling urinary catheter and 5-lead cardiac monitoring to assist in arrhythmia discrimination. A 12-lead ECG is also recorded. If the orthotopic transplant is performed with the standard technique, a remnant P wave from the native heart may be visible on the ECG or cardiac monitor (Fig. 12.17). As the native sinus node cannot conduct across the right atrial

FIGURE 12.16 Heterotopic heart transplant (LVAD configuration).

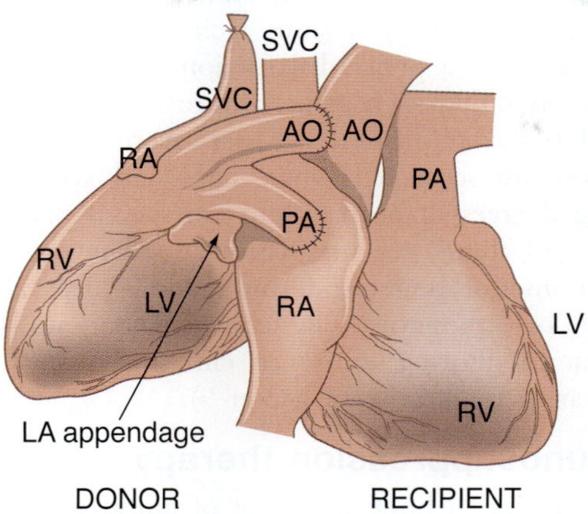

Adapted from Newcomb AE, Esmore DS, Rosenfeldt FL et al. Heterotopic heart transplantation: an expanding role in the twenty-first century? Ann Thorac Surg 2004;78(4):1345–50, with permission.

FIGURE 12.17 Rhythm strip post orthotopic transplant (standard technique).

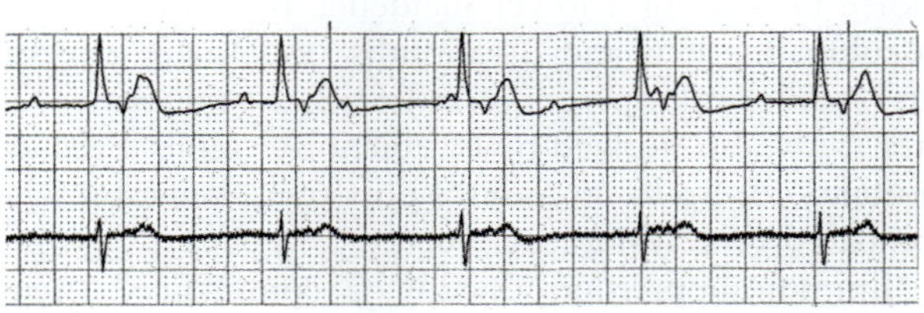

suture line, the recipient's heart rate is determined by the conduction system of the donor heart, not the native heart. Of interest, it is possible for the native heart to generate a P wave while the donor heart is in AF or other arrhythmia. (More detailed discussion of cardiac monitoring and haemodynamic management of patients with a heterotopic heart transplant is available.[111])

Monitoring data are combined with physical assessment information from all body systems to determine nursing and collaborative interventions. Intensive continuous monitoring and assessment of haemodynamic parameters according to evidence-based practices and overall clinical status allow nurses to detect and subsequently respond to emergent postoperative complications. Comprehensive guidelines for the care of heart transplant recipients, supported by the level of evidence for relevant practices, are detailed in a paper published by the ISHLT.[112] The role of nurses in cardiothoracic transplantation has evolved over the last 25 years. In order to support nurses working at the fullest extent of their education and licensure a consensus document from ISHLT provides recommendations and areas for future research.[113]

Full ventilatory support is required until the patient's haemodynamic status is stable. Respiratory status is monitored via clinical, radiological and laboratory-derived data (see Chapter 13). Enteral feeding is usually commenced on the day of admission. Renal and neurological function are closely monitored, as cyclosporin has a deleterious effect on renal function and can lead to failure as well as neurotoxicity.[114] For the small number of patients who develop allograft dysfunction requiring mechanical circulatory support (i.e. IABP, ECMO or LVAD), or acute renal failure requiring haemofiltration, hospitalisation in the critical care unit tends to last for weeks rather than for days.

The immediate period after transplantation can be a time of great hope and joy for recipients and their family and friends; however, complications and setbacks can make the path to recovery prolonged, unpredictable and difficult. The provision of psychosocial support by all members of the transplant/critical care team to family members and friends is an important part of patients' recovery from organ transplantation. Meetings with family that convey honest and open information about patient progress need to be conducted regularly. Supporting and managing patients and families following transplant is consistent with support provided to other critically ill patients (see Chapter 8). In addition, there is the issue of dealing with lost hope if the transplant fails; a very distressing time for all involved. In the immediate postoperative period, transplant recipients are at risk of developing complications that include hyperacute rejection, acute rejection, infection, haemorrhage and renal failure. In the immediate postoperative period, heart transplant recipients may experience morbidity specific to the heart transplant procedure, such as early allograft dysfunction (i.e. organ failure due to preservation injury), bleeding, right ventricular failure and acute rejection. Long-term complications include chronic renal failure, hypertension, malignancy and cardiac allograft vasculopathy. The common immediate potential complications and associated clinical management for heart recipients are discussed below.

Hyperacute rejection

Hyperacute rejection is now a rare form of humoral rejection that occurs minutes to hours after transplantation and results from ABO blood group incompatibility or the recipient having preformed, donor-specific antibodies. ABO blood group and panel reactive screening of anti-human lymphocyte antigen (anti-HLA) antibodies preoperatively minimises the possibility of hyperacute rejection, particularly in healthcare systems where blood that has been prospectively cross-matched is routinely used. If it occurs, hyperacute rejection leads to organ failure and rapid activation of the complement cascade, producing severe damage to endothelial cells, platelet activation, initiation of the clotting cascade and extensive microvascular thrombosis.[115] There is no effective treatment for hyperacute rejection apart from mechanical circulatory support or interim retransplantation.

Acute rejection

Acute rejection can be classified as either cellular or humoral.[116] Cellular rejection involves T-cell infiltration of the allograft. Cellular rejection occurs much more commonly than humoral rejection, but both may occur simultaneously.[116] Humoral or microvascular rejection is thought to be primarily mediated by antibodies. A recent review by key stakeholders has resulted in the publication of standardised nomenclature for antibody-mediated rejection.[116] Humoral rejection may occur due to the presence of a positive donor-specific cross-match or in a sensitised recipient with preformed anti-HLA antibodies. Percutaneous transvenous endomyocardial biopsy is considered the gold standard for detecting cardiac rejection. Grading of cardiac rejection has a standardised nomenclature globally.[117,118] In humoral rejection, endomyocardial biopsy reveals increased vascular permeability, microvascular thrombosis, interstitial oedema and haemorrhage, and endothelial cell swelling and necrosis.[116,119] An echocardiogram is also performed to evaluate systolic cardiac function.

Therapeutic interventions for rejection vary between centres and are based on the grade of rejection, degree of haemodynamic compromise, clinical findings and time elapsed since transplantation. Asymptomatic mild rejection (grade 1R) is rarely treated, the exception being if there is associated haemodynamic compromise; and only 20–40% of mild cases progress to moderate rejection (grade 2R), usually requiring treatment.[120] Grade 3R rejection is always treated, as it represents myocyte necrosis. Cellular rejection is usually treated with higher doses of corticosteroids, such as 'pulse' doses of methylprednisolone (1–3 g IV over 3 days), and antilymphocyte antibody agents (ATG, ATGAM or OKT3). Humoral rejection is treated with plasmapheresis, high-dose corticosteroids, cyclophosphamide therapy and antilymphocyte antibody therapy.[121] For both forms of rejection, other immunosuppressant agents such as the calcineurin inhibitor (cyclosporine, tacrolimus) and an antiproliferative cytotoxic agent (azathioprine, mycophenolate mofetil, sirolimus/rapamycin) are continued at the usual doses, assuming levels were therapeutic. It may be judicious to review the patient's medications during periods of rejection to ensure that drugs capable of reducing cyclosporin or tacrolimus serum levels, such as certain anticonvulsants and antibiotics, have not been taken. In addition to augmentation of immunosuppression therapy, fluid, pharmacological and mechanical therapeutic interventions are instituted to support cardiac function, depending on the degree of ventricular dysfunction.

Nurses have an important role in detecting acute rejection, as it is diagnosed by clinical signs and supported by histological findings from an endomyocardial biopsy. Low-grade rejection can be suspected when non-specific signs such as malaise, lethargy, low-grade fever and mood changes are present. Acute rejection causing cardiac irritation is revealed by a sinus tachycardia greater than 120 beats/min; a pericardial friction rub; or new-onset atrial arrhythmias such as premature atrial contractions, atrial flutter or fibrillation.[120] More severe forms of acute rejection are suspected when signs and symptoms of varying degrees of heart failure emerge. If patients are awake and alert, they may complain of severe fatigue, sudden onset of dyspnoea during minimal physical effort, syncope or orthopnoea. Physical assessment and haemodynamic monitoring will reveal clinical signs of left and right cardiac failure (see Chapter 9).

Immunosuppression therapy

In this section, a brief discussion of immunosuppression therapies and associated nursing implications is provided. To prevent rejection of the transplanted organ, recipients receive a triple-therapy regimen of immunosuppression agents for the remainder of their life. Triple-therapy usually consists of corticosteroids (prednisolone or prednisone), a calcineurin antagonist (cyclosporine or tacrolimus [FK506]) and an antiproliferative cytotoxic agent (mycophenolate mofetil, azathioprine or sirolimus/rapamycin).[122] For some heart patients sirolimus, also known as rapamycin, may be the cytotoxic drug of choice because of a lower incidence of cardiac allograft vasculopathy at 6 and 24 months, and lower rejection rates with sirolimus compared with azathioprine.[123] A later study also showed myco-phenolate mofetil reduced mortality for up to 36 months post-transplantation when compared to azathioprine.[123]

Immunosuppression therapy is commenced preoperatively or in the operating theatre. A maintenance immunosuppression regimen is usually instituted within hours of admission to ICU, with each patient's immunosuppressive needs individually assessed. For instance, the administration time for introduction of the selected immunosuppressive agent(s) may be delayed in patients with preexisting renal dysfunction. When the administration of the usual regimen of immunosuppression is delayed, induction therapy with antilymphocyte agents (anti-thymocyte globulin (ATG), ATGAM or OKT3) or interleukin-2 receptor antagonists (basiliximab, daclizumab) may be used in the immediate postoperative period.[95,124] Induction therapy may also be used in circumstances of primary allograft failure perioperatively, e.g. HLA mismatch (rare) or early humoral rejection, or to allow for a delay in initiating cyclosporine in patients at risk of renal failure.[124,125] A recent systematic review has found no support for the routine use of IL-2Ra therapy as routine induction therapy to achieve a survival benefit or reduction in cardiac allograft rejection.[126] The common drugs used to suppress the immune system and the nursing implications are illustrated in Table 12.5. As highlighted in Table 12.5, some immunosuppressive

TABLE 12.5
Immunosuppression medications

DRUG NAMES	TYPICAL DOSE	IMPORTANT SIDE EFFECTS	NURSING CONSIDERATIONS
Calcineurin antagonists	Maintenance		
Cyclosporin	5–10 mg/kg/day (target blood levels)	Renal impairment Hypertension Hypercholesterolaemia Abnormal liver function Headaches Gingival hypertrophy (cyclosporin only) Hirsutism (cyclosporin only) Diabetes (tacrolimus only)	Monitor renal and liver function Mix oral liquid cyclosporin with orange juice or milk in glass Do not crush tablets Time sampling of serum drug levels with dosage times
Tacrolimus	0.2–0.5 mg/kg/day (target blood levels)		
Corticosteroids	Maintenance		
Prednisolone/ prednisone	0.2–0.5 mg/kg/day Augmentation for rejection 'Pulse' of 2 g over 3 days for acute rejection	Mood change Weight gain Glucose intolerance Osteopenia Muscle weakness	Monitor blood glucose levels
Antiproliferative cytotoxic agents	Maintenance		
Azathioprine	1–2 mg/kg/day	Bone marrow suppression Gastrointestinal tract irritation (especially mycophenolate mofetil)	Cytotoxic: take full precautions when preparing, administering and disposing of drugs
Mycophenolate mofetil	2–3 g/day (adult)		
Rapamycin	Starting at 0.03 mg/kg/day (target blood levels)	Bone marrow suppression Hypercholesterolaemia Hypokalaemia	Minimise dietary cholesterol Monitor platelets and serum potassium
Interleukin-2 receptor antagonist	Induction of immunosuppression		
Basiliximab	20 mg/kg preoperatively and day 4	Few and infrequent	These drugs are often used in patients with preexisting renal dysfunction Other immunosuppression agents may be delayed with the use of these agents Little information about compatibilities: avoid concurrent administration
Daclizumab	1 mg/kg preoperatively and days 14, 28, 42, 56		
Antilymphocyte preparations	Induction or augmentation for rejection		
ATGAM/OKT3	Various, may target T lymphocyte levels	Anaphylaxis Sterile meningitis Pulmonary oedema Serum sickness	Premed of paracetamol, promethazine and hydrocortisone 30 min prior to slow infusion

Adapted from Farmer DG, McDiarmid SV, Edelstein S, et al. Induction therapy with interleukin-2 receptor antagonist after intestinal transplantation is associated with reduced acute cellular rejection and improved renal function. Transplant Proc 2004;36(2):331–2.

agents are cytotoxic (e.g. mycophenolate mofetil), requiring safety measures during preparation, delivery and disposal. Likewise, some immunosuppressive agents will be given IV (e.g. azathioprine) until patients can eat and drink as they cannot be crushed for nasogastric administration. In addition, as blood levels of some immunosuppression agents (e.g. cyclosporine, sirolimus) are taken regularly to assess efficacy, nurses need to be aware of timing blood sampling to dosage times in order to obtain accurate data to inform doses.

Infection

Infection is a major risk factor for transplant recipients due to their immunosuppressed state. The periods of greatest risk for patients are the first 3 months after transplantation, and after episodes of acute rejection when immunosuppression agents are increased.[127,128] In addition to the nosocomial bacterial infections that all surgical patients are exposed to in critical care (see Chapter 5), immunosuppressed transplant recipients are at risk of acquiring opportunistic bacterial, viral or fungal infections; latent infections acquired from the donor organ such as cytomegalovirus (CMV); or reactivation of their own latent infections (e.g. CMV or *Pneumocystis carinii*). To combat *Pneumocystis carinii*, patients receive trimethoprim with sulfamethoxazole twice weekly.[129] Despite preoperative screening for CMV, the shortage of donor organs often necessitates CMV mismatching. Effective prophylaxis for CMV infection is provided by administering CMV hyperimmune globulin to CMV-positive and CMV-negative recipients who receive a heart from a seropositive donor.[130] This commences within 24–48 hours of surgery.[124] For CMV-negative recipients of organs from seropositive donors, ganciclovir for 1–2 weeks followed by oral therapy for 3 months is required in addition to CMV hyperimmune globulin.[130,131] To prevent infection, standard precautions and meticulous handwashing (see Chapter 5) are performed, rather than isolation procedures.[132] Mandatory measures to prevent overwhelming sepsis are a high level of vigilance by clinicians for signs of infection; obtaining empirical evidence from blood, sputum, urine, wound and catheter-tip cultures; and aggressive and prompt treatment for specific organisms. Although typical signs and symptoms of infection are blunted in transplant recipients, clinicians should suspect infections when patients have a low-grade fever, hypotension, tachycardia, a high cardiac output/index, a decrease in SVR, changes in mentation, a new cough or dyspnoea.[125,133] Elevated white cell count, the presence of dysuria, purulent discharge from wounds, infiltrates on chest X-ray, sputum production or pain also indicate infection.

Prior to administering blood products, nurses must ascertain the CMV status of the patient and donor. Recipients who are seronegative for CMV and who receive a heart from a seronegative donor must receive whole blood, packed/red cells or platelets that are CMV-negative, leuco-depleted or both in order to avoid development of a primary CMV infection.[105,112,134]

Haemorrhage/cardiac tamponade

The risk of haemorrhage or cardiac tamponade is greater for heart transplant recipients than for patients undergoing CABG or valvular surgery. Preoperative anticoagulation for end-stage heart failure, insertion of LVAD for bridge to transplant or AF, impairment of hepatic function secondary to right heart failure, redo surgery, surgical suture lines connecting major vessels and atria and a larger than usual pericardium are all contributing factors. Good surgical technique is mandatory in preventing postoperative bleeding. As the promotion of haemostasis is a major therapeutic goal postoperatively, blood products, procoagulants and antifibrinolytics are commonly administered according to laboratory and clinical data. Postoperative mortality from bleeding has been reported to occur in up to 7% of cases.[133]

Early detection of haemorrhage is achieved by close monitoring of the following: haematological status; chest tube patency, drainage volume and drainage consistency; and trends in haemodynamic data that suggest cardiac tamponade (see earlier in this chapter). Our clinical experience suggests that, if patients are hypotensive sporadically for no readily apparent reason, efforts should be made to eliminate the existence of cardiac tamponade. Suspicion of cardiac tamponade may be confirmed by chest X-ray or echocardiogram if the patient's haemodynamic status is stable. Sudden cardiac arrest or haemodynamic collapse secondary to cardiac tamponade warrants an immediate return to theatre or a sternotomy in critical care.

Acute kidney injury

Acute kidney injury or varying degrees of renal dysfunction can occur in the initial postoperative period due to preexisting renal dysfunction, cyclosporin, nephrotoxic antibiotics or sustained periods of hypotension secondary to CPB or allograft dysfunction. Diuretic therapy is invariably needed in the initial postoperative period due to these factors, as well as the fluid retention effects of corticosteroids and raised filling pressures secondary to a transient loss of right and/or left ventricular compliance.[135] High doses or continuous infusions of diuretics may be required in patients who were on diuretic therapy preoperatively. Close monitoring of serum electrolyte levels will indicate the need for any supplements.

In addition to all the usual nursing and collaborative measures that are taken to prevent, detect and support renal dysfunction/failure in patients following cardiac surgery on CPB (see earlier in this chapter and Chapter 18), the type and dose of immunosuppressive agents in the postoperative period are carefully selected and initiated according to individual risk factors and clinical status. Experience suggests that early intervention with haemofiltration to support renal function is preferable to continued use of high-dose diuretics and deferred haemofiltration. This is because there is little scope to maintain low doses of renal toxic immunosuppressants for weeks given the imminent risk of rejection and resultant allograft failure.

Early allograft dysfunction and failure

Primary allograft failure is the leading cause of death in the first month and year after surgery.[136] In the immediate postoperative period, myocardial performance is depressed due to the clinical sequelae of CPB and ischaemic injury associated with surgical retrieval, hypothermic storage, prolonged ischaemic times and reperfusion. Despite a preferred time period between organ retrieval and reimplantation of 2–6 hours, the vast distances between capital cities (up to 3000 km) over which donor hearts may be transported, and a decision to accept marginal, sub-optimal organs, led Australian researchers and transplant teams to pioneer prolonged ischaemic times of up to 8 hours (New Zealand, 7 hours).

Heart transplants that encompass long distances with ischaemic periods beyond 6 hours have been, and are likely to continue to be, performed in Australia and New Zealand and other countries, as excellent short-term (30-day mortality) and long-term (ejection fraction at 1 year) outcomes have been reported. These outcomes were achieved by using innovative preservation techniques and postoperative mechanical assistance in the form of intra-aortic balloon counterpulsation and/or a right VAD.[137] Adrenaline is invariably commenced intraoperatively, irrespective of ischaemic time, to provide inotropic support to the transplanted heart.

To address these challenges at donor procurement, which have been limited by the current cold storage and heart preservation method, the TransMedics OCS has been developed. The portable, warm perfusion and monitoring system is designed to increase transplant volumes, improve patient outcomes and reduce transplant costs. Refer to OCS IFU. Also emerging, using this method, is the utilisation of hearts from DCD donors.[138]

Early allograft dysfunction can present as left, right or biventricular dysfunction. Management of cardiac dysfunction is dependent on clinical signs and underlying aetiologies that include pulmonary hypertension, acute rejection and ischaemic injury. Right ventricular dysfunction is usually secondary to pulmonary hypertension, whereas left ventricular or biventricular dysfunction results from acute rejection and ischaemic injury.

To prevent right ventricular dysfunction and failure secondary to raised pulmonary pressures, prospective heart transplant recipients are screened preoperatively for the degree and reversibility of pulmonary hypertension. Reversible pulmonary hypertension is a transpulmonary gradient less than 15 mmHg that responds to pulmonary vasodilator therapies, such as prostaglandin E1, prostacyclin or inhaled NO.[139] Right ventricular dysfunction or failure can also occur in the postoperative context due to ischaemic injury, an undersized heart (greater than 20% difference in body surface area between donor and recipient) or hypoxic pulmonary vasoconstriction.[105] Isoprenaline or milrinone, dobutamine and adrenaline are administered in this situation.[112]

Left ventricular dysfunction cannot be anticipated preoperatively, so when signs first emerge peri- or postoperatively, fluid management strategies (filling or diuresis as deemed appropriate) and inotropic agents are commenced immediately.[112] In patients with prolonged ischaemic times, mechanical assistance in the form of an IABP is invariably instituted perioperatively.

In the initial postoperative period, cardiac dysfunction can also occur as a result of a low SVR syndrome, characterised by a calculated SVR of less than 750 dynes/sec/cm^{-5} in the presence of an unsustainable high cardiac output.[92,140] The cause of low SVR syndrome is not fully understood, although it has been linked with SIRS associated with CPB (see Chapter 21), the chronic use of angiotensin-converting enzyme inhibitors for end-stage heart failure (see Chapter 10) and a deficiency of vasopressin.[140,141] Noradrenaline is titrated to achieve a calculated SVR within normal parameters and to lower the unsustainably high cardiac index. In severe cases, vasopressin may be infused at doses of 0.04–0.1 units/min concurrently with noradrenaline.[142] Experience suggests that the dose of adrenaline should be minimised in the presence of metabolic acidosis, and the noradrenaline infusion increased to achieve normotension, a calculated SVR higher than 900 dynes/sec/cm^{-5} and a sustainable cardiac index.

Patients with depressed left ventricular compliance and contractility due to cardiac dysfunction present clinically with reduced cardiac index, bradycardia, reduced tissue and end-organ perfusion (decreased mental status, oliguria, poor peripheral perfusion, slow capillary refill and raised serum lactate), low systemic venous oxygenation and dyspnoea. Bradycardia may not be evident due to chronotropic support of the denervated heart with atrial pacing and/or isoprenaline. The following discussion focuses on management of right heart dysfunction/failure and left heart dysfunction/failure (see also Chapter 10).

Right heart dysfunction/failure is suspected in patients with preexisting pulmonary hypertension or a haemodynamic profile in the intra- or postoperative context that includes a rising CVP, low-to-normal pulmonary artery diastolic/pulmonary artery wedge pressure (PAWP), high calculated pulmonary vascular resistance, raised PAPs, systemic hypotension and oliguria. The haemodynamic management of patients with right ventricular dysfunction/failure involves optimising right ventricular preload and afterload by titrating fluid and pharmacological therapies to achieve adequate tissue and end-organ perfusion. Fluid resuscitation to a CVP between 14 and 20 mmHg and inotropic therapy are necessary to ensure that the failing right ventricle continues to act as a conduit for the left ventricle. Nitric oxide by inhalation is the therapy of choice, as it provides selective pulmonary vasodilation at doses of 20–40 ppm, thereby reducing right ventricular afterload without producing systemic hypotension.[139] A secondary benefit of inhaled NO is improved oxygenation due to reduced mismatching of ventilation/perfusion.[143] If inhaled NO is not available, IV prostaglandin E1 or prostacyclin may be used to reduce right ventricular afterload when pulmonary pressures exceed 50 mmHg.[144]

Mild right ventricular dysfunction may be treated with milrinone at doses of 0.375–0.750 mcg/kg/min or drug combinations that provide afterload reduction and inotropic support (e.g. sodium nitroprusside and adrenaline). Appropriate respiratory management is essential, as hypoxaemia and metabolic or respiratory acidosis can exacerbate right ventricular failure. If pharmacological, fluid and inhaled NO therapies do not produce sustained improvement in right ventricular performance, a right VAD (e.g. Biomedicus or CentriMag® centrifugal pump) is indicated to provide temporary support for the failing right ventricle.

The immediate haemodynamic management of left ventricular dysfunction/failure secondary to acute rejection or ischaemic injury often involves fluid resuscitation to a pulmonary artery diastolic of 16–20 mmHg, high-dose inotropes, vasodilator agents and insertion of an IABP to achieve a cardiac index greater than 2.2 L/min/m^2 and adequate end-organ perfusion. The insertion of an LVAD (e.g. Biomedicus or CentriMag centrifugal pump) or full mechanical circulatory support with extracorporeal membrane oxygenation (ECMO) is indicated when aggressive therapeutic regimens fail to produce a cardiac output that provides adequate end-organ perfusion.[112,145,146] As noted earlier, augmentation of the immunosuppression regimen may also be necessary to manage the acute rejection.

Denervation

Donor heart implantation severs both afferent and efferent nervous system connections to the heart. Hence, the transplanted heart has no direct autonomic nervous system innervation but is responsive to circulating catecholamines. Denervation impairs circulatory system homeostasis, as evidenced by: a volume-expanded state; a tendency to hypertension; no sensation of angina pectoris; a high resting heart rate; a slow or absent baroreceptor reflex (to increase heart rate/cardiac output in response to hypotension); and no rises in heart rate and contractility due to hypovolaemia or vasodilation.[105] As the cardiac allograft is dependent on an adequate preload, the effects of postural changes in recipients are important. (A detailed discussion of physiology of the transplanted heart is provided elsewhere.[105])

There are four important clinical manifestations of denervation in the early postoperative period. First, drugs that act directly on the autonomic nervous system to modify heart rate (e.g. atropine, digoxin) and vagal manoeuvres (carotid sinus massage) are ineffective. Amiodarone and adenosine are effective antiarrhythmic agents. Neither amiodarone nor sotalol interact with immunosuppressive agents.[112] However, as the denervated donor sinus node is more sensitive to exogenous adenosine than a sinus node innervated in the normal way,[147] it has been suggested that adenosine be avoided.[105] That is, a usual adenosine dose may produce toxic-like effects in the context of a denervated heart. Overdrive atrial pacing is a viable alternative to drug therapy to treat a tachyarrhythmia such as atrial flutter.[148]

Second, although a high resting heart rate is possible from efferent cardiac denervation, sinus or junctional bradycardias may occur in the early postoperative period due to transient sinus node dysfunction or preoperative amiodarone. Studies suggest that sinus node dysfunction occurs in about 20% of cases,[149] although anecdotal experience suggests a higher percentage. To prevent low cardiac output secondary to bradycardias, atrial and ventricular epicardial pacing wires are inserted and atrial pacing of >90 beats/min,[112] and often at 110 beats/min, is commenced. Atrial pacing at 110 beats/min appears to 'train' the sinus node to conduct at rates of 70–100 beats/min in the long term. A resting sinus or junctional heart rate below 70 beats/min prior to hospital discharge is predictive of long-term sinus node dysfunction.[105] Insertion of a permanent pacemaker for long-term heart rate control is rarely required. Isoprenaline infusions at doses of 0.5–2 mcg/min may be used for chronotropy in combination with atrial pacing. As noted earlier, atrial arrhythmias such as atrial flutter may be an early indication of acute rejection. Ventricular arrhythmias are rare and often lethal in spite of aggressive resuscitation attempts. Persistent arrhythmias should always prompt investigation of the patient's rejection level.[112]

Third, as patients rely on circulating catecholamines, orthostatic hypotension is common. Patients are educated to sit up slowly from a lying position. Fourth, patients rarely feel anginal pain after surgery; however, there are some reports of patients regaining feelings of angina pectoris.[150] The inability of patients to feel angina pectoris is important, because all heart transplant recipients are at risk of developing accelerated allograft coronary artery disease.[151] As part of discharge education, patients are taught to identify clinical signs of angina other than chest pain, such as shortness of breath and sweating. A summary of the main clinical manifestations and nursing practice issues for patients following heart transplantation is included in Table 12.6.

Practice tip

Heart transplant patients have a denervated heart, so carotid sinus massage will not slow a tachyarrhythmia and atropine will not increase sinus node firing or atrioventricular conduction.

TABLE 12.6
Nursing care of patients after heart transplantation

CLINICAL MANIFESTATION	NURSING PRACTICE CONSIDERATIONS
Acute rejection	Detect acute rejection by clinical signs and endomyocardial biopsy Suspect low-grade rejection when malaise, lethargy, low-grade fever and mood changes are present Acute rejection is manifested by a sinus tachycardia >120 beats/min, a pericardial friction rub or new-onset atrial arrhythmias Suspect severe acute rejection with manifestations of left and right heart failure; awake patients may complain of severe fatigue, sudden onset of dyspnoea during minimal physical effort, syncope or orthopnoea
Infection	Standard infection control precautions and meticulous handwashing is required Observe for signs of infection: low-grade fever, hypotension, tachycardia, a high cardiac output/index, a decrease in SVR, changes in mentation, a new cough, dyspnoea, dysuria, sputum production or pain Monitor blood, sputum, urine, wound and catheter-tip cultures, infiltrates on chest X-ray and institute aggressive and prompt treatment for specific infective organisms Check CMV status before administering blood products
Haemorrhage/ cardiac tamponade	Monitor: haematological status; chest tube patency, drainage volume and drainage consistency; and trends in haemodynamic data that suggest cardiac tamponade Patients who are hypotensive sporadically should be assessed to eliminate cardiac tamponade as a cause
Acute renal failure	Support renal function, including titration of immunosuppressive agents to individual risk factors and clinical status, and early haemofiltration
Early allograft dysfunction	Augment the immunosuppression regimen to manage the acute rejection
Left heart failure	Observe for depressed left ventricular compliance and contractility: reduced cardiac index, possible bradycardia (may not be evident due to atrial pacing and/or isoprenaline), decreased mental status, oliguria, poor peripheral perfusion, slow capillary refill and raised serum lactate, low systemic venous oxygenation and dyspnoea Fluid resuscitate to a PAWP of 14–18 mmHg, high-dose inotropes, vasodilator agents, IABP to achieve a cardiac index >2.2 $L/min/m^2$ with adequate end-organ perfusion Insertion of full mechanical circulatory support (ECMO or LVAD) is indicated when other interventions do not provide adequate end-organ perfusion
Right heart failure	Observe for right heart dysfunction/failure: rising CVP, low-to-normal PAD/PAWP, high calculated pulmonary vascular resistance, raised PAPs, systemic hypotension and oliguria Optimise right ventricular preload and afterload: titrate fluid and medications to achieve adequate end-organ perfusion; fluid resuscitate to a CVP of 14–20 mmHg; consider inhaled NO (selective pulmonary vasodilation and improved oxygenation from reduced ventilation/perfusion mismatch), prostaglandin E1 or prostacyclin, milrinone or drug combinations with afterload reduction and inotropic support (e.g. sodium nitroprusside and adrenaline) Institute appropriate respiratory management to minimise hypoxaemia and metabolic or respiratory acidosis If no sustained improvement in right ventricular performance, a right VAD is indicated for temporary support
Denervation	Drugs with direct autonomic nervous system actions on heart rate (e.g. atropine, digoxin) and vagal manoeuvres (carotid sinus massage) are ineffective Use overdrive atrial pacing to treat tachyarrhythmias Sinus or junctional bradycardias may occur, and atrial/ventricular epicardial pacing is used to 'train' the sinus node Orthostatic hypotension is common: patients should sit up slowly from a lying position Patients rarely feel anginal pain after surgery: they need to identify other clinical signs of angina, such as shortness of breath and sweating

CMV = cytomegalovirus; CVP = central venous pressure; ECMO = extracorporeal membrane oxygenation; IABP = intra-aortic balloon pump; LVAD = left ventricular assist device; PAD = pulmonary artery diastolic; PAP = pulmonary artery pressure; PAWP = pulmonary artery wedge pressure; SVR = systemic vascular resistance.

Medium- to long-term complications

There are four long-term complications associated with heart transplantation: 1) cardiac allograft vasculopathy; 2) malignancy; 3) renal dysfunction; and 4) hypertension.[152] Cardiac allograft vasculopathy (CAV) is a diffuse, proliferative form of obliterative coronary arteriosclerosis that has experienced minimal reduction in the last 2 decades, from 32% to 29% and 46% to 40% at 5- a5- and 8-years post-transplant respectively. Notably, CAV is a leading cause of long-term mortality, accounting for up to 1 in 8 deaths beyond a year post-transplant.[153,154] Sudden death, ventricular arrhythmias and symptoms of congestive heart failure may be the first signs of significant CAV. The aetiology of CAV is multifactorial, including immunological factors (e.g. episodes of acute rejection and anti-HLA antibodies), non-immunological cardiovascular risk factors (e.g. hypertension, hyperlipidaemia, preexisting diabetes and new-onset diabetes), the surgical procedure (e.g. donor age, ischaemic time and reperfusion injury) and side effects of immunosuppression drugs such as cyclosporin and corticosteroids (e.g. CMV infection and nephrotoxicity).[112,153,154] Statins at doses less than that prescribed for hyperlipidaemia are commenced within 2 weeks of surgery irrespective of cholesterol levels to reduce episodes of rejection and CAV.[112] Standard use of cyclosporine may be augmented by mycophenolate mofetil, everolimus or sirolimus as they have been shown to reduce the onset and progression of CAV.[112] Diagnosis of CAV is difficult, due to allograft denervation, and because coronary angiogram underestimates the extent of the disease and is insensitive to early lesions.[155] Currently, intravascular ultrasound provides the most reliable quantitative information about the degree of CAV.[155] As the definitive treatment for CAV is retransplantation, ongoing research into the prevention of CAV[156] will be the most important factor in reducing the incidence and associated mortality.

All heart transplant recipients are at a greater risk of developing malignancies than the general population,[157] particularly carcinoma of the skin[157–160] and lymphoproliferative disorders,[161,162] as a consequence of long-term immunosuppression therapy.[163,164] Nurses play an important role in educating patients about how to avoid and reduce the risks of sun exposure. Treatment options in transplant recipients are the same as for the general population (e.g. chemotherapy, radiation therapy and surgical excision), in addition to a reduction in immunosuppression therapy; however, outcomes remain poor.[160]

Long-term renal dysfunction occurs primarily post-transplantation due to cyclosporin nephrotoxicity. Careful monitoring of cyclosporin levels and avoidance of hypovolaemia and other nephrotoxic drugs are important measures in reducing progression to renal failure. Importantly, findings from recent research indicate that chronic cyclosporin nephrotoxicity can be reversed by eliminating cyclosporin from immunosuppression regimens.[114] End-stage renal failure requiring dialysis or renal transplantation has been shown to be a good therapeutic option after prolonged exposure to calcineurin inhibitors (CNI) immunosuppressive medication.[165]

Systemic hypertension following transplantation has been linked with cyclosporin-induced tubular nephrotoxicity, peripheral vasoconstriction and fluid retention.[166] Lifestyle modifications such as weight loss, low sodium diet, control of diabetes and hyperlipidaemia as well as an exercise program are recommended along with optimal therapeutic doses of cyclosporin, and combinations of calcium channel blockers and angiotensin-converting enzyme inhibitors and blockers.[112] Such approaches have been reported to achieve blood pressure control in this cohort.[167]

Lifestyle issues

Following such momentous surgery, patients require sound advice regarding returning to driving, work, exercise and sexual activity. Cardiac rehabilitation with aerobic and resistance exercise is recommended to prevent short-term weight gain and glucose intolerance, as well as adverse effects of immunosuppressive therapy on skeletal muscle.[112] Return to work or education is expected and encouraged after surgery. Driving a vehicle can be considered once the patient's gait, tremor and other neurological issues are normalised, and any bradycardia managed by pacemaker implantation.[112] Pregnancy is possible after 1 year following transplantation; but only under the management of the multidisciplinary team who will explain the considerable risks involved.[112]

Summary

Primary compromise of the cardiovascular system causes patients to require admission to a critical care area and the need for specialised care including IABP and post-cardiac surgery management. Appropriate assessment and management are essential to prevent secondary complications arising. Important principles of care are summarised below.

Surgical procedures may be performed as treatment for structural abnormalities, ischaemic lesions within coronary arteries and repair or replacement of cardiac valves. Haemodynamic stability constitutes the most common challenge in the postoperative period and may be managed with fluids, cardiovascular medications, cardiac pacing and IABP. Bleeding in the postoperative period may be due to inadequate reversal or heparin, coagulopathy or surgical bleeding; therefore, appropriate diagnosis must occur before relevant treatment is instigated.

IABP is one therapy that is used to provide support in the period after cardiac surgery. Major benefits of IABP include increasing cardiac output, increasing myocardial oxygen supply and decreasing myocardial oxygen demand. Appropriate timing is essential to obtain maximum benefits, so correction of timing errors forms a central component of care. In addition, assessment of limb perfusion, with timely intervention when perfusion is inadequate, is essential to prevent limb ischaemia.

Cardiac transplantation is the gold standard of care used to provide support to the failing heart. As Cardiac Transplant centres face significant challenges with donor numbers remaining static, the increasing use of the warm perfusion method for organ retrieval has the potential to increase transplant numbers using marginal and DCD donors without relying on an increase in donor rates. Indications for heart transplantation include end-stage heart failure secondary to ischaemic heart disease and cardiomyopathy. Possible complications in the early postoperative period include acute rejection, infection, haemorrhage, renal failure, right ventricular failure and allograft dysfunction (left ventricular dysfunction/failure). A triple-therapy regimen consisting of corticosteroids, a calcineurin antagonist and an antiproliferative cytotoxic agent is used to suppress the immune system after organ transplantation. All cytotoxic agents necessitate specific administration and disposal procedures. Although early signs of low-grade rejection can be non-specific, signs of moderate rejection usually present as organ dysfunction/failure. Nursing practices for managing patients with heart transplantation focus on prevention and management of complications, maintenance of comfort and promotion of long-term recovery.

Case study

Mr Jacob is a 52-year-old patient admitted for elective aortic valve replacement due to valve stenosis (bicuspid valve). His past history includes AF, high cholesterol, and he is obese with a BMI of 34. His coronary angiography showed normal coronary arteries. Preoperative transthoracic echocardiography report revealed severe aortic valve stenosis, other valves were normal and grade II left ventricle with moderate hypertrophy but preserved systolic function.

Surgery was reported as uncomplicated. A tissue valve was used to replace the valve and CPB was used for 75 min and aortic cross-clamp time was 50 min. Continuous infusion of noradrenaline at 2 mcg/min were in progress. Patient was paced in VVI mode of 86 beats/min (due to his chronic AF), with output of 10 mA and sensitivity of 8 mV (decreased sensitivity due to oversensing issue during the case).

On admission to the ICU the patient was intubated and ventilated. He had a right radial arterial line and a right internal jugular PAC in situ. One mediastinal and one pericardial drain tube had been placed and had drained 50 mL of blood to the time of admission. A urinary catheter was also present.

Soon after the transport team had left, the ICU team including two nurses and one medical officer started to settle the patient by connecting the monitoring from transport monitor to ICU monitor, attaching chest tube to suction, adjusting the ICU ventilator and connecting the patient. Suddenly the transport monitor red alarm was activated with messages 'R-on-T' and 'ventricular tachycardia', a quick assessment of arterial waveform showed a flat line and rhythm was VT with few inappropriate pacing spikes. One nurse positioned the bed flat while looking at the pacing box, with the other nurse turning on the defibrillator and connected the pads on the patient anterior chest and charging it to 200 joules. The first defibrillation was delivered within 20 seconds of rhythm change (fortunately the transport defibrillator was still on the bed), but the patient remained in VT post shock. Immediately a second shock was delivered (same energy level) and the patient returned to pacing rhythm, rate of 86. The pacing sensitivity was adjusted to most sensitive (0.8 mV) and no further sensitivity issues (over or under sensing) were noticed. The medical officer contacted the surgical team during the events, they attended the patient immediately and at the same time theatre was put on standby just in case of return to theatre. The ICU and surgical teams reviewed the patient post-VT arrest, the cause of the arrest was narrowed down to most likely a 'R-on-T' phenomena as echocardiography ruled out bleeding, tamponade, LV dysfunction or valve issues. An arterial blood gas analysis revealed acceptable haemoglobin, electrolytes level and acid base status and a complete set of blood tests were sent to pathology. A chest X-ray confirmed ETT, PAC and chest tube placement. Left lower lobe collapse was noted (PEEP increased to 10 cmH_2O).

During the arrest, cardiac compression was not initiated as per Australian and New Zealand committee on resuscitation (ANZCOR) Guidelines 11.10: resuscitation in special circumstances: cardiac surgery.

The Guideline recommends using three stack shocks in case of a shockable rhythm arrest to minimise the potential and significant harm of external chest compression (disruption of grafts or valves) anytime in the immediate period of post-cardiac surgery (as long as the first shock is delivered within the first 20 seconds of the arrest). It is recommended for all units (ICU and cardiac) to have defibrillators accessible in the immediate vicinity of patients post-cardiac surgery.

Mr Jacob was continued on sedation for another 4 h, after that weaning started and he was extubated 8 h post-ICU admission without any neurological deficit. His intrinsic heart rate increased and maintained haemodynamic stability, pacing was turned off but still connected.

CASE STUDY QUESTIONS

1. Discuss the steps taken for the management of Mr Jacob's deterioration if the rhythm was not shockable (asystole, or bradycardia) as per ANZCOR Guidelines?
2. List the causes of cardiac arrest in the first 24 h period associated with open cardiac surgery.

RESEARCH VIGNETTE

Sigurdsson MI, Longford NT, Heydarpour M et al. Duration of postoperative atrial fibrillation after cardiac surgery is associated with worsened long-term survival. Ann Thorac Surg 2016;102(6): 2018-2026

Abstract

Background: Studies of the effects of postoperative atrial fibrillation (poAF) on long-term survival are conflicting, likely because of comorbidities that occur with poAF and the patient populations studied. Furthermore, the effects of poAF duration on long-term survival are poorly understood.

Methods: We utilized a prospectively collected database on outcomes of cardiac surgery at a large tertiary care institution between August 2001 and December 2010 with survival follow-up through June 2015 to analyze long-term survival of patients with poAF. In addition, we identified patient- and procedure-related variables associated with poAF, and estimated overall comorbidity burden using the Elixhauser comorbidity index. Survival was compared between patients with poAF (n = 513) and a propensity score matched control cohort, both for all patients and separately for subgroups of patients with poAF lasting less than 2 days (n = 218) and patients with prolonged poAF (n = 265).

Results: Patients with poAF were older and had a higher burden of comorbidities. Survival was significantly worse for patients with poAF than for the matched control group (hazard ratio 1.43, 95% confidence interval: 1.11 to 1.86). That was driven by decreased survival among patients with prolonged poAF (hazard ratio 1.97, 95% confidence interval: 1.37 to 2.80), whereas survival of patients with poAF for less than 2 days was not significantly different from that of matched controls (hazard ratio 0.91, 95% confidence interval: 0.60 to 1.39).

Conclusions: After close matching based on comorbidity burden, prolonged poAF is still associated with decreased survival. Therefore, vigilance is warranted in monitoring and treating patients with prolonged poAF after cardiac surgery.

Critique

The high prevalence of AF post cardiac surgery has been studied extensively and has been associated with increased mortality, readmission and treatment related complications such as embolic events and bleeding. This single centre prospective control study was conducted with a large sample size of 513 (30% of the 1712 patients who were screened to have adequate information for the study) postoperative patients with AF, that were propensity score matched with a control group over a period of 10 years. The participants were followed for a median of 8.5 years (range 5.9–10.9). The study concluded that the survival was worse in patients with prolonged (more than 2 days) postoperative AF (Klein test, $P < 0.001$, HR 1.97, 95% CI: 1.37–2.80) compared to control group. In addition, patients who were discharged from hospital and still in AF (n=53) had significantly worse survival than their propensity score matched control group. The length of intensive care unit stay (4 versus 2 days, $P < 0.001$) and hospital stay (12 versus 7 days, $P < 0.001$) were longer in patients with prolonged AF compared with patients with less than 2 days' AF. The study had strength in the design, definitions of study outcomes, use of propensity score matching and Elixhauser comorbidities index and that increased the validity of the results. The other strengths of this study were the number of patients enrolled into the study and the duration of follow-up that show the long-lasting adverse effects of postoperative AF. However, the major limitation of the study was use of a single centre database to collect data, reducing its generalizability.

This article gives us an insight into the survival of patients experiencing AF post cardiac surgery in addition to all other known complications associated with AF. The importance of managing AF postoperatively effectively will benefit patients in the long run.

Learning activities

1. Compare and contrast the automated and semi-automated modes of intra-aortic balloon counterpulsation.
2. Discuss with a senior colleague the main complications of IABP therapy and what strategies should be included in your care of a patient receiving IABP therapy to minimise the likelihood or impact of these complications.
3. Discuss how you would identify an intra-aortic balloon catheter rupture and immediate management.
4. Outline the principles of caring for a postoperative cardiac surgical patient during the first 4 hours of ICU admission. Provide a rationale for why these aspects of care are a priority?
5. Discuss the options available in your unit if a patient fails extubation post-cardiac surgery.
6. What haemodynamic values could assist you in deciding the choice of inotropes and vasopressors? Provide rationales.
7. Discuss the management of a patient with cardiac arrest due to pericardial tamponade post-minimally invasive cardiac surgery.

Online resources

American Heart Association, http://www.heart.org/HEARTORG

Asian Pacific Society of Cardiology, http://www.apscardio.org

Australian and New Zealand Intensive Care Society (ANZICS), www.anzics.com.au

Australian Institute of Health and Welfare, www.aihw.gov.au

Australian Organ Donor Register (AODR), www.medicareaustralia.gov.au/public/services/aodr/index.jsp

Cardiac Society of Australia and New Zealand, www.csanz.edu.au

Donate Life, www.donatelife.gov.au

National Heart Foundation of Australia, www.heartfoundation.org.au

National Heart Foundation of New Zealand, www.heartfoundation.org.nz

National Health Priorities and Quality, www.health.gov.au/internet/wcms/publishing.nsf/content/pq-cardio

The International Society for Heart and Lung Transplantation (ISHLT), www.ishlt.org

Transplant Nurses' Association (TNA), www.tna.asn.au

Transplantation Society of Australia and New Zealand (TSANZ), www.tsanz.com.au

European Society of cardiology www.escardio.org

European Heart Association, www.heartassociation.eu

Further reading

Coleman B, Blumenthal N, Currey J, et al. Adult cardiothoracic transplant nursing: an ISHLT consensus document on the current adult nursing practice in heart and lung transplantation. J Heart Lung Transplant 2015;34:139–48.

Kirklin JK, Pagani FD, Kormos RL, et al. Eighth annual INTERMACS report: special focus on faming the impact of adverse events. JHLT 2017;36(10):1080–6.

Laing C. LVAD: left ventricular assist devices for end-stage heart failure. Nurse Pract 2014;39:42–7.

Pellegrino V, Hockings LE, Davies A. Veno-arterial extracorporeal membrane oxygenation for adult cardiovascular failure. Curr Opin Crit Care 2014;20:484–92.

Zimpfer D, Netuka I, Schmitto JD, et al. Multicentre clinical trial experience with the HeartMate 3 left ventricular device: 30-day outcomes. Eur J Cardiothoroacic Surg 2016;50:548–54.

References

1. World Heart Federation. RHD Global Status Report 2015–17. World Heart Federation, 2016.
2. Wilkins E, Wilson L, Wickramasinghe K, et al. European cardiovascular disease statistics 2017. Brussels: European Heart Network; 2017.
3. Australian Institute of Health and Welfare (AIHW). Australia's health 2016. Australia's health series no. 15. AIHW, ed. Canberra: AIHW; 2016.
4. Australian Institute of Health and Welfare (AIHW). Cardiovascular disease: Australian facts 2011. Canberra: AIHW; 2011.
5. Australian Institute of Health and Welfare (AIHW). Rheumatic heart disease and acute rheumatic fever in Australia: 1996-2012. Canberra: AIHW; 2013.
6. Urden L, Stacy K, Lough M. Critical care nursing: diagnosis and management. 8th ed. St Louis: Mosby; 2018.
7. Gaudino M, Burzotta F, Bakaeen F, et al. The radial artery for percutaneous coronary procedures or surgery? J Am Coll Cardiol 2018;71(10):1167–75.
8. Di Santo P, Harnett DT, Simard T, et al. Photoplethysmography using a smartphone application for assessment of ulnar artery patency: a randomized clinical trial. CMAJ 2018;190(13):E380–8.
9. Doenst T, Diab M, Sponholz C, et al. The opportunities and limitations of minimally invasive cardiac surgery. Dtsch Arztebl Int 2017;114(46):777–84.
10. Kikuchi K, Mori M. Minimally invasive coronary artery bypass grafting: a systematic review. Asian Cardiovasc Thorac Ann 2017;25(5):364–70.
11. Taggart DP, Altman DG, Gray AM, et al. Effects of on-pump and off-pump surgery in the Arterial Revascularization Trial. Eur J Cardiothorac Surg 2015;47(6):1059–65.
12. Pettinari M, Navarro E, Noirhomme P, et al. The state of robotic cardiac surgery in Europe. Ann Cardiothorac Surg 2017;6(1):1–8.
13. İyigün T, Kaya M, Gülbeyaz SÖ, et al. Patient body image, self-esteem, and cosmetic results of minimally invasive robotic cardiac surgery. Int J Surg 2017;39:88–94.
14. Bush B, Nifong LW, Alwair H, et al. Robotic mitral valve surgery – current status and future directions. Ann Cardiothorac Surg 2013;2(6):814–17.
15. The Task Force on Myocardial Revascularization of the European Society of Cardiology (ESC) and the European Association for Cardio-Thoracic Surgery (EACTS). Guidelines on myocardial revascularization. Eur Heart J 2010;31:2501–55.
16. Curiel-Balsera E, et al. Mortality and complications in elderly patients undergoing cardiac surgery. J Crit Care 2013;28:397–404.
17. Chieffo A, Buchanan GL, Van Meighem NM, et al. Transcatheter aortic valve implantation with the Edwards SAPIEN versus the Medtronic CoreValve Revalving system devices: a multicenter collaborative study: the PRAGMATIC Plus Initiative (Pooled-RotterdAm-Milano-Toulouse in Collaboration). J Am Coll Cardiol 2013;61(8):830–6.
18. Popma JJ, Adams DH, Reardon MJ, et al. Transcatheter aortic valve replacement using a self-expanding bioprosthesis in patients with severe aortic stenosis at extreme risk for surgery. J Am Coll Cardiol 2014;63(19):1972–81.
19. Marshall L, Griffin R, Mundy J. Frailty assessment to predict short term outcomes after cardiac surgery. Asian Cardiovasc Thorac Ann 2016;24(6):546–54.
20. Belov A, Katkov K, Vinokuroz IA, et al. Cardiopulmonary bypass duration as predictor of immediate results after cardiac surgery. Khirurgiia 2015;5:4–13.
21. Wang G, Xiao S, Gao C. The effects of cardiopulmonary bypass on pulmonary function during robotic cardiac surgery. Perfusion 2015;30(3):213–18.
22. Hashim S, Chin LY, Krishnasamy S, et al. Effect of sternal closure with biological bone adhesive on pain visual analogue score and serum cytokine. J Cardiothorac Surg 2015;10(1):32.
23. Fuchigama T, Nishioka M, Akashige T, et al. Staged delayed sternal closure using a binder clip after pediatric cardiac surgery. J Card Surg 2016;31(7):464–6.
24. Motomatsu Y, Imasaka K, Tayama E, et al. Midterm results of sternal band closure in open heart surgery and risk analysis of sternal band removal. Artif Organs 2016;40(2):153–8.

25. Currey J, Browne J, Botti M. Haemodynamic instability after cardiac surgery: nurses' perceptions of clinical decision-making. J Clin Nurs 2006;15(9):1081–90.
26. St Andre AC, DelRossi A. Hemodynamic management of patients in the first 24 hours after cardiac surgery. Crit Care Med 2005;33(9):2082–93.
27. Inaiane Marlisse de Carvalho IM, et al. Systematization of nursing care in mediate post-operative of cardiac surgery. Revista de Pesquisa: Cuidado e Fundamental 2016;8(4):5062–7.
28. Broch O, Bein B, Grunewald M, et al. Accuracy of cardiac output by nine different pulse contour algorithms in cardiac surgery patients: a comparison with transpulmonary thermodilution. Biomed Res Int 2016;Article ID 3468015.
29. Epting CL, McBride ME, Wald EL, et al. Pathophysiology of post-operative low cardiac output syndrome. Curr Vasc Pharmacol 2016;14(1):14–23.
30. Currey J, Botti M. The haemodynamic status of cardiac surgical patients in the initial 2-h recovery period. Eur J Cardiovasc Nurs 2005;4(3):207–14.
31. Martin CG, Turkelson SL. Nursing care of the patient undergoing coronary artery bypass grafting. J Cardiovasc Nurs 2006;21(2):109–17.
32. Demirci C, Zeman F, Schmid C, et al. Early postoperative blood pressure and blood loss after cardiac surgery: a retrospective analysis. Intensive Crit Care Nurs 2017;42:122–6.
33. Balzer F, Aronson S, Campagna JA, et al. High postoperative blood pressure after cardiac surgery is associated with acute kidney injury and death. J Cardiothorac Vasc Anesth 2016;30(6):1562–70.
34. Soto-Ruiz KM, Peacock WF, Varon J. Perioperative hypertension: diagnosis and treatment. Neth J Crit Care 2011;15(3):143–8.
35. Sponholz C, Schelenz C, Reinhart K, et al. Catecholamine and volume therapy for cardiac surgery in Germany - results from a postal survey. PLoS ONE 2014;9(8):1–8.
36. Skhirtladze K, Base EM, Lassnigg A, et al. Comparison of the effects of albumin 5%, hydroxyethyl starch 130/0.4 6%, and Ringer's lactate on blood loss and coagulation after cardiac surgery. Br J Anaesth 2014;112(2):255–64.
37. Foroughi M, Conte AH. Cardiovascular complications and management after cardiac surgery, in postoperative critical care for cardiac surgical patients. In: Dabbagh A, Esmailian F, Aranki SF, editors. Postoperative critical care for cardiac surgical patients. Berlin: Springer; 2014. p. 197–211.
38. Ristic AD, Imazio M, Adler Y, et al. Triage strategy for urgent management of cardiac tamponade: a position statement of the European Society of Cardiology Working Group on Myocardial and Pericardial Diseases. Eur Heart J 2014;(July):1–6.
39. You SC, Shim YC, Hong GR, et al. Incidence, predictors, and clinical outcomes of postoperative cardiac tamponade in patients undergoing heart valve surgery. PLoS ONE 2016;11(11):e0165754.
40. Mastropietroa CW, et al. Clinical response to arginine vasopressin therapy after paediatric cardiac surgery. Cardiol Young 2013;23(3):387–93.
41. Wagner GS, Strauss DG. Marriott's practical electrocardiography. 12th ed. Baltimore: Lippincott, Williams & Wilkins; 2014.
42. Dennis MJ. ECG criteria to differentiate pulmonary artery catheter irritation from other proarrhythmic influences as the cause of ventricular arrhythmias [abstract]. Am Coll Cardiol 2002;39(9 Suppl.B):2B.
43. Sigurdsson MI, et al. Duration of postoperative atrial fibrillation after cardiac surgery is associated with worsened long-term survival. Ann Thorac Surg 2016;102(6):2018–26.
44. Nair SG. Atrial fibrillation after cardiac surgery. Ann Card Anaesth 2010;13:196–205.
45. Peretto G, et al. Postoperative arrhythmias after cardiac surgery: incidence, risk factors, and therapeutic management. Cardiol Res Pract 2014;1–15.
46. Bansal S, Thai HM, Hsu CH, et al. Fast track extubation post coronary artery bypass graft: a retrospective review of predictors of clinical outcomes. World J Cardiovasc Surg 2013;3:81–6.
47. Fitch ZW, Debesa O, Ohkuma R, et al. A protocol-driven approach to early extubation after heart surgery. J Thorac Cardiovasc Surg 2014;147(3):1344–50.
48. Badhwar V, Esper S, Brooks M, et al. Extubating in the operating room following adult cardiac surgery safely improves outcomes and lowers costs. J Thorac Cardiovasc Surg 2014;148(6):3101–9.
49. LaPar DJ, Hawkins RB, McMurry TL, et al. Preoperative anemia versus blood transfusion: which is the culprit for worse outcomes in cardiac surgery? J Thorac Cardiovasc Surg 2018;156(1):66–74.e2.
50. Craver C, Belk KW, Myers GJ. Measurement of total hemoglobin reduces red cell transfusion in hospitalized patients undergoing cardiac surgery: a retrospective database analysis. Perfusion 2018;33(1):44–52.
51. De Santo LS, et al. Age and blood transfusion: relationship and prognostic implications in cardiac surgery. J Thorac Dis 2017;9(10):3719–27.
52. Patel NN, Murphy GJ. Evidence-based red blood cell transfusion practices in cardiac surgery. Transfus Med Rev 2017;31(4):230–5.
53. Bolliger D, Tanaka KA. Point-of-care coagulation testing in cardiac surgery. Semin Thromb Hemost 2017;43(4):386–96.
54. Ranucci M, Baryshnikova E, Pistuddi V, et al. The effectiveness of 10 years of interventions to control postoperative bleeding in adult cardiac surgery. Interact Cardiovasc Thorac Surg 2017;24(2):196–202.
55. Sharma S, Kumar S, Tewari P, et al. Utility of thromboelastography versus routine coagulation tests for assessment of hypocoagulable state in patients undergoing cardiac bypass surgery. Ann Card Anaesth 2018;21(2):151–7.

56. Taneja R, Berry L, Pappu U, et al. Protamine requirements in cardiac surgery: effect of changes in the heparin reference standard. J Cardiothorac Vasc Anesth 2014;28(5):1227–32.
57. Hällgren O, Svenmarker S, Appelblad M. Implementing a statistical model for protamine titration: effects on coagulation in cardiac surgical patients. J Cardiothorac Vasc Anesth 2017;31(2):516–21.
58. Suárez Cuenca J, Gayoso Diz P, Gude Sampedro F, et al. Method to calculate the protamine dose necessary for reversal of heparin as a function of activated clotting time in patients undergoing cardiac surgery. J Extra Corpor Technol 2013;45(4):235–41.
59. Côté CL, Yip AM, MacLeod JB, et al. Efficacy of intraoperative cell salvage in decreasing perioperative blood transfusion rates in first-time cardiac surgery patients: a retrospective study. Can J Surg 2016;59(5):330–6.
60. Marcinkiewicz A, Jaszewski R, Piestrzeniewicz K, et al. Cardiac tamponade and para-aortic hematoma post elective surgical myocardial revascularization on a beating heart – a possible complication of the Lima-stitch and sequential venous anastomosis. BMC Cardiovasc Disord 2014;14(72).
61. Harirforoosh S, Asghar W, Jamali F. Adverse effects of nonsteroidal antiinflammatory drugs: an update of gastrointestinal, cardiovascular and renal complications. J Pharm Sci 2013;16(5):821–47.
62. Nussmeier NA, Whelton AA, Brown MT, et al. Complications of the COX-2 inhibitors parecoxib and valdecoxib after cardiac surgery. New Engl J Med 2005;352(11):1081–91.
63. Gjeilo KH, Stenseth R, Klepstad P. Risk factors and early pharmacological interventions to prevent chronic postsurgical pain following cardiac surgery. Am J Cardiovasc Drugs 2014;14:335–42.
64. Bjørnnes AK, Parry M, Lie I, et al. Pain experiences of men and women after cardiac surgery. J Clin Nurs 2016;25(19–20):3058–68.
65. Mohammadzadeh A, Towfighi F, Jafari N. Effect of magnesium on arrhythmia incidence in patients undergoing coronary artery bypass grafting. ANZ J Surg 2017;88(6):612–15.
66. Bradley D, Cresswell LL, Hogue CW Jr, et al. Pharmacologic prophylaxis: American College of Chest Physicians guidelines for the prevention and management of postoperative atrial fibrillation after cardiac surgery. Chest 2005;128(2 Suppl.):S39–47.
67. Tavares Gomes E, Muniz da Silva Bezerra SM. Anxiety and depression in the preoperative period of cardiac surgery. Rev Bras Enferm Nordeste 2017;18(3):420–7.
68. King K. Emotional and functional outcomes in women with coronary heart disease. J Cardiovasc Nurs 2001;15(3):54–70.
69. Hamester L, Souza EN, Cielo C, et al. Effectiveness of a nursing intervention in decreasing the anxiety levels of family members of patients undergoing cardiac surgery: a randomized clinical trial. Rev Lat Am Enfermagem 2016;24:1–8.
70. Heilmann C, Stotz U, Burbaum C, et al. Short-term intervention to reduce anxiety before coronary artery bypass surgery–a randomised controlled trial. J Clin Nurs 2016;25(3–4):351–61.
71. Fiabane E, Giorgi I, Candura SM, et al. Psychological and work stress assessment of patients following angioplasty or heart surgery: results of 1-year follow-up study. Stress Health 2015;31(5):393–402.
72. Mendonça KMB, de Andrade TM. Patient's perception about coronary artery bypass grafting. Braz J Cardiovasc Surg 2015;30(5):544–51.
73. Hou D, Yang F, Hou X. Clinical application of intra-aortic balloon counterpulsation in high-risk patients undergoing cardiac surgery. Perfusion 2018;33(3):178–84.
74. Deppe A-C, Weber C, Liakopoulos OJ, et al. Preoperative intra-aortic balloon pump use in high-risk patients prior to coronary artery bypass graft surgery decreases the risk for morbidity and mortality – A meta-analysis of 9,212 patients. J Card Surg 2017;32(3):177–85.
75. Shah M, Patnaik S, Patel B, et al. Trends in mechanical circulatory support use and hospital mortality among patients with acute myocardial infarction and non-infarction related cardiogenic shock in the United States. Clin Res Cardiol 2018;107(4):287–303.
76. Parissis H, Graham V, Lampridis S, et al. IABP: history-evolution-pathophysiology-indications: what we need to know. J Cardiothorac Surg 2016;11(1):122.
77. Schampaert S, et al. Modeling the interaction between the intra-aortic balloon pump and the cardiovascular system: the effect of timing. ASAIO J 2013;59(1):30–6.
78. Siriwardena M, Pilbrow A, Frampton C, et al. Complications of intra-aortic balloon pump use: does the final position of the IABP tip matter? Anaesth Intensive Care 2015;43(1):66–73.
79. de Jong MM, Lorusso R, Al Awami F, et al. Vascular complications following intra-aortic balloon pump implantation: an updated review. Perfusion 2018;33(2):96–104.
80. Pucher PH, Cummings IG, Shipolini AR, et al. Is heparin needed for patients with an intra-aortic balloon pump? Interact Cardiovasc Thorac Surg 2012;15:136–40.
81. Onorati F, et al. How should I wean my next intra-aortic balloon pump? Differences between progressive volume weaning and rate weaning. J Thorac Cardiovasc Surg 2013;145(5):1214–21.
82. Rogers L, et al. What is the optimum method of weaning intra-aortic balloon pumps? Interact Cardiovasc Thorac Surg 2016;23(2): 310–13.
83. Yarham G, Clements A, Morris C, et al. Fiber-optic intra-aortic balloon therapy and its role within cardiac surgery. Perfusion 2013;28(2):97–102.
84. Mihatov N, Dudzinski DM. Intraaortic balloon pump rupture. J Invasive Cardiol 2015;27(9):E203.
85. Chapman JR. Transplantation in Australia –50 years in progress. Med J Aust 1992;157(1):46–50.
86. McBride M, Chapman JR. An overview of transplantation in Australia. Anaesth Intensive Care 1995;2391:60–4.

87. Connellan M, Dhital K. Donor procurement from the Donation after Circulatory Death Pathway. Oper Tech Thorac Cardiovasc Surg 2017;22:58–67.
88. Page AA, Messer S, Tsui SS, et al. Large. Early results using donation after circulatory death (DCD) donor hearts. Curr Transplant Rep 2016;3(3):199–206.
89. Barnard CN. A human cardia transplant: an interim report of a successful operation performed at Groote Schuur Hospital, Capetown. S Afr Med J 1967;41(48):1271–4.
90. Excell L, Wride P, Russ GR Australia and New Zealand organ donation registry. Available from: http://www.anzdata.org/au/anzod/ANZODReport/2010/2010Contents.pdf;2010. [Accessed 19 August 2010].
91. Keogh A, Williams T, Pettersson R ANZCOTR 2016. Australia and New Zealand Cardiothoracic Organ Transplant Registry 2016 Report.
92. Myles PS, Leong CK, Currey J. Endogenous nitric oxide and low systemic vascular resistance after cardiopulmonary bypass. J Cardiothorac Vasc Anaesth 1997;11(5):571–4.
93. Eurotransplant International Foundation. Annual Report 2016, p 162.
94. Rose EA, Moskowitz AJ, Packer M, et al. The REMATCH trial: rationale, design and end points. Randomized Evaluation of Mechanical Assistance for the treatment of Congestive Heart Failure. Ann Thorac Surg 1999;67(3):723–30.
95. Kirklin JK, Naftel DC, Pagani FD, et al. Seventh INTERMACS annual report:15,000 patients and counting. J Heart Lung Transplant 2015;34:1495–504.
96. Wilhelm M. Longterm outcome following heart transplantation: a current perspective. J Thorac Dis 2015;7(3):549–51.
97. Australia and New Zealand Organ Donation Registry. The ANZROD Annual report 2017.
98. Mehra MR, Kobashigawa J, Starling R, et al. Listing criteria for heart transplantation: International Society for the Heart Lung Transplant guidelines for the care of cardiac transplant candidates – 2006. J Heart Lung Transplant 2006;25(9):1024–42.
99. Mandeep R, Mehra MD, Cantor CE, et al. The 2016 International Society Heart Lung Transplantation listing criteria for heart transplants: a 10-year update. JHLT 2016;3(1):1–23.
100. Goldstein DJ, Bello R, Shin JJ, et al. Outcomes of cardiac transplant in septuagenarians. JHLT 2012;31(7):679–85.
101. MacDonald P. Heart transplantation who should be considered and when? Intern Med J 2008;38(12):91–7.
102. Chan YK, Gerber T, Tuttle C, et al. Rediscovering heart failure: the contemporary burden and profile of heart failure in Australia. Melbourne: Mary MacKillop Institute for Health Research; 2015. Key findings 12.
103. The Transplantation Society of Australia and New Zealand. Clinical Guidelines for organ transplantation from deceased donors, 2018.
104. Chan YK, Gerber T, Tuttle C, et al. Rediscovering heart failure: the contemporary burden and profile of heart failure in Australia. Melbourne: Mary MacKillop Institute for Health Research; 2015. Key findings 2 and 3.
105. Kirklin JK, Young JB, Mc Giffin DC. Heart transplantation. Philadelphia: Churchill Livingstone; 2002.
106. Angermann CE, Spes CH, Tammen A, et al. Anatomic characteristics and valvular function of the transplanted heart: transthoracic versus transesophageal echocardiographic findings. J Heart Transplant 1990;9(4):331–8.
107. Kendall SWH, Ciulli F, Mullins PA, et al. Total orthotopic heart transplantation: an alternative to the standard technique. Ann Thorac Surg 1992;54:187–92.
108. Dreyfus G, Jebara V, Mihaileanu S, et al. Total orthotopic heart transplantation: an alternative to the standard technique. Ann Thorac Surg 1991;52(5):1181–4.
109. Nakatani T, Frazier OH, Lammermeier DE, et al. Heterotopic heart transplantation: a reliable option for a select group of high risk patients. J Heart Lung Transplant 1989;8(1):40–7.
110. Newcomb AE, Esmore DS, Rosenfeldt FL, et al. Heterotopic heart transplantation: an expanding role in the twenty-first century? Ann Thorac Surg 2004;78(4):1345–50, discussion 1350–1351.
111. Neerukonda SK, Schoonmaker FW, Nampalli VK, et al. Ventricular dysrthythmia and heterotopic heart transplantation. J Heart Lung Transplant 1992;11:793–6.
112. Costanzo MR, Dipchand A, Starling R, et al. The International Society of Heart and Lung Transplantation Guidelines for the care of heart transplant recipients. J Heart Lung Transplant 2010;29(8):914–56.
113. Coleman B, Blumenthal N, Currey J, et al. Adult cardiothoracic transplant nursing: an ISHLT consensus document on the current adult nursing practice in heart and lunch transplantation. J Heart Lung Transplant 2015;34(2):139–48.
114. Ahmed SB. Cardiac transplantation and cyclosporin nephrotoxicity. Kidney Int 2007;72(8):1029–33.
115. Kobashigawa J, Zuckermann A, Macdonald P, et al. Report from a consensus conference on primary graft dysfunction after cardiac transplant. J Heart Lung Transplant 2016;33(4):327–40.
116. Barry GL, Burke MM, Andersen C, et al. The 2013 International Society Heart Lung Transplant working formulation for the standardization of nomenclature in the pathological diagnosis of antibody mediated rejection in heart transplantation. J Heart Lung Transplant 2013;32(12):1147–62.
117. Billingham ME, Cary NR, Hammond ME, et al. A working formulation for the standardization of nomenclature in the diagnosis of heart and lung rejection: Heart Rejection Study Group. The International Society for Heart Transplantation. J Heart Transplant 1990;9(6):587–93.
118. Stewart S, Berry C, McMurray JJ. Revision of the 1990 working formulation for the standardization of nomenclature in the diagnosis of heart rejection. J Heart Lung Transplant 2005;24(11):1710–20.

119. Kobashigawa J. International Society Heart Lung Transplantation working formulation for pathologic diagnosis of antibody-mediated rejection in heart transplants: evolution and current status. J Heart Lung Transplant 2011;30(6):601–11.
120. Lloveras JJ, Escourrou G, Delisle MB, et al. Evolution of untreated mild rejection in heart transplant recipients. J Heart Lung Transplant 1992;11(4 Pt 1):751–6109.
121. Pajaro OE, et al. Antibody mediated rejection in heart transplantation a case presentation with a review of current international guidelines. J Transplant 2011;2:Article ID-351950.
122. Maravić-Stojković V, Stojković B, Miodrag P. Modern immunosuppressive agents after heart transplantation. Current Trends in Cardiology 2017;1(2):39–46.
123. Keogh A, Eisen HJ. Calcineurin inhibitors. J Heart Lung Transplant 2004;23(5 Suppl.):S202–6.
124. Aliabadi A, Grömmer M, Cochrane A, et al. Induction therapy in heart transplants, where are we now? Transpl Int 2013;26(7).
125. Husain S, Mooney ML, Danziger-Isakov L, et al. Working formulation for the standardization of definitions of infections in cardio-thoracic transplant recipients. J Heart Lung Transplant 2011;30:361–74.
126. Moller CH, Gustafsson F, Gluud C, et al. Interleukin-2 receptor antagonists as induction therapy after heart transplantation: systematic review with meta-analysis of randomized trials. J Heart Lung Transplant 2008;27(8):835–42.
127. Mason VF, Konicki AJ. Left ventricular assist devices as destination therapy. AACN Clin Issues 2003;14(4):488–97.
128. Miller LW, Naftel DC, Bourge RC, et al. Infection after heart transplantation: a multiinstitutional study. Cardiac Transplant Research Database Group. J Heart Lung Transplant 1994;13(3):381–92, discussion 393.
129. Hughes WT, Rivera GK, Schell MJ, et al. Successful intermittent chemoprophylaxis for Pneumocystis carinii pneumonitis. N Engl J Med 1987;316(26):1627–32.
130. Haddad F. Changing trends in infectious disease in heart transplantation. J Heart Lung Transplant 2010;29(3):306–15.
131. Winters GL. Cardiac transplant biopsies. Surg Pathol Clin 2012;5(2):371–400.
132. Walsh TR, Guttendorf J, Dummer S, et al. The value of protective isolation procedures in cardiac allograft recipients. Ann Thorac Surg 1989;47(4):539–44, discussion 544–545.
133. Luckraz H, Goddard M, Charman SC, et al. Early mortality after cardiac transplantation: should we do better? J Heart Lung Transplant 2005;24(4):401–5.
134. Bowden RA, Slichter SJ, Sayers M, et al. A comparison of filtered leukocyte-reduced and cytomegalovirus (CMV) seronegative blood products for the prevention of transfusion-associated CMV infection after marrow transplant. Blood 1995;86(9):3598–603.
135. Cooper DKC, Lidsky NM. Immediate postoperative care and potential complications. In: Cooper DKC, Miller LW, Patterson GA, editors. The transplantation and replacement of thoracic organs. Boston: Kluwer; 1996. p. 221–7.
136. Kobashigawa J. Report from consensus conference on primary graft failure after cardiac transplant. J Heart Lung Transplant 2014;33(4):327–40.
137. Esmore DS, Rosenfeldt FL, Mack JA, et al. Long ischaemic time allografts (>6 hr) further expand the transplant donor pool. Washington: International Society of Heart and Lung Transplantation Conference Abstracts; 2002.
138. Messer S, Page AA, Colah S, et al. Human heart transplantation from circulatory determined death donors using normothermic regional perfusion and cold storage. J Heart Lung Transplant 2018;37(7):865–9.
139. Senechal M, Pons J, Leblanc MH, et al. Effects of chronic sildenafil use on pulmonary haemodynamics and clinical outcomes in cardiac transplant. J Heart Lung Transplant 2012;31(12):1281–7.
140. Kristof AS, Magder S. Low systemic vascular resistance state in patients undergoing cardiopulmonary bypass. Crit Care Med 1999;27(6):1121–7.
141. Landry DW, Levin HR, Gallant EM, et al. Vasopressin deficiency contributes to the vasodilation of septic shock. Circulation 1997;95(5):1122–5.
142. Argenziano M, Choudhri AF, Oz MC, et al. A prospective randomized trial of arginine vasopressin in the treatment of vasodilatory shock after left ventricular assist device placement. Circulation 1997;96(9 Suppl.):II-286–II-290.
143. Rossaint R, Falke KJ, Lopez F, et al. Inhaled nitric oxide for the adult respiratory distress syndrome. N Engl J Med 1993;328(6):399–405.
144. Armitage JM, Hardesty RL, Griffith BP. Prostaglandin E1: an effective treatment of right heart failure after orthotopic heart transplantation. J Heart Lung Transplant 1987;6:348–51.
145. Wang SS, Ko WJ, Chen YS, et al. Mechanical bridge with extracorporeal membrane oxygenation and ventricular assist device to heart transplantation. Artif Organs 2001;25(8):599–602.
146. Karamlou T, Gelow J, Diggs BS, et al. Mechanical circulatory support pathways that maximize post-heart transplant survival. Ann Thorac Surg 2013;95(2):480–5, discussion 485.
147. Ellenbogen KA, Thames MD, DiMarco JP, et al. Electrophysiological effects of adenosine in the transplanted human heart. Evidence of supersensitivity. Circulation 1990;81(3):821–8.
148. Macdonald P, Hackworthy R, Keogh A, et al. Atrial overdrive pacing for reversion of atrial flutter after heart transplantation. J Heart Lung Transplant 1991;10(5 Pt 1):731–7.
149. Mackintosh AF, Carmichael DJ, Wren C, et al. Sinus node function in first three weeks after cardiac transplantation. Br Heart J 1982;48(6):584–8.

150. Stark RP, McGinn AL, Wilson RF. Chest pain in cardiac-transplant recipients. Evidence of sensory reinnervation after cardiac transplantation. N Engl J Med 1991;324(25):1791–4.
151. Parry A, Roberts M, Parameshwar J, et al. The management of post-cardiac transplantation coronary artery disease. Eur J Cardiothorac Surg 1996;10(7):528–32, discussion 53.
152. Shiba N, Chan MC, Kwok BW, et al. Analysis of survivors more than 10 years after heart transplantation in the cyclosporine era: Stanford experience. J Heart Lung Transplant 2004;23(2):155–64.
153. Chih S, Chong AY, Mielniczuk LM, et al. Allograft vasculopathy. The Achilles' heel of heart transplantation. J Am Coll Cardiol 2016;68(1):80–91.
154. Taylor D, Edwards L, Boucek MM, et al. Registry of the International Society of Heart Lung Transplantation: 23rd official adult heart transplant report 2006. J Heart Lung Transplant 2006;25:869–87.
155. Johnson DE, Alderman EL, Schroeder JS, et al. Transplant coronary artery disease: histopathologic correlations with angiographic morphology. J Am Coll Cardiol 1991;17(2):449–57.
156. Keogh A, Richardson M, Ruygrok P, et al. Sirolimus in de novo heart transplant recipients reduces acute rejection and prevents coronary artery disease at 2 years: a randomized clinical trial. Circulation 2004;110(17):2694–700.
157. Na R, Grulich AE, Meagher NS, et al. De novo cancer-related death in Australian liver and cardiothoracic transplant recipients. Am J Transplant 2013;13(5):1296–304.
158. Krikorian JG, Anderson JL, Bieber CP, et al. Malignant neoplasms following cardiac transplantation. JAMA 1978;240(7):639–43.
159. Ong CS, Keogh AM, Kossard S, et al. Skin cancer in Australian heart transplant recipients. J Am Acad Dermatol 1999;40(1):27–34.
160. Veness MJ, Quinn DI, Ong CS, et al. Aggressive cutaneous malignancies following cardiothoracic transplantation: the Australian experience. Cancer 1999;85(8):1758–64.
161. Armitage JM, Kormos RL, Stuart RS, et al. Posttransplant lymphoproliferative disease in thoracic organ transplant patients: ten years of cyclosporine-based immunosuppression. J Heart Lung Transplant 1991;10(6):877–86, discussion 886–887.
162. Cole WH. The increase in immunosuppression and its role in the development of malignant lesions. J Surg Oncol 1985;30(3):139–44.
163. Penn I. Cancers following cyclosporine therapy. Transplantation 1987;43(1):32–5.
164. Penn I, First MR. Development and incidence of cancer following cyclosporine therapy. Transplant Proc 1986;18(2 Suppl. 1):210–15.
165. Kushwaha SS. Kidney transplant as a therapeutic option for end stage renal disease developing after heart transplantation. J Heart Lung Transplant 2017;36(3):297–304.
166. Eisen HJ. Hypertension in heart transplant recipients: more than just cyclosporine. J Am Coll Cardiol 2003;41(3):433–4.
167. Ventura HO, et al. Mechanisms of hypertension in cardiac transplantation and the role of cyclosporine. Curr Opin Cardiol 1997;12(4):375–81.

Chapter 13

Respiratory assessment and monitoring

Mona Ringdal, Janice Gullick

Learning objectives

After reading this chapter, you should be able to:

- understand respiratory anatomy and normal physiology
- understand mechanisms contributing to altered respiratory function
- identify key principles underpinning assessment and monitoring of respiratory function
- describe nursing assessment and monitoring activities for critically ill patients with respiratory dysfunction
- discuss the importance of patient assessment skills, and the contribution of diagnostic and laboratory findings to ongoing clinical management
- outline the physiological basis for different types of monitoring
- describe common diagnostic procedures used in critical care.

KEY WORDS

arterial blood gases
capnography
diagnostic imaging
gas exchange
hypoxaemia
oxygen delivery
pulse oximetry
work of breathing

Introduction

The respiratory system ensures adequate tissue and cellular oxygenation for the body. It is responsible for gas exchange through the uptake of oxygen and excretion of carbon dioxide (CO_2); assists in optimal organ function; contributes to acid–base balance; and plays a large role in maintaining homeostasis. As respiratory conditions account for 20–26% of admissions to intensive care units (ICUs) in the USA and UK,[1] and up to 33% in Australian hospitals,[2] a thorough understanding of the anatomy, physiology and pathophysiology of this complex system is required to accurately assess critically ill patients and monitor response to treatment or early signs of deterioration.

In this chapter a comprehensive description of the principles and practice of respiratory assessment, monitoring and diagnostics is provided. These are foundational concepts underpinning timely and effective interventions for critically ill patients. Management of respiratory alterations, oxygenation and ventilation are discussed in Chapters 14 and 15.

Related anatomy and physiology

The thoracic cavity contains the trachea and bronchial tree, the two lungs, pleura and diaphragm. The mediastinum, located between the lungs, houses

FIGURE 13.1 Ventilatory structures of the chest wall and lungs, showing the ribs and lobes of the lungs.[3]

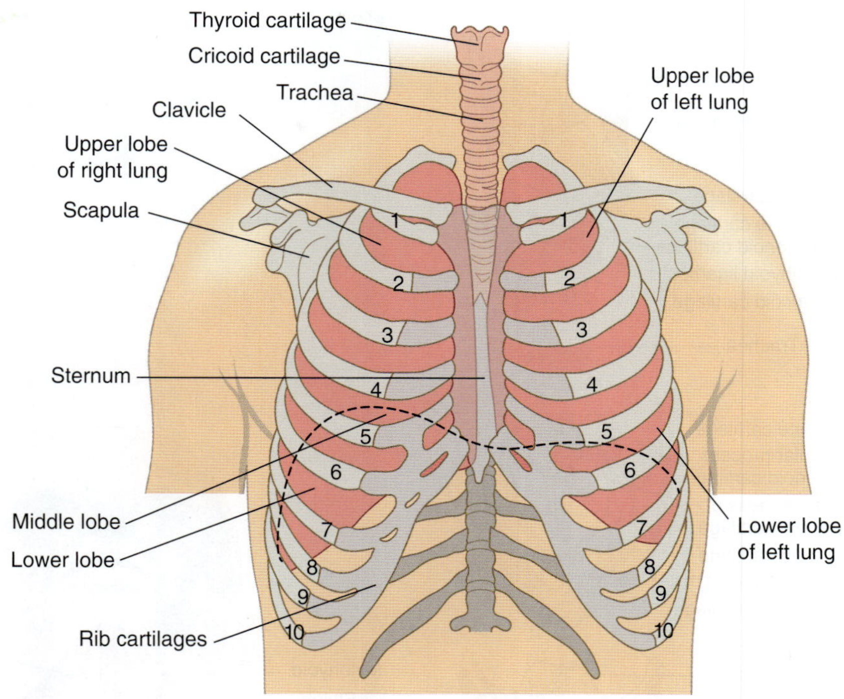

Source: Urden L, Stacy K, Lough M. Critical care nursing: diagnosis and management. 6th ed. St Louis: Mosby; 2010.

and protects the heart, great vessels and the oesophagus. Twelve pairs of ribs cover the lungs. Ten are connected to the spine posteriorly, and to the sternum or to the cartilage of the above rib anteriorly (ribs 8–10). The 11th and 12th ribs have no anterior attachment (Fig. 13.1).

The respiratory system is divided into upper and lower respiratory tracts: the upper airways consist of the nose, nasal conchae, sinus and pharynx; the lower respiratory tract includes the larynx, trachea, bronchi and lungs.[4] Larger airways are lined with stratified epithelial tissue, which has a relatively high cellular turnover rate; these cells protect and clear these large airways. Additional specialised features of this tissue include an extensive distribution of mucous/goblet cells and cilia, which facilitate the mucociliary clearance system of the airway.

Upper respiratory tract

The nasal cavities contain an extremely vascular and mucoid environment for warming and humidifying inhaled gases. To maximise exposure to this surface area, the nasal conchae create turbulent gas flow. Mucus is moved by the cilia at the top of the epithelial cells lining the conducting airways. Mucus moves towards the pharynx at a rate of 1–2 cm per min, providing filtration and cleaning of the inhaled air. One litre of mucus is produced every day with only a small part not reabsorbed by the body.[5]

The pharynx is a muscular tube that transports food to the oesophagus and air to the larynx. Inferior to the pharynx, the larynx consists mostly of cartilage attached to other surrounding structures and houses the vestibular (false) vocal folds, which do not produce any sounds but help to close the larynx during swallowing. The lower true vocal cords create the vocal sounds (Fig. 13.2).[6] The pyramid-shaped arytenoids, an important pair of cartilages within the larynx, act as attachment points for the vocal cords. This area is easily damaged by pressure from endotracheal tubes; the most significant independent risk factor for injury to the arytenoids is the length of intubation time.[5] The thyroid cartilage ('Adam's apple') and the cricoid cartilage protect the glottis and entrance to the trachea. Another cartilage in the larynx is the leaf-shaped elastic epiglottis, which protects the lower airways from aspiration of food and fluids into the lungs. The epiglottis usually occludes the inlet to the larynx during swallowing. The primitive cough, swallow and gag reflexes further protect the airway.[5] Laryngospasm is a dangerous complication caused by irritation of the vocal cords. When the muscles of the vocal cords spasm, the flow of air into the lungs is restricted leading to airway obstruction. Laryngospasm can be trigged by

FIGURE 13.2 Larynx. (**A**) Cartilages and ligaments. (**B**) Neck muscles.[7]

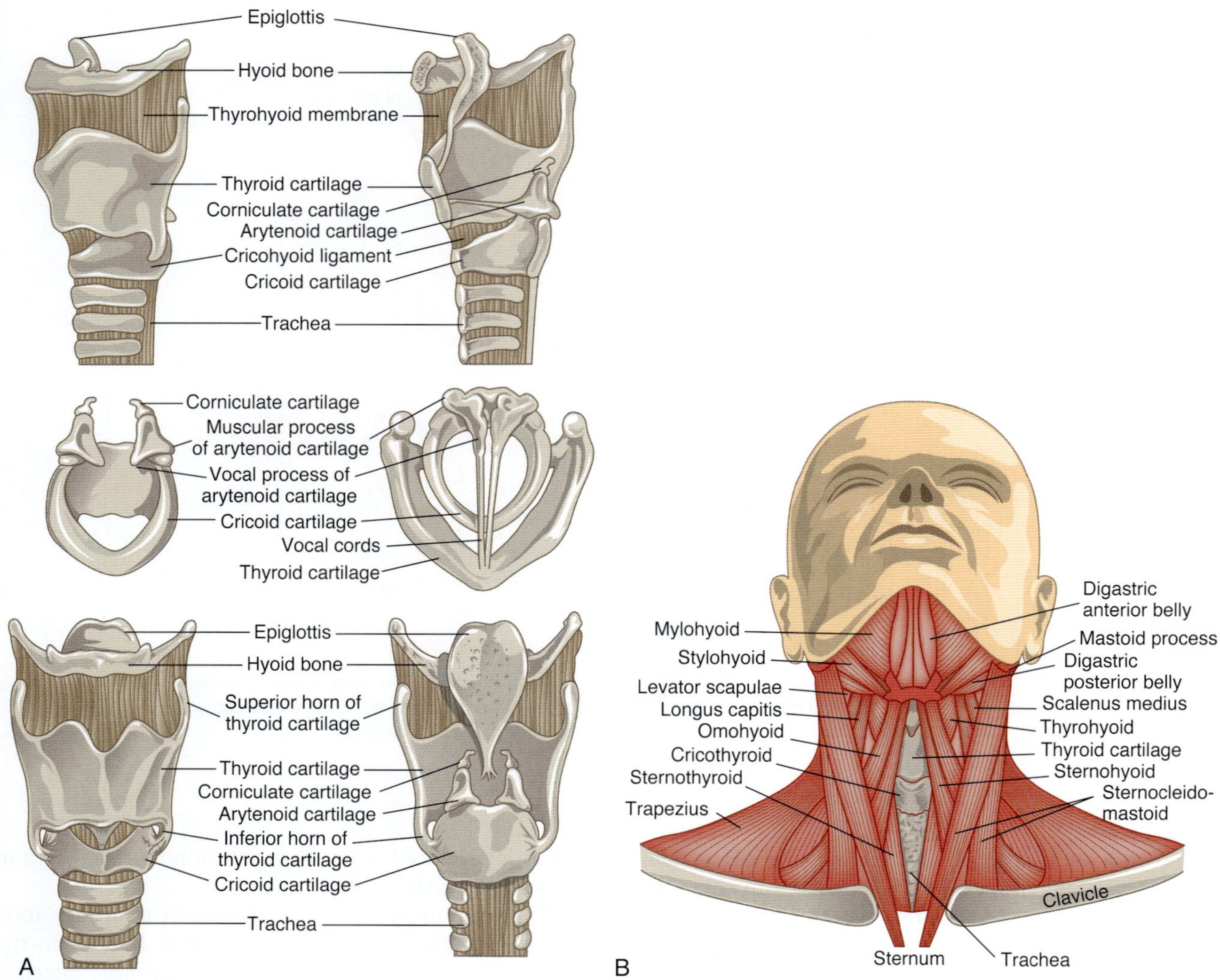

Source: Thompson J, McFarland G, Hirsch J, Tucker S. Mosby's Clinical nursing. 5th ed. St Louis: Mosby; 2012.

suctioning of the airways in non-intubated patients or when intubation is performed.[11]

Lower respiratory tract

The trachea is a hollow tube approximately 11 cm long and 2.5 cm in diameter that marks the beginning of the lower respiratory tract. The trachea is supported by 16–20 C-shaped cartilages and is another area at risk of pressure damage from artificial airways. The trachea divides at the carina into the left and right main bronchi. The bronchial tree has two mainstem bronchi that are structurally different. The right bronchus is wider and angles slightly where it divides further into the three lobes of the right lung. The most common site of aspiration of foreign objects is the right bronchus because of its anatomical position. The acutely-angled left main bronchus divides further into the two lobes of the left lung.

The airways within each lung branch further into secondary (or lobar) bronchi then tertiary (or segmental) bronchi. Further divisions within these conducting airways end with the terminal bronchioles, the smallest airways without alveoli. These conducting airways do not participate in gas exchange but form the anatomical dead space (approximately 150 mL).[8] This anatomical dead space provides the important function of humidifying and warming inspired air. It is important to remember that when a patient is mechanically ventilated, the ventilator tubing extends the dead space and may reduce the volume of fresh air that reaches the patient; this may be similar to the experience of breathing through a snorkel.

Larger airways have a greater proportion of supporting cartilage, ciliated epithelium, goblet and serous cells and, hence, a mucous layer. As the airways become smaller, the cartilage transition from C-shaped rings which hold

FIGURE 13.3 Lower airway branches.[7]

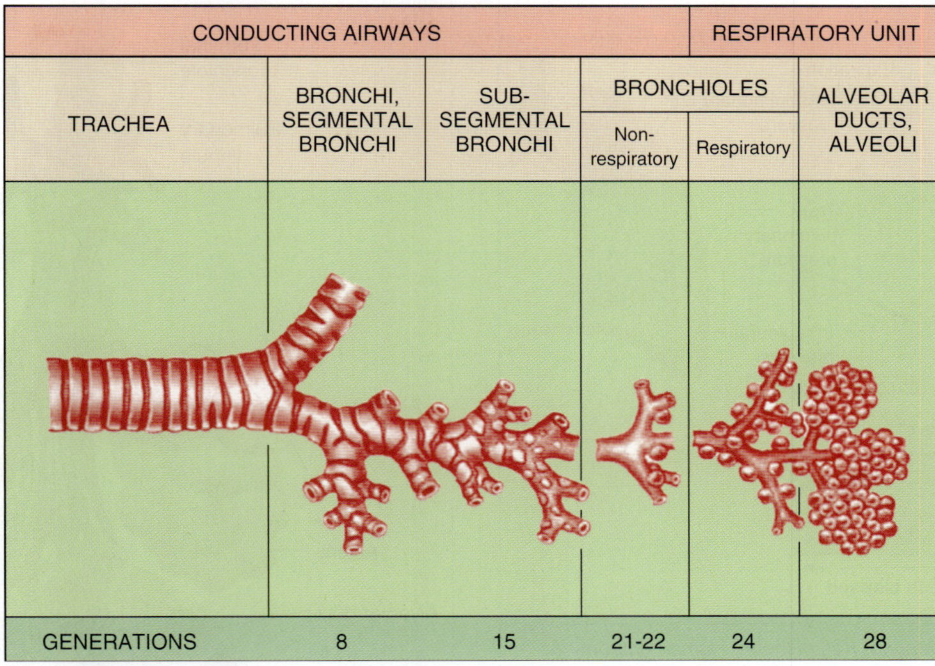

Source: Thompson J, McFarland G, Hirsch J, Tucker S. Mosby's Clinical nursing. 5th ed. St Louis: Mosby; 2012.

the trachea open, to strips of cartilage, then finally to airways with no cartilage, but with smooth muscle that forms the walls of the bronchioles. The importance of this is that the diameter of the bronchioles is, therefore, totally under autonomic nervous system control. Smooth muscle surrounds and supports the bronchioles, enabling airway diameter change and subsequent changes in airway resistance to gas flow.[9]

The number of goblet cells and amount of mucus decrease until, at the alveolar level, there is only a single layer of squamous epithelial cells. Alveolar macrophages present among these epithelial cells phagocytose any small particles that enter the alveoli.

Thorax/lungs

The lungs and heart are protected within the thoracic cage. When inspiration is triggered, expansion of the thorax creates a negative pressure causing air to flow into the lungs. The thorax then passively compresses to expel air from the lungs during expiration. The diaphragm separates the thorax from the abdomen and is the most important inspiratory muscle, performing approximately 80% of the work of breathing. Inspiration is initiated from the medulla, sending impulses through the phrenic nerve to stimulate the diaphragm to contract and flatten. The phrenic nerve originates in the cervical plexus and involves the third to fifth cervical nerves. It splits into two parts, passing to the left and right side of the heart before it reaches the diaphragm. For this reason, patients can have ventilation difficulties if phrenic nerve damage results from C3–C5 trauma.[9,10]

The conducting airways, ending in the terminal bronchioles, move inspired air towards the respiratory unit (Fig. 13.3). The respiratory unit comprises the respiratory bronchioles, alveolar ducts and alveolar sacs where the diffusion of gas molecules, or gas exchange, occurs. The pores of Kohn help to distribute gases between alveoli. The respiratory unit makes up most of the lung with a volume of 2.5–3 L during rest.[8]

Surfactant

Of particular importance to the structure and function of the respiratory system are the type I and II alveolar epithelial cells. Type I cells provide support of the alveolar unit walls. Type II cells produce an important lipoprotein, surfactant, that lines the inner alveolar surface lowering alveolar surface tension, stabilising the alveoli to optimise lung compliance and facilitating expansion during inspiration.[8] If surfactant synthesis is reduced due to pulmonary disease, lung compliance decreases and the work of breathing increases. The role of surfactant in managing the respiratory function of premature infants is well-described[11] and inactivation or dysfunction of surfactant in adults can contribute to lung disease such as acute respiratory distress syndrome (ARDS).

Pleura

Each lung is contained within a continuous thin membrane called the pleura, creating the pleural sac that surrounds each lung. The two pleural sacs, one on each side of the midline, are completely separate from each other. The parietal pleura lines the inner surface of the

FIGURE 13.4 Changes in intrapleural and intrapulmonary pressure during inspiration and expiration.[12]

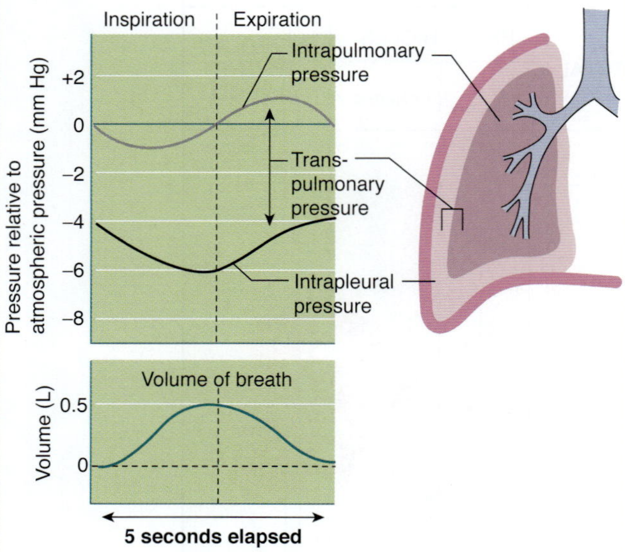

Source: Elaine N. Marieb, Katja Hoehn. Human anatomy & physiology. 8th ed. © 2010 Reprinted by permission of Pearson Education, Inc., New York.

FIGURE 13.5 Terminal ventilation and perfusion units of the lung.[13]

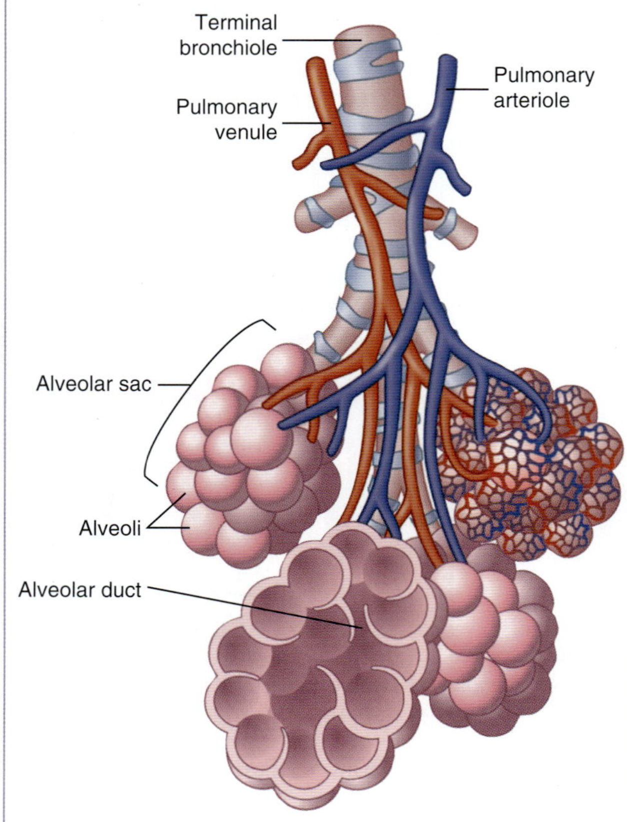

Urden LD, Stacy KM, Lough ME. Critical care nursing: diagnosis and management. 7th ed. St Louis: Mosby; 2014.

chest wall and is in close contact with the visceral pleura, which covers the lungs. The pleural space, between these two layers, contains a small amount of serous fluid, which limits friction during lung expansion.[12]

The intrapleural pressure in the pleural space under normal circumstances is always negative with a range of −4 to −10 cmH_2O; this negative pressure keeps the lungs inflated. During inhalation the pressure becomes more negative as both the lungs and the chest wall are elastic structures. These elastic fibres of the lung pull the visceral pleura inwards while the chest wall pulls the parietal pleura outward. The pressure difference between the alveolar pressure (0 cmH_2O pressure in the lungs) and the intrapleural pressure (−4 cmH_2O) across the lung wall is termed the transpulmonary pressure (+4 cm $H_2O[0 - (-4) = +4]$); and is the force that holds the lungs open[5] (Fig. 13.4).

Pulmonary circulation

The circulatory system of the lungs receives the entire cardiac output but operates as a low-pressure system; it only directs blood back to the left side of the heart (unlike the systemic circulation, which pumps blood to different regions of the entire body). Within the pulmonary circulation, the right ventricle pumps oxygen-depleted blood to the lungs via the pulmonary artery, with oxygen-rich blood returning to the left atrium via the pulmonary veins. Pulmonary blood vessels follow the path of the bronchioles, with capillaries forming a dense network in the walls of the alveoli. As illustrated in Fig. 13.5[13] the entire surface area of the alveolar wall is covered by capillaries, just large enough for a red blood cell to pass through, allowing gas exchange.

Pulmonary vessels are short and thin and have relatively little smooth muscle. The pressure inside the vessels is remarkably low (normal pulmonary artery pressure is only 25/8 mmHg; mean 15 mmHg).[8] This low-pressure system ensures that right heart workload is minimised, while promoting efficient gas exchange in the lungs (Fig. 13.6).

Bronchial circulation

The bronchial circulation, part of the systemic circulation, supplies oxygenated blood, nutrients and heat to the conducting airways (to the level of the terminal bronchioles) and to the pleura. Drainage of this deoxygenated blood is predominantly through the bronchial network, although some capillaries drain into the pulmonary arterial circulation, contributing to venous admixture or right-to-left shunt[8] (see *Pathophysiology* below for further discussion).

Control of ventilation

Normal breathing occurs automatically and is a complex function not fully understood. It is coordinated by the respiratory centre, regulated by controllers in the brain, effectors in the muscles and sensors including chemoreceptors and mechanoreceptors. There are also protective reflexes such as sneezing and coughing that respond to respiratory tract irritation by mechanical or chemical stimuli. Sneezing clears the upper respiratory tract and coughing clears the lower respiratory tract. The larynx and carina are particularly sensitive to mechanical stimuli, requiring only minor irritants to stimulate a cough. The terminal bronchioles and alveoli are responsive to chemical stimuli such as chlorine or sulphur dioxide gas.[14]

FIGURE 13.6 Comparison of pressure in the pulmonary and systematic circulations (mmHg).[8]

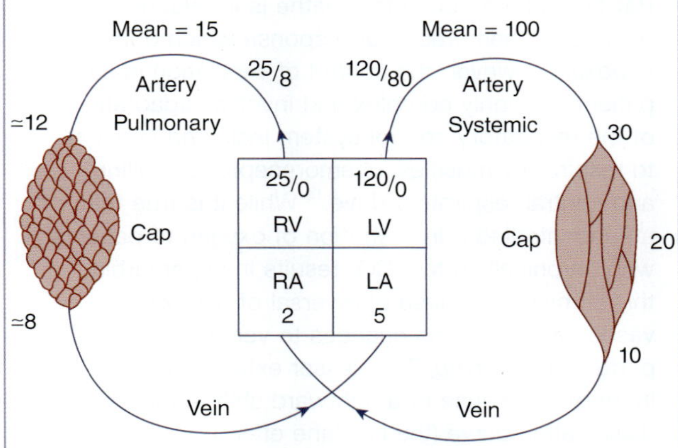

Adapted from West J, Luks A. Respiratory physiology: the essentials. 10th ed. Philadelphia: Wolters Kluwer; 2016.

Controller

In the brainstem, the medulla oblongata and the pons regulate automatic ventilation while the cerebral cortex regulates voluntary ventilation (Fig. 13.7). The respiratory rhythmic centre in the medulla can be divided into inspiratory and expiratory centres, with the following functions:[9]

- The inspiratory centre (or dorsal respiratory group) triggers inspiration.
- The expiratory centre (or ventral respiratory group) only functions during forced respiration and active expiration.
- The pneumotaxic and apneustic centre in the pons adjusts the rate and pattern of breathing.

FIGURE 13.7 Respiratory centres and reflex.[12]

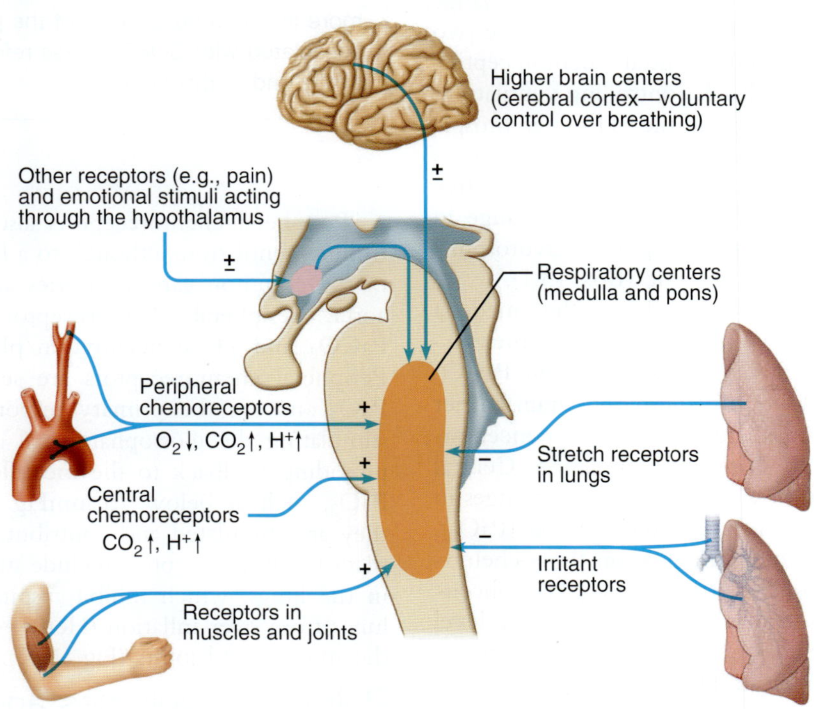

Source: Elaine N. Marieb, Katja Hoehn. Human anatomy & physiology. 8th ed. © 2010 Reprinted by permission of Pearson Education, Inc., New York.

- The cerebral cortex provides conscious voluntary control over the respiratory muscles. This voluntary control cannot be maintained when the partial pressure of carbon dioxide in the arterial blood ($PaCO_2$) and the hydrogen ion (H^+) concentration become markedly elevated; an example is the inability to hold your breath for very long.[9] Emotional and autonomic activities also affect the pace and depth of breathing.

Effectors

The diaphragm is the major muscle of inspiration, although the external intercostal muscles also contribute. The accessory muscles of inspiration (scalenes, sternocleidomastoid muscles and the pectoralis minor) are active only during exercise or strenuous breathing. Expiration is a passive act and only the internal intercostal muscles are involved at rest. During exercise, the abdominal muscles also contribute to expiration. Inspiration is triggered by stimulus from the medulla, causing downward contraction of the diaphragm, and contraction of external intercostal muscles, lifting the thorax up and out. This action lowers pressure within the alveoli (intraalveolar pressure) relative to atmospheric pressure. Air rushes into the lungs to equalise the pressure gradient. After contraction has ceased, the ribs and diaphragm relax, the pressure gradient reverses, and air is passively expelled from the lungs, which return to their resting state due to elastic recoil.

Sensors

A chemoreceptor is a sensor that responds to a change in the chemical composition of the blood; there are two types: central and peripheral. Central chemoreceptors account for 70% of the feedback controlling ventilation, and respond quickly to changes in the pH of cerebrospinal fluid and increases in $PaCO_2$.[5,10] If the $PaCO_2$ remains high for a prolonged period, as in chronic obstructive pulmonary disease (COPD), a compensatory change in bicarbonate (HCO_3^-) occurs and the pH in cerebrospinal fluid returns to its near normal value (Box 13.1).[8]

Central chemoreceptors located in the medulla respond to changes in H^+ concentration in the surrounding cerebrospinal fluid. A change in the $PaCO_2$ causes movement of CO_2 across the blood–brain barrier into the cerebrospinal fluid and alters the H^+ concentration. This increase in H^+ stimulates ventilation. Central chemoreceptors do not, however, respond to changes in the partial pressure of oxygen in arterial blood (PaO_2). Opiates also have a negative influence on these chemoreceptors, reducing sensitivity to changing H^+ concentration.[8] Hyperventilation may reduce $PaCO_2$ to a level that could cause accidental unconsciousness if the breath is held after hyperventilation. This phenomenon is well known among divers and is due to increasing levels of CO_2 as the primary trigger of breathing. If the CO_2 level is too low due to hyperventilation, the breathing reflex is not triggered until the level of oxygen has dropped below what is necessary to maintain consciousness.

BOX 13.1

Oxygen delivery in COPD

Patients with chronic respiratory conditions including COPD, often exhibit signs of hypoxia and hypercarbia, particularly during an acute exacerbation of a chronic condition. There is a strongly held belief that patients who chronically retain CO_2 no longer have a central chemoreceptor response to increased $PaCO_2$ and their drive to breathe is in relation to peripheral chemoreceptor response which detects hypoxia. However, the control of ventilation in such patients is highly complex and involves adaptations of the respiratory control system including changes to respiratory muscles, chemoreceptor signalling, and central respiratory drive.[16] While it is true that an uncontrolled administration of oxygen to patients who chronically retain CO_2 results in hypercarbia, this is mainly because of reversal of hypoxic vasoconstriction and changes to ventilation and perfusion matching. To a lesser extent arterial CO_2 increases because of a rightward shift in the CO_2 dissociation curve (the Haldane effect).[17]

Those patients most likely to develop hypercarbia associated with oxygen administration are also those with the significant hypoxaemia. For patients who chronically retain CO_2 and are hypoxic, the hypoxia must be treated and should be tailored to the patient's clinical condition. Evidence suggests that aiming for oxygen saturation between 88% and 92% results in improved patient outcome.[18,19] For more in-depth description of the physiologic changes associated with COPD please refer to *Further reading* at the end of this chapter.

Peripheral chemoreceptors also play a role in controlling ventilation, although to a lesser extent.[15] Located in the common carotid arteries and in the arch of the aorta, peripheral chemoreceptors detect changes in $PaCO_2$ and H^+ concentration/pH in arterial blood.[10] Peripheral chemoreceptors are sensitive to changes in PaO_2 and are the primary responders to hypoxaemia, stimulating the glossopharyngeal and vagus nerves and providing feedback to the medulla. In response to low PaO_2, such as below 70 mmHg (8 kilopascals [kPa]),[8] they are stimulated and contribute to maintaining ventilation. Other receptors include stretch receptors located in the lungs, which inhibit inspiration and protect the lungs from over-inflation (Hering–Breuer reflex), and in the muscles and joints (Fig. 13.7).

Pulmonary volumes and capacities

In healthy individuals, the lungs are readily distensible or compliant; when exposed to high expanding pressures or in disease states, compliance is increased or decreased. Ranges of lung volumes and capacities are illustrated in

FIGURE 13.8 For lung volume measurements, all values are approximately 25% lower in women.[21]

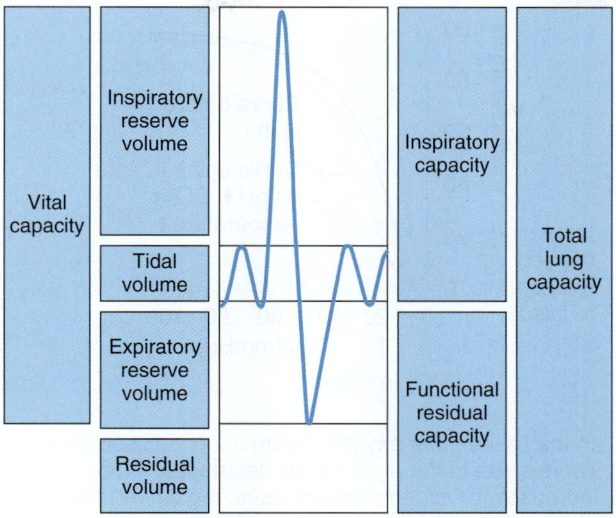

Source: Papana K, Pagana T, Pagana T. (2017). Mosby's Diagnostic and laboratory test reference. 13th ed. Philadelphia: Elsevier.

Fig. 13.8. Tidal volume is the volume of air entering the lungs during a single inspiration and is normally equal to the volume leaving the lungs on expiration (around 500 mL). During inspiration, the tidal volume of inspired air is added to the 2400 mL of air already in the lungs. This remaining volume of air in the lungs after normal expiration is the functional residual capacity[5] which:

- has an important role in keeping small alveoli open and avoiding atelectasis
- can be reduced during anaesthesia or neuromuscular blockade, most likely due to supine positioning, loss of muscle tone and resulting atelectasis[20]
- if reduced, results in the smallest alveoli closing at the end of the expiration (the 'closing volume').

The closing volume plus the residual volume is called the 'closing capacity'. The closure of the smallest airways may occur because dependent areas of the lungs are compressed, although this is not the only mechanism as these airways also close in the weightlessness of space. The closing volume is dependent on patient age: in a young healthy person it is 10% of vital capacity while for an individual aged 65 years it increases to 40%, approximating total functional residual capacity.[8]

Alveolar ventilation

Minute volume represents the volume of gas inhaled or exhaled in 1 minute and is calculated by multiplying the tidal volume by respiratory frequency (e.g. 500 mL × 12 breaths per min = 6000 mL).[22] In this example only the first 350 mL of inhaled air in each breath reaches the alveolar exchange surface, with 150 mL remaining in the conducting airways, referred to as the 'anatomic dead space'. Alveolar ventilation is the amount of inhaled air that reaches the alveoli each minute (e.g. 350 mL × 12 = 4200 mL of alveolar ventilation).[9]

Work of breathing

At rest, the energy required to breathe is minimal (less than 5% of total oxygen consumption).[8] However, changes in airway resistance and lung compliance affect the work of breathing, resulting in increased oxygen consumption.[23] Airway resistance is determined by the diameter of the airways and the airflow: laminar airflow creates lower resistance while turbulent airflow creates higher resistance. Airway resistance is not constant. Certain disease states impact airway resistance, for example during an exacerbation of asthma, where the constricted airways increase resistance.[8] As noted earlier, the lungs are very distensible, expanding during inspiration. This expansion is called the elastic or compliance work and refers to the ease with which lungs expand under pressure. Lung compliance is often monitored when patients are mechanically ventilated, and is calculated by dividing the change in lung volume by the change in transpulmonary pressure (i.e. between the alveoli and pleural space).[24] For the lung to expand, it must overcome lung viscosity and chest wall tissue (called 'tissue resistance work'). Finally, there is airway resistance work – movement of air into the lungs via the airways. The work associated with resistance and compliance is easily overcome in healthy individuals but, in pulmonary disease, both resistance work and compliance work are increased.[25,26] During exertion, when increased muscle function heightens metabolic rate, oxygen demand rises to match consumption and avoid anaerobic metabolism, and work of breathing is increased. The term 'work of breathing' is often used in critical illness, when basic respiratory processes are challenged and breathing consumes a far greater proportion of total energy.

Principles of gas transport and exchange in alveoli and tissues

Oxygen and CO_2 are transported in the bloodstream between alveoli and the tissue cells. Delivery of oxygen to tissues and transfer of CO_2 from the tissues to the capillaries occurs by diffusion and is therefore dependent on the pressure gradient between the capillary and the cell. Diffusion involves molecules moving from areas of high concentration to low concentration. Other determinants of the rate of diffusion include the thickness of the alveolar membrane, the surface area of the membrane available for gas transfer and the inherent solubility of the gas. CO_2 diffuses about 20 times more rapidly than oxygen, being much more soluble in blood.[8] At the most distal ends of the conducting airways lay an extensive network of approximately 300 million alveoli. The surface area of the lungs, if spread out flat, would be about 90 m^2 – about 40 times greater than the surface area of the skin.[5] Gas exchange occurs through the exceptionally thin alveolar membranes. Oxygen uptake takes place from the external environment via the lungs through to the blood in the adjacent alveolar capillary networks. Similarly, CO_2 diffuses from capillaries to the alveoli and is then expired.

Oxygen transport

In oxygenated blood transported by the pulmonary capillaries, there is 20 mL of oxygen in each 100 mL of blood. Oxygen is transported in two ways: dissolved in plasma (about 0.3 mL; 1.5%) with the remainder bound to haemoglobin.[9] Measured by arterial blood gases (ABGs), the 1.5% of oxygen dissolved in blood constitutes the PaO_2.[5] One gram of haemoglobin carries 1.34 mL of oxygen. The level of saturation within the total circulating haemoglobin can be measured clinically, by pulse oximetry. The amount of oxygen actually bound to haemoglobin compared with the amount of oxygen the haemoglobin can carry is commonly reported as arterial oxygen saturation (SaO_2). Oxygen is attached to the haemoglobin molecule at four haem sites. As the majority of oxygen transport is via haemoglobin, if all four sites are occupied by oxygen molecules the blood is determined to be 'fully saturated' (SaO_2 = 100%).[26]

A large reserve of oxygen is available if required, without the need for any increase in respiratory or cardiac workload. Oxygen extraction is the percentage of oxygen extracted and utilised by the tissues. At rest, just 25% of the total oxygen delivered to the tissue is extracted, although this amount does vary throughout the body, with some tissue beds extracting more and others taking less. Normally, the oxygen saturation of venous blood is 60–75%; values below this indicate that more oxygen than normal is being extracted by tissues. This can be due to a reduction in oxygen delivery to the tissues or to an increase in the tissue consumption of oxygen.[9,10]

Oxygen delivery and oxygen consumption are important considerations in the management of critically ill patients. Normal oxygen delivery in a healthy person at rest is approximately 1000 mL/min. Normal oxygen consumption is 200–250 mL/min,[10] but this can increase significantly during episodes of sepsis, fever, hypercatabolism and shivering.[26] The difference between normal delivery and normal consumption highlights the large degree of oxygen reserve available to the body.

FIGURE 13.9 Shift of the oxygen–haemoglobin dissociation curve: (**A**) to the right and (**B**) to the left.[27]

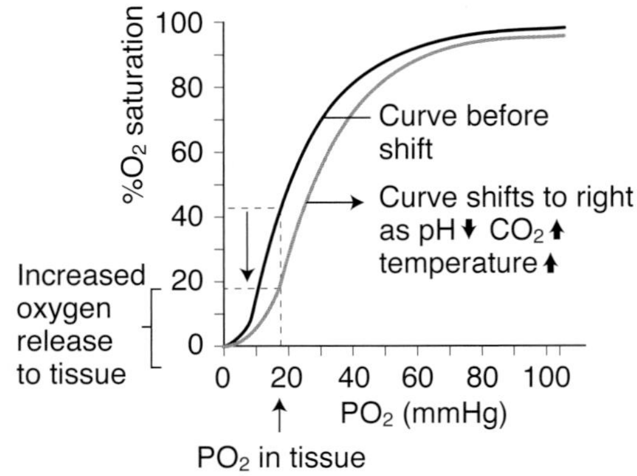

In the tissues, the oxygen–haemoglobin dissociation curve shifts to the right. As pH decreases, PCO_2 increases, or as temperature rises, the curve (black) shifts to the right (blue), resulting in an increased release of oxygen.

A

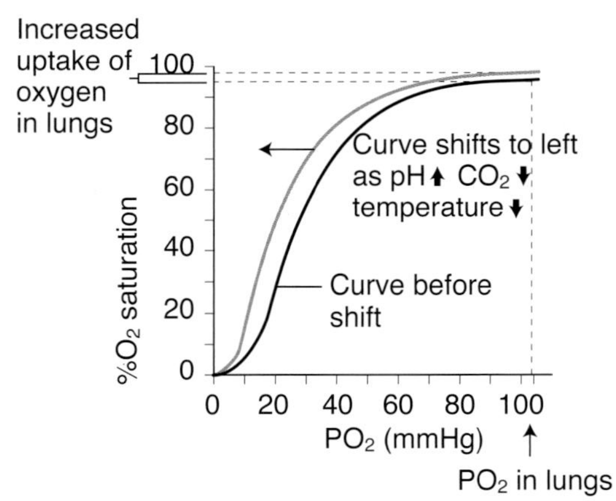

In the lungs, the oxygen–haemoglobin dissociation curve shifts to the left. As pH increases, PCO_2 decreases, or as temperature falls, the curve (black) shifts to the left (blue), resulting in an increased ability of haemoglobin to pick up oxygen.

B

Adapted from Seely R, Stephens T, Tate P. Anatomy and physiology. 7th ed. Boston: McGraw Hill; 2006.

Oxygen–haemoglobin dissociation curve

As blood is transported to the tissues and end-organs, the tendency of haemoglobin and oxygen to combine decreases, relative to the surrounding arterial oxygen tension. This relationship is illustrated by the oxygen–haemoglobin dissociation curve (Fig. 13.9). As oxygen is offloaded at the tissue level, CO_2 binds more readily with haemoglobin, to be transported back to the lungs for removal.[5]

The oxygen–haemoglobin dissociation curve relates the partial pressure of oxygen to the haemoglobin saturation in blood. While the initial part of the curve rises steeply, the latter part of the curve flattens representing the binding of oxygen to haemoglobin in the lungs. In the upper part of the curve (within the lungs), relatively large changes in the PaO_2 cause only small changes in haemoglobin saturation. Therefore, if the

PaO_2 drops from 100 to 60 mmHg (14–8 kPa), the saturation of haemoglobin changes only 7% (from a normal 97% to 90%). As long as PaO_2 remains above 60 mmHg (7.8 kPa) haemoglobin will be more than 90% saturated. The minimal changes in oxygen binding within this substantial PO_2 range allow survival at high altitudes.[9] The lower portion (steep component) of the oxygen–haemoglobin dissociation curve, between 40 and 60 mmHg (5–8 kPa), represents the release of oxygen from haemoglobin in tissue capillaries. At this point, a small drop in PaO_2 will cause a large increase in oxygen unloading. As haemoglobin is further desaturated, larger amounts of oxygen are released for tissue use, ensuring an adequate oxygen supply to peripheral tissues, even when oxygen delivery is reduced. Oxygen saturation remains at 70–75%, leaving a significant amount of oxygen in reserve. Normally only 25% of bound oxygen is unloaded during one systemic circuit. However, during exercise when the muscles need more oxygen, the PaO_2 drops and more oxygen dissociates from haemoglobin for use by muscle cells without any complementary increase in respiratory rate or cardiac output.[9]

The relationship between the two axes of this curve assumes values for haemoglobin, pH, temperature, $PaCO_2$ and 2,3-bisphosphoglycerate, a product of the breakdown of red blood cells that binds reversibly with haemoglobin, are normal. Changes to any of these values will shift the curve to the right or left and therefore reflect different values for PaO_2 and SaO_2[9] (Fig. 13.9).

Both the binding and dissociation of oxygen to haemoglobin are reversible reactions depending on the surrounding tissue. When the curve shifts to the right there is a reduced capacity for oxygen binding to haemoglobin in the lungs but oxygen is more readily released to the tissues. At a local level, in active tissue such as working muscle that generates lactic acid, acid release lowers the pH resulting in release of oxygen from haemoglobin molecules to the surrounding tissue. The same process occurs when active skeletal muscle generates heat. The increase in local temperature leads to oxygen release for use by the surrounding muscle.[9]

As blood is transported to the tissues and end-organs, the binding affinity of haemoglobin and oxygen decreases relative to the surrounding arterial oxygen tension. As oxygen is offloaded at the tissue level, CO_2 binds more readily with haemoglobin, to be transported to the lungs for removal.[5]

Carbon dioxide transport

CO_2 is transported by blood in three forms: combined with water as carbonic acid (80–90%), dissolved (5%) or attached to plasma proteins (5–10%), including haemoglobin. The dissolved CO_2 constitutes $PaCO_2$ and is measured by ABGs. The greater solubility of CO_2 compared with oxygen results in its rapid diffusion across the capillary membranes, and its easy removal.[5] As a byproduct of cellular respiration, CO_2 is produced at a rate of 200 mL/min, with only minor differences in normal concentrations in arterial (480 mL/L) and venous (520 mL/L) blood.[10]

Relationship between ventilation and perfusion

Gas exchange is the key function of the lungs, and the unique anatomy of capillaries and alveoli facilitates this process. However, because of a number of physiological factors, the ventilation to perfusion ratio (V/Q) is not matched in a 1 : 1 relationship. As normal alveolar ventilation is about 4 L/min and pulmonary capillary perfusion is about 5 L/min, the normal V/Q is 0.8.[8] In addition, pressure in the pulmonary circulation is low relative to systemic pressure, and is influenced much more by gravity and hydrostatic pressure. In the upright position, lung apices receive less perfusion compared with the bases.[8] In the supine position, apical and basal perfusions are almost equal, but the posterior (dependent) portion of the lungs receives greater perfusion than the anterior lung area. Ventilation is also uneven throughout the lung, with the bases receiving more ventilation per unit volume than the apices.[8]

Pressure within the surrounding alveoli also influences blood flow through the pulmonary capillary network. The pressure gradients between the arterial and venous ends of a capillary network normally determine blood flow. However, alveolar pressure (P_A) can be greater than venous (P_v) and/or arterial (P_a) pressure, and therefore influences blood flow and gas exchange.

For a patient in an upright position, perfusion and ventilation vary as follows:

- Zone 1 (upper area of the lungs): alveolar pressure is generally greater than both arterial and venous capillary pressure [$P_A > P_a > P_v$], and blood flow is reduced, leading to alveolar dead space (alveoli ventilated but not adequately perfused).
- Zone 2 (middle portion of the lungs): perfusion and gas exchange are influenced more by pressure differences between arterial and alveolar pressures than by the usual difference between arterial and venous pressures [$P_a > P_A > P_v$], with a normal V/Q ratio.
- Zone 3 (lung bases): alveolar pressure is lower than both arterial and venous pressures [$P_a > P_v > P_A$], and ventilation is reduced, leading to intrapulmonary shunting (alveoli perfused but not adequately ventilated)[8] (Fig. 13.10).

These physiological relationships are more complex in a critically ill patient when ventilation and/or lung perfusion is further compromised by disease processes and positive pressure ventilation, and the patient is in a supine or semi-recumbent position.[8,23]

Acid–base control: respiratory mechanisms

The respiratory system plays a vital role in acid–base balance. Changes in respiratory rate and depth can

FIGURE 13.10 The effects of gravity and alveolar pressure on pulmonary blood flow. Notice the three lung zones.[22]

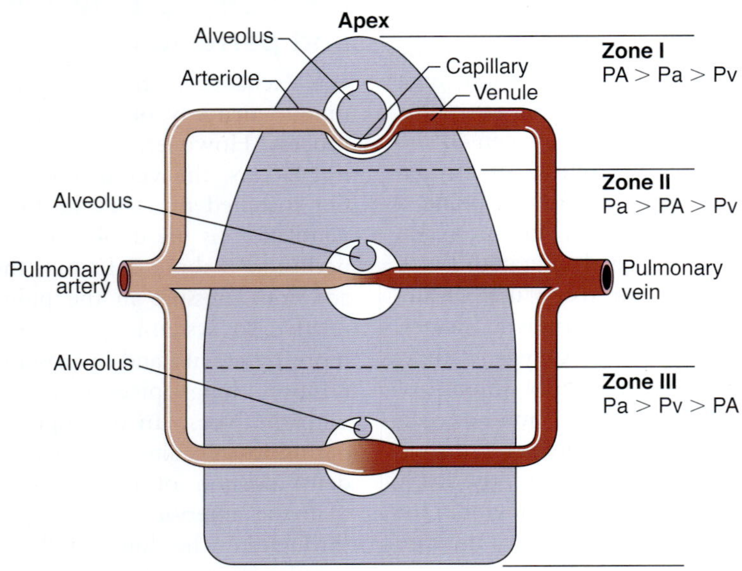

Source: Urden LD, Stacy KM, Lough ME. (2014). Critical care nursing: diagnosis and management. 7th ed. St. Louis: Mosby.

produce changes in body pH by altering the amount of carbonic acid (H_2CO_3) in the blood. The body has substantial control over acid–base balance by altering alveolar ventilation and the elimination of CO_2 through the lungs. The elimination of acid through the lungs is more than 100 times more efficient than the elimination of acid through the kidneys. If CO_2 in body water increases due to low alveolar ventilation, more H^+ will be produced because CO_2 combines with H_2O to form H_2CO_3. This breaks down to HCO_3^- and H^+ resulting in a decrease in pH.

$$CO_2 + H_2O \leftrightarrow H_2CO_3 \leftrightarrow HCO_3^- + H^+$$

The strength of the dissociation is defined by the Henderson–Hasselbalch equation, which describes the relationship between HCO_3^-, CO_2 and pH, and explains why an increase in dissolved CO_2 causes an increase in the acidity of the plasma, while an increase in HCO_3^- causes the pH to rise resulting in more alkaline plasma:

$$pH = 6.1 + \log(HCO_3^-)(CO_2)$$

where 6.1 = the negative logarithm of the acid dissociation constant in plasma for carbonic acid.[8]

Respiratory acidosis is caused by CO_2 retention and increases the denominator in the Henderson–Hasselbalch equation resulting in a decreased pH level. In a spontaneously breathing patient, this condition occurs due to hypoventilation from either shallow breaths and/or a low respiratory rate. In the acute state the body cannot compensate. If the patient develops chronic CO_2 retention over a long period, there will be a renal response to the increase in CO_2. The renal system retains HCO_3^- to return the pH to normal (i.e. respiratory acidosis is compensated).

Respiratory alkalosis occurs when a patient hyperventilates and alveolar ventilation is increased as a result of large, frequent breaths; CO_2 decreases in arterial blood and the pH rises. If this condition is maintained (e.g. walking at high altitude), the kidneys excrete HCO_3^- and the pH returns to normal (i.e. the respiratory alkalosis is compensated).[8]

Pathophysiology

Three common pathophysiological concepts that influence respiratory function in critically ill patients are hypoxaemia, inflammation and oedema. Related disease states including respiratory failure, pneumonia, ARDS, asthma and COPD are described in Chapter 14.

Hypoxaemia

Hypoxaemia describes a decrease in the PaO_2 of less than 60 mmHg (7.8 kPa).[5] This leads to less efficient anaerobic metabolism at the tissue and end-organ level, and compromised cellular function. Hypoxia is abnormally low PO_2 in the tissues, and can be due to:

- 'hypoxic' hypoxia – low PaO_2 in arterial blood due to pulmonary disease
- 'circulatory' hypoxia – reduction of tissue blood flow due to shock or local obstruction
- 'anaemic' hypoxia – reduced ability of the blood to carry oxygen due to anaemia or carbon monoxide poisoning

- 'histotoxic' hypoxia – a cellular environment that does not support oxygen utilisation due to tissue poisoning (e.g. cyanide poisoning).[8]

A hypoxic patient can show symptoms of fatigue and shortness of breath if the hypoxia has developed gradually. If the patient has severe hypoxia with rapid onset, they will have ashen skin and blue discolouration (cyanosis) of the oral mucosa, lips and nail beds. Confusion, disorientation and anxiety are other symptoms. In later stages, unconsciousness, coma and death occur.[28] Acute respiratory failure is a common patient presentation in ICU occurring in 10% of ICU admissions and it is characterised by decreased gas exchange with resultant hypoxaemia. ARDS is one such example.[29] Two different mechanisms cause acute respiratory failure: Type 1 presents with low PaO_2 and normal $PaCO_2$; Type 2 presents with low PaO_2 and high $PaCO_2$ (see Chapter 14 for further discussion).

In general, impaired gas exchange results from alveolar hypoventilation, ventilation/perfusion mismatching and intrapulmonary shunting, each resulting in hypoxaemia. Hypercapnia may also be present depending on the underlying pathophysiology.[30]

Alveolar hypoventilation occurs when the metabolic needs of the body are not met by the amount of oxygen delivered and CO_2 removed from the alveoli. Alveolar hypoventilation causing hypoxaemia is usually extrapulmonary (e.g. altered metabolism, interruption to neuromuscular control of breathing/ventilation) and is associated with hypercapnia.[31]

V/Q mismatch results when areas of lung that are perfused are not ventilated (no participation in gas exchange) because alveoli are collapsed or infiltrated with fluid from inflammation or infection (e.g. pulmonary oedema, pneumonia). This results in an overall reduction in blood oxygen levels, which is usually countered by compensatory mechanisms.[31]

Intrapulmonary shunting is an extreme case of V/Q mismatch. Shunting occurs when blood passes alveoli that are not ventilated. If there is significant intrapulmonary shunting, there may be overwhelming reductions in PaO_2.[32] CO_2 levels may still be normal but, depending on the onset and progression of respiratory pathophysiology, compensatory mechanisms may not be able to maintain homeostasis[10] (Fig. 13.11[33]).

FIGURE 13.11 Ventilation–perfusion mismatch.[33]

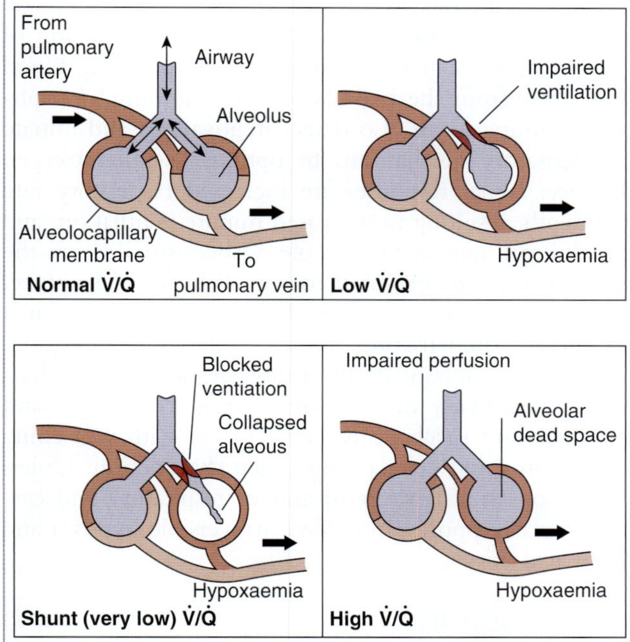

Source: Carlson K. Advanced critical care nursing. St. Louis: Saunders Elsevier; 2009.

Tissue hypoxia

There are few physiological changes with mild hypoxaemia (when oxygen saturation remains at 90% despite a PaO_2 of 60 mmHg [8 kPa]), with only a slight impairment in mental state. If hypoxaemia worsens and the PaO_2 drops to 40–50 mmHg (5.3–6.7 kPa), severe tissue hypoxia ensues. Hypoxia at the central nervous system level manifests with headaches and somnolence. Compensatory mechanisms include catecholamine release, and a decrease in renal function results in sodium retention and proteinuria.[8]

Different tissues vary in their vulnerability to hypoxia, with the central nervous system and myocardium at most risk. Hypoxia in the cerebral cortex results in a loss of function within 4–6 seconds, loss of consciousness in 10–20 seconds and irreversible damage in 3–5 minutes. In an environment that lacks oxygen, cells function by anaerobic metabolism and produce much less energy. For example, with aerobic metabolism 38 molecules of adenosine triphosphate are generated compared with two molecules of adenosine triphosphate generated in anaerobic metabolism. During anaerobic metabolism, lactic acid also increases. With less energy available, the efficiency of cellular functions such as the sodium–potassium pump, nerve conduction, enzyme activity and transmembrane receptor function is diminished.[8] The overall effect of interruption to these vital cellular activities is a reduction in organ or tissue function, which in turn compromises system and body functions.

Changes to the oxygen–haemoglobin association-dissociation curve also occur in states related to hypoxia. The curve shifts to the right when there is acidosis and/or raised levels of $PaCO_2$ as commonly seen in respiratory failure. The shift in the oxygen–haemoglobin dissociation curve to the right means that, in the lung, fewer oxygen molecules attach to the haemoglobin molecule, resulting in a decrease in arterial oxygen saturation. However, the oxygen that does attach to the haemoglobin molecule is more readily released at the tissue level.[8]

Compensatory mechanisms to optimise oxygenation

When PO_2 in the alveoli is reduced, regional hypoxic pulmonary vasoconstriction occurs, with contraction of smooth muscles in the small arterioles, directing blood flow away from the hypoxic area of the lung.[8] Peripheral chemoreceptors also detect hypoxaemia and initiate compensatory mechanisms to optimise cellular oxygen delivery. Initial responses are increased respiratory rate and depth, resulting in increased minute ventilation, and raised heart rate with possible vasoconstriction as the body attempts to maintain oxygen delivery and uptake. Increased respiratory rate is the first 'best' sign that a patient is compensating for an underlying condition. This overall upregulation cannot be sustained indefinitely, particularly in a person who is critically ill, and compensatory mechanisms begin to fail with worsening hypoxaemia and cellular and organ dysfunction. Unless the hypoxaemia is reversed and/or respiratory and cardiovascular support is provided, irreversible hypoxia and death will ensue.

Inflammation

Inflammatory processes can occur at a local level (e.g. as a result of inhalation injuries, aspiration or respiratory infections) or are secondary to systemic events (e.g. sepsis, trauma). Damage to the pulmonary endothelium and type I alveolar cells appears to play a key role in the inflammatory processes associated with ARDS.[34] Once triggered, inflammation results in platelet aggregation and complement release. Platelet aggregation attracts neutrophils, which release inflammatory mediators (e.g. proteolytic enzymes, oxygen free radicals, leukotrienes, prostaglandins and platelet-activating factor). Neutrophils also appear to play a key role in the perpetuation of ARDS.[31] As well as altering pulmonary capillary permeability, resulting in haemorrhage and leaking of fluid into the pulmonary interstitium and alveoli, mediators released by neutrophils and some macrophages precipitate pulmonary vasoconstriction. Resulting pulmonary hypertension leads to diminished perfusion to some lung areas, with dramatic alterations to both perfusion and ventilation leading to significant V/Q mismatch, and the subsequent signs and symptoms typically seen in patients with pulmonary inflammation/oedema.

Oedema

Pulmonary oedema also alters gas exchange, and results from abnormal accumulation of extravascular fluid in the lung. Two main reasons for this are an increase in hydrostatic or osmotic forces, as seen in left ventricular dysfunction or volume overload, and increased membrane permeability of the lung epithelium or endothelium, allowing accumulation of fluid. This is referred to as non-cardiogenic pulmonary oedema. ARDS may result from increased permeability of the epithelium. A more detailed discussion of ARDS is provided in Chapter 14.

Changes to respiratory function

During the early exudative phase of ARDS, tachypnoea, signs of hypoxaemia (apprehension, restlessness) and an increase in the use of accessory muscles are usually evident. These symptoms result from infiltration of fluid into the alveoli. With impaired production of surfactant during the proliferative phase, respiratory function deteriorates, and dyspnoea, agitation, fatigue and the emergence of fine crackles on auscultation are common.[31] Airway resistance is increased when oedema affects larger airways. Lung compliance is reduced as interstitial oedema interferes with the elastic properties of the lungs, and it may become challenging to adequately ventilate patients. Infiltration of type II alveolar cells into the epithelium may lead to interstitial fibrosis on healing causing chronic lung dysfunction.[35]

Respiratory dysfunction: changes to work of breathing

Without reversal of respiratory compromise, significant increases to the work of breathing will result. Clinical manifestations include tachypnoea, tachycardia, dyspnoea, low tidal volumes and diaphoresis. Hypercapnia ensues, which further compromises respiratory muscle function and precipitates diaphragmatic fatigue. Oxygen consumption during breathing can be so great that reserve capacity is reduced. If patients with pre-existing COPD (who may breathe close to the fatigue work level) experience an acute exacerbation, this can easily tip them into a fatigued state. Early identification and management of respiratory compromise before these stages improves patient outcomes.[8]

Assessment

Respiratory insufficiency is a common reason for admission to ICU, for either a potential or an actual problem, so comprehensive and frequent respiratory assessments are an essential practice role. This section outlines history taking, physical examination, bedside monitoring and diagnostic testing focused on a critically ill patient with respiratory dysfunction.

Assessment is a systematic process comprising history taking of a patient's present and previous illnesses and physical examination of their thorax, lungs and related systems. History taking and physical examination can occur simultaneously if the patient is very ill. Related diagnostic findings inform an accurate and comprehensive assessment. A thorough assessment, followed by accurate ongoing monitoring, enables early detection of changes in condition and the impact of treatment. Depending on a patient's situation, assessment can be either brief or detailed.

Patient history

History taking determines a patient's baseline respiratory status on ICU admission. If the patient is distressed only a few questions should be asked but, if the patient is able, a more comprehensive interview can be performed, focusing on four areas: the current problem, previous problems, symptoms and personal and family history. Question a family member or close friend if a patient is unable to provide their own history.

When introducing yourself, ask the patient's name, seek eye contact and create a rapport with the patient and the family. Ensure that the patient is in a comfortable position, ideally sitting up in bed. Provide privacy so that the interview is confidential. The physical examination should maintain the patient's dignity and modesty. To minimise distress for a patient who is acutely breathless, the use of short closed questions is preferable.

Practice tip

History taking by the nurse should be an interactive experience, especially the initial interview where both the patient and nurse learn a lot about each other. If the patient is too sick to be interviewed, as often is the case in ICU, the nurse can instead invite a person who is considered a 'significant other' to the patient to contribute to the patient history. This may capture important information and can contribute to patient and family-participation in care through the meaningful bringing together of patient, family and nurse.

Current respiratory problems

Begin by asking the patient about their difficulty breathing. If possible, let the patient describe the respiratory problem in his or her own words. Be focused and listen actively. Ask for location, onset and duration of the respiratory symptoms.

Previous respiratory problems

Many respiratory disorders can be chronic and pulmonary diseases may recur (e.g. tuberculosis). New diseases can complicate existing ones.[36] Problems with breathing and chest problems, number of hospitalisations, treatments and childhood respiratory diseases should be discussed with the patient.

Symptoms

Assess the onset and duration, pattern, severity and episodic or continuous nature of presenting symptoms. Also ask about the patient's perception of their respiratory problem, their opinion about its cause and, if the symptoms cause fatigue, anxiety or stress. Ask specifically about dyspnoea, cough, sputum production, haemoptysis, wheezing, chest pain or other pain, sleep disturbances and snoring.

Dyspnoea (shortness of breath) is subjective and therefore difficult to grade. The mechanism that underlies the sensation of dyspnoea is poorly understood but it is extremely uncomfortable and frightening.[36]

Assess the severity of dyspnoea by asking about breathing in relation to activities (e.g. breathlessness when dressing or walking across a room). Ask the patient how many pillows they need to sleep as this may indicate the severity of any *orthopnoea* (shortness of breath when lying flat). Orthopnoea can be a symptom of increased blood in the pulmonary circulation due to left ventricular failure, pulmonary oedema, bronchitis, asthma or obstructive sleep apnoea.

A cough can be dry or productive, episodic or continuous and, if exacerbated when the patient is lying flat, can imply heart failure. A cough can also be related to viral infections and allergies or may indicate intrathoracic disease. Ask the patient if they wake at night due to the cough, how long the cough has been present and if it is getting better or worse.

Sputum production should be considered for amount, colour or the presence of blood. Yellow or green sputum is typical in bacterial infection. Haemoptysis or sputum mixed with blood is a significant finding and can indicate tuberculosis or lung cancer. Wheezing can indicate vocal cord disorder or asthma.[36]

Chest pain can result from multiple causes; therefore, appropriate assessment is essential. Chest pain that occurs during inspiration can be due to irritation or inflammation of the pleural surface. Pleural pain is experienced mostly on one side of the chest, is knifelike in character and occurs in pneumonia, pleurisy and pneumothorax. Chest pain also occurs with fractured ribs.

The most ominous chest pain occurs as a result of myocardial ischaemia, due to poor oxygen delivery to the coronary vessels. This pain is termed angina pectoris and can arise from chronic stable angina or acute coronary syndrome[36] (see Chapter 10 for further discussion).

Sleep disturbance and snoring may be related to obstructive sleep apnoea. If the patient complains about drowsiness in the daytime, ask how many hours of continuous sleep they have at night, and whether they take a nap during the day.

Personal and family history

Family history and environment can influence pulmonary presentations. The focus of this questioning is on: tobacco use, allergies, recent travel, occupational risk, home situation and family history. Use of tobacco, current or past, is important in evaluating pulmonary symptoms. Ask the patient to quantify the amount of cigarette packs per week and how many years they have smoked. The majority of smokers have reduced lung function. Tobacco smoking is responsible for 80% of the risk of developing COPD. Exposure to second-hand smoke may also be of interest, with evidence that extended exposure is a major cause of chronic bronchitis.[37] A history of recent travel increases possible exposure to infectious respiratory diseases.[38] Recent long flights increase the possibility of deep venous thrombosis, which can lead to pulmonary embolism.[39] An occupation with exposure to allergens and toxins is important

TABLE 13.1
Description of different respiratory patterns[26]

Normal	A 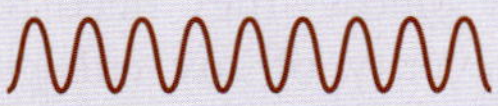 Regular and comfortable at a rate of 12–20 per min	Air trapping	B 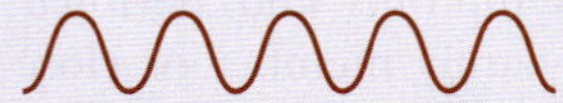 Increasing difficulty in getting breath out
Bradypnoea	C 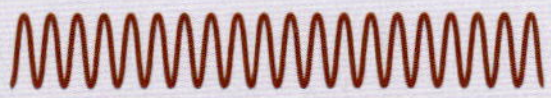 Slower than 12 breaths/min	Cheyne–Stokes	D 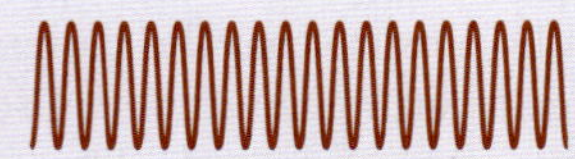 Varying periods of increasing depth interspersed with apnoea
Tachypnoea	E 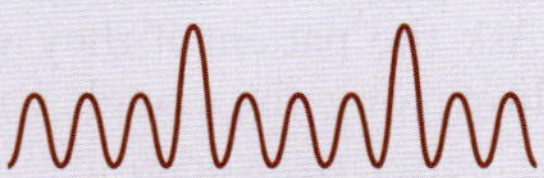 Faster than 20 breaths/min	Kussmaul	F 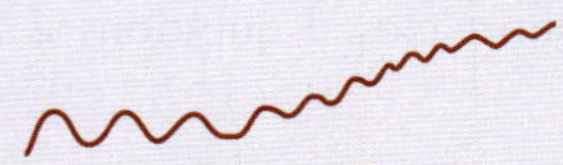 Rapid, deep, laboured
Hyperventilation (hyperpnoea)	G 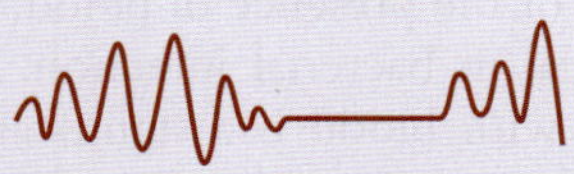 Faster than 20 breaths/min, deep breathing	Biot	H 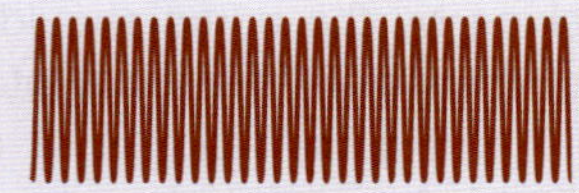 Irregularly interspersed periods of apnoea in a disorganised sequence of breaths
Sighing	I 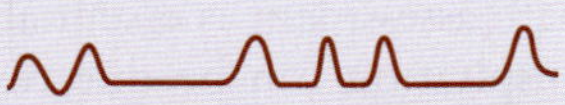 Frequently interspersed deeper breath	Ataxic	J 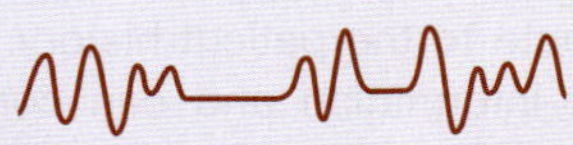 Significant disorganisation with irregular and varying depths of respiration

Adapted from: Morton P, Rempfer K. Patient assessment: respiratory system. In: Morton P, Fontaine D, eds. Critical care nursing: a holistic approach. 9th ed. Philadelphia: Wolters, Kluwer/Lippincott Williams & Wilkins; 2009.

to document as this can be associated with declining lung function.[40] Ask about the patient's home situation and whether they live with someone with an illness such as influenza or tuberculosis. Ask about children who are close to the patient, as innocuous viral infections in small children may account for severe disease in adults.[36] Also check for a family history of cancer and heart or respiratory diseases.

Physical examination

The four activities of physical examination are inspection, palpation, percussion and auscultation. Prior to commencing the examination, prepare the patient as well as possible by providing privacy, warmth, good light and quiet surroundings. Explain that the examination is a standard procedure and you will use your eyes, hands and a stethoscope. Help the patient into a comfortable sitting position in the bed if possible and have all necessary equipment easily accessible.

Inspection

Inspection involves carefully observing the patient from head to toe for signs of respiratory problems. Focus on: patient position, chest wall inspection, respiratory rate and rhythm, respiratory effort, central or peripheral cyanosis and clubbing. Note what position appears preferable for the patient; whether they look comfortable in bed, have trouble breathing or appear anxious. Observe chest wall symmetry during the respiratory cycle, anatomical structures and for the presence of scars. The most important sign of respiratory distress is respiratory rate and rhythm. The respiratory rate should be assessed over a 1-minute period so that an accurate measurement is obtained. Normal respiratory rate for adults is 12–15 per minute.[5] Abnormal breathing patterns are noted in Table 13.1.[26] Observe respiratory effort, in particular the use of accessory muscles, abdominal muscles, nasal flaring, body position and mouth-breathing.

Inspect the lips, tongue and sublingual area for central cyanosis (a late sign of hypoxia that is almost impossible to detect in a patient with anaemia).[31] Observe the extremities for oedema (can be a sign of heart failure), fingers and toes for peripheral cyanosis and clubbing of the nail beds. Peripheral cyanosis may indicate low blood flow to peripheral areas. Clubbing of finger or toe nail beds can be idiopathic or more commonly due to

FIGURE 13.12 Sequence of systematic movements for palpation, percussion and auscultation of the posterior (**A**) and anterior (**B**) chest. Comparison of the right and left sides of the chest should be performed by moving from side to side, beginning proximally and moving distally down the chest wall.[41]

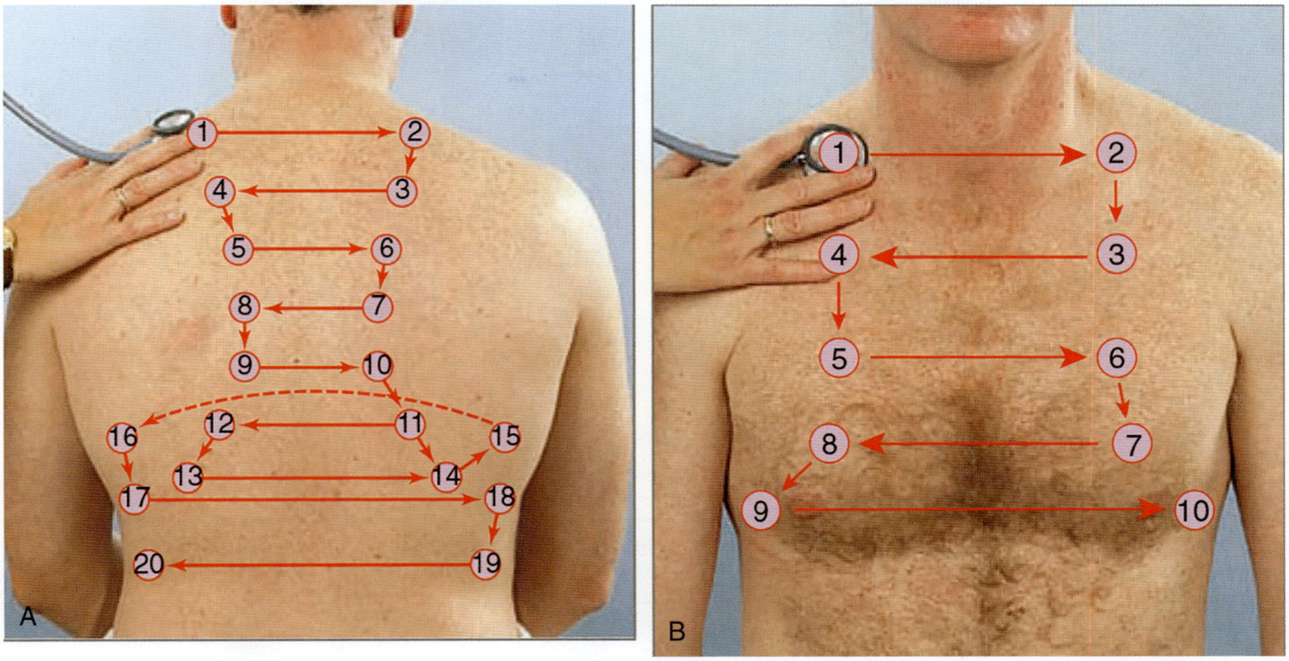

Source: Weber J, Kelly J. Health assessment in nursing. Philadelphia: Lippincott, Williams & Wilkins; 2010.

respiratory or circulatory diseases (e.g. chronic hypoxia in congenital heart disease).[36] Note also if the patient requires oxygen and record the dose. If the patient is intubated and mechanically ventilated (monitoring is explained later in this chapter), ensure the airway is adequately secured. If the patient is orally intubated, observe the mouth for the presence of lesions or pressure on the oral mucosa and lips; and observe the size of the tube, the length at the lips or teeth margin and how it is secured. If the patient has a tracheostomy, observe the stoma for signs of infection or pressure areas, the type and size of tracheostomy tube, the length at the hub if it is a tracheostomy with an adjustable flange and the manner of securement.

Palpation

Palpate the patient's chest with warm hands, focusing on: areas of tenderness, tracheal position, presence of subcutaneous emphysema and tactile fremitus. Assess for symmetry (left compared to right) and follow a systematic sequence of palpation over anterior and posterior surfaces (Fig. 13.12). Check the thorax for areas of tenderness or bony deformities and note symmetry of chest movement during breathing. Use the palm of your hand to assess skin temperature, noting clammy, hot or cold skin. To test for chest wall symmetry on inspiration, place both hands with thumbs together on the patient's posterior thorax and ask them to take a deep breath. Your thumbs should separate equally 3–5 cm during normal deep inspiration[31] (Fig. 13.13[41]). Asymmetry can occur in pneumothorax, pneumonia or other lung disorders where inspiration is affected.

Palpation of the tracheal position is useful to detect a mediastinal shift; deviation of the trachea from midline may indicate a pulmonary problem such as large pneumothorax or previous pneumonectomy.[42] The presence of subcutaneous emphysema indicates air in the subcutaneous tissue and feels like crackling under your fingers due to air pockets in the tissue.[43] This most commonly occurs in the face, neck and chest: after blunt or penetrating trauma to the chest (e.g. stabbing, gun shot, fractured ribs); facial fractures; tracheostomy; respiratory tract surgery; and in patients who are mechanically ventilated.

Palpation is also used to assess for tactile (vocal) fremitus, a normal palpable vibration. Place your hands on the patient's chest and ask them to vocalise repeatedly the term 'ninety-nine'. Fremitus is decreased (that is, impaired transmission of sounds) in pleural effusion and pneumothorax. Fremitus is increased over regions of lung where transmission is increased (e.g. pneumonia, consolidation).[36] In mechanically-ventilated patients,

FIGURE 13.13 Assessment of thoracic expansion. (**A**) Exhalation. (**B**) Inhalation.[3]

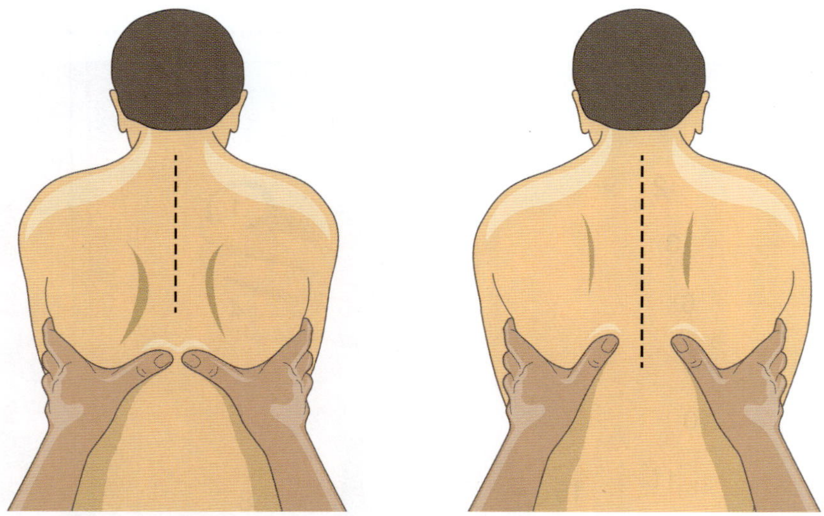

Reproduced from Urden L, Stacy K, Lough M. Critical care nursing: diagnosis and management. 6th ed. St Louis: Mosby; 2010, with permission.

fremitus can be detected when there are secretions in the airways.

Percussion

By tapping the chest with the bony structures of the hands, percussion can help to determine if the lung spaces are filled with air, fluid or sputum consolidation. Place your non-dominant hand with your middle finger extended over the area of chest to be examined. Using the middle finger of your dominant hand, tap on the distal knuckle of the finger resting on the chest wall. Starting from the upper chest wall and moving from side to side, following the same sequence as for palpation (see Fig. 13.12), compare one side to the other for variation in sound. Normally, the chest has a resonant percussion tone. A flat percussive note, soft and high-pitched, may indicate a large pleural effusion. A dull percussive note with medium intensity and pitch is heard in the presence of atelectasis, pulmonary oedema, pulmonary haemorrhage or pneumonia.[25]

Practice tip

When performing palpation or percussion of the chest with your hand and auscultation of the chest with a stethoscope, the patient will appreciate the hand and stethoscope being warmed prior to placing them on the skin.

Practice tip

When performing chest inspection, percussion and auscultation, always compare one side of the body with the other.

Auscultation

Careful interpretation of breath sounds and integration of this assessment data with other findings can provide important information about lung disorders. Use the diaphragm of the stethoscope and ensure full contact with the skin for optimal listening. For a spontaneously breathing patient, ask them to breathe through their mouth (nose breathing may alter the pitch of the breath sounds). Auscultation is performed in a systematic way so as to compare the symmetry of breath sounds (Fig. 13.12). Normal breath sounds reflect air movement through the bronchi, and sounds change as air moves from larger to smaller airways. Sounds also change when air passes though fluid or narrowed airways. Breath sounds therefore differ depending on the area auscultated. The three types of normal breath sounds are bronchial, bronchovesicular and vesicular breath sounds (Table 13.2), and these should be heard only in the areas specific to their region. If heard in the wrong place, for example bronchial breath sounds heard in the lung peripheries, it suggests consolidation.

It is important to identify and become familiar with normal breath sounds before beginning to listen for

TABLE 13.2
Characteristics of normal breath sounds

SOUND	CHARACTERISTICS
Vesicular	Heard over most of the lung field; low pitch; soft and short exhalation and long inhalation
Bronchovesicular	Heard over main bronchus area and over right posterior lung field; medium pitch; exhalation equals inhalation
Bronchial	Heard only over trachea; high pitch; loud and long exhalation

Urden L, Stacy K, Lough M. Critical care nursing: diagnosis and management. 6th ed. St Louis: Mosby; 2010.

and identify abnormal breath sounds. Abnormal breath sounds are either continuous or discontinuous. Continuous sounds include wheezes and rhonchi, while discontinuous sounds include crackles (Table 13.3). Stridor is an abnormally loud high-pitched breath sound caused by obstruction in the upper airways as a result of a foreign body, tissue or vocal cord swelling; this emergent condition requires immediate attention.[44] Absent or diminished breath sounds also require immediate treatment as it may indicate a lack of airflow through to that area of the lung.[44]

Practice tip

Use an alcohol wipe to clean the earpieces on the stethoscope prior to use to protect yourself from infection.

Identify and become familiar with normal breath sounds before beginning to listen and identify abnormal breath sounds. Abnormal breath sounds are either continuous or discontinuous. Continuous sounds include wheezes and rhonchi, while discontinuous sounds include crackles (see Table 13.3). Stridor is an abnormal, loud, high-pitched breath sound caused by obstruction in the upper airways as a result of a foreign body, tissue or vocal cord swelling; this emergent condition requires immediate attention.[46] Absent or diminished breath sounds also require immediate treatment, indicating no airflow through that area of the lung.[45]

Practice tip

Respiratory rate is an early warning sign for respiratory distress. If the patient has a high respiratory rate it can be a sign of hypoxia as the patient attempts to compensate for low PaO_2.

TABLE 13.3
Description of abnormal breath sounds[23]

ABNORMAL SOUND	DESCRIPTION	CONDITION
Absent breath sounds	No airflow to particular portion of lung	Pneumothorax Pneumonectomy Emphysematous blebs Pleural effusion Lung mass Massive atelectasis Complete airway obstruction
Diminished breath sounds	Little airflow to particular portion of lung	Emphysema Pleural effusion Pleurisy Atelectasis Pulmonary fibrosis
Displaced bronchial sounds	Bronchial sounds heard in peripheral lung fields	Atelectasis with secretions Lung mass with exudates Pneumonia Pleural effusion Pulmonary oedema
Crackles (rales)	Short, discrete popping or crackling sounds	Pulmonary oedema Pneumonia Pulmonary fibrosis Atelectasis Bronchiectasis
Rhonchi	Coarse, rumbling, low-pitched sounds	Pneumonia Asthma Bronchitis Bronchospasm
Wheezes	High-pitched, squeaking, whistling sounds	Asthma Bronchospasm
Pleural friction rub	Creaking, leathery, loud, dry, coarse sounds	Pleural effusion Pleurisy

Adapted from Urden L, Stacey K, Lough M. Critical care nursing: diagnosis and management. 6th ed. St Louis: Mosby; 2010.

Documentation and charting

Document the findings of your respiratory assessment in the patient's chart; if this is the first respiratory assessment, describe the patient's respiratory history carefully. Any abnormal findings including abnormal sounds and their characteristics should be described to enable subsequent reassessment.

Respiratory monitoring

A thorough and comprehensive assessment, with accurate ongoing monitoring, enables early detection of changes and assessment of responses to treatment for the critically ill. This section describes the main aspects of bedside respiratory monitoring and the instruments used to assess the efficiency of a patient's gas transfer mechanisms, including pulse oximetry, capnography, airway pressures and ventilator waveforms and loops.

Pulse oximetry

Pulse oximetry is a non-invasive device that measures the oxygen saturation of haemoglobin in a patient's arterial blood. The technology is common in critical and acute care areas. It is important to note that the device does not provide information on the patient's ventilatory state, but may determine oxygen saturation and detect hypoxaemia. This prompt, non-invasive detection of hypoxaemia enables detection of clinical deterioration and more rapid treatment to avoid associated complications.[47]

Pulse oximetry works by emitting two wavelengths of light, red and infrared, that pass through a pulsatile flow of blood from a diode (positioned on one side of the probe) to a photodetector (positioned on the opposite side). The signal emitted is measured over five pulses, causing a slight delay when monitoring. Oxygenated blood absorbs light differently from deoxygenated blood; the oximeter measures the amount of light absorbed by the vascular bed and calculates the percentage of haemoglobin saturation in the capillaries.

Indirect measurement of arterial oxygen saturation via the peripheral circulation using pulse oximetry is referred to as SpO_2 (the symbol 'p' denotes peripheral) and is displayed digitally on the monitor as a percentage, along with heart rate and a plethysmographic waveform. Interpreting this waveform is essential in distinguishing a true oximetry signal from one displaying dampening or artefact (Fig. 13.14). The probe is commonly placed on a finger, but can also be placed on the toe, earlobe or forehead, with forehead probes having the highest accuracy.[47,48] Change the probe position frequently to maintain adequate perfusion of the site and skin integrity.

> **Practice tip**
>
> In cool environments, wrap the hand or foot that has the sensor attached. This may improve saturation readings.

It is important to understand that pulse oximetry measures the saturation of haemoglobin as an estimate of peripheral arterial oxygen saturation (SpO_2). SpO_2 differs from PaO_2 but they are physiologically related, and this relationship is illustrated by the two axes of the oxygen–haemoglobin dissociation curve (see Fig. 13.9, and the previous physiology section for more discussion). A fit healthy adult, at sea level, with a normal haemoglobin level breathing room air would usually have a SpO_2 of 97–99%. Normal values decline with age with lower limits of normal being 96% for an 18-year-old and 94% for a 70-year-old person.[48]

> **Practice tip**
>
> Try to place the pulse oximeter on the finger of the opposite arm to where blood pressure is taken, particularly if you have no arterial line and are doing frequent non-invasive blood pressure measurements.

Limitations of pulse oximetry

- Pulse oximetry in isolation does not provide all the necessary information to evaluate oxygenation, ventilation status or acid–base balance. ABG testing is required to assess other parameters.
- Pulse oximetry readings are reasonably reliable when the SaO_2 is 90% or above; accuracy deteriorates when the SaO_2 falls below 90%.[47] When low SpO_2 readings occur and you are confident that the device is not influenced by artefact, formal ABG analysis should be conducted.
- Satisfactory arterial perfusion of the monitored tissue is required; low cardiac output states, vasoconstriction, peripheral vascular disease and hypothermia can cause inaccurate pulse signals and falsely low oxygen saturation readings. Low perfusion will result in a flattened oximetry waveform (Fig. 13.14). In such cases, confirm oxygen saturation with intermittent ABG testing. In these cases, moving the probe to another location, such as the earlobe or forehead, can improve signal quality. Forehead probes provide higher accuracy and also respond more quickly to changes in saturation. If using an earlobe probe, applying a vasodilator cream can improve both perfusion and signal quality.[48]
- Motion artefact (see Fig. 13.14), caused by patient movement or shivering, is a significant cause of erroneously low readings and false alarms.[47] Keeping the patient warm (if not contraindicated) and encouraging them to minimise movement may limit this problem. Using an ear or forehead probe may also reduce motion artefact.[48] The pulse oximetry waveform is useful to identify a true reading, versus a reading influenced by artefact.[47]
- Dark blue, green and black nail varnishes have been shown to affect SpO_2 accuracy, although the differences may not be clinically significant. There is conflicting advice as to whether placing the sensor probe sideways on the finger eliminates this

FIGURE 13.14 Common pulse oximetry waveforms.

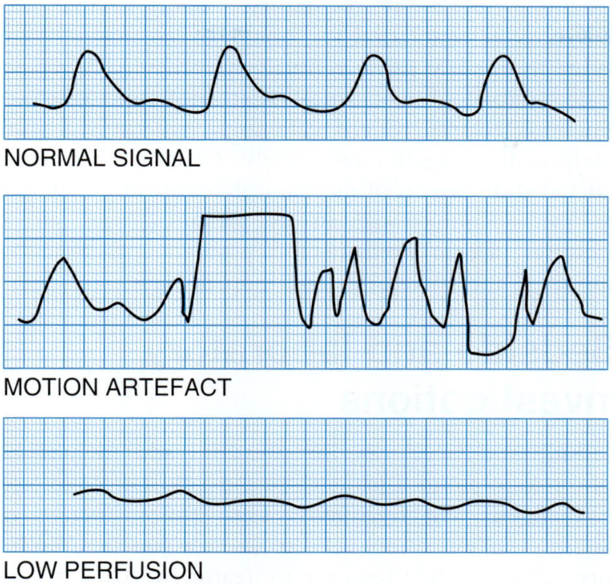

effect.[47,48] To ensure accuracy, it is recommended that nail varnish and acrylic nails be removed if possible.

- Modern pulse oximeters are relatively unaffected by light sources, the thickness of tissue or by skin pigmentation. In patients with very dark skin, oxygen saturation may be overestimated when readings are below 90%.[48]
- Conventional pulse oximetry sensors cannot differentiate between oxyhaemoglobin, carboxyhaemoglobin and methaemoglobin, and therefore provide a false estimation of oxygen saturation. An example of high levels of non-functioning haemoglobin is that of carbon monoxide poisoning; high carboxyhaemoglobin levels give a falsely high SpO_2 reading, leading to an overestimation of oxygenation. New multi-wavelength oximeters that can estimate carboxyhaemoglobin and methaemoglobin are now available but are not accurate in the presence of low SaO_2 readings and for carboxyhaemoglobin, are not necessarily interchangeable with standard laboratory tests.[47]
- In the presence of anaemia it is possible to have good oxygen saturation of available haemoglobin but poor tissue oxygenation due to a deficiency in the ability of the blood to transport oxygen.[47] In anaemia, the pulse oximetry readings may be accurate, but it is the clinician's interpretation of these readings that is important. If we are looking at SpO_2 as a marker of oxygenation, a reduced amount of functioning haemoglobin may be well saturated with oxygen but is a poor reflection of tissue oxygenation. Correction of anaemia is required to improve tissue oxygenation.
- Injection of intravenous dyes[47] may lead to a false underestimation of SpO_2 for up to 20 mins after their administration (methylene blue, indocyanine green, indigo carmine).

Practice tip

Assess the agreement between the heart rate reading displayed in the pulse oximetry section of the monitor to the heart rate calculated by the ECG. Lack of agreement may indicate that not all pulsations are being detected and the pulse oximetry reading may not be accurate.

Practice tip

Patients with COPD who are hypoxic (SpO_2 <88%) should receive supplemental oxygen. The SpO_2 targets for patients with COPD are lower with SpO_2 generally maintained at 88–92% during an exacerbation if the patient is at risk of hypercapnia.[18,19] It is important to frequently assess these patients receiving oxygen so that any compromise in breathing is noted and acted upon.

Capnography

Capnography, using infrared spectrometry, monitors expired CO_2 during the respiratory cycle and is referred to as end-tidal CO_2 ($PetCO_2$). The percentage of exhaled CO_2 at end-expiration is displayed on the monitor.

A waveform, called a capnogram is produced (Fig. 13.15), and it is important that ICU staff receive training in interpretation of capnography waveforms.[49] Continuous capnography detects subtle changes in patients' lung dynamics (i.e. changes to physiological shunting or alveolar recruitment) and can be measured in both intubated and non-intubated patients. It can be used to estimate $PaCO_2$ levels in patients with a normal ventilation–perfusion ratio (usually 1–5 mmHg less than $PaCO_2$). Levels are, however, affected by conditions common in the critically ill (e.g. low cardiac output states, elevated alveolar pressures, sepsis, hypo/hyperthermia, pulmonary embolism, alterations in tidal volume and respiratory rate), so use $PetCO_2$ to estimate $PaCO_2$ levels in these patients with caution. The amount of dead space in the circuit will also change the correlation between $PetCO_2$ and $PaCO_2$ and use of filters between the patient airway and the capnography sampling line can cause an artificially low reading.[50] Investigate any sudden changes in $PetCO_2$ levels with ABG analysis. $PetCO_2$ monitoring has many uses in the critical care unit:

FIGURE 13.15 Normal capnogram. (**A**) End inspiration; (**B**) expiratory upstroke; (**C**) expiratory plateau; (**D**) end-tidal carbon dioxide tension ($PetCO_2$).

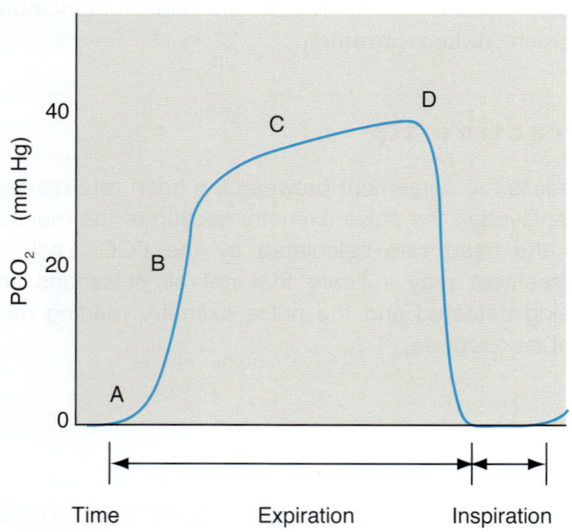

Reproduced from Miller-Keane M, O'Toole M. Miller-Keane Encyclopedia and dictionary of medicine, nursing, and allied health. 7th ed. Philadelphia: Saunders, 2003.

- indicating correct endotracheal tube placement while awaiting chest X-ray (CXR), assessing tube patency and detecting leaks or disconnection of the circuit
- monitoring ventilation status during and after weaning from mechanical ventilation
- assessing the effectiveness of cardiopulmonary resuscitation compressions and detecting return of spontaneous circulation
- monitoring ventilation continuously during sedation and anaesthesia
- assessing ventilation/perfusion status.[49]

Practice tip

The capnography monitoring line can fill with condensation, particularly if the patient has a humidified ventilator circuit. Regularly check for this and drain or replace the line as necessary. Condensation can interfere with the reading.

Capnography is recommended as a standard component of respiratory monitoring in mechanically-ventilated patients in the ICU, during transport of critically ill patients, during anaesthesia and conscious sedation, and during cardiopulmonary resuscitation.[49]

Ventilation monitoring

Mechanical ventilation is a common intervention for patients who require respiratory support in the ICU. Advances in ventilation technology have enhanced our ability to monitor many ventilator parameters. A detailed understanding of mechanical ventilation principles and functions enables patient data to be interpreted accurately and managed appropriately. Chapter 15 provides a detailed discussion of mechanical ventilation, including ventilation monitoring; airway pressures (peak airway pressure, plateau pressure and positive end-expiratory pressure); and waveforms and loop displays.

Bedside and laboratory investigations

Bedside and laboratory investigations add to available information about a patient's respiratory status and assist in diagnosis and treatment. This section focuses on common investigations used to assess a patient's respiratory status and their response to treatment: ABG analysis; blood testing; and sputum and tracheal aspirates. Given the often alien nature of the ICU environment for patients and families, explaining the purpose of respiratory monitoring procedures and devices may reduce fear and uncertainty.

Blood gas analysis

ABGs are one of the most commonly performed laboratory tests in critical care. Therefore, accurate ABG interpretation is an important clinical skill. ABG measurements enable rapid assessment of oxygenation and ventilation, and all ICUs are recommended to have a blood gas analyser as a minimum standard.[51]

Blood for ABG analysis is sampled by arterial puncture or, more commonly in critically ill patients, from an arterial catheter usually sited in the radial or femoral artery. Both techniques are invasive and only allow for intermittent analysis. The advantage of the arterial catheter is that it facilitates ABG sampling without repeated arterial punctures. Continuous blood gas monitoring is possible using an in-line fibre optic sensor as part of the arterial line, but this practice is yet to have wide application in Australasia due to cost and accuracy concerns. Questions also remain regarding the possibility for arteriovenous shunting, blood loss and infection risk with continuous systems.[52]

Sampling technique

A correct sampling technique is essential for accurate results. Prior to arterial sampling from the radial artery, a modified Allen's test should be performed. The patient should initially hold their hand high and clench their fist tightly. Occlusive pressure is then applied by the clinician's thumbs to both the ulnar and radial arteries, to obstruct blood flow to the hand. While maintaining this pressure, the patient is asked to relax their hand,

and check whether the palm and fingers have blanched. Occlusive pressure is then released on the ulnar artery only.[52] The modified Allen's test is positive if the hand flushes within 5–15 seconds, indicating that the ulnar artery has good blood flow and radial sampling is safe.

Approximately 2 mL of arterial blood is collected anaerobically and aseptically using a premixed syringe containing dry heparin.[54] If drawing the sample from an intraarterial line, a portion of blood is discarded to prevent dilution and contamination of the sample from the saline in the flush line. The discard amount is twice the dead space volume to ensure clinically accurate ABG and electrolyte measurement, and to prevent unnecessary blood loss.[55] Dead space is defined as the priming volume from the sampling port to the catheter tip; this differs depending on the arterial line setup used. Arterial blood exerts its own pressure, which is sufficient to fill the syringe to the required level; active negative pressure is to be avoided, as this causes frothing. Any excess air will cause inaccurate readings and is expelled before the syringe is capped with a hub, preventing further air contamination. The sample is analysed within 10 min if not packed in ice, or within 60 min if iced; delays cause degradation of the sample.[54] The use of ice is controversial: while it was appropriate for older style glass syringes, is it now recognised that plastic syringes become more permeable to gas at lower temperatures, allowing oxygen (but less so, carbon dioxide) to escape. For this reason, using ice to preserve samples in plastic syringes is not recommended, and this increases the importance of prompt ABG analysis.[56] Degradation also occurs if the sample is shaken; therefore, gently roll the syringe/collection tube between your fingers to mix the sample with the heparin and prevent clotting.[53] The frequency of ABG sampling should be carefully considered and based on patient need. ABG sampling may lead to losses of up to 70 mL per day and the cumulative effect may worsen anaemia and increase the need for transfusion. Evidence-based blood conservation strategies should be included in local unit guidelines. This is particularly important in the paediatric population where the use of small volume collection tubes have reduced iatrogenic blood loss.[57]

The question of whether or not to adjust the ABG analysis according to the patient's body temperature (by inputting the actual patient temperature result into the blood gas analyser) remains controversial. Hypothermia and hyperthermia can affect gas solubility, and so impact on pCO_2, pO_2 and pH. Body temperature can also shift the oxyhaemoglobin dissociation curve, as well as altering oxygen consumption and production of carbon dioxide. If local unit protocol is to adjust for temperature, it is recommended that both corrected and uncorrected ABG results are reported to avoid potentially unsafe decisions based on erroneous assumptions.[58,59]

There is a difference in the way bicarbonate is determined between an ICU-based ABG machine (which derives its value based on the pCO_2 and the pH), and a biochemistry laboratory that directly measures bicarbonate using an enzymatic assay. The true bicarbonate value is actually best determined by the Henderson–Hasselbalch equation. Any differences between an ABG machine value and that reported by a laboratory are usually within 3 mmol, and are most likely explained by pre-analytical errors or how quickly the sample was analysed, rather than one particular device being superior.[58]

Arterial blood gas analysis

ABG analysis includes measurement of the PaO_2, the $PaCO_2$, the H^+ concentration (pH) and the concentration of chemical buffer, HCO_3^-. Normal values for ABG parameters are listed in Table 13.4. Use a systematic approach when interpreting the results of ABG analysis (Table 13.5).

Assessing oxygenation: when assessing oxygenation, hypoxaemia (PaO_2 <60 mmHg or <7.8 kPa) will be the most common abnormality and may indicate the need for supplemental oxygen to maintain adequate arterial oxygenation.[60] Conversely, hyperoxia rarely occurs unless a patient is receiving supplemental oxygen therapy. Oxygen can be toxic to cells if delivered at high concentrations for a prolonged period.

Assessing the pH: the body's acid–base balance is affected by both the respiratory and metabolic systems and is evaluated by measuring the pH of arterial blood. On the pH scale of 1 to 14 (where 1 = the strongest acid and 14 = the strongest alkali), a pH of 7.4 is the middle of the normal range. Acidaemia is present with a pH of <7.35; alkalaemia is present with a pH of >7.45. The pH changes depending on the amount of H^+ or HCO_3^- in the blood with H^+ reflecting the acidic component and HCO_3^- the base or buffer.[60]

Assessing for respiratory mechanisms: $PaCO_2$ indicates the effectiveness of ventilation and rises when ventilation is sub-optimal. CO_2 combines with water to form H_2CO_3, so can alter the pH of blood.

Retention of CO_2 through hypoventilation or air trapping leads to increased H^+ ions resulting in a lower pH and development of respiratory acidosis. Alternatively, a loss of CO_2 through hyperventilation results in a higher pH and development of respiratory alkalosis. A $PaCO_2$ of >45 mmHg (6 kPa) indicates alveolar hypoventilation, due to COPD, pulmonary oedema, airway obstruction, over-sedation, narcosis, drug overdose, pain, neurological deficit or permissive hypercapnia in mechanically-ventilated patients. Conversely, a $PaCO_2$ of <35 mmHg (4.7 kPa) reflects alveolar hyperventilation, and can be due to hypoxia, pain, anxiety, pregnancy, liver failure, sepsis, early stages of asthma, permissive hypocapnia in mechanically-ventilated patients or as a compensatory mechanism for metabolic acidosis.[60]

Assessing for metabolic mechanisms: When there is a metabolic cause to a change in pH, the primary alteration will be to the HCO_3 level. This may be due to a change in alkaline substances (such as excessive intake

TABLE 13.4
Arterial blood gas normal values*

BLOOD GAS MEASUREMENT	DESCRIPTION	NORMAL VALUE
Temperature	Patient's body temperature. Analyser defaults to 37°C if not entered	37°C
Haemoglobin	Samples should be fully mixed so should be constantly agitated until analysed	Females: 115–165 g/L Males: 130–180 g/L
Acid–base status	Overall acidity or alkalinity of blood	7.35–7.45 (36–44 nmol/L)
Carbon dioxide (CO_2)	Partial pressure of arterial CO_2. A potential acid	35–45 mmHg (4.7–6.0 kPa)
Oxygen (O_2)	Partial pressure of O_2. Varies with age	80–100 mmHg (10.7–13.3 kPa)
Bicarbonate (HCO_3^-)	Standardised HCO_3^- (actual HCO_3^- minus the HCO_3^- produced by respiratory dysfunction) estimates true metabolic function. An alkali or base	22–26 mmol/L
Base excess	Measures acid–base balance. The number of molecules of acid or base required to return 1 L of blood to the normal pH (7.4)	−2 to +2 mmol/L
Oxygen saturation	Haemoglobin saturation by oxygen in arterial blood	94.5–98.2%

*Institutional norms may vary slightly.

TABLE 13.5
Steps for arterial blood gas interpretation

STEP	INTERPRETATION
1	Assess oxygenation … PaO_2 <60 mmHg (<8 kPa) indicates hypoxaemia
2	Assess the pH level … <7.35 indicates acidosis, >7.45 indicates alkalosis
3	Assess $PaCO_2$ level … <35 mmHg (<4.7 kPa) indicates respiratory alkalosis; >45 mmHg (>6.0 kPa) indicates respiratory acidosis
4	Assess HCO_3^- level … <22 indicates metabolic acidosis; >26 indicates metabolic alkalosis
5	Assess pH, CO_2 and HCO_3^-. Is there an acid–base disturbance and is it fully compensated, partially compensated or uncompensated?
6	Assess other ABG results. Are they within normal limits for the patient?

of an antacid) or a change in acid substances (such as an excess of lactic acid in the blood).[60] HCO_3^- is regulated by the renal system. A [HCO_3^-] of <22 mmol/L can lead to metabolic acidosis, caused by renal failure, ketoacidosis, lactic acidosis, diarrhoea, salicylate overdose, large volume of intravenous saline or cardiac arrest. A HCO_3^- of >26 mmol/L can lead to metabolic alkalosis, caused by severe vomiting, continuous nasogastric suction, diuretics, corticosteroids or excessive citrate administration from stored blood or renal replacement therapy.[60]

Base excess (BE) is an additional value included in the ABG report and it reflects the excess (or deficit) of base to acid in the blood. Normal BE ranges from −2 to +2. If the BE is +2 mmol/L, removal of 2 mmol of base per litre of blood is required to return the pH to 7.4. If the BE is −2 mmol/L (i.e. a base deficit), 2 mmol of base per litre of blood needs to be added to achieve a pH of 7.4. A BE greater than +3 indicates that there is more base than acid present and therefore alkalosis. A BE below −3 indicates that there is more acid than base.[60] Understanding this concept is useful as it can determine how much treatment is necessary to restore a patient's pH to normal.

Mixed disorders: Sometimes there will be both a respiratory and a metabolic cause for a disturbance in pH and this is referred to as a mixed disorder. For example, a cardiac arrest may result in a period of poor perfusion causing metabolic acidosis, and poor ventilation causing a concomitant respiratory acidosis.[60]

Assessing for compensation: the final step of interpretation is to examine the pH, CO_2 and HCO_3^- levels collectively, to determine if the patient has either fully or partially compensated the primary dysfunction, or is in an uncompensated state. With the respiratory

TABLE 13.6
Arterial blood gas findings for acid–base disturbances

	PH	$PACO_2$, MMHG (KPA)	HCO_3^-, MMOL/L
RESPIRATORY ACIDOSIS			
Uncompensated	<7.35	>45 (6.0)	Within normal limits
Partially compensated	<7.35	>45 (6.0)	>26
Fully compensated	Within normal limits	>45 (6.0)	>26
RESPIRATORY ALKALOSIS			
Uncompensated	>7.45	<35 (4.7)	Within normal limits
Partially compensated	>7.45	<35 (4.7)	<22
Fully compensated	Within normal limits	<35 (4.7)	<22
METABOLIC ACIDOSIS			
Uncompensated	<7.35	Within normal limits	<22
Partially compensated	<7.35	<35 (4.7)	<22
Fully compensated	Within normal limits	<35 (4.7)	<22
METABOLIC ALKALOSIS			
Uncompensated	>7.45	Within normal limits	>26
Partially compensated	>7.45	>45 (6.0)	>26
Fully compensated	Within normal limits	>45 (6.0)	>26

system regulating CO_2 and the metabolic system regulating HCO_3^-, restoration of normal acid–base balance and homeostasis is possible. The ability of the body to achieve homeostasis and acid–base balance depends on the ability of the respiratory and renal systems to adjust to the underlying imbalance. The degree of compensation depends on whether the pH returns to normal; full compensation results in a normal pH whereas, in partial compensation, the pH remains outside normal limits. In an uncompensated acid–base imbalance, there has been no attempt by the body to correct the acid–base imbalance and the pH, as well as either the CO_2 or HCO_3^-, is abnormal.[60]

To assess compensation, pH, CO_2 and HCO_3^- are examined in the context of a patient's clinical presentation:

- In a fully compensated state, the pH is returned to within normal limits, but the other two parameters will be outside normal limits as the body has successfully manipulated CO_2 and HCO_3^- levels to restore the pH.
- In a partially compensated state, the pH is not within normal limits, and the other parameters will also be outside of normal limits but not enough to bring the pH back to normal.
- In a non-compensated state, the pH will be outside normal limits, and the primary disruption (either CO_2 or HCO_3^-) will also be outside normal limits while the remaining parameter has not compensated for this derangement and has stayed within normal limits.

It can be difficult to differentiate the patient's primary problem from their compensatory response. As a quick guide, if the CO_2 is moving in the opposite direction to pH, then the primary disruption is respiratory; if the HCO_3^- is moving in the same direction as pH, the disruption is metabolic.[60] Table 13.6 provides a guide to ABG findings for each acid–base disorder.

Other parameters measured on the ABG sample, such as lactate, electrolytes, haemoglobin and glucose, are also considered in determining patient status. In particular, lactate, is a useful indicator of anaerobic metabolism due to poor tissue oxygenation. In healthy people, a normal lactate is 0.5–1 mmol/L, while in critically ill patients, normal lactate is considered less than 2 mmol/L. Hyperlactataemia exists where there is a persistent lactate level of 2-4 mmol/L without metabolic acidosis, and this can occur with adequate tissue perfusion. Lactic acidosis is present where a hyperlactataemia and metabolic acidosis co-exist. Hypoxic causes of lactic acidosis include respiratory failure, ischaemia, severe anaemia and shock, while non-hypoxic causes include renal or hepatic dysfunction, ketoacidosis, an excess of catecholamines and sepsis. Improved lactate levels are a useful indicator of successful therapy for these derangements.[61]

The Stewart approach

As an adjunct to traditional ABG interpretation, Peter Stewart's seminal concepts on acid–base assessment[62] suggest that, in our body's fluids, pH and HCO_3^- are merely dependent variables that cannot be directly manipulated. Stewart was particularly interested in considering the influence of resuscitation fluid management on acid–base balance. He developed six equations to assist clinicians to analyse the physiological basis of acid–base shifts, considering the impacts of strong cations, the total concentration of weak acids and CO_2.[63] Stewart's intention was not to replace traditional methods of determining acid–base balance, but to extend their usefulness and to further explain the physiological basis of complex disorders.[66] An example of the utility of Stewart's work is evident in a recent study of 300 patients with abdominal sepsis. This report demonstrated that a modification of the Stewart approach was able to identify mixed acid–base disorders which would otherwise remain undetected.[64]

Stewart's complex equations have been made more user-friendly with the development of online calculators[65] where the clinician can enter patient chemistry data online to receive an online decision support related to complex acid–base disorders (see *Online resources*). Once patient data are entered, the site offers clinicians a breakup of the relative contributions to the overall disturbance in pH by its main controlling elements. When displayed graphically, this gives the user a sense of the severity of each contributing factor, and allows input of these individual factors into virtual scenarios to predict the possible impact of specific interventions.[63]

Venous blood gas analysis

Where an arterial blood sample is difficult to collect, an alternative is to perform the same measurements on a venous blood sample. Venous blood collection may involve a peripheral venous sample using venipuncture, a central venous sample from a central line, or a mixed venous sample from the distal port of a pulmonary artery catheter. Central venous sampling has the highest evidence for correlation with ABGs. If taking a peripheral sample using venipuncture, release the tourniquet at least 1 min before the blood is drawn to reduce the impact of local ischaemia.[66]

The partial pressure of venous oxygenation (PvO_2) is not useful for measuring oxygenation, as oxygen has already been extracted at tissue level. However, ventilation and acid–base balance can be analysed using the partial pressure of carbon dioxide in venous blood ($PvCO_2$), venous pH and venous serum HCO_3. Venous oxygen saturation (SvO_2) can be used in goal-directed therapy for severe sepsis and septic shock.[67]

The minor corrections when converting venous blood gas to ABG equivalents vary slightly according to sampling site. For central sampling, add 0.03–0.05 to the pH and subtract 4–5 mmHg from the pCO_2. For peripheral samples add 0.02–0.04 to the pH and subtract 3–8 mmHg from the pCO_2. Caution should be used in patients with shock where there is poor correlation between venous and arterial samples, particularly for PCO_2 where the differences may increase by a factor of three.[66]

Continuous central venous oxygenation monitoring

SvO_2/$ScvO_2$ (mixed or central venous oxygen saturation) has been a useful assessment of oxygen delivery and consumption, particularly for patients following cardiac surgery and for those with sepsis. Continuous SvO_2/$ScvO_2$ is measured using various wavelengths of light via a pulmonary artery catheter (SvO_2) or via a central line in the superior vena cava (SvO_2) or via a peripherally inserted central line. Normal venous oxygenation is around 70–80%, meaning that healthy people consume around 25% of the oxygen available to them. When oxygen demand is higher, healthy people are able to compensate by increasing their respiratory rate and heart rate. Critically ill patients may have difficulty compensating, for increased oxygen demand, and so extract more oxygen from the tissues leading to a lower venous oxygen saturation. Causes of decreased ScvO2 include increased oxygen consumption, decreased cardiac output, decreased oxygen supply and nursing interventions such as positioning. These may indicate a need to respond through either decreasing metabolic demand, increasing inspired oxygen, correcting haemoglobin or increasing cardiac output.[67]

There are slight differences in venous oxygenation values according to the measure used. $ScvO_2$, which measures oxygen saturation from the upper part of the body, will have a value 5–10% higher than that measured using SvO_2, which uses blood returning from both the upper and lower body circulation, and from the coronary circulation. These differences correlate consistently meaning that the less invasive $ScvO_2$ monitoring, requiring only a central line, is a satisfactory surrogate.[67]

Oxygen tension-derived indices

The alveolar–arterial gradient is a marker of intrapulmonary shunting (i.e. blood flowing past collapsed areas of alveoli not involved in gas exchange). The index is calculated as $PAO_2 - PaO_2$ (where PAO_2 is the partial pressure of oxygen in the alveoli). PAO_2 is determined by a complex equation, the alveolar gas equation. PAO_2 and PaO_2 are equal when perfusion and ventilation are perfectly matched. The gradient increases with age but a value of 5–15 mmHg is normal up until approximately middle age. Despite questions about its clinical usefulness, particularly in the critically ill,[68] it is used in clinical practice as a trending tool to track intrapulmonary shunting. Simply put, the larger the gradient between PAO_2 and PaO_2, the larger the degree of intrapulmonary shunting.[69]

The ratio of PaO_2 to fraction of inspired oxygen (FiO_2), commonly referred to as the PaO_2/ FiO_2 (or P/F) ratio, was introduced as a simple way of estimating pulmonary shunting, even though it does not formally measure alveolar partial pressure. A consensus paper outlines criteria known as the *Berlin Definition*[70] to define stages of ARDS. According to this definition, a PaO_2/ FiO_2 ratio of 200–300 mmHg (≤39.9 kPa) indicates mild ARDS, a ratio of 100–200 mmHg (≤26.6 kPa) indicates moderate ARDS while a ratio of less than or equal to 100 mmHg (<13.3 kPa) indicates severe ARDS. For example, in a patient receiving a FiO_2 of 0.65 who has a PaO_2 of 90 mmHg (12 kPa), their PaO_2/ FiO_2 ratio would be 138.5 mmHg, indicating a moderate ARDS state. A diagnosis of ARDS also requires the above reductions in PaO_2/FiO_2 ratio to be present with the patient receiving at least 5 cmH_2O of positive end-expiratory pressure or continuous positive airway pressure. It requires this state to have developed within 1 week of a known clinical insult or worsening respiratory symptoms. A CXR should show bilateral opacities not fully explained by other causes and respiratory failure not fully explained by cardiac failure or fluid overload.[70]

Blood tests

Haematology and biochemistry investigations should inform treatment for patients with respiratory dysfunction. Full blood count, including a leukocyte differential count, can monitor white cell activity for patients with a confirmed or suspected infective process. When infections are severe, the full blood count will show a dramatic rise in the number of immature neutrophils. Blood cultures can also assist in diagnosis of bacterial or yeast infections and isolation of the causative organism. Viral studies may aid diagnosis for respiratory infections of unknown origin. Where pulmonary embolism is suspected, a D-dimer test can assist diagnosis of a thrombus. Routine measurement of urea and electrolytes can track renal function and acid–base status.[71]

> **Practice tip**
>
> Monitoring lactate levels is important as the levels can be used to assess the effectiveness and efficiency of resuscitative therapies. A persistently elevated lactate level is associated with higher morbidity and poorer patient outcomes. Caution should be used in interpreting lactate levels in patients with liver dysfunction; lactate clearance and normalisation is impaired for these patients during early resuscitation management.[72]

Sputum, tracheal aspirates and nasopharyngeal aspirates

Colour, consistency and volume of sputum provide useful information in determining changes in a patient's respiratory status and progress. Regular cultures of tracheal sputum reveal colonisation by opportunistic organisms, and can identify the cause of an acute chest infection or sepsis. Many ICUs have routine (weekly or twice-weekly) surveillance monitoring of tracheal aspirates in long-term mechanically-ventilated patients. In spontaneously breathing patients, sputum specimens can be collected in a sterile specimen receptacle. Specimens are best collected early in the morning. In intubated patients, using a sputum trap between the suction catheter and suction tubing assists sputum collection. A sterile technique should be maintained to reduce sample contamination.[73]

If obtaining an adequate sputum specimen in non-intubated patients is difficult, there is evidence that administration of nebulised saline (isotonic or hypertonic) may assist sputum collection. There is no evidence to support this among mechanically-ventilated patients but, anecdotally, nebulised normal saline may assist sputum production by moistening the airways and thinning secretions. Physiotherapy in the form of manual hyperinflation and head-down tilt during therapy has been shown to increase sputum production for sample collection.[73]

Instilling normal saline in an endotracheal tube to facilitate clearance and/or collection of tenacious sputum remains a controversial issue. There is no evidence that instillation facilitates secretion clearance, while there is some evidence that it increases both patient discomfort and the risk of bacterial contamination of the lower airway. Therefore, this practice is not recommended.[74]

Nasopharyngeal aspirate or swabs may be necessary to diagnose viral respiratory infections. The nasopharyngeal aspirate is collected by inserting a fine, sterile suction catheter (8 or 10 F) attached to a sputum trap through the nare and back to the nasopharynx. Suction is applied while withdrawing and slowly rotating the catheter. The catheter is flushed through to the sputum trap with sterile normal saline or transport medium if available. A nasopharyngeal swab is collected by inserting a specially designed swab to the back of the nasopharynx and rotating for 5–10 seconds. The swab is then withdrawn slowly and placed in the plastic vial containing transport medium.[75] As close contact with the patient is necessary, and the procedure can generate aerosols and droplets, personal protective equipment should be worn.[76]

Diagnostic procedures

Assessment and monitoring of the respiratory status of a critically ill patient may rely on various medical imaging tests and bronchoscopy to determine the cause

FIGURE 13.16 Chest X-ray, PA view.

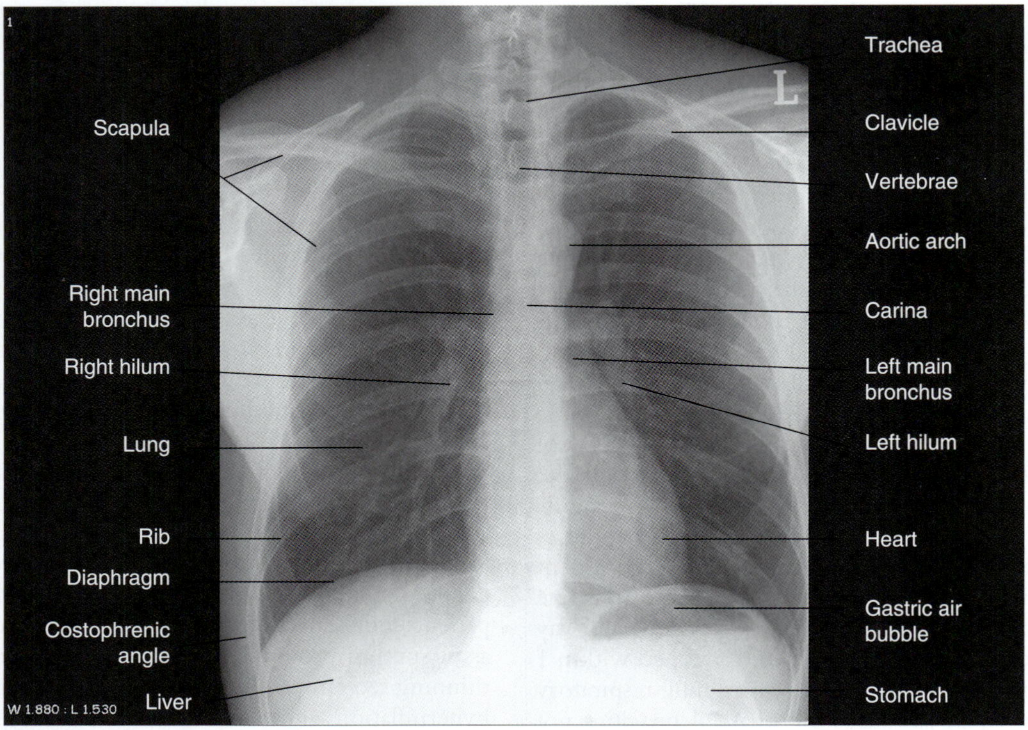

Published with permission from University of Auckland Faculty of Medical and Health Sciences.

and severity of the illness episode, relevant comorbidities and the patient's response to treatment.

Medical imaging

A range of imaging techniques may be available for supporting care of a critically ill patient with a respiratory dysfunction, depending on the level of broader health service resources available. This sub-section describes X-ray, ultrasound, computerised tomography (CT), magnetic resonance imaging and ventilation/perfusion scan techniques.

Chest X-ray

Chest radiography is a common diagnostic tool used for respiratory examination of critically ill patients. CXR allows basic information regarding abnormalities in the chest to be obtained relatively quickly. The image provides information about lung fields and other thoracic structures as well as the placement of invasive lines and tubes. In the ventilated patient, serial CXRs also enable sequential assessment of lung status in relation to therapy.[77]

In-unit X-rays of patients using portable equipment are inferior to those taken using a fixed camera in the radiology department. Patient preparation is therefore important to optimise the quality of the film.[78] Patients should ideally be positioned sitting or semi-erect; CXRs using a supine position are less effective at revealing gravity-related abnormalities such as haemothorax. Lateral view CXRs may assist identification of lesions in the thorax. Film plate location against the patient's thorax determines the view: for posteroanterior (PA) the plate is positioned against the anterior thorax (Fig. 13.16) while the anteroposterior (AP) view has the plate against the patient's back. For mobile CXRs, the AP view is used. The AP view can magnify thoracic structures and can be less distinct or even distorted, so interpret findings with caution, particularly if comparing them with previous PA images.[79]

> **Practice tip**
>
> When preparing your patient for a CXR, minimise the number of monitoring leads and unnecessary equipment in the CXR field to optimise the image. Note all lines and tubes present on the CXR request form to aid interpretation.

CXR interpretation follows a systematic process designed to identify common pathophysiological processes and the locations of lines and other items. Table 13.7 provides a comprehensive guideline for viewing

TABLE 13.7
Guide to normal chest X-ray interpretation

Technical issues	• Check X-ray belongs to correct patient; note date and time of film • Ensure you are viewing X-ray correctly (i.e. right and left markings correspond to thoracic structures) • Determine whether X-ray was taken supine or erect, and whether PA or AP • Check X-ray was taken at full inspiration (posterior aspects of 9th/10th ribs and anterior aspects of 5th/6th ribs should be visible above diaphragm) • Note the penetration of the film: dark films are overpenetrated and may require a strong light to view; white films are underpenetrated; good penetration will allow visualisation of the vertebrae behind the heart
Bones	• Check along each rib from vertebral origin, looking for fractures • Ensure clavicles and scapulas are intact
Mediastinum	• Check for presence of trachea and identify carina (approximately level of 5th – 6th vertebrae) • Check width of mediastinum: should not be more than 8 cm
Apex	• Ensure blood vessels are visible in both apices, particularly looking to rule out pneumothoraces that present as clear black shading on the X-ray. Erect X-rays are essential to facilitate visibility of pneumothoraces
Hilum	• Check for prominence of vessels in this region: it generally indicates vascular abnormalities such as pulmonary oedema or pulmonary hypertension, or congestive heart failure
Heart	• Cardiac silhouette should be not more than 50% of the diameter of the thorax, with 1/3 of heart shadow to the right of the vertebrae and 1/3 of shadow to the left of the vertebrae; this positioning helps to rule out a tension pneumothorax. It should be noted that, post-cardiac surgery, if the mediastinum is left open the heart may appear wider than this; also in AP films this may be the case due to the plate being further away from the heart
Lung	• Identify the lobes of the lungs and determine if infiltrate or collapse is present in one or more of them. Lobes are approximately located as follows: – left upper lobe occupies upper half of lung – left lower lobe occupies lower half of lung – right lower lobe occupies costophrenic portion of lung – right middle lobe occupies cardiophrenic portion of lung – right upper lobe occupies upper portion of lung
Diaphragm	• Check levels of diaphragm: right diaphragm will normally be 1–2 cm above the left diaphragm to accommodate the liver
Gastric	• Check for pneumoperitoneum and dilated loops of bowel
Catheters and lines	• Identify distal end of endotracheal tube and ensure it is placed above the carina (i.e. not in the right main bronchus) • Trace nasogastric tube along length and ensure tip is in stomach, or below stomach if nasoenteric tube • Check position of intra-aortic balloon pump and ensure it is in the descending thoracic aorta • Trace all central catheters and ensure distal tip is in correct location • Identify other lines (e.g. intercostal catheters, pacing wires) and note location

PA = posteroanterior; AP = anteroposterior.
Adapted from Lareau C, Wootton J. The 'frequently' normal chest x-ray. Can J Rural Med 2004;9(3):183–6.

and interpreting a CXR. Common abnormalities that can be detected by CXR include:

- Lobar collapse or atelectasis: loss of lung volume, displacement of fissures and vascular markings and/or diaphragmatic elevation on the affected side.
- Pneumothorax: lack of pulmonary vascular markings on the affected side so the lung field appears black. There will be mediastinal and possible tracheal shift away from the affected side in tension pneumothorax.
- Pleural effusion: in the dependent areas of the pleural spaces, costophrenic angles are blunted by fluid and there may be a mediastinal shift away from a large effusion. Effusions are best visualised

with the patient upright, and will only be evident on an AP image with 200–400 mL of fluid in the pleural space.
- Pulmonary oedema: lung fields, particularly central and perihilar areas, appear white. Kerley B lines (small horizontal lines <2 cm long) may be present in the lung periphery near the costophrenic angles.
- Pulmonary embolism: although not the optimal diagnostic tool, areas of infarction may be visualised on CXR and may be mistaken for collapse or consolidation.
- Pneumoperitoneum: free air under the diaphragm elevates the diaphragm.[79]

Ultrasound

Ultrasound imaging (sonography) is a useful bedside diagnostic tool for a select group of critically ill patients and can add to the diagnostic information provided by CXR and CT scanning. Ultrasound uses high-frequency sound waves which, when probed on the body, reflect and scatter. The advantages are that the procedure can take place within the ICU, and it is radiation-free.[81] Ultrasound is most useful for patients with fluid in the pleural space (i.e. pleural effusion, haemothorax or empyema), and provides more detailed diagnostic information than CXR alone. Ultrasound allows an estimate of the volume and exact location of the fluid present and reduces the potential for serious complications during aspiration of fluid or chest tube insertion. Newer applications of lung ultrasound technology includes assessment of lung recruitment arising from positive end-expiratory pressure, and of reaeration of the alveoli following therapy for ventilator-associated pneumonia.[82] Useful, simplified diagnostic ultrasound protocols are the BLUE-protocol (Bedside Lung Ultrasound in Emergency protocol) that guides users through signs of abnormal lung surfaces, pleural effusions, consolidation, interstitial syndrome and pneumothorax for rapid diagnosis of acute respiratory failure, and the FALLS-protocol (Fluid Administration Limited by Lung Sonography) that directs scanning activities towards identifying or ruling out causes of shock (i.e. obstructive, cardiogenic, hypovolaemic or distributive), thereby identifying which patients are most likely to benefit from fluid resuscitation.[83]

Computed tomography

CT is a diagnostic investigation that provides greater specificity in chest anatomy and pathophysiology than a plain CXR, using multiple beams in a circle around the body. These beams are directed to a specific body area and provide detailed, consecutive cross-sectional slices of the scanned regions. CT scans can be performed with or without intravenous contrast. Contrast improves diagnostic precision but is used with caution in patients with renal impairment; renal failure may preclude a patient from receiving contrast. CT scanning is useful in the detection and diagnosis of pulmonary, pleural and mediastinal disorders (e.g. pleural effusion, empyema, haemothorax, atelectasis, pneumonia, ARDS). CT scans are useful where there are discrepancies between clinical and radiographic findings, or where the patient is not responding as expected to therapy.[84] CT pulmonary angiography produces a detailed view of blood vessels and is therefore the most definitive method for diagnosing pulmonary embolism, particularly in the presence of an abnormal CXR.[85]

A significant limitation of CT scanning is that the patient is transported away from the ICU. Transport increases the risks for critically ill patients and usually requires at least two appropriately trained staff to accompany the patient. Detailed planning by the healthcare team (including imaging staff) includes ventilator support, monitoring requirements and maintenance of infusions during scanning. Portable CT scanners are available in some centres, and may reduce the risks associated with transportation of critically ill patients to fixed CT scanners.[86] See Chapter 6 for discussion of in-hospital transfers, and Chapter 23 for inter-hospital transport.

Magnetic resonance imaging

Magnetic resonance imaging (MRI) uses radiofrequency waves and a strong magnetic field rather than X-rays to provide high contrast, detailed pictures of internal organs and soft tissues that are clearer than those generated by X-ray or CT scans. It is not the imaging of choice for respiratory assessment in the critically ill, being most useful for detecting neurological or spinal cord injury and congenital heart disease. The strong magnetic field around the scanner means that ferromagnetic objects containing material that can be attracted by magnets, such as iron or steel, can become potentially fatal projectiles. MRI scans may, therefore, be unsuitable for some patients.[87] While the use of MRI is discouraged where permanent pacemakers and implantable defibrillators are in situ, recent research suggests MRIs may be safe if certain precautions are taken: MRI should only be conducted where it is absolutely necessary, and implantable devices should be checked immediately afterwards.[88] Some types of neurostimulation devices[89] and intracranial aneurysm clips[89] have been designed for safe use in MRI but careful screening should precede MRI to determine patient and device-specific risks. Dental fillings, braces and retainers are usually safe but may distort images of the face or brain.[90] MRI in people with such devices should be used where the potential benefit clearly outweighs the risks. The strong magnetic fields also have the potential to interfere with ventilators, infusion pumps and monitoring equipment.

Ventilation/perfusion scan

A V/Q scan is indicated when a mismatch of lung ventilation and perfusion is suspected, most commonly for pulmonary embolism. The ventilation scan is performed with the patient inhaling a radioisotopic gas, while the perfusion scan is performed using an intravenous radioisotope that reveals the distribution of blood flow in the pulmonary vessels. These two scans are then compared, seeking mismatches between perfusion and ventilation. In larger centres, the V/Q scan has been superseded by the CT pulmonary angiogram for detection of pulmonary embolism.[81]

Bronchoscopy

Bronchoscopy is a bedside technique used for both diagnostic and therapeutic purposes. The bronchoscope can be either rigid or flexible, with the flexible fibre optic bronchoscope most widely used in critical care. A flexible fibre optic bronchoscope allows direct visualisation of respiratory mucosa and thorough examination of the upper airways and tracheobronchial tree. The scope is passed into the trachea via the oropharynx or nares. In mechanically-ventilated patients, the scope can be passed quickly and easily down the endotracheal or tracheostomy tube using a specially adapted valve that allows passage of the scope without disconnection of mechanical ventilation. During bronchoscopy, supplemental oxygen can be administered in non-intubated patients and FiO_2 can be increased in intubated patients. Accurate continuous monitoring during the procedure includes continuous pulse oximetry, electrocardiography, respiratory rate, heart rate and blood pressure. Equipment for advanced airway management, suctioning, cardiac defibrillation and advanced life support medications is immediately available. In intubated patients, one person is responsible for security of the airway to reduce the risk of displacement during the procedure.

When performed by an experienced operator, fibre optic bronchoscopy is a relatively safe procedure in critically ill patients. In mechanically-ventilated patients, the correct diameter of bronchoscope relative to the endotracheal tube diameter is important to avoid decreases in tidal and minute volumes, decreased PaO_2 and increased $PaCO_2$. Serious complications such as bleeding, bronchospasm, arrhythmia, pneumothorax and pneumonia occur rarely.[91] Patient preparation may include CXR; haemoglobin and coagulation profile, particularly if a biopsy is to be performed; baseline ABGs; and fasting or cessation of feeds for 4–6 hours prior.

Diagnostic indications for bronchoscopy include further investigation of poor gas exchange; evaluation of haemoptysis; collection of specimens (e.g. bronchoalveolar lavage, bronchial washings, bronchial brushings, lung biopsy); diagnosis of infection, interstitial lung disease, rejection post lung transplantation, malignancy; and diagnosis of airway injury due to burns, aspiration or chest trauma. Therapeutic indications include removal of mucous plugs; removal of foreign bodies; treatment of atelectasis; assistance during tracheostomy; airway dilation and stenting for tracheobronchomalacia and tracheobronchial stenosis; and lung volume reduction for emphysema.[91]

Summary

In this chapter a comprehensive overview of assessment and monitoring of a patient with respiratory dysfunction to aid clinical decision making is provided. Acute respiratory dysfunction is a major cause for admission to a critical care unit. Whether due to a primary or secondary condition, compromise of the respiratory system can be a life-threatening situation. The related respiratory physiology, pathophysiology, assessment and respiratory monitoring, bedside laboratory investigations and medical imaging are outlined:

- Critical care nurses are in a prime position to provide systematic and dynamic bedside assessments of a patient's respiratory status including past and presenting respiratory history, and physical examination of the thorax and lungs using inspection, palpation and auscultation techniques.
- Monitoring a patient's respiratory function includes pulse oximetry and capnography. Bedside and laboratory investigations including ABG analysis, blood tests and sputum and tracheal aspirates add to available information and assists in both diagnosis and treatment. ABG testing is common and ABG interpretation is an important clinical skill for critical care nurses.
- CXR is the most common diagnostic imaging tool in the ICU. CXR interpretation follows a systematic process to identify common pathologies and to locate lines and other items. Bronchoscopy is a useful bedside diagnostic and therapeutic device. CT provides greater specificity than CXR. Ultrasound imaging is useful to diagnose fluid in the pleural space. MRI and V/Q scans are more sophisticated diagnostic tools.

Careful patient assessment is essential, as respiratory dysfunction can be immediately life-threatening. Contemporary critical care practice involves comprehensive clinical assessment skills and use of a range of monitoring devices and diagnostic procedures. This challenges critical care nurses to be adaptable and willing to embrace new skills and knowledge.

Case study

Presenting history: Lisa is a 59-year-old woman who presented to the emergency department with an 18-day history of worsening dyspnoea, fever and cough. Lisa was transferred to a medical ward where she was administered oxygen at 2 L/min which resulted in an oxygen saturation of 92–94%. The next day Lisa had increased respiratory effort and the nurse on the ward initiated a rapid response call due to vital signs exceeding the threshold criteria. After consultation with the medical consultant, Lisa was transferred to the ICU.

Past medical history: Lisa has been a healthy woman who presented to her General Practitioner (GP) for a cough 2.5 weeks ago. She ceased smoking in 1998.

Medications: No medications

Social history: Lisa works as an optician, lives alone and has two adult daughters.

ON ADMISSION

Inspection: On arrival to the ICU, Lisa was speaking in short sentences. Her respiratory rate (RR) was 45 breaths/min, temperature 39.6°C and her SpO_2 was 80% on room air. Lisa appeared to have an increased respiratory effort and was using accessory muscles of respiration. She reported no pain.

Palpation: Lisa had a regular pulse, rate 105 beats/min. When the ECG trace was reviewed her rhythm was identified as sinus tachycardia. Her blood pressure (BP) was 150/70 mmHg. The nurse noted no pedal oedema but Lisa's peripheries were cold up to her knees and her capillary refill time was more than 5 seconds suggesting poor tissue oxygenation. Vocal fremitus was difficult to determine but chest wall expansion was good.

Percussion: There appeared to be dullness over the bases.

Auscultation: There were bilateral bronchial breath sounds over the bases and a mild expiratory wheeze.

Initial management: Non-invasive ventilation with high flow nasal cannula FiO_2 0.45 was commenced. The medical officer ordered a CT of the thorax, an arterial blood gas after insertion of an arterial line and suggested a target SpO_2 range of >90%.

Other assessment findings: C-reactive protein 28 mg/L (normal range is <5 mg/L). An elevated result is a marker for inflammation.

Arterial blood gases: PaO_2 = 56 mmHg (7.5 kPa), pH = 7.41, $PaCO_2$ = 45 mmHg (6.0 kPa), BE= 3, SaO_2 = 90%. The low PaO_2 indicates hypoxia. While the pH is normal, the $PaCO_2$ is in the upper range of normal and the BE is slightly elevated, suggesting a compensatory mechanism. Lisa's hypoxia suggests her ventilation is deteriorating, and so her ABGs need monitoring and consideration within her broader clinical picture.

Chest imaging: The CT of the thorax showed 'ground glass' opacities in both lungs.

Assessment plan: More blood cultures were ordered to look for Legionella, human immunodeficiency virus or pneumococcal-antigen. A sputum specimen was collected for culture and sensitivity testing. Hourly urine measure and daily weight were commenced.

Management plan: Lisa was assessed as having multifactorial Type 1 respiratory failure, including non-specific pneumonia. Lisa was commenced on a broad-spectrum intravenous antibiotic.

DAY 1

Inspection: During the first night in the ICU, Lisa had further deterioration. While her FiO_2 was increased, this did not improve her oxygen saturation. Her RR was 40 breaths/min and an increased work of breathing was noted despite increasing non-invasive ventilation parameters.

Vital signs: Temperature 40.0°C, sinus tachycardia rate 140 beats/min and BP 100/50 mmHg.

Palpation: Lisa's feet remained cold with no oedema.

Auscultation: Widespread wheezes and reduced air entry at the bases.

Management plan: During the morning, Lisa was intubated and intravenous propofol and fentanyl were initiated. She was commenced on volume-controlled mandatory mechanical ventilation with a FiO_2 of 0.8, RR of 16, PEEP 5 cmH_2O.

ONGOING PROGRESS

The next day Lisa was sedated to a score of −3 on the Richmond Agitation and Sedation Scale (RASS) due to agitation. She was positioned supine and in a Trendelenburg position. After 4 days with no improvement in respiratory function, Lisa had a tracheostomy. She was managed with pressure support ventilation, FiO_2 0.45. Her RR was 25–30 breaths/min. The next day, Lisa was mobilised with in-bed cycling and was sitting in a chair, receiving nasogastric feeding and respiratory physiotherapy.

A week later Lisa remained in ICU with improved ventilation. Her pressure support ventilation continued with a FiO_2 of 0.4 with a speech valve connected to her tracheostomy. However, Lisa was experiencing hallucinations and displayed signs of critical illness neuropathy. The following day Lisa was extubated, was able to eat some ice-cream while sitting in bed, and had oxygen via high flow nasal cannula at FiO_2 0.40. Unfortunately, 2 days later Lisa's RR increased to 40 breaths/min with an increase in mucus production. Her heart rate increased to 145 beats/min, her SpO_2 dropped to 90% and her temperature was 39.5C°. Lisa had a new tracheostomy inserted and mechanical ventilation (MV) with pressure support ventilation was recommenced at 20 cmH_2O with an FiO_2 of 0.55. Lisa was also sedated. The next day further parameters that suggested infection included a C-reactive protein of 115 mg/L and her CXR showed further deterioration of the lungs with increased atelectasis and infiltrate which explained Lisa's increased work of breathing. The plan was to continue with broad spectrum antibiotics, intravenous steroids, and light sedation, mobilisation and pressure support ventilation of 20 cmH_2O, PEEP 5 cmH_2O and FiO_2 0.50. The nurse had the ABG goal value of PaO_2>68 mmHg (9 kPa) and $PaCO_2$ <68 mmHg (9 kPa) to consider when careful weaning guided by respiratory monitoring was initiated. Lisa received frequent physiotherapy.

Over time, nurses were able to reduce Lisa's FiO_2. Her PaO_2 and $PaCO_2$ began to slowly normalise and she was given a small and simple ventilator; a so-called 'home ventilator' sometimes used in ICU. After 2 months, Lisa was extubated and discharged to the ward. After 3 weeks on the ward, she returned home with a small amount of oxygen via nasal cannulae. She was in good spirits given her situation, appeared to have no neurological deficits and good mental health. Follow-up was arranged with respiratory and general medicine physicians and physiotherapy and home-care arrangements were made. Lisa's daughter moved in with her for the first weeks after discharge. Her discharge diagnosis was unspecified pneumonia with an autoimmune component.

DISCUSSION POINTS

- What strategies can a nurse use to collect assessment and history data when a patient like Lisa is entering ICU in respiratory distress? What sort of questions may help to clarify the diagnosis?
- The prone position can improve oxygenation and functional residual capacity but there are also safety issues to consider.
- Stewart's approach can be another way of getting more information of ABG. Discuss the advantages and disadvantages of this test.

CASE STUDY QUESTIONS

1. What is the significance of Lisa speaking in short sentences?
2. Given that Lisa was only able to speak in short sentences, what other sources of information could be valuable in accessing important health and social history?
3. If a nurse anticipated Lisa might have areas of pulmonary consolidation, what changes would he/she expect to *feel* with vocal fremitus and *hear* using percussion compared to normal areas of the lungs?
4. Lisa's first blood gas sample is taken prior to insertion of an arterial line. What important test should precede radial access to arterial blood?
5. What is Lisa's final ABG indicating prior to intubation? PaO_2 53 mmHg, pH = 7.39, $PaCO_2$ = 44 mmHg (6.0 kPa), BE= 2.
6. What are two possible triggers for the decision to intubate Lisa?

7 On admission, Lisa's peripheries were cold up to her knees and her capillary refill time was more than 5 seconds. While poor tissue oxygenation from respiratory failure was suggested as one likely cause, what is a second possible cause given she is febrile?

8 On recommencement of Lisa's MV her CXR showed atelectasis. What breath sounds might the nurse hear on auscultation as a result of atelectasis?

9 Several signs on Lisa's CXR are attributed to her increased work of breathing. What are other important contributors to increased work of breathing?

10 On admission, Lisa's C-reactive protein was elevated – a marker for inflammation. What are the possible sequelae of serious pulmonary inflammation?

RESEARCH VIGNETTE

Haugdahl H, Dahlberg H, Klepstad P, Storli SL. The breath of life. Patients' experiences of breathing during and after mechanical ventilation. Intensive Crit Care Nurs 2017; 40: 85–93

Abstract

Introduction: Breathlessness is a prevalent and distressing symptom in intensive care, underestimated by nurses and physicians. Therefore, to develop a more comprehensive understanding of this problem, the study had two aims: to compare patients' self-reported scores of breathlessness obtained during mechanical ventilation (MV) with experiences of breathlessness later recalled by patients and: to explore the lived experience of breathing during and after MV.

Method: A qualitatively driven sequential mixed method design combining prospective observational breathlessness data at the end of a spontaneous breathing trial (SBT) and follow-up data from 11 post-discharge interviews.

Findings: Four out of six patients who reported breathlessness at the end of an SBT did not remember being breathless in retrospect. Experiences of breathing intertwined with the whole illness experience and were described in four themes: existential threat; the tough time; an amorphous and boundless body; and getting through.

Conclusion: Breathing was not always a clearly separate experience, but intertwined with the whole illness experience. This may explain the poor correspondence between patients' and clinicians' assessments of breathlessness. The results suggest patients' own reports of breathing should form part of nursing interventions and follow-up to support patients' quest for meaning.[92]

Critique

This Norwegian study combined qualitative and quantitative data to explore the phenomenon of objectively measured, versus experienced and remembered, breathlessness among people who had been mechanically ventilated. This qualitatively driven, sequential mixed-methods design means that the theoretical drive is primarily inductive (exploring/discovering from the data) rather than the deductive (confirming a theory from the data); deductive approaches are more aligned to quantitative studies. The introduction provides a well-rounded exploration of the concept of breathlessness, and the authors point to their earlier publications that conclude substantial breathlessness is commonly perceived during trials of spontaneous breathing for mechanically-ventilated patients. They also note the apparent disconnect between clinician and patient ratings of breathlessness.[92]

The authors applied maximum variation sampling (i.e. a good range) for the variables of high versus low breathlessness scores, age, gender and duration of ventilation. While maximum variation sampling is a sound criterion for rigour, seeking such heterogeneity in a sample on so many elements does challenge data saturation, meaning the sample size and method of determining saturation needs to be well-described and justified. Data saturation, as a means of sample size determination, has not been discussed in this report.

The sampling strategy describes choosing respondents from the extremes of the breathlessness experience (as per their breathlessness scores). While seeking extremes makes sense in capturing the breadth of patient experience, and this likely skewed sample has a methodological purpose (i.e. to help understand each end of the breathlessness continuum), then that needs to be considered when discussing the results and drawing conclusions, given the sample may not be broadly representative of the population of mechanically-ventilated patients.

The researchers collected a high-quality data set with audio-recording and verbatim transcription of interviews. Participants drawn from three sites and having more than one author involved in the analysis strengthens the quality of the work. Elements of comprehensive qualitative reporting that are missing are whether the interviews were conducted face-to-face or by telephone, whether an interview guide was used, whether the interviewer was trained in interview techniques, whether there were others present during the interview, whether anyone declined to participate and why, and the median duration of interviews to get a sense of the richness of the data set. It is also usual to note any preexisting relationship with participants, such as having provided direct clinical care, which could make people feel either obliged to participate or obliged to provide a complimentary account of their experiences. Reporting guidelines such as the Consolidated Criteria for Reporting Qualitative Research (COREQ) for qualitative work, or the Good Reporting of a Mixed Methods Study (GRAMMS) are useful tools when designing and writing up these types of studies.

In the methods section, the authors have carefully described how the qualitative and quantitative data sets worked together to address the research aim, with a clear diagram provided. However, in the results section, there is not a strong integration of these results. The authors could have gone further in reporting the interplay between the quantitative and qualitative findings. For example, while almost half the participants had low breathlessness scores (0–3/10), there was no qualitative data that corroborated this finding and this would seem important to discuss. Good integration of data sets is a common challenge in mixed-methods reporting, and is made more challenging here by the small sample size provided for the quantitative data.

The strongest mixed-methods studies have high quality data in both study arms. Had this report included the quantitative findings from their whole data set of 100 patients (from an earlier phase of their research), rather than only reporting the demographic and clinical characteristics of their sample of 11 patients, this quantitative data would be more generalisable, and perhaps easier to make sense of when combined with the qualitative work. This would not preclude the additional reporting of the 11 patients' characteristics. It should be acknowledged that researchers are often faced with difficult decisions about how to best present their work: fitting all research into a single paper does not always allow for comprehensive reporting, and it may only have been after their initial, larger study that these authors considered the need for this further work.

Assuming the interviews were conducted in Norwegian, it is not clear how translation accuracy was ensured. This is a particular issue for interpretative qualitative approaches where there is already a high level of meaning-making during analysis. Back-translation from English to Norwegian by a second researcher is one way the authors could check the accuracy of their translation.

The study instruments (those concepts measured with a numerical rating scale) would benefit from a more detailed description: while 'breathlessness' and 'feeling secure' are reasonably self-explanatory, the concept of 'breathing progress' could be more clearly described. The authors' use of a diagram to convey their dichotomous data (yes/no in response remembered breathlessness in the ICU and persistent breathing problems several months after ICU) gives the reader an excellent grasp of these findings. It is not clear, however, whether those with ongoing breathing problems had a preexisting respiratory morbidity that would account for their ongoing breathlessness.

In the discussion, the authors note contradictory findings; that the four participants with high breathlessness scores during their trial for spontaneous breathing did not recall feeling breathless. The authors propose this could be due to ICU patients' difficulty in distinguishing generally between breathing and the illness experience. It seems equally likely that this is due to 'recall bias', where the time between events and data collection (in this case, between 5 and 14 months) impacts on the completeness of the person's recollections. The authors' strategy of seeking concrete examples for discussion, i.e. 'Can you tell me about a time when you felt breathless?' is a good way to help participants focus on and explore a specific remembered event that may have been powerful for them.

Finally, the authors propose two major influences for their phenomenological framing. The phenomenological approach, guided by the writings of van Manen and Gadamer, situate this work as interpretative, rather than descriptive. This means the authors bring a higher level of abstraction, with a focus on co-creation of meaning between researcher and participants, compared to descriptive approaches that tend to stay closer to the data. Consequently, their findings are powerfully and creatively described. With such rich influences underpinning the work it would be usual to provide greater explanation of this framing in the methods section, and then to discuss how this framing informed the analysis in the discussion section. Instead, a third existential philosopher, Merleau-Ponty, provides the lens for the discussion section which challenges the coherence of the authors' philosophical stance.

Despite some omissions in reporting, these authors have provided a rich account of participant experience. Their themes of *an existential threat*; a *tough time*; *an amorphous and boundless body* and patient's strategies for *getting through*[92] give a sense of the researchers' deep engagement with the data and an ability to co-create meaning with their participants in a way that connects with important existential elements of lived experience. Importantly, the tension between a nurse's quest for objective, easily-documented measures of dyspnoea, and a patient's nuanced and embodied experience of feeling breathless is confirmed in these findings. That the patient is frequently unable to self-report these nuanced symptoms, and that breathlessness is not a separate phenomenon, but is rather intertwined with their broader experience of being a critically ill person, is an important consideration for nurses conducting respiratory assessments in the ICU.

Online resources

Acidbase.org, www.acidbase.org

American Association for Respiratory Care, www.aarc.org

ARDS Network, www.ardsnet.org

Asian Pacific Society of Respirology, www.apsresp.org

Australian & New Zealand Society of Respiratory Science, www.anzsrs.org.au

Australian Lung Foundation, www.lungnet.org.au

Australian Resuscitation Council. Arterial blood gas analysis workshop, https://resus.org.au/download/als2_instructor/clinical/skill_stations/arterial_blood_gas_analysis/abg-workshop-guidance-jun-2016.pdf.

Basic Lung Sounds Tutorial, https://www.littmann.com.au/3M/en_AU/littmann-stethoscopes-au/education-center/training/

Become an expert in spirometry, www.spirxpert.com

Capnography: a comprehensive educational website, www.capnography.com

Chest X-rays, www.learningradiology.com

Critical Care Medicine Tutorials, www.ccmtutorials.com

European Respiratory Journal, erj.ersjournals.com

Lung Health Promotion Centre, The Alfred Hospital, Victoria, www.lunghealth.org

Respiratory Care online, www.rcjournal.com

Respiratory Research, http://respiratory-research.com

Thoracic Society of Australia and New Zealand, www.thoracic.org.au

Thorax: An International Journal of Respiratory Medicine, http://thorax.bmj.com

Further reading

Abdo WF, Heunks LMA. Oxygen-induced hypercapnia in COPD: myths and facts. Crit Care 2012;16:323.

Barbara, R-R, Thomas, EA. Interpretation of chest radiographs. InnovAiT 2018. Royal College of General Practitioners. Online. Available from: http://journals.sagepub.com/doi/abs/10.1177/1755738017735864. [Accessed 24 February 2018].

Blanch L, Villagra A, Sales B, et al. Asynchronies during mechanical ventilation are associated with mortality. Intensive Care Med 2015;41(4):633–41.

Brochard L, Martin GS, Blanch L, et al. Clinical review: respiratory monitoring in the ICU – a consensus of 16. Crit Care 2012;16(2):219. http://doi.org/10.1186/cc11146.

Dempsey JA, Smith CA. Pathophysiology of human ventilator control. Eur Respir J 2014;44:495–512.

Haugdahl H, Storli S, Meland B, et al. Underestimation of patient breathlessness by nurses and physicians during a spontaneous breathing trial. Am J Respir Crit Care Med 2015;192(12):1440–8.

Jacono FJ. Control of ventilation in COPD and lung injury. Respir Physiol Neurobiol 2013;189:371–6.

Kallet, R. Dyspnoea and asynchrony during mechanical ventilation. Crit Care April 2016 Online. Available from: https://www.ahcmedia.com/articles/137506-dyspnea-and-asynchrony-during-mechanical-ventilation. [Accessed 24 February 2018].

Martin, P. 6 mechanical ventilation nursing care plans. Nurseslabs, 2016. Online. Available from: https://nurseslabs.com/6-mechanical-ventilation-nursing-care-plans/5/. [Accessed 24 February 2018].

Metkus TS, Kim BS. Bedside diagnosis in the Intensive Care Unit. Is looking overlooked? Ann Am Thorac Soc 2015;12(10):1447–50.

Spiegel J. End-tidal carbon dioxide: the most vital of vital signs. Anesthesiology News, October 2013. Online. Available from: http://www.anesthesiologynews.com/download/Capnography_ANSE13_WM.pdf; [Accessed 30 July 2014].

References

1. Wunsch H, Angus D, Harrison D, et al. Comparison of medical admissions to intensive care units in the United States and United Kingdom. Am J Respir Crit Care Med 2011;183:1666–73.
2. Hillman K, Bristow PJ, Chey T, et al. Duration of life-threatening antecedents prior to intensive care admission. Intensive Care Med 2002;28:1629–34.
3. Urden L, Stacy K, Lough M. Critical care nursing: diagnosis and management. 6th ed. St Louis: Mosby; 2010.
4. Stanfield C. Principles of human physiology. 6th ed. Harlow: Pearson Education; 2016.
5. Marieb E, Wilhelm P, Mallatt J. Human anatomy. Global ed. London: Pearson Education; 2017.
6. Shier D, Butler J, Lewis R. Hole's human anatomy and physiology. 14th International ed. New York: McGraw Hill; 2016.
7. Thompson J, McFarland G, Hirsch J, et al. Mosby's clinical nursing. 5th ed. St Louis: Mosby; 2002.
8. West J, Luks A. Respiratory physiology: the essentials. 10th ed. Philadelphia: Wolters Kluwer; 2016.
9. Martini F, Ober W, Nath J, et al. Visual anatomy and physiology. 3rd Global ed. Harlow: Pearson Education; 2018.
10. Amerman E. Human anatomy and physiology. Global ed. Harlow: Pearson Education; 2016.
11. Aly H, Mohamed M, Wung J. Surfactant and continuous positive airway pressure for the prevention of chronic lung disease: history, reality, and new challenges. Semin Fetal Neonatal Med 2017;22:348–53.
12. Marieb E, Hoehn K. Human anatomy and physiology. 8th ed. San Francisco: Benjamin Cummings Pearson; 2010.
13. Stacy K. Pulmonary anatomy and physiology. In: Urden L, Stacy K, Lough M, eds. Critical care nursing: diagnosis and management. Maryland Heights: Elsevier; 2014.
14. Hall JE. Regulation of respiration. In: Hall JE, Guyton AC, editors. Guyton and Hall Textbook of medical physiology. 13th ed. Philadelphia: Elsevier; 2014.
15. Shier D, Butler J, Lewis R. Hole's human anatomy and physiology. 13th International ed. New York: McGraw Hill; 2013.
16. Jacono F. Control of ventilation in COPD and lung injury. Respir Physiol Neurobiol 2013;189:371–6.
17. Abdo W, Heunks L. Oxygen-induced hypercapnia in COPD: myths and facts. Crit Care 2012;16:323.
18. O'Driscoll B, Howard L, Earis J, et al. BTS guideline for oxygen use in adults in healthcare and emergency settings. Thorax 2017;72:ii1–90.
19. Beasley R, Chien J, Douglas J, et al. Thoracic Society of Australia and New Zealand oxygen guidelines for acute oxygen use in adults: 'Swimming between the flags'. Respirology 2015;20:1182–91.
20. Saraswat V. Effects of anaesthesia techniques and drugs on pulmonary function. Indian J Anaesth 2015;59:557–64.
21. Papana K, Pagana T, Pagana T. Mosby's diagnostic and laboratory test reference. 13th ed. Philadelphia: Elsevier; 2017. p. 648–750.
22. Urden LD, Stacy KM, Lough ME. Critical care nursing: diagnosis and management. 7th ed. St Louis: Mosby; 2014.
23. Hall JE. Guyton and Hall Textbook of medical physiology. 13th ed. Philadelphia: Saunders; 2015.
24. Lumb A. Nunn's applied respiratory physiology. 8th ed. New York: Elsevier; 2017.
25. Fox S. Human physiology. 13th ed. New York: McGraw Hill; 2012.
26. Morton P, Rempher K. Patient assessment: respiratory system. In: Morton P, Fontaine D, editors. Essentials of critical care nursing: a holistic approach. 10th ed. 2013.
27. Seely R, Stephens T, Tate P. Anatomy and physiology. 7th ed. Boston: McGraw Hill; 2006.

28. Luks A, Schoene R, Swenson E. High altitude. In: Mason R, Ernst J, King TJ, et al, editors. Murray and Nadel's Textbook of respiratory medicine [Internet]. 6th ed. Philadelphia: Elsevier Saunders; 2016.
29. Bellani G, Laffey J, Pham T, et al. Epidemiology, patterns of care, and mortality for patients with acute respiratory distress syndrome in Intensive Care Units in 50 countries. JAMA 2016;15:788–800.
30. Hill N. Acute ventilatory failure. In: Mason R, Ernst J, King TJ, et al, editors. Murray and Nadel's Textbook of respiratory medicine [Internet]. Philadelphia: Elsevier Saunders; 2016.
31. Urden L, Stacy K, Lough M. Critical care nursing: diagnosis and management. 8th ed. St Louis: Mosby; 2018.
32. Powell F, Wanger P, West J. Ventilation, blood flow and gas exchange. In: Mason R, Ernst J, King TJ, et al, editors. Murray and Nadel's Textbook of respiratory medicine. 6th ed. Philadelphia: Elsevier Saunders; 2016.
33. Carlson K. Advanced critical care nursing. St Louis: Saunders Elsevier; 2009.
34. Sakka S. Extravascular lung water in ARDS patients. Minerva Anestesiol 2013;79:274–84.
35. Matthay M, Murray J. Pulmonary edema. In: Mason R, Ernst J, King TJ, et al, editors. Murray and Nadel's Textbook of respiratory medicine [Internet]. 6th ed. Philadelphia: Elsevier Saunders; 2016.
36. Davis L, Murray J. History and physical examination. In: Mason R, Ernst J, King TJ, et al, editors. Murray and Nadel's Textbook of respiratory medicine [Internet]. 6th ed. Philadelphia: Elsevier Saunders; 2016.
37. MacNee W, Vestbo J, Agusti A. COPD: pathogenesis and natural history. In: Mason R, Ernst J, King TJ, et al, editors. Murray and Nadel's Textbook of respiratory diseases [Internet]. Philadelphia: Elsevier Saunders; 2016.
38. Trimble A, Moffatt V, Collins A. Pulmonary infections in the returned traveller. Pneumonia 2017;9.
39. Chen L, Han P, Wilson M, et al. Self-reported illness among Boston-area international travelers: a prospective study. Travel Med Infect Dis 2016;14:604–13.
40. Kreiss K. Occupational causes of constrictive bronchiolitis. Curr Opin Allergy Clin Immunol 2013;13:167–72.
41. Weber J, Kelly J. Health assessment in nursing. Philadelphia: Lippincott, Williams and Wilkins; 2010.
42. Light R. Pneumothorax, chylothorax, hemothorax and fibrothorax. In: Mason R, Ernst J, King TJ, et al, editors. Murray and Nadel's Textbook of respiratory medicine [Internet]. 6th ed. Philadelphia: Elsevier Saunders; 2016.
43. Cheng G, Varghese T, Park D. Pneumonemiastinum and mediastinitis. In: Mason R, Ernst J, King TJ, et al, editors. Murray and Nadel's Textbook of respiratory medicine [Internet]. 6th ed. Philadelphia: Elsevier Saunders; 2016.
44. Bidkar P, Prabhakar H. Stridor. In: Prabhakar H, editor. Complications of neuroanesthesia. Cambridge, MA: Academic Press; 2016. p. 237–46.
45. Sarkar M, Madabhavi I, Niranjan N, et al. Auscultation of the respiratory system. Ann Thorac Med 2015;10:158–68.
46. Zochios V, Protopapas A, Valchanov K. Stridor in adult patients presenting from the community: an alarming clinical sign. J Intensive Care Soc 2015;16:272–3.
47. Jubran A. Pulse oxymetry. Crit Care 2015;19:272.
48. Pretto J, Roebuck T, Beckert L, et al. Clinical use of pulse oximetry: official guidelines from the Thoracic Society of Australia and New Zealand. Respirology 2014;19:38–46.
49. Whitaker D, Benson J. Capnography standards for outside the operating room. Curr Opin Anaesthesiol 2016;29:485–92.
50. Walsh B, Crotwell D, Restrepo R. AARC clinical practice guideline. Capnography/capnometry during mechanical ventilation: 2011. Respir Care 2011;56:503–9.
51. Joint Faculty of Intensive Care Medicine. Minimum standards for transport of critically ill patients. Melbourne: Joint Faculty of Intensive Care Medicine; 2010.
52. Gelsomino S, Lorusso R, Livi U, et al. Assessment of a continuous blood gas monitoring system in animals during circulatory stress. BMC Anesthesiol 2011;11(1):https://doi.org/10.1186/1471-2253-11-1. [Accessed February 2018].
53. Theodore A, Manaker S, Finlay G. Arterial Blood Gases. UpToDate. Online. Available from: https://www.uptodate.com/contents/arterial-blood-gases. [Accessed 9 July 2018].
54. Danckers M. Arterial Blood Gas Sampling Technique. Medscape. Online. Available from: https://emedicine.medscape.com/article/1902703-technique. [Accessed 20 February 2018].
55. Wiegand DE. AACN procedure manual for high acuity, progressive, and critical care. 7th ed. Philadelphia: Elsevier Health Sciences; 2017. p. 531.
56. Baird G. Preanalytical considerations in blood gas analysis. Biochem Med (Zagreb) 2013;23:1927.
57. Ullman A, Keogh S, Coyer F, et al. 'True blood' the critical care story: an audit of blood sampling practice across three adult paediatric and neonatal intensive care settings. Aust Crit Care 2016;29:90–5.
58. Yartsev A The actual bicarbonate value. Online. Available from: http://www.derangedphysiology.com/main/. [Accessed 17 February 2018].
59. Higgins C Temperature correction of blood gas and pH measurement - an unresolved controversy. Online. Available from: https://acutecaretesting.org/en/articles/temperature-correction-of-blood-gas-and-ph-measurement–an-unresolved-controversy (2016, accessed 17 February 2018).
60. McLeod A. Arterial blood gas analysis - making it easy. Cumbria: M & K Update; 2016.

61. Gunnerson K, Pinsky M. Lactic Acidosis. Medscape. Online. Available from: https://emedicine.medscape.com/article/167027-overview (2017, accessed 18 February 2018).
62. Stewart P. How to understand acid-base A quantitative acid-base primer for biology and medicine. New York: Elsevier; 1981.
63. Morgan T. The Stewart Approach – One clinician's perspective. Clin Biochem Rev 2009;30:41–54.
64. Ahmed S, Maheshwari P, Agarwal S, et al. Evaluation of the efficacy of simplified Fencl-Stewart equation in analyzing the changes in acid base status following resuscitation with two different fluids. Int J Crit Illn Inj Sci 2013;3:206–10.
65. Elbers P, Gatz R. Acidbase.org: Bringing Stewart to the bedside. Online. Available from: http://www.acidbase.org/. [Accessed 23 July 2014].
66. Theodore A, Manaker S, Finlay G. Venous blood gases and other alternatives to arterial blood gases. UpToDate. Available from: https://www.uptodate.com/contents/arterial-blood-gases. [Accessed 18 February 2018].
67. Reyer E. The hemodynamic and physiological relevance of continuous central venous oxygenation monitoring: moving beyond sepsis. Online. Available from: http://www.icumed.com/media/402627/m1-1430-reyer-scvo2-oximetry-white-paper-rev02-web.pdf. [Accessed 17 February 2018].
68. Doorduin J, Haans A, van der Hoeven J, et al. Difficult weaning: principles and practice of a structured diagnostic approach. Netherlands J Crit Care 2013;17(4):11–15.
69. Maiden J. Pulmonary diagnostic procedures. In: Urden L, Stacy K, Lough M, editors. Critical care nursing: diagnosis and management. 7th ed. St Louis. 2014. p. 505–13.
70. The ARDS Definition Taskforce. Acute Respiratory Distress Syndrome: the Berlin definition. JAMA 2012;307:2526–33.
71. The Royal College of Pathologists of Australia. RCPA manual. The Royal College of Pathologists of Australia. Online. Available from: http://rcpamanual.edu.au/index.php?option=com_pttests&task=show_test&id=268&Itemid=77&msg=425. [Accessed 16 July 2010].
72. Sterling S, Puskarich M, Jones A. The effect of liver disease on lactate normalization in severe sepsis and septic shock: a cohort study. Clin Exp Emerg Med 2015;2:197–202.
73. Shepherd E. Specimen collection 4: procedure for obtaining a sputum specimen. Nurs Times 2017;113:49–51.
74. Intensive Care Coordination & Monitoring Unit. Suctioning an adult ICU patient with an artificial airway: a clinical practice guideline. Chatswood: Agency for Clinical Innovation; 2014. Available from: https://www.aci.health.nsw.gov.au/__data/assets/pdf_file/0010/239554/ACI14_Suction_2-2.pdf. [Accessed 26 Feb 2019].
75. BD Diagnostics. Nasopharyngeal specimen collection. Sparks, USA: Becton, Dickinson and Company, 2014.
76. NSW Health. Collection of nasal and throat swabs for respiratory virus testing. North Sydney: NSW Ministry of Health. Available from: https://www.health.nsw.gov.au/Infectious/Influenza/Documents/resp-video-instructions.pdf, 2011.
77. Ganapathy A, Adhikari N, Spiegelman J, et al. Routine chest x-rays in intensive care units: a systematic review and meta-analysis. Crit Care 2012;16:R68.
78. Canadian Agency for Drugs and Technologies in Health. Portable versus fixed X-ray equipment: a review of the clinical effectiveness, cost-effectiveness, and guidelines. Online. Available from: https://www.ncbi.nlm.nih.gov/books/NBK350586/. [Accessed 9 July 2018].
79. Cadogan M. CXR Interpretation. Online. Available from: https://lifeinthefastlane.com/investigations/cxr-interpretation/. [Accessed 24 February 2018].
80. Cukor D, Coplan J, Brown C, et al. Depression and anxiety in urban hemodialysis patients. Clin J Am Soc Nephrol 2007;2:484–90. doi:10.2215/cjn.00040107.
81. Tintalli J. Tintalli's Emergency medicine: a comprehensive study guide. New York: McGraw Hill Education; 2016.
82. Brochard L, Martin G, Blanch L, et al. Clinical review: respiratory monitoring in the ICU – a consensus of 16. Crit Care 2012;16:219.
83. Lichtenstein D. BLUE-Protocol and FALLS-Protocol: two applications of lung ultrasound in the critically ill. Chest 2015;147:1659–70.
84. Bentz M, Primack SL. Intensive care unit imaging. Clin Chest Med 2015;36:219–34.
85. Schramm K. Acute pulmonary embolism (Helical CT), (2016, accessed 24 February 2018).
86. Xie Z, Liao X, Kang Y, et al. Radiation exposure to staff in intensive care unit with portable CT scanner. Biomed Research International, https://www.hindawi.com/journals/bmri/2016/5656480/ (2016, accessed 24 February 2018).
87. Godfrey E. Magnetic resonance imaging. In: Falter F, Screaton N, editors. Imaging the ICU patient. London: Springer; 2014. p. 35–46.
88. Eyal A, Roguin A. Magnetic resonance imaging in patients with cardiac implantable electronic devices. Circulation 2015;132:e176–8.
89. De Andres J, Martinez-Sanjuan V, Fabregat-Cid G, et al. MRI-compatible spinal cord stimulator device and related changes in patient safety and imaging artifacts. Pain Med 2014;15:1815–19.
90. American College of Radiology and the Radiological Society of North America. Magnetic Resonance Imaging (MRI). RadiologyInfoorg, http://www.radiologyinfo.org/en/safety/index.cfm?pg=sfty_mr. [Accessed 9 July 2018].
91. Kabadayi S, Bellamy M. Bronchospcopy in critical care. BJA Educ 2017;17:48–56.
92. Haugdahl H, Dahlberg H, Klepstad P, et al. The breath of life. Patients' experiences of breathing during and after mechanical ventilation. Intensive Crit Care Nurs 2017;40:85–93.

Chapter 14

Respiratory alterations and management

Ana Hutchinson, Jennifer McGaughey

Learning objectives

After reading this chapter, you should be able to:

- discuss the underlying pathophysiology and evidenced-based management of acute respiratory failure
- differentiate between hypoxaemic and hypercapnoeic respiratory failure
- critically review the incidence of respiratory alterations in the critical care context
- discuss the aetiology, pathophysiology, clinical manifestations and management of common respiratory disorders managed in intensive care, specifically pneumonia, pandemic respiratory infections, asthma, chronic obstructive pulmonary disease, pneumothorax and pulmonary embolism
- describe the evidence base for key components of nursing and collaborative practice involved in the management of patients with acute respiratory failure in the intensive care unit
- outline the principles and immediate postoperative management for lung transplant recipients.

KEY WORDS

acute respiratory distress syndrome
acute respiratory failure
asthma
chronic obstructive pulmonary disease
lung transplant
respiratory infections

Introduction

The most common reason why patients require admission to an intensive care unit (ICU) is for support of the respiratory system. Use of mechanical ventilation is high with almost half of all patients admitted to ICU requiring this level of support.[1] Utilisation of mechanical ventilation increased from 178.8 cases per 100,000 US adults (341,164 cases) in 1993 to 310.9 per 100,000 (723,310 cases) in 2009.[2] Failure or inadequate function of the respiratory system occurs as a result of direct or indirect pathophysiological conditions. The process of mechanical ventilation may also injure a patient's lungs, further impacting functioning of the respiratory system. Preventing or minimising ventilator-associated lung injury is therefore also a primary goal of patient care.

In Chapter 13 the relevant assessment and monitoring practices for a patient with life-threatening respiratory dysfunction are described. In this chapter the incidence, pathophysiology, clinical manifestations and management of common respiratory disorders that result in acute respiratory failure are described. Specific conditions such as pneumonia, pandemic respiratory infections, asthma, chronic obstructive pulmonary disease (COPD), respiratory failure, acute respiratory distress syndrome (ARDS), pulmonary embolism, pneumothorax and lung transplantation are discussed. Respiratory support strategies including oxygenation and ventilation to support respiratory function during a critical illness are presented in Chapter 15.

Incidence of respiratory alterations

Respiratory diseases are common and affect significant numbers of people. They are among the leading causes of death worldwide.[3] In 2015, the Global Burden of Disease study estimated that lower respiratory tract infections were the fifth-leading cause of death worldwide and the leading infectious cause of death.[3] Although mortality associated with lower respiratory tract infections has decreased overall, the ageing population has resulted in a greater burden of disease and more disability-adjusted life-years (DALYS) lost in the over 70 years age group.[3] Between 1990 and 2015 the global prevalence of obstructive lung diseases has increased, with the prevalence of COPD increasing by 44% and asthma by 12.6%.[4] In 2011, in Australia, respiratory conditions were ranked as the sixth leading contributor to total disease burden; with COPD contributing (43%), asthma (29%) and upper respiratory conditions (20%) of the total burden of respiratory disease.[5]

Respiratory diseases are also the most common illnesses responsible for emergency admissions to hospital and visits to general practitioners and represent the most frequently reported long-term illnesses in children.[6] Infective processes, such as influenza and pneumonia, COPD, asthma and community-acquired pneumonia (CAP) represent the three largest groups of non-elective presentations requiring hospital admission. Conditions such as pneumothorax, pulmonary embolus and pulmonary oedema are relatively small groups. It should be noted, however, that these conditions often evolve throughout the course of an illness and may not, therefore, be included as the reason for admission.[7] Common respiratory alterations managed in ICU are discussed in the following sections.

Respiratory failure

Respiratory failure occurs when there is a reduction in the body's ability to maintain either oxygenation or ventilation, or both. It may occur acutely, as observed in pneumonia, or it may persist in chronic form, as observed in asthma and COPD.

Aetiology of respiratory failure

For the respiratory system to function effectively, the rate and depth of breathing has to be controlled appropriately by the brain, the chest wall must expand adequately, air needs to flow easily through the airways and effective exchange of gases needs to occur at the alveolar level. Conditions that impact one or more aspects of normal physiological functioning of the respiratory system can cause respiratory failure. The mortality associated with admission to hospital with acute respiratory failure varies according to the cause, but overall US data suggest a 20% risk of death.[8]

Respiratory failure is classified on the basis of onset (acute, chronic or acute on chronic) or on blood gas (hypoxaemic, hypercarbic or combined oxygen and ventilatory failure).[9] Acute respiratory failure is characterised by life-threatening alterations in function, the manifestations of chronic respiratory failure are more subtle and potentially more difficult to diagnose. Patients with chronic respiratory failure often experience acute exacerbations of their disease, also resulting in the need for intensive respiratory support.[10]

Pathophysiology

Respiratory failure occurs when the respiratory system fails to achieve one or both of its essential gas exchange functions – oxygenation or elimination of carbon dioxide – and can be described as hypoxaemic respiratory failure, which is primarily a failure of oxygenation, or hypercapnoeic respiratory failure, which is primarily a failure of ventilation.[9]

Hypoxaemic respiratory failure: failure to oxygenate

A patient with hypoxaemic respiratory failure presents with a low partial pressure of oxygen (PaO_2) and a normal or low partial pressure of carbon dioxide ($PaCO_2$). It is defined as hypoxaemia that is refractory to supplemental oxygen (PaO_2 <8 kPa/<60 mmHg).[9,11] Hypoxaemic respiratory failure may be caused by a reduction in inspired oxygen pressure as might occur at extreme altitude, alveolar hypoventilation, impaired oxygen diffusion or ventilation–perfusion mismatch (V/Q mismatch) (Fig. 14.1).[12]

Most major respiratory alterations can cause hypoxaemic respiratory failure, usually as a result of alveolar collapse or consolidation as occurs in severe pneumonia, or excess fluid in the lungs (decompensated chronic heart failure, renal failure or ARDS).[9] These alterations disrupt the ability of lung tissue to transfer oxygen across the alveolar membrane and hypoxaemia ensures. A severe form of mismatch known as intrapulmonary shunting occurs when adequate perfusion exists but there are sections of lung tissue that are not ventilated. In these alveoli, the oxygen content is similar to that of the mixed venous blood and the carbon dioxide (CO_2) is elevated. In other instances, ventilation may be adequate but perfusion is impaired (e.g. pulmonary embolus). In its severe form, this is known as dead space ventilation as the lungs continue to be ventilated but there is limited or no perfusion, and therefore no gas exchange. In this

FIGURE 14.1 Ventilation–perfusion mismatches.[3] Ventilation–perfusion (V/Q) ratio displays the normal balance (*star*) between alveolar ventilation and vascular perfusion allowing for proper oxygenation. When ventilation is reduced, the V/Q ratio decreases, in the most extreme case resulting in pure shunt, where V/Q = 0. When perfusion is reduced, the V/Q ratio increases, in the most extreme case resulting in pure dead space, where V/Q = infinite (∞).

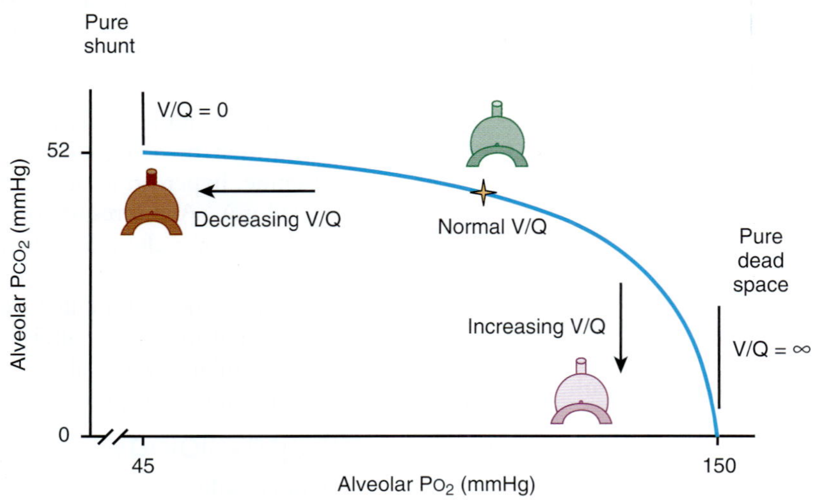

Adapted from Broaddus VC, Ernst JD, King TE, et al. Nadel's Textbook of respiratory medicine, 2-volume set. 6th ed. Philadelphia: Elsevier, 2016, with permission.

situation, the alveolar oxygen content is similar to that of the inspired gas mixture and the carbon dioxide is minimal (see Chapter 13 for further discussion).[9-13]

Hypercapnoeic respiratory failure: failure to ventilate

A patient with hypercapnoeic respiratory failure presents with a high $PaCO_2$, defined as a $PaCO_2$ >6.7 kPa/ > 50 mm Hg.[9,11] This failure is caused by alveolar hypoventilation, where the respiratory effort or minute ventilation is insufficient to allow adequate exchange of oxygen and CO_2. This may be caused by conditions that reduce respiratory drive (sedation, head injury, central nervous system infection), abnormalities of the spinal cord, neuromuscular diseases (Guillain–Barré syndrome, muscular dystrophies), chest wall abnormalities (flail chest, kyphoscoliosis), severe airflow obstruction (exacerbations of asthma or COPD) or increased CO_2 production (sepsis, burns).[11,12] COPD is one of the most common causes of hypercapnoeic acute respiratory failure[9] with 44% of patients admitted with acute exacerbations showing a degree of hypercapnia.[10]

Clinical manifestations

Patient presentations in acute respiratory failure can be quite diverse and are dependent on the underlying pathophysiological mechanism, the specific aetiology and any comorbidities that may exist.[11-14] Specific clinical manifestations for the disorders discussed in this chapter are provided in each section. Dyspnoea is the most common symptom associated with acute respiratory failure;[14] this is often accompanied by an increased rate and reduced depth of breathing and the use of accessory muscles with the notable exception of hypoventilation caused by impaired neural respiratory drive, typically from drugs such as narcotics.[15] Patients may also present with cyanosis, anxiety, confusion and/or sleepiness.[10,12]

A systematic approach to clinical assessment and management of patients with acute respiratory failure is crucial, given the large number of possible causes. Clinical investigations to assess the cause of respiratory failure vary depending on the suspected underlying aetiology and the progression of disease. Arterial blood gas (ABG) analysis, the measurement of PaO_2, $PaCO_2$, alveolar–arterial PO_2 difference and patient response to supplemental oxygen are key elements in determining the cause of acute respiratory failure. Continuous monitoring of oxygen saturation using pulse oximetry, ABG analysis and analysis of chest X-rays (CXR) are used in almost all cases of respiratory failure. Other more specialised tests such as computed tomography (CT), magnetic resonance imaging (MRI), pulmonary angiography, and other specialised investigations may be used in specific circumstances[16] (see Chapter 13).

Patient management

The primary survey (airway, breathing and circulation) and immediate management form initial routine practice.[17] Frequent assessment and monitoring of respiratory function, including a patient's response to supplemental oxygen and/or ventilatory support, is the focus. Patient comfort and compliance with the ventilation mode, ABG analysis and pulse oximetry guide any titration of respiratory support. The key goals of management are to treat the primary cause of respiratory failure, maintain adequate gas exchange and prevent or minimise the potential complications of positive pressure mechanical ventilation.[12,13,17] Comorbidities add to the complexity of managing a patient's primary condition and increase the risk of additional organ dysfunction or failure. Chronic respiratory conditions can have a significant impact on the severity of respiratory infections, while cardiovascular and renal diseases impact on disease severity and the management of many respiratory alterations. Other factors such as smoking and alcohol use, living conditions and lifestyle impact on the predisposition and clinical course of an illness.[2]

Maintaining oxygenation

The therapeutic aim is to titrate the fraction of inspired oxygen (FiO_2) to achieve a PaO_2 of 9.3 kPa/70 mmHg and to maintain minute ventilation to achieve $PaCO_2$ within normal limits where possible.[12,13,18] In acute hypoxaemic respiratory failure the use of high flow nasal cannula appears to be superior to traditional oxygen delivery systems in improving oxygenation and lung mechanics and lowering intubation rate.[19-22] Use of high flow nasal oxygen therapy can therefore be considered in patients who do not achieve target oxygen levels with traditional supplemental oxygen delivery devices.

Oxygen administration targets should be adjusted for patients with chronic hypercapnia and the administration of controlled oxygen therapy should be used to achieve a target saturation of 88–92% in all causes of acute hypercapnoeic respiratory failure. Trials of non-invasive ventilation should be started when pH<7.35 and $PaCO_2$ >6.5 kPa/49 mmHg persist or develop despite optimal medical therapy.[18]

The use of non-invasive ventilation (NIV) for the management of patients with COPD and acute hypercapnoeic respiratory failure is now considered to be standard care[23] and has been demonstrated to decrease the need for endotracheal intubation and patient mortality. A management plan should provide measures to be taken in the event of NIV failure.

Nursing staff in ICU are commonly responsible for titration of oxygen therapy to maintain a specific PaO_2 or SpO_2.[17] One concern that often arises, particularly with patients who require high concentrations of oxygen, is the risk of oxygen toxicity. The link between prolonged periods of oxygen concentrations approaching 100% and oxidant injuries in airways and lung parenchyma has been established, although mostly from animal research.[25] Although it remains unclear how these data apply to human populations, most consensus groups have argued that FiO_2 values less than 0.4 are safe for prolonged periods of time and that FiO_2 values of greater than 0.8 should be avoided if possible[25] (see Chapter 15 for further detail on assessment and management of oxygenation).

Supporting ventilation

Ventilator-associated lung injury is also a concern when managing patients with acute respiratory failure. A lung can be injured when it is stretched excessively as a result of tidal volume settings that generate high pressures, often referred to as barotrauma. The most common injury is that of alveolar rupture and/or air in the pleural space resulting in a pneumothorax. An approach known as 'lung protective ventilation' aims to minimise over-distension of the alveoli through careful monitoring of tidal volumes and airway pressures. This method of ventilation recommends targeted tidal volumes of 4–8 mL/kg per breath, based on predicated body weight, and plateau pressures <30 cmH_2O for all ventilated patients[26] (see Chapter 15 for further discussion).

Development of ventilator-associated respiratory muscle weakness has been reported as a significant issue when the respiratory muscles are rendered inactive through adjustment of ventilator settings and administration of pharmacotherapy.[27,28] A higher rate of weaning failure and mortality is associated with diaphragm dysfunction.[29,30] While it is not yet possible to provide precise recommendations for interventions to avoid this, clinicians are advised to select ventilator settings that provide for some respiratory muscle use.[27]

Prevention or minimisation of complications associated with positive pressure mechanical ventilation remains a major focus of nursing practice.[31] These complications may relate to the patient–ventilator interface (artificial airway and ventilator circuitry), infectious complications or complications associated with sedation and/or immobility. Some common complications and the appropriate management strategies are briefly outlined in Table 14.1 and are discussed further in Chapter 15.

A patient with acute respiratory failure requires extensive multidisciplinary collaboration between nurses, physiotherapists, specialist medical staff, speech and occupational therapists, dieticians, social workers, radiologists and radiographers, pharmacists and microbiologists.[32,35] Patients may require intervention to improve capacity for oxygen delivery through an adequate haemoglobin level and a cardiac output sufficient to supply oxygenated blood to the tissues.[25,26] At times this may require blood transfusion and/or the use of vasoactive medications (see Chapters 11 and 21). Extracorporeal CO_2 removal may be considered in patients with refractory respiratory failure where expertise exists.[36]

Chest physiotherapy is a routine activity for managing patients with acute respiratory failure. This involves positioning, manual hyperinflation, percussion and vibration and suctioning. The evidence base for these techniques is limited, however, with a systematic review reporting no improvement in mortality for patients with

TABLE 14.1
Complications of mechanical ventilation and associated management strategies[12,32-34]

PATIENT–VENTILATOR INTERFACE COMPLICATION	MANAGEMENT STRATEGIES
Airway dislodgement/disconnection	Endotracheal tube or tracheostomy tube is secured to optimise ventilation and prevent airway dislodgement or accidental extubation
Circuit leaks	Cuff pressure assessment Circuit checks Exhaled tidal volume measurement
Airway injury from inadequate heat/humidity	Maintain humidification of the airway using either a heat–moisture exchanger or a water-bath humidifier
Obstructions from secretions	Assess the need for suctioning regularly and suction as required
Tracheal injury from the artificial airway	Assessment of airway placement and cuff pressure (minimal occlusion method)
INFECTIOUS COMPLICATION	**MANAGEMENT STRATEGIES**
Ventilator-associated pneumonia (VAP)	Alcohol-based hand hygiene Appropriate antibiotic therapy Oral decontamination Selective digestive decontamination Semi-recumbent positioning, 30–45° Daily sedation holds Peptic ulcer disease prophylaxis Minimising interruptions to ventilator circuit (e.g. closed suctioning technique) Use of oropharyngeal vs nasopharyngeal feeding tubes Drainage of sub-glottic secretions Small bowel feeding rather than gastric feeding Aerosolised antibiotics for patients who are colonised Weaning and discontinuation of ventilatory support as soon as possible, including using nurse-led weaning protocols Early tracheostomy Prophylactic probiotics
COMPLICATION ASSOCIATED WITH IMMOBILITY/SEDATION	**MANAGEMENT STRATEGIES**
Gastrointestinal dysfunction	Prokinetic medication Constipation – bowel therapy regimen
Muscle atrophy	Passive limb movements, foot splints (see Chapter 5) and early activity/mobility (see Chapter 5)
Pressure injuries	Pressure-relieving mattresses, regular repositioning Assessment of risks and management of pressure injuries by wound care specialists, nutrition advice

Source: Broaddus et al. 2016, Yang et al. 2013, Kalanuria et al. 2014, Elliot et al. 2018.

pneumonia.[32] Guidelines for physiotherapy assessment have enabled identification of patient characteristics for treatments to be prescribed and modified on an individual basis. Table 14.2 provides an outline of management interventions for patients with respiratory failure, particularly those who may require prolonged mechanical ventilation.

Medications

Medications commonly prescribed in respiratory failure include inhalation/intravenous steroids and bronchodilators, antibiotic therapy, analgesia and sedation to maintain patient–ventilator synchrony. A patient's condition, comorbidities and the above-mentioned pharmacological therapy may also be supported with inotropic and other

TABLE 14.2
Long-term patient management in respiratory failure[12,32]

MANAGEMENT	BEST PRACTICE
Timing of tracheostomy insertion	The need for tracheostomy should be individualised.[18] Where mechanical ventilation is expected to be 10 days or more, tracheostomy should be performed as soon as identified. Early tracheostomy is associated with less nosocomial pneumonia, reduced ventilation time and shorter ICU stay
Weaning protocols	Specific plan is patient-dependent; better outcomes are achieved when there is an agreed and well communicated weaning plan
Nutrition	Consider adequate nutrition for physiological needs – important to not overfeed as this increases CO_2 production – and the need to have a balance of vitamins and minerals
Swallow assessment	Assess for dysphagia
Mobilisation	Sitting out of bed, mobilising
Communication	Communication aids, speaking valves
Activities	Activity plan/routine, entertainment (TV/films), visitors, outings
Sleep	Clustering cares, reducing stimuli to promote sleep
Family support	Importance of providing physical, emotional and/or spiritual support to family members
Tracheostomy follow-up	Outreach team: follow-up care by nurses experienced in tracheostomy care can prevent complications and improve outcomes
End-of-life decisions in acute respiratory failure	When clinically appropriate, the withholding and withdrawal of life-sustaining therapy is supported by ethical and legal principles

Source: Broaddus et al. 2016, Yang et al. 2013.

resuscitation therapies (see Chapters 11 and 21). As the use of medications will vary depending on the underlying cause of respiratory failure, these are discussed separately in the sections below.

Practice tip

Obesity hypoventilation syndrome

Obstructive sleep apnoea is a major health and social problem and rising prevalence as obesity becomes more common.[37] Patients who are obese require controlled oxygen therapy to achieve a target saturation of 88–92% and may require NIV similar to hypercapnoeic respiratory failure. As the risk of acute respiratory failure is high it is recommended that these patients are managed in a high dependency area with expertise in the use of continuous positive airway pressure, bi-level positive airway pressure and NIV.[18]

Pneumonia

Pneumonia is infection of the lung. Depending on the type and severity of the infection and the overall health of the person, it may result in acute respiratory failure. Pneumonia can be caused by most types of microorganisms, but is most commonly a result of bacterial or viral infection. In critical care the key distinctions in assessing and managing a patient with pneumonia relate to the specific aetiology or causative organism.[38] In this section the pathophysiology, aetiology, clinical presentation and management of two types of pneumonia are reviewed:

1 CAP
2 ventilator-associated pneumonia (VAP) and ventilator-associated events (VAE).

As a result of the complexity and ambiguity associated with previous definitions of VAP, there has been a significant shift towards measuring VAE as a way of monitoring ventilator-associated complications more broadly.[38] A

Practice tip

Respiratory failure in the elderly

The elderly have ageing organs and systems and other comorbidities that may exacerbate respiratory dysfunction. Frail hospitalised patients with acute respiratory failure may be at greater risk of mortality and prolonged length of hospital stay. Identification of frail patients who are at risk during hospitalisation is important to facilitate cognitive and physical rehabilitation interventions designed to improve long-term outcomes.[19]

VAE is said to have occurred when a decline in respiratory function occurs (defined by a significant increase in FiO_2 or positive end-expiratory pressure [PEEP]) in a ventilated patient after a period of initial stability. Patients who are identified as having had a VAE are then reviewed to determine if clinical signs and symptoms meet the criteria for an infective ventilator-associated complication. Ventilator-associated tracheobronchitis refers to ventilated patients who develop signs of a lower respiratory tract infection without a distinct area of consolidation of CXR. Further investigation of microbiological culture results then determines if the definition of VAP or ventilator-associated tracheobronchitis applies.[38]

Pathophysiology

The normal human lung was previously considered to be sterile; however, recent developments in microbiological diagnostics using molecular gene sequencing techniques have demonstrated that the healthy lung is colonised with microorganisms.[39] The term 'lung microbiome' refers to every organism (not only bacteria, but also archaea, fungi and viruses) that are present in the lower respiratory tract and lung tissues. Understanding how the lung microbiome affects human health and disease is an emerging area of research.[40] Current research has established that healthy lungs have characteristic flora that is not observed in individuals with chronic respiratory conditions such as asthma and COPD. A range of predominantly non-pathogenic bacteria are present at low levels in the lungs of healthy individuals, in contrast in diseased states colonies of potentially pathogenic bacteria become more dominant.[39-41]

A number of defence mechanisms exist to prevent microorganisms entering the lungs, such as particle filtration in the nostrils, sneezing and coughing to expel irritants, and mucus production to trap dust and infectious organisms and move particles out of the respiratory system. Infection occurs when one or more of these defences are not functioning adequately or when an individual encounters a large number of microorganisms at once and the defences are overwhelmed.[41,42] An invading pathogen provokes an immune response in the lungs, resulting in the following pathophysiological processes:

- alteration in alveolar-capillary permeability that leads to an increase in protein-rich fluid in the alveoli; this impacts on gas exchange and causes the patient to breathe faster in an effort to increase oxygen uptake and remove carbon dioxide
- mucus production increases and mucous plugs may develop that block off areas of the lung, further reducing capacity for gas exchange
- consolidation occurs in the alveoli, which fill with fluid and debris; this occurs particularly with bacterial pneumonia where debris accumulates from the large number of white blood cells involved in the immune response.[41,42]

Aetiology

Pneumonia is caused by a variety of microorganisms, including bacteria, viruses, fungi and parasites. In many cases, the causative organism may not be known and current practice in many cases is to initiate antimicrobial treatment as soon as possible, based on symptoms and patient history, rather than waiting for microorganism culture results. Antibiotic stewardship guidelines recommend early review of antibiotic therapy and adjustment of therapy based on microbiological results.[43,44] Different ages and characteristics of patients are often associated with different causative organisms. Viral pneumonias, especially influenza, are most common in young children, while adults are more likely to have pneumonia caused by bacteria such as *Streptococcus pneumoniae*, *Haemophilus influenzae*, *Mycoplasma pneumoniae*, *Chlamydophila pneumoniae* or other respiratory viruses. As the causative organism for CAP is frequently unidentified and there are regional differences in the prevalence of different causative organisms; use of local guidelines is recommended to guide the selection of antibiotic treatment.[43-45]

> **Practice tip**
>
> **Pneumonia in the elderly**
>
> Pneumonia is a particular concern among elderly adults as they experience an increase in the frequency and severity of pneumonia. This is largely due to the decline in immune system response that is associated with age and with the presence of comorbid disease, such as cardiac and respiratory disease. CAP is a major cause of morbidity and mortality in elderly patients. *Streptococcus pneumoniae* is the most common causative organism, with an increase in drug-resistance being reported more widely in the over-65 age group. Immunisation with pneumococcal and influenza vaccines is beneficial in the prevention of pneumonia in elderly patients.[46]

Community-acquired pneumonia

CAP is an acute infection of the pulmonary parenchyma where the infection has been contracted by the patient while in the community. Approximately 25% of patients with CAP require hospitalisation with the incidence increasing with age.[47] Clinical assessment, especially patient history, is important in distinguishing the aetiology and likely causative organism in patients with CAP. Specific information regarding exposure to animals, travel history, nursing home residency and any occupational or unusual exposure may provide the key to diagnosis. Personal habits such as smoking and alcohol consumption increase the risk of developing pneumonia and should be explored. Many patients admitted to hospital with CAP have comorbidities, suggesting that those who are chronically ill have an increased risk of developing acute respiratory failure. The most common chronic illnesses involved are respiratory disease, including smoking history, COPD and asthma, congestive cardiac failure and diabetes mellitus. Table 14.3 outlines aspects of the clinical history associated with particular causative organisms in CAP.[12]

Clinical manifestations

Symptoms for pneumonia are both respiratory and systemic. Common characteristics include fever, sweats, rigours, cough, sputum production, pleuritic chest pain, dyspnoea, tachypnoea, pleural rub, inspiratory crackles on auscultation, plus radiological evidence of infiltrates or consolidation. Cough is the most common finding in CAP and is present in up to 80% of all patients.[50]

Diagnosis

Routine screening of patients with suspected pneumonia continues to rely on microscopy and culture of lower respiratory tract specimens, blood cultures, detection of antigens in urine and serology. Methods for detection of antigens are now widely available for several pneumonia pathogens, particularly *S. pneumoniae*, *Legionella* and some respiratory viruses. Culture of respiratory secretions may be limited due to difficulty in obtaining sputum samples. For this reason, nasopharyngeal aspirates or swabs for respiratory virus detection using polymerase chain reaction techniques may be taken as part of the routine screening for CAP.[44,51,52]

Severity assessment scoring

International guidelines recommend a severity-based approach to management of CAP, in relation to the initial site of treatment (e.g. home, hospital ward, ICU), and appropriate level of intervention, including antibiotic therapy.[50] Several severity scores have been developed and validated; however, to date there is no agreement on the optimal tool or an agreed definition of the term 'severe pneumonia'. CUR65/CURB65 and the Pneumonia Severity Index (PSI) are the most widely recommended systems that produce scores and assess severity based on patient demographics, risk factors, comorbidities, clinical presentation and laboratory results[50] (Box 14.1). The Australian CAP Collaboration team devised and validated the SMART-COP scoring system for predicting the need for intensive respiratory or vasopressor support in patients with CAP. The acronym relates to the factors: low **S**ystolic blood pressure, **M**ultilobar involvement, low **A**lbumin level, high **R**espiratory rate, **T**achycardia, **C**onfusion, poor **O**xygenation and low arterial **p**H.[53] One prospective cohort study found that the SMART-COP scoring system was superior to CURB-65 and PSI in predicting the need for mechanical ventilation and inotropic support.[54]

Hospital-acquired and ventilator-associated pneumonia

Hospital-acquired pneumonia is defined as pneumonia occurring more than 48 hours after hospital admission. It is the second most common nosocomial infection and the leading cause of death from infection acquired in hospital. VAP is a form of hospital-acquired pneumonia that occurs in patients who are mechanically ventilated. The incidence of VAP is reported at 10–30% among patients who require mechanical ventilation for more than 48 hours.[38]

Critically ill ventilated patients commonly experience chest colonisation as a result of microaspiration of oropharyngeal secretions into the lower airways around the endotracheal tube (ETT) or via contamination of the ventilator circuit. This may lead to clinical signs of infection. The patient's severity of disease, physiological reserve and comorbidities influence the development of infection and the likely causative organisms. The likely causative organisms also differ between early onset (<5 days after intubation) and later (>5 days) onset VAP. In early onset VAP *Streptococcus pneumoniae, Haemophilus*

TABLE 14.3
Clinical history/comorbidities associated with particular causative organisms in community-acquired pneumonia[12,48,49]

CONDITION	CAUSATIVE ORGANISMS
Individual factors	
Alcoholism	*S. pneumoniae* (including penicillin-resistant), anaerobes, gram-negative bacilli (possibly *K. pneumoniae*), tuberculosis
Poor dental hygiene	Anaerobes
Elderly	Group B streptococci, *M. catarrhalis, H. influenzae, L. pneumophila*, gram-negative bacilli, *C. pneumoniae* and polymicrobial infections
Smoking (past or present)	*S. pneumoniae, H. influenzae, M. catarrhalis, Aspergillus* spp.
IV drug use	*S. aureus*, anaerobes, *M. tuberculosis, S. pneumoniae*

Continued

TABLE 14.3
Clinical history/comorbidities associated with particular causative organisms in community-acquired pneumonia—cont'd

CONDITION	CAUSATIVE ORGANISMS
Comorbidities	
COPD	*S. pneumoniae, H. influenzae, M. catarrhalis, Aspergillus* spp.
Post-influenza pneumonia	*S. pneumoniae, S. aureus, H. influenzae*
Structural disease of lung (e.g., bronchiectasis, cystic fibrosis)	*P. aeruginosa, P. cepacia* or *S. aureus*
Sickle cell disease, asplenia	Pneumococcus, *H. influenzae*
Previous antibiotic treatment and severe pulmonary comorbidity, (e.g. bronchiectasis, cystic fibrosis, and severe COPD)	*P. aeruginosa*
Malnutrition-related diseases	Gram-negative bacilli
Environmental exposure	
Air conditioning	*L. pneumophila*
Residence in nursing home	*S. pneumoniae*, gram-negative bacilli, *H. influenzae, S. aureus, C. pneumoniae*; consider *M. tuberculosis*; consider anaerobes, but less common
Homeless population	*S. pneumoniae, S. aureus, H. influenzae, C. gattii*: caused by inhalation of spores while sleeping, associated with red gum trees (Australia, Southeast Asia, South America)
Suspected bioterrorism	Anthrax, tularaemia, plague
Animal exposure	
Bat exposure	*H. capsulatum*
Bird exposure	*C. psittaci, C. neoformans, H. capsulatum*
Rabbit exposure	*F. tularensis*
Exposure to farm animals or parturient cats	*C. burnetii* (Q fever)
Travel history	
Travel to southwestern USA	Coccidioidomycosis; hantavirus in selected areas
Travel to southeast Asia	Severe acute respiratory syndrome (coronavirus), *M. tuberculosis*, melioidosis
Residence or travel to rural tropics	Melioidosis (*B. pseudomallei*)
Travel to area of known epidemic	Avian influenza (H5N1), swine influenza (H1N1) and severe acute respiratory syndrome (coronavirus)

COPD = chronic obstructive pulmonary disease; IV = intravenous; *B. pseudomallei* = *Burkholderia pseudomallei*; *C. burnetii* = *Coxiella burnetii*; *C. gattii* = *Cryptococcus gattii*; *C. neoformans* = *Cryptococcus neoformans*; *C. pneumoniae* = *Chlamydophila pneumoniae*; *C. psittaci* = *Chlamydia psittaci*; *F. tularensis* = *Francisella tularensis*; *H. capsulatum* = *Histoplasma capsulatum*; *H. influenzae* = *Haemophilus influenzae*; *K. pneumoniae* = *Klebsiella pneumoniae*; *L. pneumophila* = *Legionella pneumophila*; *M. catarrhalis* = *Moraxella catarrhalis*; *M. tuberculosis* = *Mycobacterium tuberculosis*; *P. aeruginosa* = *Pseudomonas aeruginosa*; *P. cepacia* = *Pseudomonas cepacia*; *S. aureus* = *Staphylococcus aureus*; *S. pneumoniae* = *Streptococcus pneumoniae*.
Source: Broaddus et al. 2016, King et al. 2018, Fink et al. 2011.

BOX 14.1

Severity scoring in CAP

CURB65/CUR65

The score is an acronym for each of the risk factors measured. One point is allocated for each risk factor present, with maximum scores of 5 and 4, respectively:

- C – **c**onfusion: a new onset of confusion, defined as an abbreviated mental test score of 8 or less
- U – **u**rea: blood urea nitrogen level >19 mg/dL
- R – **r**espiratory rate: ≥30 breaths/min
- B – **b**lood pressure: ≤90 mmHg systolic or ≤60 mmHg diastolic (not measured as part of CUR65 scoring system)
- 65 – age: ≥**65** years

Pneumonia severity index

The PSI considers a range of patient characteristics, comorbid diseases, signs and symptoms, and laboratory findings with the intent of classifying the severity of a patient's pneumonia at a risk level ranging from I to V, with V being the most severe. An online PSI calculator (see *Online resources* for link) is available to assist clinicians in applying the scoring system.

- PSI risk class I – patient can be sent home on oral antibiotics
- PSI risk class II–III – patient should be treated with IV antibiotics and may need to be monitored in hospital for 24 h
- PSI risk class IV–V – patient should be hospitalised for treatment

Adapted from Singanayagam A, Chalmers JD, Hill AT. Severity assessment in community-acquired pneumonia: a review. QJM 2009; 6:379–88.

influenzae and methicillin-sensitive *Staphylococcus aureus* are frequent. By contrast, in late-onset VAP *Pseudomonas aeruginosa, Acinetobacter baumannii*, methicillin-resistant *S. aureus* and other Gram-negative bacilli become more common.[38]

Diagnosis

VAP can be difficult to diagnose, as clinical features can be non-specific and other conditions may cause infiltrates on CXR. In addition to this, ambiguity in the definition of VAP has led to inconsistencies in interpretation and application of the definition, which has meant that comparison of incidence and/or treatment effects has been difficult. The current consensus definition developed by a joint international consortium of experts focuses on more objective data.[38] VAP is suspected when additional support is required to maintain oxygenation, such as increased FiO_2 or higher PEEP, clinical signs of infection begin to develop, including new onset of pyrexia or raised white blood cell counts, or when indicated by microbiological culture.[55]

Specific risk factors associated with increased mortality in VAP have been identified over the past decade. The most widely-recognised risk-minimisation factor is the provision of appropriate antibiotic treatment, which has reduced mortality and the rate of complications. Timeliness of antibiotic administration is an independent risk factor for mortality – mortality was increased where administration of antibiotics was delayed for more than 24 hours after diagnosis.[38,56] When VAP is suspected there are two diagnostic strategies that are commonly used to guide antibiotic prescribing:

1. Clinical strategy: involves treatment of patients with new antibiotics, based on patient risk factors and the local microbiological and resistance patterns. Antibiotic therapy is adjusted based on culture results and the patient's response to treatment.
2. Invasive strategy: involves collection and quantitative analysis of respiratory secretions from samples obtained by fibreoptic bronchoscopy or mini-bronchoalveolar lavage to confirm the diagnosis and causative organism. Antibiotic therapy is then guided by specific protocols.

Findings from a systematic review of these strategies did not demonstrate any differences in patient outcome measures including mortality, length of ICU stay or length of ventilation period.[52] Current guidelines recommend that where possible invasive strategies are used to collect samples from the distal lower airways, as this decreases contamination with upper airway secretions and may help minimise inappropriate antibiotic use.[38]

Patient management

VAP prevention strategies

Prevention of VAP is a key emphasis in the care of all mechanically-ventilated patients and involves a number of interventions. VAP prevention has a focus on decreasing the risk of aspiration of upper airway secretions, decreasing microorganism load in the oropharynx and decreasing the introduction of microorganisms into the lower airways from the use of contaminated equipment.

One approach in encouraging the implementation of VAP prevention was the combination of key aspects of patient management into an evidence-based guideline, the *Ventilator Care Bundle*. Components of the *Ventilator Care Bundle* include semirecumbent positioning, sedation holds, stress ulcer disease prophylaxis, deep vein thrombosis prophylaxis, minimising the duration of mechanical ventilation, regular oropharyngeal suctioning, and provision of mouth care and the use of closed in-line suctioning equipment to decrease contamination of the ventilator circuit.[55,57-63] A number of recent studies have demonstrated that using a structured approach to implementation of a VAP Care Bundle improved adherence to implementation of key preventative strategies between 7% and 80%.[58-60] There is level III evidence that successful implementation of a care bundle can also result in decreased VAP rates.[55,58-62]

Regular oral hygiene and frequent removal of oropharyngeal secretions can reduce the risk of microaspiration around the ETT cuff.[64,65] Despite the reported benefits, there is currently a debate about the safety of using chlorhexidine mouthwash in intubated patients.[38,66] Two recent systematic reviews have found non-statistically significant upward trends in patient mortality associated with the use of chlorhexidine mouthwash.[66,67] There is current debate as to whether its use is associated with microaspiration and subsequent acute lung injury. In response to the emerging evidence surrounding the increased mortality associated with the use of chlorhexidine in mouth care, the joint international guidelines do not currently recommend its use in intubated patients.[38,38] Tooth brushing is essential to maintaining the basic hygiene needs of the patient and current evidence supports the role of tooth brushing in the improvement of oral health and subsequent removal of dental plaques.[68] While there is no identified evidence of harm there is no definitive evidence that tooth brushing decreases the occurrence of VAP.

Selective oral or digestive decontamination involves prevention of colonisation by potentially pathogenic microorganisms, such as gram-negative aerobic microorganisms and methicillin-sensitive *Staphylococcus aureus* and yeasts, from the oropharyngeal and intestinal tracts.[38,69] In settings with low levels of antibiotic resistance selective decontamination may be associated with reductions in VAP and mortality.[69] Current guidelines recommend that in ICUs with low levels of antibiotic resistance, selective oral decontamination with non-absorbable antibiotics may be beneficial.[38] Although this strategy has been shown to be effective in reducing morbidity and mortality,[69] it is yet to be widely adopted in clinical practice.[67] Recent review of nursing considerations for administration of selective digestive decontamination highlights the importance of a comprehensive education program and an implementation plan that considers patient safety issues as well as the impact on nursing practice.[70]

Several other new strategies have been suggested and evaluated for their effectiveness in reducing VAP rates. Specialised ETT tubes that allow for aspiration of subglottic secretions,[71,72] and ETT tubes with silver antimicrobial coating have been shown to reduce VAP rates, but need further evaluation before practice recommendations can be made.[73] ETT tubes with modified cuff shapes and devices to continuously maintain ETT cuff pressure have been shown to improve maintenance of cuff pressures but there is no evidence of change in VAP rates.[74,75]

Management

Early recognition of pneumonia, timely administration of appropriate antibiotic therapy and supportive care are key aspects in pneumonia management. Supportive ventilation is a key focus for managing patients with pneumonia. In some instances, this may include increased oxygen delivery and PEEP to maintain oxygenation and prevent alveolar collapse. Chest physiotherapy remains a key component of management of all ventilated patients.[76] However, its contribution towards improving mortality in patients with pneumonia is unclear.[75] Upright positioning[77] and early mobilisation[78] are important elements of both prevention and management of pneumonia. The evidence supporting use of additional strategies, such as beds with a continuous lateral rotation or a vibration function, is limited and has been associated with complications, so recommendations for their use cannot be made.[79] See Chapter 15 for further discussion.

Medications

Antibiotic administration is fundamental to a patient's clinical progress. As noted earlier, the importance of accurate and timely administration of antibiotics directly impacts on patient outcome. In particular, in critically ill patients the first dose of antibiotics should be administered within an hour of the diagnosis of pneumonia being made.[56] Antibiotic cover for pneumonia depends on the causative organism and sensitivity to drugs (Table 14.4). The need for ongoing antibiotic therapy should be reviewed on a regular basis and de-escalation of antibiotic treatment considered once the clinical signs of infection have resolved.[80]

> **Practice tip**
>
> **Pneumonia during pregnancy**
>
> Pneumonia is a leading cause of maternal and fetal morbidity and mortality. It also increases the likelihood of the complications of pneumonia, including requirement for mechanical ventilation. Bacterial pneumonia is the most common type experienced in pregnancy although diagnosis is often delayed as a result of the reluctance to obtain a CXR. Management is similar to a non-pregnant patient with antibiotic therapy adjusted to consider the impact on the fetus.

Respiratory pandemics

Serious outbreaks of respiratory infections that spread rapidly on a global scale are termed pandemics. Their spread is rapid because the infection is usually associated with the emergence of a new virus where the majority of the population has no immunity. These infections are characterised by extremely rapid transmission with concurrent outbreaks throughout the globe; the occurrence of disease outside the usual seasonality, including during the summer months; high attack rates in all

TABLE 14.4
Preferred antimicrobial agents in pneumonia[12]

TYPE OF INFECTION	PREFERRED AGENT(S)
Community-acquired pneumonia	
Streptococcus pneumoniae	Penicillin-susceptible organisms: penicillin G, amoxicillin, clindamycin, doxycycline, telithromycin Penicillin-resistant organisms: cefotaxime, ceftriaxone, vancomycin, fluoroquinolone
Mycoplasma	Doxycycline, macrolide
Chlamydophila pneumoniae	Doxycycline, macrolide
Legionella	Azithromycin, fluoroquinolone (including ciprofloxacin), erythromycin (rifampicin)
Haemophilus influenzae	Second- or third-generation cephalosporin, clarithromycin, doxycycline, beta-lactam/beta-lactamase inhibitor, trimethoprim/sulfamethoxazole, azithromycin, telithromycin
Moraxella catarrhalis	Second- or third-generation cephalosporin, trimethoprim–sulfamethoxazole, macrolide doxycycline, beta-lactam–beta-lactamase inhibitor
Neisseria meningitidis	Penicillin
Streptococci (other than *S. pneumoniae*)	Penicillin, first-generation cephalosporin
Anaerobes	Clindamycin, beta-lactam–beta-lactamase inhibitor, beta-lactam+ metronidazole
Staphylococcus aureus Methicillin-susceptible Methicillin-resistant	Oxacillin, nafcillin, cefazolin; all + rifampin or gentamicin Vancomycin, rifampicin or gentamicin
Klebsiella pneumoniae and other Enterobacteriaceae (excluding Enterobacter spp.)	Third-generation cephalosporin or cefepime (all + aminoglycoside), carbapenem
Hospital-acquired infections	
Enterobacter spp.	Carbapenem, beta-lactam–beta-lactamase inhibitor, cefepime, fluoroquinolone; all + aminoglycoside in seriously ill patients
Pseudomonas aeruginosa	Anti-pseudomonal beta-lactam + aminoglycoside, carbapenem + aminoglycoside
Acinetobacter	Aminoglycoside + piperacillin or a carbapenem

Source: Broaddus VC EJ, King TE, Mason RJ, et al. Murray & Nadel's Textbook of respiratory medicine, 2-volume set. 6th ed. Elsevier; 2016.

age groups, with high levels of mortality particularly in healthy young adults; and multiple waves of disease immediately before and after the main outbreak'.[81]

Several severe respiratory infections have progressed to become pandemics in recent years; these have been associated with the coronavirus and influenza viruses.[82] Prediction of the interval between pandemics is difficult, but occurrence is likely to continue and therefore requires that the healthcare community be well prepared. The InFACT H1N1 Research Collaborative is a global initiative aimed at reducing the mortality associated with H1N1 through clinical research groups and professional organisations working together to gain a rapid understanding of the epidemiology and clinical presentation of the disease, and the identification of effective management strategies.[83]

Influenza epidemics

Epidemics of influenza occur regularly and are associated with high morbidity and mortality.[83] A feature of the influenza virus that explains why it continues to be associated with epidemic and pandemic disease is its high frequency of antigenic variation. This occurs in two of the external glycoproteins and is referred to as antigenic drift or antigenic shift, depending on the extent of the variation. The result of this is that new viruses are introduced into the population and, due to the absence of immunity to the virus, a pandemic of influenza results.[81]

Pandemics of influenza were observed a number of times in the 20th century and were believed to have involved viruses circulating in humans that originated from influenza A viruses in birds. The most recent influenza pandemic was declared by the World Health Organization in 2009 when a novel H1N1 influenza A virus emerged in Mexico and the USA. The disease spread globally with millions of cases reported and resulted in over 16,000 deaths by March 2010.[82] Australian and New Zealand communities had a high proportion of cases of H1N1 influenza A infection, with 856 patients being admitted to ICU, 15 times the incidence of influenza A in other recent years.[84,85]

Priorities for prevention and management of future influenza pandemics involve development of an international surveillance and response network for early detection and containment of the disease, local preparation for controlling the spread of the infection and further development of vaccines and antiviral agents.[81,83]

Patient management

Vaccination

Influenza vaccines are formulated annually based on current and recent viral strains. Success in protecting an individual against influenza requires that the virus strains included in the vaccine are the same as those currently circulating in the community. Vaccines are commonly effective in preventing influenza in 70–90% of healthy adults younger than 65 years of age. Efficacy appears lower in elderly people. Healthcare workers are a key target group for the influenza vaccine, at the very least to reduce absenteeism over what is often the busiest period for most health services and to reduce the risk of nosocomial influenza infections in hospitalised patients.[86,87]

Isolation precautions and personal protective equipment

Key aspects of infection control in an epidemic or pandemic situation focus on limiting opportunities for nosocomial spread and the protection of healthcare workers.[88] Guidelines for institutional management of these infections involve designing and implementing appropriate isolation procedures and recommending appropriate personal protective equipment.[89] Specific infection control guidelines are usually developed for individual institutions, based on government recommendations for management of staff, appropriate personal protective equipment and isolation procedures. This topic is covered in detail in Chapter 6.

Acute respiratory distress syndrome

ARDS is an acute, diffuse inflammatory lung injury, characterised by hypoxemia, bilateral infiltrates, and decreased lung compliance leading to non-hydrostatic pulmonary oedema.[90]

TABLE 14.5
Direct and indirect causes of acute lung injury[93]

DIRECT LUNG INJURY	INDIRECT LUNG INJURY
Pneumonia	Sepsis
Aspiration of gastric contents	Multiple trauma
Pulmonary contusion	Cardiopulmonary bypass
Fat, amniotic fluid or air embolus	Drug overdose
Near drowning	Acute pancreatitis
Inhalational injury (chemical or smoke)	Transfusion of blood products
Reperfusion pulmonary oedema	

Source: Adapted from Thompson BT, Chambers RC, Liu KD. Acute respiratory distress syndrome. N Engl J Med 2017;377(19):1904–5.

Aetiology

ARDS is a characteristic inflammatory response of the lung to a wide variety of insults. Epidemiological studies show a variable incidence of ARDS. Population-based estimates of ARDS range from 10 to 86 cases per 100,000, with the highest rates reported in Australia and the USA.[91] A multicentred prospective cohort study (LUNG SAFE) involving 29,144 patients from 50 countries showed that 10% of all patients admitted to the ICU had ARDS with a 46% mortality for those with severe ARDS.[92] Reasons for this variation may include differences in demographics, healthcare delivery systems and clinical coding practices. Clinical disorders that are commonly associated with ARDS can be separated into those that directly or indirectly injure the lung (Table 14.5).[93]

The most common cause of indirect injury resulting in ARDS is sepsis, followed by severe trauma and haemodynamic shock states. ARDS arising from direct injury to the lung is most commonly seen in patients with pneumonia. The risk of developing ARDS increases significantly when more than one predisposing factor is present.

Pathophysiology

Inflammatory damage to alveoli from locally or systemically released inflammatory mediators causes a change in pulmonary capillary permeability, with resulting fluid and protein leakage into the alveolar space and pulmonary infiltrates. Dilution and loss of surfactant causes diffuse alveolar collapse and a reduction in pulmonary compliance and may also impair the defence mechanisms of the lungs. Intrapulmonary shunt is confirmed when hypoxaemia does not improve despite supplemental oxygen administration.[93,94] The characteristic course of ARDS is described as having three phases:

1. Exudative phase: injury to the alveolar-capillary membrane results in an accumulation of protein-rich fluid within the alveolus impairing

gaseous exchange. This phase is characterised by migration of neutrophils into the alveolar compartment, releasing a variety of substances including proteases, gelatinases A and B and reactive nitrogen and oxygen species that damage the alveoli. Further damage is caused by resident alveolar macrophages and release of proinflammatory cytokines that amplify the inflammatory response in the lung. Significant ventilation–perfusion (intrapulmonary shunt) mismatch evolves, causing hypoxaemia and reduced lung compliance.

2 Proliferative phase: begins after 1–2 weeks as pulmonary infiltrates resolve and fibrosis and remodelling occurs to re-establish epithelial integrity or may progress to fibroproliferation phase. This phase is characterised by reduced alveolar ventilation and pulmonary compliance and ventilation–perfusion mismatch. Reduced compliance causes further atelectasis in the mechanically ventilated patient as alveoli are damaged by increased volume and/or pressure on inspiration.

3 Fibrotic phase: the final phase where alveoli become fibrotic and the lung is left with emphysema-like alterations which is linked to prolonged mechanical ventilation.

Diagnosis

Diagnosis of ARDS is based on the Berlin definition (2012)[95] developed by the European Society of Intensive Care Medicine. This definition established three risk categories (mild, moderate, severe) that are based on the degree of hypoxemia (PaO_2/FiO_2 ratio) measured with at least 5 cmH_2O of applied PEEP (Table 14.6).[92,95] The timing of acute onset was defined as less than 7 days from the predisposing clinical insult or new or worsening symptoms. To date no diagnostic biomarkers are available and definitions rely on clinical presentation and chest imaging. Chest radiograph or computed tomography to confirm the presence of bilateral opacities and respiratory failure not explained by fluid overload, (evidenced by objective assessment such as echocardiography), are diagnostic of ARDS.

TABLE 14.6

ARDS Definition Taskforce. Acute respiratory distress syndrome: the Berlin definition[95]

THE BERLIN DEFINITION OF ACUTE RESPIRATORY DISTRESS SYNDROME	
Timing	Within 1 week of a known clinical insult or new or worsening respiratory symptoms
Chest imaging[a]	Bilateral opacities – not fully explained by effusions, lobar/lung collapse, or nodules
Origin of oedema	Respiratory failure not fully explained by cardiac failure or fluid overload
Need objective assessment (e.g. echocardiography) to exclude hydrostatic oedema if no risk factor present	
Oxygenation[b]	
Mild	200 mmHg $<PaO_2/FiO_2 \leq$ 300 mmHg with PEEP or CPAP $\geq$ 5 cmH_2O[c]
Moderate	100 mmHg $<PaO_2/FiO_2 \leq$ 200 mm Hg with PEEP or CPAP $\geq$ 5 cmH_2O
Severe	$PaO_2/FiO_2 \leq$ 100 mmHg with PEEP $\geq$ 5 cmH_2O

CPAP = Continuous positive airway pressure; FiO_2 = fraction of inspired oxygen; PaO_2 = partial pressure arterial oxygen; PEEP = positive end-expiratory pressure.
[a]Chest radiograph or computed tomography scan.
[b]If altitude is higher than 1000 m, the correction factor should be calculated as follows: $PaO_2/FiO_2 \times$ (barometric pressure/760).[118]
[c]This may be delivered non-invasively in the mild acute respiratory distress syndrome group.
Source: Adapted from Ranieri VM, Rubenfeld GD, Thompson BT, et al. Acute respiratory distress syndrome: the Berlin Definition. Jama 2012;307(23):2526–33.

Clinical manifestations

Although no specific test exists to determine whether a patient has ARDS, it should be considered in any patient with a predisposing risk factor who develops severe hypoxaemia, reduced compliance and diffuse pulmonary infiltrates on CXR.[93-96] ARDS usually occurs 72 hours following onset of a presenting condition and is characterised by rapid clinical deterioration. Common symptoms include severe dyspnoea, dry cough, cyanosis, hypoxaemia requiring rapidly escalating amounts of supplemental oxygen and persistent coarse crackles on auscultation.

Assessment

A patient with ARDS requires ongoing monitoring of oxygenation and ventilation through pulse oximetry, serum lactate and ABG analysis, especially $PaCO_2$ to monitor permissive hypercapnia.[96,97] Monitoring of ventilatory pressures and volumes ensures that additional lung injury is prevented.[98,99] As many patients with ARDS require cardiovascular support, assessment of haemodynamics and peripheral perfusion is important to ensure oxygen delivery to cells is achieved.

Patient management

Despite decades of research, treatment options for ARDS are limited.[93,94] The key principles of management are treatment of the precipitating cause and providing supportive care during the period of respiratory failure. The most significant advances in the supportive care of ARDS patients have been associated with improved ventilator management.[100] Several clinical trials have shown that a large number of pharmacological strategies have not been effective in reducing mortality.[101,102]

Other supportive strategies include cautious fluid management, adequate nutrition, prevention of VAP, prophylaxis for deep vein thrombosis and gastric ulcers, weaning of sedation and mechanical ventilation as early as possible, and physiotherapy and rehabilitation. Management involves a coordinated collaborative approach including supportive ventilation, patient positioning and medication administration.[103]

Ventilation strategies

The goals of mechanical ventilation for ARDS are to prevent ventilator-induced lung injury and refractory hypoxaemia. Lung-protective strategies that used lower tidal volumes (6 mL/kg) and higher levels of PEEP reduced mortality as a result of lower plateau pressures (<30 cmH_2O).[97-99] However, systematic review evidence suggests that 10–15% of patients received tidal volumes higher than 8 mL/kg body weight, highlighting the difficulty of achieving lung protective ventilation in practice.[98,100] A conservative oxygenation (PaO_2 9.3 kPa/70 mmHg, SaO_2 90–95%) is recommended along with a higher inspiratory/expiratory ratio and respiratory rate, prone positioning and neuromuscular blockade, inhaled vasodilator therapies, and conservative fluid therapy.[95-97] The use of lung recruitment manoeuvres to improve patient outcomes remain unclear as there is conflicting research evidence. A large multisite clinical trial found an increased risk of barotrauma and 28-day all-cause mortality with a lung recruitment manoeuvre and PEEP titration compared with low PEEP;[104] while a systematic review comparing open lung ventilation to standard care found a reduction in ICU mortality with no differences in risk of barotrauma or 28-day mortality.[105]

The use of rescue therapies, when refractory hypoxaemia does occur, is controversial due to the risk of barotrauma.[106] Meta-analysis of randomised controlled trials on the use of high-frequency oscillatory ventilation in ARDS has shown no mortality benefit and a possible increased mortality risk compared to conventional lung-protective strategy ventilation.[107,108] High-frequency oscillatory ventilation is currently not recommended in patients with ARDS.[90]

Some therapies have demonstrated improved oxygenation, which may be an important goal in many patients who experience severe hypoxaemia. The key focus of rescue ventilator strategies is alveolar recruitment.[109] Strategies to support gas exchange, such as the use of extracorporeal membrane oxygenation,[110] may be used in patients with ARDS but to date systematic review evidence suggests that insufficient high-quality data is available comparing extracorporeal membrane oxygenation versus conventional therapy to determine the benefits or harms.[109] This strategy is described in more detail in Chapter 15.

Prone positioning

The use of prone position ventilation results in better oxygenation than supine ventilation largely due to the prevention of ventilator-induced lung injury and should be first-line therapy for patients with moderate-to-severe ARDS.[111] The result is a more homogeneous ventilation of the lungs and improved ventilation–perfusion matching. Systematic review evidence suggests that use of prone positioning improved survival in ARDS patients who underwent a longer duration of prone ventilation and lung-protective ventilation strategy.[112,113] In severe respiratory failure, prone positing for at least 12 hours per day is recommended.[90,96] See Chapter 15 for further discussion.

Medications

A number of non-ventilatory strategies may form part of the treatment of patients with ARDS. Neuromuscular blocking agents are used to promote patient–ventilator synchrony, especially when non-conventional modes of ventilation are used.[114] Improvements in oxygenation are usually observed and may be attributed to a reduction in oxygen consumption and improved chest wall compliance. This beneficial effect has been evidenced in short-term use of cisatracurium which showed a reduction in 28-day mortality and barotrauma with no effect on the duration of mechanical ventilation or ICU-acquired weakness for critically ill adults with ARDS.

The use of inhaled nitric oxide or prostacyclins to improve oxygen has shown no benefit in reducing mortality in ARDS and may even be associated with harmful adverse events.[115] A number of drug therapies continue to be investigated to treat ARDS in acute and subacute exudative phases. These include agents that target neutrophil recruitment and activation (neutrophil elastase inhibitors), activation of the coagulation cascade (heparin, aspirin and statins), microvascular injury and leak ($beta_2$ agonists, angiotensin-converting-enzyme inhibitors; low-dose corticosteroids), and tissue regeneration (growth factors, stem cell therapy).[101,102,116] The evidence on the role of these pharmacological agents remains unclear, although an improvement in oxygenation has been reported, improvements in other outcomes such as duration of mechanical ventilation, length of ICU stay or improved survival have not been shown.[101] The use of antiplatelet therapy has been associated with a moderately improved survival, reduced incidence of ARDS and need for mechanical ventilation in a recent systematic review, although there is a need for further robust research in this area.[117]

Asthma and chronic obstructive pulmonary disease

Asthma is primarily a chronic inflammatory disease where airflow limitation may be fully or partially reversible either spontaneously or with treatment.[118] COPD is

FIGURE 14.2 Obstructive lung diseases: overlap between asthma, chronic bronchitis and emphysema.

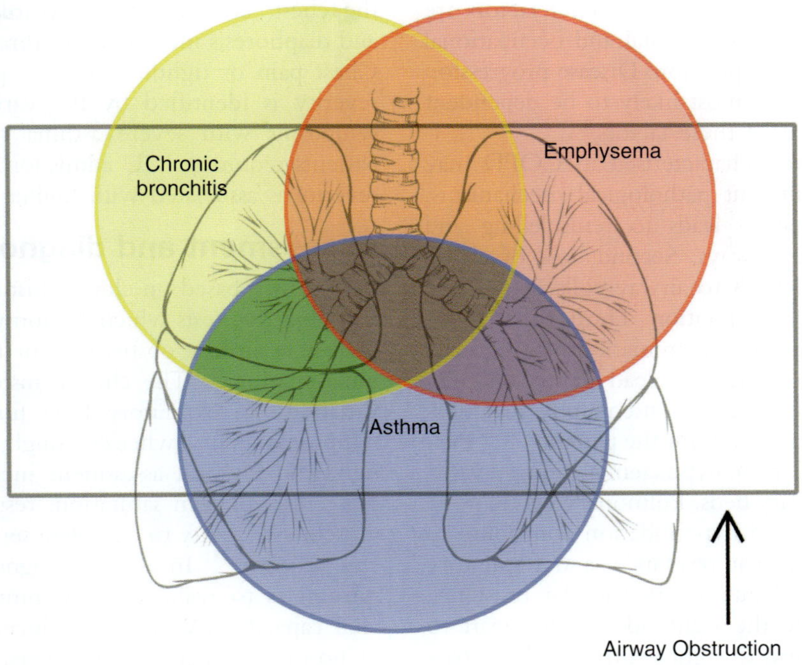

Reproduced from Des Jardins T, Burton GG. Clinical manifestations and assessment of respiratory disease. 8th ed. Elsevier, 2020.

a chronic respiratory condition where airflow limitation is progressive and not fully reversible although there may be some reversibility of airflow limitation with bronchodilators.[119] The partial airflow responsiveness to therapy in COPD results in a clinical overlap between COPD and asthma, as well as chronic bronchitis and emphysema (Fig. 14.2). Each disease is increasingly recognised as a complex of multiple phenotypes/endotypes with different pathogenic mechanisms (type 2 inflammation, viral infection, bacterial colonisation or impaired lung growth) requiring specific treatment.[120] Increasingly the co-existence of asthma and COPD is recognised as asthma-COPD overlap, which describes chronic airflow limitation in adults over 40 years with different forms of airways disease and frequent exacerbations.[121] It is, however, important to differentiate between COPD and asthma as they have different management and illness trajectories.[119-121,123]

Asthma affects approximately 300 million individuals worldwide, with prevalence rates ranging from 1% to 18% in different countries.[122] Most asthma deaths occur in lower- and middle-income countries with 383,000 deaths worldwide each year.[123] The prevalence of COPD has not declined in recent years with an estimated 3 million people in the UK[124] and 7.5% of Australians over 40 years with COPD.[125] COPD is predicted to become the fourth leading cause of death worldwide.[125]

Pathophysiology

Asthma is a complex syndrome of unknown aetiology. However, it is known to be influenced by genetic, immunological and environmental factors, and epidemiological studies show strong associations with respiratory pathogens.[122] The factors that contribute to asthma lead to infection and allergic responses, airway inflammation, airway hyper-responsiveness, bronchoconstriction and oedema that result in wheezing, breathlessness and coughing. The pathophysiology of life-threatening asthma involves constriction of the bronchioles and subsequent air-trapping in the alveoli beyond the constriction, leading to hyperinflation, expiratory airflow limitation and generation of intrinsic PEEP. This is exacerbated by increased resistance in expiratory gas flow due to a loss of elastic recoil and rapid respiratory rates. The patient increases the work of breathing, becomes rapidly fatigued and anxious and there is diminished gas exchange. These factors reduce carbon dioxide elimination while increasing its production and eventually will progress to muscle fatigue and respiratory failure.[126]

In contrast to asthma, COPD is a preventable and treatable disease associated with an inflammatory response to harmful gases or particles. Inflammation causes significant airflow narrowing that result in a permanent and progressive condition. Smoking (both active and passive) is the cardinal risk factor and continuation is the most significant determinant for disease progression.[119] However, only 25% of smokers actually develop clinically significant COPD suggesting that other factors are also involved including environmental and occupational pollutants and genetic predisposition. Disease progression in susceptible individuals is most likely to be dependent on the synergistic effects of these factors.[119,127,128]

The airflow limitation characterised in COPD may be a result of three different pathological mechanisms. First, chronic inflammation leads to remodelling and narrowing of the small airways. Second, loss of elastic support and lung recoil leads to airway collapse because the small airways close on expiration. Third, the mucous and plasma exudate from the inflammation obstructs the airway lumen. These mechanisms lead to air trapping and lung hyperinflation, which consequently produces dyspnoea and exercise limitation for the patient.[129,130] Perfusion abnormalities arise from hypoxaemia-induced vasoconstriction of the capillary beds. Pulmonary ventilation/perfusion abnormalities and hyperinflation contribute to increased pulmonary vascular resistance, and respiratory muscle fatigue. Increased pulmonary vascular resistance and hypoxaemia require the right side of the heart to work harder and may lead to right ventricular hypertrophy, dysfunction and failure (cor pulmonale).[131,132]

Pulmonary hypertension is a common complication in COPD. Its presence and severity is closely related to disease prognosis.[133,134] The incidence of right ventricular hypertrophy is approximately 40% for patients with moderate levels of COPD (i.e. forced expiratory volume $[FEV]_1$ <1000 mL).[119] The left ventricle may also be compromised by hyperinflation, which generates increased afterload.[134] Pulmonary hypertension, coronary artery disease and arrhythmias are therefore a frequent concomitant condition with COPD.[119] Impaired ventilation and perfusion leads to hypoxaemia and mechanical dysfunctions, with the primary cause of adverse lung mechanics being hyperinflation (see Chapter 11 for further discussion).

COPD is not just a disease of the lungs. COPD and systemic inflammation have been widely studied and inflammation has been considered an important key linking the disease and systemic manifestations.[123-126,129,130,133] It has been established that systemic inflammation is present during both stable phases and acute exacerbations of COPD.[135,136] Increased numbers of leucocytes, acute phase response proteins, cytokines and tumour necrosis factor are found in the blood of COPD patients. COPD is associated with quite significant systemic abnormalities including kidney and hormonal imbalances, malnutrition, muscle-wasting, osteoporosis and anaemia.[137]

Clinical manifestations

With asthma and COPD, a patient may present with expiratory wheeze, chest tightness, cough and/or dyspnoea. History and physical assessment are fundamental to determining the severity of presentation. Presence of diminished or silent breath sounds, central cyanosis, an inability to speak, an altered level of consciousness, use of accessory muscles of respiration, hyperinflation of the chest, tachypnoea, tachycardia, an upright posture and diaphoresis indicate a life-threatening case.[118,124,126,138] Chest pain or tightness may be present. The degree of severity is identified by the various clinical signs and symptoms with severe asthma representing 5–10% of patients requiring ICU admission.[139] Underestimation of severity is associated with higher mortality.[140]

Assessment and diagnostics

Diagnosis is based on clinical history, physical assessment and objective tests which demonstrate evidence of either reversible airflow obstruction or the presence of airway inflammation.[131] The clinical history provides details of variability in expiratory lung function and respiratory symptoms such as wheeze, cough, breathlessness or chest tightness. Physical assessment includes details regarding pulse rate, oxygen saturation, respiratory rate, accessory muscle use, ability to complete sentences and equal bilateral air entry.[141] In asthma, diagnosis is confirmed using spirometry to evaluate airway limitation (FEV_1 to forced vital capacity [FVC] ratio reduced >0.75–8.0 in adults) or positive bronchodilator reversibility test indicated by an increase in FEV_1 of 200 mL or greater and 12% or greater from baseline after inhalation of short-acting $beta_2$ agonists.[118,122,138] Severe asthma is associated with a recurring and severe inflammatory condition often resistant to usual therapies and often with fixed airflow obstruction.[126,142] Severe asthma exacerbations are evidenced by a >20% decrease in FEV_1 or >30 ml decrease in peak expiratory flow rate on two or more consecutive days. Respiratory alkalosis is the most common abnormality found during asthma exacerbations, but as bronchoconstriction worsens, hypercarbia and respiratory acidosis develop.[143]

In COPD a post-bronchodilator of FEV_1/FVC ratio <0.7 confirms the presence of persistent airflow limitation.[119] Further diagnostic tests and procedures involve peak flow monitoring, assessment of physical activity, oximetry, radiology and ABGs.[143] Forward-planning for potential deterioration and constant assessment of respiratory, cardiovascular and neurological systems are fundamental in determining optimal clinical progress for these patients.[119,124,144]

Patient management

In 2014, the International European Respiratory Society/American Thoracic Society published guidelines on the definition, evaluation and treatment of severe asthma targeted mainly to respiratory specialists.[142] In common with previous guidelines, they do not address issues of management in intensive care. In this respect, the *Australian Asthma Handbook* and the British Thoracic Society are more specific in their recommendations, recommending admission to ICU or a high dependency unit for deteriorating respiratory function, oxygenation and reduced level of consciousness.[118,138] Contemporary management of asthma follows a step-wise asthma management plan to minimise acute exacerbation and any subsequent respiratory arrest.[139] Many presentations will be managed in the emergency department (see Chapter 23 for further discussion) and do not require inpatient acute admission.

Large longitudinal datasets for Australia and New Zealand, the UK and Saudi Arabia show asthma hospital survival rates ranging from 90% to 100%, largely due to the reversibility of the condition.[145] Hypoxaemic patients with acute severe asthma require administration of supplementary oxygen titrated to maintain an SpO_2 level of 94–98%.[138] For patients requiring ventilatory support, NIV is increasingly used as mechanical ventilation is associated with increased mortality, barotrauma, VAP and increased length of ICU stay.[146,147]

Contemporary management of COPD includes providing care for patients in a community setting wherever possible.[144,148] NIV is increasingly used as an alternative method of respiratory support in patients with increasing hypercapnia and respiratory acidosis as a strategy to help avoid intubation, positive pressure ventilation and ICU admission.[138] However, as the mortality of COPD patients who develop acute hypercapnic respiratory failure remains high, advanced care planning prior to exacerbations is crucial.[124,144] In patients with COPD who are mechanically ventilated, a weaning strategy that includes NIV has been shown to reduce mortality and VAP without increasing the risk of re-intubation or weaning failure.[149]

Medications

First-line management of acute exacerbations of COPD includes administration of beta-2 agonists (salbutamol), muscarinic receptor antagonists (ipratropium), controlled oxygen therapy and systemic glucocorticosteroids. Antibiotic therapy is used if the patient has purulent sputum. Bronchodilators can be given by pressurised metered-dose inhaler and spacer, or by jet nebulisation. The dose interval is titrated to the response and can range from hourly to 6-hourly.[144]

First-line management of severe or life-threatening asthma exacerbations includes administration of oxygen therapy and high dose $beta_2$ agonists via continuous nebulisation, with intravenous administration considered for patients not responding to nebulised medication.[118] Systemic corticosteroids are the mainstay of treatment which have reduced mortality and ICU admission rates of asthma.[126] Patients with features of life-threatening asthma should be given magnesium sulfate.[141] See Table 14.7 for key medications used in the treatment of asthma and COPD.

Once the acute exacerbation of both asthma and COPD has resolved it is important that the severity of the individual's condition is reassessed and they are educated about the importance of maintenance therapy to prevent future severe exacerbations.[118,119]

Pneumothorax

Pneumothorax describes air that has escaped from a defect in the pulmonary tree and is trapped in the potential space between the two pleura. A pneumothorax can be classified as spontaneous, traumatic or iatrogenic and can be life-threatening. A spontaneous pneumothorax can be primary (in persons without lung disease) or secondary (in persons with lung disease). A pneumothorax is traumatic if caused by a blunt or penetrating injury, or iatrogenic if caused by complications from diagnostic or therapeutic interventions.[151]

In some cases, the amount of air trapped increases markedly if the defect in the pulmonary tree functions as a one-way valve. In this case, air enters the pleural cavity on inspiration but is unable to exit on expiration, leading to increasing intrapleural pressure. This is termed a tension pneumothorax. A patient with tension pneumothorax can present with symptoms similar to asthma, including respiratory distress, wheeze, tachycardia, tachypnoea, desaturation, hyper-expansion, agitation and decreased air entry.[151] Fortunately tension pneumothorax is a far less common condition, and the patient is more likely to report additional chest pain. The actual incidence of tension pneumothorax is relatively unexamined, but it is more likely to occur in a ventilated patient where a pneumothorax has been missed on assessment.[151]

Pathophysiology

Tension pneumothorax occurs when a one-way valve forms, allowing air to flow into the pleural space but stopping air from flowing out. The volume of intrapleural air increases with each inspiration. Consequently, pressure rises within the thoracic cavity, the lung collapses and hypoxaemia ensues. Further pressure causes a mediastinal shift that subsequently compresses the lung (causing further hypoxaemia) and the superior and inferior vena cava entering the right atrium of the heart (causing compromised venous return). Untreated, the hypoxaemia, metabolic acidosis and decreased cardiac output lead to cardiac arrest and death.[151,152]

Clinical manifestations

Severe presentations are identified by history and clinical examination (respiratory distress, cyanosis, tachycardia, tracheal shift and unilateral movement of the chest). They are also detected on CXR with a translucent appearance of the air and absence of lung markings[153] (see Chapter 13 for information on CXR interpretation).

Patient management

It is essential to check airway, breathing and circulation in all patients with chest trauma. Upright positioning may be beneficial if there is no contraindication. Penetrating wounds should be covered immediately with an occlusive or pressure bandage. If a tension pneumothorax is suspected, a thin needle can be used to relieve the pressure and allow the lung to re-inflate. If this is

TABLE 14.7
Key medications in an acute episode of asthma[126,141,150]

TYPE OF DRUG	GENERIC MEDICATION	ACTION	NURING CONSIDERATIONS
Controlled oxygen therapy	Oxygen	Increases supply of oxygen for uptake	Titrate FiO_2 to SaO_2 (aim 92–98%)
Inhaled beta$_2$ agonist	Salbutamol	Produces relaxation of bronchial smooth muscle and airflow improvement by action at beta$_2$ receptors	Metered-dose inhaler – 1–2 puffs (100–200 mcg) 4-hourly and as required. Also, continuous nebulisation via ultrasonic nebuliser and intravenous administration Side effects include muscle tremor, tachycardia and palpitations
Systemic corticosteroids	Hydrocortisone	Rapid onset (5 –6 h after administration) Increases beta-responsiveness of airway smooth muscle	Glucocorticoid dramatically reduces inflammation by its profound effects on concentration, distribution and function of peripheral leucocytes and a suppressive effect on inflammatory cytokines and chemokines 4 mg/kg initially, followed by a maintenance dose of 3 mg/kg every 6 h
	Prednisolone	Decreases inflammatory response Decreases mucus secretion	A synthetic adrenal steroid with similar glucocorticoid activity, but considerably less severe sodium and water retention effects than those of hydrocortisone (20–40 mg daily)
Methylxanthine	Aminophylline	Bronchodilator Inhibits the inflammatory phase in asthma Stimulates the medullary respiratory centre	Administration can be in oral or intravenous form plasma concentrations of 5–10 mg/L. The half-life is variable dependent on age, liver and thyroid function Intravenous theophylline should be reserved for patients who fail to respond or are intolerant of β_2-adrenoreceptor agonists Side effects include headache, nausea and vomiting
Muscarinic antagonists	Ipratropium bromide 500 mcg q.i.d.	Competitively inhibit the action of acetylcholine at the muscarinic receptors, blocking airway smooth muscle contraction	Anticholinergics exert an additional bronchodilator effect to that provided by β_2-adrenoreceptor agonists
	Magnesium sulfate	Inhibit calcium influx into airway smooth muscle, causing bronchodilation	Single dose of MgSO4 (1.2–2 g intravenously over 20 min) Dose should not be repeated as hypermagnesaemia is associated with muscle weakness and respiratory failure

Source: Tuxen et al. 2014, Bayes et al. 2016, Bonini et al. 2016.

unsuccessful, insertion of a thoracic underwater seal drain will allow the collapsed lung to re-expand.[154] If a haemothorax is present, suction on the underwater seal drain (20–60 mmHg) will expedite drainage and re-expansion of the lung. There are no reported differences in short- and long-term health outcomes between insertion of an underwater seal drainage system and simple aspiration of the air for patients with a spontaneous primary pneumothorax. Pain management and facilitation of respiratory care with oxygen therapy, non-invasive or invasive ventilation, positioning and deep breathing and coughing, and the monitoring of the chest tube and drainage for the presence of air leak and serous drainage, are key to recovery without development of further complications.[152] Chapter 12 discusses chest tube management in more detail.

Medications

Management of pain associated with chest trauma is guided by the presence of comorbidities. Epidural or intravenous opioids are the most effective pain management strategies (Table 14.8).

Pulmonary embolism

Deep vein thrombosis and pulmonary embolism (PE) are two aspects of the disease process known as venous thromboembolism (VTE). Acute PE is the most serious clinical presentation of VTE.[144] Most PEs are caused by obstruction of the pulmonary arteries by thrombi originating from the deep veins of the lower limbs or pelvis in 90% of affected patients.[152] Certain factors lead

TABLE 14.8

Common medications prescribed with chest injury: pneumothorax[154]

TYPE OF DRUG	GENERIC MEDICATION	ROUTE/ACTIONS	NURSING CONSIDERATIONS
Opioids	Morphine	Intravenous Activates opioid receptors in the brain and spinal cord Depresses respiratory centre and cough reflex Alters pain perception and CNS modulation of painful stimuli	Sedative effect with respiratory depression, decreased cough reflex, bradycardia Histamine release may lead to flushing of face or hypotension, nausea and vomiting Reduces gastrointestinal motility Reversed by naloxone
	Fentanyl	Epidural and intravenous A synthetic phenylpiperidine derivative Pharmacological actions are similar to those of morphine, but action is prompter and less prolonged, and fentanyl appears to have less emetic activity	Sedative effect with respiratory depression Can obscure the clinical course of patients with head injury Slow intravenous injection reduces the risk of respiratory muscle rigidity Use with caution in patients with renal and hepatic impairment, as action will be prolonged Respiratory depression can be reversed by naloxone. Bradycardia can be reversed by atropine
Antibiotic	Cephalosporin (first generation) for 24 h	Intravenous Bactericidal as a result of inhibition of bacterial cell wall synthesis	Active against a wide range of gram-positive and gram-negative bacilli. Highly active against *Staphylococcus aureus*, including strains resistant to penicillin

CNS = central nervous system.

Adapted from Adrales G, Huynh T, Broering B, et al. A thoracostomy tube guideline improves management efficiency in trauma patients. J Trauma 2002;52(2):210–16.

to higher incidence, immobilisation (due to long bone, pelvic and spinal fractures) and closed head injury in particular (see Table 14.9 for a list of risk factors).[155-158] In addition, critically ill patients have many additional risk factors, such as the need for surgery, catheters, immobility and use of sedatives and paralytic agents. However, in as many as 30% of the patients with PE, no provoking factors can be detected.[155]

It is estimated that over 370,000 deaths across six countries in Europe were related to venous thromboembolism.[155] Three predisposing risk factors for thrombosis are venous stasis, vein wall injury and hypercoagulability (obesity, disseminated intravascular coagulation, hormone therapy) of blood. Clinical risk factors are immobility, surgery, trauma, malignancy, pregnancy or genetic conditions (thrombophilia).[155,157] PE may have no clinical consequence or it may be catastrophic, causing sudden death. PE is stratified based on mortality risk into massive (systolic blood pressure <90 mmHg for >15 min, signs of shock or requires vasopressor support) or, submassive (systolic blood pressure >90 mmHg, right heart strain, ECG changes, elevated biomarker or ischaemia) and low risk (normotensive and no right heart dysfunction or dilation).[157,159] A number of European and international clinical practice guidelines have been published to address this significant health issue.[155,163]

Clinical manifestations

In most cases, PE is a consequence of deep vein thrombosis, therefore clinical manifestations should be considered together.

The consequences of acute PE are primarily haemodynamic. Pulmonary artery obstruction causes release of vasoactive agents with subsequent increase in pulmonary vascular resistance and right ventricular afterload.[157] Systemic vasoconstriction increases the pulmonary artery pressure resulting in increased contractility and tachycardia as the right ventricle dilates and left ventricle filling is impeded. This reduces coronary blood flow and cardiac output resulting in systemic hypotension, haemodynamic instability and hypoxaemia as a result of ventilation–perfusion mismatch.[155,157]

Early recognition is of utmost importance, but may be difficult in the ICU setting. In the mechanically-ventilated patient, difficulty to wean or sudden incidences of hypotension, tachycardia and hypoxia may be a consequence of an undetected PE. PE is suspected if patients develop dyspnoea (most common), pleuritic chest pain, cough, substernal chest pain, fever, syncope and haemoptysis.[152,155,157] Physical signs of tachypnoea, fever, tachycardia and right ventricular dysfunction may also be present if a massive PE has occurred; the patient will exhibit

TABLE 14.9
Risk factors for venous thromboembolism[155-158]

Individual	Age >70 years Previous venous thromboembolism Pregnancy and the puerperium Active or occult malignancy Varicose veins Obesity Prolonged severe immobility (bed rest, long haul flights) Oestrogen therapy (hormone replacement therapy or oral contraceptives) Inherited or acquired thrombophilia
Medical	Acute or acute on chronic chest infection Heart failure Myocardial infarction Cardiovascular disease Diabetes Some forms of cancer chemotherapy Malignancy Acute inflammatory bowel disease Nephrotic syndrome
Surgical	All surgical procedures, especially abdominal, pelvic, thoracic, orthopaedic general anaesthesia >30 min Leg trauma that requires surgery or prolonged immobilisation
ICU	Presence of central venous catheters Sepsis Respiratory or cardiac failure Mechanical ventilation Pharmacological sedation Vasopressor use End-stage renal failure

Source: Zamorano et al. 2014, Deng et al. 2015, Sista et al. 2017, Alhassan et al. 2017.

hypotension with pale, mottled skin and peripheral and/or central cyanosis.[155]

Assessment and diagnostics

Diagnosis of DVT includes assessment of risk factors, presenting symptoms and physical examination to determine probability of DVT and determine the need for further testing.[155,160] Two validated clinical prediction tools are widely used to estimate the probability that a PE has developed: 1) Modified Wells Scoring System;[161] and 2) Revised Geneva Scoring System.[152,162] These tools are based on a list of criteria of known risk factors and clinical signs: points are assigned to each criterion to produce a score indicating clinical probability of a PE. Evidence-based literature supports the practice of using these tools before proceeding to diagnostic testing. Diagnostic investigations include: compression ultrasonography for a suspected deep vein thrombosis, pathology test for elevated levels of D-dimer in plasma and CT pulmonary angiography scan and V/Q scan for PE.[160]

Patient management

Due to the high risk of venous thromboembolism in the critically ill, ICUs should have a policy for thromboembolic prophylaxis.[163] Recommended VTE prophylactic interventions include pharmacological prophylaxis with low-molecular-weight heparin or, for patients with a high risk of bleeding, mechanical prophylaxis with either graduated anti-embolic compression stockings alone or stockings combined with intermittent pneumatic compression devices.[152] It is recommended that patients undergo a risk assessment prior to initiating preventative therapies. A prognostic assessment strategy using a simplified Pulmonary Embolism Severity Index to predict 30-day mortality considers risk, clinical status and comorbidities to determine risk-adjusted management strategies.[164] Assessment of right ventricular dysfunction (echocardiography, CT or B-type natriuretic peptide) or ischaemia (troponin level) is suggested by the European Society of Cardiology guidelines to aid risk stratification.[155] Stratification and scientific guidelines allow early identification and intervention of higher risk patients.

In ICU the management of PE can be complex, hence the need for an ongoing risk assessment. For example, multisystem organ failure (particularly of the liver and kidney) and the need for invasive procedures or surgery may complicate decisions on anticoagulant therapy.[165] Providing there are no absolute contraindications (active bleeding, ischaemic stroke within 2 months, and a history of haemorrhagic stroke), the first line of treatment for patients at low or intermediate risk is subcutaneous or intravenous heparin or non-heparin-based anticoagulant therapy.[152] In patients at high risk with haemodynamic instability thrombolysis should be considered as it restores pulmonary perfusion more rapidly than anticoagulation.[155] Acute right ventricular failure with resulting low systemic output is the leading cause of death in patients with high-risk PE.[152,155] Haemodynamic and respiratory support include administration of oxygen, mechanical ventilation with low tidal volumes (6 mL/kg per body weight) and plateau pressures <30 cmH_20 and modest (500 mL) fluid challenge. If anticoagulation therapy is absolutely contraindicated or has failed, surgical pulmonary embolectomy or percutaneous catheter embolectomy can be used in high-risk patients. A further technique that can be used if thrombolysis is contraindicated is the deployment of a filter in the inferior vena cava.[157] Inhaled nitric oxide and extracorporeal membrane oxygenation are considered in patients unresponsive to standard treatment.[148,152]

Medications

Medications commonly prescribed for PE include inotropes, analgesics, thrombolytic and anticoagulant therapy. Supportive treatment of acute right ventricular failure and hypotension is vital. Inotropic drugs

TABLE 14.10
Medications for pulmonary embolism[155,165]

TYPE OF DRUG	GENERIC MEDICATION	ACTION	NURSING CONSIDERATIONS
Opioid	Morphine	Pain relief	See Table 14.8
Anticoagulant	Unfractionated heparin	A strongly acidic mucopolysaccharide with rapid anticoagulant effects Inhibits thrombin and potentiates naturally occurring inhibitors of coagulation, antifactor X (Xa) and antithrombin III No effect on existing thrombi Standard heparin has a molecular weight of 5000–30,000 daltons	Primary reperfusion indicated and renal impairment (creatinine clearance <30 mL/min) or severe obesity Dosing adjusted based on partial thromboplastin time (aPPT) Short half-life and reversed by protamine sulfate Efficacy controlled by monitoring antifactor Xa
	Low-molecular-weight (LMW) heparin	LMW heparin ranges from 1000–10,000 daltons, resulting in distinct properties LMW heparin binds less strongly to protein, has enhanced bioavailability, interacts less with platelets and yields a very predictable dose response, eliminating the need to monitor aPPT	Initial anticoagulation in PE Lower risk of inducing major bleeding Administered subcutaneously Fondaparinux contraindicated in renal failure (creatinine clearance <30 mL/min) as accumulates increasing risk of haemorrhage
Thrombolysis	Recombinant tissue-type plasminogen activator (rt-PA) alteplase, urokinase and streptokinase	Thrombolysis results in restoration of pulmonary arterial blood flow and is urgently required in massive pulmonary embolism to minimise right ventricular failure	The risks of therapy include haemorrhage. Safety and monitoring of the patient's clinical state are paramount

Source: Zamorano et al. 2014, Minet et al. 2015.

such as adrenaline, noradrenaline and dobutamine need to be carefully administered because of associated peripheral vasodilation, which may exacerbate the problem. In general, anticoagulation treatment plays the major role in patient therapy. Rapid anticoagulation is achieved with intravenous unfractionated heparin, subcutaneous low-molecular weight heparin or subcutaneous fondaparinux, an indirect factor Xa inhibitor.[152] In high-risk PE with cardiogenic shock, peripheral venous administration of thrombolytic therapy, for example streptokinase, urokinase, alteplase or recombinant tissue plasminogen activator, is the first line of treatment.[152] Table 14.10 outlines some of the key medications recommended and prescribed for patients with PE.

Lung transplantation

Transplantation is a life-saving and cost-effective form of treatment that enhances the quality of life for people with chronic respiratory disease.[166] Lung transplantation is facilitated by organ donation from patients with brain death or donation after cardiac death. Donation after cardiac death significantly increased the number of organs available for lung transplantation.[167,168] Encouragingly, results of a large multicentre study demonstrate early and intermediate patient outcomes for patients with transplants arising from organ donation after cardiac death are equivalent to outcomes for donation after brain death. A retrospective analysis of the International Society for Heart and Lung Transplantation DCD registry for transplants performed between 2003 and 2013 found that there was no difference in 1-year (88/89%) or 5-year (61%) survival between lung recipients of brain dead donors versus donation after cardiac death.[169]

Patients have received lung transplants in Australasia since the early 1990s.[170] Lung transplantation can be either single or double, depending on a patient's underlying disease state. In the postoperative period, clinicians need to carefully balance fluid management to optimise respiratory function without causing haemodynamic compromise or renal dysfunction.[166] As severe pain, particularly for transverse thoracotomy incisions, can compromise recovery significantly, effective analgesic regimens to facilitate physiotherapy are critical.[171]

Indications

The main criteria for lung transplantation in Australia are: COPD (including individuals with alpha-1 antitrypsin disorder, a genetic abnormality associated with early onset emphysema); cystic fibrosis; idiopathic pulmonary fibrosis; pulmonary arterial hypertension (PAH); and severe bronchiectasis. Among individuals receiving single-lung transplants, approximately 65% have COPD, 27% idiopathic pulmonary fibrosis and 8% have other conditions. For those receiving bilateral lung transplants, 34% have COPD and 31% cystic fibrosis.[170]

In terms of quality of life, prospective lung transplant recipients usually struggle to perform activities of daily living, may be oxygen-dependent and have New York Heart Association functional class III or IV symptoms. As a result, most patients presenting for surgery are at risk of being debilitated and may be malnourished or over-nourished, and therefore require specific interventions by health team members.[172,173] Previous studies have found that, although no specific nutritional deficit was predictive of long-term adverse outcomes, preoperative hypoalbuminaemia as a marker of malnutrition (and critical illness) was associated with poorer survival and postoperative infections; thus optimising nutritional state is critical.[162] A recent study also reported that in patients with cystic fibrosis, nutritional status is a significant predictor of postoperative lung function.[174]

Description

The four possible forms of lung transplantation, indications for each form of surgery and salient nursing implications are outlined in Table 14.11. Currently, lung transplantation takes two main forms: bilateral sequential lung transplantation (BSLTx) and single-lung transplantation (SLTx). BSLTx is the most common form of

TABLE 14.11

Comparison of the four standard lung replacement techniques, including their common indicators[175]

	HEART–LUNG	BILATERAL SEQUENTIAL LUNG	SINGLE LUNG	LIVE DONOR LOBAR
Incision	Midline sternotomy	Transverse sternotomy, i.e. horizontal 'clam shell'	Lateral thoracotomy	Transverse sternotomy, i.e. horizontal 'clam shell'
Anastomoses	Tracheal Right atrial Aortic	Left and right bronchial 'Double' left atrial Right and left pulmonary artery	Bronchial Left atrial Pulmonary artery	Lobar bronchus to bronchus Lobar vein to superior pulmonary vein Lobar artery to main pulmonary artery
Advantages	Airway vascularity All indications	Access to pleural space No cardiac allograft Less cardiopulmonary bypass	Easiest procedure Increases recipients	Increases donors Can be performed 'electively'
Disadvantages	Cardiac allograft Organ 'consumption'	Airway complications Postoperative pain severe	Airway complications Poor reserve	Complex undertaking Donor morbidity
Common indications	Congenital heart disease with pulmonary hypertension Heart and lung disease Primary pulmonary hypertension	Cystic fibrosis Bullous emphysema Primary pulmonary hypertension bronchiectasis	Emphysema COPD Pulmonary fibrosis Primary pulmonary hypertension	Cystic fibrosis Pulmonary fibrosis Primary pulmonary hypertension
Nursing considerations	Recipients may be malnourished and debilitated Rarely performed due to use of three organs. If native heart from heart–lung recipient is transplanted into another patient ('domino'), it is judicious to have relatives in separate waiting rooms during surgery (i.e. complex issues may arise)	Pain must be optimally managed to facilitate physiotherapy and timely recovery Postoperative management requires careful optimisation of haemodynamic, respiratory and renal function	Risk of pulmonary dynamic hyperinflation in obstructive disorders Complex ventilatory issues Postoperative management requires careful optimisation of haemodynamic, respiratory and renal function	Complex ethical issues

COPD = chronic obstructive pulmonary disease.

Adapted from Williams TJ, Snell GI. Lung transplantation. In: Albert RK, Spiro SG, Jett JR, editors. Clinical respiratory medicine. St Louis: Mosby; 2004, pp 831–45, with permission.

lung transplantation and has a survival advantage over and above SLTx. However, the advantage of SLTx over BSLTx is that twice as many people receive life-saving surgery. For SLTx recipients with COPD, there is an increase in the complexity of postoperative respiratory management and, for this reason, some centres may perform BSLTx for patients with COPD. SLTx is also utilised for patients with idiopathic pulmonary fibrosis and other forms of interstitial lung disease who have a high waiting-list mortality.[166]

Clinical manifestations

Postoperative management of all lung transplant recipients involves intensive clinical monitoring similar to that required for heart transplant recipients, with a focus on the stabilisation and optimisation of haemodynamic, respiratory and renal status. Great skill by clinicians is required to manage this complex interplay.[167] Respiratory dysfunction can develop due to severe dysfunction of the transplanted lung resulting from ischaemia–reperfusion injury, pulmonary oedema, hyperacute rejection and pulmonary venous or arterial anastomotic obstruction.[176] Other major complications in the early postoperative period that affect respiratory management include severe pain, diaphragmatic dysfunction, acute rejection and infection. Patients who receive an SLTx for COPD are at risk of developing pulmonary dynamic hyperinflation, requiring independent lung ventilation.[177] Haemodynamic function can be compromised in the early postoperative phase due to cardiac and respiratory problems;[178,179] renal and gastrointestinal dysfunction is also prevalent.[180] Long-term respiratory complications include airway anastomotic problems (stricture and dehiscence), suboptimal exercise performance and chronic rejection manifesting as bronchiolitis obliterans syndrome.[181,182]

Respiratory dysfunction

Respiratory dysfunction within the first 24–48 hours postoperatively is usually caused by primary graft dysfunction (PGD), a syndrome characterised by non-specific alveolar damage, lung oedema and hypoxaemia. PGD may be aggravated by factors associated with the donor (e.g. trauma, mechanical ventilation, aspiration, pneumonia and hypotension), cold ischaemic storage or inadequate preservation and disruption of pulmonary lymphatics. Clinical signs of PGD range from mild hypoxaemia with infiltrates on CXR to severe ARDS requiring high-level ventilatory support, pharmacological support and extracorporeal membrane oxygenation.[184,185] There is emerging evidence that in the early postoperative period the severity and incidence of PGD may be decreased by minimising the use of crystalloid fluids, and using vasopressors as the first-line treatment to maintain blood pressure if cardiac output is adequate.[186,187] Lung transplant recipients should be ventilated using lung-protective strategies similar to those used for patients with ARDS.[187]

Respiratory dysfunction beyond 72 hours is likely to be due to infection or hemidiaphragm paralysis secondary to phrenic nerve damage.[186,188] Although BSLTx is usually performed without cardiopulmonary bypass, for those patients who require cardiopulmonary bypass for surgery, it is recognised that there is a higher incidence of PGD.[189]

Patient management

Severity of allograft dysfunction is assessed by ABG analysis, respiratory function and patient comfort, CXR, bronchoscopy and haemodynamic parameters.[186] A careful balance in the management of haemodynamic, respiratory and renal status is vital in the first 12 hours, and their optimisation should be achieved with inotropes (e.g. adrenaline, noradrenaline) and judicious use of colloids to ensure adequate end-organ perfusion without causing pulmonary overload.[186,187] Fluid management should aim to keep filling pressures low to normal in light of a recent retrospective review that found a high central venous pressure (>7 mmHg) was associated with prolonged mechanical ventilation and high mortality.[185] Importantly, there was no evidence of renal complications associated with these low filling pressures. Fluid resuscitation should include products to correct anaemia and preoperative low plasma protein levels.

For patients who have required intraoperative cardiopulmonary bypass, high doses of inotropes are often needed to overcome a transient relative hypovolaemia. Additionally, gentle rewarming measures are needed to re-establish normothermia in order to prevent haematological and peripheral perfusion impairments associated with hypothermia. Gentle rewarming, and close monitoring of cardiac output/index and pulmonary haemodynamics should minimise the development of pulmonary oedema at this time. For patients with allograft dysfunction accompanied by high pulmonary pressures, inhaled nitric oxide is useful in decreasing high pulmonary pressures and reducing intrapulmonary shunting.[189] Continuous monitoring of cardiac output, haemodynamic parameters and urine output assists in guiding haemodynamic therapeutic interventions (see Chapter 9).

To assess the causes and progress of allograft dysfunction, CXR provides vital information about line placement, ETT position, lung expansion, lung size, position of the diaphragm and mediastinum and the presence of pneumothorax, oedema and atelectasis. Allograft dysfunction due to ischaemia–reperfusion injury appears on CXR as a rapidly developing diffuse alveolar pattern of infiltration that is greater in the lower regions, most commonly seen on the first postoperative day but may occur up to 72 hours following surgery. The presence of rapidly worsening pulmonary infiltrates (especially if associated with low cardiac indices) should, however, prompt urgent echocardiography to assess cardiac function and pulmonary venous anastomosis patency. Beyond 72 hours, alveolar and interstitial infiltration may indicate either acute rejection or an infective process.

FIGURE 14.3 Mechanism of pulmonary dynamic hyperinflation: distribution of inspiratory gas.

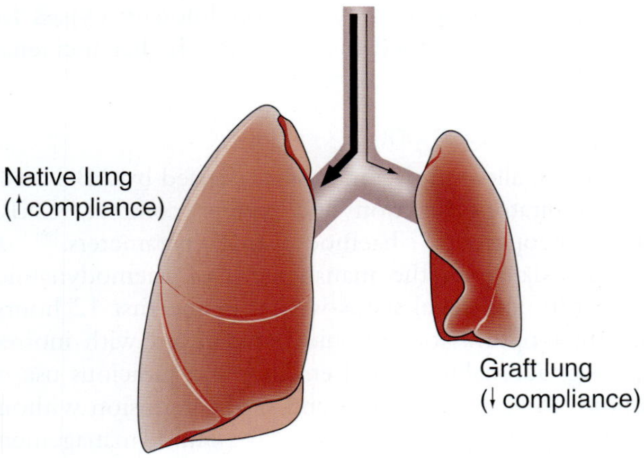

This information is combined with other respiratory and haemodynamic data to inform appropriate collaborative interventions.

Commonly, ventilatory settings and respiratory weaning are guided by pH rather than $PaCO_2$ levels.[178] A modest degree of hypercarbia is anticipated postoperatively and resolves over time. Given that lung-protective ventilation has been shown to have a positive impact on recovery and long-term outcomes in patients with ARDS, it is now recommended that SLTx and BSLTx recipients receive similar ventilator settings.[187] In SLTx recipients, ventilation/perfusion mismatches can also be improved by inhaled nitric oxide and by positioning patients regularly with the allograft uppermost.

Allograft dysfunction can develop in SLTx recipients with a remaining native COPD lung who are ventilated via a single-lumen ETT, due to gas trapping in the over-distensible native lung; a condition known as pulmonary dynamic hyperinflation (PDH) (Fig. 14.3). Any condition that lowers the compliance of the allograft can lead to PDH in these patients. Nurses need to be aware of the patients who can potentially develop PDH and to remain hypervigilant, as early signs and opportunities to stabilise patients' haemodynamic and respiratory status quickly can be easily missed. Initial presentation of PDH is usually an ABG showing inadequate ventilation (hypercapnoea) and oxygenation (hypoxaemia). For many critically ill patients the response to this clinical presentation might be to increase respiratory rate, tidal volume or PEEP. However, in the patient who has received a lung transplant and exhibits PDH, these actions will exacerbate the degree of native lung hyperinflation. A more appropriate strategy would be to reduce minute ventilation. Other common presenting cues of PDH include a haemodynamic profile of cardiac tamponade, tracheal deviation, obvious hyperinflation of the native lung with or without mediastinal shift on CXR, decreased air entry to the allograft on auscultation and pneumothorax. The early stages of PDH in a patient with a left SLTx for COPD can be seen on the CXR in Fig. 14.4.

FIGURE 14.4 Chest X-ray of a patient with left single-lung transplant for COPD who has developed PDH.

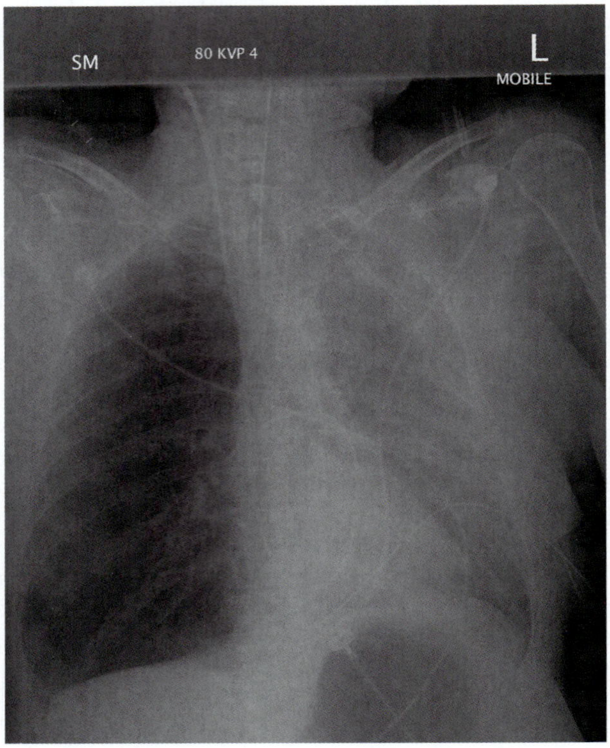

Immediate management of the condition requires attempts to minimise hyperinflation with altered ventilatory settings and bronchodilators.[187] If this fails, insertion of a dual-lumen ETT is required. Precise positioning and secure placement of the tube is vital, to avoid slight movement of the position and consequent displacement of correct cuff placement (see Fig. 14.5 for correct positioning of a dual-lumen ETT).

Independent lung ventilation is then established to ensure that the native lung receives no PEEP and a minimal tidal volume and rate. The allograft may require high levels of PEEP to provide adequate oxygenation. Ongoing assessment of respiratory function determines the timing of weaning independent lung ventilation (i.e. replacement of the dual-lumen ETT with a single-lumen ETT) and return to standard ventilatory practice. If PDH is not recognised until the patient has a cardiac arrest, the single-lumen ETT should be pushed into the bronchus of the transplanted lung in order to selectively ventilate the allograft until the patient's condition is stable and a dual-lumen ETT can be safely inserted.

Patients with allograft dysfunction are always assessed for the emergence of rejection and pulmonary infection using transbronchial biopsy and bronchoalveolar lavage in critical care. Evidence of rejection will be treated with changes in the immunosuppression regimen and

FIGURE 14.5 Correct positioning of a double-lumen endotracheal tube for pulmonary dynamic hyperinflation.

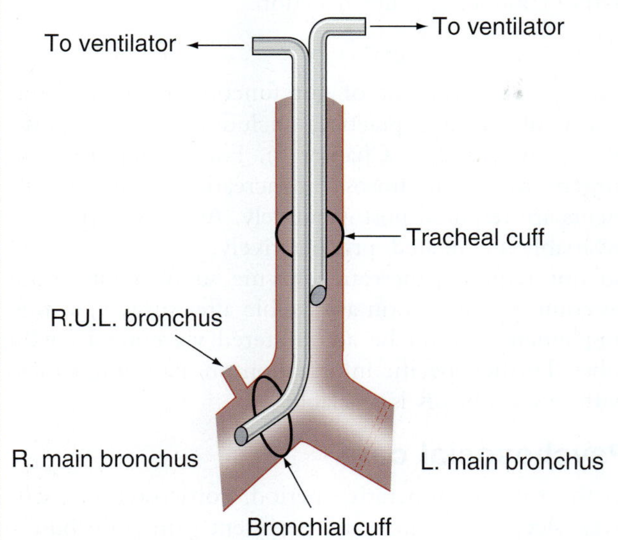

appropriate ventilatory and haemodynamic support. Many patients with rejection in the immediate post-operative period may not exhibit classic signs of rejection such as abrupt onset of dyspnoea, cough and chest tightness while mechanically ventilated. Subtle changes in respiratory effort, gas exchange and minute ventilation may be the only signs to alert the nurse to respiratory dysfunction secondary to rejection or infection during mechanical ventilation.

Classic clinical signs of pulmonary infection include a low-grade fever, increasing dyspnoea and sputum production, cough and infiltrates on a CXR. Hypotension, a reduced cardiac index and subtle changes in respiratory parameters during mechanical ventilation noted above may also be present. Pulmonary infections may be acquired through nosocomial, community or donor means, with recipient-colonised and opportunistic infections prevalent. Regardless of the means of acquisition, all infections are treated promptly with specific antibiotic, antifungal or antiviral therapies. The risk of developing cytomegalovirus and *Pneumocystis carinii* in lung transplant recipients is somewhat higher than in heart transplant recipients, so prophylactic therapies for both infections are provided. Clinicians play an important role in preventing the transmission of infection between patients and cross-contamination within patients. Meticulous handwashing between patients and between procedures as well as minimising traffic into and out of patient care areas are important measures in reducing infection rates.[190]

Pain

All recipients of lung transplantation can experience severe pain afterwards due to the incisions and chest drains.[171] However, recipients of BSLTx in particular experience extremely severe postoperative pain secondary to the transverse sternotomy (clam-shell incision) and presence of four chest tubes. The recent use of a minimally invasive thoracotomy rather than transverse sternotomy for patients with obstructive respiratory illnesses may reduce the postoperative pain experienced by recipients. Thoracic epidural analgesia has been demonstrated to improve acute postoperative pain control, decrease duration of mechanical ventilation and reduce ICU length of stay.[191,192] Ideally, all lung transplant recipients should receive epidural analgesia; however, the insertion of an epidural catheter at the time of surgery may be contraindicated due to preoperative anticoagulation therapy. In these circumstances, epidural analgesia should be instituted as soon as appropriate after surgery. Higher failure rates of transition from epidural to oral analgesia have been reported in lung transplant recipients than in other thoracotomy patients, and it is not uncommon for BSLTx recipients to require opiate analgesia for a month after surgery in order to perform activities of daily living and physiotherapy.

Patient management

Consultation with pain services to ensure that patients receive optimal analgesic regimens should be an integral component of patients' postoperative management (see Chapters 7 and 26). Paracetamol is beneficial in relieving mild-to-moderate pain, and may be used as an adjunct to centrally-acting analgesics for moderate-to-severe pain. The use of non-steroidal anti-inflammatory drugs should be avoided, due to their detrimental effects on renal and gastrointestinal function.[192]

The nursing management of intercostal chest tubes is similar to that for cardiac surgical patients[193] (see Chapter 12), with a few additional considerations. Recipients of SLTx have one apical and one basal chest tube, whereas BSLTx recipients have four chest tubes: two apical and two basal. Both BSLTx and SLTx recipients have one pleural space, so the amount and consistency of drainage from basal tubes will vary depending on patient positioning. Apical chest tubes are removed prior to basal tubes. Once lung expansion is optimal and any pneumothoraces have resolved, the apical tubes are removed. Basal chest tubes are removed once drainage is considered minimal in volume (approximately 250 mL/day) and serous in nature.[194]

Haemodynamic instability

As noted earlier, all lung transplant patients can experience haemodynamic compromise and renal impairment postoperatively as a result of strategies to manage respiratory function. Potential causes of a low cardiac output are outlined in Table 14.12. Patients with pulmonary hypertension must be carefully managed in the early postoperative period because of impaired cardiac output and changes in right ventricular dynamics. Prior to surgery, prolonged periods of a high right ventricular afterload lead to right ventricular thickening and stiffness, accompanied by limited wall motion of the left ventricle.

TABLE 14.12

Possible causes of low cardiac output in the first week after lung transplantation[193]

CARDIOVASCULAR
Hypovolaemia
Haemorrhage
Hypothermia
Acute myocardial infarction
Pulmonary venous or arterial anastomosis obstruction (embolism, clot, stitch, torsion)
Pulmonary embolism (thrombus or air)
Non-specific left ventricular dysfunction
Arrhythmias
Coronary artery air embolism
PULMONARY
Pulmonary dynamic inflation of native lung in single-lung transplantation
Pneumothorax
Oversized pulmonary allograft
OTHER
Sepsis/infection (especially line or occult gut)
Sedatives
Analgesics (especially epidural)
Transfusion reaction
Anaphylaxis
Hyperacute rejection (rare)

Adapted from Birsan T, Kranz A, Mares P, et al. Transient left ventricular failure following bilateral lung transplantation for pulmonary hypertension. J Heart Lung Transpl 1999;18(1):4–9.

Patient management

During arousal from anaesthesia and patient activity, fluctuations in oxygenation and systemic and pulmonary pressures exacerbate haemodynamic instability. When weaning from mechanical ventilation, as ventilation pressures fall, increases in preload may precipitate acute pulmonary oedema, even days after surgery.[183] Conversely, if the patient is hypovolaemic at the time of weaning, right ventricular outflow obstruction may occur. These potential events confirm that careful titration of fluid and inotropic therapies, guided by frequent, accurate monitoring of invasive haemodynamic parameters, is required in patients with preoperative pulmonary hypertension.

Renal and gut dysfunction

Reasons for renal dysfunction in lung transplant recipients in the early postoperative period are similar to those for heart recipients. The situation is, however, compounded in lung recipients due to aminoglycoside and non-steroidal anti-inflammatory drug use preoperatively, the high number of patients with diabetes and a requirement for 'dry' lungs postoperatively. Fortunately, the use of interleukin-2 receptor antibody drugs can assist in lowering the doses of calcineurin inhibitor agents to offer some early protection to the kidneys without inducing acute rejection.

Patient management

Routine management of gut function is an important aspect of nursing practice, including the prevention of constipation (see Chapter 6). For patients receiving surgery for cystic fibrosis, pancreatic enzyme supplements are required postoperatively. As these patients are invariably debilitated preoperatively, enteral feeds that do not require pancreatic enzyme supplements should be commenced as soon as possible after surgery, as these supplements cannot be administered via enteral feeding tubes. Further specific information on managing patients with cystic fibrosis is available.

Psychosocial care

In the early postoperative period, corticosteroids, sedatives, sleep deprivation and persistent pain contribute to acute organic brain syndrome. Rejection episodes can be emotionally demanding, and the requirement for higher doses of corticosteroids can lead to irritability, insomnia, profound depression, mania or psychosis.

Although lung transplantation offers recipients relief from shortness of breath and increased exercise tolerance, many patients have to continue managing other aspects of their underlying disease (e.g. cystic fibrosis). Thus, the burden of living with a chronic illness remains. Conversely, some recipients experience wellness for the first time in their life, and this can alter family and relationship dynamics. Lung transplant recipients are at higher risk than the general population of experiencing persistent symptoms of depression and anxiety. Heightened levels of depression and anxiety have been associated with decreased survival, highlighting the need for ongoing psychosocial support for lung transplant recipients.[195]

Follow-up studies have demonstrated that lung transplant improves health-related quality of life and confers a survival benefit to the majority of recipients; however, the median survival of 5.8 years is lower than for other solid tumour transplant recipients.[196] In circumstances where lung function deteriorates after initial success, patients and families experience feelings of devastation and hopelessness. Counselling services are essential in both the preoperative and the postoperative phase.[197]

Long-term sequelae

Long-term sequelae for lung transplant recipients include renal impairment, hypertension and increased risk of malignancies, like those with heart transplantations. Further information about long-term complications specific to lung transplantation, such as bronchiolitis obliterans syndrome and other non-pulmonary complications, is available.[197]

Summary

Respiratory alterations, whether a primary condition or a secondary complication of comorbidity, are a common reason for ICU admission. Vigilant assessment, monitoring and provision of a rapid response to a deteriorating state are central to critical care nursing practice. Contemporary approaches to respiratory support focus on preserving a patient's respiratory function, including use of NIV, using less-controlled ventilation when appropriate and consideration of weaning from mechanical ventilation at the earliest opportunity. The current evidence base supports strategies to prevent VAP, using daily checklists or care bundles.

Case study

A 45-year-old man with a history of hypertension and allergic rhinitis (known allergy to rye grass) presents to the emergency department (ED) with acute onset of severe shortness of breath. Over the previous 24 h there has been a rapid change in environmental weather conditions, with the weather changing from a warm spring day with high ambient pollen counts and gusty winds followed by a sudden drop in temperature and thunderstorms. On presentation to ED the patient is tachypnoeic (respiratory rate 40 breaths/min), tachycardic (heart rate > 120 beats/min), and he is speaking in short sentences. On chest auscultation he has an audible end-expiratory wheeze. In the ED he is treated with salbutamol nebulisers (2 × 5 mg at a time), oxygen to drive the nebulisers, and intravenous hydrocortisone.[118]

His response to treatment is reassessed after 5 min of continuous nebulised bronchodilator therapy; on assessment the patient is no longer able to speak, use of accessory muscle has increased and on chest auscultation his breath sounds are difficult to hear. The patient's oxygen saturation decreased to 92–93%. ABGs were obtained and showed a PaO_2 of 8.7 kPa/65 mmHg, $PaCO_2$ 8.9 kPa/67 mmHg, and a pH 7.32. Salbutamol nebuliser was continued, and ipratropium bromide nebuliser added to treat ongoing bronchospasm. A stat dose of intravenous hydrocortisone was administered. In addition to continuing pharmacological management of the patient's bronchospasm, NIV was commenced to support ventilation and manage his respiratory failure.

After 1 hour of NIV the patient's respiratory rate was 45 breaths/min, his work of breathing and use of accessory muscles had increased, and he had signs of retrosternal contraction. ABGs showed a PaO_2 of 7.3 kPa/55 mmHg, $PaCO_2$ 10.0 kPa/75 mmHg, and a pH 7.28. The patient had a rapid sequence intubation and commenced on intermittent positive pressure ventilation for acute respiratory failure.

Following intubation intravenous 10 mmol of magnesium sulfate was administered over 20 min. The patient was then transferred to ICU for management.

DISCUSSION

This patient presented with an acute-onset, severe asthma attack precipitated by an acute thunderstorm event. Although this individual does not have a known diagnosis of asthma, patients with allergic rhinitis and grass pollen allergies are susceptible to the phenomena known as 'thunderstorm asthma'.[198] In 2016, there was a thunderstorm asthma event in Melbourne, Australia that resulted in unprecedented demand on emergency response and acute health services. The majority of patients were effectively managed in the ED; however, a smaller proportion of patients required ICU admission for asthma management and there were 10 deaths associated with this event.

Severe asthma exacerbations require rapid escalation of care, intensive bronchodilator therapy and access to ICU services for management of acute respiratory failure.

CASE STUDY QUESTIONS

1. Review the severe asthma management guidelines and outline the dose and frequency of salbutamol and ipratropium nebulisers that you would consider using in this case. What would be the criteria to commence intravenous bronchodilator therapy?
2. Consider the available evidence for NIV for patients with asthma exacerbations and outline whether CPAP or BiPAP would be the most effective strategy to use in this case.
3. Interpret the results from the patient's ABG analysis.
4. Explain whether the ventilation–perfusion mismatch in this patient is due to alveolar hypoventilation, intrapulmonary shunting, dead-space ventilation or a combination of these factors.

RESEARCH VIGNETTE

Hew M, Lee J, Susanto NH, et al. The 2016 Melbourne thunderstorm asthma epidemic: risk factors for severe attacks requiring hospital admission. Allergy 2019; 74(1):122-130

Abstract

Background: The world's most catastrophic and deadly thunderstorm asthma epidemic struck Melbourne, Australia, on November 21, 2016.

Objective: Among thunderstorm-affected patients presenting to emergency rooms (ERs), we investigated risk factors predicting severe attacks requiring admission to hospital.

Methods: Thunderstorm-affected patients were identified from ER records at the eight major Melbourne health services and interviewed by telephone. Risk factors for hospital admission were analyzed.

Results: We interviewed 1435/2248 (64%) of thunderstorm-affected patients, of whom 164 (11.4%) required hospital admission. Overall, rhinitis was present in 87%, and current asthma was present in 28%. Odds for hospital admission were higher with increasing age (odds ratio 1.010, 95% CI 1.002, 1.019) and among individuals with current asthma (adjusted odds ratio [aOR] 1.87, 95% CI 1.26, 2.78). Prior hospitalization for asthma in the previous 12 months further increased the odds for hospital admission (aOR 3.16, 95% CI 1.63, 6.12). Among patients of Asian ethnicity, the odds for hospital admission were lower than for non-Asian patients (aOR 0.59, 95% CI 0.38, 0.94), but higher if born in Australia (OR = 5.42, 95% CI 1.56, 18.83).

Conclusions: In epidemic thunderstorm asthma patients who presented to the ER, higher odds for hospital admission among patients with known asthma were further amplified by recent asthma admission, highlighting the vulnerability conferred by suboptimal disease control. Odds for hospital admission were lower in Asian patients born overseas, but higher in Asian patients born locally, than in non-Asian patients; these observations suggest susceptibility to severe thunderstorm asthma may be enhanced by gene-environment interactions.

Critique

This study was conducted to investigate the risk factors which might predict the development of severe asthma which occurs as a result of thunderstorm(s) which exacerbate asthma in multiple individuals. The authors examined patients with acute asthma who presented to the ED following the world's most catastrophic and deadly thunderstorm asthma epidemic. Data from the eight major metropolitan health services in Melbourne, Australia were used to inform this study and demonstrate a strength of this work in that the individual health services demonstrated a unified approach to this work, which contributes to our knowledge about these episodic events. The clinical presentations of all patients who presented with asthma were reviewed to confirm consistency with the diagnosis of asthma.

Clinical questionnaires were developed as no previously developed or validated questionnaires to explore this issue were available. In addition to general demographic data and ethnicity, information was sought about the patient's current symptoms, their location during the event, previous history of asthma (or symptoms suggestive of undiagnosed asthma), level of control prior to the event, pharmacological management of asthma, concurrent allergies and smoking status. Characteristics of patients discharged home from the ED and those who were admitted to hospital were analysed.

Of 2242 records of thunderstorm asthma presentations to the eight health services, data were available for 64% (1435). Of these patients, 43% were known to have or had asthma and 26% had symptoms suggesting that they may have asthma. For the patients with current asthma over half (55%) reported symptoms that were not well-controlled and 58% did not have a current asthma action plan. A higher percentage (68%) were not prescribed a preventer medication (corticosteroid) prior to the thunderstorm or, if it was prescribed, used this less than five times per week. Hospital utilisation of patients with current asthma suggested low rates of non-urgent review by primary care physicians and higher rates of emergency presentations (40%) and overnight hospital admission (30%). For these patients, hospital admission in the 12 months prior to the event was associated with a higher odds of hospital admission for thunderstorm asthma.

Data suggested that age, current asthma, ethnicity and birthplace all influenced the likelihood of a severe attack which required hospitalisation. Although birthplace was not statistically significant (p=0.05) the authors none-theless stratified data by location of birth. Asian patients who were born overseas had a lower odds of admission compared with those who were born in Australia. The authors suggest the possibility that susceptibility to severe thunderstorm asthma may be enhanced by gene-environment interactions.

The authors are to be commended for the collaborative work in this area to further our knowledge of these infrequent but devastating events. Individual level data is important to understanding potential risk factors but the nature of the study precluded the authors from obtaining important information regarding exposure and local meteorological conditions that may have impacted timing, intensity and duration of exposure to the allergens. While the data suggest that people of Asian descent who were born in Australia were more likely to require hospitalisation, it should be acknowledged that statistical significance was not achieved and that the ethnicity strata sample was small. Further work will be required to validate to confirm the findings reported here.

Learning activities

1. A 56-year-old male patient is admitted to your ICU with difficulty breathing. He has a history of diabetes and has recently had the flu. His BMI is 46. How might you manage this patient given his clinical condition?
2. The rate of VAP has recently increased in your ICU. What strategies might be implemented to reduce the rate of this hospital-acquired complication?
3. Describe and compare the differences between a simple, persistent and reoccurring pneumothorax.
4. What rescue therapies might be implemented for the patient with ARDS and refractory hypoxaemia?
5. When initiating and managing respiratory support what patient assessment should be considered to optimise this therapy?
6. Chlorhexidine mouthwash has been commonly used as a strategy to prevent VAP. Why is its use no longer recommended?

Online resources

American Association for Respiratory Care, www.aarc.org

NHLBI ARDS Network, www.ardsnet.org

Asthma Australia, www.asthmaaustralia.org.au

Asthma UK, www.asthma.org.uk

Australian and New Zealand Society of Respiratory Science Ltd, www.anzsrs.org.au

Australian Lung Foundation, www.lungfoundation.com.au

British Thoracic Society, www.brit-thoracic.org.uk

Centers for Disease Control and Prevention, www.cdc.gov

National Confidential Enquiry into Patient Outcome and Death. Acute non-invasive ventilation: inspiring change (2017). https://www.ncepod.org.uk/2017niv.html

Lung Health Promotion Centre, www.lunghealth.org

Organ and Tissue Authority: Donate Life Australia, www.donatelife.gov.au

PSI/PORT Score: Pneumonia Severity Index for CAP, https://www.mdcalc.com/psi-port-score-pneumonia-severity-index-cap

Respiratory Care online, www.rcjournal.com

Respiratory Research, http://respiratory-research.biomedcentral.com

Thoracic Society of Australia and New Zealand, www.thoracic.org.au

World Health Organization, www.who.int

Further reading

Mac Sweeney R, McAuley DF. Acute respiratory distress syndrome. Lancet 2016;388:2416–30. http://dx.doi.org/10.1016/S0140-6736(16)00578-X.

Monro-Somerville T, Sim M, Ruddy J, et al. The effect of high-flow nasal cannula oxygen therapy on mortality and intubation rate in acute respiratory failure: a systematic review and meta-analysis. Crit Care Med 2017;45(4):e449–56. doi:10.1097/CCM.0000000000002091.

Narendra DK, Hess DR, Sessler CN, et al. Update in management of severe hypoxemic respiratory failure. Chest 2017;152(4):867–79. http://dx.doi.org/10.1016/j.chest.2017.06.039.

Paolone S. Extracorporeal membrane oxygenation (ECMO) for lung injury in severe acute respiratory distress syndrome (ARDS): review of the literature. Clin Nurs Res 2017;26(6):747–62. http://doi:10.1177/1054773816677808.

References

1. Wunsch H, Wagner J, Herlim M, et al. ICU occupancy and mechanical ventilator use in the United States. Crit Care Med 2013;41(12):2712–19.
2. Mehta AB, Syeda SN, Wiener RS, et al. Epidemiological trends in invasive mechanical ventilation in the United States: a population-based study. J Crit Care 2015;30(6):1217–21.
3. Global Burden of Disease [GBD]. Estimates of the global, regional, and national morbidity, mortality, and aetiologies of lower respiratory tract infections in 195 countries: a systematic analysis for the Global Burden of Disease Study 2015. Lancet Infect Dis 2017;17(11):1133–61.
4. Global Burden of Disease [GBD] 2015 Chronic Respiratory Disease Collaborators. Global, regional, and national deaths, prevalence, disability-adjusted life years, and years lived with disability for chronic obstructive pulmonary disease and asthma, 1990-2015: a systematic analysis for the Global Burden of Disease Study 2015. Lancet Respir Med 2017;5(9):691–706.
5. Australian Institute of Health and Welfare. The burden of chronic respiratory conditions in Australia: a detailed analysis of the Australian Burden of Disease Study 2011. Australian Burden of Disease Study 2017; BOD 15.(series no. 14.).
6. Forum of International Respiratory Societies. The global impact of respiratory disease –Second Edition. European Respiratory Society 2017.
7. Victorian Government. Department of Health (Victoria) Report: 10 year review of critical care services in Victoria 2002 to 2010. November 2014.
8. Stefan MS, Shieh MS, Pekow PS, et al. Epidemiology and outcomes of acute respiratory failure in the United States, 2001 to 2009: a national survey. J Hosp Med 2013;8(2):76–82.
9. Lamba TS, Sharara RS, Singh AC, et al. Pathophysiology and classification of respiratory failure. Crit Care Nurs Q 2016;39(2):85–93.
10. Gadre SK, Duggal A, Mireles-Cabodevila E, et al. Acute respiratory failure requiring mechanical ventilation in severe chronic obstructive pulmonary disease (COPD). Medicine (Baltimore) 2018;97(17):e0487.
11. Belda FJ, Soro M, Ferrando C. Pathophysiology of respiratory failure. Trends Anaesth Crit Care 2013;3(5):265–9.
12. Broaddus VC, Mason RJ, Ernst JD, et al. Murray & Nadel's textbook of respiratory medicine, 2-Volume set. 6th ed. Elsevier; 2016.
13. Creagh-Brown B. Respiratory failure. Medicine (Baltimore) 2016;44(6):342–5.
14. West JB, Luks AM. West's respiratory physiology. The essentials. 10th ed. Philadelphia: Wolters Kluwer; 2015.
15. Jolley CJ, Bell J, Rafferty GF, et al. Understanding heroin overdose: a study of the acute respiratory depressant effects of injected pharmaceutical heroin. PLoS ONE 2015;10(10):e0140995.
16. Pasin L, Zanon M, Moreira J, et al. Magnetic resonance imaging of pulmonary embolism: diagnostic accuracy of unenhanced MR and influence in mortality rates. Lung 2017;195(2):193–9.
17. Nettina SM. Lippincott manual of nursing practice. 11th ed. Philadelphia: Lippincott, Williams & Wilkins; 2013.
18. Davidson AC, Banham S, Elliott M, et al. BTS/ICS guideline for the ventilatory management of acute hypercapnic respiratory failure in adults. Thorax 2016;71(Suppl. 2).
19. Hope AA, Adeoye O, Chuang EH, et al. Pre-hospital frailty and hospital outcomes in adults with acute respiratory failure requiring mechanical ventilation. J Crit Care 2018;44:212–16.
20. Mauri T, Turrini C, Eronia N, et al. Physiologic effects of high-flow nasal cannula in acute hypoxemic respiratory failure. Am J Respir Crit Care Med 2017;195(9):1207–15.
21. Renda T, Corrado A, Iskandar G, et al. High-flow nasal oxygen therapy in intensive care and anaesthesia. Br J Anaesth 2018;120(1):18–27.

22. Mauri T, Alban L, Turrini C, et al. Optimum support by high-flow nasal cannula in acute hypoxemic respiratory failure: effects of increasing flow rates. Intensive Care Med 2017;43(10):1453–63.
23. Schreiber A, Fusar Poli B, Bos LD, et al. Noninvasive ventilation in hypercapnic respiratory failure: from rocking beds to fancy masks. Breathe (Sheff) 2018;14(3):235–7.
24. Osadnik CR, Tee VS, Carson-Chahhoud KV, et al. Non-invasive ventilation for the management of acute hypercapnic respiratory failure due to exacerbation of chronic obstructive pulmonary disease. Cochrane Database Syst Rev 2017;(7):CD004104.
25. MacIntyre NR. Supporting oxygenation in acute respiratory failure. Respir Care 2013;58(1):142–50.
26. Narendra DK, Hess DR, Sessler CN, et al. Update in management of severe hypoxemic respiratory failure. Chest 2017;152(4):867–79.
27. Schellekens WJ, van Hees HW, Doorduin J, et al. Strategies to optimize respiratory muscle function in ICU patients. Crit Care 2016;20(1):103.
28. Dres M, Dube BP, Mayaux J, et al. Coexistence and impact of limb muscle and diaphragm weakness at time of liberation from mechanical ventilation in medical intensive care unit patients. Am J Respir Crit Care Med 2017;195(1):57–66.
29. Dres M, Demoule A. Diaphragm dysfunction during weaning from mechanical ventilation: an underestimated phenomenon with clinical implications. Crit Care 2018;22(1):73.
30. Demoule A, Molinari N, Jung B, et al. Patterns of diaphragm function in critically ill patients receiving prolonged mechanical ventilation: a prospective longitudinal study. Ann Intensive Care 2016;6(1):75.
31. Tobin MJ. Physiologic basis of mechanical ventilation. Ann Am Thorac Soc 2018;15(Supplement_1):S49–52.
32. Yang M, Yan Y, Yin X, et al. Chest physiotherapy for pneumonia in adults. Cochrane Database Syst Rev 2013;(2):CD006338.
33. Kalanuria AA, Ziai W, Mirski M. Ventilator-associated pneumonia in the ICU. Crit Care 2014;18(2):208.
34. Elliot ZJ, Elliot SC. An overview of mechanical ventilation in the intensive care unit. Nurs Stand 2018;32(28):41–9.
35. Kim MM, Barnato AE, Angus DC, et al. The effect of multidisciplinary care teams on intensive care unit mortality. Arch Intern Med 2010;170(4):369–76.
36. Morelli A, Del Sorbo L, Pesenti A, et al. Extracorporeal carbon dioxide removal (ECCO2R) in patients with acute respiratory failure. Intensive Care Med 2017;43(4):519–30.
37. Jehan S, Zizi F, Pandi-Perumal SR, et al. Obstructive sleep apnea and obesity: implications for public health. Sleep Med Disord 2017;1(4).
38. Torres A, Niederman MS, Chastre J, et al. International ERS/ESICM/ESCMID/ALAT guidelines for the management of hospital-acquired pneumonia and ventilator-associated pneumonia: guidelines for the management of hospital-acquired pneumonia (HAP)/ ventilator-associated pneumonia (VAP) of the European Respiratory Society (ERS), European Society of Intensive Care Medicine (ESICM), European Society of Clinical Microbiology and Infectious Diseases (ESCMID) and Asociacion Latinoamericana del Torax (ALAT). Eur Respir J 2017;50(3).
39. Moffatt MF, Cookson WO. The lung microbiome in health and disease. Clin Med (Lond) 2017;17(6):525–9.
40. Smith AD, Zhang Y, Barber RC, et al. Common lung microbiome identified among mechanically ventilated surgical patients. PLoS ONE 2016;11(11):e0166313.
41. Huffnagle GB, Dickson RP, Lukacs NW. The respiratory tract microbiome and lung inflammation: a two-way street. Mucosal Immunol 2017;10(2):299–306.
42. Moldoveanu B, Otmishi P, Jani P, et al. Inflammatory mechanisms in the lung. J Inflamm Res 2009;2:1–11.
43. Prina E, Ranzani OT, Torres A. Community-acquired pneumonia. Lancet 2015;386(9998):1097–108.
44. Postma DF, van Werkhoven CH, Oosterheert JJ. Community-acquired pneumonia requiring hospitalization: rational decision making and interpretation of guidelines. Curr Opin Pulm Med 2017;23(3):204–10.
45. Song JH, Huh K, Chung DR. Community-acquired pneumonia in the Asia-Pacific region. Semin Respir Crit Care Med 2016;37(6):839–54.
46. Dyda A, Karki S, Hayen A, et al. Influenza and pneumococcal vaccination in Australian adults: a systematic review of coverage and factors associated with uptake. BMC Infect Dis 2016;16(1):515.
47. Jain S, Self WH, Wunderink RG, et al. Community-acquired pneumonia requiring hospitalization among U.S. adults. N Engl J Med 2015;373(5):415–27.
48. King J, Chandrasekar PH. Cryptococcosis; 2018. Available from: https://emedicine.medscape.com/article/215354-overview.
49. Nair GB, Niederman MS. Community-acquired pneumonia. In: Vincent JL, Abraham E, Moore FA, et al, editors. Textbook of critical care. 7th ed. London: Elsevier; 2017.
50. Singanayagam A, Chalmers JD, Hill AT. Severity assessment in community-acquired pneumonia: a review. QJM 2009;102(6):379–88.
51. van Someren Greve F, Ong DS, Cremer OL, et al. Clinical practice of respiratory virus diagnostics in critically ill patients with a suspected pneumonia: a prospective observational study. J Clin Virol 2016;83:37–42.
52. Berton DC, Kalil AC, Teixeira PJ. Quantitative versus qualitative cultures of respiratory secretions for clinical outcomes in patients with ventilator-associated pneumonia. Cochrane Database Syst Rev 2014;(10):CD006482.
53. Charles PG, Wolfe R, Whitby M, et al. SMART-COP: a tool for predicting the need for intensive respiratory or vasopressor support in community-acquired pneumonia. Clin Infect Dis 2008;47(3):375–84.

54. Babu A, Jose N, Jose J. A prospective observational study to evaluate the severity assessment scores in community-acquired pneumonia for adult patients. Indian J Respir Care 2017;6(2):820–3.
55. Okgun Alcan A, Demir Korkmaz F, Uyar M. Prevention of ventilator-associated pneumonia: use of the care bundle approach. Am J Infect Control 2016;44(10):e173–6.
56. Levy MM, Evans LE, Rhodes A. The surviving sepsis campaign bundle: 2018 update. Crit Care Med 2018;46(6):997–1000.
57. Gao F, Wu YY, Zou JN, et al. Impact of a bundle on prevention and control of healthcare associated infections in intensive care unit. J Huazhong Univ Sci Technol Med Sci 2015;35(2):283–90.
58. Parisi M, Gerovasili V, Dimopoulos S, et al. Use of ventilator bundle and staff education to decrease ventilator-associated pneumonia in intensive care patients. Crit Care Nurse 2016;36(5):e1–7.
59. Reper P, Dicker D, Damas P, et al. Improving the quality of the intensive care follow-up of ventilated patients during a national registration program. Public Health 2017;148:159–66.
60. Shitrit P, Meirson M, Mendelson G, et al. Intervention to reduce ventilator-associated pneumonia in individuals on long-term ventilation by introducing a customized bundle. J Am Geriatr Soc 2015;63(10):2089–93.
61. DeLuca LA Jr, Walsh P, Davidson DD Jr, et al. Impact and feasibility of an emergency department-based ventilator-associated pneumonia bundle for patients intubated in an academic emergency department. Am J Infect Control 2017;45(2):151–7.
62. Khan R, Al-Dorzi HM, Al-Attas K, et al. The impact of implementing multifaceted interventions on the prevention of ventilator-associated pneumonia. Am J Infect Control 2016;44(3):320–6.
63. Nyeo HQ, Ting KCTP. Reduce ventilator-associated pneumonia rate in the coronary care unit - an evidence based implementation project. Singapore Nursing J 2016;43(2):28–34.
64. Haghighi A, Shafipour V, Bagheri-Nesami M, et al. The impact of oral care on oral health status and prevention of ventilator-associated pneumonia in critically ill patients. Aust Crit Care 2017;30(2):69–73.
65. Chacko R, Rajan A, Lionel P, et al. Oral decontamination techniques and ventilator-associated pneumonia. Br J Nurs 2017;26(11):594–9.
66. Klompas M, Speck K, Howell MD, et al. Reappraisal of routine oral care with chlorhexidine gluconate for patients receiving mechanical ventilation: systematic review and meta-analysis. JAMA Intern Med 2014;174(5):751–61.
67. Price R, MacLennan G, Glen J. Selective digestive or oropharyngeal decontamination and topical oropharyngeal chlorhexidine for prevention of death in general intensive care: systematic review and network meta-analysis. BMJ 2014;348:g2197.
68. Hua F, Xie H, Worthington HV, et al. Oral hygiene care for critically ill patients to prevent ventilator-associated pneumonia. Cochrane Database Syst Rev 2016;(10):CD008367.
69. Daneman N, Sarwar S, Fowler RA, et al. Effect of selective decontamination on antimicrobial resistance in intensive care units: a systematic review and meta-analysis. Lancet Infect Dis 2013;13(4):328–41.
70. Marshall AP, Weisbrodt L, Rose L, et al. Implementing selective digestive tract decontamination in the intensive care unit: a qualitative analysis of nurse-identified considerations. Heart Lung 2014;43(1):13–18.
71. Huang XA, Du YP, Fu BB, et al. Influence of subglottic secretion drainage on the microorganisms of ventilator associated pneumonia: a meta-analysis for subglottic secretion drainage. Medicine (Baltimore) 2018;97(28):e11223.
72. Hubbard JL, Veneman WL, Dirks RC, et al. Use of endotracheal tubes with subglottic secretion drainage reduces ventilator-associated pneumonia in trauma patients. J Trauma Acute Care Surg 2016;80(2):218–22.
73. Tokmaji G, Vermeulen H, Muller MC, et al. Silver-coated endotracheal tubes for prevention of ventilator-associated pneumonia in critically ill patients. Cochrane Database Syst Rev 2015;(8):CD009201.
74. Monsel A, Le Corre M, Deransy R, et al. Modification of tracheal cuff shape and continuous cuff pressure control to prevent microaspiration in an ex vivo pig tracheal two-lung model. Crit Care Med 2017;45(12):e1262–9.
75. Deem S, Yanez D, Sissons-Ross L, et al. Randomized pilot trial of two modified endotracheal tubes to prevent ventilator-associated pneumonia. Ann Am Thorac Soc 2016;13(1):72–80.
76. Castro AA, Calil SR, Freitas SA, et al. Chest physiotherapy effectiveness to reduce hospitalization and mechanical ventilation length of stay, pulmonary infection rate and mortality in ICU patients. Respir Med 2013;107(1):68–74.
77. Wang L, Li X, Yang Z, et al. Semi-recumbent position versus supine position for the prevention of ventilator-associated pneumonia in adults requiring mechanical ventilation. Cochrane Database Syst Rev 2016;(1):CD009946.
78. Agency for Healthcare Quality and Research. Early mobility guide for reducing ventilator-associated events in mechanically ventilated patients. Agency for Healthcare Quality and Research.; 2017.
79. Coppadoro A, Bittner E, Berra L. Novel preventive strategies for ventilator-associated pneumonia. Crit Care 2012;16(2):210.
80. Tiszai-Szucs T, Mac Sweeney C, Keaveny J, et al. Feasibility of antimicrobial stewardship (AMS) in critical care settings: a multidisciplinary approach strategy. Med Sci (Basel) 2018;6(2).
81. McIntosh K, Perlman S. Coronaviruses, including Severe Acute Respiratory Syndrome (SARS) and Middle East Respiratory Syndrome (MERS). In: Bennett JE, Dolin R, Blaser MJ, editors. Mandell, douglas, and Bennett's principles and practice of infectious diseases. 8th ed. Philadelphia: Churchill Livingstone; 2015.
82. Neumann G, Noda T, Kawaoka Y. Emergence and pandemic potential of swine-origin H1N1 influenza virus. Nature 2009;459(7249): 931–9.
83. InFACT Global H1N1 Collaboration. InFACT: a global critical care research response to H1N1. Lancet 2010;375(9708):11–13.

84. Webb SA, Pettila V, Seppelt I, et al. Critical care services and 2009 H1N1 influenza in Australia and New Zealand. N Engl J Med 2009;361(20):1925–34.
85. The ANZIC Influenza Investigators. Critical care services and the H1N1 (2009) influenza epidemic in Australia and New Zealand in 2010: the impact of the second winter epidemic. Crit Care 2011;15(3):R143–R.
86. Knowler P, Barrett M, Watson DAR. Attitudes of healthcare workers to influenza vaccination. Infect Dis Health 2018;23(3):156–62.
87. De Serres G, Skowronski DM, Ward BJ, et al. Influenza vaccination of healthcare workers: critical analysis of the evidence for patient benefit underpinning policies of enforcement. PLoS ONE 2017;12(1):e0163586.
88. Public Health England. Seasonal influenza: guidance for adult critical care units. In: Medicine. TFoIC, ed: PHE Publications; 2017.
89. Public Health England. Infection control precautions to minimise transmission of acute respiratory tract infections in healthcare settings. PHE publications; 2016.
90. Fan E, Brodie D, Slutsky AS. Acute respiratory distress syndrome: advances in diagnosis and treatment. JAMA 2018;319(7):698–710.
91. Villar J, Blanco J, Kacmarek RM. Current incidence and outcome of the acute respiratory distress syndrome. Curr Opin Crit Care 2016;22(1):1–6.
92. Bellani G, Laffey JG, Pham T, et al. Epidemiology, patterns of care, and mortality for patients with acute respiratory distress syndrome in intensive care units in 50 countries. JAMA 2016;315(8):788–800.
93. Thompson BT, Chambers RC, Liu KD. Acute respiratory distress syndrome. N Engl J Med 2017;377(19):1904–5.
94. Yadav H, Thompson BT, Gajic O. Fifty years of research in ARDS. Is acute respiratory distress syndrome a preventable disease? Am J Respir Crit Care Med 2017;195(6):725–36.
95. Ranieri VM, Rubenfeld GD, Thompson BT, et al. Acute respiratory distress syndrome: the Berlin definition. JAMA 2012;307(23):2526–33.
96. Howell MD, Davis AM. Management of ARDS in adults. JAMA 2018;319(7):711–12.
97. Yadam S, Bihler E, Balaan M. Acute respiratory distress syndrome. Crit Care Nurs Q 2016;39(2):190–5.
98. Brower RG, Matthay MA, Morris A, et al. Ventilation with lower tidal volumes as compared with traditional tidal volumes for acute lung injury and the acute respiratory distress syndrome. N Engl J Med 2000;342(18):1301–8.
99. Bein T, Grasso S, Moerer O, et al. The standard of care of patients with ARDS: ventilatory settings and rescue therapies for refractory hypoxemia. Intensive Care Med 2016;42(5):699–711.
100. Jaswal DS, Leung JM, Sun J, et al. Tidal volume and plateau pressure use for acute lung injury from 2000 to present: a systematic literature review. Crit Care Med 2014;42(10):2278–89.
101. Tongyoo S, Permpikul C, Mongkolpun W, et al. Hydrocortisone treatment in early sepsis-associated acute respiratory distress syndrome: results of a randomized controlled trial. Crit Care 2016;20(1):329.
102. Jeon K. Pharmacotherapy for acute respiratory distress syndrome: limited success to date. Tuberc Respir Dis (Seoul) 2017;80(3):311–12.
103. Perner A, Citerio G, Bakker J, et al. Year in review in intensive care medicine 2014: II. ARDS, airway management, ventilation, adjuvants in sepsis, hepatic failure, symptoms assessment and management, palliative care and support for families, prognostication, organ donation, outcome, organisation and research methodology. Intensive Care Med 2015;41(3):389–401.
104. Cavalcanti AB, Suzumura EA, Laranjeira LN, et al. Effect of lung recruitment and titrated positive end-expiratory pressure (PEEP) vs low PEEP on mortality in patients with acute respiratory distress syndrome: a randomized clinical trial. JAMA 2017;318(14):1335–45.
105. Hodgson C, Goligher EC, Young ME, et al. Recruitment manoeuvres for adults with acute respiratory distress syndrome receiving mechanical ventilation. Cochrane Database Syst Rev 2016;(11):CD006667.
106. Adhikari NK, Dellinger RP, Lundin S, et al. Inhaled nitric oxide does not reduce mortality in patients with acute respiratory distress syndrome regardless of severity: systematic review and meta-analysis. Crit Care Med 2014;42(2):404–12.
107. Tonelli AR, Zein J, Adams J, et al. Effects of interventions on survival in acute respiratory distress syndrome: an umbrella review of 159 published randomized trials and 29 meta-analyses. Intensive Care Med 2014;40(6):769–87.
108. Maitra S, Bhattacharjee S, Khanna P, et al. High-frequency ventilation does not provide mortality benefit in comparison with conventional lung-protective ventilation in acute respiratory distress syndrome: a meta-analysis of the randomized controlled trials. Anesthesiology 2015;122(4):841–51.
109. Tramm R, Ilic D, Davies AR, et al. Extracorporeal membrane oxygenation for critically ill adults. Cochrane Database Syst Rev 2015;(1):CD010381.
110. Paolone S. Extracorporeal membrane oxygenation (ECMO) for lung injury in severe acute respiratory distress syndrome (ARDS): review of the literature. Clin Nurs Res 2017;26(6):747–62.
111. Guerin C, Baboi L, Richard JC. Mechanisms of the effects of prone positioning in acute respiratory distress syndrome. Intensive Care Med 2014;40(11):1634–42.
112. Sud S, Friedrich JO, Adhikari NK, et al. Effect of prone positioning during mechanical ventilation on mortality among patients with acute respiratory distress syndrome: a systematic review and meta-analysis. CMAJ 2014;186(10):E381–90.
113. Lee JM, Bae W, Lee YJ, et al. The efficacy and safety of prone positional ventilation in acute respiratory distress syndrome: updated study-level meta-analysis of 11 randomized controlled trials. Crit Care Med 2014;42(5):1252–62.
114. Alhazzani W, Alshahrani M, Jaeschke R, et al. Neuromuscular blocking agents in acute respiratory distress syndrome: a systematic review and meta-analysis of randomized controlled trials. Crit Care 2013;17(2):R43.

115. Fuller BM, Mohr NM, Skrupky L, et al. The use of inhaled prostaglandins in patients with ARDS: a systematic review and meta-analysis. Chest 2015;147(6):1510–22.
116. MacSweeney R, McAuley DF. Acute respiratory distress syndrome. Lancet 2016;388(10058):2416–30.
117. Mohananey D, Sethi J, Villablanca PA, et al. Effect of antiplatelet therapy on mortality and acute lung injury in critically ill patients: a systematic review and meta-analysis. Ann Card Anaesth 2016;19(4):626–37.
118. National Asthma Council Australia. The Australian asthma handbook. 1.3 ed. Australia; 2017.
119. Global Initiative for Chronic Obstructive Lung Disease. Global strategy for diagnosis, management and prevention of chronic obstructive pulmonary disease. 2018 Report; 2018.
120. Hizawa N. Clinical approaches towards asthma and chronic obstructive pulmonary disease based on the heterogeneity of disease pathogenesis. Clin Exp Allergy 2016;46(5):678–87.
121. Yanagisawa S, Ichinose M. Definition and diagnosis of asthma-COPD overlap (ACO). Allergol Int 2018;67(2):172–8.
122. Global Initiative for Asthma (GINA). Global strategy for asthma management and prevention 2018; 2018. Available from: www.ginasthma.org.
123. World Health Organization. Fact sheets: Asthma; 2017. Online. Available from: https://www.who.int/news-room/fact-sheets/detail/asthma.
124. National Institute for Health and Care Excellence (NICE). Chronic obstructive pulmonary disease in adults; 2019.
125. Toelle BG, Xuan W, Bird TE, et al. Respiratory symptoms and illness in older Australians: the Burden of Obstructive Lung Disease (BOLD) study. Med J Aust 2013;198(3):144–8.
126. Tuxen D, Naughton M. Acute severe asthma. In: Bersten AD, editor. Oh's intensive care manual. 7th ed. Oxford: Elsevier; 2014. p. 401–13.
127. Zhao J, Li M, Chen J, et al. Smoking status and gene susceptibility play important roles in the development of chronic obstructive pulmonary disease and lung function decline: a population-based prospective study. Medicine (Baltimore) 2017;96(25):e7283.
128. King PT. Inflammation in chronic obstructive pulmonary disease and its role in cardiovascular disease and lung cancer. Clin Transl Med 2015;4(1):68.
129. Caramori G, Casolari P, Barczyk A, et al. COPD immunopathology. Semin Immunopathol 2016;38(4):497–515.
130. Barnes PJ. Cellular and molecular mechanisms of asthma and COPD. Clin Sci 2017;131(13):1541–58.
131. de Miguel Díez J, Morgan JC, García RJ. The association between COPD and heart failure risk: a review. Int J Chron Obstruct Pulmon Dis 2013;8:305–12.
132. Rossi A, Aisanov Z, Avdeev S, et al. Mechanisms, assessment and therapeutic implications of lung hyperinflation in COPD. Respir Med 2015;109(7):785–802.
133. Barnes PJ, Celli BR. Systemic manifestations and comorbidities of COPD. Eur Respir J 2009;33(5):1165–85.
134. Naughton M, Tuxen DV. Acute respiratory failure in chronic obstructive pulmonary disease. In: Bersten AD, editor. Oh's intensive care manual. 8th ed. Elsevier; 2019. p. 388–401.
135. Bozinovski S, Uddin M, Vlahos R, et al. Serum amyloid A opposes lipoxin A(4) to mediate glucocorticoid refractory lung inflammation in chronic obstructive pulmonary disease. Proc Natl Acad Sci USA 2012;109(3):935–40.
136. Bozinovski S, Hutchinson A, Thompson M, et al. Serum amyloid a is a biomarker of acute exacerbations of chronic obstructive pulmonary disease. Am J Respir Crit Care Med 2008;177(3):269–78.
137. Nussbaumer-Ochsner Y, Rabe KF. Systemic manifestations of COPD. Chest 2011;139(1):165–73.
138. British Thoracic Society. SIGN 153. British guideline on the management of asthma. A national clinical guideline. Revised edition 2016. revised 2012 2016.
139. Canonica GW, Senna G, Mitchell PD, et al. Therapeutic interventions in severe asthma. World Allergy Organ J 2016;9(1):40.
140. Kelly AM, Holdgate A, Keijzers G, et al. Epidemiology, prehospital care and outcomes of patients arriving by ambulance with dyspnoea: an observational study. Scand J Trauma Resusc Emerg Med 2016;24(1):113.
141. Bayes HK, Thomson NC. Acute severe asthma in adults. Medicine (Baltimore) 2016;44(5):297–300.
142. Chung KF, Wenzel SE, Brozek JL, et al. International ERS/ATS guidelines on definition, evaluation and treatment of severe asthma. Eur Respir J 2014;43(2):343–73.
143. Fergeson JE, Patel SS, Lockey RF. Acute asthma, prognosis, and treatment. J Allergy Clin Immunol 2017;139(2):438–47.
144. Yang IA, Brown JL, George J, et al. COPD-X Australian and New Zealand guidelines for the diagnosis and management of chronic obstructive pulmonary disease: 2017 update. Med J Aust 2017;207(10):436–42.
145. Gibbison B, Griggs K, Mukherjee M, et al. Ten years of asthma admissions to adult critical care units in England and Wales. BMJ Open 2013;3(9):e003420.
146. Pallin M, Naughton MT. Noninvasive ventilation in acute asthma. J Crit Care 2014;29(4):586–93.
147. Stefan MS, Nathanson BH, Lagu T, et al. Outcomes of noninvasive and invasive ventilation in patients hospitalized with asthma exacerbation. Ann Am Thorac Soc 2016;13(7):1096–104.
148. Jeppesen E, Brurberg KG, Vist GE, et al. Hospital at home for acute exacerbations of chronic obstructive pulmonary disease. Cochrane Database Syst Rev 2012;(5):CD003573.
149. Burns KE, Meade MO, Premji A, et al. Noninvasive ventilation as a weaning strategy for mechanical ventilation in adults with respiratory failure: a Cochrane systematic review. CMAJ 2014;186(3):E112–22.

150. Bonini M, Usmani OS. Drugs for airway disease. Medicine (Baltimore) 2016;44(5):271–80.
151. Roberts DJ, Leigh-Smith S, Faris PD, et al. Clinical presentation of patients with tension pneumothorax: a systematic review. Ann Surg 2015;261(6):1068–78.
152. Yamamoto T. Management of patients with high-risk pulmonary embolism: a narrative review. J Intensive Care 2018;6:16.
153. Padley SPG. Imaging the chest. In: Bersten A, editor. Oh's intensive care manual. 7th ed. Oxford: Elsevier; 2014. p. 445–60.
154. Adrales G, Huynh T, Broering B, et al. A thoracostomy tube guideline improves management efficiency in trauma patients. J Trauma 2002;52(2):210–14, discussion 4–6.
155. Zamorano JL, Achenbach S, Helmut H, et al. 2014 ESC guidelines on the diagnosis and management of acute pulmonary embolism. Eur Heart J 2014;35(43):3033–73.
156. Deng X, Li Y, Zhou L, et al. Gender differences in the symptoms, signs, disease history, lesion position and pathophysiology in patients with pulmonary embolism. PLoS ONE 2015;10(7):1–9.
157. Sista AK, Kuo WT, Schiebler M, et al. Stratification, imaging, and management of acute massive and submassive pulmonary embolism. Radiology 2017;284(1):5–24.
158. Alhassan S, Pelinescu A, Gandhi V, et al. Clinical presentation and risk factors of venous thromboembolic disease. Crit Care Nurs Q 2017;40(3):201–9.
159. Pelliccia F, Schiariti M, Terzano C, et al. Treatment of acute pulmonary embolism: update on newer pharmacologic and interventional strategies. Biomed Res Int 2014;2014:410341.
160. Alhassan S, Leap J, Popuri A, et al. Diagnostic considerations of venous thromboembolic disease. Crit Care Nurs Q 2017;40(3):210–18.
161. Douma RA, Gibson NS, Gerdes VE, et al. Validity and clinical utility of the simplified wells rule for assessing clinical probability for the exclusion of pulmonary embolism. Thromb Haemost 2009;101(1):197–200.
162. Klok FA, Mos IC, Nijkeuter M, et al. Simplification of the revised Geneva score for assessing clinical probability of pulmonary embolism. Arch Intern Med 2008;168(19):2131–6.
163. Duranteau J, Taccone FS, Verhamme P, et al. European guidelines on perioperative venous thromboembolism prophylaxis: intensive care. Eur J Anaesthesiol 2018;35(2):142–6.
164. Jimenez D, Aujesky D, Moores L, et al. Simplification of the pulmonary embolism severity index for prognostication in patients with acute symptomatic pulmonary embolism. Arch Intern Med 2010;170(15):1383–9.
165. Minet C, Potton L, Bonadona A, et al. Venous thromboembolism in the ICU: main characteristics, diagnosis and thromboprophylaxis. Crit Care 2015;19(1):1–9.
166. Nair P, Jansz P, Plit M. Lung transplantation. In: Bersten AD, Handy JM, editors. Oh's intensive care manual. 8th ed. Oxford: Elsevier; 2019. p. 1244–55.
167. Inci I. Donors after cardiocirculatory death and lung transplantation. J Thorac Dis 2017;9(8):2660–9.
168. Erasmus ME, van Raemdonck D, Akhtar MZ, et al. DCD lung donation: donor criteria, procedural criteria, pulmonary graft function validation, and preservation. Transpl Int 2016;29(7):790–7.
169. Cypel M, Levvey B, Van Raemdonck D, et al. International society for heart and lung transplantation donation after circulatory death registry report. J Heart Lung Transplant 2015;34(10):1278–82.
170. Paraskeva MA, Levin KC, Westall GP, et al. Lung transplantation in Australia, 1986-2018: more than 30 years in the making. Med J Aust 2018;208(10):445–50.
171. Richard C, Girard F, Ferraro P, et al. Acute postoperative pain in lung transplant recipients. Ann Thorac Surg 2004;77(6):1951–5, discussion 5.
172. Chamogeorgakis T, Mason DP, Murthy SC, et al. Impact of nutritional state on lung transplant outcomes. J Heart Lung Transplant 2013;32(7):693–700.
173. Shah P, Orens JB. Impact of nutritional state on lung transplant outcomes: the weight of the evidence. J Heart Lung Transplant 2013;32(8):755–6.
174. Staufer K, Halilbasic E, Hillebrand P, et al. Impact of nutritional status on pulmonary function after lung transplantation for cystic fibrosis. United European Gastroenterol J 2018;6(7):1049–55.
175. Williams TJ, Snell GI. Lung transplantation. In: Albert RK, Spiro SG, Jett JR, editors. Clinical respiratory medicine. St Louis: Mosby; 2004.
176. Laubach VE, Sharma AK. Mechanisms of lung ischemia-reperfusion injury. Curr Opin Organ Transplant 2016;21(3):246–52.
177. Singhal A, Reed RM. Pitfalls of single lung transplantation (SLT) for chronic obstructive pulmonary disease. BMJ Case Rep 2014;2014.
178. Batra K, Chamarthy MR, Reddick M, et al. Diagnosis and interventions of vascular complications in lung transplant. Cardiovasc Diagn Ther 2018;8(3):378–86.
179. Grignola JC, Domingo E. Acute right ventricular dysfunction in intensive care unit. Biomed Res Int 2017;2017:8217105.
180. Quon BS, Mayer-Hamblett N, Aitken ML, et al. Risk of post-lung transplant renal dysfunction in adults with cystic fibrosis. Chest 2012;142(1):185–91.
181. Tabarelli W, Bonatti H, Tabarelli D, et al. Long term complications following 54 consecutive lung transplants. J Thorac Dis 2016;8(6):1234–44.
182. Langer D. Rehabilitation in patients before and after lung transplantation. Respiration 2015;89(5):353–62.

183. Chambers DC, Yusen RD, Cherikh WS, et al. The Registry of the International Society for Heart and Lung Transplantation: thirty-fourth adult lung and heart-lung transplantation report-2017; focus theme: allograft ischemic time. J Heart Lung Transplant 2017;36(10):1047–59.
184. Altun GT, Arslantaş MK, Cinel İ. Primary graft dysfunction after lung transplantation. Turk J Anaesthesiol Reanim 2015;43(6):418–23.
185. Currey J, Pilcher DV, Davies A, et al. Implementation of a management guideline aimed at minimizing the severity of primary graft dysfunction after lung transplant. J Thorac Cardiovasc Surg 2010;139(1):154–61.
186. Potestio C, Jordan D, Kachulis B. Acute postoperative management after lung transplantation. Best Pract Res Clin Anaesthesiol 2017;31(2):273–84.
187. Barnes L, Reed RM, Parekh KR, et al. Mechanical ventilation for the lung transplant recipient. Curr Pulmonol Rep 2015;4(2):88–96.
188. Shintani Y, Minami M, Inoue M, et al. Diaphragmatic plication for patients with acute phase phrenic nerve paralysis following lung transplantation: a case report. Open J Organ Transplant Surg 2016;6(1):5.
189. Meloni F. aMSM. Early peri-operative care. In: Fisher AJ, Verleden GM, Massard G, editors. Lung transplantation European respiratory society monographs. 2009.
190. Walsh TR, Guttendorf J, Dummer S, et al. The value of protective isolation procedures in cardiac allograft recipients. Ann Thorac Surg 1989;47(4):539–44, discussion 44–5.
191. Pottecher J, Falcoz PE, Massard G, et al. Does thoracic epidural analgesia improve outcome after lung transplantation? Interact Cardiovasc Thorac Surg 2011;12(1):51–3.
192. Schug SA, Palmer GM, Scott DA, et al. SE Working Group. Acute pain management: scientific evidence. 4th ed. Melbourne: Australian and New Zealand College of Anaesthetists and Faculty of Pain Medicine; 2015.
193. Birsan T, Kranz A, Mares P, et al. Transient left ventricular failure following bilateral lung transplantation for pulmonary hypertension. J Heart Lung Transplant 1999;18(1):4–9.
194. Gao S, Zhang Z, Aragon J, et al. The Society for Translational Medicine: clinical practice guidelines for the postoperative management of chest tube for patients undergoing lobectomy. J Thorac Dis 2017;9(9):3255–64.
195. Smith PJ, Blumenthal JA, Trulock EP, et al. Psychosocial predictors of mortality following lung transplantation. Am J Transplant 2016;16(1):271–7.
196. Singer JP, Katz PP, Soong A, et al. Effect of lung transplantation on health-related quality of life in the era of the Lung Allocation Score: a U.S. prospective cohort study. Am J Transplant 2017;17(5):1334–45.
197. Thabut G, Mal H. Outcomes after lung transplantation. J Thorac Dis 2017;9(8):2684–91.
198. Thien F, Beggs P, Csutoros D, et al. The Melbourne epidemic thunderstorm asthma event 2016: an investigation of environmental triggers, effect on health services, and patient risk factors. Lancet Planet Health 2018;2(6):e255–63.

Chapter 15

Ventilation and oxygenation management

Louise Rose, Frederique Paulus

KEY WORDS

artificial airway
oxygen therapy
mechanical ventilation
non-invasive ventilation
weaning

Learning objectives

After reading this chapter, you should be able to:

- describe oxygen therapy, including low-flow and high-flow devices, complications associated with oxygen therapy, and management priorities
- state nursing priorities for airway management strategies including laryngeal masks, endotracheal tubes and tracheostomy tubes
- summarise current knowledge on the physiological benefits, indications for use, associated monitoring priorities, complications, modes, settings, and interfaces for non-invasive ventilation
- state the indications for use, associated monitoring priorities, complications, classification framework, modes and settings for invasive mechanical ventilation
- outline the weaning continuum and current evidence for optimising safe and efficient weaning from mechanical ventilation
- discuss ventilation management strategies for refractory hypoxaemia
- discuss ventilation management strategies for severe airflow limitation.

Introduction

Support of oxygenation and ventilation are two of the most common interventions in intensive care; in 2015–2016, approximately 35% of adult patients in Australian and New Zealand intensive care units (ICUs) received invasive mechanical ventilation.[1] Similar numbers of critically ill patients receive ventilation in the UK,[2] whereas in the USA reported numbers range from 21% to 39%.[3] The technology available for supporting oxygenation and ventilation is complex, ranging from simple interventions, such as nasal cannulae through to invasive mechanical ventilation and extracorporeal support. Additionally, the meaning of ventilator terminology is often unclear and terms may be used interchangeably. Critical care nurses must have a strong knowledge of the underlying principles of oxygenation and ventilation that will facilitate an understanding of respiratory support devices, associated monitoring priorities and risks.

Oxygen therapy

Oxygen is required for aerobic cellular metabolism and ultimately for human survival, with some cells, such as those in the brain, being more sensitive to hypoxia than others. Refer to Chapter 13 for discussion of oxygen delivery and consumption, the oxyhaemoglobin dissociation curve, hypoxaemia and tissue hypoxia; this material provides rationales for clinical decisions regarding the administration of oxygen therapy or ventilation strategies. Oxygen therapy should be considered for patients with a significant reduction in arterial oxygen levels, irrespective of diagnosis and especially if the patient is drowsy or unconscious.

Indications

Indications for oxygen therapy include:

- cardiac and respiratory arrest
- type I respiratory failure
- type II respiratory failure
- chest pain or acute coronary syndrome with hypoxia (i.e. SpO_2 less than 93%) or evidence of shock[4]
- low blood pressure, cardiac output
- increased metabolic demands
- carbon monoxide poisoning

Complications

Administration of oxygen, regardless of the delivery device, has potential adverse effects. High concentrations of oxygen cause nitrogen washout, resulting in absorption atelectasis.

Hypoventilation and CO_2 narcosis

High-dose oxygen therapy may lead to hypoventilation, hypercapnia, and CO_2 narcosis in a small proportion of patients with chronic obstructive pulmonary disease (COPD). The processes underpinning these physiological changes are described in Chapter 13. These patients require close monitoring of $PaCO_2$ levels when oxygen therapy is instituted or increased. Although COPD patients frequently may have a lower baseline SpO_2 (88–94% compared with 96–100% in patients with no lung pathology), treatment of hypoxia is still essential, and oxygen should not be withheld or withdrawn while hypoxia remains, even if hypercapnia worsens.[5,6]

Practice tip

Oxygen should not be withheld or withdrawn while hypoxia remains, even if hypercapnia worsens.

Oxygen toxicity

Administration of high oxygen concentrations may lead to oxygen toxicity; symptoms include non-productive cough, substernal pain, reduced lung compliance, interstitial oedema, and pulmonary capillary haemorrhage. These symptoms may be mistakenly attributed to the underlying illness, especially in a sedated and ventilated patient. Many of the symptoms abate once the fraction of inspired oxygen (FiO_2) is reduced, although irreversible pulmonary fibrosis may occur (Box 15.1). The concentration and duration of oxygen exposure that induces oxygen toxicity varies between patients;[7] the lowest possible FiO_2 should therefore be used to achieve the target partial pressure of oxygen in arterial blood (PaO_2) or peripheral oxygen saturation (SpO_2).

BOX 15.1

Signs and symptoms of oxygen toxicity

Central nervous system:

- nausea and vomiting
- anxiety
- visual changes
- hallucinations
- tinnitus
- vertigo
- hiccups
- seizures

Pulmonary:

- dry cough
- substernal chest pain
- shortness of breath
- pulmonary oedema
- pulmonary fibrosis

Oxygen administration devices

Initial management of hypoxia in a spontaneously-breathing patient with an intact airway is low- or variable-flow oxygen via nasal cannulae (up to 6 L/min) or face mask (up to 15 L/min). Although oxygen devices have traditionally had FiO_2 ascribed to specific flow rates, the FiO_2 delivered to the alveoli is variable due to the influence of:

- patient factors: inspiratory flow rate, respiratory rate, tidal volume (V_T), respiratory pause
- oxygen device factors: oxygen flow rate, volume of mask/reservoir, mask exhalation port size, tightness of fit.

Normal inspiratory flow in a healthy adult ranges between 25 and 35 L/min. Patients with respiratory failure tend to increase their flow demand from 50 up to 300 L/min. Patients in respiratory distress are characterised by high respiratory rates and low V_Ts[7,8] that can significantly decrease the FiO_2 available via an oxygen delivery device, depending on the type in use.

All oxygen delivery devices use some type of reservoir to support oxygen delivery and prevent CO_2 rebreathing. For face masks, the reservoir is the mask; for nasal cannulae it is the patient's pharynx. Patients with high inspiratory flow demand will deplete the reservoir faster than it can be replenished, resulting in air entrainment and dilution of the oxygen concentration.

Variable-flow devices

A range of low or variable-flow oxygen delivery devices are available. These devices range from nasal cannulae and oxygen masks with different features, through to bag–mask ventilation.

Low-flow nasal cannulae

Traditional low-flow nasal cannulae sit at the external nares and deliver 3–4 L/min of oxygen. Higher flows may cause discomfort and damage from the drying effect on respiratory mucosa. Increased flow demand with respiratory distress dilutes the oxygen, reducing the FiO_2 to the alveoli.

High-flow nasal cannulae

High-flow nasal cannulae have slightly larger prongs that facilitate oxygen flow of up to 60 L/min leading to less air entrainment than with other oxygen delivery systems.[8,9] High-flow nasal cannulae generate low levels of end-expiratory pressure, though this is dependent on the flow rate, trachea size, and mouth closing,[10] and can therefore reduce tachypnoea and work of breathing.[11,12] The high gas flow may flush CO_2 from the anatomical dead space preventing CO_2 rebreathing and thereby decreasing $PaCO_2$, although this is not well supported by the literature.[13,14] These systems are generally well-tolerated, but must be used with heated humidification to avoid drying the respiratory mucosa.[12] High-flow nasal cannulae are now used frequently in many areas of clinical practice to avoid, or as an alternative to more invasive therapies.[15] Current evidence indicates high-flow nasal cannulae are more effective than conventional oxygen therapy and non-inferior to non-invasive ventilation (NIV). Furthermore high-flow nasal cannulae are better tolerated than NIV giving the advantages of patient comfort and therefore better tolerance of prolonged device use.[16]

Oxygen masks

Loose-fitting oxygen masks include simple (Hudson) face masks, aerosol masks used in combination with heated humidification and nebuliser treatments, tracheostomy masks and face tents. All are considered low-flow or variable-flow devices, with the delivered FiO_2 varying with patient demand. Flow rates $\geq$5 L/min minimise CO_2 rebreathing. The addition of 'tusks' to a Hudson mask may increase the oxygen reservoir,[17] but does not guarantee a consistent FiO_2 and has probably been superseded by high-flow systems.[18]

Partial rebreather and non-rebreather masks have an attached reservoir bag that enables delivery of higher levels of FiO_2. Both mask types have a one-way valve precluding expired gas entering the reservoir bag. A non-rebreather mask has two one-way valves preventing air entrainment.[19] The maximum FiO_2 delivery with non-rebreather masks is 0.85 with low flow demand, with a steep decline in alveolar oxygen concentration as minute volume increases. Non-rebreather masks may perform worse than a Hudson mask without a reservoir bag.[7]

Venturi systems

Venturi systems use the venturi effect to entrain gas via a narrow aperture via a side port increasing gas speed and gaining kinetic energy. FiO_2 concentration can be altered by widening or narrowing the Venturi device aperture to a maximum FiO_2 of 0.6. The FiO_2 concentration using a Venturi system is less affected by changes in respiratory pattern and demand in comparison to other low-flow oxygen devices.[7]

Bag–mask ventilation

Bag–mask ventilation with a self-inflating bag (and reservoir), non-return valve and mask delivers assisted ventilation at a FiO_2 of 1.0. Addition of a positive end-expiratory pressure (PEEP) valve will improve oxygenation. Manual ventilation requires a good seal between the patient's face and the mask; this may be difficult to achieve as a single operator. One person should hold the mask and lift the patient's chin, while another squeezes the bag. Effective bag–mask ventilation is confirmed when the chest visibly rises as the bag is squeezed as well as improved oxygen saturations.[20] Bag–mask ventilation may cause gastric insufflation, increasing the risk of vomiting and subsequent aspiration.

> **Practice tip**
>
> Transparent face masks are recommended for bag–mask ventilation as they allow immediate recognition if a patient vomits.

Airway support

The most common cause of partial airway obstruction in an unconscious patient is loss of oropharyngeal muscle tone, particularly of the tongue. This may be alleviated by tilting the head slightly back and lifting the chin, or thrusting the jaw forward. The head-tilt/chin-lift manoeuvre is not used if cervical spine injury is suspected.[21] The jaw-thrust manoeuvre may require two hands to maintain.[22] If more prolonged support is required, an oro- or nasopharyngeal airway can be used that may also facilitate bag–mask ventilation.

FIGURE 15.1 Nasopharyngeal airways.

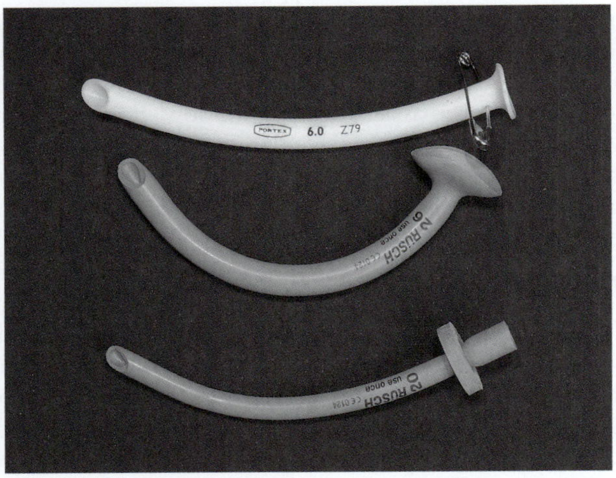

Reproduced from Davey AJ, Diba A. Ward's Anaesthetic equipment. 5th ed. London: Elsevier Saunders; 2005.

FIGURE 15.2 Laryngeal mask airways.

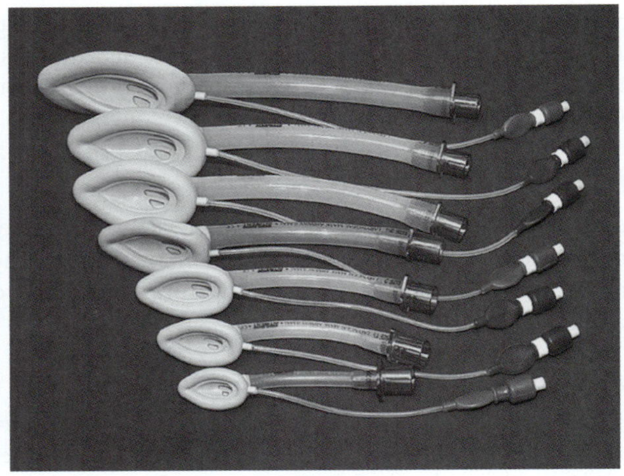

Reproduced from Davey AJ, Diba A. Ward's Anaesthetic equipment. 5th ed. London: Elsevier Saunders; 2005.

Oro- and nasopharyngeal airways

The Guedel oropharyngeal airway is available in various sizes (a medium-sized adult requires a size 4). The airway is inserted into the patient's mouth past the teeth, with the end facing up into the hard palate, then rotated 180°, taking care to bring the tongue forward and not push it back. Oropharyngeal airways are poorly tolerated in conscious patients and may cause gagging and vomiting.[20]

A nasopharyngeal airway (Fig. 15.1) is inserted through the nares into the oropharynx; it can be difficult to insert and requires generous lubrication to minimise trauma. This type of airway should not be used for patients with a suspected head injury. As well as opening the airway, suction catheters can be passed to facilitate secretion clearance. Once inserted these airways are better tolerated than an oropharyngeal airway.

Laryngeal mask airway and insertion

The classic laryngeal mask airway (cLMA) (Fig. 15.2) is positioned blindly into the pharynx to form a low-pressure seal against the laryngeal inlet. It is easier and quicker to insert than an endotracheal tube, and is particularly useful for operators with limited airway skills; the cLMA does not carry the same potentially fatal complications such as oesophageal intubation although the risk of aspiration remains.[23]

Mechanical ventilation can be delivered with low-airway pressures (less than 20 cmH_2O) via a cLMA. This device is widely used in elective general anaesthesia,[21] and can be used in critical care as an alternative to bag–mask ventilation[23] or endotracheal intubation when initial attempts at intubation have failed.[24] The 'intubating' LMA is most commonly used when a difficult intubation is anticipated or encountered. This device has a handle and is more rigid, wider and curved than the cLMA, enabling passage of a purpose-made endotracheal tube.[25]

Combitube

The Combitube is more widely used in North America for emergency situations than in Australia and the UK.[21] It is a dual-lumen, dual-cuff oesophageal-tracheal airway that enables ventilation if inserted into either the oesophagus or trachea. Inexperienced operators may find a Combitube more difficult to insert correctly than a cLMA.[25] Complications may occur in up to 40% of patients and include aspiration pneumonitis, pneumothorax, airway injuries and bleeding, oesophageal laceration and perforation and mediastinitis.[26]

Endotracheal tubes

Endotracheal intubation is the 'gold standard' for airway support, providing airway protection in the presence of airway oedema, absent gag, cough or swallow reflex. Intubation facilitates mechanical ventilation and pulmonary secretion clearance.[22]

Endotracheal tubes (ETT) have common design characteristics, are generally made from polyvinyl chloride, are available with internal diameters ranging from 2–10 mm (common adult sizes are 7–9 mm), and are up to 30 cm long. A longitudinal radio-opaque line allows visualisation of tube placement on a chest X-ray. Markings at 1 cm intervals indicate the length from the distal end, a design feature that facilitates the ability to gauge insertion depth and monitor tube movement.[27] Tubes are available with and without a distal cuff, an inflatable balloon that seals the trachea, facilitates positive-pressure ventilation and prevents aspiration of oropharyngeal contents. Cuffs come in a range of profiles and volumes, but are commonly high-volume, low-pressure enabling application of a safe pressure over a larger surface area

FIGURE 15.3 Endotracheal tubes.

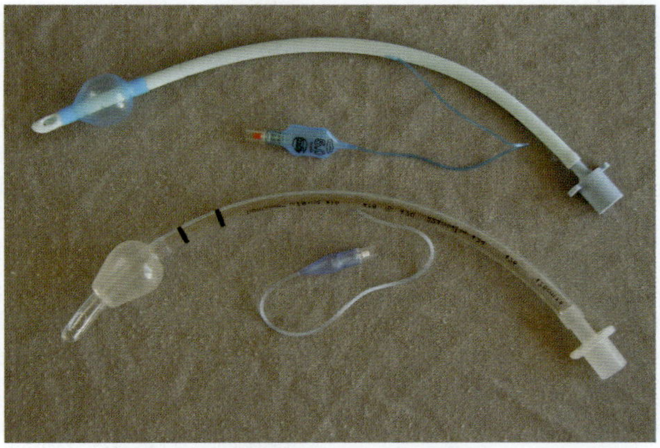

Lewis S, Heitkemper M, Dirksen S. Medical-surgical nursing. 5th ed. St Louis: Mosby; 2000.

(Fig. 15.3). A smaller inflatable balloon, attached to the cuff via a pilot line, provides a tactile gauge of cuff pressure and a small air reservoir to prevent minor changes in cuff pressure.[28]

Endotracheal tubes reinforced with a wire coil embedded within the plastic along the entire tube length prevent kinking and occlusion. These tubes are more commonly used in the operating room.[29] The wire coils can be irreversibly compressed by a strong bite occluding the airway. Reinforced tubes also increase the risk of tracheal damage and should be replaced with a standard ETT on ICU arrival. Most ETTs have a 'Murphy eye', an oval-shaped hole in the side of the tube between the cuff and the tube end that provides a patent aperture if the distal opening is occluded.[30]

Double lumen endotracheal tubes (DLT) enable independent lung ventilation (ILV) using two ventilators. ILV was initially developed for thoracic surgical procedures to allow ventilation of one lung while performing surgery on the other. ILV is also used in the critical care setting for isolation of a lung in patients with unilateral lung injury.[31] DLTs have a tracheal and a bronchial lumen, the bronchial lumen can be right or left- sided. A left-sided DLT is used most commonly because positioning is easier. Fiberoptic bronchoscopy guidance is required to confirm proper placement. DLTs have a large overall diameter but separate lumens are smaller when compared with single lumen ETT, leading to increased airway resistance. Secretion clearance through DLTs can be problematic and special care is needed to prevent tube dislocation and cuff overinflation.[31]

Preparation for intubation

Adequate preparation of the patient, equipment and environment, as well as knowledge of emergency procedures is important to ensure safe and efficient intubation. Up to 50% of patients undergoing endotracheal intubation in the ICU experience complications; around one-third will have a serious complication, including hypoxaemia, circulatory collapse, cardiac arrhythmia, cardiac arrest, oesophageal intubation, aspiration and death.[32]

Patient preparation

If appropriate, and time permits, explain the procedure to the patient and family. Prepare the patient with:

- reliable intravenous access established to allow rapid fluid and drug administration
- accurate blood pressure monitoring (preferably intraarterial)
- continuous oxygen saturation and ECG monitoring
- nasogastric tube (if in situ) should be aspirated and placed on free drainage
- positioned supine in the 'sniff' position.

Equipment and drugs

All equipment should be available and checked immediately prior to intubation, including:

- oxygen supply
- suction supply, with a range of Yankauer and y-suction catheters/closed suction device
- laryngoscope blades and compatible holder, with a functioning light, including second laryngoscope in case of device failure
- appropriately-sized face mask
- manual ventilation with a bag valve mask (e.g. Ambu® resuscitator) attached to oxygen supply
- ETT inflation checked using sterile water to ensure no leaks and even inflation, with additional ETT tubes available if needed
- water-based lubrication of tube and cuff (while maintaining sterility)
- capnography (chemical CO_2 detectors are often used in emergency situations)
- ventilator and circuit
- emergency/resuscitation trolley at bedside
- gloves, eye protection
- drugs (sedative and muscle relaxant; note sedatives should be administered before a muscle relaxant so that the patient is unaware of paralysis)

Practice tip

During intubation, know who to call for help, and do not hesitate to do so.

Procedure

The patient is preoxygenated to minimise desaturation during apnoea and laryngoscopy, commonly via bag and mask, although other methods such as NIV,[33] heated and humidified nasal oxygen,[34] and flush rate oxygen by face mask may improve preoxygenation compared to traditional face mask.[35] The practice of apnoeic oxygenation during endotracheal intubation through the administration of 15 L per minute via nasal cannula has become popular in emergency departments. To date there is insufficient evidence to recommend its routine use during endotracheal intubation in the critically ill. Intubation in ICU is usually performed via laryngoscopy with insertion of an oral ETT. Intubation may be performed using a fibreoptic bronchoscope when difficulty is encountered, or for nasal intubation.

Oral vs nasal intubation

Oral intubation is preferred unless there are specific indications for nasal intubation. Oral intubation is easier to perform and allows use of a larger diameter ETT. While nasal intubation provides better splinting for the ETT and facilitates oral hygiene, it can damage nasal structures, is contraindicated in skull fractures, and due to increased risk of maxillary sinusitis and ventilator-associated pneumonia (VAP), is not recommended for ventilation longer than 24 hours.[36]

Cricoid pressure

The cricoid cartilage, situated below the thyroid prominence, is a closed tracheal ring which, when compressed, closes the oesophagus while the trachea remains open. Cricoid pressure is performed by placing the thumb on one side of the patient's trachea, middle finger on the other side and index finger directly on the cricoid.[37] Although widely used, its efficacy is questionable as technique is frequently poor,[38] and there is wide anatomical variation in the exact orientation of the oesophagus in relation to the trachea.[39]

Backwards, upwards, rightward pressure manoeuvre

The backwards, upwards, rightward pressure (BURP) manoeuvre on the thyroid cartilage was introduced in the mid-1990s to improve visualisation during difficult laryngoscopy. The patient's jaw is thrust forward, so the head is in the 'sniffing' position. The thumb and third finger are placed on either side of the thyroid cartilage and the index finger on top. Pressure is applied in the sequence *b*ackwards (towards the spine), *u*pwards (towards the head), *r*ightward (towards the patient's right side). This is easier to perform following administration of muscle relaxants.

Cuff management

Endotracheal and tracheostomy tube cuffs prevent airway contamination by pharyngeal secretions and gastric contents and loss of V_T during mechanical ventilation. The cuff does not secure the tube in the trachea.

Confirmation of tube position

The correct position of the ETT distal end is 3–5 cm above the carina. A lip level of 20 cm for women and 22 cm for men should prevent endobronchial intubation, with the proximal end fixed at either the centre or side of the mouth.[40] Confirmation of the ETT position via chest X-ray is required immediately following intubation and at regular intervals thereafter as tube movement can occur.

Chest auscultation and observation of chest expansion to confirm ETT position is unreliable, as the chest may appear to rise with oesophageal intubation. Conversely the chest may not rise with a correctly positioned tube if the patient is obese or has a rigid chest wall. Patients with left main bronchus intubation may exhibit bilateral breath sounds.[41] End-tidal CO_2 monitoring is the 'gold standard' method for confirming ETT placement (see Chapter 13 for further information on end-tidal CO_2 monitoring). Disposable devices that change colour in the presence of CO_2 are inexpensive and easy to use, but may be inaccurate during cardiopulmonary resuscitation, or if contaminated. Capnography is the most reliable technique to identify ETT placement in both arrest and non-arrest situations.[24] Continuous end-tidal CO_2 monitoring during intubation is recommended as a minimum standard by the College of Intensive Care Medicine of Australia and New Zealand.[42]

> **Practice tip**
>
> Always ensure there is someone who is skilled at intubation immediately available when extubating a patient.

Tracheostomy

Tracheostomy may be required for upper airway obstruction, although it is most commonly performed for ICU patients requiring prolonged mechanical ventilation. The advantages of tracheostomy over endotracheal intubation include decreased risk of laryngeal damage and subglottic stenosis, reduced airway resistance and deadspace, which decreases the work of breathing and therefore supports weaning,[43] and improved patient tolerance enabling sedation reduction. The optimum time to perform tracheostomy remains contentious, and is often influenced by patient diagnosis.[44]

Procedure

Tracheostomy can be performed using a surgical or percutaneous dilatational technique. Percutaneous dilatation is contraindicated in patients with anatomical anomalies of the neck and serious bleeding disorders, and should be undertaken with caution in patients who are obese, have a cervical spine injury, coagulopathy, difficult airway or require high levels of ventilatory support.[45] Percutaneous dilatation is more commonly performed than the surgical technique in Australian and New Zealand ICUs.[45]

A variety of tracheostomy tubes are available that facilitate secretion clearance, communication and differing patient anatomy. Inner cannulas (reusable or disposable) prevent secretion build up on the internal surface of the tracheostomy tube, while fenestrated and talking tracheostomies facilitate communication, as do one-way speaking valves, such as the Passy-Muir® valve, used with the cuff deflated.

Tracheostomy care

The aim of tracheostomy care is to keep the stoma free of infection, and prevent tube blockage or dislodgement. The stoma should be assessed at least every 24 hours for trauma, infection or inflammation and fixation devices are changed with two nurses required to safely perform changes.[46] Velcro tapes are easier to change and more comfortable than cotton tape.[47] Lint-free or superabsorbent foam dressings are used under the flange to absorb secretions. Adequate humidification and suctioning will usually prevent tube obstruction (see later in this chapter). The use of inner cannulae has obviated the need for frequent tracheostomy tube changes. Single lumen (no inner cannula) tracheostomy tubes are recommended to be changed every 7–10 days.[46]

Minitracheostomy

A minitracheostomy, a small bore tracheal cannula with a diameter of 4 mm, can be inserted percutaneously in patients with an ineffective cough to facilitate respiratory secretion clearance via endotracheal suctioning. A minitracheostomy is generally used after tracheostomy removal but may be used in patients for secretion clearance that have not required tracheostomy such as those with neurological compromise. The minitracheostomy preserves glottic function and maintenance of phonation but does not provide airway protection and therefore cannot be used for invasive ventilation. Complications associated with use of a minitracheostomy occur infrequently, those complications that do occur are associated with difficulty inserting and positioning the tube.[48,49]

Complications of endotracheal intubation and tracheostomy

Tube blockage, tube dislodgement and aspiration are major complications. Partial ETT or tracheostomy tube dislodgement can cause greater harm than complete removal because of delays in diagnosis and resultant aspiration and worsening gas exchange. Tube dislodgement is most likely to occur when turning the patient, in agitated patients or when nursing staff are distracted or on breaks.[50] While physical restraint may be considered to prevent tube dislodgement, multiple studies noted patients were restrained when self-extubation or device removal occurred.[51-54] Appropriate levels of analgesia and sedation are therefore required for minimising self-extubation risk (see Chapter 6).

Complications during, and immediately after, endotracheal intubation and tracheostomy include cardiovascular compromise, bleeding, tracheal wall injury, vocal cord damage, pneumothorax, pneumomediastinum and subcutaneous emphysema. Late complications of tracheostomy include tracheal stenosis, tracheomalacia and tracheo-oesophageal fistula and infection. As noted earlier, damage to the trachea is exacerbated by high cuff pressures.[55] Percutaneous tracheostomy results in fewer wound infections, decreased incidence of bleeding and reduced mortality compared to surgical tracheostomy.[56]

Managing endotracheal and tracheostomy tubes

Tracheal suction

Patients with an ETT or tracheostomy tube require tracheal suction to remove pulmonary secretions that can lead to atelectasis or airway obstruction and impair gas exchange.[57] Suction should be performed as clinically indicated, with assessment of visible or audible secretions, rising inspiratory pressure, decreasing V_T or increased work of breathing.[58] A sawtooth pattern on the flow–volume waveform may also indicate the need for suction (discussed later in this chapter).[59]

Preoxygenation using a FiO_2 of 1.0 for approximately 60 seconds prior to suctioning is commonly performed though not supported by strong evidence unless the patient is experiencing hypoxia or has compromised cerebral circulation.[60] Preoxygenation of patients without hypoxia should be avoided as it may cause harm associated with oxygen toxicity. If a patient's oxygen saturation declines to an unacceptable level during suctioning, the FiO_2 should be increased to 1.0. Manual hyperinflation should be discouraged due to the risk of haemodynamic compromise, derecruitment, barotrauma, and lack of evidence of benefit.[61] Similarly, installation of saline is not supported due to the adverse effect on oxygen saturation.[62]

Methods

The three methods of suctioning are:

- Open suction: a suction catheter is passed under aseptic technique directly into the ETT/tracheostomy after disconnection from the ventilator circuit. Disadvantages include loss of PEEP resulting in alveolar derecruitment and increased risk of transmission of infective organisms. A surgical mask and protective eyewear should be worn.[63]
- Semi-closed suction: a suction catheter is passed through a swivel connector with a self-sealing rubber flange.
- Closed suction: in-line system is attached between the ETT/tracheostomy tube and the ventilator circuit where the suction catheter is contained in an integrated plastic sleeve. Alveolar derecruitment occurs to a lesser degree than with open suction.

There is no difference between techniques in relation to development of VAP and quantity of secretions removed.

The suction catheter diameter should not be greater than half the airway diameter, using the formula: suction catheter size [French] = (ETT size [mm] − 1) × 2. The suction catheter should be inserted to just above the carina, then withdrawn 2 cm before suction is applied to prevent damage. Suction should only last 15 seconds, using continuous, rather than intermittent, suction. Suction pressure should be set as low as possible with <150 mmHg recommended for adults and <100 mmHg for neonates.[58] Use of ETTs or tracheostomy tubes with integrated subglottic suction ports may assist in preventing VAP, especially when performed with other prevention strategies such as semirecumbant positioning and good cuff seal management.

Adverse effects

Adverse effects of suctioning include hypoxaemia, introduction of infective organisms, tracheal trauma, bradycardia, hypertension and increased intracranial pressure. Tracheal suctioning causes discomfort, and should therefore be performed only when clinically indicated, such as audible presence of secretions, desaturation and when a sawtooth pattern is observed on the flow–time scalar and flow/volume loop.[60,61]

Securing endotracheal and tracheostomy tubes

The purpose of ETT and tracheostomy tube fixation is to maintain the tube in the correct position, prevent unintended extubation or dislodgement and facilitate mechanical ventilation while maintaining skin integrity and oral hygiene.[64] ETT fixation methods include:

- tying cotton tape around the tube, then around the neck
- taping the tube to the face using medical adhesive tape
- commercial tube holders of varying designs.

There is no evidence supporting a preferred method[65] with each having specific strengths and weaknesses. A manikin study comparing cotton tapes with the Thomas Endotracheal Tube Holder demonstrated less ETT movement with the commercial tube holder.[66] Two nurses are required to prevent ETT dislodgement during fixation. Although there is also no evidence recommending a preferred frequency, ETT fixation is generally changed at least daily, to allow assessment of the underlying skin with particular attention to the ears and corners of the mouth and to facilitate oral hygiene.[64] The ETT position in the mouth is alternated at this time. ETT fixation devices including cotton ties, if applied too tightly can compress the internal or external jugular veins, which increases intracranial pressure due to reduced vascular drainage.[67] Avoid compression of internal or external jugular veins with tight cervical collar or tight tape fixation of the endotracheal tube that would impede cerebral venous drainage and result in an increase in the ICP.

> **Practice tip**
>
> Adhesive devices may become dislodged as facial hair grows under them.

Cuff pressure management

Cuff inflation pressures should be maintained at 20–30 cmH_2O (15–22 mmHg). Tracheal wall damage may occur if cuff pressure exceeds tracheal capillary perfusion pressure (27–40 cmH_2O/20–30 mmHg). Cuff inflation pressures ≤20 cmH_2O (15 mmHg) are associated with an increased risk of aspiration and an increase in VAP.[68]

There are four methods for assessing cuff inflation:

1. minimal occluding volume
2. minimal leak test
3. cuff pressure measurement
4. palpation.

Palpation of the pilot balloon is perhaps the most available and easy technique for monitoring cuff inflation but is highly subjective and inaccurate, therefore use of a manometer to measure cuff pressure is recommended.[69] In Australia and New Zealand, cuff pressure measurement is most commonly used,[70] in contrast to the UK[71] and North America[72] where it is used less frequently. Cuff pressure measurement requires a manometer attached to the pilot balloon. Cuff pressure varies with head and body position, tube position and airway pressures.[73,74] The optimum frequency of cuff pressure monitoring is unclear; at a minimum it should be done postintubation, on arrival in ICU and once per nursing shift. Recently, continuous cuff pressure measurement has been shown to reduce VAP.[75] Even with appropriate cuff inflation microaspiration occurs via the longitudinal folds in the cuff.[76]

If performing minimal occluding volume and minimal leak test, aspiration should be prevented by semirecumbent positioning, suctioning the back of the mouth (as far back as tolerated), aspiration of the nasogastric tube and discontinuation of feeds before cuff deflation.

Subglottic secretion management

For the intubated patient, oropharyngeal secretions drain into the subglottic space, pool above the cuff, and gradually leak via the longitudinal cuff folds to the lungs increasing the risk of pneumonia. Subglottic secretion drainage (SSD), a dedicated lumen within the ETT dorsal wall that exits above the cuff, enables removal of subglottic secretions either continuously via low pressure suction, or intermittently either via suction or a syringe. Tracheal mucosa injuries induced by suctioning may occur with both continuous and intermittent suctioning in up to 27% of patients.[77,78] A recent systematic review and meta-analysis found SSD to reduce the risk of VAP and the duration of ventilation though there was no evidence of effect on ICU or hospital mortality or length of stay.[79]

Managing emergencies associated with endotracheal and tracheostomy tubes

Pilot tube

If the pilot tube for the ETT or tracheostomy tube is accidentally cut or a hole is suspected in the tubing or balloon, cannulate the tubing with a 23- or 24-gauge needle to reinflate the cuff and clamp the tubing. If using a clamp with serrations, place gauze between the tube and the clamps to avoid further damage to the pilot tube.

Cuff herniation

ETT cuff herniation occurs infrequently with low-pressure high-volume cuffs, may be difficult to diagnose, but can cause life-threatening bronchial obstruction.[80] If cuff herniation is suspected (profound desaturation, loss of breath sounds), deflate and reinflate the cuff, checking the cuff pressure is within normal range. If the problem persists the tube will need changing.

Persistent cuff leaks

Cuff leaks may be categorised as leaks around an intact cuff or those due to structural damage to the cuff.[81] Structural damage generally requires replacement of the tube, particularly if leaks are large and ventilation is ineffective.

> **Practice tip**
>
> A persistent cuff leak as indicated by bubbling or other noises suggestive of gas leak and loss of V_T or cuff pressures of ≥30 cmH_2O (22 mmHg) indicating failure to generate a seal should be reviewed, check ETT position for migration and refer to medical staff.

Extubation

Following successful weaning from mechanical ventilation (see later in this chapter), assessment of the patient prior to extubation should indicate adequate gas exchange, respiratory rate and work of breathing on minimal support, respiratory muscle strength; the ability to cough and clear secretions spontaneously; and a stable haemodynamic status and mental status.[82] Serious postextubation complications of laryngospasm and stridor cannot be reliably predicted,[83] so the ease/grade of intubation should be considered prior to extubation and provision made for immediate reintubation.[84]

Mechanical ventilation

The largest international study of mechanical ventilation practices, reporting data from 8151 patients in 494 ICUs and 37 countries found the median duration of ventilation was 5 days (interquartile range 3–10 days).[85] In this patient cohort, the three most common reasons for mechanical ventilation were postoperative respiratory failure, coma and pneumonia.

A study describing ventilation and weaning practices of 55 ICUs in Australia and New Zealand in 2005 reported a similar profile as international studies for the most common indications for mechanical ventilation.[86]

Principles of mechanical ventilation

Mechanical ventilation describes the application of positive or negative pressure breaths using non-invasive or invasive techniques. Indications for initiation of mechanical ventilation are discussed below. Table 15.1 lists the patient parameters typically observed in acute and chronic respiratory failure that may influence the decision to ventilate. During positive-pressure ventilation, the type of ventilation used most commonly in critical care, the ventilator delivers a flow of gas into the lungs during inspiration using a pneumatic system. Expiration is passive.

The equation of motion

The equation of motion for the respiratory system is a mathematical model that relates pressure, volume and flow during breath delivery, with the pressure required to deliver a volume of gas determined by the elastic and resistive properties of the respiratory system[87] (Table 15.2).

Compliance and elastance

Compliance refers to the ease with which lung units distend. Elastance is the tendency of the lung units to return to their original form once stretched. Compliance is defined as the change in volume that occurs due to a change in pressure and is expressed as $C=\Delta V/\Delta P$.

Lung tissue and the surrounding thoracic structures contribute to respiratory compliance. Normal compliance for a mechanically ventilated patient ranges from 35–50 mL/cmH_2O.[88]

Resistance

Resistance refers to the forces that oppose airflow. Resistance in the airways is influenced by large and small airway diameter including the artificial airway, airway length, the gas flow rate and the density and viscosity of the inspired gas. For example, narrowing of airways causes increased resistance as does higher gas flows due to turbulent flow. During mechanical ventilation, bronchospasm, airway oedema, endotracheal tube lumen size, increased secretions, and inappropriate setting of flow rates can influence airway resistance. Normal resistance for intubated patients is 6 $cmH_2O/(L/sec)$.[88]

Ventilator graphics

Analysis of ventilator graphics provides clinicians with the ability to assess patient–ventilator interaction, appropriateness of ventilator settings and lung function.

TABLE 15.1
Physiological indications suggesting the need for mechanical ventilation

PARAMETER	NORMAL VALUES	ARF	CRF	ASSOCIATED SIGNS AND SYMPTOMS
Respiratory rate	12–20	≥28	≥30	Dyspnoea, increased activation of accessory muscles and active expiration
pH	7.35–7.45	<7.30 No compensatory changes	7.35–7.40 May be normal due to metabolic compensation	Failure to adequately ventilate: elevated $PaCO_2$, acidic pH, headache, confusion or other mental status change, tachypnoea (RR >30), flushed skin
$PaCO_2$	35–45 mmHg	>50 mmHg and rising	>50 mmHg and rising	
PaO_2	80–100 mmHg	<65 mmHg and falling	<50 mmHg and falling Hb/HCT elevated as compensatory mechanism	Failure to adequately oxygenate: decreased PaO_2 and SpO_2, tachycardia, hyper- or hypotension, dyspnoea, gasping, nasal flaring, use of accessory muscles, anxiety, agitation and altered mental status, cyanosis
HCO_3^-	22–26 mmol/L	Within normal limits	If chronic hypercapnia, then HCO_3^- >26 mmol/L is a compensatory mechanism If CRF is primarily failure to oxygenate, then HCO_3^- will be within normal limits	

ARF = acute respiratory failure; CRF = chronic respiratory failure; HCT = haematocrit; RR = respiratory rate.

TABLE 15.2
Equation of motion

EQUATION:	$P_T\ (P_{airway} + P_{muscle}) = V_T/C + V_T/T_I \times R + PEEP_T$
Abbreviations	P_T = total pressure – the sum of the pressure in the proximal airway and the pressure generated by the respiratory muscles V_T = tidal volume C = compliance T_I = inspiratory time R = resistance $PEEP_T$ = total positive end-expiratory pressure – alveolar pressure at the end of expiration and is the sum of PEEP applied by the ventilator and any intrinsic (auto) PEEP
Notes	V_T/C: describes the elastic properties of the respiratory system V_T/T_I: reflects flow in the system $V_T/T_I \times R$: resistance of the respiratory system

Scalars: pressure/time, flow/time, volume/time

Many ventilators now offer integrated graphic displays as waveforms that plot one of three parameters, pressure, flow or volume, on the vertical (*y*) axis against time, measured in seconds, on the horizontal (*x*) axis referred to as scalars. Examination of scalars can assist with assessment of patient–ventilator synchrony, patient triggering, appropriateness of inspiratory/expiratory times, presence of gas trapping, appropriateness and adequacy of flow, lung compliance and airway resistance and circuit leaks.[89-92]

Pressure vs time scalar

The morphology of this waveform depends on the control variable (volume or pressure), breath type (mandatory or spontaneous), and whether the breath is initiated by the ventilator or the patient's inspiratory effort.[91] Pressure–time waveforms reflect airway pressure (P_{aw}) during inspiration and expiration and can be used to evaluate peak and plateau inspiratory pressures and end-expiratory pressures, inspiratory and expiratory times, and appropriateness of flow (Fig. 15.4). The peak pressure represents the maximum pressure achieved during inspiration. The plateau pressure is measured during an inspiratory hold and represents the pressure applied to the small airways and alveoli. The expiratory pressure is the pressure measured once the patient has expired. Pressure–time scalars

FIGURE 15.4 Pressure, flow, volume and time waveforms.

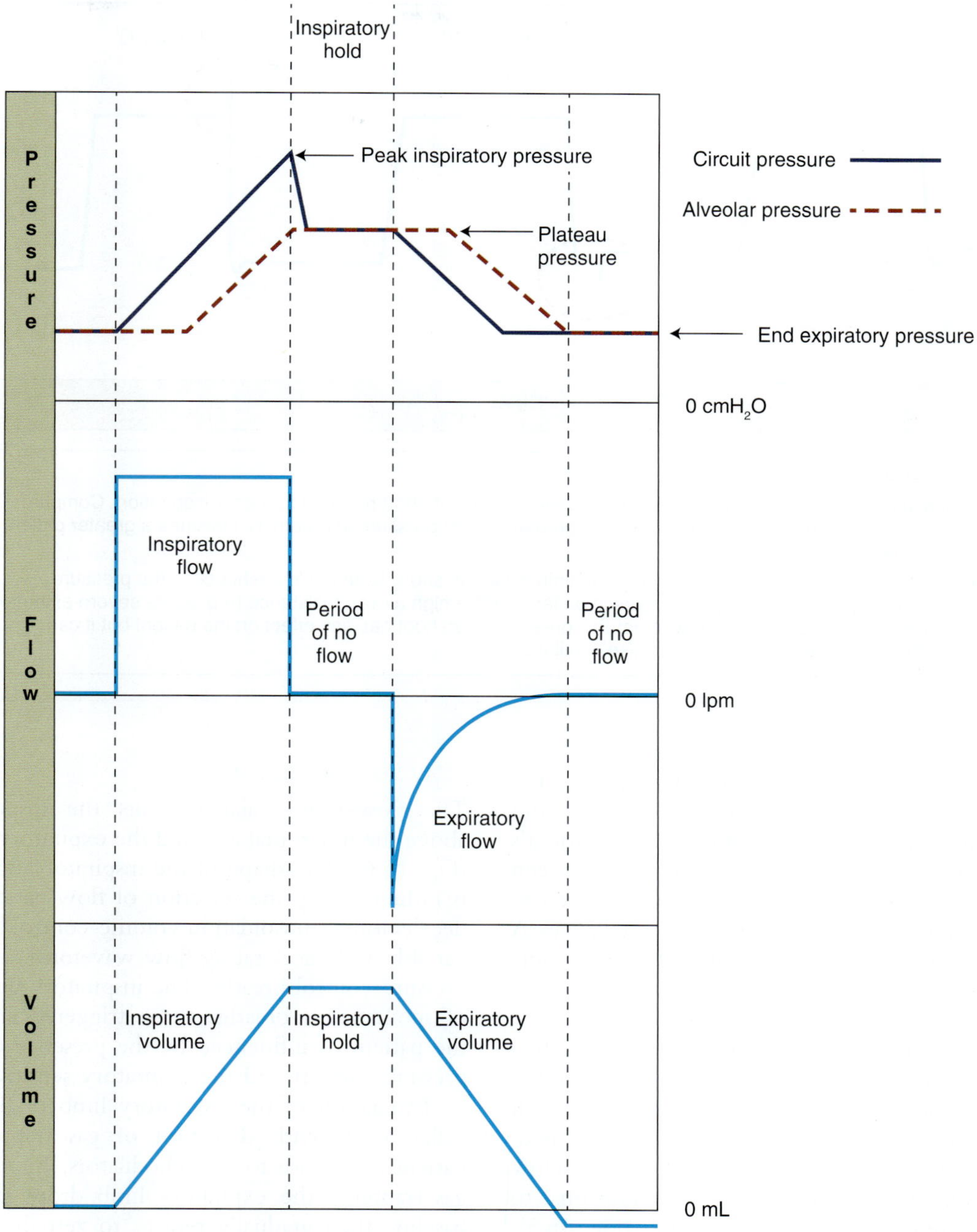

vary in appearance depending on the control variable (volume vs pressure). In *volume-control breaths* (Fig. 15.4), the inspiratory waveform continues to rise until peak inspiratory pressure is achieved according to V_T set. If an inspiratory hold is applied a plateau pressure will be generated. As the patient expires, airway pressure will drop back to the set PEEP level. *In pressure-control breaths*, the inspiratory waveform reaches its peak at the beginning of inspiration and remains at this elevation until cycling to expiration.

When interpreting the pressure waveform, it is important to recognise that the graphic waveforms display circuit pressure which does not always represent alveolar pressure. Periods of no flow (inspiratory and expiratory holds/pauses) are required to estimate alveolar pressure. The plateau pressure is a more reliable estimate of inspiratory alveolar pressure than the peak inspiratory pressure. An expiratory hold is required to determine end-expiratory alveolar pressure. Estimating alveolar pressure may be useful to assess the patient's

FIGURE 15.5 Triggering and rise time.

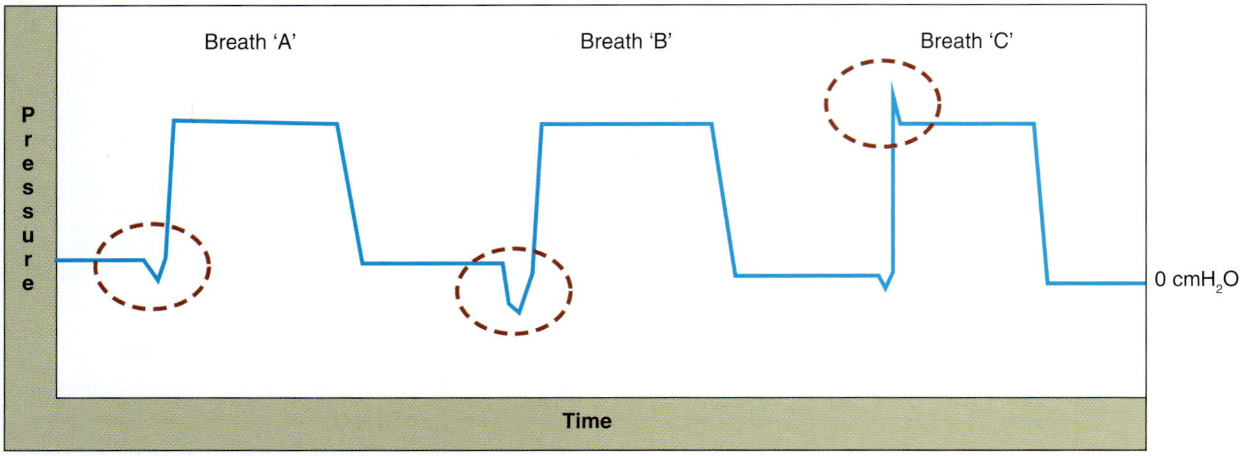

Pressure–time scalar demonstrating:

1) negative dips in pressure prior to the breath are indicative of patient effort required to trigger inspiration. Compare the drop in pressure in breath 'A' to breath 'B'. The greater drop in pressure in breath 'B' indicates a greater patient effort to trigger gas flow.
2) the effect on the pressure time scalar when the rise time is set too short. Note the 'overshootx' in the pressure waveform on breath 'C'. This sometimes occurs in patients with a high airway resistance (e.g. acute severe asthma) and a short rise time. It is questionable whether this pressure overshoot has any effect on the patient but it can trigger the high-pressure alarm and compromise ventilation.

respiratory resistance and compliance. Comparing the difference between the peak inspiratory pressure and plateau pressure can give an indication of the patient's inspiratory resistance. Comparing the difference between the plateau pressure and the end-expiratory pressure can provide information about the patient's compliance. A large difference between peak and plateau pressures indicates high airway resistance. An elevated plateau pressure indicates reduced compliance.

Spontaneous triggering of ventilation can be identified by examination of the pressure–time scalar at the beginning of inspiration. A small negative deflection indicates patient effort. When pressure triggering is used, a breath is triggered when the pressure drops below baseline. The depth of the deflection is proportional to patient effort required to trigger inspiration (Fig. 15.5). A flow-triggered breath occurs when the flow rises above baseline, although this is frequently accompanied by a small negative deflection in the pressure–time scalar. Patient inspiratory attempts that fail to trigger the ventilator can also be identified as negative deflections in the pressure waveform without corresponding responses from the ventilator.[92] Appropriateness of flow can be detected from the pressure–time scalar. If the flow is set too high or the rise time too short this can be seen as a sharp peak in the waveform (see Fig. 15.5). Conversely if flow is inadequate or the rise time too long, the incline of the inspiratory portion of the pressure waveform may be dampened or even negative.[89]

Flow vs time scalar

The flow–time scalar presents the inspiratory phase above the horizontal axis and the expiratory phase below (Fig. 15.6). The shape of the inspiratory flow waveform is influenced by the selection of flow pattern (constant, decelerating, sinusoidal) in volume-control breaths or the variable and decelerating flow waveform associated with pressure-control breaths. The inspiratory flow waveform of spontaneous breaths, those triggered and cycled by the patient, is influenced by the presence or absence of pressure support and the expiratory sensitivity.[89]

Evaluation of the expiratory limb of the flow–time scalar assists with detection of gas trapping and the patient's response to bronchodilators. In the absence of gas trapping, the expiratory limb drops sharply below baseline then gradually returns to zero before the next breath. Failure to return to baseline indicates gas trapping whereby the inspired gas is not totally expired. Gas trapping results in development of intrinsic or 'auto-PEEP'. This can adversely affect a patient's haemodynamic status and cause patient–ventilator asynchrony.[93] Gas trapping may occur in patients with airflow limitation such as those with COPD and asthma. Consequences of gas trapping include dynamic hyperinflation, reduced respiratory compliance and respiratory muscle fatigue.[94] Evaluation of the expiratory flow waveform also enables evaluation of the effects of bronchodilator therapy as, if efficacious, the expiratory flow waveform will return to baseline (Fig. 15.7).[93] Patient–ventilator asynchrony can

FIGURE 15.6 Flow vs time waveform.

Unbel	Flow wave pattern	Description
(Rectangular, square)	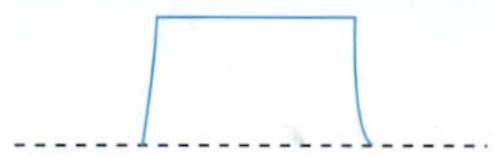	Peak flow rate is delivered immedately at the onset of inspiration, maintained throughout the inspiratory phase, and abruptly terminated at the onset of expiration.
		Common default pattern with volume-targeted modes.
Sinusoidal	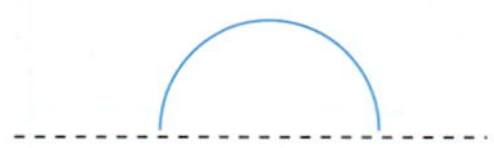	Inspiratory flow rate gradually accelerates to peak flow and then tapers off.
		Believed to mimic spontaneous inspiratory patterns.
		May increase peak inspiratory pressure (PIP).
Accelerating (ascending ramp)	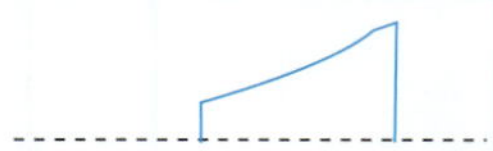	Flow gradually accelerates in a linear fashion to the set peak flow rate.
Decelerating (descending ramp)	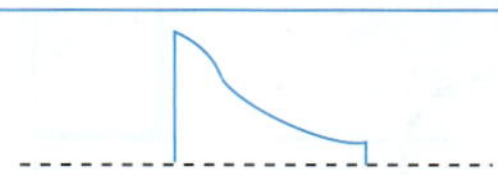	Flow is at peak at onset of inspiration and gradually decelerates throughout inspiratory phase.
		Flow ceases and ventilator cycles to expiratory phase when flow decays to a percentage of peak flow, usually 25% but varies by ventilator model. Terminal flow criteria may be adjustable in some newer ventilators.
		Rapid intial flow raises mean airway pressure and may assist in alveolar recruitment.
		May improve the distribution of gases when there is inhomogeneity of alveolar ventilation.
		Decreases dead space, increases arterial oxygen tension, and reduces PIP.

Reproduced from Pierce LNB. Management of the mechanically ventilated patient. 2nd ed. St Louis: Saunders Elsevier; 2007, Table 6.3, p. 195.

be detected in the flow waveform as abrupt decreases in expiratory flow in the expiratory limb and abrupt increases in flow in the inspiratory limb.[92]

Volume vs time scalar

The volume-time waveform originates from the functional residual capacity (baseline), rises as inspiratory flow is delivered to reach the maximum inspiratory V_T, then returns to baseline during expiration. The volume waveform is useful in troubleshooting circuit leaks (Fig. 15.8) as it will fail to return to baseline if a leak in the circuit–patient interface is present.

Loops: pressure/volume, flow/volume

Most contemporary critical care ventilators allow for monitoring of pressure, flow and volume parameters integrated into graphic loops enabling measurement of airway resistance, chest wall and lung compliance.

Pressure–volume loops

The two parameters, P_{aw} and V_T are plotted against each other, with P_{aw} on the *x* axis. For mandatory breaths, the loop is drawn counter clockwise (Fig. 15.9). Spontaneous (triggered and cycled) breaths are drawn in a clockwise fashion. When low gas flow is delivered and the patient is unable to initiate ventilation, pressure–volume loops may be used to identify the lower and upper inflection points. The lower inflection point begins near the beginning of inspiration as the P_{aw} starts to rise with little change in V_T. As P_{aw} continues to rise, the V_T increases exponentially as alveoli are recruited, resulting in a marked increase in the inspiratory limb

FIGURE 15.7 Auto-PEEP and gas trapping.

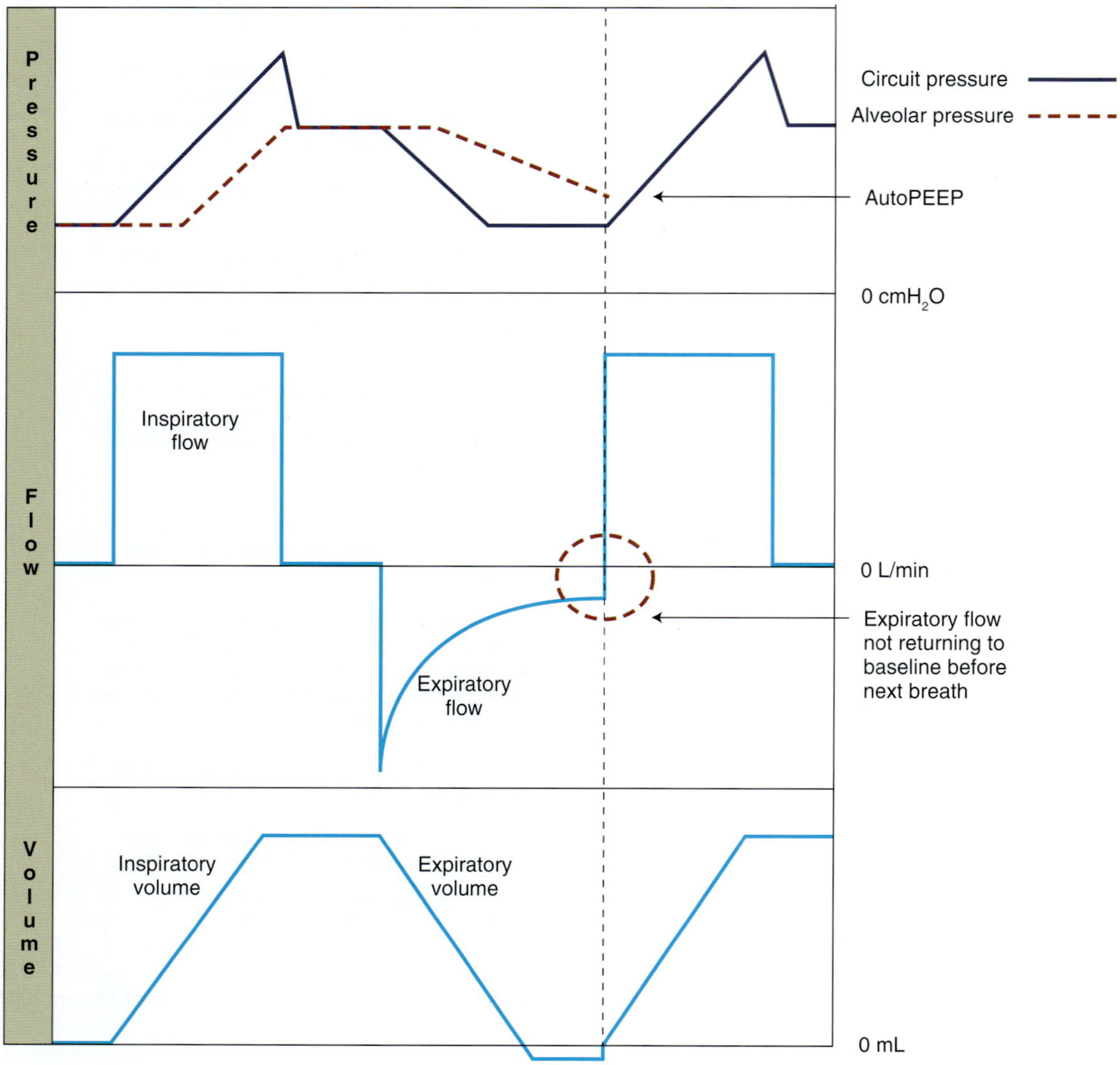

This diagram demonstrates the use of the flow pressure scalar to identify the presence of autoPEEP. In the area highlighted by the circle with the dashed line the expiratory flow has not returned to zero before the onset of the next breath. This indicates that gas trapping has occurred and the pressure in the alveoli is greater than the pressure in the ventilator circuit. This indicates the presence of 'autoPEEP'

slope. This point represents alveolar recruitment and is referred to as the lower inflection point, and may be used to guide PEEP selection.[95,96] The inspiratory limb continues until peak inspiratory pressure and maximal V_T are achieved. The bend in the inspiratory limb towards the end of inspiration is referred to as the upper inflection point, and denotes the point at which small volume increases produce large pressure increases indicating lung overdistension.[95] The expiratory limb represents lung derecruitment and is also useful in guiding PEEP selection.[97,98]

For patient-triggered mandatory breaths, the initial part of the loop occurs to the left of the *y* axis and flows in a clockwise fashion, reflecting patient effort. The loop then shifts to the right of the *y* axis and moves in a counter-clockwise fashion as the ventilator assumes the work of breathing.[88] Pressure–volume loops reflect dynamic compliance between the lungs and the

FIGURE 15.8 Tidal volume vs time, with and without leak.

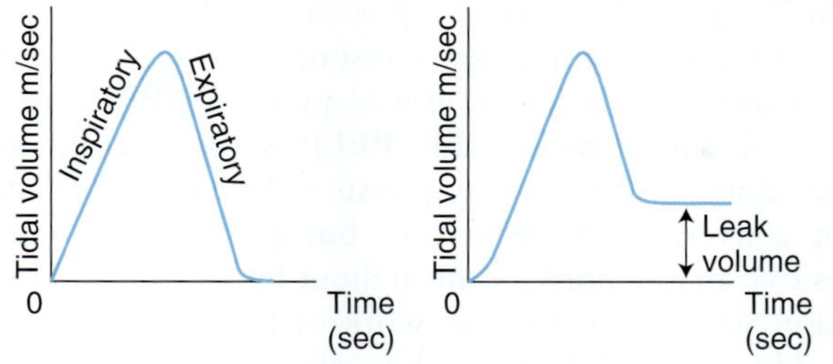

FIGURE 15.9 Pressure–volume loop.

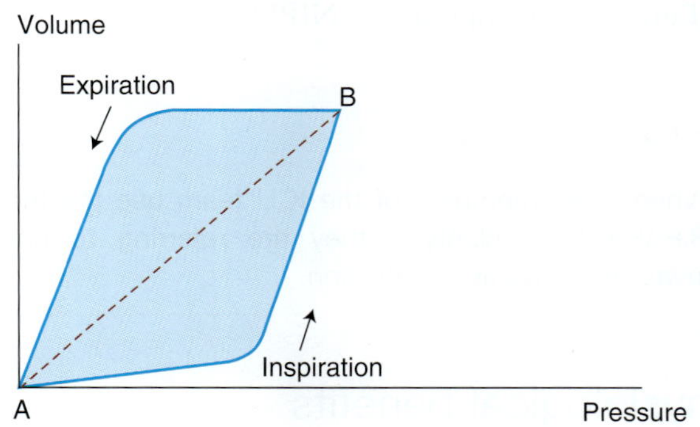

Adapted from Dräegerwerk AG & Co. http://www.draeger.com/sites/assets/Publixhingimages/Products/savina-300/UK/9097421-Fibel-Curves_Loops-en.pdf, p 26, with permission.

ventilator circuit. Decreased compliance requires greater pressure to achieve V_T and is reflected in a flattened pressure–volume loop.[99] The area between the loops represents the resistance to inspiration and expiration, known as hysteresis. As resistance increases, less V_T is delivered resulting in a shorter and wider loop; conversely, as resistance decreases, a longer, wider loop is generated (Fig. 15.10).[100]

Flow–volume loops

Flow–volume loops recorded during positive-pressure ventilation depict inspiration above the baseline and expiration below it. These loops are useful in determining response to bronchodilators and examining changes in airway resistance.

Ventilator circuits

Delivery of mechanical ventilation requires a ventilator circuit to transport gas flow to the patient. To prevent condensation from cooling of warm humidified

FIGURE 15.10 Pressure–volume loop representing resistance changes.

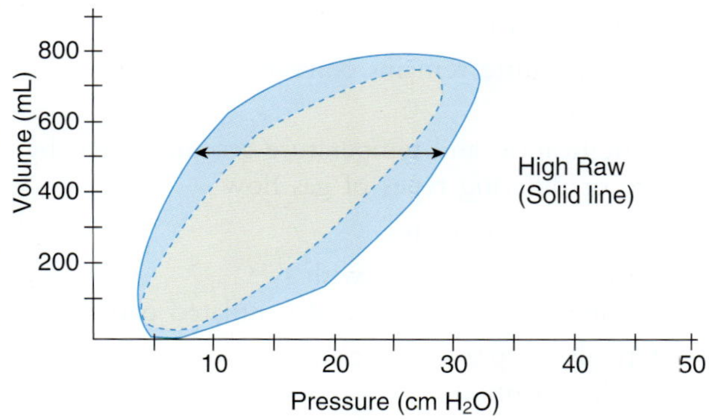

*Dashed line depicts normal Raw

Reproduced from Pierce LNB. Management of the mechanically ventilated patient. 2nd ed. St Louis: Saunders Elsevier; 2007, Table 8.18, p. 284.

gas, inspired gas is heated via a wire inside the circuit wall in either the inspiratory limb alone or both the inspiratory and expiratory limbs.[101] Historically ventilator circuits were changed frequently (48–72 h) to decrease the risk of VAP.[102] Current guidelines and recommendations for VAP prevention found evidence that the frequency of ventilator circuit changes did not reduce VAP incidence, indeed frequent changes may increase VAP due to circuit manipulation. Therefore, routine circuit changes were not necessary and circuits should only be changed when soiled or damaged.[103,104]

Humidification

Humidification warms and moistens gas to facilitate cilia action and mucus removal as well as to prevent drying and irritation of respiratory mucosa and solidification of secretions. During endotracheal intubation and mechanical ventilation, the normal humidification processes of the nasopharynx are bypassed. This, in combination with the use of dry medical gas at high-flow rates, means alternative methods of humidification are required. The best conditions for mucosal health and function over prolonged periods are when inspired gas is warmed to core body temperature and is fully saturated with water.[105]

Absolute and relative humidity

Absolute humidity refers to the amount of water vapour in a given volume of gas at a given temperature. Absolute humidity rises with increasing temperature; during mechanical ventilation gas is heated to increase the amount of water vapour it will hold. Relative humidity is expressed as a percentage, and is the actual amount of water vapour in a gas compared to the maximum amount this gas can hold (ratio of absolute to maximal humidity). Ideal humidification is achieved when the:

1 inspired gas delivered into the trachea is at 37°C with a water content of 30–43 g/m^3 (relative humidity is 100% at 37°C in the bronchi)
2 set temperature remains constant without fluctuation
3 humidification and temperature are unaffected by large or differing types of gas flow
4 device is simple to use
5 humidifier can be used with spontaneously-breathing and ventilated patients
6 safety alarms prevent overheating, overhydration and electrocution
7 resistance, compliance and dead space characteristics do not adversely affect spontaneous breathing modes
8 sterility of the inspired gas is not compromised.[106]

Humidification is applied using either a heat–moisture exchanger (HME) or a heated water bath reservoir device in combination with a heated ventilator circuit.

Heat–moisture exchanger

HMEs conserve heat and moisture during expiration enabling inspired gas to be heated and humidified. Two types of HMEs exist: hygroscopic and hydrophobic. Hygroscopic HMEs absorb moisture onto a chemically impregnated foam or paper material and have been shown to be more effective than hydrophobic HMEs.[107] HMEs are placed distally to the circuit Y-piece in line with the ETT and increase dead space by an amount equal to their internal volume.[108] HMEs should be changed every 24 hours or when soiled with secretions and are usually reserved for short-term humidification.

Heated humidification

Generally, heated humidification is used for patients requiring greater than 24 hours of mechanical ventilation. Various models of heater bases and circuits are on the market and we recommend their use in accordance with manufacturer instructions. A recent systematic review and meta-analysis reported no overall effect on artificial airway occlusion, mortality, pneumonia, or respiratory complications when HMEs were compared to heated humidification, although it noted that the $PaCO_2$ and minute ventilation were increased and body temperature was lower with the use of HMEs.[109]

Non-invasive ventilation

Non-invasive ventilation (NIV) is an umbrella term describing the delivery of mechanical ventilation without the use of an invasive airway, via an interface such as an oronasal, nasal, or full-face mask or helmet. NIV techniques include both negative and positive-pressure ventilation, although in critical care positive-pressure ventilation is primarily used.

Terminology

Positive-pressure NIV can be further categorised as non-invasive positive-pressure ventilation (NIPPV) or continuous positive airway pressure (CPAP). NIPPV is the provision of inspiratory pressure support, also referred to as inspiratory positive airway pressure (IPAP) usually in combination with PEEP. PEEP is also referred to as expiratory positive airway pressure (EPAP). CPAP does not actively assist inspiration but provides a constant positive airway pressure throughout inspiration and expiration which can decrease work of breathing.[110]

The terms biphasic (or bilevel) positive airway pressure (BiPAP) and non-invasive pressure support ventilation (NIPSV) are also used to refer to NIPPV.[111] The acronym BiPAP® is registered to Respironics (Murrayville, PA), a company that produces non-invasive ventilators including the BiPAP® Vision which is commonly used in the ICU. The acronym NIPSV is primarily used in European descriptions of NIPPV.

> **Practice tip**
>
> When other members of the ICU team use the term BiPAP/BIPAP, clarify if they are referring to non-invasive or invasive ventilation.

Physiological benefits

The efficacy of NIV in patients with acute respiratory failure is, at least in part, related to avoidance of inspiratory muscle fatigue through the addition of inspiratory positive pressure thus reducing inspiratory muscle work.[112] Application of positive pressure during inspiration increases transpulmonary pressure, inflates the lungs, augments alveolar ventilation and unloads the inspiratory muscles.[113] Augmentation of alveolar ventilation, demonstrated by an increase in V_T, increases CO_2 elimination and reverses acidaemia. High levels of inspiratory pressure may also relieve dyspnoea.[114]

The main physiological benefit in patients with congestive heart failure (CHF) is attributed to the increase in functional residual capacity associated with the use of PEEP that reopens collapsed alveoli and improves oxygenation.[115] Increased intrathoracic pressure associated with the application of positive pressure also may improve cardiac performance by reducing myocardial work and oxygen consumption through reductions to ventricular preload and left ventricular afterload.[115-117] NIV also preserves the ability to speak, swallow, cough and clear secretions, and decreases risks associated with endotracheal intubation.[118]

Indications for NIV

The success of NIV treatment is dependent on appropriate patient selection.[119] Table 15.3 outlines indications and contraindications to NIV.

TABLE 15.3
Indications and contraindications for non-invasive ventilation

INDICATIONS	
Bedside observations	Increased dyspnoea; moderate-to-severe tachypnoea: >24 breaths per min [obstructive] >30 breaths per min [restrictive] Signs of increased work of breathing, accessory muscle use and abdominal paradox
Gas exchange	Acute or acute-on-chronic ventilatory failure (best indication), $PaCO_2$ >45 mmHg, pH <7.35 Hypoxaemia (use with caution), PaO_2/FiO_2 ratio <200
CONTRAINDICATIONS	
Absolute	Respiratory arrest Unable to fit mask
Relative	Medically unstable: hypotensive shock, uncontrolled cardiac ischaemia or arrhythmia, uncontrolled upper gastrointestinal bleeding Agitated, uncooperative Unable to protect airway Swallowing impairment Excessive secretions not managed by secretion clearance techniques Multiple (i.e. two or more) organ failure Recent upper airway or upper gastrointestinal surgery

$PaCO_2$ = partial pressure of carbon dioxide in arterial blood; PaO_2 = partial pressure of oxygen in arterial blood; PaO_2/FiO_2 = ratio of partial pressure of oxygen in arterial blood to fraction of inspired oxygen.
Reproduced from Nava S, Hill N. Non-invasive ventilation in acute respiratory failure. Lancet 2009; 374(9685): 250–59.

Acute respiratory failure

Evidence supporting the role of NIV in patients with hypoxaemic respiratory failure is limited and conflicting.[115] For patients with community-acquired pneumonia, NIV has been shown to reduce intubation rates, ICU length of stay and 2-month mortality but only in the subgroup of patients with COPD.[120] Pneumonia also has been identified as a risk factor for NIV failure.[121]

Acute exacerbation of COPD and CHF

Strong evidence exists to support the use of NIV for patients with acute exacerbation of COPD and CHF. The most recent systematic review of NIV for patients with hypercapnic respiratory failure due to COPD that includes 17 trials enrolling 1264 patients found NIV as a first line intervention reduced the risk of mortality by 46% and the risk of endotracheal intubation by 65%.[122] COPD patients most likely to respond favourably to NIV include those with an unimpaired level of consciousness, moderate acidaemia, a respiratory rate of <30 breaths/minute and who demonstrate an improvement in respiratory parameters within two hours of commencing NIV.[112,123]

Early use of NIV in combination with standard therapy for patients with CHF has also been shown to reduce intubation rates and mortality when compared to standard therapy alone.[124-126] The most recent meta-analysis including 32 trials found NIV reduced hospital mortality and reintubation rates by nearly 50% compared to standard medical care and no increased risk of acute myocardial infarction.[127] The authors recommended CPAP may be considered as the first option for NIV due to more robust evidence for its effectiveness, safety and lower cost compared with NIV.[127] Practice surveys indicate CPAP may be the preferred method of NIV for patients with CHF in Australia and internationally.

NIV in weaning

NIV may be used as an adjunct to weaning to reduce the duration of invasive ventilation and associated complications.[128] Patients are extubated directly to NIV and then weaned to standard oxygen therapy. This use of NIV differs from its role in preventing reintubation in patients that develop, or who are at high risk of, postextubation respiratory failure.[129] A recent systematic review and meta-analysis of 16 trials with 994 participants (mostly COPD) using NIV immediately after extubation reported reductions in mortality, weaning failure, VAP, tracheostomy, reintubation, ICU and hospital lengths of stay, and total duration of ventilation.[130] Conversely, the effectiveness of NIV for postextubation failure is not so clear. The largest study of NIV use in postextubation respiratory failure reported worsened survival rates hypothesised to be as a result of delayed reintubation.[131] A subsequent meta-analysis suggested NIV may have a role in preventing the development of respiratory failure postextubation for those at risk, but should be used with caution once respiratory failure has developed and should not delay the decision to reintubate.[114]

Other indications

Other indications for NIV include:

- asthma[132,133]
- pulmonary infiltrates in immunocompromised patients
- neuromuscular disorders (e.g. muscular dystrophy, amyotrophic lateral sclerosis)
- fractured ribs
- obesity and central hypoventilation syndromes
- palliation.[134]

Patient section

Selection of patients to receive NIV depends on the presence of an indications listed above as well as bedside observations and gas exchange parameters found in Table 15.3.

Interfaces and settings

NIV requires an interface that connects the patient to either a ventilator, portable compressor or flow generator with a CPAP valve. The selection of an appropriate interface can influence NIV success or failure. Oronasal masks cover both the mouth and nose and are the preferred mask type for the management of acute respiratory failure.[135] Nasal masks enable speech, eating and drinking, and therefore are used more frequently for long-term NIV use. An oronasal mask enables delivery of higher ventilation pressures with less leak and greater comfort for the patient.[136] Other interfaces include full-face masks[136] that seal around the perimeter of the face and cover the eyes as well as the nose and mouth, nasal pillows, mouthpieces that are placed between the patient's lips, and helmets that cover the whole head and consist of a transparent plastic hood attached to a soft neck collar. These alternative interfaces may increase patient tolerance by reducing pressure ulceration, air leaks and patient discomfort.[137]

Initiation and monitoring priorities

Successful initiation of NIV is dependent on patient acceptance and tolerance. Patient acceptance may be aided by a brief explanation of the procedure and its benefits. Strategies to enhance patient tolerance include: use of an interface that fits the patient's facial features, commencing with low pressure levels, holding the mask gently in position prior to securing with the straps/headgear, and ensuring straps prevent major leaks but are not so tight they increase discomfort. Once NIV is commenced, the patient should be monitored for respiratory and haemodynamic stability, response to NIV treatment, ongoing tolerance, and presence of air leaks (Table 15.4). Arterial blood gas analysis should be performed at baseline and within the first 1–2 hours of commencement.[138] During the initiation and stabilisation period, patients should be monitored using a nurse-to-patient ratio of 1:1 with ongoing coaching to promote NIV tolerance throughout the early stabilisation period.

TABLE 15.4
Monitoring priorities for non-invasive ventilation

PRIORITY	ASSESSMENT
Patient comfort	Restlessness Mask tolerance Anxiety level Dyspnoea score Pain score
Conscious level	Glasgow Coma Scale
Work of breathing	Chest wall motion Accessory muscle activation RR
Gas exchange parameters	Continuous SpO_2 Arterial blood gas analysis (baseline and 1–2 hourly subsequently) Patient colour
Haemodynamic status	Continuous heart rate Intermittent blood pressure
Ventilator parameters	Air leak around mask Adequacy of PS (V_T, pH, $PaCO_2$) Adequacy of peak end-expiratory pressure (SpO_2, PaO_2)

$PaCO_2$ = partial pressure of carbon dioxide in arterial blood; PaO_2 = partial pressure of oxygen in arterial blood; PS = pressure support; RR = respiratory rate; SpO_2 = saturation of peripheral oxygen; V_T = tidal volume.
Adapted from Rose L, Gerdtz M. Use of non-invasive ventilation in Australian emergency departments. Int J Nurs Stud 2009;46(5):617–23, with permission.

Practice tip

NIV tolerance may be promoted with a simple explanation of the therapy, reassurance and constant monitoring for your patient. During initiation, allow them to take short breaks from the mask if they are in discomfort or experiencing claustrophobia.

Potential complications

Masks need to be tight-fitting to reduce air leaks; however, this contributes to pressure ulceration on the bridge of the nose or above the ears (due to mask straps/headgear). Air leaks may cause conjunctival irritation and the high flow of dry medical gas results in nasal congestion, oral or nasal dryness and insufflation of air into the stomach. Claustrophobia associated with the NIV interface may also lead to agitation reducing the efficacy of NIV treatment due to poor coordination of respiratory cycling between the patient and NIV unit.[112] More serious, yet infrequent, complications include aspiration pneumonia, haemodynamic compromise associated with increased intrathoracic pressures and pneumothorax.[113]

Detecting NIV failure

Failure to respond to NIV within 1–2 hours of commencement is demonstrated by unchanged or worsening gas exchange, as well as ongoing or new onset of rapid shallow breathing and increased haemodynamic instability.[136] Decreased level of consciousness may be indicative of imminent respiratory arrest.

Weaning from NIV

Existing guidelines provide little guidance on weaning of NIV.[139] In many cases, NIV may be simply withdrawn as opposed to weaned. For those commencing on high levels of IPAP and/or EPAP, these may need weaning based on ongoing assessment of dyspnoea, chest wall movement, as well as ventilation and oxygenation parameters. Another weaning method may be progressive extension of time off NIV, while monitoring tolerance.

Invasive mechanical ventilation

Critically ill patients with persistent respiratory insufficiency (hypoxaemia and/or hypercapnia), due to drugs, disease or other conditions, may require intubation and mechanical ventilation to support oxygenation and ventilatory demands. Clinical criteria for intubation and ventilation should be based on individual-patient assessment and patient response to measures aimed at reversing hypoxaemia. Box 15.2 describes some specific considerations for mechanical ventilation of the elderly patient.

> **BOX 15.2**
>
> **Mechanical ventilation of the elderly patient**
>
> - Elderly survivors of mechanical ventilation may have a greater increase in disability than those hospitalised and not requiring ventilation, which is information that should be shared with patients and family members when considering treatment options
> - Frail elderly are at increased risk of delirium resulting in prolonged mechanical ventilation

Indications

Indications for intubation and mechanical ventilation include:

- apnoea
- inability to protect airway; e.g. loss of gag/cough reflex; decreased Glasgow Coma Scale score
- clinical signs indicating respiratory distress: e.g. tachypnoea,[140] activation of accessory and expiratory muscles, abnormal chest wall movements,[141] tachycardia and hypertension
- inability to sustain adequate oxygenation for metabolic demands; e.g. cyanosis, SpO_2 <88%, with supplemental $FiO_2 \geq 0.5$
- respiratory acidosis (e.g. acute decrease in pH <7.25)
- postoperative respiratory failure
- shock.

The goals of mechanical ventilation are to achieve and maintain adequate pulmonary gas exchange, minimise the risk of lung injury, reduce patient work of breathing and optimise comfort.

Mechanical ventilators

Contemporary ventilators use sophisticated microprocessor controls with sensitive detection, response and control of pressure and gas flow characteristics. These ventilators are more sensitive to patient ventilatory demands, enabling improved patient–ventilator synchrony during both inspiratory and expiratory breath phases. Parameters commonly manipulated during mechanical ventilation are detailed in Table 15.5. Parameters often observed and documented are discussed below.

Phases of breath delivery

The respiratory cycle comprises both inspiratory and expiratory phases (Fig. 15.11). Pressure, flow, volume and time are parameters used to describe or classify mechanical ventilator breaths during the phases of inspiration. Ventilator breaths are classified by 1) the mechanism (ventilator or patient) that 'triggers' the start of inspiration; 2) the parameter that is 'targeted' (also referred to as 'controlled' or 'limited') during inspiration; and 3) the parameter that 'cycles' the breath from inspiration to expiration.[142]

Pressure vs volume delivery

Traditionally, clinicians have favoured volume-control ventilation (VCV) due to the ability to regulate minute ventilation (VE) and CO_2 elimination with straightforward manipulation of respiratory rate and V_T.[143] VCV provides consistent V_T delivery, independent of lung mechanics. The set V_T and flow rates used in VCV means that the ventilator is unable to increase volume or flow rates in response to the patient's inspiratory demands during mandatory breaths. This inability to respond to patient's inspiratory flow requirements can lead to dyssynchrony. Another disadvantage of VCV is the lack of control over peak airway pressure that

TABLE 15.5
Set ventilator parameters

PARAMETER	DESCRIPTION
Fraction of inspired oxygen (FiO_2)	The fraction of inspired oxygen delivered on inspiration to the patient
Tidal volume (V_T)	Volume (mL) of each breath
Set breath rate (f)	The clinician-determined set rate of breaths delivered by the ventilator (beats/min)
Inspiratory trigger or sensitivity	Mechanism by which the ventilator senses the patient's inspiratory effort. May be measured in terms of a change in pressure or flow
Inspiratory pressure (P_{insp}, P_{high})	Clinician-determined pressure that is targeted during inspiration
Inspiratory time (T_{insp})	The duration of inspiration (s)
Inspiratory : expiratory ratio (I:E)	The ratio of the inspiratory time to expiratory time
Flow ($\dot{V}$)	The speed gas travels during inspiration (L/min)
Pressure support (PS)	The flow of gas that augments a patient's spontaneously initiated breath to a clinician-determined pressure (cmH_2O)
Positive end-expiratory pressure (PEEP)	Application of airway pressure above atmospheric pressure at the end of expiration (cmH_2O)
Rise time	Time to achieve maximal flow at the onset of inspiration for pressure-targeted breaths
Expiratory sensitivity	During a spontaneous breath, the ventilator cycles from inspiration to expiration once flow has decelerated to a percentage of initial peak flow
Minute volume (V_E)	Generally not set directly but is determined by V_T and f settings. Tidal volume multiplied by the RR over 1 minute (L/min)
Airway pressure (P_{aw})	The pressure measured in cmH_2O by the ventilator in the proximal airway
Plateau pressure (P_{plat})	The pressure, measured in cmH_2O, applied to the small airways and alveoli. P_{plat} is not set but can be measured by performing an inspiratory hold manoeuvre

RR = respiratory rate.

changes in response to altered compliance and resistance. Elevated plateau pressure may cause alveolar overdistension, barotrauma and haemodynamic effects such as reduced venous return and cardiac output resulting in hypotension and thus decreased organ perfusion.[144] Clinicians need to carefully monitor ventilation to avoid injurious pressures. In VCV the peak airway pressure is achieved towards the end of inspiration, and only for a short duration, therefore distribution of gas may not be optimised and shearing stress can occur.[145] This can be overcome with use of a decelerating waveform and an inspiratory time that produces an inspiratory hold.

Pressure-control ventilation (PCV) allows control over the peak inspiratory pressure and inspiratory time. Clinicians must monitor minute ventilation and gas exchange due to the lack of a guaranteed V_T and possible changes in respiratory compliance and resistance. The variable flow and V_Ts means that there is the potential for greater interaction between patient efforts and ventilator breaths than is present in volume-controlled ventilation. The variable and decelerating inspiratory gas flow pattern of PCV enables rapid alveolar filling and more even gas distribution compared to the constant flow pattern that may be used with volume control. This decelerating flow pattern also results in improved gas exchange, decreased work of breathing and prevention of overdistension in healthy alveoli.[146-149] During PCV, the set inspiratory pressure is achieved at the beginning of the inspiratory cycle and maintained for the set inspiratory time. This promotes recruitment of alveoli with high opening pressures and long time-constants.

Ventilator parameters

Fraction of inspired oxygen

The FiO_2 is expressed as a decimal, between 0.21 and 1.0, when supplemental oxygen is applied. Room air has an oxygen content of 0.21 (21%). Ventilation is commonly

FIGURE 15.11 Phases of breath delivery.

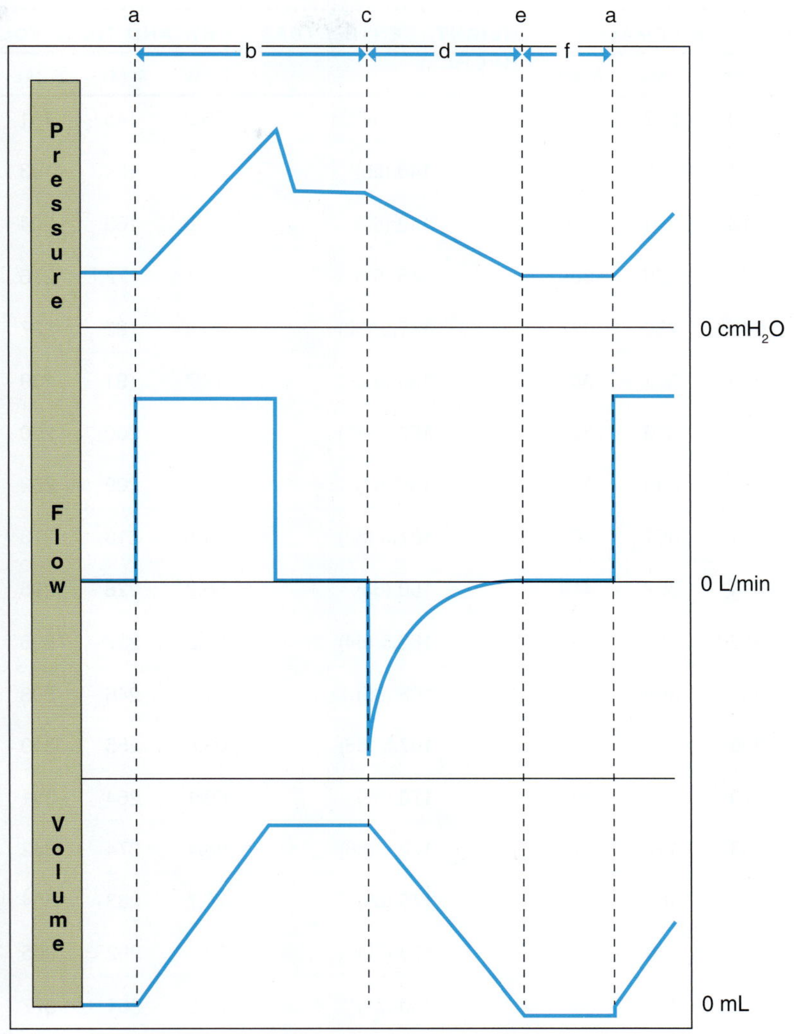

a)	start of ventilator inspiration
b)	inspiration
c)	cycle from inspiration to expiration
d)	expiration
e)	end of expiration
f)	between inspiration and expiration

commenced on a high FiO_2 setting, but as noted earlier, clinicians should consider the risks of oxygen toxicity which include disruption to the alveolar-capillary membrane and alveolar wall fibrosis.[150]

Tidal volume

V_T is the volume, measured in mL, of each breath. Set or targeted V_T is calculated using the patient's predicted body weight using height and gender-specific tables[151] to achieve 6–8 mL/kg (Table 15.6). Strong evidence indicates a mortality benefit for using 6 mL/kg in patients with acute respiratory distress syndrome (ARDS).[152] Recent professional society clinical practice guidelines recommend targeting 4-8 mL/kg predicted body weight targeting lower inspiratory pressures (plateau pressure 30 cmH_2O).[153] Evidence indicates protective lung ventilation

TABLE 15.6

ARDSnet tables for predicted body weight for females and males

PBW AND TIDAL VOLUME FOR FEMALES						HEIGHT, CENTIMETRES (INCHES)	PBW AND TIDAL VOLUME FOR MALES					
PBW	4 ML	5 ML	6 ML	7 ML	8 ML		PBW	4 ML	5 ML	6 ML	7 ML	8 ML
31.7	127	159	190	222	254	137 (54)	36.2	145	181	217	253	290
34	136	170	204	238	272	140 (55)	38.5	154	193	231	270	308
36.3	145	182	218	254	290	142 (56)	40.8	163	204	245	286	326
38.6	154	193	232	270	309	145 (57)	43.1	172	216	259	302	345
40.9	164	205	245	286	327	147.5 (58)	45.4	182	227	272	318	363
43.2	173	216	259	302	346	150 (59)	47.7	191	239	286	334	382
45.5	182	228	273	319	364	152.5 (60)	50	200	250	300	350	400
47.8	191	239	287	335	382	155 (61)	52.3	209	262	314	366	418
50.1	200	251	301	351	401	157.5 (62)	54.6	218	273	328	382	437
52.4	210	262	314	367	419	160 (63)	56.9	228	285	341	398	455
54.7	219	274	328	383	438	162.5 (64)	59.2	237	296	355	414	474
57	228	285	342	399	456	165 (65)	61.5	246	308	369	431	492
59.3	237	297	356	415	474	167.5 (66)	63.8	255	319	383	447	510
61.6	246	308	370	431	493	170 (67)	66.1	264	331	397	463	529
63.9	256	320	383	447	511	172.5 (68)	68.4	274	342	410	479	547
66.2	265	331	397	463	530	175 (69)	70.7	283	354	424	495	566
68.5	274	343	411	480	548	178 (70)	73	292	365	438	511	584
70.8	283	354	425	496	566	180 (71)	75.3	301	377	452	527	602
73.1	292	366	439	512	585	183 (72)	77.6	310	388	466	543	621
75.4	302	377	452	528	603	185.5 (73)	79.9	320	400	479	559	639
77.7	311	389	466	544	622	188 (74)	82.2	329	411	493	575	658
80	320	400	480	560	640	190.5 (75)	84.5	338	423	507	592	676
82.3	329	412	494	576	658	193 (76)	86.8	347	434	521	608	694
84.6	338	423	508	592	677	195.5 (77)	89.1	356	446	535	624	713
86.9	348	435	521	608	695	198 (78)	91.4	366	457	548	640	731

PBW = predicted body weight.
The formulae, when using height in centimetres, are:

- Females = 45.5 + 0.91 × (height in cm − 152.4)
- Males = 50 + 0.91 × (height in cm − 152.3).

Source: Adapted with information from NIH/NHLBI ARDS Network. http://www.ardsnet.org.

using 6 mL/kg as a target for patients without ARDS is associated with improved clinical outcomes.[154,155] As increasing evidence confirms high V_T causes harm[156] clinicians should consider aiming for 6–8 mL/kg in all ventilated patients.

Respiratory rate

Mandatory frequency (f) or respiratory rate (RR) is set with consideration of the patient's own respiratory effort, anticipated ventilatory requirements and the effect on the I:E ratio. Use of high doses of sedation with or without neuromuscular blockade requires setting a mandatory rate that facilitates adequate gas exchange and meets ventilation requirements. A lower frequency can be set for a patient able to breathe spontaneously in modes such as synchronised intermittent mandatory ventilation (SIMV) and assist control (A/C) (see below) to enable spontaneous triggering. Physiologically normal RRs are 12–20 breaths per min. Patients with hypoxaemic respiratory failure generally breathe 20–30 breaths per min.[157]

Triggering of inspiration

Depending on the ventilation mode, breaths are triggered by the ventilator or patient in various sequences. A breath may be triggered by the ventilator in response to time elapsed in modes with clinician-determined set frequency such as controlled mandatory ventilation (CMV), and in A/C and SIMV in the absence of spontaneous effort. Patient triggering requires the ventilator to sense the patient's inspiratory effort. Most modern generation ventilators now use flow triggering, as evidence indicates that flow triggering may be more responsive to patient effort than pressure triggering.[158] Pressure triggering requires the patient to create a negative pressure within the ventilator circuit of sufficient size to enable the ventilator to sense the effort and commence flow of gas. Flow triggering is used in conjunction with a predetermined flow of gas, usually 5–10 L/min, referred to as the bias (or base) flow, that travels continuously through the ventilator circuit. When the patient makes an inspiratory effort, they divert flow that is sensed by the ventilator. If the flow diversion reaches a clinician-determined set value, a breath is initiated.[159] The flow trigger is usually set at 1–3 L/min (1 L/min represents less patient effort and 3 L/min represents greater patient effort). Despite advances in ventilator technology, various studies continue to identify missed patient triggers that contribute to patient–ventilator asynchrony.[160] Conversely, 'auto-triggering' is ventilator triggering in the absence of spontaneous inspiratory effort. Auto-triggering is sometimes observed in patients with an increased cardiac output, such as those fulfilling brain death criteria.

Rise time

The rise time controls how quickly the ventilator reaches the clinician-determined inspiratory pressure (P_{insp}) for mandatory breaths and pressure support for spontaneous breaths. Reducing the rise time to its lowest value will enable the ventilator to reach target pressure in the shortest time frame resulting in a more rapid delivering of flow in the early phase of inspiration. This reduces work of breathing and improves synchrony. In patients with a high airway resistance e.g. severe asthma, a short inspiratory time may cause oscillation and overshoot of the pressure waveform. The clinical relevance of this is questionable but it produces an abnormal pressure waveform and results in alarm violations. Increasing the rise time may alleviate this problem. In other patients, an increased rise time may unnecessarily increase their work of breathing.[161]

Inspiratory time and inspiratory:expiratory ratio

The total time available for each mandatory breath is determined by the set inspiratory time and breath frequency. Normal inspiratory time is 0.8–1.2 seconds. Total breath time comprises the inspiratory (I) and expiratory (E) time that can be expressed as a ratio (I:E). In normal spontaneous breathing, expiratory time is approximately twice the inspiratory time (1:2 ratio). Gas flow also influences inspiratory time, with higher gas flows resulting in decreased time to achieve the target V_T. The I:E ratio can be manipulated to create an inverse relationship (1:1, 2:1, 4:1) with the goal of increased mean airway pressure resulting in alveolar recruitment and improved oxygenation. Prolonging the inspiratory time beyond normal or using inverse ratio ventilation in any mode can result in patient–ventilator dyssynchrony and increased risk of barotrauma.[162]

Inspiratory flow and flow pattern

The flow rate refers to the speed of gas, is measured in litres per minute (L/min), and generally delivered at speeds of 30–60 L/min. Higher flow rates cause turbulent gas flow, resulting in increased peak airway pressures. Lower flow rates result in laminar flow, increased inspiratory time, improved gas distribution, and lower peak airway pressures.[163] The flow of inspiratory gas can be delivered in three styles: constant or square wave, decelerating ramp, and sinusoidal pattern (see Fig. 15.6). In a constant flow pattern, the peak flow is achieved at the beginning of inspiration and is held constant throughout the inspiratory phase. This may result in higher peak airway pressures. Using a decelerating ramp, the gas flow is highest at the beginning of inspiration and tapers throughout the inspiratory phase. Sinusoidal gas flow resembles spontaneous ventilation.

Peak airway pressure

Airway pressures vary across the respiratory cycle with a number of pressures identifiable (e.g. peak inspiratory, end-expiratory). The airway pressure (P_{aw}) is an important parameter in assessing respiratory compliance and patient–ventilator synchrony, and will vary depending on V_T, RR, ventilator flow pattern, dynamic compliance and airway resistance. In pressure-targeted modes the peak inspiratory pressure is equivalent to the P_{insp}. In volume-targeted modes the peak inspiratory pressure is determined by the set V_T and patient compliance and resistance.

Positive end-expiratory pressure

PEEP is the pressure applied at the end of the expiratory cycle to prevent alveolar collapse. PEEP increases residual lung volume thereby recruiting collapsed alveoli, improving ventilation/perfusion match and enhancing movement of fluid out of the alveoli.[164,165] PEEP was originally introduced by Ashbaugh and colleagues[166] in the 1960s as a technique for treating refractory hypoxaemia in patients with ARDS. Ventilator-associated lung injury may be prevented using PEEP by recruiting atelectatic alveoli and bronchioles and preventing cyclic opening and closing of alveoli.[167] PEEP may be beneficial, however, only if the lung is recruitable such as in collapsed, as opposed to consolidated, lung.[164] Selection of optimal PEEP remains controversial. A systematic review and meta-analysis of individual-patient data suggests that higher levels of PEEP may be associated with lower hospital mortality for patients with moderate-to-severe ARDS.[168] However, there is no mortality benefit for patients without ARDS when ventilation is commenced; but some evidence of lower ARDS incidence and hypoxemia.[169] Recent professional society guidelines for ARDS management give a conditional recommendation for use of high PEEP.[153] In patients without ARDS or other causes of significant atelectasis, high PEEP levels should be used with caution.[170]

Pressure support

When triggered by the patient, the ventilator delivers flow to achieve the clinician-determined set pressure support. The flow is variable, depending on the patient demand. The V_T achieved with pressure support is dependent on chest and lung compliance as well as airway and ventilator resistance. Pressure support is generally set at 5–20 cmH_2O. Increasing the level of pressure support will result in increased V_T, and improvements in gas exchange if compliance and resistance remain constant.

Expiratory sensitivity

Expiratory sensitivity describes the percentage of decay in peak flow reached during the inspiratory phase that signals the ventilator to cycle to expiration for spontaneous breaths. In some ventilator models this is predetermined at 25%, while others allow clinician selection. Premature termination of a breath will increase inspiratory muscle workload whereas delayed breath termination increases expiratory muscle load.[171] Reducing the expiratory sensitivity in patients with COPD may prolong the inspiratory time thereby increasing the V_T and reducing the RR and gas trapping.[172]

> **Practice tip**
>
> The P_{insp} setting reflects a different value on different ventilators. P_{insp} equals total pressure including PEEP on some ventilators and P_{insp} above PEEP on others. Use the pressure–time scalar to confirm.

Ventilator modes

The mode of ventilation describes inspiratory phase variables; how the ventilator controls pressure, volume, and flow during a breath; as well as describing how breaths are sequenced. All breaths have trigger, limit and cycle inspiratory phase variables.[173] Each breath is triggered (started) either by the patient or by the ventilator. During inspiration, the breath is limited to a set target of pressure, volume, or flow. This target cannot be exceeded during each breath. The cycling variable determines the end of the inspiratory phase. Again this variable may be pressure, flow, volume, or time. Gas delivery during each breath is described by the control variable. There are five control variables: pressure, volume, flow, time and dual control (such as used in the mode pressure-regulated volume control). Breath sequencing refers to the sequence of mandatory and spontaneous breath. A spontaneous breath is one during which inspiration is both started (triggered) and stopped (cycled) by the patient. Spontaneous breaths may be assisted, as with pressure support, or unassisted. Mandatory breaths are either triggered or cycled by the ventilator.[174] A complete mode description should include: 1) the control variable; 2) the breath sequence; and 3) the targeting scheme (limit variable).

Commonly employed ventilation modes

Contemporary ventilators now provide a range of modes to facilitate mechanical ventilation. See Table 15.7.

Controlled mandatory ventilation

CMV is a mandatory mode, and is the original and most basic mode of ventilation.[175] CMV delivers all breaths at a clinician-determined set frequency (rate); the patient's spontaneous effort is not acknowledged by the ventilator.[176] VCV requires clinician selection of the frequency, PEEP, FiO_2, tidal volume, flow waveform, peak inspiratory flow and either the inspiratory time or I:E ratio. PCV requires clinician selection of rate, PEEP, FiO_2, inspiratory pressure, as opposed to tidal volume, and inspiratory time or I:E ratio depending on the ventilator type. Peak inspiratory flow and the flow waveform are manipulated by the ventilator, to achieve the clinician-selected inspiratory pressure within the set inspiratory time. The inability to breathe spontaneously during CMV contributes to diaphragm muscle

TABLE 15.7
Ventilator modes

MODE	DESCRIPTION	CLINICAL IMPLICATIONS
Controlled mandatory ventilation (CMV)	All breaths are mandatory, no patient triggering is enabled. Also called volume-controlled ventilation (volume targeted) (VCV) and pressure-controlled ventilation (pressure targeted) (PCV)	Patients with respiratory effort require sedation and neuromuscular blockade Potential for respiratory muscle atrophy due to disuse
Assist control (A/C)	Breaths may be either machine or patient triggered but all are cycled by the ventilator. Assist control may be delivered as volume (AC-VC) or pressure (AC-PC) targeted	Activation of the diaphragm with patient triggering Potential for respiratory alkalosis if tachypnoea develops
Synchronised intermittent mandatory ventilation (SIMV)	Mandatory breaths are delivered using a set rate and volume (SIMV-VC) or pressure (SIMV-PC). Mandatory breaths are synchronised with patient triggers within a timing window. Between mandatory breaths the patient can breathe spontaneously	Reduced need for sedation Activation of the diaphragm with patient triggering
Pressure support ventilation (PSV)	All breaths are patient triggered and cycled. Pressure applied by the ventilator during inspiration (PS) augments patient effort	Reduced need for sedation Facilitates ventilator weaning Level of PS can be adjusted to achieve desired V_T Sustains respiratory muscle tone and decreases work of breathing
Continuous positive airway pressure (CPAP)	All breaths are patient triggered and cycled. Positive pressure is applied throughout inspiratory and expiratory phases of the respiratory cycle	Requires intact respiratory drive and patient ability to maintain adequate tidal volumes
Volume support (VS)	Spontaneous mode with clinician pre-set target tidal volume delivery achieved with the lowest inspiratory pressure	Requires intact respiratory drive
Pressure-regulated volume control (PRVC)	Mandatory rate and target tidal volume are set, and the ventilator then delivers the breaths using the lowest achievable pressure	Dual control of volume and pressure enables guarantee of volume and pressure
Airway pressure release ventilation (APRV)	Ventilator cycles between two pre-set pressure levels for defined time periods. I:E ratio is inverse, often with a prolonged inspiratory time (4 s) and shortened expiratory time (0.8 s). Patient can breathe spontaneously at both pressure levels	Reduced need for sedation Activation of the diaphragm with patient triggering Promotes alveolar recruitment Considered a rescue mode in ARDS when used with extreme inverse ratio
Biphasic positive airway pressure (BiPAP/ BILEVEL/ Bivent)	As with APRV, the ventilator cycles between two pre-set pressure levels for defined time periods and the patient can breathe spontaneously at both pressure levels. The inspiratory time is generally shorter than, or the same length, as the expiratory time	Reduced need for sedation Activation of the diaphragm with patient triggering Promotes alveolar recruitment
Mandatory minute ventilation (MMV)	The patient's spontaneous minute ventilation is monitored by the ventilator. When the minute ventilation falls below the clinician-determined target, the ventilator increases the mandatory rate or size of tidal volumes to regain the desired minute ventilation	Guarantees minute ventilation for patients with fluctuating respiratory drive and muscle innervation such as patients awakening from anaesthesia and those with Guillain–Barré

Continued

TABLE 15.7
Ventilator modes—cont'd

MODE	DESCRIPTION	CLINICAL IMPLICATIONS
Proportional assist ventilation (PAV)[269]	Delivers positive pressure throughout inspiration in proportion to patient generated effort, and dependent on the set levels of flow assist (offsets resistance) and volume assist (offsets elastance)[268]	Requires intact respiratory drive Patients with high respiratory drive as the ventilator may over-assist and continue to apply support when the patient has stopped inspiration[269]
Proportional assist ventilation (PAV+™)	Clinician only sets a percentage of work for the ventilator. The ventilator assesses total work of breathing by randomly measuring compliance and resistance every 4–10 breaths	Requires intact respiratory drive Decreases work of breathing and improves patient–ventilator synchrony Potential for use as a weaning mode
Adaptive support ventilation (ASV)	Automatic adaptation of RR and pressure levels based on a clinician-set desired percentage of minute ventilation[270]	Automatically sets all ventilator settings except PEEP and FiO_2 Potential for use as a weaning mode
Volume- assured PS (VAPS)	The ventilator switches from pressure control to volume control, or PS to volume control during inspiration	Enables maintenance of a pre-set minimum V_T and reduces work of breathing

RR = respiratory rate.

dysfunction and atrophy which may result in difficulty weaning from the ventilator.[177]

Assist control

In A/C the patient can trigger the ventilator; however, unlike SIMV, every patient-initiated breath is assisted to the same clinician-determined V_T (volume targeted) or inspiratory pressure (pressure targeted). All breaths are cycled by the ventilator irrespective of being patient- or ventilator-triggered. In the absence of spontaneous breathing, A/C resembles CMV.

Synchronised intermittent mandatory ventilation

SIMV delivers breaths at a set frequency (rate), and can be either pressure- or volume-targeted. Setting of the ventilator is similar to setting VCV or PCV. The availability of patient triggering with SIMV facilitates provision of gas flow in recognition of a patient's spontaneous effort. SIMV uses a timing window to deliver mandatory breaths in synchrony with patient inspiratory effort.[178] Additional spontaneous breaths occurring outside of the timing window may be assisted with pressure support to augment the patient's spontaneous effort to a pre-set pressure level.

Pressure support ventilation

Pressure support ventilation (PSV) is a spontaneous mode in which the patient initiates all breaths, with support of the patient's inspiratory effort by the ventilator using rapid acceleration of flow to achieve a pre-set (by clinician) level of inspiratory pressure. Unlike CMV, SIMV or A/C, PSV does not require setting of ventilator (mandatory) breaths. PSV is usually employed with PEEP, which maintains partial inflation of alveoli during the expiratory phase to promote alveolar recruitment and oxygenation. As the support provided in PSV is fixed i.e. 10 cmH_2O, the ventilator cannot respond to changing patient inspiratory demands.

Continuous positive airway pressure

CPAP applies a set baseline positive pressure throughout the inspiratory and expiratory phase. In this spontaneous breathing mode, unlike PSV, no additional positive pressure is provided to the patient during inspiration. Due to nomenclature used on some ventilator models, PSV is frequently misrepresented as CPAP.

Volume targeted pressure-control breaths

A number of hybrid ventilator modes are commercially available that use an algorithm to target a set V_T by regulating the inspiratory pressure during pressure-controlled breaths based on the patient's resistance, compliance and inspiratory effort. Examples include pressure-regulated volume control, available on the Servo 300 and Servo I (Maquet, Solna, Sweden) and SIMV with autoflow (Dräger, Lübeck, Germany). On initiation of these modes the ventilator delivers a number of breaths during a 'learning period' to establish an estimate of the pressure required to achieve the targeted V_T. The patient's resistance, compliance and inspiratory effort continue to influence the pressure and flow delivered to attain the targeted V_T. The ventilator constantly regulates inspiratory pressure based on the pressure/volume calculation of the previous breaths and the clinician-determined target tidal volume. Volume Control (VC+) on the Puritan Bennett 980 ventilators provides a mandatory, pressure-controlled breath with unrestricted flow during the inspiratory phase. The inspiratory pressure target is again automatically adjusted from breath to breath based on changing lung conditions to achieve the desired tidal volume.

Airway pressure release ventilation, biphasic positive airway pressure, and BiLevel

Airway pressure release ventilation (APRV), BiPAP and BiLevel are ventilator modes that allow unrestricted spontaneous breathing independent of ventilator cycling, using an active expiratory valve that allows patients to exhale even in the inspiratory phase.[179,180] These modes are pressure-limited and time-cycled. In the absence of spontaneous breathing, these modes resemble conventional pressure-limited, time-cycled ventilation.[176] In North America the acronym BiPAP® is registered to Respironics non-invasive ventilators (Murrayville, PA). Therefore, ventilator companies have developed brand names such as BiLevel (Puritan Bennett, Pleasanton, CA; GE Healthcare, Madison, WI), Bivent (Maquet, Solna, Sweden), DuoPaP (Hamilton Medical, Rhäzüns, Switzerland), PCV+ (Dräger Medical, Lübeck, Germany) or BiPhasic (Viasys, Conshocken, PA) to describe essentially equivalent modes. BiLevel, available on Puritan Bennett ventilators (Pleasanton, CA, GE Healthcare, Madison, WI), can provide additional pressure support or automatic tube compensation (see below) during spontaneous breaths. Ambiguity exists in the criteria that distinguish APRV and BiPAP. When applied with the same I:E ratio, no difference exists between the two modes. APRV as opposed to BiPAP, however, is more frequently described with an extreme inverse ratio, i.e. an inspiratory time of 4 seconds and expiratory time of 0.5 seconds, and is advocated as a method to improve oxygenation in refractory hypoxemia.[180]

Automatic tube compensation

Automatic tube compensation is active during spontaneous breaths and is designed to compensate for the work of breathing associated with ETT resistance via closed-loop control of continuously calculated tracheal pressure.[181,182] During spontaneous inspiration, a pressure gradient exists between the proximal and distal ends of the ETT due to resistance created by the tube. A reduced pressure at the proximal end of the tube means a patient needs to produce a greater inspiratory force (greater negative pressure) to generate an adequate V_T.[183] Higher flow rates generate larger pressure gradients and greater resistance. Automatic tube compensation requires the airway type and size to be selected on the ventilator as well as the percentage of automatic tube compensation to be applied. Automatic tube compensation may have some role in assisting with weaning success.[184]

Neurally adjusted ventilatory assist

Neurally Adjusted Ventilatory Assist (NAVA®) is available on the Servo-i ventilator (Maquet, Solna, Sweden) and uses the electrical activity of the diaphragm to control patient–ventilator interaction.[185] Electrical activity of the diaphragm, measured using an oesophageal catheter, should result in optimal patient–ventilator synchrony as it represents the endpoint of neural output from the respiratory centres and thus is the earliest signal of patient inspiratory trigger and expiratory cycling. Pressure delivered to the airways is proportional to inspiratory diaphragmatic electrical activity using a clinician-determined proportionality factor set on the ventilator.[186] NAVA provides breath-by-breath assist in synchrony with, and in proportion to, respiratory demand.[187] NAVA improves patient–ventilator synchrony[188] and shows some promise as a weaning adjunct.[189]

Proportional assist ventilation (PAV) and proportional assist ventilation plus (PAV+™)

Proportional assist ventilation (PAV) is a spontaneous breathing mode that varies pressure support (assist) generated by the ventilator on a breath-by-breath basis based on patient's ventilator demand.[190] PAV+ is an extension of PAV whereby the ventilator measures compliance and resistance every 4–10 breaths to calculate elastance and work of breathing. The ventilator adjusts the level of support based on these measurements to meet a clinician-set level of assistance (e.g. 80%). As with NAVA, both modes may promote patient comfort and ventilator synchrony[188] and may have a role in ventilator weaning though further studies are required.[191]

Managing the mechanically-ventilated patient

Management of refractory hypoxaemia

Refractory hypoxaemia may require strategies in addition to conventional lung-protective mechanical ventilation.[152] These include recruitment manoeuvres (RMs), high frequency oscillatory ventilation (HFOV), extracorporeal membrane oxygenation (ECMO) and nitric oxide (NO).

Recruitment manoeuvres

RMs refer to brief application of high levels of PEEP to raise the transpulmonary pressure to levels higher than achieved during tidal ventilation with the goals of opening collapsed alveoli, recruiting slow opening alveoli, preventing alveolar derecruitment, and reducing shearing stress.[192] The most common RM is elevation of PEEP to achieve a peak pressure of 40 cmH_2O

for a sustained period of 40 seconds, although studies report peak pressure elevations ranging from 25–50 cmH_2O for durations ranging from 20–40 seconds.[193] Effective recruitment may be difficult to assess with the potential for either alveolar overdistension or failure to recruit.[194] Once the RM is terminated, derecruitment may occur rapidly. Adverse effects, including hypotension, acidosis and desaturation have been noted during RMs due to increased intrathoracic and intrapulmonary pressures resulting in reductions in venous return and cardiac output; however, most do not result in serious sequelae.[192] A large randomised controlled trial of 1010 patients with moderate-to-severe ARDS enrolled from 120 ICUs found RM and titrated PEEP compared with low PEEP increased 28-day all-cause mortality indicating RMs should not be routine care and must be used with caution.[195]

High frequency oscillatory ventilation

HFOV requires a specialised ventilator and manipulation of four variables: mean airway pressure (cmH_2O), frequency (Hz), inspiratory time, and amplitude (or power [ΔP]).[196] Alveolar overdistension is limited through the use of sub-deadspace tidal volumes whereas alveolar cyclic collapse is prevented by maintenance of high end-expiratory lung pressures.[197,198] High frequency (between 3 and 15 Hz) oscillations at extremely fast rates (300–420 breaths/min) create pressure waves enabling CO_2 elimination.[197] Oxygenation is facilitated through application of a constant mean airway pressure via the bias flow (rate of fresh gas).[199] In adults, recommendations for the initiation of HFOV state mean airway pressure should be set 5 cmH_2O above the peak airway pressure achieved with conventional ventilation.[200] The recommended frequency range is 3–10 Hz with 5 Hz conventionally used to initiate HFOV. Inspiratory time is set at 33% and the amplitude setting is determined by adequate CO_2 elimination.[199] Increased CO_2 elimination is achieved by lowering the frequency and increasing the amplitude.

HFOV is generally considered a rescue mode for adult patients with ARDS experiencing refractory hypoxaemia and failing conventional ventilation.[199] Two large, multicentre, randomised, controlled trials of early as opposed to rescue HFOV demonstrated either increased mortality with HFOV[201] or no effect compared to usual ventilatory care in patients undergoing mechanical ventilation for ARDS.[202] For these reasons routine use of HFOV in ARDS is not recommended.[153]

Extracorporeal membrane oxygenation

ECMO improves total body oxygenation using an external (extracorporeal) oxygenator, while allowing intrinsic recovery of lung pathophysiology by resting the lung. Indications for ECMO include acute severe cardiac or respiratory failure such as severe ARDS[203,204] and refractory shock or as a bridge to transplantation.[205] There are two types of ECMO. A veno-venous ECMO circuit drains venous blood, oxygenates the blood, and pumps the blood back into the same venous compartment.[206] A veno-arterial ECMO circuit removes deoxygenated blood from a central vein or the right atrium, oxygenates the blood, and returns oxygenated blood to the arterial side of the circulation, typically to the aorta. This form of ECMO partially supports the cardiac output as the flow through the ECMO circuit is in addition to the normal cardiac output. Veno-arterial ECMO is required for cardiac support whereas both veno-arterial or veno-venous ECMO can be used for respiratory support.[205]

Bleeding as a complication of anticoagulation is a major risk of ECMO, with cerebral bleeds being the most catastrophic.[207] Another serious complication is limb ischaemia when the femoral artery is used.

ECMO consists of three key components:

1. blood pump (either a simple roller or centrifugal force pump)
2. membrane oxygenator (bubble, membrane or hollow fibre)
3. countercurrent heat exchanger, where the blood is exposed to warmed water circulating within metal tubes.

In addition, essential safety features include bubble detectors that detect gas in the arterial line and shut the pump off; arterial line filters between the heat exchanger and arterial cannula, to trap air thrombi and emboli; pressure monitors placed before and after the oxygenator, that measure the pressure within the circuit and detect rising circuit pressures commonly caused by thrombus or circuit or cannulae occlusion; and continuous venous oxygen saturation and temperature monitoring. On commencement of ECMO the circuit is primed with fresh blood. The acid–base balance and blood gas of the primer is adjusted to ensure that the pH is within the normal range (7.35–7.45) and PaO_2 is adequate. ECMO can be delivered via veno-arterial access which requires cannulation of an artery. This method bypasses the pulmonary circulation while providing cardiac support to the systemic circulation and achieves a higher PaO_2 with lower perfusion rates. The alternative is veno-venous access, used for patients in respiratory failure with adequate cardiac function as there is no support of systemic circulation. Perfusion rates are higher, the mixed venous PO_2 is elevated and the PaO_2 is lower.[208]

Nitric oxide

NO is an endothelial smooth muscle relaxant. Inhaled NO is effective for dilation of pulmonary arteries resulting in reduced pulmonary shunting and reduced right ventricular afterload due to reduced pulmonary artery tone. Pulmonary shunting refers to failure of uptake of alveolar gas by the pulmonary vascular bed due to vascular constriction or interstitial oedema. Inhaled NO has a role in the management of pulmonary hypertension and was previously thought to have a role in management of refractory hypoxaemia for patients with ARDS. However, the most recent systematic review and meta-analysis of NO in ARDS, comprising 14 RCTs and 1275 participants, reported no effect on overall mortality despite a statistically significant improvement in oxygenation in the first 24 hours.[209]

Prostacyclin

Prostacyclin, both inhaled and intravenous, is also used to treat pulmonary hypertension. Although inhaled prostacyclin may offer some advantage by providing the drug directly to the target organ, high doses cannot be administered due to airway irritant effects.[210]

Aerosol therapy

The delivery of inhaled aerosols to invasively ventilated patients via pressurised metered-dose inhalers (pMDI) and nebulisers is a common practice in the ICU.[211] Inhalation aerosols include bronchodilators, corticosteroids, antibiotics, mucolytics and vasodilators. Jet, ultrasonic, and vibrating mesh are the common nebulisers used. Administration during invasive mechanical ventilation is challenging, factors influencing effective aerosol delivery are related to medication type, inhalation device used, type of airway humidification and the placement of the device in the circuit.[212] Deposition of aerosolised drugs in the lungs is as low as 38% with a pMDI and lower than 20% with nebulisers.[211] At present, there are no high-quality trials that prove the effectiveness of aerosol therapy in the different disease conditions.

Positioning

Regular repositioning of critically ill patients is essential for lung recruitment, prevention of atelectasis and maintenance of skin integrity (see Chapter 5).

Head of bed elevation

Supine positioning has been associated with aspiration of abnormally colonised oropharyngeal and gastric contents[213] and increased incidence of VAP compared with a semirecumbent position, defined as backrest elevation at 45°.[214] Guidelines and care bundles for VAP prevention recommend semirecumbent positioning for all mechanically-ventilated patients.[215,216] A more recent trial has, however, questioned the feasibility of 45° semirecumbent positioning as this backrest elevation was only achieved for 15% of study observations.[217] A 2016 Cochrane systematic review of 10 trials involving 878 participants concluded semirecumbent position (≥ 30°) may reduce clinically suspected VAP in comparison to a 0 to 10° supine position, although the evidence is weak due to trials with high risk of bias.[218]

Contraindications to backrest elevation include:

- suspected or existing spinal injury
- intracranial hypertension (for 45° elevation)
- unstable pelvic fractures
- prone positioning
- haemodynamic support devices (intra-aortic balloon pumps, left ventricular assist devices and ECMO)
- femoral catheterisation for continuous renal replacement therapy
- large abdominal wounds
- following femoral sheath removal.

BOX 15.3

Mechanical ventilation and the bariatric patient

- Bariatric patients are at increased risk of atelectasis and have decreased chest wall compliance due to the weight of the abdomen
- Avoid the supine position as this will further decrease lung volumes
- Bariatric patients may require higher airway pressures to generate adequate tidal volumes
- Recruitment manoeuvres may improve oxygenation
- Frail elderly may experience difficult weaning due to the presence of comorbidities such as CHF, ischaemic heart disease, and COPD

As some degree of semirecumbent positioning is preferable to supine positioning, especially for bariatric patients (Box 15.3), patients with suspected or existing spinal injury, pelvic fractures or who are being managed with prone positioning can have the head elevated by tilting the whole bed. Patients with femoral cannulation and large abdominal wounds can usually achieve 25°–30° positioning.

Clinical practice audits conducted internationally and in Australia and New Zealand indicate that compliance with a 45° semirecumbent position rarely occurs, even when taking into consideration contraindications.[219-222] Similarly, interventions to improve compliance failed to demonstrate adherence to the 45° semirecumbent position that can be sustained by the patient over time.[223]

Practice tip

Backrest elevation is difficult to estimate accurately. Use an objective measurement device such as an inclinometer or protractor.

Lateral positioning

Patients with unilateral lung disease experience a mismatch of ventilation to perfusion if the consolidated or atelectatic lung is placed in the dependent position.[224] Temporary and early positioning of the affected lung in the dependent position, among other strategies such as avoiding manual hyperinflation, for patients with unilateral pneumonia or following aspiration may be beneficial in preventing the movement of bacteria or acidic gastric contents into the non-affected lung.[225] This theory has been coined 'propagation prevention'. While appealing, as yet there have been no adequately powered randomised controlled trials to support its use. Continuous lateral rotational therapy is a positioning therapy advocated for the prevention and management of respiratory complications associated with immobility.[226] The multicentre, randomised, controlled trial found a significant reduction in VAP and shorter durations of ventilation and ICU stay in a mixed ICU population.[227] Some evidence also suggests a role in patients with severe thoracic trauma.[228] Continuous lateral rotation therapy requires a special bed system enabling rotation of the upper part of the body to a maximum angle of 90°.

Prone positioning

Prone positioning has been shown to improve oxygenation and intrapulmonary shunt fraction when compared with rotational turning in patients with ARDS.[229] Prone positioning may also decrease the risk of VAP due to improved bronchial secretion drainage, limitation of colonisation of distal lung, decreased atelectasis and increased alveolar recruitment but may increase spread of pathogens in the lung and may increase the risk of aspiration.[230,231]

Prone positioning results in changes to the distribution of ventilation and pulmonary blood flow. Pleural pressures are lower in non-dependent regions and higher in dependent regions due to gravitational forces, the weight of the overlying lung and mismatch between the local physical structures of the lung and chest wall.[232] The weight of the overlying lung increases in ARDS due to parenchymal oedema and fluid within the alveoli.[231] This gradient in pleural pressures means transpulmonary pressure is higher in non-dependent lung regions, compared to dependent regions. Perfusion also increases from previously non-dependent to dependent lung regions resulting in optimal matching of ventilation and perfusion to promote gas exchange.[233]

Increased pleural pressure in the dependent dorsal regions in the supine position can result in airway closure, atelectasis and hypoxaemia.[234] The difference in pleural pressures from non-dependent and dependent lung regions is greater in the supine compared to the prone position. In the supine position, the heart and abdominal contents also compress lung bases and decrease functional residual capacity, whereas in prone positioning, the weight of these structures are lifted from the lung.

Recent systematic review and meta-analyses that included 11 randomised controlled trials[235,236] found reduced mortality and improved oxygenation for patients with ARDS managed with protective lung ventilation. Prone positioning is now recommended for adult patients with severe ARDS for more than 12 hours per day.[153] Adverse events related to prone positioning were increased risk of decubitus ulcer formation, endotracheal obstruction and thoracotomy tube dislodgement.

Implementing prone positioning requires forward planning to ensure eye care and protection, mouth care, wound dressings, and tracheal suction are attended to before positioning the patient prone. Intravenous lines, electrocardiogram leads, urinary catheter drainage, chest drains and ostomy bags need to be secured and repositioned appropriately once the patient is positioned.[237] Prone positioning can be achieved by manual handling of the patient, requiring up to five staff, although commercial devices are available that facilitate the turning and positioning.

Complications of mechanical ventilation

Physiological complications associated with mechanical ventilation include ventilator-associated lung injury and nosocomial infection, including VAP.[238,239] Ventilator-associated lung injury occurs through alveolar overdistension and cyclic opening and closing of alveoli resulting in diffuse alveolar damage, increased permeability, pulmonary oedema, cell contraction and cytokine production.[240,241] VAP substantially increases the duration of ICU stay and is associated with an attributable mortality of 13%.[242] Additional complications associated with mechanical ventilation are listed in Table 15.8. Complications can occur due to inappropriate application of mechanical ventilation. This may result in extraalveolar gas causing pneumothoraces or subcutaneous emphysema due to high peak P_{insp}, and alveolar stretch and oedema formation as the result of large V_Ts.[243]

Weaning from mechanical ventilation

Weaning traditionally occurs via clinician-directed adjustments to the level of support provided by the ventilator, culminating in a spontaneous breathing trial (SBT) comprising either low-level pressure support or a T piece trial.

Current recommendations

No ventilation strategy is more lung-protective than the timely and appropriate discontinuation of mechanical ventilation. Weaning refers to the transition from ventilatory support to spontaneous breathing.[244] Evidence-based consensus guidelines published for weaning in 2001[178] and 2007[245] emphasise the importance of preventing unnecessary delays in the weaning process, early recognition of a patient's ability for spontaneous breathing and the use of a systematic method to identify the potential for extubation.

Weaning predictors

Clinician judgement regarding prediction of weaning readiness is known to be imperfect, with unnecessary prolongation of ventilation[246,247] or high rates of

TABLE 15.8
Complications of mechanical ventilation

ITEM	COMPLICATION(S)
Barotrauma	Pneumothorax Pneumomediastinum Pneumopericardium Pulmonary interstitial emphysema Subcutaneous emphysema
Volutrauma	Shearing stress, endothelial and epithelial cell injury, fluid retention and pulmonary oedema, perivascular and alveolar haemorrhage, alveolar rupture
Biotrauma	Activation of systemic and local inflammatory mechanisms
Ventilation/perfusion mismatch	Alveolar distension causes compression of the adjacent pulmonary capillaries resulting in dead space ventilation
↓ Cardiac output	Resulting in hypotension, ↓ cerebral perfusion pressure (CPP), ↓ renal and hepatic blood flow
↑ Right ventricular afterload	Due to ↑ intrathoracic pressure may result in ↓ left ventricular compliance and preload
↓ Urine output	Due to ↓ glomerular filtration rate, ↑ sodium reabsorption and activation of the renin–angiotensin–aldosterone system
Fluid retention	Due to above renal factors as well as ↑ antidiuretic hormone and ↓ atrial natriuretic peptide
Impaired hepatic function	Due to ↑ pressure in the portal vein, ↓ portal venous blood flow, ↓ hepatic vein blood flow
↑ Intracranial pressure	Due to ↓ cerebral venous outflow
Oxygen toxicity	Alterations to lung parenchyma similar to those found in ARDS
Pulmonary emboli and deep vein thrombosis	Due to immobility
Ileus, diarrhoea	Due to alterations in gastric motility
Gastrointestinal haemorrhage	Gastritis and ulceration may occur due to stress, anxiety and critical illness
ICU-acquired weakness	Neuropathies and myopathies develop in association with critical illness, corticosteroids and neuromuscular blockade
Psychological issues	Delirium, anxiety, depression, agitation and post-traumatic stress disorder may be experienced by critically ill ventilated patients in the acute and recovery phases

reintubation as resultant consequences, both of which are associated with adverse outcomes.[248] An evidence-based review evaluating over 50 objective physiological measurements for determining readiness for weaning and extubation found most had only a modest relationship with weaning outcome; no single factor or combination of factors demonstrating superior accuracy.[249] Of all predictors studied, the respiratory frequency to tidal volume ratio (f/V_T) appears to be most accurate.[250] However, inclusion of the f/V_T as part of a weaning protocol was found in one randomised study to increase, as opposed to decrease, the duration of weaning.[251] At present, consensus guidelines[245] do not recommend routine inclusion of weaning predictors.

Weaning methods

Various studies have attempted to identify the best weaning method. Two of the most frequently-cited studies have produced conflicting results. Brochard and colleagues[252] compared PSV, T piece trial and SIMV, and concluded that PSV reduced the duration of mechanical ventilation compared with the other methods. Esteban and colleagues[253] compared PSV, T piece trials, CPAP and progressive reduction of SIMV support, and found a once-daily T piece trial led to extubation three times more quickly than SIMV and nearly twice as quickly as PSV. A systematic review comparing trials of PSV and T piece found no clear evidence of a difference between these weaning strategies for weaning success.[254]

Spontaneous breathing trials

SBTs incorporate a focused assessment of a patient's capacity to breathe prior to extubation[255,256] and are recommended as the major diagnostic test to determine extubation readiness.[245] Recent professional society guidelines on liberation from mechanical ventilation recommend use of PSV with 5–8 cmH_2O rather than T piece of CPAP trials.[257] Generally, SBTs should need to last only 30 min.[258] Formal SBT testing is less common in Australian and New Zealand, in contrast to international findings.[259]

Weaning protocols

Implementation of various organisational strategies, such as weaning teams and non-physician-led weaning protocols, may assist in the timely recognition of weaning and extubation readiness.[260] Coupling of a sedation and weaning protocol was found to result in a three-day reduction in the duration of ventilation compared with standard care in four North American hospitals.[261] Use of protocols to minimise sedation enabling timely liberation from mechanical ventilation is another recent professional society recommendation.[257] A systematic review and meta-analysis of 17 weaning protocol trials including 2434 patients demonstrated a reduction in the duration of mechanical ventilation.[260] However, the authors cautioned that the effect of weaning protocols may vary according to the ICU organisational characteristics such as an intensivist-led ICU model, high levels of physician staffing, structured ward rounds, collaborative discussion and more frequent medical review; all characteristics reported for ICUs in Australia and New Zealand.[262-264]

Automated weaning

Automated computerised systems potentially enable more efficient weaning by providing improved adaptation of ventilatory support through continuous monitoring and real-time intervention.[265] One such system, SmartCare™/PS, monitors three respiratory parameters, f, V_T and end-tidal carbon dioxide concentration, every 2 or 5 min and periodically adapts pressure support (PS).[266,267] SmartCare™/PS establishes a respiratory status diagnosis, based on evaluation of the three parameters, and may either decrease or increase PS, or leave it unchanged to maintain the patient in a defined 'respiratory zone of comfort'.[267,268] Once SmartCare™/PS has successfully minimised the level of PS, a 1-hour observation period occurs. For patients who remain within the respiratory zone of comfort throughout the observation period, SmartCare™/PS recommends to 'consider separation', indicating the patient's respiratory status now suggests the patient will tolerate extubation.

A recent meta-analysis of automated weaning systems has shown that SmartCare™/PS may reduce the duration of weaning, total ventilation and ICU length of stay when compared to protocolised or usual care weaning.[268]

The difficult-to-wean patient

International reports indicate patients that require mechanical ventilation for ≥21 days account for approximately 10% of all mechanically-ventilated patients, but occupy 40% of ICU bed days and accrue 50% of ICU costs.[269,270] A recommendation from the National Association for Medical Direction of Respiratory Care states that prolonged mechanical ventilation should be defined as '≥21 consecutive days of ventilation required for ≥6 hours per day'.[178] Prolonged weaning has been defined as greater than 7 days of weaning after the first SBT or more than three SBTs.[245] Little evidence defines the optimal method for managing the difficult-to-wean patient. One trial found no difference in weaning duration or success when comparing tracheostomy trials to low-level PS in patients with COPD experiencing weaning difficulty.[271] A randomised controlled trial demonstrated increased weaning success with use of a once-daily progressive tracheostomy mask trial in comparison to PS weaning.[272] These patients are most likely to benefit from an individualised and structured approach to weaning using progressive lengthening of tracheostomy trials with supportive ventilation in between in combination with early physical therapy.

Patients requiring prolonged mechanical ventilation often experience retention of airway secretions due to ineffective cough and reduced mucociliary transport.[273] Retained secretions can lead to atelectasis and may promote ventilator-associated lung injury, which impair successful weaning. Techniques designed to enhance airway secretion clearance include manually-assisted cough and mechanically-assisted cough using a mechanical insufflation-exsufflation (MI-E) device. Manually-assisted cough consists of a cough timed with an abdominal or lateral costal compression. MI-E devices such as the CoughAssist™ (Philips Respironics Corp, Millersville, PA) or the NIPPY Clear-way (B&D Electromedical, Stratford-Upon-Avon, Warwickshire) alternate positive pressure (insufflation) aimed at expanding the lungs to approximately 90% of capacity[274] and negative pressures (rapid exsufflation) delivered via the ETT, tracheostomy or mask. Although some evidence suggests these techniques reduce reintubation and are safe in the critically ill, further studies are required.[275]

> **Practice tip**
>
> Tachypnoea and decreased V_T during weaning are indicators that a patient is not ready for extubation.

Summary

Support of oxygenation and ventilation during critical illness are key activities for nurses in ICU. Oxygen therapy promotes aerobic metabolism but has adverse effects that need to be considered. Various oxygen delivery devices provide low or variable flows of oxygen.

Strong evidence supports the use of NIV for COPD and CHF, but caution is required when used for other diagnoses such as pneumonia. NIV success is dependent on patient tolerance, with common complications including pressure ulcers, conjunctival irritations, nasal congestion, insufflation of air into the stomach and claustrophobia.

Airway support can be provided with oro- or nasopharyngeal airways, LMAs and endotracheal intubation; oral intubation is the preferred method. For a patient with an ETT, the key points for practice are:

- ETT placement should be confirmed with end-tidal CO_2 monitoring
- the aim of endotracheal cuff management is to prevent airway contamination and enable positive-pressure ventilation
- closed suctioning reduces alveolar derecruitment compared to open suctioning
- instillation of normal saline is not recommended during routine tracheal suctioning.

The optimal timing of tracheostomy remains uncertain; however, tracheostomy should be considered for patients experiencing weaning difficulty.

The goals of mechanical ventilation are to promote gas exchange, minimise lung injury, reduce work of breathing and promote patient comfort:

- despite its life-saving potential, mechanical ventilation carries the risk of serious physical and psychological complications
- humidification of dry medical gas is required during mechanical ventilation to prevent drying of secretions, mucous plugging and airway occlusion
- the pressure required to deliver a volume of gas into the lungs is determined by elastic and resistive forces
- contemporary ventilators now provide a range of modes to facilitate mechanical ventilation
- analysis of ventilator graphics provides clinicians with the ability to assess patient–ventilator interaction, appropriateness of ventilator settings and lung function
- semirecumbent positioning at 45° elevation has been shown to reduce VAP but compliance is poor
- RMs, HFOV, ECMO and prone positioning are strategies that may facilitate management of refractory hypoxaemia, although new evidence suggests RM and HFOV may worsen outcomes.

Case study

A 60-year-old female (Martha) was admitted to the ICU with acute respiratory failure due to community-acquired pneumonia. Martha was morbidly obese (190 kg) with extensive central obesity and a body mass index of 74.2. She had a history of COPD; however, was not prescribed steroids and had not been investigated for sleep apnoea.

Martha was commenced on broad spectrum antibiotic cover in the emergency department. Martha had a trial of NIV with FiO_2 0.7, PEEP 7 cmH_2O (EPAP 7 cmH_2O) and PS 5 cmH_2O (IPAP 12 cmH_2O) to reduce her work of breathing and improve gas exchange. The NIV trial was discontinued as Martha's dyspnoea was unrelieved, and hypoxia and hypercapnia persisted. She was intubated with a size 7 oral ETT and a bronchial alveolar lavage was performed to obtain samples for bacterial and viral screening. Nasopharyngeal swabs were also obtained. Ventilator settings following intubation were A/C, FiO_2 1.0, RR 16 breaths per min, P_{insp} 30 cmH_2O, PEEP 15 cmH_2O, and inspiratory time of 1.1 seconds. Initial blood gases were as follows: pH 7.07, PaO_2 71 mmHg, $PaCO_2$ 71 mmHg, HCO_3 16.4 mmol, base excess –9.5, sodium 123 mmol, chloride 94 mmol, lactate 0.7, SpO_2 94%, and PaO_2/FiO_2 (PF) ratio 71. Dynamic compliance was 25.6 mL/cmH_2O, resistance was 8.6 cmH2O/(L/sec). A chest X-ray showed bilateral pulmonary infiltrates and a lobular pneumonia. Chest auscultation revealed bilateral crackles, late in the inspiratory phase.

Nursing assessment indicated the following issues:

1 Notable audible cuff leak on inspiration despite a cuff pressure of 30 cmH_2O.
2 Atelectasis as evidenced by decreased air entry in lung bases, reduced compliance, diminished gas exchange, and obliteration of costophrenic angles on the chest X-ray.

To address the cuff leak, nursing staff connected rigid manometer tubing between the cuff pressure gauge and the ETT pilot tube to enable continuous cuff pressure measurement. Cuff pressure did not decrease over time, indicating that the ETT cuff was intact. Therefore, the audible air leak was not caused by a leaking ETT cuff but was due to an air leak around the cuff. On careful examination of the chest X-ray the ETT cuff was found to be above the level of the vocal cords and therefore needed repositioning.

To address the atelectasis, Martha was repositioned in a high semi-fowler position (≥45° HOB elevation). This change in positioning resulted in an immediate improvement in compliance from a baseline of 25.6 to 38.4 mL/cmH_2O. V_T also increased from 300 mL to 400 mL. These improvements enabled rapid downward titration of FiO_2 to 0.7 while maintaining a SpO_2 >90%. A RM using 40 cmH_2O for 40 seconds was performed with further improvement of Martha's oxygenation indicating her lungs were responsive to this strategy. The ventilator mode was changed to APRV with a P_{insp} of 27 cmH_2O for 6 seconds and an expiratory pressure of 5 cmH_2O for 0.4 seconds. Further improvements in oxygenation were noted (PaO_2 180 mmHg and PF ratio 225).

DISCUSSION

A cuff leak may be assumed to be secondary to a hole in the either the cuff or pilot tube; however, this is relatively rare. Audible cuff leaks are more frequently due to a malpositioned ETT. It is important to note that each time cuff pressure is measured, a small volume of gas leaves the cuff to pressurise the pressure gauge. Repeated cuff pressure measurement may cause reduced cuff pressure over time which may be falsely assumed to indicate the cuff is losing volume due to other causes. Attaching rigid tubing between the cuff and pressure gauge eliminates this problem and facilitates continuous cuff pressure measurement. This is a useful strategy for assessing cuff leak problems. In this case scenario, careful trouble shooting averted the need for ETT replacement and avoided unnecessary risk to the patient.

Patient positioning is extremely important in managing the bariatric patient. Central obesity causes cephalic displacement of the diaphragm resulting in a positive pleural pressure and subsequent alveolar collapse. Inspiratory crackles late in the inspiratory phase indicate late alveolar opening and an increased potential for lung injury due to cyclic alveolar inflation and deflation. Positive pleural pressure decreases transpulmonary pressure and often necessitates the use of higher levels of PEEP to prevent collapse. Positioning in the high semi-fowler position can have a dramatic and positive effect on lung mechanics for these patients evidenced by the increase in compliance in this case study. RMs typically have a limited period of effectiveness i.e. derecruitment generally occurs following the manoeuvre. APRV maintains the higher level of pressure for a prolonged time thus sustaining alveolar recruitment. In this case study APRV and position changes appeared to promote recruitment and improved oxygenation enabling downwards titration of the FiO_2. When considering extubation for the bariatric patient, maintaining PEEP at a high level prior to extubation and using CPAP following extubation, may prevent alveolar derecruitment.

CASE STUDY QUESTIONS

1 Why should the lowest possible FiO_2 be used to achieve a target partial pressure of oxygen in arterial blood (PaO_2) or peripheral oxygen saturation (SpO_2)?
2 Name three advantages of high-flow nasal cannulae compared to low-flow nasal cannulae.
3 What is the most reliable method for confirming ETT placement after intubation?
4 Volume-control ventilation (VCV) is a controlled mode of ventilation in which the respirator delivers a pre-set volume. Name two disadvantages of VCV.
5 Mechanical ventilation can cause several serious complications including ventilator-associated pneumonia and ventilator-associated lung injury. What is the best way to prevent these complications?
6 Prone positioning should be maintained for a maximum of 6 hours for patients with severe ARDS; true or false?

RESEARCH VIGNETTE

Clarissa C, Salisbury L, Rodgers S, Kean S. Early mobilisation in mechanically ventilated patients: a systematic integrative review of definitions and activities. J Intensive Care, BioMed Central, 2019;7:3. CC BY 4.0.

Abstract

Background: Mechanically ventilated patients often develop muscle weakness post-intensive care admission. Current evidence suggests that early mobilisation of these patients can be an effective intervention in improving their outcomes. However, what constitutes early mobilisation in mechanically ventilated patients (EM-MV) remains unclear. We aimed to systematically explore the definitions and activity types of EM-MV in the literature.

Methods: Whittemore and Knafl's framework guided this review. CINAHL, MEDLINE, EMBASE, PsycINFO, ASSIA, and Cochrane Library were searched to capture studies from 2000 to 2018, combined with hand search of grey literature and reference lists of included studies. The Critical Appraisal Skills Programme tools were used to assess the methodological quality of included studies. Data extraction and quality assessment of studies were performed independently by each reviewer before coming together in sub-groups for discussion and agreement. An inductive and data-driven thematic analysis was undertaken on verbatim extracts of EM-MV definitions and activities in included studies.

Results: Seventy-six studies were included from which four major themes were inferred: (1) *non-standardised definition*, (2) *contextual factors*, (3) *negotiated process* and (4) *collaboration between patients and staff*. The first theme indicates that EM-MV is either not fully defined in studies or when a definition is provided this is not standardised across studies. The remaining themes reflect the diversity of EM-MV activities which depends on patients' characteristics and ICU settings; the negotiated decision-making process between patients and staff; and their interdependent relationship during the implementation.

Conclusions: This review highlights the absence of an agreed definition and on what constitutes early mobilisation in mechanically ventilated patients. To advance research and practice an agreed and shared definition is a pre-requisite.

Critique

Recovery from critical illness can occur over days, months and years. Survival rates for critical illness have continued to improve with advancements in patient management. However, recovery can often be challenging with many patients experiencing both physical and psychological challenges. For those critically ill patients who require prolonged mechanical ventilation, the risk of developing ICU-acquired weakness (ICU-AW) exists and this can contribute to the development of post-intensive care syndrome (PICS). Early mobilisation has shown promise in terms of preventing or minimising ICU-AW and reports in the literature suggest that it is both feasible and safe; however, there are many barriers to this being consistently implemented in ICUs worldwide. Because of the potential benefit for early mobilisation of ventilated patients, there has been intense interest in this area from both a clinical and a research perspective.

One of the challenges in using a generated body of research in this area is the lack of standardised definitions. This makes it difficult to see the transferability of research to clinical practice and to compare bodies of work that examine the effectiveness and safety of early mobilisation. The authors of this review are to be commended for looking to the literature to address two key questions in this area:

1. How is early mobilisation in mechanically ventilated patients defined across studies?
2. What types of early mobilisation activities in mechanically ventilated patients are reported in the literature?

An integrative review approach was used, which included research using either quantitative or qualitative study designs. A detailed systematic approach to searching the literature was undertaken using a variety of bibliographic databases as well as key websites known to house clinical practice guidelines. Hand searching was used to ensure potential studies included in reference lists were not overlooked. Details of the search strategy are such that this search could be replicated with the search published a priori on the PROSPERO website. It is possible that some literature may not have been identified because of the subsequently identified heterogeneity in language used to describe early mobilisation in mechanical ventilation. Independent screening by two authors against clear and specific inclusion and exclusion criteria is evident. Language bias may be present, although the authors included literature published in both English and German. The assessment of full texts of included articles was also undertaken by two authors, to ensure rigour in study identification. A systematic approach to data extraction and quality appraisal is detailed with an inductive approach to data analysis used to identify a rich array of sub-themes and themes inherent in the definitions and activities of early mobilisation in mechanical ventilation.

In total, 76 studies were included in the review, most of which used quantitative approaches in their research. Most of the quantitative studies were cohort studies (n=33) and there were 18 randomised controlled trials. Eight qualitative studies were included. Most studies originated in the USA (n=27) although there were 12 studies undertaken in Australia and/or New Zealand. An increase in the frequency of publications addressing early mobilisation in mechanical ventilation is evident with 20 publications occurring within the 2-year period 2016–2018.

In this high-quality review the authors demonstrated the variability in definitions used for early mobilisation in mechanical ventilation. Terminology of both mobilisation and rehabilitation are used, which may be referring to different concepts; mobilisation being more focused on varying degrees of ambulation while rehabilitation seemed to focus more on functional ability. Definitions could also be either broad or narrow. The broad definitions introduce heterogeneity while the narrower definitions may challenge transferability of results. For clinicians, this diversity in the research base makes application of findings challenging. For example, it is not clear what is 'early' and while most studies have provided detail about the time when early mobilisation was commenced, this did vary across studies. Many studies were conducted by multidisciplinary teams, which is logical given the nature of the intervention; however, disciplinary language and views may further compound a lack of clarity in definitions used. Agreement in terminology is certainly needed for this body of research to continue to move forward and to be translated into clinical practice.

Learning activities

1. Describe how the terms IPAP and EPAP used on some NIV ventilators correlate with the more generic terms of PEEP and pressure support (PS).
2. Why is it important to consider the patient's respiratory rate and tidal volume when using a low flow (variable flow) oxygen delivery device?
3. How do increasing PEEP and recruitment manoeuvres increase oxygenation?
4. Identify some of the potential risks of recruitment manoeuvres and the nursing observations to detect signs of deterioration.
5. Explain how a reduction in the FiO_2 from 1.0 to 0.8 can increase the SpO_2.

Online resources

American Association for Respiratory Care, http://www.aarc.org/resources/

American Thoracic Society, http://www.thoracic.org/statements/

Anaesthesia UK, http://www.frca.co.uk/default.aspx

Australian and New Zealand Intensive Care Society, https://www.anzics.com.au/

ARDS network, http://www.ardsnet.org/

Canadian Society of Respiratory Therapists, Respiratory Resource, http://www.respiratoryresource.ca/

College of Intensive Care Medicine of Australia and New Zealand, https://www.cicm.org.au/

Covidien education resources, http://www.nellcor.com/educ/OnlineEd.aspx

Critical Care Medicine Tutorials, http://www.ccmtutorials.com/

Department of Anaesthesia and Intensive Care, Chinese University of Hong Kong, http://aic-server4.aic.cuhk.edu.hk/web8/

Intensive Care New South Wales, https://www.aci.health.nsw.gov.au/networks/icnsw

National Institute for Health and Care Excellence, https://www.nice.org.uk/

Thoracic Society of Australia and New Zealand, http://www.thoracic.org.au/

Vent World, http://www.ventworld.com/

Further reading

Branson RD, Gomaa D, Rodriquez D Jr. Management of the artificial airway. Respir Care 2014;59(6):974–89.

Canadian Critical Care Trials Group/Canadian Critical Care Society Noninvasive Ventilation Guidelines Group. Clinical practice guidelines for the use of noninvasive positive-pressure ventilation and noninvasive continuous positive airway pressure in the acute care setting. CMAJ 2011;183(3):E195–214.

Chatburn RL, Khatib ME, Mireles-Cabodevila E. A taxonomy for mechanical ventilation: 10 fundamental maxims. Respir Care 2014;59(11):1747–63.

Dhand R. How should aerosols be delivered during invasive mechanical ventilation? Respir Care 2017;62(10):1343–67.

Fan E, Brodie D, Slutsky AS. Acute respiratory distress syndrome: advances in diagnosis and treatment. JAMA 2018;319(7):698–710.

Ferrer M, Sellares J, Torres A. Noninvasive ventilation in withdrawal from mechanical ventilation. Semin Respir Crit Care Med 2014;35(4):507–18.

Jiang JR, Yen SY, Chien JY, et al. Predicting weaning and extubation outcomes in long-term mechanically ventilated patients using the modified Burns Wean Assessment Program scores. Respirol 2014;19(4):576–82.

Suzumura EA, Figueiró M, Normilio-Silva K, et al. Effects of alveolar recruitment maneuvers on clinical outcomes in patients with acute respiratory distress syndrome: a systematic review and meta-analysis. Intensive Care Med 2014;40(9):1227–40.

References

1. Australian and New Zealand Intensive Care Society. Centre for Outcome and Resource Evaluation (ANZICS CORE) Annual Report 2017. Melbourne: Australian and New Zealand Intensive Care Society; 2017.
2. Shahin J, Harrison D, Rowan K. Is the volume of mechanically ventilated admissions to UK critical care units associated with improved outcomes? Intensive Care Med 2014;40:353–60.
3. Wunsch H, Wagner J, Herlim M, et al. ICU occupancy and mechanical ventilator use in the United States. Crit Care Med 2013;41:2712–19.
4. Chew D, Aroney C, Aylward P, et al. 2011 Addendum to the National Heart Foundation of Australia/Cardiac Society of Australia and New Zealand Guidelines for the management of acute coronary syndromes (ACS) 2006. Heart Lung Circ 2011;20(8):487–502.
5. Hoiland RL, Mladinov S, Barak OF, et al. Oxygen therapy improves cerebral oxygen delivery and neurovascular function in hypoxaemic chronic obstructive pulmonary disease patients. Exp Physiol 2018.
6. Naughton M, Tuxen D. Acute respiratory failure in chronic obstructive pulmonary disease. In: Bersten A, Soni N, editors. Oh's intensive care manual. 7th ed. Philadelphia: Butterworth Heineman Elsevier; 2013. p. 354–464.
7. Wagstaff T, Soni N. Performance of six types of oxygen delivery devices at varying respiratory rates. Anaesthesia 2007;62:492–503.
8. Wagstaff A. Oxygen therapy. In: Bersten A, Soni N, editors. Oh's intensive care manual. 7th ed. Philadelphia: Butterworth Heineman Elsevier; 2013. p. 327–41.
9. Sim M, Dean P, Kinsella J, et al. Performance of oxygen delivery devices when the breathing pattern of respiratory failure is simulated. Anaesthesia 2008;63:938–40.
10. Chanques G, Riboulet F, Molinari N, et al. Comparison of three high flow oxygen therapy delivery devices: a clinical physiological cross-over study. Minerva Anestesiol 2013;79(12):1344–55.
11. Corley A, Caruana LR, Barnett AG, et al. Oxygen delivery through high-flow nasal cannulae increase end-expiratory lung volume and reduce respiratory rate in post-cardiac surgical patients. Br J Anaesth 2011;107(6):998–1004.
12. Kernick J, Magary J. What is the evidence for the use of high flow nasal cannula oxygen in adult patients admitted to critical care units? A systematic review. Aust Crit Care 2010;23:53–70.
13. Fisher and Paykel Healthcare New Zealand. Respiratory and acute care, nasal high flow. Auckland: Fisher and Paykel Healthcare New Zealand; 2010. Available from: http://www.fphcare.com/rsc/adult-care/nasal-high-flow.html. [Accessed 26 September 2010].

14. Papazian L, Corley A, Hess D, et al. Use of high-flow nasal cannula oxygenation in ICU adults: a narrative review. Intensive Care Med 2016;42(9):1336–49.
15. Peters S, Holets S, Gay P. High-flow nasal cannula therapy in do-not-intubate patients with hypoxemic respiratory distress. Respir Care 2013;58(4):597–600.
16. Helviz Y, Einav S. A systematic review of the high-flow nasal cannula for adult patients. Crit Care 2018;22(1):71.
17. Hnatiuk O, Moores L, Thompson J, et al. Delivery of high concentrations of inspired oxygen via tusk mask. Crit Care Med 1998;26:1032–5.
18. Peruzzi W, Smith B. Oxygen delivery: tusks versus flow. Crit Care Med 1998;26:986.
19. Boumphrey S, Morris E, Kinsella S. 100% inspired oxygen from a Hudson mask – a realistic goal? Resuscitation 2003;57:69–72.
20. Davies JD, Costa BK, Asciutto AJ. Approaches to manual ventilation. Respir Care 2014;59(6):810–22, discussion 22–4.
21. Cook T, Hommers C. New airways for resuscitation? Resuscitation 2006;69:371–87.
22. Joynt G, Choi G. Airway management and acute upper-airway obstruction. In: Bersten A, Soni N, editors. Oh's intensive care manual. 7th ed. Philadelphia: Butterworth Heineman Elsevier; 2013. p. 341–54.
23. Donatelli J, Gupta A, Santhosh R, et al. To breathe or not to breathe: a review of artificial airway placement and related complications. Emerg Radiol 2015;22(2):171–9.
24. Nolan J, Hazinski M, Billi J, et al. Part 1: executive summary: 2010 international consensus on cardiopulmonary resuscitation and emergency cardiovascular care science with treatment recommendations. Resuscitation 2010;81:e1–25.
25. Wahlen B, Roewer N, Lange M, et al. Tracheal intubation and alternative airway management devices used by healthcare professionals with different level of pre-existing skills: a manikin study. Anaesthesia 2009;64:549–54.
26. Vézina M-C, Trépanier C, Nicole P, et al. Complications associated with the esophageal-tracheal Combitube® in the pre-hospital setting. Can J Anesth 2007;54:124–8.
27. Haas C, Eakin R, Konkle M, et al. Endotracheal tubes: old and new. Respir Care 2014;59(6):933–52.
28. Haas C, Branson R, Folk L, et al. Patient-determined inspiratory flow during assisted mechanical ventilation. Respir Care 1995;40(7): 716–21.
29. Ball J, Platt S. Obstruction of a reinforced oral tracheal tube. Brit J Anaesthesia 2010;105:699–700.
30. Davies R. The importance of a Murphy eye. Anaesthesia 2001;56:906–24.
31. Anantham D, Jagadesan R, Tiew P. Clinical review: independent lung ventilation in critical care. Crit Care 2005;9(6):594–600.
32. Jaber S, Amraoui J, Lefrant J-Y, et al. Clinical practice and risk factors for immediate complications of endotracheal intubation in the intensive care unit: a prospective, multiple-center study. Crit Care Med 2006;34:2355–61.
33. Weingart SD. Preoxygenation, reoxygenation, and delayed sequence intubation in the emergency department. J Emerg Med 2011;40(6):661–7.
34. Vourc'h M, Asfar P, Volteau C, et al. High-flow nasal cannula oxygen during endotracheal intubation in hypoxemic patients: a randomized controlled clinical trial. Intensive Care Med 2015;41(9):1538–48.
35. Mosier J, Hypes C, Sakles J. Understanding preoxygenation and apneic oxygenation during intubation in the critically ill. Intensive Care Med 2016;43(2):226–8.
36. Holzapfel L, Chastang C, Demingeon G, et al. A randomized study assessing the systematic search for maxillary sinusitis in nasotracheally mechanically ventilated patients. Influence of nosocomial maxillary sinusitis on the occurrence of ventilator-associated pneumonia. Am J Resp Crit Care Med 1999;159:695–701.
37. Beavers R, Moos D, Cuddeford J. Analysis of the application of cricoid pressure: implications for the clinician. J Perianesth Nurs 2009;24:92–102.
38. Brisson P, Brisson M. Variable application and misapplication of cricoid pressure. J Trauma 2010;69:1182–4.
39. Priebe H. Cricoid pressure: an expert's opinion. Minerva Anestesiol 2009;75:710–14.
40. Sitzwohl C, Langheinrich A, Schober A, et al. Endobronchial intubation detected by insertion depth of endotracheal tube, bilateral auscultation, or observation of chest movements: randomised trial. BMJ 2010;341:c5943.
41. Rudraraju P, Eisen L. Confirmation of endotracheal tube position: a narrative review. J Intensive Care Med 2009;24:283–92.
42. College of Intensive Care Medicine of Australia and New Zealand. IC-1 Minimum standards for intensive care units. Melbourne: College of Intensive Care Medicine of Australia and New Zealand; 2016. Available from: https://www.cicm.org.au/CICM_Media/CICMSite/CICM-Website/Resources/Professional%20Documents/IC-1-Minimum-Standards-for-Intensive-Care-Units_2.pdf. [Accessed 3 May 2018].
43. Mallick A, Bodenham A. Tracheostomy in critically ill patients. Eur J Anaesthesiol 2010;27:676–82.
44. De Leyn P, Bedert L, Delcroix M, et al. Tracheotomy: clinical review and guidelines. Eur J Cardiothorac Surg 2007;32:412–21.
45. Australian and New Zealand Intensive Care Society. Percutaneous Dilatational Tracheostomy Consensus Statement. Melbourne: ANZICS; 2010. Available from: www.anzics.com.au/safety-quality?start=2. [Accessed 30 January 2011].
46. Russell C. Providing the nurse with a guide to tracheostomy care and management. Brit J Nur 2005;14:428–33.
47. Dennis-Rouse M, Davidson J. An evidence-based evaluation of tracheostomy care practices. Crit Care Nurs Q 2008;31:150–60.
48. Beach L, Denehy L, Lee A. The efficacy of minitracheostomy for the management of sputum retention: a systematic review. Physiotherapy 2013;99(4):271–7.

49. Abdelaziz M, Naidu B, Agostini P. Is prophylactic minitracheostomy beneficial in high-risk patients undergoing thoracotomy and lung resection? Interac Cardiovasc Thorac Surg 2011;12(4):615–18.
50. Thomas A, McGrath B. Patient safety incidents associated with airway devices in critical care: a review of reports to the UK National Patient Safety Agency. Anaesthesia 2009;64:358–65.
51. Ai ZP, Gao XL, Zhao XL. Factors associated with unplanned extubation in the intensive care unit for adult patients: a systematic review and meta-analysis. Intensive Crit Care Nurs 2018;47:62–8.
52. Curry K, Cobb S, Kutash M, et al. Characteristics associated with unplanned extubations in a surgical intensive care unit. Am J Crit Care 2008;17(1):45–51, quiz 2.
53. Chao CM, Lai CC, Chan KS, et al. Multidisciplinary interventions and continuous quality improvement to reduce unplanned extubation in adult intensive care units: a 15-year experience. Medicine (Baltimore) 2017;96(27):e6877.
54. Chuang ML, Lee CY, Chen YF, et al. Revisiting unplanned endotracheal extubation and disease severity in intensive care units. PLoS ONE 2015;10(10):e0139864.
55. Engels P, Bagshaw S, Meier M, et al. Tracheostomy: from insertion to decannulation. Can J Surg 2009;52:427–33.
56. Brass P, Hellmich M, Ladra A, et al. Percutaneous techniques versus surgical techniques for tracheostomy. Cochrane Database Syst Rev 2016;(7):Cd008045.
57. Fernandez M, Piacentini E, Blanch L, et al. Changes in lung volume with three systems of endotracheal suctioning with and without pre-oxygenation in patients with mild-to-moderate lung failure. Intensive Care Med 2004;30:2210–15.
58. AARC. AARC Clinical Practice Guidelines. Endotracheal suctioning of mechanically ventilated patients with artificial airways. Respir Care 2010;55:758–64.
59. Sole ML, Bennett M, Ashworth S. Clinical indicators for endotracheal suctioning in adult patients receiving mechanical ventilation. Am J Crit Care 2015;24(4):318–24, quiz 25.
60. Chaseling W, Bayliss S-L, Rose K, et al. Suctioning an adult ICU patient with an artificial airway, version 2. Chatswood, NSW: Agency for Clinical Innovation NSW Government; 2014.
61. Paulus F, Binnekade J, Vroom M, et al. Benefits and risks of manual hyperinflation in intubated and mechanically ventilated intensive care unit patients: a systematic review. Crit Care 2012;16(4):R145.
62. Ayhan H, Tastan S, Iyigun E, et al. Normal saline instillation before endotracheal suctioning: 'What does the evidence say? What do the nurses think?': multimethod study. J Crit Care 2015;30(4):762–7.
63. National Health and Medical Research Council. Australian guidelines for the prevention and control of infection in healthcare. Canberra: Commonwealth of Australia; 2010.
64. Intensive Care Coordination and Monitoring Unit. Stabilisation of an endotracheal tube for the adult intensive care patient. NSW Health statewide guidelines for intensive care. Sydney: New South Wales Health; 2007. Available from: http://intensivecare.hsnet.nsw.gov.au/state-wide-guidelines. [Accessed 23 January 2011].
65. Gardner A, Hughes D, Cook R, et al. Best practice in stabilisation of oral endotracheal tubes: a systematic review. Aust Crit Care 2005;18:158–65.
66. Murdoch E, Holdgate A. A comparison of tape-tying versus a tube-holding device for securing endotracheal tubes in adults. Anaesth Intensive Care 2007;35(5):730–5.
67. Haddad S, Arabi Y. Critical care management of severe traumatic brain injury in adults. Scand J Trauma Resusc Emerg Med 2012;20:12.
68. Hockey CA, van Zundert AA, Paratz JD. Does objective measurement of tracheal tube cuff pressures minimise adverse effects and maintain accurate cuff pressures? A systematic review and meta-analysis. Anaesth Intensive Care 2016;44(5):560–70.
69. Bulamba F, Kintu A, Ayupo N, et al. Achieving the recommended endotracheal tube cuff pressure: a randomized control study comparing loss of resistance syringe to pilot balloon palpation. Anesthesiol Res Pract 2017.
70. Rose L, Redl L. Survey of cuff management practices within Australia and New Zealand. Am J Crit Care 2008;17:428–35.
71. Vyas D, Inweregbu K, Pittard A. Measurement of tracheal tube cuff pressure in critical care. Anaesthesia 2002;57:275–7.
72. Sole M, Byers J, Ludy J, et al. A multisite survey of suctioning techniques and airway management parctices. Am J Crit Care 2003;12:220–30.
73. Sole M, Penoyer D, Su X, et al. Assessment of endotracheal cuff pressure by continuous monitoring: a pilot study. Am J Crit Care 2009;18:133–43.
74. Lizy C, Swinnen W, Labeau S, et al. Cuff pressure of endotracheal tubes after changes in body position in critically ill patients treated with mechanical ventilation. Am J Crit Care 2014;23(1):e1–8.
75. Lorente L, Lecuona M, Jiménez A, et al. Continuous endotracheal tube cuff pressure control system protects against ventilator-associated pneumonia. Crit Care 2014;18(2):R77.
76. Fernandez J, Levine S, Restrepo M. Technologic advances in endotracheal tubes for prevention of ventilator-associated pneumonia. Chest 2012;142(1):231–8.
77. Seguin P, Perrichet H, Pabic E, et al. Effect of continuous versus intermittent subglottic suctioning ontracheal mucosa by the Mallinckrodt TaperGuard Evac Oral Tracheal Tube in intensive care unit ventilated patients: a prospective randomized study. Indian J Crit Care Med 2018;22(1):1–4.

78. Suys E, Nieboer K, Stiers W, et al. Intermittent subglottic secretion drainage may cause tracheal damage in patients with few oropharyngeal secretions. Intensive Crit Care Nurs 2013;29(6):317–20.
79. Mao Z, Gao L, Wang G, et al. Subglottic secretion suction for preventing ventilator-associated pneumonia: an updated meta-analysis and trial sequential analysis. Crit Care 2016;20(1):353.
80. Bitgani M, Madineh H. Intraoperative atelectasis due to endotracheal tube cuff herniation: a case report. Acta Med Iran 2012;50(9):652–4.
81. El-Orbany M, Salem M. Endotracheal tube cuff leaks: causes, consequences, and management. Anesth Analg 2013;117:428–34.
82. AARC. AARC clinical practice guideline: removal of the endotracheal tube – 2007 revision & update. Respir Care 2007;52:81–93.
83. Schnell D, Planquette B, Berger A, et al. Cuff leak test for the diagnosis of post-extubation stridor. J Intensive Care Med 2017;885066617700095.
84. Pluijms WA, van Mook WN, Wittekamp BH, et al. Postextubation laryngeal edema and stridor resulting in respiratory failure in critically ill adult patients: updated review. Crit Care 2015;19:295.
85. Esteban A, Frutos-Vivar F, Muriel A, et al. Evolution of mortality over time in patients receiving mechanical ventilation. Am J Respir Crit Care Med 2013;188(2):220–30.
86. Rose L, Presneill J, Johnston L, et al. Ventilation and weaning practices in Australia and New Zealand. Anaeth Intensive Care 2009;37:99–107.
87. Hess D. Ventilator waveforms and the physiology of pressure support ventilation. Respir Care 2005;50:166–86.
88. Pilbeam S, Cairo J. Mechanical ventilation: physiological and clinical applications. 4th ed. St Louis: Mosby Elsevier; 2006.
89. Burns S. Working with respiratory waveforms: how to use bedside graphics. AACN Clin Issues 2003;14:133–44.
90. Rittner F, Doring M. Curves and loops in mechanical ventilation. Hong Kong: Draeger Medical Asia Pacific.
91. Zanella A, Bellani G, Pesenti A. Airway pressure and flow monitoring. Curr Opin Crit Care 2010;16(3):255–60.
92. Nilsestuen J, Hargett K. Using ventilator graphics to identify patient-ventilator asynchrony. Respir Care 2005;50:202–34.
93. Yang S, Yang S. Effects of inspiratory flow waveforms on lung mechanics, gas exchange, and respiratory metabolism in COPD patients during mechanical ventilation. Chest 2002;122:2096–104.
94. Blanch L, Bernabé F, Lucangelo U. Measurement of air trapping, intrinsic positive end-expiratory pressure, and dynamic hyperinflation in mechanically ventilated patients. Respir Care 2005;50:110–23.
95. Lu Q, Rouby J-J. Measurement of pressure-volume curves in patients on mechanical ventilation: methods and significance. Crit Care 2000;4:91–100.
96. Bonetto C, Calo M, Delgado M, et al. Modes of pressure delivery and patient–ventilator interaction. Respir Care Clin N Am 2005;11: 247–63.
97. Maggiore S, Jonson B, Richard J, et al. Alveolar derecruitment at decremental positive end-expiratory pressure levels in acute lung injury: comparison with the lower inflection point, oxygenation, and compliance. Am J Respir Crit Care Med 2001;164:795–801.
98. Hickling K. Best compliance during a decremental, but not incremental, positive end-expiratory pressure trial is related to open-lung positive end-expiratory pressure: a mathematical model of acute respiratory distress syndrome lungs. Am J Respir Crit Care Med 2001;163:69–78.
99. Brochard L. What is a pressure-volume curve? Crit Care 2006;10(4):156.
100. Lucangelo U, Bernabé F, Blanch L. Respiratory mechanics derived from signals in the ventilator circuit. Respir Care 2005;50:55–65.
101. Al Ashry HS, Modrykamien AM. Humidification during mechanical ventilation in the adult patient. Biomed Res Int 2014;2014:715434.
102. Branson R. The ventilator circuit and ventilator-associated pneumonia. Respir Care 2005;50:774–85.
103. Muscedere J, Dodek P, Keenan S, et al. Comprehensive evidence-based clinical practice guidelines for ventilator-associated pneumonia: prevention. J Crit Care 2008;23:126–37.
104. Hellyer T, Ewan V, Wilson P, et al. The Intensive Care Society recommended bundle of interventions for the prevention of ventilator-associated pneumonia. J Intensive Care Soc 2016;17(3):238–43.
105. Kilgour E, Rankin N, Ryan S, et al. Mucociliary function deteriorates in the clinical range of inspired air temperature and humidity. Intensive Care Med 2004;30:1491–4.
106. Bersten A. Humidication and inhalation therapy. In: Bersten A, Soni N, Oh T, editors. Oh's intensive care manual. 5th ed. Oxford: Butterworth-Heinemann; 2003.
107. Lellouche F, Taille S, Lefrancois F, et al. Humidification performance of 48 passive airway humidifiers: comparison with manufacturer data. Chest 2009;135(2):276–86.
108. Wilkes AR. Heat and moisture exchangers and breathing system filters: their use in anaesthesia and intensive care. Part 1 - history, principles and efficiency. Anaesthesia 2011;66(1):31–9.
109. Kelly M, Gillies D, Todd D, et al. Heated humidification versus heat and moisture exchangers for ventilated adults and children. Cochrane Database Syst Rev 2010;(4):CD004711.
110. Nava S, Hill N. Non-invasive ventilation in acute respiratory failure. Lancet 2009;374:250–9.
111. Rose L, Gerdtz M. Review of non-invasive ventilation in the emergency department: clinical considerations and management priorities. J Clin Nurs 2009;18:3216–24.
112. Mehta S, Hill N. Noninvasive ventilation: state of the art. Am J Respir Crit Care Med 2001;163:540–77.

113. Hill N. Noninvasive positive pressure ventilation. In: Tobin M, editor. Principles and practoce of mechanical ventilation. New York: McGraw-Hill; 2006.
114. L'Her E, Deye N, Lellouche F, et al. Physiologic effects of noninvasive ventilation during acute lung injury. Am J Respir Crit Care Med 2005;172:1112–18.
115. Hill N, Brennan J, Garpestad E, et al. Noninvasive ventilation in acute respiratory failure. Crit Care Med 2007;35:2402–7.
116. Schulze V, Meyer C, Eickholt C, et al. Impact of continuous positive airway pressure on left ventricular systolic loading and coronary flow reserve in healthy young men. Heart Lung Circ 2018;27(3):344–9.
117. Kaye D, Mansfield D, Naughton MT. Continuous positive airway pressure decreases myocardial oxygen consumption in heart failure. Clin Sci 2004;106:599–603.
118. Pladeck T, Hader C, Von Orde A, et al. Non-invasive ventilation: comparison of effectiveness, safety, and management of acute heart failure syndromes and acute exacerbations of chronic obstructive pulmonary disease. J Physiol and Pharmacol 2007;58:539–49.
119. Caples S, Gay P. Noninvasive positive pressure ventilation in the intensive care unit: a concise review. Crit Care Med 2005;33:2651–8.
120. Carrillo A, Gonzalez-Diaz G, Ferrer M, et al. Non-invasive ventilation in community-acquired pneumonia and severe acute respiratory failure. Intensive Care Med 2012;38(3):458–66.
121. Antonelli M, Conti G, Moro M, et al. Predictors of failure of noninvasive positive pressure ventilation in patients with acute hypoxemic respiratory failure; a multi-center study. Intensive Care Med 2001;27:1718–28.
122. Osadnik C, Tee V, Carson-Chahhoud K, et al. Non-invasive ventilation for the management of acute hypercapnic respiratory failure due to exacerbation of chronic obstructive pulmonary disease. Cochrane Database Syst Rev 2017;(7):CD004104.
123. Confalonieri M, Garuti G, Cattaruzza M, et al. A chart of failure risk for noninvasive ventilation in patients with COPD exacerbation. Eur Respir J 2005;25:348–55.
124. Masip J, Roque M, Sanchez B, et al. Noninvasive ventilation in acute cardiogenic pulmonary edema. JAMA 2005;294:3124–30.
125. Peter JV, Moran JL, Phillips-Hughes J, et al. Effect of non-invasive positive pressure ventilation (NIPPV) on mortality in patients with acute cardiogenic pulmonary oedema: a meta-analysis. Lancet 2006;367(9517):1155–63.
126. Winck JC, Azevedo LF, Costa-Pereira A, et al. Efficacy and safety of non-invasive ventilation in the treatment of acute cardiogenic pulmonary edema–a systematic review and meta-analysis. Crit Care 2006;10(2):R69.
127. Vital F, Ladeira M, Atallah A. Non-invasive positive pressure ventilation (CPAP or bilevel NPPV) for cardiogenic pulmonary oedema. Cochrane Database Syst Rev 2013;(5):CD005351.
128. Juern JS. Removing the critically ill patient from mechanical ventilation. Surg Clin North Am 2012;92(6):1475–83.
129. Agarwal R, Aggarwal A, Gupta D, et al. Role of noninvasive positive-pressure ventilation in postextubation respiratory failure: a meta-analysis. Respir Care 2007;52:1472–9.
130. Burns K, Meade M, Premji A, et al. Non-invasive positive pressure ventilation as a weaning strategy for intubated patients with respiratory failure. Cochrane Database Syst Rev 2013;(12):CD004127.
131. Esteban A, Frutos F, Ferguson ND, et al. Noninvasive positive pressure ventilation for respiratory failure after extubation. New Engl J Med 2004;350:2452–60.
132. Lim WJ, Mohammed Akram R, Carson KV, et al. Non-invasive positive pressure ventilation for treatment of respiratory failure due to severe acute exacerbations of asthma. Cochrane Database Syst Rev 2012;(12):Cd004360.
133. Pallin M, Naughton M. Noninvasive ventilation in acute asthma. J Crit Care 2014;29(4):586–93.
134. Quill C, Quill T. Palliative use of noninvasive ventilation: navigating murky waters. J Palliat Med 2014;17(6):657–61.
135. Ozsancak Ugurlu A, Sidhom SS, Khodabandeh A, et al. Use and outcomes of noninvasive positive pressure ventilation in acute care hospitals in Massachusetts. Chest 2014;145(5):964–71.
136. Evans TW. International Consensus Conferences in Intensive Care Medicine: non-invasive positive pressure ventilation in acute respiratory failure. Organised jointly by the American Thoracic Society, the European Respiratory Society, the European Society of Intensive Care Medicine, and the Societe de Reanimation de Langue Francaise, and approved by the ATS Board of Directors, December 2000. Intensive Care Med 2001;27(1):166–78.
137. Esquinas Rodriguez AM, Papadakos PJ, Carron M, et al. Clinical review: helmet and non-invasive mechanical ventilation in critically ill patients. Crit Care 2013;17(2):223.
138. Davidson AC, Banham S, Elliott M, et al. BTS/ICS guideline for the ventilatory management of acute hypercapnic respiratory failure in adults. Thorax 2016;71(Suppl. 2):ii1–35.
139. Keenan S, Sinuff T, Burns K, et al. Clinical practice guidelines for the use of noninvasive positive-pressure ventilation and noninvasive continuous positive airway pressure in the acute care setting. CMAJ 2011;183(3):E195–214.
140. Laghi F, Tobin M. Indications for mechanical ventilation. In: Tobin M, editor. Principles and practice of mechanical ventilation. 3nd ed. New York: McGraw-Hill; 2012.
141. Tobin M, Guenther S, Perez W, et al. Konno-Mead analysis of ribcage-abdominal motion during successful and unsuccessful trials of weaning from mechanical ventilation. Am Rev Respir Dis 1987;135:1320–8.
142. Chatburn R, Volsko T, Hazy J, et al. Determining the basis for a taxonomy of mechanical ventilation. Respir Care 2012;57(4):514–24.
143. Rose L. Advanced modes of mechanical ventilation: implications for practice. AACN Adv Crit Care 2006;17:145–58.

144. Neto AS, Jaber S. What's new in mechanical ventilation in patients without ARDS: lessons from the ARDS literature. Intensive Care Med 2016;42(5):787–9.
145. Habashi N. Other approaches to open-lung ventilation: airway pressure release ventilation. Crit Care Med 2005;33(3):S228–40.
146. Marik P, Krikorian J. Pressure-controlled ventilation in ARDS: a practical approach. Chest 1997;112:1102–6.
147. Esteban A, Alia I, Gordo F, et al. Prospective randomized trial comparing pressure-controlled ventilation and volume-controlled ventilation in ARDS. Chest 2000;117:1690–6.
148. Campbell R, Davis B. Pressure-controlled versus volume-controlled ventilation: does it matter? Respir Care 2002;47:416–26.
149. Jiang J, Li B, Kang N, et al. Pressure-controlled versus volume-controlled ventilation for surgical patients: a systematic review and meta-analysis. J Cardiothorac Vasc Anesth 2016;30(2):501–14.
150. Asfar P, Singer M, Radermacher P. Understanding the benefits and harms of oxygen therapy. Intensive Care Med 2015;41(6):1118–21.
151. Martin D, Richards G. Predicted body weight relationships for protective ventilation – unisex proposals from pre-term through to adult. BMC Pulm Med 2017;17:85.
152. ARDSnet. Ventilation with lower tidal volumes compared with traditional tidal volumes for acute lung injury and the acute respiratory distress syndrome. N Engl J Med 2000;342:1301–8.
153. Fan E, Del Sorbo L, Goligher E, et al. SoCC. An official American Thoracic Society/European Society of Intensive Care Medicine/Society of Critical Care Medicine clinical practice guideline: mechanical ventilation in adult patients with acute respiratory distress syndrome. Am J Respir Crit Care Med 2017;195(9):1253–63.
154. Serpa Neto A, Simonis F, Schultz M. How to ventilate patients without acute respiratory distress syndrome? Curr Opin Crit Care 2015;21(1):65–73.
155. Serpa Neto A, Cardoso S, Manetta J, et al. Association between use of lung-protective ventilation with lower tidal volumes and clinical outcomes among patients without acute respiratory distress syndrome: a meta-analysis. JAMA 2012;308:1651–9.
156. Neto A, Simonis F, Barbas C, et al. Lung-protective ventilation with low tidal volumes and the occurrence of pulmonary complications in patients without acute respiratory distress syndrome: a systematic review and individual patient data analysis. Crit Care Med 2015;43(10):2155–63.
157. Holets S, Hubmayr R. Setting the ventilator. In: Tobin M, editor. Principles and practice of mechanical ventilation. 2nd ed. New York: McGraw-Hill; 2006.
158. Khalil M, Elfattah N, El-Shafey M, et al. Flow versus pressure triggering in mechanically ventilated acute respiratory failure patients. Egypt J Bronchol 2015;9(2):198–201.
159. Hill L, Pearl R. Flow triggering, pressure triggering, and autotriggering during mechanical ventilation. Crit Care Med 2000;28:579–81.
160. Murias G, Villagra A, Blanch L. Patient-ventilator dyssynchrony during assisted invasive mechanical ventilation. Minerva Anestesiol 2013;79:434–44.
161. Murata S, Yokoyama K, Sakamoto Y, et al. Effects of inspiratory rise time on triggering work load during pressure-support ventilation: a lung model study. Respir Care 2010;55:878–84.
162. Amato M, Marini J. Pressure-controlled and inverse-ratio ventilation. In: Tobin M, editor. Principles and practice of mechanical ventilation. 2nd ed. New York: McGraw-Hill; 2006. p. 251–72.
163. Pierce L. Management of the mechanically ventilated patient. 2nd ed. St Louis: Saunders: Elsevier; 2007.
164. Gattinoni L, Caironi P, Carlesso E. How to ventilate patients with acute lung injury and acute respiratory distress syndrome. Curr Opin Crit Care 2005;11:69–76.
165. Kallet R. Evidence-based management of acute lung injury and acute respiratory distress syndrome. Respir Care 2004;49:793–809.
166. Ashbaugh D, Bigelow D, Petty T, et al. Acute respiratory distress in adults. Lancet 1967;2:319–23.
167. Vasques F, Duscio E, Cipulli F, et al. Determinants and prevention of ventilator-induced lung injury. Crit Care Clin 2018;34(3):343–56.
168. Briel M, Meade M, Mercat A, et al. Higher vs lower positive end-expiratory pressure in patients with acute lung injury and acute respiratory distress syndrome: systematic review and meta-analysis. JAMA 2010;303(9):865–73.
169. Serpa Neto A, Filho R, Cherpanath T, et al. Associations between positive end-expiratory pressure and outcome of patients without ARDS at onset of ventilation: a systematic review and meta-analysis of randomized controlled trials. Ann Intensive Care 2016;6(1):109.
170. Serpa Neto A, Schultz M. Optimizing the settings on the ventilator: high PEEP for all? JAMA 2017;317(14):1413–14.
171. Hess D, Kacmarek R. Essentials of mechanical ventilation. 2nd ed. New York: McGraw-Hill; 2002.
172. MacIntyre N. Patient-ventilator interactions: optimizing conventional ventilation modes. Respir Care 2011;56(1):73–84.
173. Chatburn R. Classification of ventilator modes: update and proposal for implementation. Respir Care 2007;52:301–23.
174. Chatburn R. Understanding mechanical ventilators. Expert Rev Respir Med 2010;4:809–19.
175. Kacmarek R, Branson R. Should intermittent mandatory ventilation be abolished? Respir Care 2016;61(6):854–66.
176. Chatburn R, El-Khatib M, Mireles-Cabodevila E. A taxonomy for mechanical ventilation: 10 fundamental maxims. Respir Care 2014;59(11):1747–63.
177. Haitsma J. Diaphragmatic dysfunction in mechanical ventilation. Curr Opin Anaesthesiol 2011.
178. MacIntyre NR. Evidence-based guidelines for weaning and discontinuing ventilatory support. Chest 2001;120(6):375S–95S.

179. Jain S, Kollisch-Singule M, Sadowitz B, et al. The 30-year evolution of airway pressure release ventilation (APRV). Intensive Care Med Exp 2016;4(1):11.

180. Daoud E, Farag H, Chatburn R. Airway pressure release ventilation: what do we know? Respir Care 2012;57(2):282–92.

181. Lago A, Goncalves E, Silva E, et al. Comparison of energy expenditure and oxygen consumption of spontaneous breathing trial conducted with and without Automatic Tube Compensation. J Clin Med Res 2015;7(9):700–5.

182. L'Her E. Automatic tube compensation: is it worthwhile? Respir Care 2012;57(5):813–14.

183. Unoki T, Serita A, Grap M. Automatic tube compensation during weaning from mechanical ventilation: evidence and clinical implications. Crit Care Nurse 2008;28:34–42.

184. Figueroa-Casas J, Montoya R, Arzabala A, et al. Comparison between automatic tube compensation and continuous positive airway pressure during spontaneous breathing trials. Respir Care 2010;55(5):549–54.

185. Demoule A, Clavel M, Rolland-Debord C, et al. Neurally adjusted ventilatory assist as an alternative to pressure support ventilation in adults: a French multicentre randomized trial. Intensive Care Med 2016;42(11):1723–32.

186. Verbrugghe W, Jorens P. Neurally adjusted ventilatory assist: a ventilation tool or a ventilation toy? Respir Care 2011;56(3):327–35.

187. Brander L, Sinderby C, Lecomte F, et al. Neurally adjusted ventilatory assist decreases ventilator-induced lung injury and non-pulmonary organ dysfunction in rabbits with acute lung injury. Intensive Care Med 2009;35:1979–89.

188. Schmidt M, Kindler F, Cecchini J, et al. Neurally adjusted ventilatory assist and proportional assist ventilation both improve patient-ventilator interaction. Crit Care 2015;19:56.

189. Ferreira J, Diniz-Silva F, Moriya H, et al. Neurally Adjusted Ventilatory Assist (NAVA) or Pressure Support Ventilation (PSV) during spontaneous breathing trials in critically ill patients: a crossover trial. BMC Pulm Med 2017;17(1):139.

190. Kacmarek R. Proportional assist ventilation and neurally adjusted ventilatory assist. Respir Care 2011;56(2):140–8.

191. Tirupakuzhi Vijayaraghavan B, Hamed S, Jain A, et al. Evidence supporting clinical use of proportional assist ventilation: a systematic review and meta-analysis of clinical trials. J Intensive Care Med 2018.

192. Suzumura E, Amato M, Cavalcanti A. Understanding recruitment maneuvers. Intensive Care Med 2016;42(5):908–11.

193. Hodgson C, Goligher E, Young M, et al. Recruitment manoeuvres for adults with acute respiratory distress syndrome receiving mechanical ventilation. Cochrane Database Syst Rev 2016;(11):CD006667.

194. Suarez-Sipmann F, Bohm S, Tusman G, et al. Use of dynamic compliance for open lung positive end-expiratory pressure titration in an experimental study. Crit Care Med 2007;35:214–21.

195. Writing Group for the Alveolar Recruitment for Acute Respiratory Distress Syndrome Trial (ART) Investigators, Cavalcanti A, Suzumura É, et al. Effect of lung recruitment and titrated positive end-expiratory pressure (PEEP) vs low PEEP on mortality in patients with acute respiratory distress syndrome: a randomized clinical trial. JAMA 2017;318(4):1335–45.

196. Rose L. Clinical application of ventilation modes: ventilatory strategies for lung protection. Aus Crit Care 2010;23:71–80.

197. Facchin F, Fan E. Airway pressure release ventilation and high-frequency oscillatory ventilation: potential strategies to treat severe hypoxemia and prevent ventilator-induced lung injury. Respir Care 2015;60(10):1509–21.

198. Goffi A, Ferguson N. High-frequency oscillatory ventilation for early acute respiratory distress syndrome in adults. Curr Opin Crit Care 2014;20(1):77–85.

199. Hager D. High-frequency oscillatory ventilation in adults with acute respiratory distress syndrome. Curr Opin Anaesthesiol 2012;25(1):17–23.

200. Ip T, Mehta S. The role of high-frequency oscillatory ventilation in the treatment of acute respiratory failure in adults. Curr Opin Crit Care 2012;18(1):70–9.

201. Ferguson N, Cook D, Guyatt G, et al. High-frequency oscillation in early acute respiratory distress syndrome. N Engl J Med 2013;368(9):795–805.

202. Young D, Lamb S, Shah S, et al. High-frequency oscillation for acute respiratory distress syndrome. N Engl J Med 2013;368(9):806–13.

203. Combes A, Hajage D, Capellier G, et al. Extracorporeal membrane oxygenation for severe acute respiratory distress syndrome. N Engl J Med 2018;378(21):1965–75.

204. Serpa Neto A, Schmidt M, Azevedo L, et al. Associations between ventilator settings during extracorporeal membrane oxygenation for refractory hypoxemia and outcome in patients with acute respiratory distress syndrome: a pooled individual patient data analysis: mechanical ventilation during ECMO. Intensive Care Med 2016;42(11):1672–84.

205. Makdisi G, Wang I. Extra Corporeal Membrane Oxygenation (ECMO) review of a lifesaving technology. J Thorac Dis 2015;7(7):E166–76.

206. Lindholm J. Cannulation for veno-venous extracorporeal membrane oxygenation. J Thorac Dis 2018;10(Suppl. 5):S606–12.

207. Murphy D, Hockings L, Andrews R, et al. Extracorporeal membrane oxygenation-hemostatic complications. Transfus Med Rev 2015;29(2):90–101.

208. Zangrillo A, Landoni G, Biondi-Zoccai G, et al. A meta-analysis of complications and mortality of extracorporeal membrane oxygenation. Crit Care Resusc 2013;15(3):172–8.

209. Gebistorf F, Karam O, Wetterslev J, et al. Inhaled nitric oxide for acute respiratory distress syndrome (ARDS) in children and adults. Cochrane Database Syst Rev 2016;(6):CD002787.

210. Hill N, Preston I, Roberts K. Inhaled therapies for pulmonary hypertension. Respir Care 2015;60(6):794–802.

211. Dugernier J, Ehrmann S, Sottiaux T, et al. Aerosol delivery during invasive mechanical ventilation: a systematic review. Crit Care 2017;21(1):264.
212. Dhanani J, Fraser J, Chan H, et al. Fundamentals of aerosol therapy in critical care. Crit Care 2016;20(1):269.
213. Burk R, Grap M. Backrest position in prevention of pressure ulcers and ventilator-associated pneumonia: conflicting recommendations. Heart Lung 2012;41(6):536–45.
214. Drakulovic M, Torres A, Bauer T, et al. Supine body position as a risk factor for nosocomial pneumonia in mechanically ventilated patients: a randomised trial. Lancet 1999;354:1851–8.
215. Torres A, Niederman M, Chastre J, et al. International ERS/ESICM/ESCMID/ALAT guidelines for the management of hospital-acquired pneumonia and ventilator-associated pneumonia: guidelines for the management of hospital-acquired pneumonia (HAP)/ ventilator-associated pneumonia (VAP) of the European Respiratory Society (ERS), European Society of Intensive Care Medicine (ESICM), European Society of Clinical Microbiology and Infectious Diseases (ESCMID) and Asociación Latinoamericana del Tórax (ALAT). Eur Respir J 2017;50(3).
216. Kalil A, Metersky M, Klompas M, et al. Executive summary: management of adults with hospital-acquired and ventilator-associated pneumonia: 2016 clinical practice guidelines by the infectious diseases society of America and the American Thoracic Society. Clin Infect Dis 2016;63(5):575–82.
217. van Nieuwenhoven C, Vandenbroucke-Grauls C, van Tiel F, et al. Feasibility and effects of the semirecumbent position to prevent ventilator-associated pneumonia: a randomized study. Crit Care Med 2006;34:396–402.
218. Wang L, Li X, Yang Z, et al. Semi-recumbent position versus supine position for the prevention of ventilator-associated pneumonia in adults requiring mechanical ventilation. Cochrane Database Syst Rev 2016;(1):CD009946.
219. Rose L, Baldwin I, Crawford T, et al. A multicenter, observational study of semirecumbent positioning in mechanically ventilated patients. Am J Crit Care 2010;19:e100–8.
220. Wolken R, Woodruff R, Smith J, et al. Observational study of head of bed elevation adherence using a continuous monitoring system in a medical intensive care unit. Respir Care 2012;57(4):537–43.
221. Liu J, Song H, Wang Y, et al. Factors associated with low adherence to head-of-bed elevation during mechanical ventilation in Chinese intensive care units. Chin Med J 2013;126(5):834–8.
222. Llaurado-Serra M, Ulldemolins M, Fernandez-Ballart J, et al. Related factors to semi-recumbent position compliance and pressure ulcers in patients with invasive mechanical ventilation: an observational study (CAPCRI study). Int J Nurs Studies 2016;61:198–208.
223. Rose L, Baldwin I, Crawford T. The use of bed-dials to maintain recumbent positioning for critically ill mechanically ventilated patients (the RECUMBENT study): multicentre before and after observational study. Int J Nurs Studies 2010;47:1425–31.
224. Hewitt N, Bucknall T, Faraone N. Lateral positioning for critically ill adult patients. Cochrane Database Syst Rev 2016;(5):CD007205.
225. Marini J, Gattinoni L. Propagation prevention: a complementary mechanism for 'lung protective' ventilation in acute respiratory distress syndrome. Crit Care Med 2008;36(12):252–3258.
226. Wanless S, Aldridge M. Continuous lateral rotation therapy - a review. Nurs Crit Care 2012;17(1):28–35.
227. Staudinger T, Bojic A, Holzinger U, et al. Continuous lateral rotation therapy to prevent ventilator-associated pneumonia. Crit Care Med 2010;38:486–90.
228. Schieren M, Piekarski F, Dusse F, et al. Continuous lateral rotational therapy in trauma-A systematic review and meta-analysis. J Trauma Acute Care Surg 2017;83(5):926–33.
229. Beitler J, Shaefi S, Montesi S, et al. Prone positioning reduces mortality from acute respiratory distress syndrome in the low tidal volume era: a meta-analysis. Intensive Care Med 2014;40(3):332–41.
230. Guerin C, Baboi L, Richard J. Mechanisms of the effects of prone positioning in acute respiratory distress syndrome. Intensive Care Med 2014;40(11):1634–42.
231. Kallet R. A comprehensive review of prone position in ARDS. Respir Care 2015;60(11).
232. Gattinoni L, Taccone P, Carlesso E, et al. Prone position in acute respiratory distress syndrome. Rationale, indications, and limits. Am J Respir Crit Care Med 2013;188(1):1286–93.
233. Jozwiak M, Monnet X, Teboul J. Optimizing the circulation in the prone patient. Curr Opin Crit Care 2016;22(3):239–45.
234. Fessler H, Talmor D. Should prone positioning be routinely used for lung protection during mechanical ventilation? Respir Care 2010;55:88–99.
235. Sud S, Friedrich J, Adhikari N, et al. Effect of prone positioning during mechanical ventilation on mortality among patients with acute respiratory distress syndrome: a systematic review and meta-analysis. CMAJ 2014;186(10):E381–90.
236. Bloomfield R, Noble D, Sudlow A. Prone position for acute respiratory failure in adults. Cochrane Database Syst Rev 2015;(11): CD008095.
237. Dickinson S, Park P, Napolitano L. Prone-positioning therapy in ARDS. Crit Care Clin 2011;511–23.
238. Sutherasan Y, D'Antini D, Pelosi P. Advances in ventilator-associated lung injury: prevention is the target. Expert Rev Respir Med 2014;8(2):233–48.
239. Torres A, Niederman M, Chastre J, et al. Summary of the international clinical guidelines for the management of hospital-acquired and ventilator-acquired pneumonia. ERJ Open Res 2018;4(2):pii: 00028-2018.

240. Gattinoni L, Pi A, Caironi P, et al. Ventilator-induced lung injury: the anatomical and physiological framework. Crit Care Med 2010;38(10 Suppl.):S539–48.
241. Slutsky A, Ranieri V. Ventilator-induced lung injury. N Engl J Med 2013;369(22):2126–36.
242. Melsen W, Rovers M, Groenwold R, et al. Attributable mortality of ventilator-associated pneumonia: a meta-analysis of individual patient data from randomised prevention studies. Lancet Infect Dis 2013;13(8):665–71.
243. Kao J, Kao H, Chen Y, et al. Impact and predictors of prolonged chest tube duration in mechanically ventilated patients with acquired pneumothorax. Respir Care 2013;58(12):2093–100.
244. Thille A, Cortés-Puch I, Esteban A. Weaning from the ventilator and extubation in ICU. Curr Opin Crit Care 2013;19(1):57–64.
245. Boles J-M, Bion J, Connors A, et al. Weaning from mechanical ventilation. Eur Respir J 2007;29:1033–56.
246. Shaikh H, Morales D, Laghi F. Weaning from mechanical ventilation. Semin Respir Crit Care Med 2014;35(4):451–68.
247. Thille A, Boissier F, Ben Ghezala H, et al. Risk factors for and prediction by caregivers of extubation failure in ICU patients: a prospective study. Crit Care Med 2015;43(3):613–20.
248. Cavallone L, Vannucci A. Review article: extubation of the difficult airway and extubation failure. Anesth Analg 2013;116(2):368–83.
249. Meade M, Guyatt G, Cook D, et al. Predicting success in weaning from mechanical ventilation. Chest 2001;120(6 Suppl.):400S–24S.
250. Kheir F, Myers L, Desai N, et al. The effect of flow trigger on rapid shallow breathing index measured through the ventilator. J Intensive Care Med 2015;30(2):103–6.
251. Tanios M, Nevins M, Hendra K, et al. A randomized, controlled trial of the role of weaning predictors in clinical decision making. Crit Care Med 2006;34:2530–5.
252. Brochard L, Rauss A, Benito S, et al. Comparison of three methods of gradual withdrawal from ventilatory support during weaning from mechanical ventilation. Am J Respir Crit Care Med 1994;150:896–903.
253. Esteban A, Frutos F, Tobin MJ, et al. A comparison of four methods of weaning patients from mechanical ventilation. Spanish Lung Failure Collaborative Group. New Engl J Med 1995;332:345–50.
254. Ladeira M, Vital F, Andriolo R, et al. Pressure support versus T-tube for weaning from mechanical ventilation in adults. Cochrane Database Syst Rev 2014;(5):CD006056.
255. Pellegrini J, Moraes R, Maccari J, et al. Spontaneous breathing trials with T-Piece or pressure support ventilation. Respir Care 2016;61(12):1693–703.
256. Rose L. Strategies for weaning from mechanical ventilation: a state of the art review. Intensive Crit Care Nurs 2015;31(2):189–95.
257. Ouellette D, Patel S, Girard T, et al. Liberation from mechanical ventilation in critically ill adults: an official American College of Chest Physicians/American Thoracic Society Clinical Practice Guideline: inspiratory pressure augmentation during spontaneous breathing trials, protocols minimizing sedation, and noninvasive ventilation immediately after extubation. Chest 2017;151(1):166–80.
258. Figueroa-Casas J, Connery S, Montoya R. Changes in breathing variables during a 30-minute spontaneous breathing trial. Respir Care 2015;60(2):155–61.
259. Burns K, Raptis S, Nisenbaum R, et al. International practice variation in weaning critically ill adults from invasive mechanical ventilation. Ann Am Thorac Soc 2018;494–502.
260. Blackwood B, Burns K, Cardwell C, et al. Protocolized versus non-protocolized weaning for reducing the duration of mechanical ventilation in critically ill adult patients. Cochrane Database Syst Rev 2014;(11):CD006904.
261. Girard T, Kress J, Fuchs B, et al. Efficacy and safety of a paired sedation and ventilator weaning protocol for mechanically ventilated patients in intensive care (Awakening and Breathing Controlled trial): a randomised controlled trial. Lancet 2008;371:126–34.
262. Bellomo R, Stow P, Hart G. Why is there such a difference in outcome between Australian intensive care units and others? Curr Opin Anaesthesiol 2007;20:100–5.
263. Rose L, Nelson S, Johnston L, et al. Workforce profile, organisation structure and role responsibility for ventilation and weaning practices in Australia and New Zealand intensive care units. J Clin Nur 2008;17:1035–43.
264. Rose L, Blackwood B, Burns S, et al. International perspectives on the influence of structure and process of weaning from mechanical ventilation. Am J Crit Care 2011;20(1):e10–18.
265. Branson R. Automation of mechanical ventilation. Crit Care Clin 2018;34(2):383–94.
266. Rose L, Presneill J, Cade J. Update in computer-driven weaning from mechanical ventilation. Anaesth Intensive Care 2007;35:213–21.
267. Burns K, Lellouche F, Nisenbaum R, et al. Automated weaning and SBT systems versus non-automated weaning strategies for weaning time in invasively ventilated critically ill adults. Cochrane Database Syst Rev 2014;(9):CD008638.
268. Rose L, Schultz M, Cardwell C, et al. Automated versus non-automated weaning for reducing the duration of mechanical ventilation for critically ill adults and children. Cochrane Database Syst Rev 2014;(6):CD009235.
269. Rose L, Fowler R, Fan E, et al. Prolonged mechanical ventilation in Canadian intensive care units: a national survey. J Crit Care 2015;30(1):25–31.
270. Iwashyna T, Hodgson C, Pilcher D, et al. Timing of onset and burden of persistent critical illness in Australia and New Zealand: a retrospective, population-based, observational study. Lancet Respir Med 2016;4(7):566–73.
271. Vitacca M, Vianello A, Colombo D, et al. Comparison of two methods for weaning patients with chronic obstructive pulmonary disease requiring mechanical ventilation for more than 15 days. Am J Respir Crit Care Med 2001;164(2):225–30.

272. Jubran A, Grant B, Duffner L, et al. Effect of pressure support vs unassisted breathing through a tracheostomy collar on weaning duration in patients requiring prolonged mechanical ventilation: a randomized trial. JAMA 2013;309(7):671–7.

273. Gonçalves M, Honrado T, Winck J, et al. Effects of mechanical insufflation-exsufflation in preventing respiratory failure after extubation: a randomized controlled trial. Crit Care Med 2012;16:R48.

274. Gomez-Merino E, Sancho J, Marin J, et al. Mechanical insufflation-exsufflation: pressure, volume, and flow relationships and the adequacy of the manufacturer's guidelines. Am J Phys Med Rehab 2002;81(8):579–83.

275. Rose L, Adhikari N, Leasa D, et al. Cough augmentation techniques for extubation or weaning critically ill patients from mechanical ventilation. Cochrane Database Syst Rev 2017;(1):CD011833.

Chapter 16

Neurological assessment and monitoring

DaiWai M. Olson, Leila Kuzmiuk

KEY WORDS

afferent neuron
autonomic nervous system
central nervous system
correlative neuroanatomy
decerebrate (extensor)
decorticate (flexor)
efferent neuron
intracranial pressure
neurological assessment
parasympathetic nervous system
posttraumatic amnesia
peripheral nervous system
sympathetic nervous system

Learning objectives

After reading this chapter, you should be able to:

- describe the anatomy and physiology of the nervous system
- differentiate between the central and peripheral nervous systems
- describe the techniques used for neurological assessment
- explain the importance and process of serial neurological assessment in the brain-injured patient
- identify the distinction between normal and abnormal neurological responses
- state the determinants of intracranial pressure and describe compensatory mechanisms
- relate the procedures of selected neurodiagnostic tests to nursing implications for patient care.

Introduction

The nervous system is the major controlling, regulatory and communicating system in the body. It accounts for a mere 3% of total body weight, yet utilises 15–20% of the body's metabolic resources.[1] The brain is the centre of all mental activity, including thought, learning, memory, communication, and planning. Because the brain can neither store oxygen nor effectively engage in anaerobic metabolism, any interruption in the blood or oxygen supply to the brain rapidly leads to clinically observable signs and symptoms. Glucose is virtually the sole energy substrate for the brain, and it is entirely oxidised (i.e. consumed to produce energy). Without oxygen and glucose, brain cells continue to function normally for approximately 10 seconds. The brain can be seen as an almost exclusive glucose-processing machine, producing water (H_2O) and carbon dioxide (CO_2). Together with the endocrine and immune systems, the nervous system is responsible for regulating and maintaining homeostasis for all the organs in the body. Through its receptors, the nervous system responds to the environment, both external and internal. Diseases and disorders of the nervous system are common in the critical care unit, both as primary processes and as complications of multiple organ dysfunction in the critically ill patient. An understanding of basic neurophysiology and neuroanatomy is important if these disorders are to be recognised and treated. This chapter provides an overview of neurological anatomy and physiology, and outlines the elements of a comprehensive neurological assessment.

Neurological anatomy and physiology

All the sensory details that incorporate a body's own information systems are related to neurological anatomy and physiology. Composed of central and peripheral components, with the brain as the command centre, the nervous system is responsible for the body's most fundamental activities. Nerves, which are made up of bundles of fibres, deliver impulses to various parts of the body, including the brain. The brain translates the information delivered by the impulses, which then enables the person to react.[2] This section discusses the main components of the nervous system starting from neurons and nervous system transmission. Then the central nervous system and the peripheral nervous system are examined and related to neurological assessment.

Components of the nervous system

The central nervous system (CNS) consists of the spinal cord and the brain and is responsible for integrating, processing and coordinating sensory data and motor commands (Fig. 16.1).[3] The CNS is linked to all parts of the body by the peripheral nervous system (PNS), which transmits signals to and from the CNS. The PNS is composed of 43 pairs of spinal nerves, and 12 pairs of cranial nerves that emerge from the base of the brain. All branch and diversify prolifically as they distribute to the tissues and organs of the body. The peripheral nerves carry input to the CNS via their sensory afferent fibres and deliver output from the CNS via the efferent fibres. Specific physiology of the CNS and PNS is discussed in detail later in the chapter. First, however, neuron cell anatomy and physiology are examined.

FIGURE 16.1 The functional divisions of the nervous system.

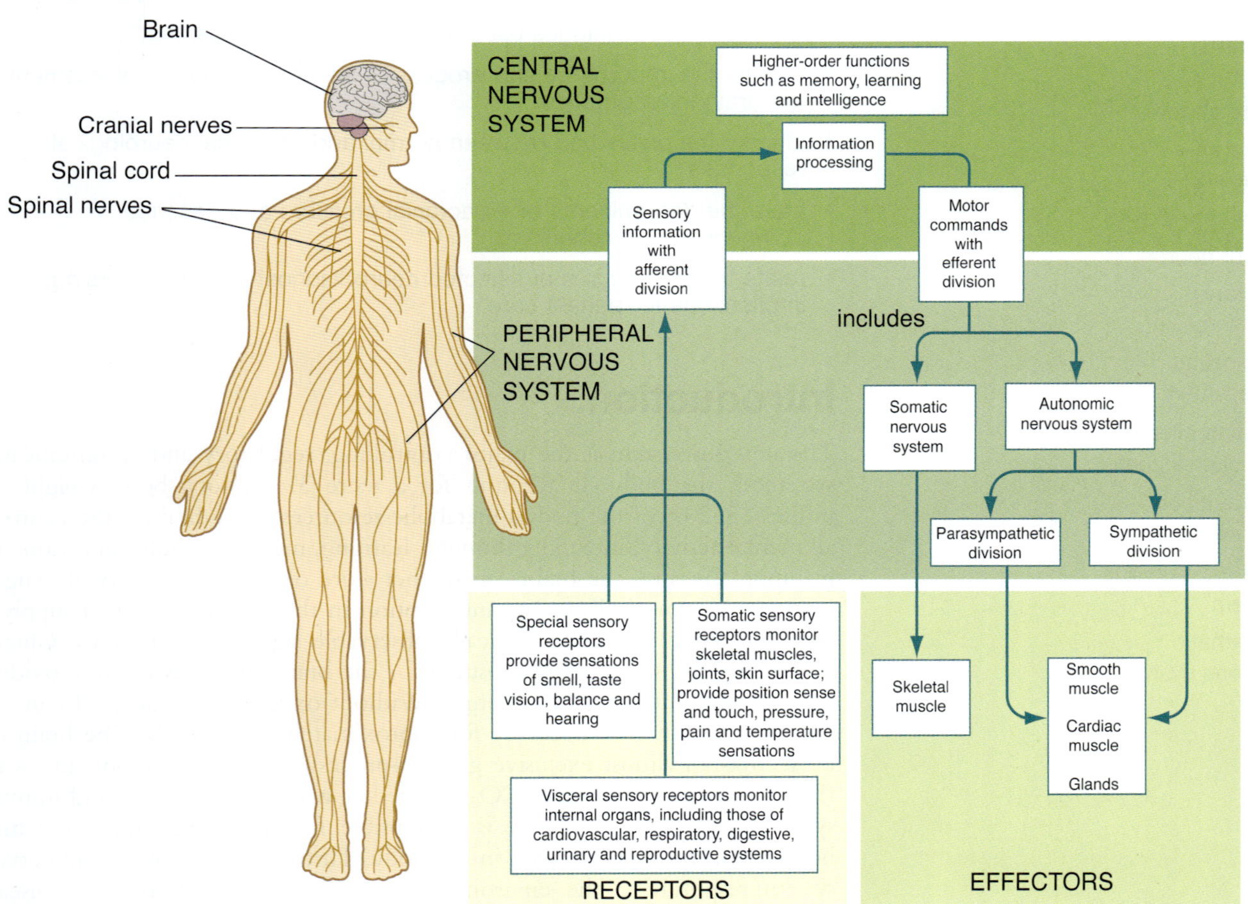

Adapted from Martini F, Nath JL, Bartholomew EF. Fundamentals of anatomy & physiology. 11th ed. Pearson; 2018.[73]

Neurons

Neurons are specialised cells in the nervous system; each is comprised of a dendrite, cell body (soma) and axon.[4] Each neuron uses biochemical reactions to receive, process and transmit information. Most synaptic contacts between neurons are either axodendritic (excitatory) or axosomatic (inhibitory). A neuron's dendritic tree is connected to many neighbouring neurons and receives positive or negative charges from other neurons. The input is then passed to the soma (cell body).[5] The primary role of the soma and the enclosed nucleus is to perform the continuous maintenance required to keep the neuron functional. Most neurons lack centrioles, important organelles involved in the organisation of the cytoskeleton and the movement of chromosomes during mitosis. As a result, typical CNS neurons cannot divide and cannot be replaced if lost to injury or disease. The fuel source for the neuron is glucose; insulin is not required for cellular uptake in the CNS.[4]

A myelin sheath, consisting of a lipid-protein casing, covers the neuron.[6] Myelin is not a continuous layer but has gaps called nodes of Ranvier (Fig. 16.2A). The myelin provides protection to the axon and speeds the transmission of impulses along nerve cells from node to node (see Fig. 16.2B). Each synaptic knob contains mitochondria, portions of the endoplasmic reticulum and thousands of vesicles filled with neurotransmitter molecules. Breakdown products of neurotransmitter released at the synapse are reabsorbed and reassembled at the

FIGURE 16.2 (**A**) Afferent and (**B**) efferent neurons, showing the soma or cell body, dendrites and axon. Arrows indicate the direction for conduction of action potentials.

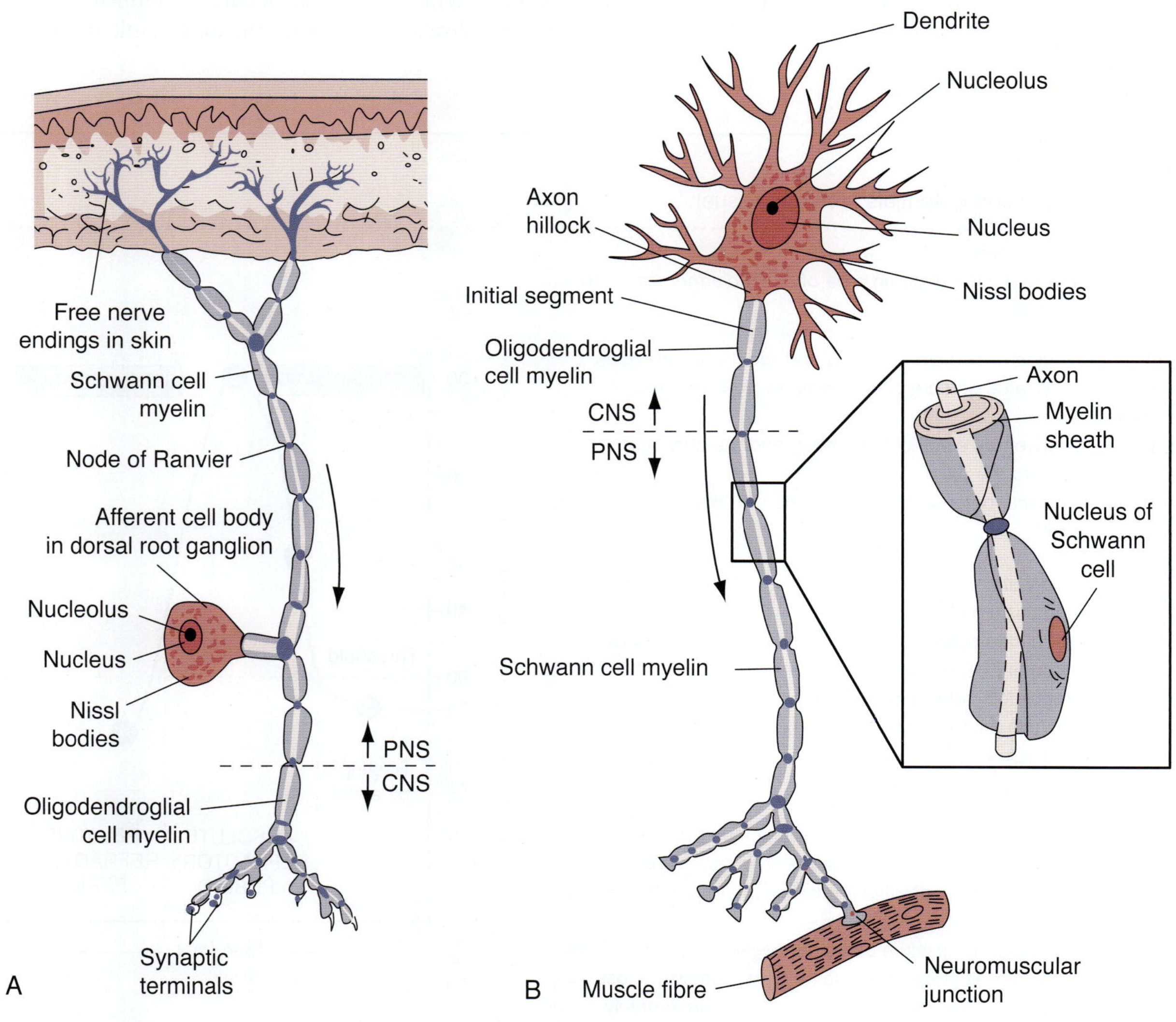

Adapted from Porth C. Pathophysiology concepts of altered health states. 9th ed. Philadelphia: Lippincott, Williams and Wilkins; 2013.

synaptic knob. The synaptic knob receives a continuous supply of neurotransmitter synthesised in the cell body, along with enzymes and lysosomes. The movement of materials between the cell body and synaptic knobs is called axoplasmic transport. Some materials travel slowly, at rates of a few mm per day. This transport mechanism is known as the 'slow stream'. Vesicles containing neurotransmitter move much more rapidly, travelling in the 'fast stream' at 5–10 mm per hour, which increases synaptic activity. Axoplasmic transport occurs in both directions. The flow of materials from the cell body to the synaptic knob is anterograde flow. At the same time, other substances are being transported towards the cell body in retrograde flow ('retro' meaning backward). If debris or unusual chemicals appear in the synaptic knob, retrograde flow soon delivers them to the cell body. The arriving materials may then alter the activity of the cell by turning appropriate genes on or off. Retrograde flow is the means of transport for viruses, pathogenic bacteria, heavy metals and toxins to the CNS, with resulting disease such as tetanus, viral encephalitis and lead intoxication. Defective anterograde transport seems to be involved in certain neuropathies, including critical illness neuropathies.[7]

Synapses

The human brain contains at least 100 billion neurons, each with the ability to influence many other cells. Although there are many kinds of synapses within the brain, they can be divided into two general classes: electrical synapses and chemical synapses. Electrical synapses permit direct, passive flow of electrical current from one neuron to another in the form of an action potential; they are described in Table 16.1. The current flows through gap junctions, which are specialised membrane channels that connect the two cells. Chemical synapses, in contrast, enable cell-to-cell communication via the secretion of neurotransmitters; the chemical agents released by the presynaptic neurons produce secondary current flow in postsynaptic neurons by activating specific receptor molecules (Fig. 16.3).

Myelin increases conduction velocity. Demyelination of peripheral nerves, as occurs in Guillain–Barré syndrome, slows conduction and may result in conduction

TABLE 16.1

Generation of action potentials (nervous tissue)

STEP 1: Depolarisation A graded depolarisation brings an area of excitable membrane to threshold (–60 mV)
STEP 2: Activation of sodium channels and rapid depolarisation The voltage-regulated sodium channels open (sodium channel activation) Sodium ions, driven by electrical attraction and the chemical gradient, flood into the cell The transmembrane potential goes from –60 mV, the threshold level, towards +30 mV
STEP 3: Repolarisation: inactivation of sodium channels and activation of potassium channels The voltage-regulated sodium channels close (sodium channel inactivation occurs) at +30 mV The voltage-regulated potassium channels are now open, and potassium ions diffuse out of the cell Repolarisation begins
STEP 4: Return to normal permeability The voltage-regulated sodium channels regain their normal properties in 0.4–1.0 ms. The membrane is now capable of generating another action potential if a larger-than-normal stimulus is provided The voltage-regulated potassium channels begin closing at –70 mV. Because they do not all close at the same time, potassium loss continues, and a temporary hyperpolarisation to approximately –90 mV occurs At the end of the relative refractory period, all voltage-regulated channels have closed, and the membrane is back to its resting state

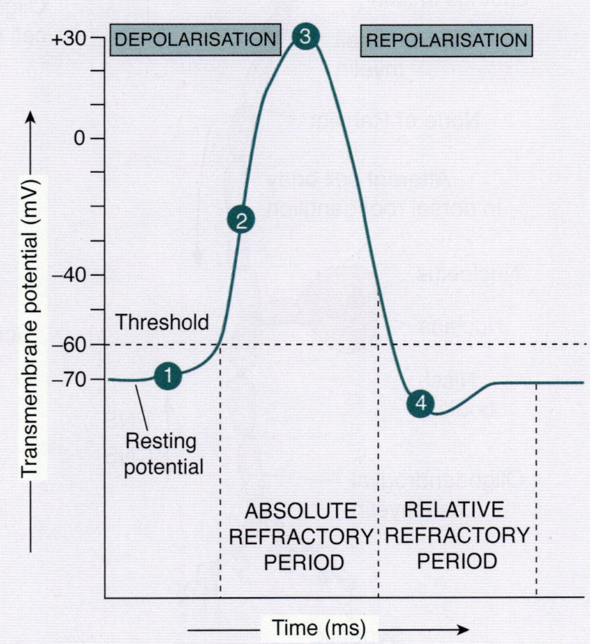

FIGURE 16.3 Sequence of events involved in transmission at a typical chemical synapse.

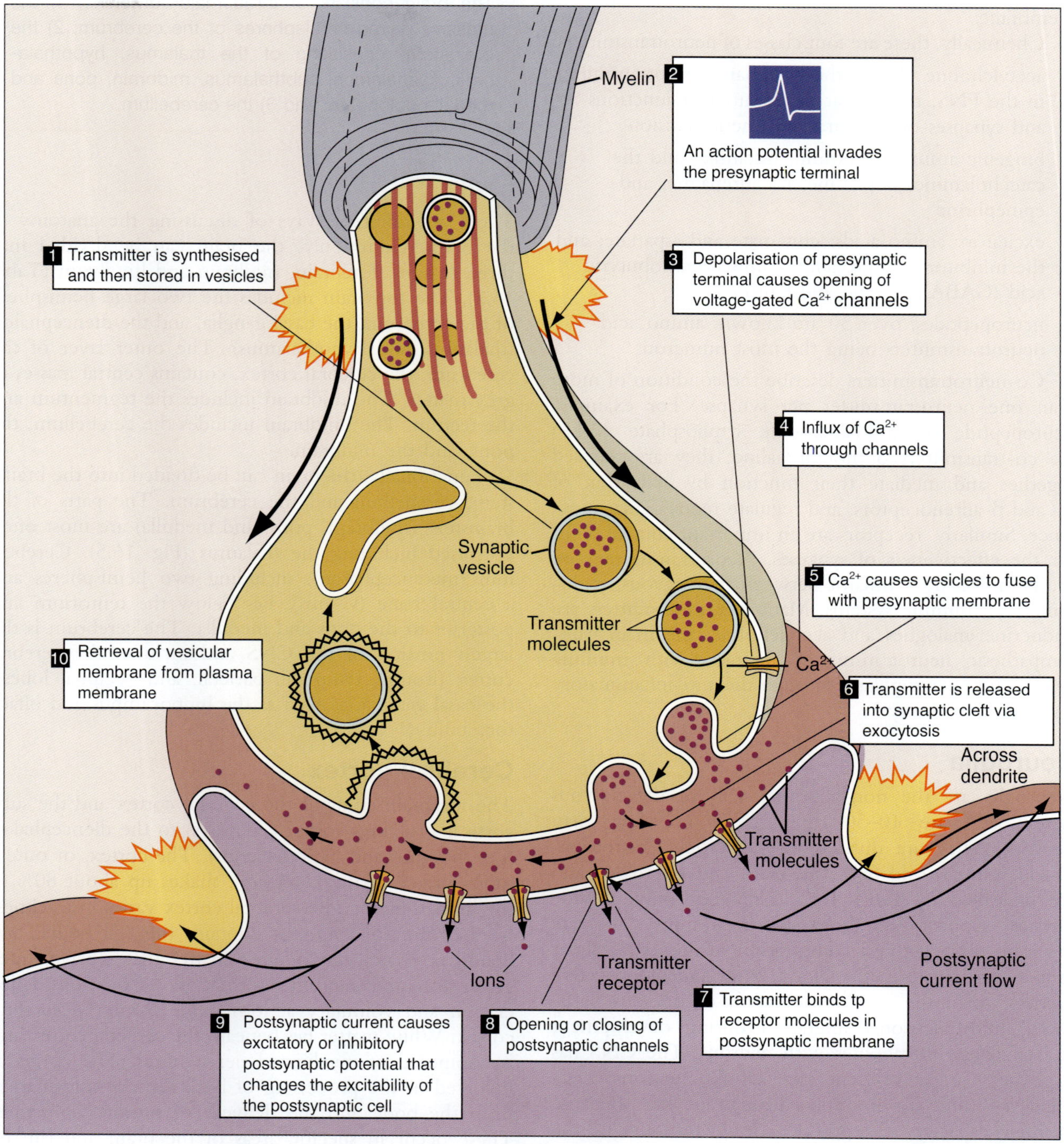

Adapted from Purves D, Augustine G, Hall W, et al. Neuroscience. 5th ed. New York: Sinauer Associates; 2012, Oxford University Press.

block, which manifests clinically as weakness.[8] Consequently, chronically demyelinated axons become vulnerable, with axon loss being a major cause of disability. In time, remyelination may occur, requiring the generation of myelin-competent oligodendrocytes, but most often it does not fully recapitulate developmental myelination.

Neurotransmitters

Neurotransmitters are chemicals that act as messengers to relay information between neurons.[9] Neurotransmitters are either inhibitory or excitatory.[10] The majority of neurotransmitters are produced in the cell body of neurons in the brain and stored in vesicles. When released, they travel across the synaptic junction and bind to specific neuroreceptor sites on the postsynaptic membrane.[11]

Chemically, there are four classes of neurotransmitters:

1 acetylcholine (ACh): the dominant neurotransmitter in the PNS, released at neuromuscular junctions and synapses of the parasympathetic division
2 biogenic amines: serotonin, histamine and the catecholamines dopamine, noradrenaline, and epinephrine
3 excitatory amino acids: glutamate and aspartate; and the inhibitory amino acids: gamma-aminobutyric acid (GABA), glycine and taurine
4 neuropeptides: over 50 are known, amino acid neurotransmitters being the most numerous.

Co-neurotransmitters describe the condition of more than one neurotransmitter per synapse. For example, neuropeptide Y and adenosine triphosphate (ATP) are co-transmitters of noradrenaline; they are released together and mediate their function by activation of α- and β-adrenoceptors, and regulate renovascular resistance. Similarly, receptors are an important control point for the effectiveness of synapses. Neurotransmitters are the common denominator between the nervous, endocrine and immune systems. Many neurotransmitters are endocrine analogues and acetylcholine, the main parasympathetic neurotransmitter, interacts with immune cells such as macrophages through the anti-inflammatory cholinergic pathway.[7]

Neuroglia

Neuroglia are the non-neuronal cells of the nervous system and are 10–50 times more prevalent than neurons. They are divided into macroglia (astrocytes, oligodendroglia and Schwann cells) and microglia, and are described in Table 16.2. They not only provide physical support but also respond to injury, regulate the ionic and chemical composition of the extracellular milieu, participate in the blood–brain and blood–retina barriers, form the myelin insulation of nervous pathways, guide neuronal migration during development and exchange metabolites with neurons. The CNS has a greater variety of neuroglia. Unlike neurons, neuroglia continue to multiply throughout life. Because of their capacity to reproduce, most tumours of the nervous system are tumours of neuroglial tissue and not of nervous tissue itself.

Central nervous system

The CNS is composed of the brain and spinal cord (Fig. 16.4). The primary purpose is to acquire, coordinate and disseminate information about the body and its environment. This section describes the anatomy and physiology of the brain and spinal cord.

> **Practice tip**
>
> The brain consists of three major divisions: 1) the massive paired hemispheres of the cerebrum; 2) the brainstem, consisting of the thalamus, hypothalamus, epithalamus, subthalamus, midbrain, pons and medulla oblongata; and 3) the cerebellum.

Brain

There are different ways of discussing the anatomy of the brain. Commonly, the brain can be divided into three regions: forebrain, midbrain and hindbrain (Table 16.3). The forebrain includes the two large hemisphere of the cerebrum, the basal ganglia, and the diencephalon (thalamus, and hypothalamus). The outer layer of the cerebrum, the cerebral cortex, contains central masses of grey matter. The midbrain includes the tegmentum and the tectum. The hindbrain includes the cerebellum, the pons, and the midbrain.

Functionally, the brain can be divided into the brainstem, cerebellum and the cerebrum. The parts of the brainstem (midbrain, pons, and medulla) are most often visualised including the thalamus (Fig. 16.5). Cerebellum (metencephalon), including two hemispheres and a central zone (vermis), lies below the tentorium and posterior to the pons and medulla. The cerebrum is the largest portion of the CNS and includes the cerebral cortex (frontal, temporal, parietal, and occipital lobes), the basal ganglia, as well as the hippocampus and olfactory bulb.

Cerebral cortex

The forebrain contains the cerebral cortex and the subcortical structures rostral (sideways) to the diencephalon (i.e. thalamus and hypothalamus). The cortex, or outermost surface of the cerebrum, makes up about 80% of the human brain. The cerebral cortex varies in thickness from 2 mm to 4 mm. It contains the cell bodies and dendrites of neurons or grey matter that receive, integrate, store and transmit information.[12] Conscious deliberation and voluntary actions come from the cerebral cortex. White matter lies beneath the cerebral cortex and is composed of myelinated nerve fibres. The cortex is involved in the processing of both sensory information from the body and the delivery of motor commands. These occur in specific areas of the brain and can be mapped. Topographically, the cerebral cortex is divided into areas of specialised functions, including the primary sensory areas for vision (occipital cortex), hearing (temporal cortex), somatic sensation (postcentral gyrus), and primary motor area (precentral gyrus). As shown in Fig. 16.6, these well-defined areas comprise only a small fraction of the surface of the cerebral cortex.

The majority of the remaining cortical area is known as the association cortex, where the processing of extensive and sophisticated neural information is performed.

TABLE 16.2

Neuroglia, their location and role as supporting nervous tissue

CELL TYPE	LOCATION	MAIN FUNCTION
Astrocytes 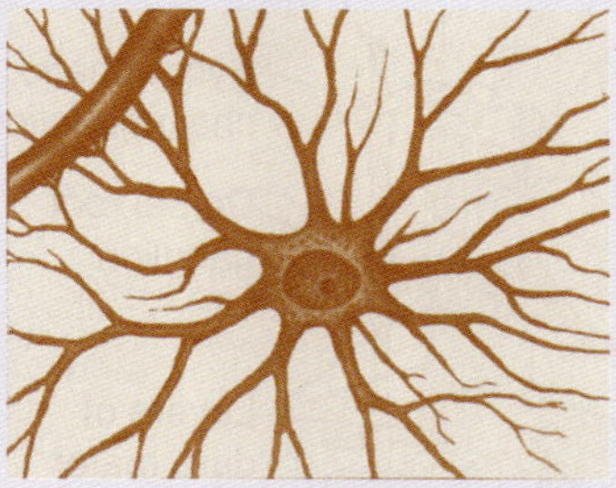	CNS: the largest and most numerous neuroglial cells in the brain and spinal cord	Astrocytes are considered as important as the neuron in communication and brain regulation They regulate communication, extracellular ionic and chemical environments between neurons They respond to injury and have an important role in cerebral oedema
Ependymal cells 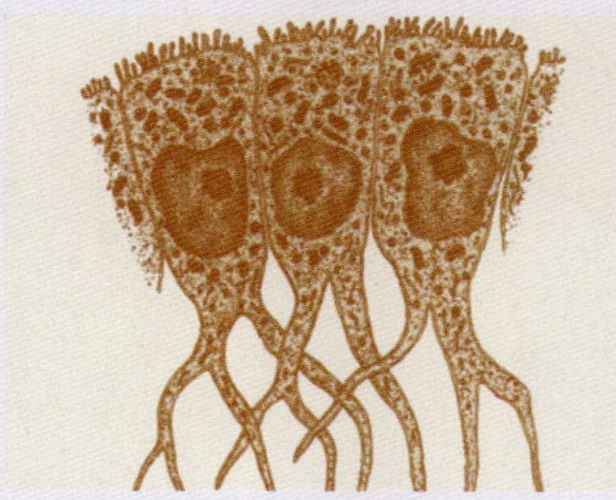	CNS: line the ventricular system of the brain and central cord of the spinal canal	Transport of CSF and brain homeostasis Phagocytotic defence against pathogens Store glycogen for brain tissue
Microglia 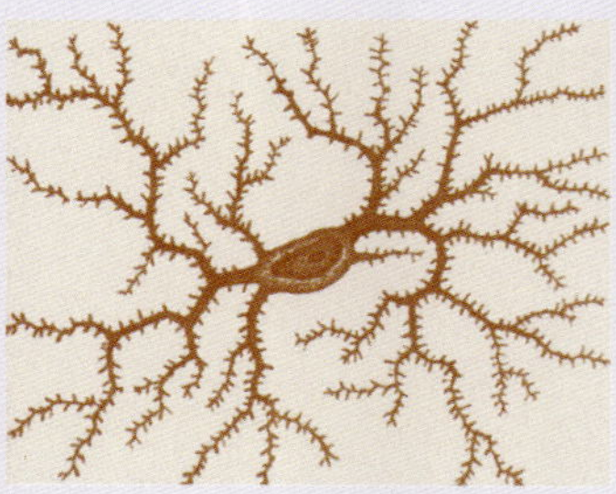	CNS: located within the brain parenchyma behind the blood–brain barrier	Wander between the peripheral immune system and the CNS as a defence to infection Displace synaptic input in injured neurons
Oligodendrocytes 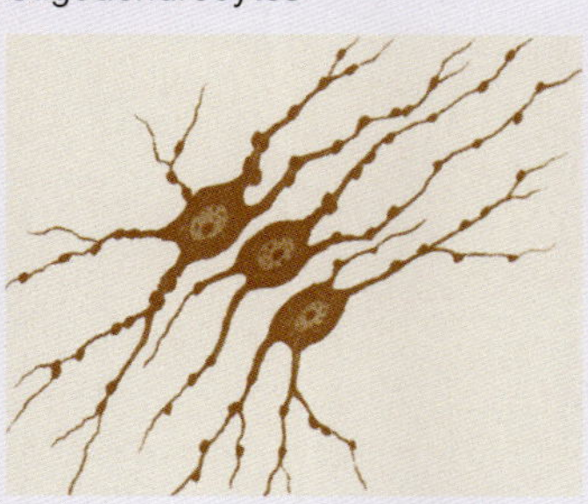	CNS: spiral around an axon to form a multilayered lipoprotein coat in both the white and grey matter in the brain and spinal cord PNS: Schwann cells are the supporting cells of the PNS	Responsible for the formation of myelin sheaths surrounding axons Oligodendrocytes wrap themselves around numerous axons at once Schwann cells wrap themselves around peripheral nerve axons Unlike oligodendrocytes, a single Schwann cell makes up a single segment of an axon's myelin sheath

The association areas are also sites of long-term memory, and they are critical to human functions such as language acquisition, speech, musical ability, mathematical ability, complex motor skills, abstract thought, symbolic thought and other cognitive functions. Association areas interconnect and integrate information from the primary sensory and motor areas via intra-hemispheric connections. The parietal–temporal–occipital association cortex integrates neural information contributed by visual, auditory and somatic sensory experiences. The prefrontal association cortex is extremely important as the coordinator of emotionally motivated behaviours, by virtue of its connections with the limbic system.

The prefrontal cortex receives neural input from the other association areas and regulates motivated behaviours by direct input to the premotor area, which serves as the association area of the motor cortex. Sensory and motor functions are controlled by cortical structures in the

FIGURE 16.4 The subdivisions and components of the CNS.

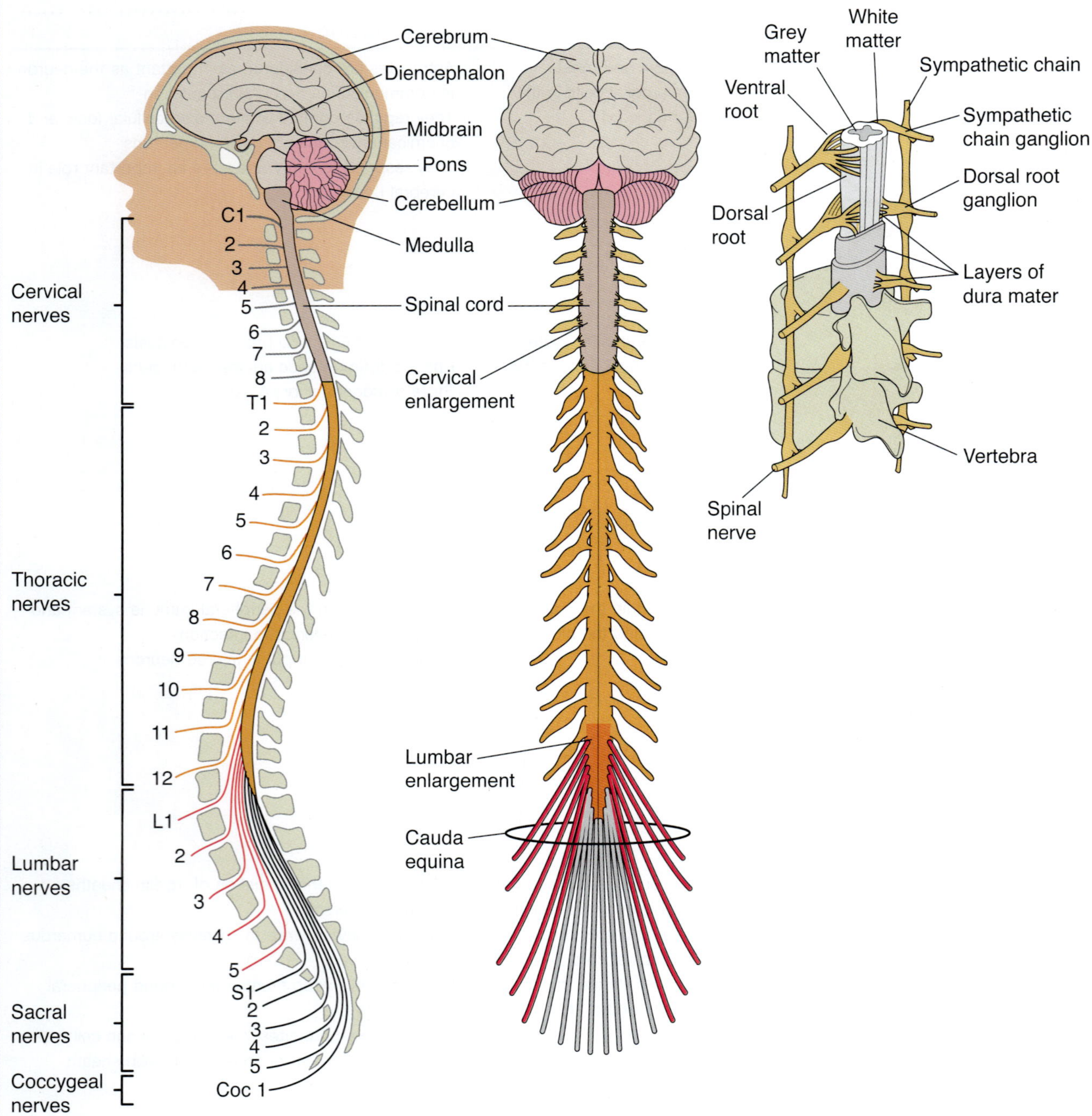

Adapted from Purves D, Augustine G, Hall W, et al. Neuroscience. 5th ed. New York: Sinauer Associates; 2012, Oxford University Press.

contralateral hemisphere. Particular cognitive functions or components of these functions may be lateralised to one side of the brain.

The cerebral cortex receives sensory information, relayed through the thalamus, from many different sensory organs and processes the information. The two hemispheres receive the information from the opposite sides of the body. Parts of the cortex that receive this information are called primary sensory areas and cross at various points in the sensory pathway, because the cerebral cortex operates on a contralateral basis. The discriminative touch system crosses high, in the medulla. The pain system crosses low, in the spinal cord. The proprioceptive sensory system that guards balance and position goes to the cerebellum, which works ipsilaterally and therefore does not cross. Almost every region

TABLE 16.3
Organisation of the brain

DIVISION	DESCRIPTION	FUNCTIONS
Forebrain		
Cerebrum 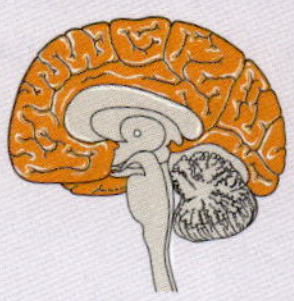	Largest and uppermost portion of the brain. Divided into two hemispheres, each subdivided into the frontal, parietal, temporal and occipital lobes	Cortex (outer layer) is the site of conscious thought, memory, reasoning and abstract mental functions, all localised within specific lobes
Diencephalon 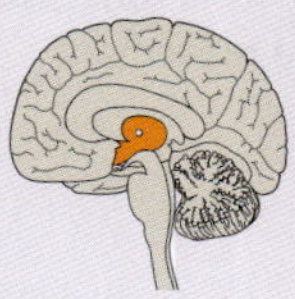	Between the cerebrum and the brainstem. Contains the thalamus and hypothalamus	Thalamus sorts and redirects sensory input; hypothalamus controls visceral, autonomic, endocrine and emotional function, and the pituitary gland. Contains some of the centres for coordinated parasympathetic and sympathetic stimulation, temperature regulation, appetite regulation, regulation of water balance by antidiuretic hormone (ADH) and regulation of certain rhythmic psychobiological activities (e.g. sleep)
Brain stem	Anterior region below the cerebrum: the medulla, pons and midbrain compose the brainstem	Connects cerebrum and diencephalon with spinal cord
Midbrain		
Midbrain 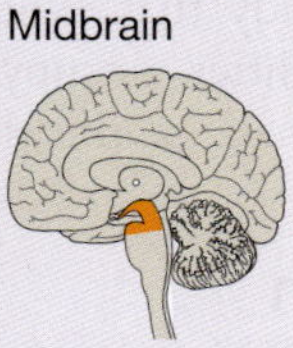	Below the centre of the cerebrum	Has reflex centres concerned with vision and hearing; connects cerebrum with lower portions of the brain. It contains sensory and motor pathways and serves as the centre for auditory and visual reflexes
Basal ganglia or corpus striatum 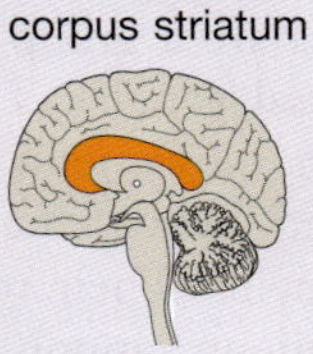	The mass of grey matter in the midbrain beneath the cerebral hemispheres. Borders the lateral ventricles and lies in proximity to the internal capsule	An important role in planning and coordinating motor movements and posture. Complex neural connections link the basal ganglia to the cerebral cortex. The major effect of these structures is to inhibit unwanted muscular activity; disorders of the basal ganglia result in exaggerated, uncontrolled movements
Pons 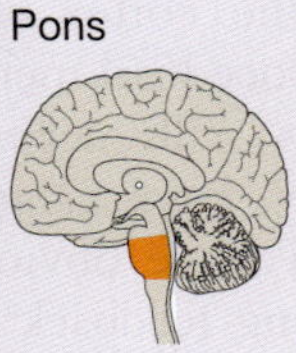	Anterior to the cerebellum	Connects the cerebellum with other portions of the brain; contains motor and sensory pathways; helps to regulate respiration; axons from the cerebellum, basal ganglia, thalamus and hypothalamus; portions of the pons also control the heart, respiration and blood pressure. Cranial nerves V–VIII connect the brain in the pons
Hindbrain	Contains a portion of the pons, the medulla oblongata and the cerebellum	
Reticular activation system (RAS) 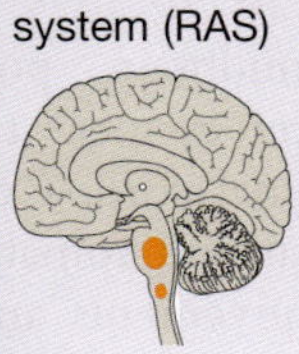	The reticular formation networks run through the brainstem core, known as the tegmentum	Activity of the cerebral cortex is dependent on both specific sensory input and non-specific activating impulses from the RAS, and is critical to the existence of the conscious state, states of alertness and arousal

Continued

TABLE 16.3
Organisation of the brain—cont'd

DIVISION	DESCRIPTION	FUNCTIONS
Midbrain		
Medulla oblongata 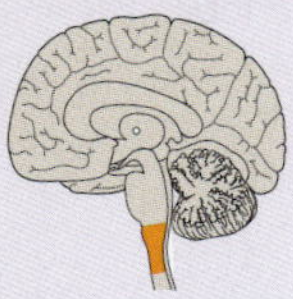	Between the pons and the spinal cord	The medulla oblongata contains motor fibres from the brain to the spinal cord and sensory fibres from the spinal cord to the brain. Most of these fibres cross at this level. Cranial nerves IX–XII connect to the brain in the medulla, which has centres for control of vital functions, such as respiration and the heart rate
Cerebellum 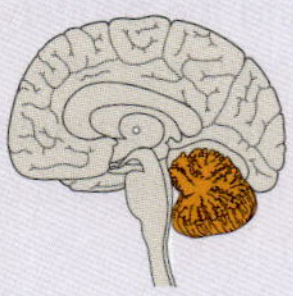	Below the posterior portion of the cerebellum. Divided into two hemispheres	Coordinates voluntary muscles; maintains balance and muscle tone; has both excitatory and inhibitory actions. It also controls fine movement, balance, position sense and integration of sensory input

FIGURE 16.5 Lateral view of the brainstem showing thalamus, midbrain, pons, and medulla.

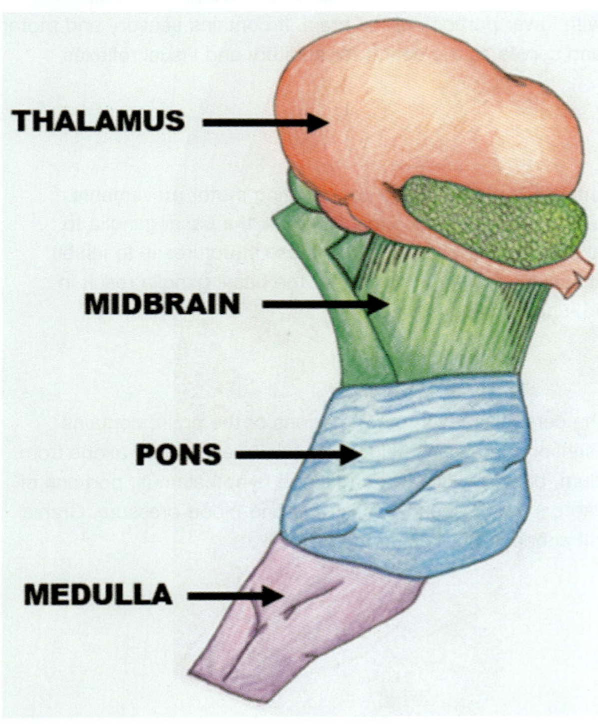

Courtesy Taylore Jansen.

of the body is represented by a corresponding region in both the primary motor cortex and the somatic sensory cortex.

The homunculus (Fig. 16.7) Is a visual representation of correlative neuroanatomy. Different areas of the body are shown by the corresponding areas in brain hemispheres. The body on the right side of Fig. 16.7 is the motor homunculus and on the left, the sensory homunculus. Representations of parts of the body that exhibit fine motor control and sensory capabilities occupy a greater amount of space than those that exhibit less precise motor or sensory functions.

Basal ganglia and cerebellum

The olfactory bulb, nucleus accumbens, putamen, globus pallidus, caudate, ventral pallidum, subthalamic nucleus and projections from the substantia nigra are a group of nuclei that collectively make up the basal ganglia. The basal ganglia play an important role in movement, as evidenced by the hypokinetic/rigid and hyper-kinetic disorders seen with lesions of related nuclei. Their role in the initiation and control of movement cannot be isolated from the motor activities of the cortex and brainstem centres discussed previously. Procedural memories for motor and other unconscious skills depend on the integrity of the premotor cortex, basal ganglia and cerebellum. The cerebellum plays a more obvious role in coordinating movements by giving feedback to the motor cortex, as well as by providing important influences on eye movements through brainstem connections, and on postural activity through projections down the spinal cord.

Brainstem

The brainstem is composed of the midbrain, pons and medulla oblongata.[10] These structures connect the cerebrum and diencephalon with the spinal cord. Collectively, these integrate vestibular, visual and somatosensory inputs for the control of eye movements and, through projections to the spinal cord, provide for postural adjustments. For example, these centres keep the images on matching regions of the retinas when the

FIGURE 16.6 (**A**) Major anatomical landmarks on the surface of the left cerebral hemisphere. The lateral sulcus has been pulled apart to expose the insula. (**B**) The left hemisphere usually contains the general interpretive area and the speech centre. The prefrontal cortex of each hemisphere is involved with conscious intellectual functions. (**C**) Regions of the cerebral cortex as determined by histological analysis. Several of the 47 regions described by Brodmann are shown for comparison with the results of functional mapping.

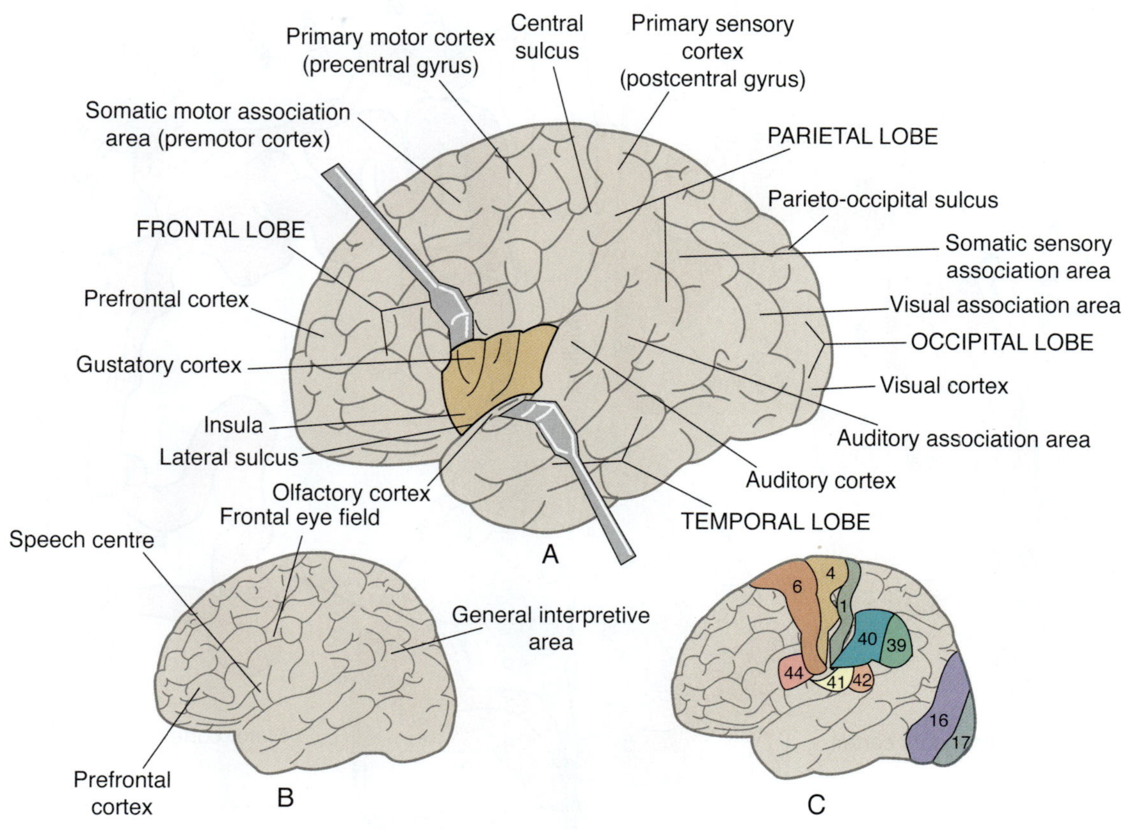

Source: Martini F, Nath JL, Bartholomew EF: Fundamentals of anatomy & physiology. 11th ed. ©2018. Printed and Electronically reproduced by permission of Pearson Education, Inc., New York, New York.

head moves by causing conjugate eye movements in the opposite direction to which the head is turned. This is the basis for the oculocephalic reflex test in neurological assessment, in which the head is rapidly turned and the eyes move conjugately in the opposite direction, demonstrating the integrity of much of the brainstem. The sequence of sleep states is governed by a group of brainstem nuclei that project widely throughout the brain and spinal cord.

The midbrain, inferior to the centre of the cerebrum, forms the superior part of the brainstem. It contains the reticular formation (which collects input from higher brain centres and passes it on to motor neurons), the substantia nigra (which regulates body movements – damage to the substantia nigra causes Parkinson's disease) and the ventral tegmental area (which contains dopamine-releasing neurons that are activated by nicotinic acetylcholine receptors). White matter in the anterior midbrain conducts impulses between the higher centres of the cerebrum and the lower centres of the pons, medulla, cerebellum and spinal cord. The midbrain contains autonomic reflex centres for pupillary accommodations to light (Edinger–Westphal nucleus), which receive stimuli via the optic nerve (CN-II) and send signals via the oculomotor nerve (CN-III) to cause pupillary constriction and accommodation of the lens. Hence, damage to CN-III will also produce a dilated pupil. It also contains the ventral tegmental area, packed with dopamine-releasing neurons that synapse deep within the forebrain and seem to be involved in pleasure: amphetamines and cocaine bind to the same receptors that it activates, and this may account at least in part for their addictive qualities.

The pons Varolii (pons) lies between the medulla oblongata and the midbrain (mesencephalon). It contains pneumotaxic and apneustic respiratory centres and fibre tracts connecting higher and lower centres, including the cerebellum. The pons seems to serve as a relay station,

FIGURE 16.7 Somatosensory and motor homunculi. Note that the size of each region of the homunculi is related to its importance in sensory or motor function, resulting in a distorted-appearing map.

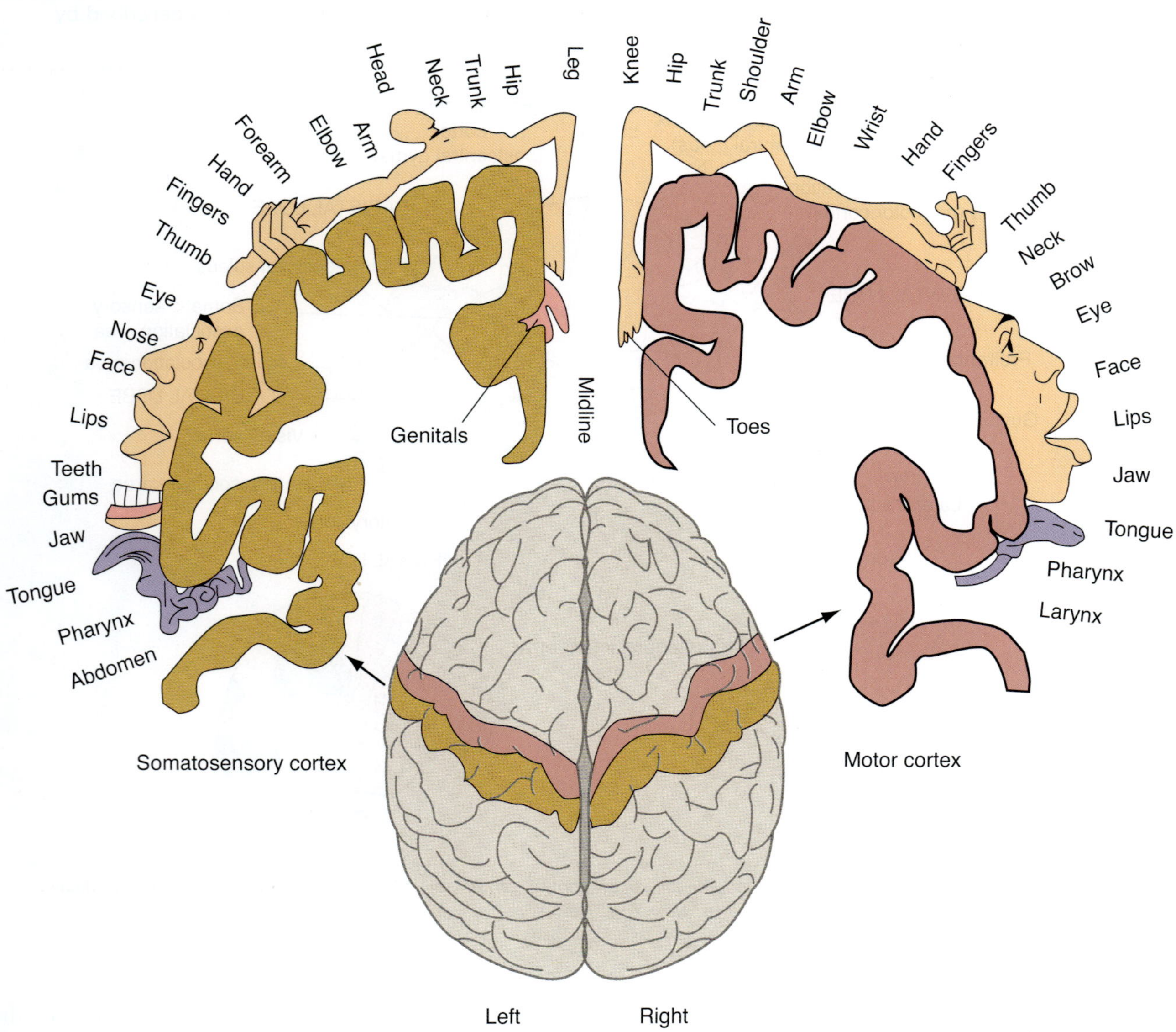

Adapted from Blumenfeld H. Neuroanatomy through clinical cases. New York: Sinauer Associates; 2010.

carrying signals from various parts of the cerebral cortex to the cerebellum. Nerve impulses coming from the eyes, ears and touch receptors are sent on to the cerebellum. The pons also participates in the reflexes that regulate breathing. Table 16.4 contains a description of the cranial nerves including their type of tract, their function and location of origin.

The medulla oblongata lies between the pons and the spinal cord and looks like a swollen tip to the spinal cord. Running down the ventral aspect of the medulla are the pyramids, which contain corticospinal fibres. The medulla oblongata controls automatic functions (e.g. breathing and heart rate) and relays nerve messages from the brain to the spinal cord. Processing of interaural time differences for sound localisation occurs in the olivary nuclei. The neurons controlling breathing have μ-receptors, the receptors to which opiates bind. This accounts for the suppressive effect of opiates on breathing. Impairment of any of the vital functions or reflexes involving these cranial nerves suggests medullary damage.

Limbic system

The limbic system includes the hypothalamus, the cingulate gyrus of the cortex, the amygdala and hippocampus in the temporal lobes and the septum and interconnecting nerve fibre tracts. The hypothalamus and limbic system, which are closely linked to homeostasis, act to

TABLE 16.4
The cranial nerves, their locations and functions

CRANIAL NERVE	TRACT(S)	FUNCTION	LOCATION OF ORIGIN
I Olfactory	Sensory	Sense of smell	Diencephalon
II Optic	Sensory	Vision	Diencephalon
III Oculomotor	Parasympathetic	Muscles that move the eye and lid, pupillary constriction, lens accommodation	Midbrain
	Motor	Elevation of upper eyelid and four of six extraocular movements	
IV Trochlear	Motor	Downward, inward movement of the eye (superior oblique)	Midbrain
V Trigeminal	Motor	Muscles of mastication and opening jaw	Pons
	Sensory	Tactile sensation to the cornea, nasal and oral mucosa and facial skin	
VI Abducens	Motor	Lateral deviation of eye (lateral rectus)	Pons
VII Facial	Parasympathetic	Secretory for salivation and tears	Pons
	Motor	Movement of the forehead, eyelids, cheeks, lips, ears, nose and neck to produce facial expression and close eyes	
	Sensory	Tactile sensation to parts of the external ear, auditory canal and external tympanic membrane	
		Taste sensation to the anterior two-thirds of the tongue	
VIII Vestibulocochlear	Sensory	Vestibular branch: equilibrium Cochlear branch: hearing	Pons
IX Glossopharyngeal	Parasympathetic	Salivation	Medulla
	Motor	Voluntary muscles for swallowing and phonation	
	Sensory	Sensation to pharynx, soft palate and posterior one-third of tongue	
		Stimulation elicits gag reflex	
X Vagus	Parasympathetic	Autonomic activity of viscera of thorax and abdomen	Medulla
	Motor	Voluntary swallowing and phonation	
		Involuntary activity of visceral muscles of the heart, lungs and digestive tract	
	Sensory	Sensation to the auditory canal and viscera of the thorax and abdomen	
XI Accessory	Motor	Sternocleidomastoid and trapezius muscle movements	Medulla
XII Hypoglossal	Motor	Tongue movements	Medulla

regulate endocrine secretion and the autonomic nervous system, and to influence behaviour through emotions and drives. The hypothalamus integrates information from the forebrain, brainstem, spinal cord and various endocrine systems. This area of the brain also contains some of the centres for coordinated parasympathetic and sympathetic stimulation, as well as those for temperature regulation, appetite regulation, regulation of water balance by antidiuretic hormone (ADH) and regulation of certain rhythmic psychobiological activities (e.g. sleep). The release of stored serotonin from axon terminals in the diencephalon suppresses activation of the ascending reticular activating system (ARAS). The ARAS controls sleep, waking, and fight-vs-flight responses. Suppression of the ARAS results in increased sleep or sleep-like states. The hypothalamus contains a plethora of neurotransmitters. These are found in the terminals of axons that originate from neurons outside the hypothalamus, but most are synthesised within the hypothalamus itself. The list of chemicals thought to act as neurotransmitters includes the 'classic' transmitters ACh, GABA, glutamate, serotonin, dopamine and noradrenaline, as well as literally dozens of peptides that have been identified in recent years.

Protection and support of the brain

The brain occupies the cranial cavity and is covered by membranes, fluid and the bones of the skull. The delicate tissues of the brain are protected from mechanical forces by 1) the bones of the cranium, 2) the cranial meninges and 3) cerebrospinal fluid. In addition, the neural tissue of the brain is biochemically isolated from the general circulation by the blood–brain barrier.

> **Practice tip**
>
> Openings in the fourth ventricle permits cerebrospinal fluid to enter subarachnoid spaces surrounding both the brain and the spinal cord.

FIGURE 16.8 Circulation of the cerebrospinal fluid (CSF): sagittal section indicating CSF presence (light blue), and routes of circulation of CSF (arrows).

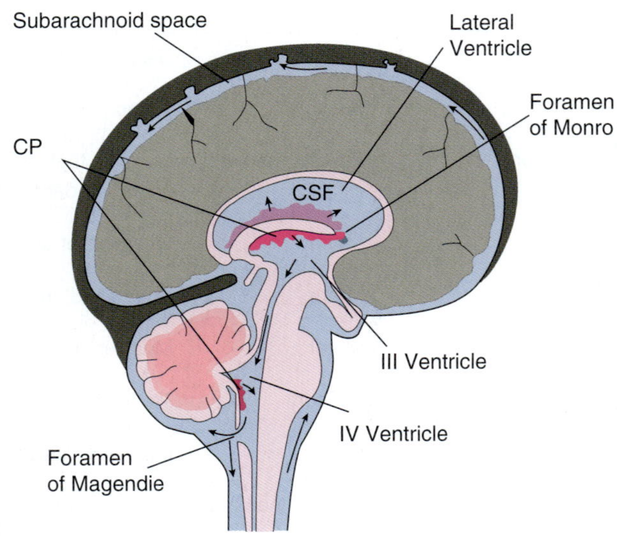

Source: Santos CRA, Duarte AC, Quintela T, et al. The choroid plexus as a sex hormone target: Functional implications. Front Neuroendocrinol 2017;44:103–121.

Cerebral spinal fluid

Cerebral spinal fluid (CSF) is an ultrafiltrate of blood plasma composed of 99% water with other constituents, making it close to the composition of the brain extracellular fluid. Approximately 500 mL of CSF is secreted each day, but only approximately 150 mL is in the ventricular system at any one time, meaning that the CSF is continuously being absorbed. The CSF produced in the ventricles must flow through the interventricular foramen, the third ventricle, the cerebral aqueduct and the fourth ventricle to exit from the neural tube.

Three openings, or foramina, allow the CSF to pass into the subarachnoid space (Fig. 16.8). Approximately 30% of the CSF passes down into the subarachnoid space that surrounds the spinal cord, mainly on its dorsal surface, and moves back up to the cranial cavity along its ventral surface. Reabsorption of CSF into the vascular system occurs through a pressure gradient. The normal CSF pressure is approximately 10 mmHg in the lateral recumbent position, although it may be as low as 5 mmHg or as high as 15 mmHg in healthy persons. The microstructure of the arachnoid villi is such that, if the CSF pressure falls below approximately 3 mmHg, the passageways collapse and reverse flow is blocked. Arachnoid villi function as one-way valves, permitting CSF outflow into the blood but not allowing blood to pass into the arachnoid spaces. The pressure in the CSF manifests as normal intracranial pressure (ICP).

Blood–brain–CSF barrier

The CNS is richly supplied with blood vessels that bring oxygen and nutrients to its cells. However, many substances cannot easily be exchanged between blood and brain because the endothelial cells of the vessels and the astrocytes of the CNS form extremely tight junctions, collectively referred to as the blood–brain barrier (BBB). In particular, small non-charged, lipid-soluble molecules can cross the BBB with ease. Evidence suggests that the BBB maintains the chemical environment for neuronal function and protects the brain from harmful substances. Substances in the blood that gain rapid entry to the brain include glucose, the important source of energy, certain ions that maintain a proper medium for electrical activity and oxygen for cellular respiration. Small fat-soluble molecules, like ethanol, pass through the BBB. Some water-soluble molecules pass into the brain carried by special proteins in the plasma membrane of the endothelial cells. Excluded molecules include proteins, toxins, most antibiotics and monoamines (e.g. neurotransmitters). Some of these unwanted molecules are actively transported out of the endothelial cells. When injured (by force or infection or oxidative processes), the permeability of the BBB is disrupted, allowing a proliferation of various chemicals and molecules – even bacteria – into the brain parenchyma, with at times devastating consequences.

Cerebral circulation

The brain must maintain a constant flow of blood in order for brain activity to occur. The arterial cerebral blood flow (CBF) to the brain consists of approximately 20% of the cardiac output (Fig. 16.9). Normal CBF is 750 mL/min. The brain autoregulates CBF over a wide range of blood pressures by vasodilation or vasoconstriction of the arteries. In response to decreased arterial flow, the arteries that make up the circle of Willis can act as a protective mechanism by shunting blood from one side to the other or from the anterior to posterior portions of the brain. This compensatory mechanism delays neurological deterioration in patients.

The cerebral veins drain into large venous sinuses and then into the right and left internal jugular veins (Fig. 16.10). The venous sinuses are found within the folds of the dura mater. Unlike most veins in the body, the veins and sinuses of the brain do not have valves, so the blood flows freely by gravity. The face and scalp veins

FIGURE 16.9 The major arteries of the brain: (**A**) ventral view: the enlargement of the boxed area showing the circle of Willis; (**B**) lateral and (**C**) mid-sagittal views showing anterior, middle and posterior cerebral arteries; (**D**) idealised frontal section showing the course of middle cerebral artery.

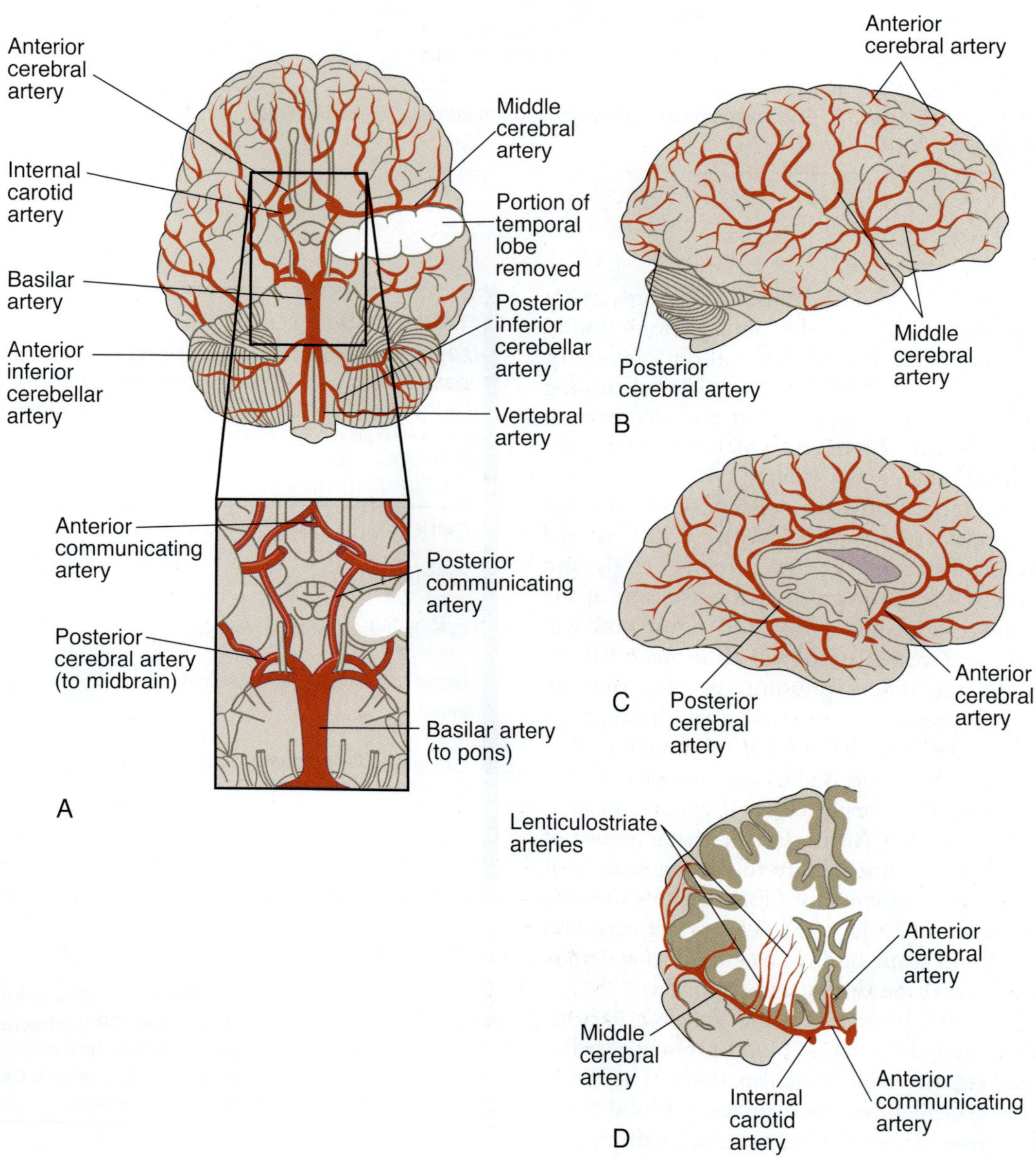

Source: Purves D, Augustine G, Hall W, et al. Neuroscience. 5th ed. New York: Sinauer Associates; 2012, Oxford University Press.

FIGURE 16.10 Cerebral venous drainage.

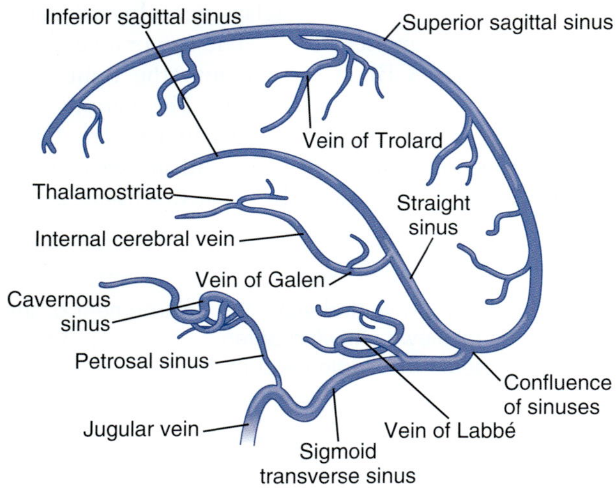

Source: Hemmings HC, Egan TD. Pharmacology and physiology for anesthesia: foundations and clinical application. 2nd ed. Philadelphia: Elsevier; 2019.

can flow into the brain venous sinuses; therefore, infection can easily be spread into the dural venous sinuses and then enter the brain. Patient position can prevent or promote venous drainage from the brain. Head turning and tilting may kink the jugular vein and decrease or stop venous flow from the brain, which will then raise the pressure inside the cranial vault.

CBF is the cerebral perfusion pressure (CPP) divided by cerebrovascular resistance (CVR). CVR is the amount of resistance created by the cerebral vessels, and it is controlled by the autoregulatory mechanisms of the brain. Specifically, vasoconstriction (and vasospasm) will increase CVR, and vasodilation will decrease CVR. It is influenced by the inflow pressure (systole), outflow pressure (venous pressure), cross-sectional diameter of cerebral blood vessels and ICP. CVR is similar to systemic vascular resistance but, due to the lack of valves in the venous system of the brain, cerebral venous pressure also influences the CVR. An important characteristic of the cerebral circulation is its ability to autoregulate; that is, the ability to maintain constant CBF despite variations in perfusion pressure (Table 16.5). This is important in protecting the brain from both ischaemia during hypotension and haemorrhage during hypertension.

CBF is affected by extrinsic and intrinsic factors. Extrinsic factors include systemic blood pressure, cardiac output, blood viscosity and vascular tone. The body responds to these demands with changes in blood flow. Aerobic metabolism requires oxygen in order to process glucose for normal energy production (production of adenosine triphosphate [ATP]). The brain does not store energy and therefore requires a constant source

TABLE 16.5

Changes in cerebrovascular and cerebrometabolic parameters when various cerebral variables are reduced with and without intact autoregulation

PRIMARY REDUCTION IN THESE VARIABLES	CBF	CBV (ICP)	$AVDO_2$
$CMRO_2$	↑	↓	–
CPP (autoregulation intact)	–	↑	–
CPP (autoregulation defective)	↓	↓	↑
Blood viscosity (autoregulation intact)	–	↓	–
Blood viscosity (autoregulation defective)	↑	–	↓
$PaCO_2$	↓	↓	↑
Conductive vessel diameter (vasospasm above ischaemic threshold)	↓	↑	↑

$AVDO_2$ = arteriovenous O_2 difference; CBF = cerebral blood flow; CBV = cerebral blood volume; ICP = intracranial pressure; $CMRO_2$ = cerebral metabolic rate of oxygen; CPP = cerebral perfusion pressure; $PaCO_2$ = arterial CO_2 tension; ↑ = increase; ↓ = decrease; – = no change.

FIGURE 16.11 The spinal cord and spinal meninges: (**A**) posterior view of the spinal cord, showing the meningeal layers, superficial landmarks and distribution of grey matter and white matter; (**B**) sectional view through the spinal cord and meninges, showing the peripheral distribution of spinal nerves.

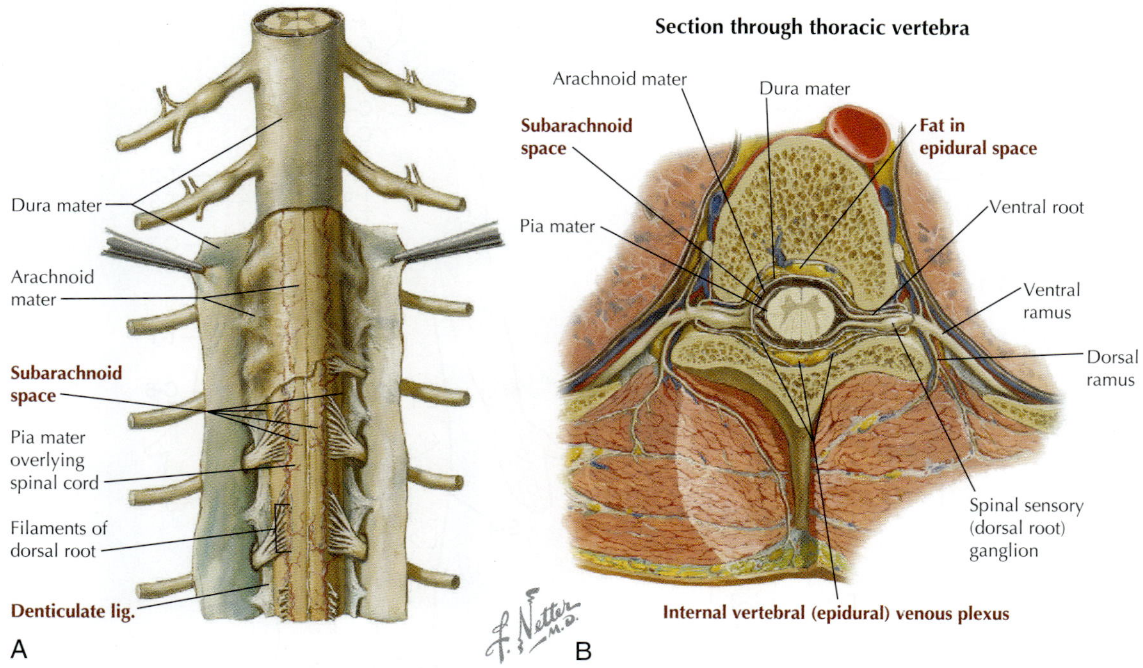

Source: Hansen JT. Netter's Clinical anatomy. 4th ed. Philadelphia: Elsevier; 2019.

of oxygen and energy, its supply from CBF can be exhausted within 3 min. Intrinsic factors include $PaCO_2$ (pH), PaO_2 and ICP. The vessels dilate with increases in $PaCO_2$ (hypercarbia) or low pH (acidosis) and with decreases in PaO_2 (hypoxia). This vasodilation increases CBF. The vessels constrict with decreases in $PaCO_2$ or high pH and with increases in local PaO_2. This vasoconstriction will decrease the CBF. In addition, intrinsic factors can change the extrinsic factors by altering the metabolic mechanisms. These changes can lead to an alteration in the CBF. For example, there can be a change from aerobic to anaerobic metabolism, which increases the concentrations of other end-products such as lactic acid, pyruvic acid and carbonic acid, which causes a localised acidosis. These end-products result in a decrease in pH that will cause an increase in CBF. Other factors that can affect CBF include pharmacological agents (anaesthetic agents and some antihypertensive agents), rapid-eye-movement sleep, arousal, pain, seizures, elevations in body temperature and cerebral trauma.

Spinal cord

The spinal cord is the link between the PNS and the brain.[13] The spinal cord has a small, irregularly shaped internal section of unmyelinated tissue (grey matter) surrounded by a larger area of myelinated axons (white matter). The grey matter is arranged so that it extends up and down dorsally in a column; one on each side; another column is found in the ventral region on each side (Fig. 16.11).

The spinal cord is an essential component of both the sensory and motor divisions of the nervous system. The first of the primary functions of the spinal cord is to transmit sensory impulses along the ascending tracts to the brain and transmit motor impulses down the descending tracts away from the brain. The second primary function of the spinal cord is to house and regulate spinal reflexes.[5] Receipt of sensory impulses may cause a reaction anywhere in the body; alternatively, the signal might be stored in the memory to be used at some stage in the future. Within the motor division of the nervous system the spinal cord helps to control the various bodily activities, including skeletal muscle activity, smooth muscle activity and secretion by both endocrine and exocrine glands.

Sensory neurons from all over the skin, except for the skin of the face and scalp, feed information into the spinal cord through the spinal nerves. As shown in Fig. 16.12, the skin surface can be mapped into distinct

FIGURE 16.12 (**A**) Anterior and (**B**) posterior distributions of dermatomes on the surface of the skin.

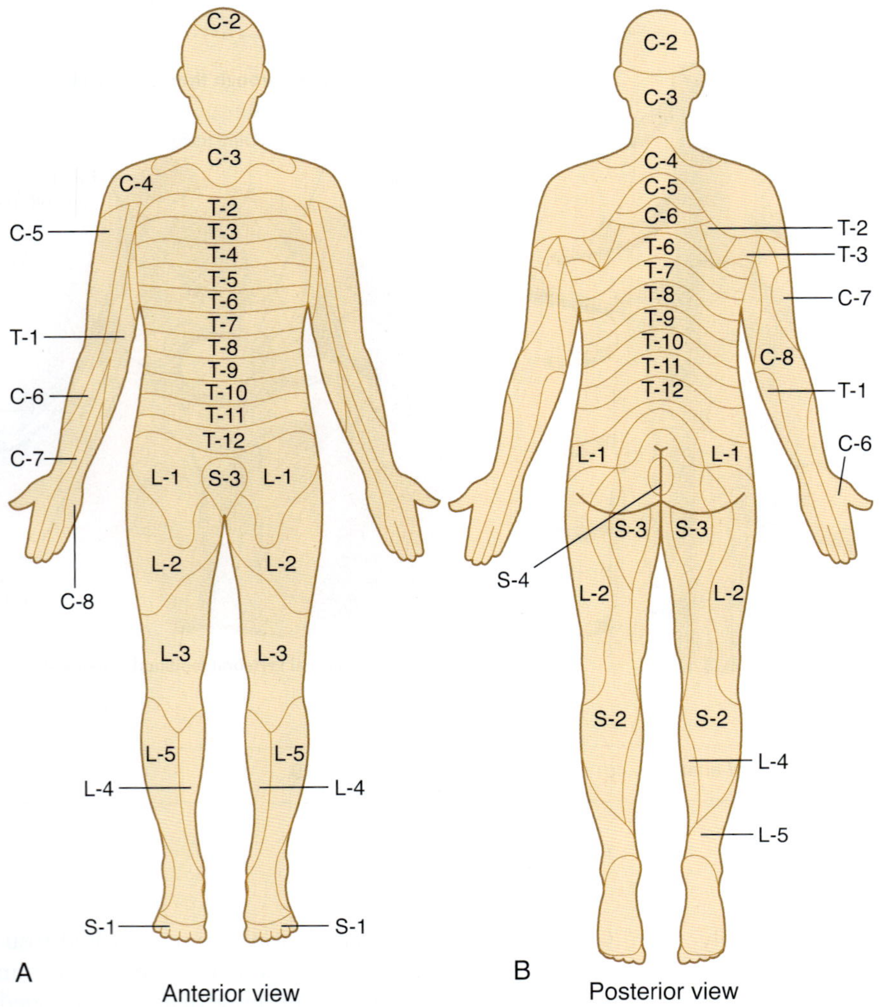

regions called dermatomes. Each dermatome corresponds to a single spinal nerve. Sensation from a given dermatome is carried over its corresponding spinal nerve. This information can be used to identify the spinal nerve or spinal segment that is involved in an injury. In some areas, the dermatomes are not absolutely distinct. Some dermatomes may share a nerve supply with neighbouring regions. For this reason, it is often necessary to numb adjacent dermatomes to achieve adequate anaesthesia.

The blood supply to the spinal cord arises from branches of the vertebral arteries and spinal radicular arteries. The mid-thoracic region, at approximately T4–T8, lies between the lumbar and vertebral arterial supplies and is a vulnerable zone of relatively decreased perfusion. This region is most susceptible to infarction during periods of hypotension, thoracic surgery or other conditions, causing decreased aortic pressure and potentially leading to ischaemic spinal injury with devastating consequences.

Peripheral nervous system

The PNS consists of 12 pairs of cranial nerves, 31 pairs of spinal nerves, and all neural structures lying outside the spinal cord and brainstem. The cranial nerves have previously been discussed regarding their role in brainstem function (see Table 16.4). The PNS has both motor and sensory components. The former includes the motor neuron cell body in the anterior horn of the spinal cord and its peripheral axonal process travelling through the ventral root and eventually the peripheral nerve. The motor nerve terminal, together with the muscle endplate and the synapse between the two, comprises the neuromuscular junction. The peripheral sensory axon, beginning at receptors in cutaneous and deep structures, as well as muscle and tendon receptors, travels back through peripheral nerves to its cell body located in the dorsal root ganglion. Its central process, travelling through the dorsal root, enters the spinal cord in the region of the dorsal horn. All commands for movement, whether reflexive or voluntary, are ultimately conveyed to the muscles by the activity of the lower motor neurons.

Motor control

Movements can be divided into three main classes: voluntary activity, rhythmic motor patterns and reflex responses. The highest-order activity, voluntary movement, allows for expression of the will and a purposeful response to the environment (e.g. reading, speaking, performing calculations). Such activity is goal-directed and largely learned, and improves with practice. In rhythmic motor patterns, the initiation and termination may be voluntary, but the rhythmic activity itself does not require conscious participation (e.g. chewing, walking, running). Reflex responses are simple, stereotyped responses that do not involve voluntary control (e.g. deep tendon reflexes or withdrawal of a limb from a hot surface). Motor control is carried out in a hierarchical, yet parallel, fashion in the cerebral cortex, the brainstem and the spinal cord. Modulating influences are provided by the basal ganglia and cerebellum through the thalamus.

Sensory control

The sensory control is responsible for detecting, interpreting and transmitting external signals. There are several different types of sensory neurons and these can be encapsulated or they can be non-encapsulated; both extend to the periphery (i.e. skin) and primarily respond to pressure, vibration, or temperature. A very light pressure may be interpreted as light touch where as a focalised high pressure may be interpreted as pain. The processing of sensory stimuli begins with a combination of mechanical and chemical signalling that causes ion channels (sodium) to open. The change in polarity becomes an electrical signal that is transmitted along the nerve and processed in the brain as pain, touch, tension, temperature, or vibration.

Autonomic nervous system

The autonomic nervous system, with its three major divisions (sympathetic, parasympathetic and enteric), is largely an involuntary system and is part of the efferent division, as shown in Fig. 16.1. The autonomic nervous system allows the body to adjust to rapidly changing external events (the 'flight or fight' response of the sympathetic division) and to regulate internal activities (blood pressure, temperature, airway and breathing, urinary function, digestion by the parasympathetic and enteric divisions). Whereas the major controlling centres for somatic (i.e. voluntary) motor activity are the primary and secondary motor cortices in the frontal lobes and a variety of related brainstem nuclei, the major locus of central control in the visceral motor system is the hypothalamus and the complex circuitry that it controls in the brainstem tegmentum and spinal cord.[5] The status of both divisions of the visceral motor system is modulated by descending pathways from these centres to preganglionic neurons in the brainstem and spinal cord, which in turn determine the activity of the primary visceral motor neurons in autonomic ganglia.[5]

The postganglionic neurons of the sympathetic system, with few exceptions, act on their effectors by releasing the neurotransmitter adrenaline and the related compound noradrenaline. This system is therefore described as adrenergic, which means 'activated by adrenaline'. The autonomic regulation of various organ systems of particular importance in clinical practice is illustrated in Fig. 16.13.

Neurological assessment and monitoring

This section explores the complex issues surrounding cerebral haemodynamics and assessment. The objective of assessment is to determine the extent of neurological injury, recognise fluctuations in condition and imminent deterioration and assist in maintaining cerebral perfusion as part of multimodal monitoring.

Physical examination

The neurological exam begins at the onset of patient contact, and the priorities are defined by a primary survey and vital signs. The patient's history and contact with family help to inform the clinical examination. The history should include the patient's normal baseline status and past neurological symptoms such as syncope or seizures. Additional information about medication use and other substance use should be included in the history.[10]

Specific areas tested during the initial neurological exam include level of consciousness, general behaviour, memory, attention and concentration, abstract thought or judgement, motor function, sensory function, and cranial nerve function. Not every aspect of the examination will be relevant in all critical care situations and therefore may not be tested. Nevertheless, the clinician should understand how all components are integrated and how they influence priority decision making for patient care.

While the essential components of the neurological exam are similar, components of the exam should be individualised to the patient's ability. It may be necessary to modify assessment techniques; for example, intubated patients who are otherwise awake and aware may gesture or write answers to questions instead of verbalising them. In addition, when patients are the recipients of very frequent neurological assessment over an extended period of time (including arousal and awareness, pupil and motor response), sleep and sensory rest deprivation is common.[14,15] Sleep deprivation and sensory overload may confound assessment accuracy. Consideration needs to be given in regard to the priorities of assessment and rest; a plan needs to implemented to promote rest

FIGURE 16.13 Sympathetic and parasympathetic divisions of the autonomic nervous system. Sympathetic outputs (**left**) arise from thoracolumbar spinal cord segments and synapses in paravertebral and prevertebral ganglia. Parasympathetic outputs (**right**) arise from craniosacral regions and synapses in ganglia in or near effector organs.

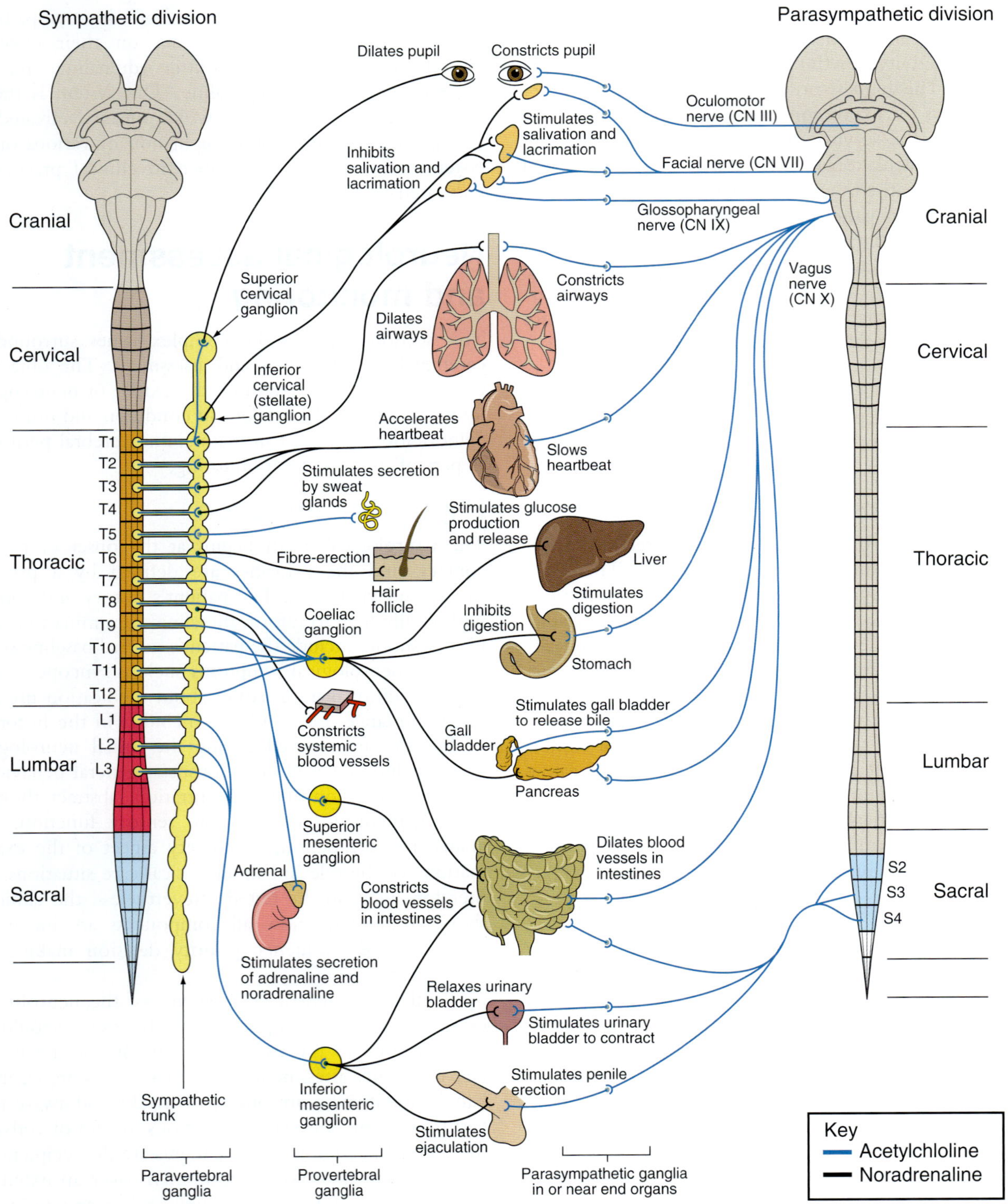

Adapted from Blumenfeld H. Neuroanatomy through clinical cases. New York: Sinauer Associates; 2010.

as neurological injury requires rest and sleep for restoration.[16] See *Online resources* for links to a full neurological assessment and physical examination protocol.

> **Practice tip**
>
> Evaluation of the level of consciousness and mentation are the most important parts of the neurological examination. A change in either is often the first clue to CNS dysfunction.

Conscious state

Consciousness can be defined in terms of an individual's internal awareness of self and external awareness of environment. Hence, awareness, arousal, and responsiveness are fundamental constituents of consciousness and should be evaluated and documented repeatedly for trend analysis. Changes in the level of consciousness are often the first sign of neurological deterioration.[17,18]

Arousal or responsiveness assessment

Evaluation of arousal typically scores the patient's response to stimuli. The Alert, Verbal, Pain, Unresponsive (AVPU) scale, the Richmond Agitation Sedation Scale (RASS), and the Glasgow Coma Scale (GCS) each have elements that assess the patient's ability to respond to stimuli.[19-22] The advanced trauma life support course recommends an initial assessment during initial resuscitation based on the response to stimulation: **A**wake, **V**erbal, **P**ain, **U**nresponsive (AVPU). Observe the patient's response (verbal or motor). If there is no response to voice or light touch, painful stimulus is needed to assess neurological status. Central pain should be used first and applied with care. Sternal rub, supraorbital pressure (least used), trapezius pinch (most used) or pinching the fleshy portion of the upper arm near the axilla are methods for introducing central pain. Hand grasp is a reflex and is unreliable to test motor strength or cognitive capacity. If the patient does not respond to verbal stimulus but moves spontaneously in a purposeful manner (picks at linen, pulls at tubes), the patient is localising. Localising is purposeful and intentional movement intended to eliminate a noxious stimulus, whereas withdrawal is a 'smaller' movement used to 'get away from' noxious stimulus. Painful stimulus is not required if spontaneous localisation has been observed. Watch for symmetry. Abnormal flexion differs from withdrawal in that the flexion is rigid and looks abnormal. Abnormal extension is a rigid movement with extension of the limbs.[23,24]

> **Practice tip**
>
> When a patient opens their eyes when you call their name, it is an indication that their reticular activating centre (brainstem) functioning is intact but it does not tell you if they are awake or aware.

> **Practice tip**
>
> Awareness means that the cerebral cortex is working in conjunction with the reticular activating system (arousal) and that the patient can interact with and interpret their environment.

Assessment of awareness and responsiveness

Awareness and responsiveness can be assessed using the GCS or the Full Outline of UnResponsivness (FOUR) score.[25,26] The GCS was developed to establish an objective, quantifiable measure to describe the prognosis of a patient with a traumatic brain injury (TBI) and includes scoring of separate subscales related to eye opening, verbal response and motor response (Table 16.6). Originally, the

TABLE 16.6
Glasgow Coma Scale

The Glasgow Coma Scale is scored between 3 and 15, 3 being the worst, and 15 the best. It comprises three parameters: best eye response, best verbal response and best motor response. The definition of these parameters is given below

THE GLASGOW COMA SCALE FOR ADULTS	PAEDIATRIC VERSION OF THE GLASGOW COMA SCALE
Best eye response (4)	Best eye response (4)
1 No eye opening	1 No eye opening
2 Eye opening to pain	2 Eye opening to pain
3 Eye opening to verbal command	3 Eye opening to verbal command
4 Eyes open spontaneously	4 Eyes open spontaneously
Best verbal response (5)	Best verbal response (5)
1 No verbal response	1 No vocal response
2 Incomprehensible sounds	2 Occasionally whimpers and/or moans
3 Inappropriate words	3 Cries inappropriately
4 Confused	4 Less than usual ability and/or spontaneous irritable cry
5 Orientated	5 Alert, babbles, coos, words or sentences to usual ability
Best motor response (6)	Best motor response (6)
1 No motor response	1 No motor response to pain
2 Extension to pain	2 Abnormal extension to pain (decerebrate)
3 Flexion to pain	3 Abnormal flexion to pain (decorticate)
4 Withdrawal from pain	4 Withdrawal to painful stimuli
5 Localising pain	5 Localises to painful stimuli or withdraws to touch
6 Obeys commands	6 Obeys commands or performs normal spontaneous movements

GCS was developed as three separate response areas and reported as such.[21] Contemporary use of the GCS automatically adds the three best response scores and easily loses the information given from the separate response areas. Reporting the GCS as three numbers and then the total gives a broader assessment interpretation.

The advantage of the GCS is that it allows rapid serial comparisons and categorisation of basic neurological function over time.[27] However, it has several recognised weaknesses, including poor prediction of outcome beyond survival, poor inter-rater reliability and inconsistent use in the prehospital and hospital settings. GCS accuracy will be affected if the patient is receiving anaesthetic agents or sedation and noxious stimuli should be avoided. Furthermore, the rare event of a *locked-in syndrome*, where a patient is neurologically aware and awake but not responding, is poorly represented by the GCS. Also, interpretation of response in regard to language used or a previous communication disability is important for assessment accuracy.[27] See *Online resources* for a link to a full GCS procedure.

The FOUR score (Fig. 16.14) is an accurate predictor of outcome in TBI.[27] It is easy to learn, remember and administer. The four components of the FOUR score are: 1) best eye response, 2) best motor response, 3) best brainstem response, and 4) evaluation of the respiratory pattern. Component sub-scores range from 0 (worst) to 4 (best), and can be rated in intubated patients, with equal weight given to each component. Best eye response is voluntary eye movement or tracking and worst eye response is no eye opening to painful stimuli. Best motor response is the ability to follow commands and worst is the absence of any motor response to painful stimuli. Best brainstem response is intact pupillary light reflex and corneal reflex, worst is the absence of pupil, corneal and cough reflexes. Respiratory pattern further evaluates brainstem function. Regular rate of respirations receives a score of 4, irregular a score of 3, Cheyne–Stokes respirations a score of 2. The intubated patient who breathes spontaneously or triggers the ventilator will receive a score of 1 and the patient who fails to trigger the ventilator (no spontaneous breaths) receives a score of 0. If all four components are graded at zero, brain death testing is suggested. The FOUR score may help the examiner to localise lesions and diagnose the patient with locked-in syndrome.

The administration of the FOUR offers a few specific advantages over utilising the GCS.[28] The FOUR adds to the eye opening of the GCS by testing eye tracking, thus incorporating midbrain and pontine functions. It allows for testing of afferent language processing and remains testable regardless of endotracheal intubation, aphasia, aphonia or trauma to the vocal apparatus. It adds to the motor score of the GCS, incorporating hand gestures into the evaluation. The bulk of the motor score is similar to the GCS except that no difference is delineated between flexor posturing and normal flexion to pain. Specific testing of brainstem reflexes via pupillary, corneal and cough reflexes further allows the clinician to localise lesions and track progression of cerebral injury, specifically by addressing unilateral fixed mydriasis, a sign alerting to uncal herniation.[28,29]

FIGURE 16.14 The Full Outline of UnResponsiveness (FOUR) Score.

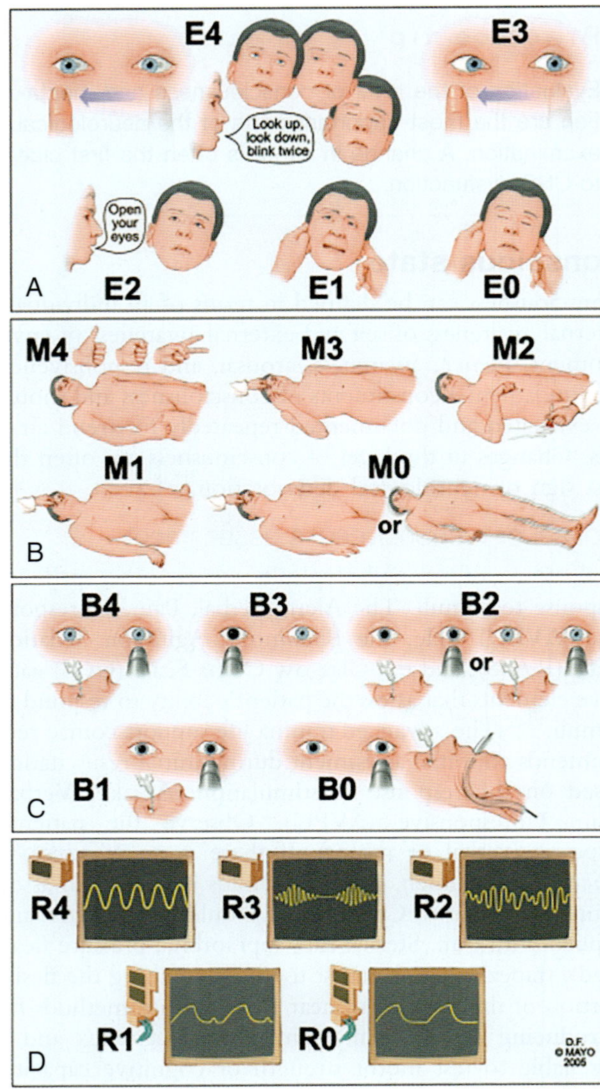

Adapted from Wijdicks EF, Bamlet WR, Maramattom BV, et al. Validation of a new coma scale: The FOUR score. Ann Neurol 2005;58(4):585-593, with permission.

Eye and pupil assessment

Pupillary responses, including pupil size and reaction to light, are important neurological observations and localise cerebral disease to a specific area of the brain. The immediate constriction of the pupil in response to light is referred to as the direct light reflex or pupillary light reflex (PLR). Removal of the light should result in dilation of the pupil. Introduction of the light into one eye should cause a similar constriction to occur in the other pupil (consensual light reaction).[30]

Other points to consider when conducting pupillary observations include the following:

- Pinpoint non-reactive pupils are associated with opiate use.
- Non-reactive pupils may also be caused by local damage.
- Atropine will cause dilated pupils.
- One dilated or fixed pupil may be indicative of an expanding or developing intracranial lesion, compressing the oculomotor nerve on the same side of the brain as the affected pupil.[31]
- A sluggish pupil may be difficult to distinguish from a fixed pupil and may be an early focal sign of an expanding intracranial lesion and raised ICP. A sluggish response to light in a previously reacting pupil must be reported immediately.[32,33]

Assessment of pupillary function focuses on three areas: 1) estimation of pupil size and shape; 2) evaluation of pupillary reaction to light; and 3) assessment of eye movements. Metabolic disturbances rarely cause pupillary changes, so abnormal pupillary findings are usually due to a nervous system lesion. Irregular-sized pupils are normal for some people and eye prostheses are common; it is important to establish and document these findings so a trend can be established to distinguish normal from altered states. However, subjective observations of pupillary function by human observers are not reliable.[32]

Handheld automated pupillometry is now widely available and provides objective scores for the pupillary light reflex previously unobtainable by subjective assessment. Pupillometry provides an objective score of the initial pupil size, latency in responding to light, constriction velocity, pupil size at maximum constriction, and pupil dilation velocity.[34] Current pupillometers also provide an indexed value to compare the observed result to known normal values. Lower indexed pupillometer values have been associated with higher ICP values.[35] See *Online resources* for a link to completing a pupillometry assessment.

> **Practice tip**
>
> Localising to painful stimuli is purposeful and intentional movement intended to eliminate a noxious stimulus, whereas withdrawal is a 'smaller' movement used to 'get away from' a noxious stimulus.

Eye and eyelid movements

Patients who are comatose will exhibit no eye opening. In patients with bilateral thalamic damage, there may be normal consciousness, but an eye-opening apraxia (i.e. non-paralytic motor abnormality characterised by difficulty initiating the act of lid elevation after lid closure) may mimic coma.[36] If the patient's eyes are closed, the clinician should gently raise and release the eyelids. Brisk opening and closing of the eyes indicates that the pons is grossly intact. If the pons is impaired, one or both eyelids may close slowly or not at all. In the patient with intact frontal lobe and brainstem functioning, the eyes, when opened, should be pointed straight ahead and at equal height. If there is awareness, the patient should look towards stimuli after eye opening. Eye deviation indicates either a unilateral cerebral or brainstem lesion. If the eyes deviate laterally, gently turn the head to see if the eyes will cross the midline to the other side. A pattern of spontaneous, slow and random movements (usually laterally) is termed 'roving-eye movements'. This indicates that the brainstem oculomotor control is intact but awareness is significantly impaired.[37]

Limb movement

Assessment of extremities and body movement (or motor response) provides valuable information about the patient with a decreased level of consciousness. The clinician must observe the patient's spontaneous movements, muscle tone and response to tactile stimuli. Decorticate (flexor) posturing is seen when there is involvement of a cerebral hemisphere and the brain stem. It is characterised by adduction of the shoulder and arm, elbow flexion and pronation and flexion of the wrist while the legs extend.[38] In terms of the GCS motor score, the *withdrawal flexor* scores higher (4/6) than a *spastic flexor* movement (3/6). Decerebrate (extensor) posturing is seen with severe metabolic disturbances or upper brainstem lesions. It is characterised by extension and pronation of the arm(s) and extension of the legs. Patients may have an asymmetrical response and may posture spontaneously or to stimuli.[39]

Motor tone is first assessed by flexing the limbs and noting increased or absent tone. If no tone is present, the hand is lifted approximately 30 cm above the bed and carefully dropped while protecting the limb from injury. The test is repeated with all extremities. Typically, the lower the level of consciousness, the closer to flaccid the limb(s) will be. An asymmetrical examination may indicate a lesion in the contralateral hemisphere or brainstem.

The next assessment, *peripheral reflex response*, is response to tactile stimuli peripherally and usually elicits a reflex response rather than a central or brain response. It is important to apply stimuli in a progressive manner, *using the least noxious stimuli necessary to elicit a response.* If there is no response to light or firm pressure, the clinician must use noxious stimuli. Each extremity is assessed individually. The typical technique for peripheral noxious stimuli involves pressure on the nail beds for asserting a peripheral stimulus. The triple-flexion response is a withdrawal of the limb in a straight line with flexion of the wrist–elbow–shoulder or the ankle–knee–hip. This response is considered a spinal reflex and is not an indication of brain involvement in the movement. The triple-flexion response is common in patients with severe neurological impairment and may be seen in patients who progressed to brain death. Care must be taken to avoid confusion between brain and spinal-mediated responses. If the patient has any other motor activity to peripheral extremity noxious stimuli, it is an indication of higher brain function.

If a noxious stimulus is applied *centrally* through a sternal rub, trapezius pinch or supraorbital nerve pressure and the patient moves an extremity, it is an indication of brain involvement in the movement and not a spinal reflex. The movement should be noted as normal, decorticate (flexor: either withdrawal or spastic) or decerebrate (extensor) and documented accordingly. It should be noted that careful consideration should be given to the choice of noxious stimuli with trapezius pinch the preferred choice as both sternal rub and supraorbital nerve pressure can be traumatic when applied. In ventilated patients, endotracheal suction can also be a substitute for a central noxious stimulus, but the choice of stimulus needs to be consistent.

Practice tip

The ability to cough with suctioning can be tested in an intubated patient and implies an intact cranial nerve X.

Facial symmetry

Subtle facial symmetry may be difficult to appreciate in patients with oedema, endotracheal tube tape and nasogastric tubes. An asymmetric response is indicative of a lesion of the facial cranial nerve (CN VII). Complete hemi-facial involvement is typically seen in peripheral dysfunction (Bell's palsy), whereas superior division (forehead) sparing weakness indicates a pontine/medullary (central) involvement. It is important to refrain from supraorbital pressure until after pupillary responses have been assessed because this noxious stimulation may cause alteration in pupillary reactivity.

Corneal reflexes

Corneal reflexes are routinely assessed only in the unconscious patient. The corneal reflex is a protective mechanism (protect the eye) and therefore improper testing could result in damage to the eye. This tests the sensory portion of the trigeminal nerve (CN V) and motor portion of the facial nerve (CN VII). To test this reflex in the unconscious patient, gently hold the eye open and allow a drop of sterile saline (may use isotonic eye drops) to land on the cornea. The patient with an intact reflex will blink (also termed 'blink to threat') in response. Due to the risk of corneal abrasion, the practice of touching the cornea with a wisp of cotton should be limited to the outer canthus.

Oropharyngeal reflexes

The oropharyngeal reflex (also called gag reflex) tests the sensory and motor function of the vagus nerve (CN X) and glossopharyngeal nerve (CN IX). The gag reflex is important in providing protection to the airway (avoid aspiration). Ask the awake patient to open their mouth and then use a soft-tipped applicator or suction catheter to lightly touch the soft palate in the back of their throat. The patient should gag if this reflex is intact. In the less responsive patient, this manoeuvre is often performed when providing oral hygiene, and the patient is assessed for elevation of the uvula when the soft palate is stimulated.

Practice tip

Sluggish pupils are found in conditions that compress the third cranial nerve, such as cerebral oedema and herniation.

Posttraumatic amnesia scale

Posttraumatic amnesia (PTA) is a disorder after brain injury that is classified as a traumatic delirium and may even be found in patients who rate a GCS of 15.[40] The incidence of delirium after a brain injury event is high, especially with severe injuries and loss of consciousness. Delirium is discussed in detail in Chapter 8; however, traumatic delirium historically has been referred to in the literature as posttraumatic amnesia. Posttraumatic amnesia is defined as the 'time elapsed from injury until recovery of full consciousness and the return of ongoing memory'. It is the initial stage of recovery from brain injury and is characterised by anterograde (formation of new memory) and retrograde (memory before injury) amnesia, disorientation and rapid forgetting. Brief periods of PTA can occur after minor concussion and may be the only clinical sign of any brain injury. This is when PTA is useful for defining the severity of injury and alerting the clinician in regard to greater surveillance and investigation, as described in Table 16.7. Patients often progress directly from coma into delirium without a clearly-defined stupor stage, so using a tool to measure PTA can be useful to gauge the actual condition of the patient in the delirium state. Duration of PTA is extremely variable, ranging from minutes to months. Although the early stages of PTA are easily recognised, identifying the end point is difficult and complex.

The duration of PTA is the best indicator of the extent of cognitive and functional deficits after TBI. The two most common means of assessing PTA are the Galveston Orientation and Amnesia Test (GOAT) and the Westmead PTA scale.[40-42] GOAT features 10 questions that assess temporal and spatial orientation, biographical recall and memory. The test consists of 10 items that involve the recall of events that occurred right before and after the injury, as well as questions

TABLE 16.7
Posttraumatic amnesia scale used to determine severity of brain injury

PTA SCORE	SEVERITY
1–4 hours	Mild brain injury
≤1 day	Moderate brain injury
2–7 days	Severe brain injury
1–4 weeks	Very severe brain injury
1–6 months	Extremely severe brain injury
>6 months	Chronic amnesia state

about disorientation. Scores of 75 or more on this scale (out of a total possible score of 100) correspond to the termination of the PTA episode. In the Westmead PTA scale, four pictures, one with the examiner's face and name, are to be recalled by the patient on the next day. Those with severe PTA will have difficulty completing such short-term memory tasks. The duration of PTA correlates well with the extent of diffuse axonal injury and with functional outcomes. A person is said to be absolved of PTA if they can achieve a perfect score for three consecutive days.[42]

Assessment of the injured brain

The primary aims of managing patients with acute brain injury in the critical care unit are to limit the risk of secondary brain injury and maintain cerebral perfusion. There is little that can be done to reverse the primary damage caused by an insult. Secondary insults may be subtle and can remain undetected by routine systemic physiological monitoring. Continuous monitoring of the CNS in the intensive care unit (ICU) serves three functions:

1. determination of the extent of the primary injury
2. early detection of secondary cerebral insults so that appropriate interventions can be instituted
3. monitoring of therapeutic interventions to provide feedback.

Despite technological advances, computerised tomography (CT), magnetic resonance imaging (MRI), and functional MRI are all limited in that they reflect the brain status at a single moment in time and are not able to provide continuous real-time data.[43] Continuous data can be provided, such as intraarterial blood pressure, pulse oximetry (SpO2), end-tidal carbon dioxide (EtCO2), and temperature; however, these data are considered surrogates and may not directly reflect changes in intracranial pathology. Advanced continuous monitoring include partial pressure of brain tissue oxygen (PbtO2) and CBF, which require invasive technology.

TABLE 16.8
The brain and related structures in CT

STRUCTURE/FLUID/SPACE	GREY SCALE
Bone, acute blood	Very white
Enhanced tumour	Very white
Subacute blood	Light grey
Muscle	Light grey
Grey matter	Light grey
White matter	Medium grey
Cerebrospinal fluid	Medium grey to black
Air, fat	Very black

Serial neurological evaluation with the GCS or FOUR score can and should be performed routinely. The use of emerging technology through continuous EEG, signal-processed EEG (bispectral index), cerebral oximetry, and transcranial Doppler is actively being investigated.

Brain imaging techniques

Computed tomography

CT is the primary neuroimaging technique in the initial evaluation of the acute brain injury patient and uses a computer to digitally construct an image based upon the measurement of the absorption of X-rays through the brain.[43] Table 16.8 generally summarises the white to black intensities seen for selected tissues in CT. The advantages of CT are: 1) it is rapidly performed, which is especially important in neurological emergencies; 2) it clearly shows acute and subacute haemorrhages into the meningeal spaces and brain; and 3) it is less expensive than an MRI. Disadvantages include: 1) it does not clearly show acute or subacute infarctions or ischaemia, or brain oedema, but only shows injury; 2) it does not differentiate white from grey matter as clearly as an MRI; and 3) it exposes the patient to ionising radiation. Despite these limitations it is still the most prevalent form of neurological imaging.

Practice tip

The mnemonic '**S**ometimes **B**lood **C**an **B**e **V**ery **B**ad' (**S**ymmetry, **B**lood, **C**isterns, **B**one, **V**entricles, **B**rain) provides a routine approach when looking at brain CT scans.

Magnetic resonance imaging

The tissues of the body contain large amounts of protons (nuclei of hydrogen atoms) that function like tiny spinning magnets. Normally, these protons are arranged randomly in relation to each other due to the constantly fluctuating magnetic field produced by the associated electrons. However, when placed in a superconducting magnet, the magnetic moments of the protons will tend to align along the direction of this external field. MRI uses this characteristic of protons to generate images of the brain and body.[43] The advantages of MRI are: 1) it can be manipulated to visualise a wide variety of abnormalities within the brain; and 2) it can show much of the detail of the brain in normal and abnormal states. The disadvantages of MRI are: 1) it does not show acute or subacute haemorrhage into the brain in any detail; 2) the time frame and enclosed space required to perform and prepare a patient for the procedure are not advantageous for neurological emergencies; 3) it is relatively more expensive compared with CT; 4) the loud noise of the procedure needs to be considered in patient management; 5) equipment for life support and monitoring needs to be non-magnetic due to the magnetic nature of the procedure; and 6) patients with metal objects such as implantable medical devices (pacemakers), shrapnel (e.g. military TBI wounds), or metal shavings (e.g. from welding) may be at increased risk and unable to undergo MRI.

Functional magnetic resonance imaging

Functional magnetic resonance imaging (fMRI) is similar to MRI but uses deoxyhaemoglobin as an endogenous contrast, which serves as the source of the magnetic signal for fMRI.[44] It can determine precisely which part of the brain is handling critical functions such as thought, speech, movement and sensation; help assess the effects of stroke, trauma or degenerative disease on brain function; monitor the growth and function of brain tumours; and guide the planning of surgery or radiation therapy for the brain.

Cerebral angiography

Cerebral angiography involves cannulation of cerebral vessels and the administration of intraarterial contrast agents and medications for conditions involving the arterial circulation of the brain. This procedure also has the benefit of using non-invasive CT or MRI with or without contrast to guide the accuracy of the procedure. For example, intracranial aneurysms and arteriovenous malformations can be accurately diagnosed and repaired without surgical intervention.

Cerebral perfusion imaging techniques

Numerous imaging techniques have been developed and applied to evaluate brain haemodynamics, perfusion and blood flow. The main advanced imaging techniques dedicated to brain haemodynamics are positron emission tomography (PET), single photon emission computed tomography (SPECT), xenon-enhanced computed tomography (XeCT), dynamic perfusion computed tomography (PCT), MRI dynamic susceptibility contrast (DSC) and arterial spin labelling (ASL). All of these techniques give similar information about brain haemodynamics in the form of parameters such as CBF or cerebral blood volume (CBV). However, each technique relies upon different technical aspects, contrasts, processing, and duration of imaging. Moreover, due to cost, few institutions have invested in providing all of the aforementioned imaging techniques. Hence, the inter-rater reliability for measuring CBF or CBV using one technology versus the other is not well defined.

ICP monitoring

Invasive measures for monitoring ICP are commonly used in patients with a severe head injury or after neurological surgery. Normal ICP varies with age, body position and clinical condition. The normal ICP is 7–15 mmHg in a supine adult, 3–7 mmHg in children and 1.5–6 mmHg in term infants. The definition of intracranial hypertension depends on the specific pathology and age, although ICP >20 mmHg is generally considered to be abnormal. Significantly increased ICP may cause a reduction in CPP and CBF, if uncorrected, this may lead to secondary ischaemic cerebral injury. Although studies have shown that high ICP is associated with poor outcome, there is no agreed upon threshold at which treatment should be initiated to reduce ICP and no agreed upon best intervention. Recent evidence supports that because ICP varies widely over a short period of time, nurses should observe ICP for at least 5 minutes prior to documenting an ICP value.[45]

ICP varies with arterial pulsation and is not a static pressure. Fluctuations can be seen with breathing and during coughing and straining. Each of the intracranial constituents occupies a certain volume and, being essentially liquid, is incompressible. ICP cannot be reliably estimated from any specific clinical feature or CT finding and must actually be measured. Different methods of monitoring ICP have been described but two methods are commonly used in clinical practice: intraventricular catheters and intraparenchymal fibre optic microtransducer systems. The traditional reference point for the transducer is the foramina of Monro (the duct joining the lateral and third ventricle that is in alignment with the middle of the ear) although, in practical terms, the external auditory meatus is often used.[46]

When ICP monitoring is required, the use of ventriculostomy catheters (external ventricular drainage [EVD] catheters) provides similar accuracy to intraparenchymal fibre optic systems. Fibre optic systems provide a reflection of ICP in the brain tissue (parenchyma) and EVD systems provide a reflection of ICP in the ventricular system. The EVD system includes an external drainage system connected to a strain gauge transducer. The drainage system and pressure transducer are primed on insertion with sterile preservative-free saline. The pressure transducer must be calibrated (also termed zero-referencing, zero-balancing, or simply zeroing) to a known value. Commonly, atmospheric pressure is used as a zero-value reference.

Monitoring ICP through an EVD has the advantage of providing a pathway to divert CSF out of the skull to reduce ICP. Alternatively, the EVD catheter may provide a pathway to instil medication into the ventricular system. The primary disadvantage to monitoring ICP through an EVD is the increased risk of infection. When there is a significant amount of blood in the ventricular system, the EVD is also prone to clogging; this loss of patency obliterates the ability to monitor ICP. Ventricular collapse may occur through overdrainage or cerebral oedema. Because the EVD relies upon a continuous column of fluid, this loss of patency affects the accuracy of ICP values. Current evidence supports a higher risk of complications when the EVD is left open to drain for extended periods of time.[47] In addition, limiting ventricular drainage per hour using gravity and three-way taps to 5–10 mL/h has been used to avoid excessively rapid CSF drainage.

Fibre optic catheter systems are becoming increasingly common. The tip of this catheter is inserted into the intraparenchymal space and provides a continuous record of ICP. Because of the lower complication rate, critical care physicians and advance practice nurses are now placing fibre optic catheters where previously only neurosurgeons placed invasive ICP monitoring. Many fibre optic catheter systems are now part of multimodal monitoring systems that provide intracranial temperature, partial pressure of brain tissue oxygen (PbtO2) and CBF.

While Brain Trauma Foundation guidelines suggest ICP monitoring for head injury patients with GCS scores <9, there is growing controversy regarding the efficacy of ICP monitoring to improve outcome from severe TBI.[48,49] A review of neurocritical care and outcome from TBI suggested that ICP/CPP-guided therapy may benefit patients with severe head injury, including those presenting with raised ICP in the absence of a mass lesion and also patients requiring complex interventions.

Practice tip

The fixed volume of brain parenchyma, CSF and intravascular blood contained within the rigid, non-expandable cranium determines ICP. Brain tissue accounts for 80% of this volume whereas blood and CSF each account for about 10%.

FIGURE 16.15 The intracranial pressure waveforms. **A** Depicts the situation of a compliant system; **B** a high-pressure wave recorded from a non-compliant system in which P2 exceeds the level of the P1 waveform, due to a marked decrease in cerebral compliance. The lower tracing **C** is an example of an ICP waveform from a patient monitoring system in which can be identified the three distinct components, as indicated in the text.

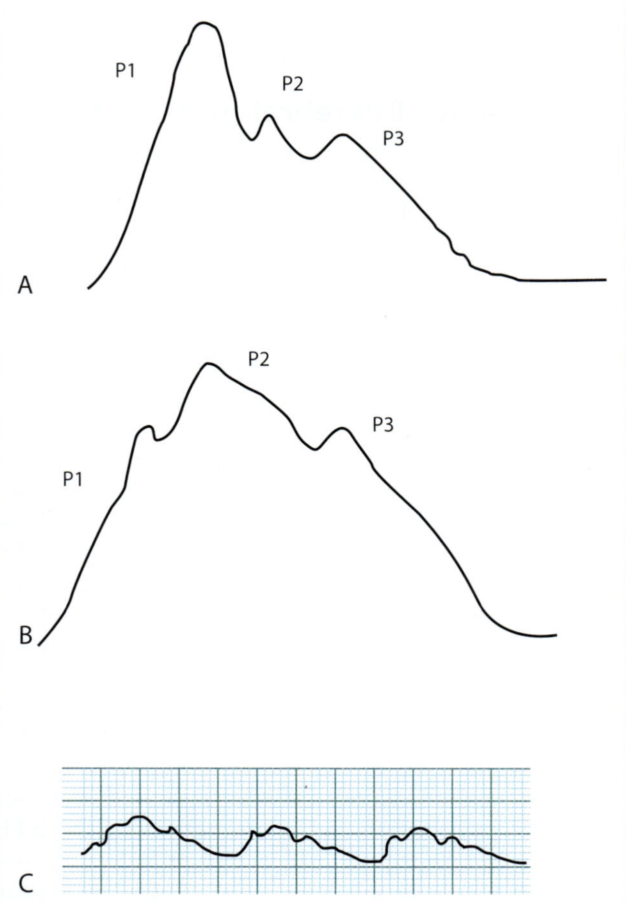

Pulse waveforms

Interpretation of waveforms that are generated by the cerebral monitoring devices is important in the clinical assessment of intracranial adaptive capacity (the ability of the brain to compensate for rises in intracranial volume without raising the ICP). Brain tissue pressure and ICP increase with each cardiac cycle and, thus, the ICP waveform is a modified arterial pressure wave (Fig. 16.15). The cardiac waves reach the cranial circulation via the choroid plexus and resemble the waveforms transmitted by arterial catheters, although the amplitude is lower.

There are three distinct peaks seen in the ICP waveform:[50]

- P1, the percussion wave, which is sharp and reflects the cardiac pulse as the pressure is transmitted from the choroid plexus to the ventricle
- P2, the tidal wave, which is more variable in nature and reflects cerebral compliance and increases in amplitude as compliance decreases
- P3, which is due to the closure of the aortic valve and is known as the dicrotic notch. Of recent importance is that the elevation of P3 may indicate low global cerebral perfusion.

It is important that the waveform be continuously observed, as changes in mean pressure or in waveform shape usually require immediate attention.[50] In acute states such as head injury and subarachnoid haemorrhage, ICP depends greatly on the link between monitoring and therapy, so close inspection of the trend in the ICP and the details derived from the waveform is extremely important. Simple ongoing visual assessment of the ICP waveform for increased amplitude, elevated P2 and rounding of the waveform provides non-specific information suggestive of decreased intracranial adaptive capacity and altered intracranial dynamics.

Assessment of cerebral perfusion

CPP is calculated as the mean arterial pressure minus the ICP and represents the pressure gradient across the vessel that drives CBF:

$$CPP = MAP - ICP$$

CPP is a pressure-based surrogate of oxygen and metabolite delivery. There is no evidence for the optimum level of CPP, and it is likely that emerging evidence will support different CPP thresholds based on injury pathology. Higher CPP has been associated with increased lung water and acute respiratory distress syndrome. Furthermore, mortality rises approximately 20% for each 10-mmHg loss of CPP. In those studies where CPP was maintained above 70 mmHg, the reduction in mortality was as much as 35% for those with severe head injury.[51] The Brain Trauma Foundation (BTF) provides a Level II B recommendation for CPP goal of 60–70 mmHg despite the lack of definitive data.[52] These guidelines also include a Level III recommendation to avoid aggressive attempts to raise CPP >70 mmHg because of the risk for respiratory failure. Despite noting associations between measured decreases in cerebral oxygenation and worse outcomes, the BTF guidelines find inadequate evidence to provide a recommendation for or against intracranial oxygen or jugular bulb oxygen monitoring.[52]

Assessment of cerebral oxygenation

The three main factors determining cerebral oxygenation are CBF, arterial oxygen content and cerebral metabolic rate of oxygen consumption.[53] In clinical practice monitoring of arterial blood gas tensions is routine in most critically ill patients. Measurement of cerebral metabolic rate of oxygen consumption is, however, not commonplace as it is technically difficult and cumbersome. Therefore, the predominant monitoring strategy in clinical practice has relied on measurements of CBF and its surrogates. This section will outline those modalities.

Jugular venous oximetry

Jugular venous catheterisation is used for deriving oxygen-based variables. It facilitates the assessment of jugular venous oxygenation ($SjvO_2$), cerebral oxygen extraction (CEO_2) and arteriovenous difference in oxygen ($AVDO_2$). All of these variables indicate changes in cerebral metabolism and blood flow, and therefore the catheter generates continuous data that reflect the balance between supply and demand of cerebral oxygen.[54] The catheter is inserted in the right jugular vein, as it is slightly larger than the left and provides readings that are more representative of overall brain function. The catheter tip is advanced so that the tip sits in the bulb of the internal jugular vein. The normal requirement for cerebral oxygen delivery is consumption at 35–40% of available oxygen, giving a normal $SjvO_2$ of 60–65%. Changes in $SjvO_2$ reflect changes in cerebral metabolic rate and CBF; however, as it is a global measure, it does not detect regional ischaemia.[53] $SjvO_2$ is also highly sensitive to operator error, requires frequent recalibration and patient positioning (e.g. changes in head or neck position), may alter the signal quality and require medical intervention to reposition the catheter. For these reasons, $SjvO_2$ is becoming increasingly less common.

Partial pressure of brain tissue oxygenation monitoring

Changes in ICP values alone may not accurately depict poor CBF or oxygenation deficits to brain tissue and may be late signs, occurring hours later when damage cannot be reversed.[55,56] Consequently, brain tissue hypoxaemia may occur during the first 24 h after injury despite controlled brain pressures. Monitoring the partial pressure of oxygen in brain tissue ($PbtO_2$) as an adjunct to ICP monitoring may provide more accurate and timelier cerebral oxygen delivery and demand than ICP alone.[53,57] Normal $PbtO_2$ (20–25 mmHg) emerges as a critical determinant of outcome, with values <20 mmHg associated with higher risk of poor functional outcomes. A $PbtO_2$ value <10 mmHg for more than 10 minutes carries a higher risk of death. Alterations in cerebral metabolic rate can also change tissue oxygen levels. Increased adherence to guidelines and reducing the patient's energy consumption via reduced noise and/or distractions, and increasing their protein caloric intake to complement their increased stress state, may improve tissue oxygenation.[58]

Cerebral microdialysis

Cerebral microdialysis remains primarily as a research tool for investigating the metabolic status of one area of brain tissue.[55,59] The microdialysis probe is inserted into the cerebral tissue where substances in the extracellular fluid surround the semipermeable membrane at the tip of the catheter. Following equilibration of the tissue metabolites with the perfusion fluid, the dialysate can be analysed for concentrations of products of energy metabolism (glucose, lactate, pyruvate, and glutamate) as indicators of hypoxia and ischaemia. In addition, interstitial glycerol can be determined, which is a parameter of lipolysis and/or cell membrane damage.[60] The products of metabolism are sampled hourly and the trends in values for each metabolite are explored as correlates of changes cerebral metabolic function. Because of limited outcome data, cerebral microdialysis is primarily used in conjunction with clinical research.

Non-invasive assessment

Invasive methods of measuring ICP, CBF and $PbtO_2$ are associated with complications. Because of this, many patients with low- or moderate-grade TBI are not monitored.[55,56] Patients benefit from non-invasive means of detecting episodes of cerebral hypoxia and ischaemia that could lead to poor outcomes, and these are detailed in the following section.

Transcranial Doppler

Transcranial Doppler (TCD) ultrasound has proved to be a safe, reliable and relatively inexpensive technology for measuring cerebrovascular blood velocities and evaluating cerebral circulation and haemodynamics.[61] A handheld transducer is used to direct pulses of ultrasound towards the cerebral arteries at the base of the skull.[62] Velocities from the cerebral arteries, the internal carotids, the basilar and the vertebral arteries can be sampled by altering the transducer location, angle and the instrument's depth setting. The commonest windows in the cranium are located in the orbit (of the eye) and in the temporal and suboccipital regions. TCD measures systolic, diastolic and mean velocity in middle cerebral artery (MCA) flow; as well as providing pulsatility index (PI), a derived value. Changes in the PI are sometimes used to identify the threshold of autoregulation. In subarachnoid haemorrhage (SAH) and TBI this may be due to vasospasm or impaired autoregulation or abnormal intracranial compliance.

Continuous electroencephalography

Electroencephalography (EEG) is used to display and record electrical activity produced by the firing of neurons within the brain. Both scalp (sensors placed on the surface of the scalp) and depth (sensors placed into brain tissue) electrodes are used in EEG monitoring. Continuous EEG (cEEG) has the advantage of being continuous and non-invasive and carries the potential to detect alterations in brain physiology at a reversible stage, which may trigger treatment before permanent brain injury occurs.[63] Currently, the main applications of cEEG are diagnosing and localising seizure, non-convulsive status epilepticus, monitoring and guiding the treatment of status epilepticus and detecting delayed cerebral ischaemia from vasospasm in SAH patients.[64–66] Other applications may include monitoring of reperfusion after interventions for acute stroke patients and detection of intracranial hypertension. Clinically unrecognised electrographic seizures and periodic epileptiform discharges have been shown to be frequent and associated with poor outcome in patients with severe brain injury from different aetiologies, including TBI, ischaemic and haemorrhagic strokes and CNS infection.[67]

The EEG becomes substantially abnormal (suppressed) when CBF declines to 20–30 mL/100 g/min. More subtle abnormalities accompany lesser degrees of hypoperfusion, including initial loss of beta activity, slowing to the theta range and then to the delta range. Irreversible injury to brain tissue occurs at cerebral flows of about 10–12 mL/100 g/min. Thus, EEG sensitivity to ischaemia allows its use in situations where cerebral perfusion is at risk. Changes over time in quantitative EEG (qEEG) parameters can trigger remote reading, focused neurological examination, imaging studies and early treatment.[68] Subtle EEG changes may be difficult to interpret in isolation, but may be better understood when interpreted along with other components of a multimodality monitoring (neurological exam, ICP, CBF, and $PbtO_2$).

Near-infrared spectroscopy

Near-infrared spectroscopy (NIRS) is a non-invasive method of monitoring continuous trends of cerebral oxygenated and deoxygenated haemoglobin by utilising an infrared light beam transmitted through the skull.[69] Oxygenated and deoxygenated haemoglobin moieties have different absorption spectra, and cerebral oxygenation and haemodynamic status can be determined by their relative absorption of near-infrared light.[70] NIRS allows interrogation of the cerebral cortex using reflectance spectroscopy via optodes, light transmitting and detecting devices, placed on the scalp. Normal saturation is 70%. Because NIRS interrogates arterial, venous and capillary blood within the field of view, the derived saturation represents regional tissue oxygenation (rSO_2) measured from these three compartments and can be used to identify tissue hypoxia and ischaemia in the brain cortex. Although promising, the clinical and bedside use of NIRS is constrained by sources of error including contamination of the signal by the extracerebral circulation (such as in the scalp), extraneous light and the presence of extravascular blood arising from subarachnoid or subdural haemorrhage.

Bispectral index monitoring

Bispectral index (BIS) monitoring is a neurophysiological monitoring device that continually analyses brain activity non-invasively through the electroencephalogram (EEG).[71] Traditionally used within the operating theatre environment to monitor a patient's level of sedation, it is now used within the intensive care environment to assess brain activity or level of consciousness. Alterations in metabolic activity or metabolic stability within the brain will be reflected on the machine's EEG. The BIS number ranges from 0 to 100.[72] A BIS number of 100 indicates a conscious patient (high metabolic activity); a BIS number of 40–60 indicates a sedation level for general anaesthesia and a BIS number of 0 indicates no brain activity detected (isoelectric/markedly decreased or absent metabolic activity).

Summary

An overview of anatomy and physiology in the context of and as applied to neurological assessment of the critically ill is provided in this chapter. Priorities of clinical assessment are described and include determining the extent of the neurological injury, recognising fluctuations in the patient's condition and assisting in the maintenance of cerebral perfusion as part of multimodal monitoring. Imaging techniques and assessment incorporate the therapeutics of ICP, CPP, CBF, $PbtO_2$, cEEG, transcranial Doppler and cerebral perfusion imaging. A report on a prospective, repeated measures, multisite national trial on differences in CPP values by measurement location is supplied in the *Research vignette*. The clinical case demonstrates neurological assessment priorities in an unstable, TBI patient. Clinical, non-invasive and invasive assessment techniques are described within the context of this patient's care.

Case study

Sam, a 52-year-old male, was driving home after visiting family interstate and was involved in a high-speed collision. At the scene, Sam was found upside down and unconscious with an initial GCS of 3. Vomit was present and suspicion of aspiration had occurred. A scalp haematoma and periorbital bruising and scalp laceration were present. His right elbow and arm were deformed. His pupils were 3 mm in diameter and were equal and reacting to light. No obvious motor, neural, abdominal or thorax injures were seen. He was extricated from the vehicle with cervical collar fitted; intravenous access was obtained and Sam was transported to the nearest Base Hospital for stabilisation.

EMERGENCY DEPARTMENT

The ambulance arrived 45 minutes later to the emergency department (ED) and bypassed triage to the resuscitation area where the trauma team conducted primary and secondary surveys. On presentation, Sam's vital signs were: heart rate 130 beats/min, respirations 35 breaths/min, blood pressure 137/77 mmHg, SpO_2 93%, temperature 36.4°C, GCS 5.

Primary survey: Sam's primary survey revealed the following details:

- Airway: patent, not protected. Vomitus and blood present – upper airway cleared. Cervical spine: status unknown, hard cervical collar in situ
- Breathing: equal air entry. Spontaneously breathing on 6 L/min at 28 breaths/min, decreased bilaterally, no tracheal deviation. Pulse oximetry 70%
- Circulation: tachycardic, normotensive. Abdomen soft and non-tender. Pulses present on palpation, temperature centrally warm, well perfused, skin pink in colour, peripherally cool; capillary refill 3 s
- Disability: GCS 5 (eye opening 1, verbal 2, motor 2); pupils equal and reactive, size 3 mm. Mobile trauma series performed – chest and pelvis X-ray and lung ultrasound

Secondary survey: The secondary survey revealed the following details:

- Head: a trauma CT was conducted and revealed traumatic intracranial haemorrhage with evidence of subarachnoid haemorrhage, parenchymal contusion, left tentorium subdural haemorrhage and cerebral oedema. A very large left parietal haematoma is present. No traumatic injury was evident within the spine, abdomen or pelvis.

CT revealed acute subarachnoid and subdural haemorrhages, parenchymal contusions and generalised cerebral oedema. No underlying fractures are present:

- Face: periorbital bruising with no obvious facial deformity. A small laceration to the front scalp. No rhinorrhoea or otorrhoea.
- Neck: no obvious lacerations observed around neck area; no evidence of tracheal deviation. Cervical spine CT found no bony injury, assessment of spine clearance not yet undertaken.
- Chest: distress on left anterior chest prior to intubation – suspected fractures ribs. Equal air entry with no crepitus. Left intercostal catheter in situ for suspected pneumothorax.
- Pelvis/abdomen: orogastric tube present. Abdomen soft with no abnormal distension. No intra-abdominal free fluid. Indwelling catheter inserted – no haematuria present.

- Back: no lacerations or bruising present. Rectal tone present.
- Upper limbs: right arm deformity. Moving both limbs in response to pain. X-ray revealed right radial, ulna and radial head fractures, pulses present.
- Lower limbs: moving both limbs. No obvious musculoskeletal injury.

The plan was for immediate intubation due to an unprotected airway and low GCS, and retrieval transfer by helicopter to the nearest trauma and neuro centre. The physician had three attempts before intubation was successful due to the presence of vomitus and blood. An arterial line was inserted and morphine and midazolam infusions were commenced.

EMERGENCY SURGERY

On arrival Sam was immediately transferred to operating theatre for a craniectomy and evacuation of the acute subarachnoid and subdural and haemorrhages and insertion of an EVD.

Following surgery, he was admitted to the ICU for further management (Table 16.9). Sam's family were notified by the local police. His family rang the ICU and spoke with the treating medical team. His family are unaware of any advanced care directivities that had been developed but stated that Sam would want active measures taken. Verbal consent was obtained from his sister (NOK) for further invasive lifesaving interventions. The Social Worker made contact and has organised emergency accommodation and would provide ongoing support on arrival.

ICU MANAGEMENT

Day 1: On arrival to the ICU, Sam's condition was critical. His vital signs were: heart rate sinus tachycardia 125 beats/min; intubated and mechanically ventilated at 16 breaths/min, Vt 640–760 mL, FiO_2 0.6, PEEP 12 cmH_2O; blood pressure 128/85 mmHg (MAP 98) with noradrenaline support for a CPP of 65; SaO_2 97%; temperature 37.9°C; pupils 3/3 mm (R/L), sluggish sequential reaction. He was heavily sedated and unresponsive with a Glasgow Coma Scale (GCS) of 3T (eye opening 1, verbal 1 [T = intubated], motor 1). His EVD system monitor displayed an ICP of 18 mmHg. He required paralysis with intermittent boluses of vecuronium and with the need for increasing levels of sedation, noradrenaline and hypertonic saline bolus to control his ICP and CPP. Normal saline was infused for maintenance fluid. Pain stimulation for neurological assessment under these conditions was only performed during endotracheal suction.

The initial arterial blood gas revealed: pH 7.28; $PaCO_2$ 47.8; PaO_2 112; HCO_3 21.9; BE –4.7; Hb 157; K^+ 4.9; Na^+ 137; Lactate 2.9; BGL 10.9

Days 2–22: Sam's clinical parameters and assessment are depicted in Table 16.9. Initially his ICP and CPP were unstable with increasing need for sedation and intermittent paralysis. Bolus doses of hypertonic saline (23.4% NaCl) were administered and increased drainage from the EVD (42 mL in 24 hours) was noted. Sam's serum sodium levels elevated to hypernatraemic state with a sodium (Na^+) range of 148–156 mmol/L (normal range is 136–144 mmol/L). He was administered free water boluses of 200 mL four times a day by orogastric tube. Targeted temperature management was initiated for elevated temperatures of 38.9°C.

Day 9: Open reduction and internal fixation to right radial and ulna fractures and surgical tracheostomy performed.

Day 11: Sputum and central venous catheter tip cultures grew *Serratia* and commenced antibiotic sensitive therapy.

Day 13: Persistent poor neurology with no eye opening or interactions. MRI performed that revealed scattered petechial haemorrhages throughout the brain stem, corpus callosum and cerebral hemispheres, consistent with diffuse axonal injury.

Day 22: Sam was discharged to ward with tracheostomy and plans were made to transfer him to his home city hospital.

CASE STUDY QUESTIONS

1 Noxious stimulus applied centrally is an assessment of what functions?
2 What effect will an elevated temperature have on a patient with an elevated ICP?
3 Discuss the relationship between ICP, CPP and secondary brain injury.
4 Discuss the physiological effects of how hypertonic 23.4% saline reduces ICP.

TABLE 16.9
Overview of Sam's clinical parameters and assessment, days 1–6

	DAY OF ADMISSION					
Parameter	1	2	3	4	5	6
Pupils (mm)						
Right	3S	2S	2+	3+	3+	3+
Left	3S	2S	2+	3+	3+	3+
GCS	3 T (E1V1(T)M1)	3 T (E1V1(T)M1)	3 T (E1V1(T)M1)	3 T (E1V1(T)M1)	5 T (E1V1(T)M3) Moving right side only	5 T (E1V1(T)M3) Moving right side only
CSF drainage (mL/24 h)	12	26	42	22	6*	
ICP range (mmHg)	11–32	8–28	12–20	9–12	6–10	
Sedation infusion	Morphine/ midazolam	Morphine/ midazolam	Morphine/ midazolam	Morphine/ midazolam		
Paralysing agent	Vecuronium intermittent	Vecuronium intermittent	Vecuronium intermittent	Vecuronium intermittent		
Noradrenaline (mcg/min)	5–18	5–16	4–14	4–9	Nil	Nil
Heart rate range (bpm)	110–135	88–110	85–99	68–90	60–90	62–87
MAP range (mmHg)	60–95	75–92	72–88	85–98	85–98	78–92
CPP range (mmHg)	49–63	64–67	60–68	59–86	79–88	63–90*
Temperature	37.9°C	37.9°C	38.9°C Thermal cooling initiated. Target 36.0°C	36.1°C	36.2°C	36.0°C*

CPP = cerebral perfusion pressure; CSF = cerebrospinal fluid; E = eye opening; GCS = Glasgow Coma Scale; ICP = intracranial pressure; M = motor; MAP = mean arterial pressure; V = verbal; (T) = intubated; * = ICP external ventricular drain /thermal cooling removed.

RESEARCH VIGNETTE

Reprinted with permission of Springer Nature. McNett MM, Bader MK, Livesay S, et al. A national trial on differences in cerebral perfusion pressure values by measurement location. Neurocritical care (Epub: Oct, 2017) doi: 10.1007/s12028-017-0467-7

Abstract

Background: Cerebral perfusion pressure (CPP) is a key parameter in management of brain injury with suspected impaired cerebral autoregulation. CPP is calculated by subtracting ICP from mean arterial pressure (MAP). Despite consensus on importance of CPP monitoring, substantial variations exist on anatomical reference points used to measure arterial MAP when calculating CPP. This study aimed to identify differences in CPP values based on measurement location when using phlebostatic axis (PA) or tragus as anatomical reference points. The secondary study aim was to determine impact of differences on patient outcomes at discharge.

Methods: This was a prospective, repeated measures, multisite national trial. Adult ICU patients with neurological injury necessitating ICP and CPP monitoring were consecutively enrolled from seven sites. Daily MAP/ICP/CPP values were gathered with the arterial transducer at the PA, followed by the tragus as anatomical reference points.

Results: A total of 136 subjects were enrolled, resulting in 324 paired observations. There were significant differences for CPP when comparing values obtained at PA and tragus reference points ($p < 0.001$). Differences remained significant in repeated measures model when controlling for clinical factors (mean CPP-PA = 80.77, mean CPP-tragus = 70.61, $p < 0.000$). When categorising CPP as binary endpoint, 18.8% of values were identified as adequate with PA values, yet inadequate with CPP values measured at the tragus.

Conclusion: Findings identify numerical differences for CPP based on anatomical reference location and highlight importance of a standard reference point for both clinical practice and future trials to limit practice variations and heterogeneity of findings.

Critique

This is a non-randomised nursing research study that examined a fundamental question of interest to nurses who provide care to patients with (ICP) monitoring. More precisely, this study was designed to examine how much difference in cerebral perfusion pressure (CPP) scores can be attributed to which anatomical reference point (level) the nurse uses when obtaining an intraarterial blood pressure (ABP) measurement. It is unlikely that randomisation would alter the results because each patient served as both control and intervention. However, the use of a pragmatic design has limitations. An intraarterial pressure (art-line) was an inclusion criteria and art-lines are typically used on more critically ill patients; hence the sample may be biased. Similarly, the study team did not adjust the head of bed (HOB) angle; it is unknown if certain patients (e.g. those with high ICP) were more likely to have their HOB >30 elevation. The sample size is large enough to provide observe for differences in this diverse sample, but it is unknown if similar results would be noted if the sample were restricted to a specific population (e.g. only patients with intracerebral haemorrhage (ICH)).

Critical care units all have different practices. Some ICUs level the ABP transducer at the PA (4th intercostal space along the mid-anterior/posterior chest circumference). When monitoring ICP, some ICUs level the ABP transducer at the tragus because this is the same reference point for levelling the ICP transducer. 324 paired readings were obtained from 136 patients at 7 different hospitals. The ICP was always transduced at the tragus, and the ABP was transduced first at the PA and second at the tragus to produce a paired reading. The authors found that although measures taken at the PA and measures at the tragus were highly correlated, there were, however, clinically and statistically significant differences in the CPP based on where the ABP transducer was levelled. Moreover, the study identified that if there were more than two episodes in which the tragus-levelled CPP value was <60 mmHg and the paired phlebostatic value was >60 mmHg, subjects were more likely to be discharged to a skilled nursing facility (29.1% vs 18.8%). Surprisingly, there was no standardised difference between CPP values taken with the transducer at either level. Hence, a formula or computational correction is not reliable (e.g. adding 10 mmHg if the transducer is at the PA).

Learning activities

The first three activities refer to the *Research vignette*.

1 What are the theoretical advantages to standardising nursing practice for establishing a reference point for the arterial line transducer?

2 Discuss the potential complications related to unmeasured or unrecognised low CPP.

3 What are the physiologic mechanisms that might influence the difference in CPP when the intraarterial blood pressure (ABP) is transduced at the tragus compared with ABP transduced at the PA?

4 Which brain structure coordinates endocrine and nervous system activities?
5 Which component of the brain controls the cardiac centres, the vasomotor centres and the respiratory rhythm centre?
6 What information does the FOUR score provide? What does the FOUR score predict?
7 A noxious stimulus is applied to the nail bed of the middle finger to test motor response. The unconscious patient elicits a flexion withdrawal response of the wrist, arm and shoulder. Explain what this response means in terms of central or peripheral response.
8 What is the pathophysiological basis for the rise in ICP? How would this manifest on the ICP waveform?
9 A patient recovering from a subarachnoid haemorrhage cannot remember events prior to the haemorrhage event. What type of amnesia is this?

Online resources

Adult Neurological Observation Chart: Education Package, www.aci.health.nsw.gov.au/__data/assets/pdf_file/0018/201753/AdultChartEdPackage.pdf

American Association of Neuroscience Nurses (AANN), www.aann.org

Australasian Neuroscience Nurses' Association, www.anna.asn.au

Brain Explorer, www.brainexplorer.org

Brain Injury Association of America, www.biausa.org

Cranial Nerves, www.youtube.com/watch?v=sAFaTaavmO8

FOUR score for Neuro Assessments, http://w3.rn.com/News/clinical_insights_details.aspx?Id=29828

GCS Part 1, www.youtube.com/watch?v=T93Ah9ZkurI&feature=player_detailpage

GCS Part 2, www.youtube.com/watch?v=_jTTPjZ_ruE

Neurocritical Care Society, www.neurocriticalcare.org

Neurological Foundation of New Zealand, www.neurological.org.nz

Official Journal of the American Academy of Neurology (AAN), http://neurology.org

Pupillometer in Critical Care, https://neuroptics.com/resource-center-neurocritical-care/

Physical Examination and Neurological Assessment, www.neurologyexam.com

Posttraumatic amnesia protocol, www.psy.mq.edu.au/pta

Society for Neuroscience, http://web.sfn.org

The Brain Trauma Foundation, www.braintrauma.org

World Health Organization Neurotrauma, www.who.int/violence_injury_prevention/road_traffic/activities/neurotrauma/en

Further reading

Berlin T. Technology. In: Bader MK, Littlejohns LR, Olson DM, editors. AANN core curriculum for neuroscience nursing. 6th ed. Glenview, IL: American Association of Neuroscience Nurses; 2016. p. 135–68.

Blumenfeld H. Neuroanatomy through clinical cases. 2nd ed. Sunderland, MA: Sinauer Associates; 2018.

Carney N, Totten AM, O'Reilly C, et al. Guidelines for the management of severe traumatic brain injury. Neurosurgery 2016;80(1):6–15.

Greenberg MS. General neurocritical care. In: Greenberg MS, editor. Handbook of neurosurgery. 8th ed. New York: Thieme Medical; 2016. p. 126–31.

Hickey JV, Kanusky JT. Overview of neuroanatomy and neurophysiology. In: Hickey JV, editor. The clinical practice of neurological and neurosurgical nursing. 7th ed. Philadelphia: Wolters Kluwer/Lipincott Williams & Wilkins; 2014. [Chapter 5].

Shank CD, Walters BC, Hadley MN. Management of acute traumatic spinal cord injuries. Handb Clin Neurol 2017;140:275–98.

Stewart-Amidei C. Assessment. In: Bader MK, Littlejohns LR, Olson DM, editors. AANN core curriculum for neuroscience nursing. 6th ed. Glenview: American Association of Neuroscience Nurses; 2016. p. 63–96.

Wijdicks EF. The scope of neurology of critical illness. Handb Clin Neurol 2017;141:443–7.

References

1. Malloy R, March K. Intracranial dynamics. In: Bader MK, Littlejohns LR, Olson DM, editors. AANN core curriculum for neuroscience nursing. 6th ed. Glenview: American Association of Neuroscience Nurses; 2016. p. 57–62.
2. Hickey JV, Kanusky JT. Overview of neuroanatomy and neurophysiology. In: Hickey JV, editor. The clinical practice of neurological and neurosurgical nursing. 7th ed. Philadelphia: Wolters Kluwer/Lipincott Williams & Wilkins; 2014.
3. Porth C. Pathophysiology concepts of altered health states. 9th ed. Philadelphia: Lippincott, Williams & Wilkins; 2014.
4. Hall JE. Transport of substances through cell membranes. Guyton and Hall Textbook of medical physiology. 13th ed. Philadelphia: Elsevier; 2016. p. 47–60.
5. Wehrwein EA, Orer HS, Barman SM. Overview of the anatomy, physiology, and pharmacology of the autonomic nervous system. Compr Physiol 2016;6(3):1239–78.
6. Armstrong RC, Mierzwa AJ, Marion CM, et al. White matter involvement after TBI: clues to axon and myelin repair capacity. Exp Neurol 2016;275(Pt 3):328–33.
7. Preliminary report: effect of encainide and flecainide on mortality in a randomized trial of arrhythmia suppression after myocardial infarction. The Cardiac Arrhythmia Suppression Trial (CAST) investigators. N Engl J Med 1989;321(6):406–12.
8. Head VA, Wakerley BR. Guillain-Barre syndrome in general practice: clinical features suggestive of early diagnosis. Br J Gen Pract 2016;66(645):218–19.
9. Kandel ER. Principles of neural science. New York: McGraw Hill; 2013.
10. Hickey JV. The clinical practice of neurological and neurosurgical nursing. 7th ed. Philadelphia: Wolters Kluwer/Lipincott Williams & Wilkins; 2014.
11. Rudolph LM, Cornil CA, Mittelman-Smith MA, et al. Actions of steroids: new neurotransmitters. J Neurosci 2016;36(45):11449–58.
12. Blumenfeld H. Cerebral hemispheres and vascular supply. In: Blumenfeld H, editor. Neuroanatomy through clinical case. 2nd ed. Sunderland, MA: Sinauer Associates; 2018. p. 391–458.
13. Blumenfeld H. Neuroanatomy through clinical cases. 2nd ed. Sunderland, MA: Sinauer Associates; 2018.
14. Grossman MN, Anderson SL, Worku A, et al. Awakenings? Patient and hospital staff perceptions of nighttime disruptions and their effect on patient sleep. J Clin Sleep Med 2016.
15. Beltrami FG, Nguyen XL, Pichereau C, et al. Sleep in the intensive care unit. J Bras Pneumol 2015;41(6):539–46.
16. Steaphen A, Olson DM, Stutzman SE. Nurses perceptions of a novel protocol addressing uniform periods of minimum assessment times. J Neurosci Nurs 2017;49(5):302–6.
17. Whyte J. Disorders of consciousness: the changing landscape of treatment. Neurology 2014;82(13):1106–7.
18. Brogan ME, Provencio JJ. Spectrum of catastrophic brain injury: coma and related disorders of consciousness. J Crit Care 2014;29(4):679–82.
19. Prottengeier J, Moritz A, Heinrich S, et al. Sedation assessment in a mobile intensive care unit: a prospective pilot-study on the relation of clinical sedation scales and the bispectral index. Crit Care 2014;18(6):615.
20. Sessler CN, Gosnell MS, Grap MJ, et al. The Richmond agitation-sedation scale: validity and reliability in adult intensive care unit patients. Am J Respir Crit Care Med 2002;166(10):1338–44.
21. Teasdale G, Jennett B. Assessment of coma and impaired consciousness. A practical scale. Lancet 1974;2(7872):81–4.
22. McNarry AF, Goldhill DR. Simple bedside assessment of level of consciousness: comparison of two simple assessment scales with the Glasgow Coma scale. Anaesthesia 2004;59(1):34–7.
23. Reith FC, Brennan PM, Maas AI, et al. Lack of standardization in the use of the Glasgow Coma Scale: results of international surveys. J Neurotrauma 2016;33(1):89–94.
24. Mattar I, Liaw SY, Chan MF. A study to explore nurses' knowledge in using the Glasgow Coma Scale in an acute care hospital. J Neurosci Nurs 2013;45(5):272–80.
25. Stead LG, Wijdicks EF, Bhagra A, et al. Validation of a new coma scale, the FOUR score, in the emergency department. Neurocrit Care 2009;10(1):50–4.
26. Wijdicks EF, Bamlet WR, Maramattom BV, et al. Validation of a new coma scale: the FOUR score. Ann Neurol 2005;58(4):585–93.
27. Wijdicks EF, Kramer AA, Rohs T Jr, et al. Comparison of the Full Outline of UnResponsiveness score and the Glasgow Coma Scale in predicting mortality in critically ill patients*. Crit Care Med 2015;43(2):439–44.

28. McNett MM, Amato S, Philippbar SA. A comparative study of Glasgow Coma Scale and Full Outline of Unresponsiveness Scores for predicting long-term outcome after brain injury. J Neurosci Nurs 2016;48(4):207–14.
29. Kasprowicz M, Burzynska M, Melcer T, et al. A comparison of the Full Outline of UnResponsiveness (FOUR) score and Glasgow Coma Score (GCS) in predictive modelling in traumatic brain injury. Br J Neurosurg 2016;30(2):211–20.
30. Greenberg MS. Handbook of neurosurgery. 8th ed. New York: Thieme Medical; 2016.
31. Chen JW, Vakil-Gilani K, Williamson KL, et al. Infrared pupillometry, the Neurological Pupil index and unilateral pupillary dilation after traumatic brain injury: implications for treatment paradigms. Springerplus 2014;3:548.
32. Olson DM, Stutzman S, Saju C, et al. Interrater reliability of pupillary assessments. Neurocrit Care 2016;24(2):251–7.
33. Kerr RG, Bacon AM, Baker LL, et al. Underestimation of pupil size by critical care and neurosurgical nurses. Am J Crit Care 2016;25(3):213–19.
34. Olson DM, Stutzman SE, Atem F, et al. Establishing normative data for pupillometer assessment in neuroscience intensive care: the 'END-PANIC' registry. J Neurosci Nurs 2017;49(4):251–4.
35. McNett M, Moran C, Janki C, et al. Correlations between hourly pupillometer readings and intracranial pressure values. J Neurosci Nurs 2017;49(4):229–34.
36. Bledsoe BE, Casey MJ, Feldman J, et al. Glasgow Coma Scale scoring is often inaccurate. Prehosp Disaster Med 2015;30(1):46–53.
37. Spinello IM. Brain death determination. J Intensive Care Med 2015;30(6):326–37.
38. Woischneck D, Skalej M, Firsching R, et al. Decerebrate posturing following traumatic brain injury: MRI findings and their diagnostic value. Clin Radiol 2015;70(3):278–85.
39. Baumann JJ, Blissitt PA, Stewart-Amidei C. Assessment. In: Bader MK, Littlejohns LR, Olson DM, editors. AANN core curriculum for neuroscience nursing. 6th ed. Glenview: American Association of Neuroscience Nurses; 2016. p. 63–96.
40. Shores EA, Marosszeky JE, Sandanam J, et al. Preliminary validation of a clinical scale for measuring the duration of post-traumatic amnesia. Med J Aust 1986;144(11):569–72.
41. Levin HS, O'Donnell VM, Grossman RG. The Galveston Orientation and Amnesia Test. A practical scale to assess cognition after head injury. J Nerv Ment Dis 1979;167(11):675–84.
42. Davidoff G, Doljanac R, Berent S, et al. Galveston Orientation and Amnesia Test: its utility in the determination of closed head injury in acute spinal cord injury patients. Arch Phys Med Rehabil 1988;69(6):432–4.
43. LeBihan D. Elementary particles. Looking inside the brain : the power of neuroimaging. Princeton: Princeton Univ. Press; 2015. p. 4–21.
44. Ramezani M, Abolmaesumi P, Marble K, et al. Fusion analysis of functional MRI data for classification of individuals based on patterns of activation. Brain Imaging Behav 2015;9(2):149–61.
45. Rogers M, Stutzman SE, Atem FD, et al. Intracranial pressure values are highly variable after cerebral spinal fluid drainage. J Neurosci Nurs 2017;49(2):85–9.
46. Olson DM, Batjer HH, Abdulkadir K, et al. Measuring and monitoring ICP in Neurocritical Care: results from a national practice survey. Neurocrit Care 2014;20(1):15–20.
47. Chung DY, Leslie-Mazwi TM, Patel AB, et al. Management of external ventricular drains after subarachnoid hemorrhage: a multi-institutional survey. Neurocrit Care 2017;26(3):356–61.
48. O'Phelan K, Shepard SAI, DeJesus-Alvelo I. Controversies in intracranial pressure monitoring. In: Koenig M, editor. Cerebral herniation syndromes and intracranial hypertension. New Brunswick, New Jersey: Rutgers University Press; 2016.
49. Chesnut R, Videtta W, Vespa P, et al. Intracranial pressure monitoring: fundamental considerations and rationale for monitoring. Neurocrit Care 2014;21(2):64–84.
50. Hawthorne C, Piper I. Monitoring of intracranial pressure in patients with traumatic brain injury. Front Neurol 2014;5:121.
51. Johnston AJ, Steiner LA, Coles JP, et al. Effect of cerebral perfusion pressure augmentation on regional oxygenation and metabolism after head injury. Crit Care Med 2005;33(1):189–95, discussion 255–7.
52. Carney N, Totten AM, O'Reilly C, et al. Guidelines for the management of severe traumatic brain injury, fourth edition. Neurosurgery 2016.
53. Vos PE, Diaz-Arrastia R. Traumatic brain injury. Chichester: John Wiley.; 2015.
54. Wijayatilake DS, Talati C, Panchatsharam S. The monitoring and management of severe traumatic brain injury in the United Kingdom: is there a consensus?: A national survey. J Neurosurg Anesthesiol 2015;27(3):241–5.
55. Korbakis G, Vespa PM. Multimodal neurologic monitoring. Handb Clin Neurol 2017;140:91–105.
56. Le Roux P, Menon DK, Citerio G, et al. Consensus summary statement of the International Multidisciplinary Consensus Conference on Multimodality Monitoring in Neurocritical Care : a statement for healthcare professionals from the Neurocritical Care Society and the European Society of Intensive Care Medicine. Neurocrit Care 2014.
57. Okonkwo DO, Shutter LA, Moore C, et al. Brain oxygen optimization in severe traumatic brain injury phase-II: a phase II randomized trial. Crit Care Med 2017;45(11):1907–14.
58. Saherwala AA, Bader MK, Stutzman SE, et al. Increasing adherence to Brain Trauma Foundation Guidelines for hospital care of patients with traumatic brain injury. Crit Care Nurse 2018;38(1):e11–20.
59. Pinczolits A, Zdunczyk A, Dengler NF, et al. Standard-sampling microdialysis and spreading depolarizations in patients with malignant hemispheric stroke. J Cereb Blood Flow Metab 2017;37(5):1896–905.

60. Carpenter KL, Young AM, Hutchinson PJ. Advanced monitoring in traumatic brain injury: microdialysis. Curr Opin Crit Care 2017;23(2):103–9.
61. Kumar G, Shahripour RB, Harrigan MR. Vasospasm on transcranial Doppler is predictive of delayed cerebral ischemia in aneurysmal subarachnoid hemorrhage: a systematic review and meta-analysis. J Neurosurg 2016;124(5):1257–64.
62. Valdueza JM, Schreiber SJ, Roehl JE, et al. Neurosonology and neuroimaging of stroke : a comprehensive reference. 2nd ed. New York: Thieme; 2017.
63. Herman ST, Abend NS, Bleck TP, et al. Consensus statement on continuous EEG in critically ill adults and children, part II: personnel, technical specifications, and clinical practice. J Clin Neurophysiol 2015;32(2):96–108.
64. Francoeur CL, Mayer SA. Management of delayed cerebral ischemia after subarachnoid hemorrhage. Crit Care 2016;20(1):277.
65. Gollwitzer S, Groemer T, Rampp S, et al. Early prediction of delayed cerebral ischemia in subarachnoid hemorrhage based on quantitative EEG: a prospective study in adults. Clin Neurophysiol 2015;126(8):1514–23.
66. Picetti E, Rossi I, Caspani ML. Continuous electroencephalographic monitoring and vasospasm. Crit Care Med 2013;41(10):e296.
67. Ko SB. Multimodality monitoring in the neurointensive care unit: a special perspective for patients with stroke. J Stroke 2013;15(2):99–108.
68. Swisher CB, Sinha SR. Utilization of quantitative EEG trends for critical care continuous EEG monitoring: a survey of neurophysiologists. J Clin Neurophysiol 2016;33(6):538–44.
69. Yucel MA, Selb JJ, Huppert TJ, et al. Functional near infrared spectroscopy: enabling routine functional brain imaging. Curr Opin Biomed Eng 2017;4:78–86.
70. Boas DA, Elwell CE, Ferrari M, et al. Twenty years of functional near-infrared spectroscopy: introduction for the special issue. Neuroimage 2014;85(Pt 1):1–5.
71. Olson DM, Zomorodi MG, James ML, et al. Exploring the impact of augmenting sedation assessment with physiologic monitors. Aust Crit Care 2013.
72. Mitchell-Hines T, Ellison K, Willis S. Using bispectral index monitoring to gauge depth of sedation/analgesia. Nursing 2016;46(4):60–3.
73. Martini F, Nath JL, Bartholomew EF. Fundamentals of anatomy & physiology. 11th ed. Pearson; 2018.

Chapter 17

Neurological alterations and management

Suzanne Bench, Elaine McGloin

Learning objectives

After reading this chapter, you should be able to:

- describe alterations in consciousness, and in motor, sensory and autonomic nerve function
- differentiate cerebral hypoxia from cerebral ischaemia and focal from global ischaemia
- differentiate between primary and secondary brain insults due to brain injury
- describe the characteristics of spinal cord trauma
- explain the characteristics of central nervous system infection and inflammation
- outline neuromuscular disorders that may be present in critically ill patients
- relate the procedures of selected neurodiagnostic tests to nursing implications for patient care
- discuss the rationale for medical and nursing management in the care of the brain-injured patient.

KEY WORDS

cerebral perfusion
coma
Guillain–Barré
intracranial hypertension
myasthenia gravis
meningitis
neuroprotection
seizures
spinal cord injury
stroke
subarachnoid haemorrhage
traumatic brain injury

Introduction

Numerous conditions encountered in critical care areas relate to serious neurological dysfunction. While most are associated with critical illness, or are at least well defined, several others occur infrequently and are not addressed extensively in this chapter. The effects of a primary illness frequently obscure the onset of an abrupt neurological complication. For example, a metabolic disorder producing encephalopathy or the use of sedation to allow better synchrony with a mechanical ventilator can delay recognition of an intracerebral haemorrhage. Neurological alterations are generally defined by problems that derive from the acute aspects of diseases such as stroke, brain and spinal cord injury and status epilepticus. This chapter discusses the concepts that underlie neurological abnormalities and addresses current management techniques and modalities.

Neurological dysfunction

This section discusses the concepts of neurological dysfunction including altered levels of consciousness, motor and sensory function and cerebral metabolism and perfusion.

Alterations in consciousness

Impaired consciousness is often the first sign of a severe pathological process. Consciousness is the recognition of self and the environment, which requires both arousal and awareness. Decreased consciousness can range from mild depression to coma, the most severe form of absolute unconsciousness.

Altered cognition and coma

Coma is a state of unresponsiveness from which the patient, who appears to be asleep, cannot be aroused by verbal and physical stimuli to produce any meaningful response. Therefore, the diagnosis of coma implies the absence of both arousal and consciousness.[1] Coma must be considered a symptom with numerous causes and several management modes. Stupor is a state of unconsciousness from which the patient can be awakened, but produces inadequate responses to verbal and physical stimuli. Somnolence is a state of unconsciousness from which the patient can be fully awakened.

Although there are many specific causes of unconsciousness, the sites of cerebral affection are either the bilateral cerebral cortex or the brainstem reticular activating system. The commonest causes of bilateral cortical disease are deficiencies of oxygen, metabolic disorders, physical injury, toxins, post-convulsive coma and infections.[2] The reticular activating system maintains the state of wakefulness through continuous stimulation of the cortex. Any interruption may lead to unconsciousness. The reticular activating system can be affected in three principal ways: by supratentorial pressure, by infratentorial pressure and by intrinsic brainstem lesions. Supratentorial and infratentorial lesions produce impaired consciousness by enlarging and displacing tissue. Lesions that affect the brainstem itself damage the reticular activating system directly.

Practice tip

The first principle of management of a person found unconscious is to maintain their airway.

Recently acquired confusion, severe apathy, stupor or coma implies dysfunction of the cerebral hemispheres, the diencephalon and/or the upper brainstem.[3] Focal lesions in supratentorial structures may damage both hemispheres, or may produce swelling that compresses the diencephalic activating system and midbrain, causing transtentorial herniation and brainstem damage. Primary infratentorial (brainstem or cerebellar) lesions may compress or directly damage the reticular formation anywhere between the level of the mid-pons and (by upward pressure) the diencephalon. Metabolic or infectious diseases may depress brain functions by a change in blood composition or the presence of a direct toxin. Impaired consciousness may also be due to reduced blood flow (as in syncope or severe heart failure) or a change in the brain's electrical activity (as in epilepsy). Concussion, anxiolytic drugs and anaesthetics impair consciousness without producing detectable structural changes in the brain.

Many of the enzymatic reactions of neurons, glial cells and specialised cerebral capillary endothelium in the brain is catalysed (i.e. accelerated) by the energy-yielding hydrolysis of adenosine triphosphate to adenosine diphosphate and inorganic phosphate. Without a constant and generous supply of adenosine triphosphate, cellular synthesis slows or stops, neuronal functions decline or cease, and cell structures quickly fall apart.[4] The use of lactate for oxidative metabolism becomes prominent when extracellular brain lactate concentration increases to supraphysiological levels, inducing a sparing of cerebral glucose. The brain depends entirely on the process of glycolysis and respiration within its own cells to provide its energy needs. Even short interruptions of blood flow, and thereby of the oxygen and glucose supply, threatens tissue vitality.

Seizures

A seizure is an uninhibited, abrupt discharge of ions from a group of neurons resulting in epileptic activity.[5] The majority of patients experiencing seizures in the intensive care unit (ICU) do not have preexisting epilepsy, and their chances of developing epilepsy in the future are usually more dependent on the cause than on the number or intensity of seizures that they experience. However, because of the other deleterious neuronal and systemic effects of seizures, their rapid diagnosis and suppression during a period of critical illness is necessary.

Seizures are classified depending on how they start as: 1) partial or focal seizures; 2) generalised or full body seizures involving both cerebral hemispheres; or 3) partial seizures with secondary generalisation. Patients may be conscious during a partial seizure whereas during generalised seizures they are not. As partial seizures may not always progress to tonic–clonic movement or alteration in consciousness, partial seizure represents one of the most elusive diagnoses in neurology and is often misdiagnosed. One of the most helpful points in the history of a partial seizure patient is the pre-epileptic event, the aura. The patient will describe the aura as a virtually identical sensation every time.

Seizures may either prompt the patient's admission to ICU (because of status epilepticus) or develop as a complication of another illness.[6] Seizures can be due to vascular, infectious, neoplastic, traumatic, degenerative, metabolic, toxic or idiopathic causes. Factors influencing the development of posttraumatic epilepsy include an early posttraumatic seizure, depressed skull fracture, intracranial haematoma, dural penetration, focal neurological deficit and posttraumatic amnesia over 24 hours with the presence of a skull fracture or haematoma. Seizures in critically ill patients are most commonly due to drug effects; metabolic, infectious or toxic disorders; or intracranial mass lesions, although they may be due to trauma or neoplasm.[7] Conditions producing seizures tend either to increase neuronal excitation or to impair neuronal inhibition. A few generalised disorders (e.g. non-ketotic hyperglycaemia) may produce partial or focal seizures.

Alterations in motor, sensory and autonomic nerve function

Alterations in motor and sensory function include skeletal muscle weakness and paralysis. They result from lesions in the voluntary motor and sensory pathways, including the upper motor and sensory neurons of the corticospinal and corticobulbar tracts, or the lower motor and sensory neurons that leave the central nervous system (CNS) and travel by way of the peripheral nerves to the muscle and sensory receptors.

Muscle tone, which is a necessary component of muscle movement, is a function of the muscle spindle (myotatic) system and the extrapyramidal system, which monitors and buffers input to the lower motor neurons by way of the multisynaptic pathways.[8] Upper motor neuron lesions produce spastic paralysis, and lower motor neuron lesions produce flaccid paralysis. Damage to the upper motor and sensory neurons of the corticospinal, corticobulbar and spinothalamic tracts is a common component of stroke.[9] Polyneuropathies involve multiple peripheral nerves and produce symmetrical sensory, motor and mixed sensori-motor deficits:

- Lesions of the corticospinal and corticobulbar tracts result in weakness or total paralysis of predominantly distal voluntary movement. Babinski's sign (i.e. dorsiflexion of the big toe and fanning of the other toes in response to stroking the outer border of the foot from heel to toe) and spasticity (increased muscle tone and exaggerated deep tendon reflexes) often characterise these lesions.
- Disorders of the basal ganglia (extrapyramidal disorders) do not cause weakness or reflex changes. Their hallmark is involuntary movement (dyskinesia), causing increased movement (hyperkinesias) or decreased movement (hypokinesia) and changes in muscle tone and posture.
- Cerebellar disorders cause abnormalities in the coordination of movement and fine motor skills. Strength is minimally affected. Critical illness myopathy and polyneuropathies are the most common causes of neuromuscular weakness in the intensive care setting. Causes include long-term mechanical ventilation, with risks increased by specific disease processes, female gender and high glucose levels.[10] See Chapter 8 for more information about these conditions.

Dysfunctions of the autonomic nervous system or autonomic dysreflexia result from failure or imbalance of the sympathetic or parasympathetic components of the autonomic nerve dysfunction with resultant signs such as: 1) increased (>120/min) or decreased (<50/min) heart rate; 2) increased respiratory rate (>24/min); 3) raised temperature (>38.5°C); 4) increased (>160 mmHg) or decreased (<85 mmHg) systolic blood pressure; 5) increased muscle tone; 6) decerebrate (extensor) or decorticate (flexor) posturing; and 7) profuse sweating. For example, in spinal injury the presence of a noxious stimulus can be transmitted from the periphery to the spinal cord and activate a dysfunctional sympathetic response.

Autonomic nervous system dysfunctions reflect the numerous interactions among the CNS, peripheral nervous system (both sympathetic and parasympathetic branches), the endocrine system and the immune system.[11] Dysfunctions range from alterations in the sympathetic–parasympathetic balance to almost complete cessation of activity as occurs in spinal cord injury. As the autonomic nervous system controls organ function, dysfunction affects all organs. The immune system is connected to the nervous system through the autonomic nervous system, thus many patients with infections, systemic inflammatory response and multi-organ failure exhibit autonomic nerve dysfunction. Autonomic nerve dysfunction can be assessed by time and spectral domain heart rate variability.[12]

Alterations in cerebral metabolism and perfusion

Neuronal cell death occurs in both high and low oxygenated states during injury. Cerebral metabolism and perfusion are compromised by diverse injury processes and biochemical patterns of ischaemia and mitochondrial dysfunction, forming the basis of secondary brain injury processes.[13]

Cerebral ischaemia and mitochondrial dysfunction

Ischaemia (inadequate delivery of oxygen) and the inadequate removal of carbon dioxide from the cell causes an increase in the production of intracellular lactic acid. Ischaemia can be caused by an increase in nutrient utilisation by the brain in a hyperactive state, a decrease in delivery related to either cerebral or systemic complications and/or a mismatch between delivery and demand.[14] The ischaemic cascade is described in Fig. 17.1 and covered in detail elsewhere.[15] Inflammation together with oxidative stress, excitotoxicity, failure of ionic homeostasis including disrupted calcium, sodium and potassium homeostasis, and energy failure are the key pathological changes in ischaemic brain damage.[16]

FIGURE 17.1 Ischaemic cascade. In cerebral ischaemia, energy failure causes depolarisation of the neuronal membrane, and excitatory neurotransmitters such as glutamate are released together. A marked influx of Ca^{2+} into neurons then occurs, which provokes the enzymatic process leading to irreversible neuronal injury. Inflammation is also a contributing factor in the development of ischaemic damage.

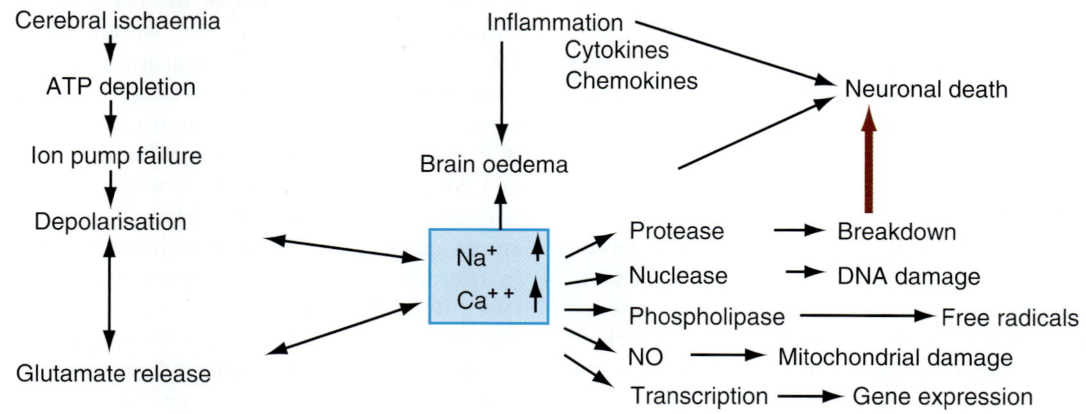

There is a significant inflammatory response in the ischaemic brain with significant changes in the peripheral immune system. When cerebral blood flow (CBF) falls to about 40% of normal, electroencephalography (EEG) slowing occurs. When CBF falls below 10 mL/100 g/min (i.e. 20%), the function of ionic pumps fails, which leads to membrane depolarisation. Cerebral ischaemia and reperfusion injury contribute to the cascade of physiological events that is termed secondary brain injury.[17]

Mitochondrial dysfunction occurs in the secondary phase of brain injury and is often associated with normal oxygen levels after reperfusion in the brain. Mitochondria are sensitive to the high levels of free glutamate that are the product of injury and reperfusion. Free calcium and nitrous oxide promote excessive production of reactive oxygen species and mitochondrial membrane permeability. Degradation of deoxyribonucleic acid and essential proteins follows and results in neuronal cell death.[17]

Cerebral oedema

Cerebral oedema is defined as increased brain water content. The brain is particularly susceptible to injury from oedema because of its confined space and limitation of expansion. There are no lymphatic pathways within the CNS to carry away the fluid that accumulates. The Monro–Kellie hypothesis states that the contents of the cranium, which is about 80% brain tissue, 10% blood and 10% cerebral spinal fluid (CSF), are incompressible and thus an increase in volume in one of the components without a corresponding decrease in another component causes a rise in pressure.[18]

After brain injury, alterations in ionic gradients cause a stepwise progression from cytotoxic to vasogenic oedema.[19] Ischaemia leads to the cessation of primary active transport via the sodium–potassium pump. As a result, co-transporters (secondary active transport) and passive transporters (via ion channels) attempt to maintain cellular processes.[19] By doing so, neurons and neuroglia accumulate active solutes that cause cellular swelling and eventually passage of fluid into the extracellular space. While the classifications of oedema are useful to define specific treatments, they are somewhat arbitrary, as cytotoxic and vasogenic oedema often occur concurrently. In fact, each of these processes may cause the other. Ultimately, these changes can lead to raised intracranial pressure (ICP) and herniation.

Cytotoxic oedema, also termed intracellular oedema, is reversible in its early phases. Cellular swelling, usually of astrocytes in the grey matter, generally occurs following a cerebral ischaemia event such as cardiac arrest.[19] The resulting hypoxia or anoxia causes a reduction of the production of adenosine triphosphate (ATP) leading to a failure of the sodium–potassium pump and the influx of Na^+ into the cell. This in turn increases the intracellular osmolarity triggering the movement of extracellular water into the cell, increasing the cell volume. The blood–brain barrier remains intact and capillary permeability is not impaired. However, eventually, endothelial and neuroglial dysfunction impairs the ability to maintain the integrity of the blood–brain barrier and vasogenic oedema ensues.

Vasogenic oedema, sometimes termed extracellular oedema, is caused by increased capillary permeability.[19] Rises in brain water content are often quite dramatic because the fluid that results from increased capillary permeability is usually rich in proteins, resulting in the spread of oedema and brain ischaemia. This can lead to further cytotoxic oedema, and to the progressive breakdown of both astrocytes and neurons.[19]

Interstitial oedema occurs as a result of hydrocephalus, when the pressure within the ventricles is higher than the capacity of the ependymal cells to confine the CSF within the ventricles. The ventricular ependymal lining ruptures allowing CSF into the extracellular space, most commonly the periventricular white matter. Causes of interstitial oedema include obstructing masses, meningitis, subarachnoid haemorrhage and normal pressure hydrocephalus.

Hydrocephalus

Hydrocephalus is the result of an imbalance between the formation and drainage and/or reabsorption of CSF. Reduced absorption most often occurs when one or more passages connecting the ventricles become blocked, preventing movement of CSF to its drainage sites in the subarachnoid space just inside the skull. This type of hydrocephalus is called 'non-communicating'. Reduction in absorption rate, called 'communicating hydrocephalus', can be caused by damage to the arachnoid villi, for example following a subarachnoid haemorrhage. Both types lead to an elevation of the CSF pressure in the brain. A third type of hydrocephalus, 'normal pressure hydrocephalus' is marked by ventricle enlargement without an apparent rise in CSF pressure and can be misdiagnosed.[20]

Hydrocephalus may be caused by congenital brain defects, haemorrhage in either the ventricles or the subarachnoid space, CNS infection (syphilis, herpes, meningitis, encephalitis or mumps) or tumours. Treatment includes ventriculostomy drainage of CSF in the short term or a surgical shunt for those with chronic conditions. Either is predisposed to blockage and infection.

> **Practice tip**
>
> The clinical features of idiopathic normal pressure hydrocephalus are abnormal gait, cognitive impairment and urinary incontinence. In older people, these can be misdiagnosed as dementia.

Intracranial hypertension

ICP is the pressure exerted by the contents of the brain within the confines of the skull and the blood–brain barrier. ICP incurs changes to the compensatory reserve and pulse amplitude, as illustrated in Fig. 17.2.[21] Normal ICP is 0–10 mmHg. Sustained pressure of >15 mmHg is termed intracranial hypertension, with implications for CBF.[22] Areas of reduced CBF and focal ischaemia appear when ICP is >20 mmHg and global ischaemia occurs at >50 mmHg. The ICP waveform contains valuable information about the nature of cerebrospinal pathophysiology. Both autoregulation of CBF and compliance of the cerebrospinal system are reflected in the ICP waveform.[23] Waveform analysis of ICP is described in Chapter 16.

Initially, intracranial compliance allows compensation for rises in intracranial volume by means of shunting CSF down the thecal sac, increased reabsorption of CSF and vasoconstriction of the cerebral venous vessels reducing the volume of blood within the cranial vault. These mechanisms of autoregulation enable a constant CBF to be maintained over a range of arterial perfusion pressures. During a slow continuous rise in volume, the ICP rises to a plateau level at which the increased level of CSF absorption keeps pace with the rise in volume with ample compensatory reserve. When these compensatory mechanisms become exhausted, pressure begins to rise and the patient exhibits signs and symptoms of raised ICP. The time taken to overcome these protective processes depends on how quickly the rise of intracranial volume occurs and is expressed as an index, as shown in Fig. 17.3.[24] Intermittent expansion (which in health can be caused by Valsalva manoeuvres such as coughing and straining) causes only a transient rise in ICP at first. When sufficient CSF has been absorbed to accommodate the volume, the ICP returns to normal.

If the ICP rises to the level of arterial pressure, this itself begins to rise, accompanied by bradycardia or other disturbances of heart rhythm, termed Cushing's response. Dilation of the small pial arteries and some slowing of venous flow, which is followed by pulsatile venous flow, also occurs. The respiratory changes associated with increased ICP depend on the level of brainstem involved. A midbrain involvement results in Cheyne–Stokes respiration. When the midbrain and pons are involved, there is sustained hyperventilation. There are rapid and shallow respirations with upper medulla involvement, with ataxic breathing in the final stages (Fig. 17.4).[25] Neurogenic pulmonary oedema may also occur due to increased sympathetic activity because of the effects of elevated ICP on the hypothalamus, medulla or cervical spinal cord.

The causes of intracranial hypertension are classified as acute or chronic. Acute causes include brain trauma, ischaemic injury and intracerebral haemorrhage. Infections such as encephalitis or meningitis may also lead to intracranial hypertension. Chronic causes include many intracranial tumours, such as ependymomas, or hydrocephalus that may gradually impinge on CSF pathways and interfere with CSF outflow and circulation. As the ICP continues to increase, the brain tissue becomes distorted, leading to herniation and additional vascular injury.[26]

Neurological therapeutic management

This section explores the management of cerebral perfusion. The objective is to identify deficits in perfusion allowing the initiation of strategies aimed at preventing

FIGURE 17.2 The volume–ICP curve relationship.

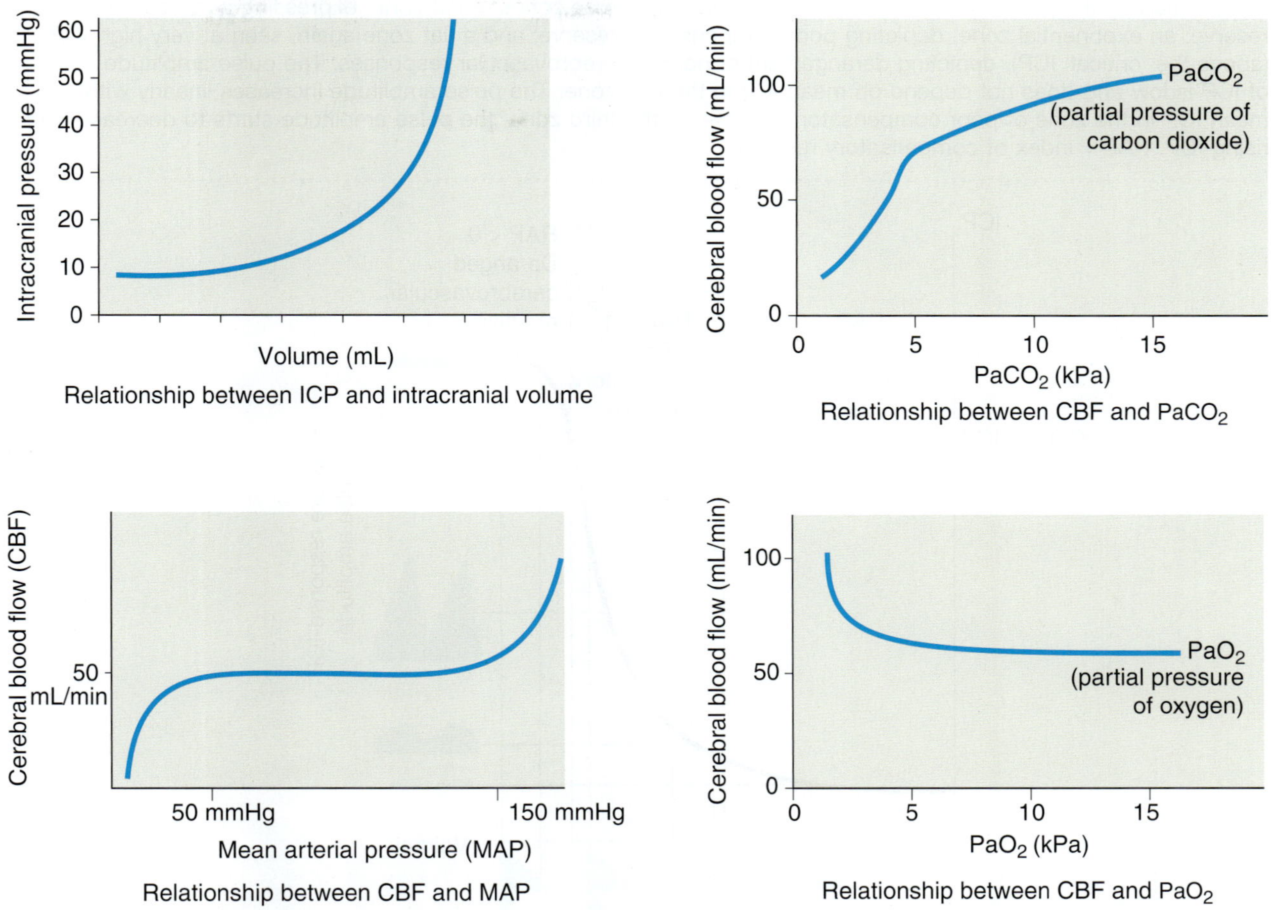

Source: McLeod A. Traumatic injuries to the head and spine, 2: nursing considerations. Br J Nurs 2004;13(17):1041–9, with permission.

secondary insults and further ischaemia. The modalities of neuroprotection, including the management of intracranial hypertension and cerebral ischaemia are discussed and nursing interventions, based on published guidelines for the prevention of secondary insults and promotion of cerebral perfusion, are considered.

Optimising cerebral perfusion

Intracranial hypertension and cerebral ischaemia are the two most important secondary injury processes that can be anticipated, monitored and treated in the ICU. This applies to all aetiologies of brain injury including trauma. Advanced cerebral monitoring techniques are described in Chapter 16. Episodes of brain hypoxia are common and may occur even when ICP and cerebral perfusion pressure (CPP) are normal, emphasising the value of multimodal monitoring that integrates data from several physiological monitors.[27] These observations can help clinicians to better understand the complex pathophysiology of the brain after an acute insult, evaluate autoregulation and identify optimal physiological targets and the utility of therapeutic interventions. The selection of oxygenation monitoring focuses on the appropriateness of focal or global monitoring, the location of the monitor in relation to the injury and the intermittent or continuous nature of the monitoring device.

Practice tip

Cerebral perfusion pressure (CPP) = mean arterial pressure (MAP) − ICP. So, if ICP is increased, MAP must be increased to maintain CPP.

Management of intracranial hypertension

Intracranial hypertension is treated by removing mass lesions and/or increasing the space available for expansion of injured tissue.[28] This may be achieved by

FIGURE 17.3 In a simple model, pulse amplitude of intracranial pressure (ICP) (expressed along the *y*-axis on the right side of the panel) results from pulsatile changes in cerebral blood volume (expressed along the *x*-axis) transformed by the pressure–volume curve. This curve has three zones: a flat zone, expressing good compensatory reserve; an exponential zone, depicting poor compensatory reserve; and a flat zone again, seen at very high ICP (above the 'critical' ICP), depicting derangement of normal cerebrovascular responses. The pulse amplitude of ICP is low and does not depend on mean ICP in the first zone. The pulse amplitude increases linearly with mean ICP in the zone of poor compensatory reserve. In the third zone, the pulse amplitude starts to decrease with rising ICP. RAP = index of compensatory reserve.

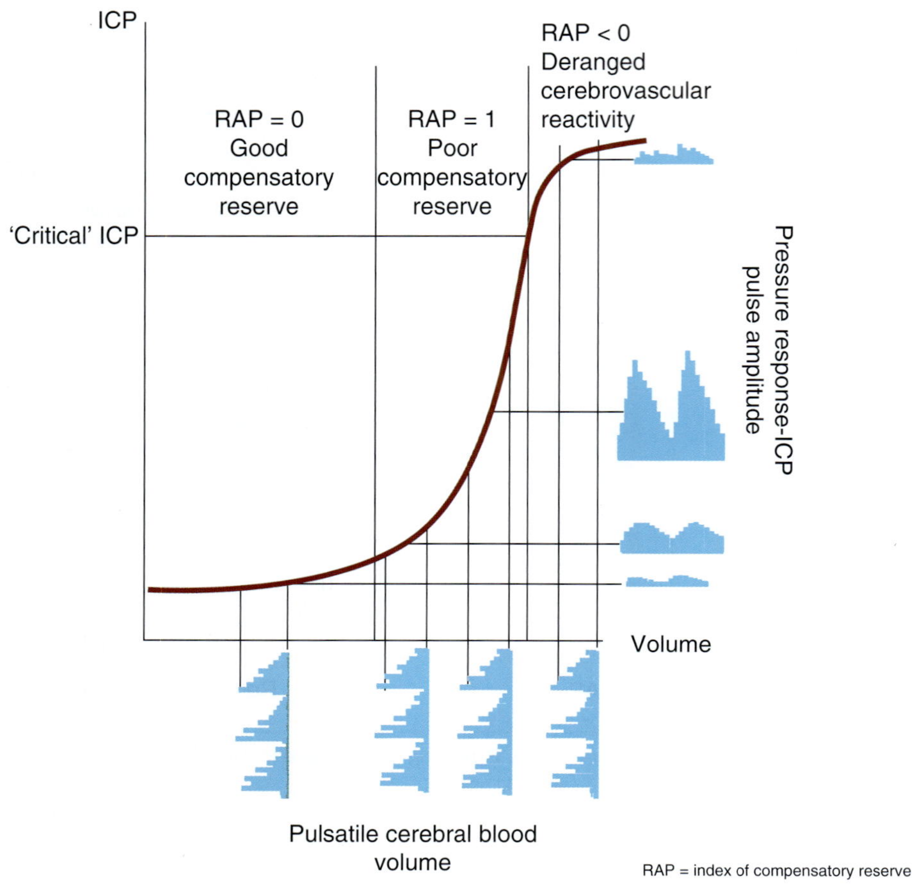

Source: Czosnyka M, Pickard J. Monitoring and interpretation of intracranial pressure. J Neurol Neurosurg Psychiat 2004;75(6):813–21, with permission from BMJ Publishing Group Ltd.

reducing one of the other available intracranial fluid volumes such as:

1 CSF via ventricular drainage
2 cerebral blood volume by hyperventilation, osmotic diuretic therapy or hypothermia
3 brain tissue water content by osmotic diuretic therapy
4 removing swollen and irreversibly injured brain
5 increasing cranial capacity by craniotomy decompression.

The application of these concepts to the following therapeutic strategies is important in the management of intracranial hypertension.[28]

Practice tip

In brain injury, position the patient at 45° head-up to maximise cerebral perfusion and minimise cerebral oedema.

External ventricular drainage

External ventricular drains allow both the monitoring of ICP levels and the drainage of CSF. The use of continuous versus intermittent drainage systems remains variable, with little evidence to guide practice in the adult population. Open systems, where drainage is continuous, risk sudden drops in ICP, which can be life-threatening,

FIGURE 17.4 Injury to the brainstem can result in various abnormal respiratory patterns.

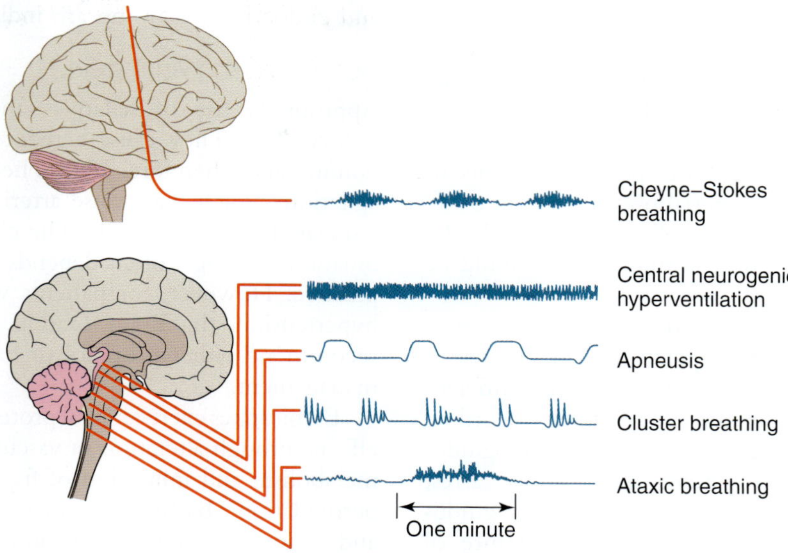

Reproduced from Porth C, Martin G. Essentials of pathophysiology; concepts of altered health states. 3rd ed. Philadelphia: Lippincott, Williams & Williams 2011 with permission.

while also allowing only for intermittent ICP monitoring. In contrast, closed systems, where ICP is continuously monitored, have to be intermittently opened to allow for CSF drainage. The Brain Trauma Foundation guidelines recommend a continuous drainage system, zeroed at the level of the midbrain, based on moderate levels of evidence.[29] Both systems carry a high risk of infection.

Ventilation therapies

Hyperventilation reduces $PaCO_2$. It will reduce ICP by vasoconstriction induced by alkalosis, but it also decreases CBF. The fall in ICP parallels the fall in cerebral blood volume. Hyperventilation decreases regional blood flow to hypoperfused areas of the brain. Thus, generally $PaCO_2$ should be maintained in the low normal range of about 35-45 mmHg (4.6–6 kPa). Hyperventilation should be utilised only when ICP elevations are refractory to other treatments and when brain tissue oxygenation is in the normal range.[29] The Brain Trauma Foundation Guidelines recommend hyperventilation therapy only be used as a temporising measure to treat a critically elevated ICP, which is refractory to other therapies, and with cerebral oxygen monitoring to allow measurement of oxygen delivery levels. The Brain Trauma Foundation also recommend that it should be avoided during the acute phase (i.e. 24 hours).[29]

Osmotherapy

Acute administration of an osmotic such as mannitol or hypertonic saline produces a potent anti-oedema action, primarily on undamaged brain regions with an intact blood–brain barrier. This treatment causes the movement of water from the interstitial and extracellular space into the intravascular compartment, thereby improving intracranial compliance or elastance. In addition to causing 'dehydration' of the brain, osmotic agents have been shown to exert beneficial non-osmotic cerebral effects, such as augmentation of CBF (by reducing blood viscosity, resulting in enhanced oxygen delivery), free radical scavenging and diminishing CSF formation and enhancing CSF reabsorption.[30]

There is insufficient evidence available to recommend one type of hyperosmolar agent over another, but the Brain Trauma Foundation acknowledges the increasing use of hypertonic saline.[29] Both intravenous hypertonic saline (3%) and 20% mannitol can help reduce ICP and maintain haemodynamic status. But, mannitol also has a diuretic effect, which is relatively contraindicated in patients with both traumatic brain injury (TBI) and hypovolaemia as it may worsen intravascular volume depletion and decrease cerebral perfusion.[30] A recent systematic review and meta-analysis found no mortality benefit or effect on controlling ICP with the use of hypertonic saline compared to other solutions.[31]

Targeted temperature management

Targeted temperature management may be used to prevent fever, to maintain normothermia, or to reduce core temperature. Hyperthermia is common in brain-injured patients and is independently associated with increased morbidity and mortality, partly due to its effects on ICP. Temperature elevations as small as 1–2°C above normal can aggravate ischaemic neuronal injury and exacerbate brain oedema.[32]

ICP falls significantly at brain temperatures below 37°C and CPP peaks at 35–36°C. However, at temperatures below 35°C, both oxygen delivery and oxygen consumption decrease. Cardiac output also decreases progressively with hypothermia.[33] Temperatures lower than 34°C substantially increase the volume of intravenous (IV) fluid infusion and inotrope requirements to maintain an adequate mean arterial pressure and at 31°C serum potassium, white blood cell count and platelet counts are diminished.[34] Thus, normothermia should be the standard of care.

In some patients (e.g. those following cardiac arrest or with a TBI) lower target temperatures may be used to reduce intracranial hypertension and maintain sufficient CPP.[35] The target temperature may differ according to the situation. For example, international guidelines recommend cooling patients post-cardiac arrest to 32–36°C.[36–38] In contrast, the 2017 French guidelines recommend maintaining a target temperature of 35–37°C in severe TBI, lowered to 34–35°C for those with refractory hypertension.[36] They further suggest considering targeted temperature management at 32–35°C in patients with refractory status epilepticus.

The optimal length of time or the best method by which to actively cool someone remains unknown although some studies suggest longer-term cooling for up to 5 days may be most beneficial.[39] Active cooling may be initiated using paracetamol, cooling blankets, evaporative cooling and other innovative cooling technologies. Care should be taken to avoid complications such as hypokalaemia and hyperaemia (increased blood flow), which may occur during rewarming, resulting in dysrhythmias, acute brain swelling and rebound intracranial hypertension.[39] It is also important to avoid shivering, which can be counterproductive. Canadian guidelines recommend a continuous method of temperature assessment, such as oesophageal monitoring.[36]

Corticosteroids

Excessive inflammation has been implicated in the progressive neurodegeneration that occurs in multiple neurological diseases, including cerebral ischaemia. The efficacy of glucocorticoids is well established in ameliorating oedema associated with brain tumours and in improving the outcome in subsets of patients with bacterial meningitis. Despite encouraging experimental results, clinical trials of glucocorticoids in ischaemic stroke, intracerebral haemorrhage, aneurysmal subarachnoid haemorrhage (aSAH) and TBI have not shown a definite therapeutic effect. Furthermore, the CRASH (**c**orticosteroid **r**andomisation **a**fter **s**ignificant **h**ead injury) trial reported that risk of death was higher in the treatment group than in the control group.[40] Thus, high-dose steroids are not indicated for use in TBI. However, anterior pituitary insufficiency is an under-recognised problem in patients with severe TBI, particularly in elderly people or those who have diffuse axonal injury and skull base fracture. In these instances, administration of hydrocortisone in physiological doses and endocrine follow-up are indicated.[41]

Sedatives and analgesics

Appropriate use of sedatives and analgesics can help reduce ICP. They cause a reduction in cerebral blood volume and, therefore, ICP. They also reduce pain and agitation, which may cause arterial hypertension and an associated increase in ICP. The choice of drug (or combination of drugs) often depends on local protocols and practice. However, for patients with severe intracranial hypertension, the Brain Trauma Foundation guidelines recommend either propofol or barbiturates for first-line management.[29]

Barbiturates exert cerebral protective and ICP-lowering effects through alteration in vascular tone, suppression of metabolism and inhibition of free radical-mediated lipid peroxidation. Barbiturates may effectively lower CBF and regional metabolic demands, which in turn decrease CBF and cerebral volume. This results in beneficial effects on ICP and global cerebral perfusion. However, barbiturates can cause significant hypotension and should only be used to control elevations in ICP, which are refractory to other interventions, once haemodynamic stability has been achieved.[29]

Propofol has a rapid onset and short duration of action and is commonly used to help lower ICP. At higher doses (>5 mg/kg/h), propofol can also induce EEG burst suppression, that can effectively treat status epilepticus.[42] However, there is no evidence that it improves mortality or 6-month outcomes and high doses are associated with significant adverse effects, including hypotension. Many other commonly used sedatives, analgesics and anaesthetic agents can also induce hypotension, potentially reducing CPP and increasing ICP. Careful bedside monitoring and titration is therefore required.

Surgical interventions

The European TBI Guidelines suggest that operative management be considered for large intracerebral lesions within the first 4 hours of injury. The use of unilateral craniectomy after the evacuation of a mass lesion, such as an acute subdural haematoma or traumatic intracerebral haematoma, is accepted practice. Surgery is also recommended for open compound depressed skull fractures that cause a mass effect.[43] Mass effect on computerised tomography (CT) scan is defined as distortion, compression and/or displacement of intracranial contents; dislocation or obliteration of the fourth ventricle; compression or loss of visualisation of the basal cisterns or the presence of obstructive hydrocephalus.

Decompressive craniectomy (removal of a portion of the skull) for refractory intracranial hypertension has been performed since 1977, with a significant reduction in ICP for both TBI [43] and ischaemic stroke.[44] However, in 2011, a multicentre trial of early decompressive craniectomy in patients with severe TBI (the DECRA trial) reported that, although an early bifrontotemporoparietal decompressive craniectomy in adults with severe diffuse TBI and refractory intracranial hypertension decreased ICP and length of stay in the ICU, it was associated with more unfavourable outcomes at both 6 and 12 months.[45] The subsequent **r**andomised **e**valuation of **s**urgery with **c**raniectomy for **u**ncontrollable **e**levation of ICP (RESCUEicp) trial[46] used a higher threshold for intervention than did the DECRA trial, and included patients with mass lesions and unilateral or bilateral decompressive craniectomy. Nevertheless, conclusions remain the same and indicate that while decompressive craniectomy lowers mortality, survivors have poorer functional outcomes than those treated conservatively.

Fundamental nursing care considerations

Nurses should consider the impact of the environment and interventions on a patient's ICP and take proactive steps to avoid unnecessary rises, while promptly recognising and treating any increases that do occur, as described in Table 17.1. Clustering of care activities can produce a cumulative and resistant effect on ICP, which can be difficult to return to baseline, resulting in decreased CPP. ICP monitoring allows the clinician to assess the effect of interventions on a patient's ICP and CPP and to individualise care. In the case of uncontrollable ICP rises, non-essential interventions should be terminated and the ICP allowed to return to baseline. Care should be taken to limit noxious stimuli, such as environmental noise and pain as these can increase ICP and adequate sedation and analgesia administered to keep the patient calm and pain free. Even though a patient may not be able to respond, nurses should always assume they can hear and understand; address them by name and explain all procedures. Adapting the environment, for example by dimming lights and consideration to family visitation and its effects on a patient's ICP should be made.

Maintaining head position at 30° facilitates cerebral venous drainage while having no adverse effects on CPP, although the results of a trial comparing acute stroke patients nursed flat with those nursed at a minimum of 30° head-up did not show any difference in disability outcomes.[47] Extreme hip flexion, the Trendelenburg position and lateral flexion of the neck should, however, be avoided as these positions increase intrathoracic pressure and thus ICP.[48] Chest physiotherapy and suctioning are important as they improve gas exchange, helping to maintain CPP, but they also increase ICP.[49]

A head to toe skin assessment should be carried out every shift. The use of a pressure-relieving mattress should be considered, although for patients who have either a confirmed or suspected spinal injury, the use of an alternating pressure air mattress is contraindicated as the neutral alignment of the spinal column cannot be guaranteed. Deep vein thrombosis prevention should also be in place, noting that the use of graduated compression stockings may be contraindicated in some patients, e.g. following stroke. Hygiene interventions should include regular oral, eye and hair care and a bowel regimen to avoid constipation, which can increase intraabdominal pressure and ICP.[48] These essential nursing cares and others are described in Chapter 5. Regular repositioning of nasogastric and endotracheal tubes will help prevent the development of pressure injury, which could be a source of pain and thus increase ICP. Care should also be taken to avoid overtightening endotracheal tubes, which can restrict venous drainage.

Central nervous system disorders

CNS disorders include brain and/or spinal injury from trauma, infection or immune conditions. The pathophysiology and aetiology of these disorders are discussed here, including management of these conditions.

Traumatic brain injury

TBI has replaced the former term 'head injury' and is defined as an alteration in brain function, or other evidence of brain pathology, caused by an external force, which can affect the scalp, skull or brain.[50] The range of severity of TBI is broad, from concussion through to post-coma unresponsiveness. The incidence of TBI is increasing worldwide, though estimates vary considerably between countries.[50,51] Reviewers of the global literature agree that the incidence of TBI is highest in countries of low to middle income; in males and in those aged 15–25 years. Rates in older populations (over 65 years) are also increasing. Outcome data from long-term follow-up of TBI cohorts support that physical and neuropsychological difficulties are common and it is estimated that there are at least 13 million people living with TBI-related disability in the USA and the European Union.[50]

Aetiology

Falls are the leading cause of TBI (35.2%), followed by being struck by/against an object and motor vehicle collisions or traffic accidents.[51,52] However, road traffic accidents and gunshot wounds to the head lead to the most TBI fatalities. In contrast, sporting accidents and falls account for a far greater percentage of mild injuries. Infants and toddlers up to 4 years of age, older adolescents aged 15–19 years and adults older than 65 years of age are the highest risk age groups for TBI.[53] This trimodal distribution has been demonstrated for most ethnic and racial groups studied, as well as in global studies of TBI. Most studies have found that the highest age-specific incidence is in the young adult years. Injury and debility in this age group also carries significant morbidity, with many more years of potential life lost and lost productivity for injuries incurred in young people. For every age group studied, males are more likely to

TABLE 17.1
Nursing interventions for the brain-injured patient with intracranial hypertension

AIM	GOAL	INTERVENTIONS
Maintain adequate oxygenation and ventilation	PaO_2 100 mmHg (13.3 kPa) $PaCO_2$ 35–40 mmHg (4.6–5.3 kPa) PaO_2/FiO_2 ratio >350 SaO_2 98% SjO_2 50–75% $PbtO_2$ >20 Airway patent Lungs clear on auscultation Prevention of ventilator-associated pneumonia (VAP)	• Maintain airway – will require intubation for Glasgow Coma Scale <8 or diaphragmatic respiratory insufficiency • Assess bilateral chest movement: listen for airway obstruction or ET cuff leak; auscultate for air entry • Assess chest X-ray • Consider pre-oxygenation prior to suction/repositioning/other interventions • Obtain ABG and manipulate set FiO_2 and ventilator settings to meet parameter goals • Monitor end-tidal CO_2 continuously • Be aware of the impact of increasing levels of PEEP on ICP levels. Chest physiotherapy and suction patient as needed • Use frequent subglottal suctioning, and maintain head of bed elevation at 30° or more to prevent aspiration • In recovery: assess for upper airway weakness and reflex (prevent aspiration), sputum retention and atelectasis
Maintain haemodynamic stability and CBF	MAP: ≥90 mmHg Stroke: thrombolytic, embolic and ICH, MAP 90–120 mmHg $PbtO_2$ <20 CVP 5–10 mmHg CPP 60–70 mmHg Haematocrit 33% or haemoglobin content 80–100 g/L	• Maintain euvolaemia • Give prescribed intravenous fluids (avoiding dextrose solutions) as prescribed to maintain CVP and PCWP within parameters • Use noradrenaline once euvolaemic in order to optimise MAP • Observe $PbtO_2$ for sedation-induced hypotension • Transfuse with red blood cells as appropriate • Monitor BP, CVP and other hemodynamic parameters • Monitor closely for signs and symptoms of neurogenic pulmonary oedema, especially in patients with cardiac history • Transcranial Doppler image to check for vasospasm • Non-traumatic aSAH, administer IV nimodipine infusion to prevent vasospasm as prescribed; consider components of HH therapy • Ischaemic stroke, administer tPA within 3 h of event • ICH, prevent rebleeding; administer prescribed haemostatic medications, reduce hypertension
Maintain ICP and CPP within target range	ICP <20 mmHg CPP 50–70 mmHg	• Elevate head of bed above the level of the heart to obtain optimal level of ICP and CPP. Monitor ICP, CPP and $PbtO_2$ to ensure optimal level for your patient (15–30°) • Avoid Trendelenburg position, extreme hip flexion and lateral flexion of neck • Position body with neck straight and no knee elevation in order to maintain venous outflow • If patient has a ventriculostomy, drain per prescription • Individualise care to control ICP; terminate non-essential interventions if ICP rises above set parameters • Administer prescribed hypertonic saline or mannitol infusions • Consider paralytics if positioning, cooling, sedation and mannitol does not resolve increased ICP • Prepare for surgical craniotomy if indicated • Drainage of CSF via EVD
Maintain normothermia	Core temperature 35–37°C	• Continuous monitoring of temperature e.g. via oesophageal monitoring or indwelling urinary catheter • Administration of paracetamol • Instigate the use of cooling blankets or other devices as necessary • Avoid shivering of the patient as this can increase ICP

TABLE 17.1
Nursing interventions for the brain-injured patient with intracranial hypertension—cont'd

AIM	GOAL	INTERVENTIONS
Maintain environment/ reduce stimulation	A calm and stress-free environment	• Group necessary interventions in a timely manner to allow adequate rest • Limit noxious stimuli; minimise noise and lighting • Avoid overstimulation and limit interventions if ICP is precarious • Assess the need for and administer analgesia and sedation (e.g. propofol, morphine, fentanyl, lorazepam/midazolam) as prescribed • Speak to patient using their name and explain procedures even if unconscious • Sensitively manage visitors remembering the importance of contact with family and friends
Maintain nutrition		• Promote early enteric feeding • Oral enteric feeding tube (nasogastric contradicted in TBI) • Dietitian referral for metabolic requirements
Essential care	Patient integument maintained and infection free: skin, mucous membranes, cornea, wounds, invasive lines Patient safety enabled, preventing nosocomial infection, secondary brain injury, self-harm	• Head to toe assessment of skin integrity, corneas, mucous membranes • Provide regular eye, oral and hair care • Instigate a bowel care protocol to avoid constipation • Deep vein thrombosis prevention as appropriate to patient's condition • Ensure ETT ties are secure but not too tight which can impede intracranial venous outflow and lead to raised ICP. • Consider the use of alternate ETT securement, such as taped to the face, when ICP is refractory to treatment • Regular repositioning for pressure area care and chest management • Consider a pressure-relieving mattress • Consider need for kinetic therapy, e.g. rotation/percussion therapy bed (within spinal precautions where necessary) • Maintain infection control interventions and closely monitor for infection related to invasive devices and wounds • Use of chemical and physical restraint after assessment and prescription, within institutional policy • Ensure effective verbal and written communication with other health professionals
Psychological/ family	Family and significant others informed and supported Psychological wellbeing of patient maintained The patient feels safe	• Refer and coordinate information and service provision from other health professionals • The provision of quality, informed and inclusive care to the patient provides family and significant others with the confidence that the nurse advocates for the patient in their place • Ensure psychological assessment and administer prescribed therapy for delirium and posttraumatic stress • Nursing interventions planned to allow for rest and recovery • Administer coordinated rehabilitation strategies

ABG = arterial blood gas; BP = blood pressure; aSAH = aneurysmal subarachnoid haemorrhage; CBF = cerebral blood flow; CPP = cerebral perfusion pressure; CVP = central venous pressure; ET = endotracheal; $ETCO_2$ = end-tidal carbon dioxide; ETT = endotracheal tube; FiO_2 = fraction of inspired oxygen; HH = hypervolaemic hypertensive; ICH = intracerebral haemorrhage; ICP = intracranial pressure; IV = intravenous; MAP = mean arterial pressure; $PaCO_2$ = partial pressure of alveolar carbon dioxide; PaO_2 = partial pressure of alveolar oxygen; $PbtO_2$ = brain tissue oxygenation; PCWP = pulmonary capillary wedge pressure; PEEP = positive end-expiratory pressure; SaO_2 = arterial oxygen saturation; SjO_2 = jugular venous oxygen saturation; TBI = traumatic brain injury; tPa = tissue plasminogen activator; VAP = ventilator-associated pneumonia suffer TBI than females. Among young people, males are up to seven times more likely to suffer a TBI. People of colour and those of lower socioeconomic strata also suffer rates of TBI 30% to 50% higher than the majority of individuals. Alcohol is involved in 50% of cases of TBI, either because of intoxicated drivers or pedestrians, increased risk of falls, suicide attempts or interpersonal violence.[53,54]

The transfer of energy to the brain tissue causes the damage and is a significant determinant in the severity of injury. The introduction of safer car designs, airbags and other road traffic initiatives (e.g. redesigning hazardous intersections, driver education campaigns, random breath testing and reducing speed limits) have decreased the overall number of road fatalities; improvements in retrieval, neurosurgery and intensive care in the past few decades have enabled many people to survive injuries that would previously have been fatal.

Pathophysiology

TBI is a heterogeneous pathophysiological process (Fig. 17.5). The mechanisms of injury forces inflicted on the head produce a complex mixture of diffuse and focal lesions within the brain.[55] Damage resulting from an injury can be immediate (primary) or secondary in nature. Secondary injury results from disordered autoregulation and other pathophysiological changes within the brain in the days immediately after injury. Urgent neurosurgical intervention for intracerebral, subdural or extradural haemorrhages can mitigate the extent of secondary injury. Scalp lesions can bleed profusely and quickly lead to hypovolaemic shock and brain ischaemia. Cerebral oedema, haemorrhage and biochemical response to injury, infection and increased ICP are among the commonest physiological responses that can cause secondary injury. Tissue hypoxia is also of major concern and airway obstruction immediately after injury contributes significantly to secondary injury. Poor CBF, due to direct (primary) vascular changes or damage, can lead to ischaemic brain tissue, and eventually neuronal cell death.[56] Systemic changes in temperature, haemodynamics and pulmonary status can also lead to secondary brain injury (Fig. 17.6). In moderate-to-severe, and occasionally in mild injury CBF is altered in the initial

FIGURE 17.5 Pathophysiology of traumatic brain injury.

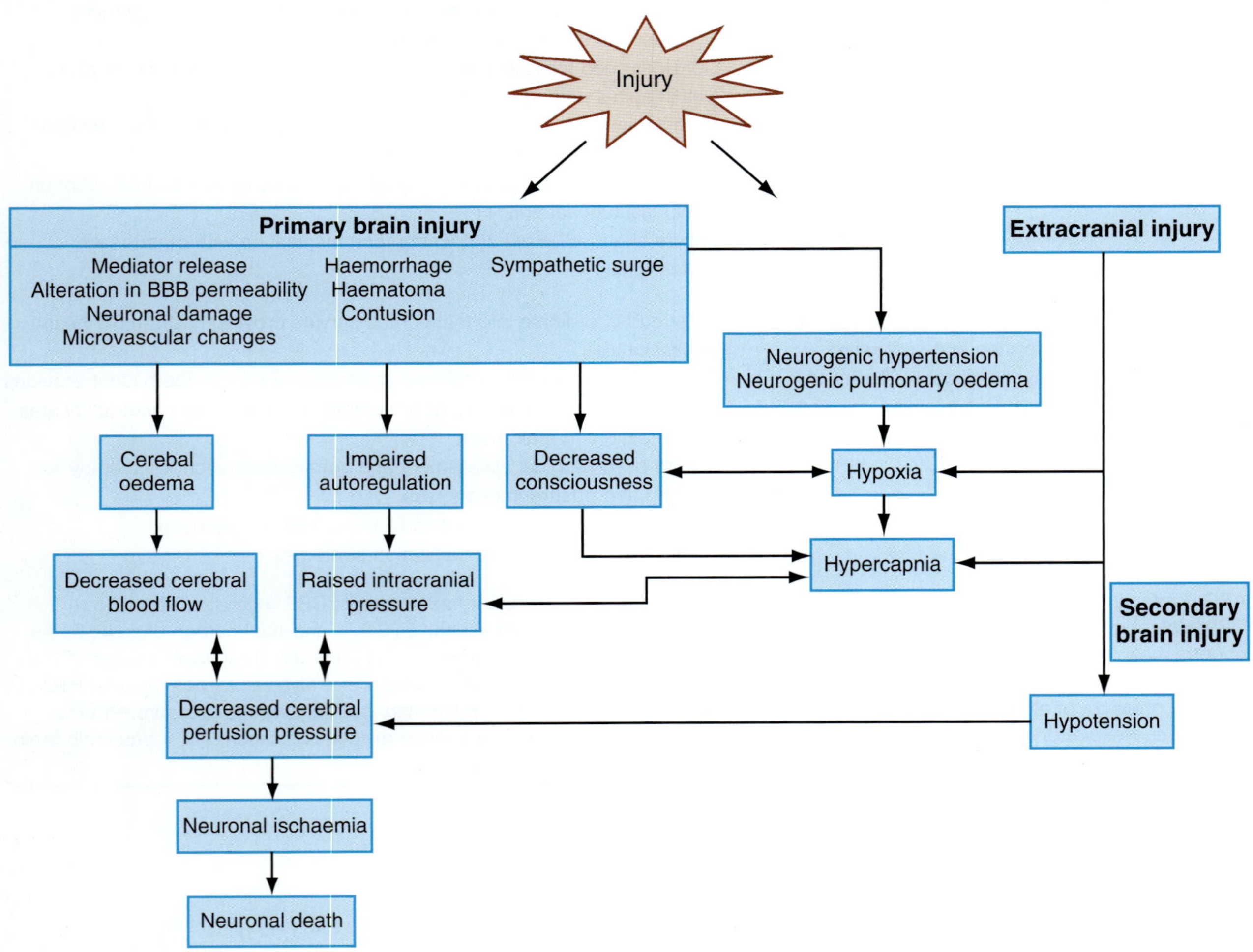

FIGURE 17.6 Conceptual changes in cerebral blood flow (CBF) and intracranial pressure (ICP) over time following traumatic brain injury: (**A**) cytotoxic oedema; (**B**) vasogenic oedema; (**C**) CBF. CPP = cerebral perfusion pressure; MAP = mean arterial pressure.

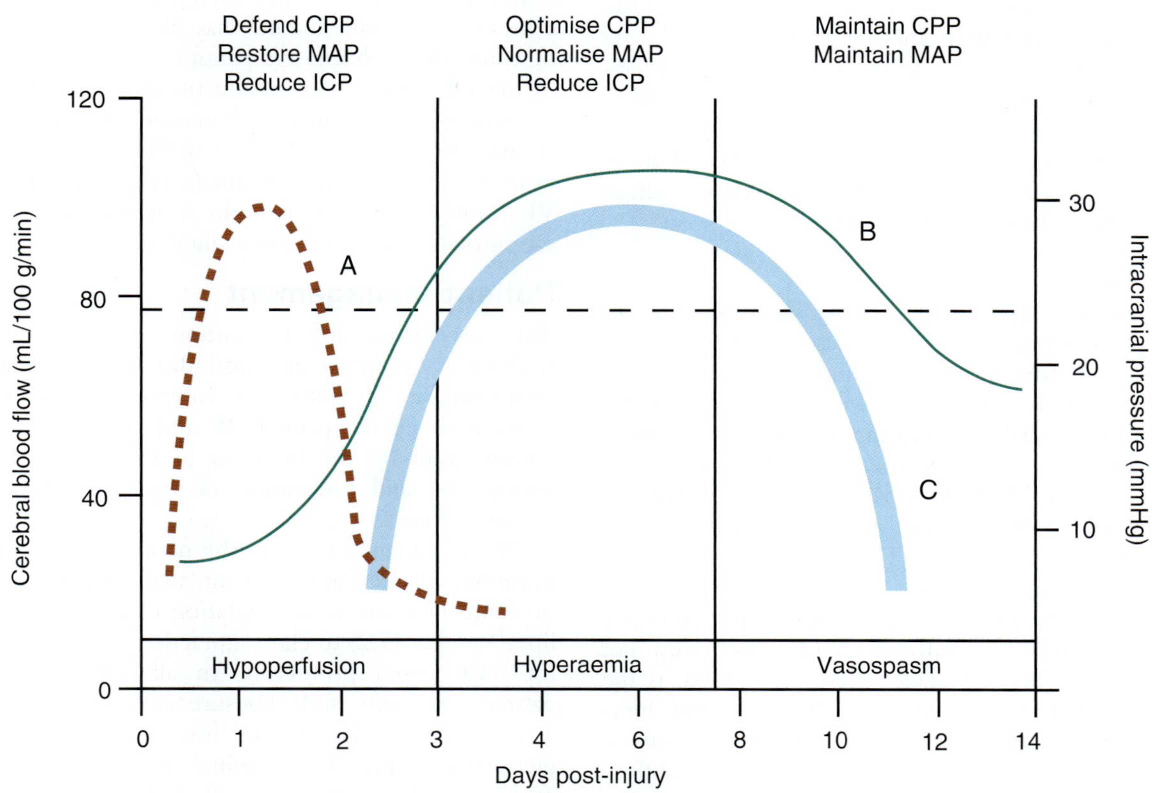

2–3 days, followed by a rebound hyperaemic stage (days 4–7) leading to a precarious state (days 8–14) of cerebral vessel unpredictability and vasospasm.[57] More than 30% of TBI patients have autonomic nerve dysfunction characterised by episodes of increased heart rate, respiratory rate, temperature, blood pressure, muscle tone, decorticate or decerebrate posturing and profuse sweating.[58] Lack of insight into these processes and implementing early weaning of supportive therapies can lead to significant secondary insults.

Classification

Mild TBI is usually defined as when someone has a Glasgow Coma Scale (GCS) score of 13 to 15. It often presents as a component of multi-trauma or sports injury and can be overlooked at the expense of other peripheral injuries.[59] Clinical symptoms such as dizziness, confusion, posttraumatic amnesia, nausea and vomiting which persist at 4 hours post-injury require continued observation. Routine head CT is recommended to exclude mass lesions and diffuse axonal injury. Moderate TBI presents with a GCS of 9–12. Patients will require an early CT scan and should be admitted to hospital for at least 24 hours for close observation. A GCS of 8 or less is considered a severe TBI requiring resuscitation, early intubation to prevent hypoxaemia and early CT scan to guide management.

Primary vs secondary injury

Brain injury associated with TBI can be divided into primary and secondary injury. Primary injury is the damage that occurs at the time of the trauma and is a result of mechanical forces being applied to the brain tissue. The mechanisms of injury are contact (coup), acceleration-deceleration (contrecoup) and rotational acceleration-deceleration (diffuse axonal), which result in shearing, compression and stretching (tensile) of the structures of the brain. Secondary injury is the damage occurring after the primary impact and, unlike primary injury, can be prevented and treated. The mechanisms of secondary injury include an inflammatory cascade response, neurotoxicity due to the release of glutamate, and electrolyte imbalances caused by the breakdown of the sodium–potassium pump. Hypoxia, hypotension, intracranial hypertension and changes to CBF will further exacerbate secondary injury. Careful monitoring of the patient is required to reduce or prevent the incidence of secondary injury.

Focal injury

Because of the shape of the inner surface of the skull, focal injuries are most commonly seen in the frontal and temporal lobes, but they can occur anywhere. Contact phenomena or a local blow to the head, or the head coming into contact with another item with force, are commonly superficial and can generate contusional haemorrhages through coup and contrecoup mechanisms.[59] Cerebral contusions are readily identifiable on CT scans, but may only become visible on CT on days 2 or 3. Deep intracerebral haemorrhages can result from either focal or diffuse damage to the arteries.

Diffuse injury

Diffuse (axonal) injury refers to the shearing of axons and supporting neuroglia; it may also traumatise blood vessels and can cause petechial haemorrhages, deep intracerebral haematomas and brain swelling.[59] Diffuse injury results from the shaking, shearing and inertial effects of a traumatic impact as often seen in high speed motor vehicle accidents. Mechanical damage to small venules as part of the blood–brain barrier can also trigger formation of haemorrhagic contusions. This vascular damage may increase neuronal vulnerability, causing post-traumatising perfusion deficits and the extravasation of potentially neurotoxic blood-borne substances. The most consistent effect of diffuse brain damage, even when mild, is the presence of altered consciousness. The depth and duration of coma provide the best guide to the severity of the diffuse damage. The majority of patients with diffuse injury will not have any CT evidence to support the diagnosis. Other clinical markers of diffuse injury include the high speed or force strength of injury, absence of a lucid interval and prolonged retrograde and anterograde amnesia. Fig. 17.7 contrasts CT scans with haematoma formation and diffuse axonal injury.

Skull fractures

Skull fractures are present on CT scans in about two-thirds of patients after TBI. Skull fractures can be linear, depressed or diastatic, and may involve the cranial vault or skull base. In depressed skull fractures the bone fragment may cause a laceration of the dura mater, resulting in a cerebrospinal fluid leak or become embedded in the parenchyma requiring surgery to elevate or remove the bone fragment.[59] Basal skull fractures include fractures of the cribriform plate, frontal bones, sphenoid bones, temporal bone and occipital bones. The clinical signs of a basal skull fracture may include: CSF otorrhoea or rhinorrhoea, haemotympanum or presence of blood in the tympanic cavity of the middle ear, postauricular ecchymoses, periorbital ecchymoses and injury to the cranial nerves – VII (weakness of the face), VIII (loss of hearing), olfactory (loss of smell), optic (vision loss) and VI (double vision). CSF leaks from the nose and ears can also be detected using a glucometer.

FIGURE 17.7 Extradural haematoma and a subtle subdural haematoma (**left**), subdural haematoma (**middle left**), diffuse axonal injury (**middle right**) and combination injuries (**right**).

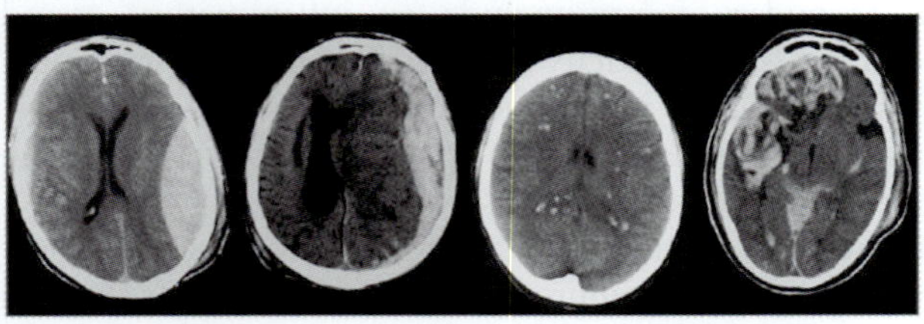

Patient management

The surveillance and prevention of secondary injury is the key to improving morbidity and mortality outcomes in patients with TBI. Interventions are targeted at maintaining adequate CBF and minimising oxygen consumption by the brain to prevent ischaemia. The anticipation and prevention of systemic complications are also crucial.

Nursing management of the neurologically impaired, immobilised, mechanically ventilated patient is described in Table 17.1 and is an adaptation of the current guidelines[29] (Table 17.2) to clinical practice (see *Online resources* for TBI-related protocols). In all TBI multi-trauma patients, disability and exposure/environmental control assessment includes further investigations with complete CT scans. Until spinal injury is definitively excluded, TBI management should also include spinal precautions.

Spinal cord trauma

Traumatic spinal cord injury (SCI) is estimated to have a global-incidence rate of 23 cases per million of the population.[60,61] This translates to almost 180,000 cases per year. Traffic-related accidents are the leading cause of traumatic SCI in developed countries, accounting for one-third to one-half of cases.[62] Falls are the next most common cause, with rates increasing in the elderly in particular. In developing countries, traumatic SCI is most often caused by falls at home or in the workplace, with rates as high as 63%.[63] The highest proportion of violence-related traumatic SCI occurs in areas of armed conflict or high availability of weapons. Recreational injuries occur most often with snowboarding, rugby and diving accidents. A systematic review of 13 studies from around the world indicated that in most regions there are peak rates of traumatic SCI in young adults (15–29 years) and that in older age groups the incidence rate increased steadily with increasing age.[64] A predominance of males is also evident.

Of all SCI cases, 51% result in complete tetraplegia (loss of function in the arms, legs, trunk and pelvic organs). The predominant risk factors for SCI include age, gender, and alcohol and drug use.[63] The vertebrae most often involved in SCI are the 5th, 6th and 7th

TABLE 17.2
Summary of Brain Trauma Foundation guidelines of the management of severe traumatic brain injury[29]

ITEM	LEVEL I EVIDENCE	LEVEL II EVIDENCE	LEVEL III EVIDENCE
BP and oxygenation	None	BP should be monitored and hypotension (SBP <90 mmHg) avoided	Oxygenation should be monitored and hypoxia (PaO_2 <60 mmHg/8 kPa or O_2 saturation <90%) avoided
Hyperosmolar therapy	None	Mannitol is effective for control of raised ICP at doses of 0.25 gm/kg to 1 g/kg body weight. Arterial hypotension (SBP <90 mmHg) should be avoided Hypertonic saline evidence is limited on the use, concentration and method of administration for the treatment of traumatic intracranial hypertension	Restrict mannitol use prior to ICP monitoring to patients with signs of transtentorial herniation or progressive neurological deterioration not attributable to extracranial causes
Prophylactic hypothermia	Insufficient data	Insufficient data	Prophylactic hypothermia is not significantly associated with decreased mortality Prophylactic hypothermia is associated with significant higher Glasgow Outcome Scale scores
Infection prophylaxis	Insufficient data	Peri-procedural antibiotics for intubation should be administered to reduce the incidence of pneumonia – but does not change length of stay or mortality	Routine ventricular catheter or prophylactic antibiotic use for ventricular catheter placement is not recommended to reduce infection
		Early tracheostomy – reduces mechanical ventilation days	Early extubation in qualified patients, without increased risk of pneumonia
Deep vein thrombosis prophylaxis	Insufficient data	Insufficient data	Graduated compression stockings or intermittent pneumatic compression stockings until ambulatory Low-molecular-weight heparin or low unfractionated heparin in combination with above. Risk of expansion of intracranial haemorrhage
Indications for ICP monitoring	Insufficient data	ICP monitoring recommended for patients with GCS score of 3–8 with abnormal CT	Normal CT with two or more of the following: • Age 40+ years • Motor posturing • SBP <90 mmHg • GCS score 9–15 with abnormal CT at prescription discretion
ICP monitoring technology	Insufficient data	Insufficient data	Insufficient data The ventricular catheter with external strain gauge, most accurate low-cost, reliable ICP device Can also be recalibrated in situ Parenchymal ICP cannot be recalibrated. Negligible drift

Continued

TABLE 17.2

Summary of Brain Trauma Foundation guidelines of the management of severe traumatic brain injury—cont'd

ITEM	LEVEL I EVIDENCE	LEVEL II EVIDENCE	LEVEL III EVIDENCE
ICP treatment threshold	Insufficient data	Treatment initiated ICP above 20 mmHg	A combination of ICP values, clinical and brain CT should be used to determine the need for treatment
Cerebral perfusion	Insufficient data	Aggressive attempts to maintain CPP above 70 mmHg with fluids and pressors due to risk of ARDS	CPP of <50 mmHg should be avoided The CPP value to target lies within the range of 50–70 mmHg Patients with intact pressure autoregulation tolerate higher CPP values Ancillary monitoring of cerebral parameters that include blood flow, oxygenation or metabolism facilitates CPP management
Brain oxygen monitoring and thresholds	Insufficient data	Insufficient data	Jugular venous oxygenation (<50%) or brain tissue oxygen tension (<15 mmHg) are treatment thresholds and are to be avoided
Anaesthetics, analgesics and sedatives	Insufficient data	Manage pain and agitation High-dose barbiturate may be used in haemodynamically stable patients refractory to other ICP treatments. Propofol for the control of ICP. High-dose propofol can produce significant morbidity	None advised
Nutrition	Insufficient data	Full caloric replacement by Day 7 post-injury	None advised
Anti-seizure prophylaxis	Insufficient data	Phenytoin or valproate is not recommended for preventing late posttraumatic seizures Anticonvulsants are indicated to decrease the incidence of early posttraumatic seizures	None advised
Hyperventilation	Insufficient data	Prophylactic hyperventilation ($PaCO_2$ <25 mmHg/3.3 kPa) is not recommended	Use hyperventilation for temporary reduction of elevated ICP Hyperventilation should be avoided during the first 24 h after injury when CBF is often critically reduced If hyperventilation used: SjO_2 or $PbrO_2$ measures recommended to monitor oxygen delivery
Steroids	Not recommended	None advised	None advised

ARDS = acute respiratory distress syndrome; BP = blood pressure; CBF = cerebral blood flow; CPP = cerebral perfusion pressure; CT = computerised tomography (scan); GCS = Glasgow Coma Scale; ICP = intracranial pressure; $PaCO_2$ = partial pressure of alveolar carbon dioxide; PaO_2 = partial pressure of alveolar oxygen; $PbrO_2$ = brain tissue oxygenation; SBP = systolic blood pressure; SjO_2 = jugular venous oxygen saturation.

Adapted from Brain Trauma Foundation, American Association of Neurological Surgeons, Joint Section on Neurotrauma and Critical Care. Guidelines for management of severe head injury. New York: Brain Trauma Foundation; 2007.

cervical (neck), the 12th thoracic and the 1st lumbar. These vertebrae are the most susceptible because there is a greater range of mobility in the vertebral column in these areas. Damage to the spinal cord ranges from transient concussion or stunning (from which the patient fully recovers) to contusion, laceration and compression of the cord substance (either alone or in combination) to complete transection of the cord (which renders the patient paralysed below the level of the injury).[64]

Mechanisms of injury

Cervical injury can occur from both blunt and penetrating trauma but in reality is a combination of different mechanisms of acceleration and deceleration, with and without rotational forces and axial loading.[63] An illustrative example is a diving injury, caused by a direct load through the head and cervical spine. Cervical trauma is produced by a combination of the mechanisms listed below:

- Hyperflexion: usually results from forceful deceleration and often seen in patients who have sustained trauma from a head-on motor vehicle collision or diving accident. The cervical region is most often involved, especially at the C5–C6 level.
- Vertical compression or axial loading: typically occurs when a person lands on the feet or buttocks after falling or jumping from a height. The vertebral column is compressed, causing a fracture resulting in damage to the spinal cord.
- Hyperextension: is the most common type of injury. Hyperextension injuries can be caused by a fall, a rear-end motor vehicle collision or hit on the head (e.g. during a boxing match). Hyperextension of the head and neck may cause contusion and ischaemia of the spinal cord without vertebral column damage. Whiplash injuries are the result of hyperextension. Violent hyperextension with fracture of the pedicles of C2 and forward movement of C2 on C3 produces the 'Hangman's fracture'.
- Extension–rotation: rotational injuries result from forces that cause extreme twisting or lateral flexion of the head and neck. Fracture or dislocation of vertebrae may also occur. The spinal canal is narrower in the thoracic segment relative to the width of the cord so, when vertebral displacement occurs, it is more likely to damage the cord. Until the age of 10, the spine has increased physiological mobility due to lax ligaments, which affords some protection against acute SCI. Elderly patients are at a higher risk due to osteophytes and narrowing of the spinal canal.

Classification of spinal cord injuries

SCI can be broadly classified as complete or incomplete.[64] The diagnosis of complete SCI cannot be made until spinal cord shock resolves. There are four incomplete SCI syndromes as follows:

- Anterior cord syndrome: injury to the motor and sensory pathways in the anterior parts of the spine. Patients are able to feel crude sensation, but movement and detailed sensation are lost in the posterior part of the spinal cord. Clinically, the patient usually has complete motor paralysis below the level of injury (corticospinal tracts) and loss of pain, temperature and touch sensation (spinothalamic tracts), with preservation of light touch, proprioception and position sense. The prognosis for anterior cord syndrome is the worst of all the incomplete syndrome prognoses.
- Posterior cord syndrome: is usually the result of a hyperextension injury at the cervical level and is not commonly seen. Position sense, light touch and vibratory sense are lost below the level of the injury.
- Central cord syndrome: injury to the centre of the cervical spinal cord, producing weakness, paralysis and sensory deficits in the arms but not the legs. Hyperextension of the cervical spine is often the mechanism of injury, and the damage is greatest to the cervical tracts supplying the arms. Clinically, the patient may present with paralysed arms but with no deficit in the legs or bladder.
- Brown-Séquard syndrome: this involves injury to the left or right side of the spinal cord. Movements are lost below the level of injury on the injured side, but pain and temperature sensation are lost on the side opposite to the injury. The clinical presentation is one in which the patient has either increased or decreased cutaneous sensation of pain, temperature and touch on the same side of the spinal cord at the level of the lesion. Below the level of the lesion on the same side, there is complete motor paralysis. On the patient's opposite side, below the level of the lesion, there is loss of pain, temperature and touch because the spinothalamic tracts cross soon after entering the cord.

Pathophysiology

SCI can be separated into two categories: primary injuries and secondary injuries. Primary injuries are the result of the initial insult or trauma, and are usually permanent. The force of the primary insult produces its initial damage in the central grey matter of the cord. Secondary injuries are usually the result of a contusion or tear injury, in which the nerve fibres begin to swell and disintegrate. Secondary neural injury mechanisms include ischaemia, hypoxia and oedema, cellular and molecular inflammatory injury and cell death. Ischaemia, the most prominent post-SCI event, may occur up to 2 hours post-injury and is intensified by the loss of autoregulation of the spinal cord microcirculation.[65] This will decrease blood flow, which is then dependent on the systemic arterial pressure in the presence of hypotension or vasogenic spinal shock. Oedema develops at the injured site and spreads into adjacent areas. Hypoxia may occur because of inadequate airway maintenance and ventilation. Immune cells, which normally do not enter the spinal cord, engulf the area after a SCI and release regulatory chemicals, some of which are harmful to the spinal cord. Highly reactive oxidising agents (free radicals) are produced, which damage the cell membrane and disrupt the sodium–potassium pump.

Free radical production and the formation of reactive oxygen and nitrogen species or lipid peroxidation lead to vasoconstriction, increased endothelial permeability and increased platelet activation. A secondary chain of events produces ischaemia, hypoxia, oedema and haemorrhagic lesions, which in turn result in the destruction of myelin and axons. Autoregulation of spinal cord blood flow may be impaired in patients with severe lesions or substantial oedema formation. These secondary reactions, believed to be the principal causes of spinal cord degeneration at the level of injury, are thought to be reversible 4–6 hours after injury. Therefore, if the cord has not suffered irreparable damage, early intervention is needed to prevent partial damage from developing into total and permanent damage.[66,67]

Spinal shock occurs with physiological or anatomical transection or near-transection of the spinal cord. It occurs immediately or within several hours of a SCI and is caused by the sudden cessation of impulses from the higher brain centres.[68] It is characterised by the loss of motor, sensory, reflex and autonomic function below the level of the injury, with resultant flaccid paralysis. Loss of bowel and bladder function also occurs. In addition, the body's ability to control temperature is lost (i.e. poikilothermia) and the patient's temperature tends to equilibrate with that of the external environment.

Neurogenic spinal shock occurs as a result of mid- to upper-level cervical injuries and is the result of sympathetic vascular denervation and peripheral vasodilation. The loss of spinal cord vasculature autoregulation occurs, causing the blood flow to the spinal cord to be dependent on the systemic blood pressure. Signs and symptoms include hypotension, severe bradycardia and loss of the ability to sweat below the level of injury. The same clinical findings pertaining to disruption of the sympathetic transmissions in spinal shock occur in neurogenic shock (see Chapter 21).[68]

Systemic effects of spinal cord injury

The traumatic insult causing the SCI is associated with an immediate stimulation of central and peripheral sympathetic tone. Initially, the elevated sympathetic activity raises systemic arterial blood pressure and induces cardiac dysrhythmias. At the stage of spinal shock with loss of neuronal conduction, the sympathetic excitation is closely followed by decreases in systemic vascular resistance, arterial hypotension and venous pooling. Lesions above the level of T5 additionally present with severe bradycardia and cardiac dysfunction. The decreases in cardiac output combined with systemic hypotension further aggravate spinal cord ischaemia in tissues with defective autoregulation.[66]

SCI may produce respiratory failure. The extent of respiratory complications is related to the level of the injured segments. Injuries above the level of C4–C5 produce complete paralysis of the diaphragm, with substantial decreases in tidal volume and consecutive hypoxia. With lesions below C6, the function of the diaphragm is maintained and there is incomplete respiratory failure due to paralysed intercostal and abdominal musculature. As a consequence, arterial hypoxia and hypercapnia occur, both of which promote neuronal and glial acidosis, oedema and neuroexcitation.[68]

Patient management

SCI should be suspected in patients with neck pain, sensory and motor deficits, unconsciousness, intoxication, spondylitis or rheumatoid arthritis, all major trauma, distracting injuries, head injury and facial fractures. Where a SCI is suspected or cannot be excluded, the patient must be placed on a spine board with the head and neck immobilised in a neutral position to reduce the risk of neurological deterioration from repeated mechanical insults.[69] Spinal injury patients are susceptible to pressure injuries (see Chapter 5), so time must be considered when hard surfaces are used for immobilisation. Total neck immobilisation should not interfere with maintenance of the airway, and inadequate respiratory function must be avoided.[64]

Practice tip

It is important to appropriately size and fit rigid cervical spine collars, which may be difficult in patients with excess adipose tissue. Collars that are too short or tall can lead to cervical spine flexion or extension. The use of a collar also increases the chances of the patient developing a pressure injury. Care must be taken to assess the skin integrity beneath the collar, particularly on the occiput, chin and across the clavicles.

Resuscitation

Initial treatment aims for decompression of the spinal cord and reversal of neurogenic shock and respiratory failure. Spinal shock is associated with decreases in systemic vascular resistance, arterial hypotension, venous pooling, severe bradycardia and decreased myocardial contractility. Consequently, treatment of neurogenic shock includes fluid replacement to maintain arterial blood pressure, circulatory volume, renal function and tissue oxygenation. Lower-limb compression assists with venous return. Infusion of free water must be avoided, as this decreases plasma osmolarity and promotes spinal cord oedema. Atropine may be administered to reverse bradycardia and increase cardiac output. Administration of vasopressors (e.g. noradrenaline) prior to correction of the intravascular volume status may increase systemic vascular resistance (left ventricular afterload) and further impair myocardial contractility. Therefore, careful volume replacement is the first step, and administration of vasopressors the second step, in the treatment of arterial hypotension and low cardiac output after acute cervical SCI.

The major early cause of death in patients with acute cervical SCI is respiratory failure. Tracheal intubation may be indicated in unconscious patients, in patients with shock or those with other major associated injuries and during cardiovascular and respiratory distress. It is also indicated in conscious patients presenting with the following criteria: maximum expiratory force below 20 cmH_2O, maximum inspiratory force below 20 cmH_2O, vital capacity below 1000 mL and presence of atelectasis, contusion and infiltrate.[66]

Investigations

Following the initial assessment of the patient, detailed CT diagnostic radiography defines the bone damage and compression of the spinal cord. Cervical spine fractures occur predominantly at two levels, at the level of C2 and at the level of C6 or C7. Unfortunately, 20–30% of these fractures can be missed on plain radiographs. Current recommendations are to consider use of multidetector-row CT as the initial screening examination in suspected cervical trauma instead of radiographs or standard CT. Specific radiological procedures such as cervical myelography, high-resolution CT scan or magnetic resonance imaging (MRI) will identify fractures, dislocation of bony fragments and spinal cord contusion.[69]

Neuroprotective and regenerative strategies

In patients with a dislocated cervical fracture, decompression and anatomical bony realignment may be achieved with traction forces applied manually, or with halo or Gardner–Wells systems under radiological control. If the anatomical bony alignment procedures and traction forces fail to decompress the cord, surgical intervention to remove the lesion is required. The timing of surgical intervention remains controversial. While urgent surgical decompression or internal stabilisation should be performed in all patients with deteriorating neurological status, surgical treatment may be deferred in patients with stable neurological deficits.[70]

The most promising neuroprotective reparative therapeutic strategies undergoing investigation include riluzole, hypothermia, granulocyte colony-stimulating factor, glibenclamide, minocycline, Cethrin (VX-210), and anti-Nogo-A antibody.[70] Apart from hypothermia, most others have not been successful, which has been attributed to attempting to block only one molecular pathway of a complex range of SCI molecular mechanisms. There has been renewed interest in regeneration, which involves stem cell transplantation or similar restorative approaches designed to optimise spontaneous axonal growth and myelination, but human research remains in its infancy due to limiting legislation in some countries.

Collaborative care interventions

Patients with acute cervical SCI require ICU monitoring, observation and support of ventilation, a nasogastric tube to reduce abdominal distension and risk of aspiration (if there is no risk related to TBI and basal skull fracture), a urinary catheter and thermal maintenance. In addition, the following should be noted:[67]

- Tracheostomy is indicated in high cervical spine injury and ischaemia, sometimes temporarily while the early oedema is resolving.
- Spinal alignment and immobilisation requires careful positioning with dedicated neck support by experienced clinicians.
- Shoulder and lumbar support pillows are often prescribed. Pressure-relief mattresses must be suitably designed for spine immobilisation and, when prescribed, can be tilted to facilitate ventilation.
- Meticulous integument and bowel care is indicated with daily protocols for regular stool softeners and peristaltic stimulants essential for the prevention of autonomic dysreflexia (i.e. strong sensory input from the bowel to the spinal cord that evokes a massive reflex sympathetic surge) and autonomic nerve dysfunction.
- Early nutritious feeding is essential, whether oral or enteric; however, aspiration must be prevented. The supplementation of feeding with high-energy protein fluids to match the catabolic state assists with recovery (see Chapter 19).
- Both hyper- and hypoglycaemia must be avoided.[71]
- The concepts of pain relief and sedation in patients with SCI are based on the maintenance of coupling between metabolism and spinal cord blood flow while achieving hypnosis, analgesia and a 'relaxed cord'. These concepts include maintenance of normal to high systemic perfusion pressures, normoxia and normocapnia.
- Psychological and empathetic support is essential and appropriate referral for grieving and stress is paramount. Rehabilitation counselling and planning starts at the acute stage to give the family unit future focus and hope.

See *Online resources* for specific protocols related to spinal injury.

Cerebrovascular disorders

Cerebral vascular disorders include cerebrovascular disease and cerebral vascular incidents (stroke). A stroke (acute brain injury of vascular origin) is defined as an interruption of the blood supply to any part of the brain, resulting in damaged brain tissue.

According to the World Health Organization, stroke claims 6.2 million lives each year and globally is the second most common cause of death, exceeded only by coronary heart disease.[72] The incidence of stroke in the USA is about 7.2 million[73] and in the UK, approximately 152,145 people suffer a stroke per annum.[74] Stroke is also the primary cerebrovascular disorder in Australia and New Zealand.[75] The age-adjusted incidence of stroke is higher in men than women in all countries. Those over 65 years are also most at risk.[72]

Stroke is divided into two major categories: ischaemic (85%), in which vascular occlusion and significant hypoperfusion occur; and haemorrhagic (15%), in which there is extravasation of blood into the brain. Although there are some similarities between the two broad types of stroke, the aetiology, pathophysiology, medical management, surgical management and nursing care differ.

Aetiology

Hypertension is the leading risk factor for stroke. Other risk factors include diabetes, cardiac disease, previous cerebrovascular disease (transient ischaemic attack or stroke or myocardial infarction), age, sex, lipid disorders, excessive ethanol ingestion, elevated haematocrit, elevated fibrinogen and cigarette smoking.[73] Cerebral arteriosclerosis predisposes individuals to both ischaemic and haemorrhagic stroke. Smoking is the strongest risk factor for aSAH. Atrial fibrillation, endocarditis and medications containing supplemental oestrogen are risk factors for embolic stroke. Seizures develop in approximately 10% of cases, usually appearing in the first 24 hours and more likely to be focal than generalised. Occurrence of seizures within 24 hours of stroke is associated with higher 30-day mortality, which may be a reflection of severe neuronal damage.[75]

Ischaemic stroke

Ischaemic stroke compromises blood flow and energy supply to the brain, which triggers mechanisms that lead to cell death, and are embolic or thrombotic in origin. Infarction occurs rapidly in the region of most severe ischaemia (termed ischaemic penumbra) and expands at the expense of the surrounding hypoxic tissue, from the centre to the periphery. Therapeutic strategies in acute ischaemic stroke are based on the concept of arresting the transition of the penumbral region into infarction, thereby limiting ultimate infarct size and improving neurological and functional outcome. Ischaemic stroke can be further categorised as middle cerebral artery occlusion, acute basilar occlusion and cerebellar infarcts.[76]

The management of an ischaemic stroke comprises four primary goals: restoration of CBF (reperfusion), prevention of recurrent thrombosis, neuroprotection and supportive care.[76] The timing of each element of clinical management needs to be implemented in a decisive manner. For eligible patients, IV tissue plasminogen activator should be administered with a dose of 0.9 mg/kg (maximum of 90 mg), with 10% of the total dose administered as an initial bolus and the remainder infused over 60 min, provided that treatment is initiated within 4.5 hours of clearly defined symptom onset.[76] The recommendation assumes a relatively higher value on long-term functional improvement and a relatively lower value on minimising the risk of intracerebral haemorrhage in the immediate peristroke period.

Endovascular clot retrieval is increasingly being used as a reperfusion therapy following ischaemic stroke. This involves the use of a mechanical device to remove the blockage. This therapy can be used in conjunction with IV tissue plasminogen activator. As cardiac dysrhythmias such as atrial fibrillation predispose to embolic events, cardiac monitoring for at least 24 hours should be carried out. Table 17.3 shows the classification and treatment strategies, and the *Online resources* reflect specific ischaemic stroke protocols.

Practice tip

For consideration of ischaemic stroke lysis, the timing of the onset of symptoms needs to be very clearly defined. In particular, if a patient wakes from sleep with stroke symptoms, the timing of onset must be assumed to be when they were last well – that is, the time when they went to sleep.

TABLE 17.3
Classification and type of ischaemic stroke and treatment options

CLASSIFICATION	TREATMENT OPTIONS
Middle cerebral artery occlusion	Intravenous or intraarterial tissue plasminogen activator (tPA) Exclusion criteria: >3 h elapsed from stroke onset and widespread early infarct changes on CT scan Tolerate autoprotective hypertension for perfusion of the ischaemic penumbra
Acute basilar occlusion	Anticoagulation with intravenous heparin Thrombolysis up to 12 h after onset
Cerebellar infarcts	May be difficult to recognise because of the slow evolution of brainstem and cerebellar signs Aspirin, antihypertensives and conventional cerebral oedema strategies

Haemorrhagic stroke

Haemorrhagic stroke is divided into two main categories, intracerebral haemorrhage and spontaneous subarachnoid haemorrhage.

Intracerebral haemorrhage

Intracerebral haemorrhage (ICH) comprises 10–15% of all strokes with an incidence of 24.6 per 100,000 person-years, with a growing incidence associated with the use of anticoagulation, antiplatelet agents and an ageing population.[77] Despite this, ICH remains the last stroke type without a definitive treatment and contributes to significant morbidity and mortality. Up to half of patients die within 30 days, often despite extensive stays in the ICU. Moreover, those who survive have a high degree of long-term disability.[77] Pathogenesis of ICH include hypertension, vascular malformations, brain tumours, bleeding disorders, or the use of drugs such as cocaine or amphetamines, which elevate blood pressure. Ideally, patients with acute ICH should be admitted to an ICU based on the need for close monitoring of neurological and haemodynamic condition and the risk for early deterioration from haematoma expansion, cerebral oedema, hydrocephalus or airway compromise. Many ICHs continue to grow and expand over several hours after onset of symptoms.

As with all emergency management, initial assessment of airway, breathing and circulation is critical. Until the diagnosis of ICH is made from neuroimaging, airway and haemodynamic management proceeds in a common pathway with other stroke subtypes. Because many ICH patients are obtunded or comatose, airway management (specifically the need for intubation for airway protection) should be considered throughout the early treatment course. Following the diagnosis of ICH, immediate consideration should be given to the need for 1) acute control of elevated blood pressure; 2) correction of coagulopathy because of medications or underlying medical conditions; and 3) the need for urgent surgical haematoma evacuation.[78] Over 90% of patients have acute hypertension, whether or not there is a history of preexisting hypertension. It remains unclear whether this response is adaptive (to maintain perfusion to an ischaemic penumbra surrounding the haematoma) or potentially harmful (resulting in rebleeding, peri-haematoma oedema expansion, or both).[78] The American Heart Association/American Stroke Association 2015 guidelines recommend that for patients with a systolic pressure between 150 and 220 mmHg and without contraindication to acute blood pressure (BP) treatment, acute lowering to 140 mmHg is safe and can improve functional outcome.[78] They further advise that for patients presenting with a systolic >220 mmHg, it may also be reasonable to consider aggressive reduction of BP with a continuous intravenous infusion and frequent BP monitoring.

Use of antithrombotic medications are a risk factor for the occurrence of ICH, as well as for haematoma expansion if an ICH occurs. As there is a broad range of antithrombotic medications, including warfarin, heparin, antiplatelet agents such as aspirin and clopidogrel and agents such as dabigatran and rivaroxaban, the specific risks and interventions to reverse coagulopathy vary. Also, coagulopathies may be due to underlying medical conditions, such as liver disease or haematological malignances.[79] Patients with ICH should have intermittent pneumatic compression for prevention of venous thromboembolism as compression stockings are not recommended for use in this population.[79] Most of the brain injury and swelling that happens in the days after ICH is the result of inflammation caused by thrombin and other coagulation end-products.[80] Dysautonomia, in the form of central fever, hyperventilation, hyperglycaemia and tachycardia or bradycardia, is common. Hyperglycaemia at the time of hospital admission is associated with early mortality and poor outcome in ICH patients.[81]

Subarachnoid haemorrhage

Subarachnoid haemorrhage (SAH) is defined as a bleed into the subarachnoid space, which can be spontaneous or associated with a TBI. Spontaneous SAH is most commonly due to vascular abnormalities such as cerebral or brain aneurysm. Admission to the ICU is required for grade 4 aneurysmal SAH (aSAH) based on the World Federation of Neurosurgical Societies Scale[82] (Table 17.4). This level of severity is at greater risk of systemic complications and clinical deterioration.[83] Resuscitation is directed towards maintaining CPP by ensuring adequate arterial BP (often with the use of inotropes to produce relative hypertension although reactive hypertension is often present), ensuring euvolaemia and producing relative haemodilution.[84]

Hypovolaemia occurs in 30–50% of patients and hyponatraemia in 30% of patients.[84] In the first 6 days, plasma volume decreases of greater than 10% can occur following aSAH, thus increasing the risk of delayed

TABLE 17.4
World Federation of Neurosurgical Societies scale for aneurysmal subarachnoid haemorrhage (aSAH)[82]

GRADE	GLASGOW COMA SCALE	MOTOR DEFICIT
I	15	Absent
II	14–13	Absent
III	14–13	Present
IV	12–7	Present or absent
V	6–3	Present or absent

Source: Teasdale GM, Drake CG, Hunt W, et al. A universal subarachnoid hemorrhage scale: report of a committee of the World Federation of Neurosurgical Societies. J Neurol Neurosurg Psychiatry. 1988;51(11):1457, with permission from BMJ Publishing Group Ltd.

cerebral ischaemia and vasospasm.[85] Women have been found to have more significant drops in blood volume than men following aSAH. 'Third space' loss, insensible losses and blood loss account for this drop in fluid volume, as well as electrolyte disturbances.[86]

> **Practice tip**
>
> Fever is the most common medical complication in patients suffering from aSAH and is associated with neurological deterioration.

In the acute stages, other aspects of management include suitable analgesia, seizure control and treatment with nimodipine to prevent delayed cerebral ischaemia and vasospasm.[84] Acute hydrocephalus secondary to aSAH is usually managed by external ventricular drainage and is associated with neurological improvement. ICP monitoring and drainage of CSF via ventriculostomy is also indicated.[85]

Increased sympathetic activation from the presence of haemoglobin in the subarachnoid space results in elevated catecholamine levels. This is characterised by hypothalamically mediated changes including increased sympathetic and parasympathetic activity that causes cardiac and pulmonary complications (neurogenic pulmonary oedema).[87] Manifestations include electrocardiographic changes, dysrhythmias, impaired cardiac contractility, elevated troponin levels and myocardial necrosis. Cardiac and pulmonary complications are associated with delayed cerebral ischaemia and poor outcome after aSAH. As cardiac function is one of the determinants for adequate CBF, it is essential to identify such occurrences early and treat them accordingly.

Hyponatraemia occurs from alterations in atrial natriuretic factor in response to sympathetic nervous system activation. The syndrome of inappropriate secretion of antidiuretic hormone is primarily responsible for hyponatraemia in those with aSAH, as is cerebral salt-wasting syndrome; however, both mechanisms are still relatively misunderstood.

Prevention of delayed cerebral ischaemia and cerebral vasospasm

Delayed cerebral ischaemia can occur as a result of aSAH. It is defined as the occurrence of focal neurological impairment (such as hemiparesis, aphasia, apraxia, hemianopia or neglect) or a decrease of at least two points on the GCS (on either the total score or one of its individual components of eye, motor, verbal). This drop in GCS should last for at least 1 hour, and is not apparent immediately after aneurysm occlusion and cannot be attributed to other causes by means of clinical assessments, cerebral CT or MRI scanning, and appropriate laboratory studies.[88] Delayed cerebral ischaemia occurs in about 30% of patients surviving the initial haemorrhage, mostly between days 4 and 10 after aSAH. The known clinical symptoms, such as decrease in the level of consciousness and focal signs, e.g. aphasia and hemiparesis, may be reversible or otherwise progress to cerebral infarction resulting in an unfavourable outcome or even death. A diagnosis of delayed cerebral ischaemia is made after exclusion of other causes (such as infection, hypotension, hyponatraemia and others), and is especially difficult in patients who are comatose or sedated.[89] The latter are typically patients with a high grade on the World Federation of Neurosurgical Societies Scale (grade 4–5), approximately 40–70% of the patient population with ruptured aneurysms.[90] The Fisher scale is also used to classify the amount of subarachnoid blood seen on CT scan and can help predict the likelihood of vasospasm.[91] Early brain injury and cell death, blood–brain barrier disruption and initiation of an inflammatory cascade, microvascular spasm, microthrombosis, cortical-spreading depolarisations and failure of cerebral autoregulation have all been implicated in the pathophysiology of delayed cerebral ischaemia.

Cerebral vasospasm is a self-limited vasculopathy that develops 4–21 days after SAH (Fig. 17.6). Vasospasm occurs when the clot undergoes lysis (dissolution), increasing the chances of rebleeding. About one-third of aSAH patients develop symptomatic vasospasm, which is associated with neurological signs and symptoms of ischaemia. Post-TBI cerebral vasospasm occurs in approximately 10–15% of patients. Oxyhaemoglobin, a product of haemoglobin (Hb) breakdown, probably initiates vasoconstriction, leading to smooth-muscle proliferation, collagen remodelling and cellular infiltration of the vessel wall. The resulting vessel narrowing can lead to delayed cerebral ischaemia. The initial proinflammatory effect elicited by Hb and Hb-bound cells initiates an inflammatory cascade and cortical-spreading depolarisation involving an increase of cytokines, leukocytes and cell adhesion molecules characterising the inflammatory process. The symptoms are poorly localised and develop gradually over hours, suggesting a progressing, global disease process.

Calcium antagonists have not been effective in TBI SAH with vasospasm. However, nimodipine has demonstrated effectiveness in the treatment of vasospasm in aSAH, reducing the incidence of delayed cerebral ischaemia and poor outcome by 40%, without ameliorating vasospasm.[92]

Despite its widespread use as a mainstay therapy for cerebral vasospasm, research evidence does not support the use of 'Triple H' therapy (hypervolaemia, hypertension, haemodilution).[92] Clinical studies reveal that hypervolaemia results in pulmonary oedema, as well as haemodilution, and with it a decrease in arterial oxygen and oxygen-carrying capacity. Anaemia has also been associated with a worse outcome after aSAH. Thus, haemodilution has been eliminated from 'Triple H' therapy and the target is now euvolaemia rather than hypervolaemia. These changes, along with the established hypertensive therapy, are the mainstays in clinical practice recommended in the Neurocritical Care Society aSAH guidelines.[93]

It is believed that early open surgical clipping or wrapping and endovascular coil embolisation prevent rebleeding and that removal of blood from the basal cisterns around the major cerebral arteries may prevent vasospasm.[94] In aSAH, endovascular therapies should be considered in patients at risk for vasospasm-related ischaemia prior to the development of delayed cerebral ischaemia. Prophylactic angioplasty done without the presence of angiographic arterial narrowing exposes patients to risk of vessel rupture and death without clear benefit in outcome.[93] Thus, routine prophylactic cerebral angioplasty is not recommended.[93]

Cerebral venous thrombosis

Compared to cerebral infarctions from arterial sources, cerebral venous infarctions are less common, with reported incidence of 0.22 to 1.57 per 100,000.[95,96] It is particularly important to recognise cerebral venous thrombosis because there is general consensus that early anticoagulation can result in good clinical outcomes. MRI and CT vascular imaging have made it easier to establish the diagnosis, but close monitoring of the patient is essential, as late deterioration can occur.

Patient management

Expected outcomes for patients with acute ischaemic and haemorrhagic stroke include prevention of secondary injury and of airway and respiratory complications, and maintenance of haemodynamic stability. Timely assessment and intervention are paramount in the management of ischaemic stroke, especially regarding interventional pharmacology and prevention of cerebral haemorrhage.[83] See *Online resources* for specific protocols related to stroke.

Atrial fibrillation and deep vein thrombosis prevention (in ischaemic stroke) both require anticoagulation control. In haemorrhagic stroke, a sequential compression device and stockings are indicated as anticoagulants are a risk factor for rebleeding. Maintenance of bowel and bladder function and prevention of integument complications, malnutrition, seizures and increasing neurological deficits are important goals. Environmental precautions are implemented to provide a non-stimulating environment, preventing rises in ICP and further bleeding.

Sensory perceptual and motor alterations need to be assessed in regard to effective communication and pain management. Rehabilitation and psychological support for the patient and significant others are integrated into the acute care phase for a smooth transition.

Infection and inflammation

The CNS infections of major interest in the ICU are divided into those that affect the meninges (meningitis) and those that affect the brain parenchyma (encephalitis), which may be viral or bacterial in aetiology. Many medical conditions can mimic viral encephalitis. Particular attention should be given to the possibility of such non-viral infections as cerebral malaria, which may be rapidly fatal if not treated early. Metabolic conditions, such as liver and renal failure and diabetic complications, may also cause confusion due to the manifestation of cerebral oedema. The possible role of alcohol and drug ingestion should also be considered.

Meningitis

Meningitis is inflammation of the pia and arachnoid layers of the meninges. Acute community-acquired meningitis can develop within hours to days and is usually viral or bacterial. Viral meningitis usually has a good prognosis, whereas bacterial meningitis is associated with significant rates of morbidity and death, so it is critical to recognise and differentiate them promptly.[97] The incidence, mortality and morbidity from acute community-acquired meningitis has decreased significantly, especially in high-income countries, probably as a result of vaccination and better antimicrobial and adjuvant therapy, but the disease still has a high toll.[97,98] Table 17.5 shows the CSF profiles for acute meningitis and encephalitis and Table 17.6 shows the classification, treatment and clinical presentation of meningitis.

Complications of meningitis vary according to the aetiological organism, the duration of symptoms prior to initiation of appropriate therapy and the age and immune status of the patient. Temporary problems include development of haemodynamic instability and disseminated intravascular coagulopathy, particularly in meningococcal infection, syndrome of inappropriate secretion of antidiuretic hormone or other dysregulation of the hypothalamic–pituitary axis (e.g. diabetes insipidus), and an acute rise in ICP.

> **Practice tip**
>
> The dose of antimicrobial drug required for treating meningitis is usually higher than normal as penetration across the blood–CSF barrier is poor.

Focal neurological signs may develop in the early stages of meningitis, but are more common later. The development of subdural empyema, brain abscess and acute hydrocephalus may require surgical intervention. Bacterial meningitis with accompanying bacteraemia can lead to a marked systemic inflammatory response with septic shock and acute respiratory distress syndrome.

Encephalitis

Encephalitis indicates inflammation of the brain substance (parenchyma) and can range from being a mild and self-limiting condition to a serious, life-threatening illness. Inflammation of the meninges (meningoencephalitis) or spinal cord (encephalomyelitis) may also be present.

Herpes simplex virus encephalitis is the most common sporadic viral encephalitis worldwide, with an annual incidence of 1 in 250,000–500,000.[99] Without treatment, herpes simplex virus encephalitis is fatal in up to 80% of cases, and leaves up to 50% of survivors with long-term sequelae.[100] Other common causes

TABLE 17.5
Typical profiles of cerebrospinal fluid in acute meningitis and encephalitis

		MENINGITIS		ENCEPHALITIS
INVESTIGATION	REFERENCE RANGE	BACTERIAL	VIRAL	BACTERIAL/VIRAL
Opening pressure	<30 mmH_2O	Raised	Normal	Raised
White cells				
Total count	<5 × 10^6/L	Greatly raised	Moderately raised	Moderately raised
Differential	Lymphocytes (60–70%), monocytes (30–50%), no neutrophils or red blood cells	Neutrophils predominate	Lymphocytes predominate	Lymphocytes predominate
Glucose concentration	2.8–4.4 mmol/L	Lowered	Normal	Normal
CSF: serum glucose ratio	>60%	Lowered	Normal	Normal
Protein concentration	<0.45 g/L	Raised	Normal or slightly raised	Normal or slightly raised

include enteroviruses, influenza virus and *Mycoplasma pneumoniae*, with geographical location, history of travel, animal exposure and vaccination determining the likely pathogen. *Mycobacterium tuberculosis, Cryptococcus neoformans and Treponema pallidum (syphilis)* can also affect the brain parenchyma, but they usually result in chronic or subacute meningitis.

In the majority of encephalitis cases, the offending organism finds access to the brain via the nasopharyngeal epithelium and the olfactory nerve system. Arboviruses are transmitted from infected animals to humans through the bite of infected animals.[100] The cytokine storm results in neural cell damage, as well as the apoptosis of astrocytes. The disruption of the blood–brain barrier progresses to septic shock, disseminated intravascular coagulopathy and multi-organ failure. Encephalitis may present with progressive headache, fever and alterations in cognitive state (confusion, behavioural change, dysphasia) or consciousness. Focal neurological signs (paresis) or seizures (focal or generalised) may also occur. Upper motor signs (hyper-reflexia and extensor–plantar responses) are often present, but flaccid paralysis and bladder symptoms may occur if the spinal cord is involved.[101] Associated movement disorders or the inappropriate secretion of antidiuretic hormone may be seen. The most sensitive type of imaging for diagnosis of encephalitis is MRI; in HSV encephalitis, CT scans may initially appear normal, but MRI usually shows involvement of the temporal lobes and thalamus.[102] Examination of CSF can assist in differential diagnosis. Refer to Table 17.6 for CSF profiles. EEG is less sensitive but may be helpful if it shows characteristic features (e.g. lateralising periodic sharp and slow-wave patterns).

Patient management

Neurological derangement often coexists with circulatory insufficiency, impaired respiration, metabolic derangement and seizures. Protecting the patient from injury secondary to raised ICP and seizure activity is essential. Prevention of complications associated with immobility, such as decubitus and pneumonia, is required. It is important to institute droplet infection control precautions in those attending the patient until 24 hours after the initiation of antibiotic therapy (oral and nasal discharge is considered infectious). See *Online resources* for infection control protocols relating specifically to meningitis.

Support in an ICU is often required in encephalitis to maintain ventilation, protect the airway and manage complications, such as cerebral oedema. The management of acute viral encephalitis includes aggressive airway, ventilation, sedation, seizure, haemodynamic and fluid and nutritional support. Clinical deterioration is usually the result of severe cerebral oedema with diencephalic herniation or systemic complications, including generalised sepsis and multiple organ failure. The use of ICP monitoring in acute encephalitis remains controversial but should be considered if there is a rapid deterioration in the level of consciousness, and if imaging suggests raised ICP. Prolonged sedation may be necessary. Decompressive craniotomy may be successful in cases where there is rapid swelling of a non-dominant temporal lobe, as poor outcome is otherwise likely.[102]

Neuromuscular disorders

Generalised muscle weakness can manifest in several disorders that require ICU admission or complicate the

TABLE 17.6
Classification of acute meningitis

ACUTE MENINGITIS	BACTERIAL – NOTIFIABLE DISEASE	VIRAL
Aetiology	*Neisseria* meningitis • Serogroups A, B, C – 90% invasive isolates • Serogroup B – most disease • Serogroup A – epidemic disease and indigenous *Haemophilus influenzae* type B, *Streptococcus pneumoniae*, *Listeria monocytogenes*	Enteroviruses: 85–95% of cases Herpes simplex 1 and 2 Varicella zoster Cytomegalovirus Epstein–Barr HIV infection can also present as aseptic meningitis Post-infectious encephalomyelitis: may occur following a variety of viral infections, usually of the respiratory tract. *Cryptococcus neoformans* Fungal isolates
Pathophysiology	Rapid recognition and diagnosis of meningitis is imperative Quick and insidious progress of disease Colonisation of mucosal surfaces (nasopharynx) Haematogenous or contiguous spread Specific antibodies important defence Bacterial invasion of meninges: inflammatory response, breakdown of the BBB, cerebral oedema, intracranial hypertension Vasculitis, spasm and thrombosis in cerebral blood vessels	The physical signs are not so marked and the illness is not as severe and prolonged as bacterial meningitis Viral infection of mucosal surfaces of respiratory or gastrointestinal tract Virus replication in tonsillar or gut lymphatics Viraemia with haematogenous dissemination to the CNS Meningeal inflammation, BBB breakdown, cerebral oedema, vasculitis and spasm
Clinical presentation and progression	Presents with sepsis: headache, fever, photophobia, vomiting, neck stiffness, alteration of mental status Meningococcaemia is characterised by an abrupt onset of fever (with petechial or purpuric rash) Progresses to purpura fulminans, associated with the rapid onset of hypotension, acute adrenal haemorrhage syndrome and multi-organ failure Kernig's sign Brudzinski's sign Cranial nerve palsy (III, IV, VI, VII) uncommon and develop after several days Focal neurological signs in 10–20% cases Seizures in 30% of cases Signs of intracranial hypertension: coma, altered respiratory status Leads to hypertension and bradycardia before herniation, or brain death, leads to irreversible septic shock	Presents with non-specific symptoms, viral respiratory illness, diarrhoea, fever, headache, photophobia, vomiting, anorexia, rash, cough and myalgia Occurs in summer or late autumn Enteroviral, pleurodynia, chest pain, hand-foot-mouth disease HSV-2: acute genital herpes
Treatment	If meningococcal infection is suspected, the best way to reduce mortality is to administer empirical IV therapy immediately Ceftriaxone 2 g IV 12-hourly or cefotaxime 2 g IV 6-hourly or immediately Consequent dose, times and type of antibiotic need to be modified after full investigation and a detailed examination have taken place Dexamethasone may be prescribed: needs to be at same time as antibiotic as outcome neurologically is reduced if given after antibiotic. Reduces BBB permeability Supportive treatment and resuscitation Management of intracranial hypertension/ischaemia	Administer intravenous aciclovir Dexamethasone may be prescribed: reduces BBB permeability Supportive treatment and resuscitation Management of intracranial hypertension/ischaemia

BBB = blood–brain barrier; CNS = central nervous system

clinical course of patients. These may involve motor neuron disease, disorders of the neuromuscular junction, peripheral nerve conduction and muscular contraction. These disorders manifest as Guillain–Barré syndrome, myasthenia gravis and critical illness polyneuropathies and myopathy.

Guillain–Barré syndrome

Guillain–Barré syndrome (GBS) is an immune-mediated disorder resulting from generation of autoimmune antibodies and/or inflammatory cells that cross-react with epitopes on peripheral nerves and roots, leading to demyelination or axonal damage or both, and autoimmune insult to peripheral nerve myelin. Estimates of GBS incidence range from 0.8 to 1.9 cases per 100,000 person-years, are higher in males and increase with age.[103] Of all patients, 85% recover with minimal residual symptoms; severe residual deficits occur in up to 10%. Residual deficits are most likely in patients with rapid disease progression, those who require mechanical ventilation or those 60 years of age or over. Death occurs in 3–8% of cases, resulting from respiratory failure, autonomic dysfunction, sepsis or pulmonary emboli.[104]

Aetiology

The diagnosis of GBS is confirmed by the findings of cytoalbuminological dissociation (elevation of the CSF protein without concomitant CSF pleocytosis), and by neurophysiological findings suggestive of an acute (usually demyelinating) neuropathy. These abnormalities may not be present in the early stages of the illness.[103] There are two forms of GBS. The demyelinating form, the more common one, is characterised by demyelination and inflammatory infiltrates of the peripheral nerves and roots. In the axonal form the nerves show Wallerian degeneration (the fatty degeneration of a nerve fibre after it has been severed from its cell body) with an absence of inflammation. Discrimination between the axonal and demyelinating forms relies mainly on electrophysiological methods. There is a close association between GBS and a preceding infection, suggesting an immune basis for the syndrome. The commonest infections are due to *Campylobacter jejuni*, cytomegalovirus and Epstein–Barr virus.

Pathophysiology

GBS is the result of a cell-mediated immune attack on peripheral nerve myelin proteins. The Schwann cell is spared, allowing for remyelination in the recovery phase of the disease. With the autoimmune attack there is an influx of macrophages and other immune-mediated agents that attack myelin, cause inflammation and destruction and leave the axon unable to support nerve conduction. This demyelination may be discrete or diffuse, and may affect the peripheral nerves and their roots at any point from their origin in the spinal cord to the neuromuscular junction. The weakness of GBS results from conduction block and concomitant or primary axonal injury in the affected motor nerves. Pain and paraesthesias are the clinical correlates of sensory nerve involvement.

Clinical manifestations

Onset is rapid, and approximately 20% of cases lead to total paralysis, requiring prolonged intensive therapy with mechanical ventilation. The therapeutic window for GBS is short, and the current optimal treatment with whole plasma exchange or immunoglobulin therapy lacks immunological specificity and only halves the severity of the disease.[103] GBS has three phases – acute, plateau and recovery – each stage lasting from days to weeks and in recovery to months and years. The patient presents with:

- symmetrical weakness, diminished reflexes and upward progression of motor weakness; a history of a viral illness in the previous few weeks suggests the diagnosis
- changes in vital capacity and negative inspiratory force, which are assessed to identify impending neuromuscular respiratory failure.

Indications for ICU admission include the following: ventilatory insufficiency, severe bulbar weakness threatening pulmonary aspiration, autonomic instability or coexisting general medical factors,[104] and often a combination of factors, are present. About 30% of patients have respiratory failure that requires mechanical ventilation. Ventilatory failure is primarily caused by inspiratory muscle weakness, although weakness of the abdominal and accessory muscles of respiration, retained airway secretions leading to pulmonary aspiration and atelectasis are all contributory factors. The associated bulbar weakness and autonomic instability reinforce the need for control of the airway and ventilation.

> **Practice tip**
>
> In Guillain–Barré syndrome vital capacity less than 20 mL/kg is a sign of respiratory fatigue. Early intubation leads to earlier extubation and a better prognosis.

Acute motor and sensory axonal neuropathy, the acute axonal form of GBS, usually presents with a rapidly developing paralysis over hours and a rapid development of respiratory failure requiring tracheal intubation and ventilation. $PaCO_2$ may remain constant until just before intubation, emphasising the importance of not relying purely on arterial blood gas (ABG) analysis to make decisions regarding intubation.

Sensory involvement in relation to pain has been studied asserting the clinical observation of pain ranging from mild to severe in the acute and rehabilitant phases. Chronic pain is often present in survivors of GBS.[105]

There may be total paralysis of all voluntary muscles of the body, including the cranial musculature, the ocular muscles and the pupils. Prolonged ventilatory support is likely in GBS patients who experience rapid disease progression, bulbar dysfunction, bilateral facial weakness or autonomic nerve dysfunction. Tracheostomy is usually performed within 2 weeks, and mechanical ventilation is delivered in a supportive mode with minimal yet adequate sedation and pain management.[106]

Patient management

Assessment and understanding of neuromuscular weakness through motor and sensory neurological assessment is vital in the acute care and rehabilitation of GBS patients (see *Online* resources for published guidelines):

- Comprehensive respiratory assessment (level of overall patient comfort, frequency and depth of breathing, forced vital capacity, use of accessory muscles, presence of paradoxical respiration and integrity of upper airway reflexes), ABG data and chest radiography determine levels of fatigue in both the acute stage (for intubation and ventilation) and rehabilitation (weaning) stage. Long-term ventilation increases the risk of ventilator-associated pneumonia, requiring routine surveillance.
- Cardiovascular assessment is important, as serious tachyarrhythmias and bradyarrhythmias and destabilising fluctuations in BP caused by autonomic impairment are prevalent. This feature is common during fatigue, sleep and states of dehydration. Often, autonomic dysfunction is worst in the early stages of a nosocomial infection.[107]
- Cranial nerve assessment and dermatome (for sensory) and muscle strength assessment assist in mapping the progression, severity and rehabilitation of the disease and determining the risk of aspiration. Pain (especially neuropathic) is particularly common in GBS during changes in myelination, and can be difficult to treat.[108]

A structured care plan, involving the patient and family is essential for continuity of care, particularly in the long-term recovery phase. The provision of sleep, good nutrition and prevention of the complications of immobility (nosocomial infections, deep vein thrombosis, integument and muscular weakening, adequate nutrition and constipation) are important.[106] The following points also need consideration:[106,108]

- Endotracheal and pharyngeal suction can be demanding (weakened upper airway reflexes), and sputum plugging and retention requires frequent repositioning and physiotherapy.
- Routine daily gentle exercise as part of a flexible program improves wellbeing and strength.
- Fatigue must be avoided, as autonomic nerve dysfunction, deafferent pain syndromes, muscle pain and depression can be exacerbated.
- Suctioning, coughing, bladder distension, constipation and the Valsalva manoeuvre can also aggravate autonomic nerve dysfunction instability.
- Therapeutic massage, warm and cold packs and careful positioning contribute to comfort and pain management.
- The patient's surroundings should be pleasant and presentable, especially during long recovery.
- Communication techniques need to be refined to prevent fatigue and frustration.
- Patience, tolerance, empathy, humour and family involvement assist the patient in psychological resilience and recovery.

Intravenous immunoglobulin administration may cause low-grade fever, chills, myalgia, diaphoresis, fluid imbalance, neutropenia, nausea and headaches, and at times acute tubular necrosis. Administration and assessment require adherence to transfusion protocols.[106] Transfusion nurse specialists in collaboration with the patient's nurse perform plasmapheresis.

In the acute phase, accurate diagnosis and timely ventilatory support are provided by effective communication between primary and in-hospital care providers.[106] Multidisciplinary case management is utilised after stabilisation in the acute phase, especially when the level of severity is determined. Recovery and rehabilitation process information is provided to the patient and family so that consultation and communication are effective in recovery.

Myasthenia gravis

Myasthenia gravis is an autoimmune disorder caused by autoantibodies against the nicotinic acetylcholine receptor on the postsynaptic membrane at the neuromuscular junction. It is characterised by weakness and fatigability of the voluntary muscles. For women, it peaks in the second and third decades of life, while for men it tends to occur in the sixth to eighth decades of life. Although a relatively rare disease, prevalence rates have been rising steadily over recent decades, probably due to decreased mortality, longer survival and higher rates of diagnosis.[109] Approximately 20% of patients will experience a myasthenic crisis, typically within 2 years of diagnosis, which can lead to the development of respiratory failure, progressive bulbar weakness failure of airway protection and severe limb and truncal weakness causing extensive paralysis, requiring an admission to ICU.[109]

Aetiology

Myasthenic crisis occurs when weakness from acquired myasthenia gravis becomes severe enough to necessitate intubation for ventilatory support or airway protection. Myasthenic crisis is most likely in patients whose history includes previous crisis, oropharyngeal weakness or thymoma. Possible triggers include infections, aspiration, physical and emotional stress and changes in medications.[110] Most antibiotics have a trigger effect and should be carefully prescribed. Median duration of hospitalisation for crisis is 1 month. The patient usually spends half of this time intubated in the ICU. About

25% of patients are extubated on hospital day 7, 50% by hospital day 13, and 75% by hospital day 31. The mortality rate during hospitalisation for crisis has fallen from nearly 50% in the early 1960s to between 3% and 10% today. With the incidence of crisis remaining stable over the past 30 years, this fall in mortality rates probably reflects improvements in the ICU management of these patients.[111]

Pathophysiology

In myasthenia gravis both structural changes in the architecture of the neuromuscular junction and dynamic alterations in the turnover of acetylcholine receptors erode the safety margin and efficiency of neuromuscular transmission. Of all patients with myasthenia gravis, 80–85% have an identifiable and quantifiable antibody found in the immunoglobulin G fraction of plasma, which is responsible for blocking receptors to the action of acetylcholine at the neuromuscular junction.[111] Therefore, successful neuromuscular transmission is markedly affected by small and subtle changes in acetylcholine release and other triggers (as above), and this gives rise to the decrement in transmission with repetitive stimulation and the characteristic fatigable muscle weakness. Diagnosis is usually by clinical examination and serology testing for antibodies. The 'Tensilon' test, which involves the injection of IV edrophonium and observing the patient for increased eyelid muscle strength, may also be used, although can cause adverse reactions such as bronchospasm and bradycardia, and false-positive results. Pharmacological management for myasthenia gravis includes the use of anticholinesterases (pyridostigmine), steroids, azathioprine and cyclophosphamide. Thymectomy reduces the antibodies responsible for acetylcholine blockade and is often performed early in the disease.[110,112] Plasmapheresis and IV immunoglobulin are also used in the short term for myasthenic crisis and are especially useful for preventing respiratory collapse or assisting with weaning.

Clinical manifestations

In a myasthenic crisis, vital capacity falls, cough and sigh mechanisms deteriorate, atelectasis develops and hypoxaemia results.[110] Ultimately, fatigue, hypercarbia and ventilatory collapse occur. Commonly, superimposed pulmonary infections lead to increased morbidity and mortality. Assessment for triggers begins with a careful review of systems, with attention to recent fevers, chills, cough, chest pain, dysphagia, nasal regurgitation of liquids and dysuria. Detailed history taking should note any trauma, surgical procedures and medication use. General assessment includes vital signs; ear, nose and throat inspection; chest auscultation; and abdominal check. In addition to supportive care and the removal of triggers, management of myasthenic crisis includes treatment of the underlying myasthenia gravis. An experienced neurologist, who will ultimately provide the patient's care outside the ICU, should be part of the care team. Options for treatment during crisis include: use of acetylcholinesterase inhibitors, plasma exchange, IV immunoglobulins and immunosuppressive drugs, including corticosteroids.[111] Cholinergic crisis and myasthenic crisis are due to two different situations although both cause muscle weakness. Cholinergic activity can increase only if the enzymes that break down acetylcholine are deactivated. This can happen when the patient is taking drugs like neostigmine or pyridostigmine.

Patient management

Careful and accurate assessment in the presenting myasthenic crisis patient determines the triggers of the event and incorporates a history, including infections and prescribed medications. These medications can exacerbate acetylcholine receptor blockade, and respiratory demand proves too much for the patient. Awareness by the nurse of trigger medications ensures advocacy for the patient (see *Online* resources for published guidelines).

- Respiratory and cardiovascular assessment incorporates upper and lower airway muscle weakness. ABGs are a poor marker for intubation and ventilation because these values change late in the decompensation cycle. Being able to recognise fatigue (inability to speak, poor lung expansion, vital capacity below 1 L, shoulder and arm weakness) in patients with neuromuscular weakness and air hunger is important.[112]
- Non-invasive ventilation can be difficult to administer safely, with the potential for aspiration due to insidious upper airway weakness; however, the option should be considered with careful assessment of gag, swallow and cough reflexes in order to prevent intubation.[112]
- Neuromuscular blockade should be avoided (residual long-term paralysis), with the use of glottal local anaesthetic spray for emergency intubation and ventilation.
- Placement of small-bore duodenal tubes decreases the risk of aspiration and may be more comfortable than regular nasogastric tubes.
- Tracheostomy is generally not needed, as the duration of intubation is often less than two weeks.
- Cardiac assessment needs to include assessment for both atrial and ventricular dysrhythmias due to autonomic nerve dysfunction.[111] These can be insidious and can be provoked by subtle changes in electrolytes.
- Nursing care will relate to the needs of long-term immobilised, intubated, ventilated patients with neuromuscular alterations.

Myasthenia gravis patients have similar care needs to those of patients with GBS (refer to *Patient management* for GBS). Fatigue and the structure and timing of care are very important. Flexibility of care is important, as energy fluctuates on an hourly basis.[112] Despite having a shorter recovery time than GBS, weaning and recovery in myasthenia gravis is still a slow process and impulsive extubation is discouraged. Therapy should be tailored on an individual basis using best clinical judgement.

Status epilepticus

Status epilepticus is defined as enduring seizure activity that is not likely to stop spontaneously. The traditional definition is 30 min of continuous seizure activity (updated to 5 min to indicate the point at which treatment should be started) or two or more seizures without full recovery of consciousness between seizures.[113] There are as many types of status epilepticus as there are types of seizures. The distinction between convulsive and non-convulsive status epilepticus depends on clinical observation and on a clear understanding of typology.[114] Estimates of the overall incidence have varied from 9.9 to 41 per 100,000 person-years, depending on the population studied and the definitions used.[115] Over half the cases are acute symptomatic, emphasising the importance of identifying an acute precipitant. In adults, low anti-epileptic drug levels, cerebrovascular accident, hypoxia, metabolic causes and alcohol represent the main acute causes. Mortality is about 20%; most patients die of the underlying condition rather than the status epilepticus itself. Status epilepticus can result in permanent neurological and mental deterioration; the risks of morbidity greatly increase with longer duration of the episode. Status epilepticus in the ICU falls into two main groups: those transferred to the ICU because of uncontrolled (refractory) status epilepticus and those who are admitted to the ICU for another reason and have status epilepticus as an additional finding.[116]

Pathophysiology

At a cellular level, status epilepticus results from a failure of normal inhibitory pathways, primarily mediated by gamma-aminobutyric acid acting via gamma-aminobutyric acid A receptors. This loss of inhibitory drive allows the activation of excitatory feedback loops, leading to repetitive, synchronous firing of large groups of neurons. As seizure activity continues, there is a further decline in gamma-aminobutyric inhibitory tone that counterbalances neuronal excitation function. Continued excitatory input mediated primarily by glutamate leads to neuronal cell death.[116]

Clinical manifestations

Convulsive status epilepticus is a medical emergency. The initial consequence of a prolonged convulsion is a massive release of plasma catecholamines, which results in a rise in heart rate, BP and plasma glucose. During this stage cardiac dysrhythmias are often seen, and may be fatal. CBF is greatly increased, and thus glucose delivery to active cerebral tissue is maintained. As the seizure continues, hyperthermia above 40°C with lactic and respiratory acidosis continues to intensify, especially without adequate resuscitation and control of the seizure.

The status epilepticus may then enter a second, late phase in which cerebral and systemic protective measures progressively fail. The main characteristics of this phase are: a fall in BP; a loss of cerebral autoregulation, resulting in the dependence of CBF on systemic BP; and hypoglycaemia due to the exhaustion of glycogen stores and increased neurogenic insulin secretion. ICP can rise precipitously. The combined effects of systemic hypotension and intracranial hypertension may result in a compromised cerebral circulation and cerebral oedema. Intracranial pressure monitoring is advisable in prolonged cases when raised ICP is suspected. Further complications that can occur include rhabdomyolysis leading to acute tubular necrosis, hyperkalaemia and hyponatraemia.[117]

Patient management

The online resources describe management of seizures in general; however, the following specific status epilepticus aspects of patient management should be considered:

- Resuscitation
- Specific post-status epilepticus patient assessment
- Pharmacological patient management.

Status epilepticus requires control of the seizure and then investigation regarding the cause. Airway protection is often difficult in the seizing patient, so the first line of treatment includes basic life-support measures followed by the administration of IV propofol, midazolam or, in refractory cases, phenytoin. Neuromuscular blockade will be required to facilitate intubation in patients who continue to have tonic–clonic seizure activity despite these pharmacological interventions. A short-acting, non-depolarising muscle relaxant that is devoid of significant haemodynamic effects and does not raise ICP is the preferred agent (e.g. rocuronium). Succinylcholine should be avoided if possible, as the patient may be hyperkalaemic as a consequence of possible rhabdomyolysis. Prolonged neuromuscular blockade should be avoided as it only stops the motor response, hence masking the altered neuronal activity. Once the seizures are controlled, intubation and ventilation can protect the airway and potentially reverse the acidosis.

Practice tip

The three most crucial factors determining the outcome from status epilepticus are the underlying aetiology, the speed of anti-seizure treatment and the age of the person. Older aged individuals with status epilepticus frequently have a symptomatic cause, possess a more limited reserve to recover due to comorbidities and have a higher mortality rate.

Neurological assessment is limited in the sedated patient. Pupillary response is usually sluggish and reflects the medication prescribed. Routine monitoring in an ICU is essential, with CT and MRI to exclude mass lesions. Blood glucose levels should be checked immediately by bedside testing. Blood should be tested for electrolytes, magnesium, phosphate, calcium, liver and renal function, haematocrit, white blood cell count, platelet count, anti-epileptic drug levels, toxic drugs and substances (particularly salicylates) and alcohol.

EEG monitoring in the ICU for refractory status epilepticus is essential, as a patient may enter a drug-induced coma with little outward sign of convulsions yet have ongoing electrographic epileptic activity. Furthermore, continuous recording will give an indication of worsening of generalised convulsions regardless of the presence or absence of sedating drugs or paralysing agents. This manifests as bilateral EEG ictal discharges on the monitor. Deeper sedation and anaesthesia are then indicated and can be titrated to EEG results.[118]

The goal of pharmacological therapy is to achieve the rapid and safe termination of the seizure, and to prevent its recurrence without adverse effects on the cardiovascular and respiratory systems or without altering the level of consciousness. Diazepam, lorazepam, midazolam, phenytoin and phenobarbitone have all been used as first-line therapy for the termination of status epilepticus. The best regimen to use will depend on the cause of the seizure and previous anti-epileptic drug therapy. A patient who develops status epilepticus during alcohol withdrawal may not need continued medication following the withdrawal process. In contrast, patients with for example, encephalitis or trauma may require high doses of anti-epileptic medication to control seizure activity.

Summary

A description and application of neurological alterations and their management are provided in this chapter, beginning with an overview of neurological dysfunction, specifically pathophysiological alterations of consciousness, alterations in motor and sensory function and alterations in cerebral perfusion and metabolism. Cerebral oedema is related to ICP preceding the therapeutic management of these conditions. Intracranial hypertension is discussed in association with cerebral perfusion and metabolic events. CNS disorders including traumatic brain and spinal injury, their aetiology, clinical pathophysiology and management are covered. Cerebrovascular disorders that focus on ischaemic stroke, intracerebral haemorrhage and subarachnoid haemorrhage are described. Meningitis and encephalitis are included in the section on infection and inflammation with GBS, myasthenic crisis and status epilepticus in the neuromuscular alterations' component.

Case study

Eleanor, a 49-year-old female, was cleaning her kitchen at around midday when she suddenly fell to the floor. Her husband called an ambulance, which arrived approximately 9 min later. The paramedics found Eleanor unresponsive and pale on the kitchen floor in a pool of vomitus and urine, GCS was 3, pupils were equal size 3 mm and reactive. Respiratory rate was 23 breaths/min, SpO_2 96%, heart rate 115 beats/min and a BP of 143/89 mmHg. Eleanor's husband denied any seizure-like activity. Over a period of approximately 12 min, Eleanor's GCS gradually improved to 11 (E3, V4, M4). She was noted to have a right-sided motor deficit (i.e. no movement in right upper limb but with some limited spontaneous movements of lower limb). A 20-gauge IV cannula was inserted, and ondansetron 4 mg IV was given. Oxygen at 6 L via a face mask was applied and Eleanor was transported to the Emergency Department (ED) with a suspected left-sided stroke. A history of hypertension and smoking were noted. No known drug allergies.

On arrival in the ED at 12:48, a stroke call was activated. An initial CT scan showed a SAH with blood in the left ventricle. Both internal carotid arteries showed approximately 50% stenosis with moderate-to-severe microvascular disease. As the hospital Eleanor did not provide a neurovascular surgery service, Eleanor was transferred to a nearby tertiary hospital.

A second higher resolution CT/CT angiogram performed on arrival to the second hospital again demonstrated an acute SAH with a small amount of blood in the occipital horn of the left ventricle and slightly more pronounced hydrocephalus. It also showed two aneurysms, one at the left middle cerebral artery and another at the left anterior aneurysm. Based on Eleanor's clinical presentation and CT scans, her haemorrhage was deemed to be a World Federation of Neurosurgical Societies grade 2, Fisher grade 4.

Eleanor became agitated, slightly combative and hypertensive (systolic BP (SBP) 185 mmHg). She was intubated and transferred to the ICU to await emergency surgery for insertion of an external ventricular drain due to the likelihood of a progressive hydrocephalus.

DAY 0

Eleanor was sedated using propofol and fentanyl infusions and commenced on a nimodipine infusion as per protocol. She was ventilated on synchronised intermittent mandatory ventilation (SIMV) with settings of 5 cmH_20 positive end-expiratory pressure (PEEP) and 8 cmH_20 of pressure support (PS), fraction of inspired oxygen (FiO_2) 0.35, tidal volumes of 350 mL and a respiratory rate of 14 breaths/min. On return from theatre for insertion of a right frontal external ventricular drain at 20:20, the postoperative orders were:

- External ventricle drain at 15 cm above the reference points and on free drainage – draining 8–16 mL/h of blood-stained CSF
- SBP limits <140 mmHg due to unsecured aneurysm

A routine electrocardiogram showed ST depression in leads V4–6, with a rise in troponin level. Despite an initial plan to wean sedation to allow for neurological assessment, to maintain the SBP limits below 140 mmHg Eleanor required a greater depth of sedation. Digital subtraction angiography ± coiling was booked for the following day.

DAYS 1–2

In theatre, the left middle cerebral artery aneurysm was coiled using balloon assistance as this was felt to be the aneurysm which had ruptured and was therefore at greater risk of rebleeding. The angiogram was also suggestive of widespread atheromatous disease and there were multiple points of vasospasm in the vessels supplying the left frontal and parietal lobes. The procedure took approximately 6 h.

Given the vasospasm, on return to ICU the SBP limits were changed to 140–160 mmHg. Eleanor's GCS was 10 (E3, V1(t), M6, pupils equal and reacting to light (PEARL)), but a new deficit was noted with nil movement of the right arm. The neurosurgeons therefore set a new SBP target of 160–200 mmHg requiring the commencement of a noradrenaline infusion. Concern was raised regarding the unsecured aneurysm but the real risk of ischaemic damage outweighed the potential risk of rupture of another aneurysm. Throughout this time Eleanor's ICP remained within normal limits (3–9 mmHg). Troponin levels continued to rise from 93 to 237, but a transthoracic echocardiogram showed no abnormalities. Nasogastric feeding was commenced. A meeting was held between Eleanor's husband Michael, her son and the medical teams to discuss the findings and treatment. As with all meetings with family members, the nurse caring for the patient attended.

Over the next 12 h, noradrenaline requirements increased. Eleanor remained euvolaemic with a central venous pressure of 10–14 mmHg. Vasopressin was therefore added enabling the noradrenaline infusion to be reduced. Eleanor continued to obey commands when the propofol was held for hourly neurological assessments. Eleanor could now move her upper arm with gravity eliminated but still had no movement in her hand. A CT brain showed a decrease in the size of the ventricles but no evidence of infarction or new haemorrhage.

DAYS 3–7

A repeat brain CT and angiogram carried out on day 3 showed a region of hypodensity of the left middle frontal gyrus in keeping with an area of infarction probably related to vasospasm. The angiogram showed the coiled aneurysm and moderate-severe left-sided vasospasm, which was treated with intraarterial administration of nimodipine and verapamil.

The noradrenaline and vasopressin infusions were slowly reduced while still maintaining the elevated SBP limits set by the neurosurgeons. The ventilation mode was changed to a spontaneous mode, and the PEEP and PS settings reduced with a view to extubation, which was carried out on day 4.

Attempts to switch the nimodipine infusion to the nasogastric tube route proved unsuccessful due to the profound hypotensive episodes which occurred approximately 15 min following administration. During this time, Eleanor continued to obey commands but the strength in her right upper limb fluctuated. The SBP parameters continued to be 160–200 mmHg with the noradrenaline titrated to the movement of the right upper limb, i.e. the aim was for an SBP of 160 mmHg but higher if the deficit became more pronounced.

DAYS 8–14

On day 8 Eleanor was extubated on to high flow nasal oxygen; this time successfully. Post extubation, Eleanor was found to have a GCS of 13–14 (E3-4, V4, M6, PEARL), movement of left upper and lower limbs against gravity and resistance, movement of right upper limb with gravity eliminated and right lower limb against gravity but not resistance.

Over the course of the next 3 days, several attempts to reduce the SBP limits to below 160 mmHg resulted in a deterioration of Eleanor's neurological condition, increased drowsiness and confusion, and a more pronounced weakness of the right upper limb, all of which improved when the SBP was increased to >160 mmHg using inotropes.

Repeat CT/CT angiogram carried out on day 14 showed expected progression of the left middle frontal gyrus infarct and a small amount of residual blood in the occipital horns of the lateral ventricles. The external ventricular drain was clamped with the proviso that it be returned to free drainage if the ICP became >20 mmHg and/or there was a deterioration in Eleanor's neurological condition.

Eleanor was reviewed by the speech pathologist who initially placed her on a dysphagia soft diet and mildly thick fluids, upgraded eventually to a normal diet and then fluids.

DAY 15–49

The SBP limits were relaxed to >140 mmHg which, given Eleanor's history of hypertension, required no pharmacological intervention. While a number of attempts were made to clamp the external ventricular drain, they resulted in increased confusion and drowsiness. Another CT scan was carried out which showed hydrocephalus. On day 24, a decision was then made to convert to an internal ventricle–peritoneal shunt.

Eleanor was moved to the neurosurgical ward where she continued to make progress and was later transferred to a rehabilitation institution. A 6-month readmission date was set for coiling of her remaining intracranial aneurysm. Eleanor remained in the rehabilitation facility for 10 days before discharge home. Her only deficit on discharge was a residual mild weakness of her right hand.

CASE STUDY QUESTIONS

1. With a brain injury to the left side of the brain, what deficits would you expect to see in your patient? What potential communication problems may be encountered and why?
2. From your reading of the *Case study*, discuss Eleanor's risk factors for SAH and cerebral ischaemia/infarction following the haemorrhage.
3. Explain the pathophysiology process for why patients with a SAH are at risk of developing hydrocephalus?
4. What clinical signs are indicative of vasospasm?
5. Why are patients with a SAH at risk of developing ST changes? Describe the process.

RESEARCH VIGNETTE

Mohamed WRA, Leach MJ, Reda NA et al. The effectiveness of clinical pathway-directed care on hospitalisation-related outcomes in patients with severe traumatic brain injury: a quasi-experimental study. J Clin Nurs 2018; 27:e820–e832

Abstract

Aims and objectives: To compare the effectiveness of clinical pathway-directed care to usual care on hospitalisation-related outcomes in patients with severe traumatic brain injury (STBI).

Background: Severe traumatic brain injury is a major cause of disability and mortality in young adults. Clinical pathways endeavor to bring evidence and clinical practice closer together to foster the delivery of best practice and to improve patient outcomes.

Design: Quasi-experimental study.

Methods: The study was conducted in a trauma intensive care unit of a large teaching hospital in Egypt. Patients aged 18–60 years with a diagnosis of STBI, a Glasgow Coma Scale score between 3–8 and a nonpenetrating head injury were consecutively assigned to 15 days of care. The outcomes assessed were complications related to hospitalization, clinical variances, length of intensive care unit (ICU) stay, ICU readmission rate and patient/family satisfaction.

Results: Sixty participants completed the study (30 in each arm). Apart from age, there were no significant differences between groups in baseline characteristics. The clinical pathway group demonstrated statistically significantly fewer cases of hospitalization-related complications on day 15, and a significantly shorter length of ICU stay, lower ICU readmission rate and a high level of patient/family satisfaction when compared with the usual care group. The effect of the intervention on fever, pressure ulceration, hyperglycaemia and readmission to the ICU was no longer statistically significant after controlling for age.

Conclusions: The findings of the current study suggest that the implementation of a clinical pathway for patients with severe TBI may be helpful in improving the patient experience as well as some hospitalization-related outcomes.

Critique

This study compared the effectiveness of clinical pathway-directed care to usual care in adults with severe traumatic brain injury (TBI). Authors provide a strong rationale for the study, based on a current lack of robust evidence and report a statistically significant difference in outcomes in favour of the intervention group. So, based on these data, should we recommend the use of clinical pathway-directed care for patients with severe TBI?

The process of developing the intervention was rigorous and included a comprehensive review of the literature. In accordance with best practice, pilot work tested the feasibility of the intervention and the study protocol prior to conducting a definitive trial. The sample size (*n*=60, 30 in each study arm) was also informed by a power calculation using data from the pilot work and the two groups were well matched except for age. In addition, monitoring delivery of the intervention ensured fidelity increasing the internal validity of the study.

Randomised controlled trials (RCTS) are the gold standard design for establishing cause and effect relationship; however, investigators in this study used a single centre open-label quasi-experimental design. Quasi-experimental designs increase the risk of selection bias; commonly because, as in the case of this study, they do not randomise participants to a study group and because they do not blind researchers and/or those delivering care to a participant's assigned group (clinical pathway or usual care). Contamination between groups may also have been possible. Additionally, there is inadequate description of the data collection tools and methods and the extent of any attrition. These factors further increase the risk of bias.

The level of statistical significance was set at a conventional $P < 0.05$; however, there is no mention of any clinical significance testing. While statistical significance implies that the difference seen in the sample also exists in the population, measures of clinical significance can provide information about whether any differences are clinically important.

Overall, this study suggests that implementation of clinical pathway-directed care for severe TBI is unlikely to cause harm. However, the extent to which its use has a positive impact on experiences and outcomes needs further investigation using a multi-centre RCT before making any strong recommendations for practice.

Learning activities

1 What are the main causes of raised ICP?

2 Describe the management of a patient with raised ICP.

3 Explain the differences between the various types of stroke and briefly outline the management of each.

4 Describe the possible complications associated with a subarachnoid haemorrhage.
5 Explain the treatments available for a patient admitted with an ischaemic stroke.
6 A patient has been admitted following a high-speed motor vehicle accident which resulted in a C4–C5 SCI.
   a Describe the mechanisms of injury to the spinal cord involved with this type of accident.
   b Outline the initial management of this patient.
7 What is the clinical management of a patient who presents in status epilepticus?
8 Define hydrocephalus and the possible causes of the development of this condition.
9 Describe the differences between bacterial and viral meningitis in terms of presentation and treatment.

Online resources

TRAUMATIC BRAIN INJURY

AACN Clinical Practice Guideline series. Care of the patient undergoing intracranial pressure monitoring/ external ventricular drainage or lumbar drainage, http://files.mmintensivecare.webnode.pt/200000471-ad055ad4d0/Intracranial%20Pressure%20Monitoring.pdf

Brain Trauma Foundation, https://braintrauma.org/guidelines/guidelines-for-the-management-of-severe-tbi-4th-ed#/

BMJ Best practice. Assessment of traumatic brain injury, acute, http://bestpractice.bmj.com/topics/en-gb/515#referencePop1

Centers for Disease Control and Prevention: Traumatic brain injury & concussion, www.cdc.gov/traumaticbraininjury

CSF drainage and ICP monitoring system, www.youtube.com/watch?v=MPpH8MnXhb8&list=PLH9gpVKlHL6p09M1Pz8Upo qggfwLsfxzA

National Resource Centre for Traumatic Brain Injury, www.brainlink.org.au

SPINAL CORD INJURY

BMJ Best Practice: Acute cervical spine trauma, http://bestpractice.bmj.com/topics/en-gb/944

National Institute for Health and Care Excellence (NICE) Guideline NG41. Spinal injury: assessment and initial management, https://www.nice.org.uk/guidance/ng41/evidence/full-guideline-2358425776

Academy Spinal Cord Injury Nurses (ASCIP), www.academyscipro.org

Cervical collars, www.youtube.com/watch?v=cYxnp6ml8mE

International Spinal Cord Society (ISCoS), http://www.iscos.org.uk/

Emergency Neurological Life Support Traumatic Spine Injury Protocol, 2016, http://enlsprotocols.org/files/TSI.pdf

STROKE

AHA/ASA GUIDELINE 2018. Guidelines for the early management of patients with acute ischemic stroke: a guideline for healthcare professionals from the American Heart Association/American Stroke Association, http://stroke.ahajournals.org/content/49/3/e46

AHA/ASA GUIDELINE 2015. Guidelines for the management of spontaneous intracerebral hemorrhage. A guideline for healthcare professionals from the American Heart Association/American Stroke Association, http://stroke.ahajournals.org/content/early/2015/05/28/STR.0000000000000069

AHA/ASA GUIDELINE 2012. Guidelines for the management of aneurysmal subarachnoid hemorrhage. A guideline for healthcare professionals from the American Heart Association/American Stroke Association, http://stroke.ahajournals.org/content/early/2012/05/03/STR.0b013e3182587839

BMJ Best practice; Ischaemic stroke, http://bestpractice.bmj.com/topics/en-gb/1078

BMJ Best practice; Haemorrhagic stroke, https://bestpractice.bmj.com/topics/en-gb/1079

National Institute for Health and Care Excellence (NICE) Stroke pathways, https://pathways.nice.org.uk/pathways/stroke

Australian Institute of Health and Welfare publication: Stroke and its management in Australia: an update, www.aihw.gov.au/publication-detail/?id=60129543613

National Stroke Foundation of Australia publication, www.strokefoundation.com.au

INFECTIONS

BMJ Best practice. Bacterial meningitis, http://bestpractice.bmj.com/topics/en-gb/539

British Infection Association. Published guidelines, https://www.britishinfection.org/guidelines-resources/published-guidelines/

Centers for disease control and prevention. Guideline for isolation precautions: preventing transmission of infectious agents in healthcare settings, https://www.cdc.gov/infectioncontrol/guidelines/isolation/appendix/transmission-precautions.html

GUILLAIN-BARRÉ/MYASTHENIA GRAVIS

BMJ Best practice. Guillain-Barré syndrome, http://bestpractice.bmj.com/topics/en-gb/176

GBS/CIDP Foundation International, https://www.gbs-cidp.org/

Myasthenia Gravis Foundation America. International consensus guidance for management of myasthenia gravis, http://n.neurology.org/content/neurology/early/2016/06/29/WNL.0000000000002790.full.pdf

STATUS EPILEPTICUS

American Epilepsy Society. Resources and guidelines, https://www.aesnet.org/clinical_resources/guidelines

BMJ Best practice. Status epilepticus, https://bestpractice.bmj.com/topics/en-gb/464

Further reading

Hachem LD, Ahuja CS, Fehlings MG. Assessment and management of acute spinal cord injury: from point of injury to rehabilitation. J Spinal Cord Med 2017;40(6):665–75.

Hickey J. The clinical practice of neurological and neurosurgical nursing. 7th ed. Philadelphia: Lippincott & Wilkins; 2014.

Hussein MTEL, Zettel S, Suykens AM. The ABCs of managing increased intracranial pressure. J Nurs Educ Pract 2017;7(4):6–14.

References

1. Cavanna AE, Shah S, Eddy CM, et al. Consciousness: a neurological perspective. Behav Neurol 2011;24(1):107–16.
2. Edlow JA, Rabinstein A, Traub SJ, et al. Diagnosis of reversible causes of coma. Lancet 2014;384(9959):2064–76.
3. Cavanna AE, Cavanna SL, Servo S, et al. The neural correlates of impaired consciousness in coma and unresponsive states. Discov Med 2010;9(48):431–8.
4. Strosznajder RP, Czubowicz K, Jesko H, et al. Poly(ADP-ribose) metabolism in brain and its role in ischemia pathology. Mol Neurobiol 2010;41(2–3):187–96.
5. Huff JS, Fountain NB. Pathophysiology and definitions of seizures and status epilepticus. Emerg Med Clin North Am 2011;29(1):1–13.
6. Varelas PN, Spanaki MV, Mirski MA. Status epilepticus: an update. Curr Neurol Neurosci Rep 2013;13(7):357.
7. Veening JG, Barendregt HP. The regulation of brain states by neuroactive substances distributed via the cerebrospinal fluid; a review. Cerebrospinal Fluid Res 2010;6(7):1.
8. Winhammar J, Rowe D, Henderson R, et al. Assessment of disease progression in motor neuron disease. Lancet Neurol 2005;4(4): 229–38.
9. Di Pino G, Pellegrino G, Assenza G, et al. Modulation of brain plasticity in stroke: a novel model for neurorehabilitation. Nat Rev Neurol 2014;10(10):597–608.
10. Shepherd S, Batra A, Lerner DP. Review of critical illness myopathy and neuropathy. Neurohospitalist 2017;7(1):41–8. doi:10.1177/1941874416663279.
11. Silverman MN, Heim CM, Nater UM, et al. Neuroendocrine and immune contributors to fatigue. PM R 2010;2(5):338–46.
12. Guan L, Collet JP, Mazowita G, et al. Autonomic nervous system and stress to predict secondary ischemic events after transient ischemic attack or minor stroke: possible implications of heart rate variability. Front Neurol 2018;(9):90. doi:10.3389/fneur.2018.00090. eCollection 2018.
13. Bulstrode H, Nicoll JAR, Hudson G, et al. Mitochondrial DNA and traumatic brain injury. Ann Neurol 2014;75(2):186–95.
14. Trendelenburg G. Molecular regulation of cell fate in cerebral ischemia: role of the inflammasome and connected pathways. J Cereb Blood Flow Metab 2014;34(12):1857–67.

15. Jhelum P, Karisetty BC, Kumar A, et al. Implications of epigenetic mechanisms and their targets in cerebral ischemia models. Curr Neuropharmacol 2017;15(6):815–30.
16. Kumar VSS, Gopalakrishnan A, Nazirog'lu M, et al. Calcium ion – the key player in cerebral ischemia. Curr Med Chem 2014;21(18):2065–75.
17. Giacino JT, Fins JJ, Laureys S, et al. Disorders of consciousness after acquired brain injury: the state of the science. Nat Rev Neurol 2014;10(2):99–114.
18. Partington T, Farmery A. Intracranial pressure and cerebral blood flow. Anaes Intens Care Med 2014;15(4):189–94.
19. Stokum JA, Gerzanich V, Simard JM. Molecular pathophysiology of cerebral edema. J Cereb Blood Flow Metab 2016;36(3):513–38.
20. Kiefer M, Unterberg A. The differential diagnosis and treatment of normal-pressure hydrocephalus. Dtsch Arztebl Int 2012;109(1–2):15–26.
21. McLeod A. Traumatic injuries to the head and spine, 2: nursing considerations. Br J Nurs 2004;13(17):1041–9.
22. Cummings BM, Yager PH, Murphy SA, et al. Managing edema and intracranial pressure in the intensive care unit. In: Lo EH, Lok J, Ning MM, et al, editors. Vascular mechanisms in CNS trauma. New York: Springer; 2014. p. 363–78.
23. Di Ieva A, Schmitz EM, Cusimano MD. Analysis of intracranial pressure: past, present, and future. Neuroscientist 2013;19(6):592–603.
24. Czosnyka M, Pickard J. Monitoring and interpretation of intracranial pressure. J Neurol Neurosurg Psychiat 2004;75(6):813–21.
25. Porth C, Gaspard K. Essentials of pathophysiology: concepts of altered health states. 4th ed. Philadelphia: Wolters Kluwer; 2015.
26. Latronico N. The relationship between the intracranial pressure – volume index and cerebral autoregulation. Intensive Care Med 2013;1:153.
27. Kirkman MA, Smith M. Multimodality neuromonitoring. Anesthesiol Clin 2016;34(3):511–23.
28. Stocchetti N, Maas AI. Traumatic intracranial hypertension. N Engl J Med 2014;370(22):2121–30.
29. Brain Trauma Foundation. Guidelines for the management of severe traumatic brain injury. 4th ed. Online. Available from: www.braintrauam.org.
30. Kheirbek T, Pascual J. Hypertonic saline for the treatment of intracranial hypertension. Curr Neurol Neurosci Rep 2014;14(9):1–6.
31. Berger-Pelleiter E, Émond M, Lauzier F, et al. Hypertonic saline in severe traumatic brain injury: a systematic review and meta-analysis of randomized controlled trials. CJEM 2016;18(2):112–20.
32. Yenari MA, Colbourne F, Hemmen TM, et al. Therapeutic hypothermia in stroke. Stroke Res Treat 2011;2011:157969. doi:10.4061/2011/157969.
33. Akbari Y, Mulder M, Razmara A, et al. Cool down the inflammation: hypothermia as a therapeutic strategy for acute brain injuries. In: Chen J, Hu X, Stenzel-Poore M, et al, editors. Immunological mechanisms and therapies in brain injuries and stroke. Springer Series in Translational Stroke Research 6. New York: Springer; 2014. p. 349–75.
34. Marion DW, Regasa LE. Revisiting therapeutic hypothermia for severe traumatic brain injury ... again. Crit Care 2014;18(3):160.
35. Kirkman MA. Targeted temperature management and acute brain injury: an update from recent clinical trials. Current Anesthesiology Reports 2016;6(3):214–22.
36. Cariou A, Payen JF, Asehnoune K, et al; for the Société de Réanimation de Langue Française (SRLF) and the Société Française d'Anesthésie et de Réanimation (SFAR) in conjunction with the Association de Neuro Anesthésie Réanimation de Langue Française (ANARLF), the Groupe Francophone de Réanimation et Urgences Pédiatriques (GFRUP), the Société Française de Médecine d'Urgence (SFMU), and the Société Française Neuro-Vasculaire (SFNV). Targeted temperature management in the ICU: guidelines from a French expert panel. Ann Intensive Care 2017;7(70):1–14.
37. Howes D, Gray SH, Brooks SC, et al. Canadian guidelines for the use of targeted temperature management (therapeutic hypothermia) after cardiac arrest: a joint statement from The Canadian Critical Care Society (CCCS), Canadian Neurocritical Care Society (CNCCS), and the Canadian Critical Care Trials Group (CCCTG). Resuscitation 2016;98:48–63.
38. Donnino MW, Andersen LW, Berg KM, et al; the ILCOR ALS Task Force. Temperature management after cardiac arrest. Resuscitation 2016;98:97–104.
39. Povlishock JT, Wei EP. Posthypothermic rewarming considerations following traumatic brain injury. J Neurotrauma 2009;26(3):333–40.
40. Edwards P, Arango M, Balica L, et al. Final results of MRC CRASH, a randomised placebo-controlled trial of intravenous corticosteroid in adults with head injury-outcomes at 6 months. Lancet 2005;365(9475):1957–9.
41. Tritos NA, Yuen KC, Kelly DF, et al. American Association of Clinical Endocrinologists and American college of endocrinology disease state clinical review: a neuroendocrine approach to patients with traumatic brain injury. Endocr Pract 2015;21:823.
42. Adembri C, Venturi L, Pellegrini-Giampietro DE. Neuroprotective effects of propofol in acute cerebral injury. CNS Drug Rev 2007;13:333–51.
43. Li LM, Timofeev I, Czosnyka M, et al. Review article: the surgical approach to the management of increased intracranial pressure after traumatic brain injury. Anesth Analg 2010;111(3):736–48.
44. Vibbert M, Mayer SA. Early decompressive hemicraniectomy following malignant ischemic stroke: the crucial role of timing. Curr Neurol Neurosci Rep 2010;10(1):1–3.
45. Cooper JD, Rosenfeld JV, Murray L, et al. Decompressive craniectomy in diffuse traumatic brain injury. N Engl J Med 2011;364(16):1493–502.
46. Hutchinson PJ, Kolias AG, Timofeev IS, et al; for the RESCUEicp Trial Collaborators. Trial of decompressive craniectomy for traumatic intracranial hypertension. N Engl J Med 2016;375:1119–30.
47. Anderson CS, Arima H, Lavados P, et al; for the HeadPoST Investigators and Coordinators. Cluster-randomized, crossover trial of head positioning in acute stroke. N Engl J Med 2017;376:2437–47.

48. Haddad SH, Arabi YM. Critical care management of severe traumatic brain injury in adults. Scand J Trauma Resusc Emerg Med 2012;20(12):1–15.
49. Ferreira LL, Valenti VE, Vanderlei LCM. Chest physiotherapy on intracranial pressure of critically ill patients admitted to the intensive care unit: a systematic review. Rev Bras Ter Intensiva 2013;25(4):327–33.
50. Roozenbeek B, Maas AI, Menon DK. Changing patterns in the epidemiology of traumatic brain injury. Nat Rev Neurol 2013;9(4):231–6.
51. Nguyen R, Fiest KM, McChesney J, et al. The international incidence of traumatic brain injury: a systematic review and meta-analysis. Can J Neurol Sci 2016;43(6):774–85.
52. National Center for Injury Prevention and Control. Rates of TBI-related hospitalizations by age group – United States, 2001–2010 [online]. Atlanta: Centers for Disease Control and Prevention; 2014.
53. Peeters W, van den Brande R, Polinder S, et al. Epidemiology of traumatic brain injury in Europe. Acta Neurochir (Wien) 2015;157(10): 1683–96.
54. Myburgh JA, Cooper DJ, Finfer SR, et al. Epidemiology and 12-month outcomes from traumatic brain injury in Australia and New Zealand. J Trauma 2008;64(4):854–62.
55. Soustiel JF, Sviri GE, Mahamid E, et al. Cerebral blood flow and metabolism following decompressive craniectomy for control of increased intracranial pressure. Neurosurgery 2010;67(1):65–72.
56. Badruddin A, Taqi MA, Abraham MG, et al. Neurocritical care of a reperfused brain. Curr Neurol Neurosci 2011;11(1):104–10.
57. Choi HA, Jeon S-B, Samuel S, et al. Paroxysmal sympathetic hyperactivity after acute brain injury. Curr Neurol Neurosci Rep 2013;13(8):1–10.
58. Zakharova N, Kornienko V, Potapov A, et al. Mapping of cerebral blood flow in focal and diffuse brain injury. In: Zakharova N, Kornienko V, Potapov A, et al, editors. Neuroimaging of traumatic brain injury. Switzerland: Springer International Publishing; 2014. p. 107–23.
59. Rabinowitz AR, Li X, Levin HS. Sport and nonsport etiologies of mild traumatic brain injury: similarities and differences. Annu Rev Psychol 2014;65:301–31.
60. Fitzharris M, Cripps RA, Lee BB. Estimating the global incidence of traumatic spinal cord injury. Spinal Cord 2014;52(2):117–22.
61. Singh A, Tetreault L, Kalsi-Ryan S, et al. Global prevalence and incidence of traumatic spinal cord injury. Clin Epidemiol 2014;6:309–31.
62. Jazayeri SB, Beygi S, Shokraneh F, et al. Incidence of traumatic spinal cord injury worldwide: a systematic review. Eur Spine J 2014;1–14.
63. Wilson JR, Cho N, Fehlings MG. Acute traumatic spinal cord injury: epidemiology, evaluation, and management. In: Patel VV, Patel AP, Harrop JS, et al, editors. Spine surgery basics. Berlin: Springer-Verlag; 2014. p. 399–409.
64. Silva NA, Sousa N, Reis RL, et al. From basics to clinical: a comprehensive review on spinal cord injury. Prog Neurobiol 2014;114:25–57.
65. Evans LT, Lollis SS, Ball PA. Management of acute spinal cord injury in the neurocritical care unit. Neurosurg Clin N Am 2013;24(3):339–47.
66. Lo V, Esquenazi Y, Han MK, et al. Critical care management of patients with acute spinal cord injury. J Neurosurg Sci 2013;57(4):281–92.
67. Eckert MJ, Martin MJ. Trauma: spinal cord injury. Surg Clin North Am 2017;97(5):1031–45.
68. Pimentel L, Diegelmann L. Evaluation and management of acute cervical spine trauma. Emerg Med Clin North Am 2010;28(4):719–38.
69. National Institute for Health and Care Excellence (NICE) Spinal injury: assessment and initial management. NG41. 2016; https://www.nice.org.uk/guidance/ng41.
70. Ulndreaj A, Badner A, Fehlings MG. Promising neuroprotective strategies for traumatic spinal cord injury with a focus on the differential effects among anatomical levels of injury. F1000Res 2017;6(F1000 Faculty Rev):1907. doi:10.12688/f1000research.11633.1.
71. Kramer AH, Roberts DJ, Zygun DA. Optimal glycemic control in neurocritical care patients: a systematic review and meta-analysis. Crit Care 2012;16(5):R203.
72. World Health Organization. The top ten causes of death. 2017. [online] http://www.who.int/mediacentre/factsheets/fs310/en/.
73. American Heart Association (AHA). Statistical Update. Heart disease and stroke statistics- 2018 Update. A report from the American Heart Association. Circulation 2018;137:e67–492.
74. Townsend N, Wickramasinghe K, Bhatnagar P, et al. Coronary heart disease statistics 2012 edition. London: British Heart Foundation; 2012.
75. Chung JM. Seizures in the acute stroke setting. Neurol Res 2014;36(5):403–6.
76. Powers WJ, Rabinstein AA, Ackerson T, et al; on behalf of the American Heart Association Stroke Council. Guidelines for the early management of patients with acute ischemic stroke: a guideline for healthcare professionals from the American Heart Association/American Stroke Association. Stroke 2018;[Epub ahead of print].
77. Van Asch CJ, Luitse MJ, Rinkel GJ, et al. Incidence, case fatality, and functional outcome of intracerebral haemorrhage over time, according to age, sex, and ethnic origin: a systematic review and meta-analysis. Lancet Neurol 2010;9:167–76.
78. Hemphill JC, Greenberg SM, Anderson CS, et al. Guidelines for the management of spontaneous intracerebral hemorrhage. A guideline for healthcare professionals from the American Heart Association/American Stroke Association. Stroke 2015;46(7):2032–60.
79. Steiner T, Al-Shahi Salman R, Beer R, et al. European Stroke Organisation guidelines for the management of spontaneous intracerebral hemorrhage. Int J Stroke 2014;9(7):840–55.
80. Zhou Y, Wang Y, Wang J, et al. Inflammation in intracerebral hemorrhage: from mechanisms to clinical translation. Prog Neurobiol 2014;115:25–44.
81. Tan X, He J, Li L, et al. Early hyperglycaemia and the early-term death in patients with spontaneous intracerebral haemorrhage: a meta-analysis. Internal Med J 2014;44(3):254–60.

82. Teasdale GM, Drake CG, Hunt W, et al. A universal subarachnoid hemorrhage scale: report of a committee of the World Federation of Neurosurgical Societies. J Neurol Neurosurg Psychiatry 1988;51(11):1457.
83. Helbok R, Kurtz P, Vibbert M, et al. Early neurological deterioration after subarachnoid haemorrhage: risk factors and impact on outcome. J Neurol Neurosurg Psychiatry 2013;84(3):266–70.
84. Connolly ES, Rabinstein AA, Carhuapoma JR, et al; American Heart Association Stroke Council; Council on Cardiovascular Radiology and Intervention; Council on Cardiovascular Nursing; Council on Cardiovascular Surgery and Anesthesia; Council on Clinical Cardiology. Guidelines for the management of aneurysmal subarachnoid hemorrhage: a guideline for healthcare professionals from the American Heart Association/American Stroke Association. Stroke 2012;43(6):1711–37.
85. Tagami T, Kuwamoto K, Watanabe A, et al. Effect of Triple-h prophylaxis on global end-diastolic volume and clinical outcomes in patients with aneurysmal subarachnoid hemorrhage. Neurocrit Care 2014;21(3):462–9.
86. Hamdan A, Barnes J, Mitchell P. Subarachnoid hemorrhage and the female sex: analysis of risk factors, aneurysm characteristics, and outcomes. J Neurosurg 2014;121(6):1367–73.
87. Moussouttas M, Lai EW, Huynh TT, et al. Association between acute sympathetic response, early onset vasospasm, and delayed vasospasm following spontaneous subarachnoid hemorrhage. J Clin Neurosci 2014;21(2):256–62.
88. de Rooij NK, Rinkel GJ, Dankbaar JW, et al. Delayed cerebral ischemia after subarachnoid hemorrhage: a systematic review of clinical, laboratory, and radiological predictors. Stroke 2013;44(1):43–54.
89. Brathwaite S, Macdonald RL. Current management of delayed cerebral ischemia: update from results of recent clinical trials. Transl Stroke Res 2014;5(2):207–26.
90. Sarrafzadeh AS, Vajkoczy P, Bijlenga P, et al. Monitoring in neurointensive care – the challenge to detect delayed cerebral ischemia in high grade aSAH. Front Neurol 2014;5:34.
91. Fisher C, Kistler J, Davis J. Relation of cerebral vasospasm to subarachnoid hemorrhage visualized by computerized tomographic scanning. Neurosurgery 1980;6(1):1–9.
92. Luoma A, Reddy U. Acute management of aneurysmal subarachnoid haemorrhage. Contin Educ Anaesth Crit Care Pain 2013;13(2):52–8.
93. Diringer MN, Bleck TP, Claude Hemphill J 3rd, et al. Neurocritical Care Society. Critical care management of patients following aneurysmal subarachnoid hemorrhage: recommendations from the Neurocritical Care Society's Multidisciplinary Consensus Conference. Neurocrit Care 2011;15:211–40.
94. Sandström N, Yan B, Dowling R, et al. Comparison of microsurgery and endovascular treatment on clinical outcome following poor-grade subarachnoid hemorrhage. J Clin Neurosci 2013;20(9):1213–18.
95. Coutinho JM, Zuurbier SM, Aramideh M, et al. The incidence of cerebral venous thrombosis: a cross-sectional study. Stroke 2012;43:3375.
96. Devasagayam S, Wyatt B, Leyden J, et al. Cerebral venous sinus thrombosis incidence is higher than previously thought: a retrospective population-based study. Stroke 2016;47:2180–2.
97. Kasanmoentalib ES, Brouwer MC, van de Beek D. Update on bacterial meningitis: epidemiology, trials and genetic association studies. Curr Opin Neurol 2013;26(3):282–8.
98. World Health Organization (WHO) Meningococcal meningitis. [online] http://www.who.int/en/news-room/fact-sheets/detail/meningococcal-meningitis.
99. Bradshaw M, Venkatesan A. Herpes simplex virus-1 encephalitis in adults: pathophysiology, diagnosis, and management. Neurother 2016;13(3):493–508.
100. Hills SL, Rabe IB, Fischer M. Chapter 3: Infectious Diseases Related to Travel. Japanese encephalitis. Centers for Disease Control and Prevention (CDC). 2018. Available from: https://wwwnc.cdc.gov/travel/yellowbook/2018/infectious-diseases-related-to-travel/japanese-encephalitis.
101. Middleton D, Pallister J, Klein R, et al. Hendra virus vaccine, a one health approach to protecting horse, human, and environmental health. Emerg Infect Dis 2014;20(3):372.
102. Rozenberg F. Acute viral encephalitis. Handb Clin Neurol 2013;112:1171–81.
103. Vellozzi C, Iqbal S, Stewart B, et al. Cumulative risk of Guillain–Barré syndrome among vaccinated and unvaccinated populations during the 2009 H1N1 influenza pandemic. Am J Public Health 2014;104(4):696–701.
104. Bhagat H, Dash HH, Chauhan RS, et al. Intensive care management of Guillain–Barré syndrome: a retrospective outcome study and review of literature. J Neuroanaesth Crit Care 2014;1(3):188.
105. Ruts L, Drenthen J, Jongen JLM, et al. Pain in Guillain–Barré syndrome: a long-term follow-up study. Neurology 2010;75(16):1439–47.
106. BMJ Best Practice. Guillain-Barré syndrome. 2017 [online]. Available from: http://bestpractice.bmj.com/topics/en-gb/176/pdf/176.pdf.
107. Yuki N, Hartung H-P. Guillain–Barré syndrome. N Engl J Med 2012;366(24):2294–304.
108. van den Berg B, Walgaard C, Drenthen J, et al. Guillain–Barré syndrome: pathogenesis, diagnosis, treatment and prognosis. Nature Rev Neurol 2014;10(8):469–82.
109. Spilane J, Higham E. Myasthenia gravis. BMJ 2012;345:e8497.
110. Vacca V. Myasthenia gravis and myasthenic crisis. Nurs 2018 Crit Care 2017;12(5):38–46.
111. Sakaguchi H, Yamashita S, Hirano T, et al. Myasthenic crisis patients who require intensive care unit management. Muscle Nerve 2012;46(3):440–2.

112. Bhagat H, Grover V, Jangra K. What is optimal in patients with myasthenic crisis: invasive or non-invasive ventilation? J Neuroanaesth Crit Care 2014;1(2):116.

113. Sánchez S, Rincon F. Status epilepticus: epidemiology and public health needs. J Clin Med 2016;5(8):71.

114. Huff JS, Fountain NB. Pathophysiology and definitions of seizures and status epilepticus. Emerg Med Clin North Am 2011;29(1):1–13.

115. Neligan A, Sander JW. Epidemiology of seizures and epilepsy. Epilepsy 2013;28–32.

116. Hocker S, Wijdicks EF, Rabinstein AA. Refractory status epilepticus: new insights in presentation, treatment, and outcome. Neurol Res 2013;35(2):163–8.

117. Fernandez A, Claassen J. Refractory status epilepticus. Curr Opin Crit Care 2012;18(2):127–31.

118. Claassen J, Taccone FS, Horn P, et al. Recommendations on the use of EEG monitoring in critically ill patients: consensus statement from the neurointensive care section of the ESICM. Intensive Care Med 2013;39(8):1337–51.

Chapter 18

Support of renal function

Ian Baldwin, Susan Dirkes

KEY WORDS

acute kidney injury
acute renal failure
continuous renal replacement therapy
extracorporeal circuit
dialysis history
urine production

Learning objectives

After reading this chapter, you should be able to:

- summarise the physiology of urine production
- differentiate between acute and chronic renal failure and describe the most likely causes of kidney injury in the critically ill adult
- outline treatment approaches in managing acute kidney injury in critical illness
- describe the indications for renal replacement therapy in critical care
- understand the circuit and key components included for dialysis support and renal replacement therapy in the critically ill
- appreciate the unique and purpose-made fluids utilised to achieve this along with the importance of fluid balance in the anuric patient
- understand the role of newer biomarkers for identification of kidney injury
- understand the principles and challenges associated with nursing management of continuous renal replacement therapy in critical care.

Introduction

Deterioration of kidney function as a result of physiological injury to the point where there is retention of nitrogenous wastes is a common manifestation of critical illness and is often associated with failure of other organs. Acute kidney injury (AKI) is a syndrome with numerous causes and associated factors, including glomerulonephritis, prerenal azotaemia, urinary tract obstruction, vasculitis, shock and sepsis. Acute tubular necrosis is a collective term commonly used in the past to describe acutely deteriorating renal function, reflecting pathological changes from various renal insults of a nephrotoxic or ischaemic origin. Factors that cause renal function to deteriorate are not always ischaemic or necrotic in origin, and a syndrome with degrees of deterioration prior to an anuric state and failure is often evident. Functional impairment correlates poorly with structural injury to the kidneys[1] and is insufficient to define AKI as it is occurring. Therefore, a consensus definition and classification system has been established that focuses on incremental organ injury rather than end-stage organ failure.[2,3] AKI is defined as a rapid decrease in kidney function, resulting in an inability to maintain acid–base, fluid and electrolyte balance, and to excrete nitrogenous wastes. This new approach describes staging of AKI severity and embraces the concept and dynamics of organ failure where a dynamic spectrum is found, from small indiscrete changes in function that are immediately reversible, through to gross acute signs and irreversible organ failure.[3] With this change of conceptual focus in recent years new consensus guidelines have been released in an effort to better guide clinical understanding and decision making, the most comprehensive being from the Kidney Disease: Improving Global Outcomes (KDIGO) group.[4] Three stages of AKI are defined by the 2012 KDIGO Clinical Practice Guidelines for Acute Kidney Injury and are based on the elevation in serum creatinine and/or decline in urinary output, which correlates with prognosis.[4] On average, 5% of hospital admissions and 30% of intensive care unit (ICU) admissions carry a diagnosis of AKI, and it will develop in 25% of hospitalised patients. Patients with AKI of any type are at higher risk for all-cause mortality according to prospective cohorts, whether or not there is substantial renal recovery. The rates of AKI in the hospital setting have increased steadily since the 1980s and continue to rise.[5]

FIGURE 18.1 Kidney and urinary drainage system.

Organs and structures of the urinary system

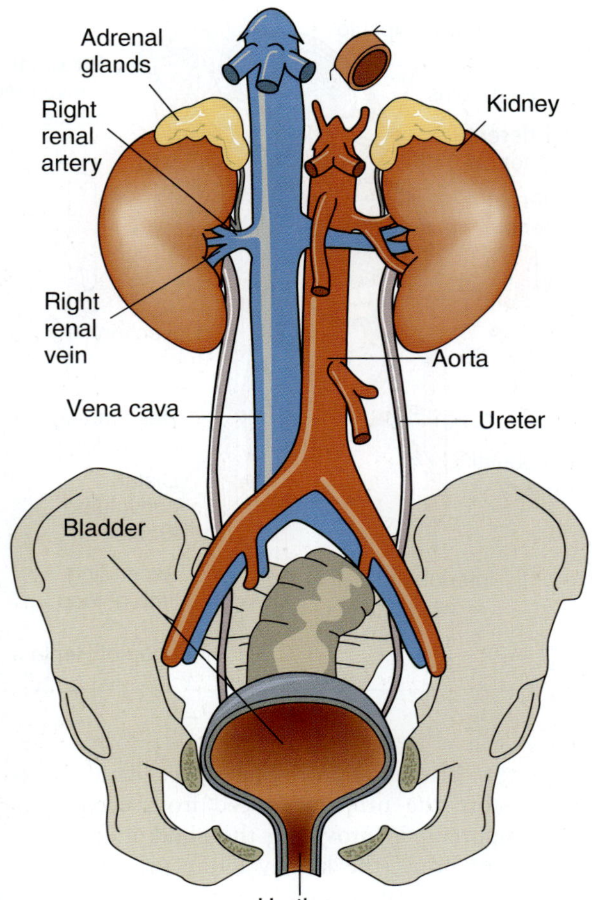

Frontal section of kidney

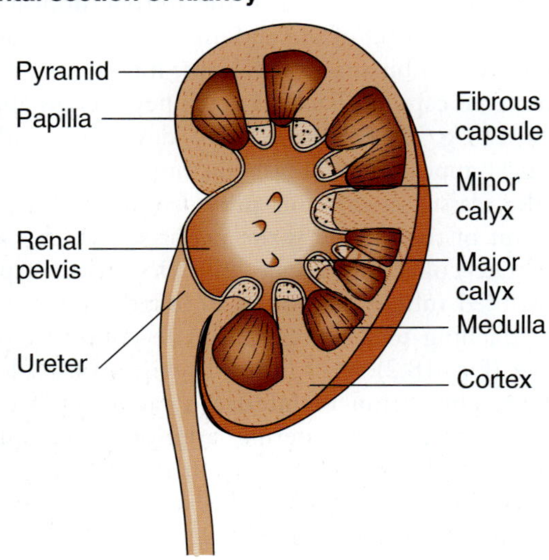

Related anatomy and physiology

The renal system has a number of key functions, including regulation and maintenance of fluid and electrolyte balance, clearance of metabolic and other waste products, an indirect role in the maintenance of blood pressure, acid–base balance and an endocrine function. An appreciation of renal function, in critical illness is essential as it relates to fluid management, blood pressure, electrolyte and acid–base function.

Regulation and maintenance of the extracellular fluid and electrolyte constituents occur principally via the process of filtration and reabsorption. The kidneys receive approximately 25% of the cardiac output each minute, and excrete approximately 180 L/day of glomerular filtrate. Fortunately, tubular reabsorption accounts for approximately 178.5 L/day of the original filtrate, allowing for a modest daily fluid intake or retention of 1.5 L for fluid homeostasis.[6] During this process of filtration and reabsorption, metabolic by-products and electrolyte and other wastes (including many drugs) are also excreted and maintained in balance. As with all body organ systems, an adequate blood pressure and supply of oxygen to the kidneys is paramount in maintaining the fluid and electrolyte regulatory role.

Anatomy of the kidney, nephron and urinary drainage system

The functional anatomy of the renal system includes the two kidneys, ureters, bladder and urethra (Fig. 18.1).

FIGURE 18.2 Nephron and glomerulus.

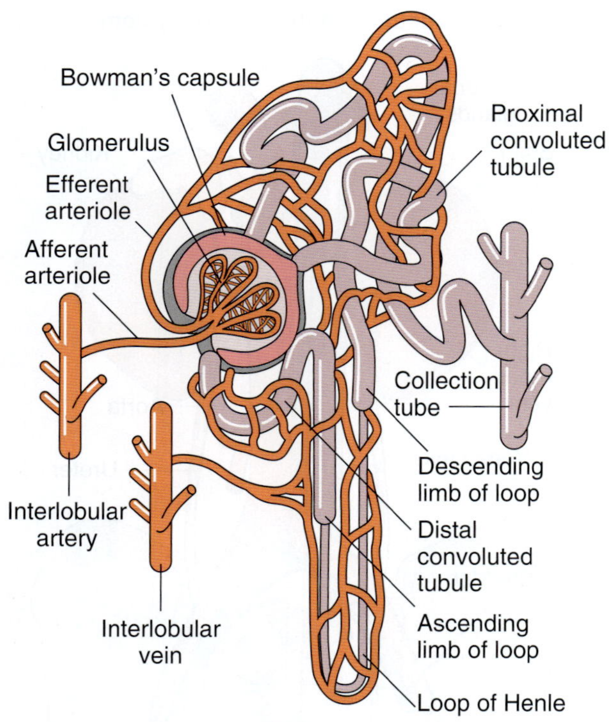

The ureters, bladder and urethra collect, drain and temporarily store the urine produced from each kidney.[7] While important in providing the conduit for the final excretion of urine, the kidney is the primary organ of interest in the renal system, particularly in critical care practice, and hence will be described in more detail from the anatomical and physiological perspectives.

The kidneys are located in the retroperitoneal space on the posterior wall of the abdominal cavity, encased in a protective combination of the ribs, muscle, fat, tendon and the renal capsule. Each adult kidney weighs approximately 140 g. The kidneys may develop a different anatomical appearance, or vary in number and location from the classic description provided here. The functional unit of the kidney is the nephron, which consists of a filtrate-collecting device (the Bowman's capsule), a convoluted tubule that varies in length and diameter, finally attaching to a common filtrate-collecting tubule and duct (Fig. 18.2). Within the Bowman's capsule rests the glomerulus, a tuft of interlaced capillaries that arise from the afferent or entering arteriole. The efferent arteriole then drains and exits from the glomerulus, via a closely entwined network called the peritubular capillaries, until these collect in the venous network of the kidney.[7]

The glomeruli and nephrons lie in the cortical area of the kidney, while the collecting ducts gather together into the renal pyramids, which lie in the medulla of the kidney. The pyramids drain into the calyces of the kidney, which then drain into the renal pelvis where urine is gathered to drain into the ureter. The major blood vessels of the kidney, the renal artery and veins also enter the renal capsule through the pelvis of the kidney.[7]

Urine production, regulation of glomerular filtration rate and filtrate reabsorption in the nephron

Urine production consists of a three-stage process, which occurs in the nephron: glomerular filtration, tubular reabsorption and tubular secretion (Fig. 18.3). As previously noted, the production of urine is highly dependent on delivery of blood under pressure to the glomerulus. This results in the first step of the urine production process, glomerular filtration. The glomerular filtration rate (GFR) is about 125 mL/min under normal conditions. Changes in the diameter of the afferent and efferent arteriole help regulate glomerular blood flow, and subsequent filtration flow, but this is unable to compensate for large variations of mean blood pressure. Filtration rates may rise or fall markedly over the course of a day.[8]

The filtrate is essentially plasma water and anything dissolved therein. Proteins, blood cells are not dissolved in the plasma water and do not enter the tubule system as filtrate. As the filtrate transgresses the glomerulus it is collected into the Bowman's capsule and delivered into the nephron proximal convoluted tubule, loop of Henle and then the distal convoluted tubule, where a number of processes result in the reabsorption of about 99% of the glomerular filtrate. The remaining fluid within the tubule drains into the collecting tubule to form urine. This fluid has substantially different properties from the original glomerular filtrate, as fluid and many electrolytes and glucose are reabsorbed by the peritubular capillaries.

Despite the tremendous permeability of the glomerular membrane, it has a high degree of selectivity for the size of molecules it allows to pass through. The molecular weight of even the smallest plasma protein is almost too high to pass through. Ionic charge (+ve/−ve) also changes the filtrate composition and reabsorption and negatively charged molecules are filtered less than positively charged molecules of equal size.[6] Disease and certain conditions can change or affect this physiology resulting in higher protein losses, poor reabsorption of essential amino acids and proteinuria. Red blood cells, like proteins also are too large to pass through the membrane such that the glomerular filtrate is almost the same composition as the plasma water.[6]

Along with blood pressure, the sodium content of the extracellular fluid is critical in maintaining fluid balance, as it constitutes the major electrolyte and osmotic agent of the glomerular filtrate. It is imperative that sodium intake and loss are equally balanced, as excessive losses will result in associated fluid loss and excessive intake will result in fluid retention. If sodium balance is not

FIGURE 18.3 Urine formation: filtration, reabsorption and excretion.

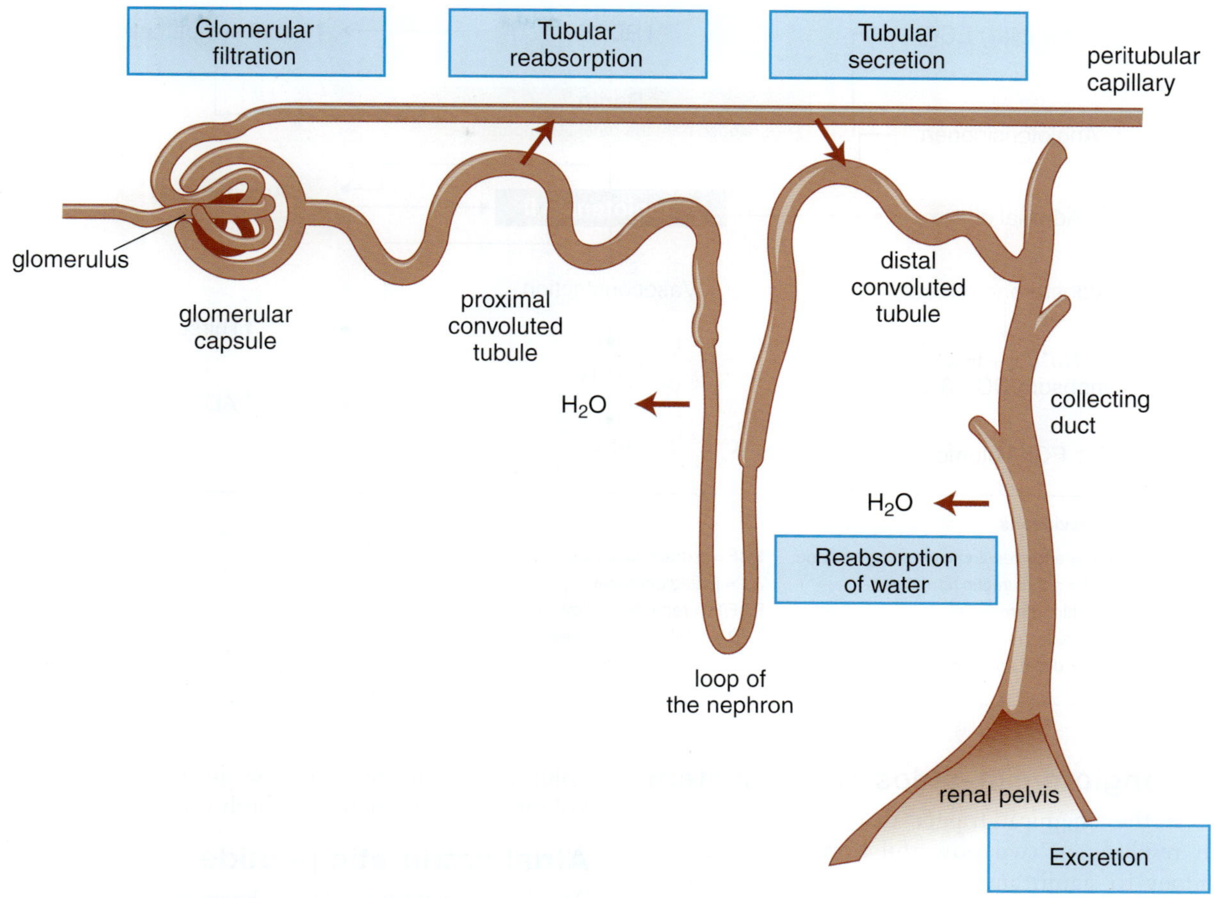

Adapted from Mader S. Inquiry into life. 11th ed. New York: McGraw-Hill; 2006.

maintained, other compensations such as a rise in blood pressure may result to restore fluid balance. As blood pressure rises, the excretion of sodium also increases by way of additional glomerular filtrate. In this way, water and sodium balance are inextricably linked.[6]

Hormonal and neural regulation of renal function

Various feedback mechanisms exist that assist in precisely adjusting the final amount of fluid and electrolyte to be excreted from the kidney. These include the sympathetic nervous system response, angiotension II, aldosterone, antidiuretic hormone and atrial natriuretic peptide. All these mechanisms work in synchrony with blood pressure and sodium balance in ensuring a highly regulated circulating and extracellular fluid volume.[6]

Sympathetic nervous system

Stimulation of the sympathetic nervous system by loss of blood volume occurs by reflex via the low-pressure volume sensors in the pulmonary and venous circulations. This is complemented by further stimulation if arterial pressure falls. The sympathetic nervous system widely innervates the kidney and is able to reduce the filtration rate by constricting the afferent arteriole of the glomerulus, thus inhibiting blood flow and pressure necessary to create the GFR. This stimulation of the sympathetic nervous system also increases the reabsorption of salt and water in the tubule and stimulates the release of renin.

Antidiuretic hormone

The antidiuretic hormone is excreted from the pituitary gland under regulation of hypothalamic osmoreceptors (thirst centre), and reduces kidney diuresis (the excretion of water). By enhancing the kidney's ability to concentrate urine, it ensures that the excretory functions of waste products and electrolytes continue while limiting fluid loss. Antidiuretic hormone is essential to surviving limited periods of fluid deprivation and fine-tuning the urine volume production on a continuous basis.

FIGURE 18.4 Renin–angiotensin–aldosterone system (RAAS).

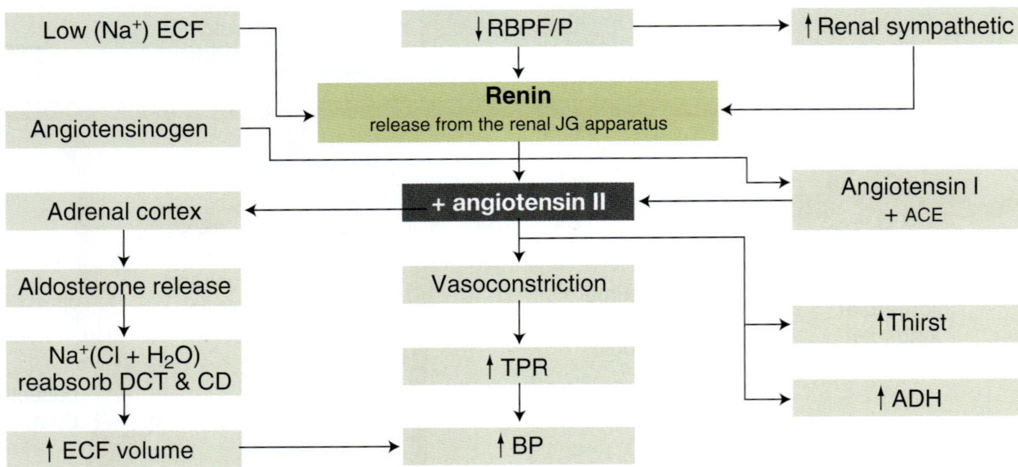

Abbreviations

ACE = angiotension-converting enzyme
ADH = antidiurectic hormone
BP = blood pressure
CD = collecting duct
DCT = distal collecting duct
ECF = extracellular fluid
JG = juxtaglomerular
RBF/P = renal blood flow/pressure
TPR = total peripheral resistance

Renin–angiotensin–aldosterone system

Renin is the chemical trigger that initiates a cascade system resulting in two powerful hormones acting on the kidney to significantly influence sodium and water excretion (Fig. 18.4). Renin is produced and released from the juxtaglomerular apparatus, a collection of cells in the macula densa of the distal tubule, and the adjacent afferent arteriole next to the glomerulus, which monitors blood sodium concentration. When released, renin stimulates the activation of angiotensin I from circulating but inactive angiotensinogen. Under the influence of coenzyme A, angiotensin I converts to angiotensin II, a potent vasoconstrictor and stimulus to reabsorb sodium and water. The vasoconstrictor effect raises blood pressure and flow to the glomerulus, inhibiting further renin release (a negative feedback mechanism) as perfusion pressure normalises. This allows the return of natriuresis (sodium excretion) and diuresis. This response is essential in assisting with retaining fluid in the event of falling blood pressure, or boosting fluid excretion as blood pressure rises. It also responds effectively to a rise in sodium intake by reducing angiotensin II formation and allowing a larger natriuresis, resulting in maintenance of sodium balance, a key to tissue fluid distribution and balance.[6]

Aldosterone is a mineralocorticoid excreted from the adrenal cortex in response to angiotensin II. Aldosterone increases the reabsorption of sodium, and hence water, in the cortical-collecting tubules and increases the rate of potassium excretion. This has a dual effect of regulating sodium balance and extracellular fluid volume. As fluid volume accumulates, the rise in GFR self-limits the volume effect by increasing both diuresis and natriuresis.

Atrial natriuretic peptide

Atrial natriuretic peptide is a hormone released from the atria of the heart in response to atrial stretching during periods of increased circulating fluid volume. Atrial natriuretic peptide is therefore often described as having an antagonising effect to the renin–angiotensin–aldosterone system (which acts primarily to preserve sodium and water). These natriuretic, and hence diuretic, effects are mild and self-limiting, and occur in response to mild rises in GFR and reductions in sodium reabsorption. As blood pressure falls, the drop in GFR compensates for the effect of atrial natriuretic peptide, ensuring that excessive loss of sodium and water does not occur.[6]

Regulation of acid–base and electrolyte balance

The kidney assists in the management of body pH by regulation of the excretion of hydrogen (H(+)) and bicarbonate (HCO_3^-) ions. While the renal response to alkalosis or acidosis is slow in comparison with plasma buffers and respiratory regulation (see Chapter 13), it does result in a net loss of H^+ ions or recovery of HCO_3^- ions, which are the basis of human pH balance (Fig. 18.5). During acidosis the kidney raises H^+ secretion by active transport to combine with ammonia in the renal tubule to form ammonium, which is unable to be reabsorbed. Coincidentally, raised H^+ excretion

FIGURE 18.5 Hydrogen ion regulation in the kidney.

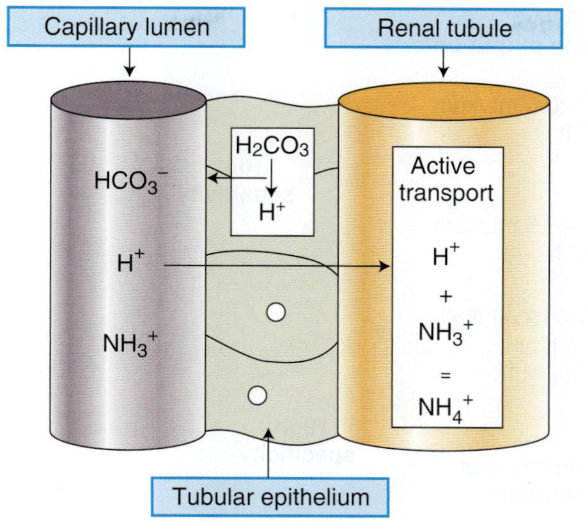

increases the reabsorption of sodium, which increases the alkalotic ion, HCO_3^- Conversely, during alkalosis the reabsorption of hydrogen ions is increased. These changes in hydrogen ion concentration in the renal filtrate alter the pH of the urine down to a maximum level of four.[6,8] The buffering of H^+ with ammonia reduces the acidifying effect of the hydrogen ions, particularly as some ammonium combines with chloride to form ammonium chloride.[6]

Role as an endocrine organ

The kidney has two homeostatic roles as an endocrine organ. Although neither has effects relevant to acute illness, patients with chronic renal dysfunction often need supplementation to overcome the loss of renal endocrine support. Erythropoietin is important in stimulating the generation of new red blood cells and is released from the kidney in response to a sustained drop in arterial blood oxygen levels. The kidney also produces the active form of vitamin D, 1,25-Dihydroxy vitamin D3, also known as calcitriol. Calcitriol helps regulate the absorption of calcium from the gut, which in turn promotes bone resorption of calcium and the reabsorption of calcium in the kidney. This active form is necessary for the maintenance of body calcium levels.[6]

Pathophysiology and classification of renal failure

Diseases of the kidneys affect the structure and therefore the function of the nephrons in some way. Pathology such as this, if untreated, may not cause complete and terminal loss of renal function or end-stage renal disease (ESRD), but depending on extent of nephron damage or 'injury' occurring at the time, and any previous illness that resulted in undetected kidney damage.[3,4] By focusing on factors that resulted in kidney injury, both individually and collectively, more serious damage that may result in failure can be averted. This concept is more clearly described in the later section on acute tubular damage and AKI, which includes classification as the RIFLE (see Fig. 18.6A) and KDIGO Criteria (see Fig. 18.6B).[3,4] In addition, AKI has a significant effect on mortality and increased health risks.[9] A systematic review of 25 studies with data from 254,408 adults, of whom 55,150 had AKI[10] demonstrated that AKI was associated with an 86% increase in cardiovascular mortality and a 38% increased risk of cardiovascular events such as congestive heart failure, acute MI, and stroke. AKI was also associated independently with a 58% increase in the risk of congestive heart failure and a 40% increase in the risk of acute myocardial infarction (MI).

The conventional classification of AKI is based on the perceived causative mechanisms:[3,5]

- prerenal
- intrarenal (intrinsic)
- postrenal.

Irrespective of the causative mechanism, should kidney injury progress to failure, the same renal replacement therapies are suitable to support life until recovery may occur.

Prior to considering whether a critically ill patient has suffered acute injury, it has been recommended the effects of intraabdominal hypertension be considered.[11] As it is possible that up to half of mechanically-ventilated patients will have this to some degree, measures to relieve the pressure should be considered as changes in renal function can result due to either direct pressure on the kidney and/or drainage system or increased pressure within the venous circulation of the kidney. Intraabdominal hypertension also clouds the assessment of haemodynamic parameters and cardiovascular performance, making it difficult to assess fluid needs and responsiveness to fluid resuscitation.[11] For a more detailed discussion of intraabdominal hypertension, please refer to Chapter 20.

Prerenal causes

Prerenal causes are the most common aetiology of AKI, accounting for 40–80% of cases, depending on the population studied. Prerenal azotemia is due to renal hypoperfusion, which is an appropriate physiologic change. If reversed quickly with restoration of renal blood flow, renal parenchymal damage often does not occur. If hypoperfusion persists, ischaemia can result, causing intrinsic kidney injury. Prerenal factors affecting blood supply to the kidneys, such as hypovolaemia, cardiac failure or hypotension/shock are the most common causes of AKI.[12] The mechanism and outcome are easily related.

Decreased renal perfusion can occur in several ways, such as a decrease in intravascular volume, a change in vascular resistance, or low cardiac output. Causes of volume depletion include haemorrhage, gastrointestinal

FIGURE 18.6 (**A**) Criteria for diagnosis of acute kidney injury (AKI): the risk, injury and failure criteria with outcomes of loss and end-stage renal disease (RIFLE). (**B**) Criteria for AKI diagnosis: three stages.

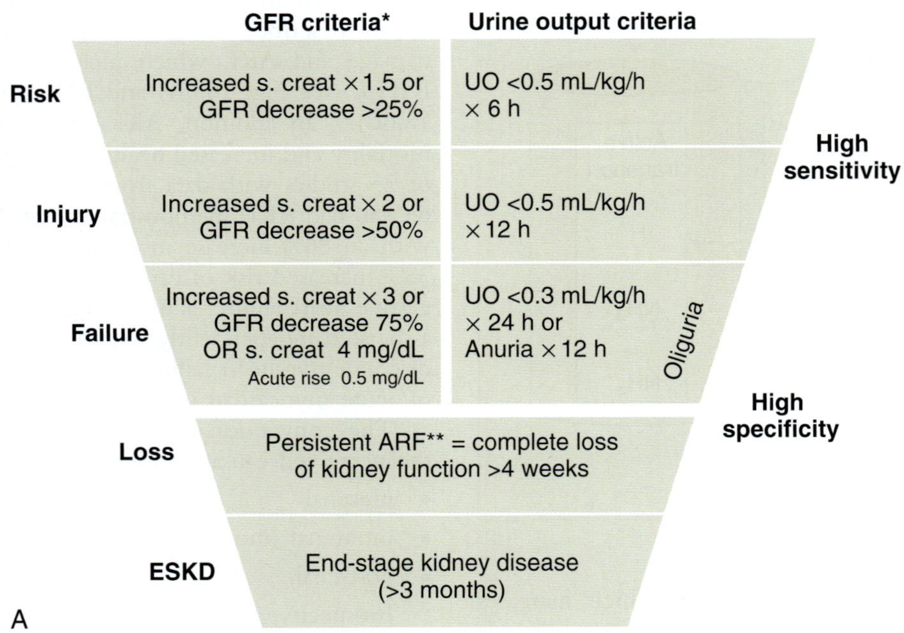

A

Staging of AKI

Stage	Serum creatinine	Urine output
1	1.5–1.9 times baseline OR ≥ 0.3 mg/dl (≥ 26.5 μmol/l) increase	<0.5 ml/kg/h for 6–12 hours
2	2.0–2.9 times baseline	<0.5 ml/kg/h for ≥12 hours
3	3.0 times baseline OR Increase in serum creatine to ≥4.0 mg/dl (≥353.6 μmol/l) OR Initiation of renal replacement therapy OR, In patients <18 years decrease in eGFR to <35ml/min per 1.73 m^2	<0.3 ml/kg/h for ≥24 hours OR Anuria for ≥12 hours

B

Source (B): Section 2: AKI Definition. Kidney International Supplements, Volume 2, Issue 1, 19–36. With permission from Elsevier.

losses, dehydration, excessive diuresis, extravascular space sequestration, pancreatitis, burns, trauma, and peritonitis. Low cardiac output is a state of low effective renal arterial blood flow. This occurs in states of cardiogenic shock, heart failure, pulmonary embolism, and pericardial tamponade. Arrhythmias and valvular disorders can also reduce cardiac output. In the ICU setting, positive pressure ventilation will decrease venous return, also decreasing cardiac output.

As blood flow to the kidneys is reduced, there is a lower rate of glomerulofiltration, urine production diminishes, and wastes accumulate. This state can be

FIGURE 18.7 Neuroendocrine response to shock, resulting in oliguria.

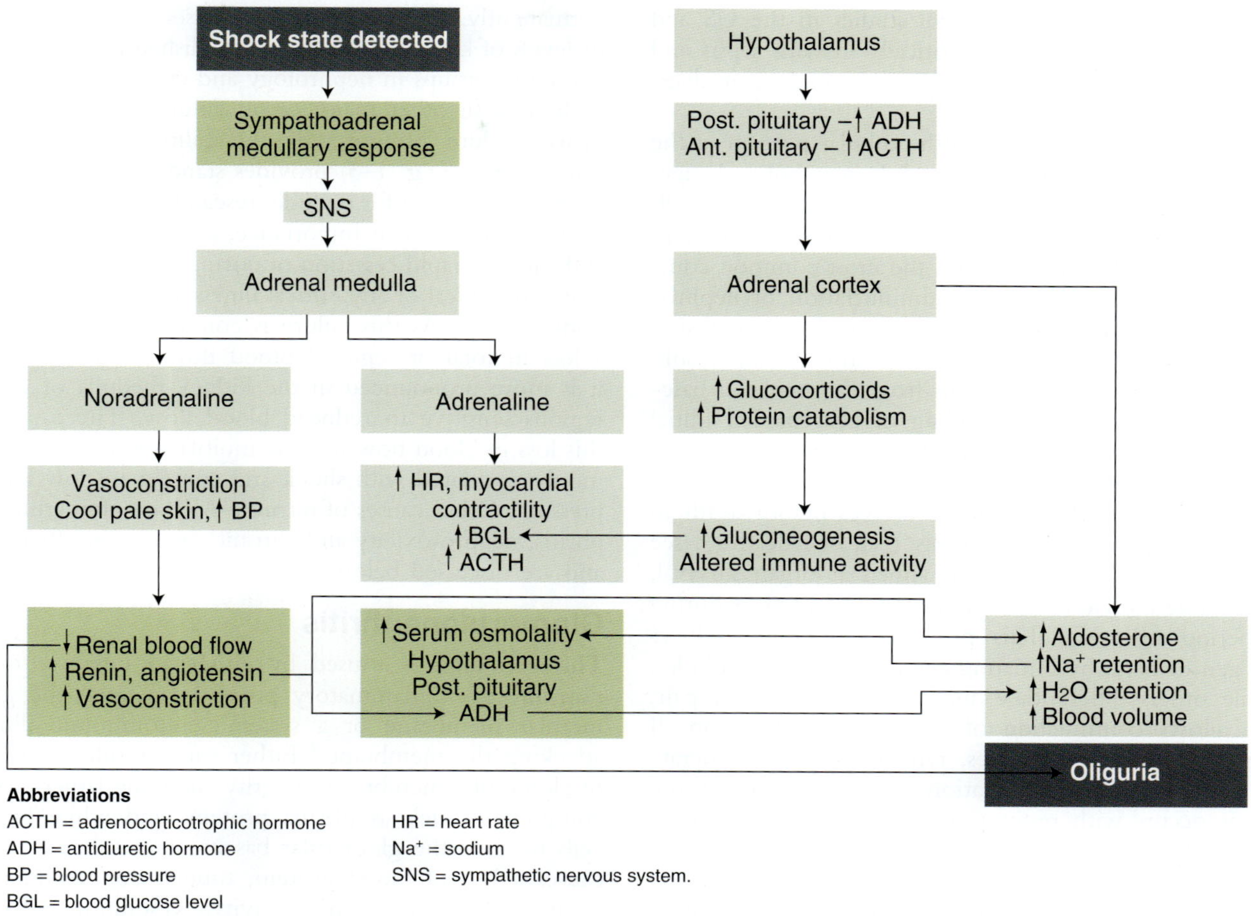

reversed by restoration of blood volume or blood pressure. In the short term (1–2 h), nephrons remain structurally normal and respond by concentrating urine for the excretion of waste products. The physiological process combines neuroendocrine control of the hypothalamus and the sympathomimetic response, which then regulates both antidiuretic hormone secretion and stimulation of the renin–angiotensin–aldosterone system (Fig. 18.7). This process is highly influenced by any preexisting illness or concurrent factors such as diabetes and systemic infection.[9] Treatment of prerenal insults depends entirely on the causes, but achievement of euvolaemia, attention to serum electrolytes, and avoidance of nephrotoxic drugs are benchmarks of therapy. This involves careful assessment of volume status, cardiac function, diet, and drug usage.[5]

Intrarenal (intrinsic) causes

Intrinsic damage to the nephron structure and function can be due to infective or inflammatory illness, toxic drugs, toxic wastes from inflammation in sepsis, vascular obstructive thrombus or emboli. In differentiating this type of AKI, an unexpected process of elimination has been suggested where failure of kidney function persists, despite and after restoration of adequate perfusion (blood flow). Surprisingly this state also appears where no loss of perfusion has occurred, and there is no obstruction to urine flow.[9] Diagnosis is made by exclusion of other causes. This pathology is termed acute tubular necrosis (ATN).

AKI such as this accounts for approximately 85% of intrinsic AKI. The two major causes of ATN are ischaemia and nephrotoxin exposure. Ischaemic AKI is characterised not only by inadequate GFR but also by renal blood flow inadequate to maintain parenchymal cellular perfusion. Renal tubular damage with low effective arterial blood flow to the kidney can result in tubular necrosis and apoptosis. This occurs in the setting of prolonged hypotension or hypoxemia, such as volume depletion or shock. Underlying sepsis can also be an independent risk factor for ATN. Major surgical procedures can involve prolonged periods of hypoperfusion, which are exacerbated by vasodilating anaesthetic agents.[5]

The precise causative pathology of ATN is not easily identifiable in critically ill patients with multiple comorbidities, for example diabetes, advanced age, investigations requiring radio-opaque dye administration, potent and nephrotoxic drug administration, sepsis or major surgery with an inflammatory state due to an underlying infection. Several studies in the US and Europe showed that in the critically ill with sepsis and AKI, mortality ranges from 28–90% depending on diagnostic criteria or definition.[13-15]

ATN describes damage to the tubular portion of the nephron and may range from subtle metabolic changes to total dissolution of cell structure, with tubular cells 'defoliating' or detaching from the tubule basement membrane.[9,16] In critical illness, the most common combination causing AKI is the administration of nephrotoxic agents in association with prolonged hypoperfusion or ischaemia.[16-18] Tubular cells suffer an ischaemic insult, causing a shedding of the cells from the nephron basement membrane. This shedding of cells has an initial loss of cell polarity, and then cell death, with a 'patchy' occurrence along the tubule basement membrane.[16] In addition, some cells detach themselves before death in a response known as apoptosis (cell self-death)[16] (see Chapter 22). The response is aimed at organ survival, with some individual cells 'sacrificing' themselves during a period of crisis. This protective response reduces oxygen demand by initiating cell death in some tubules, while others differentiate and/or proliferate for repair, and allows continuation of some normal function. If the causative process abates, remaining cells regenerate by epithelial cell differentiation and proliferation, tissue repair occurs with restoration of normal epithelium in some tubules and nephron function returning.

During this period cellular 'debris' collects in the tubule loops, causing obstruction of tubular flow, with back-leak of filtrate occurring through the 'patchy' exposed tubular membrane surface. An inflammatory process is also stimulated due to release of cell adhesion factors and leucocyte activation,[19] which in turn causes further vasoconstriction and ischaemia[20] in the acute stage. The back leakage and static tubular fluid creates a concentrate that, by diffusion, raises blood levels of wastes such as urea, creatinine and other toxins. Along with the cessation of urine flow, toxicity occurs due to high serum levels of wastes such as urea, creatinine, potassium and undefined toxins.[19] This is the clinical state associated with the pathology of AKI that better describes the total 'picture' of pre-illness status, immediate causative events and degree of injury determined by patient serum creatinine or urine output.[2-4]

In the past authors have often employed the term ATN to describe this type of obstructive and ischaemic AKI,[21] using it as a surrogate for AKI in the acute setting, as it focuses on the pathophysiology of tubular damage, recognising this damage as a final outcome of all causative factors. However, more recently, with the development of a consensus definition for AKI describing stages of illness severity, the term AKI is now used reflecting pathophysiology, the outcome of many causative factors and the clinical context where small derangements may be evident with reversibility of dysfunction and recovery, through to irreversible damage with kidney failure, and cessation of function permanently.[16-18] This acronym is associated with stages or levels of kidney dysfunction established by expert and consensus groups in nephrology and critical care.[2-4] This is done with other major organ failures such as heart[22] or liver failure.[23] Importantly, the ability to describe AKI using staging (e.g. 1–3) provides standard clinical reference and language for bedside, research and publications.

KI is of particular importance, as it is abrupt in onset and causes a rapid cessation of normal nephron function, a picture typical of any critical illness and failure of other body organs.[3] As this failure is commonly mediated by a loss in total or regional blood flow to the kidney,[19] it is more pronounced in the kidney medulla or outer regions sensitive to reduced blood flow. The cause of this loss in blood flow may be multifactorial but is commonly associated with shock and consequent low blood pressure. Other causes of intrinsic AKI are glomerulonephritis, nephrotoxicity and chronic vascular insufficiency and are discussed below.

Glomerulonephritis

This condition is caused by either an infective or a non-infective inflammatory process damaging the glomerular membrane or a systemic autoimmune illness attacking the membrane.[9] Either cause results in a loss of glomerular membrane integrity, allowing larger blood components such as plasma proteins and white blood cells to cross the glomerular basement membrane. This causes a loss of blood protein, tubular congestion and failure of normal nephron activity. Resolution is based on treating the cause, such as an infection or autoimmune inflammatory illness.[24]

Nephrotoxicity

Nephrotoxicity occurs as a result of damage to nephron cells from a wide range of agents, including many drugs used in critical care (e.g. antibiotics, anti-inflammatory agents, cancer drugs, radio-opaque dyes). Toxic products of muscle breakdown in severe illness and trauma, commonly called rhabdomyolysis (see Chapter 23),[9,25] blood product administration reactions and blood cell damage associated with major surgery are also causative agents.[26] As these agents may often be given concurrently, a cumulative effect, along with intermittent falls in renal perfusion, may result in the development of intrinsic AKI.

Aminoglycosides cause some degree of ATN in up to 25% of hospitalised patients receiving therapeutic levels of the drugs. Non-oliguric kidney injury typically occurs after 5–10 days of exposure. Predisposing factors include underlying kidney damage, volume depletion, and advanced age. Aminoglycosides can remain in renal tissues for up to a month, so kidney function may not recover for some time after stopping the medication. Monitoring of peak and trough levels is important, but trough levels are more helpful in predicting renal toxicity. Gentamycin, tobramycin, vancomycin, intravenous acyclovir and several cephalosporins are nephrotoxic; streptomycin is the least nephrotoxic of the aminoglycosides.[27]

Radiographic contrast media may be directly nephrotoxic. Contrast-induced nephropathy is the third leading cause of new-onset AKI in hospitalised patients. It results from a combination of direct renal tubular epithelial cell toxicity and renal medullary ischaemia.[28] Predisposing factors include patient comorbidities, amount of contrast administered, concomitant medication use such as non-steroidal anti-inflammatory agents and angiotensin converting enzyme inhibitors. Lower volumes of contrast with lower osmolality agents are recommended in high-risk patients. Toxicity usually occurs within 24–48 hours after the radiocontrast study.[28]

Vascular insufficiency

One-third of patients who develop AKI in the ICU have chronic renal dysfunction.[29] This chronic dysfunction may be undiagnosed prior to the critical illness, and may be related to diabetes, the ageing process and/or long-term hypertension. These factors create a reduction in both large and microvasculature blood flow into and within the kidney, therefore reducing glomerular filtration activity and affecting the reabsorption and diffusive process of the nephron. This reduction in blood flow is exacerbated by degenerative vessel obstruction with atheromatous plaque, particularly pronounced in diabetic patients due to ineffective glucose metabolism. Diabetic patients are more likely to develop AKI associated with medical care in hospital from what may otherwise seem to be a relatively trivial insult to the kidneys in a younger, healthy patient. The event may be enough to move the patient from kidney injury to ESRD, as they lack any degree of 'renal reserve' or tolerance to events such as low blood pressure or administration of nephrotoxic drugs normally filtered by the kidney.[15]

Postrenal causes

Urinary tract obstruction is the primary postrenal cause of AKI, and is uncommon in the critical care setting as it is rarely associated with acute onset renal failure.[9] Postrenal causes are the least common reason for AKI, accounting for approximately 5–10% of cases, but are important to detect because of their reversibility. Postrenal azotaemia occurs when urinary flow from both kidneys, or a single functioning kidney, is obstructed. Occasionally, postrenal uropathies can occur when a single kidney is obstructed if the contralateral kidney cannot adjust for the loss in function, (e.g. in a patient with advanced chronic kidney disease (CKD)). Obstruction leads to elevated intraluminal pressure, causing kidney parenchymal damage, with marked effects on renal blood flow and tubular function, and a decrease in GFR.

Postrenal causes include urethral obstruction, bladder dysfunction or obstruction, and possibly obstruction within the ureters and renal pelvises. In men, benign prostatic hyperplasia is the most common cause. Patients taking anticholinergic drugs are at risk for urinary retention. Obstruction can also be caused by bladder, prostate, and cervical cancers, retroperitoneal fibrosis and neurogenic bladder. Less common causes are blood clots in the urine pathway, bilateral ureteral stones, urethral stones or strictures, and bilateral papillary necrosis.[5]

The kidneys are vital human body organs essential to sustaining life. An important interrelationship of the kidneys and other body organs exists, called 'organ crosstalk' with the brain, heart, liver and lungs dependent on receiving 'clean' blood to function. As toxins and fluid rapidly accumulate due to AKI during critical illness, these changes contribute to organ dysfunction. AKI induces remote organ injury in the heart, brain, lungs, liver and gut involving multiple inflammatory pathways, including increased expression of soluble pro-inflammatory mediators, innate and adaptive immunity, cellular apoptosis, physiologic derangements and genomic changes.[30]

Treatment

Treatment is aimed at hastening recovery and avoiding complications. Preventive measures should be taken to avoid volume overload and hyperkalaemia, both of which occur in the kidney with impaired function. Widespread use of diuretics in critically ill patients with AKI should be encouraged only in states of volume overload and with caution and close attention to responsiveness. Disabling side effects of supranormal diuretic dosing include hearing loss and cerebellar dysfunction. This is mainly due to peak frusemide levels; this risk can be minimised using a frusemide drip. A starting dose of 0.1–0.3 mg/kg/h is appropriate, increasing to a maximum of 0.5–1 mg/kg/h. A bolus of 1–1.5 mg/kg should be administered at the beginning of each dose escalation. Intravenous thiazide diuretics can be used to augment urinary output; chlorothiazide, 250–500 mg intravenously every 8–12 hours, is a reasonable choice. Another good choice to augment diuresis is metolazone at doses of 2.5–5 mg given orally once to twice daily, 30 minutes prior to loop diuretics. Metolazone is less expensive than intravenous chlorothiazide and has reasonable bioavailability.[5]

AKI: clinical and diagnostic criteria for classification

Clinical assessment

Clinical assessment of the patient with impending renal failure can involve myriad tests and investigations; however, the majority of these are not used to assess the critically ill patient. The clinical history is important in differentiating preexisting renal disease and cataloguing the numerous factors already discussed that can contribute to AKI. The key assessments used in monitoring renal function are urine output, serum creatinine and urea levels, combined with more general measures including heart rate, blood pressure, fluid balance, gas exchange, chest radiology and daily weight. These measures are essential for the critically ill patient, and alterations provide the diagnostic key. They also link into the wider assessment of fluid and electrolyte balance, as described in Chapters 9 and 21.

Biomarkers for the detection of AKI

Numerous biomarkers have been identified in the last several years that can indicate if kidney injury is occurring and when damage has been done. Serum creatinine, a marker of kidney function but not kidney injury,[31] has been a benchmark for decades to determine loss of renal function, a guide to treatment and renal support techniques, but it has limitations. Normal creatinine is variable and influenced by age, race, and sex and a rise in serum creatinine may not occur until there is a marked decrease in the GFR.[30,32] Also, creatinine is not adequate for an early identification of reduced GFR and it does not allow differentiation between hemodynamically mediated changes in renal function and intrinsic renal failure or obstructive nephropathy. Most importantly, serum creatinine does not differentiate between quickly reversible, volume-sensitive reductions in GFR.

Practice tip

Serum creatinine reflects the real value of GFR under steady-state conditions, but not when renal function is deteriorating. Critically ill patients are not in a steady state so the use of serum creatine in this patient population as a marker of renal function may be limited.[1,33]

The search for a sensitive and clinically useful biomarker continues, and this is a big difference in early detection and predictive management for AKI when compared to the utility of cardiac enzymes and troponin with cardiac ischaemia. Four biomarkers being investigated for the detection and or management of AKI are outlined briefly as examples.

Neutrophil gelatinase-associated lipocalin

Neutrophil gelatinase-associated lipocalin, a protein of the lipocalin family, is expressed at very low constant levels in different cell types. It is highly expressed after ischaemic or toxic kidney injury in humans and in many animals. The elevation of neutrophil gelatinase-associated lipocalin is detectable as early as 3 hours after the injury and peaks approximately 6–12 h after injury, depending on the severity of injury. The elevation can persist up to 5 days after the initial injury when the injury is severe.[34] Neutrophil gelatinase-associated lipocalin can rise days before sepsis causing elevation in serum creatinine and can be influenced by several factors including baseline renal function, sepsis and urinary tract infection.[35]

Kidney Injury molecule-1

Kidney Injury molecule-1 is a transmembrane glycoprotein which is expressed at low levels in the normal kidney as well as in other organs but is influenced by comorbidities and therefore may lack specificity.[36,37] Kidney Injury molecule-1 has a protective effect in the kidney in ischaemia/repercussion injury and has been proposed to play an important role in kidney recovery and tubular regeneration because it mediates the phagocytosis of cell debris into cultured renal epithelial cells.[38,39]

Tissue inhibitor of metalloproteinases-2 (TIMP-2) and insulin-like growth factor binding protein-7 (IGFBP-7)

Tissue inhibitor of metalloproteinases-2 (TIMP-2) and insulin-like growth factor binding protein-7(IGFBP- 7) are two biomarkers studied that can increase in response to a wide variety of insults (inflammation, oxidative stress, ultraviolet radiation, drugs and toxins). These two biomarkers relate to a cellular defence mechanism known as cell-cycle arrest. In the setting of ischaemic or septic kidney injury, renal epithelial cells have been shown to undergo cell-cycle arrest.[40] Each phase of the cell cycle has a specific function that is required for appropriate cell proliferation. In order for cells to divide and begin the process of repair, they must enter and exit each phase of the cell cycle on schedule. If the cell exits a phase too soon, or stays in a phase too long, or if DNA is damaged within the cell, the normal repair and recovery process can become affected and DNA damage can occur.[41] In patients undergoing coronary artery bypass surgery (CABG), at four time-points where these biomarkers were measured, the biomarkers decreased at the end of the surgery but increased again at the 4-hour time-point after CABG, and further the next postoperative day.[42]

Proenkephalin

Proenkephalin (penKid) has been recently described as a valuable plasma biomarker of AKI in acutely ill patients, including those with sepsis and heart failure.[43-45] Proenkephalin represents a stable analyte of labile enkephalins, which affects kidney function. In a recent study proenkephalin showed a significant higher association with AKI compared to other biomarkers.[46] Biomarkers continue in development and clinical evaluation for the detection and management of AKI.

Complications of AKI and kidney failure

Uraemic complications

Uraemic complications are influenced by the rate of urea accumulation and vary from patient to patient. As serum urea levels rise rapidly (e.g. over a few days), above

20 mmol/L blood coagulation can be affected. A rash and related itchiness can occur. As blood levels continue to rise, neurological function can be affected and level of consciousness will deteriorate. In some cases high levels of urea can result in encephalopathy.[47]

Cardiovascular alterations

Cardiovascular alterations can occur as a result of AKI[48] as a result of direct effects on the myocardium but also because of fluid accumulation and electrolyte disturbance. The greatest concern is fluid overload as a consequence of failure to excrete the excess quantities of fluid used in resuscitating critically ill patients and the necessity to provide adequate nutrition in the form of parenteral or enteral nutrition.[49] Without appropriate management heart failure and pulmonary oedema can develop. Refer to Chapter 11 for a more detailed discussion of cardiac arrhythmias associated with electrolyte disturbances.

Respiratory alteration

As noted earlier, fluid accumulation will invariably result in inadequate clearance of the pulmonary interstitial space by the pulmonary lymphatics, resulting firstly in interstitial oedema and moving on to overt pulmonary oedema and serious impairment of pulmonary gas exchange. Respiratory rate may also increase as patients develop metabolic acidosis both through renal injury and associated critical illness.

Haematological alterations

The primary haematological concern in AKI is related to the anticoagulatory effects of rapidly increasing serum urea. While the kidney accounts for 90% of circulating erythropoietin production,[12] the acute nature of severe AKI does not influence anaemia to the extent of more common causes such as haemorrhage related to trauma or surgery or even iatrogenic blood loss.

Neurological alterations

Changes to central nervous system function can be related to accumulating urea, fluid and disruption of sodium balance. In the most severe form these can result in loss of consciousness and fitting.

Diagnosis

The management of AKI begins with the diagnosis, based on the patient's presenting signs and symptoms linked to a patient history. A long-term history of renal disease involving urinary tract infections, diabetes, cardiac failure and systemic inflammatory illnesses are all highly relevant.[21] Immediate history of presentation to a hospital involving surgery or any life-threatening illness with associated shock is also highly relevant in association with reduced urine output volumes over time.

Nurses in the critical care setting, who measure urine output hourly, readily recognise a key sign of impending renal dysfunction. Oliguria in the absence of catheter obstruction should be responded to quickly, as this suggests inadequate kidney blood flow and, to some extent, is a delayed observation considering the continual moderation of kidney function producing urine output. Persisting oliguria or the onset of anuria with associated rises in blood creatinine fulfils the injury phase of AKI. This sequence of events can be identified in the well-established classification known as the 'RIFLE' criteria – i.e. the **r**isk, **i**njury, **f**ailure, and outcome criteria of **l**oss and **e**nd-stage disease. This has provided the basis for a widely-accepted approach to diagnosing and classifying AKI.[2,4]

Consensus definitions and classification for AKI: the RIFLE criteria and KDIGO staging

The RIFLE criteria are shown in Fig. 18.6A, and use rising creatinine and falling urine output as highly sensitive and specific indicators for a continuum of renal failure. This useful classification system established in the year 2000 by a dialysis quality group provides grading for loss of kidney function, reflecting stages of injury to the kidney before failure occurs. Without this, the small but important losses of kidney function before the failure state are not adequately considered.[1] This approach provides a consensus definition for loss of kidney function that is useful for clinical practice and research into this area, with clinicians all talking the same 'language' when comparing patients and/or results from clinical trials. The shape of the diagram indicates that more people will develop symptoms of AKI linked to kidney 'injury' and be considered 'at risk' (high sensitivity) than those at the bottom of the definition, who are fewer in number but need to fulfil strict criteria (high specificity).

Since this time and as a progression in AKI understanding, in 2012 a European consensus group established the KDIGO initiative and combined the work of another expert North American group, the Acute Kidney Injury Network[50,51] and published an AKI staging of severity with three stages (i.e. 1–3). The Acute Kidney Injury Network and KDIGO expert groups provide many helpful clinical care guidelines[50,51] for identification and care of patients with AKI.

Practice tip

A reduction in urine output is an important sign of impending AKI; however, checking a catheter for blockage is also important. A bladder scanner may also reveal a full bladder where no catheter is in place. The use of newer digital urine output monitoring systems is helpful to maintain vigilance in urine output monitoring by using alarms when urine output falls less than 0.5 mL/kg/h and can function by automatically[52,53] documenting hourly into the electronic medical record.

Management of the patient with AKI

Reducing further insults to the kidneys

After diagnosis, the next management principle is to remove or modify any cause that may exacerbate the pathological process associated with AKI. Further interventions and investigations are performed in relation to findings from the history and hospital presentation. These may include:[9]

- further intravenous fluid resuscitation (despite an oligo-anuric state) and restoration of blood pressure using inotropic/vasoactive drugs
- physical or diagnostic assessment for renal outflow obstruction and alleviation if present
- avoiding contrast-enhanced radiological investigations
- ceasing or modifying the dose of any nephrotoxic drugs or agents and treating infection with alternative, less toxic antibiotics.

Initial management strategies for the early stages of AKI remain conservative, with careful management of fluid (once adequate circulating volume is assured) and haemodynamics, encouraging diuresis if present, monitoring blood profiles for changes in urea and electrolytes and limiting or reformulating administration of agents that may contribute to the accumulation of urea and electrolytes (e.g. enteral or intravenous nutritional supplements). The use of agents such as mannitol, dopamine and frusemide, while popular in practice, have not been shown to be of any value in improving outcome in patients at risk of AKI.[9,54]

Despite these efforts, life-threatening biochemistry may arise in AKI, such as severe acidosis and hyperkalaemia (pH <7.1 and serum potassium >6.5 mmol/L), that requires immediate treatment and is an indication for beginning renal replacement therapy (RRT) without elevation of serum creatinine and oliguria and fluid overload.[55]

Fluid balance

As oliguria and anuria are key diagnostic and clinical signs of renal dysfunction, reducing fluid intake is necessary to prevent intravascular overload and tissue oedema until renal recovery begins or a type of RRT is started. Reducing or restricting fluid intake can be a challenge in the critically ill as it is not uncommon for these patients to be administered 3 L of fluid in 24 hours.[56] A balance state for this degree of fluid administration suggests a urine output at 3–4 mL/kg/h without considering other insensible losses will rarely cause intravascular volume depletion.[57-59] Strategies can be considered to minimise fluid intake such as preparing drug infusions without diluent and in a concentrated version of the usual preparation. Pharmacists may assist with this requirement and offer advice for drug preparation and delivery. Restriction of oral fluids can be implemented and monitored using a fluid chart, with the aim of adhering to the prescribed volume. Nutrition therapy is important for optimising patient outcome but can also contribute to increased fluid intake. Enteral feeding is preferred for most critically ill patients and standard enteral feeding formulas can contribute about 1.5 L of fluid intake per day in an adult.[60] Nutrition is very important in the patient experiencing AKI where growth and repair is needed with damaged kidney cells and protein depletion avoided. Calorie-dense enteral feeding formulas (2 kcal/mL) can be considered as a strategy to minimise fluid intake associated with enteral feeding (see Chapter 19 for further discussion on nutrition in critical illness). Fluid balance charting and a clear understanding of the maximum fluid intake per day is vital for managing AKI at this stage, and a maximum intake of 1.5 L per day is a common target in the adult patient.[61] An inability to prevent a positive fluid balance, largely due to meeting nutritional requirements, is often the reason RRT is initiated.[62] Care should also be taken to prevent fluid overload with AKI at this time. Studies in children show increased morbidity and mortality in fluid overloaded patients.[43] Fluid volume loading leads to organ congestion and a resultant decrease in renal blood flow.[63-65]

Electrolyte balance

Managing serum electrolytes, in particular potassium, is essential for patient stability as low or high levels are more likely to be associated with life-threatening arrhythmias.[66] However, phosphate, calcium and sodium may also be abnormal and require strategies to reduce, supplement or control the serum level away from toxicity. Hyponatraemia, for example, may be associated with altered mental state, impaired consciousness and even seizures.[67]

Acid–base balance

Control of the acid–base balance is another essential function of the healthy kidneys and, with failure, metabolic acidosis will develop due to decreased buffering and accumulation of many acids not excreted.[39] An increased minute ventilation may be observed in the patient, representing a physiological attempt to control acidaemia. This requires additional energy and caloric consumption and is another indication that RRT should be implemented using bicarbonate fluids to control the acidaemia.[68]

Pharmacotherapy and altered pharmacokinetics

The modification of drug regimens to effect changes to excretion and volume of distribution is a further aspect of clinical management during the onset of AKI. Drugs are excreted from the body after hepatic and other organ metabolism, which converts them to a water-soluble form such that they appear in the urine. Therefore, modification of dose (through reduction or frequency of administration) and monitoring for serum levels helps to prevent further renal insult while ensuring the desired clinical effect.[27]

Aminoglycosides are a key group of antibiotics requiring adjustment and monitoring in AKI, if not ceasing and substituting for another appropriate but less nephrotoxic antibiotic.[40] Other drugs administered in the ICU that warrant attention include narcotics, histamine-2 receptor antagonists and beta-blockers. Pharmacy product information attached with packaging and/or local pharmacy information usually provides helpful suggestions and guidelines for relevant drug use in AKI. If RRT is started, and is functioning continuously with efficiency, the clearance and toxicity of drugs is of less concern and dosing may resume to normal for some drugs with close monitoring continuing.[68]

If conservative measures fail, ongoing management of the patient with AKI requires RRT. This enables control of blood biochemistry, prevents toxin accumulation, and allows removal of fluids so that adequate nutrition can be achieved, but importantly this is a support system and not a treatment for AKI. The criteria and indications for initiating RRT are listed in Box 18.1. One indication is enough to initiate RRT, while two or more make RRT urgent. Combined derangements can create the necessity to commence therapy before individually-defined limits have been reached. Early initiation of treatment is widely advocated and may confer more rapid renal recovery, but timing and illness progression and outcomes for best practice is currently of high interest.

BOX 18.1

Proposed criteria for the initiation of renal replacement therapy in adult critically ill patients[14]

- Oliguria (urine output <200 mL/12 h)
- Anuria/extreme oliguria (urine output <50 mL/12 h)
- Hyperkalaemia (K + >6.5 mmol/L)
- Severe acidaemia (pH <7.1)
- Azotaemia (urea >30 mmol/L)
- Clinically significant organ (esp. lung) oedema
- Uraemic encephalopathy
- Uraemic pericarditis
- Uraemic neuropathy/myopathy
- Severe dysnatraemia (Na + >160 or <115 mmol/L)
- Hyperthermia
- Drug overdose with dialysable toxin

Approaches to renal replacement therapy

A brief review of the historical perspectives associated with the development of modern-day dialysis and RRT provided in the ICU is helpful in understanding key concepts and methods for RRT and in particular as a continuous (C) method or CRRT (continuous renal replacement therapy).

History

Dialysis is a term describing RRT and refers to the purification of blood through a membrane by diffusion of waste substances.[69] Table 18.1 outlines historical events during the development of dialysis in Europe and the USA.

The original rotating drum kidney (Fig. 18.8) provided limited effective waste clearance and prompted design and development of a new membrane for solute exchange that had a greater surface area and required less blood volume. This led to the development of the hollow-fibre filter membrane structure in the 1960s, which became the ‘artificial kidney’.[70]

The combination of an extracorporeal circuit (EC), blood pump and filter membrane and the associated nursing management are now commonly known as haemodialysis. With industrial and scientific developments, such as plastics moulding and electronics, current dialysis techniques are safe, effective and a life-sustaining treatment for the millions of people who suffer acute and chronic kidney failure.[71,72]

Nursing of dialysis patients has developed into a specialist field of knowledge and skill, with nurses combining their holistic view of patient management with the specialist needs of patients with renal failure, from the outpatient setting to the ICU, including a collaborative approach to further adaptations of dialysis best suited to the critically ill.[73–75]

Development of renal replacement therapy in critical care

Historically, AKI was treated in the ICU with the use of peritoneal dialysis (PD), which did not require specialist nurses or doctors. This simple technique removes wastes by infusing a dialysis fluid into the abdomen, allowing diffusion and osmosis to occur between the peritoneum and fluid before draining out again in repeated cycles.[76] This was performed by the ICU nurse and prescribed by ICU doctors, but was inadequate in its clearance of waste and fluid volume, and was associated with infection, limitation of respiratory function and exacerbated glucose intolerance.[9,76] Today, PD is rarely, if ever, used in the management of renal failure in the critical care setting.

In 1977 Peter Kramer, a German ICU doctor, developed a new dialytic technique called continuous arteriovenous haemofiltration (CAVH), which was specifically intended for use in the critically ill patient. It was later

TABLE 18.1
Historical events in the development of dialysis

TIME PERIOD AND DEVELOPER	DESCRIPTION
1854: Thomas Graham, Scottish chemist	First used the term 'dialysis' to describe the transport of solutes through an ox bladder, which drew attention to the concept of a membrane for solute removal from fluid
1920s: George Haas, German physician	First human dialysis was carried out, performing six treatments on six patients. Haas failed to make further progress with the treatment but is recognised as an early pioneer of dialysis
1920–30s	Synthetic polymer chemistry allowed development of cellulose acetate, a membrane integral to the further development of dialysis treatments
1940s: Willem Kolff, Dutch physician	The discovery of heparin, an anticoagulant, enabled further development of dialysis during World War II, the Kolff rotating drum kidney (Fig. 18.8)
1940–50s: Kolff and Allis-Chalmers, USA	Further modification of the Kolff dialyser and the development of improved machines
1950s: Fredrik Kiil, Norway	Developed the parallel plate dialyser made of a new cellulose, cuprophane. This required a pump to push the blood through the membrane and return the blood to the patient
1950–60s	Dialysis began to be widely used to treat kidney failure
1960s: Richard Stewart and Dow Chemical, USA	The hollow-fibre membrane dialyser used a membrane design of a cellulose acetate bundle, with 11,000 fibres providing a surface area of 1 m^2
1970s	Use of the first CAVH circuits for diuretic-resistant oedema by Kramer
1980s	First continuous therapies using blood pump and intravenous pumps to control fluid removal and substitution: Australia and New Zealand led the way
1990s	New purpose-built machines used; Gambro Prisma, Baxter BM 11 + 14 to provide pump-controlled therapies with integrated automated fluid balance using scales to measure fluids. Cassette circuits, automated priming; new membranes
2000	Further purpose-built machines using direct measurement for waste and substitution fluids via Hygieia–Kimal machine. Introduction of high fluid exchange rates for sepsis treatment. Introduction of dialysis-based machines in ICU for daily 'hybrid' treatments: SLEDD and SLEDDf
2010	Multiple CRRT machines; more advanced graphics interface and smart alarms. Waste disposal systems. High flux, porous membranes
2020	Further advances with CRRT machines enabling mode changes during treatment, increased safety alarms for fluid 'balance', treatment data storage and transmission. Automated citrate anticoagulation software

CAVH = continuous arteriovenous haemofiltration; CRRT = continuous renal replacement therapy; SLEDD = sustained low-efficiency daily dialysis; SLEDDf = sustained low-efficiency daily diafiltration.

renamed slow continuous ultrafiltration (SCUF), as it enabled the removal of plasma water in addition to dissolved wastes (convective clearance of solutes) at a flow rate of 200–600 mL/h by passive drainage from the membrane as blood flowed through it.[77] This marked the beginning of continuous RRT in the ICU as an intervention prescribed and managed by ICU nurses and doctors for patients with AKI.

Refinement of renal replacement therapy

Today, a dialysis blood pump enables a much more efficient technique for therapeutic benefit in the ICU patient with AKI. The use of roller blood pumps to generate pressure and a reliable flow of blood, thus eliminating the need for arterial puncture and access,

FIGURE 18.8 The Kolff Rotating Drum Dialyser. Historical in the development of dialysis.

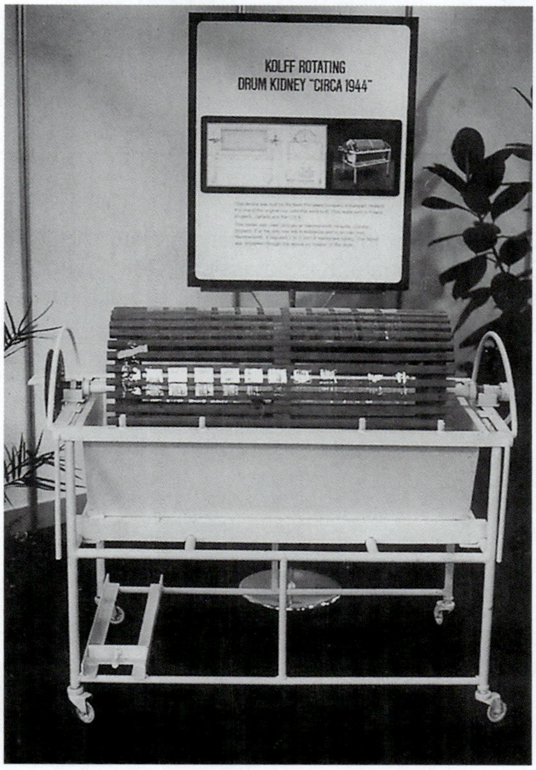

Reproduced from Thomas N, ed. Renal nursing. 2nd ed. London: Baillière Tindall, 2002.

was introduced. This is termed continuous veno-venous haemofiltration (CVVH), and can reliably pump blood at a constant rate and achieve ultrafiltration volumes of 1000 mL/h. With further modifications to the circuit and filter set-up, a diffusive component was added to the therapy by running a dialysate volume through the haemofilter, flowing between the membrane fibres and counter-current to blood flow. This was termed continuous veno-venous haemodiafiltration (CVVHD(f)).[78]

Principles of extracorporeal CRRT

Both intermittent haemodialysis and CRRT require a machine to pump blood and fluids; pressure and flow devices to monitor treatment; a tubing and filter membrane set that together create an EC (outside the body blood pathway); and a catheter connecting the patient's circulation to the circuit (see Fig. 18.9). This catheter enables blood to be drawn from and returned to the patient (known as 'access'). Access can be achieved by three different techniques:

- temporary catheters inserted via a skin puncture into an artery for drawing blood and a vein to return the blood (arteriovenous access)

FIGURE 18.9 Renal replacement therapy blood path circuit common to all approaches. EC: extracorporeal circuit.

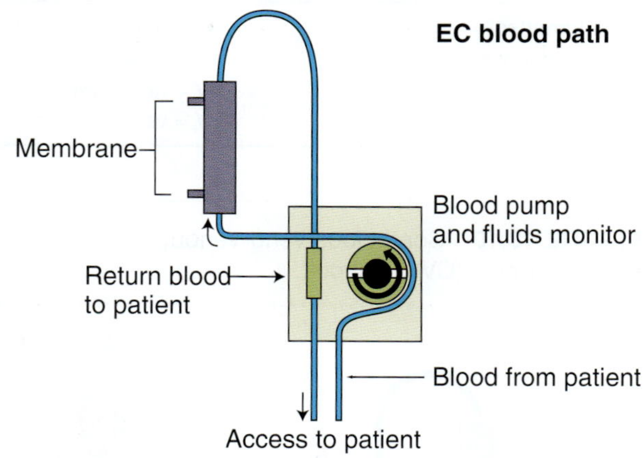

- a surgical joining of an artery and vein (usually in the forearm), making a large vessel that is punctured with needles to both draw and return the blood (arteriovenous fistula)
- a catheter with two lumens to draw and return blood via a large central vein (a dual veno-venous access catheter).

In the acute renal failure setting and where temporary treatment is anticipated, the two-lumen catheter is recommended.[79,80]

Haemodialysis, haemofiltration and haemodiafiltration

Haemodialysis, haemofiltration and haemodiafiltration are three common techniques used to achieve artificial kidney support in AKI. The basic blood path or circuit for these therapies is indicated in Fig. 18.9 and is a useful review to understand each therapy and where the RRT fluids are then applied to the circuit, differentiating them as techniques.

The extracorporeal component is a common factor in all these different circuit designs. The difference between treatments is how the solutes such as urea, creatinine and other waste products and the solvent or plasma water are removed from the blood as it passes through the filter membrane (artificial kidney), and the intermittent versus continuous prescription of the therapy. The three physical mechanisms of fluid and solute management are convection, diffusion and ultrafiltration. Table 18.2 lists the commonly-used abbreviations to describe the timing of treatment, blood access for the therapy and mode of solute removal.

Convection

Convection is the process whereby dissolved solutes are removed along with plasma water as it is filtered through the dialysis membrane. The word is derived from the

TABLE 18.2
Abbreviations describing modes of renal replacement therapy

TIMING OF THERAPY	ROUTE OF ACCESS	MECHANISM OF SOLUTE REMOVAL
I = intermittent	A = arterial	H (or HF) = haemofiltration – convection
C = continuous	V = venous	D (or HD) = haemodialysis – dialysis
S = slow	AV = arteriovenous	HDF = haemodiafiltration – diffusion and convection
	VV = veno-venous	UF = ultrafiltration – plasma water removal

FIGURE 18.10 Continuous veno-venous haemofiltration (CVVH) circuit.

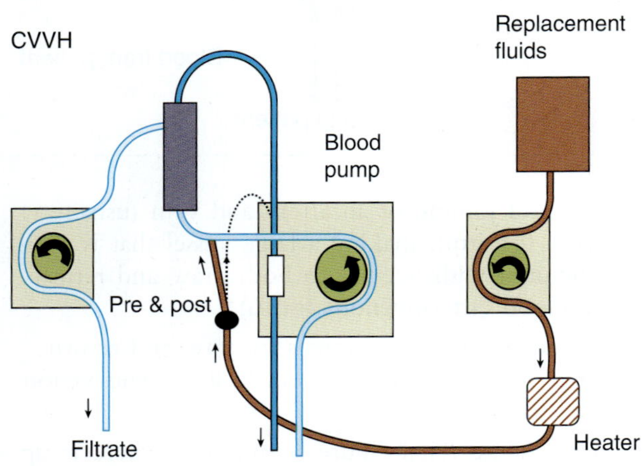

FIGURE 18.11 Intermittent dialysis circuit (IHD). HCO_3^-: bicarbonate; K+: potassium; Qdf: flow of dialysis fluid; RO (reverse osmosis); UF: ultrafiltrate.

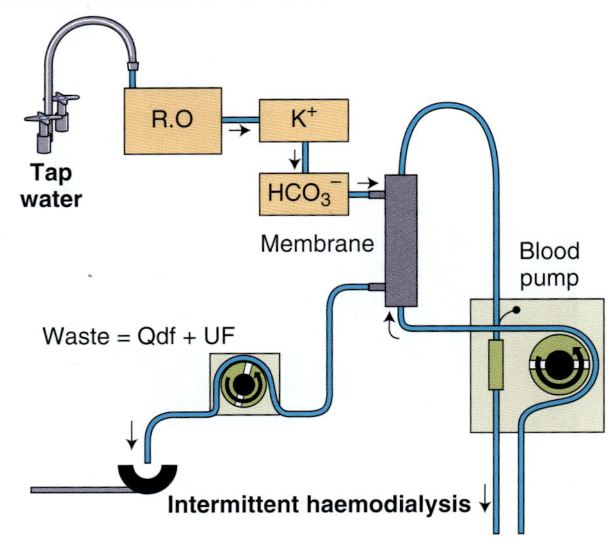

Latin *convehere*, meaning 'to remove or to carry along with'.[81] This process is similar to that occurring in the native kidney glomerulus, as plasma water is filtered across the nephron tubule via the Bowman's capsule. In RRT, the plasma water with the dissolved wastes is discarded; the deficit is then replaced with commercially manufactured artificial plasma water in equal or slightly lower amounts to achieve a desired fluid balance. This blood purification process is commonly known as haemofiltration. When applied on a continuous basis in the ICU, haemofiltration can adequately replace essential renal functions, and is particularly effective in managing fluid balance.[55,82] Fig. 18.10 illustrates the circuit and set-up for continuous veno-venous hemofiltration.

Diffusion

Diffusion refers to the physical movement of solutes across a semipermeable membrane from an area of high concentration to that of a relatively low concentration; that is, solutes move across a concentration gradient.[83] A higher concentration gradient results in a greater rate of diffusive clearance. As blood passes through the dialysis membrane, dialysate fluid, reflecting normal blood chemistry, is exposed to blood on the opposing side of the membrane fibre. Diffusive clearance is continuous as solute exchange occurs with the dialysate fluid and the blood continually moving in and out of the membrane. As waste-laden blood enters the hollow membrane fibre and fresh dialysate is in continuous supply, this process performs an effective waste-removal function. Blood and dialysate are established in a counter-current or opposing flow to each other to maximise the diffusive process,[84] mimicking the normal nephron function of the kidneys.[85]

A diffusive clearance technique can be performed with increasing intensity and effect by making both blood and dialysate flow faster, with technical problems delivering the high fluid and blood flow being the limiting factor increasing clearance. The two flows need to be maintained in relation to each other; for the diffusive clearance to be efficient the dialysate flow must always equal or exceed the blood flow. A common setting for an intermittent dialysis treatment would be a blood flow and dialysate fluid flow of 300 mL/min each. When applied on an intermittent basis, as is normal for patients receiving RRT for chronic renal failure, this is called intermittent haemodialysis.[86] Fig. 18.11 illustrates the circuit set-up for intermittent haemodialysis.

Ultrafiltration

Ultrafiltration is the process that allows plasma water to leave the blood, achieving body fluid or water loss.[85]

Dialysis (or Nephrology) nurses measure a fluid loss by weighing the patient before and after a treatment. This process is primarily used to achieve fluid balance, an important function of the kidneys. The only difference between this process and the convective clearance of solutes is that this fluid is not replaced, and is therefore not considered to be an adequate solute management method. Ultrafiltration cannot be undertaken in large amounts without fluid replacement, as it would cause hypovolaemia. It is implemented during a dialysis period by removing small amounts each hour (e.g. 250 mL/h for 4 h) during the intermittent treatment cycle.

There are different therapeutic effects from each form of RRT and different operational prescriptions of blood and fluid flow. Combinations of convection and diffusion can be used, known as CVVHDf.[86] An increase in the diffusive component (i.e. raising the dialysate flow rate in CVVHDf) will increase the removal of small-molecular-weight substances such as potassium and assist with hydrogen ion exchange via buffer solution. This can also be achieved via increasing filtration fluid flow (convective clearance), which will also add an increase in clearance of larger molecules, for example those associated with severe infection and systemic inflammation or sepsis. Fig. 18.12 illustrates the circuit and set-up for CVVHDf. These different modes or methods to achieve solute clearance, acid–base control and fluid balance and supporting the patient with failing kidneys are applied with similar success and outcome. Large randomised controlled trials[60,87] or meta-analysis reviews[88] investigating anticoagulation methods report similar patient demographics, and outcomes for ICU stay, morbidity and mortality. There are some physician preferences for mode choice with CRRT and this is possibly associated with training pathways in medicine.[89]

FIGURE 18.12 Continuous veno-venous haemodiafiltration (CVVHDf) circuit.

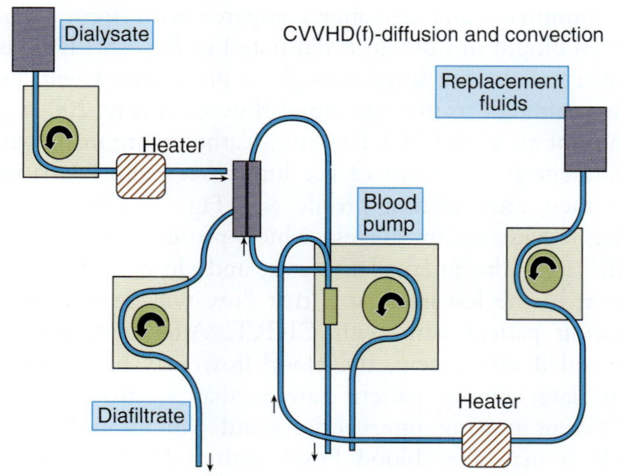

Delivering CRRT

To correctly understand the different variants of RRT, how each achieves waste removal and fluid balance along with knowledge of how to 'troubleshoot' the machine providing RRT, nurses benefit from a clear understanding of major circuit components, their functions and the blood pathway known as the EC. For the treatment or therapy, physicians prescribe this as a 'dose' and is the volume of fluid removed as waste in respective modes, as outlined in Fig. 18.10 and Fig. 18.12. Estimated or actual patient weight can be used, and 25 mL/kg/h is common in adults for the effluent and waste removal. That is, for an 80-kg patient this would be prescribed and set at 2L/h and automatically controlled by the machine pumps and software.

Importantly and precisely linked to this fluid removal and dose is the volume replaced or substituted and dictated by the mode used. In diffusive mode such as CVVHD: as dialysate fluid. In a convective mode, known as CVVH, fluids are administered into the blood pathway and can be before or after the membrane. Fluid administration before the membrane is termed pre-dilution and after the membrane is referred to as post-dilution. Any fluid administered pre-dilution changes the blood haematocrit and, unless the blood flow is increased to compensate, subsequent solute clearance within the membrane reduces. This aspect of clearance and the effect of fluids administered and blood flow is known as filtration fraction.[90] However, the dilution does help to prevent clotting within the membrane and is considered clinically beneficial.[91] If the waste-removal rate is increased in either mode for a negative fluid balance, the dose is increased as a result and depending on the amount per hour.[90]

Membranes

The filter or haemofilter (blood filter) is the primary functional component of the RRT system, responsible for separating plasma water from the blood and/or allowing the exchange of solutes across the membrane by diffusion. The filter is made of a plastic casing, containing a synthetic polymer inner structure arranged in longitudinal fibres. A schematic diagram of a haemofilter is shown in Fig. 18.13. The fibres are hollow and have pores along their length with a size of 15,000–30,000 daltons. This allows plasma water to pass through, carrying dissolved wastes out of the blood (most of which have a molecular weight <20,000 daltons), while larger plasma proteins and blood cells (at least 60–70,000 daltons) are retained.[92] Plasma water separated from the blood in this way is carried away from the filter by a side exit port and a pump, where it is measured and directed into a collection bottle or bag as waste; this convective clearance of solutes is similar to urine produced by the normal kidneys. The plasma water loss is replaced in equal volume with a commercially manufactured plasma water substitute, as previously stated is

FIGURE 18.13 Haemofilter (dialysis membrane). Cross-sectional view indicating longitudinal synthetic fibres conveying blood into and out of the plastic casing outer structure. Plasma water is removed via the side ultrafiltrate port during CVVH applying convective clearance. In CVVHDf, the blood is exposed to fluid via the membrane fibres so that diffusive clearance can occur.

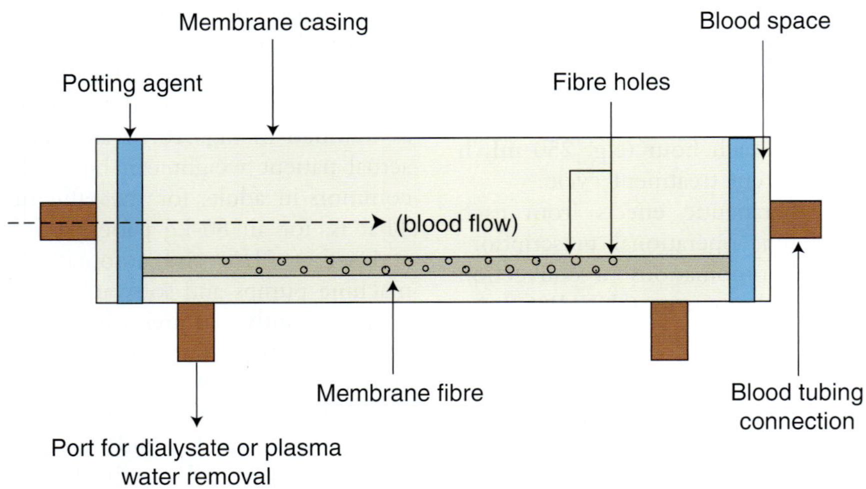

either post-dilution and after the 'filtered' blood exits the haemofilter or pre-dilution, prior to the blood entering the haemofilter, or can be both at the same time (pre- and post-dilution). The plasma water replacement contains no metabolic wastes and achieves blood purification as it is continuously replaced.[82,93]

Filter membrane polymers are made of different materials: AN69 (acrylonitrile/sodium methallyl sulfonate), polyacrylonitrile, polyamide and polysulfone;[94] or polyethersulfone. All demonstrate similar artificial kidney effects and are generally chosen according to the supplier circuit provided or, when this is not fixed, by the vendor or prescribing preference.[95] The most important characteristics of filters used in continuous modes of therapy are: 1) a high plasma water clearance rate at low blood flow rates and circuit pressures; and 2) high permeability to middle-sized molecular weight substances (500–15,000 daltons, e.g. inflammatory cytokines), which are often encountered in critical illness.[95]

Vascular access

As previously noted, to establish CRRT it is necessary to create a blood flow outside the body using the EC.[80] Blood is most commonly accessed from the venous circulation of the critical care patient via a catheter placed in a central vein (e.g. femoral). Blood is both withdrawn from the vein and returned to the same vein – that is, veno-venous access by means of a double (dual)-lumen catheter. When the same procedure is carried out by accessing blood from the patient's systemic circulation via an artery and returning it to a vein, the term arteriovenous is used.[96] In this system there is no mechanical blood pump required, as the patient's arterial blood pressure provides a flow of blood in the EC. Veno-venous haemofiltration has the advantages of requiring only a single venipuncture, a reliable blood flow delivered from a blood pump and alternative venous access sites if there is site infection or access is difficult. While it is easy to establish flow within arteriovenous-driven circuits and no complex system of blood pumps and pressure sensors are necessary, this method is susceptible to flow problems associated with low patient arterial blood pressure and high venous pressures, a common occurrence in critically ill patients and the method is now almost obsolete.[97,98]

The dual-lumen catheter used for veno-venous access has an internal diameter of 1.5–3 mm and catheter lumens are sufficiently separated from each other at their tip to prevent filtered blood from mixing with unfiltered blood when used in the recommended sequence.[99] This ensures that filtered blood does not simply pass back through the EC and artificial kidney, where there would be minimal waste clearance compared with 'fresh' unfiltered blood; this design is illustrated in Fig. 18.14A. The catheter must be small enough to place into a vein but large enough to provide blood flow of at least 200 mL/min for an adult CRRT circuit. Catheters are made with different arrangement of the lumens revealing variation in their cross-section profile (see Fig. 18.14B). There is no evidence to suggest which profile is better, but the larger the internal diameter, and closer to the right heart,[100] the less likely it is that flow will be obstructed during patient care with CRRT. After a catheter is threaded into a vein, the blood flow may be adequate, but later during patient care it may obstruct due to different nursing interventions and patient movement, which may alter blood flows within the low-pressure venous system.[101]

FIGURE 18.14 (**A**) Vascular-access catheters for CRRT. Dual-lumen, Bard® Niagara™ and Gambro Dolphin Protect™ catheters; (**B**) concept diagram of catheter lumen profiles used for dual-lumen CRRT catheters.

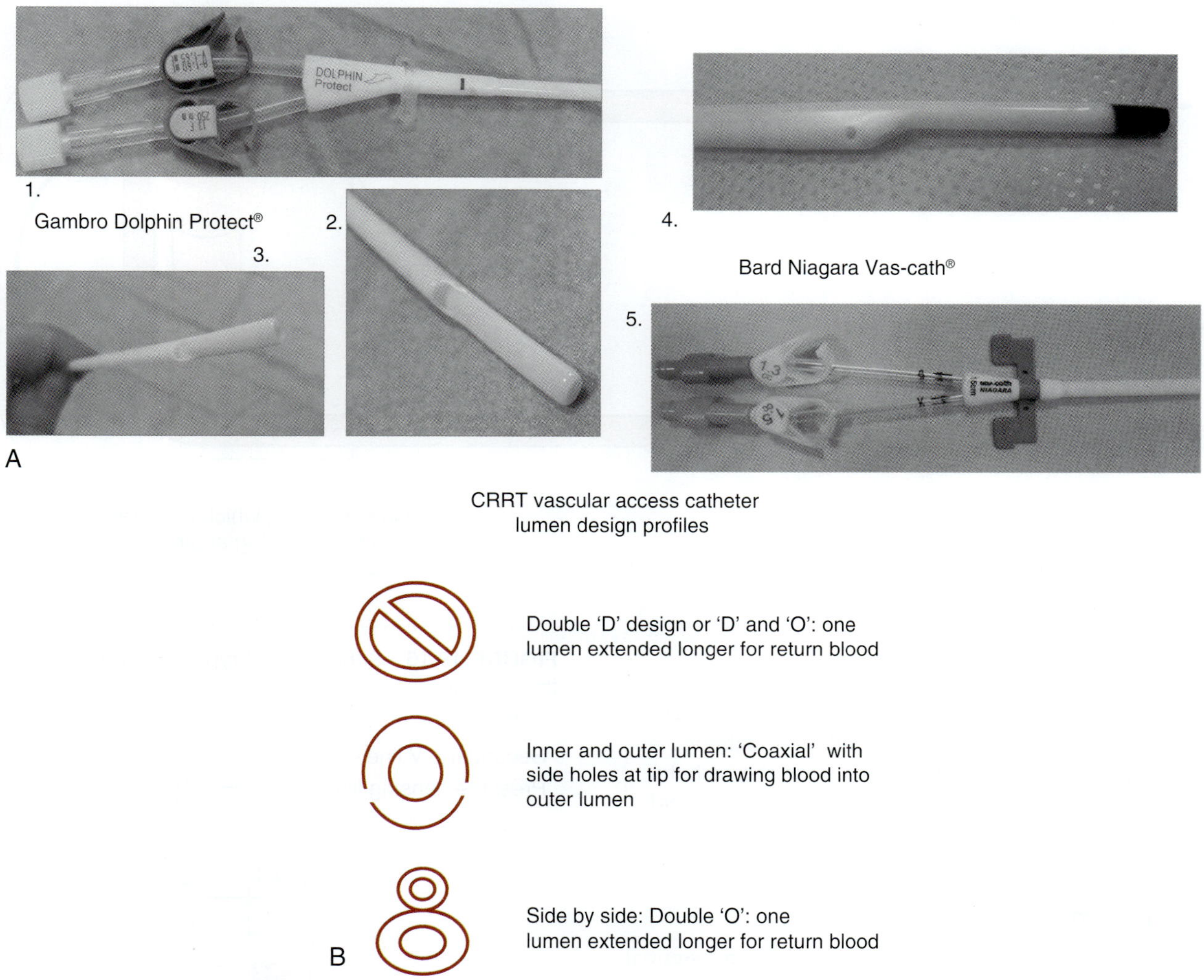

Insertion sites may be affected by nursing care interventions. Placement of the catheter is usually in the femoral or internal jugular vein, and less often, the subclavian.[102] In short-term haemodialysis catheterisation, femoral and internal jugular central venous access routes have similar risks for catheter-related complications except internal jugular central venous access routes can be associated with higher risk of mechanical complications.[103] The right internal jugular vein is the vessel of choice for CRRT because it is the shortest, most direct vascular route to the right atrium and therefore provides potentially better blood flow.[103] The left internal jugular vein can also be used, but it has a longer and less direct route to the right atrium. Anecdotally, the subclavian position is more easily managed for dressing and securing, continuous observation and patient comfort, but is more problematic in terms of flow reliability. KDIGO practice guidelines[4] do not support use of the subclavian vein. Intrathoracic pressure changes associated with physiotherapy or spontaneous patient coughing and breathing, coupled with the upright position of patients, may hinder blood flow from the subclavian-sited access catheter. While these issues are not encountered with a femoral-placed catheter, flow problems can arise due to side-lying and flexion at the groin or hip.[97,101,103]

The flow performance of any vascular-access catheter can be affected by the patient's position in bed, spontaneous movement and repositioning activities as part of routine nursing care in the critically ill for pressure-area prevention. Catheter lumen outlet or inlet obstruction can be due to contact with the vessel wall, or to the formation of a sharp bend due to the patient's movement. These factors contribute to compromising blood flow in the EC, and have been identified to occur without awareness, and contribute to clotting. Moderate flow reductions have been detected by an ultrasound Doppler flow probe attached to the circuit tubing during clinical care and CRRT use validating this problem.[97]

FIGURE 18.15 Roller pump for RRT.

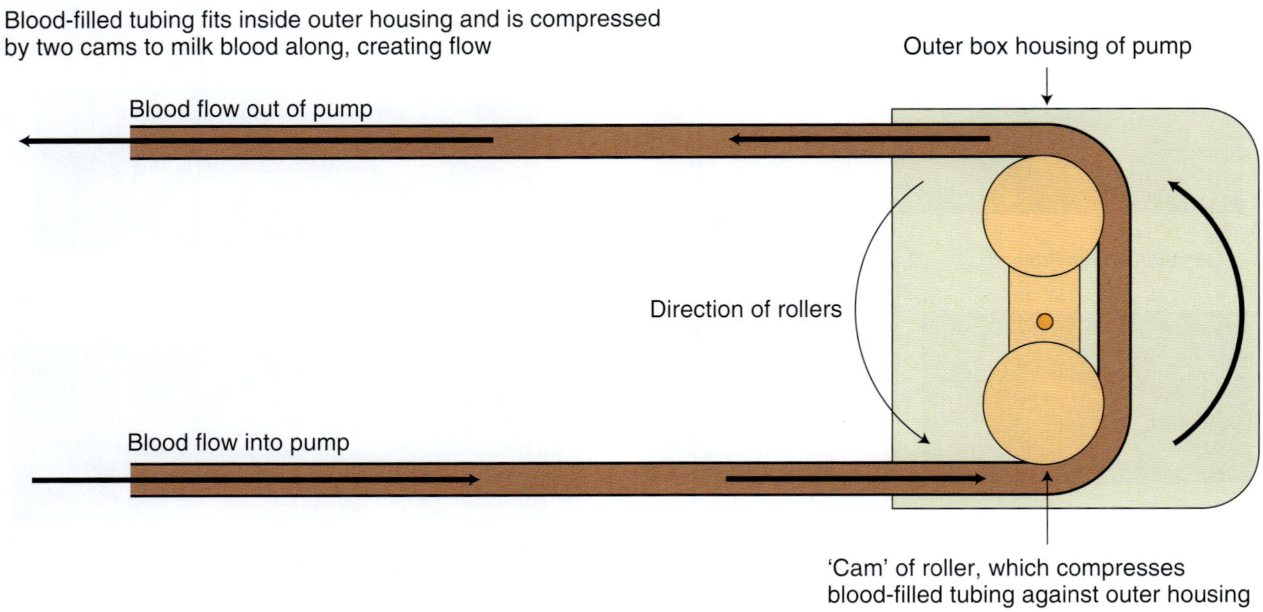

Practice tip

If CRRT circuits clot or fail, remember, if this is associated with failure of the access catheter, restarting a new treatment is also likely to fail unless the catheter is changed or re-sited. The solution or response is not to prompt an increase in anticoagulant dose.

Blood pump

In veno-venous modes, a pump component is essential as part of the patient's blood volume flows externally to the body via the EC. Blood flow is maintained by a 'roller pump' (Fig. 18.15), which propels blood along the tubing in a peristaltic fashion (milking along by compression of the tubing), compressing the blood-filled tubing but having no contact with the blood itself. This roller rotates at a rate providing a flow of fresh unfiltered blood to the haemofilter, enabling it to clear metabolic waste products. This roller pump allows compression of tubing to move the blood forward.

The compression is not continuous, as there is a short time (<0.5 s) when there is no compression to allow the tubing to refill with fresh blood. The compressed tubing re-expands behind the rotating roller and fills with fresh blood from the access and will be compromised if the catheter is obstructed in any way.

Venous return line bubble trap chamber

The purpose of using a bubble trap chamber is to prevent any gas bubbles in the EC from entering the patient's circulation by allowing them to rise to the top of a small, vertically positioned collection reservoir (Fig. 18.16). Venous pressure is commonly measured via a tubing connection into the top of this venous chamber, and additional intravenous fluids can be administered into this chamber via a secondary tube connection. The level of blood in the chamber must be below the top, to prevent spillage into the pressure monitoring line. It

FIGURE 18.16 Schematic of typical venous bubble trap design.

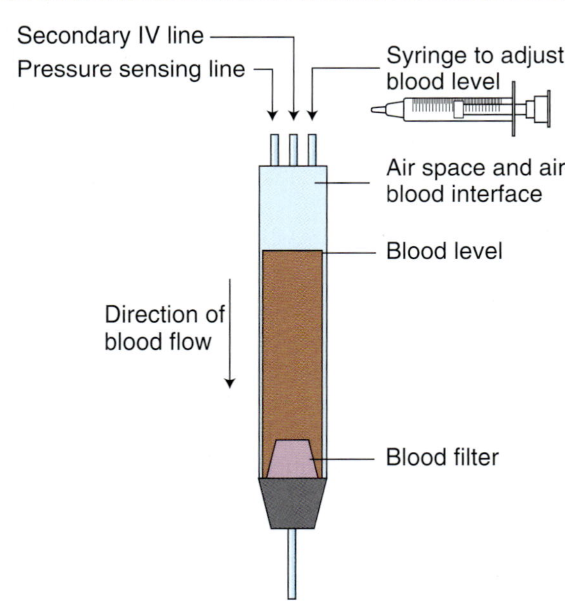

is advised that the blood level be adjusted to near full but allow for visual inspection of incoming blood flow and to ensure that any air or gas bubbles are trapped here.[104,105] As this creates a gas–blood interface within the venous chamber there is a potential source of venous chamber clotting and hence circuit failure.[104] Addition of replacement fluids into this chamber when using post-dilution fluid administration can cause a plasma fluid layer to develop above the blood level and may reduce clotting by stopping blood foaming on its surface and eliminates air or gas contact with the blood.[104] Newer CRRT machine designs such as the NxStage® System[106] (NxStage Medical Inc., Lawrence, MA) do not incorporate a bubble trap since the air detector on the venous bloodline is extremely precise at detecting any air coming out of the haemofilter or dialyser. In addition, the presence of a bubble trap in traditionally designed machines increases the likelihood of clot formation as there is a gas–blood interface.

Anticoagulation

There are several different drugs utilised to prevent blood clotting in the EC; heparin, prostacyclin, thrombin inhibitors and sodium citrate have been used separately or in various combinations and each has potential complications or side effects (Table 18.3).[107,108] As blood comes into contact with the plastic tubing and the polymer fibres of the filter, various clotting systems are activated. This is a normal action of blood when exposed to non-biological surfaces. The aim of anticlotting drugs is to delay clot formation while the blood is outside the body, particularly when within the densely-packed fibres of the filter. As calcium, blood platelet cells and thrombin are vital in clot formation, these drugs are targeted to one of these elements. This targeting must not be too pronounced, as the patient may begin to bleed when the blood returns from the EC to the body.

Heparin is the most commonly-used agent for the prevention of clotting, as it is inexpensive, widely available and easily reversed by another drug, protamine.[109] Heparin is usually administered into the EC before the blood enters the filter, although the optimal place to administer any anticoagulant drug during CRRT is not agreed upon.[110,111] A bolus is often given prior to circuit connection, either in the circuit prime or via the venous access catheter. A maintenance dose (5–15 units/kg/h) is then adjusted against the relevant laboratory tests and a visual inspection for clotting in the EC is undertaken, particularly noting the venous bubble trap.

Citrate is another popular anticoagulant for CRRT as an alternative to heparin, but use is increasing to replace heparin as a first line anticoagulant in many ICUs. Citrate buffers pH and chelates calcium, inducing anticoagulation of blood by reducing serum ionised calcium level. For anticoagulation, the dose and administration rate of citrate are commonly set to achieve a reduction in the CRRT circuit blood ionised calcium level to <0.3 mmol/L.[112] As ionised calcium is essential

TABLE 18.3
Commonly-used anticlotting agents for CRRT

DRUG	BENEFITS	PRECAUTIONS
Heparin	Inexpensive, wide experience, easily reversed, easily monitored, short half-life	Sensitivity reactions, heparin-induced thrombocytopenia, to be effective means increased risk of bleeding systemically
Low-molecular-weight heparin (LMWH)	Moderately inexpensive, increasing experience, less likely to result in sensitivity reactions	Difficult to monitor, not easily reversed, longer half-life, dosing varies between types of LMWH
Prostacyclin	Very short-acting, has a physiological role in inhibiting platelet activity, does not exacerbate other drug reactions	Expensive, no measure of effectiveness, narrow dose range with associated hypotension, individual patients sensitive to haemodynamic effects, unstable in solution
Citrate-based solutions or citrate concentrate – as infusion	Limit anticlotting effect to extracorporeal circuit (EC) – 'regional anticoagulation'; results suggest very effective in prolonging circuit life	Substantial metabolic effect if not adequately managed (serum ionised calcium must be monitored closely); requires additions to EC to administer and reverse and use of specialised replacement/dialysate solutions Not useful when liver failure present, citrate is converted to bicarbonate by the liver providing the necessary buffer for renal replacement therapy (RRT). Acidosis may occur in liver failure
No anticlotting agent (with saline flushes)	No side effects, no exacerbation of unstable haematological status, liver failure	May encounter very short circuit life that consumes remaining haematological components, risk of fluid overload if saline flushes not part of fluid balance. No evidence saline flushes have any benefit

for the progression of the coagulation cascade to form a stable clot, an anticoagulant effect is achieved when the calcium is bound or chelated.[112] A continuous infusion of citrate is administered into the CRRT circuit, as patient blood enters the circuit, similar to heparin administration. A new approach in Australia includes citrate as an additive to commercially prepared CRRT replacement fluids. When circuit blood returns to the patient circulation, it mixes with systemic blood and the calcium concentration is restored to normal; free citrate not binding to calcium is metabolised by the liver to provide carbon dioxide and bicarbonate as a necessary buffer.[113] However, citrate-bound calcium is lost in the waste fluid removed and requires replacement by a separate calcium infusion to maintain serum calcium levels to normal, at 1.0–1.3 mmol/L.[112,113] Due to the complex nature of the citrate-based anticoagulation approach a number of different protocols have been proposed to aid in management.[114] Not all methods will be applied in the one ICU, and local expertise development of one method and an alternative is common. Recent reviews provide a good synopsis of each method as they are different depending on CVVH or CVVHDF mode.[108]

Thrombin inhibitors are another type of anticoagulant that can be used in CRRT. They inhibit free and clot-bound thrombin and do not react with antibodies to heparin.[115] Thrombin inhibitors such as argatroban are useful in patients who have heparin-induced thrombocytopenia associated with heparin anticoagulation.[116] These inhibitors are more expensive than heparin but provide effective anticoagulation. The KDIGO guidelines[4] recommend the use of thrombin inhibitors rather than other anticoagulants or no anticoagulant. Argatroban is cleared by the liver and has a half-life of 31 to 59 min.[117] Dosage includes a loading and a maintenance dose adjusted to keep the aPTT 1–3 times the reference level.[115]

If bleeding occurs during anticoagulation with argatroban, the infusion can be turned off. In an ex vivo study, the effects of argatroban were able to be reversed using recombinant-activated factor VII. In patients with hepatic failure or with multiple organ dysfunction syndrome and sepsis, the clearance of argatroban may be markedly reduced.[117]

The use of frequent isotonic fluid flushes to prevent clotting

One approach to prevention of clot and protein collection within the membrane and 'clotting' is to flush the circuit or infuse small bolus volumes of saline or crystalloid solution throughout continuous treatment e.g. 100 mL each hour. However, small and single centre studies of flushing with physiological saline have shown mixed benefits to prevent circuit clotting. Saline flushes might be a better option for patients with a high risk for bleeding or low platelet count, a prolonged activated partial thromboplastin time, or international normalised ratio. This fluid flush if used requires a change to fluid loss settings and attention to fluid removal accordingly.

Normal clotting time, a laboratory test designed to measure the time taken for blood to clot under laboratory conditions, is used as a reference to determine a suitable therapeutic range of the anticlotting drug during CRRT. Different tests are applicable to different medications and their site of action in the clotting cascade. When using any anticlotting agent, a balance is required between the benefits of increased coagulation suppression and the higher risk of patient systemic bleeding.

Fluids and fluid balance

Fluid used during any form of CRRT is a commercially manufactured product with an electrolyte composition similar to blood plasma.[93,118] This provides a solution useful as a replacement solution for plasma water removed in convective mode such as CVVH, or as a dialysate solution in diffusive mode or CVVHDf.[119] These respective applications allow for plasma water replacement with 'clean' and buffered plasma water following toxin-laden plasma water removal or, during CVVHDf, for plasma water to be exposed to the whole blood across the membrane fibres so that toxins and molecules will diffusively exchange from blood into the fluid. The additives or recipe for three commonly-used commercial fluids are listed in Table 18.4 together with saline solution and normal blood plasma chemistry for comparative analysis. The key additives of note in commercial fluids[93] are the elevated level of bicarbonate and a variable concentration of potassium (no potassium option also), providing an effective buffer for the acidaemia and hyperkalaemia associated with AKI.

Throughout the course of a continuous treatment with CRRT, hypokalaemia may occur and a higher potassium-added solution may be required to correct and maintain normal serum levels. First-generation commercial fluids used lactic acid as the buffer additive, requiring liver metabolism to produce bicarbonate in vivo.[118] This preparation is now not used in favour of a bicarbonate-added fluid, prepared just prior to using a two-compartment bag (Fig. 18.17) as the two fluids are unstable in long-term storage. The higher cost, problems with reconstituting bicarbonate solution bags and manual handling of large (5 L) fluid bags did increase interest in 'online' fluid production from tap-water at the bedside. This approach can be less expensive, requires no bag changing or reconstituting by nurses,[120] but does require the installation of a complex and expensive reverse osmosis machine, the cost of which would be offset if large volumes of fluid were then consumed from this online manufacture. This approach is used in some centres for these reasons, and is applied as ICU 'daily dialysis' or extended dialysis modes and are the therapy of choice.[120,121]

Fluid balance monitoring and adjustment to machine settings is a key nursing responsibility in managing a patient treated with CRRT.[122] This requires an operator

TABLE 18.4
Blood plasma chemistry compared with commonly-used commercial CRRT fluids

	BLOOD – PLASMA (A)	SALINE (BAXTER, TOONGABBIE, AUSTRALIA)	BAXTER ACCUSOL	GAMBRO HEMOSOL B0 (GAMBRO, LUND, SWEDEN)	BAXTER HAEMOFILTRATION CITRATE SOLUTION (BAXTER, TOONGABBIE, AUSTRALIA)
Sodium (mmol/L)	136–145	150	140	140	152
Chloride (mmol/L)	98–07	150	113.5	109.5	99
Potassium (mmol/L)	3.5–5.1	0	4.0 or 2.0	4.0 or 2.0	5
Bicarbonate (mmol/L)	22–29	0	35	32	0
Calcium	2.15–2.55	0	1.75	1.75	0
Magnesium	0.66–1.07	0	0.5	0.5	0
Citrate (mmol/L)	0	0	0	0	18
Lactate	0.5–2.2		0	3.0	0.0
pH (range)	7.35–7.45	4.0–7.0	7.4	7.0–8.5	5–6.5
mOsm/kg (listed or estimated)	280–300	300	300.3	287	270

Adult ranges from: http://www.austinpathology.org.au/test-directory.

FIGURE 18.17 Two-compartment bicarbonate bag.

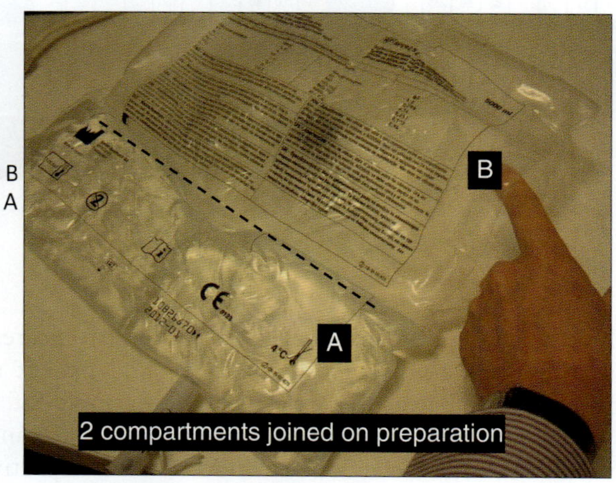

of the machine to enter a rate of fluid removal each hour, or for a longer set time period, and the machine is intended to achieve this target for the set time. It is important to remember this volume of fluid removed is simply the machine-prescribed loss of fluid removed, commonly determined by electronic scales in the machine, or the balancing chambers and does not equate to the overall fluid balance of the patient.[123] A simple fluid balance calculation accounts for addition of all intakes, plus small physician-ordered volume loss, minus outputs each hour. The set volume removal each hour to achieve a desired fluid state must be determined in context for the entire clinical status of a patient where verbal communication and written prescribing orders must be clear to differentiate 'machine loss – setting' from patient net 'loss' or balance per hour.[122] Despite simple software for setting the desired fluid loss or removal per hour during treatment, mistakes and errors occur.[122] In

FIGURE 18.18 Screen dump of a bedside e-fluid balance chart.

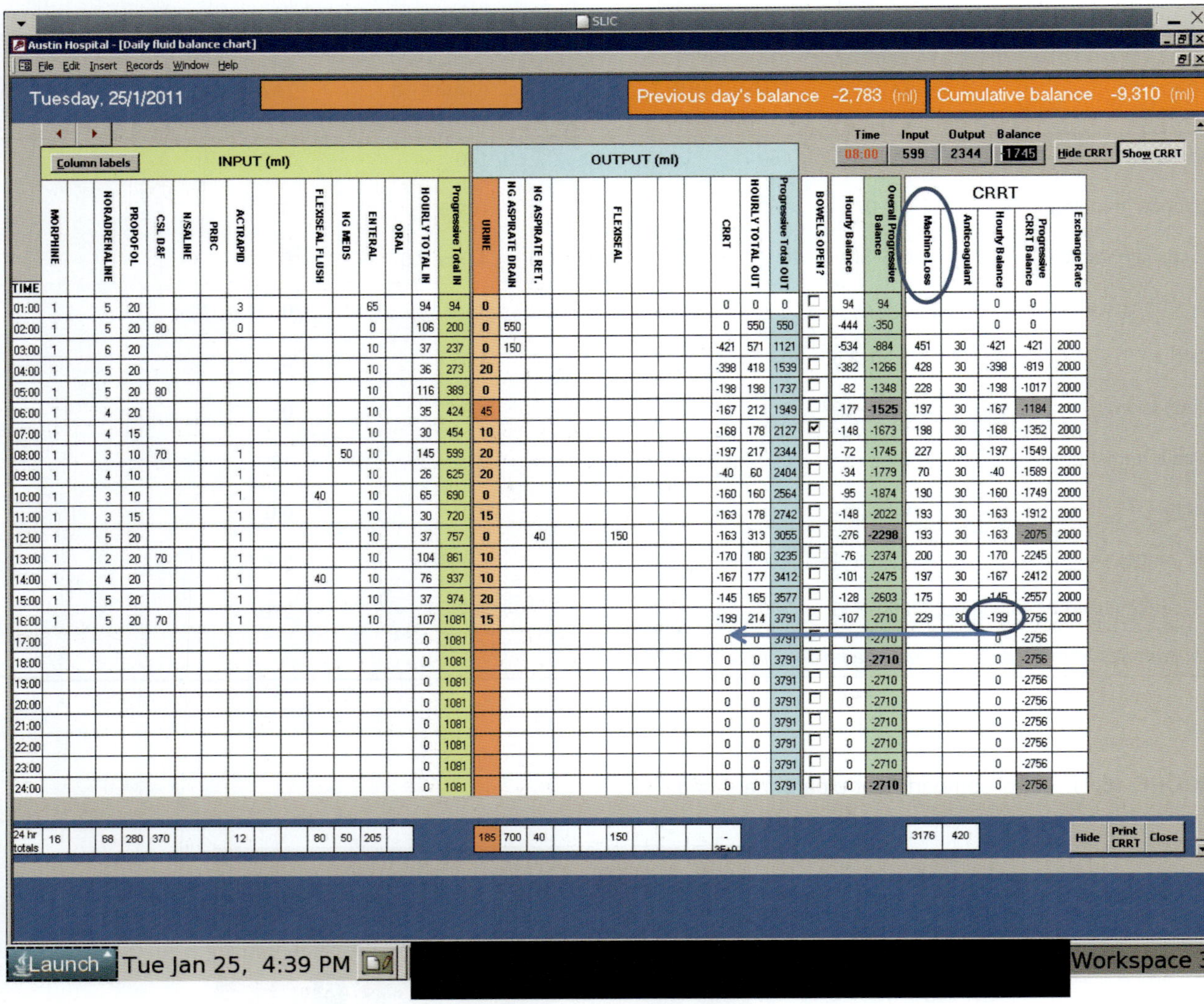

TIME	MORPHINE		NORADRENALINE	PROPOFOL	CSL D&F	N/SALINE	PRBC	ACTRAPID			FLEXISEAL FLUSH	NG MEDS	ENTERAL	ORAL	HOURLY TOTAL IN	Progressive Total IN
01:00	1		5	20				3					65		94	94
02:00	1		5	20	80			0					0		106	200
03:00	1		6	20									10		37	237
04:00	1		5	20									10		36	273
05:00	1		5	20	80								10		116	389
06:00	1		4	20									10		35	424
07:00	1		4	15									10		30	454
08:00	1		3	10	70			1				50	10		145	599
09:00	1		4	10				1					10		26	625
10:00	1		3	10				1			40		10		65	690
11:00	1		3	15				1					10		30	720
12:00	1		5	20				1					10		37	757
13:00	1		2	20	70			1					10		104	861
14:00	1		4	20				1			40		10		76	937
15:00	1		5	20				1					10		37	974
16:00	1		5	20	70			1					10		107	1081
17:00															0	1081
18:00															0	1081
19:00															0	1081
20:00															0	1081
21:00															0	1081
22:00															0	1081
23:00															0	1081
24:00															0	1081
24 hr totals	16		68	280	370			12			80	50	205			

TIME	URINE	NG ASPIRATE DRAIN	NG ASPIRATE RET.			FLEXISEAL				CRRT	HOURLY TOTAL OUT	Progressive Total OUT	BOWELS OPEN?	Hourly Balance	Overall Progressive Balance	CRRT: Machine Loss	Anticoagulant	Hourly Balance	Progressive CRRT Balance	Exchange Rate
01:00	0									0	0	0	☐	94	94			0	0	
02:00	0	550								0	550	550	☐	-444	-350			0	0	
03:00	0	150								-421	571	1121	☐	-534	-884	451	30	-421	-421	2000
04:00	20									-398	418	1539	☐	-382	-1266	428	30	-398	-819	2000
05:00	0									-198	198	1737	☐	-82	-1348	228	30	-198	-1017	2000
06:00	45									-167	212	1949	☐	-177	-1525	197	30	-167	-1184	2000
07:00	10									-168	178	2127	☑	-148	-1673	198	30	-168	-1352	2000
08:00	20									-197	217	2344	☐	-72	-1745	227	30	-197	-1549	2000
09:00	20									-40	60	2404	☐	-34	-1779	70	30	-40	-1589	2000
10:00	0									-160	160	2564	☐	-95	-1874	190	30	-160	-1749	2000
11:00	15									-163	178	2742	☐	-148	-2022	193	30	-163	-1912	2000
12:00	0		40			150				-163	313	3055	☐	-276	-2298	193	30	-163	-2075	2000
13:00	10									-170	180	3235	☐	-76	-2374	200	30	-170	-2245	2000
14:00	10									-167	177	3412	☐	-101	-2475	197	30	-167	-2412	2000
15:00	20									-145	165	3577	☐	-128	-2603	175	30	-145	-2557	2000
16:00	15									-199	214	3791	☐	-107	-2710	229	30	-199	-2756	2000
17:00										0	0	3791	☐	0	-2710			0	-2756	
18:00										0	0	3791	☐	0	-2710			0	-2756	
19:00										0	0	3791	☐	0	-2710			0	-2756	
20:00										0	0	3791	☐	0	-2710			0	-2756	
21:00										0	0	3791	☐	0	-2710			0	-2756	
22:00										0	0	3791	☐	0	-2710			0	-2756	
23:00										0	0	3791	☐	0	-2710			0	-2756	
24:00										0	0	3791	☐	0	-2710			0	-2756	
24 hr totals	185	700	40			150				-3E+0						3176	420			

some cases, particularly in small children and babies, this can be fatal.[124,125] Most machines now provide limits for the amount of accumulative fluid balance error (+ve or –ve) before an alarm will sound with a display message to advise the nurse. Such errors can occur due to fluid bags remaining clamped, or fluid pathway lines kinked or clamped. Logically, the machine is removing or infusing fluid but the machine scales or balancing chambers are not detecting a weight change. The fluids infused as replacement or removed as waste plus additional fluid for a loss are usually all recorded on a fluid balance formula in electronic charting at the bedside. This is presented as inputs and outputs charting, with the difference between these amounts understood as the balance; usually a negative in the context of a patient with AKI, anuric, and in the ICU setting, is commonly set for a negative balance overall. This fluid balance is achieved easily with recent electronic records included in ICU clinical information and patient management systems. See Fig. 18.18 as an example of such a spreadsheet chart from a bedside computer and software used.

Irrespective of patient acuity, when CRRT is used, individual patient assessment for fluid status must occur at least twice a day. Subtle temperature changes in the patient, surgical drain losses, diarrhoea and variable fluid intake all contribute to a more precise fluid balance.[126] Regular weighing of patients may assist in assessing overall patient condition, in addition to regular physical and clinical assessment of the patient. Electrolyte disturbances may also occur despite use of balanced replacement solutions. Particular attention should focus on regular assessment of fluid and electrolytes, especially potassium, sodium, phosphate and magnesium levels. See Fig. 18.19 for a sample hourly fluid loss calculation.

> **Practice tip**
>
> Fluid removal during CRRT is prescribed by doctors and usually to a time frame or target aim for the day. The nurse needs to calculate the rate per hour for the target and perform a recalculation if CRRT is off and there is no treatment for any time.

Patient management

Nursing protocols have previously been focused on machine priming, patient preparation and use of a CRRT system as this was the essential training pathway for nurses learning the operator–machine–patient interface.[127] Current CRRT machines are highly automated and have advanced software with instructional on-screen coloured pictures, circuit diagrams and text prompts providing a sequential step-by-step approach for priming, patient connection and key alarms. Nonetheless, the clinical knowledge, psychomotor skills and the responsibility for managing an EC to efficiently and safely treat a critically ill patient should not be understated.[128] The nurse-to-patient ratio for CRRT is commonly 1:1 worldwide, acknowledging the attention and focus required despite the advances in machine automation.[128,129] This is a reasonable approach as CRRT in the ICU is very different to the use of dialysis for chronic renal failure where a nurse may oversee three or four patients on dialysis under their care and with different start times (overlapping) for a 3–4-hour treatment in each case. In the ICU these patients are usually in a multi-organ failure state, are intubated and require mechanical ventilation, cardiovascular support, enteral feeding, need many intravenous drugs and infusions and have reduced neurological function with or without sedation. This is a picture mandating both technical and cognitive tasks in addition to comprehensive nursing care, including full hygiene and all care for the bedridden, and often unconscious patient.

Monitoring correct machine function for reliable flow of blood, continuous changing of bags as substitution fluids empty and waste bags fill, adjustment and constant review for stability with anticoagulation agents and the overall monitoring and response to other parameters of patient metabolic stability with electrolyte, acid–base and temperature management represent some of the work associated with the nursing care required.[79,82,130] Machine and circuit preparation, connection and, when required, stopping and disconnecting a treatment are further skill and knowledge sets for ICU nurses. It is in the key interest of both doctors and nurses in the ICU that the treatment be 'continuous' as frequent stopping and restarting is a lot of work for nurses and may cause instability in the patient.[131]

In Table 18.5 a summary of key nursing practice and interventions for bedside use is provided making this information a suitable reference for nursing knowledge

FIGURE 18.19 CRRT hourly fluid balance calculation example.

CRRT Typical Fluid Balance Calculation

All intakes (tube feeds, IVs IVBPs, flushes) mL	**A**	**110**
MD ordered net loss	**B**	**+50mL**
Total		**160mL**
All outputs (nasogastric tube, chest drain(s), urine output or stool)	**C**	**--10**
	D	**150 mL**
Actual fluid pumped mL	**E**	**142**

Actual Fluid Balance = A - C – E = 42mL

Most e-charting will automatically calculate fluid balance

TABLE 18.5
Troubleshooting guide: key nursing practice and interventions for CRRT

	POTENTIAL PROBLEM (NUMBERED LIST)	KEY NURSING INTERVENTIONS REQUIRED, REFERENCED TO LISTED NUMBER
Patient and machine/ system preparation before use	1 Machine alarms and technical failure on starting treatment 2 Air entrainment during prime 3 Fluid setting errors 4 Fluids/electrolytes incorrect 5 Machine and patient too far apart or machine placed out of staff view	1 Machine self-test and/or checklist completed 2 Double-check all circuit lines around circuit, particularly for clamps ON or OFF as required 3 Treatment orders cross-checked with settings 4 Double-check fluids used, e.g. any additives required 5 Position machine according to access catheter site: at feet for femoral line, at bedside for subclavian and at bed head for jugular with screen faced to staff desk or charts/computer Recommendation: • Have your own pre-start check routine (paper document list)

Continued

TABLE 18.5
Troubleshooting guide: key nursing practice and interventions for CRRT—cont'd

	POTENTIAL PROBLEM (NUMBERED LIST)	KEY NURSING INTERVENTIONS REQUIRED, REFERENCED TO LISTED NUMBER
Connection to the system and initiation of therapy	1 Access catheter obstruction/failure 2 Hypotension on start	1 Prepare access connections with antiseptic, aspirate any instilled drug and test easy flush return (venous) lumen and aspirate outflow (arterial) lumen 2 Connect both circuit lines to access catheter administering priming volume to patient a Increase vasoactive drugs if necessary to increase MAP b Start blood pump slowly with small increases until blood fills all of the circuit Recommendations: • Use two nurses for connection routine. Start fluid replacement and removal only after blood circuit is full and at prescribed speed, stay with patient until stable ≈ first 15 min Patient in bed, supine position and MAP >70 mmHg, stable
In-use troubleshooting alarms and maintenance, fluid balance	1 Excessive negative pressure >–100 mmHg: 'arterial alarm' 2 High pressure >+100 mmHg: 'venous alarm' 3 High TMP alarm 4 Air-detected alarm 5 Hypothermia 6 Fluid balance errors 7 Electrolyte imbalance	1 & 2 Maintain access catheter alignment, preventing kinks in access and circuit lines 1 & 2 Do not place extra connections or taps between access catheter and circuit lines 3 Suggests filter clotting or blood flow too slow for fluids settings 4 Ensure venous chamber is filled with blood, bubbles are removed regularly with post-dilution fluid into the chamber 5 Heater set to 37°C or greater to compensate for heat loss from EC 6 Use fluids charting or similar to account for all fluid inputs including anticoagulant volume. Clarify orders to set machine 'loss' in respect of this. Commonly a net negative. Orders and settings should not be prescribed to administer fluid – no net positive 7 Potassium additive to CRRT fluid is often required after 24–48 h of treatment; some patients are hypokalaemic despite acute renal failure. Phosphate monitoring and correction is important Recommendations: • Assess and reset fluid balance settings hourly, particularly in unstable patients and for inexperienced staff • Fluid gain or positive fluid balance using CRRT should be considered an adverse event or complication of use
Monitoring and adjustment to anticoagulation	1 Premature clotting in circuit and filter	1 Check and monitor effect of anticoagulant therapy according to local policy. With heparin use this could be after first 6 h and then daily a Maintain adequate dose to therapeutic range b Use pre-dilution fluid administration c Use blood flow greater than 150 mL/min d Use large-bore access catheter and take care not to obstruct or kink catheter e Keep blood pump operating: minimise stops >30 s Recommendation: • If frequent failure (clotting <4 h), always check for blood flow obstruction before more, or alternative, anticoagulation; e.g. review to consider change or replacement of access catheter
Access care and dressings	1 Access dislodgement 2 Access catheter infection 3 Access catheter obstruction	1 Ensure catheter sutured in place and well secured with dressing; single or double ('sandwich' technique) biofilm–polyurethane 2 Use asepsis when flushing or connecting to access catheter; monitor site for infection and patient for suspected line sepsis. Use catheter site alcohol patch, e.g. chlorhexadine-impregnated dressing 3 Use heparin to fill catheter dead-space when not in use for >4 h and label accordingly Recommendation: • Use flexible dressing with application to both sides along catheter allowing movement away off skin surface, preventing obstruction during patient care/ positioning and lifting or tearing off dressing

TABLE 18.5
Troubleshooting guide: key nursing practice and interventions for CRRT—cont'd

	POTENTIAL PROBLEM (NUMBERED LIST)	KEY NURSING INTERVENTIONS REQUIRED, REFERENCED TO LISTED NUMBER
Vital sign monitoring	**1** Arrhythmias, hypotension, temperature	**1** Monitor vital signs hourly, consider any links between changes, and use of RRT; e.g. low CVP and excessive fluid removal, temperature fluctuations when CRRT OFF and ON Recommendation: • CVP readings should be performed 2–4-h during CRRT; CVP can be used as a target for daily fluid loss prescription. Weigh the patient if possible. Do frequent blood gas and electrolytes commonly associated with ICU care
Assessment of filter function and patency	**1** Filter clotting abruptly with inability to return circuit blood to the patient **2** Inadequate solute removal	**1** If TMP or pre-filter pressure (P-IN) >250 mmHg is diagnostic of filter clotting consider electively returning blood by crystalloid infusion into outflow limb of circuit and ceasing treatment – follow local policy: **a** Observe for venous chamber clot development. If excessive and venous pressure >150 mmHg, consider electively returning blood – cease treatment **2** Assess patient's solute levels: urea and creatinine should be reducing or stable Recommendations: • Predicting circuit or filter clotting can be difficult. TMP and P-IN can rise quickly after being stable or within normal range. If there is a trend upwards reflecting diagnosis of clotting, cease treatment electively to avoid blood flow 'standstill' and a failure to restart and blood loss • Nurses may document these pressures hourly or check the machine frequently, but they must respond quickly to cease treatment
Cessation of treatment and disconnection from the extracorporeal circuit	**1** Blockage and/or clotting in access catheter **2** Inadvertent blood loss **3** Infectious risk	**1** Use concentrated heparin (other anticoagulant) to fill dead-space of catheter when not in use >4 h. Use heparin 1000 IU/mL and follow manufacturer specifications for volume required **2** Always attempt to cease a circuit before it clots and always return patient blood if possible **3** Use asepsis for disconnection procedure Recommendation: • Access catheter should not be used for other purposes/infusions when RRT is not connected
Temporary disconnection for procedures	**1** Maintenance of circuit before reconnection **2** Infection **3** Inadvertent fluid administration	**1** Flush out any excess blood residue in circuit, keep blood pump operational with saline (prime) in circuit **2** Circuits in use for >24 h before disconnection or not restarted after 6 h following temporary disconnection, consider discarding **3** After restarting circuit, increase fluid loss to remove fluid used to re-establish RRT Recommendation: • Re-use of circuits in this context is not desirable and with prior planning should be avoidable e.g. plan for radiology, surgery etc when circuit off or restart new circuit around these interventions. If this is done, consider adding heparin 5000 IU to circuit when temporarily disconnected unless contraindicated, but flush this out with 200–300 mL prime solution before reconnection; always use additive label indicating heparin added

CRRT = continuous renal replacement therapy; CVP = central venous pressure; EC = extracorporeal circuit; MAP = mean arterial pressure; TMP = transmembrane pressure.

FIGURE 18.20 Shift checklist for CRRT.

Shift check list CRRT as CVVH: Infomed HF 440

Check	Rationale
Machine position relative to patient with blood lines not too tight - stretched	Patient movement could cause excess drag on vascath site and securing tape
Brakes ON	Machine must have brakes on to prevent inadvertent movement and risk of above
Fluids: correct for K^+ and both bags hanging from same point – height, both line clamps open	Fluids should empty at similar rate, minimise mixing, scales and balance alarms more likely if the bags hanging at different heights
Flush line connected, correct fluid, clamped as close to blood path as possible. Date this bag.	Fluid to return patient blood; this may be required any time. Clamp close to blood path prevent blood tracking back up this line and clotting, only to be flushed in with use
Waste bottle hanging stable and waste pump hose with end plug ready, coiled on machine holder.	This bottle will weigh > 16 Kg on full. Needs to hang with stability to prevent scales alarms. Hose ready for use with end cap to prevent drips
Venous – bubble chamber full and inspect for clot	Adjust this up slowly, with syringe attached. Keep full to trap gas / air and allow for the level to fall during use with gas entry associated with bicarbonate fluids (CO_2) when heated
Luer syringe (10 ml), 3 way tap and dead end cap(red) in line - for chamber adjustment	Luer syringe will not fall / slip off during use; red cap blocks pathway between venous blood chamber and UF pathway if 3 way tap was accidently opened to both chambers.
Screen settings & Alarms	
Blood flow - speed	200 mls/min. standard
UF flow	2000 ml/hr standard CVVH
Manual Pre-dilution %	50:50 for CVVH (Citrate use 70% pre)
'Weight loss' – Fluid loss rate ml/hr	Check orders – fluid loss target
Next intervention (hr:min)	Time until fluids bag change or bottle empty
Temperature setting	Default at 37°, maybe ↑↓ to patient need
Venous +10 ---- + 150 mmHg (influenced by blood flow rate and chamber clotting, access function – blue lumen)	This pressure always positive, measured on the return limb of circuit. ~ 50 – 100 mmHg
Arterial -150 ---- -10 mmHg (influenced by blood flow rate and access function – red lumen)	This pressure always negative, measured on the outflow limb of circuit. ~ -50 – -100 mmHg
Trans-membrane pressure (TMP) (Pin + Pv)/2 - Puf	Indicative of clotting / clogging in the membrane. Set at 200 mmHg initially. When 250^+ mmHg, usually terminate treatment.
Anticoagulation and Prescription orders	Check drug dose and orders correct

and skills associated with CRRT use in the ICU. Practice recommendations are also included. This information is general to any CRRT machine, and does not include a detailed anticoagulation protocol. Anticoagulation technique for CRRT usually dominates any policy and is viewed more frequently in comparison to the psychomotor skills component for machine preparation, connection and fluids bags management. Nursing practice policies can also be supplemented with machine-specific and quick reference 'one page' lists for shift check or anticoagulation method. See Fig. 18.20 as an example of a shift checklist.

Continuous renal replacement machines

There are many machines available for CRRT in the ICU. How to identify the machine that a particular ICU should use or purchase is a common question from nurses, and there is limited literature available providing

TABLE 18.6
Machine design and build approaches

MACHINE TYPE	WASTE COLLECTION	MEMBRANE	CIRCUIT	PRESSURE MEASUREMENT	PRIMING PREPARATION AND SOFTWARE OPTION(S)
A	One 5 L or 10 L bag, empty when full, change bag(s)	AN69, prefitted, not changeable	Cartridge kit-based, multipurpose; all modes	In-line pressure transducers	Fully automated, software for management of citrate anticoagulation
B	One 5 L or two bags, empty when full, change bags	Different membranes possible – polyethersulfone or others	Cartridge kit-based, multipurpose; all modes	In-line pressure transducers	Fully automated, intelligence software for fluid management
C	Drain to bedside outlet; no bag collection required	Company provided membrane in kit	Cartridge kit-based, multipurpose; all modes	In-line and other pressure transducers	Fully automated, intelligence software for fluid management

comparisons of their technical characteristics.[132,133] Table 18.6 outlines the major differences in machines or system approaches. Three machines adopting common design features from Table 18.6 are shown in Fig. 18.21 (Prismaflex; Hospal, Lyon, France), Fig. 18.22 (Aquarius, Nikkiso, Sydney, Australia), and Fig. 18.23 (NxStage®, Lawrence MA), each highlighting the major technical differences in how CRRT machines are presented and used.

Teaching and training CRRT

Since introduction of CRRT to the ICU in the 1980s and early 1990s, medical companies as machine vendors have developed and expanded their offerings for teaching and training nurses in the use of CRRT machines and the broader aspects of AKI and patient care. More commonly, where CRRT is imbedded in use for many years, the education focus is with smaller groups teaching new procedures and methods, updates, orientation for new staff and specialist training in association with postgraduate certification. These didactic session topics may be scheduled in the sequence and over several weeks to become more powerful when supplemented with simulation activities linked to live patient care and bedside clinical support.[127,134] A recent report suggests that, when simulation is added to didactic CRRT education programs, an improvement in CRRT functional time (filter 'life') is observed – a direct benefit to users, lessening cost and better for patients.[134]

The key to successful CRRT education and training is to develop nurses with clinical experience managing CRRT regularly in the ICU and encouraging these experts to teach others around them when they can. Educators may already be in place for broader aspects of ICU education and postgraduate trainees but, for any staffing structure with or without dedicated teaching roles, identifying a small number of nurses as CRRT 'champions' for training and ongoing support when CRRT is in progress is a common and successful approach to provide learning for others over the 24/7 context in ICU.

Quality and measures of success

Maintaining quality and nursing expertise for CRRT in the ICU will be related to the frequency of use and the size of the user group. When there are long periods between CRRT use, and/or when the ICU has a large staff number, ensuring competency may be challenging. Regular competency checks and staff assessments can be performed[128,135] depending upon resource allocation for this task. Shift allocation of the nurse to a patient with AKI and treatment with CRRT care may benefit from predetermined skill sets as a guide to best match the individual nurse's competency with the CRRT-treated patient and ensure safety.[128] The most useful measure for quality when using CRRT is the progressive 'life' of the circuit or filter.[82] This data point may be recorded on bedside charts alongside hourly observations (see concept in Fig. 18.24) or electronically into an ICU clinical information system and provides an instant audit for each circuit used and throughout the patient treatment. This variable is most commonly used to compare efficacy of different anticoagulation techniques, but may also be considered a measure of access catheter and blood flow reliability, machine technical function and staff user competence.[90,135] Circuit or filter life (these terms are used interchangeably) is reported widely in the literature and, despite lacking a clear bedside definition, published data from large randomised trials indicate that a median life of 21 hours is common.[87] Poor circuit life at 4–6 hours reflects clinical problems and an interprofessional review before the next treatment begins is warranted.

FIGURE 18.21 Prismaflex CRRT machine.

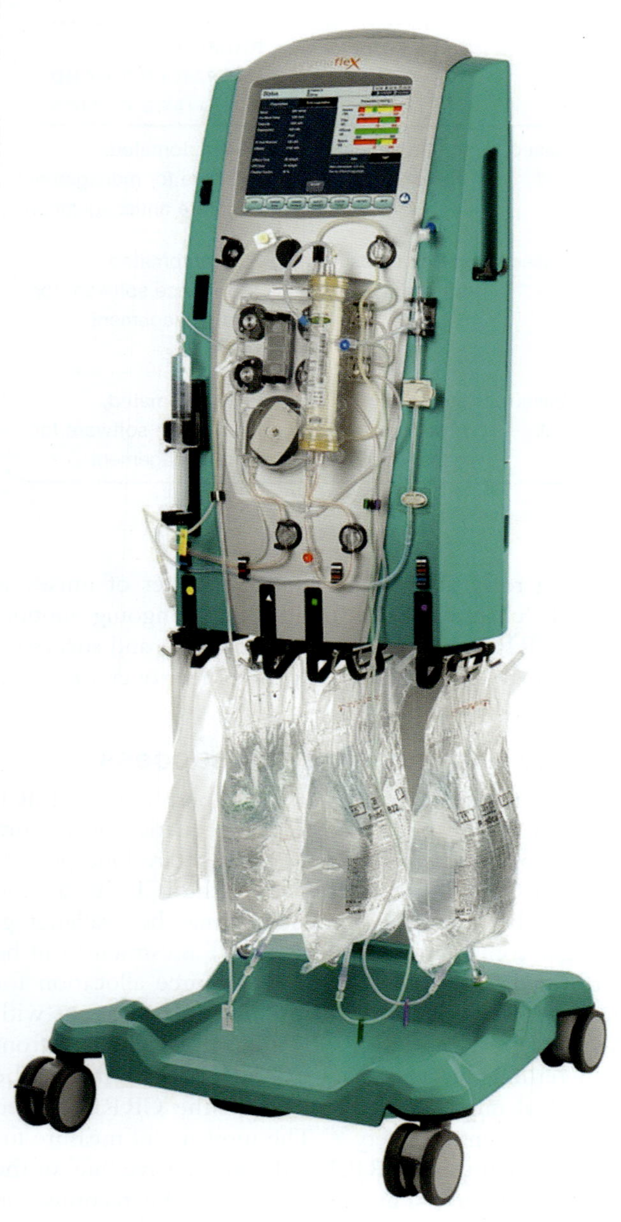

Source: © Baxter Healthcare.

FIGURE 18.22 Aquarius CRRT Machine, Nikkiso, Sydney, Australia.

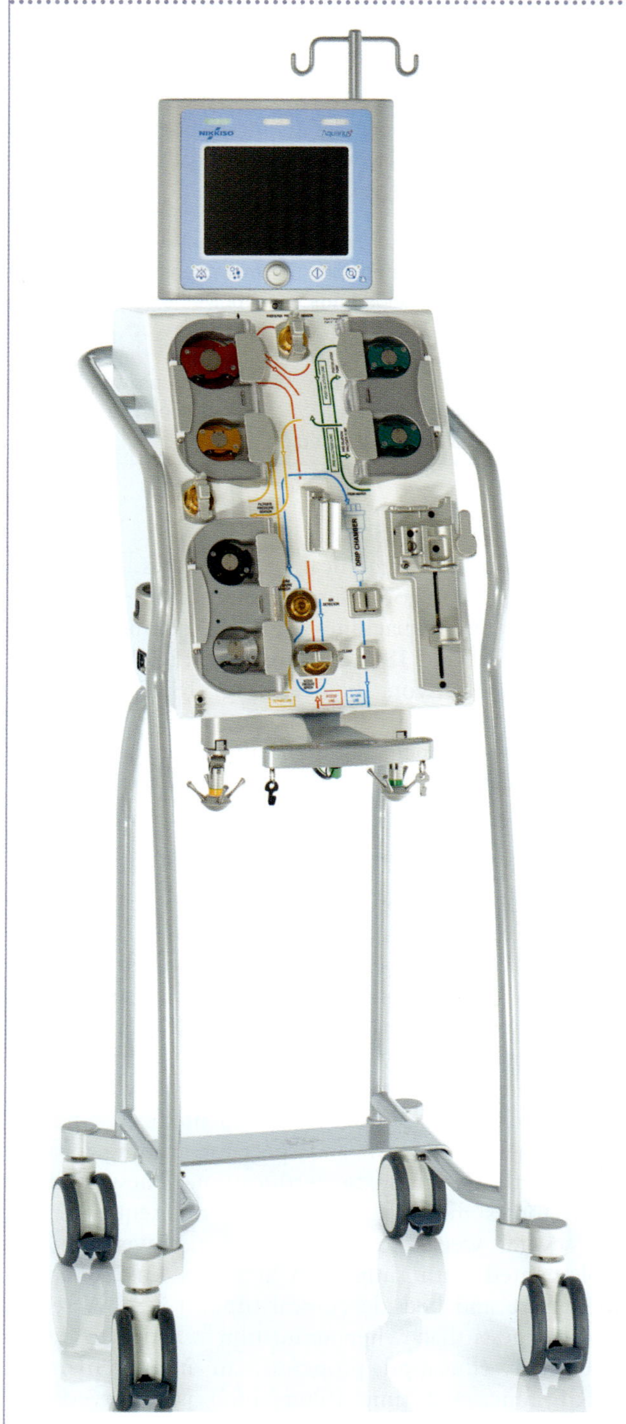

Source: © Nikkiso ANZ.

Special considerations

Paediatrics: babies and small children of 3–30 kg body weight

The use of dialysis and haemofiltration in babies and small children is a specialty area; however, many aspects of adult CRRT apply, particularly for those patients >15 kg.[136] Key differences, depending on size and weight, for this patient group are: 1) a smaller membrane surface area (size), and smaller circuit tubing to reduce priming and circuit volume; 2) a smaller access catheter (<7 Fr) depending on body weight and often placed in the femoral vein; 3) blood flow rate 3–5 mL/kg/min; 4) fluids flow (dialysate or substitution) rates – variable depending on mode but 2 L/1.73 m^2/h is common; 5) increased prevention of hypothermia as this problem is

FIGURE 18.23 NxStage System One CRRT machine, NxStage, Lawrence, MA.

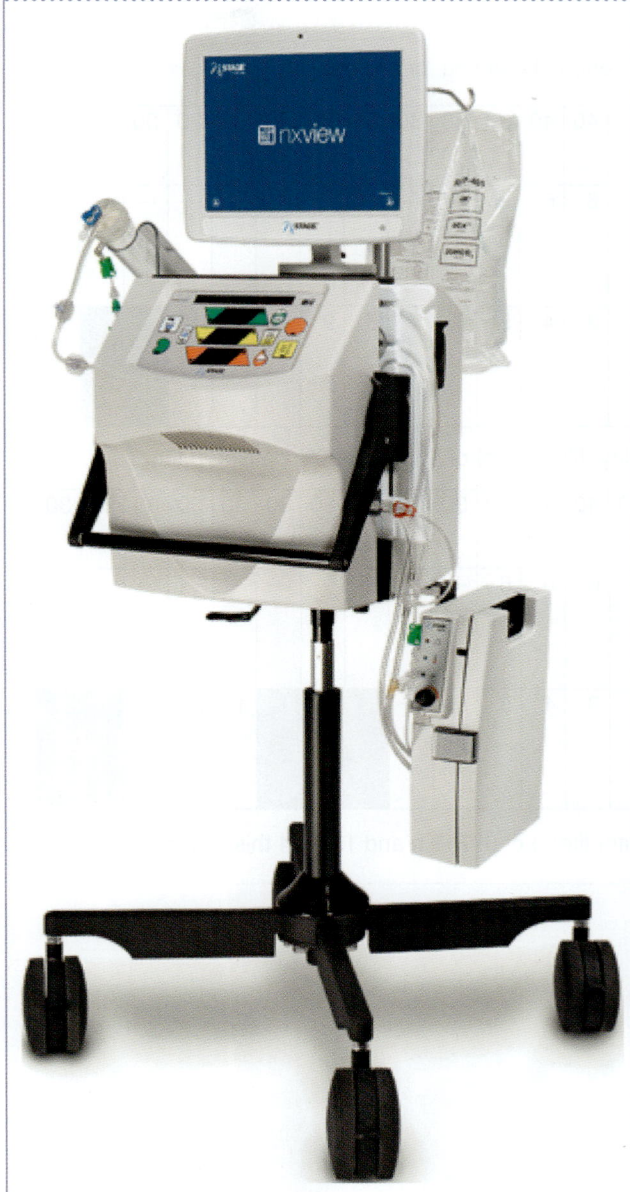

Courtesy NxStage Medical, Lawrence, MA, USA

exacerbated in babies and small infants.[137] Anticoagulation is the same as for adults but with reduced drug doses for the size of the infant or child.[137]

Extracorporeal membrane oxygenation

Increasingly, extracorporeal membrane oxygenation (ECMO) is applied for those with refractory hypoxaemia in association with respiratory failure or used in the context of right heart failure and combined heart-lung failure.[138] These critically ill patients frequently have AKI and require CRRT.[139] It is convenient and often necessary to connect the CRRT circuit into the ECMO circuit as the patient may have other access sites used for multiple cannulation. In any case, the high blood flow associated with ECMO and the placement of the circuit tubing allows for a connection of the CRRT circuit at many places. The preferred attachment site is pre-oxygenator.[140] The only limiting factor is the positive pressure in the ECMO circuit, which is not compatible with the normally negative access pressure when using venous access with a CRRT machine. Some machines provide a software option to select access pressure +ve, allowing this use with ECMO, others do not and may require some alarm override or restrictive device to create negative pressure for the outflow from the ECMO into the CRRT line. Some simple techniques used for insertion of a CRRT circuit into the ECMO circuit can be used to prevent excess pressure alarms.[141]

The anticoagulation provided for the use of ECMO is a convenient state for the successful use of the CRRT and much of this is usually controlled by a perfusionist or a cardiac anaesthetist overseeing the ECMO support in conjunction with the ICU nurse.[139]

Blood purification

This term can be used for all and any mode or technique associated with an EC and removal of wastes and or toxins by diffusion, convection (or both) or by removal and discard of whole plasma with equal replacement (plasma exchange or apheresis).[142] In some approaches, plasma is removed or separated from the blood and pumped through a highly adsorptive membrane to remove toxins or protein bound drugs, and the clean plasma returned to the EC and patient.[142] In other blood purification methods, different membranes are used to be more selective for larger molecules and target various blood mediators associated with a target illness; sepsis for example.[143] These are known as high flux or high sieving coefficient membranes[144] and are useful when rhabdomyolysis is treated. This condition occurs secondary to trauma and particularly crush injury with a high release of myoglobin and myoglobinuria presenting, which is toxic to the kidney and a cause of AKI.[145]

Operating theatre

There are some circumstances when CRRT is useful in the operating theatre. This is in association with any prolonged surgical case where AKI exists in association with a critical illness and specific surgery such as hepatic transplant. Local factors related to ICU staffing, and the surgical and anaesthetic teams' working relationship with the ICU, will influence exactly how this is achieved. The literature in this area is sparse;[146] however, retrospective and small data sets reflect that CRRT in the operating theatre is achievable and safe.[147]

FIGURE 18.24 Bedside charts concept image with consecutive filter life hours associated with hourly vital signs and charting in the ICU. Time on and off treatment easily identified. In addition to total hours delivered each day (h and % of 24).

First entry at 0100 h, beginning a 24-h period of charting or e-recording

Infusion A (mg/hr)	30	30	30	30	30	40	40	40	40	40	40	40	40	30	30	30	30	30	30	30	30	30	30	30
Infusion B (mg/hr)	5	5	5	5	5	5	5	5	6	6	6	6	6	6	---	---	---	---	---	---	---	---	---	---
CRRT filter 'life' h cumulative	28	29	30	31	32	33	34	35		1	2	3	4	5	6	7	8	9	10	11	12			1

The above charting concepts shows continuity from previous day: filter life(s) of 35, 12 h, 90% delivered time

Infusion A (mg/hr)	30	30	30	30	30	40	40	40	40	40	40	40	40	30	30	30	30	30	30	30	30	30	30	30
Infusion B (mg/hr)	5	5	5	5	5	5	5	5	6	6	6	6	6	6	---	---	---	---	---	---	---	---	---	---
CRRT filter 'life' h cumulative	---	---	---	1	2	3	4	5		1	2	3	4	5	6	7				1	2	3		

The above charting concepts shows CRRT starting day, and filter life(s) of 5, 7, 3 h and 15 h/24 this day. 62%

Summary

In this chapter a review of the important physiological functions of the kidney is provided and the context of kidney failure is also defined as an injury, or AKI, and this can be considered in stages of severity and is the basis of classification as for other organ failures. Management of patients with AKI is discussed and includes diagnosis and biomarkers associated, prevention of further injury, fluid and electrolyte balance and aspects of nutrition and pharmacy before consideration of an artificial support or RRT. There are now established criteria for stages of AKI indicating when an artificial kidney support should begin replacing the functions of the kidney. This support is broadly termed dialysis but is provided in the many variants of RRT, and as a continuous therapy in the ICU setting as CRRT. The history of dialysis is relevant as nurses have always played an important role in providing this treatment that, when integrated into the care of the critically ill, requires substantial clinical knowledge and technical skills. The machine and circuit for CRRT are useful to understand as these assist preparation, connection to the patient and then troubleshooting during use. The major failing of CRRT is clotting of the EC, and anticoagulation approaches are the key preventive strategy. When clotting occurs, delays occur, and time is lost before restarting and this is a key communication time with prescribers to prevent a secondary failure of treatment, e.g. a positive fluid balance. Teaching CRRT and quality review are very important for a successful program in the ICU. Finally, the concept of blood purification techniques is introduced and the use of CRRT in special considerations is briefly discussed, which includes use in the operating theatre, with small children and use with ECMO.

Case study

A 27-year-old woman was admitted with advanced intrahepatic cholangiocarcinoma and two days ago she underwent a right hepatectomy. During this surgery, she experienced intraabdominal bleeding and became hypotensive requiring several units of blood products and vasopressor therapy. She has also now developed AKI and requires CRRT.

Neuro: She is currently intubated and sedated, and receiving intravenous fentanyl for pain and sedation management.

Cardiovascular: Vasopressin is being administered to maintain the mean arterial pressure >60 mmHg. Her electrolytes are normal.

Pulmonary: She had one episode of desaturation overnight and remains on positive end-expiratory pressure 10 mmHg. Her chest X-ray is normal but lung sounds are diminished at the bases, and occasional rhonchi are heard.

Renal: She is currently on CRRT, CVVHD, net loss of 100 mL. Dialysate fluid 2.5 L/ h, blood flow rate 250 mL/min. Albumin 25 g of 25% has been ordered to improve blood pressure and replace volume. Intermittent catheterisation is undertaken every 48 h. Vancomycin levels require monitoring.

Gastrointestinal: A nasoduodenal tube is in place for enteral feeding. She is currently being fed at goal rate.

Infectious diseases: She has evidence of right groin wound cellulitis. Her white blood cell count is decreasing and she continues on broad spectrum antibiotics meropenem, vancomycin and tobramycin.

Endocrine: She has experienced episodes of hypoglycaemia, which have been managed with intravenous dextrose 10%, titrated to blood glucose levels.

Hematology: A full blood count is taken every 6 h including assessment of coagulation factors and fibrinogen. She is receiving vitamin K 10 mg once daily.

Skin: Her skin is intact, except for her groin wound, which is dressed.

Lines: She has a right subclavian double lumen central venous catheter, a right internal jugular dialysis catheter, and a right radial arterial line.

CASE STUDY QUESTIONS

1. Is CRRT (continuous treatment) or intermittent haemodialysis three times a week most appropriate for this patient?
2. You note that the ordered net fluid loss removal via CRRT of 100 mL/h seems to be creating fluctuations in heart rate; her blood pressure is not stable with hypotension (systolic less than 80 mmHg, frequently). What could you do in this case?
3. Is a blood flow rate of 250 mL/min too high? Why do you think it is ordered at this rate?
4. Should this patient be on anticoagulation to keep the CRRT circuit patent?

RESEARCH VIGNETTE

A retrospective review of fluid balance control in CRRT. Davies H, Leslie GD, Morgan D. Aust Crit Care 2017;30(6):14-319

Introduction: An effect of severe acute kidney injury (AKI) is the development of oliguria and subsequent retention of fluid. Recent studies have reported an association between fluid overload and increased mortality in critically ill patients. Achieving fluid balance control through haemofiltration is an important part of dialysis dose delivery in continuous renal replacement therapy (CRRT).

Aims: 1) Compare the prescribed dose with the delivered dose of dialysis and haemofiltration for CRRT. 2) Identify how interruptions and delays in treatment delivery impact on fluid balance management.

Method: A retrospective cohort study was undertaken of daily fluid balance and fluid removal for patients who required CRRT. Each observation chart and prescription order for every treatment day was reviewed. Each patient was exposed to the same treatment mode, predilutional continuous veno-venous haemodiafiltration (CVVHDf). A comparison was made of fluid balance control delivered to the patient over 24 h against the dose of fluid removal prescribed.

Results: The observation charts of 46 consecutive patients were reviewed for total of 288 treatment days. Median number of days patients received CRRT was 5 (range 1–31). Median circuit life was 16 h (range 0–66). Fluid removal targets did not occur in 75 (26%) treatment days. Median daily fluid removal shortfall was 300 mL (range 25–3800 mL). Mean number of daily treatment interruptions 1.25, SD±0.49. The most frequent cause of treatment downtime was circuit clotting (45%). Mean length of treatment downtime was 3.71, SD±4.36h excluding delays attributed to assessment of renal function.

Conclusion: In over a quarter of treatment days, prescribed fluid removal was not achieved. Frequency of interruptions and delays in resumption of treatment compromised fluid balance control. Daily targets for fluid removal which are not achieved contribute to fluid overload and may compromise the outcome of patients who require CRRT.

Critique

Fluid administration, urine output and 'balance' assessment are vital throughout all stages of kidney failure. As with normal renal function, monitoring the fluid loss or 'urine output' during CRRT hourly is also necessary to ensure this aspect of renal replacement is being achieved. Prescribing a loss and delivering this are not always completed. Nursing provides the essential role to identify the patient fluid status, report and communicate this to the medical team, and then follow the prescribing goal. However, nurses using this technology must adapt and respond to the frequent and many interruptions and changes to the equation associated with interventions and care of a critically ill patient throughout the day and night.

Davies, Leslie and Morgan provide a useful publication and good example of nursing research where data and evidence can improve nursing practice and develop safer care. They report their findings from an adult intensive care where positive fluid balance during CRRT was frequent and fluid balance targets were not being achieved. This finding was at a time where others were reporting the association between positive fluid balance during AKI and mortality.

The authors conducted a retrospective review over a 4-month period using a convenience sample design. Data was collected for case demographics and patients with AKI treated with CRRT, and primary research aims were assessment of fluid balance control. Key aims were to review prescribed and delivered dose or effective treatment time and to identify interruptions and delays with treatment. This approach provided a new and important understanding for the cause of positive fluid balance when treatments are stopped unexpectedly and with delay before restart. Unless the fluid loss settings are increased and 'catch up' thinking and a change to hourly fluid removal and loss settings is applied, targets are not met. In addition, the task or target for the next day may then be increased and more difficult; the authors termed this a 'carry over' effect.

Two hundred and eighty-eight charts (24h) were reviewed including 46 patients. This data reflected the use of 277 CRRT circuits with a median life or time before clotting/stopping of 15.5 h. Clotting was associated with 45%. Delay before restart was 3.71 h and was up to 26 h. Overall, 26% of all treatments did not achieve daily fluid balance and a median shortfall of 300 mL. For the last day of a treatment, 37% of the patients assessed remained in a positive fluid balance.

Some important conclusions and discussion were the 'carry over' effect for fluid balance targets where nurses need to identify this, report and discuss with medical prescribers and change the settings accordingly. As prescribing is usually with forecast or expected status for each 24-h period, continuity and minimal interruption to CRRT is essential and not well recognised. The 'off-time' is a further, and also underrated, aspect of CRRT use, acknowledging nursing is the primary role to minimise this. Charting for fluid balance has been an hourly nursing task when managing CRRT, but evaluation of the overall 'balance' (input and output calculation) was less frequent; e.g. every 6 or 12 h. If the balance assessment is provided each hour when charting is undertaken, any prescribing and failure of delivery and imbalance can be identified and changes made.

More recent adoption of electronic charting software may provide this improvement in fluid balance management and prompt more frequent response with improved outcomes. Finally, weighing patients in the ICU is useful on admission and daily throughout their stay, helping to identify positive fluid state by weight gain.

Learning activities

1. Review the filter or circuit 'life' and the 'off time' in your ICU and compare to the data presented in the *Research vignette*.
2. Suggest further research for this area of fluid balance and prescribed compared with delivered 'dose' and achievement of control.
3. Audit your patient during CRRT and assess for any fluid removal shortfall.
4. Consider and suggest ideas to prevent any daily fluid removal shortfall; a policy or practice change for your ICU.

Online resources

Acute Dialysis Quality Initiative, www.ADQI.org

Continuous renal replacement therapies, www.ccrtonline.com

Pediatric continuous renal replacement therapy, www.pcrrt.com

Further reading

Bellomo R, Vaara ST, Kellum JA. How to improve the care of patients with acute kidney injury. Intensive Care Med 2017;43:727–9.

Cerdá J, Baldwin I, Honore P, et al. Role of technology for the management of AKI in critically ill patients: from adoptive technology to precision continuous renal replacement therapy. Blood Purif 2016;42:248–65.

Dunn W, Shyamala S. Filter lifespan in critically ill adults receiving continuous renal replacement therapy: the effect of patient and treatment-related variables. Crit Care Resusc 2014;16(3):225–31.

Fealy N, Aitken L, du Toit E, et al. Continuous renal replacement therapy: current practice in Australian and New Zealand intensive care units. Crit Care Resusc 2015;17:83–91.

Fuhrman DY, Kellum JA. Biomarkers for diagnosis, prognosis and intervention in acute kidney injury. Contrib Nephrol 2016;187:47–54.

Kellum JA, Bellomo R, Ronco C. Does this patient have acute kidney injury? An AKI checklist. Intensive Care Med 2016;42:96–9.

Kellum JA, Sileanu FE, Murugan R, et al. Classifying AKI by urine output versus serum creatinine level. J Am Soc Nephrol 2015;26(9):231–8.

Legrand M, Darmon M, Joannidis M, et al. Management of renal replacement therapy in ICU patients: an international survey. Intensive Care Med 2013;39:101–8.

Rewa OG, Villeneuve PM, Lachance P, et al. Quality indicators of continuous renal replacement therapy (CRRT) care in critically ill patients: a systematic review. Intensive Care Med 2017;43(6):50–763.

Schneider AG, Baldwin I, Freitag E, et al. Estimation of fluid status changes in critically ill patients: fluid balance chart or electronic bed weight? J Crit Care 2012;27(6):45, e7–12.

Zhang L, Baldwin I, Zhu G, et al. Automated electronic monitoring of circuit pressures during continuous renal replacement therapy: a technical report. Crit Care Resusc 2015;17(1):1–54.

References

1. Murugan R, Kellum J. Acute kidney injury: what's the prognosis? Nat Rev Nephrol 2011;7(4):209–17.
2. Kellum JA, Bellomo R, Ronco C. Definition and classification of acute kidney injury. Nephron Clin Pract 2008;109:c182–7.
3. Kellum JA, Bellomo R, Ronco C. The concept of acute kidney injury and the RIFLE criteria. In: Ronco C, Bellomo R, Kellum J, editors. Contributions to nephrology, vol. 156. Basel: Karger; 2007. p. 10–16.
4. Kidney Disease: Improving Global Outcomes (KDIGO) Acute Kidney Injury Work Group. KDIGO clinical practice guideline for acute kidney injury. Kidney Int Suppl (2011) 2012;2:1–138.
5. Dirkx TC, Woodell T, Watnick S. Kidney disease. In: Papadakis M, McPhee S, editors. Current medical diagnosis and treatment. New York: McGraw-Hill; 2018.
6. The kidneys and body fluids. In: Guyton AC, Hall JE, editors. Textbook of medical physiology. 13th ed. Philadelphia: WB Saunders; 2016.
7. Gray's anatomy of the human body: the Bartleby.com edition. Available from: http://www.bartleby.com/107/253.html. [Accessed August 2014].
8. Bellomo R, Kellum JA, Ronco C. Acute kidney injury. Lancet 2012;380:756–66.
9. Chalkias A, Xanthos T. Acute kidney injury (Letter). Lancet 2012;380:1904.A.
10. Odutayo A, Wong CX, Farkouh M, et al. AKI and long-term risk for cardiovascular events and mortality. J Am Soc Nephrol 2017;28(1): 377–87.
11. Hendenstierna G, Larsson A. Influence of abdominal pressure on respiratory and abdominal organ function. Curr Opin Crit Care 2012;18: 80–5.
12. Blantz RC, Singh P. Analysis of the prerenal contributions to acute kidney injury. Contrib Nephrol 2011;174:4–11.
13. Zimmerman JL, Shen MC. Rhabdomyolysis. Chest 2013;144(3):1058–65.
14. Weisbord SD, Gallagher M, Jneid N, et al. Outcomes after angiography with sodium bicarbonate and acetylcystine. N Engl J Med 2017.
15. Mei M, Zhao HW, et al. Efficacy of acetylecystine in preventing acute kidney injury after cardiac surgery: a meta -analysis. J Invest Surg 2018;31(1).
16. Sheridan A, Bonventre J. Pathophysiology of ischaemic acute renal failure. Contrib Nephrol 2001;132:7–21.
17. Han SS, Kim S, Ahn SY, et al. Duration of acute kidney injury and mortality in critically ill patients: a retrospective observational study. BMC Nephrol 2013;14:133.
18. Uchino S, Bellomo R, Bagshaw SM, et al. Transient azotaemia is associated with a high risk of death in hospitalized patients. Nephrol Dial Transplant 2010;25(6):1833–9. doi:10.1093/ndt/gfp624. [Epub 2010 Jan 6].
19. Bonventre JV. Pathophysiology of ischemic acute renal failure. Inflammation, lung-kidney cross talk, and biomarkers. Contrib Nephrol 2004;144:19–30.
20. Bonventre JV. Dedifferentiation and proliferation of surviving epithelial cells in acute renal failure. J Am Soc Nephrol 2003;14(Suppl. 1):S55–61.
21. Endre ZH. Acute renal failure. In: Whitworth JA, Lawrence JR, Kincaid-Smith P, editors. Textbook of renal disease. 2nd ed. Edinburgh: Churchill Livingstone; 1994.
22. Krum H, Abraham WT. Heart failure. Lancet 2009;373:941–55.
23. Kamath PS, Kim WR, Advanced Liver Disease Study Group. The model for end-stage liver disease (MELD). Hepatology 2007;45(3): 797–805. Review.
24. Cumming AD. Acute renal failure: definitions and diagnosis. In: Ronco C, Bellomo R, editors. Critical care nephrology. Dordrecht: Kluwer Academic; 1998.
25. Myers BD, Moran SM. Haemodynamically mediated acute renal failure. N Engl J Med 1986;314:97–105.
26. Iaina A, Peer G. Post surgery/polytrauma and acute renal failure. In: Ronco C, Bellomo R, editors. Critical care nephrology. Dordrecht: Kluwer Academic; 1998.
27. Jamal JA, Mueller BA, Choi GYS, et al. How can we ensure antibiotic dosing in critically ill patients receiving different types of renal replacement therapy? Diagn Microbiol Infect Dis 2015;82:92–103.
28. Möckel M, Radovic M, Kühnle Y, et al. Acute renal haemodynamic effects of radiocontrast media in patients undergoing left ventricular and coronary angiography. Nephrol Dial Transplant 2008;23(5):1588–94.
29. Endre ZH. Post cardiac surgery acute renal failure in the 1990s. Aust N Z J Med 1997;25:278–9.
30. White LE, Hassoun HT. Inflammatory mechanisms of organ crosstalk during ischemic acute kidney injury. Int J Nephrol 2012;2012:505197.
31. Waikar SS, Betensky RA, Emerson SC, et al. Imperfect gold standards for biomarker evaluation. Clin Trials 2013;10(5):696–700.
32. Andreucchi M, Faga T, Pisani A, et al. The ischemic/ nephrotoxic acute kidney injury and the use of biomarkers in clinical practice. Eur J Intern Med 2017;39:1–8.
33. Pakula AM, Skinner RA. Acute kidney injury in the critically ill patient: a current review of the literature. J Intensive Care Med 2016;m31(5): 319–24.
34. Mishra J, Ma Q, Prada A, et al. Identificationof neutrophil gelatinase-associated lipocalin as a novel early urinary biomarker for ischemic renal injury. J Am Soc Nephrol 2003;14:2534–43.

35. Mishra J, Dent C, Tarabishi R, et al. Neutrophil gelatinase-associated lipocalin (NGAL) as a biomarker for acute renal injury after cardiac surgery. Lancet 2005;365(9466):1231–8.
36. Parikh CR, Coca SG, Thiessen-Philbrook H, et al. Postoperative biomarkers predict acute kidney injury and poor outcomes after adult cardiac surgery. J Am Soc Nephrol 2011;22(9):1748–57.
37. Schmidt-Ott KM. Neutrophil gelatinase-associated lipocalin as a biomarker of acute kidney injury–where do we stand today? Nephrol Dial Transplant 2011;26:762–4.
38. Ichimura T, Hung CC, Yang SA, et al. Kidney injury molecule-1: a tissue and urinary biomarker for nephrotoxicant-induced renal injury. Am J Physiol Renal Physiol 2004;286(3):F552–63.
39. Parravicini E. The clinical utility of urinary neutrophil gelatinase-associated lipocalin in the neonatal ICU. Parravicini E. Curr Opin Pediatr 2010;22(2):146–50.
40. Lamiere N, Vanholder R, vanBiesen W. How to use biomarkers efficiently in acute kidney injury. Kidney Int 2011;1047–50.
41. Liu Y, Guo W, Zhang CF, et al. Urinary interlukin-18 is a marker for human acute tubular necrosis. Am J Kidney Dis 2004;43(3):405–14.
42. Sjostrom P, Tidman M, Jones I. Determination of the production rate and non-renal clearance of cystatin-C and estimation of the glomerular filtration rate for the serum concentratin of cystatin-C in humans. Scand J Clin Lab Invest 2005;65(2):111–24.
43. Honore PM, Nguyen BH, Gong M, et al. Urinary tissue inhibitor of mettalopro-teinases-2 and insulin-like growth factor binding protein-7 for risk stratification of acute kidney injury in patients with sepsis. Crit Care Med 2016;44(10):1851–60.
44. Kellum JA, Chawla LS. Cell-cycle arrest and acute kidney injury: the light and the dark sides. Nephrol Dial Transplant 2016;31(1):16–22.
45. Marino R, Struck J, Hartmann O, et al. Diagnostic and short-term prognostic utility plasma pro-enkephalin (pro-ENK) for acute kidney injury in patients admitted with sepsis to the emergency department. J Nephrol 2015;28:717–24.
46. Sezen SF, Kenigs VA, Kapusta DR. Renal excretory responses produced by the delta opioid agonist BW373U86 in conscious rats. J Pharmacol Exp Ther 1998;287:238–45.
47. Seifter JL, Samuels MA. Uremic encephalopathy and other brain disorders associated with renal failure. Semin Neurol 2011;31(2):139–43.
48. Gams ME, Rabbs H. The distal organ effect of acute kidney injury. Kidney Int 2012;81:942–8. doi:10.1038/ki.2011.241.
49. Schrier RW. Fluid administration in critically ill patients with acute kidney injury. Clin J Am Soc Nephrol 2010;5(4):733–9.
50. Levey AS, Eckardt KU, Tsukamoto Y, et al. Definition and classification of chronic kidney disease: a position statement from Kidney Disease: Improving Global Outcomes (KDIGO). Kidney Int 2005;67(6):2089–100.
51. Ronco C, Levin A, Warnock DG, et al; AKIN Working Group. Improving outcomes from acute kidney injury (AKI): report on an initiative. Int J Artif Organs 2007;30(5):373–6.
52. Gayat E, Touchard C, Hollinger A, et al. Back-to-back comparison of penKid with Nephrocheck to predict acute kidney injury at admission in the intensive care unit: a brief report. Crit Care 2018;22:24.
53. Meersch M, Schmidt C, Van Aken H, et al. Urinary TIMP-2 and IGFBP7 as early biomarkers of acute kidney injury and renal recovery following cardiac surgery. PLoS ONE 2014;9:e93460.
54. Cole L, Bellomo R, Silvester W, et al. A prospective, multicenter study of the epidemiology, management and outcome of severe acute renal failure in a 'closed' ICU system. Am J Respir Crit Care Med 2000;162:191–6.
55. Bellomo R, Ronco C, Kellum J, et al; ADQI working group. Acute renal failure: definition, outcome measures, animal models, fluid therapy and information technology needs: the Second International Consensus Conference of the Acute Dialysis Quality Initiative (ADQI) Group. Crit Care 2004;8(4):R204–12.
56. Finfer S, Norton R, Bellomo R, et al; on behalf of the SAFE Study Investigators. The SAFE study: saline versus albumin for fluid resuscitation in the critically ill patient. Vox Sang 2004;87(Suppl. 2):S123–31.
57. Irfan M, Idris A. Overview of PES biocompatible / hemodialysis membranes: PES blood interactions and modification techniques. Mater Sci Eng C Mater Biol Appl 2015;56:574–92.
58. Koyner JL, Shaw AD, Chawla LS, et al. TIMP*IGFBP7 biomarker panel accurately predicts acute kidney injury in high risk surgical patients. J Trauma Acute Care Surg 2016;80(2):243–9.
59. Otero A, Apalkov A, Fernández R, et al. A new device to automate the monitoring of critical patients' urine output. Biomed Res Int 2014;2014:Article ID 587593. http://dx.doi.org/10.1155/2014/587593.
60. The RENAL Replacement Therapy Study Investigators. An observational study for fluid balance and patient outcomes in the randomized evaluation of normal vs. augmented level of replacement therapy trial. Crit Care Med 2012;40:1753–60.
61. Peake SL, Chapman MJ, Davies AR, et al; George Institute for Global Health; Australian and New Zealand Intensive Care Society Clinical Trials Group. Enteral nutrition in Australian and New Zealand intensive care units: a point-prevalence study of prescription practices. Crit Care Resusc 2012;14(2):148–53.
62. Fiaccadori E, Cremaschi E, Regolisti G. Nutritional assessment and delivery in renal replacement therapy patients. Semin Dial 2011;24(2):169–75.
63. Bellomo R, Prowle J. Diuretic therapy in fluid overloaded and heart failure patients. Contrib Nephrol 2010;164:153–63.
64. Alobaidi R, Morgan C, Basu RK, et al. Association between fluid balance and outcomes in critically ill children: a systematic review and meta-analysis. JAMA Pediatr 2018;172(3):257–68.
65. Prowle JR, Echeverri JE, Ligabo EV, et al. Fluid balance and acute kidney injury. Nat Rev Nephrol 2010;6(2):107–15.

66. Bellomo R, Ronco C. Indications and criteria for initiating renal replacement therapy in the intensive care unit. Kidney Int 1998;53(S66):s106–9.
67. Ostermann M, Dickie H, Tovey L, et al. Management of sodium disorders during continuous haemofiltration. Crit Care 2010;14:418.
68. Choi G, Gomersall CD, Tain Q, et al. Principles of antibacterial dosing in continuous real replacement therapy. Crit Care Med 2009;37: 2268–82.
69. Medline Plus. Online Medical Dictionary. Online. Available from: https://medlineplus.gov/ency/patientinstructions/000707.htm. [Accessed March 2019].
70. Vienken J, Diamantoglou M, Henne W, et al. Artificial dialysis membranes: from concept to large scale production. Am J Nephrol 1999;9:355–62.
71. Cameron JS. Practical haemodialysis began with cellophane and heparin: the crucial role of William Thalhimer (1884–1961). Nephrol Dial Transplant 2000;15:1086–91.
72. Ronco C, La Greca G. The role of technology in hemodialysis. Contrib Nephrol 2002;137:1–12.
73. Baldwin I, Elderkin T. Continuous hemofiltration: nursing perspectives in critical care. New Horiz 1995;3(4):738–47.
74. Martin R, Jurschak J. Nursing management of continuous renal replacement therapy. Semin Dial 1996;9(2):192–9.
75. Mehta R, Martin R. Initiating and implementing a continuous renal replacement therapy program. Semin Dial 1996;9(2):80–7.
76. Wild J. Peritoneal dialysis. In: Thomas N, editor. Renal nursing. 2nd ed. London: Baillière Tindall; 2002.
77. Kramer P, Wigger W, Rieger J, et al. Arteriovenous haemofiltration: a new and simple method for treatment of overhydrated patients resistant to diuretics. Klin Wochenschr 1977;55:1121–2.
78. Ronco C, Brendolan A, Bellomo R. Current technology for continuous renal replacement therapies. In: Ronco C, Bellomo R, editors. Critical care nephrology. Dordrecht: Kluwer Academic; 1998.
79. Baldwin I, Fealy N. Nursing for renal replacement therapies in the intensive care unit: historical, educational, and protocol review. Blood Purif 2009;27:174–81.
80. Davenport A, Mehta S. The acute dialysis quality initiative – Part VI: access and anticoagulation in CRRT. Adv Ren Replace Ther 2002;9(4):273–81.
81. Ofsthun NJ, Colton CK, Lysaght MJ. Determinants of fluid and solute removal rates during hemofiltration. In: Henderson LW, Quellhorst G, Baldamus CA, et al, editors. Hemofiltration. Berlin: Springer-Verlag; 1986.
82. Baldwin I, Fealy N. Clinical nursing for the application of renal replacement therapies in the intensive care unit. Semin Dial 2009;22(2): 189–93.
83. Thomas N. Haemodialysis. In: Thomas N, editor. Renal nursing. 2nd ed. London: Baillière Tindall; 2002.
84. Baldwin I, Baldwin M, Fealy N, et al. Concurrent versus counter-current dialysate flow during CVVHD. A comparative study for creatinine and urea removal. Blood Purif 2016;41:171–6.
85. Ronco C, Bellomo R. Basic mechanisms and definitions for continuous renal replacement therapies. Int J Artif Organs 1996;19:95–9.
86. Bellomo R, Ronco C, Mehta R. Technique of continuous renal replacement therapy: nomenclature for continuous renal replacement therapies. Am J Kidney Dis 1996;28(5 Suppl. 3):s2–7.
87. VA/NIH Acute Renal Failure Trial Network, Palevsky PM, Zhang JH, et al. Intensity of renal support in critically ill patients with acute kidney injury. N Engl J Med 2008;359(1):7–20.
88. Bai M, Zhou M, He L, et al. Citrate versus heparin anticoagulation for continuous renal replacement therapy: an updated meta-analysis of RCTs. Intensive Care Med 2015;41(12):2098–110.
89. Bellomo R, Cole L, Reeves J, et al. Who should manage CRRT in the ICU? The intensivist's viewpoint. Am J Kidney Dis 1997;30(5 Suppl. 4):S109–11.
90. Boyle M, Baldwin I. Understanding the continuous renal replacement therapy circuit for acute renal failure support; a quality issue in the intensive care unit. AACN Adv Crit Care 2010;21(4):365–75.
91. Uchino S, Fealy N, Baldwin I, et al. Pre-dilution vs. post-dilution during continuous veno-venous hemofiltration: impact on filter life and azotemic control. Nephron Clin Pract 2003;94(4):94–8.
92. Clark WR, Gao D, Lorenzin A, et al. Membranes and sorbents. Contrib Nephrol 2018;194:70–9.
93. Godden J, Spexarth F, Dahlgren M. Standardization of continuous renal-replacement therapy fluids using a commercial product. Am J Health Syst Pharm 2012;69(9):786–93.
94. Relton S, Greenberg A, Palevsky P. Dialysate and blood flow dependence of diffusive solute clearance during CVVHD. ASAIO J 1992;38(3): M691–6.
95. Honore PM, Jacobs R, Joannes-Boyau O, et al. Newly designed CRRT membranes for sepsis and SIRS-a pragmatic approach for bedside intensivists summarizing the more recent advances: a systematic structured review. ASAIO J 2013;59:99–106.
96. Davenport A, Mehta S. The acute dialysis quality initiative – Part VI: access and anticoagulation in CRRT. Adv Ren Replace Ther 2002;9(4): 273–81.
97. Honore PM, Spapen HD. Evolution of vascular access and anticoagulation. Contrib Nephrol 2018;194:15–24.
98. Baldwin I, Bellomo R, Koch B. A technique for the monitoring of blood flow during continuous hemofiltration. Intens Care Med 2002;28: 1361–4.

99. Kox WJ, Rohr U, Wauer H. Practical aspects of renal replacement therapy. Int J Artif Organs 1996;19(2):100–5.
100. Morgan D, Ho K, Murray C, et al. A randomized trial of catheters of different lengths to achieve right atrium versus superior vena cava placement for continuous renal replacement therapy. Am J Kidney Dis 2012;60(2):272–9.
101. Baldwin I, Bellomo R, Koch W. Blood flow reductions during continuous renal replacement therapy and circuit life. Intensive Care Med 2004;30:2074–9.
102. Fealy N, Aitken L, du Toit E, et al. Continuous renal replacement therapy: current practice in Australian and New Zealand intensive care units. Crit Care Resusc 2015;17:83–91.
103. Crosswell A, Brain MJ, Roodenburg O. Vascular access site influences circuit life in continuous renal replacement therapy. Crit Care Resusc 2014;16(2):127–30.
104. Baldwin I. Factors affecting circuit patency and filter life. In: Ronco C, Bellomo R, Kellum J, editors. Contributions to nephrology, vol. 156. Basel: Karger; 2007. p. 178–84.
105. Baldwin I, Fealy N, Carty P, et al. Bubble trap chamber clotting during continuous renal replacement therapy: vertical versus horizontal blood flow entry. Blood Purif 2012;34:213–18.
106. Clarke WR, Turk JE. Approaches to quotidian analysis: the NxStage system one. Semin Dial 2004;17(2):167–70.
107. Dirkes S, Wonnacott R. Continuous renal replacement therapy and anticoagulation: what are the options? Crit Care Nurse 2016;36(2): 34–41.
108. Tolwani AJ, Wille K. Anticoagulation for continuous renal replacement therapy. Semin Dial 2009;22(2):141–5.
109. Karakala N, Tolwani A. We use heparin as the anticoagulant for CRRT. Semin Dial 2016;29(4):272–4.
110. Baldwin I, Tan HK, Bridge N, et al. Possible strategies to prolong circuit life during hemofiltration: three controlled studies. Ren Fail 2002;24(6):839–48.
111. Leslie G, Jacobs I, Clarke G. Proximally delivered high volume heparin does not improve circuit life in continuous venovenous haemodiafiltration (CVVHD). Intensive Care Med 1996;22:1261–4.
112. Tolwani A, Wille KM. Regional citrate anticoagulation for continuous renal replacement therapy: the better alternative? Am J Kidney Dis 2012;59(6):745–7.
113. Schneider AG, Journois D, Rimmelé T. Complications of regional citrate anticoagulation: accumulation or overload? Crit Care 2017;21(1):281.
114. Davies H, Morgan D, Leslie GD. A regional citrate anticoagulation protocol for pre-dilutional CVVHDf: the 'Alabama concept'. Aust Crit Care 2008;21(3):154–6.
115. Grouzi E. Update on argatroban for the prophylaxis and treatment of heparin-induced thrombocytopenia type II. J Blood Med 2014;5: 131–41.
116. Link A, Girndt M, Selejan S, et al. Argatroban for anticoagulation in continuous renal replacement therapy. Crit Care Med 2009;37(1): 105–10.
117. Saugel B, Phillip V, Moessmer G, et al. Argatroban therapy for heparin induced thrombocytopenia in ICU patients with multiple organ dysfunction syndrome: a retrospective study. Crit Care 2012;16(2):415.
118. Aucella F, Di Paolo S, Gesualdo L. Dialysate and fluid composition for CRRT. Contrib Nephrol 2007;156:287–96.
119. Davenport A. Replacement and dialysate fluids for patients with acute renal failure treated by continuous veno-venous haemofiltration and/or haemodiafiltration. Contrib Nephrol 2004;144:317–28.
120. Baldwin I, Bellomo R. Sustained low efficiency dialysis in the ICU. Int J Intensive Care 2002;Winter:177–87.
121. Zhang L, Yang J, Eastwood GM, et al. Extended daily dialysis versus continuous renal replacement therapy for acute kidney injury: a meta-analysis. Am J Kidney Dis 2015;66(2):322–30.
122. Davies H, Leslie GD, Morgan D. A retrospective review of fluid balance control in CRRT. Aust Crit Care 2017;30(6):314–19.
123. Davies H, Leslie GD, Morgan D, et al. A comparison of compliance in the estimation of body fluid status using daily fluid balance charting and body weight changes during continuous renal replacement therapy. Aust Crit Care 2018;pii: S1036-7314(17)30286-2.
124. Sutherland SM, Zappitelli M, Alexander SR, et al. Fluid overload and mortality in children receiving continuous renal replacement therapy: the prospective pediatric continuous renal replacement therapy registry. Am J Kidney Dis 2010;55:316–25.
125. Bouchard J, Soroko SB, Chertow GM, et al; and the PICARD group. Fluid accumulation, survival and recovery of kidney function in critically ill patients with acute kidney injury. Kidney Int 2009;76:422–7.
126. Murugan R, Hoste E, Mehta RL, et al; Acute Disease Quality Initiative (ADQI) Consensus Group. Precision fluid management in continuous renal replacement therapy. Blood Purif 2016;42(3):266–78.
127. Baldwin I. Training, management and credentialling for CRRT in critical care. Am J Kidney Dis 1997;30(5):S112–16.
128. Graham P, Lischer E. Nursing issues in renal replacement therapy: organization, manpower assessment, competency evaluation and quality improvement processes. Semin Dial 2011;24(2):183–7.
129. Przybyl H, Evans J, Haley L, et al. Training and maintaining: developing a successful and dynamic continuous renal replacement therapy program. AACN Adv Crit Care 2017;28(1):41–50.
130. Dirkes S, Hodge K. Continuous renal replacement therapy in the adult intensive care unit: history and current trends. Crit Care Nurse 2007;27(2):61–6, 68–72, 74–80.

131. Fealy N, Baldwin I, Bellomo R. The effect of circuit down time on uraemic control during continuous veno-venous haemofiltration. Crit Care Resusc 2002;4:266–70.
132. Ronco C. Machines used for continuous renal replacement therapy. In: Kellum J, Bellomo R, Ronco C, editors. Continuous renal replacement therapy. New York: Oxford University Press; 2010.
133. Clark WR, Villa G, Neri M, et al. Advances in machine technology. Contrib Nephrol 2018;194:80–9.
134. Mottes T, Owens T, Niedner M, et al. Improving delivery of continuous renal replacement therapy: impact of a simulation-based educational intervention. Pediatr Crit Care Med 2013;14(8):747–54.
135. Rewa OG, Villeneuve PM, Lachance P, et al. Quality indicators of continuous renal replacement therapy (CRRT) care in critically ill patients: a systematic review. Intensive Care Med 2017;43(6):750–63.
136. Ricci Z, Goldstein SL. Pediatric continuous renal replacement therapy. Contrib Nephrol 2016;187:121–30.
137. Askenazi DJ, Goldstein SL, Koralkar R, et al. Continuous renal replacement therapy for children ≤10 kg: a report from the prospective pediatric continuous renal replacement therapy registry. J Pediatr 2013;162(3):587–92, e3.
138. Combesa A, Bacchettab M, Brodieb D, et al. Extracorporeal membrane oxygenation for respiratory failure in adults. Curr Opin Crit Care 2012;18(1):99–104.
139. Combes A, Brodie D, Bartlett R, et al. Position paper for the organization of extracorporeal membrane oxygenation programs for acute respiratory failure in adult patients. Am J Respir Crit Care Med 2014;190(5):488–96. doi:10.1164/rccm.201404-0630CP.
140. Seczynska B, Krolikowski W, Nowak I, et al. Continuous renal replacement therapy during extracorporeal membrane oxygenation in patients treated in medical intensive care unit: technical considerations. Ther Apher Dial 2014;18(6):523–34.
141. Sandoval CP, Garwood C, et al. Continuous renal replacement therapy case vignettes. AACN Adv Crit Care 2017;28(1):64–73.
142. Lemaire A, Parquet N, Galicier L, et al. Plasma exchange in the intensive care unit: technical aspects and complications. J Clin Apher 2017;32(6):405–12.
143. Clark E, Molnar AO, Joannes-Boyau O, et al. High-volume hemofiltration for septic acute kidney injury: a systematic review and meta analysis. Crit Care 2014;18(1).
144. Ronco C, Clark WR. Haemodialysis membranes. Nat Rev Nephrol 2018;14(6):394–410.
145. Esposito P, Estienne L, Serpieri N, et al. Rhabdomyolysis-associated acute kidney injury. Am J Kidney Dis 2018;71(6):A12–14.
146. Parmar A, Bigam D, Meeberg G, et al. An evaluation of intraoperative renal support during liver transplantation: a matched cohort study. Blood Purif 2011;32(3):238–48.
147. Douthitt L, Bezinover D, Uemura T, et al. Perioperative use of continuous renal replacement therapy for orthotopic liver transplantation. Transplant Proc 2012;44(5):1314–17.

Chapter 19

Nutrition assessment and therapeutic management

Andrea Marshall, Teresa Williams

KEY WORDS

anabolism
catabolism
enteral nutrition
glycaemic control
hypermetabolism
total parenteral nutrition

Learning objectives

After reading this chapter, you should be able to:

- describe the changes in metabolism associated with critical illness
- describe the consequences of malnutrition and how they influence recovery from critical illness
- identify appropriate nutrition assessment strategies and critique methods of determining nutritional requirements in critical illness
- apply theoretical knowledge of nutritional requirements, assessment of and potential for malnutrition in critical illness
- rationalise selected nutritional support strategies for specific clinical conditions
- critically analyse the role of glycaemic control in the context of critical illness.

Introduction

Critical illness is associated with increased catabolism that occurs at a time when oral intake may be difficult or impossible. Failure to provide adequate nutrition during this time will result in an accumulated energy deficit, muscle wasting and decreased lean body mass, which are associated with adverse outcomes. During critical illness optimising protein and energy intake is important because inadequate nutrition, which results in an overall nutrition deficit, is associated with increases in morbidity and mortality. Enteral nutrition (EN) is the preferred method of nutrition therapy for the critically ill although some patients might require parenteral nutrition (PN) or a combination of EN and PN.

As part of the interdisciplinary team, nurses play an important role in achieving optimal nutrition and are responsible for monitoring achievement of nutrition goals and implementing strategies to optimise nutrition intake. In this chapter an overview of metabolism and the consequences of malnutrition are provided. This is followed by discussion of nutritional assessment and delivery strategies where an emphasis is placed on nutrition therapy through the provision of EN. Tailoring nutrition to specific disease states is also included in this chapter. Lastly, we discuss the importance of glycaemic control in critical illness.

Metabolism

The body requires energy in order to support normal body and cellular function. Energy is derived from the metabolism of macronutrients including carbohydrate, protein and fat. Following consumption of food, carbohydrates are broken down and stored as glycogen in the liver and skeletal muscle, and fat, stored in adipose tissue, is available for long-term energy requirements. Proteins and amino acids, however, are not stored and reduced protein intake can result in catabolism of body protein.[1]

The breakdown of food to produce energy is carried out in three phases: 1) the digestion of large macromolecules into simple subunits; 2) intracellular breakdown of subunits to acetyl CoA and production of small amounts of adenosine triphosphate (2 molecules); and 3) production of ATP through oxidative phosphorylation[1] (Fig. 19.1).

Effect of critical illness on metabolism

The stress and injury associated with critical illness triggers the hypothalamus, sympathetic nervous system and adrenal medulla to initiate a response that results in hypercatabolism.[2] Hormones released from the gut and adipose tissue may further trigger the stress response in critically ill patients.[3] Mediators of this response include cytokines including interleukin-1, interleukin-6 and tumour necrosis factor-α and production of counter-regulatory hormones such as catecholamines, cortisol, glucagon and growth hormone induce catabolism (Fig. 19.2) This increased catabolism that occurs in response to these mediators varies across the course of critical illness and can persist well beyond the initial period of critical illness or injury;[4,5] the clinical consequences are outlined in Table 19.1.[6]

> **Practice tip**
>
> Metabolic rate fluctuates throughout an episode of critical illness and can vary significantly between patients. Generally, the sicker a patient is the higher their metabolic rate. These changes in metabolic rate might influence how practitioners decide to prescribe nutrition support.

To maintain normal cellular function, body cells require adequate amounts of the six basic nutrients: carbohydrates, fats and proteins to provide energy, and vitamins, minerals and water to catalyse metabolic processes. How best to provide this nutrition support to critically ill patients remains an area of controversy and requires additional basic and clinical research to inform our understanding of this complex area.[7]

Malnutrition

Malnutrition in critical illness is an important consideration with a reported prevalence of between 38% and 75%.[8,9] In critical illness, malnutrition can be preexisting[10] and the result of chronic starvation without inflammation or associated with chronic disease with mild-to-moderate degrees of inflammation. Malnutrition can also occur as the result of recent and acute disease with marked inflammatory response.[11] Determining the extent of preexisting malnutrition in critical care is challenging because of the heterogeneous patient populations and use of different criteria to characterise malnutrition.[8] Preexisting malnutrition in critical illness can increase the absolute risk of 90-day postdischarge mortality and is also a significant predictor of unplanned 30-day hospital readmission.[10]

Critically ill patients are also at risk of developing iatrogenic or hospital-acquired malnutrition with the prescription and delivery of nutrition contributing factors. Consequently, accurate assessment of nutritional requirements and strategies to ensure the prescribed nutrition is delivered is vital. The patient's clinical presentation can also have an impact on nutritional adequacy with surgical patients receiving less nutrition than medical patients.[12]

> **Practice tip**
>
> Critically ill patients, particularly the elderly, can present to the intensive care unit (ICU) with existing malnutrition. Obtaining information on pre-admission nutrition status from the patient and/or their family can help determine whether there is increased nutrition risk.

Consequences of malnutrition

Historically, the provision of nutrition to critically ill patients was considered a supportive strategy which could help provide exogenous macronutrients during periods of critical illness to minimise loss of muscle mass. Nutrition is now considered a therapy which can help attenuate stress metabolism, prevent oxidative cellular injury and modulate immune responses.[13]

Patients who experience malnutrition during critical illness often experience unfavourable outcomes including increased infectious morbidity, multiple-organ dysfunction, prolonged hospitalisation and disproportionate mortality.[13] Longer term malnutrition can contribute to loss of muscle mass and reduced functional recovery. The extent to which the provision of artificial nutrition ameliorates these complications is unclear.[7] The degree of critical illness and hypercatabolism varies between patients and is often difficult to determine. For this reason, it is necessary to assess, as accurately as possible, the nutritional requirements of each individual patient,

FIGURE 19.1 Three phases of catabolism.[1]

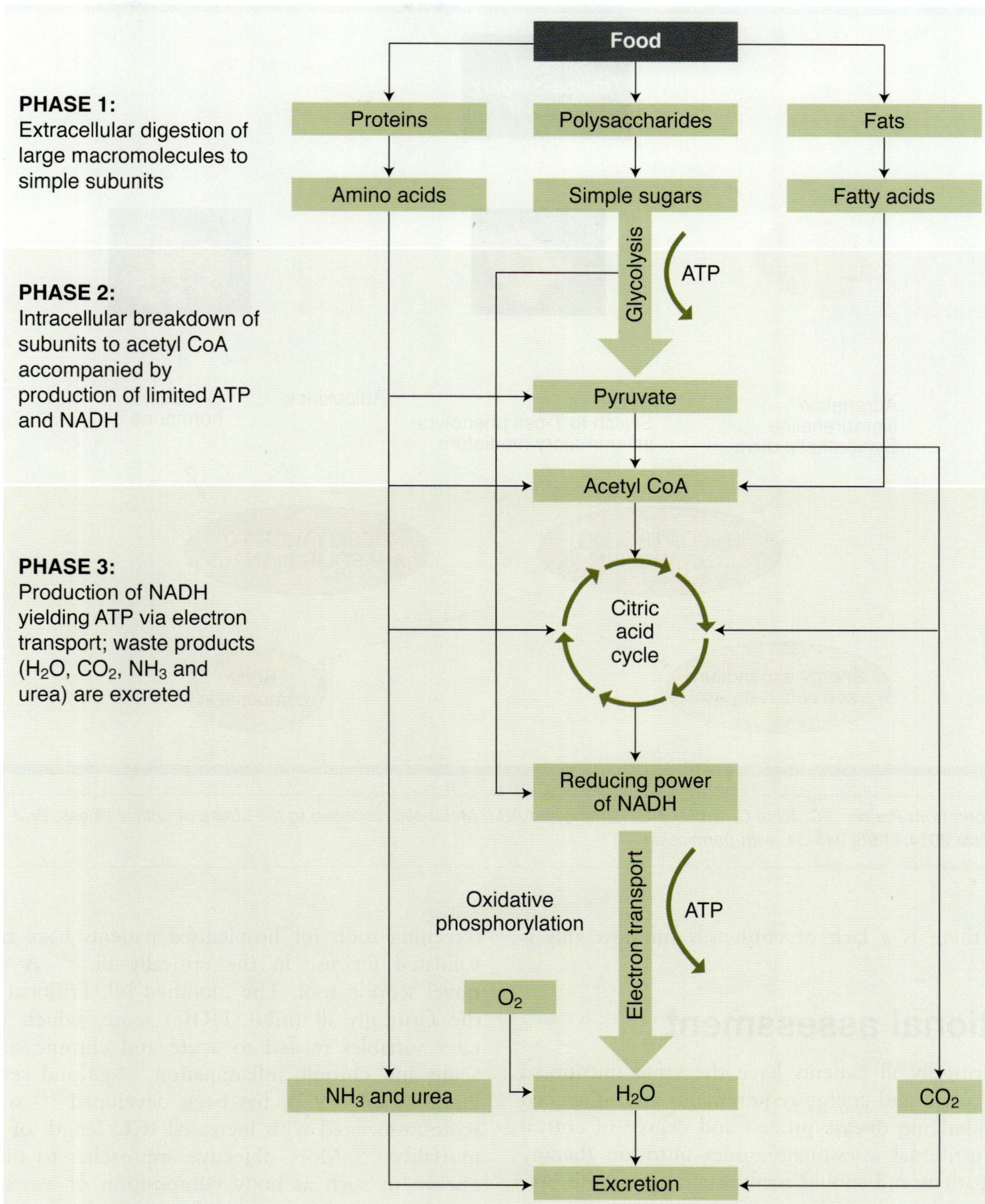

Adapted from McCance KL, Huether SE, Brashers VL, Rote NS, editors. Pathophysiology: the biologic basis for disease in adults and children. 7th ed. Maryland Heights: Elsevier; 2015, Figure 1-24, p. 26, with permission.

FIGURE 19.2 The metabolic response to stress.

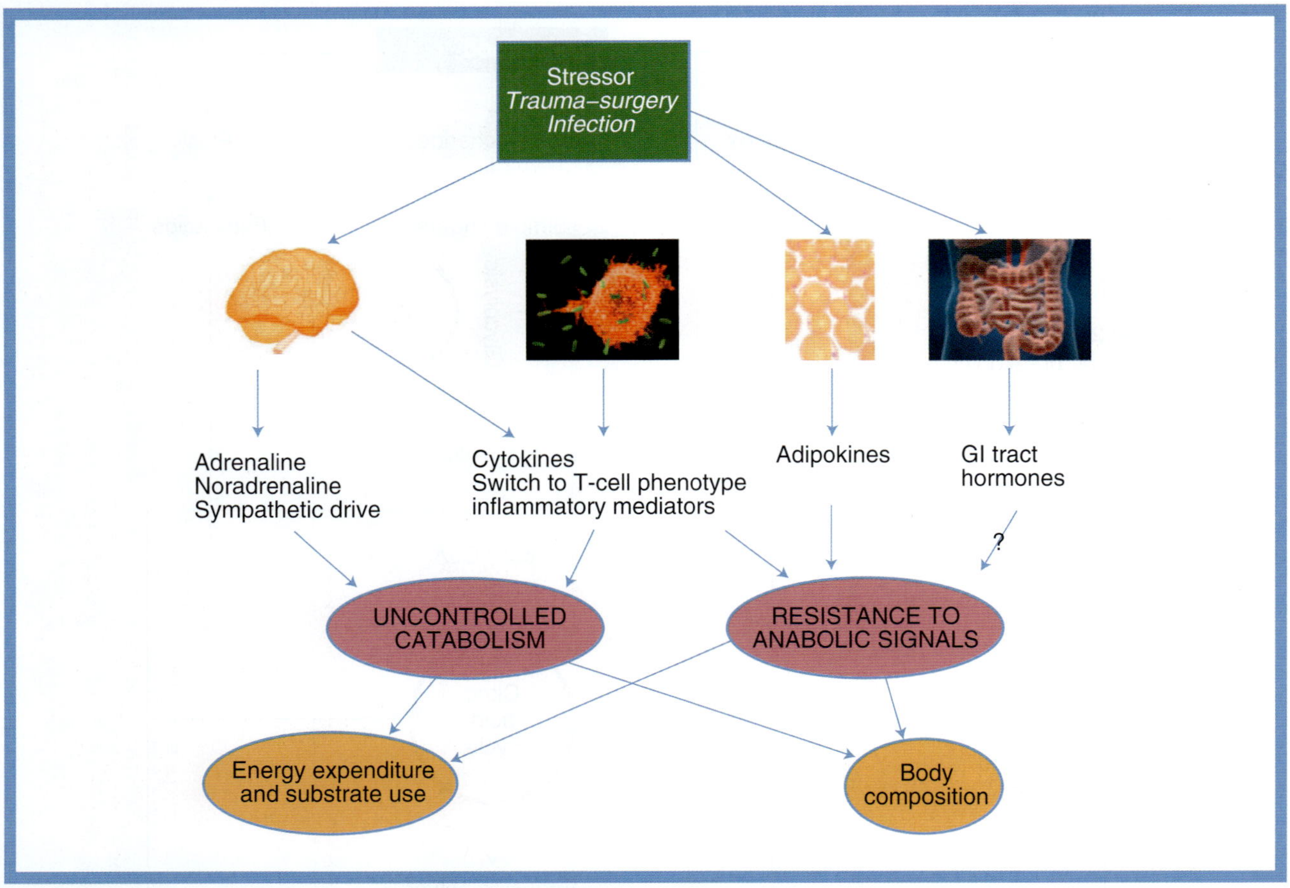

Reproduced from Preiser J-C, Ichai C, Orban J-C, Groeneveld ABJ. Metabolic response to the stress of critical illness. Br J Anaesthesia 2014;113(6):945-54, with permission.

although there is a lack of consensus on how this is best done.[14]

Nutritional assessment

Not all critically ill patients have the same nutritional needs.[15] Protein and energy requirements are influenced by the underlying disease process and degree of critical illness. Nutritional assessment guides nutrition therapy for each patient and should incorporate patient history, clinical diagnosis, physical examination, anthropometric data, laboratory tests, dietary assessment and functional outcomes.[16] The degree of acute or chronic inflammation is an important contributing factor to the development of malnutrition.[17,18]

Not all critically ill patients are alike with variations in nutrition risk. Energy expenditure varies and is reported to range from 22 to 34 kcal/kg/day.[2] Assessing which patients might be at greatest nutritional risk is important to identify those who are likely to benefit most from nutrition therapy. Existing nutrition screening tools for hospitalised patients have not been validated for use in the critically ill.[19,20] A validated novel scoring tool, The modified NUTritional Risk in the Critically ill (mNUTRIC) score, which incorporates variables related to acute and chronic starvation, acute and chronic inflammation,[21] age and severity of illness (Table 19.2), has been developed[22-24] with high scores associated with increased ICU length of stay and mortality.[23,25] More objective approaches to nutritional assessment such as body composition or assessment of muscle mass using computed tomography,[26] ultrasound[27] or bioelectirc impedence[28] have been explored but have practical limitations or are yet to be well validated in the critically ill.[13] Further work is needed to refine this or other tools to identify nutrition risk in critically ill patients to determine which patients are most likely to benefit from nutrition therapy.

Determining nutritional requirements

Determining caloric requirements is largely dependent on energy expenditure, influenced by patient activity,

TABLE 19.1
Clinical consequences of the metabolic response to stress[6]

CONSEQUENCE	DESCRIPTION
Energy expenditure (EE)	In the early phase of critical illness/injury the EE is usually lower than before the illness/injury; EE increases in the later phases of critical illness/injury. In chronic critical illness the EE is more difficult to predict and is influenced by physiological changes and therapeutic interventions
Use of energy substrates	The use of proteins, lipids and carbohydrates as energy sources changes during critical illness. Metabolism of macronutrients can be influenced by absorption, intracellular metabolism and substrate oxidation. In the early phases, carbohydrate oxidation is increased. As illness progresses glucose utilisation decreases and there is increased use of fats and proteins. this can result in loss of muscle which may impact functional recovery
Stress hyperglycaemia	Metabolism of carbohydrates are changed in critical illness and results in rapid use of glycogen stores as well as increased endogenous glucose production; both result in increased plasma glucose concentrations. Hormone release (catecholamines, growth hormone, cortisol and cytokines) Increase glucose production by the liver and contribute to insulin resistance
Lactate as a substrate	Lactate can be converted to glucose and is possibly a fuel used by organs under conditions of stress. Lactate may be a useful, if not obligatory, substrate used by organs such as the brain and heart, during stress conditions
Lipids	Lipids as an energy source require large amounts of oxygen in order to be converted to ATP by the mitochondria. Metabolism of lipids can be increased but complete oxidation is only possible if the mitochondria are fully functional, although mitochondrial function may be impaired during critical illness
Proteins	Protein breakdown can exceed synthesis after stress. Stress metabolism can result in increased degradation of protein and contribute to depletion of skeletal muscles and ICU-acquired weakness
Changes in body composition	Changes include loss of lean body mass and preservation of fat tissue and increased lipid storage. Body cell mass is decreased and extracellular fluid is increased

stage of illness, type of injury and previous nutritional status.[4] Resting energy expenditure (REE) is the primary consideration when prescribing energy intake because it is the largest component of total energy expenditure for hospitalised patients.[29] Determining REE can be measured using indirect calorimetry or estimated using one of many different predictive equations. Two randomised clinical trials have demonstrated that protein and energy intake is increased when indirect calorimetry is used;[30,31] however, evidence quality is limited and further research in this area is needed. Both approaches to determining energy requirements are used in ICUs and have advantages and limitations.

Practice tip

For severely malnourished patients, improving nutrition support can cause refeeding syndrome to occur. In this syndrome metabolic disturbances occur that are characterised by electrolyte disorders, particularly hypophosphataemia.

Indirect calorimetry

Indirect calorimetry is the 'gold standard' and most precise way of determining energy expenditure in critical illness[32] but is infrequently used because of financial and resources constraints.[33] Through indirect calorimetry, energy expenditure is calculated using oxygen consumption and carbon dioxide production.[34] Measurement accuracy can be affected by many factors including instrument performance, ambient temperature and volume leaks that might occur through the calorimeter, endotracheal tube or chest drains.[35] Patient-related factors also can influence measurement of REE, such as physical activity, food consumption and physiological stress such as pain. To obtain the most accurate measurement of REE it is recommended that these measurements be taken under steady-state conditions,[35] that is where there is at least a 5-minute period with ≤10% coefficient of variance in the oxygen consumption and carbon dioxide production.[36] However, metabolic equilibrium is not well defined and variation in how steady state is determined exists.[29] Comprehensive discussions of practical aspects of indirect calorimetry are published elsewhere.[35]

TABLE 19.2
Conceptual model and variables included in the NUTritional Risk in the Critically ill (NUTRIC) score[22]

CONCEPTS	PROPOSED VARIABLES	VARIABLES RETAINED IN FINAL SCORE
Acute starvation	Decreased oral intake over the last week	No
	Pre-ICU hospital admission	Yes
Chronic starvation	Weight loss over the last 6 months	No
	BMI <20	No
Acute inflammation	IL-6	Yes
	PCT	No
	CRP	No
Chronic inflammation	Comorbid illness	Yes
Severity of illness	Age	Yes
	APACHE II score	Yes
	SOFA score	Yes

APACHE = Acute physiology and chronic health evaluation; BMI = body mass index; CRP = C-reactive protein; IL-6 = interleukin-6; PCT = procalcitonin; SOFA = sequential organ failure assessment.

TABLE 19.3
Predictive equations for estimating energy expenditure in critically ill patients[37]

American College of Chest Physicians	25 × weight If BMI 16–25 kg/m^2 use usual body weight If BMI > 25 kg/m^2 use ideal body weight If BMI <16 kg/m^2 use existing body weight for the first 7×10 days then ideal body weight
Harris–Benedict equation	Men: 66.4730 + (13.7516 × weight) + (5.0033 × height) − (6.7550 × age) Women: 655.0955 + (9.5634 × weight) + (1.8496 × height) − (4.6756 × age)
Ireton-Jones 1992 equation	1.925 − (10 × age) + (5 × weight) + (281 for males) + (292 if trauma present) + (851 if burns present)
Ireton-Jones 1997 equation	(5 × weight) − (11 × age) + (244 for males) + (239 if trauma present) + (840 if burns present) + 1784
Penn State 1998	(1.1 × value from Harris–Benedict equation) + (140 × T_{max}) + (32 × VE) − 5340
Penn State 2003	(0.85 × value from Harris–Benedict equation) + (175 × T_{max}) + (33 × VE) − 6433
Swinamer 1990	(945 × body surface area) − (6.4 × age) + (108 × temperature) + 24.2 × respiratory rate) + (817 × V_T) − 4349

BMI = body mass index.
Source: Walker RN, Heuberger RA. Predictive equations for energy needs for the critically ill. Respir Care 2009;54(4):509-21, with permission.

Predictive equations

Because indirect calorimetry is not available in many ICUs, it is common practice to use predictive equations (Table 19.3) to determine energy requirements.[37] The accuracy of predictive equations is poor compared to measurement of REE using indirect calorimetry; however, some predictive equations perform better in critical illness than do others. Some equations use only static variables (such as height, weight, age and sex) to predict REE. Others use more dynamic variables (such as body temperature, minute ventilation, heart rate) in an attempt to account for the metabolic variation that occurs in critical illness.[38]

Although the accuracy of predictive equations compared to indirect calorimetry has been evaluated in many studies, no single equation is identified as being superior.[39-41] With over 200 predictive equations described in the literature[13] and variable accuracy of these equations it makes selection challenging particularly because of influencing factors such as body mass index (BMI),[41] sex[39] and age.[42]

While most predictive equations are likely to underestimate measured energy expenditure in the critically ill, wide variations in predicted energy expenditure have been reported and may contribute to both over and underfeeding.[43] A recent systematic review of-18 studies it was demonstrated that, at a patient level, predictive equations underestimated energy requirements in between 13% and 90% of patients; overestimation of energy requirements was observed in up to 88% of patients.[43] Despite the variable accuracy of predictive equations they may provide some guidance for nutrition prescription in the absence of indirect calorimetry but should be used alongside other assessments of nutritional requirements.

Practice tip

Ongoing patient assessment should be undertaken throughout the critical illness trajectory to ensure nutrition prescription closely matches patient requirements.

FIGURE 19.3 Nutrition support during recovery from critical illness.

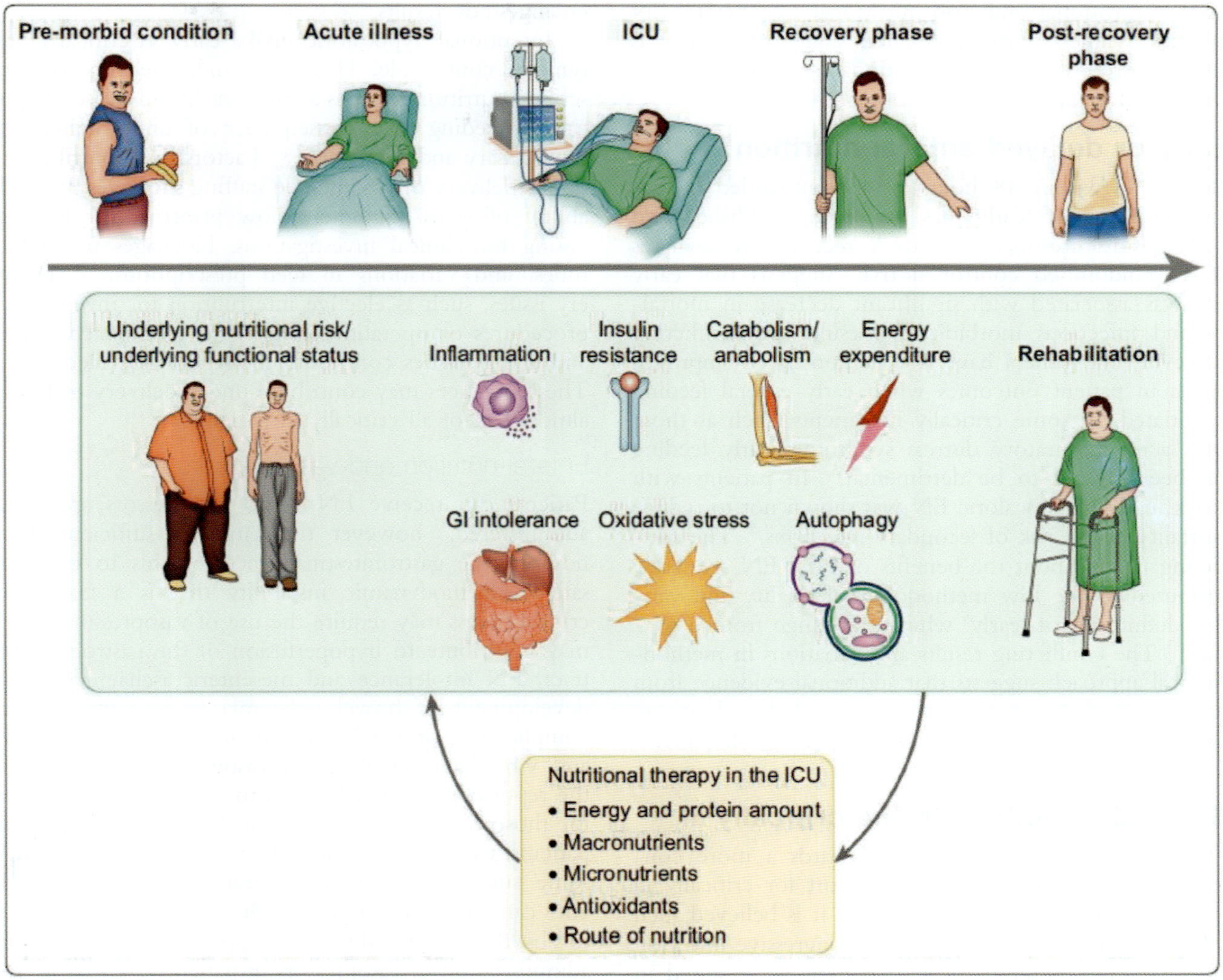

Reprinted by permission of Springer Nature, Arabi YM, et al. The intensive care medicine research agenda in nutrition and metabolism. Intensive Care Med 2017; 43(9): 1239-1256.

Nutrition support

Prevention, detection and correction of malnutrition are important components of optimal nutritional support in critical illness. Nutrition support is instituted to optimise the patient's metabolic state, reduce morbidity and improve recovery. Additional benefits of nutrition support include attenuation of the metabolic response to stress, restriction of oxidative cellular injury and moderation of the immune response.[44,45] Most critically ill patients cannot consume food or fluids orally and in these situations EN is the preferred method of feeding for patients.[13,46] For some patients PN alone or combined with EN may also be required to provide optimal nutrition support.[13] Nutrition support is important throughout the trajectory of recovery from critical illness requirements and nutrition support interventions are likely to vary throughout[15] (Fig. 19.3).

Enteral nutrition

EN has benefits beyond simply the supply of nutrients to the body[47] and any amount is beneficial. EN increases gastric mucosal blood flow, stimulates brush border enzymes, preserves epithelial tight cell junctions[48] and provides gut-derived mucosal immunity.[49,50] Major effects of EN are: preservation of intestinal epithelium, mucosal mass and microvilli height; prevention of bacterial translocation; and a positive effect on the gut-associated lymphoid tissue, the source of most mucosal immunity in humans.[3] Septic complications are decreased when EN is provided.[51] Stimulating and improving gastrointestinal immune function is an important goal of early EN[52] with the gut microbiome maintained in part by luminal nutrient stimulation which in turn enhances microbial diversity.[53] While there is still much to learn in relation to the nutritional and non-nutritional benefits to EN in critical illness, current research suggests that EN is the preferred strategy of nutritional support for most critically ill patients.

Early or delayed enteral nutrition?

Early EN (within 48 hours) is recommended[13,46] but the definition of 'early' has not been established and study results are inconsistent. A recent meta-analyses of 21 randomised controlled trials suggests that early EN was associated with significant decrease in mortality and infectious morbidity.[13] Results are conflicting however, and others have not demonstrated improvements in patient outcomes when early enteral feeding is initiated. In some critically ill patients, such as those with acute respiratory distress syndrome, early feeding has been shown to be detrimental.[54] In patients with shock, early normocaloric EN was shown not to reduce mortality or the risk of secondary infections.[55] The conflicting results about the benefits of early EN are likely attributed to the low methodological quality and variable definitions of 'early' which can range from 3 to 7 days.[15] The conflicting results and variations in methodological approach suggests that additional evidence from large, high-quality, randomised, controlled trials investigating optimal timing of EN in critically ill patients is needed.

Hypocaloric intake in the critically ill

There has been a recent trend towards a more conservative approach to nutrition support for critically ill patients at low nutrition risk because it is believed such patients are unlikely to benefit from aggressive nutrition therapy.[13] The potential lack of benefit has resulted in recommendations that specialised nutrition therapy in the first week in ICU is not required for low risk patients.[13] However, others have recommended implementation of strategies to optimise delivery of nutrition in critically ill patients[56] and hypocaloric feeding in the first few days of critical illness remains controversial.[57] Initial starvation for a brief period to support autophagy is encouraged by some researchers[58,59] while others advocate for more aggressive approaches to nutrition therapy.[60-62]

In several observational studies[63-66] the reduced provision of energy and protein were associated with worse outcomes. Observational studies may be confounded by many factors including severity of illness, where patients who were less sick and tolerated enteral nutrition better were more likely to be adequately fed and have better outcomes.[44] Conversely, two randomised controlled trials demonstrated that if early EN exceeded actual energy expenditure it was likely to be harmful and should be avoided,[67,68] findings that have not been demonstrated in other studies.[69-71] The differences in recommendations regarding EN dose in the early stages of critical illness can be influenced by the evidentiary base drawn on when formulating recommendations with differing methodological design and patient characteristics influencing study results.[56]

Intentional hypocaloric intake early in critical illness remains contestable. However, under-delivery of prescribed nutrition remains a concern. In most cases, hypocaloric feeding as a consequence of under-delivery is unnecessary and avoidable.[72,73] Factors that contribute to under-delivery of EN include staffing shortages, unavailability of feeds/equipment, low priorities for feeding, fasting for clinical investigations, blockages in feeding tubes, and variations in feed prescriptions.[74,75] Delivery issues, such as elective interruption for investigative procedures or operations, high gastric residual volumes and airway issues contribute to hypocaloric feeding.[76,77] These practices may contribute under-delivery of EN in almost half of all critically ill patients.[78]

Enteral nutrition and vasopressors

Patients can receive EN while vasopressors are being administered;[13] however, there must be sufficient blood flow to the gastrointestinal tract for this to be done safely. Haemodynamic instability that is a feature of critical illness may require the use of vasopressors which may contribute to hypoperfusion of the gastrointestinal tract, EN intolerance and mesenteric ischaemia.[79] The development of bowel ischaemia is, however, a rare complication of EN.[80] In patients receiving early EN and who had low doses of vasopressors administered, the reported ICU and hospital mortality was lower than for those receiving late EN; the benefit was greater in patients treated with multiple vasopressors.[81] There is some suggestion that administration of enteral nutrients can improve gut blood flow enabling the bowel to absorb nutrients during vasopressor therapy.[81,82] The administration of vasopressors in patients with sepsis and shock, however, is associated with both improved and diminished perfusion. Mentec et al[83] reported gastric intolerance was higher in patients receiving vasopressor therapy while others found patients tolerated EN.[77]

Practice tip

Nurses should regularly assess for barriers to achieving daily nutritional goals and work with the interdisciplinary team to ensure nutrition intake is optimised.

Enteral nutrition protocols

EN protocols improve the delivery of enteral feeds and clinical outcomes.[13,77] Protocol variability exists because of the lack of robust research in the management of EN.[13,46] In the absence of strong research evidence, rituals are embraced and rarely challenged.[73] Furthermore, the implementation and sustainability of guidelines are influenced by multiple factors such as clinician preference, patient population, clinical contexts and content of guidelines.[84] Decisions of what to include may be challenged by the variation in guideline recommendations.[56]

Management of enteral feeding

Routes of enteral feeding

Wide-bore nasogastric or orogastric tubes are most commonly used in the critically ill in the early stages of EN. Should prolonged EN be anticipated (longer than 1 month), or where patients have gastric intolerance then gastrostomy, duodenostomy or jejunostomy tubes may be used. Postpyloric feeding is useful if patients are not tolerating gastric feeding,[85] but has not been shown to be superior to gastric feeding. Postpyloric enteral access is recommended for patients deemed to be at high risk for aspiration. Improved nutrient delivery and reduced risk of pneumonia were reported in meta-analyses of RCTs comparing postpyloric and gastric EN.[13] However there is insufficient evidence to demonstrate whether gastric or small bowel feeding results in better nutritional adequacy.[86]

For some critically ill patients, gastric secretions may increase when small bowel feeding is initiated.[87] A double-lumen tube is available, one lumen for gastric aspiration and decompression and the second for simultaneous jejunal feeding, but these tubes are not widely used in the clinical setting.[88]

Assessment of enteral feeding tube placement

The correct placement of enteral feeding tubes is crucial to promote adequate nutrition and avoid adverse events. The correct insertion of enteral feeding tubes in the critically ill can be challenging because these patients often have a reduced cough reflex, altered sensorium and receive sedative and narcotic medications.[89] Misplacement of the feeding tube into the tracheobronchial tree is a potential complication of tube insertion.[90] Complications such as infusion of tube feedings, pneumothorax, pneumonitis, hydropneumothorax, bronchopleural fistula, empyema and pulmonary haemorrhage have also been reported.[91] Confirmation of tube placement is routinely done with radiography (Fig. 19.4). Bedside techniques are also used to estimate the tube location during insertion and to reassess placement thereafter.[92] Variations in approaches to (re)assessing feeding tube placement have been reported and some nurses may be unaware of the limitations of bedside techniques in assessing feeding tube placement.[93] Less reliable methods of confirming tube placement include the use of pH, observation of the colour of gastric aspirates, auscultation, and monitoring length of tube.[94]

New and novel techniques being investigated to confirm correct placement of the nasogastric tube[95] include:

- Ultrasonographic visualisation of the upper oesophagus[96-98]
- Real-time image-guided placement using Kangaroo with IRIS Technology[99,100]
- Colorimetric capnometry method[96]
- Non-invasive, real-time localisation system uses passive magnetic tracking techniques with a small permanent magnet embedded at the tip of the NG tube with the position ascertained from embedded sensors worn around the neck.[101,102]

While all have problems with their ability to correctly identify placement of the nasogastric tube in the critically ill patient in the ICU, future research is promising.

Assessment of feeding tube placement by auscultation of air insufflated into the stomach remains a common clinical practice although auscultation should NOT be used as the sole method to determine placement of the gastric tube because it is unreliable. Other limited practices include:

- Nasogastric aspirate from critically ill patients receiving continuous feedings may have the appearance of unchanged formula, regardless of the site of the feeding tube.[103]
- A pH of 0–5 may be used to indicate gastric placement of enteral feeding tubes, although this technique may be problematic for patients receiving histamine-2-receptor antagonists or proton pump inhibitors. Aspirated fluid with a low pH may be assumed to originate from the stomach but fluid from an infected pleural space can also be acidic.[104]
- Capnometry and capnography measuring end-tidal carbon dioxide can indicate respiratory placement of the tube through an increase in carbon dioxide[105] and might be useful in assessing placement of nasogastric tubes in mechanically ventilated patients.[96] It is important to recognise that this technique does not help differentiate oesophageal, gastric or intestinal placement.
- Measuring the concentrations of pepsin and trypsin in feeding tube aspirates can be used as a method of predicting tube placement; however, methods to measure pepsin and trypsin at the bedside are currently unavailable.[106]

Ongoing assessment of feeding tube placement is essential, as feeding tubes may migrate after initial placement. Marking the feeding tube at the point where it exits the nose and measurement of tube length protruding from the anterior nares will facilitate detection of migration of the enteral tube. Radio-opaque tubes have markers to enable accurate measurement and documentation of tube position. They should be used with the methods previously described for ongoing assessment.

In the absence of X-ray, several approaches should be used in combination to verify tube position. Metheny et al[103] found measuring: 1) length of tubing extending from the insertion site, 2) volume of aspirate from the feeding tube, 3) appearance of the aspirate and 4) pH of the aspirate were able to correctly differentiate between

FIGURE 19.4 Correct placement of a nasogastric tube.[92]

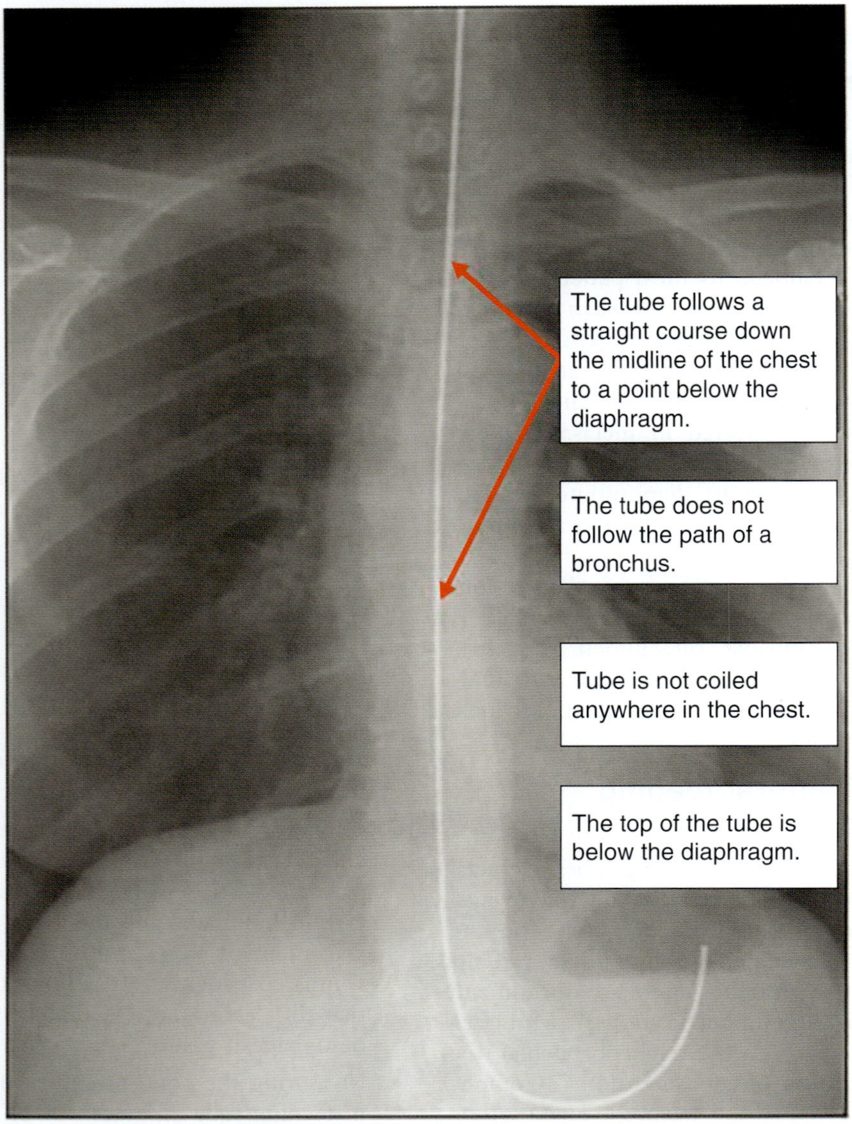

Source: © Pennsylvania Patient Safety Authority

gastric and bowel tube placement during continuous feedings in 81% of predictions.

Practice tip

Radiographic assessment of feeding tube placement is the gold standard. When this is not available feeding tube placement should be confirmed using more than one method.

Feeding regimens

Once the enteral feeding tube is successfully placed, administration of the feeding solution can begin using a variety of methods, including bolus, intermittent and continuous enteral feeding (Table 19.4). Bolus enteral feeding is rarely used in ICU. It is less clear whether intermittent or continuous feeding is more beneficial.[107,108] Concerns about increased risk of aspiration with intermittent enteral feeding has not been substantiated in the literature;[109] however, the research in this area is limited in both quantity and quality. Because of

TABLE 19.4
Methods of feed delivery

METHOD	DESCRIPTION
Bolus	• Delivery of a large volume of tube feed into the stomach over a short period of time (>100 mL) • Associated with complications, such as aspiration and vomiting
Intermittent	• A several-hour infusion a few times a day (e.g. 150 mL/h for 3 hours, three times per day), or delivered over a longer period (12–16 hours) with an 8–12-hour rest period • Allows gastric acidity and therefore limits bacterial overgrowth • Requires a higher hourly rate to meet caloric requirements
Continuous	• The delivery of small amounts of formula per hour over a 24-hour period • May make caloric requirements more achievable • Continuous dilution of gastric acid may contribute to bacterial overgrowth

inconclusive evidence regarding feeding regimens, decisions are based on individual patient assessment and the clinician's clinical judgement.

Commencing enteral nutrition

For most critically ill patients, EN can be safely commenced. There are relatively few absolute contraindications to commencing enteral feeding including ileus, intestinal obstruction, active gastrointestinal haemorrhage and haemodynamic instability.[110] Relative contraindications may also be present and may require a mixed approach incorporating EN and PN as a nutrition support strategy.

For many years a functioning bowel was considered necessary before EN could be commenced and there were perceptions that bowel rest was necessary. This approach is questionable because bowel function is not inhibited by starvation[44] and outcomes of gastrointestinal disorders traditionally treated with bowel rest are improved with EN.

Patients should not have EN withheld if they have absent bowel sounds, postoperative ileus[44] or after gastrointestinal surgery.[46] The risk of anatomic leaks and fistulas in patients who have had bowel surgery and also receive early EN is lower in comparison to delayed feeding or PN.[46] EN following gastrointestinal surgery is associated with a significantly lower risk of infection and reduced hospital length of stay.[46] Bowel sounds are indicative of contractility, and may not relate to mucosal integrity, barrier function, or absorptive capacity. Nevertheless, a high number of signs of intolerance necessitate further clinical evaluation.[13]

The appropriate starting rate for EN is controversial and there are no empirical data on which to base the decision. Feeding is often started at 30 mL/h, but may range from 10 to 100 mL/h. Increasing the rate of enteral feeding is equally variable, but strategies to progress patients towards meeting their daily caloric requirements should be employed. There is insufficient evidence to suggest commencing at goal rate is beneficial for patients who are not at increased nutrition risk.[13] When nutrition risk is not present, trophic feeds (20–20 kcal/hour) may be sufficient to prevent gastric mucosal atrophy and maintain integrity of the gut. Findings from recent clinical trials[69,70] suggest that there are no differences in mortality or other key clinical outcomes when patients received underfeeding (40–60% of calculated caloric requirements) or standard feeding (70–100% of calculated caloric requirements). Recognising that these data were obtained in young, medical and well-nourished patients it is not surprising that a benefit was not observed. It is also possible that insufficient calories were delivered to patients in the standard feeding group.[111]

For patients who have experienced a prolonged period of starvation or total PN, some clinicians may use a more conservative approach to enteral feeding because risk of refeeding syndrome is increased.[112] Although reported risk factors associated with refeeding syndrome vary, low BMI, unintentional weight loss, starvation, history of alcohol abuse and low initial electrolyte concentrations are thought to be contributing factors.[113] Although not common, this syndrome is associated with severe derangement in fluid and electrolyte levels (particularly hypophosphataemia, hypomagnesaemia and hypokalaemia), and may result in significant morbidity and mortality.[114]

Managing complications of enteral nutrition

Once EN is established, it is important to assess for such complications as feeding intolerance that can result in gastric distension, vomiting, diarrhoea and increased gastric residual volume.[115] Pulmonary aspiration, hyperglycaemia, hypercarbia, electrolyte imbalances and feed contamination are also complications that should be monitored daily and interventions implemented to minimise their occurrence. Monitoring tolerance to EN through the measurement of gastric residual volume is viewed as an important aspect of nursing management, although consensus on what constitutes a high gastric residual and any recommendations for interventions remain controversial.[116] Current guidelines[13] recommend that the gastric residual volume (GRV) should not be used as part of routine care to monitor ICU patients receiving EN. For those ICUs where GRVs are still utilised, withholding EN for GRVs <500 mL in the absence of other signs of intolerance should be avoided. Critically ill patients exhibit elevated GRV for a variety of reasons including feeding intolerance[117] and reduced gastric motility.[118] Tube diameter, tube position, type of gastric access and the patient's position can also influence GRV measurement accuracy.[44] High GRVs do not predict aspiration, and low GRVs do not mean that aspiration will not occur. Studies[119,120] have shown no difference in risk for pulmonary aspiration between low and high GRV groups. It is assumed that measuring GRV is accurate and useful but GRV does not correlate with clinical or radiological abdominal findings.[121]

The amount of GRV considered excessive varies in clinical practice and there are insufficient data to guide the development of recommendations in this area.[116] While some suggest assessment of GRVs is not required, the value of this practice is likely patient-dependent. In surgical patients a threshold of 200 mL is suggested as a marker for adjusting the EN delivery rate while higher GRVs are recommended in critically ill patients with a volume of between 250 and 500 mL considered acceptable.[116] After aspiration of gastric residual volume the gastric aspirate is either returned or discarded. The evidence for discarding gastric aspirate is weak,[122] and refeeding GRVs up to a maximum of 250 mL or discarding GRVs may be acceptable.[123] Enteral feeding is interrupted when the GRV exceeds a prescribed threshold for acceptable GRV; however, there are no data to support this practice. Ceasing feeds in response to GRV is questionable,[120] particularly as a balanced enteral diet in itself has a prokinetic effect.[124]

Practice tip

In determining feeding intolerance, a single high GRV in the absence of physical examination or radiographic findings should not result in the cessation of enteral feeding. Persisting with enteral feeding has demonstrated benefits.

Practice tip

When evaluating GRV in relation to the rate of enteral feeding, remember to take into account the production of gastric secretion, which can be as much as 2500 mL/day.

Development of diarrhoea is another complication for enterally fed patients,[125] and is a common reason why enteral feeding is reduced or ceased while other contributing factors may be unrecognised. Diarrhoea may contribute to fluid and electrolyte disorders, patient (and nursing) distress and a higher cost of patient care.[113] Unfortunately, defining diarrhoea is problematic, as it is a subjective assessment that relies on nursing interpretation rather than on quantifiable assessment of stool weight.[126,127] EN should not be automatically interrupted for diarrhoea;[13] feeds should be continued while evaluating the aetiology of diarrhoea to determine appropriate treatment. There are many reasons for diarrhoea in critically ill patients who receive EN,[125] often occurring simultaneously, including:

- underlying disease[128]
- medications including antibiotics due to side effects, toxicity and disruption to gut microbiota[5]
- hypoalbuminaemia[129]
- use of histamine-2-receptor antagonists[130]
- contamination of enteral feeding solution.[131,132]

Enteral feeding solutions present an excellent medium for the growth of microorganisms and bacterial contamination of enteral feeds is common.[131] Strategies to limit bacterial contamination of enteral feeding solutions include:

- meticulous preparation of feeding solutions and equipment[133]
- commercially prepared formula in closed systems used in preference to decanted feeds[134]
- limiting the time feeding solution is kept at room temperature once opened and hang times[134]
- meticulous attention to handwashing and limiting manipulation of the EN bags and delivery system at the bedside.[133]

The use of probiotics in critically ill patients has been suggested as a strategy for managing diarrhoea in enterally fed, critically ill patients. Probiotics are viable microorganisms which may be beneficial when ingested in adequate amounts. During critical illness changes in the commensal microbiota can contribute to gastrointestinal dysfunction. Administration of probiotics is theoretically sensible; however, there is inadequate research to demonstrate benefit to the general ICU patient population.[135] While there are potential benefits of using probiotics, such as reduced infections including ventilator-associated pneumonia, there are currently no data to demonstrate that the use of probiotics has any impact on diarrhoea.[136]

Practice tip

Nurses may be tempted to stop EN in the presence of diarrhoea but there is no evidence to support withholding enteral feeding in critically ill patients. The only exception may be if there are significant disturbances in fluid and/or electrolyte balance.

Prevention of pulmonary aspiration

An important complication of enteral feeding is the development of pulmonary aspiration and nosocomial pneumonia. Determining whether aspiration has occurred is difficult, even for experienced clinicians.

High GRVs have been linked to the potential for pulmonary aspiration, although this has not been shown in research.[120] Oropharyngeal secretions can contribute to nosocomial pneumonia and subglottic aspiration has improved outcomes.[137] Nursing strategies to improve gastric emptying include elevation of the head of the bed 30–45° (unless otherwise contraindicated), because the likelihood of gastro-oesophageal reflux is reduced;[138,139] however, this recommendation is based on weak evidence.[13] With a lack of strong evidence, experts recommend the head of the bed of mechanically ventilated patients be elevated 30° to 45° provided there are no contraindications to doing so.

Clinical judgement should be exercised when using semi-upright positioning in the critically ill because the evidence to support this practice is not compelling and the balance between benefits and harm is unknown. Nursing patients semi-recumbent at 45° can be difficult because the patient often slides down and the position can be uncomfortable for the patient. Experimental models also suggest that the semi-recumbent position may enhance the flow of mucous into the lungs with an increased risk of bacterial colonisation and pneumonia.[140] Until further evidence is available to guide practice decisions, patient positioning should be at the discretion of clinicians.

Prokinetic agents, such as erythromycin and metoclopramide, can improve gastric emptying and feeding tolerance, and avoid gastro-oesophageal reflux and pulmonary aspiration.[141] These prokinetic agents do, however, have undesirable effects. Use of erythromycin is associated with the development of bacterial resistance, and metoclopramide is associated with numerous systemic side effects.[142] Because of the limitations created by adverse effects of these promotility agents, further work is being done to identify alternative pharmacologic agents to improve gut motility and gastric emptying.[143]

Assessment of pulmonary aspiration

Despite preventive strategies, pulmonary aspiration may still occur in some patients, and accurate assessment is essential. Common methods performed easily at the bedside to identify possible aspiration of gastric contents and/or enteral feeding formula include:

- The efficacy of the dye method is no longer recommended for accuracy and safety concerns.[13] Blue dye is poorly standardised and has a low sensitivity in detecting microaspiration.[144] There are significant safety concerns using either blue food colouring or methylene blue because of the potential to induce mitochondrial toxicity and interfere with oxidative phosphorylation.[145]
- Measurement of glucose in tracheobronchial secretions is another method to detect pulmonary aspiration but is no longer recommended..[145,146] Tracheobronchial secretions normally contain <5 mg/dL glucose, higher amounts of glucose may suggest aspiration of glucose-rich enteral feeding formula. Differences in enteral feeding solutions affect the sensitivity of this method, with low glucose solutions being more difficult to detect. Also, patients not receiving enteral feeding can have detectable glucose in aspirates.[146] This is further confounded by the presence of blood, which is closely associated with glucose values >20 mg/dL; consequently, any blood in the respiratory tract could contribute to a false-positive result.
- Measurement of pepsin in tracheobronchial secretions has been used in an animal study that suggested that the detection of pepsin, a component of gastric secretions, may be useful in determining pulmonary aspiration.[147] Further investigation in acutely ill patients receiving enteral feeding is necessary.

> **Practice tip**
>
> Nursing patients with the head of the bed elevated is common in ICU; however, more evidence is needed to demonstrate that this practice prevents pulmonary aspiration.

Parenteral nutrition

EN is the preferred method of nutritional support because it has physiological advantages, and is associated with fewer infectious and metabolic complications. EN as a nutrition therapy is also less expensive than PN and the use of PN in the context of critical illness remains controversial. PN bypasses the gastrointestinal system and the crucial role that hormones and nutrients play in regulating gut function, metabolic pathways and hepatic function.[44] In addition there are metabolic, immunological, endocrine and infective complications from infusing solutions of high glucose concentration and fat globules intravenously.[148] PN impairs humoral and cellular immunological defences and the association of PN with increased free radical formation may be important for patients who are critically ill.[44] One avoidable complication of PN is exceeding the energy target, and this is more likely to occur in those patients who are also receiving pharmacological therapy containing lipids or glucose, if these are not also taken into account when determining nutrition prescription.

Studies report conflicting results on the benefit of PN for the nutrition support of critically ill patients with early studies reporting worse clinical outcomes.[149] More recently studies have supported the use of parenteral nutrition.[51,150] In a randomised clinical audit, Harvey et al[51] compared enteral and parenteral nutrition and found no significant differences in mortality or infection rate. Recent guidelines[13] recommend that EN is supplemented with PN in patients who cannot commence early EN or until target nutrition goals are achieved.

McClave et al[13] recommend PN be initiated after 1 week, unless the patient is severely malnourished. The EPaNIC study showed that late, rather than early, initiation of PN in patients who could not achieve caloric requirements using EN alone was associated with fewer complications and faster recovery.[151] However, another study[152] demonstrated that supplemental PN in the first week of critical illness resulted in a reduction in late infections. With conflicting evidence, it is necessary for clinicians to carefully assess the patient to determine which patients are most likely to benefit from more aggressive nutrition therapy early in their ICU stay.

PN solutions contain carbohydrates, lipids, proteins, electrolytes, vitamins and trace elements (Table 19.5). PN, whether supplementary or complete, provides daily allowances of nutrients and minerals. The addition of vitamins and trace elements to PN solutions is necessary, particularly as water-soluble vitamins and trace elements are rapidly depleted (Table 19.6).[153] Standardised PN formulations, although as effective as custom-made PN in providing caloric requirements, are less likely to achieve estimated protein requirements and have been noted to be associated with hyponatraemia.[154] Glucose is the primary energy source in PN solutions. Concentrations of 10–70% glucose may be used in PN solutions although the final concentration of the solution should be no more than 35%. The high concentration of PN solutions can cause thrombosis so PN is normally

TABLE 19.5
Components of PN solutions

COMPONENT	RECOMMENDATION	GRADE*
Carbohydrate	The minimal amount of carbohydrate required is about 2 g/kg of glucose per day	B
	Hyperglycemia (glucose >10 mmol/L) contributes to death in the critically ill patient and should also be avoided to prevent infectious complications	B
	Reductions and increases in mortality rates have been reported in ICU patients when blood glucose is maintained between 4.5 and 6.1 mmol/L. No unequivocal recommendation on this is therefore possible at present	C
	There is a higher incidence of severe hypoglycaemia in patients treated to the tighter limits	A
Lipids	Lipids should be an integral part of PN for energy and to ensure essential fatty acid provision in long-term ICU patients	B
	Intravenous lipid emulsions (LCT, MCT or mixed emulsions) can be administered safely at a rate of 0.7 g/kg up to 1.5 g/kg over 12 to 24 h	B
	The tolerance of mixed LCT/MCT lipid emulsions in standard use is sufficiently documented. Several studies have shown specific clinical advantages over soybean LCT alone but require confirmation by prospective controlled studies	C
	Olive oil-based PN is well tolerated in critically ill patients	B
	Addition of EPA and DHA to lipid emulsions has demonstrable effects on cell membranes and inflammatory processes. Fish oil-enriched lipid emulsions probably decrease length of stay in critically ill patients	B
Amino acids	When PN is indicated, a balanced amino acid mixture should be infused at approximately 1.3–1.5 g/kg ideal body weight/day in conjunction with an adequate energy supply	B
	When PN is indicated in ICU patients the amino acid solution should contain 0.2–0.4 g/kg/day of L-glutamine (e.g. 0.3–0.6 g/kg/day alanyl-glutamine dipeptide)	A
Micronutrients	All PN prescriptions should include a daily dose of multivitamins and of trace elements	C

*Grade of recommendation – the grade of recommendation is based on the quality of the evidence where A is high, B is moderate, C is low and D is very low (as quoted in Guyatt GH, Oxman AD, Vist GE, et al. GRADE: an emerging consensus on rating quality of evidence and strength of recommendations. BMJ 2008; 336:924–6).
DHA = docosahexaenoic acid; EPA = eicosapentaenoic acid; LCT = long chain triglycerides; MCT = medium chain triglycerides.
Adapted from Singer P, Berger MM, Van den Berghe G, et al. ESPEN Guidelines on parenteral nutrition: intensive care. Clin Nutr 2009;28(4):387-400, with permission.

infused via a central venous catheter. Catheter insertion, ongoing care and replacement are similar to that with any other central venous catheter and although delivering nutrient rich solutions, there are insufficient data to suggest whether patients receiving PN are at higher risk of developing a catheter-related bloodstream infection.[155] Although the evidence-base is weak, expert recommendations suggest that a dedicated central venous catheter, or lumen of a multilumen catheter, should be used to deliver PN.[156] Manipulation of the catheter and tubing should be avoided to minimise infection of the catheter. Peripheral administration can be considered when the final solution concentration is 10–12%,[157] but is not usually used in the context of critical illness because high volumes of PN would be required to meet caloric requirements. Routine monitoring of the patient's fluid balance, glucose, biochemical profile, full blood count, triglycerides, trace elements and vitamins is necessary. The patient is also assessed for signs of complications associated with the administration of PN (Table 19.7).

TABLE 19.6
Trace elements in TPN[153]

TRACE ELEMENT	ACTION
Zinc	Wound healing
Iron	Haemoglobin synthesis
Copper	Erythrocyte maturation and lipid metabolism
Manganese	Calcium and phosphorus metabolism
Cobalt	Essential constituent of vitamin B12
Iodine	Thyroxine synthesis
Chromium	Glucose utilisation

Practice tip

PN solutions are high in glucose and therefore require vigilance in preventing catheter-related infection.

Transition to oral diet and fluids

The patient's condition, length of stay in ICU and their ability to swallow will influence when and how quickly oral nutrition can commence. Accurate identification of swallowing disorders in ICU patients is crucial to determine the safety and type of oral nutrition. Dysphagia that occurs in ICU patients following extubation is usually an ICU-acquired disorder,[158] although it is also possible for patients to have an undiagnosed swallowing disease. The prevalence of swallowing disorders in patients with acute respiratory failure who are extubated is unknown. The estimated prevalence of dysphagia ranges between 3% and 62% for patients recovering from critical illnesses.[159] Six potential mechanisms can cause patients in the ICU to develop dysfunctional swallowing. Endotracheal and tracheostomy tubes can cause direct trauma, focal ulceration and inflammation.[158] Neuromyopathy resulting in muscular weakness can also cause postextubation dysphagia.[160] The third mechanism for dysphagia is the development of dysfunctional oropharyngeal and laryngeal sensation. Sensation abnormalities can result from either critical illness polyneuropathy or local oedema.[161] Swallowing dysfunction in critical illness can be related to impaired sensorium as a result of ICU-acquired delirium, underlying critical illness or the effects of sedating medications.[162] Gastro-oesophageal reflux is disordered swallowing in critically ill patients and some of the pathophysiological processes responsible for gastro-oesophageal reflux are likely to continue in the immediate postextubation period.[158]

Swallowing dysfunction can also occur because of dyssynchronous breathing and swallowing in patients

TABLE 19.7
Short-term metabolic complications associated with total PN

COMPLICATION	CAUSE	DETECTION AND TREATMENT
Hyperosmolar coma	Occurs acutely if a rapid infusion of hypertonic fluid is administered. Infusion can cause severe osmotic diuresis, resulting in electrolyte abnormalities, dehydration and malfunction of the central nervous system	Daily blood samples, accurate measurements of fluid balance, routine blood samples Reduce infusion rate, correct electrolyte imbalances
Electrolyte imbalance	Disturbances in serum electrolytes, particularly sodium potassium, urea and creatinine, may occur early in the treatment of TPN. Electrolyte imbalances can be caused by the patient's underlying medical condition; requirements vary with individual patients' needs. Can be caused by inadequate or excessive administration of intravenous fluids	Daily blood samples taken early in treatment to detect abnormalities Replacement fluid as required, extra intravenous fluids may be required during the stabilisation period

Continued

TABLE 19.7
Short-term metabolic complications associated with total PN—cont'd

COMPLICATION	CAUSE	DETECTION AND TREATMENT
Hyperglycaemia	Critically ill patients may be resistant to insulin because of the secretion of ACTH and adrenaline. This promotes the secretion of glycogen, which inhibits the insulin response to hyperglycaemia	Monitor the patient's blood sugar 4-hourly after commencement of treatment or as required. Monitor daily urinalysis for glucose and ketones An insulin infusion may be required to keep blood sugar levels within prescribed limits
Rebound hypoglycaemia	May occur on discontinuation of TPN because hyperinsulinism may occur after prolonged intravenous nutrition. A rise in serum insulin occurs with infusion, and thus sudden cessation of infusion can result in hypoglycaemia	Glucose infusion rate should be gradually reduced over the final hour of infusion before discontinuing. Some patients may receive a 10% glucose solution after cessation of TPN
Hypophosphataemia	Glucose infusion results in the continuous release of insulin, stimulating anabolism and resulting in rapid influx of phosphorus into muscle cells. The greatest risk is to malnourished patients with overzealous administration of feeding. Patients who are hyperglycaemic, who require insulin therapy during TPN or who have a history of alcoholism or chronic weight loss may require extra phosphate in the early stages of treatment	Monitor phosphate levels daily. Hypophosphataemia will usually appear after 24–48 h of feeding Reduce the carbohydrate load and give phosphate supplementation
Lipid clearance	Lipids are broken down in the bloodstream with the aid of lipoprotein lipase found in the epithelium of capillaries in many tissues. A syndrome known as fat overload syndrome can occur when infusion of lipid is administered that is beyond the patient's clearing capacity, resulting in lipid deposits in the capillaries	Blood samples should be taken after the first infusion commences (within 6 h) to observe for lipid in the blood
Side effects of lipid infusion	Some patients suffer symptoms either during or after an infusion of lipid mix PN. The exact cause is unknown. The patient may complain of headache, nausea or vomiting, and generally feels unwell	Treat mild symptoms. If tolerated, the TPN solution of non-protein calories can be given in the form of glucose. However, it is essential that the regimen includes some fat to prevent the development of fatty acid deficiency
Anaphylactic shock	This is a rare complication but may occur as a reaction to the administration of a lipid	It may be necessary to administer adrenaline and/or steroids, and to provide supportive therapy as required
Glucose intolerance	TPN using glucose as the main source of calories is associated with a rise in oxygen consumption and CO_2 production. The workload imposed by the high CO_2 production may precipitate respiratory distress in susceptible patients, particularly those requiring mechanical ventilation	Observe patients for signs of respiratory distress. Provide non-protein calories in the form of glucose lipid mix. Slow initial rate of infusion
Liver function	Abnormalities with liver function can be associated with TPN. May be attributable to hepatic stenosis with moderate hepatomegaly; patients may also develop jaundice. Liver function tests often return to normal after cessation of therapy; however, TPN can lead to severe hepatic dysfunction in neonates	Monitor liver function tests twice weekly. There are several factors that may contribute to development of abnormal liver function tests. These most often occur after a period of time and appear to be more of a problem when there is an excess calorie intake or in glucose-based regimens

ACTH = adrenocorticotrophic hormone; TPN = total parenteral nutrition; PN = parenteral nutrition.

with underlying respiratory impairment and tachypnoea. The study of those factors that increase the risk for impaired swallowing in awake, recently extubated patients without strokes or neuromuscular diseases is less advanced. Specific risk factors for this type of postextubation dysphagia have been reported in a few epidemiological studies.[159,163,164] Risk factors for the development of dysphagia postextubation include time of orotracheal intubation, age, altered vocal quality and degree of voice impairment.[165] There are some data to suggest that critically ill patients who have required prolonged intubation may be at increased risk of dysphagia but are also less likely to be referred for screening.[166,167] Comparisons of studies are limited by biased patient selection, heterogeneous study populations and differing diagnostic protocols.

The most common diagnostic test to evaluate for postextubation dysphagia is a bedside swallow evaluation performed by a speech language pathologist. Although the components of this examination are not standardised and can vary by practitioner,[158] patients usually undergo an interview, a structural and functional evaluation of their mouth and their cough response and an assessment of swallowing function with different food textures and liquid thicknesses. The bedside swallow evaluation has been criticised for poor sensitivity as well as poor inter- and intra-rater reliability.[168] Despite not being validated against gold standard tests, a seven-point scale that incorporates the perceived aspiration risk and subsequent dietary recommendations is often used to grade the severity of dysphagia.[169] Additional tests may be ordered to assist in the diagnosis of postextubation dysphagia. A videofluoroscopic swallow study, often referred to as a modified barium swallow, is highly sensitive and specific for aspiration.[159] The other gold standard instrumental procedure to evaluate for postextubation dysphagia is a fibre optic endoscopic swallow study.[170]

Nutrition intake following ICU admission is important as this is a time where it is recognised that the patient may be at increased nutrition risk. In an observational study of 50 critically ill patients, oral intake was inadequate in the week following extubation with no patients consuming more than 50% of daily requirements.[171] Patients who are being weaned from nutrition support may have oral nutrition slowly introduced. For longer stay patients, particularly those who have ICU-acquired weakness, weaning from enteral or PN onto oral nutrition may commence with a trial of oral feeding by day supplemented by nutrition support at night.

Many patients resume oral intake after discharge from ICU. Strategies to support nutritional intake of patients on an oral diet typically target organisational or patient level factors designed to improve volitional nutritional intake. Use of oral nutrition supplements (ONS) is an additional strategy that can be used to increase protein and calorie intake and may be of benefit to those patients who continue to be at high nutrition risk and who have decreased nutritional intake. In a recent mega review of 13 systematic reviews published over the last decade,[172] the use of ONS was associated with a reduction in mortality, particularly in acutely ill patients compared with routine care (OR 0.61, 95 % CI 0.40–0.78 for hospitalised patients; OR 0.65 95 % CI 0.41–1.02 for long-term care patients). A reduction in infections and pressure ulcers was also seen with the use of ONS especially in acutely ill or elderly patients, following hospital discharge. Other novel strategies are being evaluated to address the issue of malnutrition and underfeeding throughout the critical illness recovery trajectory including complex interventions that incorporate family partnerships.[173,174]

Practice tip

Patients who have been intubated for prolonged periods are at risk for developing dysphagia. Swallowing screening and swallowing assessment might be necessary prior to commencing oral intake. Strategies should be employed to ensure swallowing assessment is undertaken quickly so nutrition intake is not negatively impacted.

Nutrition in specific clinical conditions

Not all critically ill patients are the same. Age, severity of illness, BMI and specific clinical presentations can each influence nutritional requirements and the nutrition support required. Approaches to nutrition therapy may be similar regardless of clinical presentation, such as the timing and route of feeding and techniques used to monitor nutritional status and tolerance of nutrition. However, every patient should be individually assessed, and nutrition therapy approaches targeted to their specific clinical condition. There are some general recommendations for specific clinical presentations that can serve as a guide for selecting optimal nutrition in some patient groups.

Obesity

As the proportion of the population with obesity increases so too does the number of obese patients admitted to critical care areas. The key difference for obese patients is the accumulation of body fat. There can also be an increase in muscle mass because of the effort of carrying extra body weight.[175] However, increased muscle mass is not uniformly present in all obese patients and those whose movement is severely restricted, are older or who have chronic illness may have loss of skeletal muscle mass.[176]

As most predictive equations of energy expenditure are weight based it is necessary to adjust to ideal body weight to avoid overfeeding. It is important to recognise that although body weight increases, the energy expenditure does not increase to the same extent.[177] When the BMI is >40 the increase in energy expenditure is only 14%, less than those patients with a BMI <30 or between 30 and 40 where the increase is approximately 25%.

Assessment of the obese critically ill patient should incorporate assessment of central adiposity, metabolic syndrome and sarcopenia.[13] Understanding how obesity influences energy expenditure can help guide nutrition prescription. Attention has been given to hypocaloric feeding for critically ill obese patients as a strategy to improve outcome.[178] It is suggested that a high protein hypocaloric approach to feeding be implemented in obese ICU patients as a strategy to preserve lean body mass, mobilise adipose stores and minimise metabolic complications of overfeeding.[13] This is based on the premise that nitrogen balance does not deteriorate during hypocaloric feeding[179] and that energy expenditure is more difficult to accurately determine in obese patients – so overfeeding is more likely. Overfeeding can also contribute to increased carbon dioxide production and therefore increase respiratory load, which may not be accommodated by the critically ill obese patient.[180] Despite these physiological rationales there is a lack of evidence to suggest hypocaloric feeding of the critically ill obese patient is beneficial.

Practice tip

Effective monitoring of nutrition therapy is essential in the critically ill obese patient to avoid complications such as hyperglycaemia, dyslipidaemia, hypercapnia, fluid overload and hepatic stenosis.

Protein requirements are another important consideration for the critically ill obese patient. In critical illness protein requirements are usually increased[175] and most recommendations are for 1.2–1.5 g/kg/day protein although these recommendations can be as high as 2.0 g protein/kg ideal body weight.[175] For the critically ill obese patient protein prescription should be based on ideal body weight with adjustments for increasing body weight. Whether other specific nutrients, such as arginine, glutamine and leucine, are beneficial for the critically ill obese patient is unclear.[13]

Practice tip

Obese critically ill patients might have increased GRVs because of increased intraabdominal pressure, which inhibits gastric emptying.

Sepsis

The incidence of sepsis is on the increase worldwide and, although mortality rates have improved in recent years, these can still be high.[181] Sepsis results in an overwhelming cytokine-mediated, proinflammatory response to the presence of infection and is characterised by widespread inflammation, vasodilation, leukocyte accumulation and increased microvascular permeability.[182]

There is a dearth of literature which specifically addresses the nutritional needs of patients with sepsis and many studies of critically ill patients include a limited number of septic patients.[183] The current Surviving Sepsis Guidelines have nutrition-specific recommendations for the patient with sepsis:[184] 1) early PN (alone or in combination with EN) is not recommended; 2) early initiation of EN should be commenced when patients are able to be fed enterally;[184] 3) EN should be advanced as tolerated. With the low quality of available evidence the use of omega-3 fatty acids as an immune supplement is not recommended.[185] There are no contraindications to administering EN in patients with sepsis and shock; however, it is recommended that initial resuscitation be achieved before EN is commenced.[13] A clear approach for how nutrition support might be provided is lacking because studies using different methodologies and different patient populations have produced conflicting results.

Renal failure

Critically ill patients with renal failure have widely variable metabolic patterns and nutritional requirements, making decisions about patient-specific nutritional requirements and goals challenging. The optimal nutrition requirements for patients with acute kidney injury are unclear and assessment of nutritional requirements is complicated not only by fluctuating fluid balance and body weight[186] but also by the underlying disease and type and intensity of renal replacement therapy.[187] For critically ill patients who require renal replacement therapy, there can be additional loss of glucose, amino acids, proteins, trace elements and vitamins that are water soluble and have a low molecular weight.[188] These losses can be pronounced when highly efficient renal replacement therapy such as continuous veno-venous haemofiltration or prolonged intermittent strategies such as sustained low-efficiency dialysis are used.

Although each patient requires nutritional assessment and tailored nutritional prescription, it is suggested that a calorie intake of 25–30 kcal/kg/day is required for patients with renal failure.[13] Because protein catabolism and a sustained negative nitrogen balance are often present in acute kidney injury, protein supplementation becomes important to prevent lean muscle loss. Optimal intake of proteins and amino acids for the patient with acute kidney injury who may require renal replacement therapy is often hotly debated. Recommendations range from 1.2–2 g/kg/day[13] up to 2.5 g/kg/day.[189] Increased protein provision is particularly important if the patient is receiving continuous renal replacement therapy as this is associated with significant amino acid loss of between 10 g/d and 15 g/d.[190] In addition to protein and calorie replacement, the use of pharmaconutrients with anti-inflammatory effects, such as glutamine and omega-3 fatty acids, might play a role preventing further deterioration of renal function and assisting with improvement in renal function following acute kidney injury, although there are insufficient data at present that demonstrate such an approach improves outcomes in these patients.[186]

Pancreatitis

Severe acute pancreatitis is a disease associated with increased morbidity and mortality.[191] Severe acute pancreatitis causes both local and systemic complications and results in increased catabolism and hypermetabolism, although the severity of clinical presentations can vary widely.[192]

Patients with moderate to severe acute pancreatitis should have intragastric EN commenced at a trophic rate using a standard polymeric formula which is advanced to goal when fluid resuscitation is complete.[13] There is no benefit to jejunal feeding in patients with severe acute pancreatitis.[193] The use of PN in severe acute pancreatitis should be avoided because EN confers greater benefit. Previous meta-analysis suggest that in severe acute pancreatitis the use of EN as the nutrition therapy results in reduced infectious morbidity, hospital length of stay,[194] need for surgical intervention,[195] multiple organ failure and mortality.[196]

Trauma and surgery

Nutritional recommendations for trauma patients are generally the same as those for all critically ill patients. Like data from more heterogeneous critically ill patients, early EN has a demonstrated mortality benefit.[197] Nasogastric feeding is suitable for most trauma patients although small bowel feeding might be required for those patients who require longer periods of nutrition support.[198]

Critically ill surgical patients do require special attention because they are at the highest risk of hospital-acquired malnutrition.[12] Prolonged periods of inadequate oral nutrition are associated with higher mortality and, even for those patients who are well nourished at time of surgery, should they be unable to eat for more than 7 days, nutritional support is indicated.[198]

Postoperative patients may, however, continue to receive little or no nutrition following surgery. Postoperative ileus is often a concern, which means some clinicians do not provide EN. Instead, gastric aspiration is implemented and the patient is given intravenous fluids. However, studies of gut motility demonstrate that small bowel peristalsis returns within hours following a laparotomy.[44] Therefore, interruption of nutritional intake is not necessary following surgery, even for patients who have undergone gastrointestinal surgery. A meta-analysis of 15 studies that included 1240 patients demonstrated that early postoperative nutrition was associated with significant reductions in complications and there was no evidence of negative outcomes that commonly concern clinicians, including anastomotic dehiscence.[199]

Enteral feeding may often be withheld in those patients with abdominal compartment syndrome who have a decompressive celiotomy because of the concerns about bowel dysfunction.[44] However, early EN has been shown to be feasible in these situations and is associated with improved outcomes.[46] In the absence of bowel injury it is also possible to provide EN to the patient with an open abdomen.[200]

Existing malnutrition can be a significant concern for surgical patients because of the association with complication rates, delayed recovery and longer ICU and hospital stay.[201] Preconditioning may be required and is usually best delivered by the enteral route.

Burns

Shortly after injury severe burns are associated with a high degree of hypermetabolism and hypercatabolism.[202] Burns can also result in destruction of skeletal muscle.[203] The hypermetabolic and hypercatabolic response to severe burn injury can result in significant caloric deficits and weight loss that may lead to immune dysfunction, decreased wound healing, severe infections and death.[202] Comprehensive nutritional assessment is important for patients with severe burns[204] and helps to inform nutrition therapy strategies (Table 19.8). Assessing caloric requirements can be challenging and indirect calorimetry is the preferred method of determining REE.[205] When this equipment is unavailable, burns-specific predictive equations should be used. Predictive equations developed before improvements to burn management may result in an overestimation of requirements. Of the predictive equations used in burns, the Toronto Formula is

TABLE 19.8
Comprehensive nutrition assessment in the patient with severe burns[211]

HISTORY AND PHYSICAL EXAMINATION	PREEXISTING MALNUTRITION
	Malabsorption
	Paralytic ileus
	Severe shock
	Bowel obstruction
	Diffuse peritonitis
Laboratory measurements	Serum albumin and prealbumin
	Nitrogen balance
	Tests for immune function
Clinical examination	Anthropometric measurements
	Fluid intake and output
Metabolic assessment	Indirect calorimetry

TABLE 19.9

Predictive equations for estimating caloric requirements in patients with burns[208]

AGE, Y	NAME	FORMULA
0–1	Galveston Infant	2100 kcal/m^2 + 1000 kcal/m^2 burn
1–11	Galveston Revised	1800 kcal/m^2 + 1300 kcal/m^2 burn
12–16	Galveston Adolescent	1500 kcal/m^2 + 1500 kcal/m^2 burn
16–59	Curreri formula	25 kcal/kg body weight + (40) TBSA
	Toronto formula	−4343 + (10.5 × TBSA) + (0.23 × CI) + (0.84 × HBE) + (114 × T) − (4.5 × PBD)
≥60	Curreri formula	20 kcal/kg body weight + 65 (TBSA)

CI = total calorie intake the previous day; HBE = Harris–Benedict estimates; PBD = number of postburn days to the day preceding the estimation; T = average of core temperatures (°C) the previous day; TBSA = burn size in total body surface area.

Source: Rodriguez NA, Jeschke MG, Williams FN, et al. Nutrition in burns: Galveston contributions. JPEN J Parenter Enteral Nutr 2011;35(6):704-14. PubMed PMID: 21975669. Pubmed Central PMCID: 3778650.

the most complicated and likely difficult within a busy clinical setting (Table 19.9).

Early EN (within 4–6 h of injury) should be provided to patients with burns when oral intake is not possible or inadequate.[13] PN can be used with EN and/or oral intake is not possible. Protein requirements are similar to that for other critically ill patients and recommendations are for patients with burn injury to receive 1.5–2g/kg/day of protein.[206] There are several benefits to early and continuous EN including a decreased hypermetabolic response; decreased levels of circulating catecholamines, cortisol and glucagon;[207] preservation of gut mucosal blood flow and mucosal integrity; and improved gut motility.[208] Administering specific micronutrients may improve immune function and positively influence septic morbidity and mortality.[209] Many pharmaconutrients have been studied in the context of nutrition support for the patient with burns although their benefit is yet to be clearly demonstrated.[210]

Glycaemic control in critical illness

Hyperglycaemia and increased insulin resistance are characteristics of the body's stress response and activation of the sympathetic and adrenal and hypothalamic–pituitary–adrenal axis responses to critical illness.[3] Hyperglycaemia has been considered a beneficial adaptive response to stress to provide energy substrate to the organs involved in the 'fight or flight' response.[211] There is some, although inconsistent, evidence of an association of hyperglycaemia with high mortality and morbidity.[212-214]

The complexity of the physiological processes associated with hyperglycaemia in critical illness and the sophisticated research required to generate valid information render clinical decision making related to glycaemic control challenging. Nevertheless, the concept of glycaemic control is accepted but there are variations in the recommended range of acceptable values for glucose levels.[13] The Society for Critical Care Medicine recommends a range of 150–180 mg/dL[215] and the American Association of Parenteral and Enteral Nutrition recommends 140–180 mg/dL.[13] Initial single-centre clinical trials evaluating glycaemic control in critical illness demonstrated improvements in short-term morbidity and mortality[216,217] but these same benefits have not been demonstrated in larger clinical trials.[212] The optimal target for glycaemic control in critical illness is not clear[218] although it is recognised that the lower the target the more likely are adverse events associated with hypoglycaemia. The discrepancies in these studies have been attributed to many factors including the variability in target ranges for blood glucose, methods of blood glucose measurement, difficulty for some studies to achieve separation of the treatment and control groups, compliance with the therapy and employment of different nutritional strategies.[218]

Insulin infusions are used to control high blood glucose levels and nurses have an integral role in the management of these patients. It is recommended that blood glucose values are monitored every 1–2 h until glucose values and insulin infusion rates are stable, then every 4 h thereafter.[123] The continuation of insulin infusions in patients who have their EN decreased or ceased requires more frequent blood glucose monitoring because of the risk for hypoglycaemia.[219]

The use of intravenous insulin for tight glycaemic control can contribute to rapidly changing blood glucose levels; therefore, vigilant monitoring is required. Increased frequency of blood glucose measurement may impact on the provision of patient care or, if not attended, contribute to underdetection of hypoglycaemia. Nursing fatigue has also been associated with increased hypoglycaemia.[220]

Validity of blood glucose measurement is also an important consideration. Formal laboratory testing is considered the 'gold standard' for blood glucose measurement but point-of-care testing of blood glucose is common in the critical care setting. Blood glucose may be sampled from arterial, venous and capillary blood. The use of capillary blood in testing blood glucose may be problematic, particularly in those patients for whom hypoperfusion is an issue.[221] It is recommended that point-of-care testing using capillary blood is interpreted with caution because the measurements may not accurately estimate arterial blood or plasma glucose values.[123]

It is clear that hyperglycaemia should be avoided. However, the inconsistencies in published studies mean that an agreed specified target for blood glucose in the critically ill patient population is difficult to achieve. The optimal target blood glucose level is unknown and may differ depending on the patient's clinical presentation.

Summary

Critically ill patients are at increased risk of malnutrition because of increased metabolic requirements coupled with challenges in delivering prescribed nutrition. Critical care nurses play a pivotal role in ensuring nutritional adequacy and are well positioned to coordinate interdisciplinary collaboration to optimise nutrition therapy. Optimising nutrition in critical illness is assisted by accurate assessment of nutritional requirements and prescribing nutrition that closely matches the patient's individual needs. Delivery of prescribed nutrition is the role of the nurse and attention should be given to minimising interruptions to nutrition therapy. During recovery from critical illness and when the patient resumes oral intake, nutritional risk can be increased because of factors that impact on the patient's ability to eat. Assessment of the ability to safely resume oral intake might be necessary for those patients at risk of dysphagia. Attention to nutritional requirements should commence on admission to the ICU and extend beyond both ICU and hospital discharge.

Case study

David, a 57-year-old builder, was admitted to ICU with necrotising fasciitis which developed in a lower leg wound. He was admitted with sepsis and haemodynamic stability was achieved with fluid resuscitation and vasoactive agents. His admission weight was 127 kg and he was 190 cm tall. His BMI was 38.0 (class 2 obesity).

David was intubated and mechanically ventilated in ICU for 10 days during which he underwent seven operative procedures for debridement of the necrotic tissues. On arrival to ICU a nasogastric tube was inserted and he was commenced on enteral feeding at 60 mL/h of a standard polymeric enteral feeding formula of 1.28 kcal/mL and 6.3g protein /100 mL. During his stay in ICU enteral feeding was repeatedly discontinued for surgical procedures, sometimes for as long as 6 hours per day.

David was extubated on day 11 of his ICU stay and his nasogastric tube was removed. He was discharged to the ward the following day.

DISCUSSION

Critically ill patients often have increased nutritional requirements either as a result of preexisting malnutrition or because of decreased nutritional intake that is insufficient to meet the increased energy expenditure that is typical in critical illness. There are a number of key issues relating to nutritional status and the provision of nutrition that are central to this case study. These include preexisting obesity, sepsis, hypotension and shock requiring vasopressors.

Obesity: It can be challenging to accurately determine nutritional requirements for critically ill patients and this is particularly the case in the context of obesity. While obese patients do accumulate increased body fat they can also have an increased amount of muscle mass because of the need to carry extra body weight. Most ICUs do not have the benefit of a metabolic cart to measure energy expenditure so predictive equations are often used to determine caloric requirements. Most of these equations are weight based; therefore, adjustment needs to be made so ideal body weight is used in the equation, otherwise overfeeding might result. Hypocaloric and high protein EN should be used for obese patients. Based on the nutrition prescription for this patient David would have received 91 g of protein per day. This is less than the recommended *minimum* protein intake of 104 g/day (based on 1.2g/kg/day – ideal body weight 87 kg). The nutrition prescription of 60 mL/h is insufficient to deliver goal calories as well. Using an ideal body weight of 87 kg (BMI 24) and a caloric prescription of 25 kcal/kg/day, the enteral feeding rate should be adjusted to deliver 2175 kcal/day (rate of 71 mL/h). It is possible that the estimation of his energy expenditure could have led to either over- or underfeeding. Indirect calorimetry, where available, could assist with more accurate measures of energy expenditure and caloric requirements.

Hypotension: Hypotension and the use of vasopressors can reduce splanchnic perfusion and is sometimes perceived as a contraindication to EN. Enteral nutrients have been shown to increase gut blood flow, which allows the bowel to absorb nutrients during vasopressor therapy. There is insufficient evidence to suggest whether EN should continue or be withheld when vasopressors are being administered with the results from a limited number of studies being inconsistent. Individual patient assessment is required to guide clinical practice in this area. In this case study EN was commenced despite vasopressor therapy and the patient did not exhibit any signs of gastric intolerance.

Sepsis: The approach to nutrition support for critically ill patients with sepsis is similar to that for any other critically ill patient. The fluctuations in metabolic rate that would have occurred during recovery from critical illness may have made assessment of nutrition needs challenging. The metabolic response to critical illness changes as critical illness progresses. In the first few days of critical illness, endogenous glucose production may be sufficient to meet energy needs of critically ill patients. However, it would have been projected that this patient's ICU length of stay would be longer than for most other patients which places him at increased nutrition risk. Ongoing assessment of energy expenditure using indirect calorimetry may have been beneficial as a component of ongoing nutrition assessment.

Surgical intervention: Repeated surgical interventions for debridement of necrotic tissue was necessary. As David remained intubated and mechanically ventilated there was no need to discontinue enteral feeding prior to surgery. The repeated discontinuation of EN would have resulted in a significantly lower energy and protein adequacy and this would have a negative impact on long-term recovery. Maintaining lean body mass is critical to improved functional recovery following critical illness and patients for whom nutrition is optimised are more likely to be discharged home following hospitalisation.

CASE STUDY QUESTIONS

1. On admission, what information might you request from the family to help you to assess whether David was nutritionally at risk prior to admission?
2. In the case study the patient presented with moderate obesity and sepsis, treated with vasoactive agents. Discuss how these two factors might influence tolerance of EN.
3. In the transition from EN to oral nutrition, what strategies could be used to ensure optimal nutrition intake during recovery?

RESEARCH VIGNETTE

Reignier J, Boisrame-Helms J, Brisard L, et al. Enteral versus parenteral early nutrition in ventilated adults with shock: a randomised, controlled, multicentre, open-label, parallel-group study (NUTRIREA-2). Lancet 2018;391(10116):133-43

Background

Whether the route of early feeding affects outcomes of patients with severe critical illnesses is controversial. We hypothesised that outcomes were better with early first-line enteral nutrition (EN) than with early first-line parenteral nutrition (PN).

Methods: In this randomised, controlled, multicentre, open-label, parallel-group study (NUTRIREA-2 trial) done at 44 French intensive care units (ICUs), adults (18 years or older) receiving invasive mechanical ventilation and vasopressor support for shock were randomly assigned (1:1) to either PN or EN, both targeting normocaloric goals (20–25 kcal/kg per day), within 24 h after intubation. Randomisation was stratified by centre using permutation blocks of variable sizes. Given that the route of nutrition cannot be masked, blinding of the physicians and nurses was not feasible. Patients receiving PN could be switched to EN after at least 72 h in the event of shock resolution (no vasopressor support for 24 consecutive hours and arterial lactate <2 mmol/L). The primary endpoint was mortality on day 28 after randomisation in the intention-to-treat-population. This study is registered with ClinicalTrials.gov, number NCT01802099.

Findings: After the second interim analysis, the independent Data Safety and Monitoring Board deemed that completing patient enrolment was unlikely to significantly change the results of the trial and recommended stopping patient recruitment. Between 22 March 2013 and 30 June 2015, 2410 patients were enrolled and randomly assigned; 1202 to the enteral group and 1208 to the parenteral group. By day 28, 443 (37%) of 1202 patients in the enteral group and 422 (35%) of 1208 patients in the parenteral group had died (absolute difference estimate 2.0%; [95% CI 1.9–5.8]; p=0.33). Cumulative incidence of patients with ICU-acquired infections did not differ between the enteral group (173 [14%]) and the parenteral group (194 [16%]; hazard ratio [HR] 0.89 [95% CI 0.72–1.09]; p=0.25). Compared with the parenteral group, the enteral group had higher cumulative incidences of patients with vomiting (406 [34%] vs 246 [20%]; HR 1.89 [1.62–2.20]; p<0.0001), diarrhoea (432 [36%] vs 393 [33%]; 1.20 [1.05–1.37]; p=0.009), bowel ischaemia (19 [2%] vs five [<1%]; 3.84 [1.43–10.3]; p=0.007), and acute colonic pseudo-obstruction (11 [1%] vs three [<1%]; 3.7 [1.03–13.2; p=0.04).

Interpretation: In critically ill adults with shock, early isocaloric EN did not reduce mortality or the risk of secondary infections but was associated with a greater risk of digestive complications compared with early isocaloric PN.

Critique

Several studies have examined the effect of EN versus PN on patient outcomes. The results have been inconsistent with variations in the design, sample size, timing of feeding, number of calories delivered and outcomes measured. This well-designed randomised controlled trial of adult patients in shock who were receiving mechanical ventilation and vasopressors randomised 2410 patients from 44 French ICUs.[55] The study concentrated on the route of feeding comparing EN versus PN. The results did not show a difference in major clinical outcomes (mortality and infection) between these two groups. There were fewer gut-related complications in patient who received PN. Rates of bowel ischaemia and acute colonic pseudo-obstruction were evaluated, both of which were higher in patients receiving EN. However, the method of assessment by unblended adjudication committees may introduce potential bias. The rates of some of these complications were also quite rare. Tian and Doig suggest that 85 patients would need to be treated with PN to prevent one case of bowel ischaemia.[222] While PN resulted in improved outcomes such as vomiting, diarrhoea, bowel obstruction and hypoglycaemia), for the clinically important outcomes of pneumonia, duration of mechanical ventilation, ICU stay and mortality, improved outcomes associated with PN were not evident. The economic impact of PN was substantively higher with estimated costs of PN four times higher than those for EN.[222]

In NUTRIREA-2 EN was commenced at target dose of 20–25 kcal/kg/day. Others have suggested that early hypocaloric nutrition intake may be more appropriate, particularly in patients with shock. The use of vasopressors may contribute to hypoperfusion of the gastrointestinal tract, EN intolerance and mesenteric ischaemia.[79] Because of the association with improved outcomes, clinical practice guidelines currently recommend commencing EN within 24–48 hours of resuscitation or when hemodynamic stability is reached (defined as adequate perfusion pressure, stable doses of vasoactive drugs, stabilised or decreasing levels of lactate and metabolic acidosis, and mean arterial pressure ≥60 mmHg).[223] The early and aggressive approach to EN in patients with shock may explain the higher rates of gastrointestinal complications.

The study was stopped early after the second interim analysis. Random variation often causes large treatment effects at the beginning of the trial but lessens as the trial progresses.[224] The investigators acknowledged that stopping the trial early was a limitation. Trials that stop early (truncated trials) are likely to overestimate the size of the effect. The apparent compelling results in such trials may fast track the process of publication, clinical practice guideline development and quality assurance initiatives[225] but the investigators argued that the results were similar to those of the interim analyses and that it was unlikely that the inclusion of the 444 patients to meet their sample size target were unlikely to have changed the results. The other limitation of the trial is that neither the patients nor the ICU staff were masked to treatment allocation, but the investigators argued that blinding was not possible considering the nature of the treatments. The investigators noted that enteral feeding may cause gut ischaemia but research is needed to confirm this finding. Van Dyck and Casaer in their recent commentary note that early EN does not save lives in the ICU.[15,226] They suggest that a better endpoint for clinical trials is the reduction of the burden of long-term limitations in physical function.[226]

Learning activities

1 Review your patients' notes and calculate what their total daily caloric intake was for the previous day. Once you have obtained this figure, compare this with the prescribed intake. If patients have not received their total daily caloric intake, consider what factors may have contributed to this and how these might be overcome in future.

2 Review the notes of two medical and two elective surgical patients admitted to your ICU. Which patients demonstrated some evidence of preexisting nutrition risk?

3 Should critically ill patients who have had gastrointestinal surgery not receive EN postoperatively?

4 Your patient has been in ICU for the past 14 days and is now ready to be discharged to the ward. During the patient's ICU stay there has been progressive loss of lean body mass. In handover to the nurses on the ward what key points would you make to ensure that nutrition optimisation is a priority on the ward?

5 On admission to the ICU a nasogastric tube is placed and position confirmed on X-ray. Enteral feeding is subsequently commenced. What strategies do you take to ensure safe feeding throughout the patient's ICU stay?

6 During the initial admission period to ICU your patient was not tolerating EN well. GRVs were high and the patient's gut was distended. PN has been the nutrition support strategy used for this patient and today the decision was made to reintroduce EN. How will you manage this transition from PN to EN?

Online resources

American Society for Parenteral and Enteral Nutrition, www.nutritioncare.org

Australasian Society for Parenteral and Enteral Nutrition, www.auspen.org.au

Critical Care Nutrition, www.criticalcarenutrition.com

The European Society for Clinical Nutrition and Metabolism, www.espen.org

Further reading

Ayers P, Guenter P, Holcombe B, et al, editors. A.S.P.E.N. Parenteral nutrition handbook. Maryland: The American Society for Parenteral and Enteral Nutrition; 2014.

Berger MM. Critical care nutrition therapy for non-nutritionists. New York: Springer; 2017.

Corkins MR, editor. The A.S.P.E.N. Pediatric Nutrition Support Core Curriculum. 2nd ed. Maryland: The American Society for Parenteral and Enteral Nutrition; 2015.

Farber P, Siervo M. Nutrition in critical care. Cambridge: Cambridge University Press; 2014.

Seres DS, Van Way CW III, editors. Nutrition support for the critically ill. Cham: Humana Press; 2016.

Singer P. Nutrition in intensive care medicine: beyond physiology. In: Koletzko B, editor. World review of nutrition and dietetics, vol. 105. Basel: Karger; 2013.

References

1. McCance KL. Cellular biology. In: McCance KL, Huether SE, Brashers VL, et al, editors. Pathophysiology: the biologic basis for disease in adults and children. 7th ed. St Louis: Elsevier Health Sciences; 2015. p. 1–48.
2. Singer P. From mitochondrial disturbances to energy requirements. In: Singer P, editor. Nutrition in intensive care medicine: beyond physiology. World Rev Nutr Diet. vol. 105. Basel: Karger; 2013. p. 1–11.
3. Preiser JC, van Zanten AR, Berger MM, et al. Metabolic and nutritional support of critically ill patients: consensus and controversies. Crit Care 2015;19:35.
4. Stanojcic M, Finnerty CC, Jeschke MG. Anabolic and anticatabolic agents in critical care. Curr Opin Crit Care 2016;22(4):325–31.
5. Btaiche IF, Chan LN, Pleva M, et al. Critical illness, gastrointestinal complications, and medication therapy during enteral feeding in critically ill adult patients. Nutr Clin Pract 2010;25(1):32–49.

6. Preiser JC, Ichai C, Orban JC, et al. Metabolic response to the stress of critical illness. Br J Anaesth 2014;113(6):945–54.
7. Sundstrom M, Rehal M, Tjader I, et al. Nutritional needs for the critically ill in relation to inflammation. Curr Opin Clin Nutr Metab Care 2016;19(2):138–43.
8. Lew CCH, Yandell R, Fraser RJL, et al. Association between malnutrition and clinical outcomes in the intensive care unit: a systematic review [formula: see text]. JPEN J Parenter Enteral Nutr 2017;41(5):744–58.
9. Hudson L, Chittams J, Griffith C, et al. Malnutrition identified by Academy of Nutrition and Dietetics/American Society for Parenteral and Enteral Nutrition is associated with more 30-day readmissions, greater hospital mortality, and longer hospital stays: a retrospective analysis of nutrition assessment data in a major medical center. JPEN J Parenter Enteral Nutr 2018;doi:10.1002/jpen.1021. [Epub ahead of print].
10. Mogensen KM, Horkan CM, Purtle SW, et al. Malnutrition, critical illness survivors, and postdischarge outcomes: a cohort study. JPEN J Parenter Enteral Nutr 2017;148607117709766.
11. Jensen GL, Mirtallo J, Compher C, et al. Adult starvation and disease-related malnutrition: a proposal for etiology-based diagnosis in the clinical practice setting from the International Consensus Guideline Committee. JPEN J Parenter Enteral Nutr 2010;34(2):156–9.
12. Drover JW, Cahill NE, Kutsogiannis J, et al. Nutrition therapy for the critically ill surgical patient: we need to do better! JPEN J Parenter Enteral Nutr 2010;34(6):644–52.
13. McClave SA, Taylor BE, Martindale RG, et al. Guidelines for the provision and assessment of nutrition support therapy in the adult critically ill patient: Society of Critical Care Medicine (SCCM) and American Society for Parenteral and Enteral Nutrition (A.S.P.E.N.). JPEN J Parenter Enteral Nutr 2016;40(2):159–211.
14. Garcia NM, McClave SA, Bozeman MC, et al. Emerging concepts in critical care nutrition and the provision of enteral nutrition support. Curr Surg Rep 2015;3(11):34.
15. Arabi YM, Casaer MP, Chapman M, et al. The intensive care medicine research agenda in nutrition and metabolism. Intensive Care Med 2017;43(9):1239–56.
16. Correia M. Nutrition screening vs nutrition assessment: what's the difference? Nutr Clin Pract 2017;884533617719669.
17. Kozeniecki M, Codner P, Heyland DK. Identifying nutritional risk in critical illness. Curr Pulmonol Rep 2017;6(1):48–53.
18. Compher C, Chittams J, Sammarco T, et al. Greater protein and energy intake may be associated with improved mortality in higher risk critically ill patients: a multicenter, multinational observational study. Crit Care Med 2017;45(2):156–63.
19. Coltman A, Peterson S, Roehl K, et al. Use of 3 tools to assess nutrition risk in the intensive care unit. JPEN J Parenter Enteral Nutr 2015;39(1):28–33.
20. van Bokhorst-de van der Schueren MA, Guaitoli PR, Jansma EP, et al. Nutrition screening tools: does one size fit all? A systematic review of screening tools for the hospital setting. Clin Nutr 2014;33(1):39–58.
21. Jensen GL, Wheeler D. A new approach to defining and diagnosing malnutrition in adult critical illness. Curr Opin Crit Care 2012;18(2):206–11.
22. Heyland DK, Dhaliwal R, Jiang X, et al. Identifying critically ill patients who benefit the most from nutrition therapy: the development and initial validation of a novel risk assessment tool. Crit Care 2011;15(6):R268.
23. de Vries MCH, Koekkoek WAC, Opdam MH, et al. Nutritional assessment of critically ill patients: validation of the modified NUTRIC score. Eur J Clin Nutr 2018;72:428–35.
24. Rahman A, Hasan RM, Agarwala R, et al. Identifying critically-ill patients who will benefit most from nutritional therapy: further validation of the 'modified NUTRIC' nutritional risk assessment tool. Clin Nutr 2016;35(1):158–62.
25. Kalaiselvan MS, Renuka MK, Arunkumar AS. Use of Nutrition Risk in Critically Ill (NUTRIC) Score to assess nutritional risk in mechanically ventilated patients: a prospective observational study. Indian J Crit Care Med 2017;21(5):253–6.
26. Moisey LL, Mourtzakis M, Kozar RA, et al. Existing equations to estimate lean body mass are not accurate in the critically ill: results of a multicenter observational study. Clin Nutr 2017;36(6):1701–6.
27. Paris MT, Mourtzakis M, Day A, et al. Validation of bedside ultrasound of muscle layer thickness of the quadriceps in the critically ill patient (VALIDUM Study). JPEN J Parenter Enteral Nutr 2017;41(2):171–80.
28. Kuchnia A, Earthman C, Teigen L, et al. Evaluation of bioelectrical impedance analysis in critically ill patients: results of a multicenter prospective study. JPEN J Parenter Enteral Nutr 2017;41(7):1131–8.
29. Schoeller DA. Making indirect calorimetry a gold standard for predicting energy requirements for institutionalized patients. J Am Diet Assoc 2007;107(3):390–2.
30. Singer P, Anbar R, Cohen J, et al. The tight calorie control study (TICACOS): a prospective, randomized, controlled pilot study of nutritional support in critically ill patients. Intensive Care Med 2011;37(4):601–9.
31. Saffle JR, Larson CM, Sullivan J. A randomized trial of indirect calorimetry-based feedings in thermal injury. J Trauma 1990;30(7):776–82, discussion 82-3.
32. McClave SA, Martindale RG, Kiraly L. The use of indirect calorimetry in the intensive care unit. Curr Opin Clin Nutr Metab Care 2013;16(2):202–8.
33. Guttormsen AB, Pichard C. Determining energy requirements in the ICU. Curr Opin Clin Nutr Metab Care 2014;17(2):171–6.
34. Haugen HA, Chan LN, Li F. Indirect calorimetry: a practical guide for clinicians. Nutr Clin Pract 2007;22(4):377–88.
35. Schlein KM, Coulter SP. Best practices for determining resting energy expenditure in critically ill adults. Nutr Clin Pract 2014;29(1):44–55.

36. McClave SA, Spain DA, Skolnick JL, et al. Achievement of steady state optimizes results when performing indirect calorimetry. JPEN J Parenter Enteral Nutr 2003;27(1):16–20.
37. Walker RN, Heuberger RA. Predictive equations for energy needs for the critically ill. Respir Care 2009;54(4):509–21.
38. Cooney RN, Frankenfield DC. Determining energy needs in critically ill patients: equations or indirect calorimeters. Curr Opin Crit Care 2012;18(2):174–7.
39. Kross EK, Sena M, Schmidt K, et al. A comparison of predictive equations of energy expenditure and measured energy expenditure in critically ill patients. J Crit Care 2012;27(3):321 e5–12.
40. Faisy C, Guerot E, Diehl JL, et al. Assessment of resting energy expenditure in mechanically ventilated patients. Am J Clin Nutr 2003;78(2):241–9.
41. Frankenfield DC, Coleman A, Alam S, et al. Analysis of estimation methods for resting metabolic rate in critically ill adults. JPEN J Parenter Enteral Nutr 2009;33(1):27–36.
42. Siervo M, Bertoli S, Battezzati A, et al. Accuracy of predictive equations for the measurement of resting energy expenditure in older subjects. Clin Nutr 2013.
43. Tatucu-Babet OA, Ridley EJ, Tierney AC. Prevalence of underprescription or overprescription of energy needs in critically ill mechanically ventilated adults as determined by indirect calorimetry: a systematic literature review. JPEN J Parenter Enteral Nutr 2016;40(2):212–25.
44. Marik PE. Enteral nutrition in the critically ill: myths and misconceptions. Crit Care Med 2014;42(4):962–9.
45. Hermsen JL, Sano Y, Kudsk KA. Food fight! Parenteral nutrition, enteral stimulation and gut-derived mucosal immunity. Langenbecks Arch Surg 2009;394(1):17–30.
46. Reintam Blaser A, Starkopf J, Alhazzani W, et al. Early enteral nutrition in critically ill patients: ESICM clinical practice guidelines. Intensive Care Med 2017;43(3):380–98.
47. Slack E, Balmer ML, Macpherson AJ. B cells as a critical node in the microbiota-host immune system network. Immunol Rev 2014;260(1):50–66.
48. Mittal R, Coopersmith CM. Redefining the gut as the motor of critical illness. Trends Mol Med 2014;20(4):214–23.
49. Martindale RG, Warren M. Should enteral nutrition be started in the first week of critical illness? Curr Opin Clin Nutr Metab Care 2015;18(2):202–6.
50. McClave SA, Martindale RG, Rice TW, et al. Feeding the critically ill patient. Crit Care Med 2014;42(12):2600–10.
51. Harvey SE, Parrott F, Harrison DA, et al. Trial of the route of early nutritional support in critically ill adults. N Engl J Med 2014;371(18):1673–84.
52. Schorghuber M, Fruhwald S. Effects of enteral nutrition on gastrointestinal function in patients who are critically ill. Lancet Gastroenterol Hepatol 2018;3(4):281–7.
53. Ralls MW, Miyasaka E, Teitelbaum DH. Intestinal microbial diversity and perioperative complications. JPEN J Parenter Enteral Nutr 2014;38(3):392–9.
54. Peterson SJ, Lateef OB, Freels S, et al. Early exposure to recommended calorie delivery in the intensive care unit is associated with increased mortality in patients with acute respiratory distress syndrome. JPEN J Parenter Enteral Nutr 2017;148607117713483.
55. Reignier J, Boisrame-Helms J, Brisard L, et al. Enteral versus parenteral early nutrition in ventilated adults with shock: a randomised, controlled, multicentre, open-label, parallel-group study (NUTRIREA-2). Lancet 2018;391(10116):133–43.
56. Patel JJ, Lemieux M, McClave SA, et al. Critical care nutrition support best practices: key differences between Canadian and American guidelines. Nutr Clin Pract 2017;32(5):633–44.
57. Patel JJ, Martindale RG, McClave SA. Controversies surrounding critical care nutrition: an appraisal of permissive underfeeding, protein, and outcomes. JPEN J Parenter Enteral Nutr 2017;148607117721908.
58. Schetz M, Casaer MP, Van den Berghe G. Does artificial nutrition improve outcome of critical illness? Crit Care 2013;17(1):302.
59. Marik PE, Hooper MH. Normocaloric versus hypocaloric feeding on the outcomes of ICU patients: a systematic review and meta-analysis. Intensive Care Med 2016;42(3):316–23.
60. Lee ZY, Barakatun-Nisak MY, Noor Airini I, et al. Enhanced protein-energy provision via the enteral route in critically ill patients (PEP uP Protocol): a review of evidence. Nutr Clin Pract 2016;31(1):68–79.
61. McClave SA, Saad MA, Esterle M, et al. Volume-based feeding in the critically ill patient. JPEN J Parenter Enteral Nutr 2015;39(6):707–12.
62. Wischmeyer PE, Hasselmann M, Kummerlen C, et al. A randomized trial of supplemental parenteral nutrition in underweight and overweight critically ill patients: the TOP-UP pilot trial. Crit Care 2017;21(1):142.
63. Weijs PJ, Stapel SN, de Groot SD, et al. Optimal protein and energy nutrition decreases mortality in mechanically ventilated, critically ill patients: a prospective observational cohort study. JPEN J Parenter Enteral Nutr 2012;36(1):60–8.
64. Alberda C, Gramlich L, Jones N, et al. The relationship between nutritional intake and clinical outcomes in critically ill patients: results of an international multicenter observational study. Intensive Care Med 2009;35(10):1728–37.
65. Allingstrup MJ, Esmailzadeh N, Wilkens Knudsen A, et al. Provision of protein and energy in relation to measured requirements in intensive care patients. Clin Nutr 2012;31(4):462–8.
66. Faisy C, Llerena MC, Savalle M, et al. Early ICU energy deficit is a risk factor for Staphylococcus aureus ventilator-associated pneumonia. Chest 2011;140(5):1254–60.
67. Casaer MP, Van den Berghe G. Nutrition in the acute phase of critical illness. N Engl J Med 2014;370(25):2450–1.

68. Weijs PJ, Looijaard WG, Beishuizen A, et al. Early high protein intake is associated with low mortality and energy overfeeding with high mortality in non-septic mechanically ventilated critically ill patients. Crit Care 2014;18(6):701.
69. National Heart Lung, and Blood Institute Acute Respiratory Distress Syndrome Clinical Trials Network, Rice TW, Wheeler AP, et al. Initial trophic vs full enteral feeding in patients with acute lung injury: the EDEN randomized trial. JAMA 2012;307(8):795–803.
70. Arabi YM, Aldawood AS, Haddad SH, et al. Permissive underfeeding or standard enteral feeding in critically ill adults. N Engl J Med 2015;372(25):2398–408.
71. Petros S, Horbach M, Seidel F, et al. Hypocaloric vs normocaloric nutrition in critically ill patients: a prospective randomized pilot trial. JPEN J Parenter Enteral Nutr 2016;40(2):242–9.
72. Lee ZY, Ibrahim NA, Mohud-Yusof BN. Prevalence and duration of reasons for enteral nutrition feeding interruption in a tertiary intensive care unit. Nutrition 2018;53:26–33.
73. Marshall AP, Cahill NE, Gramlich L, et al. Optimizing nutrition in intensive care units: empowering critical care nurses to be effective agents of change. Am J Crit Care 2012;21(3):186–94.
74. Cahill NE, Jiang X, Heyland DK. Revised questionnaire to assess barriers to adequate nutrition in the critically ill. JPEN J Parenter Enteral Nutr 2016;40(4):511–18.
75. Williams TA, Leslie GD, Leen T, et al. Reducing interruptions to continuous enteral nutrition in the intensive care unit: a comparative study. J Clin Nurs 2013;22(19–20):2838–48.
76. Kuslapuu M, Jogela K, Starkopf J, et al. The reasons for insufficient enteral feeding in an intensive care unit: a prospective observational study. Intensive Crit Care Nurs 2015;31(5):309–14.
77. McCall ME, Adamo A, Latko K, et al. Maximizing nutrition support practice and measuring adherence to nutrition support guidelines in a Canadian tertiary care ICU. J Intensive Care Med 2018;33(3):209–17.
78. Cahill NE, Dhaliwal R, Day AG, et al. Nutrition therapy in the critical care setting: what is 'best achievable' practice? An international multicenter observational study. Crit Care Med 2010;38(2):395–401.
79. Patel JJ, Codner P. Controversies in critical care nutrition support. Crit Care Clin 2016;32(2):173–89.
80. McClave SA, Chang WK. Feeding the hypotensive patient: does enteral feeding precipitate or protect against ischemic bowel? Nutr Clin Pract 2003;18(4):279–84.
81. Khalid I, Doshi P, DiGiovine B. Early enteral nutrition and outcomes of critically ill patients treated with vasopressors and mechanical ventilation. Am J Crit Care 2010;19(3):261–8.
82. Berger MM, Berger-Gryllaki M, Wiesel PH, et al. Intestinal absorption in patients after cardiac surgery. Crit Care Med 2000;28(7):2217–23.
83. Mentec H, Dupont H, Bocchetti M, et al. Upper digestive intolerance during enteral nutrition in critically ill patients: frequency, risk factors, and complications. Crit Care Med 2001;29(10):1955–61.
84. Cahill NE, Murch L, Cook D, et al. Improving the provision of enteral nutrition in the intensive care unit: a description of a multifaceted intervention tailored to overcome local barriers. Nutr Clin Pract 2014;29(1):110–17.
85. Jones K, Maxwell PJ, McClave S, et al. Optimizing enteral nutrition in medical intensive care patients. Curr Pulmonol Rep 2017;6:64–9.
86. Saran D, Brody RA, Stankorb SM, et al. Gastric vs small bowel feeding in critically ill neurologically injured patients: results of a multicenter observational study. JPEN J Parenter Enteral Nutr 2015;39(8):910–16.
87. Ho KM, Dobb GJ, Webb SA. A comparison of early gastric and post-pyloric feeding in critically ill patients: a meta-analysis. Intensive Care Med 2006;32(5):639–49.
88. Silk DB, Quinn DG. Dual-purpose gastric decompression and enteral feeding tubes rationale and design of novel nasogastric and nasogastrojejunal tubes. JPEN J Parenter Enteral Nutr 2015;39(5):531–43.
89. McGinnis CM, Worthington P, Lord LM. Nasogastric versus feeding tubes in critically ill patients. Crit Care Nurse 2010;30(6):80–2.
90. Miller KR, McClave SA, Kiraly LN, et al. A tutorial on enteral access in adult patients in the hospitalized setting. JPEN J Parenter Enteral Nutr 2014;38(3):282–95.
91. Blumenstein I, Shastri YM, Stein J. Gastroenteric tube feeding: techniques, problems and solutions. World J Gastroenterol 2014;20(26):8505–24.
92. Metheny NA, Stewart BJ, Mills AC. Blind insertion of feeding tubes in intensive care units: a national survey. Am J Crit Care 2012;21(5):352–60.
93. Bourgault AM, Heath J, Hooper V, et al. Methods used by critical care nurses to verify feeding tube placement in clinical practice. Crit Care Nurse 2015;35(1):e1–7.
94. Santos SC, Woith W, Freitas MI, et al. Methods to determine the internal length of nasogastric feeding tubes: an integrative review. Int J Nurs Stud 2016;61:95–103.
95. Fan EMP, Tan SB. Nasogastric tube placement confirmation: where we are and where we should be heading. Proc Singapore Healthc 2017;26(3):189–95.
96. Wong KW, Chan HH, Wong CP, et al. Using color flow detection of air insufflation to improve accuracy in verifying nasogastric tube position. Am J Emerg Med 2017;35(2):333–6.
97. Deshpande R, Akhtar S, Haddadin AS. Utility of ultrasound in the ICU. Curr Opin Anaesthesiol 2014;27(2):123–32.
98. Gok F, Kilicaslan A, Yosunkaya A. Ultrasound-guided nasogastric feeding tube placement in critical care patients. Nutr Clin Pract 2015;30(2):257–60.

99. Mizzi A, Cozzi S, Beretta L, et al. Real-time image-guided nasogastric feeding tube placement: a case series using Kangaroo with IRIS Technology in an ICU. Nutrition 2017;37:48–52.
100. Chau JP, Lo SH, Thompson DR, et al. Use of end-tidal carbon dioxide detection to determine correct placement of nasogastric tube: a meta-analysis. Int J Nurs Stud 2011;48(4):513–21.
101. Bear DE, Champion A, Lei K, et al. Electromagnetically guided bedside placement of post-pyloric feeding tubes in critical care. Br J Nurs 2017;26(18):1008–15.
102. Koopmann MC, Kudsk KA, Szotkowski MJ, et al. A team-based protocol and electromagnetic technology eliminate feeding tube placement complications. Ann Surg 2011;253(2):287–302.
103. Metheny NA, Schnelker R, McGinnis J, et al. Indicators of tubesite during feedings. J Neurosci Nurs 2005;37(6):320–5.
104. DiVietro ML, Huggins JT, Angotti LB, et al. Pleural fluid analysis in chronic hemothorax: a mimicker of infection. Clin Med Insights Case Rep 2015;8:71–6.
105. Lavillegrand JR, Offenstadt G, Maury E, et al. Colorimetric capnometry and feeding tube placement. In: Rajendram R, Preedy VR, Patel VB, editors. Diet and nutrition in critical care. New York: Springer; 2015.
106. Metheny NA, Stewart BJ, Smith L, et al. pH and concentrations of pepsin and trypsin in feeding tube aspirates as predictors of tube placement. JPEN J Parenter Enteral Nutr 1997;21(5):279–85.
107. Patel JJ, Rosenthal MD, Heyland DK. Intermittent versus continuous feeding in critically ill adults. Curr Opin Clin Nutr Metab Care 2018;21(2):116–20.
108. Di Girolamo FG, Situlin R, Fiotti N, et al. Intermittent vs continuous enteral feeding to prevent catabolism in actuely ill adult and pediatric patients. Curr Opin Clin Nutr Metab Care 2017;20(5):390–5.
109. Kadamani I, Itani M, Zahran E, et al. Incidence of aspiration and gastrointestinal complications in critically ill patients using continuous versus bolus infusion of enteral nutrition: a pseudo-randomised controlled trial. Aust Crit Care 2014;27(4):188–93.
110. Seron-Arbeloa S, Zamora-Elson M, Labarta-Monzon L, et al. Enteral nutrition in critical care. J Clin Med Res 2013;5(1):1–11.
111. Heyland DK. Should we PERMIT systematic underfeeding in all intensive care unit patients? Integrating the results of the PERMIT study in our clinical practice guidelines. JPEN J Parenter Enteral Nutr 2016;40(2):156–8.
112. Bally MR, Blaser Yildirim PZ, Bounoure L, et al. Nutritional support and outcomes in malnourished medical inpatients: a systematic review and meta-analysis. JAMA Intern Med 2016;176(1):43–53.
113. Friedli N, Stanga Z, Sobotka L, et al. Revisiting the refeeding syndrome: results of a systematic review. Nutrition 2017;35:151–60.
114. Owers EL, Reeves AI, Ko SY, et al. Rates of adult acute inpatients documented as at risk of refeeding syndrome by dietitians. Clin Nutr 2014.
115. Blaser AR, Starkopf J, Kirsimagi U, et al. Definition, prevalence, and outcome of feeding intolerance in intensive care: a systematic review and meta-analysis. Acta Anaesthesiol Scand 2014.
116. Elke G, Felbinger TW, Heyland DK. Gastric residual volume in critically ill patients: a dead marker or still alive? Nutr Clin Pract 2015;30(1):59–71.
117. DeLegge MH. Managing gastric residual volumes in the critically ill patient: an update. Curr Opin Clin Nutr Metab Care 2011;14(2):193–6.
118. Deane A, Chapman MJ, Fraser RJ, et al. Mechanisms underlying feed intolerance in the critically ill: implications for treatment. World J Gastroenterol 2007;13(29):3909–17.
119. Reignier J, Mercier E, Le Gouge A, et al. Effect of not monitoring residual gastric volume on risk of ventilator-associated pneumonia in adults receiving mechanical ventilation and early enteral feeding: a randomized controlled trial. JAMA 2013;309(3):249–56.
120. McClave SA, Lukan JK, Stefater JA, et al. Poor validity of residual volumes as a marker for risk of aspiration in critically ill patients. Crit Care Med 2005;33(2):324–30.
121. Landzinski J, Kiser TH, Fish DN, et al. Gastric motility function in critically ill patients tolerant vs intolerant to gastric nutrition. JPEN J Parenter Enteral Nutr 2008;32(1):45–50.
122. Juve-Udina ME, Valls-Miro C, Carreno-Granero A, et al. To return or to discard? Randomised trial on gastric residual volume management. Intensive Crit Care Nurse 2009;25(5):258–67.
123. Dhaliwal R, Cahill N, Lemieux M, et al. The Canadian critical care nutrition guidelines in 2013: an update on current recommendations and implementation strategies. Nutr Clin Pract 2014;29(1):29–43.
124. Metheny NA, Schallom ME, Edwards SJ. Effect of gastrointestinal motility and feeding tube site on aspiration risk in critically ill patients: a review. Heart Lung 2004;33(3):131–45.
125. de Brito-Ashurst I, Preiser JC. Diarrhea in critically ill patients: the role of enteral feeding. JPEN J Parenter Enteral Nutr 2016;40(7): 913–23.
126. Lordani CR, Eckert RG, Tozetto AG, et al. The knowledge of intensive care professionals about diarrhea. Rev Bras Ter Intensiva 2014;26(3):299–304.
127. Whelan K, Judd PA, Taylor MA. Defining and reporting diarrhoea during enteral tube feeding: do health professionals agree? J Hum Nutr Diet 2003;16(1):21–6.
128. Chang SJ, Huang HH. Diarrhea in enterally fed patients: blame the diet? Curr Opin Clin Nutr Metab Care 2013;16(5):588–94.
129. Tan M, Zhu JC, Yin HH. Enteral nutrition in patients with severe traumatic brain injury: reasons for intolerance and medical management. Br J Neurosurg 2011;25(1):2–8.

130. Buendgens L, Bruensing J, Matthes M, et al. Administration of proton pump inhibitors in critically ill medical patients is associated with increased risk of developing Clostridium difficile-associated diarrhea. J Crit Care 2014;29(4):696 e11–15.
131. Akers KS, Shields BA, Akers ME, et al. Microbial contamination of enteral nutrition mixtures in a hyperthermal environment: a follow-up investigation. Nutr Clin Pract 2015;30(4):582–4.
132. Okuma T, Nakamura M, Totake H, et al. Microbial contamination of enteral feeding formulas and diarrhea. Nutrition 2000;16(9):719–22.
133. Lyman B, Williams M, Sollazzo J, et al. Enteral feeding set handling techniques. Nutr Clin Pract 2017;32(2):193–200.
134. Perry J, Stankorb SM, Salgueiro M. Microbial contamination of enteral feeding products in thermoneutral and hyperthermal ICU environments. Nutr Clin Pract 2015;30(1):128–33.
135. Bo L, Li J, Tao T, et al. Probiotics for preventing ventilator-associated pneumonia. Cochrane Database Syst Rev 2014;(10):CD009066.
136. Manzanares W, Lemieux M, Langlois PL, et al. Probiotic and synbiotic therapy in critical illness: a systematic review and meta-analysis. Crit Care 2016;19:262.
137. Muscedere J, Rewa O, McKechnie K, et al. Subglottic secretion drainage for the prevention of ventilator-associated pneumonia: a systematic review and meta-analysis. Crit Care Med 2011;39(8):1985–91.
138. Metheny NA, Frantz RA. Head-of-bed elevation in critically ill patients: a review. Crit Care Nurse 2013;33(3):53–66. quiz 7.
139. Schallom M, Orr J, Metheny N, et al. Gastroesophageal reflux in critically ill patients. Dimens Crit Care Nurs 2013;32(2):69–77.
140. Bassi GL, Zanella A, Cressoni M, et al. Following tracheal intubation, mucus flow is reversed in the semirecumbent position: possible role in the pathogenesis of ventilator–associated pneumonia. Crit Care Med 2008;36(2):518–25.
141. Lewis K, Alqahtani Z, McIntyre L, et al. The efficacy and safety of prokinetic agents in critically ill patients receiving enteral nutrition: a systematic review and meta-analysis of randomized trials. Crit Care 2016;20(1):259.
142. van Zanten ARH. Do we need new prokinetics to reduce enteral feeding intolerance during critical illness? Crit Care 2016;20:294.
143. Chapman MJ, Deane AM, O'Connor SL, et al. The effect of camicinal (GSK962040), a motilin agonist, on gastric emptying and glucose absorption in feed-intolerant critically ill patients: a randomized, blinded, placebo-controlled, clinical trial. Crit Care 2016;20(1):232.
144. Metheny NA, Dahms TE, Stewart BJ, et al. Efficacy of dye-stained enteral formula in detecting pulmonary aspiration. Chest 2002;122(1):276–81.
145. Maloney JP, Ryan TA, Brasel KJ, et al. Food dye use in enteral feedings: a review and a call for a moratorium. Nutr Clin Pract 2002;17(3):169–81.
146. Maloney JP, Ryan TA. Detection of aspiration in enterally fed patients: a requiem for bedside monitors of aspiration. JPEN J Parenter Enteral Nutr 2002;26(6 Suppl.):S34–41. discussion S-2.
147. Hallal C, Chaves VS, Borges GC, et al. Acid and weakly acidic gastroesophageal reflux and pepsin isoforms (A and C) in tracheal secretions of critically ill children. Chest 2015;148(2):333–9.
148. Casaer MP, Ziegler TR. Nutritional support in critical illness and recovery. Lancet Diabetes Endocrinol 2015;3(9):734–45.
149. Heyland DK, MacDonald S, Keefe L, et al. Total parenteral nutrition in the critically ill patient: a meta-analysis. JAMA 1998;280(23): 2013–19.
150. Doig GS, Simpson F, Sweetman EA, et al. Early parenteral nutrition in critically ill patients with short-term relative contraindications to early enteral nutrition: a randomized controlled trial. JAMA 2013;309(20):2130–8.
151. Casaer MP, Mesotten D, Hermans G, et al. Early versus late parenteral nutrition in critically ill adults. N Engl J Med 2011;365(6):506–17.
152. Heidegger CP, Berger MM, Graf S, et al. Optimisation of energy provision with supplemental parenteral nutrition in critically ill patients: a randomised controlled clinical trial. Lancet 2013;381(9864):385–93.
153. Strachan S. Trace elements. Curr Anaesth Crit Care 2010;21(1):44–8.
154. Blanchette LM, Huiras P, Papadopoulos S. Standardized versus custom parenteral nutrition: impact on clinical and cost-related outcomes. Am J Health Syst Pharm 2014;71(2):114–21.
155. Gavin NC, Button E, Keogh S, et al. Does parenteral nutrition increase the risk of catheter-related bloodstream infection? A systematic literature review. JPEN J Parenter Enteral Nutr 2017;41(6):918–28.
156. Gavin NC, Button E, Castillo MI, et al. Does a dedicated lumen for parenteral nutrition administration reduce the risk of catheter-related bloodstream infections? A systematic literature review. J Infus Nurs 2018;41(2):122–30.
157. Worthington PH, Gilbert KA. Parenteral nutrition: risks, complications, and management. J Infus Nurs 2012;35(1):52–64.
158. Macht M, Wimbish T, Bodine C, et al. ICU-acquired swallowing disorders. Crit Care Med 2013;41(10):2396–405.
159. Skoretz SA, Flowers HL, Martino R. The incidence of dysphagia following endotracheal intubation: a systematic review. Chest 2010;137(3):665–73.
160. Goldsmith T. Evaluation and treatment of swallowing disorders following endotracheal intubation and tracheostomy. Int Anesthesiol Clin 2000;38(3):219–42.
161. Hermans G, De Jonghe B, Bruyninckx F, et al. Clinical review: critical illness polyneuropathy and myopathy. Crit Care 2008;12(6):238.
162. Leder SB, Suiter DM, Lisitano Warner H. Answering orientation questions and following single-step verbal commands: effect on aspiration status. Dysphagia 2009;24(3):290–5.
163. Rousou JA, Tighe DA, Garb JL, et al. Risk of dysphagia after transesophageal echocardiography during cardiac operations. Ann Thorac Surg 2000;69(2):486–9.

164. Hogue CW Jr, Lappas GD, Creswell LL, et al. Swallowing dysfunction after cardiac operations. Associated adverse outcomes and risk factors including intraoperative transesophageal echocardiography. J Thorac Cardiovasc Surg 1995;110(2):517–22.
165. Oliveira ACM, Friche AAL, Salomao MS, et al. Predictive factors for oropharyngeal dysphagia after prolonged orotracheal intubation. Braz J Otorhinolaryngol 2017.
166. Brodsky MB, Huang M, Shanholtz C, et al. Recovery from dysphagia symptoms after oral endotracheal intubation in acute respiratory distress syndrome survivors. A 5-year longitudinal study. Ann Am Thorac Soc 2017;14(3):376–83.
167. Daly E, Miles A, Scott S, et al. Finding the red flags: swallowing difficulties after cardiac surgery in patients with prolonged intubation. J Crit Care 2016;31(1):119–24.
168. Ramsey DJ, Smithard DG, Kalra L. Early assessments of dysphagia and aspiration risk in acute stroke patients. Stroke 2003;34(5):1252–7.
169. Mullen R. Evidence for whom?: ASHA's national outcomes measurement system. J Commun Disord 2004;37(5):413–17.
170. Scheel R, Pisegna JM, McNally E, et al. Endoscopic assessment of swallowing after prolonged intubation in the ICU setting. Ann Otol Rhinol Laryngol 2016;125(1):43–52.
171. Petersen S, Tsai AA, Scala CM, et al. Adequacy of oral intake in critically ill patients 1 week after extubation. J Am Diet Assoc 2010;110(3):427–33.
172. Somanchi M, Tao X, Mullin GE. The facilitated early enteral and dietary management effectiveness trial in hospitalized patients with malnutrition. JPEN J Parenter Enteral Nutr 2011;35(2):209–16.
173. Marshall AP, Wake E, Weisbrodt L, et al. A multi-faceted, family-centred nutrition intervention to optimise nutrition intake of critically ill patients: the OPTICS feasibility study. Aust Crit Care 2016;29(2):68–76.
174. Marshall AP, Lemieux M, Dhaliwal R, et al. Novel, family-centered intervention to improve nutrition in patients recovering from critical illness: a feasibility study. Nutr Clin Pract 2017;32(3):392–9.
175. Dickerson RN, Patel JJ, McClain CJ. Protein and calorie requirements associated with the presence of obesity. Nutr Clin Pract 2017;32(1_suppl):86S–93S.
176. Gallagher D, DeLegge M. Body composition (sarcopenia) in obese patients: implications for care in the intensive care unit. JPEN J Parenter Enteral Nutr 2011;35(5 Suppl.):21S–8S.
177. Frankenfield DC. Obesity. In: Singer P, editor. Nutrition in intensive care medicine: beyond physiology. Basel, Switzerland: 2013.
178. Choban P, Dickerson R, Malone A, et al. A.S.P.E.N. Clinical guidelines: nutrition support of hospitalized adult patients with obesity. JPEN J Parenter Enteral Nutr 2013;37(6):714–44.
179. Frankenfield DC, Smith JS, Cooney RN. Accelerated nitrogen loss after traumatic injury is not attenuated by achievement of energy balance. JPEN J Parenter Enteral Nutr 1997;21(6):324–9.
180. Porhomayon J, Papadakos P, Singh A, et al. Alteration in respiratory physiology in obesity for anesthesia-critical care physician. HSR Proc Intensive Care Cardiovasc Anesth 2011;3(2):109–18.
181. Stevenson EK, Rubenstein AR, Radin GT, et al. Two decades of mortality trends among patients with severe sepsis: a comparative meta-analysis. Crit Care Med 2014;42(3):625–31.
182. Gotts JE, Matthay MA. Sepsis: pathophysiology and clinical management. BMJ 2016;353:i1585.
183. Elke G, Heyland DK. Enteral nutrition in critically ill septic patients-less or more? JPEN J Parenter Enteral Nutr 2014.
184. Rhodes A, Evans LE, Alhazzani W, et al. Surviving sepsis campaign: international guidelines for management of sepsis and septic shock: 2016. Intensive Care Med 2017;43(3):304–77.
185. Lu C, Sharma S, McIntyre L, et al. Omega-3 supplementation in patients with sepsis: a systematic review and meta-analysis of randomized trials. Ann Intensive Care 2017;7(1):58.
186. Fiaccadori E, Regolisti G, Maggiore U. Specialized nutritional support interventions in critically ill patients on renal replacement therapy. Curr Opin Clin Nutr Metab Care 2013;16(2):217–24.
187. Druml W. The renal failure patient. In: Singer P, editor. Nutrition in intensive care medicine: beyond physiology. Basel: Karger; 2013. p. 126–35.
188. Wiesen P, Van Overmeire L, Delanaye P, et al. Nutrition disorders during acute renal failure and renal replacement therapy. JPEN J Parenter Enteral Nutr 2011;35(2):217–22.
189. Lopez Martinez J, Sanchez-Izquierdo Riera JA, Jimenez Jimenez FJ, et al. Guidelines for specialized nutritional and metabolic support in the critically-ill patient: update. Consensus SEMICYUC-SENPE: acute renal failure. Nutr Hosp 2011;26(Suppl. 2):21–6.
190. Honore PM, De Waele E, Jacobs R, et al. Nutritional and metabolic alterations during continuous renal replacement therapy. Blood Purif 2013;35(4):279–84.
191. Sundararajan K, Schoeman T, Hughes L, et al. Predictors and outcomes of acute pancreatitis in critically ill patients presenting to the emergency department of a tertiary referral centre in Australia. Emerg Med Australas 2017;29(2):184–91.
192. Portelli M, Jones CD. Severe acute pancreatitis: pathogenesis, diagnosis and surgical management. Hepatobiliary Pancreat Dis Int 2017;16(2):155–9.
193. Singh A, Chen M, Li T, et al. Parenteral nutrition combined with enteral nutrition for severe acute pancreatitis. ISRN Gastroenterol 2012;2012:791383.
194. McClave SA, Chang WK, Dhaliwal R, et al. Nutrition support in acute pancreatitis: a systematic review of the literature. JPEN J Parenter Enteral Nutr 2006;30(2):143–56.

195. Marik PE, Zaloga GP. Meta-analysis of parenteral nutrition versus enteral nutrition in patients with acute pancreatitis. BMJ 2004;328(7453):1407.
196. Cao Y, Xu Y, Lu T, et al. Meta-analysis of enteral nutrition versus total parenteral nutrition in patients with severe acute pancreatitis. Ann Nutr Metab 2008;53(3–4):268–75.
197. Doig GS, Heighes PT, Simpson F, et al. Early enteral nutrition reduces mortality in trauma patients requiring intensive care: a meta-analysis of randomised controlled trials. Injury 2011;42(1):50–6.
198. Weimann A. The surgical/trauma patient. In: Singer P, editor. Nutrition in intensive care medicine: beyond physiology. Basel: Karger; 2013. p. 106–15.
199. Osland E, Yunus RM, Khan S, et al. Early versus traditional postoperative feeding in patients undergoing resectional gastrointestinal surgery: a meta-analysis. JPEN J Parenter Enteral Nutr 2011;35(4):473–87.
200. Burlew CC, Moore EE, Cuschieri J, et al. Who should we feed? Western Trauma Association multi-institutional study of enteral nutrition in the open abdomen after injury. J Trauma Acute Care Surg 2012;73(6):1380–7.
201. Rosenthal MD, Vanzant EL, Martindale RG, et al. Evolving paradigms in the nutritional support of critically ill surgical patients. Curr Probl Surg 2015;52(4):147–82.
202. Lundy JB, Chung KK, Pamplin JC, et al. Update on severe burn management for the intensivist. J Intensive Care Med 2016;31(8):499–510.
203. Garcia de Lorenzo y Mateos A, Ortiz Leyba C, Sanchez SM, et al. Guidelines for specialized nutritional and metabolic support in the critically-ill patient: update. Consensus SEMICYUC-SENPE: critically-ill burnt patient. Nutricion hospitalaria 2011;26(Suppl. 2):59–62.
204. Hayhoe R, Maniatis K, Shahrokhi S, et al. Nutrition support in burn injury. In: Hickson M, Smith SK, Whelan K, editors. Advanced nutrition and dietetics in nutrition support. Oxford: Wiley-Blackwell; 2018.
205. Dickerson RN. Estimating energy and protein requirements of thermally injured patients: art or science? Nutrition 2002;18(5):439–42.
206. Gibran NS, Committee on O, Delivery of Burn Care ABA. Practice guidelines for burn care, 2006. J Burn Care Res 2006;27(4):437–8.
207. McDonald WS, Sharp CW Jr, Deitch EA. Immediate enteral feeding in burn patients is safe and effective. Ann Surg 1991;213(2):177–83.
208. Rodriguez NA, Jeschke MG, Williams FN, et al. Nutrition in burns: Galveston contributions. JPEN J Parenter Enteral Nutr 2011;35(6):704–14.
209. Nordlund MJ, Pham TN, Gibran NS. Micronutrients after burn injury: a review. Journal of Burn Care & Research 2014;35(2):121–33.
210. Tan HB, Danilla S, Murray A, et al. Immunonutrition as an adjuvant therapy for burns. Cochrane Database Syst Rev 2014;(12):CD007174.
211. Robinson LE, van Soeren MH. Insulin resistance and hyperglycemia in critical illness: role of insulin in glycemic control. AACN Clin Issues 2004;15(1):45–62.
212. Investigators N-SS, Finfer S, Chittock DR, et al. Intensive versus conventional glucose control in critically ill patients. N Engl J Med 2009;360(13):1283–97.
213. Arabi YM, Dabbagh OC, Tamim HM, et al. Intensive versus conventional insulin therapy: a randomized controlled trial in medical and surgical critically ill patients. Crit Care Med 2008;36(12):3190–7.
214. De La Rosa Gdel C, Donado JH, Restrepo AH, et al. Strict glycaemic control in patients hospitalised in a mixed medical and surgical intensive care unit: a randomised clinical trial. Crit Care 2008;12(5):R120.
215. Jacobi J, Bircher N, Krinsley J, et al. Guidelines for the use of an insulin infusion for the management of hyperglycemia in critically ill patients. Crit Care Med 2012;40(12):3251–76.
216. van den Berghe G, Wouters P, Weekers F, et al. Intensive insulin therapy in critically ill patients. N Engl J Med 2001;345(19):1359–67.
217. Van den Berghe G, Wilmer A, Hermans G, et al. Intensive insulin therapy in the medical ICU. N Engl J Med 2006;354(5):449–61.
218. Gunst J, Doig GS. The optimal blood glucose target in critically ill patients: more questions than answers. Intensive Care Med 2017;43(1):110–12.
219. Preiser JC, Devos P, Ruiz-Santana S, et al. A prospective randomised multi-centre controlled trial on tight glucose control by intensive insulin therapy in adult intensive care units: the Glucontrol study. Intensive Care Med 2009;35(10):1738–48.
220. Louie K, Cheema R, Dodek P, et al. Intensive nursing work schedules and the risk of hypoglycaemia in critically ill patients who are receiving intravenous insulin. Qual Saf Health Care 2010;19(6):e42.
221. Dellinger RP, Levy MM, Rhodes A, et al. Surviving sepsis campaign: international guidelines for management of severe sepsis and septic shock: 2012. Crit Care Med 2013;41(2):580–637.
222. Tian F, Doig GS. NUTRIREA-2 trial finds that early enteral nutrition and early parenteral nutrition do not differ with regard to major clinical outcomes. J Thorac Dis 2018;10(3).
223. Ortiz Leyba C, Montejo Gonzalez JC, Vaquerizo Alonso C, et al. [Guidelines for specialized nutritional and metabolic support in the critically-ill patient. Update. Consensus of the Spanish Society of Intensive Care Medicine and Coronary Units-Spanish Society of Parenteral and Enteral Nutrition (SEMICYUC-SENPE): patient with sepsis]. Med Intensiva 2011;35(Suppl. 1):72–6.
224. Bassler D, Briel M, Montori VM, et al. Stopping randomized trials early for benefit and estimation of treatment effects: systematic review and meta-regression analysis. JAMA 2010;303(12):1180–7.
225. Guyatt GH, Briel M, Glasziou P, et al. Problems of stopping trials early. BMJ 2012;344:e3863.
226. Van Dyck L, Casaer MP. Nutrition in the ICU: sometimes route does matter. Lancet 2018;391(10116):98–100.

Chapter 20

Gastrointestinal, metabolic and liver alterations

Andrea Marshall, Adam Riedlinger

Learning objectives

After reading this chapter, you should be able to:

- describe the changes in gastrointestinal physiology and metabolism associated with critical illness
- identify patients at risk for the development of stress ulcers and rationalise therapeutic interventions for their prevention
- identify patients at risk for the development of intraabdominal hypertension and abdominal compartment syndrome and suggest management strategies to decrease intraabdominal pressure
- describe the physiological changes that occur during diabetic ketoacidosis and rationalise assessment and treatment strategies
- discuss the effects of critical illness on hepatic function and evaluate the consequences of liver dysfunction
- describe the treatment of liver failure, including liver support therapies and transplantation.

KEY WORDS

diabetic ketoacidosis
extracorporeal liver support
hepatic encephalopathy
hepatorenal syndrome
hyperosmolar hyperglycaemic state
intraabdominal hypertension
liver failure
liver transplantation
stress-related mucosal disease

Introduction

During episodes of critical illness, patients often experience disturbance in their metabolic and/or endocrine function. In the previous chapter, the changes to metabolism that occur during critical illness and the role of the gastrointestinal system in nutrition were outlined. The gastrointestinal system is also involved in many other important functions including immunity and protection.

Effective gastrointestinal function requires an adequate blood supply to ensure oxygen and nutrients are available at the cellular level. However, in critical illness splanchnic circulation may be compromised without overt signs being evident. This alteration in regional blood flow and tissue oxygen delivery can compromise normal metabolic and endocrine function.

In this chapter the effect of gastrointestinal physiology on critical illness is discussed. Gastrointestinal dysfunction, including the development of stress-related mucosal diseases and development of increased intraabdominal pressure, is discussed. A major component of this chapter is dedicated to organ specific gastrointestinal compromise including liver dysfunction, liver transplantation, alcoholic liver disease and pancreatitis. An overview of the assessment and management of diabetic ketoacidosis is also provided.

Gastrointestinal physiology

As described in Chapter 19, digestion and absorption of nutrients such as carbohydrates, amino acids, minerals and water are key functions of the gastrointestinal system. Another important role of the gastrointestinal tract is immunity. Part of this immunity is the established barrier between the gastrointestinal tract and the blood supply. There are a number of different mechanisms by which the gastrointestinal system prevents the movement of substances (other than nutrients, water and electrolytes) into the systemic circulation and these are outlined in Table 20.1. In the setting of critical illness, gastrointestinal hypoperfusion may be present, resulting in decreased oxygen and nutrient delivery at the cellular level, and this in turn can lead to decreased effectiveness of these protective functions.[8]

Alterations to normal gastrointestinal physiology in critical illness

During critical illness, there are a number of alterations that can occur to gastrointestinal physiology. The intestinal epithelium consists of one layer of cells separating the gut lumen from the rest of the body. These cells are responsible for nutrient absorption, and important immune functions including a barrier to pathogens, secreting hormones, cytokines and antimicrobial peptides.[6] During critical illness changes to gut epithelium, the immune system and gut microbiome may occur. Although nutrient absorption may be altered[3,8] including the ability of the small intestine to absorb nutrients,[9] most critically ill patients appear to be able to tolerate enteral nutrition, making the clinical significance of impaired absorption unclear. Alterations in the defence

TABLE 20.1
Protective mechanisms of the gastrointestinal system and impacts of critical illness

MECHANISM	ACTION
Motility	Propels bacteria through the GI tract. In critical illness, motility may be altered because of enteric nerve impairment and altered smooth muscle function, inflammation (mediated by cytokines and nitric oxide), gut injury, hypoperfusion, medications (opioids, dopamine), electrolyte disturbances, hyperglycaemia, sepsis and increased intracranial pressure[1]
Hydrochloric acid secretion	Reduces gastric acidity and destroys bacteria. Parietal cells in the stomach produce hydrochloric acid and keep the intragastric environment relatively acidic (pH approx. 4.0). An acidic pH has bactericidal and bacteriostatic properties,[2] thus limiting overgrowth in the stomach
Bicarbonate	Bicarbonate ions bind with hydrogen ions to form water and carbon dioxide, preventing the hydrogen ions (acid) from damaging the duodenal wall[3]
Bile salts	Bile salts provide protection against bacteria by breaking down the liposaccharide portion of endotoxins, thereby detoxifying gram-negative bacteria in the gastrointestinal tract. The deconjugation of bile salts into secondary bile acids inhibits the proliferation of pathogens and may destroy their cell walls[4]
Mucin production	Prevents the adhesion of bacteria to the wall of the GI tract. Mucous cells secrete large quantities of very thick, alkaline mucus (approximately 1 mm thick in the stomach). Glycoproteins present in the mucus prevent bacteria from adhering to and colonising the mucosal wall[5]
Epithelial cell shedding	Limits bacterial adhesion. The mucosal lining of the entire gastrointestinal tract is composed of epithelial cells that create a physical barrier to bacterial invasion. These cells are replaced approximately every 3–5 days,[5] limiting bacterial colonisation
Zona occludens (tight junctions surrounding each cell in the epithelial sheet)	The junctions between epithelial cells provide a barrier to microorganisms. Intermediate junctions (zonula adherens) function primarily in cell–cell adhesion, while the tight junctions (zonula occludens) limit the movement of bacteria and toxins across the gut wall[6]
Gut-associated lymphoid tissue	Protection against bacterial invasion is provided by gut-associated lymphoid tissue, capable of cell-mediated and humoral-mediated immune responses[6]
Kupffer cells	Kupffer cells in the liver and spleen provide a back-up defence against pathogens that cross the barrier of the gastrointestinal wall and enter the systemic circulation[7]

mechanisms of the gastrointestinal tract may also occur and contribute to the development of multiple organ dysfunction in critical illness.[10] The changes to gut function in critical illness are complex and there are likely many factors contributing to the development of gut dysfunction.

Gut permeability can change as a result of critical illness. Intestinal epithelial cells undergo accelerated programmed cell death, the tight junctions between epithelial cells are compromised and as a result microbes can permeate the barrier that is the intestinal wall.[6] Thinning of the mucus layer of the intestinal tract can also occur as a result of critical illness.[11] A thinner mucus layer can lead to autodigestion and destruction of the intestinal epithelium, which may allow pancreatic enzymes to enter intestinal lymphatic channels and this may result in tissue injury and multiple organ failure.[12]

More recently, significant attention has been focused on the gut microbiome and how changes in intestinal homeostasis can contribute to worsening clinical outcomes.[13] While our understanding of the role of the gut microbiome is evolving it is recognised that the microbial ecosystems of the gut changes substantially in critical illness. Physiological changes in critical illness together with treatment strategies may contribute to imbalance in the introduction, elimination, and reproduction of microbes and this may contribute to changes in the gut microbiome (Table 20.2).

Stress-related mucosal damage

The reported incidence of stress-related mucosal damage is variable and complicated by variable definitions and difficulty in measurement of end points, and the heterogeneity of patient populations.[29] It is estimated that the majority of critically ill patients will develop evidence of stress-related mucosal erosion and subepithelial haemorrhage on endoscopy within 72 hours of admission to the intensive care unit (ICU).[30] Occult abnormalities have been observed in approximately one-third of critically ill patients on mechanical ventilation; the most common of these are gastritis and mucosal erosion from the nasogastric tube.[31] Gastrointestinal bleeding occurs in 2–5% of patients[32] and is associated with worse patient outcomes.[33] The incidence of clinically significant bleeding, that is bleeding associated with hypotension, tachycardia and a drop in haemoglobin level necessitating transfusion, is estimated to be 1% and 6%.[34] Over time the incidence of stress-related mucosal damage has continued to decrease and this is largely attributed to overall advances and improvements in the management of critically ill patients. Aggressive fluid resuscitation, improved ventilatory management, which minimises increased lung pressures, and preferential use of enteral nutrition have likely all contributed to reduced incidence of stress-related mucosal disease in the critically ill.[35]

Factors influencing the development of stress-related mucosal damage include splanchnic hypoperfusion, which may influence mucosal ischaemia and reperfusion injury.[36] The mucus–bicarbonate gel layer[26] and decreased prostaglandin levels, which impair mucus replenishment, and increased nitric oxide synthase contribute to reperfusion injury and cell death.[6] The protective mechanisms and factors that promote injury are detailed in Table 20.3.

A number of risk factors are associated with the development of stress-related mucosal damage. These include, but are not limited to: shock where vasopressors or inotropes are required to maintain blood pressure, need for intermittent or continuous renal replacement therapy, mechanical ventilation for more than 24 hours, acute coagulopathy, history of coagulopathy within the previous 6 months, treatment with an anticoagulant, and history of chronic liver disease.[43]

Preventing stress-related mucosal damage

Prophylaxis for stress-related mucosal damage is often part of the care of the critically ill, although evidence demonstrating an added benefit when this therapy is applied to those patients who are not identified as at risk for developing stress-related mucosal damage is limited in both quantity and quality.[44] The most frequently prescribed medications to prevent stress-related mucosal damage include proton pump inhibitors and histamine-2 receptor antagonists, although proton pump inhibitors are often preferred and considered more effective in preventing gastrointestinal bleeding.[45] A positive impact on mortality and intensive care length of stay associated with stress-ulcer prophylaxis is also yet to be established.[44] There is also some emerging evidence that the use of proton pump inhibitors may contribute to increased infection risk[46] and cardiovascular events[47] in critically ill patients.

It is common for the majority of critically ill patients to receive some form of stress-ulcer prophylaxis during their episode of critical illness, likely because of recommendations from influential groups such as the Surviving Sepsis Campaign.[48] With the risk for clinical substantial bleeding being low, it is important to consider whether stress-ulcer prophylaxis is always warranted, especially considering the pharmacological therapy is not risk-free and is associated with economic consequences.[49] There are a variety of pharmacological strategies that can be used to prevent stress ulcers from developing and, most commonly, proton pump inhibitors (PPIs) and histamine-2-receptor antagonists (H_2RAs) are used as first-line therapy.[45] A number of clinical trials are underway (PEPTIC in Australia and New Zealand and SUP-ICU in Europe) to further evaluate treatment effectiveness.

Histamine-2-receptor antagonists

H_2RAs inhibit the production of gastric acid by binding to the histamine-2 receptor on the basement membrane

TABLE 20.2
Ecological effects of critical illness on the gastrointestinal microbiome

PATHOPHYSIOLOGICAL PROCESSES	MICROBIAL IMMIGRATION	MICROBIAL ELIMINATION	ENVIRONMENTAL GROWTH CONDITIONS
Decreased oral intake	Decreased immigration of food-associated microbiota[14]	No direct effect	Shift to stress conditions of nutrient scarcity and altered nutritional substrate[14]
Altered oropharyngeal microbiota	Increased immigration of Proteobacteria and potential pathogens[15]	No direct effect	No direct effect
Intestinal dysmotility	No direct effect	Decreased elimination, increased upper gastrointestinal community burden	No direct effect
Systemic hyperglycaemia and electrolyte disturbances	No direct effect	Decreased elimination (intestinal dysmotility)[16]	No direct effect
Gut hypoperfusion, reperfusion injury, impaired mucosal integrity	No direct effect	Increased elimination via translocation to mesenteric lymphatics[17]	Increased mucosal inflammation, increased free radical concentrations and nitrate availability,[21] shift from commensal anaerobes to Proteobacteria and select Firmicutes[22]
Decreased bile salt concentration	No direct effect	Decreased elimination of bile-sensitive species[4]	Selective overgrowth of bile-sensitive species[4]
Endogenous opioid production	No direct effect	Decreased elimination (intestinal dysmotility)	Selective increase in virulence of opioid-responsive species,[23] disruption of stabilising commensal relationships[24]
Endogenous catecholamine and inflammatory cytokine production	No direct effect	Decreased elimination (intestinal dysmotility)[18]	Selective promotion of growth and virulence of potential pathogens,[25] increased mucosal inflammation via splanchnic hypoperfusion, decreased oxygen tension and pH
Disruption of intestinal mucus layer	No direct effect	Increased elimination via translocation to mesenteric lymphatics[19]	Altered nutrient supply, altered oxygen gradients,[26] loss of mucus reservoir of antibacterial peptides[27]
Impaired mucosal immunity: decreased IgA and defensing production	No direct effect	Decreased elimination of potential pathogens, increased elimination via translocation to mesenteric lymphatics[20]	Loss of growth inhibition for potential pathogens, decreased abundance of commensal Bacteroidetes[28]

Adapted from Dickson RP. The microbiome and critical illness. Lancet 2016; 4: 59-72.

of the parietal cell.[29] However, gastric acid secretion may also occur through stimulation of the acetylcholine or gastrin receptors present in parietal cells;[2] therefore, complete blocking of gastric acid production does not occur when H_2RAs are used (Fig. 20.1). Further limitations of H_2RAs are that tachyphylaxis can occur quickly[29] and tolerance may develop within 48 hours of administration.[2] Nevertheless, this pharmacological strategy to prevent stress-related mucosal disease remains commonplace in critical care. The decrease in gastric acidity as a result of H_2RA use may be beneficial from the perspective of preventing stress-related mucosal disease, but changes in gastric pH could lead to bacterial overgrowth in the stomach, micro-aspiration and, consequently, an increase in the incidence of nosocomial pneumonia. Further research is required to develop a more comprehensive understanding of the benefits and adverse effects of H_2RAs.[44]

TABLE 20.3
Factors contributing to stress-related mucosal disease

FACTORS	MECHANISM	ACTION
Protective mechanisms	Mucosal prostaglandins	Protect the mucosa by stimulating blood flow, mucus and bicarbonate production[6] Stimulate epithelial cell growth and repair
	Mucosal bicarbonate barrier	Forms a physical barrier to acid and pepsin, preventing injury to the epithelium[2]
	Epithelial restitution and regeneration	Epithelial cells rapidly regenerate but the process is highly metabolic and may be impaired by physiological stress[6]
	Mucosal blood flow	Mucosal blood flow helps remove acid from the mucosa, supplies bicarbonate and oxygen to the mucosal epithelial cells[37]
	Cell membrane and tight junctions	Tight junctions between mucosal epithelial cells prevent the back diffusion of hydrogen ions[6]
Factors promoting injury	Acid	Gastric acid secretion may be a contributing factor to the development of stress-related mucosal injury although gut ischaemia as a consequence of hypotension, use of vasoconstrictors or inflammatory mediators are also contributing factors[38]
	Pepsin	May cause direct injury to the mucosa[39] Facilitates the lysis of clots[40]
	Mucosal hypoperfusion	Reduced mucosal blood flow results in reduced oxygen and nutrient delivery, making epithelial cells susceptible to injury[41] Contributes to mucosal acid–base imbalances
	Reperfusion injury	Nitric oxide, which causes vasodilation and hyperaemia, is released during hypoperfusion and results in an increase in cell-damaging cytokines[42]
	Intramucosal acid–base balance	The mucus layer protects the epithelium and traps bicarbonate ions that neutralise acid, thus a decrease in bicarbonate secretion results in intramucosal acidosis and local injury[2]
	Systemic acidosis	Results in increased intramucosal acidity
	Free oxygen radicals	Generated as a result of tissue hypoxia, free oxygen radicals cause oxidative injury to the mucosa[41]
	Bile salts	Bile salts reflux from the duodenum into the stomach and may have a role in stress-related damage although the exact mechanism is uncertain[4]
	Helicobacter pylori	Conflicting results exist about the role of *H. pylori* as a cause of stress-induced mucosal disease in the critically ill[38]

Reproduced from Marshall AP. The gut in critical illness. In: Carlson K, editor. AACN Advanced critical care nursing. Philadelphia: Elsevier; 2009, Table 29-3, with permission

Practice tip

In patients with renal failure who are receiving H_2RAs an adjustment to the dose may be required because H_2RAs are excreted via the kidney. Ranitidine is the most common H_2RA administered in ICU and it can potentiate the action of midazolam and increase plasma levels of theophylline and phenytoin.

Proton pump inhibitors

PPIs have a greater ability to maintain an increased intragastric pH than H_2RAs. These drugs work by irreversibly binding to the proton pump, effectively blocking all three receptors responsible for gastric acid secretion by the parietal cell (see Fig. 20.1).[2] PPIs are also able to limit vagally-mediated gastric acid secretion.[50]

FIGURE 20.1 Mechanism of action of stress-ulcer prophylaxis agents.

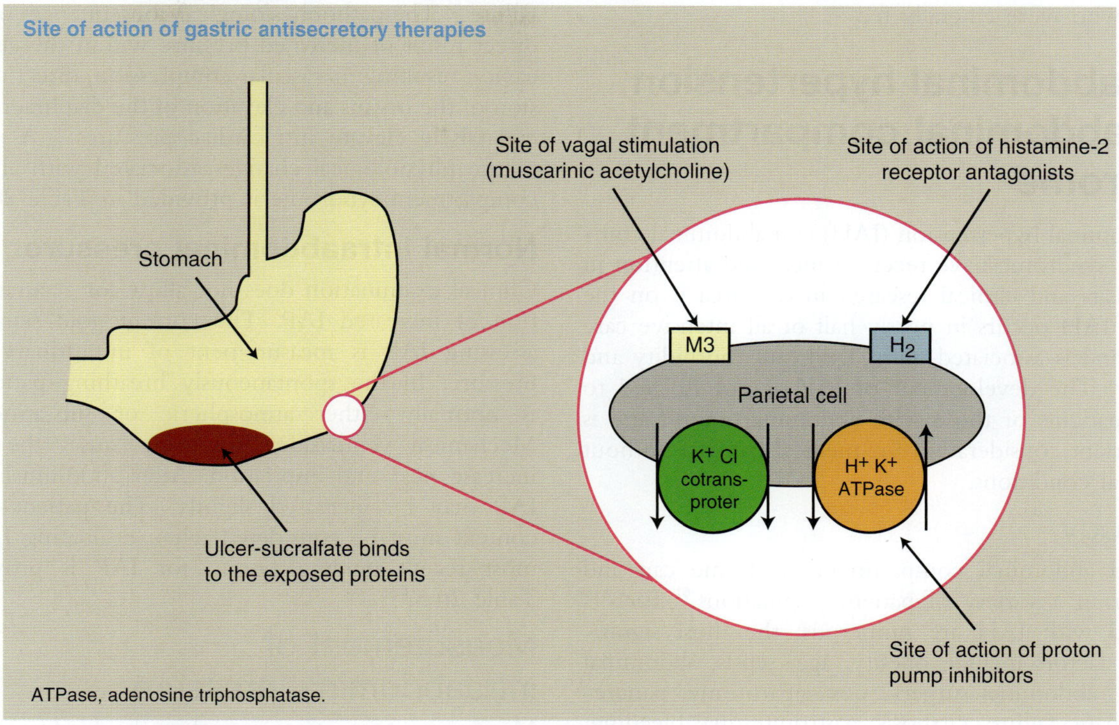

Reproduced from Whitman Z, O'Neil DHR. Gastric disorders: modifications of gastric content, antacids and drugs influencing gastric secretions and motility. Anaesthesia and Intensive Care Medicine 2017;19(1):25-9, with permission.

PPIs are more effective than H_2RAs in reducing clinically important bleeding and do not appear to increase the risk of nosocomial pneumonia.[51] Clinical evaluation of the efficacy of PPIs is, however, somewhat limited; few studies have specifically studied the prophylactic use of PPIs for stress-related mucosal damage and many have methodological limitations. Intravenous PPIs may be more effective than H_2RAs in raising the gastric pH but it is unclear whether this translates to a clinically important effect.[2] PPIs are, however, associated with an increased risk of developing *Clostridium difficile* infection.[52]

PPIs that may be administered intravenously include omeprazole, esomeprazole and pantoprazole. Omeprazole has the highest potential for drug interactions and interferes with the metabolism of some drugs commonly used in intensive care, including cyclosporine, diazepam, phenytoin and warfarin.[53]

Sucralfate

Sucralfate provides protection against stress-related mucosal disease through a number of mechanisms. Sucralfate provides a protective barrier on the surface gastric epithelium, stimulates mucus and bicarbonate secretion, stimulates epithelial renewal, improves mucosal blood flow and enhances prostaglandin release.[21] Given orally or via a nasogastric tube, sucralfate is well tolerated and may be as effective as H_2RAs in decreasing clinically significant bleeding[54] but may not be as effective as PPIs.[55] It is possible that sucralfate may also reduce the risk of ICU-acquired pneumonia, compared with H_2RAs although stronger quality of evidence may be required.

Enteral nutrition

It is postulated that enteral nutrition has a role in stress-ulcer prophylaxis because its administration can buffer gastric acid and increase intragastric pH,[29] improve gastric mucosal blood flow[56] and promote the release of protective substances such as prostaglandins and mucus.[57] In critically ill patients, enteral nutrition administration is more effective at increasing intragastric pH than either H_2RAs or PPIs.[58] A recent randomised controlled exploratory study has investigated whether enteral nutrition alone may prevent stress-related gastrointestinal bleeding in mechanically ventilated patients.[59] Although this study is small and has some methodological limitations the data suggest that in patients who are tolerating early enteral nutrition, there is no additional benefit to providing stress-ulcer prophylaxis (pantoprazole). The findings of this study are supported by a recent systematic review and meta-analysis of seven randomised controlled trials comparing stress-ulcer prophylaxis to either placebo or no prophylaxis in enterally-fed critically ill patients. Although further research is needed in this area, no benefit to stress-ulcer prophylaxis was observed in patients who were enterally fed.[60]

Intraabdominal hypertension and abdominal compartment syndrome

Intraabdominal hypertension (IAH) and abdominal compartment syndrome have received increased attention in recent years and clinical research in this area is on the increase. IAH occurs in nearly half of all intensive care patients and is associated with significant morbidity and mortality. The development of IAH is not isolated to surgical patients or those with abdominal injury, and is an important consideration for medical patients without abdominal conditions.

Aetiology

IAH and abdominal compartment syndrome can and do occur in a variety of patient populations.[61] Factors associated with IAH are numerous; the most significant risk factors include obesity, age, sepsis, abdominal infection, abdominal surgery, post-laparotomy, pancreatitis, hepatic failure, cirrhosis, gastrointestinal bleeding, ileus and liver dysfunction.[62] Risk factors that are more specific to critically ill patients include obesity, sepsis, abdominal surgery and ileus. Abdominal compartment syndrome is potentially fatal. Consequently, it is imperative that all clinicians be aware of the underlying physiological changes, assessment and management in at-risk patients. Rates of IAH have decreased in recent years as approaches to fluid resuscitation have become less aggressive.[63]

> **Practice tip**
>
> The critically ill obese patient is at higher risk of developing intraabdominal hypertension and abdominal compartment syndrome and may benefit from intraabdominal pressure monitoring.

Pathophysiology

Increased intraabdominal pressure (IAP) results from an increase in pressure within the confined anatomic space of the abdominal cavity. When IAP rises in this closed anatomic space, blood flow may be reduced and tissue viability threatened.[64]

This increase in pressure may result from causes such as intraperitoneal bleeding, peritonitis, ascites or distention of the gas-filled bowel. Clinical data show that increases in IAP result in physiological changes in vital organ function.[61] Early detection of increases in IAP can be challenging, and it is a sustained increase in abdominal pressure or the development of IAH that affects regional blood flow and impairs tissue perfusion, contributing to the development of multiple organ failure.[65] The pathophysiological consequences occur as a direct result of increased pressure within the abdominal cavity, resulting in vascular compression, direct compression of the organs and elevation of the diaphragm, which can falsely elevate intracardiac pressures.[66] A summary of the physiological changes associated with abdominal compartment syndrome is provided in Table 20.4.

Normal intraabdominal pressure

Clinical examination does not allow for accurate detection of increased IAP. The current gold standard for assessing IAP is measurement of intraurinary bladder pressure. In the spontaneously breathing patient, IAP is normally either atmospheric or sub-atmospheric. Mechanical ventilation, however, causes the IAP to increase near end-inspiration. After abdominal surgery, IAP may be increased slightly. The patient's clinical context must be considered when evaluating IAP. The most recent grading system for IAP is provided in Table 20.5.[69]

Measurement of intraabdominal pressure

Measurement of pressure within the bladder has been validated as closely approximating IAP[70] and is the recommended standard approach for the measurement of intraabdominal pressure.[71] This technique can, however, be influenced by the measurement technique. For example, air bubbles in the system and changes in transducer positions may influence pressure measurement, with wide variations in IAP being noted.[72]

There are a variety of techniques for measuring IAP described in the literature[61,71] and the direct peritoneal catheter measurement is the most ideal but not the most practical. IAP measurements should be performed when patients exhibit one or more of the risk factors and the trans-bladder technique is the measurement technique recommended by the World Society of the Abdominal Compartment Syndrome.[69] The reliability of other methods, such as intragastric measurement, is not well demonstrated in clinical practice.[73]

> **Practice tip**
>
> The trans-bladder technique is the most common method used for measuring IAP. Attention should be given to consistent and accurate measurement to track trends.

IAP measurement should be accurate and reproducible. There are a number of commercial devices now available to aid the measurement of IAP; however, these are not required and a measurement system can easily be created from existing equipment normally available

TABLE 20.4
Physiological changes associated with abdominal compartment syndrome

SYSTEM	PHYSIOLOGICAL EFFECTS
Respiratory[66]	Cephalad deviation of diaphragm leads to decreased lung and chest wall compliance Peak inspiratory pressures increase Functional residual volume and lung capacity are reduced, resulting in ventilation/perfusion mismatching Hypoxia and hypercarbia may result, necessitating mechanical ventilation Pulmonary vascular resistance increases
Cardiovascular[66,67]	Inferior vena cava and portal vein compression results in decreased venous return Decreased left ventricular compliance Artificially increased right atrial pressure, pulmonary artery occlusion pressure Decreased cardiac index Elevated systemic vascular resistance from arteriolar vasoconstriction and increased intraabdominal pressure (IAP)
Renal[68]	Oliguria (IAP 15–20 mmHg) Anuria (IAP >30 mmHg) May be a consequence of decreased cardiac output, compression of renal vessels, increased renal vascular resistance or redistribution of blood flow to renal medulla
Gastrointestinal[61,62]	Decreased splanchnic perfusion and tissue hypoxia Increased GI mucosal acidosis Reduced hepatic blood flow Abnormalities in normal gut mucosal barrier function that may permit bacterial translocation Decreased abdominal wall blood flow Increased pressure on oesophageal varices may result in bleeding
Neurological[61]	Increased intracranial pressure because of impaired venous return

Reproduced from Marshall AP. The gut in critical illness. In: Carlson K, editor. AACN Advanced critical care nursing. Philadelphia: Elsevier; 2009, Table 29-4, with permission.

TABLE 20.5
Intraabdominal hypertension grading system[69]

GRADE	BLADDER PRESSURE (MMHG)
I	12–15
II	16–20
III	21–25
IV	>25

Adapted from Kirkpatrick AW, Roberts DJ, De Waele J, et al. Intra-abdominal hypertension and the abdominal compartment syndrome: updated consensus definitions and clinical practice guidelines from the World Society of the Abdominal Compartment Syndrome. Intensive Care Med 2013;39(7):1190–206.

in most ICUs. The procedures for IAP measurement techniques may differ; however, the key principles for performing measurements are outlined in Table 20.6.[61,74]

Management of intraabdominal hypertension and abdominal compartment syndrome

Surveillance for IAH and abdominal compartment syndrome requires close observation of the patient to identify potential risk factors and relevant changes to physiological parameters. For those patients who are at risk, close monitoring of IAP is required and pre-emptive measures are instituted. For example, a decision may be made to delay closure of the abdomen or to use an alternative means of abdominal content coverage. For the non-surgical patient, optimal resuscitation may be important in preventing IAH; over-resuscitation needs to be avoided. The approach to managing the patient with IAH or abdominal compartment syndrome is dependent on their clinical presentation. The World Society of the Abdominal Compartment Syndrome has developed evidence-based management algorithms that are useful in guiding clinical management (Figs 20.2 and 20.3).[69]

TABLE 20.6

Key principles for measuring intraabdominal pressure (IAP)[61]

	RECOMMENDATION
Measurement techniques	• IAP should be measured in mmHg • Measurement should be recorded at end-expiration • The transducer should be zeroed at the mid-axillary line at the level of the iliac crest • Determine measurement 30-60 s after instillation of saline to allow bladder detrusor muscle to relax • Monitor IAP every 4-6 h. Monitoring can be ceased when IAP is <12 mmHg for several hours and the patient is clinically improving
Instillation volume	• A maximum of 25 mL sterile saline should be used as the instillation volume in adults • In children the volume instilled should be 3 mL/kg[74]
Patient position	• IAP should be measured in supine position, where possible • IAP is significantly increased when the head of bed is elevated more than 20° • If head-of-bed elevation is required, consider the reverse Trendelenburg position during IAP measurement to minimise compression of the abdomen by the chest

Adapted from Kirkpatrick AW, Roberts DJ, De Waele J, et al. Intra-abdominal hypertension and the abdominal compartment syndrome: updated consensus definitions and clinical practice guidelines from the World Society of the Abdominal Compartment Syndrome. Intensive Care Med 2013;39(7):1190–206

The critically ill patient with diabetes

Diabetes is a major cause of morbidity and mortality worldwide.[75] The prevalence of diabetes internationally is rising and follows a global trend and over one-third of adults with diabetes live in the Western Pacific region. Reasons for this include an increase in the rates of obesity, physical inactivity, the ageing population, better detection of diabetes and longer survival of affected individuals.[76] The prevalence of diagnosed diabetes continues to increase worldwide, in adults as well as youth. In 2015, a reported 415 million people worldwide had diabetes and this number is projected to increase to 640 million by the year 2040.[77] Worryingly, reports of undiagnosed diabetes are on the increase with type 2 diabetes remaining undetected for many years, particularly in developing countries.[77]

Aetiology of diabetes

Diabetes mellitus is a disorder of metabolism that is characterised by glucose intolerance. Diabetes is not a single disease per se, but a group of heterogeneous disorders where the aetiology of glucose disturbance is multifactorial.[77] Ongoing effect of poor glycaemic control can ultimately contribute to the development of end-organ damage. In the long term, diabetes is associated with increased morbidity and mortality but acute complications of diabetes, such as diabetic ketoacidosis and hyperosmolar hyperglycaemic state, may necessitate patient management in the ICU.[78]

Acute complications of diabetes

Diabetic ketoacidosis (DKA) and hyperosmolar hyperglycaemic state (HHS) are two extremes of what can occur when a deficiency in insulin is present.[79] DKA is a metabolic derangement resulting from a relative or absolute insulin deficiency, characterised by hyperglycaemia (>11.0 mmol/L), metabolic acidosis (pH <7.3) and ketosis (raised blood ketone bodies or ketonuria).[80] It is usually precipitated, in insulin- and non-insulin-dependent diabetics, by infection or the omission (or inadequate dosing) of insulin.[81] It may also be the cause of the first presentation in new-onset diabetes. Additionally, DKA is increasingly being identified in patients with type 2 diabetes.[82]

HHS is seen more often in older patients with type 2 diabetes, and is characterised by hyperglycaemia and the pathological consequences of extreme dehydration. Unlike DKA, where there is insufficient insulin, in HHS insulin excretion is maintained, so lipolysis and ketoacidosis do not feature. Although DKA and HHS are considered separate entities, DKA and HHS may co-exist in about a third of cases, especially among older patients.[79]

While these are often considered two distinct states, they can present simultaneously. DKA usually occurs much more quickly with the onset of HHS being more insidious. Both complications are characterised by polyuria, polydipsia and weight loss. Patients with DKA can also present with nausea and vomiting.[83] A comparison of DKA with HHS is provided in Table 20.7.[84]

Pathophysiology

Inadequate production (or administration) of insulin to meet metabolic need (or a rise in metabolic demand resulting from the stress of infection, trauma or surgery, for instance) is associated with a rise in the secretion of the counter-regulatory hormones glucagon, the catecholamines and cortisol[83] (Box 20.1). When insulin is deficient, hyperglycaemic results from gluconeogenesis, accelerated glycogenolysis and impaired glucose use by peripheral tissues.[81] Lipase results in the breakdown of triglycerides into glycerol and free fatty acids which are

FIGURE 20.2 Intraabdominal hypertension and abdominal compartment syndrome management algorithm.[69]

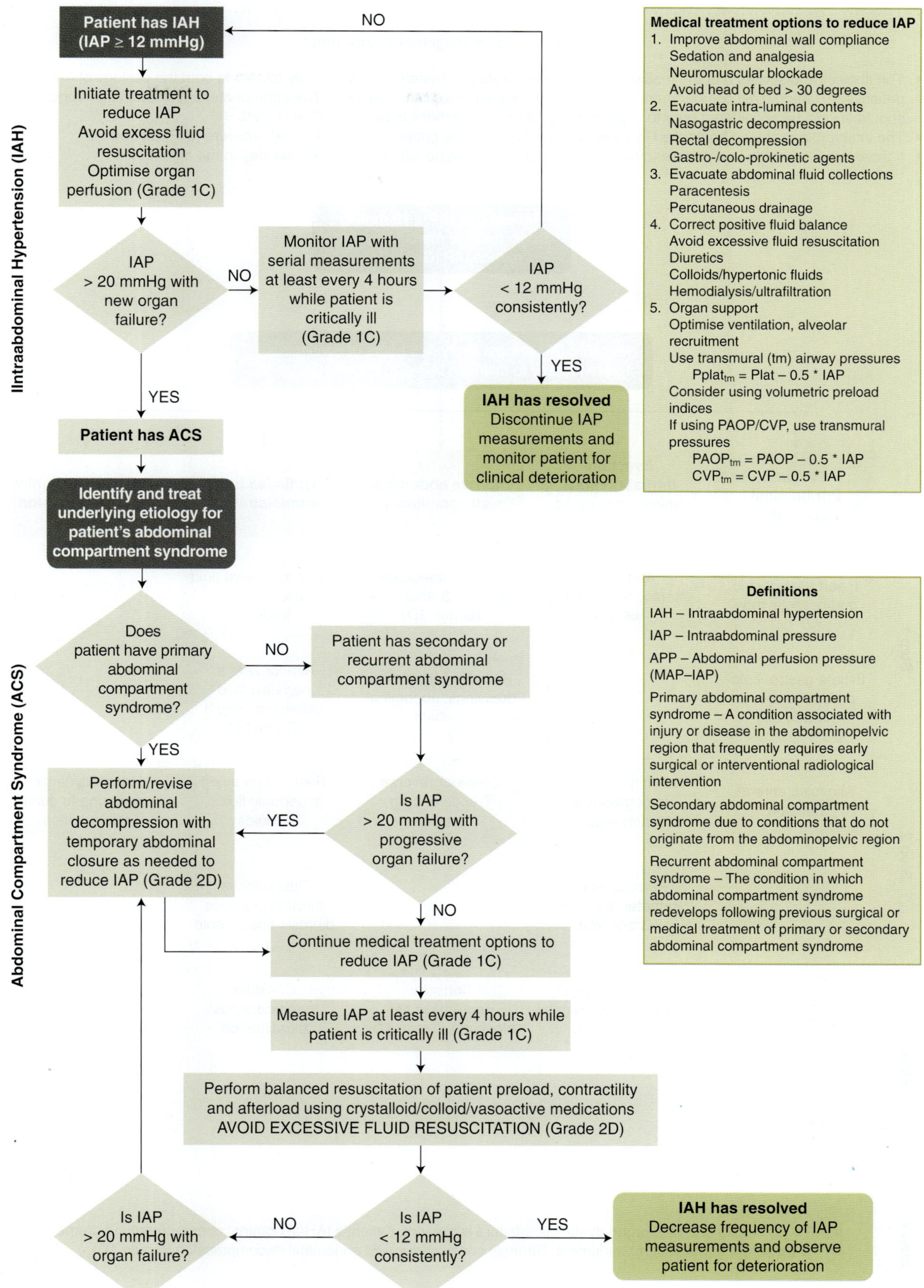

Reprinted with permission of Springer Nature. Kirkpatrick AW, Roberts DJ, De Waele J, Jaeschke R, Malbrain ML, De Keulenaer B, et al. Intra-abdominal hypertension and the abdominal compartment syndrome: updated consensus definitions and clinical practice guidelines from the World Society of the Abdominal Compartment Syndrome. Intensive Care Med 2013;39(7):1190–206

FIGURE 20.3 Intraabdominal hypertension and abdominal compartment syndrome medical management algorithm.[69]

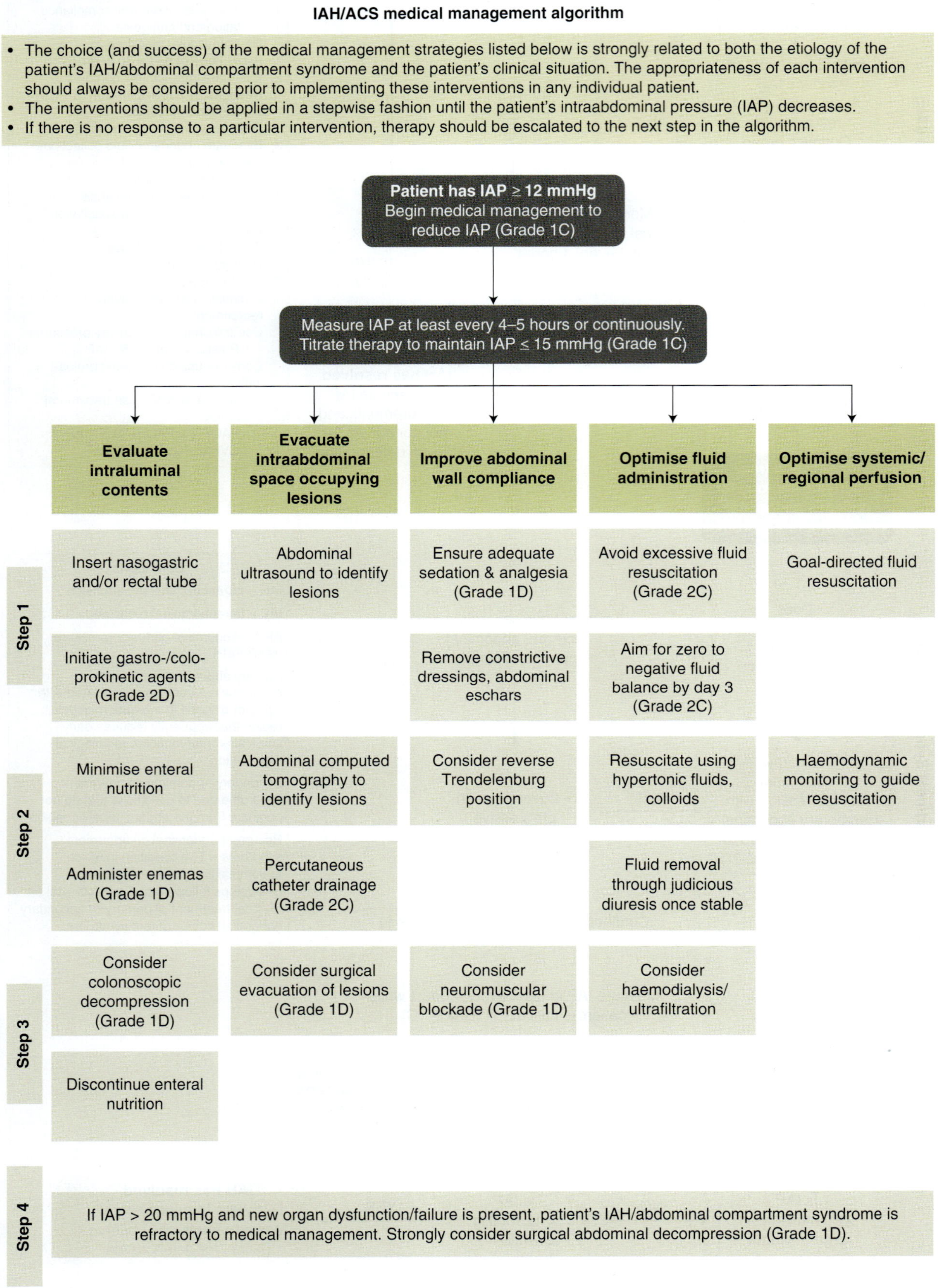

Reprinted with permission of Springer Nature. Kirkpatrick AW, Roberts DJ, De Waele J, Jaeschke R, Malbrain ML, De Keulenaer B, et al. Intra-abdominal hypertension and the abdominal compartment syndrome: updated consensus definitions and clinical practice guidelines from the World Society of the Abdominal Compartment Syndrome. Intensive Care Med 2013;39(7):1190–206

TABLE 20.7

Comparison of presentation and electrolyte deficits in DKA and HHS[81, 84]

PRESENTATION	DKA	HHS
Prodromal illness	Days	Weeks
Diabetes type	More common in T1D	More common in T2D
Coma	++	+++
Blood glucose	++	+++
Ketone	+++	0 or +
Acidaemia	+++	0 or +
Anion gap	++	0 or +
Osmolality	++	+++
Signs	Polydipsia Polyuria Weakness Weight loss Nausea Vomiting Abdominal pain	Polydipsia Polyuria Weakness Weight loss
Symptoms	Hypothermia Tachycardia Tachypnoea Kussmaul breathing Ileus Acetone breath Altered sensorium	Hypothermia Hypotension Tachycardia Altered sensorium
TYPICAL DEFICITS		
Total water (litres)	6	9
Water (mL/kg)	100	100–200
Na^+ (mmol/kg)	7–10	5–13
Cl^- (mmol/kg)	3–5	5–15
K^+ (mmol/kg)	3–5	4–6
PO_4 (mmol/kg)	5–7	3–7
Mg^{2+} (mmol/kg)	0.5–1.0	0.5–1.0
Ca^{2+} (mmol/kg)	0.5–1.0	0.5–1.0

T1D: type 1 diabetes; T2D: type 2 diabetes.
Source: Fayfam et al., 2017; Keays et al., 2009.

subsequently oxidised into ketone bodies in the liver.[81] As ketone bodies accumulate serum bicarbonate concentration decreases and metabolic acidosis results. In the HHS, insulin levels are higher and this inhibits ketogenesis and metabolic acidosis (Fig. 20.4).

BOX 20.1

Effects of counter-regulatory hormones in DKA[83]

- Catecholamines:
  - Promote lipolysis, resulting in the production of FFA and glycerol; FFA and glycerol used as precursors for gluconeogenesis
- Glucagon:
  - Stimulates gluconeogenesis
- Cortisol:
  - Promotes lipolysis
  - Promotes protein breakdown and release of amino acids
  - Promotes hepatic gluconeogenesis

DKA = diabetic ketoacidosis; FFA = free fatty acids.
Source: Nyenwe EA, Kitabchi AE. The evolution of diabetic ketoacidosis: An update of its etiology, pathogenesis and management. Metabolism 2016;65(4):507–21.

Management of diabetic ketoacidosis and hyperosmolar hyperglycaemic state

Management of DKA involves rehydration and electrolyte replacement, insulin administration, correction of acidosis and treatment of the precipitating factor.[83] Although historically the approach to managing DKA has been variable, there is evidence to suggest that a standardised approach can have a positive impact on patient outcome.[85]

Management of HHS is similar to that for DKA and includes: respiratory support; fluid replacement; insulin treatment to turn off ketogenesis and the accompanying metabolic derangement; electrolyte replacement; monitoring for and prevention of complications of hypoglycaemia, hypokalaemia, hyperglycaemia and fluid volume overload; and patient teaching and support. Ongoing assessment of blood glucose levels is essential.[86]

Effectiveness of treatment is usually assessed by resolution of the acidosis (in DKA) and the control of hyperglycaemia. Regular testing of arterial blood gases, blood sugar and electrolytes (especially potassium) is vital until the blood sugar has stabilised and the ketosis and acidosis resolves.[81] Considering that fewer patients are now admitted to ICU with DKA and HHS, understanding the management of these patients is vital and protocols have been developed to guide practice.

Blood ketones (beta-hydroxybutyrate) can now easily be measured using blood from a finger prick with a bedside handheld monitor. It has been suggested that blood ketone monitoring allows for insulin titration with reference to ketones in addition to usual blood sugar monitoring.[86] Fig. 20.5 provides an algorithm to guide the management of DKA and HHS.[87]

FIGURE 20.4 Pathogenesis of hyperglycaemic emergencies.[81]

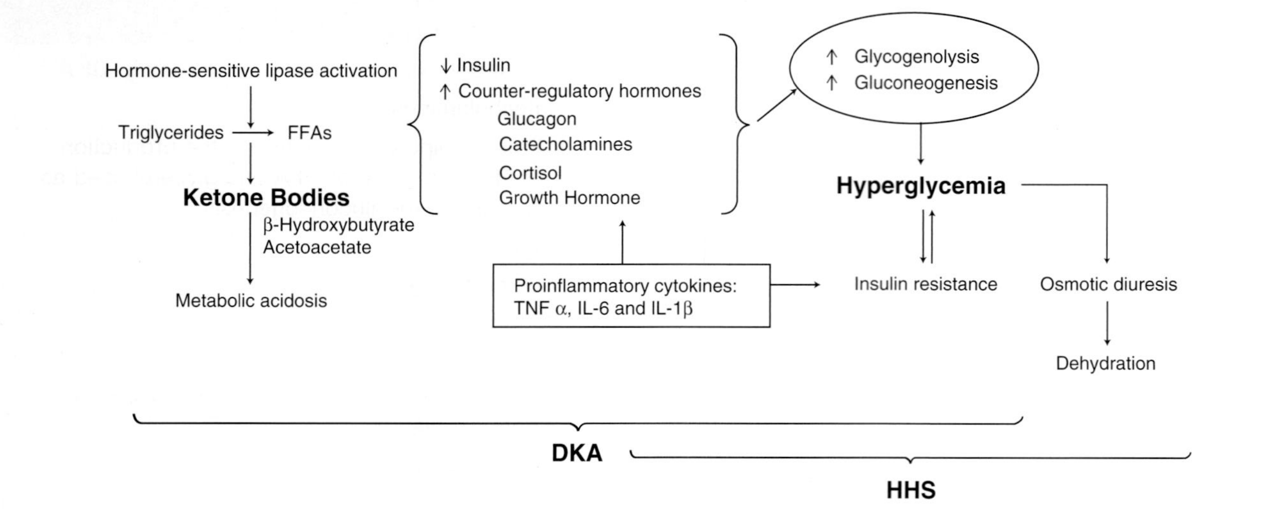

Reproduced with permission from Fayfman M, Pasquel FJ, Umpierrez GE. Management of hyperglycemic crises: diabetic ketoacidosis and hyperglycemic hyperosmolar state. Med Clin North Am 2017;101(3): 587-606, Figure 1, p. 592.

FIGURE 20.5 Treatment of DKA.[87]

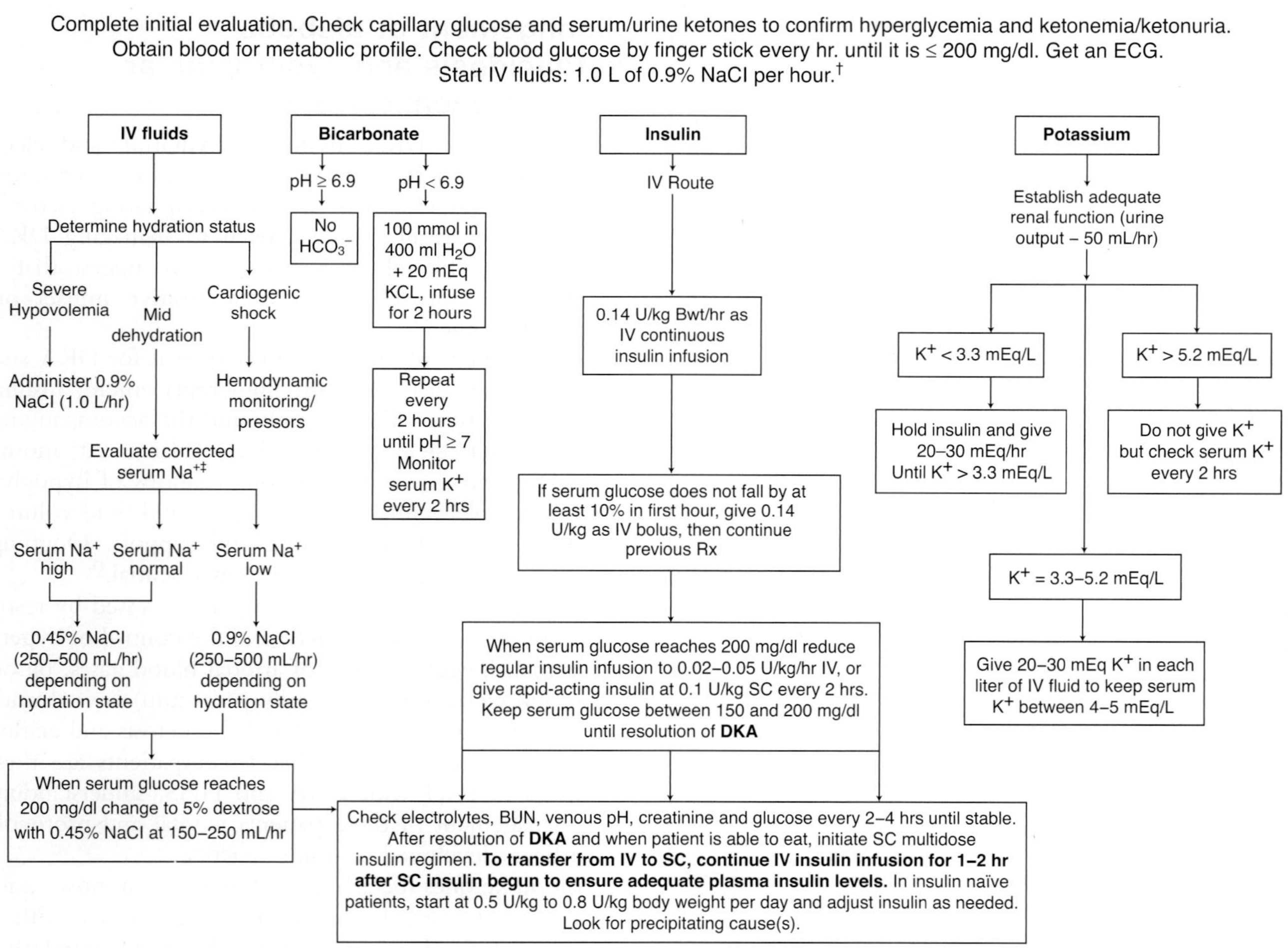

**DKA diagnostic criteria: blood glucose > 250 mg/dl, arterial pH < 7.3, bicarbonate < 15, mEq/l, and moderate ketonuria or ketonemia.*
‡Serum Na should be corrected for hyperglycemia (for each 200 mg/dl glucose, add 1.6 mEq to sodium value for corrected serum value)
Source: Nyenwe EA, Kitabchi AE. The evolution of diabetic ketoacidosis: An update of its etiology, pathogenesis and management. YMETA; ISSN – 0026-0495. 2016. Elsevier Inc.

Pancreatitis

The pancreas has many key endocrine and exocrine functions. Regulating blood glucose through the production of the hormones insulin, glucagon, and somatostatin, as well as producing enzymes to aid digestion in the gut. If pancreatic function is inhibited through injury or disease, this can have significant effects on systemic function.

In normal function, digestive enzymes are in an inactive form in the pancreas, only becoming active when in the presence of other substances found in the duodenum. Pancreatitis occurs when a known or unknown cause stimulates these digestive enzymes to become active while still inside the pancreas leading to autodigestion of pancreatic tissue and inflammation. Common causes of acute pancreatitis are alcohol, gallstones, or this can often be idiopathic. Pancreatitis is diagnosed by the presence of two of three of the following findings: abdominal pain consistent with the condition (acute, persistent, severe epigastric pain often radiating to the back); raised serum lipase or amylase (at least three times the upper limit of normal); and characteristic findings on contrast enhanced computerised tomography scanning.[88]

Acute pancreatitis is subdivided into two types, interstitial oedematous pancreatitis and necrotising pancreatitis. These are broadly differentiated by the condition of the pancreatic and surrounding tissues as inflamed or necrotic. There are two phases of the disease, early and late, with peaks of mortality at either point. The early phase is characterised by systemic inflammation, and the late phase when this persists longer than 1–2 weeks. Three classifications of severity are suggested, characterised by the presence of local or systemic complications and with increasing mortality (Table 20.8).[88]

TABLE 20.8
Classifications of acute pancreatitis[88]

SEVERITY	CHARACTERISTICS
Mild acute pancreatitis	Absence of organ failure and absence of local or systemic complications
Moderately severe acute pancreatitis	Transient organ failure or local or systemic complications in the absence of persistent organ failure (<48 h)
Severe acute pancreatitis	Persistent organ failure (>48 h)

Reproduced from Banks PA, Bollen TL, Dervenis C, Gooszen HG, Johnson CD, Sarr MG, et al. Classification of acute pancreatitis – 2012: revision of the Atlanta classification and definitions by international consensus. Gut 2013;62(1):102-11 with permission of BMJ Publishing Group.

All patients with organ failure or severe acute pancreatitis should be managed in a critical care setting.[89] Acute pancreatitis should be managed with aggressive intravenous (IV) hydration to mitigate organ failure; currently there is no high-quality evidence for specific pharmacological interventions.[90] Surgical intervention is reserved for the most severe cases and is not a recommended routine treatment strategy.

Fasting can be useful initially, as pain can occur when the pancreas is stimulated to produce and release enzymes by the presence of food in the gut; however, enteral feeding should be commenced 48 hours after presentation. Some prefer the nasojejunal route to provide nutrition, with the view that postpyloric feeding may preclude the painful effects mentioned above. However, both routes have been found to be as effective and, as with most critically ill patients, enteral nutrition has been shown to be preferable to parenteral nutrition.[91] Additional information on nutrition in criticall illness is provided in Chapter 19.

Pain is a common and debilitating symptom associated with acute pancreatitis; opioids appear to be an appropriate choice for treatment,[92] with the use of patient-controlled analgesia a clinically useful option.

Liver dysfunction

The liver is responsible for a vast array of metabolic functions. It performs the vital functions of controlling metabolic pathways, participating in digestion, immunological protection, detoxifying chemicals and clearing toxins and drugs. This means that alterations to normal liver function can have broad-ranging consequences, from changes in metabolic processes (such as glucose homeostasis), failure to produce clotting factors (with resultant severe haemorrhage) to other organ effects such as brain, lung and kidney impairment and injury. Accordingly, liver dysfunction can impact substantially on the nursing care needs of the critically ill patient.

Related anatomy and physiology

The liver is the largest internal organ, weighing approximately 1200 to 1600 g in the adult. It receives approximately 25% of total cardiac output through a dual vascular supply consisting of the hepatic artery and portal vein. Approximately 75% of all hepatic blood flow arises from the portal vein with the remaining 25% from the hepatic artery. Anatomically, the liver consists of four lobes: the major left and right lobes and the minor caudate and quadrate lobes. The right lobe is considerably larger than the left. Functionally, the liver is divided into eight segments each with their own inflow and outflow blood supply and biliary drainage. Hepatic lobules, or liver *acinus*, are small units consisting of a single or double layer of hepatocytes arranged in plates interspersed with capillaries (sinusoids) that receive inflowing blood from the portal and hepatic pathways. To protect the systemic circulation from the toxins absorbed from the intestines, the sinusoids are lined with macrophages known as Kupffer cells. The hepatic vein then drains effluent blood from the liver into the general circulation.

The liver is responsible for the synthesis and drainage system for bile (used in the breakdown and absorption of lipids from the intestine). Biliary salts are formed from multiple enzymatic reactions in the hepatocytes. Bile drains from the hepatocytes into bile ducts and then into the common hepatic duct, before passing into the gall bladder via the common bile duct.[93]

The arrangement of the circulation to the liver with its rich vascular architecture enables it to perform the vital functions of carbohydrate, fat and protein metabolism; production of bile to aid in digestion; production, conjugation and elimination of bilirubin; immunological and inflammatory responses; glycogen storage; and detoxification of toxins and drugs. As the kidneys are responsible for clearance of water-soluble toxins from the body, the liver clears protein-bound (largely albumin) toxins and excretes them into the gastrointestinal tract for elimination, or reabsorption in water-soluble form for subsequent renal excretion.[93]

Mechanisms of liver cell injury

Liver cell injury and death can occur either as a direct result of injury to the cell, resulting in cell necrosis, or as a result of cellular stress and the triggering of apoptotic pathways, leading to programmed cell death. Major factors for the triggering of the apoptotic pathway are hypoxia causing ischaemia and reperfusion; reactive oxygen metabolites resulting from alcohol or drug ingestion; accumulation of bile acids resulting from cholestasis; and inflammatory cytokines such as tumour necrosis factor-alpha.[94] The apoptotic pathway results in the deconstruction of the cellular structure from the inside out, while necrosis results in cell rupture and release of cellular contents. Although these processes may overlap, it is thought that the apoptotic pathway is a way of preventing the inflammatory response that is triggered with cell necrosis. The activation of the inflammatory response results in secondary liver cell injury and contributes to the multiple organ dysfunction seen in liver failure.[94,95]

The degree and time course of liver cell damage from viral hepatitis depends on the immune response. Immune recognition and destruction of infected cells may result in either clearance of the virus or ongoing inflammation, cell death and fibrosis if the virus is not cleared. This process may progress over 20–40 years to cirrhosis and hepatocellular carcinoma.[96] Chronic excessive alcohol intake may also result in a slower chronic course of liver injury that eventually results in cirrhosis, liver failure or hepatocellular carcinoma.[97]

Liver cells may also be injured by the toxic effects of drugs or their metabolites, as in paracetamol overdose,[98] or by therapeutic doses of drugs such as non-steroidal anti-inflammatory drugs, phenytoin or antimalarial agents. Other poisoning from the ingestion of mushrooms (e.g. *Amanita phalloides*)[99] and from the use of recreational drugs such as ecstasy and amphetamines may result in liver cell death and liver failure. Diseases of the biliary system, such as primary biliary cholangitis and primary sclerosing cholangitis, also result in liver dysfunction and failure.[100,101]

The liver has a remarkable regenerative capacity. After injury and necrosis, liver cells rapidly regenerate around areas of surviving cells to restore the lost tissue while maintaining homeostasis during hepatic regeneration.[102,103] However, with chronic injury, fibrosis or scarring occurs, resulting in the loss of the functional architecture and cell mass and ultimately in cirrhosis. Cirrhosis results in destruction of the normal liver vasculature, increased resistance to blood flow and back pressure into the portal circulation. Dilation of the venous system leading into the liver results in the formation of varices.[104]

Liver cell injury may occur to such a degree that a critical amount of hepatic necrosis results in the failure of the liver to maintain metabolic, synthetic and clearance functions leading to death. Liver cell injury may also occur more slowly, giving rise to chronic liver injury.[105]

Epidemiology of viral hepatitis

Worldwide, the incidence of hepatitis B and C is estimated to be 390 million[96,106-114] with the largest proportion (approximately 240 million) being people infected with hepatitis B. A high mortality rate from hepatitis accounts for approximately 1.3 million deaths worldwide annually.[115,116] Prevalence estimates for hepatitis B indicate that a high burden of infection exists in sub-Saharan Africa and some countries in the Western Pacific region. Over time the prevalence of hepatitis B has decreased in some areas, likely because of public health measures and vaccination.[117] Regionally the seroprevalence of hepatitis C varies with highest rates observed in Central, South and East Asia, North Africa and the Middle East. The lowest prevalence of hepatitis C was observed in tropical Latin America, high-income North America and high-income Asia Pacific regions.[118] It should be noted, however, that approximately 25% of people with hepatitis C virus exposure have cleared the virus and are not chronically infected. Also, many patients can be cured of hepatitis C virus due to newer therapies; however, lack of access to antiviral therapy may limit the number of people who can be successfully treated and reducing newer infections is a major focus of health organisations.[119]

Alcohol-related liver disease

Alcohol-induced liver damage is an increasingly common cause of liver disease, particularly in the developed world.[120] The burden of alcohol attributable diseases is significant, in 2010 it was estimated to be responsible for 120,168 years of life lost in Australia.[121] The mechanisms by which alcohol causes liver damage are not entirely understood. The main factors involved in developing alcoholic fatty liver are increased production of toxic substances from alcohol metabolism, as well as ethanol having a direct effect on metabolic pathways.[122] In some individuals with alcoholic fatty livers this will progress to a marked inflammatory stage, called alcoholic steatohepatitis (or alcoholic hepatitis). This is thought to be due to several other factors including acetaldehyde-induced toxic effects leading to oxidative stress (a byproduct of ethanol metabolism), the creation of reactive oxygen species, and the release of proinflammatory cytokines.[122] Up to 40% of patients with severe alcoholic hepatitis die within 6 months after the onset of symptoms, so appropriate management is key.[123]

The onset of the clinical syndrome in alcoholic hepatitis is characterised by rapid onset jaundice, fever, ascites, and sarcopenia. Biochemically you would expect to find raised hepatic enzymes, raised white cell count, increased serum total bilirubin, and a prolonged clotting time. The presence of a raised serum creatinine is a poor prognostic marker as it usually precedes renal failure and death.[123] There are several scoring systems including Maddrey's discriminant function, the Glasgow Alcoholic Hepatitis score, and model for end-stage liver disease (MELD), used for the assessment of severity of alcoholic hepatitis and to guide treatment, all using varied selections of biochemical markers.

The treatment of alcoholic hepatitis consists of the management of associated symptoms as in any form of decompensated liver disease, and the mitigation of organ failure. Any approach should include treatment of the acute alcohol withdrawal syndrome (short-acting benzodiazepines) and the provision of adequate nutrition.[123,124] Pharmacological treatment for alcoholic hepatitis is now led by corticosteroids, as recent evidence has shown that other often-used therapies were ineffective.[125] However, despite their widespread usage there is little evidence of a survival benefit being conferred. There has been limited evidence for the use of liver transplantation for acute alcoholic hepatitis[126] but this is only in carefully selected patient groups and has yet to be replicated on a wider scale.

Liver dysfunction/failure

Liver dysfunction can be acute or chronic. Chronic liver disease is usually associated with cirrhosis and can develop from viral (hepatitis B and C), drug (alcohol), metabolic (Wilson's disease) or autoimmune (primary biliary cholangitis) conditions. Acute liver failure (ALF) is an uncommon condition associated with rapid liver dysfunction leading to jaundice, hepatic encephalopathy (HE) and coagulopathy.[127] Terminology for acute liver failure is not standardised and several terms have been proposed, including acute hepatic failure and fulminant hepatic failure. Historically, fulminant hepatic failure was used to refer to the rapid onset of liver failure accompanied by HE within 8 weeks of diagnosis in the absence of preexisting liver disease.[96] Unfortunately, this was problematic because determining the onset of jaundice and encephalopathy is often difficult and coagulation results, such as international normalised ratio, are more reliable indicators of liver failure. It has also been proposed that 'hyperacute', 'acute' and 'subacute' liver failure should be used instead, with hyperacute referring to the development of encephalopathy within 7 days of the onset of jaundice, acute related to 8–28 days from jaundice to encephalopathy and subacute liver failure when encephalopathy occurs within 5–12 weeks of the onset of jaundice.[128] It has further been proposed that acute and subacute hepatic failure should be used; however, universal acceptance of these terms has not occurred with clinical use of all of the above terms.

ALF without preexisting liver disease can result from drug reactions, toxins or viral infection, or from the effect on inflammatory mediators released in response to tissue injury. Liver failure can also occur as an acute decompensation of chronic liver disease, described as acute-on-chronic liver failure (AoCLF), or as an end-stage decompensation in chronic liver failure. AoCLF is a syndrome with heterogeneous definitions but is broadly characterised by severe acute hepatic dysfunction with associated extrahepatic organ failure and high short-term mortality, which can be precipitated by bacterial or viral infection, bleeding or intoxication, and results in a severe clinical syndrome similar to that seen in ALF; however, osmotic compensatory mechanisms that fail in ALF tend to remain effective in AoCLF therefore making the development of intracranial hypertension less common.[127] In AoCLF, the function of the residual liver cell mass may be adequate to maintain hepatic homeostasis if the precipitating event can be treated, returning the patient to a compensated phase of their underlying disease.

End-stage decompensation of chronic liver failure represents irreversible deterioration with inadequate residual function to maintain homeostasis, and liver transplantation is the only long-term viable treatment; however, short-term mortality is low if acute episodes are managed effectively.[129]

Liver dysfunction is also a common consequence of critical illness, and may be caused by inadequate perfusion leading to ischaemic injury or as a result of the inflammatory response in sepsis. Given the number of drugs that critically ill patients receive, the possibility of liver injury as a result of drug reactions and toxicity should always be considered. Causes, definitions and key points can be seen below (Fig. 20.6).[130]

Consequences of liver failure

The consequences of liver failure manifest as a syndrome of HE, renal dysfunction or hepatorenal syndrome (HRS), oesophageal and gastric varices, ascites, respiratory compromise, haemodynamic instability, susceptibility to infection, coagulopathy and metabolic derangement with notable differences in presentation and treatment between acute (without preexisting liver disease) and chronic presentations.[127]

FIGURE 20.6 Causes of liver insults, definitions and key points of intensive care acquired acute liver injury, hepatic dysfunction and acute liver failure.[124] ALP = alkaline phosphatase; ALT = alanine aminotransferase; AST = aspartate aminotransferase; γ-GT = γ-glutamyl transpeptidase; ICG-PDR = indocyanine green plasma disappearance rate; INR = international normalised ratio.

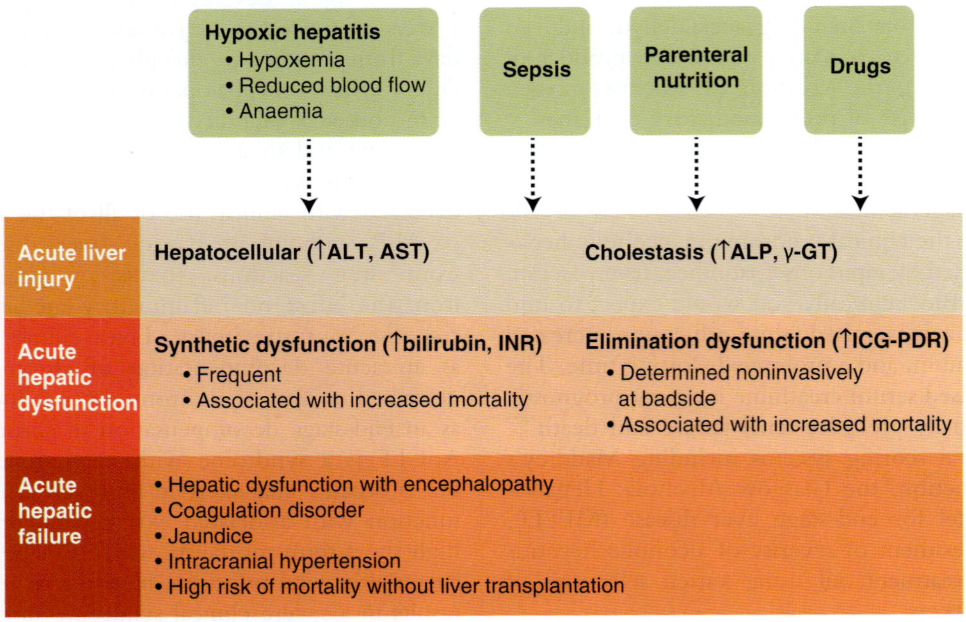

Reproduced from Lescot T, Karvellas C, Beaussier M, Magder S. Acquired liver injury in the intensive care unit. Anesthesiology: The Journal of the American Society of Anesthesiologists 2012 Oct 1;117(4):898-904.

Hepatic encephalopathy

HE is a reversible neuropsychiatric complication due to metabolic dysfunction associated with liver disease.[131] The cerebral effects of liver failure may manifest as an altered sleep–wake cycle, mild confusion/disorientation, asterixis and coma. Patients with AoCLF may develop a mild degree of cerebral oedema, while a differential feature of ALF is the risk of death from cerebral oedema and raised intracranial pressure.[132]

The exact mechanisms responsible for the development of HE are unclear, although raised ammonia levels resulting from the failure of the liver urea cycle are thought to be central to the pathogenesis. The raised ammonia levels disrupt the blood–brain barrier, which can lead to the development of cerebral oedema, a life-threatening complication in ALF. Ammonia levels also seem to be related to the disruption of neurotransmission, resulting in decreased cerebral function.[133] In addition, reactive oxidative species causing oxidative stress and inflammatory cytokine release have been suggested; however, the exact pathophysiology is yet to be fully elucidated.[102]

HE is usually classified using the West Haven criteria,[103] a four-stage scale, according to the severity of clinical signs and symptoms (Table 20.9).[134] Although used in clinical practice, the West Haven criteria have poor sensitivity and no inherent metric component, with poor interobserver reliability. For instance, in patients with grades III–IV encephalopathy, the Glasgow Coma Scale is probably a more sensitive tool for neurological assessment. A more easily used, but less specific classification is to describe symptoms as covert (West Haven grades 0–1) or overt (grades 2–4).[111,135] Other grading criteria have been proposed but are yet to be validated in large clinical trials.[112,135]

Hepatorenal syndrome

HRS is the development of renal failure in patients with severe liver disease (acute or chronic), in the absence of any other identifiable cause of renal dysfunction, this is a diagnosis of exclusion and therefore acute kidney injury should always be considered as the first potential cause of any renal dysfunction. HRS that develops rapidly in the setting of ALF or AoCLF is classified as type 1 HRS, while type 2 HRS is slowly progressing and is usually associated with diuretic-resistant ascites.[113]

The pathophysiological features of HRS appear to be caused by an inflammatory response from the injured liver, resulting in upregulation of nitric oxide production that results in splanchnic vasodilation.[114] Splanchnic vasodilation results in redistribution of circulating blood volume and a lowered mean arterial pressure. The reduction in perfusion pressure results in an enhanced

TABLE 20.9
West Haven grading of hepatic encephalopathy[134]

	GRADE	CHARACTERISTICS
Covert	MHE	Psychometric or neuropsychological alterations of tests exploring psychomotor speed/executive functions or neurophysiological alterations without clinical evidence of mental change
	I	Trivial lack of awareness Euphoria or anxiety Shortened attention span Impaired performance of simple tests, e.g. addition
Overt	II	Lethargy or apathy Subtle personality changes Inappropriate behaviour
	III	Somnolence to semi-stupor, but unresponsive to verbal stimuli Confusion Gross disorientation
	IV	Coma: unresponsive to verbal or painful stimuli

sympathetic nervous system response and local renal autoregulatory responses. The net result of these effects is a reduction in renal blood flow and increased activity of the renin–angiotensin–aldosterone system, resulting in sodium (aldosterone) and water retention (arginine vasopressin; see Chapter 18).

Practice tip

Using lactate- or citrate-buffered substitution/dialysis fluid for renal replacement therapy in patients with very severe liver dysfunction should be undertaken with caution, as they may be unable to metabolise the lactate or citrate and could develop an increasing metabolic acidosis.

Varices and variceal bleeding

The development of varices and variceal bleeding arises from portal hypertension. This manifests when blood flowing from an area of high pressure (i.e. the cirrhotic liver) to areas of lower pressure (i.e. the collateral circulation, involving veins of the oesophagus, spleen, intestines and stomach) causes the tiny, thin-walled vessels to become engorged and dilated, forming varices that are vulnerable to gastric secretions, resulting in rupture and haemorrhage.[136] Variceal haemorrhage is a major cause of acute decompensation and a reason for admission to the ICU. It is an acute clinical event characterised by severe gastrointestinal haemorrhage presenting as haematemesis, with or without melaena, and haemodynamic instability (tachycardia and hypotension).[137]

Practice tip

Coagulation state and the risk of trauma to varices should be carefully considered before insertion of nasogastric or orogastric tubes, or suctioning of the upper airway. Trauma may result in epistaxis with significant bleeding or variceal bleeding.

Ascites

Ascites is one of the most common complications of cirrhosis, arising from the same pathophysiological mechanisms underlying the formation of varices (portal hypertension). In the ICU setting it becomes an issue when abdominal pressures rise, resulting in reduced cardiac output due to decreased venous return and renal impairment. Pressure on the diaphragm causes loss of lung volume, resulting in increased work of breathing and compromised oxygenation. The presence of ascites can also lead to bacterial translocation from the gut, potentially causing spontaneous bacterial peritonitis and sepsis.[138]

Respiratory compromise

Patients with liver failure may have poor oxygen exchange, fluctuating Glasgow Coma Scale score that requires intubation for airway protection, and hepatopulmonary syndrome. Hepatopulmonary syndrome is found in up to 30% of patients with cirrhosis.[139] It is defined as heterogeneous pulmonary microvascular dilation resulting in impaired oxygenation, and it is generally assumed that vascular production of vasodilators, specifically nitric oxide, underlies the vasodilation in hepatopulmonary syndrome. It has also been hypothesised that the mechanisms that trigger hepatopulmonary syndrome are the same as those that result in the hyperdynamic circulation (low systemic vascular resistance and high cardiac output) seen in liver failure.[139] Other factors, such as pleural effusions or severe ascites, may impinge on ventilation.

Haemodynamic instability, susceptibility to infection, coagulopathy and metabolic derangement

A hyperdynamic, low vascular resistance picture, similar to that associated with sepsis, is seen in liver dysfunction. This probably results from the production, and reduction in clearance, of vasodilator substances (nitric oxide) from the inflammatory response of the injured liver cells.[140] Sepsis may also be a complication of liver dysfunction because of the failure of the liver to produce acute-phase proteins and the impaired function of Kupffer cells leading to a functional immunosuppression.[141]

Hepatocyte damage leads to a decreased production of the majority of clotting factors and, therefore, alters haemostatic function. However, conventional laboratory tests poorly correlate with actual occurrence of haemostatic complications; importantly, not only the risk of bleeding is elevated in liver dysfunction, thrombosis can also occur.[142] The presence and severity of marked coagulopathy is a strong prognostic indicator.

Disordered metabolic function and failure of synthetic function can manifest as unstable blood glucose levels.

Practice tip

Patients in ALF or AoCLF are at risk of hypoglycaemia, and blood glucose levels should be measured routinely.

Patient management

Early signs of the patient presenting with ALF are malaise, loss of appetite, fatigue, nausea, jaundice, bruising, bleeding, inflamed/enlarged liver, possibly epigastric and right-upper-quadrant pain, deranged liver function tests, fluctuating Glasgow Coma Scale score due to HE and high or low blood glucose levels.[127] Fluctuating blood glucose levels may require close monitoring, at least every 4 hours; patients may require insulin infusion or 10–50% dextrose infusion to maintain normoglycaemia. If ALF is suspected, admission to an ICU is recommended to monitor for further deterioration, and provide supportive management and airway protection. The patient presenting with AoCLF will have similar symptoms but will present with other unique characteristics. Cirrhosis and portal hypertension will often lead to oesophageal and gastric varices, ascites, renal and pulmonary dysfunction, malnutrition, bone disease, sepsis, palmar erythema, spider naevi and feminisation in males.[97] If liver failure is suspected, investigating ingestion of hepatotoxic substances, such as paracetamol, steroids and ethanol, oral or intravenous recreational drug use and any recent travel that might have exposed the patient to viral infections is required. Early referral to specialist services, especially in ALF, is key to offering all treatment options.

Neurological considerations

Cerebral oedema is present in 80% of patients with grade IV encephalopathy and is the leading cause of death due to brain herniation.[102] Patients with cerebral oedema and raised intracranial pressure due to ALF are managed primarily as patients with acute head injury (see Chapter 17); however, there are important differences in pathophysiology that must be considered as some treatment strategies used in acute brain injury may not be effective.

Assessment of liver function

Patients presenting with ALF require a careful history to establish the cause of liver injury. The well-known signs of chronic liver disease (e.g. palmar erythema, spider naevi and ascites) may not be present. Biochemical and haematological tests determine whether liver cell injury is occurring, with liver synthesis and clearance functions assessed by albumin level and prothrombin time, and bilirubin level, respectively.[143] These measures have been incorporated into a scoring system to determine liver dysfunction and prognostic information for liver transplantation suitability (MELD) (see later in this chapter under *Liver transplantation*). Liver function test values and indications are listed in Table 20.10.[144]

Treatment

ALF or AoCLF therapy often involves the support and treatment of the consequences of liver failure, such as sepsis, encephalopathy, renal failure and coagulopathy (Table 20.11). Treatments are usually directed to supportive therapy, depending on the severity of manifestation; however, liver transplantation is used according to selection criteria in ALF and several different liver support systems have been trialled without long-term survival benefits.[148]

Oesophageal balloon tamponade and transjugular intrahepatic portosystemic stent/shunt

There are several types of balloon tamponade devices available on the market: the Sengstaken–Blakemore tube, the Linton tube, and the Minnesota tube. The Sengstaken–Blakemore tube is a three-lumen tube with oesophageal and gastric balloons, and gastric aspiration port. The Minnesota tube adds a fourth lumen to allow oesophageal aspiration. The benefit of these tubes is that direct pressure can be applied to gastric and oesophageal varices by balloon inflation and traction.[149] The Linton tube has one lumen for inflation of the pear-shaped gastric balloon and two additional lumens for oesophageal and gastric aspiration.

Prior to insertion (oral or nasal), balloons are lubricated, checked for leakage and the distance to the cardio-oesophageal junction is estimated (nose to ear, then to xiphisternum). Once inserted, the gastric balloon is inflated with 50 mL air and pulled back until resistance is felt. Position (lying compressed against the cardio-oesophageal junction) is confirmed by X-ray. Then, the gastric balloon is inflated according to the manufacturer's instructions and traction is applied using skin traction, the use of a weight (500 or 1000 mL IV fluid bag) attached to rope occurs in some settings but the risk of tube migration is enhanced. Nursing care of patients involves:

- sedation for comfort
- head of the bed raised at least 30° to facilitate gastric emptying and prevent aspiration

TABLE 20.10
Liver function tests[144]

BLOOD TEST	NORMAL VALUE	DESCRIPTION
Alanine aminotransferase (ALT) and aspartate aminotransferase (AST)	ALT: <35 U/L AST: <40 U/L	• ALT and AST are enzymes that indicate liver cell damage; they are produced within the liver cells (hepatocytes) and leak out into the general circulation when the liver cells are damaged • ALT is a more specific (but less sensitive) indication of liver inflammation • In acute liver injury, ALT and AST may be elevated to the high 100s, even 1000s, of U/L • In chronic liver damage, such as hepatitis or cirrhosis, there may be mild-to-moderate elevation (100–300 U/L) • ALT and AST are commonly used to measure the course of chronic hepatitis and the response to treatments
Alkaline phosphatase (ALP) and gamma-glutamyl-transpeptidase (GGT)	ALP: 25–100 U/L GGT: males <50 U/L; females <30 U/L	• These are enzymes that indicate obstruction to the biliary system • They are produced in the liver, or within the larger bile channels outside the liver • GGT is used as the supplementary test to be sure that a rise in ALP is indeed coming from the liver or biliary tree • A rise in GGT but normal ALP may indicate liver enzyme changes induced by alcohol or medications, causing no injury to the liver • ALP and GGT are commonly used to measure bile flow obstructions due to disorders such as gallstones, a tumour blocking the common bile duct, biliary tree damage, alcoholic liver disease or drug-induced hepatitis
Bilirubin	<20 micromol/L	Results from the breakdown of red blood cells. Thus bilirubin is protein-bound and circulates in the blood in an unconjugated form. The liver processes bilirubin to a water-soluble conjugated form that is excreted in the urine and faeces. • Liver injury or cholestasis results in an elevated bilirubin level • Raised unconjugated bilirubin without an accompanying rise in conjugated bilirubin is consistent with red blood cell destruction (haemolysis) • Raised bilirubin levels result in jaundice • In cases of chronic liver disease, bilirubin levels usually remain normal until significant damage occurs and cirrhosis develops • In cases of acute liver failure (ALF), bilirubin levels will rise rapidly and result in marked jaundice; the degree of rise is indicative of the severity of illness
Albumin	32–45 g/L	• Albumin is a major protein formed by the liver; it provides a gauge of liver synthetic function (i.e. albumin levels are lowered in liver disease)

Source: Pagana KD, Pagana TJ. Mosby's Manual of Diagnostic and Laboratory Tests. 3rd ed. St Louis, Missouri: Mosby Elsevier; 2006.

- ensuring that gastric/oesophageal ports are on free drainage, with regular monitoring of type and amount of drainage
- ensuring that correct traction is maintained, with regular checking of tube migration and checking position at nares/lips at regular intervals (4/24 hours).[150]

Tamponade is generally maintained for 24 hours, then traction is removed and the balloon deflated to assess for further bleeding. If the patient is stabilised, endoscopy can be performed. If bleeding persists, the balloon(s) is/are reinflated and traction reapplied.[149]

Once the patient has been stabilised, a transjugular intrahepatic portosystemic stent/shunt, also known as TIPS, may be considered to control variceal haemorrhage. TIPS is a metal expandable stent inserted to decompress the portal venous system, diverting blood flow through an alternative path.[151]

Extracorporeal liver support

The aim of extracorporeal liver support therapy is to allow time for liver recovery or to provide support until a liver transplant is possible.[152] There are two main types of extracorporeal liver support therapy, namely artificial and bioartificial devices. The artificial devices are cell-free systems that use a combination of dialysis, mainly using albumin, and plasma exchange.[153] These systems aim to reduce toxins and have been shown to reduce bilirubin and improve HE.[154] In contrast, bioartificial extracorporeal liver support devices are biological systems utilising either porcine hepatocytes or a human

TABLE 20.11
Treatment of liver failure complications

CONDITION	TREATMENT
Hepatic encephalopathy	• Treatment revolves around general supportive therapy until liver function recovers or liver transplant is undertaken[133,145] • Cerebral oedema and raised intracranial pressure are treated as for an acute head injury (see Chapter 17) • Reduce production and absorption of ammonia by preventing/controlling upper gastrointestinal bleeding. Gastrointestinal administration of non-absorbable disaccharides such as lactulose or lactitol to remove protein derived from dietary intake or bleeding can be useful in chronic liver disease but harmful in acute aetiologies. Continuous renal replacement therapy can also be useful in the removal of circulating ammonia[103,127]
Hepatorenal syndrome (HRS)	• Liver transplant is the primary treatment for type 1 HRS in patients with cirrhosis • If transplant is contraindicated or delayed, vasoconstrictors (e.g. terlipressin) may be effective in constricting the dilated splanchnic arterial bed, thus improving renal perfusion pressure and renal function. Vasoconstrictors may be given in association with intravenous albumin in order to increase intravascular volume[146,147]
Variceal bleeding	A successful outcome, as in all cases of gastrointestinal haemorrhage, hinges on prompt resuscitation, haemodynamic support and correction of haemostatic dysfunction, preferably in the intensive care setting • The patient is intubated for airway protection • Adequate intravenous access in inserted, preferably large, wide-bore cannulas for rapid fluid resuscitation • Haemodynamic instability is corrected with volume expanders initially and then blood products • The source of bleeding is identified by endoscope, and varices are banded/ligated (latex bands placed around the varices to 'strangle' the vessel), or sclerotherapy or diathermy (heat used to cauterise bleeding vessel) is used • Terlipressin and octreotide infusions may be used to reduce portal circulation pressure • If bleeding is uncontrollable, a balloon tamponade device can be inserted
Ascites	Salt and water restrictions along with diuretic therapy are methods that have been used to control ascites in the preliminary phases of end-stage liver failure; however, in the intensive care setting these measures are impractical and usually unsuccessful • Paracentesis is very effective at reducing ascites and is a simple procedure to remove fluid and an aid in diagnosis • Correction of coagulopathy or thrombocytopenia should be considered when the international normalised ratio is greater than 2.5 or the platelet count is markedly reduced • Paracentesis may aid in determining the cause of ascites (ascites-serum albumin gradient, ascitic cytology, microscopy and culture for acid-fast bacilli, chylous ascites) and in establishing or excluding primary or secondary peritonitis in patients with ascites (ascitic white cell and neutrophil count, culture) • Litres of ascites are normally removed, and the volume is replaced with IV concentrated albumin to prevent fluid shifts and hypotension • Mean arterial pressures, central venous pressures, heart rate and urine output are carefully monitored during the procedure

hepatoblastoma cell line to sustain temporary hepatic function; however, the construction and use of these devices is complex and has been limited to specialist centres. There are continuing challenges with extracting viable hepatic cells and incorporation into the bioreactors with which the extracorporeal circuits interface, thereby limiting their use.[155]

Despite much research, the clinical use of extracorporeal liver support therapies has been difficult due to a lack of clinical guidelines about when to institute and which types of patients should be selected, and technical considerations, such as flow rate and duration of therapy, have yet to be elucidated.[152] In many cases, the definitive treatment for severe ALF is liver transplantation when irreversible liver injury has occurred;[143] however, extracorporeal liver support systems may provide sufficient liver support until transplantation is available.[152] To date, evidence suggests that artificial and bioartificial devices may be used for detoxification and biochemical improvements, but this is not accompanied by survival benefits. High volume plasmapheresis is the only treatment to demonstrate a statistically significant improvement in transplant-free survival.[152,154]

Liver transplantation

Liver transplantation is the definitive treatment for patients suffering acute and chronic end-stage liver

FIGURE 20.7 The model for end-stage liver disease (MELD/PELD) calculation.[164]

MELD

(3.78 x $\log_e$ [serum bilirubin*]) + 11.20[$\log_e$ INR] + 9.57[$\log_e$ serum creatinine*] + 6.43 (constant for liver disease aetiology)

PELD

(0.436 x age†) − (0.687 x log [albumin#]) + (0.480 x log [bilirubin*]) + (1.857 x log [INR]) + (0.667 x growth failure‡)

* measured in mg/dL
\# measured in g/dL
† Age < 1 year = 1; all others = 0
‡ Values > 2 standard deviations from the norm = 1; all others = 0

Reproduced from Protty MB, Haboubi HN, Yeoman AD. Changes in the Model of End-Stage Liver Disease (MELD) scores on day 7 predict mortality in acute on chronic liver disease: the delta-MELD project. J Hepatol 2017;55(1): S387.

failure when other supportive critical care therapies have been exhausted.[143,156] Over the past 20 years, survival after liver transplantation has improved, which has been related to better pre-transplant and postoperative therapies and increases in intraoperative surgical refinement and management. This has also reduced time in critical care and reduced overall hospital length of stay. Survival rates of all patients who have undergone liver transplantation exceed 90% at 1 year[157] with children having superior survival rates to adults.[158] ALF patients accounted for 7% in the USA and 8% in Europe of all liver transplantations with lower survival rates (68% at 5 years) in comparison to all liver transplants.[159]

Indications for transplantation

Indications for liver transplantation are patients with severe liver disease in whom alternative treatments have been exhausted. Categories consist of ALF, end-stage liver disease, metabolic liver disease and primary liver cancer.[160] Timing and patient selection is of critical importance, as this has contributed to the success of transplantation. Re-transplantation for any disorder is considered only in patients with acceptable predicted survival.[161]

Contraindications for transplantation

Patients with extrahepatic malignancy and uncontrolled systemic infection where high-dose immunosuppressive therapy is contraindicated are not suitable for transplantation. In addition, patients with alcoholic liver disease with social instability and patients with inadequate or absent social support are relative contraindications due to increased risk of non-adherence to immunosuppressive therapy.[162]

Recipient selection

Recipient selection for liver transplantation is of critical importance as it affects mortality, especially when determining patients with ALF. There are a variety of prognostic indicators and selection scoring systems, including the Kings College, Clichy, Child–Turcotte–Pugh and MELD classification systems.[143] While there are different systems, most incorporate the severity of HE and coagulation status. In Australia and New Zealand, the MELD and paediatric end-stage liver disease (PELD) scoring systems are used for liver transplantation eligibility.[162] The MELD score is a mathematical model that includes bilirubin, creatinine and the international normalised ratio, which was originally devised to predict survival after TIPS.[163] The MELD/PELD score is an excellent predictor of mortality, especially in ALF (Fig. 20.7).[164]

Once the need for transplantation is established, the decision to allocate a donor liver to a patient is based on donor and recipient blood group; donor size and size of recipient; suitability of donor liver for splitting; severity of disease; matching of functional status of donor with severity of liver disease; and hepatitis B and C status of donor and recipient. Extensive testing and consultation are part of the liver transplant process. Clinical consultation occurs with hepatologists, clinical nurse consultants, social workers, dietitians, psychiatrists, psychologists and drug and alcohol professionals, if required.

Surgical techniques

Orthotopic liver transplantation

Orthotopic liver transplantation is the replacement of the diseased liver. It was pioneered in the 1960s and has been improved considerably due to technical aspects of the surgery itself and enhanced haemodynamic stability during the procedure.[165]

Two main techniques are used for orthotopic liver transplantation: portal bypass or the piggyback technique. Portal bypass occurs where an internal temporary portocaval shunt or external veno-venous bypass is used.[166] In the piggyback technique, the recipient's inferior vena cava is left and the donor inferior vena cava is piggybacked onto the recipient's inferior vena cava. The advantages of this technique include haemodynamic stability during the anhepatic phase, reduced operating times and reduced use of blood products, enabling a shorter length of hospital stay.[166]

Split-liver transplantation

The disparity between the increasing number of people on transplant waiting lists and the shortage of donor livers available has led to several innovative strategies. Split-liver transplantation occurs when the donated organ is divided for two recipients, with the larger right segment to an adult and the smaller left lobe to a child.[167] The complication rate is higher in split-liver than whole-liver transplants due to biliary leaks and anastomosis strictures. This technique has significantly reduced the number of children waiting for liver transplantation, although little impact has been made on adult waiting lists.[167]

Auxiliary liver transplantation

This technique consists of implanting a segment of donor liver temporarily, to allow the recipient's native liver to recover. Once recovery has occurred, the donor liver may be removed, or immunosuppression ceased leading the implanted graft to atrophy. This approach is most useful in conditions known to cause reversible ALF (acute viral hepatitis, mushroom toxicity, or drug induced).[168] This therefore potentially removes the long-term requirement for immunosuppression, and thus the associated complications.

Adult living donor liver transplantation

Living donor liver transplantation is an established option for paediatric patients with end-stage liver disease.[169] This technique involves removal of the left lobe from the live donor, usually the recipient's parent, which is then transplanted into the child. It is a relatively straightforward procedure, with little risk to the donor.[169]

Postoperative management

Initial management and nursing care

The initial postoperative care of liver transplant patients on return to critical care involves stabilisation, management of positive pressure ventilation, continuous haemodynamic monitoring and physical assessment, as with all critically ill surgical patients. Oliguria is commonly related to intraoperative fluid losses and fluid shifts.

Once initial stabilisation is achieved, treatment is governed by clinical progress. Typically, the critical care stay for a routine postoperative liver transplantation does not exceed 24–48 hours; as long as physiological systems are maintained, discharge to the ward can be anticipated. An abdominal computerised tomography scan may be considered at 7–10 days postoperatively or when clinically indicated.

The initial postoperative care is similar for all liver transplant patients. However, progress, stability and discharge from critical care can be affected by the patient's preoperative condition and severity of liver failure. The unique pathophysiology inherent in the liver failure patient will predispose to varying effects on coagulopathy, cardiopulmonary, neurological, haemodynamic and metabolic functions.[170]

Blood loss and coagulopathy

The major risk during and post-surgery is massive blood loss, due to a combination of factors. The surgical process itself involves anastomosis of major arteries and veins, predisposing the patient to bleeding and hypovolaemia during surgery and anastomotic leaks post-surgery.[171] Patients are likely to be coagulopathic from hepatic synthetic dysfunction, leading to failure of synthetic clotting factors.[172] Correction of coagulopathy with blood products such as fresh frozen plasma, platelets, cryoprecipitate and factor VIIa may control minor postoperative bleeding, but if bleeding continues an exploratory laparotomy may be required. Conversely, it is not desirable to overcorrect coagulopathy, due to the potential for vascular complications such as hepatic artery thrombosis. Careful monitoring is required to identify and manage hypotension, tachycardia, excessive blood loss from drains, falling haemoglobin, abdominal swelling and oozing from insertion sites. Thrombocytopenia is a common postoperative problem, with platelet counts often falling in the first week post-transplant. If platelet counts are low, a platelet transfusion may be necessary, especially prior to removal of drains, lines, cannulae and sheaths.

Cardiovascular

Haemodynamic instability in the early postoperative period may be due to hypovolaemia or haemorrhage. Treatment includes fluid boluses to increase preload and the initiation of inotropes may be necessary with a low threshold for the introduction of advanced cardiac output monitoring. The patient may present with a hyperdynamic profile including a high cardiac output, low systemic vascular resistance and low mean arterial pressure,[173] although this usually reverses 1 week after transplantation.

Neurological

The most frequent neurological complications relate to patients with preexisting HE. In ALF patients, cerebral oedema with raised intracranial pressure is common and, after liver transplantation, cerebral oedema may take up to 48 hours to subside. Therefore, continuation of preoperative measures to reduce intracranial pressure is necessary. These include elevating the head of the bed 30°; ensuring head, neck and body alignment; maintaining endotracheal tapes so they are not constrictive to allow venous return and prevent cerebral congestion; reducing neurological stimuli; and timing activities to prevent spikes in intracranial pressure (see Chapter 17).[174]

Respiratory

Preexisting pulmonary complications associated with liver disease can affect postoperative recovery and need to be considered when weaning ventilation and maintaining adequate oxygenation. Patients post-transplant often experience bi-basal collapse and consolidation, and are prone to infection, similar to other critical care patients who undergo complex surgical procedures that are extended.[175] Incentive spirometry, chest physiotherapy, early mobilisation and adequate pain relief are recommended, with early extubation the most effective in reducing pulmonary complications.[175]

Gastrointestinal

Patients with end-stage liver disease often have malnutrition and bone disease, which may influence postoperative management. Fluid overload and ascites can quite often mask signs of malnutrition. Early nutrition is imperative in the postoperative period, and enteral feeding can supplement caloric needs (see Chapter 19). If caloric intake is inadequate, consultation with a dietitian will assist with enteral supplementation. Total parenteral nutrition is rarely required.

Renal

Renal dysfunction is a significant post-transplantation problem. Risk factors include preexisting renal disease or HRS, intraoperative hypotension, extensive transfusion of blood products, nephrotoxic drugs such as cyclosporin and tacrolimus, sepsis and graft dysfunction.[170] HRS is reversible post-transplantation. Patients who are receiving renal support such as continuous renal replacement therapy usually require continuation of renal support postoperatively for a period of time until recovery of kidney function is evident (see Chapter 18).

Graft dysfunction and rejection

Re-transplantation is required in 7–10% of liver transplants; the most common causes of early graft dysfunction are primary graft non-function and vascular complications.[161] Acute graft rejection was the most challenging obstacle in the early years of transplantation but, with the development of current immunosuppressive therapy, acute rejection can be avoided, resulting in improved success rates of transplantation.[176] Immunosuppressive therapy has improved with the use of newer drugs and patients are most commonly placed on a combination of tacrolimus or cyclosporine and steroids.[177,178]

Allograft dysfunction occurs within 48 hours of transplantation, and is characterised by varying degrees of coma, renal failure, worsening coagulopathy, poor bile production and marked elevation in the liver enzymes and worsening acidosis. The cause of allograft dysfunction is not always known; possible causes are injury to the liver, either before or during the donor operation procedure, ischaemic-reperfusion injury or graft stenosis. Acute rejection is generally evident in the second week post-transplant, and is generally suspected with an elevation in liver enzymes, a decline in bile quality (only if a T tube is present), occasional fever and tachycardia.

Primary graft non-function is defined as failure of the graft to function in the first postoperative week but this can occur much more quickly. It is manifested by failure to regain consciousness, sustained elevated transaminases, increasing coagulopathy, acidosis and poor bile production. Causes include massive haemorrhagic necrosis, ischaemia-reperfusion injury and hepatic artery thrombosis.

Management of late complications

Readmission to critical care after liver transplantation is not uncommon. Factors include cardiopulmonary dysfunction from infection or fluid overload, respiratory failure from collapse and consolidation, tachypnoea, recipient age, preoperative liver function, bilirubin, the amount of blood products administered intraoperatively, graft dysfunction, severe sepsis and postoperative surgical complications such as bleeding and biliary anastomotic leaks.[179] Outcomes are affected by intraoperative and postoperative complications, renal failure, advanced liver disease and malnutrition.[180]

Summary

The gastrointestinal system can become significantly compromised during critical illness. Alterations in the gastrointestinal system can also cause critical illness. The gastrointestinal system involves not just the gastrointestinal tract but also organs that support digestion including the pancreas and liver. Disruptions to the gastrointestinal system and normal gastrointestinal physiology can be altered during critical illness because of redistribution of blood flow away from the gut and other abdominal organs. Specifically, the gastrointestinal system can become hypoperfused and normal physiological processes responsible for digestion, absorption, immunity and protection become compromised.

Critically ill patients can be at risk of developing stress-related mucosal disease although incidence of clinically important bleeding remains relatively low. Nevertheless, it remains common practice to provide stress-ulcer prophylaxis to critically ill patients, particularly for those patients considered at high risk. During critical illness, patients may also be at risk for the development of IAH, with approximately half of all ICU patients having increased IAP. Recognising potential risk factors for the development of IAH is essential so that monitoring can be commenced and treatment initiated where necessary.

Critical illness can also result from the inability of the body to effectively use glucose in energy production. An increasing number of people worldwide have diabetes and when illness occurs this can precipitate significant alterations in blood glucose and result in the development of DKA or HHS. Because of the ensuing physiological derangements these patients often need to be admitted to a critical care area for close monitoring and treatment until they are stabilised.

Liver dysfunction causing hepatocellular injury and death can occur due to direct injury or cellular stress. This can be mediated via several avenues, such as metabolic disturbances, ischaemia, inflammatory processes or reactive oxygen metabolites from drug and alcohol ingestion. Acute failure can be acute or preceded by a chronic dysfunction. In Australia and New Zealand, high rates of hepatitis B and C predispose individuals to chronic liver dysfunction that can lead to acute hepatic decompensation. While ALF is uncommon, patients who present are often critically ill. In addition, liver failure causes major disturbances in other body systems often resulting in coagulopathy, cerebral oedema HE, sepsis, renal failure and metabolic derangement. Therapy is usually directed at multi-organ support as extracorporeal liver support therapies have not sufficiently developed to sustain liver function during the acute phase.

Liver transplantation remains the definitive treatment option for acute and chronic liver failure patients when supportive multi-organ therapy is not sustainable. Preexisting hepatic dysfunction and liver transplantation surgery can lead to a high risk of haemorrhage and coagulopathy postoperatively. Careful haematological management is required to control postoperative bleeding. Clinicians must ensure that patients receive appropriate haemodynamic management for hyperdynamic states and that measures to avoid rises in intracranial pressure are implemented.

Case study

A 54-year-old man was admitted to the ICU after presenting to the emergency department with a history of nausea, vomiting and abdominal pain. His admission weight was 132 kg and height 183 cm (BMI 39.4). His past medical history included hypertension, obesity, previous smoker, and minimal alcohol intake. On examination he had abdominal tenderness in the right upper quadrant and epigastrium.

On admission the initial blood tests showed:

White blood cells	15.9 (4–11 11.9 × 10^9/L)
Creatinine	55 (60–110 umol/L)
Blood glucose	13.2 mmol/L
Lipase	1987 (0–160 units/L)
Amylase	796 (30–220 units/L)
ALP	92 (30–110 U/L)
LD	560 IU/L (120–250 U/L)
ALT	809 (0–45 units/L)
AST	253 (0–35 units/L)
Ca	2.12 (2.10–2.60 mmol/L)
Bilirubin	70 (0–20 μmol/L)

He was diagnosed with gallstone pancreatitis and during his 7-week ICU stay he developed necrotising gallstone pancreatitis and intraabdominal collections. Sepsis and systemic inflammatory response syndrome were evident throughout admission and the patient was treated with multiple antibiotics to treat infection associated with the necrosis. Respiratory failure was a feature during this admission with invasive mechanical ventilation required several times during admission. Although extubation was possible on several occasions, the patient required endoscopy and cyst necrosectomy for removal of necrotic tissue. He developed acute kidney injury requiring dialysis and developed an intestinal ileus. Nutrition support was provided through a nasojejunal tube and the patient required administration of parenteral and enteral nutrition because of ongoing intolerance, despite use of prokinetic agents.

DISCUSSION

Severe acute pancreatitis is the most serious form of pancreatitis and is associated with a high morbidity and mortality. Initially the patient will exhibit a proinflammatory response which results in systemic inflammatory response syndrome.[181] After the first few weeks an anti-inflammatory response occurs which can lead to the development of multiple organ failure, as was the case for this patient who exhibited respiratory, renal and gut failure. As the necrosis was associated with infection this necessitated surgical removal of the tissue.

The nursing challenges associated with this patient included managing nutrition support. Obesity together with gastrointestinal inflammation and ileus made administration of enteral nutrition challenging, consequently supplemental parenteral nutrition was added.[91] Administration of enteral nutrition was also problematic because of feeds needing to be repeatedly stopped for endoscopy which was necessary for the removal of necrotic tissue.

Ongoing respiratory failure meant that mechanical ventilation was required. Ventilation can be challenging in obese patients because the increased IAPs often result in higher than normal mean airway pressures and it is difficult to deliver adequate tidal volumes. The patient's airway can also be difficult to access which may create additional challenges when repeated intubations are required for procedures. Weaning from ventilation can be more difficult if the patient has decreased respiratory drive and increased work of breathing.[182]

Ongoing patient management may require the use of specialised equipment to reposition the patient.

CASE STUDY QUESTIONS

1 When a patient is receiving enteral and parenteral nutrition simultaneously, how would you manage the transition enteral nutrition alone?
2 What consequences might prolonged critical illness and obesity have for longer term functional recovery?
3 Describe strategies to be used to prevent pressure injuries in an obese, critically ill patient.

RESEARCH VIGNETTE

Marr KJ, Abdel-Aziz S, Lam L, et al. Nutritional status and performance of multiple bedside tools for nutrition assessment among patients waiting for liver transplantation: a Canadian experience. Clin Nutr 2017; 17:68-74

Abstract

Background: Malnutrition is an important predictor of morbidity and mortality among cirrhotic patients. Our objectives were to assess protein-calorie malnutrition (PCM) in cirrhotic pre-liver transplant patients and to study the correlation between subjective global assessment (SGA) and other objective measures of malnutrition.

Methods: We recruited pre-liver transplant adult patients at our center between October 2012 and Oct 2015. Nutrition status was assessed via SGA. PCM was assessed by comparing recommended to actual protein and calorie intake. SGA was correlated with body mass index (BMI), dry BMI, handgrip strength by calibrated dynameter (HGS), and mid-arm circumference (MAC). We used non-parametric statistical methods in our analysis.

Results: Seventy patients were included in this study. Majority were males (n = 46, 66%) with a median age of 58 years (IQR: 50–61). Moderate to severe malnutrition was prevalent in our cohort (SGA-A: n = 15 (21.4%), SGA-B: n = 30 (42.9%) and SGA-C: n = 25 (35.7%)). There was a significant difference in the recommended calories consumed between SGA groups (A 98.5% vs. C 79.2%, $P = 0.03$). A similar trend was observed for the recommended protein consumed (A 85.4%, C 62.5%; $P = 0.09$). SGA correlated with BMI (A = 26.4, C = 22.4; $P<0.01$), dry BMI (A = 25.9, C = 20.4; $P<0.01$), HGS (A = 67.0, C = 47.0 PSI; $P = 0.03$), and MAC (A = 29.5 cm, C = 22.0 cm; $P<0.01$). HGS and MAC were strongly correlated (Spearman correlation 0.49, $P<0.01$).

Conclusions: Cirrhotic patients have significant protein-calorie malnutrition. Multiple malnutrition tools including BMI, dry BMI, HGS and MAC were precisely able to assess malnutrition.

Critique

Liver transplantation is a potential treatment option for patients with end-stage liver disease. Malnutrition is common in in cirrhosis, with anorexia, malabsorption and hypermetabolism being contributing factors. Changes in the way in which nutrients are used may also contribute to the development of malnutrition. Malnourished cirrhotic patients are more likely to die and experience post-transplant complications such as infection as well as increased length of ICU and hospital stay. Optimising nutrition in pre-transplant patients may be promising but identifying who is most likely to benefit from or require active nutrition therapy is complicated by challenges in assessing malnutrition. A gold standard for the assessment of malnutrition in this patient population is lacking although the Subjective Global Assessment (SGA) is most commonly used. Other methods of assessing nutrition status include BMI, dry BMI, mid-arm circumference (MAC), mid-arm muscle circumference (MAMC), triceps skin thickness and handgrip strength (HGS).

In this prospective observational study 70 adult patients on a liver transplant waiting list were enrolled and moderate to severe malnutrition was evident with over three-quarters of patients having a SGA B or SGA C. While it would be reasonable to assume that the degree of liver failure aligned with malnutrition, this was not evident and no association between the MELD score and SGA were observed. Nutritional adequacy was assessed by calculating the percent of protein and calorie requirements consumed with requirements determined based on current ESPEN nutrition guidelines in liver disease (35–40 kcal/kg/day and 1.2–1.5 g protein/day).[183] Nutritional adequacy was best in the SGA A group (98.5% consumed recommended calories; 85.4% consumed recommended protein). Patients with more severe malnutrition (SGA C) had the lowest protein/energy intake consuming 79.2% of recommended calories and 62.5% of recommended protein. Nutrition intake data was collected using a 3-day food diary completed by the patients so it is possible that intake was either over- or underestimated. Social desirability may also have been a factor if patients wanted to provide the physician nutrition specialists or dietitians in the High Risk Malnutrition Clinic with a positive impression of their nutrition status, particularly if they were concerned whether this might have influenced their eligibility for transplantation. It is also possible that these patients who were on a pre-transplant waiting list were keen to optimise their postoperative recovery and were aware of the risks associated with malnutrition; this may have led to increased nutritional intake during the study period. Although there were discrepancies between recommended and actual protein/energy intake, intake of 75% of requirements has been previously identified as adequate in a broad cohort of hospitalised patients.[184]

Nutrition assessment was undertaken with data collected to calculate the SGA, BMI, dry BMI, MAC, and HGS. Not surprisingly, BMI and dry BMI decreased with nutrition status as determined by the SGA; dry BMI had a higher diagnostic accuracy, likely because it adjusted for increased weight associated with ascites or oedema. For all nutrition assessment strategies, the diagnostic accuracy was best for males. MAC in males had a high diagnostic accuracy (Area under Receiver Operator Curve 0.87) but this was not observed in females. The positive predictive value for malnutrition using the MAC in men was 97%. It is not clear why MAC as a potential strategy for screening was not as accurate in women and it was hypothesised that muscle wasting may occur at a different timepoint in the disease. As with other nutrition studies, HGS declines in patients who are more malnourished. As with MAC, HGS had higher diagnostic accuracy in men (AUROC 0.80) compared to women (AUROC 0.56). As a pilot study, only 70 patients were enrolled and therefore type II error may have been present, meaning that detection of a statistically significant difference may not have been observed in females.[185] The study was also not designed to detect gender differences so further work would need to be undertaken to explore this aspect of nutrition assessment.

Learning activities

1. On your next clinical shift, identify what stress-ulcer prophylaxis your patient is receiving (if any) and whether they have risk factors for the development of stress-related mucosal disease.
2. When you are next in the clinical area, consider the clinical presentations of the patients in the ICU and identify which patients might most benefit from IAP monitoring.
3. Compare and contrast the physiological changes that occur in DKA and HHS. How do these differences influence the management strategy for restoring normoglycaemia?
4. A patient with acute pancreatitis is admitted to ICU. On dietitian review the recommendation is to commence enteral feeding via the nasogastric tube. Your experience has been that these patients require small bowel

feeding or parenteral nutrition. What is the current evidence base for nutrition support for patients with pancreatitis?

5 What treatment strategies should you anticipate for a patient with alcoholic hepatitis?

6 What would make liver transplantation in patients with alcoholic hepatitis most successful?

Online resources

American Diabetes Association, http://www.diabetes.org/

Australian Diabetes Council, http://www.nfpfoundation.org.au/organisation/australian-diabetes-council

European Association for the Study of the Liver, www.easl.eu

European Society for Organ Transplantation, https://www.esot.org/

International Diabetes Federation, https://www.idf.org/our-network/regions-members/europe/welcome.html

National Diabetes Education Program, http://ndep.nih.gov

Online MELD Calculator, https://optn.transplant.hrsa.gov/resources/allocation-calculators/meld-calculator/

The Australia and New Zealand Liver Transplant Registry, www.anzltr.org

The Transplantation Society of Australia and New Zealand, www.tsanz.com.au

World Society of the Abdominal Compartment Syndrome, www.wsacs.org

Further reading

Holt RIG, Cockram C, Flyvbjerg A, et al. Textbook of diabetes. 5th ed. Hoboken: Wiley Blackwell; 2017.

Lee WE, Williams R. Acute liver failure. Cambridge: Cambridge University Press; 2011.

McDonald D, Ackerman G, Khailova L, et al. Extreme dysbiosis of the microbiome in critical illness. mSphere 2016;1(4):e00199–16.

References

1. Taylor RW. Gut motility issues in critical illness. Crit Care Clin 2016;32(2):191–201.
2. Whitman Z, O'Neil DHR. Gastric disorders: modifications of gastric content, antacids and drugs influencing gastric secretions and motility. Anaesthesia Intensive Care Medicine 2017;19(1):25–9.
3. Deane AM, Rayner CK, Keeshan A, et al. The effects of critical illness on intestinal glucose sensing, transporters, and absorption. Crit Care Med 2014;42(1):57–65.
4. Begley M, Gahan CG, Hill C. The interaction between bacteria and bile. FEMS Microbiol Rev 2005;29(4):625–51.
5. Puleo F, Arvanitakis M, Van Gossum A, et al. Gut failure in the ICU. Semin Respir Crit Care Med 2011;32(5):626–38.
6. McClave SA, Lowen CC, Martindale RG. The 2016 ESPEN Arvid Wretlind lecture: the gut in stress. Clin Nutr 2018;37(1):19–36.
7. Zigmond E, Varol C. With respect to macrophages, judge the liver by its cover. Immunity 2017;47(2):219–21.
8. Meng M, Klingensmith NJ, Coopersmith CM. New insights into the gut as the driver of critical illness and organ failure. Curr Opin Crit Care 2017;23(2):143–8.
9. Nguyen NQ, Besanko LK, Burgstad C, et al. Delayed enteral feeding impairs intestinal carbohydrate absorption in critically ill patients. Crit Care Med 2012;40(1):50–4.
10. Klingensmith NJ, Coopersmith CM. The gut as the motor of multiple organ dysfunction in critical illness. Crit Care Clin 2016;32(2):203–12.
11. Mittal R, Coopersmith CM. Redefining the gut as the motor of critical illness. Trends Mol Med 2014;20(4):214–23.
12. Schmid-Schonbein GW, Chang M. The autodigestion hypothesis for shock and multi-organ failure. Ann Biomed Eng 2014;42(2):405–14.
13. Krezalek MA, DeFazio J, Zaborina O, et al. The shift of an intestinal 'microbiome' to a 'pathobiome' governs the course and outcome of sepsis following surgical injury. Shock 2016;45(5):475–82.
14. David LA, Maurice CF, Carmody RN, et al. Diet rapidly and reproducibly alters the human gut microbiome. Nature 2014;505(7484):559–63.
15. Fox JG, Boutin SR, Handt LK, et al. Isolation and characterization of a novel helicobacter species, 'Helicobacter macacae', from rhesus monkeys with and without chronic idiopathic colitis. J Clin Microbiol 2007;45(12):4061–3.

16. Bjornsson ES, Urbanavicius V, Eliasson B, et al. Effects of hyperglycemia on interdigestive gastrointestinal motility in humans. Scand J Gastroenterol 1994;29(12):1096–104.
17. Deitch EA. Gut-origin sepsis: evolution of a concept. Surgeon 2012;10(6):350–6.
18. Dive A, Foret F, Jamart J, et al. Effect of dopamine on gastrointestinal motility during critical illness. Intensive Care Med 2000;26(7):901–7.
19. Katayama M, Xu D, Specian RD, et al. Role of bacterial adherence and the mucus barrier on bacterial translocation: effects of protein malnutrition and endotoxin in rats. Ann Surg 1997;225(3):317–26.
20. Teltschik Z, Wiest R, Beisner J, et al. Intestinal bacterial translocation in rats with cirrhosis is related to compromised Paneth cell antimicrobial host defense. Hepatology 2012;55(4):1154–63.
21. Winter SE, Winter MG, Xavier MN, et al. Host-derived nitrate boosts growth of *E. coli* in the inflamed gut. Science 2013;339(6120):708–11.
22. Honda K, Littman DR. The microbiome in infectious disease and inflammation. Annu Rev Immunol 2012;30:759–95.
23. Zaborina O, Lepine F, Xiao G, et al. Dynorphin activates quorum sensing quinolone signaling in Pseudomonas aeruginosa. PLoS Pathog 2007;3(3):e35.
24. Zaborin A, Smith D, Garfield K, et al. Membership and behavior of ultra-low-diversity pathogen communities present in the gut of humans during prolonged critical illness. MBio 2014;5(5):e01361–14.
25. Alverdy J, Holbrook C, Rocha F, et al. Gut-derived sepsis occurs when the right pathogen with the right virulence genes meets the right host: evidence for in vivo virulence expression in Pseudomonas aeruginosa. Ann Surg 2000;232(4):480–9.
26. Albenberg L, Esipova TV, Judge CP, et al. Correlation between intraluminal oxygen gradient and radial partitioning of intestinal microbiota. Gastroenterology 2014;147(5):1055–63, e8.
27. Meyer-Hoffert U, Hornef MW, Henriques-Normark B, et al. Secreted enteric antimicrobial activity localises to the mucus surface layer. Gut 2008;57(6):764–71.
28. Salzman NH, Hung K, Haribhai D, et al. Enteric defensins are essential regulators of intestinal microbial ecology. Nat Immunol 2010;11(1):76–83.
29. Plummer MP, Blaser AR, Deane AM. Stress ulceration: prevalence, pathology and association with adverse outcomes. Crit Care 2014;18:213.
30. Barbateskovic M, Marker S, Jakobsen JC, et al. Stress ulcer prophylaxis in adult intensive care unit patients - a protocol for a systematic review. Acta Anaesthesiol Scand 2018.
31. Ovenden C, Plummer MP, Selvanderan S, et al. Occult upper gastrointestinal mucosal abnormalities in critically ill patients. Acta Anaesthesiol Scand 2017;61(2):216–23.
32. Krag M, Perner A, Wetterslev J, et al. Prevalence and outcome of gastrointestinal bleeding and use of acid suppressants in acutely ill adult intensive care patients. Intensive Care Med 2015;41(5):833–45.
33. Reintam Blaser A, Poeze M, Malbrain ML, et al. Gastrointestinal symptoms during the first week of intensive care are associated with poor outcome: a prospective multicentre study. Intensive Care Med 2013;39(5):899–909.
34. Bardou M, Quenot JP, Barkun A. Stress-related mucosal disease in the critically ill patient. Nat Rev Gastroenterol Hepatol 2015;12(2):98–107.
35. Buendgens L, Tacke F. Do we still need pharmacological stress ulcer prophylaxis at the ICU? J Thorac Dis 2017;9(11):4201–4.
36. Gyires K, Feher A. Stress, neuropeptides and gastric mucosa. Curr Pharm Des 2017;23(27):3928–40.
37. Qin X, Sheth SU, Sharpe SM, et al. The mucus layer is critical in protecting against ischemia-reperfusion-mediated gut injury and in the restitution of gut barrier function. Shock 2011;35(3):275–81.
38. Kubicki M, Warrillo SJ. Gastrointestinal problems in intensive care. Anaesthesia and Intensive Care Medicine 2018;19(3):93–7.
39. Allen A, Flemstrom G. Gastroduodenal mucus bicarbonate barrier: protection against acid and pepsin. Am J Physiol Cell Physiol 2005;288(1):C1–19.
40. Fennerty MB. Pathophysiology of the upper gastrointestinal tract in the critically ill patient: rationale for the therapeutic benefits of acid suppression. Crit Care Med 2002;30(6 Suppl.):S351–5.
41. Sertaridou E, Papaioannou V, Kolios G, et al. Gut failure in critical care: old school versus new school. Ann Gastroenterol 2015;28(3):309–22.
42. Santos RG, Quirino IE, Viana ML, et al. Effects of nitric oxide synthase inhibition on glutamine action in a bacterial translocation model. Br J Nutr 2014;111(1):93–100.
43. Schefold JC, Perner A, Lange T, et al. Effects of stress ulcer prophylaxis in adult ICU patients receiving renal replacement therapy (Sup-Icu RENal, SIREN): study protocol for a pre-planned observational study. Trials 2018;19(1):26.
44. Krag M, Perner A, Wetterslev J, et al. Stress ulcer prophylaxis versus placebo or no prophylaxis in critically ill patients. A systematic review of randomised clinical trials with meta-analysis and trial sequential analysis. Intensive Care Med 2014;40(1):11–22.
45. Alshamsi F, Belley-Cote E, Cook D, et al. Efficacy and safety of proton pump inhibitors for stress ulcer prophylaxis in critically ill patients: a systematic review and meta-analysis of randomized trials. Crit Care 2016;20(1):120.
46. MacLaren R, Reynolds PM, Allen RR. Histamine-2 receptor antagonists vs proton pump inhibitors on gastrointestinal tract hemorrhage and infectious complications in the intensive care unit. JAMA Intern Med 2014;174(4):564–74.
47. Charlot M, Ahlehoff O, Norgaard ML, et al. Proton-pump inhibitors are associated with increased cardiovascular risk independent of clopidogrel use: a nationwide cohort study. Ann Intern Med 2010;153(6):378–86.

48. Rhodes A, Evans LE, Alhazzani W, et al. Surviving Sepsis Campaign: international guidelines for management of sepsis and septic shock: 2016. Crit Care Med 2017;45(3):486–552.
49. Marker S, Krag M, Moller MH. What's new with stress ulcer prophylaxis in the ICU? Intensive Care Med 2017;43(8):1132–4.
50. Sesler JM. Stress-related mucosal disease in the intensive care unit: an update on prophylaxis. AACN Adv Crit Care 2007;18(2):119–26, quiz 27–8.
51. Alhazzani W, Alenezi F, Jaeschke RZ, et al. Proton pump inhibitors versus histamine 2 receptor antagonists for stress ulcer prophylaxis in critically ill patients: a systematic review and meta-analysis. Crit Care Med 2013;41(3):693–705.
52. Buendgens L, Bruensing J, Matthes M, et al. Administration of proton pump inhibitors in critically ill medical patients is associated with increased risk of developing Clostridium difficile-associated diarrhea. J Crit Care 2014.
53. Spirt MJ, Stanley S. Update on stress ulcer prophylaxis in critically ill patients. Crit Care Nurse 2006;26(1):18–20, 2–8; quiz 9.
54. Alquraini M, Alshamsi F, Moller MH, et al. Sucralfate versus histamine 2 receptor antagonists for stress ulcer prophylaxis in adult critically ill patients: a meta-analysis and trial sequential analysis of randomized trials. J Crit Care 2017;40:21–30.
55. Alhazzani W, Alshamsi F, Belley-Cote E, et al. Efficacy and safety of stress ulcer prophylaxis in critically ill patients: a network meta-analysis of randomized trials. Intensive Care Med 2018;44(1):1–11.
56. Kozar RA, Hu S, Hassoun HT, et al. Specific intraluminal nutrients alter mucosal blood flow during gut ischemia/reperfusion. JPEN J Parenter Enteral Nutr 2002;26(4):226–9.
57. Ephgrave KS, Kleiman-Wexler RL, Adair CG. Enteral nutrients prevent stress ulceration and increase intragastric volume. Crit Care Med 1990;18(6):621–4.
58. Marik PE, Vasu T, Hirani A, et al. Stress ulcer prophylaxis in the new millennium: a systematic review and meta-analysis. Crit Care Med 2010;38(11):2222–8.
59. El-Kersh K, Jalil B, McClave SA, et al. Enteral nutrition as stress ulcer prophylaxis in critically ill patients: a randomized controlled exploratory study. J Crit Care 2018;43:108–13.
60. Huang HB, Jiang W, Wang CY, et al. Stress ulcer prophylaxis in intensive care unit patients receiving enteral nutrition: a systematic review and meta-analysis. Crit Care 2018;22(1):20.
61. Rogers WK, Garcia L. Intraabdominal hypertension, abdominal compartment syndrome, and the open abdomen. Chest 2018;153(1):238–50.
62. Roberts DJ, Ball CG, Kirkpatrick AW. Increased pressure within the abdominal compartment: intra-abdominal hypertension and the abdominal compartment syndrome. Curr Opin Crit Care 2016;22(2):174–85.
63. Kirkpatrick AW, Nickerson D, Roberts DJ, et al. Intra-abdominal hypertension and abdominal compartment syndrome after abdominal wall reconstruction: quaternary syndromes? Scand J Surg 2017;106(2):97–106.
64. Maluso P, Olson J, Sarani B. Abdominal compartment hypertension and abdominal compartment syndrome. Crit Care Clin 2016;32(2):213–22.
65. Fagoni N, Piva S, Marino R, et al. The IN-PANCIA study: clinical evaluation of gastrointestinal dysfunction and failure, multiple organ failure, and levels of citrulline in critically ill patients. J Intensive Care Med 2017;885066617742594.
66. Christensen M, Craft J. The cardio-respiratory effects of intra-abdominal hypertension: considerations for critical care nursing practice. Intensive Crit Care Nurs 2018;44:53–8.
67. Malbrain MLNG, De Waele JJ, De Keulenaer BL. What every ICU clinician needs to know about the cardiovascular effects caused by abdominal hypertension. Anaesthesiol Intensive Ther 2015;47(4):388–99.
68. Malhotra A. Acute kidney injury. In: Rodriguez A, Barraco R, Ivatury R, editors. Geriatric trauma and acute care surgery. Cham: Springer; 2018.
69. Kirkpatrick AW, Roberts DJ, De Waele J, et al. Intra-abdominal hypertension and the abdominal compartment syndrome: updated consensus definitions and clinical practice guidelines from the World Society of the Abdominal Compartment Syndrome. Intensive Care Med 2013;39(7):1190–206.
70. Fusco MA, Martin RS, Chang MC. Estimation of intra-abdominal pressure by bladder pressure measurement: validity and methodology. J Trauma 2001;50(2):297–302.
71. Sugrue M, De Waele JJ, De Keulenaer BL, et al. A user's guide to intra-abdominal pressure measurement. Anaesthesiol Intensive Ther 2015;47(3):241–51.
72. Pouliart N, Huyghens L. An observational study on intraabdominal pressure in 125 critically ill patients. Crit Care 2002;6(Suppl. 1):S3.
73. Becker V, Schmid RM, Umgelter A. Comparison of a new device for the continuous intra-gastric measurement of intra-abdominal pressure (CiMon) with direct intra-peritoneal measurements in cirrhotic patients during paracentesis. Intensive Care Med 2009;35(5):948–52.
74. De Waele J, Pletinckx P, Blot S, et al. Saline volume in transvesical intra-abdominal pressure measurement: enough is enough. Intensive Care Med 2006;32:455–9.
75. Draznin B, Kahn PA, Wagner N, et al. Clinical diabetes centers of excellence: a model for future adult diabetes care. J Clin Endocrinol Metab 2018;103(3):809–12.
76. Organisation WH. Global report on diabetes. Geneva, Switzerland: World Health Organisation; 2016.
77. Federation ID. IDF diabetes atlas. Brussels, Belgium: International Diabetes Federation; 2017.
78. Moller N. Acute metabolic complications of diabetes: diabetic ketoacidosis and the hyperosmolar hyperglycemic state. In: Holt RIG, Cockram CS, Flyvbjerg A, et al, editors. Textbook of diabetes. 5th ed. Hoboken: John Wiley; 2016.

79. Anzola I, Gomez PC, Umpierrez GE. Management of diabetic ketoacidosis and hyperglycemic hyperosmolar state in adults. Expert Rev Endocrinol Metab 2016;11(2):177–85.
80. Dhatariya KK, Vellanki P. Treatment of diabetic ketoacidosis (DKA)/hyperglycemic hyperosmolar state (HHS): novel advances in the management of hyperglycemic crises (UK versus USA). Curr Diab Rep 2017;17(5):33.
81. Fayfman M, Pasquel FJ, Umpierrez GE. Management of hyperglycemic crises: diabetic ketoacidosis and hyperglycemic hyperosmolar state. Med Clin North Am 2017;101(3):587–606.
82. Kamata Y, Takano K, Kishihara E, et al. Distinct clinical characteristics and therapeutic modalities for diabetic ketoacidosis in type 1 and type 2 diabetes mellitus. J Diabetes Complications 2017;31(2):468–72.
83. Nyenwe EA, Kitabchi AE. The evolution of diabetic ketoacidosis: an update of its etiology, pathogenesis and management. Metabolism 2016;65(4):507–21.
84. Keays RT. Diabetic emergencies. In: Bersten AD, Soni N, editors. Oh's intensive care manual. 6th ed. Philadelphia: Elsevier; 2009. p. 613–20.
85. Thuzar M, Malabu UH, Tisdell B, et al. Use of a standardised diabetic ketoacidosis management protocol improved clinical outcomes. Diabetes Res Clin Pract 2014;104(1):e8–11.
86. Bhansali A, Sukumar SP. Hyperosmolar hyperglycemic state. World Clinics Diabetology: Complications of Diabetes 2016;2(1):1–10.
87. Nyenwe EA, Abbas EK. The evolution of diabetic ketoacidosis: An update of its etiology, pathogenesis and management. Metabolism 2016;65(4):507–21.
88. Banks PA, Bollen TL, Dervenis C, et al. Classification of acute pancreatitis – 2012: revision of the Atlanta classification and definitions by international consensus. Gut 2013;62(1):102–11.
89. Nesvaderani M, Eslick GD, Cox MR. Acute pancreatitis: update on management. Med J Aust 2015;202(8):420–3.
90. Moggia E, Koti R, Belgaumkar AP, et al. Pharmacological interventions for acute pancreatitis. Cochrane Database Syst Rev 2017;(4):CD011384.
91. Yao H, He C, Deng L, et al. Enteral versus parenteral nutrition in critically ill patients with severe pancreatitis: a meta-analysis. Eur J Clin Nutr 2018;72(1):66.
92. Basurto Ona X, Rigau Comas D, Urrútia G. Opioids for acute pancreatitis pain. Cochrane Database Syst Rev 2011;(7).
93. Huffmann AF. Bile acids and the enterohepatic circulation. In: Arias I, Shafnitz D, Boyer JL, et al, editors. The liver: biology and pathobiology. 5th ed. Chichester: Wiley-Blackwell; 2009.
94. Tacke F, Luedde T, Trautwein C. Inflammatory pathways in liver homeostasis and liver injury. Clin Rev Allergy Immunol 2009;36(1):4–12.
95. Guicciardi ME, Gores GJ. Apoptosis: a mechanism of acute and chronic liver injury. Gut 2005;54(7):1024–33.
96. Trey D, Davidson C. The management of fulminant hepatic failure. In: Popper H, Schaffner Fe, editors. Progress in liver disease. New York: Grune and Stratton; 1970. p. 292–8.
97. Asrani SK, O'Leary JG. Acute-on-chronic liver failure. Clin Liver Dis 2014;18(3):561–74.
98. Hodgman MJ, Garrard AR. A review of acetaminophen poisoning. Crit Care Clin 2012;28(4):499–516.
99. Santi L, Maggioli C, Mastroroberto M, et al. Acute liver failure caused by Amanita phalloides poisoning. Int J Hepatol 2012;2012:487480.
100. Lammers WJ, Kowdley KV, van Buuren HR. Predicting outcome in primary biliary cirrhosis. Ann Hepatol 2014;13(4):316–26.
101. Williamson KD, Chapman RW. Primary sclerosing cholangitis. Dig Dis 2014;32(4):438–45.
102. Rose CF. What's new in our understanding of the pathogenesis of hepatic encephalopathy? Clin Liver Dis 2017;10(2):29–31.
103. Vilstrup H, Amodio P, Bajaj J, et al. Hepatic encephalopathy in chronic liver disease: 2014 Practice Guideline by the American Association for the Study of Liver Diseases and the European Association for the Study of the Liver. Hepatology 2014;60(2):715–35.
104. Mehta G, Gustot T, Mookerjee RP, et al. Inflammation and portal hypertension – The undiscovered country. J Hepatol 2014;61(1): 155–63.
105. Rosselli M, MacNaughtan J, Jalan R, et al. Beyond scoring: a modern interpretation of disease progression in chronic liver disease. Gut 2013;62(9):1234–41.
106. Perz JF, Armstrong GL, Farrington LA, et al. The contributions of hepatitis B virus and hepatitis C virus infections to cirrhosis and primary liver cancer worldwide. J Hepatol 2006;45(4):529–38.
107. Mohd Hanafiah K, Groeger J, Flaxman AD, et al. Global epidemiology of hepatitis C virus infection: new estimates of age-specific antibody to HCV seroprevalence. Hepatology 2013;57(4):1333–42.
108. WHO. Hepatitis B fact sheet No. 204. Geneva: World Health Organisation; 2014. Contract No.: July.
109. WHO. Hepatitis C fact sheet No. 164. Geneva: World Health Organisation; 2014.
110. WHO. Prevention and control of viral hepatitis infection: framework for global action. Geneva: World Health Organisation; 2012.
111. Bajaj JS, Wade JB, Sanyal AJ. Spectrum of neurocognitive impairment in cirrhosis: implications for the assessment of hepatic encephalopathy. Hepatology 2009;50(6):2014–21.
112. Hassanein TI, Schade RR, Hepburn IS. Acute-on-chronic liver failure: extracorporeal liver assist devices. Curr Opin Crit Care 2011;17(2):195–203.
113. Lata J. Hepatorenal syndrome. World J Gastroenterol 2012;18(36):4978–84.

114. Davenport A, Sheikh MF, Lamb E, et al. Acute kidney injury in acute-on-chronic liver failure: where does hepatorenal syndrome fit? Kidney Int 2017;92(5):1058–70.
115. WHO. Hepatitis. Geneva: World Health Organisation; 2014.
116. Cowie B, MacLachlan JH, editors. The global burden of liver disease attributable to hepatitis B, hepatitis C, and alcohol: increasing mortality, differing causes. Hepatology; 2013; Washington DC.
117. Schweitzer AMD, Horn JM, Mikolajczyk RTP, et al. Estimations of worldwide prevalence of chronic hepatitis B virus infection: a systematic review of data published between 1965 and 2013. Lancet 2015;386(10003):1546–55.
118. Thrift AP, El-Serag HB, Kanwal F. Global epidemiology and burden of HCV infection and HCV-related disease. Nat Rev Gastroenterol Hepatol 2016;14:122.
119. Department of Health and Aging. Third National Hepatitis C Strategy 2010–2013 Canberra, Australia Australian Government; 2010.
120. O'Shea RS, Dasarathy S, McCullough AJ. Alcoholic liver disease. Hepatolog 2010;51(1):307–28.
121. Gao C, Ogeil R, Lloyd B. Alcohol's burden of disease in Australia. Canberra: FARE and VicHealth in collaboration with Turning Point; 2014.
122. European Association for the Study of Liver. EASL clinical practical guidelines: management of alcoholic liver disease. J Hepatol 2012;57(2):399–420.
123. Lucey MR, Mathurin P, Morgan TR. Alcoholic hepatitis. N Engl J Med 2009;360(26):2758–69.
124. Fialla AD, Israelsen M, Hamberg O, et al. Nutritional therapy in cirrhosis or alcoholic hepatitis: a systematic review and meta-analysis. Liver Int 2015;35(9):2072–8.
125. Thursz MR, Richardson P, Allison M, et al. Prednisolone or pentoxifylline for alcoholic hepatitis. N Engl J Med 2015;372(17):1619–28.
126. Mathurin P, Moreno C, Samuel D, et al. Early liver transplantation for severe alcoholic hepatitis. N Engl J Med 2011;365(19):1790–800.
127. Bernal W, Wendon J. Acute liver failure. N Engl J Med 2013;369(26):2525–34.
128. Cardoso FS, Marcelino P, Bagulho L, et al. Acute liver failure: an up-to-date approach. J Crit Care 2017;39:25–30.
129. Hernaez R, Solà E, Moreau R, et al. Acute-on-chronic liver failure: an update. Gut 2017;66:541–53.
130. Lescot T, Karvellas C, Beaussier M, et al. Acquired liver injury in the intensive care unit. Anesthesiology 2012;117(4):898–904.
131. Bismuth M, Funakoshi N, Cadranel JF, et al. Hepatic encephalopathy: from pathophysiology to therapeutic management. Eur J Gastroenterol Hepatol 2011;23(1):8–22.
132. Liotta EM, Romanova AL, Lizza BD, et al. Osmotic shifts, cerebral edema, and neurologic deterioration in severe hepatic encephalopathy. Crit Care Med 2018;46(2):280–9.
133. Frontera JA. Management of hepatic encephalopathy. Curr Treat Options Neurol 2014;16(6):297.
134. Conn HO, Leevy CM, Vlahcevic ZR, et al. Comparison of lactulose and neomycin in the treatment of chronic portal-systemic encephalopathy. A double blind controlled trial. Gastroenterology 1977;72(4 Pt 1):573–83.
135. Bajaj J, Cordoba J, Mullen K, et al. The design of clinical trials in hepatic encephalopathy – an International Society for Hepatic Encephalopathy and Nitrogen Metabolism (ISHEN) consensus statement. Aliment Pharmacol Ther 2011;33(7):739–47.
136. Rajoriya N, Tripathi D. Historical overview and review of current day treatment in the management of acute variceal haemorrhage. World J Gastroenterol 2014;20(21):6481–94.
137. Garcia-Tsao G, Abraldes JG, Berzigotti A, et al. Portal hypertensive bleeding in cirrhosis: risk stratification, diagnosis, and management: 2016 practice guidance by the American Association for the study of liver diseases. Hepatology 2017;65(1):310–35.
138. Wiest R, Lawson M, Geuking M. Pathological bacterial translocation in liver cirrhosis. J Hepatol 2014;60(1):197–209.
139. Koch DG, Fallon MB. Hepatopulmonary syndrome. Clin Liver Dis 2014;18(2):407–20.
140. Liu H, Lee SS. Acute-on-chronic liver failure: the heart and systemic hemodynamics. Curr Opin Crit Care 2011;17(2):190–4.
141. Bauer M, Press AT, Trauner M. The liver in sepsis: patterns of response and injury. Curr Opin Crit Care 2013;19(2):123–7.
142. Khoury T, Ayman AR, Cohen J, et al. The complex role of anticoagulation in cirrhosis: an updated review of where we are and where we are going. Digestion 2016;93(2):149–59.
143. Wang DW, Yin YM, Yao YM. Advances in the management of acute liver failure. World J Gastroenterol 2013;19(41):7069–77.
144. Pagana KD, Pagana TJ. Mosby's manual of diagnostic and laboratory tests. 3rd ed. St Louis: Mosby Elsevier; 2006.
145. Vaquero J, Chung C, Cahill ME, et al. Pathogenesis of hepatic encephalopathy in acute liver failure. Semin Liver Dis 2003;23(3):259–69.
146. Gines P, Quintero E, Arroyo V, et al. Compensated cirrhosis: natural history and prognostic factors. Hepatology 1987;7(1):122–8.
147. Dagher L, Moore K. The hepatorenal syndrome. Gut 2001;49(5):729–37.
148. Castaldo ET, Chari RS. Liver transplantation for acute hepatic failure. HPB (Oxford) 2006;8(1):29–34.
149. Parbhu SK, Adler DG. Endoscopic management of acute esophageal variceal bleeding. Tech Gastrointest Endosc 2017;19(2):74–8.
150. Christensen T. The treatment of oesophageal varices using a Sengstaken-Blakemore tube: considerations for nursing practice. Nurs Crit Care 2004;9(2):58–63.
151. Merola J, Fortune BE, Deng Y, et al. Transjugular intrahepatic portosystemic shunt creation for cirrhotic portal hypertension is well tolerated among patients with portal vein thrombosis. Eur J Gastroenterol Hepatol 2018;30(6):668–75.
152. Karvellas CJ, Subramanian RM. Current evidence for extracorporeal liver support systems in acute liver failure and acute-on-chronic liver failure. Crit Care Clin 2016;32(3):439–51.
153. Carpentier B, Gautier A, Legallais C. Artificial and bioartificial liver devices: present and future. Gut 2009;58(12):1690–702.

154. Larsen FS, Schmidt LE, Bernsmeier C, et al. High-volume plasma exchange in patients with acute liver failure: an open randomised controlled trial. J Hepatol 2016;64(1):69–78.

155. Zhao LF, Pan XP, Li LJ. Key challenges to the development of extracorporeal bioartificial liver support systems. Hepatobiliary Pancreat Dis Int 2012;11(3):243–9.

156. Liou IW, Larson AM. Role of liver transplantation in acute liver failure. Semin Liver Dis 2008;28(2):201–9.

157. Muller X, Marcon F, Sapisochin G, et al. Defining benchmarks in liver transplantation: a multicenter outcome analysis determining best achievable results. Ann Surg 2018;267(3):419–25.

158. Lynch SV, Balderson GA. ANZLT Registry Report 2016. Brisbane, QLD, Australia; 2016.

159. O'Grady J. Liver transplantation for acute liver failure. Best Pract Res Clin Gastroenterol 2012;26(1):27–33.

160. O'Leary JG, Lepe R, Davis GL. Indications for liver transplantation. Gastroenterology 2008;134(6):1764–76.

161. Yoo PS, Umman V, Rodriguez-Davalos MI, et al. Retransplantation of the liver: review of current literature for decision making and technical considerations. Transplant Proc 2013;45(3):854–9.

162. The Transplantation Society of Australia and New Zealand (TSANZ). Organ transplantation from deceased donors: Consensus statement on eligibility criteria and allocation protocols. TSANZ; 2010.

163. Llado L, Figueras J. Techniques of orthotopic liver transplantation. HPB (Oxford) 2004;6(2):69–75.

164. Protty MB, Haboubi HN, Yeoman AD. Changes in the Model of End-Stage Liver Disease (MELD) scores on day 7 predict mortality in acute on chronic liver disease: the delta-MELD project. J Hepatol 2017;55(1):S387.

165. Agopian VG, Petrowsky H, Kaldas FM, et al. The evolution of liver transplantation during 3 decades: analysis of 5347 consecutive liver transplants at a single center. Ann Surg 2013;258(3):409–21.

166. Doria C, Goldstein S, Marion IR. Orthotopic liver transplantation: surgical techniques. In: Doria C, editor. Contemporary liver transplantation organ and tissue transplantation. Cham: Springer; 2017.

167. Renz JF, Yersiz H, Reichert PR, et al. Split-liver transplantation: a review. Am J Transplant 2003;3(11):1323–35.

168. Boudjema K, Sulpice L. Auxiliary liver transplantation. Atlas of upper gastrointestinal and hepato-pancreato-biliary surgery. Springer; 2016. p. 569–76.

169. Miller CM, Quintini C, Dhawan A, et al. The International Liver Transplantation Society living donor liver transplant recipient guideline. Transplantation 2017;101(5):938–44.

170. Razonable RR, Findlay JY, O'Riordan A, et al. Critical care issues in patients after liver transplantation. Liver Transpl 2011;17(5):511–27.

171. Perera T, Bramhall S. Surgical aspects of liver transplantation. In: Neuberger J, Ferguson J, Newsome PN, editors. Liver transplantation: clinical assessment and management. Chichester: John Wiley; 2014.

172. Esmat Gamil M, Pirenne J, Van Malenstein H, et al. Risk factors for bleeding and clinical implications in patients undergoing liver transplantation. Transplant Proc 2012;44(9):2857–60.

173. Larsen FS, Strauss G, Knudsen GM, et al. Cerebral perfusion, cardiac output, and arterial pressure in patients with fulminant hepatic failure. Crit Care Med 2000;28(4):996–1000.

174. Živković SA. Neurologic complications after liver transplantation. World J Hepatol 2013;5(8):409–18.

175. Feltracco P, Carollo C, Barbieri S, et al. Early respiratory complications after liver transplantation. World J Gastroenterol 2013;19(48):9271–81.

176. Dienstag JL, Cosimi AB. Liver transplantation – a vision realized. N Engl J Med 2012;367(16):1483–5.

177. Gotthardt DN, Bruns H, Weiss KH, et al. Current strategies for immunosuppression following liver transplantation. Langenbecks Arch Surg 2014;doi:10.1007/s00423-014-1191-9.

178. Choudray NS, Saijal S, Shukla R, et al. Current status of immunosuppression in liver transplantation. J Clin Exp Hepatol 2013;3(2):150–8.

179. Seehofer D, Eurich D, Veltzke-Schlieker W, et al. Biliary complications after liver transplantation: old problems and new challenges. Am J Transplant 2013;13(2):253–65.

180. Bilbao I, Armadans L, Lazaro JL, et al. Predictive factors for early mortality following liver transplantation. Clin Transplant 2003;17(5):401–11.

181. Zerem E. Treatment of severe acute pancreatitis and its complications. World J Gastroenterol 2014;20(38):13879–92.

182. Formenti P, Marini JJ. Implications of obesity for mechanical ventilation. In: Esquinas A, Lemyze M, editors. Mechanical ventilation in the critically ill obese patient. Cham: Springer; 2018.

183. Plauth M, Cabré E, Riggio O, et al. ESPEN guidelines on enteral nutrition: liver disease. Clin Nutr 2006;25(2):285–94.

184. Kondrup J, Johansen N, Plum LM, et al. Incidence of nutritional risk and causes of inadequate nutritional care in hospitals. Clin Nutr 2002;21(6):461–8.

185. Halsey LG, Curran-Everett D, Vowler SL, et al. The fickle P value generates irreproducible results. Nat Methods 2015;12(3):179–85.

Chapter 21

Pathophysiology and management of shock

Margherita Murgo, Ruth Kleinpell

KEY WORDS

anaphylactic shock
cardiogenic shock
distributive shock
hypovolaemic shock
neurogenic shock
obstructive shock
sepsis
septic shock

Learning objectives

After reading this chapter, you should be able to:

- describe the clinical manifestations of shock
- differentiate the various shock states
- describe principles of shock management
- discuss end points of resuscitation
- identify appropriate monitoring for a patient with shock
- review and evaluate care for a patient with a specific shock type.

Introduction

> *It is a bad symptom when the head, hands, and feet are cold, while the belly and sides are hot, but it is a very good symptom when the whole body is equally hot.*
>
> THE BOOK OF PROGNOSTICS BY HIPPOCRATES, 400 BC[1]

Shock is an altered physiological state that affects the functioning of every cell and organ system in the body. It is a complex syndrome reflecting changing blood flow to body tissues with accompanying cellular dysfunction and eventual organ failure. Shock presents as a result of impaired nutrient delivery to the tissue:[2,3]

- when compensatory mechanisms can no longer respond to decreases in tissue perfusion
- when nutrient uptake is impaired at the cellular level.

While the cause of shock may be multifactorial, treatment focuses on optimising tissue perfusion and oxygen delivery. Shock is often classified according to the primary underlying mechanism: a disruption of intravascular blood volume, impaired vasomotor tone or altered cardiac contractility.[4] The shock syndrome is one of the most pervasive manifestations of critical illness present in intensive care patients.

Early detection and management of shock to reverse pathological processes improves patient outcomes.[5] Although the traditional hallmark of shock is hypotension – where the systolic blood pressure is <90 mmHg – this can be a late or misleading sign and is considered a medical emergency.[6] It is therefore critical that other signs and symptoms are identified early by frequent observations to detect a patient's deteriorating state and respond before irreversible shock ensues.[7] No single vital sign is adequate in determining the level or extent of shock[5] nor is there a specific laboratory test that diagnoses the cause of the shock syndrome.

In this chapter an overview of the pathophysiology of shock, the commonly described categories and associated pathologies, along with appropriate monitoring and interventions for managing a patient in shock are described.

Pathophysiology

Shock is classified by aetiology[2]: hypovolaemic, cardiogenic, distributive[8] and obstructive (Fig. 21.1).[9] Each type has a specific mechanism of action that leads to altered tissue perfusion and oxygen and nutrient uptake at the cellular level (Table 21.1). In practice, it is common for different shock types to be existent in the same presentation; for example, a patient with septic shock might also be hypovolaemic and/or have myocardial dysfunction.

Shock occurs when there is an inability of the body to meet metabolic demands of the tissues; hypoperfusion (decreased blood flow to the tissues) results in cellular dysfunction, as there is homeostatic imbalance between nutrient supply and demand, and adaptive responses can no longer accommodate circulatory changes.[8,10] These adaptive responses are moderated via numerous 'sensors' throughout the thorax and large vessels in particular, which detect subtle changes in pressure (baroreceptors) or biochemical changes (chemoreceptors). These receptors feedback to the hypothalamus, which regulates, through the pituitary gland and adrenal cortex, the release of a number of hormones including antidiuretic hormone and adrenocorticotrophic hormone to target organs such as the kidney. The adrenal cortex mediates the mineral and glucocorticoid response to counter the developing effects of shock. This concurrent direct feedback stimulates the sympathetic nervous system to act on blood vessel tone, particularly the arterioles, and organs such as the adrenal gland and kidney to respond via the release of endogenous catecholamines (adrenaline and noradrenaline), mineral and glucocorticoids (aldosterone, cortisol) and the renin–angiotensin–aldosterone system. Activation of the renin–angiotensin–aldosterone system results in synthesis of angiotensin II, a powerful vasoconstrictor that further potentiates the reduction in peripheral blood vessel capacity.

Collectively, these responses form a sympatho–endocrine–adrenal axis that moderates the systemic response to shock. The axis maintains circulation to the vital organ system and combines with the inflammatory response to limit local and systemic tissue damage and ultimately confer a survival advantage. Combined responses include profound vasoconstriction, oligoanuria (fluid retention), redirection of blood flow to vital organs, hyperglycaemia, immunomodulation and procoagulation. This universal response to impending shock is particularly effective in compensating for loss of circulating blood volume, but may be counterproductive when pump failure occurs or is 'uncoupled' in distributive shock states.

As adaptive responses fail, cardiac output becomes insufficient to provide adequate organ perfusion despite increasing tissue oxygen consumption (see Chapters 9 and 10). When oxygen is 'supply dependent', oxygen delivery is decreased and, to compensate, increased oxygen extraction occurs to enable continued tissue oxygen consumption. However, when oxygen delivery falls below a critical threshold, and extraction demand rises above the available blood oxygen levels, this compensation mechanism fails and oxygen debt results.[5]

Hypoperfusion may also exist despite a relatively normal cardiac output, and may not be immediately clinically evident.[5] This results in maldistribution of blood flow to some tissues while other areas receive more blood flow than needed[6,8,10] and is often referred to as distributive shock. This response is typical of the shock types that affect vasomotor tone, for example septic, neurogenic and anaphylactic shock. Maldistribution may leave some organ systems ischaemic for long periods leading to persistent organ dysfunction and failure.[5] There is also evidence supporting the presence of cytopathic hypoxia as a result of excessive production of cellular proinflammatory mediators such as nitric oxide and tumour necrosis factor-alpha. Adenosine triphosphate stores become depleted due to this impaired mitochondrial oxygen utilisation[11] interfering with electron transport and metabolism. Nitric oxide is associated with vascular relaxation and is a major contributor to alterations in microvasculature and capillary leak in sepsis.[12]

Organ systems have varying responses in shock and are not measured directly. Often surrogate markers of global hypoperfusion are used to indicate the severity of shock. Lactate and acid–base disturbances, such as an increase in strong ion gap, have been suggested as early markers of mitochondrial dysfunction and cellular hypoperfusion (Fig. 21.2).[7,9] These 'surrogate' biochemical markers of hypoperfusion (pH, serum lactate and standard base excess) assess acidaemia and provide some insight into the degree of shock.[13] Lactate, a strong anion with basal production of approximately 1300 mmol/day,[14] is a product of metabolism. Increased levels are present in tissue hypoxia, hypermetabolism, decreased lactate clearance, inhibition of pyruvate dehydrogenase and activation of inflammatory cells, all characteristics of developing shock (Table 21.2). Increased lactate production is a warning sign of impending organ failure, as it is indicative of anaerobic metabolism. Blood lactate levels have been directly linked to deteriorating patient outcomes in shock.[13,15]

Serum concentrations greater than 5 mmol/L in the setting of metabolic acidosis are indicative of high mortality.[14]

FIGURE 21.1 Types of shock. (**A**) Signs of tissue perfusion; (**B**) types of shock; (**C**) cardiac changes. CVP: central venous pressure; SvO_2 mixed venous oxygen saturation.

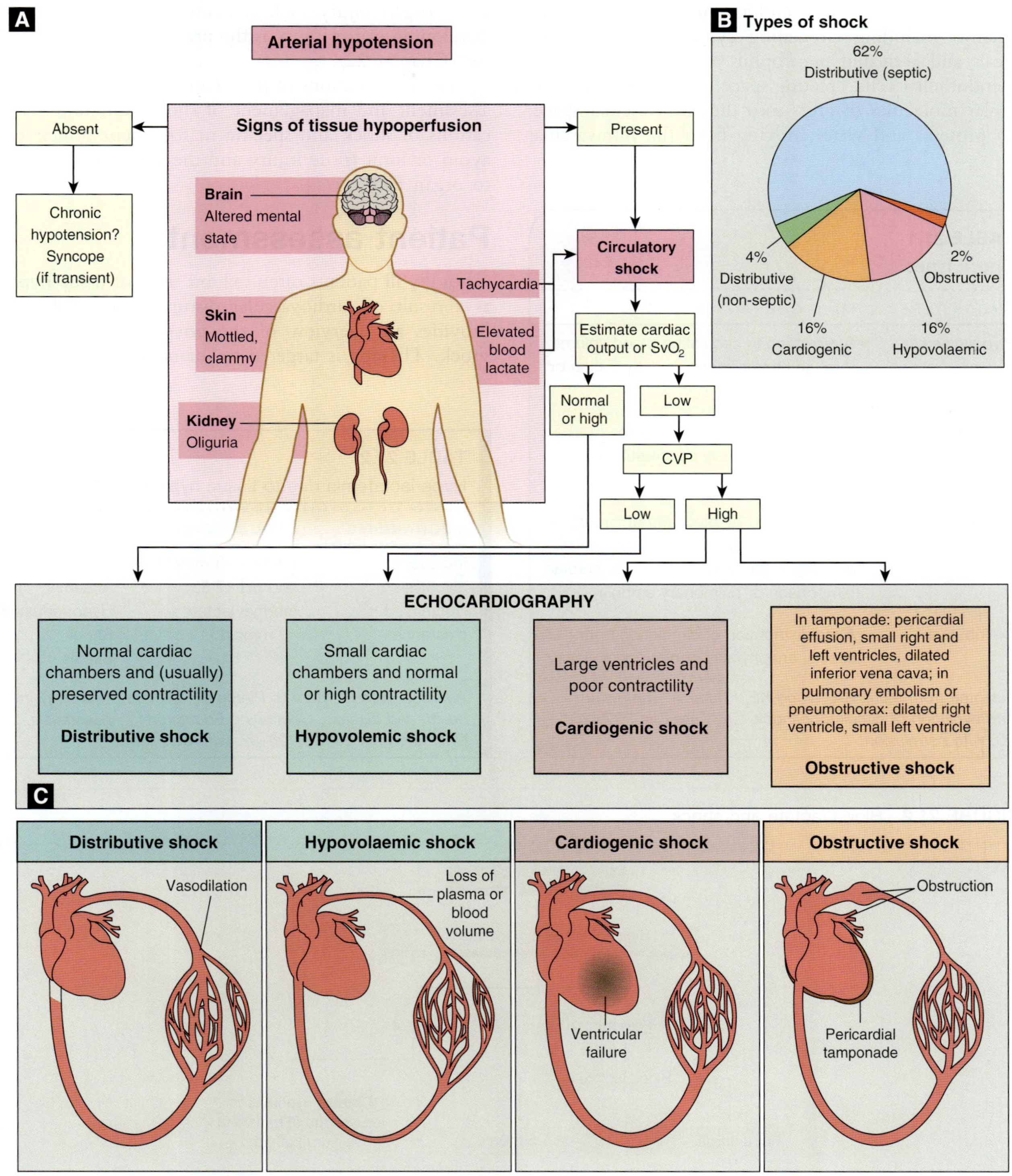

Source: From Vincent J-L, De Backer D. Circulatory shock. New Engl J Med 2013;369(18):1726–34. Copyright © (2013) Massachusetts Medical Society. Reprinted with permission from Massachusetts Medical Society.

As the shock state worsens and the body fails to compensate, organ systems begin to fail. This is complicated by 'capillary leak' or increased microvascular permeability that leads to interstitial oedema due to alterations to the vascular endothelium. Many immune mediators including circulating cytokines, oxygen-free radicals and activated neutrophils alter the structure of the endothelial cells, creating space to allow larger intravascular molecules to cross into the extravascular space, with proteins and water moving from the intravascular space into the interstitium.[16] This response mechanism improves the supply of nutrient-rich fluid to the site of injury; however, systemically, fluid shifts lead to hypovolaemia, impaired organ function and development of acute organ injury such as acute kidney injury.[16] This developing organ injury is the precedent to organ failure (see Chapter 22).

The next sections of this chapter describe the general assessment and management of shock, different classifications of shock and specific management principles to avoid or limit tissue injury and the eventual progression to organ failure.

TABLE 21.1
Shock types

SHOCK TYPE	MAIN CHARACTERISTIC
Hypovolaemic	A reduction in circulating blood volume through haemorrhage or dehydration or plasma fluid loss
Cardiogenic	Pump failure (impaired cardiac contractility) usually as a result of myocardial infarction
Obstructive	Characterised by blockage of circulation to the tissues by impedance of outflow or filling in the heart (e.g. due to cardiac tamponade or pulmonary emboli)
Distributive	A maldistribution of circulation from sepsis, anaphylaxis or neurogenic injury

Adapted from Manji RA, Wood KE, Kumar A. The history and evolution of circulatory shock. Crit Care Clin 2009;25:1–29, with permission.

Patient assessment

Critically ill patients often exhibit signs of tissue hypoxia as a result of cardiovascular disturbances.[17] Table 21.3 provides an overview of the physiological changes in shock. Therapy is targeted to maintain oxygen delivery

TABLE 21.2
Hyperlactatemia due to tissue hypoxia

MECHANISMS	SERUM LEVELS	CAUSES
Increased glycolysis Decreased clearance	Lactate >5 mmol/L and pH <7.35 (normal lactate <2 mmol/L)	Hypoxaemia Anaemia Hypoperfusion Shock Sepsis

Adapted from Phypers B, Pierce JT. Lactate physiology in health and disease. Continuing Education in Anaesthesia, Crit Care Pain 2006;6:128–32, with permission.

FIGURE 21.2 Blood lactate and shock.

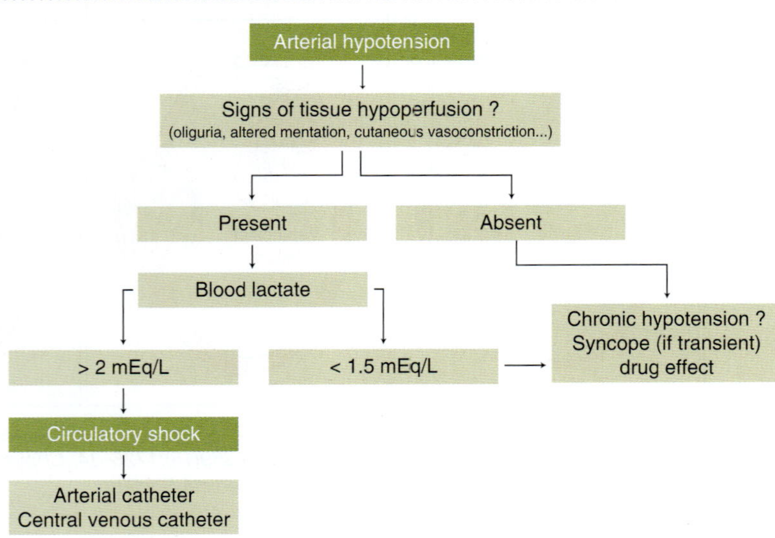

Source: Vincent J-L, Ince C, Bakker J. Clinical review: Circulatory shock – an update: a tribute to Professor Max Harry Weil. Critical Care 2012 11/20;16(6).

TABLE 21.3
Physiological changes in shock

	PHYSIOLOGICAL CHANGE				
SHOCK CLASSIFICATION	CARDIAC OUTPUT	SYSTEMIC VASCULAR RESISTANCE	CAPILLARY CIRCULATION	PULMONARY CAPILLARY PRESSURE	PULMONARY VASCULAR RESISTANCE
Hypovolaemic	↓	↑	↓	↓	↑
Cardiogenic	↓	↑	↓	↑	↑
Distributive:	↑	↓	↓	↓	↑
• septi	↓	↓	↓	↓	↓
• anaphylactic	↓/NC	↓	↓	↓	↑
• neurogenic					
Obstructive	↓	↓	↓	↑	↑

↑ = increase; ↓ = decrease; NC = no change.

to vital organs to prevent ischaemia and cell death.[17,18] Ideally, organ systems and tissues should be monitored individually;[17] however, global measures, such as perfusion pressure, cardiac output and oxygen delivery, are commonly used as surrogates to assist in treatment decision making.[19] Patient assessment and haemodynamic monitoring, including calculation of cardiac output, are used to differentiate shock states and assess progress in relation to treatment.[18,20,21] Cardiac output is seen by many clinicians as an important assessment of shocked patients as it is a major determinant of oxygen delivery.[17,18] Critically ill patients are frequently assessed clinically, although cardiac output estimations from physical examination alone are generally unreliable and patient status may change quickly.[22] Therefore, invasive techniques are most commonly used in critical care to measure cardiac output (see also Chapter 9).

Non-invasive assessment

Perfusion status is determined clinically using gross organ function such as mental status, urine output and peripheral warmth and colour (Fig. 21.3).[5,9] Basic physical assessment of cardiovascular, central nervous system and renal function is essential when assessing a patient at risk of shock. Subtle changes in mentation, urine output, heart rate and capillary refill are all signs of physiological compensation in response to altered tissue perfusion associated with shock. Regular tracking of these vital signs and trend monitoring through careful documentation can alert clinicians to impending deterioration in the shock state.

Level of consciousness may deteriorate; an early sign may be anxiety, and progress to restlessness, delirium, agitation or coma. Other assessment findings include cool, clammy skin, postural hypotension, tachycardia and decreased urine output.[9] The reliability of these measures is questionable, particularly where multiple assessments

FIGURE 21.3 Windows for assessment.

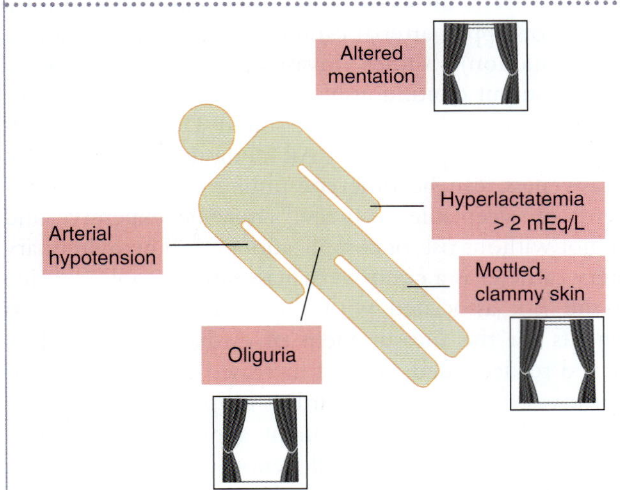

Reproduced from Vincent J-L, Ince C, Bakker J. Clinical review: Circulatory shock – an update: a tribute to Professor Max Harry Weil. Crit Care 2012;16(6):239.

by different clinicians are performed. In the intensive care unit (ICU) continuous electrocardiograph monitoring and invasive monitoring techniques are employed to assist in the objective assessment of changes in cardiovascular state. A reliable and accurate non-invasive clinical assessment technique of estimating cardiac output would be clinically useful,[20] allowing assessment of patients without invasive monitoring, or used to verify accuracy of invasive devices. While a number of non-invasive cardiac output measuring devices are available, further research and refinement is required before widespread application in critical care[23] and particularly in shocked states.[24] New technologies hold promise in aiding clinician assessment of haemodynamic status using non-invasive methods. Clinical ultrasound is being used with increasing frequency with assessment of inferior vena cava (IVC) collapsibility during respiration to assess volume status. A meta-analysis of studies comparing IVC diameter in hypotensive versus normotensive individuals demonstrated a trend towards a decreased IVC size in the hypotensive group compared to the control group. However, measures such as cardiac output or stroke volume variation were not consistently examined to assess for clinical changes based on increased IVC diameter. Additional research is warranted to evaluate the clinical application of clinical ultrasound using IVC.[25]

Invasive assessment

Continuous assessment of heart rate and blood pressure by an intraarterial catheter also enables circulatory access for frequent blood sampling to assess serum lactate levels, electrolytes and blood gas estimation, including pH.

The indicator dilution method using a thermal (thermodilution) signal (cold or hot) was traditionally the customary clinical standard for measuring cardiac output in ICU.[19] This was achieved by placement of a pulmonary artery catheter, or a central line, in conjunction with a thermistor-tipped arterial cannula (transpulmonary aortic thermodilution). Other invasive techniques measure cardiac output continuously using pulse contour or arterial pressure analysis and ultrasound Doppler methods using an oesophageal probe. All methods have degrees of invasiveness, can be time-consuming to yield measurements of acceptable accuracy,[26] may be expensive and are not without risk of complications.[20,27] The pulmonary artery catheter is a controversial assessment tool[18,21,27] due to the risk associated with the invasive device versus benefits for the measurement of cardiac output.[28] This has led to decreased use and increased interest in less or non-invasive measures of cardiac output.

A further invasive assessment approach is the continuous estimation of mixed venous oxygen saturation using a light-emitting sensor in a pulmonary artery catheter. As tissue oxygen delivery fails to meet demand and oxygen extraction rises, the residual oxygen content of blood returning to the lungs will fall; in effect, this is a surrogate indicator of failure to meet body tissue oxygen demand. This technology was used in the landmark study by Rivers and colleagues[29] to monitor early deterioration of septic shock patients presenting to the emergency department (ED) in need of resuscitation, and was part of a goal-directed approach to managing patients. This single-centre study was the subject of much interest for its claimed improvement in patient outcome, with goal-directed resuscitation being assessed in a number of major multicentre studies to verify findings within an international context and varying approaches to critical care delivery.[30] The recent publication of large clinical trials has further informed the evidence, impacting this approach and will be discussed later in the chapter.

Management principles

Managing a patient in shock focuses on treating the underlying cause, and restoration and optimisation of perfusion and oxygen delivery; this includes relevant activities using the acronym VIP.[3,31] It is also suggested that giving critically ill patients a daily 'FASTHUG', to ensure daily assessment and interventions in priority areas, improves the quality of care for patients in ICU[32] (see *Practice tips* below). Clinical management of patients with different types of shock is discussed separately below.

Practice tip

'FASTHUG' mnemonic

- **F**eeding (prevent malnutrition, promote adequate caloric intake)
- **A**nalgesia (reduce pain, improve physical and psychological wellbeing)
- **S**edation (titrate to the 3Cs – calm, cooperative, comfortable)
- **T**hromboembolic prophylaxis (prevent DVT)
- **H**ead of bed elevated (up to 45° to reduce reflux and VAP)
- **U**lcer prophylaxis (to prevent stress ulceration)
- **G**lycaemic control (to maintain normal blood glucose levels)

Source: Vincent J-L. Give your patient a fast hug (at least) once a day. Crit Care Med 2005;33:1225–9.

Practice tip

'VIP' acronym

- **V**entilation, including airway, added oxygen and ventilation
- **I**nfusion of appropriate volume expanders
- Improved heart **P**umping with drug therapy such as antiarrhythmics, inotropes, diuretics and vasodilators

Source: Weil M. Personal commentary on the diagnosis and treatment of circulatory shock states. Curr Opin Crit Care 2004;10:246–9.

Hypovolaemic shock

Hypovolaemia is a common primary cause of shock and also a factor in other shock states. Insufficient circulating blood volume is the underlying mechanism, leading to decreased cardiac output and altered perfusion.[33,34] Death related to haemorrhage is most likely in the first few hours after injury.[34] The most obvious cause is direct injury to vessels leading to haemorrhage, but there are more insidious causes such as dehydration from

TABLE 21.4
Signs and symptoms of hypovolaemic shock

PARAMETER	MILD (15–30% LOSS)	MODERATE (30–40% LOSS)	SEVERE (>40% LOSS)
Blood pressure	No change	Lowered	Hypotensive
Pulse (beats/min)	≥100	≥120	≥140
Respirations (breaths/min)	>20	>30	>40
Neurological	Normal to slightly anxious	Mildly anxious to confused	Confused, lethargic
Urine output (mL/h)	>30	20–30	5–15, negligible
Capillary refill	Normal	Reduced, >4 s	Reduced, >4 s

Source: Hooper N, Armstrong TJ. Shock, Hemorrhagic. [Updated 2017 Nov 27]. In: StatPearls [Internet]. Treasure Island (FL): StatPearls Publishing; 2018 Jan. Available from: https://www.ncbi.nlm.nih.gov/books/NBK470382/. CC BY 4.0.

prolonged vomiting or diarrhoea, sepsis and burns.[35] It is important to consider other types of shock, such as obstructive and neurogenic shock, as differential diagnoses to ensure the correct treatment of the patient.[36]

Hypovolaemic shock is often classified as mild, moderate or severe, depending on the amount of volume loss (Table 21.4). As the shock state worsens, associated compensatory mechanisms will be more pronounced, and hypovolaemic shock may deteriorate to multiple organ dysfunction syndrome if poor oxygen delivery is prolonged[33] (see Chapter 22).

Clinical manifestations

Symptoms of haemorrhage may not be present until more than 15–30% of blood volume is lost, and will deteriorate as the shock state worsens.[35] Estimating blood or plasma loss is difficult and dilutional effects of resuscitation fluids may be evident when assessing haemoglobin and haematocrit.[35] As the body compensates for the reduced circulating volume, widespread vasoconstriction occurs in most body systems apart from the heart and central nervous system. Systemic vascular resistance rises markedly in an attempt to retain a viable circulatory system; this accounts for many of the signs and symptoms associated with circulatory compensation. However, as tissues are starved of oxygen and nutrients over a prolonged ischaemic time, local mediators are released as part of the inflammatory responses, leading to organ microvasculature vasodilation, and capillaries re-open to maintain oxygen delivery and reduce hypoxia.[35] This is a hallmark of developing multiple organ dysfunction syndrome.

Patient management

Clinical management of hypovolaemia focuses on minimising fluid loss and restoration of circulating blood volume[35] once the airway and breathing are secure. More than one large-bore intravenous cannulae are usually inserted and lost circulating volume is replaced by colloids, isotonic crystalloids or blood products to

FIGURE 21.4 Physiological derangements during haemorrhage/massive transfusion. APTT: activated partial thromboplastin time; Ca: calcium; INR: international normalised ratio; PT: prothrombin time; SBE: standard base excess.

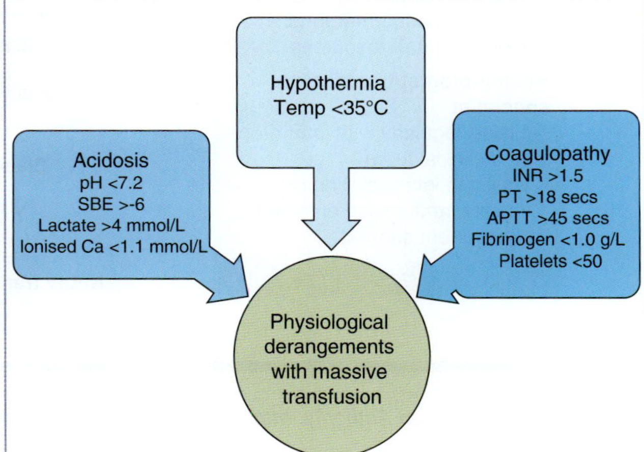

achieve haemodynamic end points, such as a mean arterial pressure >65 mmHg. Body heat can be lost rapidly due to blood loss, the rapid infusion of room temperature fluids and exposure in the pre-hospital setting or during repeated physical examination. It is therefore important to institute measures to maintain patient temperature >35°C to avoid coagulopathies and loss of thermoregulation.[37] The aim is to ameliorate the lethal triad of anaemia, coagulopathy and hypothermia, which can lead to worsening haemorrhage and eventual death (Fig. 21.4).[34,35,37] Hypothermia is an independent risk factor for death in haemorrhagic shock.[36]

Critical care nurses must be efficient and practised at initial patient assessment to establish the degree of compensation occurring in a hypovolaemic patient. Fig. 21.4 highlights clinical manifestations of haemorrhage. Careful

FIGURE 21.5 Massive transfusion protocol. APTT: activated partial thromboplastin time; FFP: fresh frozen plasma; INR: international normalised ratio; PT: prothrombin time; RBC: red blood cells.

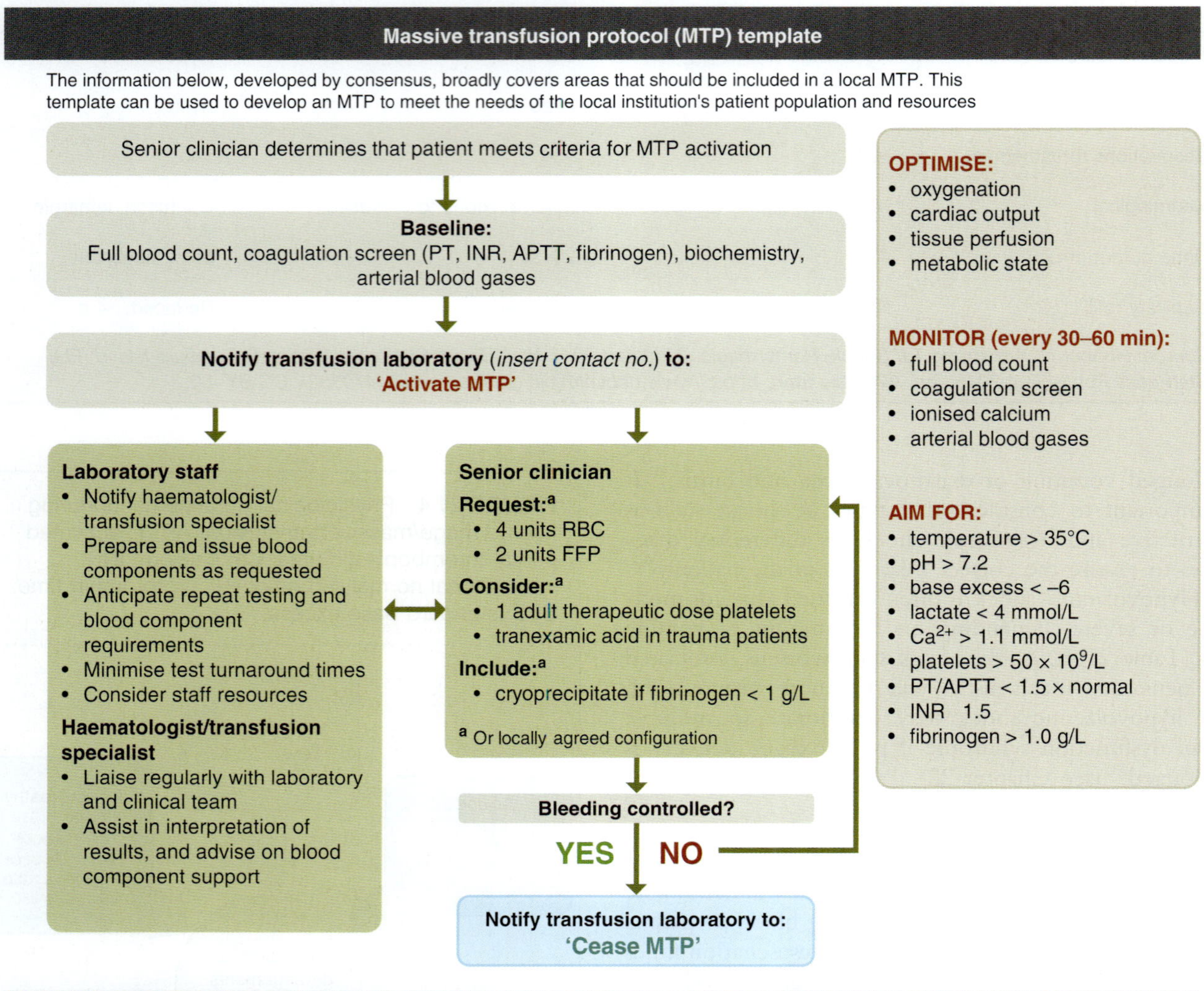

Source: National Blood Authority. http://www.blood.gov.au/system/files/documents/pbm-module1-mtp-template_0.ppt.

consideration of a patient's clinical picture will establish a hierarchy and priority of needs. Many hospitals have some level of track and trigger response that escalates care to appropriate levels such as medical emergency teams or rapid response teams. However, nurses are in a position to institute first-line management, such as establishing intravenous access, if this is a core skill. There are also many protocols and guidelines available to guide initial fluid resuscitation where a patient has indications of inadequate circulating blood volume. Although such guidelines might vary slightly, they aim to restore circulating blood volume through the administration of fluid boluses. Up to 20 mL/kg of colloid or 30–40 mL/kg crystalloid may be recommended. Critical bleeding and massive transfusion protocols (Fig. 21.5) should also be available to guide patient management. BloodSafe Australia (https://www.bloodsafelearning.org.au) has lessons available on this issue.

Fluid resuscitation

Fluid resuscitation is a first-line treatment for hypovolaemic shock; providing fluid volume increases preload and therefore cardiac output and organ perfusion. A related principle is that the fluid infused should reflect fluid loss. For example, in burns, plasma replacement might be warranted or in massive haemorrhage, fresh blood may be indicated. There has been a recent systematic review of a bundle of care for haemorrhagic shock to improve concordance between the evidence base and practice (Box 21.1). It has been suggested that fluid therapy should be managed in the same way as prescribing medication after consideration of the risks and benefits of a selected fluid.[38] Giving a fluid challenge is not always appropriate; the determining factors will be assessment of volume responsiveness, and whether the infusion will not be deleterious, causing overload, fluid shifts and

BOX 21.1

Resuscitation from haemorrhagic shock

- Commence massive transfusion protocol
- Upon arrival measure lactate and/or base deficit
- In a 1:1:1 ratio transfuse packed red blood cells, platelets and plasma
- Upon arrival measure coagulopathy using viscoelastic techniques
- Avoid large volume crystalloid resuscitation (no more than 3 L over 6 hours)

Adapted from Shafi S, Collinsworth AW, Richter KM, et al. Bundles of care for resuscitation from hemorrhagic shock and severe brain injury in trauma patients - Translating knowledge into practice. J Trauma Acute Care Surg 2016;81(4):780-94.

perpetuating inflammatory responses.[5] The fluid type, volume, rate and targeted end points should be documented;[35] and often this is structured as a bolus dose in volume/kg to achieve a measured haemodynamic variable. See Table 21.5 for a list of some of the frequently used resuscitation fluids and their compositions. When massive transfusion is required, attention should be given to product selection and this should be guided by an evidence-based protocol.

Practice tip

Fluid bolus in high risk groups

- Care should be taken when administering fluid bolus to all patients with particular attention to high risk groups such as the elderly.
- Assess regularly for signs of fluid overload and pulmonary oedema including: shortness of breath, orthopnoea, bibasal auscultation of fine end-inspiratory crackles, oedema, increased central venous pressure. Escalate signs of distress immediately for medical review.

Minimum volume resuscitation

The use of high ratios of blood products and low fluid volume during damage control resuscitation confers a survival benefit.[39] Much of the knowledge around major trauma and haemorrhage has come from military research and management of 'field trauma'.[40] Maintaining a systolic blood pressure of approximately 90 mmHg may be beneficial as clotting factors are not diluted and remaining blood volume retains its viscosity.[41] Selection of the appropriate fluid for surgical management and 'permissive hypotension' (deliberate limiting or minimising resuscitation until after adequate surgical control of haemorrhage)[35,37] will be assessed by the multidisciplinary team. This restrictive fluid regimen is a process linked to damage control surgery.[41] The goal of this management strategy is to maintain the systolic blood pressure end point using blood products in an effort to limit coagulopathy[41] and stopping the haemorrhage through direct pressure, tamponade devices and other techniques.[40]

Debate surrounds early surgical intervention prior to aggressive fluid resuscitation.[34] The premise is that allowing a lower perfusion pressure prior to achieving haemostasis with controlled or no fluid infusion results in less blood loss, as the compensatory mechanisms described earlier in this chapter are not as profound.[34] Use of medications such as factor IVa and erythropoietin also remains controversial in the setting of critical haemorrhage.[37] Guidelines for 'massive transfusion' released by the Australian National Blood Authority do not recommend use of factor IVa beyond licensed indications, although there may be an indication when conventional therapy has failed to secure haemostasis following massive blood loss and transfusion of blood products.[42] The current debate also includes dosage and thromboembolic complications associated with its use.[37] It is important to note the National Blood Authority guideline under review.

Crystalloids versus colloids

The scientific rationale for using colloids over crystalloids is to preserve plasma oncotic pressure so as to retain intravascular fluid and minimise oedema.[43] This rationale has not been supported by the research. The recently published CRISTAL study has not improved understanding around which fluid is most suitable in hypovolaemic shock as no treatment benefit between crystalloids and colloids was identified.[44] This unblinded, multicentre, randomised, controlled trial was conducted over a decade and enrolled nearly 3000 patients. The primary outcome was 28-day mortality.[44] The colloid versus crystalloid fluid resuscitation debate will continue as other large trials have also been unable to demonstrate outcome benefits except in some subsets of patients.[45,46] Crystalloids have more often been suggested in guidelines given the less harmful effects when compared to starch and gelatin containing solutions.[43,47]

If moderate-to-severe hypovolaemia is suspected, blood is often used to improve oxygen-carrying capacity. Further dilution of blood by volume expanders increases hypoxia, otherwise known as isovolaemic anaemia, and red cells are usually required. Use of isotonic saline as a volume expander is common, although resuscitation with large volumes of saline solutions can be associated with hyperchloraemic acidosis[34] and haemodilution.[40] Blood and blood components are usually considered necessary where patients exhibit signs of moderate-to-severe haemorrhage. There is no perfect resuscitation fluid, and selection is guided by patient condition and the type of fluid lost and a goal-directed, rather than liberal, approach is usually suggested.[43]

TABLE 21.5
Resuscitation fluids

VARIABLE	HUMAN PLASMA	4% ALBUMIN	COLLOIDS								CRYSTALLOIDS		
			HYDROXYETHYL STARCH						4% SUCCINYLATED MODIFIED FLUID GELATIN	3.5% UREA-LINKED GELATIN	0.9% SALINE	COMPOUNDED SODIUM LACTATE	BALANCED SALT SOLUTION
			10% (200/0.5)	6% (450/0.7)	6% (130/0.4)		6% (130/0.42)						
Trade name		**Albumex**	**Hemohes**	**Hextend**	**Voluven**	**Volulyte**	**Venofundin**	**Tetraspan**	**Gelofusine**	**Haemaccel**	**Normal saline**	**Hartmann's or Ringer's lactate**	**Plasmalyte**
Colloid source		**Human donor**	**Potato starch**	**Maize starch**	**Maize starch**	**Maize starch**	**Potato starch**	**Potato starch**	**Bovine gelatin**	**Bovine gelatin**			
Osmolarily (mOsm/L)	291	250	308	304	308	286	308	296	274	301	308	280.6	294
Sodium (mmol/L)	135-145	148	154	143	154	137	154	140	154	145	154	131	140
Potassium (mmol/L)	4.5-5.0			3.0		4.0		4.0		5.1		5.4	5.0
Calcium (mmol/L)	2.2-2.6			5.0				2.5		6.25		2.0	
Magnesium (mmol/L)	0.8-1.0			0.9		1.5		1.0					3.0
Chloride (mmol/L)	94-111	128	154	124	154	110	154	118	120	145	154	111	98
Acetate (mmol/L)						34		24					27
Lactate (mmol/L)	1-2			28								29	
Malate (mmol/L)								5					
Gluconate (mmol/L)													23
Bicarbonate (mmol/L)	23-27												
Octanoate (mmol/L)		6.4											

Note: to convert the values for potassium to milligrams per decilitre, divide by 0.2558. To convert the values for calcium to milligrams per decilitre, divide by 0.250. To convert the values for magnesium to milligrams per decilitre, divide by 0.4114.
Source: Lira A, Pinsky M. Choices in fluid type and volume during rescusitation: impact on patient outcomes. Annals of Intensive Care 2014;4:38. Springer. CC BY 4.0.

Blood and blood products

There are a number of factors to consider when administering large amounts of blood products. Massive transfusion is defined as replacement of a patient's total blood volume in less than 24 hours or 50% of blood volume in 4 hours. This equates to approximately 10 units of packed red blood cells,[40,48] although there are inconsistent descriptions in the literature.[48] A number of complications following massive transfusion can be evident such as transfusion reactions, coagulopathies, hypothermia and sepsis.[42] Massive transfusion is also associated with high mortality,[48] with human errors such as misidentification and incorrect blood component to patient also a significant risk during high stress situations.

Patients receiving massive blood transfusions require careful monitoring for signs of volume overload, metabolic derangements, hypothermia, citrate toxicity, hyperkalaemia and coagulopathies because clotting factors are often depleted. Dilution and clotting factor consumption cause microvascular bleeding, often manifesting as oozing from multiple sites even after surgical correction (disseminated intravascular coagulation).[48] The Australian and New Zealand Intensive Care Society Clinical Trials Group conducted research to determine if administration of fresher blood decreased 90-day mortality. This was based on the hypothesis that shorter storage would reduce 'storage lesion' and harm to patients. The TRANSFUSE study found that age of red cells did not affect 90-day mortality in critically ill patients.[49]

The National Blood Authority in Australia Critical Care module suggests a restrictive blood transfusion strategy.[50] This is supported by a National Safety and Quality Health Service Standard related to blood management.[51] The standard requires health services to optimise conserving the patient's own blood, document decisions about transfusion, prescribe in alignment with national criteria and report adverse events.[51] The current version of the Critical Care Module in the national guidelines outlines the deleterious effects of blood transfusion and makes clear recommendations about when red cells and other blood products are appropriate for use.[50]

Leucocyte depletion occurs during donation in many countries including Australia. This decreases upregulation of the inflammatory immune response associated with transfusion. Internationally, there are a number of organisations that produce guidelines for blood transfusion. The Council of Europe has published a high-level guide on the preparation of and quality assurance on the use of blood components. The Australian National Blood Authority has published six comprehensive and easy-to-use clinical practice guidelines (see *Practice tip*).

The Australian National Blood Authority Critical Bleeding/Massive Transfusion guideline makes clear recommendations about blood product use during haemorrhage. See Fig. 21.5 for the Massive Transfusion Protocol template.

The use of tranexamic acid, an antifibrinolytic agent, is recommended as standard practice for patients in need of massive transfusion.[52] Mortality was reduced in a large randomised controlled trial of more than 20,000 trauma patients in those patients that received tranexamic acid.[53] The survival benefit in this study was greatest when treatment occurred in the first hour. This effect was all but lost if administered more than 3 hours after injury. Even with the large sample, these results gave rise to debate about including the use of tranexamic acid in guidelines due to insufficient evidence.[54] However, common practice includes the administration of 1 g intravenously within the first hour and additional 1 g infused over next 8 hours.

> **Practice tip**
>
> **Blood product usage**
>
> Keep up-to-date and download abbreviated recommendations and tools for use at the bedside from the National Blood Authority (Australia) website as they are completed and updated (see *Online resources*). Always refer back to your local policies and guidelines before patient intervention.

Cardiogenic shock

Cardiogenic shock manifests as circulatory failure from cardiac dysfunction,[55] and is reflected in a low cardiac output (cardiac index <2.1 L/min/m^2), hypotension (systolic blood pressure <90 mmHg), severe pulmonary congestion and high central vascular filling pressures (pulmonary artery occlusion pressure >18 mmHg).[56] Additional parameters obtained through invasive monitoring include intrathoracic blood volume index >850 mL/m^2, global end-diastolic volume >700 mL/m^2 and extravascular lung volume index >10 mL/kg.[57,58] Cardiogenic shock is commonly associated with acute myocardial infarction and manifests when 40% or more of the left ventricle is ischaemic. It is also related to mechanical disorders such as acute cardiac valvular dysfunction or septal defects, deteriorating cardiomyopathies or congestive cardiac failure,[59] and trauma. Cardiogenic shock can also occur as a result of obstruction or inhibition of left ventricular ejection, also referred to as obstructive shock, such as occurs in pulmonary embolus, dissecting aneurysm or cardiac tamponade[31,59] (see Chapter 10). Myocardial depression from non-cardiac causes such as sepsis, acidosis, myocardial depressant factor, hypocalcaemia or drug impact may be so severe as to present as cardiogenic shock.

Incidence has been estimated at 3% of patients presenting with acute myocardial infarction. Mortality remains high (50–80%)[60] given death from acute myocardial infarction overall is 7%. This increased mortality occurs despite treatment advances such as emergency revascularisation.[61] Wider distribution of interventional cardiac revascularisation services has likely improved

TABLE 21.6
Obstructive shock types

TYPE	DESCRIPTION	SIGNS	AETIOLOGY	TYPICAL MANAGEMENT
Cardiac tamponade	Acute circulatory failure secondary to compression of the heart chambers by a pericardial effusion	Anxiety, hypotension, chest pain, tachypnoea, pulsus paradoxus, tachycardia, high CVP	Pericardial injury, aortic dissection, trauma, post-cardiac surgery and rarely infective causes Symptoms include right-sided diastolic collapse	Pericardial drainage
Tension pneumothorax	Progressive build-up of air within the pleural space by allowing air in but not out; pressure in the pleural space pushes the mediastinum to the opposite side, obstructing venous return to the heart	Deviated trachea away from the affected side, hyperexpansion on the side of the pneumothorax with little air movement and distended neck veins	Penetrating chest injury, blunt trauma, hospital procedures such as insertion or removal of central lines, lung biopsy	Needle thoracostomy as soon as possible (large cannula inserted to the 2nd intercostal space at the mid-clavicular line); however this procedure is not without complications and it has been suggested that the diagnosis should be confirmed on X-ray prior to the procedure, and a pleural drain will be required after
Pulmonary embolism	Thrombotic occlusion of a pulmonary artery	Increases right-sided afterload, enlarges RV and deviates septum to left, thus decreasing left ventricular volume and compliance	Shortness of breath, chest pain, haemoptysis	Thrombolysis or surgical embolectomy

CVP = central venous pressure; RV = right ventricle.
Adapted from Bodson L, Bouferrache K, Vieillard-Baron A. Cardiac tamponade. Curr Opin Crit Care 2011;17:416–24.

outcomes for patients who present early in the course of their acute disease. Current timing recommendations for treating myocardial infarction with ST elevation with primary percutaneous coronary intervention include a door-to-balloon time of 90 minutes or less to improve outcomes.[62]

Clinical signs include poor peripheral perfusion, tachycardia and other signs of organ dysfunction such as confusion, agitation, oliguria, cool extremities and dyspnoea, many of which are present in hypovolaemic shock.[55] Compensatory mechanisms are conflicting, as cardiac workload is increased on an already-failing heart, yet cardiac muscle oxygen delivery may be compromised. A careful but rapid assessment of the clinical history is helpful in differentiating the precipitant cause of this shock.

Because of similar clinical presentation, obstructive shock is at times described as cardiogenic shock. Obstructive shock is not as common as other types of shock[9] and is associated with a low cardiac output due to extra cardiac processes inhibiting circulatory flow. The two main types are associated with impedance to cardiac filling from causes such as tension pneumothorax and cardiac tamponade and factors that increase afterload such as aortic dissection or massive pulmonary embolus.[63] Examples of conditions that can lead to obstructive shock are provided in Table 21.6. Obstructive shock may be temporarily treated by maintaining preload with fluid resuscitation until definitive intervention to remove the obstruction to forward blood flow.

Managing patients with heart failure as a result of cardiogenic shock can be challenging and is often undertaken simultaneously with preparation for definitive treatment. Maintaining perfusion is difficult, as compensatory mechanisms usually cause further harm to the heart. While judicious administration of fluid is considered in terms of optimising remaining cardiac function, administration of pharmacological agents that reduce cardiac workload and improve function is paramount: dobutamine for inotropic and afterload-reducing effects via vasodilation and morphine to reduce pain, improve coronary perfusion and reduce oxygen demand. Treatment of the underlying cause is critical and may include surgery to repair obstruction to flow or percutaneous resolution of a coronary artery blockage. See Chapter 10 for a more detailed discussion of the management of acute myocardial infarction and heart failure.

> **BOX 21.2**
>
> **Clinical features of cardiogenic shock**
>
> - Low cardiac output and hypotension
> - Poor peripheral perfusion – pale, cool, clammy peripheries
> - Oliguria
> - Altered mentation, restlessness and anxiety
> - Tachycardia and arrhythmias
> - Pulmonary congestion with widespread inspiratory crackles and hypoxaemia (perhaps with frank pulmonary oedema)
> - Dyspnoea and tachypnoea
> - Respiratory alkalosis (hyperventilation) or acidosis (respiratory fatigue)
> - Lactic acidosis
> - Distended neck veins, elevated jugular venous pressure

Clinical manifestations

The clinical features of cardiogenic shock are reflective of congestive cardiac failure, although with greater severity[57] (Box 21.2). Other symptoms consistent with the cause of the cardiogenic shock may also be present, including chest pain and ST-segment changes, murmurs, features of pericardial tamponade and arrhythmias.

In the absence of invasive monitoring, the profile of hypotension, peripheral hypoperfusion and severe pulmonary and venous congestion is evident although this 'classic' profile is not universal. On initial examination, approximately 30% of patients with shock of left ventricular aetiology will have no pulmonary congestion and an estimated 9% will have no hypoperfusion.[64]

In acute left ventricular myocardial infarction, the structural or contractile abnormality impairs systolic performance resulting in incomplete left ventricular emptying. This results in subsequent progressive congestion of first the left atrium, then the pulmonary circulation, right ventricle, right atrium and finally the venous circulation.[65] When invasive haemodynamic monitoring is available, changes that may be observed include decreased cardiac output and increased systemic resistance and myocardial oxygen demand (Fig. 21.6).

A patient with cardiogenic shock is also assessed and monitored for their oxygen delivery and tissue oxygen requirements. Systemic oxygen delivery falls in proportion to a declining cardiac output, and is further exacerbated as hypoxaemia develops with pulmonary oedema. Initially, oxygen consumption may be sustained by an increase in tissue oxygen extraction ratio.[66] A quarter of delivered oxygen is extracted by tissues but, as delivery falls, tissues extract proportionally more oxygen to meet metabolic needs. Oxygen consumption can therefore be sustained until the severity of oxygen delivery deficit exceeds the ability to increase extraction. Maximal extraction is approximately 50%, and consumption falters when oxygen delivery falls to around 500–600 mL/min (cardiac index <2.2 L/min/m^2).[66,67] While use of a pulmonary artery catheter is a well-described measure of severity in cardiogenic shock (as with hypovolaemic shock), evidence of improved patient outcome is unclear.[21,28]

Once oxygen consumption falls, subsequent anaerobic metabolism leads to lactic acidosis.[17] Progressive tissue ischaemia and injury ensues, along with worsening metabolic acidosis unless oxygen delivery can be restored. Myocardial contractile performance continues to deteriorate when myocardial ischaemia develops or when existing ischaemia or infarction extends, leading to a vicious cycle of ischaemia and dysfunction.[66]

Compensatory responses effective in hypovolaemic shock are initially advantageous, but may ultimately be counterproductive when cardiogenic shock is due to myocardial infarction:

- Tachycardia offsets low stroke volume but increases myocardial oxygen consumption and decreases diastolic duration, reducing coronary perfusion time.
- Vasoconstriction limits the severity of hypotension but increases resistance to left ventricular emptying and may contribute to worsening of the cardiac output, in particular when cardiogenic shock is due to contractile dysfunction.
- An increase in cardiac workload to overcome the rise in systemic afterload increases myocardial oxygen demand, which cannot be met due to coronary artery occlusion.
- Developing pulmonary congestion is no longer contained within the pulmonary capillary and moves into the alveolar capillary space, creating pulmonary oedema, further impeding oxygen delivery to the circulation.

Patient management

Treatment of cardiogenic shock includes haemodynamic management, respiratory and cardiovascular support, biochemical stabilisation and reversal or correction of the underlying cause. This complex presentation requires a coordinated approach to the multiple aspects of care of a patient with cardiogenic shock.

A rapid response to impending deterioration associated with cardiogenic shock includes repeated assessment and measures to optimise oxygen supply and demand. Frequent, thorough assessment of the patient's status is essential, and should focus on:

1. identification of patients at risk of clinical deterioration
2. assessment of the severity of shock and identification of organ or system dysfunction

FIGURE 21.6 Sequence of haemodynamic changes in cardiogenic shock.

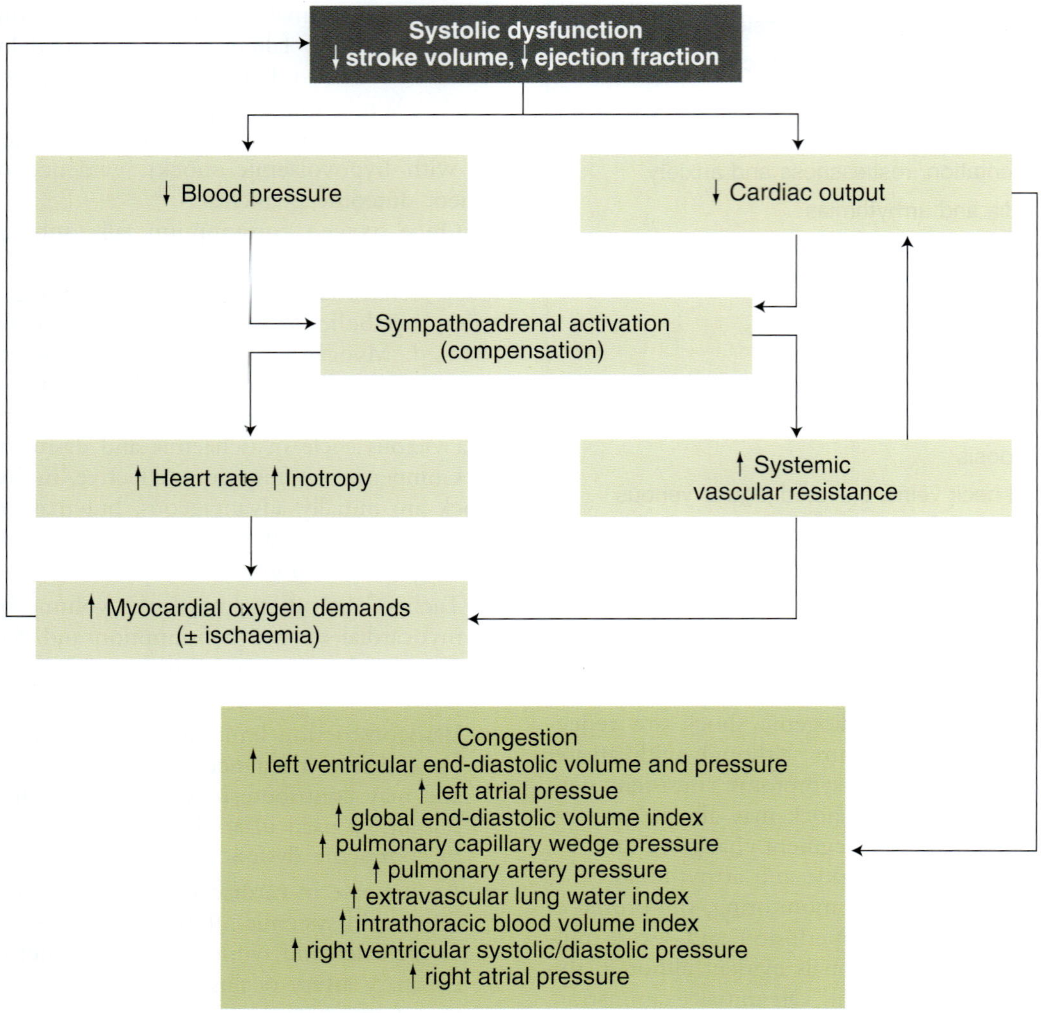

3 assessment of the impact of treatment
4 identification of complications of treatment.

Assessment follows a systematic approach and is conducted as often as indicated by the patient's condition, centering on the cardiovascular system as well as related systems that cardiac function influences, including respiratory, renal, neurological and integumentary systems.

Typical treatment regimens require preload reduction, augmentation of contractility with intravenous inotropes and afterload manipulation. These aspects are undertaken concurrently due to the potential severity of cardiogenic shock. Endotracheal intubation with mechanical ventilation is implemented if necessary, but the need for mechanical ventilation is associated with an increase in mortality.[68]

Optimising oxygen supply and demand

As cardiogenic shock is associated with an imbalance of oxygen supply and demand throughout the body, measures to optimise this balance by increasing oxygen supply and decreasing demand are essential (Box 21.3).

Preload management

Preload reduction relieves pulmonary congestion, reduces myocardial workload and improves contractility, which is in part impaired by overstretched ventricles. Careful assessment of patient fluid status is necessary prior to either the administration of small aliquots of fluid to enhance deteriorating myocardial function or enhanced diuresis to reduce circulating blood volume. Any fluid offloading is balanced against the risk of excessive blood volume depletion and depression of cardiac output and blood pressure. Desired end points of therapy may include a reduction in right atrial, pulmonary artery and pulmonary artery occlusion pressures, or improvements in intrathoracic blood volume, global end-diastolic volume and extravascular lung water, depending on available monitoring equipment.

BOX 21.3

Managing oxygen supply and demand

Strategies to increase oxygen supply include:

- positioning the patient upright to promote optimum ventilation by reducing venous return and lessening pulmonary oedema; this strategy may contribute to hypotension
- administering oxygen, continuous positive airway pressure and bi-level positive airway pressure support as required.[75]

Strategies to reduce oxygen demand include:

- limiting physical activity
- implementing measures to reduce patient anxiety, including communication, explanation and analgesic and sedative medications. Avoid those medications that are cardio-depressive.

Practice tip

Measures to reduce preload include:

- sitting a patient up with their legs either hanging over the side of the bed or in a dependent position
- IV diuretics such as frusemide usually administered as an intermittent bolus or, if necessary, as a continuous infusion
- venodilation (glyceryl trinitrate infusions at 10–200 mcg/min titrated to blood pressure)[4]
- ultrafiltration (may be considered to rapidly reduce circulating volume)
- respiratory support with continuous positive airway pressure (indicated for pulmonary relief, with the additional benefit of reducing venous return).

Additional measures to reduce pulmonary hypertension may be employed. Morphine is useful to lessen anxiety and oxygen demands during cardiogenic shock,[69] and may offer additional benefits by reducing pulmonary artery pressure and pulmonary oedema. Morphine has predictable effects and can be reversed. Other treatment options include correction of hypercapnoea, if present, and nitric oxide by inhalation.

Inotropic therapy

Intravenous positive inotropes promote myocardial contractility to improve cardiac output and blood pressure. Currently available inotropes are not uniform in their beneficial effect on cardiac output and blood pressure because of additional vasoactive actions (either vasodilation or constriction) (Table 21.7). Selection of an inotropic agent is therefore partly based on inotropic potency as well as the desired effect on vascular resistance:

- vasodilation in addition to inotropy (inodilator effect) favours cardiac output, but may compromise blood pressure[70]
- vasoconstriction in addition to inotropy (inoconstrictor effect) improves blood pressure, but may at times compromise left ventricular emptying and cardiac output.

All inotropes present a paradox in the treatment of cardiogenic shock, as they have the potential to increase heart rate and myocardial oxygen demands, and increase the frequency of arrhythmias. Monitoring is used to identify heart rate, rhythm and the development of ST-segment or T-wave changes. The best regimen for cardiogenic shock has not been established. There is controversy about using drug combinations with opposing effects; however, there is evidence that using dilators and pressors together is superior to the use of inopressors alone.[71] The vasodilation seen with inodilator agents may reduce both preload and afterload, leading to more effective myocardial pumping and an increased cardiac output. The effect on blood pressure is variable, as the opposing actions of increased contractility and vasodilation are not uniform in potency, and occur with differing effects between patients. By reducing afterload, left ventricular emptying is favoured with a reduction in cardiac contractility, reducing myocardial oxygen demand.[72-74] In a large study of more than 900 patients with cardiogenic shock requiring a vasopressor agent to maintain perfusion, short-term mortality was improved when a dilator was part of the medication regimen.[71]

Inoconstrictors constrict the vasculature, resulting in increased preload and afterload while also increasing myocardial contractility.[75] These increases, particularly in afterload, generally result in a raised blood pressure, but the impact on cardiac output is less predictable. An increase in cardiac output is often seen with these agents, but the increase in afterload may become limiting to left ventricular emptying when there is significant contractile impairment. Inoconstrictors are therefore generally selected when the afterload and resultant blood pressure are more severely compromised than the cardiac output. Vasoconstriction also further increases myocardial work and myocardial oxygen demand, and may worsen ischaemia.[71]

Dobutamine has traditionally been the inodilator of choice,[76] although accumulating evidence for levosimendan, a calcium-sensitising agent, suggests improved outcomes.[72,74] The slow onset of action time of levosimendan (hours) makes it a less suitable drug for acute resuscitation; other inotropes are therefore currently used initially and, if required, levosimendan is introduced later. The long half-life (>5 days) of levosimendan confers a lasting impact on contractility after cessation of the infusion. Milrinone is also an effective inodilator,[75] but excessive vasodilation may contribute to significant hypotension; in practice, a concurrent vasoconstrictor (e.g. noradrenaline) may be administered. Close

TABLE 21.7
Vasoactive agents

DRUG	ACTIONS	DOSE RANGE	PHYSIOLOGICAL EFFECTS	NURSING CONSIDERATIONS
Dobutamine	Synthetic adrenergic agonist β_1-agonist β_2-agonist	100–200 mcg/min	Inotropy Vasodilation ↑↑ Cardiac output ↑ Blood pressure ↑ Heart rate	CVC administration Arrhythmia risk Excess dilation may cause hypotension
Dopamine	Dopaminergic β_1-agonist α-agonist (at higher doses)	'Inotropic' dose: 5–10 mcg/kg/min 'High' dose: 10–20 mcg/kg/min	Mainly inotropic ↑ Blood pressure ↑ Cardiac output Vasoconstriction dominates ↑↑ Blood pressure	CVC administration Tachycardia Arrhythmia risk Risk peripheral vascular compromise
Levosimendan	Calcium sensitiser	Loading: 6–12 mcg/kg over 10 min Infusion: 0.05–0.2 mcg/kg/min (max 24–48 h use)	Inotropy Vasodilation ↑↑ Cardiac output	Tachycardia Arrhythmia risk Risk hypokalaemia Risk Q-T prolongation Excess dilation may cause hypotension Half-life: 5 days
Adrenaline	Sympathomimetic α-agonist β_1-agonist β_2-agonist	1–20 mcg/min or higher	Potent inotrope and constrictor ↑ Cardiac output ↑↑ Blood pressure ↑↑ Heart rate	Tachycardia common Arrhythmia risk Risk peripheral vascular compromise Myocardial work
Milrinone	Phosphodiesterase inhibitor	Loading: 50–75 mcg/kg Infusion: 0.375–0.75 mcg/kg/min	Inotropy Potent vasodilator ↑↑ Cardiac output ↓ Blood pressure	Vasodilation may be marked Observe for hypotension
Noradrenaline	Sympathomimetic α-agonist β_1-agonist Little effect on β_2-receptors	1–20 mcg/min or higher	Potent inotrope and constrictor ↑↑ Blood pressure ↑ Coronary artery blood flow	Reflex bradycardias Arrhythmia risk Risk peripheral vascular compromise
Vasopressin	Vascular (V-1) receptors Renal (V-2) receptors	0.1–0.4 mcg/min	Inotropy ↑ SVR ↑ Vasoconstriction	Check liver function

CVC = central venous catheter; SVR = systemic vascular resistance; ↑ = increase; ↓ = decrease.
Adapted from Lampard JG, Lang E. Vasopressors for hypotensive shock. Ann Emerg Med 2013;61:351–2; Magder SA. The highs and lows of blood pressure: toward meaningful clinical targets in patients with shock. Crit Care Med 2014;42:1241–51.

management of intravascular fluid volume is critical when using these agents.

Dopamine and adrenaline are the major agents in the inoconstrictor class, and are more effective at raising blood pressure than inodilators. Both agents also increase cardiac output, but when there is significant impairment of contractility the increase in afterload may cause cardiac output to suffer. Importantly, inoconstrictors increase myocardial work and oxygen demands, raise heart rate and increase the risk of tachyarrhythmias; these impacts are stronger with adrenaline than for dopamine.

Afterload control

Specific management of afterload, independent of contractility, is sometimes necessary, although caution is needed as the maintenance of blood pressure often provides little scope for further afterload reduction.

Arteriodilators such as sodium nitroprusside reduce afterload and increase cardiac output, although with limitations due to hypotension.[77] The introduction of oral angiotensin-converting enzyme inhibitors is recommended as soon as possible after stabilisation of the patient with infarct-related cardiogenic shock.[78,79]

Adjunctive therapies

A range of adjunctive therapies is available for refractory shock, when first-line treatments are ineffective, and can include the use percutaneous mechanical circulatory support devices, which are now used more frequently[80] – these include, intra-aortic balloon pump (IABP) and extracorporeal membrane oxygenation (ECMO). Initiation of mechanical ventilation and correction of metabolic disturbances are also key interventions. These strategies are discussed below in relation to cardiogenic shock.

Intra-aortic balloon pumping

Low cardiac output, pulmonary congestion, reduced mean arterial pressure and myocardial ischaemia from cardiogenic shock may all be improved by the introduction of IABP therapy (see Chapter 12). Balloon inflation during diastole raises mean arterial pressure and promotes coronary and systemic blood flow, while balloon deflation in advance of systole reduces afterload. This afterload reduction improves cardiac output and reduces left ventricular systolic pressure, lessening the oxygen demands of the ischaemic ventricle by reducing the necessary contractile force of the left ventricle. In a large trial database, IABP did not impart a survival benefit at 12 months in an open label trial comparing outcomes from patients with early revascularisation and optimal medical management.[81] The IABP-SHOCK trial had some limitations with a high crossover rate, relatively small sample size, variable insertion timing.[80]

Extracorporeal membrane oxygenation

Extracorporeal membrane oxygenation (ECMO) is an accepted treatment of cardiac failure when persistent shock is evident despite adequate fluid resuscitation and administration of vasopressors and inotropes. There is a 40% survival to discharge in patients with cardiogenic shock.[82] ECMO is defined as the temporary use of a modified cardiopulmonary bypass circuit for support of patients with potentially reversible cardiac and/or respiratory failure.[83] ECMO provides a mechanism for gas exchange as well as cardiac support thereby allowing for recovery from existing disease. This therapy is complex and should be provided in centres where adequate facilities and human resources are available to ensure optimal implementation.[83] There are recommendations set for use of ECMO on the Extracorporeal Life Support Organisation website (see *Online resources*). Management of the patient receiving ECMO is complex. Often, more than one nurse is required to provide support in the first 24 hours. Large-bore catheters are used to ensure adequate extracorporeal circulation. Apart from the infective risk, disconnection poses a risk of rapid exsanguination. While ECMO provides cardiac support and gas exchange, it is vital to continue to promote recovery by maintaining cardiac function and reducing the risk of complications.

Respiratory support

Varying degrees of pulmonary oedema accompany cardiogenic shock, causing hypoxaemia due to intrapulmonary shunt, decreased compliance and increased work of breathing. Hyperventilation with respiratory alkalosis may initially compensate for hypoxaemia and lactic acidosis, but fatigue during this increased work of breathing may cause patient progression to hypoventilation and respiratory acidosis. Oxygen is administered for hypoxaemia, but the response may be limited as the primary gas exchange defect is an intrapulmonary shunt. Non-invasive ventilatory approaches may be sufficient, but intubation and mechanical ventilation may be required in the acute phase of treatment. Continuous positive airway pressure at conventional levels of 5–15 cmH_2O is well established as a support for the spontaneously breathing patient with pulmonary oedema.[84] This respiratory support strategy improves hypoxaemia, decreases work of breathing, reduces left ventricular afterload and provides additional benefit by impeding venous return, an effect that may lessen pulmonary congestion. These benefits are weighed against the potential for hypotension.

If hypoventilation and dyspnoea continue despite the use of continuous positive airway pressure, non-invasive bi-level positive airway pressure may be considered. Additional pressure support is applied during inspiration, above existing baseline pressure, improving inspiratory efficiency, with increased tidal volume and reduced work of breathing.[85,86] Endotracheal intubation and ventilation should be undertaken when neither strategy results in improvement, or when the patient continues to deteriorate or tire. Many clinicians prefer to intubate and ventilate early, even in the absence of a specific respiratory need, to decrease the cardiovascular demands of the greater ventilatory effort. However, this approach is controversial as mechanical ventilation is associated with poorer patient outcomes[86] and disturbs cardiovascular balance as it exerts changes to intrathoracic pressures, particularly at inspiratory initiation.

Ventilation strategies largely reflect those for other compliance disorders such as adult respiratory distress syndrome and are described in more detail in Chapter 15. Initially, full mechanical ventilation with little or no contribution from the patient is appropriate to correct arterial blood gases and lessen the cardiovascular demands of the ventilatory burden. Subsequent reduction of ventilatory support, as the patient's respiratory ability improves, follows conventional processes.

Biochemical normalisation

Frequent biochemistry measurement is necessary to detect and monitor the following aspects of care:

- arterial blood gases to identify the adequacy of ventilation and oxygenation and the presence of metabolic acidosis
- lactic acid measurement to assess the level of shock and changes in patient response to treatment
- hypokalaemia or hypomagnesaemia due to aggressive diuretic use
- hyperkalaemia due to severe acidosis, especially in the presence of renal failure
- hyperglycaemia due to the stress response to acute illness, and in response to sympathomimetic administration
- decline in bicarbonate levels due to pH buffering, although replacement therapy is not routinely undertaken unless the arterial pH is life-threatening
- urea and creatinine to detect the onset of acute renal failure due to renal hypoperfusion.

Renal replacement therapies may be used for fluid and electrolyte control when renal function suffers or as a strategy for unloading fluid from the circulation (see Chapter 18).

Sepsis and septic shock

Sepsis is a leading cause of admission to ICU and has an associated high mortality. Sepsis occurs in response to infection and can lead to organ system dysfunction and circulatory shock, resulting in high morbidity and mortality rates for hospitalised patients. New definitions published in 2016 highlight the complex pathophysiology of sepsis and septic shock.[87] The new definition of sepsis identifies that sepsis is a life-threatening organ dysfunction resulting from a dysregulated host response to infection.[87] Septic shock is defined as a subset of sepsis in which circulatory, cellular, and metabolic alterations are associated with a higher mortality rate than sepsis alone.[87] The use of the systemic inflammatory response syndrome (SIRS) criteria to identify sepsis was identified as not clinically useful as SIRS criteria can be present in many hospitalised patients, including those who never develop infection. A recent study of 1,171,797 patients from 172 ICUs in Australia and New Zealand over a 14-year timeline, found that among 109,663 who had infection and organ failure, 13,278 (12.1%) did not have SIRS criteria indicative of sepsis, highlighting that 1 in 8 patients admitted with infection and new organ failure had high rates of organ failure with significant morbidity and mortality, despite not meeting the SIRS criteria for the definition of sepsis.[88]

The third consensus definition task force recommended elimination of the terms sepsis syndrome, septicaemia, and severe sepsis. New criteria for identifying organ dysfunction in the ICU was outlined including use of the Sequential (sepsis-related) Organ Failure Assessment (SOFA) score. Variables required to calculate the SOFA include PaO_2/FiO_2 ratio, Glasgow Coma Scale score, mean arterial pressure, serum creatinine or urine output, bilirubin level, platelet count, and type, dose, and rate of vasopressor therapy. Organ dysfunction is identified as being represented by an increase in the SOFA score of 2 points or more.[87] The use of the quick SOFA (qSOFA) which incorporates altered mentation, systolic blood pressure of 100 mm Hg or less, and respiratory rate of 22/min or greater, is advocated for use to identify adult patients with suspected infection outside the ICU who are likely to have poor outcome.[87]

While estimates show trends towards decreasing case fatality, the incidence of sepsis cases is increasing at a larger rate,[89] and sepsis and septic shock result in a significant number of deaths annually.[90] In a report to the 70th World Health Assembly, it was reported that there are approximately six million deaths from sepsis worldwide every year, many of which were preventable.[91] It is estimated that there are 5000 deaths annually in Australia.[92]

The Surviving Sepsis Campaign

The Surviving Sepsis Campaign is an international collaborative formed after the Barcelona Declaration in 2002 to reduce the mortality of sepsis by 25% over a 5-year period. The aims included increasing awareness and developing treatment guidelines for severe sepsis and shock, including a comprehensive list of graded recommendations (now in its fifth edition).[93-96] World-wide Sepsis Day occurs on September 13 each year to continue the push for improving outcomes. Although the first version of the sepsis guidelines was supported by many countries, the second and much expanded version was not endorsed in Australia,[97] as many of the recommendations were based on research involving non-ICU and/or non-sepsis patients.

The most recent update of the 'Surviving Sepsis Campaign Guidelines' was published in 2017 and outlines evidence-based recommendations for the management of sepsis and septic shock.[90] Various recommendations have been combined to form a bundle,[98] which includes interventions or care elements implemented together to achieve better outcomes.[99] Bundles have been introduced to change processes of care and as quality or benchmarking measures (see Chapter 3). Further research and evaluation are needed as mortality benefits of 'care bundles' may be a result of increased clinician awareness rather than the impact of treatment changes.[100] In a recent meta-analysis of the previous 6- and 24-hour sepsis bundles, a better treatment effect was seen with the 6-hour bundle.[101] The current 1-hour bundle is updated on the Surviving Sepsis website. The current suggested sepsis bundle appears in Table 21.8.

Some bundles were developed then refuted, so it is important for critical care nurses to continuously update knowledge as further evidence becomes available. An example of a refuted bundle relates to tight glycaemic control. The recommendation in the Surviving Sepsis guidelines supported tight glycaemic control in earlier versions.[102,103] The NICE-SUGAR study subsequently concluded that measures to maintain blood glucose level of <10 mmol/L increased mortality, particularly

TABLE 21.8
Surviving sepsis 1-hour bundle[98]

BUNDLE ELEMENT	GRADE OF RECOMMENDATION AND LEVEL OF EVIDENCE
Measure lactate level. Re-measure if initial lactate is >2 mmol/L	Weak recommendation, low quality of evidence
Obtain blood cultures prior to administration of antibiotics	Best practice statement
Administer broad-spectrum antibiotics	Strong recommendation, moderate quality of evidence
Rapidly administer 30 mL/kg crystalloid for hypotension or lactate ≥ 4 mmol/L	Strong recommendation, low quality of evidence
Apply vasopressors if patient is hypotensive during or after fluid resuscitation to maintain MAP ≥ 65 mmHg	Strong recommendation, moderate quality of evidence

Reprinted with permission of Springer Nature. Levy MM, Evans LE, Rhodes A. The Surviving Sepsis Campaign Bundle: 2018 update. Intensive Care Med 2018;44:925. https://doi.org/10.1007/s00134-018-5085-0.

in relation to severe hypoglycaemia.[104] A meta-analysis of 26 ICU-related 'tight glycaemic control' studies suggested that the practice could increase risk to ICU patients.[105] The more pragmatic approach of maintaining blood glucose levels close to normal without inducing hypoglycaemia and other metabolic imbalances is therefore appropriate.[103] The 2016 version of the Surviving Sepsis Campaign recommends a protocolised approach to instituting insulin to manage hyperglycaemia when two consecutive measurements are >10 mmol/L with blood glucose measured every 1–2 hours until stable and then 4-hourly, preferably using arterial sampling to target an upper blood glucose 180 mg/dL (10 mmol/L).[90]

Clinical manifestations

Septic shock results when infectious agents or infection-induced mediators in the bloodstream produce haemodynamic compromise. Primarily a form of distributive shock, it is characterised by ineffective tissue oxygen delivery and extraction associated with inappropriate peripheral vasodilation, despite preserved or increased cardiac output.[65] Hypovolaemia is also associated with septic shock due to the characteristic increased vasodilation. This presents a clinical picture of a warm, pink and apparently well-perfused patient in early stages of septic shock with an elevated cardiac output, in contrast to that seen in hypovolaemic or cardiogenic shock patients.

Unchecked, cellular dysfunction in the presence of a failing compensatory process leads to cellular membrane damage, loss of ion gradients, leakage of lysosomal enzymes, proteolysis due to activation of cellular proteases and reductions in cellular energy stores that may result in cell death. Once enough cells from vital organs have reached this stage, shock becomes irreversible and death can occur despite eradication of the underlying septic focus. About half of patients who succumb to septic shock die of failure of multiple organs.[65]

The effect of sepsis and septic shock on the cardiovascular system is profound; the haemodynamic hallmark is generalised arterial vasodilation with an associated decrease in systemic vascular resistance. Arterial vasodilation is mediated in part by cytokines that upregulate the expression of inducible nitric oxide synthase in the vasculature. Vascular response to the vasodilatory effect of nitric oxide and the activation of adenosine triphosphate-sensitive potassium channels combine to cause closure of the voltage-gated calcium channels in the cell membrane. As the vasoconstrictor effect of noradrenaline and angiotensin II depends on open calcium channels, lack of response to these pressor hormones that are central to compensatory mechanisms in shock can occur with the inevitable failure of delivery of oxygen to the functional mitochondria, resulting in lactic acidosis in patients with sepsis.[106] With high circulating levels of endogenous vasoactive hormones during sepsis, downregulation of their receptors occurs.

Early identification and diagnosis

Where a patient can respond cogently during history and physical assessment, timelines of the infective process should be documented. Sites considered as infective sources include decubitus ulcers, invasive lines, drains, wounds, sinuses, ears, teeth, throat, chest, blood, lungs, back, abdomen, perianal, genital/urinary tract, bones and joints. More invasive sampling may include bronchioalveolar lavage, cerebral spinal fluid, pleural fluid, abdominal collections or biopsy of other sites as clinically appropriate. X-rays, computerised tomography scans and surgical consultation will also be a priority.

Patient management

As with other forms of shock, initial management includes not only acting to correct physiological deterioration by initiating fluid management and frequent observation and assessment, but also addressing the underlying cause of sepsis through source (of infection) control. Goal-directed therapy includes prevention of tissue hypoxia, typically through rigorous fluid resuscitation with either crystalloids or colloids to achieve specific haemodynamic end points, such as a central venous pressure of 8–12 mmHg, mean arterial pressure of >65 mmHg, and urine output >0.5 mL/kg/h. Vasopressor and inotropic therapy may then be added to maintain adequate perfusion pressure; noradrenaline is the vasopressor of choice because of vasoconstrictor effects.[90]

Initial resuscitation

The 2016 sepsis guidelines recommend managing sepsis and septic shock as medical emergencies, and instituting immediate resuscitation.[90] Resuscitation for sepsis-induced hypoperfusion is recommended with at least 30 mL/kg of intravenous crystalloid given within the first 3 hours. Additional fluids may be indicated based on frequent reassessment of hemodynamic status. The guidelines indicate that reassessment should include a thorough clinical examination and evaluation of available physiologic variables (heart rate, blood pressure, arterial oxygen saturation, respiratory rate, temperature, urine output, and others, as available) as well as other non-invasive or invasive monitoring, as available. An initial target mean arterial pressure of 65 mmHg is recommended in patients with septic shock requiring vasopressors. Resuscitation is recommended to normalise lactate in patients with elevated lactate levels as a marker of tissue hypoperfusion.[90]

Measuring surrogate markers of preload as an indicator of volume status is a contentious issue, as central venous pressure as a measure of preload is not a good marker of volume responsiveness.[26,107] While central venous pressure was used in many older sepsis trials of early goal-directed therapy protocols[29,108-110] and is an often-documented end point of resuscitation, early goal-directed therapy was widely discussed and criticised in the literature. The ProCESS trial,[111] the ARISE trial [112] and the ProMISe trial[113] have impacted the recommendations over the iterations of the surviving sepsis guidelines. Guiding resuscitation therapy to these indices is no longer recommended. The guidelines recommend the use of dynamic measures to assess the need for additional fluid resuscitation and predicting those patients who are likely to respond to a fluid challenge by increasing stroke volume. These techniques encompass passive leg raises, fluid challenges against stroke volume measurements, or the variations in systolic pressure, pulse pressure, or stroke volume to changes in intrathoracic pressure induced by mechanical ventilation.[90] Minimum continuous monitoring also includes electrocardiogram, blood pressure, pulse oximetry and other measures to assess preload and volume responsiveness, along with regular assessment of lactate, oxygenation and markers of inflammation and coagulation.

Source control and antimicrobial therapy

Identifying and removing the source of infection and treating the infection with appropriate antimicrobial therapy are the mainstays of therapy for a patient with sepsis. Research indicates that in the ICU setting the most prevalent site of primary infection is pulmonary, followed by abdominal, together accounting for approximately 70% of cases.[114-116]

To provide patients with appropriate antimicrobial treatment for targeting the infecting organism, obtaining appropriate samples prior to instigating antimicrobial therapy is the clinical standard, although any prescribed treatment should not be delayed as time to antibiotic administration is important in severe sepsis.[117] The Surviving Sepsis guidelines recommend that, to optimise identification of causative organisms, at least two blood cultures should be obtained before antimicrobial therapy with at least one drawn percutaneously and one drawn through each vascular access device.[90,95] In a large retrospective study, every additional hour to effective antimicrobial initiation in the first 6 hours after onset of hypotension was associated with >7% decrease in survival.[117,118] Optimising dosage to achieve a therapeutic concentration is also important. Current practice depends on the mechanism of action of the antibiotic. For example, glycopeptides are often continuously infused to maintain a serum concentration above the minimum inhibitory concentration and therefore kill microbes more effectively. More recently there has been evidence that beta-lactams should also be infused.[119] Beta-lactams are time-dependent and the concentration needs to be four times higher than the minimum inhibitory concentration in order to have efficacy.[120] Aminoglycosides have an effect through rapid administration to reach target concentrations and have a 'post-antibiotic effect'.

Recently, a paradigm shift has been suggested in relation to antimicrobial therapy: to get it right the first time with high doses, while limiting the duration of therapy and the potential to increase resistance.[121] Regardless, empirical therapy should be de-escalated as soon as microbiology results support directed therapy.

Haemodynamic support and adjunctive therapy

A range of drug therapies aimed at supporting and ameliorating the signs and symptoms of septic shock is available and, while inotropes in particular provide an important adjunct in managing the acute shock phase, other drug therapies remain controversial.

Fluid therapy in sepsis

Fluid resuscitation with crystalloid or colloid has long been controversial in the critical care literature. The landmark Saline versus Albumin Fluid Evaluation (SAFE) study[45] demonstrated that, in the adult intensive care patient population, albumin can be considered safe, without demonstrating any clear advantage over sodium chloride 0.9%. In the study, 6997 patients were randomised to receive either saline (n = 3500) or albumin (n = 3497). No significant differences were noted between the two treatment groups for 28-day all-cause mortality, days in intensive care, days in hospital, days on mechanical ventilation and days of renal replacement therapy.[45] In a predefined subgroup analysis of severe sepsis patients in this study, the adjusted odds ratio for death for albumin versus saline was 0.71.[122] There have been a number of landmark studies published since SAFE but the fluid of choice remains controversial. The Crystalloid versus Hydroxyethyl Starch Trial (CHEST)[47] compared 0.9% sodium chloride with 6% hydroxyethyl starch and showed that fluid resuscitation of all-comers requiring fluid resuscitation had no significant outcome difference at 90 days but higher levels of renal injury. Nearly 29% of patients in the study were septic.[123] Hydroxyethyl starch is not recommended for patients with sepsis. This study, along with the retraction of many research papers related to prior research,[124] led to changes globally in the recommendations for use of hydroxyethyl starch. More recently, the ProCESS trial showed no significant outcome difference between three resuscitation groups including two protocol-based approaches, early goal-directed therapy and standard resuscitation, and the third group of 'usual care'.[111] A 2013 Cochrane review of eligible randomised trials in critically ill patients supports the use of crystalloids for resuscitation given the lack of clear outcome benefit of other fluids.[125]

The Surviving Sepsis Campaign guidelines do not advocate a preferred resuscitation fluid but support fluid challenge in volume responsive patients. Crystalloids are recommended as the initial fluid choice (up to 30 mL/kg) and subsequent intravascular volume replacement for patients with sepsis and septic shock. Albumin is suggested when patients require a substantial fluid resuscitation.[90]

Irrespective of fluid selection, the disruption of the vascular bed in early septic shock through widespread vasodilatation results in increased capillary permeability and rapidly developing interstitial oedema. Large amounts of fluid can be administered without seemingly improving oxygen delivery while adding to developing generalised oedema that further impairs cellular delivery of oxygen and nutrients. Fluid resuscitation alone is therefore of limited value in septic shock and other measures must be considered.

Inotropes and vasopressors

A goal of maintaining mean arterial pressure greater than 65 mmHg is common, with inotropes and vasopressors commenced when fluid resuscitation is considered adequate. Administration of these drugs requires continuous blood pressure monitoring and enables effective titration to meet the treatment goal. The Surviving Sepsis guidelines recommend noradrenaline for its specific alpha-receptor effects as the first-choice vasopressor, with use of adrenaline (added or substituted) when an additional agent is needed, with the use of vasopressin 0.03 units/min added to or substituted for noradrenaline.

Dobutamine (2.5–10 mcg/kg) may be added to support patients who show evidence of persistent hypoperfusion despite adequate fluid loading and the use of vasopressor agents.[90] Refractory hypotension, resistant to vasopressors, has been linked to downregulation of receptors. Vasopressin (0.4–0.6 units/h) has been shown to reduce the requirements of other vasopressor agents.[126]

Administration of vasopressin in vasodilatory shock may help maintain blood pressure despite the relative ineffectiveness of other vasopressor hormones.[106] Specifically, arginine vasopressin may inactivate the KATP channels and thereby lessen vascular resistance to noradrenaline and angiotensin II. It also decreases the synthesis of nitric oxide (as a result of a decrease in the expression of nitric oxide synthase) as well as cyclic guanosine monophosphate signalling by nitric oxide.[106] The sites of major arterial vasodilation in sepsis – the splanchnic circulation, the muscles and the skin – are vascular beds that contain abundant arginine vasopressin receptors. In sepsis, vasopressin stores are quickly depleted. Administration of exogenous arginine vasopressin (0.04–0.06 units/min) can raise blood pressure by 25–50 mmHg by returning plasma concentrations of antidiuretic hormones to their earlier high levels.[106]

Steroids

The use of steroid therapy in severe sepsis remains controversial. At times, steroid replacement therapy may be used when patients display resistance to increasing doses of adrenergic agonists, as might occur in adrenal insufficiency. Some research indicates that patients with septic shock who are unable to increase cortisol levels in response to a challenge may benefit from administration of low-dose corticosteroids[127] (see Chapter 22). The Surviving Sepsis guidelines recommend not using intravenous hydrocortisone to treat adult septic shock patients if adequate fluid resuscitation and vasopressor therapy are able to restore haemodynamic stability. Where this is not achievable, the use of intravenous hydrocortisone alone at a dose of 200 mg per day is recommended.

Supportive therapy

The Surviving Sepsis guidelines outline several areas of supportive therapy including blood product administration, renal replacement therapy, stress ulcer prophylaxis, deep vein thrombosis prophylaxis and nutritional support. Red blood cell transfusion is recommended only when the haemoglobin concentration decreases to <7.0 g/dL in adults in the absence of myocardial ischaemia, severe hypoxia or acute haemorrhage. The use of fresh frozen plasma to correct clotting abnormalities is not recommended in the absence of bleeding or planned invasive procedures. Additionally, prophylactic platelet transfusion is not recommended when counts are <10,000/mm^3 (10 × 109/L) in the absence of apparent bleeding and when counts are <20,000/mm^3 (20 × 109/L) if the patient has a significant risk of bleeding. Higher platelet counts (≥ 50,000/mm^3 [50 × 109/L]) are advised for active bleeding, surgery, or invasive procedures.[90]

The Surviving Sepsis guidelines recommend either continuous or intermittent renal replacement therapy for patients with sepsis and acute kidney injury. The guidelines also recommend that patients with sepsis receive pharmacologic prophylaxis (unfractionated heparin or low-molecular-weight heparin) for venous thromboembolism in the absence of contraindications to the use of these agents.[90] Translocation of gut bacteria due to splanchnic hypoperfusion and increased permeability is a factor in secondary septic insults and stress ulceration[128] (see Chapter 20). The guidelines recommend stress ulcer prophylaxis for patients with sepsis or septic shock who have risk factors for gastrointestinal bleeding using either proton pump inhibitors or histamine-2 receptor antagonists (see Chapter 20). In critically ill patients, early initiation of enteral feeding is recommended rather than a complete fast or only intravenous glucose. The use of parenteral nutrition alone or parenteral nutrition in combination with enteral feedings is not recommended for patients who can be fed enterally. Chapter 19 provides further discussion of the nutrition support relevant to patients with sepsis. Equally important to patient-specific measures is institution of diligent infection control practices in ICU.[129]

As the patient with sepsis and shock has a high mortality rate, addressing goals of care is an additional area of focus recommended in the guidelines. The guidelines outline that the prognosis for achieving goals of care and the level of certainty for the prognosis be discussed with patients and families; that treatment plans should incorporate palliative care principles and, as appropriate, end-of-life care planning; and that goals of care be addressed as early as feasible but no later than within 72 hours of ICU admission. As critical care nursing promotes patient- and family-centred care, addressing the needs of families and providing ongoing information and support are essential.

Symptom management of fever is prevalent in hospitals. Treatment with medicines that have an antipyretic effect has been considered a standard of care without the support of good evidence. Fever is an adaptive response to infection and is beneficial in activating various immune responses. The HEAT trial[130] explored if permissive hyperthermia through avoidance of paracetamol in known or suspected infection in ICU improves survival to 28 days. The intervention and control groups had similar outcomes.[131] The evidence about temperature management in shock states and sepsis is conflicting and should be managed depending on the clinical circumstances.[132]

Anaphylaxis

Anaphylaxis is the most severe, potentially life-threatening form of an allergic or hypersensitivity reaction,[133-137] and is mostly immunoglobulin E-mediated.[138] Food-induced anaphylaxis has been defined by the National Institute of Allergy and Infectious Diseases as a serious allergic reaction that is rapid in onset, typically mediated by immunoglobulin E, involving systemic mediator release from sensitive mast cells and basophils.[139] Food-induced anaphylaxis is being increasingly studied due to increasing prevalence because of both genetic and unspecified environmental factors.[140] Food anaphylaxis has the same mechanism and clinical manifestations as other allergens with sensitised mast cells and basophils. Exercise-induced anaphylaxis, where a reaction depends on the temporal association of allergen ingestion and exercise, has also been described.[139]

Allergies are common; however, anaphylaxis appears rare.[135] Although data are sporadic in the literature, 0.01–0.02% of the general population is affected.[138] Anaphylaxis appears more common in Western countries with a rising incidence,[139,141,142] but this may be related to better reporting mechanisms. The prevalence of allergy with anaphylaxis has been documented to be as high as 7% in an Australian study of children, with insect stings, oral medications or food the most often cited causes. However, in this study, less than 1% of the population actually suffered an anaphylactic reaction manifesting with generalised multisystem allergic reaction, including evidence of airway involvement, rashes, gastrointestinal and cardiovascular dysfunction.[143] The published American prevalence is based on large population surveys and estimates that anaphylaxis affects 1.6% of the population.[144] There have been more than 100 food allergens identified but there are a few responsible for most reactions and this differs based on geographical location[141,142] and cannot always be explained by genetic factors.[140] The International Collaboration in Asthma, Allergy and Immunology are developing consensus guidelines to support management.[141]

Three criteria have been established in order to rapidly diagnose anaphylaxis as set out in Box 21.4.[139] There are currently no recommended biomarkers to support clinical diagnosis although histamine and tryptase are sometimes used.[145]

Clinical manifestations

The allergic response is via a host mast-cell reaction mediated by immunoglobulin E,[133] and antibody produced in response to the allergen that is attached to basophils (mast cells). Once sensitised to an allergen, subsequent exposure may lead to an anaphylactic reaction in affected individuals. One suggested mechanism is that subsequent exposure leads to mast-cell–allergen complexes and the release of histamine.[146] Reactions to an allergen cannot be predicted, however, and subsequent exposure may lead to either an amplified or lesser response.[134] There may be an initial reaction, which subsides with treatment over about 24 hours, but there has been described a second or rebound reaction up to 8–10 hours after initial exposure to an allergen.[133]

Exposure to an allergen causes release of histamine and other mediators, with subsequent vasodilation and increased microvascular permeability – a distributive form of shock. Histamine peaks at 5–10 min and is metabolised rapidly, returning to baseline within 60 min. Other mediators have a sustained effect.[138] This makes histamine a poor clinical biomarker for anaphylaxis. The antigen–antibody reaction may directly damage vascular walls, while release of vasoactive mediators, such

BOX 21.4

Diagnostic criteria for anaphylaxis

1 Acute onset of an illness (over minutes to several hours) involving skin, mucosal tissue or both (for example, generalised hives, pruritus or flushing, swollen lips/tongue/uvula), plus either:
   a Respiratory compromise (for example, dyspnoea, wheeze/bronchospasm, stridor, reduced peak expiratory flow rate, hypoxaemia)
   b Reduced blood pressure (BP) or associated symptoms of end-organ dysfunction (for example, hypotonia [circulatory collapse], syncope, incontinence) or:
2 **Two** or more of the following that occur rapidly after exposure to a likely allergen for that patient (minutes to several hours):
   a Involvement of the skin/mucosal tissue (for example, generalised hives, itch/flush, swollen lips/tongue/uvula)
   b Respiratory compromise (for example, dyspnoea, wheeze/bronchospasm, stridor, reduced peak expiratory flow rate, hypoxaemia)
   c Reduced BP or associated symptoms of end-organ dysfunction (for example, hypotonia, syncope, incontinence)
   d Persistent GI symptoms (for example, crampy abdominal pain, vomiting) or
3 Age-related decrease in systolic BP or a greater than 30% decrease from baseline after exposure to a known allergen for that patient (minutes to several hours):
   a 1 month to 1 year: systolic BP of less than 70 mmHg
   b 1–10 years old: systolic BP of less than (70 mmHg plus twice the age)
   c 11 years to adult: systolic BP of less than 90 mmHg or greater than 30% decrease from baseline

as histamine, serotonin, bradykinins and prostaglandins, triggers a systemic response, resulting in vasodilation and increased capillary permeability, with widespread loss of fluid into the interstitial space and hypovolaemia. Blood pressure and cardiac output/index may fall with a compensatory rise in heart rate. Severe bronchospasm may also occur from mediator-induced bronchial oedema and pulmonary smooth muscle contraction. Abdominal pain is thought to be due to the inflammation of Peyer's patches, which are clusters of lymphatic tissue containing B lymphocytes, located in the mucosa and submucosa of the small intestine.[146]

A list of signs and symptoms for anaphylaxis appears in Table 21.9. It is thought that anaphylaxis is sometimes misdiagnosed because up to 20% of presentations do not have obvious cutaneous signs.[139] Anaphylaxis should be considered when there are two or more organ systems involved.[144] There is a high mortality in patients with asthma and those on beta-blocker or angiotensin-converting enzyme inhibitor medications;[134,147] these medications may limit the effectiveness of adrenaline therapy. Age and preexisting lung disease are the most important factors in relation to severity; older people and those with asthma or airways disease have a higher risk of a life-threatening reaction.[146]

Patient management

Initial management

Diagnosis of an anaphylactic reaction requires an appropriate assessment and history, including acute onset, history of allergic reaction and initial measures instituted to support airway, breathing and circulation. Removal of the causative agent, if possible, and treatment within 30 min of exposure to an allergen result in improved outcomes.

The Australian and New Zealand Anaesthetic Allergy Group have produced a consensus guideline (see *Online resources*) and devised a number of useful resources to support management of anaphylaxis during anaesthesia.[148] These guidelines are broadly applicable in critical care units. See *Practice tip* for a list of suggested anaphylaxis emergency equipment.

Practice tip

Anaphylaxis emergency box

- Adrenaline 1:1000 (consider adrenaline autoinjector availability in rural locations for initial administration by nursing staff)
- 1-mL syringes; 21-gauge needles
- Oxygen
- Airway equipment, including nebuliser and suction
- Defibrillator
- Manual blood pressure cuff
- Intravenous access equipment (including large-bore cannulae)
- Pressure sleeve (aids rapid infusion of fluid under pressure)
- At least 3 L of normal saline

Measures to assess and support airway, breathing and circulation are important, considering the rapid impact of circulating mediators and potential decline in respiratory and cardiovascular function. Securing the airway

TABLE 21.9
Symptoms of allergic reactions

ORGAN SYSTEM	IMMEDIATE SYMPTOMS	DELAYED SYMPTOMS
Cutaneous	Erythema Pruritus Urticaria Morbilliform eruption Angioedema	Erythema Flushing Pruritus Morbilliform eruption Angio-oedema Eczematous rash
Ocular	Pruritus Conjunctival erythema Tearing Periorbital oedema	Pruritus Conjunctival erythema Tearing Periorbital oedema
Upper respiratory	Nasal congestion Pruritus Rhinorrhoea Sneezing Laryngeal oedema Hoarseness Dry staccato cough	
Lower respiratory	Cough Chest tightness Dyspnoea Wheezing Intercostal retractions Accessory muscle use	Cough, dyspnoea, wheezing
GI (oral)	Angio-oedema of the lips, tongue or palate Oral pruritus Tongue swelling	
GI (lower)	Nausea Colicky abdominal pain Reflux Vomiting Diarrhoea	Nausea Abdominal pain Reflux Vomiting Diarrhoea Haematochezia Irritability and food refusal with weight loss (young children)
Cardiovascular	Tachycardia (occasionally bradycardia in anaphylaxis) Hypotension Dizziness Fainting Loss of consciousness	
Miscellaneous	Uterine contractions Sense of 'impending doom'	

Adapted from Sampson HA, Munoz-Furlong A, Campbell RL, et al. Second symposium on the definition and management of anaphylaxis: summary report – Second National Institute of Allergy and Infectious Disease/Food Allergy and Anaphylaxis Network Symposium. [Reprint in Ann Emerg Med. 2006 Apr;47(4):373-80; PMID: 16546624]. J Allergy Clin Immunol 2006;117:391–7, with permission.

TABLE 21.10
Adrenaline doses

AGE (years)	WEIGHT (kg)	VOLUME OF ADRENALINE 1:1000	ADRENALINE AUTOINJECTORS
<1	5–10	0.05–0.1 mL	
1–2	10	0.1 mL	10–20 kg (~1–5 years): 0.15 mg (green-labelled) device
2–3	15	0.15 mL	
4–6	20	0.2 mL	
7–10	30	0.3 mL	>20 kg (~>5 years): 0.3 mg (yellow-labelled) device
10–12	40	0.4 mL	
>12 and adults	>50	0.5 mL	

Reproduced with permission from the Australasian Society of Clinical Immunology and Allergy (ASCIA). The latest version of the source document can be found here www.allergy.org.au/hp/papers/acute-management-of-anaphylaxis-guideline.

and providing high oxygen concentration is vital as most anaphylactic-related deaths are due to asphyxiation.[138] Adrenaline is recommended as first-line drug treatment[134,138,146] and in a recent systematic review the evidence suggested prompt use of adrenaline to reduce the risk of death.[137] Administration is usually via intramuscular injection (to the vastus lateralis muscle or mid-outer thigh) as it leads to a more rapid increase in plasma concentration than subcutaneous administration.[137] The first dose is often given using the patient's own injecting device (e.g. Epipen or Anapen) for common food and venom allergies as they are more likely to occur out of hospital. Subsequent doses are usually required once a patient is in hospital. The Australasian Society of Clinical Immunology and Allergy Incorporated suggest intramuscular adrenaline in the doses suggested in Table 21.10.[149]

Intravenous doses of adrenaline depend on the severity and condition of the patient. If the patient is unresponsive and life support algorithms are in play, the dose of adrenaline is 1 mg as per the International Liaison Committee on Resuscitation Guidelines and the algorithms for cardiopulmonary resuscitation are followed for subsequent dosing. The dose of adrenaline administered in anaphylaxis for patients that have not been managed with Advanced Life Support algorithms is more controversial. When a continuous infusion is required for ongoing symptom management it is suggested an adrenaline infusion be prepared and administered at a dose of 0.1 mcg/kg/min with titration to maintain the desired blood pressure. The same monitoring as for any patient on an adrenaline infusion should be used including continuous blood pressure.[148,149]

Aggressive fluid resuscitation (20 mL/kg) is also usually required[148,149] as the intravascular blood volume may quickly be depleted by up to 70%. The type of fluid used in resuscitation can vary and, if a colloid is being administered to the patient and there is no known other trigger for the reaction, the colloid should cease as it may be responsible.[148] A maximum of 50 mL/kg in the first 30 min is suggested for persistent hypotension.[148,149]

Airway management

Early elective intubation is recommended for patients with airway oedema, stridor or any oropharyngeal swelling. Patients with airway swelling and/or angio-oedema are at high risk for rapid deterioration and respiratory compromise.[148] Late presentation to hospital or delayed intubation when airway swelling is present may mean that intubation and other emergency airway procedures may be extremely difficult. Multiple attempts at intubation increase laryngeal oedema or cause trauma to the airway. Early recognition of the potentially difficult airway allows planning for alternative airway management by experts in difficult airways.

Adjunctive support

Adjunctive drugs include histamine$_1$- (H_1) and $_h$istamine$_2$ (H_2)-antagonists, antihistamines, corticosteroids and other beta$_2$-agonists for airway symptoms. The H_2-antagonists are competitive antagonists of histamine at the parietal cell H_2 receptor. A systematic review assessed the evidence related to efficacy of H_2-antihistamines. The review did not find any studies based on the inclusion criteria and made no specific treatment recommendation.[136] However, it seems at this stage that it is likely to be beneficial to block both H_1 and H_2 receptors when urticaria is present.[137] H_1-antihistamines are also helpful to reduce pruritus.[137] It is important to note the use of antihistamines is not recommended for anaphylaxis crisis management.[149]

Corticosteroids (1 mg/kg up to 200 mg)[149] may be beneficial for persistent bronchospasm, asthma and severe cutaneous reactions but not in acute management,[148,149] and their use remains unproven.[149] Glucagon and noradrenaline may be required for patients on beta-blockers who may have resistant severe hypotension and bradycardia.[150] Glucagon exerts positive inotropic and chronotropic effects, independently of catecholamines, while atropine may reverse bradycardia. Vasopressin and other vasopressors such as metaraminol are suggested where shock is refractory to adrenaline.[138] Given that a second reaction (biphasic) may occur after the initial allergic response, monitoring should continue for up to 48 hours.[138]

Preventative care

There is no current cure for anaphylaxis.[141] Individuals with known allergies are taught avoidance of allergens as a first line, and then to have a management plan for inadvertent exposure including the use of emergency kits with adrenaline for intramuscular injection (Epipen).[135,141,146,151] Antihistamines are also used in food allergy to manage non-severe reactions and immune-modulating pharmacological agents are a probable future direction for management.[139] Desensitisation therapy may also reduce severity of symptoms and therefore improve quality of life.

Neurogenic/spinal shock

Neurogenic shock is a form of distributive shock caused by loss of vasomotor (sympathetic) tone from disruption to or inhibition of neural output. Characteristics include a systolic blood pressure <90–100 mmHg and a heart rate <80 beats/min without other obvious causes.[152] Note that the heart rate is within otherwise accepted normal limits. Most often it is described as a triad of hypotension, bradycardia and hypothermia. However, the precise mechanisms are unknown.[153] The primary cause is a spinal cord injury above T6, secondary to disruption of sympathetic outflow from T1–L2 and to unopposed vagal tone, leading to decreased vascular resistance and associated vascular dilation and increased activity below the injury level.[154] It may also develop after anaesthesia, particularly spinal, cerebral medullary ischaemia or when there is spinal cord complete or partial injury above the mid-thoracic region (thoracic outflow tract).

Spinal shock is a subclass of neurogenic shock, with a transient physiological (rather than anatomical) reflex depression of cord function below the level of injury and associated loss of sensorimotor functions. Incidence has been reported at 14% of patients presenting to the ED within 2 hours of injury and predominantly[152] affects up to 20% of patients with cervical damage and lasts up to 5 weeks after an injury.[154] Spinal shock can also occur with a spinal cord laceration or contusion, and is associated with varying degrees of motor and sensory deficit (see also Chapters 17 and 23). Trauma is frequently the reason for primary injury,[152] with traffic accidents, assault, falls at work and sport the most common causes and a 4:1 ratio of males to females.[155] Simultaneous injuries may also be responsible for haemodynamic compromise,[152] and neurogenic shock with hypotension may have multiple aetiologies.[153] Haemorrhagic shock in combination with neurogenic shock has a poor outcome.

Clinical manifestations

Inhibited sympathetic outflow results in dominance of the parasympathetic nervous system, with a reduction in systemic vascular resistance and lowered blood pressure. Preload to the right heart is reduced, which lowers stroke volume and subsequent cardiac output/index. The usual response to reduction in cardiac output (a raised heart rate) does not occur due to the parasympathetic nervous system and blockage of sympathetic compensatory responses, and the patient may be bradycardic and hypotensive[154]with their skin warm and dry.

In spinal shock there may be an initial rise in blood pressure due to release of catecholamines, followed by hypotension,[154] which usually resolves within 24 hours.[155] Flaccid areflexic paralysis,[155] including that of the bladder and bowel, is observed and sustained priapism may also develop. Symptoms may last hours to days, until the reflex arcs below the level of injury begin to regain function. This is a result of damage to the spinal cord, and obvious manifestations include pale, cold skin above the site of injury, and warm, pink skin below the site of injury. Anhidrosis (absence of sweating) may be present. Heart rate may be slow, requiring intervention.

Secondary injury may occur from impaired vasomotor tone, ischaemia, thrombosis, increased permeability, inflammatory and cellular dysfunction. Spinal cord oedema occurs 3–6 days after injury and may lead to a shocked state.[155]

Patient management

The extent of injury, whether complete (no sensory or motor function) or incomplete (some sensory or motor function), determines clinical medical management. Priority focuses on airway, breathing and circulation. The riskiest time is the first 7–10 days after injury.[156]

Haemodynamic support is required and is usually provided in an escalating manner with fluid first followed by pharmacological agents to maintain targets. Mean arterial pressure augmentation may be required but is the subject of ongoing debate.[156] Spinal surgery has better outcomes when performed within 24 hours of the trauma.[154]

Initial stabilisation and neck immobilisation

After neck and torso stabilisation, the patient with confirmed or suspected spinal cord injury is placed in a position that supports spinal precautions (neutral neck positioning with immobilisation) with spinal boards removed within 20 min if possible. Immobilisation may be achieved with sandbags either side of the head, the use of collars and log rolling.[155] Caution for spinal instability remains despite medical imaging clearance, due to the potential for spinal ligament damage. The patient is positioned supine, with their legs in alignment with the torso.

Elevation of the head may cause pooling of blood in the lower limbs, exacerbating hypotension,[154] and makes the patient sensitive to sudden position changes. It is important to note that while this is a standard practice it also may cause additional unintended issues for the patient such as discomfort, occipital pressure areas and impaired respiratory function. These precautions also inhibit airway interventions and increase risk of aspiration and raised intracranial pressure.[155]

Fluid therapy

Loss of sympathetic outflow requires close cardiac and haemodynamic monitoring for bradycardia and hypotension. Cardiovascular complications such as hypotension, bradycardia and arrythmias are common after spinal cord injury.[157] Symptomatic bradycardia is treated and may require cardiac pacing if unresponsive to atropine. Therapies include fluid resuscitation with the addition of inotropes, if necessary, to improve vasomotor function. This increases preload and maintains a mean arterial pressure >80–85 mmHg[156] to restore spinal cord perfusion and to prevent secondary neuronal hypoperfusion.[158] This higher (supranormal) mean arterial pressure may be targeted to improve recovery and prevent secondary injuries.[158] Volume expansion with colloids and crystalloids or blood products will vary depending on patient situation; however, subgroup analysis in the SAFE trial indicated that colloids and hypotonic solutions may not be the best options.[45]

Respiratory support

Respiratory insufficiency is common[156] and, as such, respiratory function is closely monitored to prevent or minimise atelectasis, pneumonia[158] and secretion retention. The level of injury is indicative of the potential for respiratory muscle weakness (Table 21.11). The diaphragm is innervated by the phrenic nerve (originating at C3–C5); any injury above C3 leads to complete respiratory muscle paralysis and patients will require ventilatory support.[158] Incomplete injuries between C3 and C5 may also require ventilation initially but subsequently recover some respiratory function. Intubation is complicated by any spinal cord injury as airway interventions cause some level of spinal movement and respiratory failure is an independent predictor of mortality in spinal cord injury.[155] Coughing, and therefore secretion clearance, is reliant on 'expiratory muscles' and, for patients with injuries that interfere with abdominal and intercostal muscle function, careful monitoring of the work of breathing and secretion clearance should be initiated. There will be varying levels of decreased respiratory function with substantially reduced lung volumes.

TABLE 21.11
Respiratory muscle innervation by cord level

CORD LEVEL INNERVATION	ACCESSORY MUSCLE
C3–C5 (mostly C4)	Diaphragm
C6	Serratus anterior Latissimus dorsi Pectoralis
T1–11	Intercostals
T6–L1	Abdominals

Adjunctive support

Hypothermia may be present, resulting from dilated peripheral blood vessels allowing radiant loss of heat. A patient is monitored for core temperature changes, and external warming devices may be required.

Paralytic ileus is a concern in the acute phase of injuries above T5, where disruption of integrative innervation pathways leads to unmodulated colonic functioning[159] and peristaltic hypomotility. Ileus may lead to respiratory compromise and should be managed. The patient should remain 'nil by mouth' and treatment includes gastric decompression, adequate intravenous hydration and electrolyte balance. Drug therapy with prokinetics, probiotics, aperients and intravenous neostigmine or lignocaine has been reported to be useful.

Pressure care is attended every second hour and, where Jordan frames are used, slats should be removed between use. The patient is susceptible to deep venous thrombosis[157] particularly high risk when spinal cord injury is involved, so sequential calf compression devices and other prophylaxis such as anticoagulants are initiated early with D-dimers monitored regularly.

Resuscitation end points

End points of resuscitation in shock states are similar but will differ depending on the cause. Table 21.12 outlines some of the discussed targets.

TABLE 21.12
Resuscitation end points

PARAMETER	TARGETS/RECOMMENDATIONS	PRECAUTIONS
Blood pressure	Target diastolic blood pressure ≥65 mmHg[2] Target systolic blood pressure >90 mmHg as soon as possible	This target may be higher depending on pre-morbid state and specific organ requirements such as closed head injury or haemorrhagic shock
Urine output	Target ≥0.5 mL/h	
Serum lactate levels	There is evidence that serum lactate is a clear marker for outcome in patients[176] There have been suggestions that any patient with a lactate >4 should be managed in a critical care environment Improving lactate levels to 'normal' is associated with improved survival	For patients presenting to emergency with a suspicion of sepsis it should be measured and assessed in the first hour
Arterial base deficit	In combination with lactate base deficit in shock is related to oxygen transport imbalance at the cellular level and it is a good marker with lactate level for adequacy of resuscitation[177]	A high base deficit (≥4) is indicative of abnormal oxygen utilisation and patients have a higher mortality
Oxygen monitoring	Monitoring of oxygen saturation is readily available and required when any shock state is suspected It is important to assess oxygen requirements even in the setting of acceptable oxygen saturation as increasing requirement is indicative of deterioration P/F ratio (partial pressure of oxygen-to-fraction of inspired oxygen ratio) may be used as a guide to assess the level of dysfunction given that the normal result is approximately 500 (100/0.21) Oxygenation should also be assessed through arterial blood gas sampling and utilisation assumptions may be made by comparing with a venous sample	A P/F ratio <250 in the presence of high supplemental oxygen should be regarded as indicative of serious respiratory dysfunction Any patient requiring maximum oxygen support should be investigated
Mixed venous oxygen saturation	Normal mixed venous oxygen saturation levels are between 60% and 80% It may be used to guide resuscitation but is an invasive method of monitoring Haemoglobin should be measured in conjunction with this variable	A reduced mixed venous saturation indicates increasing extraction and worsening shock state High levels may be seen that may be indicative of cellular dysfunction in relation to oxygen extraction
End-tidal carbon dioxide	End-tidal carbon dioxide monitors usually provide both numeric and graphic waveform displays of the concentration using non-invasive measurement of exhaled carbon dioxide End-tidal carbon dioxide is an estimate of the patient's alveolar ventilation status 'Stat cap' devices are standard on resuscitation trolleys for supporting confirmation of endotracheal tube placement by quickly establishing if carbon dioxide is exhaled	End-tidal carbon dioxide monitoring is unreliable in the setting of increased ventilation perfusion mismatch with worsening arterial carbon dioxide retention and increased peripheral carbon dioxide production[16]
Preload	Preload should be maximised without overstretching Usually this is achieved using fluid bolus in shock states (refer to the relevant sections)	Where preload is leading to congestion and cardiac failure, pharmacotherapy and ventilator support may be required
Right ventricular end-diastolic volume index	Provides a clinical estimate of right ventricular preload and has a normal adult parameter of 60–100 mL/m^2 Observing for changes with fluid challenge may support resuscitation by providing information about volume responsiveness[2]	

TABLE 21.12

Resuscitation end points—cont'd

PARAMETER	TARGETS/RECOMMENDATIONS	PRECAUTIONS
Afterload	Afterload reduction strategies are employed in many shocked states to improve cardiac output as increased afterload increases the work of the myocardium Afterload is affected by vascular resistance Calculations for SVR are used to measure afterload	During shock states, resistance is increased through constriction and oxygen and energy are required for function
Contractility	Contractility is not easily measured clinically but the improvement would be observed usually by increased cardiac output or other surrogate measures with the addition of inotropes	
Temperature	Thermoregulation is an essential homeostatic mechanism. Many critically ill patients will have an elevated temperature. The literature is variable about management of temperature in different shock states[132]	Treatment of temperature may differ between shock states particularly in relation to patients with traumatic brain injury, sepsis and post-cardiac arrest

P/F ratio = PaO_2/FiO_2.; SVR= systemic vascular resistance.

Summary

Shock is a generic term describing a syndrome and pervasive set of potentially life-threatening symptoms. The pathophysiological changes associated with shock feature a complex interaction of generic compensatory mechanisms that attempt to sustain perfusion and particularly oxygen delivery to the vital organ systems of the body. These protective responses are particularly strong in supporting cerebral perfusion and combine responses from the sympathetic nervous, endocrine and adrenal/renal systems. As shock develops cellular dysfunction occurs in response to the release of a large collection of systemic and local inflammatory mediators, which inevitably overwhelm cell function and lead to diffuse organ injury if shock continues unabated. The classification system described here differentiates shock into categories including hypovolaemic, cardiogenic and distributive; classification is dependent on aetiology. Distributive shock states result in impaired oxygen and nutrient delivery to the tissues as a result of failure of the vascular system (the blood distribution system). While there may be additional factors (e.g. infection) beyond simple failure to provide sufficient perfusion to the capillary bed due to widespread vascular dilation, the common factor for all underlying causes of distributive shock is widespread failure of the vasculature. The most common categories of distributive shock are associated with SIRS, anaphylaxis and neurogenic shock.

Clear assessment is required to distinguish the type of shock aids in appropriate treatment decisions, targeting the cause and managing associated symptoms. Critical care nurses are in a position to provide clear assessment and first-line emergency management of the various shock states. Collaborative integrated care is important to provide the patient with the best possible outcome.

Case study

An independent 68-year-old man, James, presented to the ED at 2330 hours with abdominal pain, diarrhoea, nausea and vomiting for the past day. James had a history of gastroenteritis, Crohn's disease with two prior surgeries for colectomies, type 2 diabetes and hypertension. His initial observations in the ED included a blood pressure of 133/75 mmHg, heart rate of 102 beats/min, temperature of 37.8°C and respiratory rate of 20 breaths/min, with an oxygen saturation of 95%. Routine blood tests were ordered and 1000 mL of intravenous balanced salt solution (lactated ringers) was given as a 'bolus' due to suspected dehydration. Intravenous metoclopramide 10 mg was administered, and blood cultures were taken after James had been in the department for approximately 4 hours.

The next set of observations included a temperature of 38.7°C. James was also noted to be drowsy with a score on the Glasgow Coma Scale (GCS) of 14. He was then transferred to the medical assessment unit pending admission to the medical ward.

The next morning James was reviewed on the ward round and he continued to be drowsy with intermittent abdominal pain and continuing but decreased episodes of diarrhoea. His observations included an increased temperature of 38.5°C, blood pressure of 120/80 mmHg and oxygen saturation of 94% on room air. His ongoing diagnosis was gastroenteritis although other types of infection were considered given his prior medical issues. A stool culture was ordered and IV metronidazole and vancomycin prescribed. A note was made in the patient's medical record to administer the antibiotics and following checking of blood culture results. An abdominal computerised tomography (CT) scan was ordered. Just after James left for the scan, the hospital microbiology department contacted the ward to report a preliminary positive blood culture for gram-positive cocci – this was not communicated to the staff in radiology or to the attending physician.

One of the scanners malfunctioned and James had to wait on a gurney in the hallway for 2 hours prior to the CT scan. During the scan, the technician noted an increase in heart rate to 118 beats/min and a blood pressure of 100/80 mmHg, respiratory rate was 22 breaths/min. A medical officer was called to review him as he was looking unwell and during the CT scan had rigours with increasing abdominal discomfort. The medical officer took additional blood cultures, ordered a stat dose of vancomycin after reviewing current blood pathology, noting the positive culture and increased white cell count of 24 $\times 10^9$/L.

When the CT scan was concluded James returned to the medical unit. He arrived after shift change and there was no handover provided. An hour after his return to the ward his observations included a temp of 39.2°C, respiratory rate of 22 breaths/min, SpO_2 88% on room air and heart rate of 122 beats/min with a decreased level of consciousness. These observations automatically triggered an immediate clinical emergency response call.

James was assessed by the medical emergency team and transferred to ICU for ongoing care. He received non-invasive ventilation to maintain oxygen saturations >94% and tolerated that for 2 hours; however, his respiratory status declined, and he required intubation and mechanical ventilation to support respiratory function and noradrenaline to support blood pressure and continuous renal replacement therapy commenced. James was persistently febrile over the next few days even with vancomycin in a therapeutic range. James also had a fluctuating GCS and repeat CT scans indicated changes consistent with multiple cerebral infarcts.

James's poor prognosis was considered by the medical team and discussed with his family. There was a decision made not to escalate interventions and to ensure James's comfort by instituting palliative measures. James died 12 days after admission.

This case study is a good example of care provided with confirmation bias towards gastroenteritis due to his history of Crohn's disease that probably led to less importance placed on providing antibiotic therapy. The delay to treatment may have been implicated in James's decline and, given his pre-admission status, every effort should have been made to prevent this. Hospital processes and transfers between services are risky times where handover may be limited or incomplete. It is important in these cases to consider the checking procedures to ensure all interventions have been performed.

CASE STUDY QUESTIONS

1 Identify possible sources of infection for James.
2 What early clinical indications are there that James's condition is progressing from sepsis to septic shock?
3 What opportunities existed during James's time in the ED to optimise his 'sepsis path'?

RESEARCH VIGNETTE

Tirkkonen et al. Outcome of adult patients attended by rapid response teams: a systematic review of the literature. Resuscitation 2017;112:43-52

Abstract

Background: An abundance of studies have investigated the impact of rapid response teams (RRTs) on in-hospital cardiac arrest rates. However, existing RRT data appear highly variable in terms of both study quality and reported uses of limitations of care, patient survival and patient long-term outcome.

Methods: A systematic electronic literature search (January 1990–March 2016) of the PubMed and Cochrane databases was performed. Bibliographies of articles included in the full-text review were searched for additional studies. A predefined RRT cohort quality score (range 0–17) was used to evaluate studies independently by two reviewers.

Results: Twenty-nine studies with a total of 157,383 RRT activations were included in this review. The quality of data reporting related to RRT patients was assessed as modest, with a median quality score of 8 (range 2–11). Data from the included studies indicate that a median 8.1% of RRT reviews result in limitations of medical treatment (range 2.1–25%) and 23% (8.2–56%) result in a transfer to intensive care. A median of 29% (6.9–35%) of patients transferred to intensive care died during that admission. The median hospital mortality of patients reviewed by RRT is 26% (12–60%), and the median 30-day mortality rate is 29% (8–39%). Data on long-term survival is minimal. No data on functional outcomes was identified.

Conclusions: Patients reviewed by rapid response teams have a high and variable mortality rate, and limitations of care are commonly used. Data on the long-term outcomes of RRT are lacking and needed.

Critique

There are many reports that demonstrate systematic hospital challenges for inpatients who develop shock and require rapid intervention to prevent cardiac arrest. The observable precursor to deterioration is the measurement of vital signs and when they fall outside of normal ranges they are associated with adverse events for patients. Track and trigger systems have been introduced in many countries to reduce the time to intervention and reduce the chance of cardiac arrest. Once an arrest has occurred the evidence suggests that every minute of delay to defibrillation leads to lower survival rates.[160]

Cardiac arrest rates were higher prior to the implementation of track and trigger systems[161,162] that address some of the systemic issues related to adverse events in hospitals. Identified issues include failure to recognise or respond to deteriorating patients, inadequate or delayed treatment, unstable patient transfers and a lack of clinical supervision at the point of care. There are various standards and performance indicators aimed at improving patient care through a rapid response system.

This recently published systematic review of the impact of rapid response teams on the cardiac arrest rate in hospitals is one of many reviews that detail the impact of track and trigger systems in the last 10 years. The change management strategies required to successfully implement recognition and response systems have been described in multiple publications and systems have been implemented successfully around the world.[163] These systems are continuing to mature in Australian hospitals and require clinical governance, education, human and other supportive resources to preserve their function.[164] There continues to be multiple publications that describe non-compliance with recognition and response processes, which means that improvements and ongoing organisational support is required for sustainability.

The results supporting implementation of rapid response systems in multiple systematic reviews and meta-analysis have been mixed. Some systematic reviews with meta-analyses conclude that the introduction of recognition and response systems has been associated with reducing in-hospital mortality and cardiac arrests.[165,166] This review and reviews from 2014 and 2016[167,168] were less supportive of rapid responses systems and prior systematic reviews had been ambivalent, reporting poor quality evidence and lack of clear patient outcome benefit.[169-172]

This systematic review used the PRISMA[173] approach although no meta-analysis was performed. The search was conducted in PubMed and Cochrane which are suitable databases. The review methodology was typical of similar articles and a quality assessment was performed on the selected literature using the RRT quality score which was produced by the author team based on ILCOR recommendations. The quality of data reporting was assessed as modest and outcome of the review asserted that patients reviewed by rapid response teams have a high and variable mortality rate and that data on the long-term outcomes of RRT are lacking.[174] Considering the large amount of research that has been undertaken in this area the fact that only 29 articles met the inclusion criteria is surprising. There were 359 articles screened. This may have been due to the limitations of only reviewing articles that led to limitations of medical treatment, ICU transfer and mortality, hospital mortality at defined end points.[174] The quality score is understandable given the type of research being conducted. There were only 17 prospective trials, and most were at a single centre with 12 of the studies from Australia.[174] The median activation rate from the included studies was 15.9/1000 admissions, which is of interest as it has been suggested that a minimum dose effect of 25 calls per 1000 admissions is necessary to maintain an adequate rapid response system.[175]

There have been advances in medical treatment over the search period, which was 16 years, and this would impact the outcomes measured. It is unlikely that there would ever be de-investment in rapid response systems and they are integral with community expectations of hospitals. The systems have allowed for a common language within a facility to describe deterioration and escalate care when a patient's clinical condition is outside of the scope of the ward or clinicians involved in care.

There are a number of limitations outlined by the authors mostly due to the heterogeneous nature of systems and research designs but there are still important lessons. The findings of this review that are of interest because they highlight the high rates of ICU transfers and limitations that are placed on patient interventions as a result of the rapid response. This has implications for improving the way in which clinicians determine goals of care with patients and appropriateness of interventions.

Learning activities

1. What are the implications for dosing patients receiving renal replacement therapies?
2. What assessments are important to obtain appropriate information for a patient presenting with signs of hypoperfusion?
3. What are key monitoring strategies to assess end-organ perfusion?
4. What are the common management strategies for all shock types?
5. What are the important considerations for managing care at the end-of-life?

Online resources

American Heart Association, www.heart.org/HEARTORG

Australian and New Zealand Anaesthetic Allergy Group, www.anzaag.com/Default.aspx

Australian and New Zealand Anaesthetic Allergy Group Anaphylaxis Management Guidelines, http://www.anzca.edu.au/resources/endorsed-guidelines

Australian Commission on Safety and Quality in Healthcare, https://www.safetyandquality.gov.au/

Australian Society of clinical immunology and allergy, https://www.allergy.org.au/health-professionals/anaphylaxis-resources

Extracorporeal life support organization: https://www.elso.org/Home.aspx

National Blood Authority Australia, www.nba.gov.au

NSW Institute for Trauma and Injury Management, https://www.aci.health.nsw.gov.au/get-involved/institute-of-trauma-and-injury-management/clinical/trauma-guidelines/Guidelines

Patient Blood Management Guidelines App: for iPad, www.blood.gov.au/pbm-ipad

Sepsis, www.ihi.org/Topics/Sepsis/Pages/default.aspx

Spinal cord injury network, http://www.spinalnetwork.org.au/

Surviving Sepsis, www.survivingsepsis.org/

Traumatic Brain Injury http://www.traumaticbraininjury.com/

World Allergy Organization, www.worldallergy.org/index.php

Further reading

Australian Commission on Safety and Quality in Health Care. National Consensus Statement: essential elements for safe and high-quality end-of-life care. Sydney: ACSQHC; 2015. Available from: https://www.safetyandquality.gov.au/wp-content/uploads/2015/05/National-Consensus-Statement-Essential-Elements-forsafe-high-quality-end-of-life-care.pdf.

Australian Commission on Safety and Quality in Health Care. National Consensus Statement: essential elements for recognising and responding to clinical deterioration. 2nd ed. Sydney: ACSQHC; 2010. Available from: https://www.safetyandquality.gov.au/wp-content/uploads/2012/01/national_consensus_statement.pdf. The third edition will be available later in the year or early next year.

Dellinger RP, Schorr CA, Levy MM. A users' guide to the 2016 Surviving Sepsis Guidelines. Crit Care Med 2017;45:381–5.

Doyle JF, Schortgen F. Should we treat pyrexia? And how do we do it? Crit Care 2016;20(1):303.

Stettler GR, Moore EE, Nunns GR, et al. Rotational thromboelastometry thresholds for patients at risk of massive transfusion. J Surg Res 2018;228:154–9.

References

1. Adams F. The book of prognostics, by Hippocrates. Adelaide: eBooks@adelaide. University of Adelaide Library; 2007.
2. Cecconi M, De Backer D, Antonelli M, et al. Consensus on circulatory shock and hemodynamic monitoring. Task force of the European Society of Intensive Care Medicine. Intensive Care Med 2014;40(12):1795–815.
3. Vincent J-L, Ince C, Bakker J. Clinical review: circulatory shock – an update: a tribute to Professor Max Harry Weil. Crit Care 2012;16(6):239.
4. Manji RA, Wood KE, Kumar A. The history and evolution of circulatory shock. Crit Care Clin 2009;25(1):1–29, vii.
5. Barbee RW, Reynolds PS, Ward KR. Assessing shock resuscitation strategies by oxygen debt repayment. Shock 2010;33(2):113–22.
6. Bangash MN, Kong ML, Pearse RM. Use of inotropes and vasopressor agents in critically ill patients. Br J Pharmacol 2012;165(7):2015–33.
7. Strehlow MC. Early identification of shock in critically ill patients. Emerg Med Clin North Am 2010;28(1):57–66, vii.
8. Bridges EJ, Dukes S. Cardiovascular aspects of septic shock: pathophysiology, monitoring, and treatment. Crit Care Nurse 2005;25(2): 14–16, 8-20, 2–4 passim; quiz 41–2.
9. Vincent JL, De Backer D. Circulatory shock. N Engl J Med 2013;369(18):1726–34.
10. Vallet B, Wiel E, Lebuffe G, editors. Resuscitation from circulatory shock: an approach based on oxygen-derived parameters. New York: Springer New York; 2005.
11. Galley HF. Oxidative stress and mitochondrial dysfunction in sepsis. Br J Anaesth 2011;107(1):57–64.
12. Fortin CF, McDonald PP, Fulop T, et al. Sepsis, leukocytes, and nitric oxide (NO): an intricate affair. Shock 2010;33(4):344–52.
13. Mikkelsen ME, Miltiades AN, Gaieski DF, et al. Serum lactate is associated with mortality in severe sepsis independent of organ failure and shock. Crit Care Med 2009;37(5):1670–7.
14. Phypers B, Pierce JMT. Lactate physiology in health and disease. Continuing Education in Anaesthesia Critical Care and Pain 2006;6(3):128–32.
15. Zhang Z, Xu X. Lactate clearance is a useful biomarker for the prediction of all-cause mortality in critically ill patients: a systematic review and meta-analysis. Crit Care Med 2014;42(9):2118–25.
16. Sherwood ER, Toliver-Kinsky T. Mechanisms of the inflammatory response. Best Pract Res Clin Anaesthesiol 2004;18(3):385–405.
17. Caille V, Squara P. Oxygen uptake-to-delivery relationship: a way to assess adequate flow. Crit Care 2006;10(Suppl. 3):S4.
18. Adams KL. Hemodynamic assessment: the physiologic basis for turning data into clinical information. AACN Clin Issues 2004;15(4): 534–46.
19. Casserly B, Read R, Levy MM. Hemodynamic monitoring in sepsis. Crit Care Clin 2009;25(4):803–23, ix.
20. Moshkovitz Y, Kaluski E, Milo O, et al. Recent developments in cardiac output determination by bioimpedance: comparison with invasive cardiac output and potential cardiovascular applications. Curr Opin Cardiol 2004;19(3):229–37.
21. Levin PD, Sprung CL. Another point of view: no swan song for the pulmonary artery catheter. Crit Care Med 2005;33(5):1123–4.

22. Boettger SF, Pavlovic D, Grundling M, et al. Comparison of arterial pressure cardiac output monitoring with transpulmonary thermodilution in septic patients. Med Sci Monit 2010;16(3):Pr1–7.
23. Boyle M, Steel L, Flynn GM, et al. Assessment of the clinical utility of an ultrasonic monitor of cardiac output (the USCOM) and agreement with thermodilution measurement. Crit Care Resusc 2009;11(3):198–203.
24. Suess EM, Pinsky MR. Hemodynamic monitoring for the evaluation and treatment of shock: what is the current state of the art? Semin Respir Crit Care Med 2015;36(6):890–8.
25. Dipti A, Soucy Z, Surana A, et al. Role of inferior vena cava diameter in assessment of volume status: a meta-analysis. Am J Emerg Med 2012;30(8):1414–9.e1.
26. Pittman J, Bar-Yosef S, SumPing J, et al. Continuous cardiac output monitoring with pulse contour analysis: a comparison with lithium indicator dilution cardiac output measurement. Crit Care Med 2005;33(9):2015–21.
27. Shah MR, Hasselblad V, Stevenson LW, et al. Impact of the pulmonary artery catheter in critically ill patients: meta-analysis of randomized clinical trials. JAMA 2005;294(13):1664–70.
28. Harvey SE, Welch CA, Harrison DA, et al. Post hoc insights from PAC-Man – the UK pulmonary artery catheter trial. Crit Care Med 2008;36(6):1714–21.
29. Rivers E, Nguyen B, Havstad S, et al. Early goal-directed therapy in the treatment of severe sepsis and septic shock. N Engl J Med 2001;345(19):1368–77.
30. Ho BC, Bellomo R, McGain F, et al. The incidence and outcome of septic shock patients in the absence of early-goal directed therapy. Crit Care 2006;10(3):R80.
31. Weil MH. Personal commentary on the diagnosis and treatment of circulatory shock states. Curr Opin Crit Care 2004;10(4):246–9.
32. Vincent JL. Give your patient a fast hug (at least) once a day. Crit Care Med 2005;33(6):1225–9.
33. Stennett AK, Gainer JL. TSC for hemorrhagic shock: effects on cytokines and blood pressure. Shock 2004;22(6):569–74.
34. Santry HP, Alam HB. Fluid resuscitation: past, present, and the future. Shock 2010;33(3):229–41.
35. Gutierrez G, Reines HD, Wulf-Gutierrez ME. Clinical review: hemorrhagic shock. Crit Care 2004;8(5):373–81.
36. Hooper N, Jan AT. Shock, Hemorrhagic; 2017. Available from: https://www.ncbi.nlm.nih.gov/books/NBK470382/. [Updated 27 Nov 2017].
37. Beekley AC. Damage control resuscitation: a sensible approach to the exsanguinating surgical patient. Crit Care Med 2008;36(Suppl. 7): S267–74.
38. Myburgh JA, Mythen MG. Resuscitation fluids. N Engl J Med 2013;369(13):1243–51.
39. Guidry C, Gleeson E, Simms ER, et al. Initial assessment on the impact of crystalloids versus colloids during damage control resuscitation. J Surg Res 2013;185(1):294–9.
40. Ball CG. Damage control resuscitation: history, theory and technique. Can J Surg 2014;57(1):55–60.
41. Duke MD, Guidry C, Guice J, et al. Restrictive fluid resuscitation in combination with damage control resuscitation: time for adaptation. J Trauma Acute Care Surg 2012;73(3):674–8.
42. Patient Blood Management Guidelines: Module 1: Critical Bleeding/Massive Transfusion [database on the Internet]. NBA. 2011.
43. Mandal M. Ideal resuscitation fluid in hypovolemia: the quest is on and miles to go! Int J Crit Illn Inj Sci 2016;6(2):54–5.
44. Annane D, Siami S, Jaber S, et al. Effects of fluid resuscitation with colloids vs crystalloids on mortality in critically ill patients presenting with hypovolemic shock: the CRISTAL randomized trial. JAMA 2013;310(17):1809–17.
45. Finfer S, Bellomo R, Boyce N, et al. A comparison of albumin and saline for fluid resuscitation in the intensive care unit. N Engl J Med 2004;350(22):2247–56.
46. Alderson P, Bunn F, Lefebvre C, et al. Human albumin solution for resuscitation and volume expansion in critically ill patients. Cochrane Database Syst Rev 2004;(4):Cd001208.
47. Myburgh JA, Finfer S, Bellomo R, et al. Hydroxyethyl starch or saline for fluid resuscitation in intensive care. N Engl J Med 2012;367(20): 1901–11.
48. Criddle LM, Eldredge DH, Walker J. Variables predicting trauma patient survival following massive transfusion. J Emerg Nurs 2005;31(3): 236–42, quiz 320.
49. Cooper DJ, McQuilten ZK, Nichol A, et al. Age of red cells for transfusion and outcomes in critically ill adults. N Engl J Med 2017;377(19): 1858–67.
50. Authority NB. Patient blood management guidelines: module 4: critical care. Canberra: NBA; 2012.
51. Australian Commission on Safety and Quality in Health Care. National Safety and Quality Health Service Standards. In: ACSQHC. 2nd ed. Sydney: 2017.
52. Rappold JF, Pusateri AE. Tranexamic acid in remote damage control resuscitation. Transfusion 2013;53(Suppl. 1):96s–9s.
53. Roberts I, Shakur H, Coats T, et al. The CRASH-2 trial: a randomised controlled trial and economic evaluation of the effects of tranexamic acid on death, vascular occlusive events and transfusion requirement in bleeding trauma patients. Health Technol Assess 2013;17(10):1–79.
54. Gruen RL, Jacobs IG, Reade MC. Trauma and tranexamic acid. Med J Aust 2013;199(5):310–11.
55. Lim N, Dubois MJ, De Backer D, et al. Do all nonsurvivors of cardiogenic shock die with a low cardiac index? Chest 2003;124(5):1885–91.
56. Bendjelid K. Five recurrent misconceptions regarding cardiogenic shock management. Cardiol Rev 2014;22(5):241–5.

57. Hofer CK, Furrer L, Matter-Ensner S, et al. Volumetric preload measurement by thermodilution: a comparison with transoesophageal echocardiography. Br J Anaesth 2005;94(6):748–55.
58. Agricola E, Bove T, Oppizzi M, et al. 'Ultrasound comet-tail images': a marker of pulmonary edema: a comparative study with wedge pressure and extravascular lung water. Chest 2005;127(5):1690–5.
59. Worthley LI. Shock: a review of pathophysiology and management. Part I. Crit Care Resusc 2000;2(1):55–65.
60. Dubey L, Sharma S, Gautam M, et al. Cardiogenic shock complicating acute myocardial infarction–a review. Acta Cardiol 2011;66(6):691–9.
61. Carnendran L, Abboud R, Sleeper LA, et al. Trends in cardiogenic shock: report from the SHOCK study. The SHould we emergently revascularize Occluded Coronaries for cardiogenic shocK? Eur Heart J 2001;22(6):472–8.
62. Menees DS, Peterson ED, Wang Y, et al. Door-to-balloon time and mortality among patients undergoing primary PCI. N Engl J Med 2013;369(10):901–9.
63. Herget-Rosenthal S, Saner F, Chawla LS. Approach to hemodynamic shock and vasopressors. Clin J Am Soc Nephrol 2008;3(2):546–53.
64. Menon V, White H, LeJemtel T, et al. The clinical profile of patients with suspected cardiogenic shock due to predominant left ventricular failure: a report from the SHOCK Trial Registry. SHould we emergently revascularize Occluded Coronaries in cardiogenic shocK? J Am Coll Cardiol 2000;36(3 Suppl. A):1071–6.
65. Topalian S, Ginsberg F, Parrillo JE. Cardiogenic shock. Crit Care Med 2008;36(Suppl. 1):S66–74.
66. Leach RM, Treacher DF. The pulmonary physician in critical care 2: oxygen delivery and consumption in the critically ill. Thorax 2002;57(2):170–7.
67. Shoemaker WC, Appel PL, Kram HB, et al. Prospective trial of supranormal values of survivors as therapeutic goals in high-risk surgical patients. Chest 1988;94(6):1176–86.
68. Lesage A, Ramakers M, Daubin C, et al. Complicated acute myocardial infarction requiring mechanical ventilation in the intensive care unit: prognostic factors of clinical outcome in a series of 157 patients. Crit Care Med 2004;32(1):100–5.
69. Khalid L, Dhakam SH. A review of cardiogenic shock in acute myocardial infarction. Curr Cardiol Rev 2008;4(1):34–40.
70. Allen JM. Understanding vasoactive medications: focus on pharmacology and effective titration. J Infus Nurs 2014;37(2):82–6.
71. Pirracchio R, Parenica J, Resche Rigon M, et al. The effectiveness of inodilators in reducing short term mortality among patient with severe cardiogenic shock: a propensity-based analysis. PLoS ONE 2013;8(8):e71659.
72. Follath F, Cleland JG, Just H, et al. Efficacy and safety of intravenous levosimendan compared with dobutamine in severe low-output heart failure (the LIDO study): a randomised double-blind trial. Lancet 2002;360(9328):196–202.
73. Mebazaa A, Barraud D, Welschbillig S. Randomized clinical trials with levosimendan. Am J Cardiol 2005;96(6a):74g–9g.
74. Moiseyev VS, Poder P, Andrejevs N, et al. Safety and efficacy of a novel calcium sensitizer, levosimendan, in patients with left ventricular failure due to an acute myocardial infarction. A randomized, placebo-controlled, double-blind study (RUSSLAN). Eur Heart J 2002;23(18):1422–32.
75. Nativi-Nicolau J, Selzman CH, Fang JC, et al. Pharmacologic therapies for acute cardiogenic shock. Curr Opin Cardiol 2014;29(3):250–7.
76. O'Connor CM, Gattis WA, Uretsky BF, et al. Continuous intravenous dobutamine is associated with an increased risk of death in patients with advanced heart failure: insights from the Flolan International Randomized Survival Trial (FIRST). Am Heart J 1999;138(1 Pt 1):78–86.
77. Opasich C, Cioffi G, Gualco A. Nitroprusside in decompensated heart failure: what should a clinician really know? Curr Heart Fail Rep 2009;6(3):182–90.
78. Annane D, Bellissant E, Pussard E, et al. Placebo-controlled, randomized, double-blind study of intravenous enalaprilat efficacy and safety in acute cardiogenic pulmonary edema. Circulation 1996;94(6):1316–24.
79. Investigators TAIREAS. Effect of ramipril on mortality and morbidity of survivors of acute myocardial infarction with clinical evidence of heart failure. Lancet (London, England) 1993;342(8875):821–8.
80. Miller PE, Solomon MA, McAreavey D. Advanced percutaneous mechanical circulatory support devices for cardiogenic shock. Crit Care Med 2017;45(11):1922–9.
81. Thiele H, Zeymer U, Neumann FJ, et al. Intra-aortic balloon counterpulsation in acute myocardial infarction complicated by cardiogenic shock (IABP-SHOCK II): final 12 month results of a randomised, open-label trial. Lancet 2013;382(9905):1638–45.
82. Organisation ELS. ELSO adult cardiac failure supplement to the ELSO general guidelines, vol. Version 13. Ann Arbor: 2013.
83. Organisation ELS. ELSO guidelines for cardiopulmonary extracorporeal life support, vol. Version 14. Ann Arbor: 2017.
84. Murray S. Bi-level positive airway pressure (BiPAP) and acute cardiogenic pulmonary oedema (ACPO) in the emergency department. Aust Crit Care 2002;15(2):51–63.
85. Agarwal R, Aggarwal AN, Gupta D, et al. Non-invasive ventilation in acute cardiogenic pulmonary oedema. Postgrad Med J 2005;81(960): 637–43.
86. Park M, Sangean MC, Volpe Mde S, et al. Randomized, prospective trial of oxygen, continuous positive airway pressure, and bilevel positive airway pressure by face mask in acute cardiogenic pulmonary edema. Crit Care Med 2004;32(12):2407–15.
87. Singer M, Deutschman CS, Seymour C, et al. The third international consensus definitions for sepsis and septic shock (sepsis-3). JAMA 2016;315(8):801–10.
88. Kaukonen KM, Bailey M, Bellomo R. Systemic inflammatory response syndrome criteria for severe sepsis. N Engl J Med 2015;373(9):881.
89. Kempker JA, Martin GS. The changing epidemiology and definitions of sepsis. Clin Chest Med 2016;37(2):165–79.

90. Rhodes A, Evans LE, Alhazzani W, et al. Surviving Sepsis Campaign: international guidelines for management of sepsis and septic shock: 2016. Crit Care Med 2017;45(3):486–552.
91. World Health Organization. Service delivery and safety. Improving the prevention, diagnosis and clinical management of sepsis. World Health Organization; 2017. Available from: https://www.who.int/servicedeliverysafety/areas/sepsis/en/.
92. The George Institute for Global Health. Stopping sepsis: a national action plan. Sydney: The George Institute for Global Health; 2017. A Health Policy Report.
93. Dellinger RP, Carlet JM, Masur H, et al. Surviving Sepsis Campaign guidelines for management of severe sepsis and septic shock. Crit Care Med 2004;32(3):858–73.
94. Dellinger RP, Levy MM, Carlet JM, et al. Surviving Sepsis Campaign: international guidelines for management of severe sepsis and septic shock: 2008. Crit Care Med 2008;36(1):296–327.
95. Dellinger RP, Levy MM, Rhodes A, et al. Surviving Sepsis Campaign: international guidelines for management of severe sepsis and septic shock: 2012. Crit Care Med 2013;41(2):580–637.
96. Rhodes A, Evans LE, Alhazzani W, et al. Surviving Sepsis Campaign: international guidelines for management of sepsis and septic shock: 2016. Intensive Care Med 2017;43(3):304–77.
97. Hicks P, Cooper DJ, Webb S, et al. The Surviving Sepsis Campaign: international guidelines for management of severe sepsis and septic shock: 2008. An assessment by the Australian and New Zealand intensive care society. Anaesth Intensive Care 2008;36(2):149–51.
98. Levy MM, Evans LE, Rhodes A. The Surviving Sepsis Campaign bundle: 2018 update. Intensive Care Med 2018.
99. Joint Commission Perspectives on Patient Safety. Raising the bar with bundles: treating patients with an all-or-nothing standard. Joint Commission on Accreditation of Healthcare Organizations 2006;6(4).
100. Finfer S. The Surviving Sepsis Campaign: robust evaluation and high-quality primary research is still needed. Crit Care Med 2010;38(2):683–4.
101. Chamberlain DJ, Willis EM, Bersten AB. The severe sepsis bundles as processes of care: a meta-analysis. Aust Crit Care 2011;24(4):229–43.
102. van den Berghe G, Wouters P, Weekers F, et al. Intensive insulin therapy in critically ill patients. N Engl J Med 2001;345(19):1359–67.
103. Van den Berghe G, Schetz M, Vlasselaers D, et al. Clinical review: intensive insulin therapy in critically ill patients: NICE-SUGAR or Leuven blood glucose target? J Clin Endocrinol Metab 2009;94(9):3163–70.
104. Finfer S, Chittock DR, Su SY, et al. Intensive versus conventional glucose control in critically ill patients. N Engl J Med 2009;360(13):1283–97.
105. Griesdale DE, de Souza RJ, van Dam RM, et al. Intensive insulin therapy and mortality among critically ill patients: a meta-analysis including NICE-SUGAR study data. CMAJ 2009;180(8):821–7.
106. Schrier RW, Wang W. Acute renal failure and sepsis. N Engl J Med 2004;351(2):159–69.
107. Marik PE, Varon J. Early goal-directed therapy: on terminal life support? Am J Emerg Med 2010;28(2):243–5.
108. Puskarich MA, Marchick MR, Kline JA, et al. One year mortality of patients treated with an emergency department based early goal directed therapy protocol for severe sepsis and septic shock: a before and after study. Crit Care 2009;13(5):R167.
109. Focht A, Jones AE, Lowe TJ. Early goal-directed therapy: improving mortality and morbidity of sepsis in the emergency department. Jt Comm J Qual Patient Saf 2009;35(4):186–91.
110. Rivers EP, Coba V, Whitmill M. Early goal-directed therapy in severe sepsis and septic shock: a contemporary review of the literature. Curr Opin Anaesthesiol 2008;21(2):128–40.
111. Yealy DM, Kellum JA, Huang DT, et al. A randomized trial of protocol-based care for early septic shock. N Engl J Med 2014;370(18):1683–93.
112. Peake SL, Delaney A, Bailey M, et al. Goal-directed resuscitation for patients with early septic shock. N Engl J Med 2014;371(16):1496–506.
113. Mouncey PR, Osborn TM, Power GS, et al. Trial of early, goal-directed resuscitation for septic shock. N Engl J Med 2015;372(14):1301–11.
114. Finfer S, Bellomo R, Lipman J, et al. Adult-population incidence of severe sepsis in Australian and New Zealand intensive care units. Intensive Care Med 2004;30(4):589–96.
115. Padkin A, Goldfrad C, Brady AR, et al. Epidemiology of severe sepsis occurring in the first 24 hrs in intensive care units in England, Wales, and Northern Ireland. Crit Care Med 2003;31(9):2332–8.
116. Brun-Buisson C, Meshaka P, Pinton P, et al. EPISEPSIS: a reappraisal of the epidemiology and outcome of severe sepsis in French intensive care units. Intensive Care Med 2004;30(4):580–8.
117. Kumar A. Optimizing antimicrobial therapy in sepsis and septic shock. Crit Care Clin 2009;25(4):733–51, viii.
118. Kumar A, Roberts D, Wood KE, et al. Duration of hypotension before initiation of effective antimicrobial therapy is the critical determinant of survival in human septic shock. Crit Care Med 2006;34(6):1589–96.
119. Taccone FS, Laterre PF, Dugernier T, et al. Insufficient beta-lactam concentrations in the early phase of severe sepsis and septic shock. Crit Care 2010;14(4):R126.
120. Dulhunty JM, Roberts JA, Davis JS, et al. A protocol for a multicentre randomised controlled trial of continuous beta-lactam infusion compared with intermittent beta-lactam dosing in critically ill patients with severe sepsis: the BLING II study. Crit Care Resusc 2013;15(3):179–85.
121. Lipman J, Boots R. A new paradigm for treating infections: 'go hard and go home'. Crit Care Resusc 2009;11(4):276–81.

122. Finfer S, McEvoy S, Bellomo R, et al. Impact of albumin compared to saline on organ function and mortality of patients with severe sepsis. Intensive Care Med 2011;37(1):86–96.
123. Bagshaw SM, Chawla LS. Hydroxyethyl starch for fluid resuscitation in critically ill patients. Can J Anaesth 2013;60(7):709–13.
124. Myburgh J. CHEST and the impact of fraud in fluid resuscitation research. Crit Care Resusc 2011;13(2):69–70.
125. Perel P, Roberts I, Ker K. Colloids versus crystalloids for fluid resuscitation in critically ill patients. Cochrane Database Syst Rev 2013;28(2):Cd000567.
126. Obritsch MD, Bestul DJ, Jung R, et al. The role of vasopressin in vasodilatory septic shock. Pharmacotherapy 2004;24(8):1050–63.
127. Lipiner-Friedman D, Sprung CL, Laterre PF, et al. Adrenal function in sepsis: the retrospective Corticus cohort study. Crit Care Med 2007;35(4):1012–18.
128. Magnotti LJ, Deitch EA. Burns, bacterial translocation, gut barrier function, and failure. J Burn Care Rehabil 2005;26(5):383–91.
129. Maragakis LL. Recognition and prevention of multidrug-resistant Gram-negative bacteria in the intensive care unit. Crit Care Med 2010;38(Suppl. 8):S345–51.
130. Young PJ, Weatherall M, Saxena MK, et al. Statistical analysis plan for the HEAT trial: a multicentre randomised placebo-controlled trial of intravenous paracetamol in intensive care unit patients with fever and infection. Crit Care Resusc 2013;15(4):279–86.
131. Young P, Saxena M, Bellomo R, et al. Acetaminophen for fever in critically ill patients with suspected infection. N Engl J Med 2015;373(23): 2215–24.
132. Doyle JF, Schortgen F. Should we treat pyrexia? And how do we do it? Crit Care 2016;20(1):303.
133. Ellis AK, Day JH. Diagnosis and management of anaphylaxis. CMAJ 2003;169(4):307–11.
134. McLean-Tooke AP, Bethune CA, Fay AC, et al. Adrenaline in the treatment of anaphylaxis: what is the evidence? BMJ 2003;327(7427): 1332–5.
135. Gold MS. EpiPen epidemic or good clinical practice? J Paediatr Child Health 2003;39(5):376–7.
136. Nurmatov UB, Rhatigan E, Simons FE, et al. H2-antihistamines for the treatment of anaphylaxis with and without shock: a systematic review. Ann Allergy Asthma Immunol 2014;112(2):126–31.
137. Dhami S, Panesar SS, Roberts G, et al. Management of anaphylaxis: a systematic review. Allergy 2014;69(2):168–75.
138. Kanji S, Chant C. Allergic and hypersensitivity reactions in the intensive care unit. Crit Care Med 2010;38(Suppl. 6):S162–8.
139. Sampson HA, Munoz-Furlong A, Campbell RL, et al. Second symposium on the definition and management of anaphylaxis: summary report–Second National Institute of Allergy and Infectious Disease/Food Allergy and Anaphylaxis Network symposium. J Allergy Clin Immunol 2006;117(2):391–7.
140. Berin MC, Sampson HA. Mucosal immunology of food allergy. Curr Biol 2013;23(9):R389–400.
141. Burks AW, Tang M, Sicherer S, et al. ICON: food allergy. J Allergy Clin Immunol 2012;129(4):906–20.
142. Sicherer SH, Sampson HA. Food allergy. J Allergy Clin Immunol 2010;125(2 Suppl. 2):S116–25.
143. Boros CA, Kay D, Gold MS. Parent reported allergy and anaphylaxis in 4173 South Australian children. J Paediatr Child Health 2000;36(1):36–40.
144. Wood RA, Camargo CA Jr, Lieberman P, et al. Anaphylaxis in America: the prevalence and characteristics of anaphylaxis in the United States. J Allergy Clin Immunol 2014;133(2):461–7.
145. Simons FE, Frew AJ, Ansotegui IJ, et al. Practical allergy (PRACTALL) report: risk assessment in anaphylaxis. Allergy 2008;63(1):35–7.
146. Brown SG. Clinical features and severity grading of anaphylaxis. J Allergy Clin Immunol 2004;114(2):371–6.
147. Pumphrey R. Anaphylaxis: can we tell who is at risk of a fatal reaction? Curr Opin Allergy Clin Immunol 2004;4(4):285–90.
148. Anaesthetists AaNZAAGaAaNZCo. Anaphylaxis management guidelines: Introduction; 2013. http://www.anzaag.com/Docs/PDF/Management%20Guidelines/Mx%20Guidelines%20Intro%20v1.1Jun13.pdf. [Accessed 29 March 2015].
149. Australian Society of Clinical Immunology and Allergy. Acute management of anaphylaxis guidelines; 2018. Available from: https://www.allergy.org.au/images/stories/pospapers/ASCIA_Guidelines_Acute_Management_Anaphylaxis_2018.pdf. [Accessed 19 January 2019].
150. Tang AW. A practical guide to anaphylaxis. Am Fam Physician 2003;68(7):1325–32.
151. Wang J, Sampson HA. Treatments for food allergy: how close are we? Immunol Res 2012;54(0):83–94.
152. Guly HR, Bouamra O, Lecky FE. The incidence of neurogenic shock in patients with isolated spinal cord injury in the emergency department. Resuscitation 2008;76(1):57–62.
153. Summers RL, Baker SD, Sterling SA, et al. Characterization of the spectrum of hemodynamic profiles in trauma patients with acute neurogenic shock. J Crit Care 2013;28(4):531.e1–531.e5
154. Hagen EM. Acute complications of spinal cord injuries. World J Orthop 2015;6(1):17–23.
155. Stevens RD, Bhardwaj A, Kirsch JR, et al. Critical care and perioperative management in traumatic spinal cord injury. J Neurosurg Anesthesiol 2003;15(3):215–29.
156. Ryken TC, Hurlbert RJ, Hadley MN, et al. The acute cardiopulmonary management of patients with cervical spinal cord injuries. Neurosurgery 2013;72(Suppl. 2):84–92.
157. Hagen EM, Rekand T, Gronning M, et al. Cardiovascular complications of spinal cord injury. Tidsskr Nor Laegeforen 2012;132(9): 1115–20.
158. Miko I, Gould R, Wolf S, et al. Acute spinal cord injury. Int Anesthesiol Clin 2009;47(1):37–54.

159. Baumann A, Audibert G, Klein O, et al. Continuous intravenous lidocaine in the treatment of paralytic ileus due to severe spinal cord injury. Acta Anaesthesiol Scand 2009;53(1):128–30.
160. Chan PS, Krumholz HM, Nichol G, et al. Delayed time to defibrillation after in-hospital cardiac arrest. N Engl J Med 2008;358(1):9–17.
161. Hughes C, Pain C, Braithwaite J, et al. 'Between the flags': implementing a rapid response system at scale. BMJ Qual Saf 2014;23(9): 714–17.
162. Corfield AR, Lees F, Zealley I, et al. Utility of a single early warning score in patients with sepsis in the emergency department. Emerg Med J 2014;31(6):482–7.
163. Beitler JR, Link N, Bails DB, et al. Reduction in hospital-wide mortality after implementation of a rapid response team: a long-term cohort study. Crit Care 2011;15.
164. Hillman KM, Chen J, Jones D. Rapid response systems. Med J Aust 2014;201(9):519–21.
165. Maharaj R, Raffaele I, Wendon J. Rapid response systems: a systematic review and meta-analysis. Crit Care 2015;19(1):254.
166. Solomon RS, Corwin GS, Barclay DC, et al. Effectiveness of rapid response teams on rates of in-hospital cardiopulmonary arrest and mortality: a systematic review and meta-analysis. J Hosp Med 2016;11(6):438–45.
167. Smith ME, Chiovaro JC, O'Neil M, et al. Early warning system scores for clinical deterioration in hospitalized patients: a systematic review. Ann Am Thorac Soc 2014;11(9):1454–65.
168. Le Lagadec MD, Dwyer T. Scoping review: the use of early warning systems for the identification of in-hospital patients at risk of deterioration. Aust Crit Care 2016.
169. Chan PS, Jain R, Nallmothu BK, et al. Rapid response teams: a systematic review and meta-analysis. Arch Intern Med 2010;170.
170. Winters BD, Weaver SJ, Pfoh ER, et al. Rapid-response systems as a patient safety strategy: a systematic review. Ann Intern Med 2013;158.
171. McNeill G, Bryden D. Do either early warning systems or emergency response teams improve hospital patient survival? A systematic review. Resuscitation 2013;84(12):1652–67.
172. Alam N, Hobbelink EL, van Tienhoven AJ, et al. The impact of the use of the Early Warning Score (EWS) on patient outcomes: a systematic review. Resuscitation 2014;85(5):587–94.
173. Liberati A, Altman DG, Tetzlaff J, et al. The PRISMA statement for reporting systematic reviews and meta-analyses of studies that evaluate health care interventions: explanation and elaboration. Ann Intern Med 2009;151.
174. Tirkkonen J, Tamminen T, Skrifvars MB. Outcome of adult patients attended by rapid response teams: a systematic review of the literature. Resuscitation 2017;112:43–52.
175. Jones D, Bellomo R, DeVita MA. Effectiveness of the medical emergency team: the importance of dose. Crit Care 2009;13.
176. Poblete GH, Nijsten MW, Bakker J. Lactate. In: Pinto Lima A, Silva E, editors. Monitoring tissue perfusion in shock. Cham: Springer; 2018.
177. Kincaid EH, Miller PR, Meredith JW, et al. Elevated arterial base deficit in trauma patients: a marker of impaired oxygen utilization. J Am Coll Surg 1998;187(4):384–92.

Chapter 22

Multiple organ dysfunction syndrome

Melanie Greenwood, Alison Juers

KEY WORDS

apoptosis
cytokines/mediators
inflammation
multiple organ dysfunction syndrome
immunoparesis
procoagulation
sepsis

Learning objectives

After reading this chapter, you should be able to:

- define the common terminology related to multiple organ dysfunction syndrome
- describe the related pathophysiology of multiple organ dysfunction syndrome
- identify the clinical manifestations of multiple organ dysfunction syndrome
- identify patients at risk of developing multiple organ dysfunction, including predictors of mortality
- initiate appropriate monitoring, care planning and evaluation strategies for the patient with multiple organ dysfunction in relation to the current evidence base
- discuss treatment strategies that promote homeostasis in the patient with multiple organ dysfunction syndrome.

Introduction

The incidence of multiple organ dysfunction syndrome (MODS) is increasing and is the most frequent cause of death in the intensive care.[1] The term MODS describes a continuum of physiological derangements and subsequent dynamic alterations in organ function that may occur during a critical illness.[2] Multiple organ failure was a term commonly used, but is somewhat misleading as normal physiological function can, in most cases, be restored in survivors of a critical illness who have temporary organ dysfunction.[3,4] Although the syndrome affects many organs, it also affects physiological systems such as the haematological, immune and endocrine systems. MODS therefore more accurately describes altered organ function in a critically ill patient who requires medical and nursing interventions to achieve homeostasis.[4]

MODS is associated with widespread endothelial and parenchymal cell injury because of hypoxic hypoxia, direct cytotoxicity, apoptosis, immunosuppression and coagulopathy.[4] Four clinical stages describe a patient with developing MODS:[5]

1 increasing volume requirements and mild respiratory alkalosis, accompanied by oliguria and hyperglycaemia

2. tachypnoea, hypocapnia and hypoxaemia, with moderate liver dysfunction and possible haematological abnormalities
3. developing shock with azotaemia, acid–base disturbances and significant coagulation abnormalities
4. vasopressor dependence with oliguria or anuria, ischaemic colitis and lactic acidosis.

Cellular damage in various organs in patients who develop MODS begins with the onset of local injury that is then compounded by activation of the innate immune system. This includes a combination of pattern recognition, receptor activation and release of mediators at the microcellular level, leading to episodes of hypotension or hypoxaemia and secondary infections.[4,5] The primary therapeutic goal for nursing and medical staff is prompt, definitive control of the source of infection or pro-inflammation[6] and early recognition of preexisting factors that may lead to subsequent organ damage away from the initial site of injury. This pre-emptive therapy is instituted to maintain adequate tissue perfusion and prevent the onset of MODS. Recognition and response to early signs of clinical deterioration are therefore important to minimise further organ dysfunction.

In this chapter the pathophysiology of inflammatory and infective conditions that may lead to multiple organ dysfunction is described. System responses and specific organ dysfunction are discussed, expanding on dialogue in previous chapters, particularly Chapter 20. Assessment of the severity of MODS and nursing considerations in the treatment of the MODS patient are presented.

Pathophysiology

The syndrome of multiple organ dysfunction is most closely related to an outcome of sepsis, which is described in Chapter 21; however, it may have many other causes, such as trauma[6] or failure of the gut.[7] MODS is a state characterised by aberrant cellular responses involving multiple organ systems and sequential processes. The pathogenesis of MODS is complex, simultaneously involving every cell type, neurohormonal axis and organ system.[8]

In brief, alterations in tissue perfusion and oxygenation at the level of the microcirculation can result in dysfunction of organs.[9] Hypoxic hypoxia results from altered metabolic regulation of tissue oxygen delivery, which contributes to further organ dysfunction. Microcirculatory injury, as a result of lytic enzymes and vasoactive substances (nitric oxide, endothelial growth factor), is compounded by the inability of erythrocytes to navigate the septic microcirculation. Mitochondrial electron transport is affected by endotoxins in sepsis, nitric oxide and tumour necrosis factor alpha (TNF-α), leading to disordered energy metabolism (Fig. 22.1). This causes cytopathic or histotoxic anoxia.[10] This context of impaired oxygen utilisation where oxygen delivery is normal[8,10] results from diminished mitochondrial production of cellular energy – adenosine triphosphate (ATP) – despite normal or even supranormal intracellular oxygen levels.[11] Cellular hypoxia increases free radicals further compounding oxidative stress, which results in calcium entering the endoplasmic reticulum and mitochondria leading to cell death.[12] Cytopathic hypoxia appears resistant to resuscitation measures, and may ultimately worsen already-existing organ dysfunction. During sepsis or ischaemia, mitochondria respond by facilitating cell death rather than the restoration of homeostasis.[8]

Apoptosis is normal physiological programmed cell death and is the main mechanism to eliminate dysfunctional cells.[13] Apoptosis involves chromatin condensation, membrane blebbing, cell shrinkage and subsequent breakdown of cellular components into apoptotic bodies. This normally orderly process is deranged in critical illness, leading to tissue or organ bed injury and MODS. Proinflammatory cytokines released in sepsis may delay apoptosis in activated macrophages and neutrophils, but in other tissues, such as gut endothelium, accelerated apoptosis occurs.[10]

In contrast, necrosis is a form of cell death characterised by cellular swelling and loss of membrane integrity as a result of hypoxia or trauma. Necrosis has been termed 'cellular energy crisis',[13] and is unregulated resulting in loss of membrane sodium/potassium/ATP-ase pumps. This loss leads to cell swelling, rupture and spillage of intracellular contents into surrounding regions creating collateral damage.[13] Necrosis therefore can involve significant amounts of tissue and organ bed damage. Apoptosis differs from necrosis in that it does not seem to involve the recruitment of inflammatory cells or mediators to complete its task. Activation of an enzyme cascade systematically cleaves proteins and degrades the cell's nuclear deoxyribonucleic acid (DNA) with the end result being death of the cell. This requires energy from mitochondria and, if not available, necrosis of the cell occurs. Apoptosis and necrosis are processes important to understand in relation to future MODS research.[13]

Increased concentrations of cell-free plasma DNA are present in various clinical conditions such as stroke, myocardial infarction and trauma – a likely result of accelerated cell death. Maximum plasma DNA concentrations correlated significantly with acute physiology and chronic health evaluation (APACHE) II scores and maximum sequential organ failure assessment (SOFA) scores (described later in this chapter), with cell-free plasma DNA concentrations higher in hospital non-survivors than in survivors. Using regression analysis, maximum plasma DNA was an independent predictor of hospital mortality.[14]

Other cellular organelles may also exhibit pathological reactions in MODS. In ischaemia/reperfusion, endoplasmic reticulum loses its ability to process proteins, which induces the expression of heat shock proteins,[8] affecting transcription of proteins necessary for

FIGURE 22.1 Pathophysiology of cellular dysfunction.

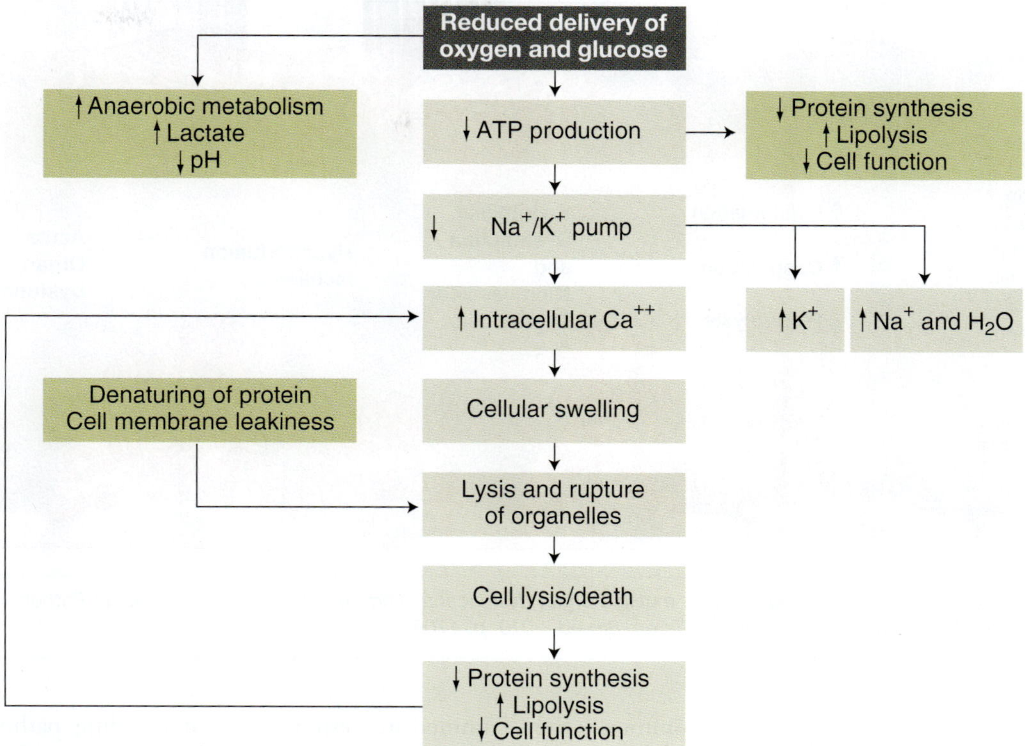

Source: McCance KL, Grey TC. Altered cellular and tissue biology. In: Pathophysiology: the biologic basis for disease in adults and children. 6th ed. St Louis: Mosby; 2010, p. 53.

organ-specific functions. For example, liver cell metabolism, renal cell function or cardiac cell contractility may be affected.[8] This has led to the concept of a mode of hibernation[8,12,15] of cells at the expense of survival of the whole organism.[8]

Cellular communication is also altered in MODS. Cells normally communicate through highly interactive bidirectional neural networks.[16] The endothelium acts as a communication interface between cells, organs and systems and is involved in orchestration of systemic responses, including haemodynamic regulation, inflammation and coagulation; oxygen and nutrient delivery; oxidative stress; and sensing of psychological stress and neuroendocrine alterations.[8,10] In critical illness, endothelia release molecules that trigger the immune and neuroendocrine systems to produce a generalised inflammatory response.[8] The combination of the pathophysiological processes involved with the development of MODS, compensatory mechanisms and the effect on target organs and systems is now discussed.

Systemic response

After an overwhelming incident such as trauma, breaches in intestinal integrity, sepsis or non-infectious inflammation, a complex range of interrelated reactions occurs that result in a cascade of responses. The complex host response generated involves the inflammatory immune systems, hormonal activation and metabolic derangements, resulting in multiple organ system involvement.[12,17] These host-responses are initially adaptive to maintain nutrient perfusion to the tissues; however, eventually organ systems become dysfunctional and fail, and the body is no longer able to maintain homeostasis[18] (Fig. 22.2).

Initially, proinflammatory mediators are released locally to fight foreign antigens and promote wound healing. Anti-inflammatory mediators are also released to downregulate the initial response to the insult.[19] If the local defence system is overwhelmed, inflammatory mediators appear in the systemic circulation and recruit additional leucocytes to the area of damage. A whole-body stress response ensues, further compounding the situation. If the proinflammatory mediators and the anti-inflammatory response are imbalanced, the patient may develop systemic inflammatory response syndrome (SIRS) and subsequent immunological dissonance[19] of organ dysfunction.[2,18]

Regardless of the trigger event, lymphocytes (T cells, B cells, natural killer cells) and macrophages are activated

FIGURE 22.2 Progression of SIRS-Sepsis-Shock-MODS.[41]

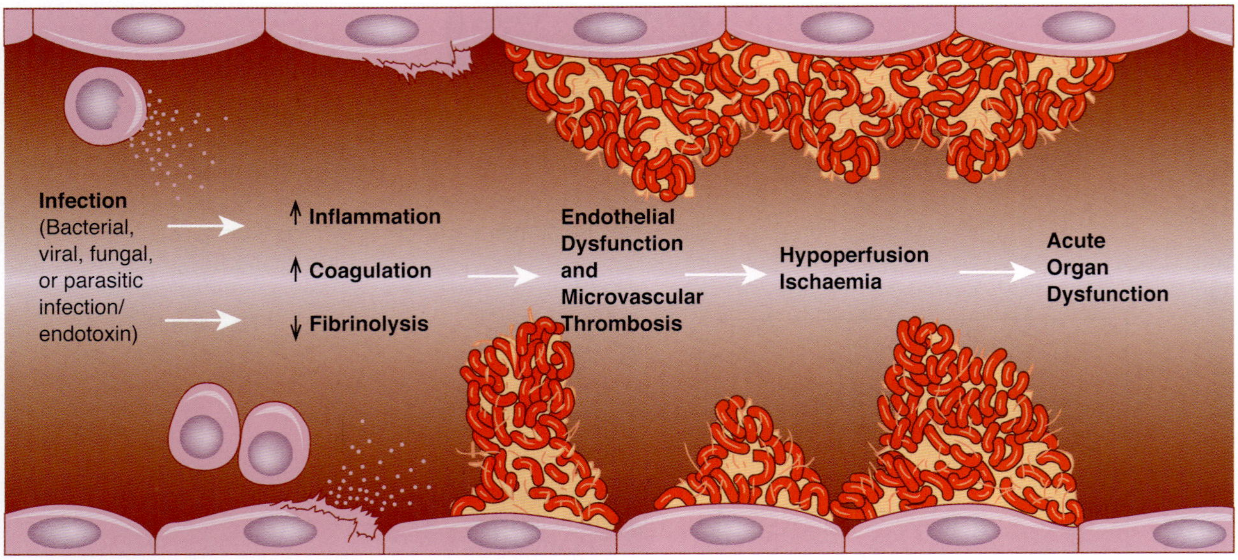

Source: Cheek DJ, Martin LL, Morris SE. Shock, multiple organ dysfunction syndrome, and burns in adults. In Pathophysiology: The Biologic Basis for Disease in Adults and Children. 6th ed. 2010, p. 1709.

by cytokines (cellular signalling agents) to commence the inflammatory or anti-inflammatory response. A number of interleukins (IL) have been identified as key cytokines in proinflammatory (e.g. IL-1, IL-6) or anti-inflammatory (e.g. IL-10, IL-6, IL-4) responses. IL-6 is unique in that it has both pro- and anti-inflammatory properties. The inflammatory response results in clinical signs of hypoperfusion, culminating in shock.

Intracellular transcription factors, in particular nuclear factor kappa B, are important in innate and adaptive immunity,[20,21] as they regulate the transcription of genes involved in the inflammatory and acute stress response, leading to expression of TNF-α, interleukins and tissue factor.[2,21] Nuclear factor kappa B therefore plays an important role in response pathways in critical states including hypoxia, ischaemia, haemorrhage, sepsis, shock and MODS.[18,22,23]

The inflammatory cascade activates a number of prostaglandins and leukotrienes that also have pro- and anti-inflammatory effects. Thromboxane A_2 plays a role in the acute phase, in part due to stimulation of platelet aggregation, leading to microvascular thrombosis and tissue injury;[18] it may also play a role in pulmonary bronchoconstriction and myocardial depression.

The specific pathophysiological concepts of inflammation, oedema and infection are discussed below.

Inflammation

Inflammation is part of innate immunity, a generic response to injury, and is normally an excellent mechanism to localise injury and promote healing.[24,25] The basis of this immune response is recognition of, and an immediate response to, an invading pathogen without necessarily having previous exposure to that pathogen.[26] Neutrophils, macrophages, natural killer cells, dendrites, coagulation and complement are the principal active components of the innate host response.[25] Compensatory anti-inflammatory response syndrome and SIRS produce cardiovascular shock, altered homeostasis, apoptosis, organ dysfunction and immune suppression.[27]

The classic signs of inflammation are:

- pain
- oedema
- erythema and heat (from vasodilation)
- leucocyte accumulation and capillary leak.[24,25]

Nitric oxide and prostaglandins (e.g. prostacyclin) are the primary mediators of vasodilation and inflammation at the injury site.[25] Injured endothelium produces molecules that attract leucocytes and facilitate movement to the tissues. White blood cells accumulate by margination (adhesion to endothelium during the early stages of inflammation) and neutrophils accumulate at the injury site, where rolling and adherence to binding molecules on the endothelium occurs with eventual movement across the endothelium into the tissues.[25] Different blood components therefore escape the intravascular space and occupy the interstitial space where they play the main role in successive phases of the inflammatory response. The endothelium thus plays a bidirectional mediating role between blood flow and the interstitial space where inflammation mainly takes place.[28] Macrophages, neutrophils and monocytes are responsible for phagocytosis and the production of toxic free radicals to kill invading pathogens.[26] The complement system, a collection of 30 proteins circulating in the blood, is also activated, with plasma and membrane proteins acting as adjuncts to inflammatory and immune processes.[26] When activated by inflammation and microbial invasion, these processes facilitate lysis (cellular destruction) and phagocytosis (ingestion) of foreign material.[7,25]

Dysfunction of organ systems often persists after the initial inflammatory response diminishes; this is largely unexplained, although dysoxia (abnormal tissue oxygen metabolism and utilisation) has been implicated.[7] Hypoxia induces release of IL-6, the main cytokine that initiates the acute phase response. After reperfusion of ischaemic tissues, tissue and neutrophil activation forms reactive oxygen species (e.g. hydrogen peroxide) as a byproduct. These strong oxidants damage other molecules and cell structures that they come into contact with,[15,25] resulting in water and sodium infiltrate and cellular oedema.

Oedema

Oedema occurs as a consequence of alterations to tissue endothelium, with increased microvascular permeability or 'capillary leak'. As noted earlier, many mediators, including circulating cytokines, oxygen free radicals and activated neutrophils alter the structure of endothelial cells, enabling larger molecules such as proteins and water to cross into the extravascular space.[25,29] This response mechanism improves supply of nutrient-rich fluid to the site of injury but, if this becomes systemic, fluid shifts can lead to hypovolaemia or third-spacing (interstitial oedema) or affect other organs (e.g. acute lung injury, acute kidney injury).[29]

Infection and immune responses

Infection exists when there is one of the following: positive culture, serology,[30] presence of polymorphonuclear leucocytes in a normally sterile body fluid except blood or clinical focus of infection such as perforated viscus or pneumonia.[31] The immune response to infection has both non-specific and specific actions, with inflammation and coagulation responses intricately linked in sepsis pathophysiology.[31-33] Tissue injury and the production of inflammatory mediators lead to:

- coagulation via the expression of tissue factor and factor VIIa complex (tissue factor pathway)[32,33]
- coagulation amplification via factors Xa and Va, leading to massive thrombin formation and fibrin clots (common coagulation pathway).[31,33]

Note that blood cell injury or platelet contact with endothelial collagen initiates the contact activation pathway.[31]

Procoagulation

Tissue factor is a procoagulant glycoprotein-signalling receptor,[34] expressed when tissue is damaged or cytokines are released from macrophages or the endothelium[35] (Fig. 22.3). Prothrombin is formed, leading to thrombin and fibrin generation from activated platelets. Resulting clots are stabilised by factor XIII and thrombin-activatable fibrinolysis inhibitor.[35] Fibrinolysis is a homeostatic

FIGURE 22.3 Tissue factor pathway.

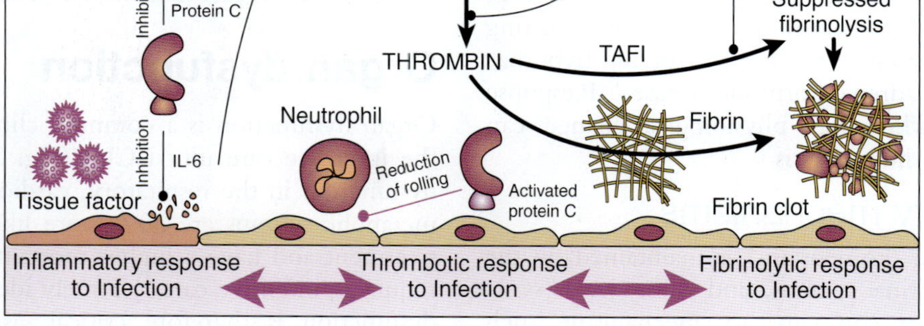

Adapted from McCance KL, Heuther SE, Brashers VL, Rote NS. Pathophysiology: the biological basis for disease in adults and children. 6th ed. Mosby Elsevier: St Louis; 2010, with permission.

process that dissolves clots via the plasminogen–tissue plasminogen activator–plasmin pathway (involving antithrombin, activated protein C and tissue factor pathway inhibitor). Activated protein C:[36]

- reduces inflammation by decreasing TNF-a and nuclear factor kappa B production
- reduces thrombin production when activated via thrombin–thrombomodulin complexes (anticoagulant action)
- inhibits thrombin-activatable fibrinolysis inhibitor and plasminogen activator inhibitor-1 (profibrinolytic action).[36]

Activated protein C is consumed in severe sepsis, and thrombomodulin is unable to activate protein C,[34-36] promoting a proinflammatory, prothrombotic state.[34]

Endocrine response

Physiological changes are triggered as a normal response to a stressor. In a critically ill patient, however, chronic activation of the stress response, including the hypothalamic–pituitary–adrenal axis and the sympathetic–adrenal–medullary axis, results in ongoing production of glucocorticoid hormones and catecholamines.[37] This response interferes with the regulation of cytokine-producing immune cells, leading to immune dysfunction. Other compensatory mechanisms are instigated in an attempt to maintain supply and perfusion to organs.[18]

These homeostatic mechanisms are activated through positive or negative feedback systems to counteract stress. When stress is extreme or prolonged, these normal homeostatic mechanisms may be insufficient and a patient may respond through a sequence of physiological changes called the stress response. The stress response occurs in three stages: the alarm reaction, the resistance reaction and exhaustion (Fig. 22.4).[35]

The alarm reaction (flight-or-fight response)[35] is initiated when stress is detected, increasing the amount of glucose and oxygen available to the brain, skeletal muscle and heart. Two-thirds of total blood volume is also redistributed to support central circulation.[35] A rise in glucose production and the breakdown of glycogen in skeletal muscle increases circulating glucose levels, providing an immediate energy source. The long-lasting second stage is a resistance reaction, involving hypothalamic, pituitary and adrenal hormone release.[37] Response exhaustion occurs when these physiological changes can no longer maintain homeostasis.

Compensatory mechanisms

Internal equilibrium (homeostasis) is maintained by the nervous and endocrine systems, and these work symbiotically with other compensatory mechanisms, such as endothelial cells, to maintain cellular perfusion. The nervous system responds rapidly to maintain homeostasis by sending impulses to organs to activate neurohormonal responses (see Chapters 16 and 21). Autonomic dysfunction reflects 'uncoupling' of neurally-mediated organ interactions in MODS[15] characterised by heart rate, baroreflex and chemoreflex variability. Endothelins (ET-1, ET-2, ET-3) are potent vasoconstrictors produced by endothelial cells that regulate arterial pressure.[22] The endocrine system works in a slow and sustained manner by secreting hormones, which travel via the blood to end-organs.

An initial acute-adaptive response is activated when an insult or stress occurs. For example, the body senses a disruption of blood flow through baroreceptor and chemoreceptor reflex actions: baroreceptors located in the carotid sinus detect changes in arterial pressure;[35] chemoreceptors co-located with the baroreceptors detect oxygen, carbon dioxide and hydrogen ion concentration. When alterations are sensed, the cardiovascular centre in the brain adjusts autonomic outflow accordingly.[35] In a patient with decreased tissue perfusion, there is increased peripheral vasoconstriction, contractility and heart rate. Blood flow is shunted to the vital organs (brain, heart, lungs), and away from less vital areas such as the gastrointestinal system, skin and reproductive organs.[35] Important hormonal regulators of blood flow are also activated from decreased blood flow to the kidneys, including adrenocorticotrophic hormone and the renin–angiotensin–aldosterone system (see Chapter 18). Adrenal medullary hormones, adrenaline and noradrenaline, vasopressin (antidiuretic hormone) and atrial natriuretic peptide also regulate blood flow to maintain adequate circulation and tissue oxygenation.[2,38,39]

Arterial pressure is a major determinant of tissue perfusion as it forces blood through the regional vasculature.[40] Hypotension (systolic blood pressure <90 mmHg or mean arterial pressure [MAP] <70 mmHg) results from either low systemic vascular resistance or a low cardiac output.[35] Glomerular filtration falls, leading to reduced urine output; low cerebral blood flow results in an altered level of consciousness; and other manifestations reflect low-flow states in other organ systems. To maintain oxygen supply, respirations and heart rate increase to meet organ oxygenation demands.[34] Heart rate variability is suggested as a strong predictor of mortality in MODS.[12] Organ dysfunction ensues if balance is not sufficiently re-established (Table 22.1).

Organ dysfunction

Organ dysfunction is a common clinical presentation in the intensive care unit (ICU) (Fig. 22.5). Patients with dysfunction in the respiratory, cardiovascular, hepatic or metabolic systems are 50% more likely to require ICU treatment and have a higher mortality than patients not requiring intensive care.[43] Timely identification of organ dysfunction is therefore critical, as early intervention reduces damage and improves recovery in organ systems. As each organ fails, the average risk of death rises by 11–23%,[44] with mortality from trauma between 67% and

FIGURE 22.4 Actions of the stress response.[41]

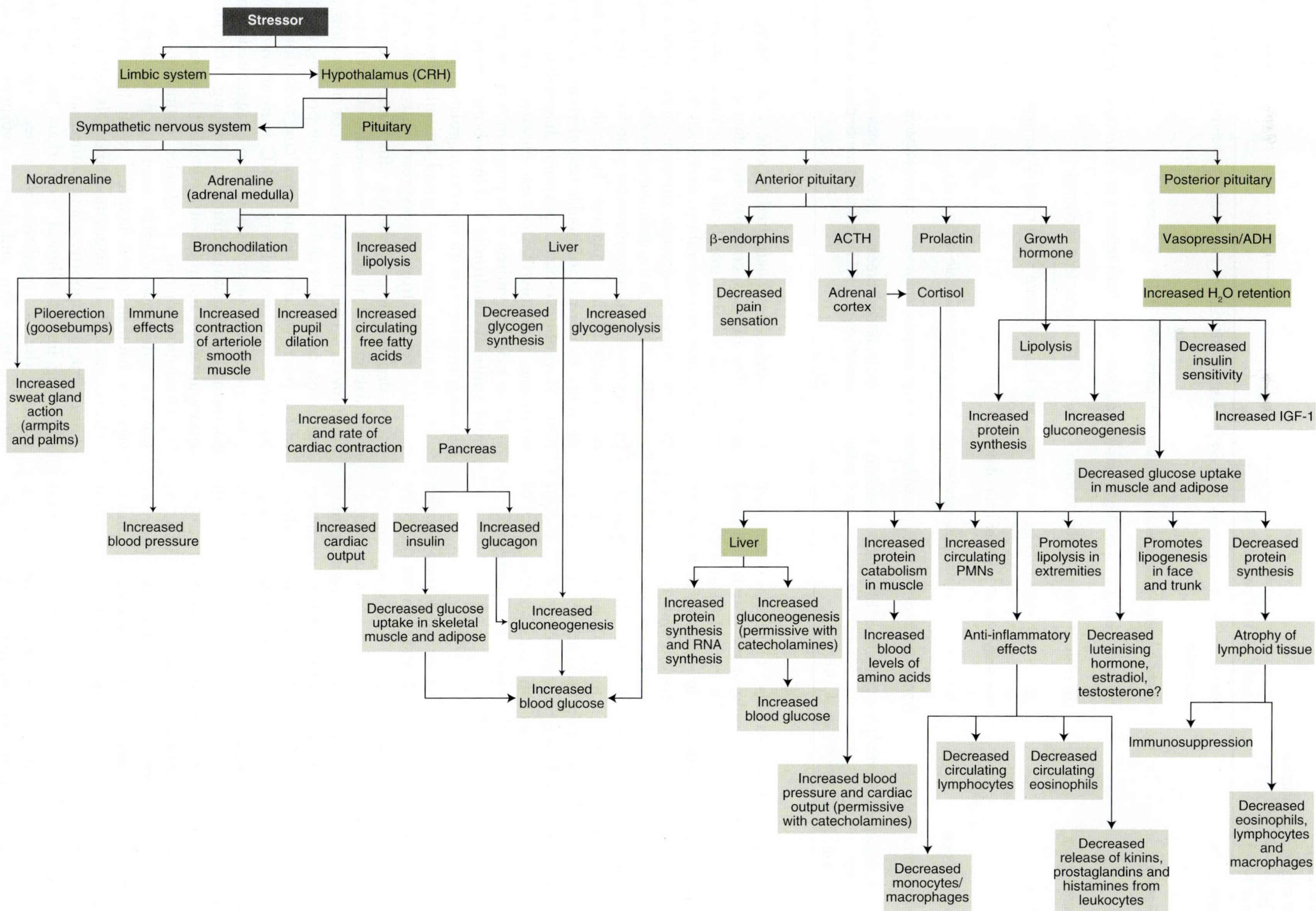

Adapted from McCance KL, Heuther SE, Brashers VL, Rote NS. Pathophysiology: the biological basis for disease in adults and children. 6th ed. St Louis: Mosby Elsevier; 2010, with permission.

TABLE 22.1
Acute organ dysfunction[41,42]

ORGAN SYSTEM	CLINICAL PARAMETERS
Cardiovascular	Patient requires vasopressor support for systolic BP <90 mmHg or MAP <70 mmHg for 1 h despite fluid bolus
Respiratory	Patient requires mechanical ventilation: PF ratio <250, PEEP >7.5 cmH_2O
Renal	Low urine output <0.5 mL/kg/h; raised creatinine >50% from baseline or requiring acute dialysis
Haematological	Low platelet count (<1,000,000/mm^3) or APTT/PTT >upper limit of normal
Metabolic	Low pH with increased lactate (pH <7.3 and plasma lactate >upper limit of normal)
Hepatic	Liver enzymes >2 × upper limit of normal
Central nervous	Altered level of consciousness/reduced Glasgow Coma Scale score
Gastrointestinal	Translocation of bacteria, possible elevated pancreatic enzymes and cholecystitis

APTT = activated partial thromboplastin time; BP = blood pressure; MAP = mean arterial pressure; PEEP = peak end-expiratory pressure; PF = PaO_2/FiO_2 = partial pressure of arterial oxygen/fraction of inspired oxygen; PTT = partial thromboplastin time.
Source: Bauer, 2005; Vincent et al., 1996.

100% as more than one organ fails.[6] The organ system that most commonly fails is the pulmonary system, followed by the cardiovascular, renal and haematological systems.[45] Organ and system dysfunctions are a result of hypoperfusion, inflammation, cellular dysfunction and oedema. Dysfunctions of the cardiovascular (Chapters 10 and 11), respiratory (Chapter 14), renal (Chapter 18) and hepatic and gastrointestinal systems (Chapter 20) have been previously addressed. The next sections address the haematological, endocrine and metabolic systems. Neurological dysfunction is also common in the patient with MODS and complements previous discussions in Chapter 17.

Haematological dysfunction

Inflammatory responses and disseminated intravascular coagulation (DIC) have pivotal and synergistic roles in the development of MODS.[45-47] The coagulopathy present in MODS results from deficiencies of coagulation system proteins such as protein C, antithrombin III and tissue factor inhibitors.[34] Inflammatory mediators initiate direct injury to the vascular endothelium, releasing tissue factor, triggering the tissue factor pathway (extrinsic coagulation cascade) and accelerating thrombin production.[34] Coagulation factors are activated as a result of endothelial damage with binding of factor XII to the subendothelial surface and activation of factors VIII, X, XI, XII, calcium and phospholipid.[34] The final pathway is production of thrombin, which converts soluble fibrinogen to fibrin. Fibrin and aggregated platelets form intravascular clots.

Inflammatory cytokines also initiate coagulation through activation of tissue factor, a principal activator of coagulation. Endotoxins increase the activity of inhibitors of clot breakdown (fibrinolysis). Levels of protein C and endogenous activated protein C are decreased in sepsis; this inhibits coagulation cofactors Va and VIIa and acts as an antithrombotic in the microvasculature.[34]

Microvascular thrombosis that leads to MODS results from two major syndromes: thrombotic microangiopathy and DIC. Thrombotic microangiopathy is characterised by formation of microvascular platelet aggregates and occasionally fibrin formation. Typically, there is history of injury to the microvascular endothelium (e.g. thrombotic thrombocytopenic purpura, haemolytic uraemic syndrome, haemolytic anaemia, elevated liver enzymes and low platelet syndromes of pregnancy or antiphospholipid antibody syndrome).[48] Thrombotic microangiopathy usually presents with normal coagulation profiles such as prothrombin times and partial thromboplastin time.[48]

DIC results from widespread activation of tissue factor-dependent coagulation, insufficient control of coagulation and plasminogen-mediated attenuation of fibrinolysis.[48] This leads to formation of fibrin clots, consumption of platelets and coagulation proteins, occlusion of the microvasculature and resultant reductions in cellular tissue oxygen delivery.[34] DIC is most commonly a result of trauma or sepsis and is an exaggerated response to normal coagulation aimed at limiting infection and exsanguination and promoting wound healing.[34]

Thrombocytopenia (a platelet count of <80,000/mm^3 or a decrease of ≥50% over the preceding 3 days) signifies haematological failure,[49] with leucocytopenia/cytosis, markers of coagulation and DIC also present.[31] Treatment is supportive and aimed at removing the triggering insults. Clinical biomarkers include a simultaneous rise in prothrombin time, activated partial thromboplastin time and thrombocytopenia.[31] A patient may exhibit bleeding from puncture sites (e.g. invasive

FIGURE 22.5 Pathogenesis of multiple organ dysfunction syndrome.[37]

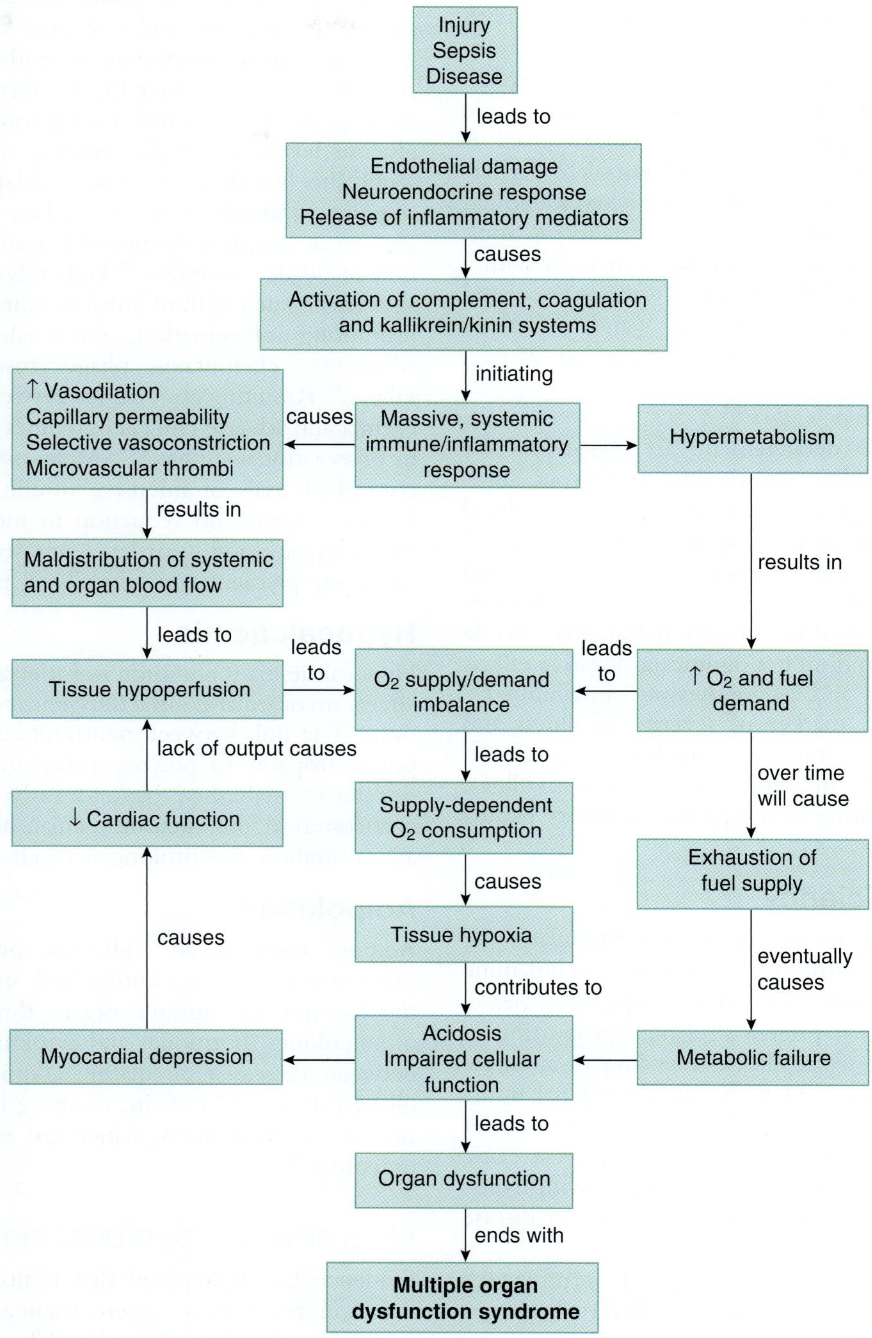

Adapted from Craft JA, Gordon CJ, Heuther SE et al. Understanding pathophysiology. 2nd ed. St Louis: Mosby Elsevier; 2018, with permission.

vascular access), mucous membranes including bowel or upper gastrointestinal tract. Bruising or other subcutaneous petechiae may be evident. The skin should be protected from trauma.

Primary therapy is directed at the cause of the insult, with SIRS, ischaemia, uraemia, hepatotoxins and sources of infection, injury or necrosis managed concurrently. Aggressive resuscitation includes crystalloid or colloid administration and replacement of blood components and clotting factors using packed cells, platelets, cryoprecipitate and fresh frozen plasma. End points for haemoglobin, platelets and coagulation levels have not been agreed upon and replacement is therefore individualised.[50]

The role of heparin or fractionated heparin is controversial in the presence of sepsis, particularly in those with overt thromboembolism or extensive fibrin deposition, such as in purpura fulminans or ischaemia in the extremities.[31] Administration of activated protein C in its role as inhibitor of the coagulation cascade is controversial. A Cochrane review of four studies involving 4911 participants (4434 adults and 477 paediatric patients) identified no reduction in risk of death (28-day mortality) in adult participants with severe sepsis, but was associated with a higher risk of bleeding.[51] Effectiveness was not associated with the degree of severity of sepsis[31] and, therefore, activated protein C is no longer recommended.

Endocrine dysfunctions

Numerous endocrine derangements are noted in critically ill patients, including abnormalities in thyroid, adrenocortical, pancreas, growth and sex hormones. Critical illness-related corticosteroid insufficiency is associated with more frequent use of vasopressors and increased mortality.[52] A high thyrotropin level is an independent predictor of non-survival in critically ill patients,[52] while subclinical hypothyroidism has significant negative effects on cardiac function and haemodynamic instability.[52,53] Hyperglycaemia is a marker of severity of illness and predictor of poor outcome in non-diabetic patients.[52] Leptin increases early in sepsis, correlating with illness severity and contributing to the proinflammatory pathogenesis of MODS.[52]

Adrenal insufficiency

The hypothalamic–pituitary–adrenal axis modulates the adaptive response to stressors[52] through catecholamine secretion, cytokine activation and vasopressin release. Adrenal insufficiency is present in a high proportion of patients with sepsis, septic shock, bleeding or multiple trauma[54-58] and is associated with chronic adrenal insufficiency and recent physiological stress, or in new-onset adrenal insufficiency.[52] Adrenal insufficiency as a cause of shock should be considered in any patient with hypotension with no signs of infection, cardiovascular disease or hypovolaemia.

Methods to diagnose acute adrenal insufficiency include: 1) a single random cortisol level check, or a change in cortisol level after exogenous adrenocorticotrophic hormone is administered; or 2) a short corticotrophin stimulation test with administration of high-dose adrenocorticotrophic hormone. A change in cortisol level (≤9 mcg/dL) is considered relative adrenal insufficiency. It is, however, argued that patients with severe sepsis may have appropriate cortisol levels, but not the reserve function to respond to the stimulation test.[59] Evaluation of adrenal function in critically ill patients is complex and assays of free cortisol levels offer an advantage over total cortisol levels in the presence of low binding proteins such as hypoalbuminaemia.[58]

Glycaemia

Hyperglycaemia is common in critically ill patients as a result of stress-induced insulin resistance and accelerated glucose production, and excessive circulating levels of glucagon, growth hormone, sympathomimetics and glucocorticoids (see Chapter 19). An increased caloric intake from parenteral or enteral nutrition may also increase glucose levels. Hyperglycaemia as a stress response in septic shock is thought to be an adaptive and beneficial response, though in some studies, maintaining blood glucose at less than 10 mmol/L resulted in 10% reduction in 90-day mortality.[60] Hyperglycaemia has undesirable effects such as fluid imbalance, immune dysfunction, promoting inflammation, abnormalities in granulocyte adherence, chemotaxis, phagocytosis and intracellular killing.[60] Resulting associations between severe hyperglycaemia and adverse clinical outcomes have been reported in observational studies.[60-62] Meta-analysis of randomised controlled trials of intensive insulin therapy for septic patients showed no reduction in mortality;[61] therefore, lower target blood sugar levels are not recommended for managing glycaemia in critically ill patients.

Hypocalcaemia

Hypocalcaemia is common in patients with MODS[63] and affects myocardial contractility and neuromuscular functions. The link between neuromuscular changes such as polyneuropathy or polymyopathy and critical illness has not been established beyond early investigations into corticosteroid use, neuromuscular blocking medication administration and prolonged mechanical ventilation.[64]

Adipokines

Adipose tissue is an endocrine organ that plays an important role in immunity and metabolism affecting the function of multiple organs through the secretion of adipokines (hormones and cytokines). There is a link between increased circulating adipokines, in particular blood resistin and visfatin, resulting in severe inflammation and critical illness, which are associated with poor outcomes.[65]

Neurological dysfunction

Evidence has highlighted that multiple organ dysfunction can result from severe traumatic brain injury or subarachnoid haemorrhage (see Chapter 17). Cardiovascular and respiratory dysfunction contribute to mortality in approximately two-thirds of all deaths following severe traumatic brain injury.[66] In non-traumatic subarachnoid haemorrhage the incidence and importance of life-threatening conditions from non-neurological physiology has been identified, including lethal arrhythmias, myocardial ischaemia and dysfunction and neurogenic pulmonary oedema.[67] The cause of cardiovascular and respiratory organ dysfunction following these acute, severe neurological events is associated with dysfunction of the sympathetic nervous system. Beta-blockers may modulate the sympathetic storm resulting from severe neurological injury.[68]

Critically ill patients may develop a syndrome of neuromuscular dysfunction characterised by generalised muscle weakness and an inability to wean successfully from mechanical ventilation. ICU-acquired weakness, including critical illness neuromyopathy syndromes, has been associated with risk factors including hyperglycaemia, SIRS, sepsis, MODS, renal replacement therapy, glucocorticoids, neuromuscular blocking agents and catecholamine administration.[69] The risk of ICU-acquired weakness is nearly 50% in patients with sepsis, MODS or protracted ventilation,[69] with short-term survival uncertain. Addressing high blood glucose levels may be a potential strategy for decreasing ICU-acquired weakness.[70]

Survivors of sepsis-induced multiple organ dysfunction may also suffer long-term cognitive impairment, including alterations in memory, attention, concentration and/or global loss of cognitive function.[71] The participation of the brain during sepsis is poorly understood; septic encephalopathy affects approximately one-third of septic patients.[72,73] In Chapter 6 the physical, psychological and cognitive sequelae for survivors of a critical illness during their recovery are described.

Multiple organ dysfunction

MODS contributes to significant morbidity and use of intensive care resources worldwide. Patients with MODS have an increased ICU length of stay when compared to high-risk patients without multiple organ involvement[43,74-77] and very high 5-year mortality.[75,78-80] Post-traumatic MODS increases with age, severity of injury, gender (increased incidence in males), presence of traumatic brain injury, massive transfusion (>6 units packed red blood cells), coagulopathy, thrombocytopaenia, hypotension on admission and hyperlactataemia.[74] Half of critically injured patients develop MODS within 3 days post-injury.[81] The epidemiology of MODS varies with North American and Australian studies in post-injury organ failure indicating a reduction in incidence.[76,77,82] Internationally, a reduction in MODS-related mortality is reported;[76,82-84] however, data from the developing world are scant. Post-injury MODS mortality rates are between 11% and 27%.[6,76,85-87] This overall decrease in mortality is occurring despite increasing patient acuity and may reflect improvements in the delivery of critical care.[74,88]

Scoring systems

Organ dysfunction can be a consequence of a primary insult or a secondary insult due to circulating mediators (e.g. the patient with acute lung injury from pneumonia that also has renal dysfunction or failure as a consequence). This is sometimes quantified by scoring systems, traditionally used for predicting mortality but increasingly being explored as clinical management tools.[6,89,90] These systems are continually being tested and modified, to assess organ dysfunction severity and prognosis in an effort to identify patients who will benefit most from timely clinical intervention.[6] Scoring systems such as APACHE, simplified acute physiology score and mortality probability models account for information relating to a 24-hour cycle of patient data (commonly in the first 24 hours of admission), but do not account for the dynamic nature of many of the factors that affect clinical outcomes, thus potentially limiting their use for early MODS diagnosis and intervention.

Specific instruments designed to assess organ dysfunction or failure include the SOFA score, the more trauma-specific Denver multiple organ failure score, the Marshall multiple organ dysfunction score and the logistic organ dysfunction score (Table 22.2).[75,91,92] The Denver score appears to be more specific for detecting trauma-related MODS; however, the SOFA score demonstrates greater sensitivity.[92,93] SOFA scores uses the worst values for six commonly measured clinical parameters within a 24-hour period: PaO_2/FiO_2 (PF ratio), an index that may be used to characterise acute respiratory distress syndrome; platelet count; bilirubin level; mean arterial blood pressure; ± inotropic support; Glasgow Coma Scale score; creatinine concentration or urine output. A score greater than 3 or higher indicates single organ dysfunction, with a total score of >5 or 2 or more single organ dysfunctions indicative of MODS.[75] A rise in baseline SOFA score (assumed to be zero in the absence of known organ dysfunction) of greater than or equal to 2 points signifies acute organ dysfunction in the setting of infection.[94] Many variations of SOFA-based models have emerged in the literature, including modification of the neurological component utilising the Richmond Agitation-Sedation scale to more accurately assess the neurological component, often problematic in the intubated, sedated patient[95] and the qSOFA score, designed to identify the potential septic patient in the non-ICU setting.[91] SOFA scoring has the advantage of ease of use, as the clinical and laboratory data required are routinely available. Other scoring systems that allow pre-hospital identification of trauma patients predisposed to MODS are also being developed.[89] Overall, there is no one universally accepted gold standard scoring system with different systems used in MODS research.[96]

Other factors

Biomarkers such as lactate, base deficit and platelet count are also being studied as indicators of occult hypoperfusion and severity of organ dysfunction.[94,98-100] Blood lactate levels are routinely collected in the early stage of ICU admission, supporting early resuscitation as a management strategy to prevent organ dysfunction. Serial lactate scores may therefore be appropriate to guide optimal oxygen delivery in early resuscitation, with hyperlactataemia a sign of impending organ dysfunction.[94,99] With the production of point-of-care lactate analysers, pre-hospital lactate levels may also identify

TABLE 22.2
Sequential organ failure assessment (SOFA) score[42,75,97]

SOFA SCORE	0	1	2	3	4
Respiration PaO_2/FiO_2	>400	≤400	≤300	≤200[a]	≤100[a]
Coagulation platelets × $10^3/mm^3$	>150	≤150	≤100	≤50	≤20
Liver bilirubin	<1.2 mg/dL >32 micromol/L	1.2–1.9 20–32	2.0–5.9 33–101	6.0–11.9 102–204	>12.0 >204
Cardiovascular hypotension	MAP >70 mmHg	MAP <70 mmHg	Dopamine ≤5 or Dobutamine (any dose)[b]	Dopamine >5 or adrenaline ≤0.1 or noradrenaline ≤0.1[b]	Dopamine >15 or adrenaline >0.1 or noradrenaline >0.1[b]
CNS Glasgow Coma Scale	15	13–14	10–12	6–9	<6
Renal creatinine or urine output	<1.2 mg/dL <110 micromol/L	1.2–1.9 110–170	2–3.4 171–299	3.5–4.9 300–440 or <500 mL/day	>5.0 >440 or <200 mL/day

[a]With respiratory support.
[b]Adrenergic agents administered for at least 1 h (doses in mcg/kg per min).
FiO_2 = fraction of inspired oxygen; MAP = mean arterial pressure; PaO_2 = partial pressure of arterial oxygen.
Source: Vincent et al., 1996; Hutchings et al., 2017; Minne et al., 2008.

patients predisposed to MODS and influence care delivery. Prospective, well-controlled studies are, however, needed to confirm the role of lactate and other biomarkers in MODS management.[101]

Variations in the human DNA sequences can affect the way a person responds to disease. Researchers have studied the gene code for plasminogen activator inhibitor 1, which is a key element in the inhibition of fibrinolysis and is active during acute inflammation[102] (the gene most studied is found at the 4G/5G insertion/deletion loci), and have found that different aspects bind as either a repressor (5G) or activator (4G) protein. For example, the 4G allele (position on the gene) of the 4G/5G gene sequence variation has been associated with increased susceptibility to community-acquired pneumonia and increased mortality in cases of severe pneumonia. It has also been reported to affect the risk of developing severe outcomes and higher mortality in meningococcal sepsis and trauma.[103,104] In trauma, damage-associated molecular patterns are released into the extracellular and vascular compartments. Mitochondrial DNA is a damage-associated molecular pattern and a potential activator of the immune response to trauma, identification of which raises its potential for therapeutic modulation.[81] Among critically ill patients with severe sepsis due to pneumonia, carriers of the plasminogen activator inhibitor 1 4G/5G genotypes have higher risk for MODS and septic shock.[102] In future, identification of genetic factors may assist selection of appropriate therapy for the patient at risk. Experimental *BRCA1* gene therapy research is showing early promising results on key cellular processes involved in stimulating DNA repair and cellular defence.[102]

Patient management

Improvement in patient survival with MODS is thought to be due to improved identification of patients predisposed to MODS, improved shock and critical care management, awareness of secondary insults and a better understanding of the risk factors associated with MODS. Current prevention and management strategies therefore focus on identifying at-risk patients via informed clinical assessment, scoring systems and biomarkers, efficient shock resuscitation, timely treatment of infection or injury, exclusion of secondary inflammatory insults and organ support.[6,93,94,96]

Effective shock resuscitation

For the critically injured patient, shock resuscitation includes permissive hypotension (with a higher arterial pressure for traumatic brain-injured patients) and reversal of hypothermia, coagulopathy and acidosis. Additionally, damage control surgery, judicious volume replacement and transfusion of blood products reduces the likelihood of MODS development.[74]

A number of interventions have been recommended to reduce mortality for patients with MODS due to

BOX 22.1

Surviving sepsis campaign

The Surviving Sepsis Campaign is an international collaborative formed in 2003 to reduce the mortality of sepsis. Guidelines for the management of severe sepsis and shock were updated in 2016 and offer a comprehensive list of graded recommendations to care for these patients.[99] Many of the recommendations for practice have implications for critical care nurses and the multidisciplinary team (see *Online resources*).

Adapted from Rhodes A, Evans L, Alhazzani W et al. Surviving Sepsis Campaign: international guidelines for management of sepsis and septic shock: 2016. Intensive Care Med 2017, 43:304-77.

sepsis. The Surviving Sepsis Campaign international guidelines are based on clinical evidence graded according to the quality of evidence available (Box 22.1). The fourth version of the guidelines released in 2017 emphasises sepsis and septic shock as medical emergencies, recommending a minimum of 30 mL/kg intravenous crystalloid resuscitation within the first 3 hours of sepsis-induced hypoperfusion, aiming for a MAP of 65 mmHg in shocked patients needing vasopressors. Further fluid resuscitation is guided by ongoing thorough clinical assessment and normalisation of elevated lactate levels.[99] See Chapter 21 for further discussion of resuscitation in shock.

Early treatment of injury/infection

In the severely injured patient, damage control surgery controls haemorrhage, minimising protracted resuscitation associated acidosis and coagulopathy. Moreover, inflammatory mediator release is attenuated. Subsequent debridement of non-viable or infected tissue reduces the likelihood of the development of MODS from sepsis, often a delayed presentation in the trauma patient.[74]

Timely treatment of infection in the patient with sepsis or septic shock, is critical in the prevention and management of MODS. In the septic patient, the incidence of early acute kidney injury increases with delays in antimicrobial therapy from the onset of hypotension[105] as does acute lung injury.[106] Mortality increases for every hour delay in administration of the first appropriate antimicrobials.[107,108] The Surviving Sepsis Campaign guidelines recommend empiric, broad-spectrum IV antimicrobials be commenced as soon as possible and within 1 hour of identification of sepsis or septic shock.[99] While there has been conjecture regarding optimal timing, subsequent, high quality studies reinforce the mortality benefit of early antimicrobial therapy particularly in septic shock.[109-114]

As early antimicrobial administration may be difficult to achieve given competing patient management priorities (e.g. airway management, volume resuscitation, vasopressor administration), systems must be developed to promote early administration.[109,115,116] Nurses are in a pivotal position to ensure these guidelines or processes are developed, implemented and evaluated.

Practice tip

Tips for promoting early antimicrobial administration in severe sepsis/septic shock[99,115-117]

- Sepsis protocol in use recognising sepsis as a time-dependent emergency.
- Ensure antimicrobial therapy high priority in sepsis protocol.
- Do not delay antimicrobial administration if difficulty sampling blood cultures (cultures need to be collected within 45 minutes of diagnosis of severe sepsis or septic shock).
- Ensure adequate supply of antimicrobials in the emergency department and ICU that fit local colonisation patterns.
- Utilise STAT orders for initial antimicrobial administration.
- Administer appropriate antibiotics that can be given via intravenous push vs longer infusion.
- Plan efficient sequencing of antimicrobial administration. Consider simultaneous delivery via multiple vascular access.
- Consider intraosseous access for first dose antimicrobial administration.
- Emphasise education of staff on the significance of early administration of initial antimicrobial.
- Consider other potential barriers to early antimicrobial administration in your facility e.g. critically analyse communication strategies within healthcare teams.

Combination antibiotic therapy may offer a survival benefit in septic shock, but may be deleterious to patients with a low mortality risk.[118] Certainly, antibiotic overuse and misuse is of concern given the emergence of antibiotic resistance.[99,119] Other factors that can lead to antibiotic failure in the critically ill include increased volume of distribution secondary to expanded extracellular volume, transient increased drug clearance due to elevated cardiac output (early sepsis) and increased free-drug levels secondary to reduced serum albumin. Maximum antibiotic dosage levels on day 1 of therapy, guided by predicted volume of distribution, are therefore recommended in life-threatening infections, as inadequate antibiotic penetration can occur due to impaired vascularity of infected tissue (inhibits delivery of antibiotic), antibiotic antagonism (uncommon but possible with combination therapy) and coexisting unrecognised bacterial infection.[99,120] Subsequent antibiotic dosing must be guided by drug clearance. This will be influenced by the associated organ dysfunction.[120] Nursing assessment of patient response to antibiotic therapy (resolution or exacerbation of signs of sepsis) and surveillance for sites of unrecognised infection are also important.

Source control (e.g. abscess drainage, removal of infected necrotic tissue or potentially infected device) is also an essential aspect of infection control and should be implemented as soon as practicable after diagnosis of sepsis. The method of source control chosen should always involve a risk/benefit analysis as source control interventions can exacerbate complications.[99] Nurses play a pivotal role in identification of infection source via astute ongoing patient assessment.[121,122]

Steroid therapy

As septic shock is a major complication of infectious processes, the relationship among the immune, coagulation and neuroendocrine systems has been explored.[46,123] The role of corticosteroids in the treatment of septic shock has led to a number of trials that suggested some survival benefit for low-dose corticosteroid therapy. More research is required, however, because of conflicting findings from individual studies.

The current surviving sepsis guidelines recommend the use of hydrocortisone in patients with septic shock after adequate fluid resuscitation and use of vasopressors without haemodynamic stability. Therapy with corticosteroids at a physiological dose, rather than a high dose, followed observations that patients with septic shock who had a reduced response to corticotropin were more likely to have increased mortality, and that pressor response to noradrenaline may be improved by the administration of hydrocortisone.[124] A trial exploring steroid use in sepsis demonstrated reduced vasopressor requirements and early lower mortality, but no difference in 1-year survival. A multicentre trial to address whether hydrocortisone therapy reduces mortality (ADRENAL) demonstrated that hydrocortisone administration did not improve survival in patients with septic shock.[54] Among patients with septic shock receiving positive pressure ventilation, a continuous infusion of hydrocortisone did not result in lower 90-day mortality than placebo.[54] Shock reversal was shorter in patients who received a hydrocortisone infusion (200 mg/d) compared to placebo, with more ventilator-free days, decreased length of stay in intensive care and it was noted that there were fewer blood transfusions in the hydrocortisone group.[54]

Long-term treatment with corticosteroids may result in an inadequate response of the adrenal axis to subsequent stress such as infection, surgery or trauma, with resulting onset or worsening of shock.[124] Critical illness alters cortisol metabolism and function; for example, renal dysfunction may prolong the half-life of circulating cortisol, and inflammatory cytokines may increase glucocorticoid receptor affinity. Corticosteroid administration is associated with hyperglycaemia and may affect patient outcomes, necessitating insulin to normalise blood glucose levels. A multicentre trial (Corticosteroids and Intensive Insulin Therapy for Septic Shock [COIITS])[55] demonstrated that intensive insulin therapy (aim for glucose level 4.5–6.0 mmol/L) did not improve in-hospital mortality for patients treated with hydrocortisone and oral fludrocortisones for septic shock.

Exclusion of secondary insults and organ support

Prevention of secondary inflammatory insults and organ support include a broad range of interventions including use of massive transfusion protocols,[125] recognition of abdominal compartment syndrome via urine catheter manometry,[126] lung protective ventilation, early nutritional support, glycaemic monitoring, and haemodynamic support using vasopressors and renal replacement therapy.[99] Routine evidence-based measures are also essential, including hygiene; bowel management; pressure area, mouth and eye care; and other processes of care (e.g. FASTHUG; see Chapter 21).

Awareness of the latest evidence that underpins management of these complex patients is important. Nurses play a key role in prevention of secondary insults by delivery of thorough, coordinated and timely nursing care.[121] Despite this, there is a surprising dearth of literature specifically addressing the complex nursing care required by a MODS patient. These patients require highly skilled nurses who are able to balance competing priorities via ongoing patient assessment, care planning, monitoring and evaluation. Contemporary research is focusing on homogeneous subgroups of critically ill patients in an effort to refine MODS treatment, as opposed to heterogeneous groups where treatment impacts may be hidden by patient diversity.[45,127] The complex care required to nurse the MODS patient is highlighted in the clinical case study.

Practice tip

Tips for detecting haematological dysfunction in the patient with MODS:[50]

- Monitor the skin for significant bruising or petechiae.
- Check the sites of invasive devices such as arterial, central venous access or urinary catheters for bleeding.
- Test urine or faeces for occult blood.
- Note oral bleeding during mouth care or from the nose when nasal cleansing.
- Detect progressive changes in coagulation or platelet profiles.

Summary

Multiple organ dysfunction is a common presentation to critical care units across the world. Critical care nurses require high-level knowledge of pathophysiology and early recognition of failure of individual organs and the antecedents to the development of organ failure. The pathophysiological consequence of the inflammatory response as a consequence of conditions such as trauma, gut failure, disease and sepsis requires understanding of individual organ function and responses to stressors. This is so that pre-emptive strategies can be initiated to prevent further organ failure and support individual organs. Patients with MODS are complex patients to manage, requiring highly skilled nursing care that involves vigilant assessment, planning of intervention priorities, monitoring and ongoing treatment evaluation. Well-developed time management skills are required to include all routine cares and required treatment. Balancing care priorities begins on patient presentation as highlighted by the importance of initial resuscitation, early antimicrobial therapy and advanced haemodynamic support.

Case study

Mr Marsh, aged 46, was admitted surgically for excision of a salivary gland tumour from the hard and soft palate, and flap reconstruction. He was noted to be allergic to erythromycin and penicillin. The surgery was uneventful and he was admitted to ICU for overnight ventilation. Intravenous cefotaxime was given intraoperatively and continued postoperatively. He was extubated the following morning, mobilised and nasogastric feeding commenced. That evening he complained of abdominal distention, nausea and experienced diarrhoea, which was noted to be malodourous. He developed a fever to 38.4°C.

On the second day after surgery diarrhoea and vomiting continued. Nasogastric feeding was withheld, intravenous fluids were increased, electrolytes were replaced and a septic screen was taken including testing for *Clostridium difficile*. Daily weighs were commenced, and he was discharged to the ward.

That evening Mr Marsh remained febrile up to 39.3°C and he was commenced on intravenous metronidazole. Computed tomography pulmonary angiography revealed no abnormalities. Day 3 he remained febrile up to 39.7°C and was reviewed by the ICU consultant, who could not identify a source of infection. His white cell count was normal. Blood cultures were repeated plus a viral polymerase chain reaction (PCR) stool test was collected. Loperamide and low-density feeding were commenced. Intravenous fluids and electrolyte replacement continued. Despite SpO_2 96% on room air, he was commenced on humidified oxygen via a tent mask due to a dry mouth.

By the fourth postoperative day Mr Marsh was afebrile and antibiotics were ceased. Diarrhoea continued and by day 5 he was again febrile with decreased urine output and an increase in serum creatinine (331 micromol/L) despite intravenous fluid therapy of 180 mL/h. On reassessment by the ICU team, transfer to ICU was arranged for more aggressive fluid resuscitation (7 kg weight loss noted since admission). It was noted that SpO_2 was 80–85% when oxygen therapy was removed.

Within 45 minutes of admission to ICU the patient developed mild hypotension (systolic blood pressure of 110–90 mmHg), tachycardia and tachypnoea. His clinical presentation was one of sepsis. New vascular access devices were inserted, a full septic screen attended and intravenous meropenem was administered within 30 min of hypotension and vancomycin was administered within 2 hours of hypotension and metronidazole ordered 2 hours later by the infectious diseases' physician. Review of pathology noted no *C. difficile* had been detected; however, a repeat stool sample was collected for testing. Urine output improved with further fluid resuscitation and creatinine levels began to fall.

On the evening of the sixth postoperative day gram-positive cocci resembling *Staphylococci* were detected in blood cultures. Mr Marsh's respiratory status deteriorated with increasing oxygen requirements, increasing thick creamy secretions and widespread transmitted sounds and crackles noted on auscultation. A chest X-ray revealed bilateral lower zone shadowing consistent with pneumonia. Due to an anticipated difficult airway, a surgical tracheostomy was planned for the morning; however, due to rapid clinical deterioration, intubation was undertaken in the ICU. Successful intubation was achieved on first attempt but Mr Marsh's oxygenation was poor (highest SpO_2 65%) and he experienced a ventricular fibrillation arrest with return of spontaneous circulation after 20 min. Mr Marsh required infusions of adrenaline, noradrenaline and vasopressin to maintain MAP >60 mmHg. He was ventilated on FiO_2 1.0, tidal volumes of 600 mL, rate 20 breaths/min, positive end-expiratory pressure of 15 cm with SpO_2 90%. Despite a transoesophageal echo showing normal left ventricular size and function and moderate right ventricular dilation, Mr Marsh now had established multi-organ dysfunction syndrome involving the respiratory, renal and gastrointestinal systems. Methicillin-resistant *Staphylococcus aureus* was identified from the sputum sample taken on readmission to ICU. *Clostridium difficile* was eventually identified from a sample collected on readmission to ICU, utilising a different testing strategy to the first sample collected. Mr Marsh continued on maximal therapy; however, treatment was withdrawn several days later due to futility.

DISCUSSION

The gut is often overlooked as an organ in relation to organ dysfunction. Increasingly in the literature, the gut is being recognised as a complex system that maintains a critical balance between the epithelium, microbiome and the immune system.[128] In this case, it is difficult to determine the degree to which the gut propagated further organ dysfunction; however, ongoing fluid loss did have an impact on the initial acute kidney injury. Despite early recognition of deterioration and administration of broad-spectrum antimicrobials on diagnosis of sepsis (first dose of meropenem administered within 30 min of hypotension), Mr Marsh only received all ordered antibiotics within 2.5 hours of hypotension. This highlights how competing priorities when managing the critically ill patient and the type of antimicrobials prescribed can impact on the speed of antimicrobial delivery. This case also reinforces the mortality that can be associated with nosocomial infection.

CASE STUDY QUESTIONS

1. Identify the organs and body systems that failed in the case of Mr Marsh.
2. Review the recommendations for preparation and administration of IV meropenem, vancomycin and metronidazole. Identify strategies to streamline administration of these drugs.
3. Develop a care plan for Mr Marsh on readmission to ICU. Ensure that you include routine cares as well as care specifically targeted at organ support. Discuss your plan with an experienced colleague.

RESEARCH VIGNETTE

Hazeldine J, Naumann DN, Toman E et al. Prehospital immune responses and development of multiple organ dysfunction syndrome following traumatic injury: a prospective cohort study. PLoS Med 2017:14(7); https://doi.org/10.1371/journal.pmed.1002338

Background: Almost all studies that have investigated the immune response to trauma have analysed blood samples acquired post-hospital admission. Thus, we know little of the immune status of patients in the immediate post-injury phase and how this might influence patient outcomes. The objective of this study was therefore to comprehensively assess the ultra-early, within 1-hour, immune response to trauma and perform an exploratory analysis of its relationship with the development of multiple organ dysfunction syndrome (MODS).

Methods and findings: The immune and inflammatory response to trauma was analysed in 89 adult trauma patients (mean age 41 years, range 18–90 years, 75 males) with a mean injury severity score (ISS) of 24 (range 9–66), from whom blood samples were acquired within 1 hour of injury (mean time to sample 42 minutes, range 17–60 minutes). Within minutes of trauma, a comprehensive leukocytosis, elevated serum pro- and anti-inflammatory cytokines, and evidence of innate cell activation that included neutrophil extracellular trap generation and elevated surface expression of toll-like receptor 2 and CD11b on monocytes and neutrophils, respectively, were observed. Features consistent with immune compromise were also detected, notably elevated numbers of immune suppressive CD16BRIGHT CD62LDIM neutrophils (82.07 x 106/l ± 18.94 control versus 1,092 x 106/l ± 165 trauma, $p < 0.0005$) and CD14+HLA-DRlow/- monocytes (34.96 x 106/l ± 4.48 control versus 95.72 x 106/l ± 8.0 trauma, $p < 0.05$) and reduced leukocyte cytokine secretion in response to lipopolysaccharide stimulation. Exploratory analysis via binary logistic regression found a potential association between absolute natural killer T (NKT) cell numbers and the subsequent development of MODS. Study limitations include the relatively small sample size and the absence of data relating to adaptive immune cell function.

Conclusions: Our study highlighted the dynamic and complex nature of the immune response to trauma, with immune alterations consistent with both activation and suppression evident within 1 hour of injury. The relationship of these changes, especially in NKT cell numbers, to patient outcomes such as MODS warrants further investigation.

Critique

The researchers set the background to the work by drawing attention to the complex nature of the acute immune response to injury and that little is known on the ultra-early immune and inflammatory response that occurs within minutes of traumatic injury. The current view on how major injury influences the immune system is based upon analysis of blood samples obtained following hospital admission, often several hours post-injury. Patients who survive initial haemorrhage may die following complications such as MODS or sepsis, with the individual's immune response to injury significantly influencing the development of these conditions. The researchers questioned the role that inflammation had on the posttraumatic immune and inflammatory response to trauma and how this influenced patient outcome, stratification for treatment and the development of novel therapies. The results from the study revealed traumatic injury resulted in immediate immune dysfunction, with evidence of concomitant immune activation and suppression detected within minutes of injury. The features detected in the blood samples taken within minutes of injury were absent from samples obtained in the following hours or days post-trauma. The authors suggest that the complex and dynamic nature of the acute immune response to injury mean that targeting one element of the immune response is unlikely to reduce the immune-paresis or the incidence of MODS.

The study was well designed, and is significant in relation to the incidence of MODS among the critically ill trauma patients who are admitted to critical care. The researchers suggest the development of a blood test to determine which patients have a response that predispose them to sepsis or MODS is an area for further investigation. The relationship of the immune response to the development of MODS and mortality outcomes for patients with trauma should encourage future prospective studies that may translate into improved healthcare outcomes for critically ill patients.

Learning activities

1. Identify five key elements essential in managing the patient with emergent MODS.
2. Outline four strategies that may facilitate the prevention of MODS.
3. Identify eight strategies that aim to minimise secondary insult and provide organ support for the MODS patient.
4. Organ dysfunction is associated with reduced cellular oxygenation. What are some of the ways in which cellular oxygen delivery can be disrupted?
5. What are the four key systemic pathophysiological responses that contribute to the development of MODS?
6. There are different scoring systems available to identify MODS and the SOFA score is one of the most common. What variables are used when determining a SOFA score?

Online resources

The Institute for Healthcare Improvement (IHI) is a non-profit organisation for advancing the quality and value of health care. Search the site for sepsis-related information about improving care and severe sepsis bundles, www.ihi.org

The Surviving Sepsis guidelines webpage provides access to full text documents, references, presentations, updated position statements and tools related to the guidelines, www.survivingsepsis.org

The US National Institutes of Health clinical trials registry. Search the site for current trials in MODS, www.clinicaltrials.gov

Further reading

Alsina M, Martin-Ancel A, Alarcon-Allen A, et al. The severity of hypoxic-ischaemic encephalopathy correlates with multiple organ dysfunction in the hypothermia era. Pediatr Crit Care Med 2017;18(3):234–40.

Estenssoro E. The central nervous system as an indicator of multiple organ dysfunction: a mini-review. J Organ Dysfunct 2007;3:3–6.

Fröhlich M, Lefering R, Probst C, et al. Epidemiology and risk factors of multiple-organ failure after multiple trauma: an analysis of 31,154 patients from the Trauma Register DGU. J Trauma Acute Care Surg 2014;76(4):921–8.

Poulose V, Koh J, Tay TR, et al. A randomised pilot study of parenteral glutamine supplementation in severe sepsis. Crit Care Shock 2017;20(3):61–7.

Sauaia A, Moore E, Johnson J, et al. Temporal trends of postinjury multiple-organ failure: still resource intensive, morbid, and lethal. J Trauma Acute Care Surg 2014;76(3):582–93.

Van Wessen KJP, Leenen LPH. Reduction in mortality rates of postinjury multiple organ dysfunction syndrome: a shifting paradigm? A prospective population-based cohort study. Shock 2018;49(1):33–8.

Vasilevskis EE, Pandharipande PP, Graves AJ, et al. Validity of a modified Sequential Organ Failure Assessment score using the Richmond Agitation-Sedation scale. Crit Care Med 2016;44(1):138–46.

Yadav H, Harrison AM, Hanson AC, et al. Improving the accuracy of cardiovascular component of the Sequential Organ Failure Assessment Score. Crit Care Med 2015;43(7):1449–57.

References

1. Ricci Z, Robmagnoli S, Ronco C, et al. From continuous renal replacement therapies to multiple organ support therapy. Contrib Nephrol 2018;194:155–69.
2. Mizock B. The multiple organ dysfunction syndrome. Disease-a-month: DM 2009;55(8):476–526.
3. Al-Khafaji A, Sharma S. Multiple organ failure of sepsis. eMedicine Critical Care [Internet]. 2010. Available from: http://emedicine.medscape.com/article/169640-overview.
4. Marshall J. The multiple organ dysfunction system. Surgical treatment: Evidence based and problem oriented. 2001. Available from: http://www.ncbi.nlm.nih.gov/bookshelf/br.fcgi?book=surg&part=A5364.
5. Deitch E. Multiple organ failure: pathophysiology and potential future therapy. Ann Surg 1992;216(2):117–34.
6. Rendy L, Sapan H, Kalesarran L. Multiple organ dysfunction syndrome (MODS) prediction score in multi-trauma patients. Int J Surg Open 2017;8:1–6.
7. Klingensmith N, Coopersmith C. The gut as the motor of multiple organ dysfunction in critical illness. Crit Care Clin 2016;32(2):203–12.
8. Papathanassoglou E, Bozas E, Giannakopoloulou M. Multiple organ dysfunction syndrome pathogenesis and care: a complex systems' theory perspective. Nurs Crit Care 2008;13(5):249–59.
9. Mitchell C. Tissue oxygenation monitoring as a guide for trauma resuscitation. Crit Care Nurse 2016;36(3):12–19.
10. Pinsky M, Al-Faresi F, Brenner B, et al. Septic shock. eMedicine Critical Care [Internet]. 2011. Available from: http://emedicine.medscape.com/article/168402-overview.
11. Mizock B. The multiple organ dysfunction syndrome. Dis Mon 2009;55(8):476–526.
12. Duran-Bedolla J, Montes de Oca-Sandoval M, Saldana-Navor V, et al. Sepsis, mitochondrial failure and multiple organ dysfunction. Clin Invest Med 2014;37(2):E58–69.
13. Henke K, Eigisti J. Self-annihilation: a cell's story of suicide. Dimens Crit Care Nurs 2005;24(3):117–19.
14. Saukkonen K, Lakkisto P, Varpula M, et al. Association of cell-free plasma DNA with hospital mortality and organ dysfunction in intensive care unit patients. Intensive Care Med 2007;33(9):1624–7.
15. Singer M. The role of mitochondrial dysfunction in sepsis induced multi-organ failure. Virulence 2014;5(1):66–72.
16. Schmidt H, Lotze U, Ghanem A, et al. Relation of impaired interorgan communication and parasympathetic activity in chronic heart failure and multiple-organ dysfunction syndrome. J Crit Care 2014;29(3):367–73.
17. Leite H, de Lima L. Metabolic resuscitation in sepsis: a necessary step beyond the haemodynamics. J Thorac Dis 2016;8(7):552–7.
18. Tsirigotis P, Chondropoulos S, Gkirkas K, et al. Balanced control of both hyper and hypo-inflammatory phases as a new treatment paradigm in sepsis. J Thoracic Dis. 2016;8(5):312–16.
19. Jastrow K, Gonzalez E, McGuire M, et al. Early cytokine production risk stratifies trauma patients for multiple organ failure. J Am Coll Surg 2009;3(209):320–31.
20. Padgett D, Glaser R. How stress influences the immune response. Trends Immunol 2003;24(8):444–8.
21. Hubbard W, Bland K, Chaudry I. The role of the mitochondrion in trauma and shock. Shock 2004;22(5):395–402.
22. Magder S, Cernacek P. Role of endothelins in septic, cardiogenic, and hemorrhagic shock. Can J Physiol Pharmacol 2003;81(6):635–43.

23. Zingarelli B, Sheehan M, Wong H. Nuclear factor-kappaB as a therapeutic target in critical care medicine. Crit Care Med 2003;31(Suppl.):S105–11.
24. Osuka A, Ogura H, Ueyama M, et al. Immune response to traumatic injury: harmony and discordance of immune system homeostasis. Acute Med Surg 2014;1:63–9.
25. Sherwood E, Toliver-Kinsky T. Mechanisms of the inflammatory response. Best Pract Res Clin Anaesthesiol 2004;18(3):385–405.
26. Weigand M, Horner C. The systemic inflammatory response syndrome. Best Prac Res Clin Anaesthesiol 2004;18(3):455–75.
27. Popa C, Rusu O, Kocsis A, et al. SIRS and MODS in acute pancreatitis. Mod Med 2015;22(1):31–8.
28. Arias J, Aller M. Surgical inflammation: a pathophysiological rainbow. J Transl Med 2009;7(9).
29. Su J, Zhang Y, Hu W. The current opinions of capillary leak syndrome. Open J Clin Diagn 2015;5:14–19.
30. Calandra T, Cohen J. The international sepsis forum consensus conference on definitions of infection in the intensive care unit. Crit Care Med 2005;33(7):1538–48.
31. Tsao C, Ho S, Wu C. Coagulation abnormalities in sepsis. Acta Anaesthesiol Taiwanica 2015;53(1):16–22.
32. Vincent J, Rello J, Marshall J, et al. International study of the prevalence of outcomes of infection in intensive care units. JAMA 2009;302(21):2323–9.
33. van Vught L, Klein Klouwenberg P, Spitoni C. Incidence, risk factors, and attributable mortality of secondary infections in the intensive care unit after admission for sepsis. JAMA 2016;315(14):1469–79.
34. Simmons J, Pittet J. The coagulopathy of acute sepsis. Curr Opin Anaethesiol 2015;28(2):227–36.
35. Craft J, Gordon C, Huether S, et al. Alterations of cardiovascular function across the lifespan. In: Understanding pathophysiology. Sydney: Mosby; 2018. p. 648.
36. Shorr A, Bernard GR, Dhainaut J, et al. Protein C concentrations in severe sepsis: an early directional change in plasma levels predicts outcome. Crit Care 2006;10:R92.
37. Preiser J, Ichai C, Orban J, et al. Metabolic response to the stress of critical illness. Br J Anaesth 2014;113(6):945–54.
38. McCance K, Heuther S, Brashers V, et al. Pathophysiology: the biological basis for disease in adults and children. 6th ed. St Louis: Mosby Elsevier; 2010.
39. Østergaard L, Granfeldt A, Secher N, et al. Microcirculatory dysfunction and tissue oxygenation in critical illness. Acta Anaesthesiol Scand 2015;59:1246–59.
40. Leone M, Asfar P, Radermacher P, et al. Optimizing mean arterial pressure in septic shock: a critical reappraisal of the literature. Crit Care 2015;19:101–8.
41. Bauer M, ed. Multiple organ failure – update on pathophysiology and treatment strategies. Euroanesthesia Conference Proceedings; 2005 May 28–31; Vienna, Austria: European Society of Anaesthesiology.
42. Vincent J, Moreno R, Takala J, et al. The SOFA (sepsis related organ failure assessment) score to describe organ dysfunction/failure. Intensive Care Med 1996;22:707–10.
43. van Wessem K, Leehan L. Reduction in mortality rates of postinjury multiple organ dysfunction syndrome: a shifting paradigm? A prospective population-based cohort study. Shock 2018;49(1):33–8.
44. Ferreira F, Bota D, Bross A, et al. Serial evaluation of the SOFA score to predict outcome in critically ill patients. JAMA 2001;286(14):1754–8.
45. Rohde J, Odden A, Bonham C, et al. The epidemiology of acute organ system dysfunction from severe sepsis outside of the intensive care unit. J Hosp Med 2013;8(5):243–7.
46. Cabera C, Manson J, Shepherd J, et al. Signatures of inflammation and impending multiple organ dysfunction in the hyperacute phase of trauma: a prospective cohort study. PLoS Med 2017;14(7):e1002352.
47. Manson J, Cole E, De'Ath H, et al. Early changes within the lymphocyte population are associated with the development of multiple organ dysfunction syndrome in trauma patients. Crit Care 2016;20:176–85.
48. Gando S. Microvascular thrombosis and multiple organ dysfunction syndrome. Crit Care Med 2010;38(2 (Suppl.)):S35–42.
49. Izak M, Bussel J. Management of thrombocytopenia. F1000Prime Rep 2014;6:45–55.
50. Bougle A, Harrois A, Duranteau J. Resuscitative strategies in traumatic haemorrhagic shock. Ann Intensive Care 2013;3(1):1–9.
51. Martí-Carvajal A, Salanti G, Cardona-Zorrilla A Human recombinant activated protein C for severe sepsis 2007. Available from: http://www2.cochrane.org/reviews/en/ab004388.html.
52. Gheorghija V, Barbu A, Gheorghiu M, et al. Endocrine dysfunction in sepsis: a beneficial or deleterious host response. Germs 2015;5(1):17–25.
53. Economidou F, Douka E, Tzanela M, et al. Thyroid function in critical illness. In: Rajendram R, Preedy VR, Patel VB, editors. Diet and nutrition in critical care. New York: Springer; 2015.
54. Venkatesh B, Finfer S, Cohen J, et al. Adjunctive glucocorticoid therapy in patients with septic shock. N Engl J Med 2018;378(9):797–808.
55. Annane D, Bellissant E, Bollaert P, et al. Corticosteroids for treating sepsis. Cochrane Database Syst Rev 2015;(12):CD002243. Available from: https://www.ncbi.nlm.nih.gov/pubmed/26633262.
56. Annane D, Pastores S, Rochwerg B, et al. Guidelines for the diagnosis and management of critical illness-related corticosteroid insufficiency (CIRCI) in critically ill patients (Part I): Society of Critical Care Medicine (SCCM) and European Society of Intensive Care Medicine (ESICM) 2017. Intensive Care Med 2017;43(12):2078–88.

57. Yang Y, Liu L, Jiang D, et al. Critical illness-related corticosteroid insufficiency after multiple traumas: a multicenter, prospective cohort study. J Trauma Acute Care Surg 2014;76(6):1390–6.
58. Hamrahian A, Fleseriu M. Evaluation and management of adrenal insufficiency in critically ill patients: disease state review. Endocr Pract 2017;23(6):716–25.
59. Annane D, Renault A, Brun-Buisson C, et al. Hydrocortisone plus fludrocortisone for adults with septic shock. N Engl J Med 2018;378(9):809–18.
60. Wernly B, Lichtenauer M, Hoppe U, et al. Hyperglycemia in septic patients: an essential stress survival response in all, a robust marker for risk stratification in some, to be messed with in none. J Thorac Dis 2016;8(7):E621–4.
61. Song F, Zhong L, Han L, et al. Intensive insulin therapy for septic patients: a meta-analysis of randomized controlled trials. Biomed Res Int 2014;2014:10.
62. van Vught LA, Wiewel MA, Klein Klouwenberg PM, et al. Admission hyperglycemia in critically ill sepsis patients: association with outcome and host response. Crit Care Med 2016;44(7):1338–46.
63. Dias C, Leite H, Nogueira P, et al. Ionized hypocalcemia is an early event and is associated with organ dysfunction in children admitted to the intensive care unit. J Crit Care 2013;28:810–15.
64. Langhans C, Weber-Carstens S, Schmidt F, et al. Inflammation-induced acute phase response in skeletal muscle and critical illness myopathy. PLoS ONE 2014;9(3):e92048.
65. Hajri T, Gharib M, Kaul S, et al. Association between adipokines and critical illness outcomes. J Trauma Acute Care Surg 2017;83(3):507–19.
66. Sonneville R, Verdonk F, Rauturier C, et al. Understanding brain dysfunction in sepsis. Ann Intensive Care 2013;3:15–25.
67. Manikandan S. Cardiovascular manifestations of subarachnoid haemorrhage. J Neuroanaesthesiol Crit Care 2017;4(S1):38–44.
68. Meyer K. Understanding paroxysmal sympathetic hyperactivity after traumatic brain injury. Surg Neurol Int 2014;5(Suppl. 13):S490–2.
69. Hodgson C, Tipping C. Physiotherapy management of intensive care unit-acquired weakness. J Physiother 2017;63(1):4–10.
70. Hermans G, van den Berghe G. Clinical review: intensive care unit acquired weakness. Crit Care 2015;19(1):274–82.
71. Calsavara A, Nobre V, Barichello T, et al. Post-sepsis cognitive impairment and associated risk factors: a systematic review. Aust Crit Care 2018;31(4):242–53.
72. Mazeraud A, Pascal Q, Verdonk F, et al. Neuroanatomy and physiology of brain dysfunction in sepsis. Clin Chest Med 2016;37:333–45.
73. Heming N, Mazeraud A, Verdonk F, et al. Neuroanatomy of sepsis-associated encephalopathy. Crit Care 2017;21:65–70.
74. Llompart-Pou J, Talayero M, Homar J, et al. Multiorgan failure in the serious trauma patient. Med Intensiva 2014;38(7):455–62.
75. Hutchings L, Watkinson P, Young J, et al. Defining multiple organ failure after major trauma: a comparison of the Denver, Sequential Organ Failure Assessment and Marshall scoring systems. J Trauma Acute Care Surg 2017;82(3):534–41.
76. Dewar D, Tarrant SK, King K, et al. Changes in the epidemiology and prediction of multiple organ failure after injury. J Trauma Acute Care Surg 2013;74(3):774–9.
77. Sauaia A, Moore E, Johnson J, et al. Temporal trends of post-injury multiple-organ failure: still resource intensive, morbid, and lethal. J Trauma Acute Care Surg 2014;76(3):582–92.
78. Herridge M, Chu L, Matte A, et al. The RECOVER Program: disability risk groups and 1-year outcome after 7 or more days of mechanical ventilation. Am J Respir Crit Care Med 2016;194(7):831–44.
79. Bingold T, Lefering R, Zacharowski K, et al. Individual organ failure and concomitant risk of mortality differs according to the type of admission to ICU – a retrospective study of SOFA score of 23,795 patients. PLoS ONE 2015;10(8):e0134329.
80. Lone N, Walsh T. Impact of intensive care unit organ failures on mortality during five years after a critical illness. Am J Respir Crit Care Med 2012;76(4):640–7.
81. Aswani A, Manson J, Itagaki K, et al. Scavenging circulating mitochondrial DNA as a potential therapeutic option for multiple organ dysfunction in trauma hemorrhage. Front Immunol 2018;9(891).
82. Suarez De La Rica A, Gilsanz F, Maseda E. Epidemiologic trends of sepsis in western countries. Ann Transl Med 2016;4(17):325–31.
83. Mayr F, Yende S, Angus D. Epidemiology of severe sepsis. Virulence 2014;5(1):4–11.
84. Fröhlich M, Lefering R, Probst C, et al. Epidemiology and risk factors of multiple-organ failure after multiple trauma: an analysis of 31,154 patients from the TraumaRegister DGU. J Trauma Acute Care Surg 2014;76(4):921–7.
85. Safari S, Shojaee M, Rahmati F, et al. Accuracy of SOFA score in prediction of 30-day outcome of critically ill patients. Turk J Emerg Med 2016;16(4):146–50.
86. Kaukonen K, Bailey M, Suzuki S, et al. Mortality related to severe sepsis and septic shock among critically ill patients in Australia and New Zealand, 2000-2012. JAMA 2014;311(13):1308–16.
87. Minei J, Cuschieri J, Sperry J, et al. The changing pattern and implication of multiple organ failure after blunt injury with hemorrhagic shock. Crit Care Med 2012;40(4):1129–35.
88. Barie P, Hydo L, Shou J, et al. Decreasing magnitude of multiple organ dysfunction syndrome despite increasingly severe critical surgical illness: a 17-year longitudinal study. J Trauma 2008;65(6):1227–35.
89. Vogel J, Liao M, Hopkins E, et al. Prediction of postinjury multiple-organ failure in the emergency department: development of the Denver Emergency Department Trauma Organ Failure Score. J Trauma Acute Care Surg 2014;76(1):140–5.

90. Anami E, Grion C, Cardoso L, et al. Serial evaluation of SOFA score in a Brazilian teaching hospital. Intensive Crit Care Nurs 2010;26(2):75–82.
91. Seymour C, Liu V, Iwashyna T, et al. Assessment of clinical criteria for sepsis: for the third international consensus definitions for sepsis and septic shock (sepsis-3). JAMA 2016;315(8):762–74.
92. Frolich M, Wafaisade A, Mansuri A, et al. Which score should be used for posttraumatic multiple organ failure? Comparison of the MODS, Denver- and SOFA-Scores. Scand J Trauma Resusc Emerg Med 2016;24(130).
93. Dewar D, White A, Attia J, et al. Comparison of post injury multiple-organ failure scoring systems: Denver versus Sequential Organ Failure Assessment. J Trauma Acute Care Surg 2014;77(4):624–9.
94. Singer M, Deutschman C, Seymour C, et al. The third international consensus definitions for sepsis and septic shock. JAMA 2016;315(80):801–10.
95. Vasilevskis E, Pandharipande P, Graves A, et al. Validity of a modified sequential organ failure assessment score using the Richmond Agitation-Sedation scale. Crit Care Med 2016;44(1):138–46.
96. McConnell K, Coopersmith C. Organ failure avoidance and mitigation strategies in surgery. Surg Clin North Am 2012;92:307–19.
97. Minne L, Abu-Hanna A, de Jonge E. Evaluation of SOFA-based models for predicting mortality in the ICU: a systematic review. Crit Care 2008;12(6):R161.
98. Montmany Vioque S, Navarro Soto S, Rebasa Cladera P, et al. Measurement of lactic acid in multiple injury patients and its usefulness as a predictor of multiorgan failure and mortality. Cir Esp 2012;90(2):107–13.
99. Rhodes A, Evans L, Alhazzani W, et al. Surviving sepsis campaign: international guidelines for management of sepsis and septic shock. Intensive Care Med 2017;43:304–77.
100. Nydam T, Kashuk J, Moore E, et al. Refractory postinjury thrombocytopenia is associated with multiple organ failure and adverse outcomes. J Trauma 2011;70(2):406–7.
101. Guyette F, Suffoletto B, Castillo J, et al. Prehospital serum lactate as a predictor of outcomes in trauma patients: a retrospective observational study. J Trauma 2011;70(4):782–6.
102. Teoh H, Quan A, Creighton A, et al. BRCA1 gene therapy reduces systemic inflammatory response and multiple organ failure and improves survival in experimental sepsis. Gene Ther 2013;20:51–61.
103. Rodrigues Filho E, Ikuta N, Simon D, et al. Prognostic value of circulating DNA levels in critically ill and trauma patients. Rev Bras Ter Intensiva 2014;26(3):305–12.
104. Papurica M, Rogobete A, Sandesc D, et al. Advances in biomarkers in critical ill polytrauma patients. Clin Lab 2016;62(6):977–86.
105. Bagshaw S, Lapinsky S, Dial S, et al. Acute kidney injury in septic shock: clinical outcomes and impact of duration of hypotension prior to initiation of antimicrobial therapy. Intensive Care Med 2009;35:871–81.
106. Iscimen R, Cartin-Ceba R, Yilmaz M, et al. Risk factors for the development of acute lung injury in patients with septic shock: an observational cohort study. Crit Care Med 2008;36(5):1518–22.
107. Kumar A, Ellis P, Arabi Y, et al. Initiation of inappropriate antimicrobial therapy results in a fivefold reduction of survival in human septic shock. Chest 2009;136(5):1237–48.
108. Ferrer R, Martin-Loeches I, Phillips G, et al. Empiric antibiotic treatment reduces mortality in severe sepsis and septic shock from the first hour: results from a guideline-based performance improvement program. Crit Care Med 2014;42(8):1749–55.
109. Gaieski D, Mikkelsen M, Band R, et al. Impact of time to antibiotics on survival in patients with severe sepsis or septic shock in whom early goal-directed therapy was initiated in the emergency department. Crit Care Med 2010;38(4):1045–53.
110. Whiles B, Deis A, Simpson S. Increased time to initial antimicrobial administration is associated with progression to septic shock in severe sepsis patients. Crit Care Med 2017;45(4):623–9.
111. Liu V, Fielding-Singh V, Greene J, et al. The timing of early antibiotics and hospital mortality in sepsis. Am J Respir Crit Care Med 2017;196(7):856–63.
112. Kethireddy S, Bilgili B, Sees A, et al. Culture-negative septic shock compared with culture-positive septic shock: a retrospective cohort study. Crit Care Med 2018;46(4):506–12.
113. Pruinelli L, Westra B, Yadav P, et al. Delay within the 3-hour Surviving Sepsis Campaign guideline on mortality for patients with severe sepsis and septic shock. Crit Care Med 2018;46(4):500–5.
114. Kalil A, Johnson D, Lisco S, et al. Early goal-directed therapy for sepsis: a novel solution for discordant survival outcomes in clinical trials. Crit Care Med 2017;45(4):607–14.
115. Amaral A, Fowler R, Pinto R, et al. Patient and organizational factors associated with delays in antimicrobial therapy for septic shock. Crit Care Med 2016;44(12):2145–53.
116. deBoisblanc B. It is about time: antibiotic delays in the treatment of septic shock. Crit Care Med 2016;44(12):2279–80.
117. Leisman D, Wie B, Doerfler M, et al. Association of fluid resuscitation initiation within 30 minutes of severe sepsis and septic shock recognition with reduced mortality and length of stay. Ann Emerg Med 2016;68(3):298–311.
118. Kumar A, Safdar N, Kethireddy S, et al. A survival benefit of combination antibiotic therapy for serious infections associated with sepsis and septic shock is contingent only on the risk of death: a meta-analytic/meta-regression study. Crit Care Med 2010;38(8):1651–64.
119. van Zanten A. The golden hour of antibiotic administration in severe sepsis: avoid a false start striving for gold*. Crit Care Med 2014;42(8):1931–2.

120. Ulldemolins M, Roberts J, Lipman J, et al. Antibiotic dosing in multiple organ dysfunction syndrome. Chest 2011;139(5):1210–20.
121. Kleinpell R, Aitken L, Schorr C. Implications of the new international sepsis guidelines for nursing care. Am J Crit Care 2013;22(3):212–22.
122. Jones J. Managing sepsis effectively with national early warning scores and screening tools. Br J Community Nurs 2017;22(6):278–81.
123. Churpek M, Zadravecz F, Winslow C, et al. Incidence and prognostic value of the systemic inflammatory response syndrome and organ dysfunctions in ward patients. Am J Respir Crit Care Med 2015;192(8):958–64.
124. Gibbison B, López-López JA, Higgins JPT, et al. Corticosteroids in septic shock: a systematic review and network meta-analysis. Crit Care 2017;21(1):78.
125. Cotton B, Au B, Nunez T, et al. Predefined massive transfusion protocols are associated with a reduction in organ failure and postinjury complications. J Trauma 2009;66(1):41–8, discussion 8-9.
126. Dewar D, Moore FA, Moore EE, et al. Postinjury multiple organ failure. Injury 2009;40(9):912–18.
127. Qin W, Zhang X, Yang S, et al. Risk factors for multiple organ dysfunction syndrome in severe stroke patients. PLoS ONE 2016;11(11):1–10.
128. Meng M, Klingensmith N, Coopersmith C. New insights into the gut as the driver of critical illness and organ failure. Curr Opin Crit Care 2017;23(2):143–8.

Section 3

Specialty practice

Chapter 23

Emergency presentations

Alister Hodge, Pauline Calleja

KEY WORDS

disaster management
envenomation
extended practice
heat illnesses
hypothermia
near-drowning
poisoning
retrieval
triage

Learning objectives

After reading this chapter, you should be able to:

- describe the uniqueness of the emergency care environment
- describe the different international triage models and outline the development of Australasian triage models
- discuss the process of initial patient assessment and triage nursing practice
- integrate emergency nursing principles and practice in initial patient care
- describe the various roles of extended nursing practice in the emergency setting
- describe the principles and practice of patient preparation for retrievals or transfers
- discuss the principles for the management of disaster victims in the emergency department (ED)
- discuss the initial nursing management of common presentations to the ED, including respiratory or neurological dysfunction, chest pain, abdominal pain, poisoning, envenomation, submersion and heat illness.

Introduction

Emergency nursing practice covers an enormous range of clinical presentations. This chapter provides an overview of emergency care provided to patients treated within an emergency department (ED) and is not specific to patients who are critically ill. In many hospitals, critical care nurses are required at times to move between the ED, ICU, cardiac and recovery units. This chapter therefore aims to aid critical care nurses who deliver patient care within the emergency setting. Please read in conjunction with Chapters 24 and 25, which describe the management of additional common presentations to the ED: trauma and resuscitation emergencies, respectively. Chapter 1 contains information on extended nursing roles relevant to emergency nursing.

In this chapter the organisational systems and processes of care in an ED environment, including triage, specifics of ED extended practice nursing roles, multiple casualties/disaster management and transport/retrieval of critically ill patients, are described. Details of a select group of the most common emergency presentations and conditions related to critical care practice are then discussed. The initial clinical assessment and incidences of these common presentations are outlined, and the likely diagnoses associated with these presentations and their initial management in the ED are identified. Ongoing management of these selected conditions is covered in this chapter.

Emergency nursing practice encompasses the holistic care of individuals of all ages who present with perceived or actual physical and/or mental health alterations and of all levels of acuity. These presentations are often undiagnosed and require a range of prompt symptomatic and definitive interventions. Emergency clinical practice is usually unscheduled, episodic and acute in its nature, and is therefore is unique in the demands it places on nursing staff.[1,2] In many instances the emergency nurse is the first healthcare professional to be in contact with an acutely ill or injured patient.[1]

Background

Emergency nursing is unique, in that it involves the care of patients with health problems that are often undiagnosed on presentation but perceived as sufficiently acute by the individual to warrant seeking emergency care in the hospital setting. As patients present with signs and symptoms rather than medical diagnoses, refined assessment skills are paramount in deciding level of acuity and urgency of the patient to facilitate assessment in a safe and timely manner. Many skills required by emergency nurses are based on a broad foundation of knowledge that serves as a guide in collecting information, making observations and evaluating data, and sorting and analysing relevant information to inform decision making.[3,4] This foundation enables an emergency nurse to communicate appropriately with other members of the healthcare team, and to implement appropriate independent and collaborative nursing interventions.

Emergency nurses are specialists in acute episodic nursing care, and their knowledge, skills and expertise encompass almost all other nursing specialty areas. Emergency nurses therefore possess a unique body of knowledge and skill sets to manage a wide variety of presentations across all age groups; this includes familiarity with general physical and emotional requirements of each age group as these relate to their presenting health needs.[1] ED nurses work collaboratively with pre-hospital emergency personnel, doctors and other healthcare providers and community agencies to provide patient care.[4,5] Roles in the ED include triage, direct patient care, patient flow, collaborative care delivery, providing emotional support during crises, documenting and arranging ongoing care, admission to the hospital, transfer to another healthcare facility or discharge into the community, often within time-pressured deadlines.[5,6] Triage ensures that patients are managed in order of clinical urgency, and that ED resources such as staff, equipment, treatment area, are utilised appropriately.[7]

History of triage

Triage was first described in 1797 during the Napoleonic wars by Surgeon Marshall Larrey, Napoleon's chief medical officer, who introduced a system of sorting casualties that presented to the field dressing stations. His aims were military rather than medical, however, so the highest priority was given to soldiers who had minor wounds and could be returned quickly to the battle lines with minimal treatment.[8]

The documented use of triage was limited until World War I, when the term was used to describe a physical area where sorting of casualties was conducted, rather than a description of the sorting or triage process itself.[9] Triage continued to develop into a formalised assessment process, with subsequent adoption of initial categorising of patient urgency and acuity within most civilian EDs.[8]

International approaches to triage

The triage process has evolved internationally, particularly over the past two decades. Four main triage scales are available and, although used in the country in which they were developed, they have also been implemented or adapted in other health services. The Canadian Emergency Department Triage and Acuity Scales (CTAS),[10] the Manchester Triage Scale (MTS)[3] and the Australasian Triage Scale (ATS)[4,11] are the most common five-level triage scales used with the ATS being reported as the most reliable,[12] although debate exists about how reliability is measured[13] and some contexts rely on other factors to determine suitability preferring the Manchester Triage System.[14,15] In the USA, three-level triage scales have historically been used but, due to poorer performance compared with five-level triage scales,[16] the five-level triage scales are now recommended for use across the USA (e.g. Emergency Severity Index or the CTAS).[17] Newer triage systems have been developed, e.g. the four-level Taiwan Triage System[18] and the Soterion Rapid Triage System.[19] These newer systems are not widely reported or implemented and require further testing.[8,19]

Characteristics of the ATS, CTAS, MTS and ESI five-level triage scales are presented in Table 23.1.[20] Although somewhat similar, there are variations in some aspects such as timeframes for which a person should wait to see a doctor. For example, the ESI does not define expected time intervals to doctor evaluation, and not all scales are adapted to specific populations, such as paediatrics, or settings, such as rural environments. The Manchester Triage System differs to the ATS, CTAS and ESI in that it uses an algorithm approach with 52 presenting complaints to derive a triage score. The other systems use a slightly different approach where a combination of observation, history taking and physical examination facilitates the nurse's judgement to apply a triage score. Updates to and computerisation of previous guidelines have been undertaken over the years.[21]

TABLE 23.1
Comparison of characteristics of the ATS, CTAS, MTS and ESI 5-level triage scales

CRITERION	CTAS	ATS	ESI	MTS
Time to triage assessment	10 min	NS	NS	NS
Time to nurse assessment	Based on initial triage	NS	NS	NS
Time to doctor assessment	Immediate/15/ 30/60/120 min	Immediate/10/ 30/60/120 min	NS	Immediate/10/ 60/120/240 min
Fractile response time (CTAS)/performance threshold (NTS)	I-98, II-95, III-90, IV-85, V-80	I-100, II-80, III-75, IV-70, V-70	NS	NS
Pain scale	10-point scale	NS	>7/10 *consider* up-triage to ESI level 2	A major factor considered for each chief complaint
Paediatrics	Used in CTAS	NS but generally recognised	Paediatric VS criteria included to help determine ESI level 2 vs 3; fever criteria for <24 months included	Not addressed in the algorithm
Sentinel diagnoses	Yes	Yes	Not used	52 chief complaints vs sentinel diagnosis
Expected admission rates	Specified	Defined using actual data from multiple sites	Benchmarking data available	NS
Education implementation material	Web-based training available for a fee	Emergency Education Triage Kit (ETEK) Workbook, resource book and quick reference guide website: http://www.health.gov.au/internet/main/publishing.nsf/Content/casemix-ED-triage+Review+Fact+Sheet+Documents	2012 edition of the Implementation Handbook Emergency Severity Index (ESI): A Triage Tool for Emergency Departments website: https://www.ahrq.gov/professionals/systems/hospital/esi/index.html	Published manual: Mackway-Jones K, Marsden J, Windle J, editors. Emergency triage. Manchester Triage Group. 3rd ed. Plymouth: Wiley Blackwell; 2013
Rural setting	Yes	NS	NS	NS
Additional comments			Uses acuity to identify level 1 and 2 patients, and resources to identify levels 3–5	Algorithmic approach that uses 52 chief complaint-based flow charts; the triage nurse then continues an algorithmic approach and assesses life threat, pain, haemorrhage, consciousness level, temperature and acuteness for each chief complaint

Note: the ATS performance thresholds have since been revised to: 100%, 80%, 75%, 70%, 70%.[26]
NS = not specified; VS = vital sign; MTS = Manchester Triage Scale.
Adapted from Fernandes CM, Tanabe P, Gilboy N, et al. Five-level triage: a report from the ACEP/ENA Five-level Triage Task Force. J Emerg Nurs 2005;31(1):39-50; quiz 118, with permission.

Educational materials to support each of the scales are available. An International Triage Scale has been proposed but requires development and testing.[21]

Development of triage processes: focus on Australia and New Zealand

Australia is a world leader in the development of emergency triage and patient classification systems. Because other triage systems (CTAS, MTS, ESI) have primarily been adapted from the Australian system,[21] the focus here is on the development of the Australian and New Zealand ATS. Since the late 1960s a number of locally developed triage systems were developed and implemented; in the early 1990s a unified scale was proposed. The National Triage Scale (NTS) was subsequently tested and demonstrated to have the essential characteristics of utility, reliability and validity.[21] In 1993, the NTS was adopted by the Australasian College for Emergency Medicine in its triage policy,[22] and subsequently renamed the ATS as it was implemented in most EDs in Australia and New Zealand (Table 23.2).[23]

The process of triage

All patients presenting to an ED should be triaged on arrival by a suitably experienced and trained registered nurse.[4,17,24,25] This assessment represents the first clinical contact and the commencement of care in the department. The ideal features of a triage area are: a well-signposted location close to the patient entrance; ability to conduct examination and primary treatment of patients in privacy; close proximity to the acute treatment and resuscitation areas; and appropriate resources including an examination table, thermometer, a sphygmomanometer, stethoscope, glucometer and pulse oximetry.[4,25,26] Access to emergency equipment, communication devices (such as telephone, emergency buzzer), standard precaution equipment (such as gloves and hand-wash) and paper/electronic recording facilities are also important.

As the first clinician in the ED to interview the patient, the triage nurse gathers and documents information from the patient, family and friends, or pre-hospital emergency personnel. Professional maturity is required to manage the stress inherent in dealing with an acutely ill patient and family members (under significant stress themselves), while rapidly making informed judgement on priorities of care for a wide range of clinical problems.[27]

The triage nurse receives and records information about the patient's reason for presentation to the ED, beginning with a clear statement of the complaint, followed by historical information and related relevant details, such as time of onset, duration of symptom/s and what aggravates or relieves the symptom/s. A brief, focused physical assessment including vital signs may be undertaken to identify the urgency and severity of the condition, and may be collected as part of the triage process to inform decision making.[25] Triage assessment generally should be no longer than 2–5 min, balancing between speed and thoroughness.[4] From the information collected, the triage nurse determines the need for immediate or delayed care,[8] and assigns the patient a 1–5 ATS category in response to the statement: *This patient should wait for medical assessment and treatment no longer than …* .[4] The patient must be then allocated to an appropriate area within the ED for care to be delivered.

Patients with acute conditions that threaten life or limb receive the highest priority while those with minor illness or injury are assigned a lower priority. It may not be possible to categorise the patient correctly in all instances, and it is better to conservatively allocate priority to ensure the patient is seen sooner, if the triage category is unclear.[4,24] Importantly, a triage allocation can be altered at any time.[4,24] If a patient's condition changes while awaiting medical assessment/treatment, or if additional relevant information becomes available that impacts on the patient's urgency, the patient should be re-triaged to a category that reflects the determined urgency. Frequent, ongoing observation and assessment of patients is therefore routine practice following the initial triage assessment.[4,24,25]

Practice tip

Triage decisions must be accurate, ensure the patient's safety and be reproducible across clinicians and departments. The decision regarding triage urgency should not be clouded by factors other than the patient's clinical condition.[7]

The premise for a triage decision is that utilisation of valuable healthcare resources should provide the greatest benefit for those most in need, and that persons in need of urgent attention always receive that care.[7] Triage encompasses the entire body of emergency nursing practice, and nurses complete a comprehensive triage education program prior to commencing this role. Formal triage training resources have been developed that provide the essential education components to promote consistency in application of the triage score, depending on the scales used.[27,28]

Triage categories

After triage assessment is undertaken on arrival, patients are allocated one of five triage categories depending on the triage scale used (see Tables 23.1 and 23.2). Prompt assessment of airway, breathing, circulation and disability remains the cornerstone of patient assessment in any clinical context, including triage.[4]

Triage assessment

Patient assessment at triage has three major components: quick, systematic and dynamic. Speed of assessment is required in life-threatening situations, with the focus on

TABLE 23.2
ATS category characteristics[4]

ATS CODE	TYPICAL DESCRIPTION
1	**Immediately life-threatening** (or imminent risk of deterioration) Patients are critically ill and require immediate transfer to a resuscitation area for initial resuscitation, with no delay at triage. The majority will arrive by ambulance, and will be suffering from: multi-trauma shock unconsciousness convulsions extreme dyspnoea cardiorespiratory arrest
2	**Imminently life-threatening** Patients 'at high risk' of critical deterioration or have very severe pain from any cause. Assessment and treatment need to commence within 10 min for: chest pain or other symptoms suggestive of myocardial ischaemia, pulmonary embolism or aortic dissection important time-critical treatment (e.g. thrombolysis, antidote) severe abdominal pain or other symptoms suggestive of ruptured aortic aneurysm severe dyspnoea from any cause altered levels of consciousness acute hemiparesis/dysphasia fever, rash, headache, suggestive of sepsis or meningitis severe skeletal trauma such as femoral fractures or limb dislocations very severe pain from any cause (practice mandates the relief of pain or distress within 10 min)
3	**Potentially life-threatening or situational urgency** Patients have significant illness or injury and should have assessment and treatment commenced within 30 min of presentation. Typical patients include those with: moderately severe pain from any cause (e.g. abdominal pain, acute headache, renal colic), but not suggestive of critical illness; practice mandates relief of severe discomfort or distress within 30 min symptoms of significant infections (e.g. lung, renal) moderate injury (e.g. Colles' fracture, severe laceration without active haemorrhage) head injury, with transient loss of consciousness persistent vomiting/dehydration
4	**Potentially serious** The patient's condition may deteriorate, or adverse outcome may result, if assessment and treatment is not commenced within 1 h of arrival. Patients have moderate symptoms, symptoms of prolonged duration or acute symptoms of low-risk preexisting conditions, including: minor acute trauma (e.g. sprained ankle) minor head injury, no loss of consciousness mild haemorrhage earache or other mildly painful conditions practice mandates relief of discomfort or distress within 1 hour there is a potential for adverse outcome if time-critical treatment is not commenced within 1 h likely to require complex work-up and consultation and/or inpatient management
5	**Less urgent** The patient's condition is minor or chronic; acute symptoms of minor illness, symptoms of chronic disease or with a duration of greater than 1 week. Symptoms or clinical outcome will not be significantly affected if assessment and treatment are delayed up to 2 h from arrival. Examples include: chronic lower back pain with mild symptoms minor wounds: small abrasion/minor lacerations most skin conditions clinical administrative presentations (e.g. results review, medical certificates, repeat prescriptions)

Source: Adapted from Australasian College for Emergency Medicine. Guidelines on the implementation of the Australasian Triage Scale in Emergency Departments Australia: Australasian College for Emergency Medicine; 2016.

airway, breathing, circulation and disability, and a quick decision on what level of intervention is required. A systematic approach to assessment is used for all patients in all circumstances, to ensure reproducibility. Finally, the triage assessment must be dynamic, in that several aspects can be undertaken at once, and acknowledges that a patient's condition can change rapidly after initial assessment. Various assessment models are available, but fundamentally they all include components of observation, history taking, primary survey and secondary survey.[27,28]

Patient history/interview

The triage interview provides the basis for data gathering and clinical decision making regarding patient acuity. After an introduction, the triage nurse asks person-specific, open-ended questions. Use of close-ended questions or summative statements enables clarification and confirmation of information received, and a means of checking understanding by the patient.[25] Privacy is important to ensure that the patient is comfortable in answering questions of a personal nature. Most EDs need to balance providing an area that is private and accessible, yet safe for staff to work in relative isolation.

A large component of the triage assessment may be based on subjective data, which are then compared and combined with objective data obtained through the senses of smell, sight, hearing and touch to determine a triage category. Although not required during every triage episode to reach an accurate decision, vital signs such as pulse, blood pressure, respiratory rate, oxygen saturation, temperature and blood glucose level can be measured to assist in estimating urgency.[4] Additional investigations that are surplus to requirement to make a triage decision should be avoided to ensure that triage does not in itself become a barrier to the patient accessing care.

Primary survey

While taking a patient history, the triage nurse also simultaneously conducts a primary survey. As noted earlier, airway, breathing, circulation and neurological function are observed. If any major problem is observed (or a patient is identified as ATS category 1 or 2), the interview is ceased and the patient is transferred immediately to the acute treatment or resuscitation area.[4]

Focused clinical assessment

A secondary survey, involving a focused, systematic physical examination, is conducted after the patient history and primary survey have been completed. This examination is not comprehensive but focuses on the presenting complaint while avoiding tunnel vision and wrong conclusions.[25] Remember that the patient may not be able to lie down or be exposed for an examination in the triage area, and may be distressed. The triage process should reflect a system of rapid assessment that is reproducible and adaptable to a variety of presentations. The secondary survey may be performed by the triage nurse if time permits or by another registered nurse who may be able to initiate appropriate investigations (such as X-rays) or initial management (such as analgesia), according to hospital protocols. Further information regarding advanced practice roles, such as the clinical initiatives nurse, is presented in Chapter 1.

TABLE 23.3
Aids to triage assessment[29]

MNEMONIC	COMPONENTS
SOAPIE	**S**ubjective data **O**bjective data **A**ssessment (to enable formulation of a ...) **P**lan (that is ...) **I**mplemented (and ...) **E**valuated (as to its success)
AMPLE	**A**llergies **M**edications **P**ast medical history **L**ast food and fluids ingested **E**nvironmental factors and **E**vents leading to presentation
PQRST	**P**rovoking or **P**recipitating factors **Q**uality and **Q**uantity (severity) of the symptom **R**egion/**R**adiation **S**ymptoms associated **T**ime of onset and duration of episode, and **T**reatment

Practice tip

The triage physical assessment should be quick, accurate and concise, focusing on the presenting complaint.

Approaches to triage assessment

A range of approaches to nursing assessment is applicable to triage assessments (Table 23.3). Body systems approach enables systematic examination of each body system to discover abnormalities (i.e. central nervous system, cardiovascular system, respiratory system, gastrointestinal system etc).[28] Detailed descriptions of systems assessment are available elsewhere in the text.[29]

Triage assessment of specific patient groups

While triage assessment is a complex process for a range of patient presentations, some specific groups are more demanding, such as mental health, paediatric, older and mass casualty patients.

TABLE 23.4
Examples of a mental health triage tool[25]

ATS		OBSERVATION	ACTION
1	Immediate	Severe behavioural disorder with immediate threat of dangerous violence to self or others	Provide continuous visual observation in safe environment Ensure adequate personnel to provide restraint/detention
2	Emergency	Severe behavioural disturbance with probable risk of danger to self and others	Provide continuous visual observation in safe environment Use defusing techniques Ensure adequate personnel to provide restraint/detention
3	Urgent	Moderate behavioural disturbance or severe distress with possible danger to self and others	Provide safe environment, frequent visual observations every 10 min
4	Semi-urgent	Semi-urgent mental health problem with no immediate risk to self or others	Regular visual observations at a maximum of every 30 min
5	Non-urgent	No behavioural disturbance or acute distress with no danger to self or others	Regular visual sighting at a maximum of 1-h intervals

Source: Adapted from Department of Health and Aging. Emergency Triage Education Kit: Department of Health 2013 [cited 2018]. Available from: http://www.health.gov.au/internet/main/publishing.nsf/Content/casemix-ED-triage+Review+Fact+Sheet+Documents.

Mental health presentations

Patients with psychiatric problems presenting to an ED should be triaged, assessed and treated as for other presenting patients, with particular attention to appropriate initial medical assessment and management.[30]

Resources outlining specific mental health triage category descriptors are readily available and relate specific aspects of mental health presentation with clinical urgency and triage categories (Table 23.4)[25] including an outline of suggested responses, such as patient placement requirements based on the level of risk and urgency.[30,31] Although the triage process has the same underlying principles, factors associated with mental health presentations may vary between geographical settings and countries where there are differences in health system structure, financing and sociocultural contexts.[25,32]

Paediatric presentations

Children presenting to the ED are assessed and assigned a triage category as for adults, although vital differences in paediatric anatomy, physiology and clinical presentations should be considered (see Chapter 27). The reliance on information from parents or primary carers and their capacity to identify deviations from normal are important, particularly in supporting recognition of often subtle indicators of serious illness in infants and young children. Paediatric triage resources are available to assist in identifying physiological alterations and applying a triage category based upon identified physiological discriminators.[25]

Practice tip

A short time is a long time in the life of a child; they may develop serious illness in a much shorter time than for an adult.

Older persons

With the ageing population globally, there is a trend towards an increase in the use of emergency services by older persons. While older persons should be triaged according to their presenting complaint, this can be complicated by various factors. It is therefore important to consider additional comorbidities, place of residence, medications and cognitive function when triaging older adults.[33] Evidence-based recommendations and policy guidelines for the management of older persons in the ED are available with additional recommendations provided by key organisations.[33,34] Important points to remember when triaging the elderly:

- Older persons have an increased medical complexity and nursing dependency.[35]
- Be attuned to the potential signs of elder abuse,[35] and the presence of pressure sores.
- Note the use of aids such as hearing aids, glasses and walking sticks that assist with activities of daily living.
- The older person (particularly if from an aged care facility) may have an advanced medical directive that should be used to ensure their wishes are respected in the event of a life-threatening illness.[35]

Practice tip

When triaging older people important considerations include other illnesses they may have, where they live, medications they are on and changes in their cognitive function.

Extended clinical skills

Within the ED, there has been an evolution of clinical roles and skill set for nurses. This has come about largely in response to an increasing number of emergency presentations, and to improve performance in patient flow, waiting times, length of stay and patient satisfaction.[36] Within the ED, new clinical roles, as discussed in more detail in Chapter 1, mean that registered nurses with extended clinical skills and knowledge can progress patient assessment and management through nurse-initiated radiology and nurse-initiated analgesia.

Nurse-initiated radiology

Nurse-initiated radiology ordering enables radiological investigations of extremities,[37] joints such as hips and shoulders, and the chest according to clinical protocols that list inclusion and exclusion criteria[38] based on findings from the patient's history and clinical examination. The inclusion criteria reflect well-established clinical indicators. While nurse-initiated radiology ordering is often undertaken as an extended triage nurse function, it can be performed by any accredited nurse. The use of nurse-initiated radiology, especially in association with extremity injuries, is safe and accurate, reducing both waiting time and department transit time and improving both patient and staff satisfaction.[38]

Nurse-initiated analgesia

Although pain is a common complaint in many patients presenting to the ED, timeliness, adequacy and appropriateness of analgesia administration have been suboptimal and contribute to poor patient satisfaction.[39] Consequently, many EDs have developed nurse-initiated analgesia protocols, standing orders or pathways to enable designated emergency nurses to implement analgesia regimens before medical assessment. These protocols are locally derived and note patient inclusion and exclusion criteria for managing mild, moderate or severe pain in both adult and paediatric patients, and often include administration of an antiemetic. A numerical pain rating scale or a visual analogue scale is used to direct the type and route of analgesia administration. Severe pain protocols outline intravenous (IV) narcotic administration, including incremental and total maximum administration dosages. After administration of the initial dose, the administering nurse gives subsequent doses in response to patient assessment of pain score and vital signs (pulse, blood pressure and respiratory rate). Protocols directed towards moderate and minor pain may include either single or incremental IV or oral analgesia. Nurse-initiated analgesia protocols are safe and effective, shortening the time ED patients wait for analgesia,[40,41] which should assist in improving patient outcomes and satisfaction.

Retrievals and transport of critically ill patients

The care of an acutely ill patient often includes transport, either within a hospital to undergo tests and procedures or between hospitals to receive a higher level of care or to access a hospital bed. The movement of critically ill patients places the patient at a higher risk of complications during the transport period[42–44] because of condition changes, inadequate availability of equipment or support from other clinicians or the physical environment in the transport vehicle. For this reason, the standard of care during any transport must be equivalent to, or better than, that at the referring clinical area.[42,43] Safe transport of patients requires planning and stabilisation by staff with appropriate skills and experience. This section focuses on the movement of critically ill patients between hospitals.

Retrievals

Although there are a variety of retrieval or transport models, most retrieval teams comprise doctors, nurses and paramedics with specialised training in critical care. The skills of the escort personnel need to match the acuity of the patient, so that they can respond to whatever clinical problems are presented.[43] Thus, retrieval team staff need to deliver high-level critical care equal to the standard of the receiving centre but need to be familiar with the challenges associated with working outside the hospital environment. Standards and guidelines for the transport of critically ill patients have been established by multiple professional associations.[43,45] There is now significant evidence that trauma systems impact positively on patient outcomes and in particular for reducing the odds of mortality for critically ill patients who have their inter-hospital transfer coordinated by a central retrieval organisation.[46]

When transporting an unstable patient, it is essential that a minimum of two people focusing solely on the clinical care aspects of the patient are present, in addition to other staff transporting the patient and equipment. The transport team leader is usually a medical officer with advanced training in critical care medicine or, for the transport of critical but stable patients, a registered nurse with critical care experience. The precise composition of the transport team can depend on the clinical circumstances in each case. The skill set includes advanced cardiac life support, arrhythmia interpretation and treatment and emergency airway management, where possible a specialised team focused only on transporting critically ill patients ensures better patient outcomes and fewer adverse events.[47,48]

Preparing a patient for inter-hospital transport

Adequate and considered preparation for the transport of a critically ill patient from one hospital area to another should be appropriately planned and not compromised by undue haste. Appropriate evaluation and stabilisation are required to ensure patient safety during transport, including assessment of airway, breathing, circulation and suitable IV access as well as safety of staff and assets.[43]

If potential airway compromise is suspected, careful consideration should be given to an elective intubation prior to transport rather than an emergency airway intervention in a moving vehicle, airborne aircraft or a radiology department. A laryngeal mask airway is not an acceptable method of airway management for critically ill patients undergoing transport because of the problems associated with movement.[43] A nasogastric or orogastric tube is inserted in all patients requiring mechanical ventilation, and especially prior to aeromedical transport.

Fluid resuscitation and inotropic support are initiated prior to transporting the patient. Planning for the trip needs to include adequate reserves of blood or other IV fluid for use during transport. If the patient is combative or uncooperative, the use of sedative and/or neuromuscular blocking agents and analgesia may be indicated, and in some cases will preclude certain types of transport at specific times of the day (e.g. patients at high risk for behavioural challenges may not be transported aeromedically at night unless sedated and paralysed due to the risk to staff and patient). A syringe pump with battery power is the most appropriate method for delivering medications for sedation and pain relief. A urinary catheter is inserted for transports of extended duration and all unconscious patients.[43]

Equipment essential for transport includes:

- equipment for airway management, sized appropriately and transported with each patient (check for operation before transport)
- portable oxygen source of adequate volume to provide for the projected timeframe, with enough of a reserve as a contingency in case of unexpected delays (this reserve requirement will depend on the type of retrieval, patient needs, and retrieval distance)
- non-rebreather mask and bag-valve-mask with oxygen reservoir of the appropriate size
- handheld spirometer for tidal volume measurement
- available high-pressure suction
- basic resuscitation drugs and supplemental medications, such as sedatives and narcotic analgesics (considered in each specific case) and other drugs as required for the patient presentation when transporting from rural/remote locations due to limited assets in these locations
- a transport monitor, displaying electrocardiogram (ECG) and heart rate, oxygen saturation, end-tidal CO_2 and as many invasive channels as required for pressure measurements.

The patient's identification bracelet should be checked and verified, medical records and relevant information such as laboratory and radiology findings are copied for the receiving facility, and other documentation includes initial medical evaluation and medical officer to medical officer communication, with the names of the accepting doctors and the receiving hospital.[43]

Patient monitoring during transport

Critically ill patients undergoing transport receive the same level of monitoring as they would have in a critical care unit. Monitoring equipment should be selected for its reliable operation under transport conditions, as monitoring can be difficult during transport; the effects of motion, noise and vibration can make even simple clinical observations (e.g. chest auscultation or palpation) difficult, if not impossible. Due to the risk of transporting ventilated patients the monitor should have a capacity for storing and reproducing patient bedside data and printouts during transport.[43] An appropriate transport ventilator provides full ventilatory support, monitors airway pressure with a disconnect alarm and should have adequate battery and gas supply for the duration of transport.[43] Adverse events during transport of critically ill patients fall into two categories: 1) equipment dysfunction, such as ECG lead disconnection, loss of battery power, loss of IV access, accidental extubation, occlusion of the endotracheal tube or exhaustion of oxygen supply (at least one team member should be proficient in operating and troubleshooting all equipment), and 2) physiological deteriorations related to the critical illness.[49] Mechanisms for audit, quality improvement and teaching purposes should be in situ to allow for feedback, performance review and service improvements.[45]

Respiratory presentations

Patients with respiratory dysfunction are common presentations to the ED and are seen across all age groups. Respiratory symptoms can be associated with a broad range of underlying pathologies. This section will discuss the initial assessment and treatment of several common respiratory diseases seen in the ED. Chapter 14 provides more detailed information regarding respiratory diseases.

Presenting symptoms and incidence

Patients presenting with respiratory complaints may display a range of symptoms. These symptoms will vary based upon the age of the patient, the underlying cause of the symptoms and the severity of the underlying condition. A list of frequently encountered respiratory signs and symptoms can be found in Box 23.1.[50]

Shortness of breath or dyspnoea is a frequent symptom or complaint on presentation to the ED. Respiratory presentations are not isolated to any one specific patient population or age group and are frequently encountered in patients across the lifespan. Dyspnoea, while commonly associated with respiratory conditions such as asthma, pneumonia, chronic obstructive pulmonary disease and cardiac conditions, has multiple aetiologies and can be caused by disease in almost any organ system. Shortness of breath is a significant symptom and is commonly associated with the need for hospital admission.[50,51]

BOX 23.1

Signs and symptoms commonly associated with respiratory presentations[50]

- Shortness of breath
- Dyspnoea (painful or difficulty breathing)
- Decreased SaO^2
- Cyanosis
- Alteration in respiratory rate – tachypnoea/bradypnoea
- Alterations in respiratory depth or pattern
- Use of accessory muscles
- Intercostal and/or subcostal recession
- Inability to speak in full sentences
- Wheeze
- Stridor (upper airway respiratory disorders)
- Alterations in level of consciousness
- Anxiety/feeling of impending doom

Assessment, monitoring and diagnostics

On arrival, patients with respiratory complaints should be quickly assessed utilising a systematic approach to determine whether there is any potentially life-threatening disturbance to the airway, breathing or circulation that requires immediate medical assessment and/or resuscitative intervention.

Initial assessment should include a thorough history focused on the presenting complaint/s. A detailed history may often identify the underlying process; however, the emergency clinician should maintain a high index of suspicion of other potential causes during the initial assessment.[50,52] The history should focus on the nature of symptoms, the timing of the onset of symptoms, associated features, the possibility of trauma or aspiration and past medical history, especially the presence of chronic respiratory conditions. After obtaining a history, a physical assessment of the respiratory system should be undertaken (see Chapter 13 for a detailed description of respiratory physical assessment).

Patients with significant respiratory symptoms are best managed in an acute monitored bed or resuscitation area of the ED. A set of observations including heart rate, respiratory rate, blood pressure, temperature and oxygen saturation should be completed and the patient's heart rate and oxygen saturation can be continuously monitored. Pulse oximetry plays an important role in the monitoring of the patient with a respiratory complaint. The recognition of hypoxaemia is significantly improved with the use of pulse oximetry.[53]

IV access should be obtained and venous blood samples may be collected for full blood count, urea, electrolytes and creatinine where clinically indicated. A chest X-ray (CXR) should be ordered in most instances. The CXR is one of the most useful investigations in the patient with a respiratory presentation. Interpretation of the CXR will not distinguish between all possible underlying pathologies and may appear normal in some instances. Therefore, interpretation of the CXR should always be performed in light of the clinical history and other examination findings.[51] An arterial blood gas (ABG) test may be indicated in patients with a significant respiratory presentation. The ABG will provide useful information that assists in identifying alterations to oxygenation, ventilation and acid–base status.[51] In many cases, a venous blood gas can be gained in lieu of ABG to avoid arterial trauma and a painful procedure for the patient. Venous blood gas values of PCO_2, pH and HCO_3^- can be interpreted to estimate the corresponding arterial values to inform decision making as if an ABG has been gained.[54] Spirometry or peak flow measurements may also be utilised in the assessment of the patient. Peak expiratory flow rate, forced vital capacity and forced expiratory volume in 1 second are useful in determining the nature of the underlying respiratory condition and, when the values are compared with predicted normal values, are useful in determining severity. These tests are, however, effort- and technique-dependent and the patient who is acutely short of breath may not be able to perform them.[51]

Oxygen therapy should be commenced early in patients presenting with signs of acute respiratory compromise, including patients known to have chronic obstructive pulmonary disease. Patients with acute hypoxia require oxygen. The often-mentioned complications associated with oxygen, especially in the patient with known chronic obstructive pulmonary disease, are uncommon. Such complications are concentration- and time-dependent, having a slow onset, which allows time for monitoring with pulse oximetry, blood gas analysis and clinical review.[51]

Patient diagnoses and management

Common diagnoses related to patients who present with shortness of breath include asthma, respiratory failure and pneumonia.[52]

Asthma

Asthma is a very common reason for patients presenting to Australasian EDs. Over 2.2 million Australians have asthma: up to 16% of children and 12% of adults are affected by the condition.[55] In other developed countries like the USA, asthma is the most common respiratory disease, affecting between 4% and 5% of the population.[56] Asthma is a chronic inflammatory disease of the airways in which many cells and cellular elements play a role, including mast cells, eosinophils, T lymphocytes, macrophages, neutrophils and epithelial cells. The inflammatory changes cause recurrent episodes of wheezing, breathlessness, chest tightness and coughing associated with widespread reversible airflow obstruction of the airways. This airflow obstruction or excessive narrowing is a result of airway smooth muscle contraction and swelling of the airway wall due to smooth muscle hypertrophy, inflammatory changes, oedema, goblet cell and mucous gland hyperplasia and mucus hypersecretion.[56,57]

Normally, airways widen during inspiration and narrow in expiration. In asthma, the above responses combine to severely narrow or close the lumen of the bronchial passages during expiration, with altered ventilation and air trapping.[56,57] The causes of asthma are related to many factors, including allergy,[58] infection (increased reaction to bronchoconstrictors such as histamine), irritants (e.g. noxious gases, fumes, dusts, dust mites, powders) or heredity, although the exact role or importance of any hereditary tendency is difficult to assess.[56]

A patient usually has a history of previous asthma attacks. Common risk factors that a patient may experience a future fatal or near fatal asthma exacerbation include a recent history of poor asthma symptom control, and a prior history of a previous near fatal asthma exacerbation requiring endotracheal intubation, mechanical ventilation and intensive care admission.[59] Often, an acute episode follows a period of exercise or exposure to a noxious substance, or a known allergen. The onset of the asthma may be characterised by vague sensations in the neck or pharynx, tightness in the chest with breathlessness, loose but non-productive cough with difficulty in raising sputum, difficulty breathing, particularly on expiration, with increasing severity as the episode continues; apprehension and tachypnoea may follow as the patient becomes hypoxic, with audible wheezing.[56,57]

The characteristics and initial assessment of acute mild, moderate and severe/life-threatening asthma in adults are outlined in Table 23.5. The associated clinical management guidelines for acute asthma are outlined in Table 23.6. Be alert to the high-risk patient whose ability to ventilate is impaired: this is a life-threatening condition. Such patients will exhibit an inability to talk, central cyanosis, tachycardia, use of respiratory accessory muscles, a silent chest on auscultation and possibly a history of previous intubation for asthma.[57,58,60]

Acute respiratory failure

Acute respiratory failure exists when the lungs do not provide sufficient gas exchange to meet the body's need for oxygen consumption, carbon dioxide elimination or both. Acute respiratory failure results from a number of causes.[61] When alveolar ventilation decreases, arterial oxygen tension falls and carbon dioxide rises. The rise in arterial carbon dioxide produces increased serum carbonic acid and pH falls, resulting in respiratory acidosis.[61] If uncorrected, low arterial oxygen combines with low cardiac output to produce diminished tissue perfusion and tissue hypoxia. Anaerobic metabolism results in increased lactic acid, aggravating the acidosis caused by carbon dioxide retention. In the process, a wide range of symptoms develop, involving the central nervous and cardiovascular systems.[57] Arterial blood gases confirm the diagnosis, with hypercarbia and a partial pressure of carbon dioxide in the arterial blood >45 mmHg and hypoxaemia evidenced by a partial pressure of oxygen in the arterial blood <60 mmHg, and a pH <7.35 evident. A CXR identifies the specific lung disease.[61]

Clinical management focuses on correction of hypercapnia, treatment of hypoxaemia, correction of acidosis and identification and correction of the specific cause[61] (see Chapter 14). For a spontaneously breathing patient, administer oxygen by Venturi mask (24%) or nasal cannula. Adjust oxygen therapy, according to arterial blood gas findings at 15–20-min intervals, to achieve a partial pressure of oxygen in the arterial blood of 85–90 mmHg. For a patient with inadequate respiratory effort, non-invasive ventilation may be instituted (see Chapter 15). In an apnoeic situation, initiate ventilatory

TABLE 23.5
Initial assessment and characteristics of acute asthma[60]

SYMPTOMS	SEVERITY OF ATTACK		
	Mild/moderate	Severe	Severe or life-threatening
Able to talk in	Sentences	Unable to finish sentence in one breath	
Physical exhaustion	No	Use of accessory muscles neck and intercostal. Tracheal tug or subcostal recession	Exhaustion or collapse. May have paradoxical chest wall movement
Pulse oximetry (room air)	>94%	90–94%	<90%
Level of consciousness	Normal	May be agitated, obvious respiratory distress	Reduced conscious level
Wheeze intensity	Variable	Moderate–soft	Often soft or absent
Central cyanosis	Absent	May be present	Cyanosis present

Source: Adapted from National Asthma Council Australia. Rapid primary assessment of acute asthma in adults and children. Australian Asthma Handbook V1.3 2017 [Access 11.1.18], http://www.asthmahandbook.org.au/acute-asthma/clinical/primary-assessment.

TABLE 23.6
Initial clinical management in acute asthma

	MILD	MODERATE	SEVERE OR LIFE-THREATENING
Hospital admission necessary	Probably not	Likely to be required	Yes, arrange immediate transfer to high-level care
Oxygen	High flow of at least 8 L/min, titrated to maintain SaO_2 >90%, preferably >94%. Monitor effect by oximetry. Frequent measurement of arterial blood gases in severe asthma if not responding		
Beta-2-agonist via a metered-dose inhaler and spacer *or* nebulised solution with 8 L/min O_2	Salbutamol 4–12 puffs via spacer. Repeat dose every 20–30 min for first hour if needed or sooner if needed	Salbutamol 8–12 puffs *or* Salbutamol 5 mg nebule if patient cannot breathe through spacer. Repeat dose every 20 min for first hour or sooner if needed	Salbutamol 10 mg via continuous nebulisation
Ipratropium bromide metered-dose inhaler via spacer *or* nebulised solution	If poor response, add 8 puffs via spacer	If poor response, add 8 puffs via spacer or 500 mcg nebule via nebuliser added to nebulised salbutamol. Give dose every 20 min for first hour, then repeat every 4–6 h as required	If poor response, add 8 puffs via spacer or 500 mcg nebule via nebuliser added to nebulised salbutamol. Give dose every 20 min for first hour, then repeat every 4–6 h as required
Steroids	Yes, oral prednisolone 37.5–50 mg)	Yes, oral prednisolone 37.5–50 mg. If oral route not possible, hydrocortisone 100 mg IV every 6 h	IV hydrocortisone 100 mg 6-hourly
Other agents	Not indicated	Not indicated	For life-threatening and no response, magnesium sulfate 10 mmol IV infusion over 20 min may help
CXR (and other investigations	Not usually necessary	Not necessary unless focal signs present, or no improvement with therapy	Necessary if no response to initial therapy or suspect pneumothorax/infection Check for hypokalaemia
Observations	Regular	Continuous	Continuous

Adapted from National Asthma Council Australia. Managing acute asthma in adults. Australian Asthma Management Handbook. V1.3 [Access 11/1/18]. Available from: www.asthmahandbook.org.au/figure/show/65.

assistance with bag–mask ventilation (see Chapter 15) prior to endotracheal intubation, and then commence mechanical ventilation.

Pneumonia

Pneumonia is an acute inflammatory condition of lung tissue caused by a variety of viral and bacterial organisms, fungi and parasites.[62] These organisms cause an inflammatory response from the cells involved in the affected segment of lung tissue. Pneumonia may occur in previously healthy patients, but more often it is associated with conditions that impair the body's defence mechanisms[63] (see Chapter 14). The predominant symptoms associated with pneumonia are a combination of cough, chest pain (usually pleuritic), dyspnoea, fever (with or without chills) and mucoid, purulent or bloody sputum, with an abrupt or gradual onset.[62] Common findings on physical exam include tachypnoea, fever, tachycardia, possible cyanosis, diminished respiratory excursion due to pleuritic pain, end-respiratory crackles or rales on auscultation with bronchial breathing over areas of consolidation[62,63] (see Chapter 14).

Investigations include a CXR, which may reveal varying infiltrates – interstitial, segmental or lobar. The CXR, however, may initially be clear until later in the illness and following adequate rehydration.[51] Venous blood samples will be analysed to identify a raised white cell count (i.e. leucocytosis). Blood cultures and sputum cultures will also be acquired to assist in identifying the causative organism. Blood gases will assist in determining the degree of impaired gas exchange. Hypoxaemia and often hypocarbia may be present.[62]

Initial treatment involves administration of oxygen therapy via face mask. Oxygen therapy should be evaluated frequently in response to pulse oximetry values. Treatment will routinely require IV fluid therapy to ensure adequate hydration, and administration of antibiotics orally or parentally in accordance with existing antibiotic guidelines or suspected infective agent (see Chapter 14). Ventilatory support may be required in some cases; in spontaneously breathing patients, non-invasive ventilation via a face mask should be utilised before invasive ventilation. Mechanical ventilation is not normally required unless there is some underlying cardiopulmonary disease.[62]

Chest pain presentations

Chest pain or chest discomfort is a common presenting complaint to the ED and can be associated with a number of different clinical conditions, several of which are associated with life-threatening pathology.[64] The identification of cardiac-related chest pain is important. During an initial assessment it may be difficult to differentiate between non-cardiac and cardiac causes of chest discomfort based on pain characteristics such as intensity, location, radiation and other associated symptoms.[65,66] Therefore, it is important to consider any presentation in which chest pain is a feature as cardiac in origin until a cardiac cause has been ruled out or another cause has been confirmed.

Description of presenting symptoms and incidence

The incidence of acute chest pain presentations appears to be increasing as patients are more aware of the importance of early treatment for myocardial infarction due to public awareness campaigns.[65] In American EDs over 5.5 million people presented in 2007–2008 with chest pain as their primary complaint.[64] The pain or discomfort associated with chest pain presentations is often described in a variety of ways in terms of onset, intensity, duration and radiation (Table 23.7).

Up to 9% of patients who will go on to be diagnosed with an acute coronary syndrome (ACS) may present with a number of these associated symptoms but without chest pain. These patients tend to be elderly, female, diabetic and non-white minorities.[67] Therefore, it is important to consider the possibility of a cardiac presentation in patients presenting with these associated symptoms even in the absence of chest pain.[67]

TABLE 23.7
Features of chest pain[67]

CHEST PAIN FEATURE	DESCRIPTION
Description	Typical: pressure, a weight on the chest, tightness, constriction about the throat, an acheing feeling Less typical: epigastric, indigestion, stabbing, pleuritic, sharp
Onset	Unprovoked or gradual With physical exertion or emotional stress
Intensity	Mild to severe
Radiation	To one or both arms, neck, jaw or back
Associated symptoms	Shortness of breath, nausea, vomiting, weakness, dizziness, anxiety, feeling of impending doom, palpitations, diaphoresis

Adapted from Dagiely S. An algorithm for triaging commonly missed causes of acute abdominal pain. J Emer Nurs 2006;32(1):9, with permission.

Assessment, monitoring and diagnostics

Any patient presenting with a complaint of chest pain requires urgent assessment, generally within 10 min of arrival to the ED. Any patient with evidence of a disturbance to airway, breathing or circulation requires close monitoring, immediate medical assessment and resuscitative interventions. The initial assessment should include a 12-lead ECG and a history of the presenting complaint including an evaluation of the pain utilising a systematic approach. The ECG should be rapidly evaluated for the presence of ST-segment elevation or a new left bundle branch block suggestive of an acute myocardial infarction (AMI) so that time-critical treatment can be initiated. If the initial ECG is non-diagnostic and symptoms continue, repeat ECGs should be performed at 15-min intervals.[67,68]

The patient should have cardiac monitoring commenced in order to identify any life-threatening arrhythmias. Supplemental oxygen should also be commenced in patients with SaO_2 <90%, patients in respiratory distress and those presenting high-risk features for hypoxia. Supplemental oxygen use for patients without hypoxia has not been proven to cause benefit or harm but has the disadvantages of cost and discomfort for the patient.[69] An IV cannula should be inserted and routine venous blood samples collected for troponin T or troponin I, which are cardiac enzymes that, when elevated, suggest myocardial injury. Cardiac enzymes are usually repeated within 6 hours of ED presentation.[70] A physical examination should also be performed. The physical examination may be of limited value in identifying cardiac causes of the pain but will be beneficial in identifying non-cardiac causes of the pain or complications associated with cardiac-related conditions.[65,67] The examination should also include assessment of the abdomen as a number of significant abdominal complaints may also present with chest pain as a feature.[66] A CXR should also be performed in order to identify any potential causes for the patient's pain.

Patient diagnoses and management

Acute coronary syndromes

Chest pain of cardiac origin results from reduced or obstructed coronary blood flow, commonly due to atherosclerosis, although coronary artery spasm or an embolism may also be involved.[65] Angina, whether stable or unstable, is a temporary condition in which there is no damage to the myocardial cells. A time-critical obstruction results in death or necrosis of a segment of myocardial cells resulting in an AMI.[66]

ACS collectively describes unstable angina and AMI. Coronary heart disease is the largest single cause of death and the commonest cause of sudden death in Australia and New Zealand.[71] It is the leading cause of premature death and disability in both countries, although death rates have fallen since the 1960s. ACS is a common life-threatening condition seen in the ED and therefore represents an important area of clinical practice in the ED. Chapters 10 and 11 provide additional information about presentations of cardiac dysfunction, including pathophysiology, clinical manifestations and treatment of cardiac conditions. This section summarises clinical management processes in the ED.[66]

The initial management of patients with suspected ACS involves risk stratification and rapid identification of patients with AMI, initiation of antithrombotic therapy, and identification of suitability for reperfusion therapy.[72] Reperfusion therapy consists of the administration of thrombolytic drugs with or without percutaneous coronary intervention (angioplasty ± stent). Percutaneous coronary intervention is generally only available to patients in larger centres where there is access to such resources. If percutaneous coronary intervention is not available, suitable patients should be managed with thrombolysis.[66]

The ongoing management in the ED for patients with ACS includes oxygen therapy in patients with SaO_2 <93%,[70] administration of aspirin 300 mg – if not already administered by pre-hospital personnel – and pain relief. Pain relief management generally includes the administration of IV morphine in small incremental doses. Pain relief may also include the administration of nitrates initially via the sublingual route; however, if pain persists despite IV morphine, the administration of IV nitrates may be indicated.[72] The patient and their family should also be provided reassurance, information and emotional support.

Patients without initial evidence of AMI are subsequently stratified into high-, intermediate- and low-risk groups based upon the presence of a number of clinical features associated with the presentation including the significance and duration of pain, ECG findings, past history, cardiovascular disease risk factors and cardiac enzyme results.[72] Specific ongoing treatment and management is then guided by the associated risk pathway.[66]

Thoracic aortic dissection

Thoracic aortic dissection (TAD) occurs when there is a tear in the intimal layer of the vessel wall. Blood passes through the tear, separates the intima from the vessel media or adventitia and results in a false channel. Shear forces lead to dissection propagation as blood flows through the false channel.[67] The incidence of TAD is quite low; ACS is 80 times more common. Identification of this life-threatening condition in the patient presenting with chest pain is important as patients often require immediate surgery. TAD is most commonly seen in men aged 50 to 70 years who have a history of hypertension. Other risk factors include Marfan's disease and other connective tissue disorders, cocaine or ecstasy use, pregnancy and aortic valve replacement.[73] TAD is associated with an acute and sudden onset of severe pain that is maximal at symptom onset. Pain is usually located in the midline and may be present in the back and rarely radiates. The pain is often described as sharp, tearing or ripping in nature.[73] Patients may also have pulse deficits or blood pressure differences (>20 mmHg) between the upper arms. CXR will be abnormal in 80–90% of cases with a widened mediastinum seen in approximately 50% of cases.[74] Patients will most commonly have the diagnosis confirmed using contrast computed tomography (CT). The management of TAD is aimed at aggressive control of blood pressure and pulse with sodium nitroprusside and beta-blockers, relief of pain with narcotic analgesia and referral and/or transport to cardiothoracic services for definitive surgical intervention.[74]

Abdominal symptom presentations

Acute abdominal pain is a common complaint, accounting for 5–10% of all presentations to the ED.[75] Specific cause for the presenting abdominal pain will not be found in 30–40% of patients of all ages;[76] for children, a diagnosis of non-specific abdominal pain accounts for up to 60% of cases.[77] About 20% of adult patients presenting will require surgical intervention and/or hospital admission.[77]

Common causes in the elderly include cholecystitis, diverticular disease, bowel obstruction and gastroenteritis.[78] Elderly patients are more likely to have catastrophic illnesses rarely seen in younger patients, including mesenteric ischaemia, leaking or ruptured abdominal aortic aneurysm and myocardial infarction.[79] Up to one-third require surgical intervention,[77] while 15% will not have a cause for their abdominal pain found. Presentations by elderly patients are often complicated by delays in seeking medical attention, atypical presentations, associated medical conditions and comorbidities, medications and cognitive function.

Assessment, monitoring and diagnostics

Patients presenting with abdominal pain are assessed quickly for any disturbance to airway, breathing or circulation requiring close monitoring, immediate medical assessment and/or resuscitative interventions. Abnormal vital signs are suggestive of clinically significant abdominal pain.[79] A thorough history includes location and

FIGURE 23.1 An algorithm for triaging commonly missed causes of acute abdominal pain.[81] AAA: abdominal aortic aneurysm; β-HCG: beta-human chorionic gonadotropin; RLQ: right lower quadrant.

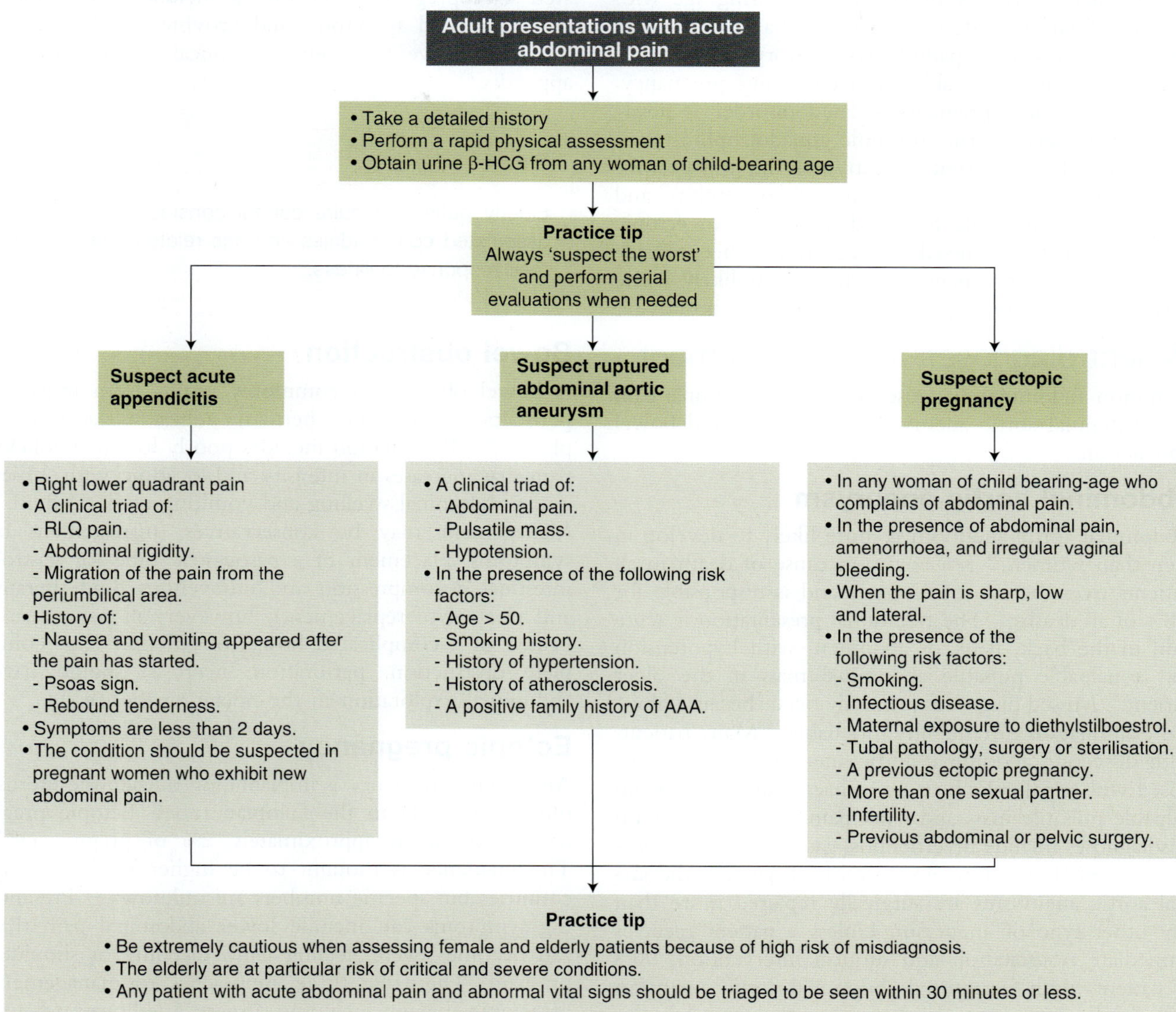

Source: Dagiely S. An algorithm for triaging commonly missed causes of acute abdominal pain. J Emer Nurs 2006;32(1):9.

timing of onset; quantity, quality and radiation of pain; associated symptoms, previous history and general state of health. A complaint-specific history and physical examination is performed for a differential diagnosis.[80] Physical assessment includes visual inspection of the abdomen with the patient in a supine position, followed by auscultation, then gentle palpation and percussion of all four quadrants of the abdomen, working towards the area of reported pain.[80] While location of the pain is important, it can be misleading, as various pathological processes can localise to different areas of the abdomen (Fig. 23.1).[81] An ECG is considered to rule out myocardial ischaemia or infarction, as some cardiac patients may present with upper abdominal pain as the predominant symptom. Myocardial ischaemia may also be caused by the physiological stress of the intraabdominal pathology.[76,81]

Administration of narcotic analgesia in acute abdominal pain does not hinder assessment or obscure abdominal findings, nor cause increased morbidity or mortality, and may allow for a better abdominal examination.[82] Incremental doses of a narcotic can minimise pain but not palpation tenderness. Analgesics enable relaxation of the patient's abdominal muscles and decrease anxiety, potentially improving information obtained from the physical examination.[40]

Venous blood samples are collected for full blood count, urea, electrolytes, creatinine, liver function tests and lipase.[83] A dipstick urinalysis can suggest specific disease. For example, leucocytes, nitrites and/or blood in the urine can suggest a urinary tract infection and haematuria can suggest renal colic, but should be considered in the context of other clinical findings and formal microscopy.[83] Women of childbearing age with abdominal pain provide the challenge of a broader range of potential causative pathologies. History and physical examination are unreliable in determining pregnancy. If pregnancy or a pregnancy-related disorder is possible, a urine beta-human chorionic gonadotrophin test is performed. Test sensitivity is extremely high; a positive finding occurs within a few days of conception, and accuracy is comparable to blood sampling. An ectopic pregnancy may be missed if pregnancy is not considered; an ectopic pregnancy is extremely unlikely if the beta-human chorionic gonadotrophin result is negative.[83]

Patient diagnoses and management

Common abdominal diagnoses for acute abdominal pain are abdominal aortic aneurysm, appendicitis and bowel obstruction.

Abdominal aortic aneurysm

Abdominal aortic aneurysm is more likely to develop in men than women,[84] is a common cause of death in all patients over the age of 65 years and is responsible for 0.8% of all deaths.[77] The traditional presentation is acute pain in the back, flank or abdomen, with hypotension and a palpable pulsatile abdominal mass in the older patient.[85] Missed diagnoses primarily occur because physical examination is frequently unreliable.[86] Many patients with dissecting abdominal aortic aneurysm are misdiagnosed with renal colic because of haematuria present, no palpable pulsatile mass and flank pain.[86] Other common misdiagnoses include diverticulitis, gastrointestinal haemorrhage, AMI and musculoskeletal back pain.[85] Abdominal aortic aneurysms are surgically repaired more than any other type of aneurysm. Unless a patient receives immediate resuscitation and surgical intervention, 90% of patients with a ruptured abdominal aortic aneurysm will die; however, even with surgery, the mortality rate is still 50%.[85]

Appendicitis

Appendicitis is the most common acute abdominal pain presentation worldwide that requires a surgical intervention. About 8% of people in Western countries will have appendicitis during their lifetime.[87] Along with pain (usually in the right lower quadrant), other presenting symptoms may include nausea and vomiting.[87] Imaging increases diagnostic accuracy and aims to decrease the negative appendectomy rate. CT is the preferred modality of imaging; however, in children and pregnant women, abdominal ultrasound is preferred.[88] Appendicitis can mimic almost all acute abdominal pain presentations, and is frequently misdiagnosed as gastroenteritis during the initial ED visit, pelvic inflammatory disease or urinary tract infection.[83] Although it is a well-studied disease, appendicitis continues to be difficult to diagnose in ED because of its varied presentations. Elderly patients require careful consideration due to associated comorbidities[87] and women of childbearing age are commonly misdiagnosed due to anatomical changes associated with pregnancy. Treatment includes management of pain-related symptoms and provision of IV hydration. Definitive treatment is surgical removal of the appendix.[89]

Practice tip

Elderly patients require careful consideration due to associated comorbidities and age-related changes to their response to illness.

Bowel obstruction

A bowel obstruction commonly results from impaired peristaltic movement, hernias, adhesions and neoplasms.[90,91] Presentation includes poorly localised colicky pain that increases in intensity and location, with subsequent abdominal swelling and vomiting of faecal fluid.[90] Management may be conservatives (management of symptoms, placement of a nasogastric tube for gastrointestinal decompression and intravenous fluid therapy and electrolyte replacement); however, all patient suspected of a complicated bowel obstruction (e.g. complete obstruction, perforation, necrosis) should have abdominal exploration in the operating theatre.[92]

Ectopic pregnancy

An ectopic pregnancy is implantation outside the uterus, most commonly in the fallopian tubes. Ectopic pregnancies occur in approximately 2% of pregnancies.[93] The incidence is thought to be higher in developing countries but specific numbers are unknown.[94] Presenting symptoms can include lower abdominal pain that can become severe, feeling faint, bleeding or shoulder tip pain. There are three approaches to management of ectopic therapy including surgery, methotrexate, and expectant management for a small proportion of women. Emergency surgery is indicated in the event of haemodynamic instability, or signs of impending or active rupture of the ectopic mass.[95]

Acute stroke

Cerebrovascular disease is highly prevalent in developed countries. In some countries that have seen continuing industrialisation (such as Asia and Africa) the increasingly unhealthy lifestyle is being reflected in diseases including cerebrovascular disease.[96] In China, different epidemiological changes, such as an ageing population, high prevalence of smoking and hypertension, are expected to result in an increase in stroke rates.[96] In Australia, cerebrovascular disease is the third-largest cause of death.[71]

The two general stroke classifications are:

- Ischaemic strokes are precipitated by disrupted blood flow to an area of the brain as a result of arterial occlusion. Acute ischaemic stroke presentations are now referred to as a 'brain attack', to promote early presentation for access to time-critical treatments[97] and because the pathophysiology and current treatment of acute ischaemic stroke mimics that of AMI. From an ED perspective, serious long-term disability can be minimised if ischaemic stroke is recognised and treated promptly; that is, within 4.5 hours of symptom onset.[98]

- Haemorrhagic strokes are caused by rupture of a blood vessel, which produces bleeding into the brain parenchyma. (Chapter 17 details the pathophysiological processes.)

For patients diagnosed with an ischaemic stroke, 13–25% will die within the first 30 days and 60% within 10 years.[99] Permanent disability requiring care in a nursing home or other long-term facility is required for around 10%.[99]

Assessment, monitoring and diagnostics

Symptoms of stroke are common amongst patients presenting to the ED; presenting signs vary from profound alterations in level of consciousness and limb hemiplegia to mild symptoms affecting speech, cognition or coordination. Symptoms may include confusion, dizziness, ataxia, visual disturbances, dysphasia or receptive and expressive aphasia, dysphagia, weakness and numbness or tingling of the face, arm or leg, which is usually unilateral.[100] Many disorders resemble a stroke presentation so emergency clinicians must quickly determine if another condition is responsible for the patient's neurological deficits. Other conditions include post-ictal phase following seizures, migraine with neurological deficits, hypoglycaemia or hyperglycaemia, systemic infections, brain tumours, hyponatraemia and hepatic encephalopathy.[101]

The aims of the initial contact phase with the patient is to ensure medical stability, to reverse any contributing conditions to the patient's problem, to identify the pathophysiologic basis for the presenting neurological symptoms, and to identify if patients experiencing an ischaemic stroke will be suitable for thrombolytic therapy.[102] The focus of initial assessment is airway, breathing, circulation and disability. Of note, for airway assessment, stroke symptoms include altered muscle function, affecting swallowing and speech functions. A patient with a Glasgow Coma Scale (GCS) score of 9 or less may require intubation to protect and secure the airway.[96] The patient's breathing pattern should be assessed and continually monitored. Supplemental oxygen should be provided to hypoxic patients to maintain oxygen saturation >94%; however, it should not be given to non-hypoxic stroke victims.[102] Hypertension is common, with the increase improving any cerebral ischaemia so this should not be lowered unless dangerously high or contraindicated.[103] Hypotension or dehydration decreases cerebral blood flow and perfusion and should be corrected, although fluid replacement is instituted with caution. Vital signs are documented every 15 min during drug therapy to identify changes suggestive of internal bleeding. Maintaining blood pressure less than 185/110 mmHg during fibrinolytic infusion decreases the risk of intracerebral haemorrhage.[97]

A thorough assessment of neurological disability should be undertaken, including a GCS (see Chapter 16). An ECG is recorded to detect any abnormal rhythm such as atrial fibrillation, which may be associated with stroke presentation.[104] IV access is obtained to administer medications, and collect blood for electrolytes, haematology and coagulation studies. Assessment of blood glucose will rule out hypoglycaemia or hyperglycaemia as a cause of the presenting symptoms. Abnormal glucose levels adversely affect cerebral metabolism.[102] After obvious alternative diagnoses are excluded, a brain CT scan determines whether a stroke is haemorrhagic or ischaemic in origin. While a new-onset ischaemic stroke may not be evident for up to 24 hours, blood in the cranial cavity will be apparent immediately. Patients with any sign of haemorrhage are excluded for fibrinolytic therapy.[105]

Management

Acute ischaemic stroke management includes timely administration of a fibrinolytic agent in appropriately selected patients (Box 23.2), which facilitates reperfusion, minimises tissue damage and reduces long-term stroke sequelae. Longer times between symptom onset and fibrinolytic infusion are associated with higher rates of morbidity and mortality.[106] Early presentation is therefore essential to instigate appropriate assessments and investigations, including CT scanning, and then thrombolytic administration and still fall within the narrow treatment window. Acute stroke unit care, with specialised teams dedicated to the rapid assessment and management of presentations, can significantly reduce death and disability[106] (see Chapter 17).

Overdose and poisoning

Poisoning is a common clinical presentation throughout the world. Worldwide up to 9% of deaths are related to drug and alcohol misuse in the age group between 15 and 29.[109,110] Suicide is a global issue and in 2015 accounted for 1.4% of deaths worldwide, with a significant number of these related to chemical ingestion.[111] In Australia and New Zealand, poisoning accounts for 1–5% of admissions to public hospitals, rates which have changed little since 1993–94.[112]

The usual types of poisoning encountered as ED presentations include self-poisoning with prescribed drugs, ingestion of illicit drugs and common dangerous substances (e.g. detergents, cleansers; psychotropic agents; analgesics; insecticides; paracetamol, aspirin).[109] A range of artificial and naturally-occurring substances can produce acute poisonings. The toxicity of a substance depends on numerous factors, such as dose, route of exposure and

BOX 23.2

Criteria for administering fibrinolytic therapy in ischaemic stroke[105]

Inclusion criteria (all must be positive):

- Age ≥18 years
- Clinical diagnosis of ischaemic stroke with measurable neurological deficit
- Time of symptom onset <4.5 h minimum and well established[107,108]

Exclusion criteria (all must be negative):

- Evidence of intracranial haemorrhage on non-contrast head CT
- Only minor or rapidly improving stroke symptoms
- High suspicion of subarachnoid haemorrhage, even with normal CT
- Active internal bleeding
- Known bleeding condition, including but not limited to platelets <100,000/mm^3
- Patient received heparin within 48 h and had an elevated activated partial thromboplastin time (PTT)
- Current use of oral anticoagulants (e.g. warfarin)
- Recent use of anticoagulant and elevated international normalised ratio (INR >1.5) or prothrombin time (>15 s)
- Intracranial surgery or serious head trauma, or previous stroke within 3 months
- Major surgery or serious trauma within 14 days
- History of intracranial haemorrhage, arteriovenous malformation, or aneurysm
- Witnessed seizure at stroke onset
- Recent AMI
- Systolic blood pressure >185 mmHg or diastolic blood pressure >110 mmHg at time of treatment

the victim's preexisting conditions. Poisoning, whether intentional or unintentional, can occur at any time, and may involve single or multiple substances.[109,110]

The vast amount of knowledge required concerning all poisons prompted the development of poison control information centres to provide specific information and guidance for healthcare providers and the general public on the management of a poisoned patient; to collect statistics on toxic substances; and to educate the public on the prevention or recognition of toxic exposures. Other initiatives to limit the incidence and severity of acute poisoning include the control of drugs, specific information on labels, the introduction of blister packs and enforced safety standards such as childproof caps.[113]

Assessment, monitoring and diagnostics

The poisoned patient may present with a wide range of clinical features from no symptoms through to a life-threatening condition or the potential to deteriorate rapidly and should always be assessed immediately. Triage decisions should be based on the potential for rapid deterioration and the need for urgent intervention. Resuscitation may be necessary before any further definitive care can be commenced. The priorities of care for all patients include the assessment and maintenance of an airway, adequate ventilation and circulation.[109,110] Successful resuscitation may require removal of the toxin, counteraction of the poisoning by an antidote if available, and the treatment or support of symptoms.[109,110] It is extremely important to note that many drugs, such as paracetamol, may have limited initial effects but serious, potentially fatal consequences if not treated in a timely manner[114]

An accurate history is often the most significant aid in directing care. If a history is unobtainable or uncertain, there are several general guidelines that may prove helpful for dealing with the patient who has an altered mental state or conscious level[109,110] (Table 23.8).

Poisoning should always be considered when dealing with a patient who has a sudden-onset, acute illness. If there is a strong suspicion of poisoning, a clinician should attempt to compare the patient's presentation with symptoms caused by the suspected toxin and the likelihood of exposure.

Accidental poisonings are the commonest cause of medical emergencies in the paediatric patient population. Childhood ingestions tend to be accidental and to involve a single substance. Intentional poisonings occur more often with adults, and are more likely to involve multiple substances.[109,110,112] Poisonings in the aged population are often complicated by co-existing medical conditions, which may exaggerate the effects or impair the excretion of the substances involved. Boys are more likely to be the victims of poisoning than girls. Adult women attempt suicide with poisons more often than men, but men's suicide intentions are associated with a higher mortality rate.[109,111,112]

Practice tip

Poisonings in the aged population are often complicated by co-existing medical conditions, which may exaggerate the effects or impair excretion of the substances involved.

Previous history

Patients with existing medical conditions often have multiple medications that could be either intentionally or unintentionally ingested. The use of multiple drugs may cause untoward reactions. A patient with a history

TABLE 23.8
Acronyms outlining potential causes of altered levels of consciousness[109,110]

ACRONYM	CAUSE	ACRONYM	CAUSE
T	**T**rauma	A	**A**lcohol/Acidosis
I	**I**nfection/Insulin (hypo-hyperglycaemia)	E	**E**ndocrine
			Encephalopathy
P	**P**sychosis		**E**lectrolyte abnormality
	Porphyria		
		I	**I**nsulin/diabetes Infection
S	**S**eizure		
	Syncope	O	**O**xygen: hypoxia of any cause
	Space-occupying lesion		**O**piates/Overdose
	Stroke	U	**U**raemia

of depression may attempt suicide with psychotropic drugs. A quick onset and acute illness or condition should raise the level of suspicion of a poisoning, especially if there is no history of previous signs or symptoms that suggest another cause.

Suspected toxin

Rescue personnel, family or friends should bring any container, plant product or suspected toxin with the patient to the hospital, as long as the substance presents no risk of contamination to the person retrieving it. A child's play area should be inspected for possible sources of toxins.[109]

Time of poisoning

History should include time of exposure, onset of symptoms and time since treatment began. Alcohol is the commonest drug taken with other intentional self-poisonings, and can potentiate a range of medication effects and increase the incidence of vomiting and potential aspiration.[109,110] Poisonings in children tend to occur most often just prior to mealtimes, when they are hungry. Adults may take substances late in the evening, fall asleep and be found several hours later.[110]

A thorough assessment may provide clues about an unconscious, uncooperative or suspicious presentation. Assess for respiratory effort, skin colour, pupil size and reactivity, reflexes and general status. Auscultation of the lung fields, the apical pulse and presence of active bowel sounds provide a baseline for further assessment and clues about current problems. Check blood pressure as often as necessary to determine cardiovascular stability. Percuss the thorax and abdomen to detect accumulations of fluid or air.[109,110] Needle marks, pill fragments, uneaten leaves or berries or drug paraphernalia assist in a diagnosis.[109,110] The presence of pressure areas on the skin may indicate how long the patient has been unresponsive. Any odours are important to note. An oily-garlicky smell may be due to pesticides.[115] Other odours may indicate chronic medical disorders (e.g. fruity odour with diabetic ketoacidosis) or neglect of personal hygiene.

Practice tip

Odours are important to note, as they may reflect not only poisoning but other medical disorders, for example a fruity odour may reflect diabetic ketoacidosis.

Toxicology screens include an analysis of serum and urine to determine the presence and amount of a substance. Laboratory levels are helpful but must be considered according to the nature of the substance and its rate of metabolism. Certain substances are sequestered in fatty tissues or are bound to serum proteins, and may be present with a misleadingly low serum level.[110] Serum electrolytes, non-electrolytes, osmolality, arterial blood gases and urine electrolytes are used to determine the patient's overall status or response to therapy. Continuous cardiac monitoring supplemented with a 12-lead ECG or invasive monitoring devices may be required to help provide symptomatic care.[109,110]

Initial and ongoing care of the victim follows three principles:[109,110]

1 preventing further absorption of the toxin
2 enhancing elimination of absorbed toxin from the body

3 preventing complications by providing symptomatic or specific treatments, including psychiatric management.

Management: preventing toxin absorption

Ingested poisons are best removed while still in the upper gastrointestinal tract when possible. Emesis and gastric lavage were used in the past to empty the stomach, although a significant body of evidence now suggests that these are relatively ineffective and effectiveness decreases rapidly after 1 hour.[109,110] Both the patient and substance should be evaluated for appropriateness of gastric emptying.[109,110]

The patient's consciousness level, gag reflex and ability to vomit while protecting the airway from aspiration should be considered. Any central nervous system depressants can obtund the protective gag or cough reflex. If the ingested substance has a rapid onset of action, such as with benzodiazepines, it is safer to avoid emetics because of the risk of a sudden fall in the level of consciousness.[109,110]

Ingested poisons

Evaluate the substance ingested to determine whether gastric emptying is appropriate. The physical properties of a drug may make it more responsive to a particular type of gastric emptying. For example, the antimuscarinic effect of tricyclic antidepressants on gut motility can prolong gastrointestinal absorption, increasing plasma levels.[116] Also, consider the effects of substances on tissue. Corrosives, such as acids, alkalis and iron supplements, produce irritation and tissue breakdown when in contact with the skin or mucous membranes. Recognition is important, as therapy may cause further injury. Emesis could be contraindicated, and a lavage tube may further traumatise injured tissue.[117] Ipecac syrup and vomiting are generally ineffective against a substance with an antiemetic property, such as phenothiazines.[109,110] Waiting for emesis also causes further delay in definitive treatment. Other substances have natural emetic qualities if taken in sufficient doses (e.g. hand soaps and liquid soap detergents).[118]

Evaluate other substances on an individual basis. There are situations, however, when the amount, character or additional chemicals present make it necessary to remove the ingested substance from the stomach. Occasionally, therapy is based on the reported amount taken or time since ingestion. Time since ingestion is important in order to rule out the benefit of therapy. The stomach tends to empty its contents after 1 hour, unless a substance that slows gastric motility has been ingested. For example, narcotics can slow peristalsis and may be found in the stomach several hours after ingestion.[109,110] A patient may also underreport the dosage to avoid an obviously unpleasant experience. Although conservative management with observation is appropriate in certain situations, the risk of not treating might be greater in others.[109,110] If a large number of tablets or pills are consumed at one time, they may clump together in the stomach and form a mass that is too large to pass out of the pylorus (e.g. aspirin).[119]

Once a substance enters the lower gastrointestinal tract, it can be absorbed into the mesenteric circulation. As absorption can vary according to substance, slow-release characteristics, rate of peristalsis and the presence of other substances, it is possible for a poison to be present in the bowel for an extended period of time. If intestinal motility can be stimulated or the toxin permanently bound until excretion, then further absorption is reduced.[109,110] Activated charcoal is a refined product with an enormous surface area that binds to a large range of substances to enhance elimination, and is the most effective decontaminating agent currently available if ingested within 1 hour of poisoning.[109,110] Unfortunately, not all poisons ingested can be bound by charcoal, such as alcohol, corrosives, hydrocarbons and heavy metals.[109,110]

Inhaled poisons

A patient poisoned by inhalation of toxic gases or powders should be removed from the source as soon as it is safe to do so. Attempts to remove the substance, which is usually a vapour, gas or fine particulate matter, from the lung are not normally useful.[109,110] The history of a patient suspected of an inhaled poison should include time of exposure, the duration of exposure, the onset of symptoms, suspected inhalant and time since treatment began.

Staff involved in direct care of the patient should take precautions to avoid unprotected contact to reduce the risk of self-contamination with unknown substances. For many inhaled poisons, clothing may contain significant amounts of the poison and serve as a continuous source of the toxin. Contaminated linen and clothes should be removed carefully, sealed in a bag and destroyed.[109,110]

Contact poisons

Contact poisons are dangerous because of their ability to enter the body via the skin or mucous membranes. All clothing and all of the toxic substance should be carefully removed, preferably with an irrigating and neutralising solution. Precautions to avoid direct skin contact and reduce the risk of self-contamination should be used. Clothing may contain significant residual amounts of the poison and serve as a continuous source of the toxin. Contaminated linen and clothes should be sealed in a bag and destroyed.[109,110]

Management: enhancing elimination of the toxin from blood

After a substance has entered the bloodstream, it is normally excreted from the body either in an unchanged form or after liver metabolism and detoxification.

TABLE 23.9
Summary of the management of poisoning victims[109,115-117,120-122]

AIM	ACTION
Prevent absorption of toxin	• Ingested toxins: activated charcoal is the most effective method of reducing adsorption • Inhaled toxins: remove victim from source of contamination and administer oxygen or provide fresh air • Contact toxins: remove any substances from the body surface, preferably with copious amounts of irrigating fluid. Remove clothing and place in a sealed bag to reduce vapour hazards. Use special caution with corrosive materials and pesticides
Enhance elimination of the toxin from the blood	Ingested or injected toxins: administer an antidote or antagonist if available (e.g. naloxone for opiates; flumazenil for benzodiazepines). Employ forced diuresis, for acidification or alkalinisation of the urine; and haemodialysis
Prevent complications by providing symptomatic or specific treatment	Carefully monitor all vital systems. Continually reassess patient for changes or response to therapy. Administer antidotes as prescribed. Provide symptomatic care as needed for: cardiac arrhythmias, CNS depression or stimulation, fluid and electrolyte imbalances, acid–base disturbances, renal function, effects of immobility

Various metabolic byproducts are eliminated in the bile and faeces or urine. Urinary excretion of substances can be enhanced by increasing the filtration process by forcing diuresis and the administration of large volumes of IV solutions and/or diuretics. Enhanced secretion can also occur by inhibiting absorption in the renal tubules or by stimulating the secretion of substances into the urine.[109,110]

Alkalinisation of urine

Manipulation of the absorption or secretion process of a drug can be assisted by chemically altering the structure of some substances. All substances break down into ions at a specific pH for that substance. Altering the pH of urine with acidifying or alkalising drugs allows the poison to be forced into an ionic state and then excreted in the urine. This ion-trapping process is effective only for substances that are primarily eliminated by the kidneys,[109,110] for example salicylates and tricyclic antidepressants.[116,120]

Haemodialysis or haemoperfusion

If a dangerous amount of a poison is present or if renal failure is evident, haemodialysis or haemoperfusion may be used to enhance excretion. Dialysis is effective in removing substances that are reversibly bound to serum proteins, or not stored in body fat, only. This is a highly invasive approach and is normally reserved for life-threatening cases (see Chapter 18 for further discussion).[110]

Management: preventing complications and specific symptomatic care

Supportive care is the key element in managing an acutely poisoned patient. Once a patient has either ingested or been exposed to many poisons, there are limited options other than to treat the symptoms as they appear or become clinically significant (Table 23.9).[109,115-117,120-123]

TABLE 23.10
Common emergency antidotes[109,115-117,120-122]

POISONING	ANTIDOTE
Benzodiazepines	Flumazenil
Opioids	Naloxone
Paracetamol	N-acetylcysteine
Organophosphates	Atropine and pralidoxime
Tricyclic antidepressants	Sodium bicarbonate
Carbon monoxide	Oxygen
Insulin	Dextrose

Antidotes act to antagonise, compete with or override the effects of the poison, although few specific antidotes exist for toxins (Table 23.10). In some cases, an absorbed toxin can be rendered benign by the use of an antidote (e.g. the interaction between naloxone and opiates). For chelating agents, such as desferrioxamine for iron poisoning, a non-toxic compound is formed that is then safely eliminated from the body.[124] The effect of an antidote may be only temporary if the antidote has a shorter half-life than the poison. Most antidotes are given either in a specific dose or at a response to dose rate.[124] For many poisonings, symptomatic care involves support and protection of vital organ systems. Routine and frequent physical assessment of respiratory, cardiovascular and renal function enables identification of potential problems. If large volumes of fluids or drugs that alter serum pH are administered, the patient's electrolyte and acid–base balance are also monitored.[109,115-117,120-123]

A poisoning may be the physical manifestation of an emergency or crisis that requires emotional support. A patient may have underlying emotional conflict/s or mental health problems, regardless of whether the poisoning was intentional or accidental. Psychological care is, therefore, an important component for all patients presenting with poisoning.[109,110] Many facilities offer the services of a mental health worker while the patient is still in the ED. If the patient's condition is stable and the poisoning has not altered their mental state, early intervention is appropriate.

For adult patients, the desire for treatment is not as important as the manner in which treatment is received. Even though patients may initially refuse care, if approached in a non-threatening way and given some form of control, they will usually comply. If threatened with force or restraints, they are placed in the position of either submitting to coercion or resisting therapy in order to 'protect' themselves. A paediatric patient may be too young either to fully understand or to effectively cooperate with staff.

Central nervous system depressants

A large number of common medications are capable of depressing levels of consciousness, thought processes or important regulatory centres located within the central nervous system (CNS). The clinical findings associated with CNS alteration can vary a great deal from drug class to class or within the same drug family, as physical effects are dependent on the chemical structure of the drug, the dose, the route of exposure, any other co-ingested drugs and the rate of drug metabolism. In addition, the chemical structure and/or purity of illicit drugs may be affected by variations or deliberate aberrations in the manufacturing process.[125,126] Drugs in this section include sedatives, hypnotics, tranquillisers and narcotics.

Assessment

The predominant observed effect is an altered level of CNS function.[125,126] A spectrum of physical findings is possible with the selective action of the specific drug on inhibitory or excitatory centres of the brain: effects can vary from mild euphoria to convulsions, or mild sedation to coma, dependence, addiction and tolerance. Narcotics constrict the pupil, and some patients experience nausea and vomiting due to a stimulation of the chemoreceptor trigger zone in the medulla.[110,125,126]

A narcotic overdose is distinctive, with a set of readily identifiable features. These features include a decreased respiratory rate and tidal volume, constriction of the pupil, hypotension and an altered level of consciousness.[125,126] Other factors may, however, affect these findings, as outlined in Box 23.3.

BOX 23.3

Factors confounding diagnosis of narcotic overdose[109,110,125,127]

- A decreased respiratory effort may produce hypercarbia, which in turn may cause pupil dilation.
- Chronic narcotic users tend to have multiple problems associated with their drug use or lifestyle, which may modify findings.
- CNS depressants in sufficiently high dose cause depression of vital regulatory centres in the brain.
- Altered respirations cause hypoventilation, stasis of secretions and atelectasis. The resultant hypoxia serves to further aggravate the sensorium and cerebral functioning.
- Narcotics may produce idiopathic pulmonary oedema
- CNS depressants often possess the ability to cause peripheral vasodilation, with a resultant hypotension and tachycardia.
- Arrhythmias may occur because of cardiac conduction effects or tissue hypoxia.

Patients with an altered level of consciousness are subject to injury from decreased sensory ability or prolonged immobilisation. Reddened areas over bony prominences or pressure points appear within a short time. Skin blisters indicate altered blood flow, usually due to excessive pressure. Actual skin breakdown can occur within 3 hours. If external pressure or altered circulation to an extremity is allowed to continue for over 4 hours, compartment syndrome may develop.[125,126]

Effects of multiple drug use

A patient who ingests a combination of drugs may experience toxicity because of additive or synergistic effects.[125,126] Illicitly produced drugs will most likely have had substances added (e.g. glucose powders, icing sugar, talcum powder) to dilute or 'cut' them, to increase the volume of their supply and thus profit to the supplier.[123,124] Users may also intentionally inject other drugs (e.g. antihistamines, amphetamines, benzodiazepines) to modify or potentiate the effects of narcotics.[125,126]

Potential for acute or active infections

The use of non-sterile solutions and equipment and the sharing of injection equipment significantly increase the likelihood of acute or active infections. Frequent exposure and a depressed immune response also predispose a patient to severe infections, such as hepatitis, osteomyelitis, infective bacterial endocarditis and encephalitis/meningitis.[125,126]

TABLE 23.11
Assessment and management of specific drug overdoses[109,116,117,119-120,122,130]

TYPE OF POISONING	GENERAL MANAGEMENT	ANTIDOTE	CLINICAL CONSIDERATIONS
CNS depressants (morphine, heroin, methadone, oxycodone)	Supportive care of airway, breathing, circulation	Naloxone hydrochloride (Narcan); specific reversal agent	Action of naloxone may be much shorter than the duration of effect of the drug; the patient may need to be observed for return of unconsciousness
CNS stimulants	Supportive care of airway, breathing, circulation	Benzodiazepines may be used to reduce symptoms	Reduce stimulation in the surrounding environment; monitor cardiovascular status and temperature[114,115,118,122,125,129]
Salicylate	Observe for hyperventilation and acid–base disturbances	Nil; charcoal may be used	Monitor electrolyte changes and increases in fever
Paracetamol	Careful history required to determine time and amount taken; initially vague symptoms	N-acetylcysteine	Antidote must be given within the specified time range; consider the effects of other drugs (i.e. paracetamol and codeine combinations); monitor for signs of hepatotoxicity
Carbon monoxide	Supportive care of airway, breathing, circulation	High concentrations of oxygen therapy	Hyperbaric oxygen may be required; monitor carboxyhaemoglobin; oxygen saturation monitors will give erroneously high readings
Organophosphates	Decontamination; supportive care of airway, breathing, circulation	Pralidoxime chloride; benzodiazepines	Maintain careful decontamination and personal safety considerations

Management

General principles for the management of a patient with ingestion of a toxic substance with a reduced level of consciousness apply. Prevent continued absorption by administering activated charcoal for oral ingestions and provide symptomatic care (Table 23.11).[125,126]

Central nervous system stimulants

CNS stimulants increase the activity of the reticular activating system, promoting a state of alertness and affecting the medullary control centres for respiratory and cardiovascular function. Many illegal stimulants are poorly manufactured, with no guarantee of purity or consistency in dosage. The possibility of overdose is therefore always present, producing profound CNS excitation.[125,126] Commonly used stimulants include amphetamines, dexamphetamine, methylphenidate, lysergic acid diethylamide (LSD), phencyclidine (PCP), caffeine, cocaine and methamphetamines.[125,126]

Assessment

Both psychological and physical symptoms are produced. A patient may demonstrate repetitive, non-purposeful movements, grind their teeth and appear suspicious of or paranoid about others. Physiological stimulation causes an increase in metabolism, with flushing, diaphoresis, hyperpyrexia, pupillary dilation and vomiting evident. Dizziness, loss of coordination, chest pains, palpitations or abdominal cramps may also occur. During the acute phase of poisoning, severe intoxication and loss of rational mental functioning may lead individuals to behave irrationally and even attempt suicide. Anxiousness and a general state of tension may also lead the affected person to attempt to harm others.[125] Death is possible from cardiovascular collapse or as a sequela to convulsions and acute drug toxicity.[125]

Management

If a patient has ingested the drug, emesis or lavage is of little value, and an individual risk–benefit assessment is required. Gastric emptying may precipitate more severe agitation with a concomitant rise in blood pressure, pulse rate and metabolism.[125] Activated charcoal and cathartics may be administered to promote elimination. Ongoing emergency management includes:[125]

- support of vital functions
- reduction of external stimulation by placing the patient in a quiet, non-threatening environment where a supportive person can attempt to calm and 'talk the person down' while observing for untoward reactions
- sedating when necessary, although it is not desirable to give more medications in a precarious situation; sedation may be needed to control seizures or keep the patient from self-harm.

> **Practice tip**
>
> Note that there are no specific antidotes for CNS stimulants.

Amphetamines and designer drugs

Amphetamines and designer drugs have been drugs of abuse for several years. Originally, many of them were designed and introduced as anaesthetic agents, decongestants or for other legitimate purposes. Amphetamines are chemically related to the anaesthetic ketamine, with a similar CNS response.[125] Most drugs in this group were discontinued or controlled because of the delirium and agitation experienced by the patients who had received them; paradoxically, these effects led to their popularity as recreational drugs.[125] Amphetamines are synthetic sympathomimetic drugs; they are available in oral, intranasal or IV forms; crystalline rock forms such as 'ice' are smoked. Death may occur from overdose, self-mutilation or dangerous activities such as diving or walking on roads.[125]

Assessment

Depending on the dose, route and time since exposure, a person exhibits characteristic behavioural and physical changes. With high-dose intoxication, the patient has pronounced CNS involvement – altered levels of consciousness, seizure activity or a loss of protective gag, corneal and swallow reflexes. Nystagmus is a classic sign, along with hypertension and an elevated body temperature. A significant rise in arterial pressure presents a risk for intracerebral haemorrhage. One of the distinguishing features of amphetamines is their ability to produce coma without affecting respirations.[125] The patient may risk dehydration and renal failure if muscle breakdown has occurred. A high urine output should be maintained and serum urea and creatinine levels monitored to detect a decrease in renal function.[125]

Lower dose intoxications do not produce unconsciousness but typically cause behavioural patterns that reflect depersonalisation and distorted perceptions of events or other people. The patient's physical and mental responses may be dulled and slow, or abusive and delusional. Intoxication is marked by paranoid thoughts, with the patient responding to therapeutic or friendly gestures with behaviours ranging from apprehension to aggressive hostility. To avoid stimulating the patient and thereby intensifying the behaviour, a quiet environment should be provided for initial assessment and treatment, although this is often difficult in the ED.[125]

> **Practice tip**
>
> Noxious environmental stimulation such as bright lighting, loud noises and activity can provoke these patients to become anxious and uncooperative.

Management

Gastric emptying is normally ineffective due to delays in seeking treatment. If a patient presents early, activated charcoal and cathartics are useful in preventing further absorption. Noises, sights and sounds provoke paranoid ideation and may present a risk to staff and other patients. 'Talking down' is usually not successful and probably only serves to exacerbate the situation. If the patient is demonstrating hostile or self-abusive forms of behaviour, chemical restraints may be needed to protect him/her and any others present. The use of physical restraints is not without danger, and they should never be used as a substitute for a more desirable environment. If the threat of danger or psychosis is significant, sedatives such as diazepam or haloperidol may be necessary to control the patient's behaviour. IV diazepam is also used to control frequent seizure activity, and along with hyperthermia should be aggressively managed.[125] Hyperthermia is managed primary using IV benzodiazepines and IV fluid resuscitation.[125] If behaviour, or hyperthermia remains significantly dangerous to patient or staff, intubation and paralysis may be required.[125]

Salicylate poisoning

Aspirin is the commonest form of salicylate in the home and is found in many over-the-counter medications, such as combination analgesic and topical ointments.[120] Aspirin may be ingested orally, absorbed through the rectal mucosa, or applied to the skin in topical preparations. Under normal circumstances, the kidneys serve as the principal organ of excretion. In Australia salicylate poisoning is relatively uncommon, due to public preference for paracetamol as the preferred analgesic and antipyretic.[120] The three common types of aspirin overdose are: accidental ingestion (more common in young children); intentional ingestion (more common in adults); and chronic toxicity (occurs in any age group).[119]

Assessment, monitoring and diagnostics

Intentional or accidental ingestion is straightforward, with a clear history of poisoning. Chronic toxicity is, however, often unrecognised.[120] Many individuals are not aware of correct dosages, may combine multiple drugs, each of which contains aspirin, or may have impaired excretion due to dehydration. The symptoms of chronic aspirin overdose include dehydration, lethargy and fever and resemble the original problem being treated, and some people will continue treating themselves with aspirin for these symptoms. Chronic toxicity has a higher mortality than acute ingestion.[120]

Toxicity may result if aspirin is ingested in amounts greater than 150 mg/kg. Aspirin toxicity can result in tachypnoea, fever, tinnitus, disorientation, coma and convulsions. Acid–base disturbances arise from a direct stimulatory effect on the respiratory centre in the CNS. An increased rate and depth of respirations causes hypocarbia and respiratory alkalosis, with renal compensation by bicarbonate elimination. However, salicylates also alter metabolic processes, resulting in metabolic acidosis. Blood gases can therefore reflect acidosis, alkalosis or a combination of the two. Tinnitus is a symptom of the effect of aspirin on the 8th cranial nerve.[110]

Aspirin interferes with cellular glucose uptake, causing initial hyperglycaemia. Cellular levels of glucose become depleted and the patient then demonstrates hypoglycaemic effects, particularly those related to the CNS. Later, serum levels may be either normal or hypoglycaemic.[110] Patients may be nauseated and vomit after ingestion, causing fluid and electrolyte imbalance.[119] Aspirin use is also associated with local tissue irritation and gastrointestinal bleeding. Normal platelet function is altered by aspirin, with an increased tendency for bleeding. Concomitant use of anticoagulants increases the risk of haemorrhage.[119]

Management

Absorption can be reduced with activated charcoal. Repeat doses should be given for patients with signs of ongoing absorption.[128] Urine alkalisation and forced diuresis can significantly increase elimination, as salicylates are weak acids excreted by the kidneys. Haemodialysis is reserved for extreme cases with profound acidosis, high blood levels, persistent CNS symptoms or renal failure.[110]

As salicylates have no known specific antidote,[128] supportive therapy includes prevention of dehydration by carefully monitoring fluid output and providing adequate fluid replacement and monitoring serum electrolytes for imbalance and replacing as needed. Evaluate arterial blood gases to determine whether the patient continues to have an effect from aspirin toxicity or is not responding to therapy. Temperature elevations should be controlled with external cooling methods if fever develops.

Paracetamol poisoning

The incidence of paracetamol, also known as acetaminophen, toxicity is associated with approximately half of all Australasian toxic ingestions, due in part to its common availability as an analgesic/antipyretic agent.[121] The drug is absorbed in the stomach and small bowel, with 98% metabolised by the liver using one of two mechanisms: most is via a pathway that breaks down into non-toxic byproducts; the second hepatic pathway usually metabolises about 4% of the drug, but the process has a toxic byproduct. The liver is capable of detoxifying the toxic byproduct by combining it with a naturally occurring substance, glutathione. In an overdose or when the minor pathway has already been stimulated (e.g. concomitant barbiturate use), more paracetamol is metabolised by the secondary pathway and the toxic byproduct accumulates, quickly consuming the available glutathione, resulting in liver tissue destruction.[121,129]

Assessment, monitoring and diagnostics

The amount of paracetamol ingested is best determined from the patient history, as serum levels, although helpful, can be easily distorted. A nomogram is used to plot measured levels against time postingestion as a relative indicator of toxicity. A relatively small dose of 200 mg/kg paracetamol is considered to be toxic, although hepatotoxicity occurs after an ingestion of 140 mg/kg or 10 g in a single dose.[121,129]

Liver function studies are helpful to recognise the development of hepatic dysfunction or damage. These include liver enzymes, serum bilirubin, protein, prothrombin time, partial thromboplastin time and platelets.[119,127] Three phases of toxic damage resulting from excess paracetamol are presented in Table 23.12.[114,121,129]

Management

Absorption can be reduced with activated charcoal when the patient presents to hospital early; however, following periods of 2 hours or greater ingestion-activated charcoal is unlikely to be very effective. Haemodialysis with a charcoal dialysate has been used in an attempt to remove unchanged paracetamol from the liver, but this does not remove the toxic byproduct. Forced diuresis is also not effective, because little paracetamol (about 2%) is removed by the kidneys.[121,129]

TABLE 23.12

Phases of toxic damage resulting from an excess of paracetamol[114,121,129]

PHASE	TIMEFRAME	SYMPTOMS
Phase 1	First 24 h	Vague symptoms of nausea, vomiting and malaise
Phase 2	24–48 h	Vague symptoms subside; onset of right upper quadrant pain due to hepatic injury; urine output may decrease as paracetamol potentiates the effect of antidiuretic hormone; liver enzymes, bilirubin, proteins and clotting studies may be abnormal
Phase 3	60–72 h	Liver impairment becomes more obvious, with jaundice, coagulation defects, hypoglycaemia and hepatic encephalopathy; renal failure or cardiomyopathy may also occur; death from hepatic failure occurs in approximately 10% of severe overdose

The specific therapy for paracetamol poisoning is administration of the antidote, N-acetylcysteine, which is structurally similar to glutathione and binds to the toxic byproduct. When given within 24 hours of an acute ingestion, N-acetylcysteine is effective in preventing hepatic damage.[121,129]

Carbon monoxide poisoning

Carbon monoxide is a gaseous byproduct of incomplete fuel combustion and is present where there is a flame in a confined space with improper ventilation or air exchange. Levels of carbon monoxide can accumulate rapidly, and the gas is dangerous as it is colourless, odourless, tasteless and non-irritating.[130] Common sources of carbon monoxide are faulty radiant heaters, kerosene lamps, cooking stoves, engine exhausts and fireplaces. Acute carbon monoxide poisoning is the commonest form of successful poisoning in three of the world's most developed countries.[130,131]

Assessment, monitoring and diagnostics

Haemoglobin has a 210–240-fold greater affinity for carbon monoxide than for oxygen and shifts the oxygen–haemoglobin curve to the left (see Chapter 13). As carbon monoxide displaces oxygen from red blood cells, the patient experiences hypoxaemia and hypoxia.[122,130,131] Headache, nausea and vague pains are often experienced at onset of poisoning, and the patient may feel increasingly tired and sleepy, have difficulty concentrating and fail to recognise the onset of poisoning. With higher levels of inhalation, the patient may be tachypnoeic, tachycardic and experience loss of consciousness. A characteristic red colour presents in the lips with skin flushing.[122,130,131] The most important factors in determining carbon monoxide poisoning are a history of exposure with an elevated blood carboxyhaemoglobin level.[122,130,131]

Management

As CO is an inhaled toxin, the patient should be removed from the contaminated environment to prevent further absorption and allowed to breathe fresh air until 100% oxygen can be administered, although this may be ineffective because of the bond between carbon monoxide and haemoglobin. High flow high concentration oxygen administration will, however, substantially reduce the half-life of carbon monoxide.[122] Hyperbaric oxygenation is used to treat severe cases of carbon monoxide poisoning, as pressurised oxygen reduces the half-life of the carboxyhaemoglobin molecule and shortens the duration of its effects. Mild-to-moderate poisoning can be managed without the use of hyperbaric oxygen, as hyperbaric oxygenation is not available at every facility. Treatment depends on carboxyhaemoglobin serum levels, time since exposure, transport time to the hyperbaric chamber and the clinical symptoms of the patient.[122,130,131] Patients should be monitored for adverse effects of hypoxia, as they may have convulsions, cardiac arrhythmias and acid–base disturbances.

Corrosive acids

Several substances are discussed here due to their similar ability to cause local tissue injury. Some common acids involved in toxic emergencies are acetic acid (vinegar), carbolic acid (phenol disinfectants), chlorine (swimming pools, sanitising agents), hydrochloric acid (pools, cleaning agents), hydrofluoric oxalic (laundry agents), sodium bisulfate (toilet cleaning agents that become acidic when added to water) and sulfuric acid (car battery acid).

Ingested corrosives can produce immediate or late life-threatening complications. In general, acids cause burn-like injuries.[117,132] Patients who ingest corrosive agents can shows signs of tachycardia, hypotension, and tachypnoea.[117] Life-threatening complications can present with ulceration and perforation of oral and oesophageal mucosa, presenting a danger for haemorrhage and mediastinitis, and also show signs of dyspnoea, chest pain, fever, subcutaneous emphysema and on auscultation a pleural rub.[117] Certain corrosive agents, like hydrofluoric acids, can have a direct effect on cardiovascular deterioration due to causing hypocalcaemia which may present as changes to the QT interval, torsades des pointes, or other arrhythmias.[132]

Assessment

Physical findings are site-specific and relate to the type of exposure – ingestion, inhalation or contact (Table 23.13). Ingested acids present as burns to the mouth and pharynx. Patients able to vocalise complain of pain, gastric irritation with vomiting and haematemesis. Fumes from an ingested substance may cause pneumonitis. Contact with skin or eyes is similar to other types of burns, with a sharply defined blister or wound, inflammation, pain and ulceration. Hypotension and cardiovascular collapse are also possible when damage occurs to underlying vital structures.[117,132]

Inhalation irritates respiratory tissues, producing direct damage, oedema and alterations in ventilation. Patients may initially experience coughing, choking, gasping for air and increased respiratory secretions. Clinicians should assess and monitor any obvious tissue injury, impaired respiratory function and subsequent effects of hypoxia and pulmonary oedema, which may occur up to 6–8 hours later.[117,132] ABGs, ventilation studies, serial CXRs and frequent physical assessments are used to monitor for changes.

Management

Contaminated clothing should be removed to prevent recontamination, care should be taken to ensure staff are not contaminated and exposed in this process. Patients with external contamination should be washed thoroughly to remove any remaining surface material that may come into contact with treating staff. For acid contact with skin or eyes, begin immediate flushing with

TABLE 23.13
Summary of assessment and management of acid and alkali exposure[117]

	CORROSIVE ACIDS OR CORROSIVE ALKALIS
Assessment	• Burns to skin, mouth, pharynx or oesophagus • Gastric irritation with nausea and vomiting
Management	• Airway • Breathing • Circulation • Decontamination
Prevent absorption	• Do not induce vomiting • Remove contaminated clothing • Flush the skin with copious amounts of water
Enhance elimination	• Administer chelating agents if they exist, such as calcium gluconate for hydrofluoric acid
Symptomatic management	• Protect burnt skin with sterile dressings • Monitor respiratory status

a non-reactive liquid and continue to do so for at least 15 min to guarantee complete removal. In most cases water will be the safest and best available liquid. Provide skin or eye protection with a sterile dressing.[117]

For ingested acids, emesis or lavage should not be attempted, as the substance will cause additional damage when ejected from the stomach. A gastric tube may also cause structural damage by penetrating or irritating friable tissues.[117,132] Do not attempt to neutralise the acid, as this may result in a chemical reaction and generate heat as a byproduct, with potential further burning and damage to the patient.[117,132] Suctioning of oral secretions should be done carefully and with as much visualisation of tissues as possible. A patient may be given water or milk to irrigate the upper gastrointestinal tract, although extreme care is required to ensure that the airway is adequately protected because there is a risk of aspiration.[117,132]

Corrosive alkalis

Alkalis produce tissue destruction on contact by interacting with tissue component fats and proteins and producing necrotic tissue. Erosion of the oesophagus and stomach occurs if ingested orally, and peritonitis or mediastinitis may develop as sequelae. Late effects are similar to those produced by acids. Oesophageal strictures due to scarring are common postingestion. About 25% of patients who ingest a strong alkali will die from the initial insult.[117,132]

Skin contact and ingestion are the commonest types of injury from an alkali; however, ingestion is the most immediately life-threatening form of contact. Alkalis involved in toxic emergencies include many substances found around the house, such as detergents and cleaning agents that contain ammonia; cement and builder's lime; low-phosphate detergents; dishwasher detergents that contain sodium carbonate; and laundry bleaches that contain sodium hypochlorite.[117,132]

Assessment

The immediate response to ingestion is increased secretions, pain, vomiting or haemoptysis. Signs of perforation include fever, respiratory difficulty or peritonitis. Approximately 98% of patients develop strictures.[117,132] Alkalis and skin contact produce a soap-like substance because of the interaction with tissue fats, giving a slimy, soapy feeling.[117,132]

Management

Induced vomiting or gastric lavage should not be attempted for ingested alkalis, as these will be neutralised by stomach acid. Lavage tubes may cause further tissue damage.[117,132] External contact with alkalis necessitates copious irrigation of the point of contact. Continue irrigation for at least 15 min; in the case of the eye, irrigation may be necessary for up to 30 min. Cover all wounds after irrigation with sterile dressings to reduce the risk of infection.

A patient should be nil by mouth until an inspection of the mouth and throat is conducted to determine the amount and extent of burns. An oesophagoscopy will identify the degree of injury and enable direct irrigation of any affected areas of mucosa.[117] Alkalis that contain phosphates may produce a systemic hypocalcaemia, and IV calcium gluconate may be required. Continue to monitor for systemic effects of perforation or tissue injury.[117]

Petroleum distillates

Petroleum distillates are common substances. Typical petroleum products are benzene, fuel oils, petrol, kerosene, lacquer diluents, lubricating oil, mineral oil, naphthalene, paint thinners and petroleum spirits. Toxicity depends on: route of exposure (ingestion or aspiration); volatility (ease with which the substance evaporates); viscosity (density or thickness); amount ingested; and presence of other toxins.[110,133]

Products with a low viscosity are more likely to be aspirated and can quickly spread over the lung surface. Substances with low viscosity and high volatility, for example benzene, kerosene, and turpentine, are toxic in doses as low as 1 mL/kg, with death from doses of 10–250 mL. Mortality is increased if an additional toxic substance is present, or if accidental aspiration occurs.[133]

Assessment

Aspiration causes pneumonitis with low-grade fever, tachypnoea, coughing, choking, gagging and pulmonary oedema as a late effect.[133] As petroleum distillates are fat solvents and rapidly cross the lipid-rich cell membrane, nerve tissue is especially sensitive to injury. A patient may exhibit local effects, such as depressed nerve conduction, or varied central effects, such as feelings of wellbeing, headache, tinnitus, dizziness, visual disturbances, through to respiratory depression, altered levels of consciousness, convulsions and coma.[117,133]

Management

In the awake and alert patient, the decision to treat is based on the physical properties of the substance, the likelihood of aspiration or other complications and the amount consumed.[131] When preventing absorption, careful consideration needs to be given to gastric emptying, as neither induced vomiting nor gastric lavage is recommended.

The patient's respiratory status should be immediately assessed for possible aspiration. A patient that is coughing, has cyanosis or appears hypoxic may have aspirated or developed chemical pneumonitis.[117] If the patient is lethargic or unconscious, an endotracheal tube must be placed for adequate airway protection, although this heightens the risk of aspiration as hydrocarbons adhere to the tube and increase the risk of chemical pneumonitis.[117]

Organophosphates

Organophosphates are a large and diverse group of chemicals used in domestic, industrial and agricultural settings (e.g. insecticides, herbicides).[115,123] The primary effect of organophosphates is binding and inactivation of acetylcholinesterase, a neurotransmitter that metabolises acetylcholine.[115,123]

Organophosphates can be absorbed through the skin, ingested or inhaled. Although most patients become symptomatic soon after ingestion, the onset and duration of action depend on the nature and type of compound, the degree and route of exposure, the mode of action of the compound, its lipid solubility and rate of metabolic degradation.[115,123]

Mortality from intentional ingestion of organophosphates causing poisoning in Australia accounted for 25.3% of coronial suicides between 2001 and 2013.[134] Men aged 30–50 years were more likely to attempt suicide with organophosphates, and were more likely to be of lower socioeconomic status and living in an agricultural area.[134] Common complications include respiratory distress, seizures and aspiration pneumonia, with respiratory failure the commonest cause of death.[123]

Assessment, monitoring and diagnostics

The clinical findings of organophosphate poisoning can be divided into three broad categories: muscarinic effects, nicotinic effects and effects on the CNS. Common muscarinic manifestations are summarised by the mnemonic SLUDGE: **S**alivation, **L**acrimation, **U**rination, **D**efecation, **G**I upset, **E**mesis.[115,123] Other symptoms include bradycardia, hypotension, bronchospasm, cough, abdominal pain, blurred vision, miosis and sweating. Nicotinic effects include muscle fasciculations, cramping, weakness and diaphragmatic failure. Autonomic effects include hypertension, tachycardia, pupillary dilation and pallor.

CNS effects include anxiety, restlessness, confusion, ataxia, seizures, insomnia, dysarthria, tremors, coma and paralysis. The three types of paralysis that may result from organophosphate poisoning are described in Table 23.14.

Laboratory diagnosis is based on the measurement of cholinesterase activity using either erythrocyte or plasma levels; erythrocyte cholinesterase is more accurate, but plasma cholinesterase is easier to test and is more widely available. Erythrocyte acetylcholinesterase is found in the grey matter of the CNS, red blood cells, peripheral nerve and muscle. Plasma cholinesterase circulates in plasma and is found in white matter of the CNS, pancreas and heart.[115,123] Mild poisoning is when the cholinesterase activity is reduced to 20–50% of normal; moderate poisoning occurs when activity is 10–20% of normal; and severe poisoning occurs at less than 10% of

TABLE 23.14
Types of paralysis that may result from organophosphate poisoning[115,123,134]

TYPE	ONSET	PRESENTATION	DURATION OF SYMPTOMS
Type 1	Occurs shortly after exposure	Acute paralysis secondary to persistent depolarisation at the neuromuscular junction	
Type 2	24–96 h after resolution of acute cholinergic poisoning	Paralysis and respiratory distress Proximal muscle groups are involved, with relative sparing of distal muscle groups	Up to 3 weeks
Type 3	2–3 weeks after exposure to large doses of certain organophosphates	Distal muscle weakness with relative sparing of the neck muscles, cranial nerves and proximal muscle groups	Up to 12 months

normal cholinesterase enzyme activity. Levels do not, however, always correlate with clinical illness.[115]

Management

Initial priorities in managing organophosphate poisoning are airway, breathing and circulation, incorporating D for danger, as organophosphates also present considerable risk to staff caring for the patient, especially during the initial phases of management. All of the patient's clothing should be removed and considered as hazardous waste. The patient's decontamination with soap and water is a priority, as soap with a high pH breaks down organophosphates.[115,123] Staff must use personal protective equipment, such as neoprene or nitrile gloves, and gowns are worn when decontaminating patients. Charcoal cartridge masks for respiratory protection are useful, although evidence suggests that the nosocomial risk to staff may not be as significant as was once thought.[135] Intubation is commonly required after significant exposure, due to respiratory distress from laryngospasm, bronchospasm or severe bronchorrhoea. Continuous cardiac monitoring and an ECG are used to check for bradycardias. Activated charcoal is used for gastric decontamination for those patients who have ingested organophosphate. The mainstay of treatment is atropine and pralidoxime, with a benzodiazepine used for seizure control.[123] Atropine blocks acetylcholine receptors and halts the cholinergic stimulation. Very large doses of atropine are usually required, 1–2 g IV, and repeated if muscle weakness is not relieved or the signs of poisoning recur. Clearing of bronchial secretions is the end point of atropine administration, not pupil size or the absolute dose.[123] Pralidoxime hydrochloride reactivates acetylcholinesterase and is effective at restoring skeletal muscle function but is less effective at reversing muscarinic signs. Over time, the bond between organophosphate and cholinesterase becomes permanent and the effectiveness of pralidoxime diminishes.[123] Benzodiazepines are clinically indicated through their binding to specific receptor sites, potentiating the effects of gamma-aminobutyrate and facilitating inhibitory transmitters for management of seizures.[115,123]

Envenomation

Venomous animals can be land-based or marine-based, and their distribution ranges from broad to very specific locations. Exposure of humans to venom produces a large and varied range of symptomatology, which often results in an emergency presentation. It is therefore important for critical care nurses to be familiar with the types of potentially venomous animals inhabiting the catchment area of their health setting. From a first aid perspective it is vital nurses are familiar with the presentation and management of specific life-threatening or injury-causing envenomation, including the use of antivenom when one exists. Most countries have local poison information centres for advice from expert toxicologists (see *Online resources*). Common envenomations across Australia and New Zealand are described below.

Redback/katipo spider bite

Description and incidence

The redback spider (*Latrodectus hasseltii*) is found throughout Australia but more commonly in temperate regions. Tasmania has the lowest frequency of reported bites, while areas around Alice Springs, Perth and Brisbane are especially infested.[136] The redback spider is easily identifiable by the presence of a red, orange or brownish stripe on its characteristic black, globular abdomen. The female is much larger than the male; generally, only the female is considered dangerous. Juveniles are smaller, more variably coloured and may lack any spots or stripes. Bites from both male and juvenile spiders may result in symptoms, although these tend to be less significant than bites from females.[136]

The redback spider has also become established outside Australia, including in New Zealand, Japan and South America.[137] Although bites are rare, small populations of redback spiders have been reported in New Zealand in Central Otago (South Island) and New Plymouth (North Island) since the early 1980s.[138] The only other venomous spider in New Zealand is the katipo (*Latrodectus katipo*) from the same genus as the redback. The katipo has a black, rounded body, slender legs and a red stripe on the abdomen. Symptoms of katipo spider bite are similar to those of the redback spider and, where indicated, redback antivenom is used to treat bites.[139]

A redback spider bite is a frequent cause for ED presentations and the most clinically significant spider bite in Australia.[140] Most bites are minor, with either minimal or no symptoms and requiring no antivenom. In approximately 20% of cases, significant envenomation occurs and antivenom administration is generally indicated, although death is extremely unlikely in untreated cases. Redback antivenom is the most commonly administered antivenom in Australia.[136]

Clinical manifestations

Envenomation by a redback spider is known as latrodectism; the venom contains excitatory neurotoxins that stimulate release of catecholamines from sympathetic nerves and acetylcholine from motor nerve endings.[136] Signs and symptoms associated with a significant envenomation are distinctive, and diagnosis is by clinical findings. Initially, there is a minor sting at the bite site, where the spider may or may not have been seen. Over the first hour the bite becomes progressively painful to severe, spreading proximally with and involving swollen and tender local lymph nodes. Localised sweating at the bite site or limb or generalised sweating may appear, associated with hypertension and malaise. Pain eventually becomes generalised and may be expressed as chest, abdominal, head or neck pain suggestive of other acute conditions such as myocardial infarction.[136]

Progression of symptoms generally occurs in less than 6 hours but may take up to 24 hours. People with minor untreated bites may experience symptoms for several weeks.[136] Other less common signs and symptoms include local piloerection, nausea, vomiting, headache, fever, restlessness/insomnia, tachycardia and neurological symptoms such as muscle weakness or twitching.[136]

Assessment

Patients presenting with pain from a bite who have the offending spider with them are straightforward in terms of initial assessment. Identification of the spider is confirmed and a history of the event obtained, including the time of the bite and any first aid initiated. A brief assessment of the bite site and the involved limb is undertaken, including the extent of pain, presence of sweating and painful tender lymph nodes, and a baseline set of vital signs. Patients are then placed in a suitable area for medical assessment and ongoing observation.[137]

Adult patients presenting with vague limb pain, or preverbal children who are 'distressed' and 'cannot be settled', may be unaware that they have been bitten by a redback. The pain may not have been felt at the time of the bite and no spider may have been seen. Thorough history taking, physical assessment and knowledge of the effects of latrodectism enable detection of a suspected spider bite.[137]

Management

There is no recommended definitive first aid for a redback spider bite. Application of cold packs to the bite site and administration of simple analgesia, such as paracetamol, may assist with local pain relief. The use of a pressure immobilisation bandage is not necessary, as symptom progression is slow and not life-threatening, and will cause further pain only in the affected limb. Remove any pressure bandage that was applied during first aid after identification of the spider is confirmed.[136]

Presence of the above symptoms (pain, swelling, localised sweating at the site) indicates systemic envenomation requiring administration of redback spider antivenom.[136] Prior to administration, the patient should be placed in a clinical area with readily available resuscitation equipment to treat any anaphylactic reaction, although this is rare. An IV cannula is inserted and adrenaline 1:1000 is prepared for the possibility of anaphylaxis.

The initial dose of redback spider antivenom is administered intramuscularly (IM) or IV, and symptoms should subside over the next 30–60 min.[136] Complete resolution of symptoms requires no specific further treatment. If there has not been complete resolution of symptoms after 2 hours further antivenom is given, although there is no evidence of this being beneficial.[136] If after a further 2 hours there is incomplete resolution of symptoms or no discernible response after 4 ampoules of antivenom, expert advice should be sought via the local poison information centre and adequate analgesia given.[136] Patients who are symptom-free after 6 hours of observation or the administration of antivenom can be discharged home with instructions to re-present should any symptoms return. Redback spider antivenom administration in various stages of pregnancy has not been associated with direct or indirect harmful effects to the fetus.[136]

Practice tip

Observations for the development or progression of symptoms of a redback envenomation focus on development of local pain that spreads proximally and increases in intensity, development of sweating (either local or generalised) and hypertension.

Funnel-web spider bite

Description and incidence

Funnel-web spiders are the most venomous spiders to humans worldwide, and Australian funnel-web spiders (*Atrax* or *Hadronyche* genera) are found primarily along the east coast. The Sydney funnel-web spider (*Atrax robustus*) is found mainly around Sydney, while other species are found in eastern New South Wales and central and southern Queensland. The spider is large, black or dark brown and approximately 3 cm long in the body. Male spiders have smaller bodies and are significantly more toxic than females.[136]

Clinical manifestations

Funnel-web spider bites are potentially rapidly lethal;[141] however, only 10–20% of bites result in systemic envenomation, with the majority being minor and not requiring antivenom. The bite is extremely painful, and fang marks are likely to be seen. Signs and symptoms of systemic envenomation may appear within 10–30 min, and include perioral tingling and tongue fasciculation, increased salivation, lacrimation, piloerection, sweating; nausea, vomiting, headache; hypertension, tachycardia; dyspnoea, pulmonary oedema; irritability, decreased consciousness and coma.[136] Regardless of the presence of symptoms, all possible funnel-web spider bites are managed as a medical emergency.[141]

Assessment

Patients with suspected funnel-web spider bites are rapidly assessed for the presence of any signs and symptoms of envenomation and allocated an ATS triage category of 1–3, based on presenting symptoms. A pressure immobilisation bandage is applied if this was not done during initial first aid.[136] Patients with signs of envenomation are moved to a resuscitation area for immediate treatment, including urgent antivenom administration and management of the clinical effects of envenomation. Monitoring and assessment for potentially serious manifestations focus on:

- airway compromise due to decreased level of consciousness, requiring airway protection with an airway adjunct or endotracheal intubation

- breathing for respiratory compromise due to pulmonary oedema, requiring continuous positive airway pressure or intubation/ventilation with positive end-expiratory pressure (see Chapter 15)
- circulatory compromise due to profound hypotension, although a late sign with hypertension more commonly seen, requires IV access and volume replacement. Circulatory compromise/failure may lead to cardiac arrest requiring cardiopulmonary resuscitation (see Chapter 25).

All patients require full monitoring with constant nursing observation. A patient with no signs of envenomation on arrival has a detailed history taken regarding the circumstances of the bite, the time of bite, a description of the spider and any first aid undertaken. The patient is then regularly assessed for any symptoms suggesting systemic envenomation. After thorough medical assessment, if there are no signs of systemic envenomation, any first aid such as a pressure immobilisation bandage is removed and the patient observed for 6 hours. With no diagnostic test for funnel-web spider envenomation and no venom detection procedure available, clinical diagnosis is based on the history and symptoms.[136]

Management

For signs of systemic envenomation, funnel-web spider antivenom is administered slowly IV over 15–20 min;[136] premedication is not required, although the patient is observed closely for anaphylaxis.[127] In severe envenomation associated with dyspnoea, pulmonary oedema or decreased level of consciousness, the initial antivenom dose may be doubled. More antivenom may be required until all major symptoms have resolved.[136] The antivenom dose for children is the same as the adult dose.[142] First aid measures such as a pressure immobilisation bandage can be removed after antivenom administration and the symptoms have stabilised; this may take several hours.[136]

Snake bites

Worldwide there are a variety of snakes that have the capacity to envenomate humans and cause life-threatening clinical features;[143] broadly these snakes fall into three groups: elapids, pit vipers and cobras. Elapids are mostly encountered throughout Australasia, pit vipers in the Americas and cobras in Africa and south Asia.

The focus of this section will be on the life-threatening Australasian elapid species.

Description and incidence

Australasia is inhabited by many snakes (over 140 recognised snakes from 30 different species; 25% of all known venomous snakes, and 40% of all dangerous front-fanged snakes or elapids).[144] New Zealand has no known venomous terrestrial snakes.[145] Australian venomous snakes are found in both rural areas and residential and metropolitan areas, especially when in close proximity to bushland and in periods of drought. Snake bite envenoming constituted 15% of admissions in Australian hospitals between 2000 and 2013;[146] mortality rates associated with those hospitalised with snake venom were twice as high as those associated with other envenomations (e.g. arthropod envenomation).[146]

Clinical manifestations

The majority of snake bites do not result in significant envenomation.[144] Bites are generally recognised by the patient at the time because of associated pain, although some bites are unrecognised. The bite site may show minimal to obvious signs of punctures or scratches, with accompanying swelling and bruising. Multiple bites are possible and are generally associated with major envenomation. Australian snake venoms contain various toxins that are responsible for the systemic effects[147] (Table 23.15). Renal damage may occur as a consequence of myoglobinuria from severe rhabdomyolysis or haemoglobinuria associated with coagulopathies, leading to acute renal failure (see Chapter 18).[147]

Assessment

Patients presenting with snake bite(s) are allocated a high priority for assessment and treatment even if they appear well on arrival. Patients who present without effective first aid measures (the application of a pressure immobilisation bandage and splint) have these applied immediately.[148] The pressure immobilisation bandage is applied with a broad (15-cm) bandage, commencing over the bite site with the same pressure that would be used for a sprained ankle. The bandage is then extended to cover the whole limb, including fingers/toes, and the limb is splinted and immobilised.[149] Correct application of the pressure bandage is important, as any benefit is lost with bandages that are too loose, not applied to the whole limb or with no splinting or immobilisation.[149] Elasticised bandages are superior to crepe bandages in obtaining and maintaining adequate pressure.[149] Do not wash the wound prior to applying the pressure immobilisation bandage, as swabbing of the bite site is used when performing venom detection. The patient should not mobilise to minimise distribution of any injected venom. Once applied, the pressure immobilisation bandage is not removed until the patient is in a healthcare location that is stocked with antivenom.[149]

> **Practice tip**
>
> Pressure immobilisation may be contraindicated or ineffective in bites from exotic snake species. Many of these non-Australasian species of snake have venoms that cause local tissue destruction. For example, pit vipers and cobras can both cause extensive localised tissue damage. Immobilisation is the mainstay of first aid.[150]

TABLE 23.15
Characteristics and clinical manifestations of snake venom[145,155]

TOXIN	EFFECTS	SIGNS AND SYMPTOMS
Neurotoxin	Blocks transmission at the neuromuscular junctions, causing skeletal and respiratory muscle flaccid paralysis, presynaptic and/or postsynaptic	Ptosis (drooping of upper eyelids) Diplopia (double vision) Ophthalmoplegia (partial or complete paralysis of eye movements) Fixed, dilated pupils Muscle weakness Respiratory weakness, paralysis
Haemotoxin	Causes coagulopathies, resulting in either: defibrination with low-fibrinogen, unclottable blood, but usually with a normal platelet count or direct anticoagulation with normal fibrinogen and platelet count Both cause an elevated prothrombin ratio and international normalised ratio	Bleeding from bite wounds Bleeding at venipuncture sites Haematuria
Myotoxin	Causes myolysis, resulting in generalised destruction of skeletal muscles with high serum creatine kinase and leading to myoglobinuria and occasionally severe hyperkalaemia	Muscle weakness Muscle pain on movement Red or brown urine, which tests positively to blood

A brief and focused history explores the time and circumstances of the bite, a description of the snake (colour, length), geographical location and the application of any first aid. The patient is assessed for general symptoms including headache, nausea, vomiting, abdominal pain, collapse, convulsions and anxiety, although these alone do not indicate envenomation.[148] Additional signs and symptoms include blurred or double vision, slurred speech, muscle weakness, respiratory distress, bleeding from the bite site or elsewhere, and pain and swelling at the bite site and associated lymph nodes.[127]

Patients with suspected snake bite are located in an acute area with full monitoring available, with symptomatic patients placed in a resuscitation area. The patient requires insertion of IV access devices and collection of blood for pathology tests including full blood count, urea, electrolytes, creatine, creatinine kinase and full coagulation studies. Unnecessary venipunctures should be avoided, including sites where it may be difficult to control bleeding should it occur. Healthcare settings without ready access to pathology services may need to perform whole blood clotting time testing at the bedside to assess for any coagulopathy; however, point of care testing is not accurate in these cases and therefore where possible the patient should be retrieved to the nearest centre for testing as soon as possible.[127]

All probable snake bites require observation for at least 12 hours, as some serious symptoms may be delayed.[148] Patients should be assessed for tachycardia, hypotension or hypertension, and falling oxygen saturation, altered respiratory rate, forced vital capacity or peak expiratory flow rate, indicating respiratory muscle paralysis. Frequent neurological observations focus on identification of muscle weakness and paralysis; clinicians should note any ptosis, diplopia, dysphagia, slurred speech, limb weakness or altered levels of consciousness. An indwelling catheter should be inserted for close monitoring of urine output and presence of any myoglobin in urine.[148]

To identify the likely snake involved and thus the correct antivenom required, a bedside snake venom detection kit is used at the bite site or with a urine sample by a trained laboratory technician. Although there are some reports of false negatives and false positives associated with the use of snake venom detection kits, these are mostly associated with operator errors.[151] Nevertheless, snake venom detection kits should be used in conjunction with clinical and biochemical examinations noting that a negative skin test does not indicate a non-venomous snake and should not alter management.[127] A swab of the washings from the bite area is collected by leaving the pressure immobilisation bandage on and creating a window over the bite site to expose the bitten area. Testing takes about 25 min. If there are signs of systemic envenomation, urine can be used to perform the test; blood should be avoided, as it is unreliable. A positive result indicates that venom from a particular snake is present, but does not mean that systemic envenomation has occurred, while a negative result does not exclude systematic envenomation.[148]

Practice tip

Whole blood clotting time is performed by drawing 1 mL venous blood and placing it in a glass test tube. If the blood has not clotted within 20 min, a coagulopathy is likely to exist, suggesting envenomation; however, this test still can fail to identify 20% of cases likely to require antivenom.[152]

In patients with known snake bite and systemic envenomation, antivenom administration is required if there is any degree of paralysis, significant coagulopathy, any myolysis (myoglobinuria or creatinine kinase >500 mcg per litre), unconsciousness and/or convulsions.[148] In an asymptomatic patient with normal pathology and a negative or positive snake venom detection result, it is likely that envenomation has not occurred. In this case, the pressure immobilisation bandage can be removed under close observation in a resuscitation area. The patient is fully reevaluated including repeat blood tests, assessing coagulation parameters, within 1–2 hours after removal of the pressure bandage. If the patient's condition remains unchanged, further observation and repeat blood tests at 6 and 12 hours are required. Patients with no evidence of envenomation after 12 hours may be discharged.[127]

Management

A patient with evidence of systemic envenomation requires antivenom administration; monovalent antivenom is used in preference to polyvalent antivenom when the identity of the snake species is known. Polyvalent antivenom is a mixture of all monovalent antivenoms, and is therefore used for severe envenomation where the identity of the snake is unknown and the patient's condition does not allow time for a snake venom detection kit result, or where there is insufficient monovalent antivenom available.[148] Expert advice from a poison information centre may assist in identifying the snake, based on known habitats and distribution as well as presenting symptoms. Antivenom is always administered IV in a diluted strength of 1:10 (or less if volume is a concern) via an infusion. Administration is commenced slowly while observing for signs of any adverse reaction. The infusion rate can be increased if no reaction occurs, with the whole initial dose administered over 15–20 min. The dose will vary depending on the type of antivenom, type of snake and number of bites; the use of 4–6 ampoules is not uncommon in severe envenomation.[148] Use of premedication before antivenom administration is controversial; at present the antivenom manufacturer does not recommend any premedication to reduce the chance of anaphylaxis. Regardless of whether a premedication is used, prepare to treat anaphylaxis.[127]

When the patient's condition has stabilised after the initial dose of antivenom, the pressure immobilisation bandage is removed, with continuous close observation for any clinical deterioration caused by the release of venom contained by the pressure bandage. If deterioration is evident, further antivenom and reapplication of the pressure immobilisation bandage may be required.[127] Patients without signs of deterioration still require ongoing observation in a high dependency unit/intensive care unit and repeat testing of coagulation at 3 and 6 hours post-antivenom administration should be done. Ongoing observation and pathology studies should occur for at least 24 hours.[148]

In children, management for snake bite is similar, with antivenom dosages the same as for an adult. Dilution volume can be reduced (from 1:10 to 1:5) for children.[145]

Box jellyfish envenomation

Chironex fleckeri (box jellyfish) is one of the world's most dangerous venomous animals.[153] The jellyfish is a cubic (box-shaped) bell measuring 20–30 cm across and weighing up to 6 kg and as it is transparent in water it can be difficult to identify. The tentacles are covered with millions of stinging nematocysts, each a spring-loaded capsule that contains a penetrating thread that discharges venom. Threads are 1 mm in length and capable of penetrating the dermis of adult skin. The tentacles also produce a sticky substance that promotes adherence to a victim's skin, causing some tentacles to be torn off and remain attached to the person, where the nematocysts remain active.[153]

Description and incidence

Most stings occur during the summer months (December, January) in the tropical waters of northern Australia, from Gladstone in Queensland around to Broome in Western Australia, on hot, calm and overcast days when the jellyfish moves from the open sea to chase prey in shallow water. The exact incidence of stings is difficult to determine, but they are common in children.[154] There have been more than 70 confirmed deaths from envenomation by *Chironex fleckeri* in northern Australia,[154] of which the last 12 were children.[155]

Clinical manifestations

Most stings are minor, with clinically significant stings occurring from larger jellyfish. Stings generally occur on the lower half of the body and are characterised by immediate and severe pain. Pain increases in severity and may cause victims, especially children, to become incoherent. While mechanisms of toxicity remain poorly understood, death is thought to occur from central respiratory failure, or cardiotoxicity leading to atrioventricular conduction disturbances or paralysis of cardiac muscle.[155] Victims may become unconscious before they can leave the water following envenomation, and death can occur within 5 min.[127]

Multiple linear lesions, which characteristically appear in a cross-hatched pattern, are seen on the area where tentacle contact occurs. A pattern of transverse bars is usually seen along the lesions, along with an intense acute inflammatory response, initially as a prompt and massive appearance of wheals, followed by oedema, erythema and vesicle formation, which can lead to partial- or full-thickness skin death.[154,155]

Assessment

Patients presenting to ED after potential box jellyfish sting are easily diagnosed based on the history, the presence of pain and their skin lesions as outlined above. Generally, some form of pre-hospital management or first aid will have been instituted. On arrival, patients with signs of clinically significant stings, alteration in consciousness, cardiovascular or respiratory function, or those with severe pain are seen immediately.

Management

Treatment focuses on appropriate first aid, administration of adequate pain relief, symptomatic management of cardiovascular and respiratory effects and the administration of box jellyfish antivenom when indicated. While Australian Resuscitation Council recommends that first aid measures include liberal application of vinegar to the sting area for 30–60 seconds, this is being questioned by researchers as not being well-evidenced,[155] with heat or ice application, depending on geographical location, a considered approach.[155,157] Vinegar inactivates the undischarged nematocysts, so removal of any remaining tentacles should occur prior to vinegar to prevent further envenomation.[156] Mild stings respond to the application of ice packs and simple oral analgesia, after the application of vinegar. Patients with moderate-to-severe pain require IV narcotic analgesia. For patients with continuing severe pain, antivenom is administered along with continued parenteral analgesia.[158]

Patients are observed for the development of cardiorespiratory symptoms, including arrhythmias. Management focuses on specific clinical effects, ranging from oxygen administration and IV fluid resuscitation through to intubation/mechanical ventilation or cardiopulmonary resuscitation.[153,158] Antivenom is indicated in patients with cardiorespiratory instability, cardiac arrest or severe pain unrelieved by narcotic analgesia. Antivenom is carried by pre-hospital personnel, and administration may occur prior to ED presentation. A 20,000-unit ampoule of box jellyfish antivenom is diluted in 100 mL normal saline and administered IV. over 20 min. The number of ampoules used varies with clinical status: at least one for cardiorespiratory instability; up to three for life-threatening situations with an inadequate response; and at least six for a cardiac arrest.[155]

While the application of a pressure immobilisation bandage to affected limbs after vinegar application was previously recommended as a first aid intervention, there is little current evidence supporting this in box jellyfish stings, and its application may promote additional venom release and therefore be potentially dangerous.[156] Some research has suggested a role for magnesium sulfate in management for patients not responding to antivenom[158] but practice is variable and not well supported with evidence.[156]

Irukandji envenomation

The Irukandji is a small marine jellyfish, with stinging tentacles capable of causing intense pain and catecholamine release.[153]

Description and incidence

Irukandji syndrome is a poorly-understood marine envenomation encountered in far northern and northwestern areas of Australia. Death is uncommon and attributed to cerebral haemorrhage and is associated with other comorbid conditions; however, Irukandji syndrome is a potentially life-threatening emergency and should be treated in a resuscitation environment.[155]

Assessment

People stung by an Irukandji may have no symptoms initially, and experience a latent time period, but may develop symptoms up to 1 hour after being stung.[153] Irukandji syndrome produces clinical features of severe lower back pain, muscle cramps; raised blood pressure, pulse; and respiratory compromise, vomiting and anxiety.[155] A patient with suspected Irukandji envenomation is placed in an acute area with full monitoring available.

Management

The mainstays of patient management are pain control and symptom management. Application of vinegar has been part of first aid treatment but, due to delay in the presentation of symptoms following a sting, this may be of limited value. Evidence is emerging indicating that washing the area with either fresh or salt water may also be effective. Pain is severe, and opioid analgesia may be required; if requirements for opioids are very high, fentanyl is considered.[155] There is anecdotal evidence that magnesium sulfate may have a role in the management of Irukandji syndrome not responsive to the above treatments, but this remains unproven.[159]

Ciguatera

Ciguatera is a type of seafood poisoning caused by the consumption of fish, especially certain tropical reef fish, which contain one or more naturally-occurring neurotoxins from the family of ciguatoxins. Ciguatera is reported as the most common form of seafood poisoning in the world, and is considered a mild non-fatal disease, affecting at least 50,000 people every year.[160] In Australia, there have been numerous outbreaks of ciguatera poisoning in many areas of the country including New South Wales.[161]

Ciguatera toxins (ciguatoxins) are among the deadliest poisons known.[162] These heat-stable toxins originate from a microorganism that attaches to certain species of

TABLE 23.16
Symptoms of ciguatera[162]

GASTROINTESTINAL	NEUROLOGICAL	CARDIOVASCULAR	OTHER SYMPTOMS
Abdominal pain	Paraesthesia in extremities and around the mouth, tingling, burning and pain	Bradycardia	Dermatitis
Nausea	Painful extremities	Tachycardia	Rash
Vomiting	Paradoxical temperature reversal where hot feels cold and cold feels hot	Hypotension	Arthralgia and myalgia
Diarrhoea	Temperature sensitivity	Hypertension	General weakness
	Vertigo	Arrhythmia	Salivation
	Dental pain where teeth feel loose		Dyspnoea
	Blurred vision		Neck stiffness
	Tremor		Headache
			Ataxia
			Sweating
			Metallic taste in the mouth

algae in tropical areas around the world; these toxins become altered after ingestion by progressively larger fish up the food chain.[162]

Clinical manifestations and diagnosis

Ciguatera poisoning typically presents as an acute gastrointestinal illness, followed by a neurological illness with classical symptoms of heat and cold reversal of sensation that may last for a few days after consumption of contaminated fish[160] (Table 23.16).

A patient may become sensitive to repeated exposure to ciguatoxins; additional exposure to poisoning from ciguatera may be more severe than the first episode. Importantly, patients exposed to ciguatera suffer recurrences following the consumption of seemingly innocuous foods (e.g. nuts, nut oils, caffeine, alcohol or animal protein foods), with relapses months or years after the initial poisoning.[162]

Diagnosis is made on a patient's history and clinical features: consumption of fish followed by an acute gastrointestinal and neurological illness. There is no conclusive diagnostic test for the presence of ciguatoxins.[162]

Management

Treatment of ciguatera poisoning is supportive care and symptom management. Mannitol is no longer recommended; therefore, IV fluids and analgesics are the mainstay of treatment, and avoidance of alcohol which is known to exacerbate symptoms is recommended.[158]

Scombroid fish poisoning

Scombroid poisoning is a form of food poisoning caused by the combination of inadequately cooled fish and the bacterial decomposition of the fish flesh resulting in a release of histamine.[158] The active component of scombrotoxin is histamine. The main groups of fish associated with this type of poisoning are the *Scombridae*, that is tuna and mackerels; however, other fish such as mahi-mahi have also been known to have illness-causing potential. Scombrotoxin is not inactivated by the cooking process.[163]

Clinical manifestations and diagnosis

People normally start feeling unwell in about 30 min after eating fish affected with scombrotoxin, with flushing, development of a rash and urticaria. This may be followed by more profound symptoms such as tachycardia, pounding headaches, difficulty breathing and collapse due to hypotension.[163] Only one death has been recorded from scombroid fish poisoning.[163]

Management

The mainstays of treatment are controlling the histamine reaction with antihistamines and supportive nursing care for symptoms. Histamine-2 receptor blockers have been shown to be useful for up to 24 hours following the development of symptoms. This prolonged treatment allows the scombrotoxin to be eliminated from the patient's system.[163] In rare cases if symptoms are severe and resistant to antihistamines, drugs such as IMI adrenaline and low-dose pressors may play a role in management.[163]

Drowning

Description and incidence

Drowning is the process of experiencing respiratory impairment due to submersion or immersion in a liquid. Near-drowning is now an obsolete term.[164] Submersion incidents are often preventable events associated with significant mortality and morbidity in both adults and children, usually necessitating an ED presentation and subsequent hospital admission. Worldwide, there are an estimated 360,000 drowning deaths annually with children, males and those with increased access to water most at risk.[165] The location of drowning varies from country to country. In the USA, artificial pools and natural bodies of freshwater were common drowning locations, particularly for children.[166] In Australia, drowning often occurred in private pools, lakes and surf beaches.[167] In Uganda, lakes and rivers were common sites, particularly for young males.[168] A bimodal distribution of deaths is seen in children, with a peak in the toddler age group (0–4 years) and a second peak in young adolescent males (15–19 years).[169,170]

It is estimated that, for every drowning death, there are 4–5 near-drowning hospital admissions and 14 ED presentations.[167,169] Near-drowning is also associated with high-impact injuries, especially boating or personal watercraft incidents and shallow-diving-related injuries. Associated cervical spine injury is seen in 0.5% of near-drowning cases.[171]

Clinical manifestations

The sequence of events in drowning has been identified primarily by animal studies, highlighting an initial phase of panic struggling, some swimming movements and sometimes a surprise inhalation. There may be aspiration of small amounts of water at this time that produces laryngospasm for a short period. Apnoea and breath-holding occur during submersion and are often followed by variable amount of aspiration of fluid, followed by apnoea. This leads to severe hypoxia, loss of consciousness and disappearance of airway reflexes, resulting in further water moving into the lungs prior to death.[171,172]

Approximately 80–90% of submersion victims aspirate water into the lungs due to loss of airway reflexes and laryngospasm. Approximately 10–15% of victims have sustained laryngospasm, and no detectable amount of water will be aspirated, with the resulting injury secondary to anoxia. The terms 'dry' vs 'wet' drowning have been discarded at the World Congress on Drowning.[169,172] Preexisting medical conditions predispose a person to drowning and should be considered during management, including seizures, arrhythmia (especially torsades de pointes associated with long Q-T interval), coronary artery disease, depression, cardiomyopathy (dilated or hypertrophic obstructive), hypoglycaemia, hypothermia, intoxication or trauma.[173]

Pulmonary manifestations after aspiration of fresh or salt water differ, as fresh water is hypotonic and when aspirated moves quickly into the microcirculation across the alveolar–capillary membrane. With fresh water aspiration, surfactant is destroyed, producing alveolar instability, atelectasis and decreased lung compliance and resulting in marked ventilation/perfusion mismatching.[169] In contrast, salt water has 3–4 times the osmolality of blood and, when aspirated, draws damaging protein-rich fluid from the plasma into the alveoli, resulting in both interstitial and alveoli oedema, with associated bronchospasm and subsequent shunting and ventilation/perfusion mismatch.[174]

Despite these different physiological effects from aspirated fresh and salt water, the resulting clinical manifestation is the same: profound hypoxaemia secondary

FIGURE 23.2 Pathophysiology of respiratory failure due to fluid aspiration.[174]

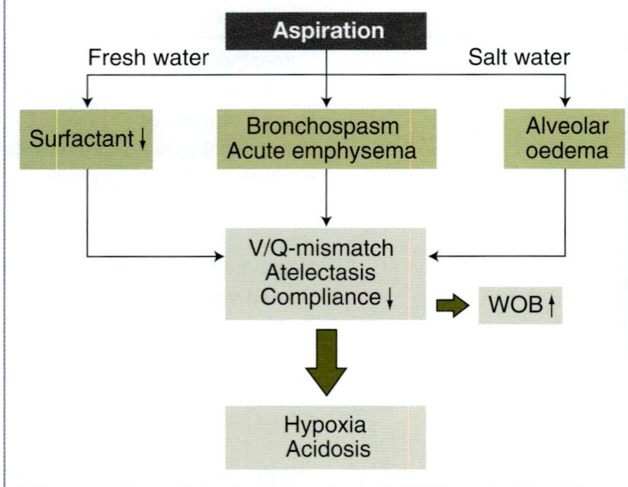

V/Q-mismatch, ventilation/perfusion mismatch; WOB, work of breathing.

to ventilation/perfusion mismatch with intrapulmonary shunting (Fig. 23.2).[174] Patients with evidence of fluid aspiration often progress to develop severe acute respiratory distress syndrome within a very short time.[169] No significant effects on electrolytes are noted in humans, as rarely more than 10 mL/kg and commonly no more than 4 mL/kg of water is aspirated, while clinically significant electrolyte disturbances occur when over 22 mL/kg has been aspirated.[174]

Cardiovascular effects are influenced by the extent and duration of hypoxia, derangement of acid–base status, the magnitude of the stress response and hypothermia.[171] Ventricular arrhythmias and asystole may result from hypoxaemia and metabolic acidosis. Acute hypoxia results in release of pulmonary inflammatory mediators, which increase right ventricular afterload and decrease contractility.[174] Hypotension is commonly seen due to volume depletion secondary to pulmonary oedema, intracompartmental fluid shifts and myocardial dysfunction.[171]

Severe hypoxic and ischaemic injury is the most important factor related to outcome and subsequent quality of life. Other factors influencing the extent of injury include water temperature and submersion time, stress during submersion and co-existing cardiovascular and neurological disease.[174,175,] Prediction of death or persistent vegetative state in the immediate period after near-drowning is difficult. Patients awake or with only blunted consciousness on presentation usually survive without neurological sequelae. A third of patients admitted in coma or after cardiopulmonary resuscitation will survive neurologically intact or with only minor deficits, while the remaining two-thirds of patients will either die or remain in a vegetative state.[171]

Hypothermia is a well-documented feature in submersion victims.[172] Incidents of submersion times of greater than 15 min where victims recovered with a good neurological outcome all occurred in very cold water (<10°C). While the exact mechanisms in these outcomes are unclear, acute cold submersion hypothermia may be protective against cerebral insult by: very rapid cooling in victims with low levels of subcutaneous fat who have aspirated a large amount of very cold water; induced muscle paralysis leading to minimal struggling and very little oxygen depletion; and the heart gradually slowing to asystole in the presence of profound hypothermia.[174,175] In these cases prolonged resuscitative efforts may be warranted, including active and aggressive re-warming interventions, that should not be abandoned until the patient has been re-warmed to at least 30°C.[174]

Assessment

Continuously monitor heart rate, blood pressure and oxygen saturation, and assess neurological status, including any seizure activity. Deterioration is evident with a falling level of consciousness, a high alveolar–arterial gradient, respiratory failure evidenced by a partial pressure of carbon dioxide in the arterial blood >45 mmHg or worsening blood gas results.[174] Caution should be taken to avoid activities that may cause a rise in intracranial pressure. A 12-lead ECG identifies any arrhythmias that result from acidosis and hypoxia rather than electrolyte abnormalities. The patient should be managed conventionally (see Chapter 11).[174] All patients require serial CXR, as lung fields often worsen in the first few hours. In clinically significant submersions, the CXR will typically show bilateral infiltrates undifferentiated from other causes of pulmonary oedema.

Management

The condition of the patient, the environment and the skill of the attending rescue personnel will influence pre-hospital management of the post-submersion patient, and the adequacy of initial basic life support at the scene is the most important determinant of outcome.[176] The Heimlich manoeuvre should not be performed in an attempt to remove aspirated water, as it is ineffective and likely to promote aspiration of gastric contents. Supplemental oxygen 100% is administered as soon as possible.[175]

For patients presenting to the ED in cardiac arrest, active resuscitation measures continue (see Chapter 25), although the need for continued cardiopulmonary resuscitation is generally associated with a poor neurological outcome; however, patients experiencing submersions in very cold water may have a better outcome.[176] The focus of management for patients with spontaneous circulation includes respiratory support and the correction of hypoxia, neurological assessment and maintenance of optimal cerebral perfusion, cardiovascular support and maintenance of haemodynamic stability, correction of hypothermia and management of other associated injuries.

All patients require 100% supplemental oxygen via a non-rebreathing mask initially, unless mechanical ventilation is required. Indications for endotracheal intubation include inability to maintain own airway, PaO_2<60 mmHg or SpO_2 <90% despite high flow oxygen, PCO_2 >50 mmHg.[177] Patients without any respiratory symptoms should be observed for 6–12 hours, until there is a normal CXR, no signs of respiratory distress and normal oxygen saturation on room air.[175] Alert patients unable to maintain adequate oxygenation should be considered for continuous positive airway pressure or bi-level positive airway pressure prior to intubation provided they are able to maintain their own airway, with its effect on circulation monitored closely (see Chapter 15).

While cerebral oedema and intracranial hypertension is often seen in hypoxic neuronal injury, only general supportive measures are recommended as there is insufficient evidence to indicate that invasive intracranial pressure monitoring and related management improve outcomes.[175] Any seizures should be promptly treated with appropriate measures (see Chapter 17). Acute respiratory distress syndrome should be managed with non-invasive ventilation if possible.[172] Barbiturate-induced coma or corticosteroids are not recommended as there is no evidence of improvement in outcome.[178]

Cardiovascular support may require a multifaceted approach, initially by improving hypoxia and correcting circulating volume. Hypotensive patients require rapid volume expansion (crystalloid or colloid) and an indwelling catheter for hourly urine measurement. Patients with persistent cardiovascular compromise may require inotropic support in conjunction with invasive haemodynamic monitoring.[175]

Patients presenting with associated high-impact or shallow-diving mechanisms should have cervical spine immobilisation instituted with the application of a rigid cervical collar, especially for complaints of neck pain or an altered level of consciousness (see Chapter 17). The management of hypothermia and re-warming methods outlined below are appropriate for the management of near-drowning.

Hypothermia

Description and incidence

Hypothermia is a core body temperature that is lower than 35°C and occurs with exposure to low ambient temperatures that are influenced by low environmental temperatures, humidity, wind velocity, extended exposure time or cold water immersion.[179] Cold injury is a common occurrence in those climates with cooler ambient conditions; however, when body heat is lower than the surrounding environmental conditions, it can easily develop so it is not an uncommon problem in Australia and New Zealand, despite the relatively warm weather zones in the former. The very young and very

TABLE 23.17
Physiological effects of hypothermia[179,180,183]

	DEGREE OF HYPOTHERMIA		
Physiological effects	Mild (32–35°C)	Moderate (28–32°C)	Severe (<28°C)
General metabolic	Shivering Raised oxygen consumption Hyperkalaemia	Raised oxygen consumption Acidosis	Normal metabolic functions fail
Cardiac	Vasoconstriction Tachycardia Increased cardiac output	Atrial arrhythmias Bradycardia	Ventricular arrhythmias Decreased cardiac output
Respiratory	Tachypnoea Bronchospasm	Decreased respiratory drive	Apnoea
Neurological	Confusion Hyperreflexia	Lowered level of consciousness Hyporeflexia	Coma Absent reflexes
Coagulation	Platelet dysfunction Impaired clotting enzyme function Increased blood viscosity	Increased haematocrit	Lower bleeding times due to failure of clotting systems

old are most susceptible to injury.[180] A normal core temperature of 37°C has a variation of 1–2°C. Temperature maintenance is essential for normal homeostatic functioning, and normal adaptive mechanisms can respond to reductions in ambient temperature.

Clinical manifestations

When skin temperature is reduced after exposure to the cold, sympathetic stimulation occurs causing peripheral vasoconstriction, decreased skin circulation and shunting of blood centrally to vital organs. Blood pressure, heart rate and respiratory rate rise, and shivering (involuntary clonic movements of skeletal muscle) stimulates metabolic activity to produce heat and blood flow to striated muscles to maintain a normal core temperature. If continued exposure to cold occurs these compensatory functions fail, and hypothermia results.[180]

Ambient temperatures need not be particularly low, as other contributing factors such as wind or a person having wet clothing may be significant. A patient with a decreased level of consciousness may present with hypothermia after lying on a cool surface. As a person's core temperature drops, progressive cardiac abnormalities occur; normal sinus rhythm may progress to sinus bradycardia, T-wave inversion, prolonged P–R and Q–T intervals, atrial fibrillation and ventricular fibrillation. A QRS abnormality, the Osborn wave, represented by a positive deflection at the junction of the QRS and ST segments, is frequently described as being characteristic of cold injury.[181]

Metabolic acidosis and blood-clotting abnormalities are common, as well as hypoglycaemia, which occurs because of depletion of glycogen stores caused by excessive shivering. Hyperglycaemia can be present because of inhibition of insulin action due to the lowered temperature.[180] The physiological alterations that accompany lowering of core temperature to below 30°C are summarised in Table 23.17.[179,182,183]

Management

A patient with severe hypothermia may appear dead: cold, pale, stiff, with no response to external stimulation. Successful resuscitation of patients has occurred at temperatures as low as 17°C, due to the low body temperature protecting vital organs from hypoxic injury.[184] This is reflected in the anecdotal phrase, 'patients are not dead until they are warm and dead'; however, core temperature of <15°C of K+ >12 mmol/L is considered unsalvageable.[180] In most cases resuscitation should continue until the patient's core temperature reaches 32°C.[180]

Practice tip

Removing wet clothing and drying the patient is an extremely important first aid measure for a cold wet patient to prevent further cooling.

Passive external re-warming (PER) is the preferred treatment in patients with mild hypothermia (32–35°C). In PER, wet clothing is removed, then the patient covered with blankets or other forms of insulation, producing a reduction in heat loss, and allowing the patient's intrinsic heat production to re-warm.

Active external warming is indicated for moderate-to-severe hypothermia (32–28°C). Shunting of cold peripheral blood to the core may lead to further chilling of the myocardium and ventricular fibrillation;[179] therefore, re-warming of the trunk should be commenced before the extremities to minimise core temperature afterdrop with associated acidemia and hypotension related to arterial vasodilation.[185] External warming using warm blankets, forced warm air blankets and heat packs in contact with the patient's body should raise body temperature by approximately 2.5°C per hour.[179] Inhalation re-warming with oxygen warmed to 42–46°C is also effective, as around 10% of metabolic heat is lost through the respiratory tract.[182]

If a patient's core temperature is <28°C, 'core re-warming' is indicated. This approach is favoured, as experimental evidence indicates that return to normal cardiovascular function is more rapid with temperature rises of up to 7.5°C per hour.[179] A number of invasive internal warming options are available, including peritoneal lavage, although the most effective of all internal methods is cardiopulmonary bypass, as it transfers heat at a rate several times faster than any other methods available, that being approximately 7.5°C per hour. While the technique is efficient, it is obviously more invasive and carries associated risks, and so is reserved for profoundly hypothermic patients.[180]

Practice tip

Always measure the blood glucose of hypothermic patients to exclude hypoglycaemia as a reason for an altered conscious state.

Hyperthermia and heat illness

Description and incidence

Potentially one of the more significant environmental fears expressed by many scientists is the issue of climate change and the consequence of heat-related illness worldwide. Global warming and events such as recurrent prolonged hot weather days have recently caused numerous deaths through Europe, the USA and Australia, and scientists are predicting the events will become more common. Heat-related illness is common in Australia and represents a significant public health risk, although there are only limited deaths compared to what has happened in the USA and Europe.[186]

Heat-related illness can affect any age group; however, it is the very young, because of their larger surface area, reduced sweating capacity and inability to access their own fluids, and the older person, who may have fluid restrictions because of other health reasons or are taking medications that affect their capacity to sweat, and a tendency to layer clothing, who are at the highest risk. The other vulnerable group is those in the younger age bracket undertaking physical activity during hot weather periods, whether because of work or sports.[186]

Alterations in thermoregulatory function cause varying degrees of heat illness, categorised as three types: heat cramps, heat exhaustion and heat stroke.[180] Excessive exposure to heat substantially increases fluid and electrolyte losses from the body.[186] The loss of both fluids and electrolytes in addition to impaired organ function leads to the complications of heat illnesses. Factors contributing to heat illness include elevated ambient temperature, increased heat production due to exercise, infection and drugs such as amphetamines, phenothiazines or other stimulants.[180]

Clinical manifestations

Environmental heat illness is more likely to develop when the ambient temperature exceeds 32–35°C and the humidity is greater than 70%.[186] Assessment of the patient's physical state and vital signs including GCS provides some evidence of hypovolaemia and potential or impending shock.

Heat exhaustion is a more severe form of heat illness and is associated with severe water or salt depletion due to excessive sweating; the patient's temperature may range between normal and below 40°C.[186] Combined water and salt losses cause muscle cramps, nausea and vomiting, headache, dizziness, weakness, fainting, thirst, tachycardia, hypotension and profuse sweating, but with normal neurological function.

Heat stroke is the most severe and serious form of heat-related illness, with temperatures above 41°C and impaired neurological function. Heat stroke is a profound disturbance of the body's heat-regulating ability, and is often referred to as 'sunstroke', although it relates to the body's inability to dissipate heat, loss of sweat function and severe dehydration rather than actual sun exposure.[180]

Management

Initial management of the hyperthermic patient focuses on airway, breathing and circulation, correction of urgent physiological states such as hypoxia, severe potassium imbalances and acidosis. A heat-stressed patient can have large fluid losses and require prompt fluid resuscitation, preferably isotonic sodium chloride solution. Total water deficit should be corrected slowly; half of the deficit is administered in the first 3–6 hours, with the remainder over the next 6–9 hours.[179]

Rapid cooling is the second priority: lowering core temperature to less than 38.9°C within 30 min improves survival and minimises end-organ damage.[179] Non-invasive external methods of cooling include removal of clothing and covering the patient with a wet, tepid sheet. Ice packs can be placed next to the patient's axillae, neck and groin. Invasive cooling measures such as iced gastric lavage and cardiopulmonary bypass are reserved for the patient who fails to respond to conventional cooling methods.[179] Core body temperature should be monitored using a continuous rectal or tympanic probe.

Multiple patient triage/disaster

Disaster triage is a process designed to provide the greatest benefit to multiple patients when treatment resources and facilities are limited. Disaster triage systems differ from the routine triage system used within the ED (e.g. the ATS, MTS): system care is focused on those victims who may survive with proper therapy, rather than on those who have no chance of survival or who will live without treatment. The system was first devised during war as a method of managing large numbers of battlefield casualties. Today it is applicable for treating multiple victims of illness or injury outside and within the hospital setting. Variations exist between states and countries regarding disaster victim triage classifications. It is therefore important to be familiar with local plans and policy.

Triage of mass victims may be necessary in common situations, for example vehicle collisions with multiple occupants, as well as other large-scale disasters, such as earthquakes, floods, bushfires, damaging storms, public transport incidents or explosions. The principles of triage vary little, though the methods used to communicate triage information and to match victims with available resources may differ. Triage at the scene of a major incident or disaster is commenced by the first qualified person to arrive, most commonly an ambulance officer of the first responding team. This person is initially responsible for performing immediate primary surveys on all victims and for determining and communicating the numbers and types of resources needed to provide initial care and transport.[187]

In Australia, New Zealand, the UK and the USA, disaster systems have up to five triage categories (depending on jurisdictional and local protocols), usually with corresponding colours. Despite slight variation, the aim is similar: to provide the best level of care and ensure the highest number of survivors. Those who are mortally injured but alive may be given a low treatment priority, though this will almost certainly ensure their death. These decisions are therefore best made by an experienced doctor. In a situation with a large number of casualties, one or more doctors should be present at the site to lead the triage effort. Further, it is not within the scope of practice of non-physician emergency personnel to pronounce a patient dead, but properly trained ambulance or rescue personnel can recognise the signs of death for the purposes of triage until doctors can formally declare death.[188]

Emergency department response to an external disaster: receiving patients

Disasters may produce mass victims on a scale that means routine processes and practices in the ED and hospital will be overwhelmed. The ED response to an external disaster forms part of the overall hospital response, outlined in a hospital disaster plan. The ED response plans also sit within the larger context of other health disciplines where there is a consideration of the prevention of, preparedness for, response to and recovery from the health problems arising from a disaster.[189] These plans are reviewed regularly for currency and practised for preparedness. The following aspects form part of ED planning and response to receiving patients from an external disaster.

Department preparation

If the disaster site is close to the hospital, a significant number of disaster victims will self-evacuate from the site and arrive at the hospital without any pre-hospital triage, treatment or decontamination before any formal notification has been received. In this instance the ED will need to declare the incident and commence the notification process required.[189] The ED may be quickly overwhelmed with arriving patients; the closest local medical facility may receive up to 50–80% of the disaster victims within 90 minutes of the incident.[65] On notification of a disaster response a number of key positions should be allocated (medical coordinator, nursing coordinator, triage nurse, medical triage officer). These personnel are senior staff with specific disaster training and knowledge of the hospital's disaster plan.[189] Nursing and medical coordinators are responsible for allocating staff to specific duties; all designated roles are outlined on action cards available for staff to read prior to commencing their roles.

The capacity of the ED to accommodate a large influx of patients needs to be maximised. Patients currently in the department are reviewed for a decision to admit. Patients requiring admission are transferred out of the department to a suitable location in the hospital. Patients suitable for discharge or referral to their local medical officer, including patients with minor complaints currently waiting, should be discharged or referred to community resources. A small number of patients may need to remain in the ED, and their care will need to be prioritised in conjunction with arriving disaster victims.[189]

Areas of the department are designated to accommodate the expected severity of the victims (e.g. resuscitation room for priority 1 patients, observation areas for priority 2). Walking wounded casualties with relatively minor injuries and who are unlikely to require admission to hospital are best accommodated in a treatment area outside the ED, as this reduces congestion and increases the capacity for more significantly-injured victims to be managed.[187]

Additional staff members are notified from the current staff lists to participate in the disaster management. Staff members are allocated to teams to manage bed spaces within designated treatment areas. Additional staff from outside the ED may be deployed to assist; these staff should be teamed with routine ED staff because of their familiarity with the layout and location of equipment and other resources. It is important to recognise the need to replace staff to avoid fatigue, especially in incidents of a protracted nature. Therefore, not all staff should be called in initially. Where possible, staff who usually work together on a daily basis should work in teams during the disaster period.[187,189]

Triage and reception

Routine, day-to-day triage and reception processes will be ineffective when receiving large numbers of disaster victims. A registration process for disaster victims generally involves collecting minimal personal information from the patients, where possible, and the allocation of a prepared disaster hospital number used for identification and ordering investigations. Triage assessments will often be undertaken by both a medical officer and a nurse, and the process will be brief and focused. Most victims will have been allocated a triage tag in the field, but are reevaluated for any changes, as their condition may have deteriorated. Triage assessment is based on observations of the nature and extent of the victims' injuries.[187] Patients present in the ED prior to disaster notification are considered part of the disaster event and triaged in the same manner.

Treatment

Treatment provided during a disaster will not reflect routine practices; priorities focus on resuscitation, identification of serious injuries, identification of patients requiring urgent surgery and stabilisation of patients for transfer out of the ED. The best overall outcomes during a disaster are achieved when the routine principles of resuscitation and management are adapted to reflect the resources available.[187]

Transfer from the ED

Patients are triaged, stabilised and transferred out to the operating theatre or other clinical areas as soon as possible using designated transfer staff and a coordinated process outlined in the hospital plan. This will maintain the effectiveness and efficiency of the department as victims continue to arrive. During and after the incident, opportunity for staff to debrief is an important aspect to manage staff psychosocial wellbeing.[186]

Chemical, biological and radiological events

Since the Japanese doomsday cult Aum Shinrikyo released sarin nerve gas on the Tokyo subway in March 1995, killing 12 people, terrorist incidents and hoaxes involving toxic or infectious agents have been on the rise. The ease of obtaining non-nuclear radioactive material may mean that 'dirty bombs'[190] are more likely to be used as an explosive device. The availability and the impact of chemical and biological threat materials are both relatively high, with potentially devastating impact.[191] Because biological and chemical agents are so dissimilar, each category will be dealt with separately but there are common elements or characteristics.

Chemical agents

Chemical agents are supertoxic chemicals used for the purpose of poisoning victims. They are similar to hazardous industrial chemicals, but hundreds of times more toxic. For example, the 1995 sarin attack in Tokyo caused 1039 injuries and at least 4000 people with psychogenic symptoms.[191] Sarin is approximately 60 times more toxic than methylisocyanate. To put this in perspective, a leak of methylisocyanate from a factory in Bhopal, India, in 1984 caused 200,000 people to be affected: 10,000 severely affected and 3300 deaths.[192] Relatively small quantities of a military grade chemical agent could have the same capability to produce large numbers of casualties (symptomatic and psychological).[191]

Table 23.18 provides a summary of the more common chemical agents, their effects, clinical presentations and treatments. It needs to be stressed that specialised personal protective equipment (PPE) and specialist training are required to manage these situations.[193,194,195]

Biological agents

The use of biological weapons is not a recent concept. Biological agents have the longest history of use, dating back to the 14th century.[195] Biological agents are living organisms or toxins that have the capacity to cause disease in people, animals or crops. Toxins are a special type of poisonous chemical categorised as biological agents because they were created by living organisms. They generally behave like chemical agents and serve the same function: to poison people.

Biological agents are relatively inexpensive to produce and have the potential to be devastating in their effects. Organisms such as anthrax, plague and smallpox have been the agents of greatest concern from a potential terrorist use perspective.[194] Table 23.19 presents an outline of biological agents, clinical presentations and treatments.[191,194,195]

Radiological agents

Radiological materials can pose both an acute and long-term hazard to humans. In many ways, they behave like some of the chemical agents in that they cause cellular damage. A major difference is that radiological agents do not necessarily have to be inhaled or come into contact with the skin to do damage.[190]

The deployment of a nuclear weapon would be catastrophic, as evidenced by events such as that in Hiroshima or industrial accidents as occurred at Chernobyl. While very different, both events produced immediate injury and had long-term effects of ionising radiation on large populations. The event of highest risk is likely to

TABLE 23.18
Summary of common chemical agents, effects, clinical presentations and treatments[194,195]

TYPE OF CHEMICAL	EFFECT	EXAMPLE	CLINICAL PRESENTATION	ANTIDOTES/TREATMENT
Nerve agent	Inhibits the activation of acetylcholinesterase	Sarin VX Soman Tabun	Muscarinic and nicotinic signs	Atropine 2-Pyridine aldoxime methyl chloride Benzodiazepines
Blood agents	Binds with cytochrome oxidase, causing hypoxia	Cyanide	Hypoxia	Cyanide kit Sodium nitrite Sodium thiosulfate
Vesicants	Chemical burns	Mustard gas Lewisite	Burns and blisters	Decontamination with soap and water
Pulmonary agents	Irritation to the respiratory tract	Chlorine phosgene	Respiratory distress Pulmonary oedema	Oxygen

TABLE 23.19
Summary of biological agents, clinical presentations and treatments[191,194,196]

BIOLOGICAL GROUP	EXAMPLE	CLINICAL PRESENTATION	TREATMENT
Virus	Smallpox (variola)		Supportive care
Bacteria	Anthrax (*Bacillus anthracis*) Plague (*Yersinia pestis*)	Inhalational • Respiratory failure • Widened mediastinum • Severe sepsis	Antibiotics
		Pneumonic plague • Respiratory failure • Haemoptysis • Painful lymph nodes	Antibiotics
Toxin	Botulism (*Clostridium botulinum*)		Supportive care Botulism immune globulin

be a ‘dirty bomb’ that combines conventional explosives with any available radioactive source.[194]

Psychological effects

A chemical, biological or radiological terrorism incident may or may not result in mass casualties and fatalities as intended. However, large numbers of psychological casualties are very likely and, therefore, regardless of the effectiveness of the attack and number of people actually exposed to the agent, there will most likely be a mass casualty situation. The psychological implications of chemical and biological weapons may be worse than the physical ones. Chemical and biological weapons are weapons of terror; part of their purpose is to wreak destruction via psychological means by inducing fear, confusion and uncertainty in everyday life. The long-term social and psychological effects of an episode of chemical or biological attack, real or suspected, would be as damaging as the acute ones, if not more so.[197]

Major challenges for chemical, biological or radiological responders

A well-delivered chemical or biological event would be catastrophic and exposure for emergency workers likely, as occurred previously when 110 staff developed signs and symptoms of exposure following the 1995 sarin attack in Tokyo.[198]

To protect staff, there must be clear procedures for dealing with potentially exposed or contaminated patients. This begins with proper assessment of a patient in need of isolation or decontamination and includes understanding of what PPE is appropriate and the capability of staff to effectively use the PPE. Emergency personnel must also have immediate access to the PPE that they need to limit their risk of exposure. However, the issue is complex: advanced levels of PPE require training and special skills to be used safely. Decontamination of patients with chemical exposure is a high-risk activity for untrained staff.[198]

Summary

An overview of important emergency systems and processes, outlining the practice of initial assessment and prioritisation of patients presenting to the ED through the unique nursing process of triage has been provided in this chapter. The role of the emergency nurse in the initial assessment, intervention and management of the patient has been described. The initial ED management of common emergency presentations was outlined, reflecting current practice and based on the latest available evidence.

The emergency environment is dynamic, and it was beyond the scope of this chapter to describe the full extent of emergency nursing practice and the clinical entities that are frequently managed. It is therefore important for a critical care nurse to be familiar with the content provided in the other chapters in this text, as well as other resources. As noted at the beginning of this chapter, other common presentations to the ED, such as trauma and cardiorespiratory arrest, are described in Chapters 24 and 25.

Emergency nursing is a demanding specialty area of practice, as are all areas of specialty practice. The challenges with emergency nursing come with the volumes of predicable patient groups, changing demographics in our community and the unpredictable or unusual presentations and volume of presentations. Emergency nurses need to prepare themselves with a broad knowledge base, adaptability to change and resilience to meet these demands.

Case study

18 MARCH 2018

1600 h: Patient Steven Turner, a 35-year-old male, was referred to the emergency department (ED) by his local doctor for management of possible early appendicitis. At triage, he did not appear to be distressed, and reported an onset of generalised abdominal pain the day before. There was no compromise to ABCD, and his vital signs were within normal parameters. He was allocated an ATS category 4 (to be seen within 1 h) and placed in the Reception area while awaiting assessment.

1630 h: While awaiting initial assessment by the treating doctor, a registered nurse (RN) initiated relevant investigations and analgesia. Early acquisition of relevant investigations means that information necessary to make a treatment or diagnostic decision will be at hand at the earliest possible time. The RN inserted a peripheral venous catheter, and gained bloods for full blood count, liver function tests, electrolytes, urea and creatinine, lipase. He also gained a urine sample to complete urinalysis, and initiated paracetamol 1 g for analgesia.

1715 h: Steven was reviewed by a doctor. On clinical exam, he had mild nausea, his abdomen was soft. There was no evidence of guarding, some mild peri-umbilical pain and no renal angle or right iliac fossa tenderness. McBurney's and Rovsing signs were negative. Visual examination did not reveal evidence of hernia or any scars from previous abdominal surgeries. He did not have nausea or vomiting, and his bowel actions were normal; there was no bleeding per rectum. His white cell count was 12×10^9/L; other bloods and urinalysis were unremarkable.

After review by an Emergency Consultant, a decision was made to not conduct a CT scan due to age and lack of overt clinical signs. It was explained to the patient that the pain may be due to an early appendicitis; however, other differential diagnoses include gastroenteritis, mesenteric adenitis or intestinal colic. The most prudent course recommended was to watch and wait. It was confirmed that Steven had support at home, and someone who could transport him easily back to the ED if necessary. A repeat set of vital signs were taken that confirmed that blood pressure, pulse, respiratory rate and temperature were within normal parameters. The patient was discharged home with explanations of signs and symptoms of concern that would require him to return to the ED.

19 MARCH 2018

1045 h: Steven Turner re-presented to triage the next morning with deterioration of abdominal pain overnight. Steven indicated to the triage nurse that the pain was worse in right lower abdomen, and any movement of his abdomen increased the pain sharply. In triage he was alert and interacting, talking in full sentences with a strong radial pulse. He was allocated an ATS category 3, to be seen within 30 min, and a non-monitored bed requested from the Nurse Unit Manager for ongoing management of the patient.

1055 h: On reaching a bed, the RN responsible for Steven's ongoing care obtained a full set of vital signs. Steven's blood pressure was 125/75 mmHg, heart rate 110 beats/min, respiratory rate 18 breaths/min, SaO_2 98% on room air, and temperature was 37.8°C.

An intravenous catheter was inserted and bloods taken for electrolytes, renal function and full blood count.

The patient stated his pain rated 8/10. The RN initiated analgesia of oxycodone 5 mg and paracetamol 1 g, and advised the patient to remain nil by mouth while waiting to be seen by either the treating doctor or nurse practitioner.

1100 h: A history and physical assessment were completed by the treating doctor. Steven described that initially the pain was generalised/central abdomen and as it deteriorated, the pain localised to his right lower abdomen. He had not felt like eating overnight and now also had nausea. On assessment, the doctor found a positive McBurney's sign, and positive Rovsing sign with rebound tenderness.

The treating doctor made a working diagnosis of appendicitis and referred the patient to the surgical registrar for review.

1230 h: The patient was still awaiting surgical review. Steven notified his nurse that his pain had worsened. On review by the RN, a deterioration in vital signs was also noted; his blood pressure was 95/50 mmHg, heart rate 130 beats/min, respiratory rate 24 breaths/min, SaO_2 98% on room air, and temperature 38.8°C.

On repeat abdominal exam, the RN found Steven to have a rigid abdomen. His deteriorating condition was escalated to the Nurse Unit Manager and senior doctor for urgent review, and the patient was moved to a resuscitation bay for closer observation.

On review by the senior doctor, the following interventions were commenced:

- A second intravascular catheter was inserted
- A fluid challenge was commenced
- IV antibiotics were commenced
- Additional investigations including a venous blood gas, blood culture, group and hold were done.

His previous blood work was reviewed and showed a white blood cell count of 18×10^9/L; renal function was normal. A request was made for urgent surgical review for acute abdomen, and possible ruptured appendix.

1300 h: Steven responded to fluid bolus with repeat vital signs and his blood pressure was now 110/75 mmHg, heart rate 110 beats/min, respiratory rate 18 breaths/min, SaO_2 98% on room air. He was considered stable enough to undergo an urgent CT of the abdomen which identified a ruptured appendix with free fluid in abdomen.

Steven was taken to the operating theatre where he had a laparoscopic appendectomy and then was transferred to the ward for ongoing IV antibiotics and observation for development of peritonitis or abscess.

CASE STUDY QUESTIONS

1. Steven presents twice to the ED with a presenting complaint of abdominal pain. What features influenced the triage nurse to allocate a different triage category for the second presentation?
2. On Steven's initial presentation, he is sent home without having definitive imaging via a CT abdomen that could possibly have identified a diagnosis of appendicitis. Why did the treating consultant decide against a CT abdomen on his first visit to the ED?
3. During management of the same disease process, Steven is at different times managed in three different areas of the ED. Why is this?
4. During Steven's second presentation, he clinically deteriorates. What are clinical manifestations of severe sepsis and septic shock that he exhibited?
5. An intravenous fluid bolus and targeted antibiotics are administered. What do each of these interventions seek to achieve?
6. Why was an urgent abdominal CT not undertaken until Steven's vital signs had improved?

RESEARCH VIGNETTE

Twibell R, Siela D, Riwitis C, Neal A. A qualitative study of factors in nurses' and physicians' decision-making related to family presence during resuscitation. J Clin Nurs 2018; 27: e320-e334

Background: Regardless of the expanding practice of family presence during resuscitation, clinicians continue to examine and debate the practice. Family presence during resuscitation is a decision made on a case by case basis as many organisations do not have a policy about this practice. While there is research into this topic, there is little clarity about the factors that influence this decision-making by clinicians.

Objectives: The aim of the study was to investigate the concurrence between factors that influence physicians' and nurses' decision making for family presence during resuscitation.

Design: Qualitative exploratory-descriptive

Setting: The study was conducted in one 350-bed Midwestern hospital in the USA.

Participants: Physicians and nurses from diverse care areas (internal medicine, emergency, surgical, critical care, family practice).

Methods: Participants responded to three set questions in writing, anonymously at set collection points in the hospital. Possible participant pool included 750 nurses, and 300 physicians.

Results: Responses were received from 325 nurses and 193 physicians. This included 328 written responses from nurses and 310 from physicians (some questions were not answered by all participants). From nursing data five themes were elicited: Trauma to the family, Family benefits, Family may disrupt, Responding to negative emotions of family, Making family presence decisions is hard. Nurses decisions were informed by how likely the family was to be traumatised from the resuscitation, the potential for disruption during the resuscitation by family members, and possible benefits to families for being included. From the physician data, five themes were also elicited: Families may disrupt, Families lack understanding, Traumatising nature of the resuscitation, Patient preference, Family benefits. The physician group's highest weighted factors included the possibility of family members compromising patient care due to disruption during resuscitation, and then the family's knowledge about resuscitations.

Conclusions: While there was some agreement on factors when deciding to include or exclude family from resuscitation, differences were about the focus of each discipline. Physician focus was on the patient primarily while nurses focused on the patient, family and resuscitation team.

Critique

This paper described the factors associated with how clinicians made decisions about why they would or would not include family during resuscitation efforts. Previous research into this area has found differences in perceptions of staff, with nurses mostly focusing on benefit over risk and physicians focused on risks over benefits. This appears to be reflected in this study where fear of risk meant the weighting of themes was very focused on risk to patient outcomes and risk to team/self by physicians, and nurses focusing more specifically on benefits to patient, family and resuscitation team. While some themes were different, some were common across groups. This includes 'Families may disrupt'. Physicians weighted this theme as the largest driving factor while for nurses it was third in the list of five. This theme is described in previous international research and is focused on the risk of resources, focus and attention being diverted from the patient to the family or being delayed because of family involvement. Clinicians in this study reported using criteria to assess for probable family disruption; however, there appear to be no specific screening tools available for this purpose. 'Traumatising nature of resuscitation' was the second shared theme in which both groups were concerned with the potential for family members to be psychologically harmed by seeing their loved one undergo the often graphic and brutal nature of resuscitation, especially if the outcome was death, and wanted to protect families from that. 'Family benefits' was another shared theme; however, it was weighted more heavily by nurses. Benefits to family was valued over risk of trauma to family for nurses. Assessment of benefits to family was unknown because it was not written down and due to methodology this was not able to be explored.

The other themes in this study which nurses and physicians differed most on included: 'Families lack understanding'. In this physician-focused theme risk was decreased significantly If they thought families could understand what was happening and would have less unrealistic expectations of resuscitation. If families were not educated about resuscitation (or had 'too much' influence on this by TV drama shows), they were less likely to invite them into the resuscitation. A theme uncovered in the nursing data called 'Responding to negative family emotions' described resources at hand to support family and the role and abilities needed for that role. 'Patient preference' a physician-only theme, described the physicians' willingness to consider patient wishes; however, noted this was not able to be considered where patients were unconscious or deteriorated quickly. 'Making family presence decisions' was a nurse-only theme as physicians did not discuss an emotional component to the decision making. This is another example for where different methodology could have provided further clarity on this disparity. Nurses discussed making these decisions was hard due to the potential consequences and high stakes of the decisions made in a time-pressured context. Consequences were discussed as those for patients, families and for clinicians as litigation was also a frequent concern.

Methods

A convenience sample of clinicians was used to collect a large amount of information as part of a larger research study. Participant recruitment was managed through multiple techniques such as announcements in staff meetings, educational sessions and by email. Consent was inferred by returning responses. Participants responded in writing to three fixed questions:

1. I would not invite family presence during resuscitation because …
2. I would invite family presence during resuscitation because …
3. Please write in this space any experiences, stories, thoughts or feelings you have about inviting families to be present during resuscitation of loved ones.

Data was analysed by thematic analysis by five members of the research team. Individual analysis occurred first then the researchers collaborated in a group session where themes were selected and refined until consensus was reached. Weighting was allocated by the researchers to the themes based on frequency of occurrence and by placing a value judgement on the impact the theme had according to the way it was referred to by participants in their written entries. While this process was robust, there are inherent limitations due to the nature of the methodology. Firstly, member checking of the themes could not occur due to the responses being anonymous, although selected nurses and physicians concurred that the themes arrived at were reasonable. Secondly, because there was no opportunity to clarify meaning which would normally occur with face to face interviews or focus groups, data depth could have been an issue; however, the researchers felt the large number of responses may have adjusted this limitation. Additionally, both data sets were analysed by the same team, which means the first data set outcomes could have influenced the analysis of the second data set. This study was conducted at a single site with specific family-centred care which could limit generalisability, additionally the site did not have a policy about family presence during resuscitation which may have influenced the decision making.

Overall, this is a good example of a well-conducted study demonstrating how a different method of data collection can give a broad sample, although depth of data had to be sacrificed for this in many of the themes.

Learning activities

1. Review your local guidelines for treatment and management of sepsis.
2. Relevant imaging can help guide a future treatment plan or surgical intervention; however, it may also represent an unacceptable risk as it is a difficult environment for resuscitation if there is a sudden clinical deterioration. What would be considered minimum physiological parameters for safe transport to imaging?

3 In abdominal pain presentations, patients may experience 'visceral' and/or 'somatic' pain depending upon which structures are involved in the disease process. Which structures experience these different types of pain, and how do they differ in symptoms?

Online resources

American Emergency Nurses Association, www.ena.org

Australasian College for Emergency Medicine, www.acem.org.au

Australian College of Emergency Nursing, https://acen.com.au

Australian Institute of Health and Welfare, www.aihw.gov.au

Australian Venom Research Unit, www.avru.org

Best Bets, www.bestbets.org

Clinical Toxinology Resources, Women's and Children's Hospital, Adelaide, www.toxinology.com

College of Emergency Nursing Australasia, www.cena.org.au

College of Emergency Nursing New Zealand, www.nzno.org.nz/groups/colleges/college_of_emergency_nurses

Commonwealth Serum Laboratories Antivenom Handbook eMedicine, www.emedicine.com

Emergency Nursing World, http://enw.org

National Asthma Council of Australia, www.nationalasthma.org.au

New Zealand Health Information Service, www.nzhis.govt.nz

New Zealand Ministry of Health, www.moh.govt.nz

Poisons Information Australia, telephone: 131126

Poisons Information New Zealand, telephone: 0800 POISON or 0800 764766

The Cochrane Centre, http://acc.cochrane.org

Further reading

White J. A clinician's guide to Australian venomous bites and stings: incorporating the updated CSL Antivenom Handbook; 2013. CSL Ltd. http://www.toxinology.com/fusebox.cfm?staticaction=generic_static_files/cgavbs_avh.html.

References

1. Domagala SE, Vets J. Emergency nursing triage: keeping it safe. J Emerg Nurs 2015;41(4):313–16.
2. Solheim J. Emergency nursing: the profession, the pathway, the practice. Inidanapolis: Sigma Theta Tau International, Honorary Society of Nursing; 2016.
3. Mackway-Jones K, Marsden J, Windle J. Emergency triage: manchester triage group. 3rd ed. Chichester: John Wiley; 2014.
4. Australasian College for Emergency Medicine. Guidelines on the implementation of the Australiasian Triage Scale in Emergency Departments Australia: Australasian College for Emergency Medicine; 2016. Available from: https://acem.org.au/getattachment/4320524e-ad60-4e7c-a96d-bdf90cd7966c/G24-Implementation-of-the-Australasian-Triage-Scal.aspx. [Accessed 2018].
5. College of Emergency Nursing Australasia. Practice standards for the emergency nursing specialist: College of Emergency Nursing Australasia; 2013. 3rd ed. Available from: https://www.cena.org.au/wp-content/uploads/2014/10/Practice_Standards_for_the_Emergency_Nurse_Specialist_June_14.pdf. [Accessed 2018].
6. Richardson D, editor. Triage. 4th ed. Edinburgh: Elsevier; 2015.
7. Hodge A, Hugman A, Varndell W, et al. A review of the uality assurance processes for the Australasian Triage Scale (ATS) and implications for future practice. Australas Emerg Nurs J 2013;16:21–9.
8. Dippenaar E, Bruijns S. Triage is easy, said no triage nurse ever. Int Emerg Nurs 2016;29:1–2.
9. McMahon M. ED triage: is a five level triage system the best? Am J Nurs 2003;103(3):61–3.
10. Canadian Association of Emergency Physicians. Implementation guidelines; 2018. Available from: http://caep.ca/resources/ctas/implementation-guidelines#triage-acuity-scale-definitions. [Accessed 5 April 2018].

11. College of Emergency Nursing Australasia. Triage and the Australaian Triage Scale: College of Emergency Nursing Australasia; 2015. Available from: http://cena.org.au/wp-content/uploads/2014/10/Position-Statement-Triage-and-the-Australasian-Triage-Scale.pdf. [Accessed 2018].
12. van der Wulp I, van Stel HF. Calculating kappas from adjusted data improved the comparability of the reliability of triage systems: a comparative study. J Clin Epidemiol 2010;63(11):1256–63.
13. Urushidani S, Nakayama T. Five-level emergency triage systems: variation in assessment of validity. Emerg Med J 2017;34(11):703–10.
14. Krey J. Triage in emergency departments. Comparative evaluation of 4 international triage systems. Med Klin Intensivmed Notfmed 2016;111(2):124–33.
15. Parenti N, Reggiani MLB, Iannone P, et al. A systematic review on the validity and reliability of an emergency department triage scale, the Manchester Triage System. Int J Nurs Stud 2014;51(7):1062–9.
16. Travers DA, Waller AE, Bowling JM, et al. Five-level triage system more effective than three-level in tertiary emergency department. J Emerg Nurs 2002;28(5):395–400.
17. Emergency Nurses Association. Triage qualifications and competency. J Emerg Nurs 2017;43(6):571.
18. Ng CJ, Hsu KH, Kuan JT, et al. Comparison between Canadian Triage and Acuity Scale and Taiwan Triage System in emergency departments. J Formos Med Assoc 2010;109(11):828–37.
19. Maningas PA, Hime DA, Parker DE, et al. The Soterion Rapid Triage System: evaluation of inter-rater reliability and validity. J Emerg Med 2006;30(4):461–9.
20. Fernandes CM, Tanabe P, Gilboy N, et al. Five-level triage: a report from the ACEP/ENA Five-level Triage Task Force. J Emerg Nurs 2005;31(1):39–50, quiz 118.
21. FitzGerald G, Jelinek GA, Scott D, et al. Emergency department triage revisited. Emerg Med J 2010;27(2):86–92.
22. Commonwealth Department of Health and Family Services and the Australian College of Emergency Medicine. Australian national triage scale: a user's manual. Pardy M, ed. Canberra: CDHFS; 1997.
23. Australasian College for Emergency Medicine. Australasian triage scale. Emerg Med 2002;14:335–6.
24. College of Emergency Nursing Australasia. Position statement: Triage and the Australasian Triage Scale Hobart, Australia: College of Emergency Nursing Australasia; 2015. Available from: http://cena.org.au/wp-content/uploads/2014/10/Position-Statement-Triage-and-the-Australasian-Triage-Scale.pdf. [Accessed 2018].
25. Department of Health and Aging. Emergency Triage Education Kit: Department of Health; 2013. Available from: http://www.health.gov.au/internet/main/publishing.nsf/Content/casemix-ED-triage+Review+Fact+Sheet+Documents. [Accessed 2018].
26. Foley A. Triage process and department practice are different. J Emerg Nurs 2017;43(2):185–6.
27. College of Emergency Nursing Australasia. Position Statement Triage Nurse; 2009. Available from: http://www.cena.org.au/. [Accessed 5 April 2018].
28. Gilboy N, Tanabe P, Travers DA, et al. The Emergency Severity Index (ESI): A triage tool for Emergency Department. Version 4 https://www.ahrq.gov/professionals/systems/hospital/esi/esi1.html2012. Available from: http://www.ncbi.nlm.nih.gov/pubmed/16126100. [Accessed April 2018].
29. Kitt S. Emergency nursing: a physiological and clinical perspective. 2nd ed. Philadelphia: WB Saunders; 1995.
30. Mental Health and Drug and Alcohol Office. Mental Health Triage Policy. Sydney: NSW Government; 2012.
31. Mental Health and Drug and Alcohol Office. Mental Health for Emergency Department – A Reference Guide. NSW Department of Health, Sydney 2009.
32. Adeosun I, Adegbohun AA, Jeje OO, et al. Urgent and nonurgent presentations to a psychiatric emergency service in Nigeria: pattern and correlates. Emerg Med Int 2014;2014:479081.
33. Australian and New Zealand Society for Geriatric Medicine. The management of older patients in the emergency department. In: Australian and New Zealand Society for Geriatric Medicine, ed. 2015.
34. Carpenter CR, Bromley M, Caterino JM, et al. Optimal older adult emergency care: introducing multidisciplinary geriatric emergency department guidelines from the American College of Emergency Physicians, American Geriatrics Society, Emergency Nurses Association, and Society for Academic Emergency Medicine. J Am Geriatr Soc 2014;62(7):1360–3.
35. Arendts G, Lowthian J. Demography is destiny: an agenda for geriatric medicine in Australasia. Emerg Med Australas 2013;25(3):271–8.
36. Hodge APL, Daly B, Hagness C, et al. Revision and evaluation of an 'advanced' nursing role in an Australian emergency department. Australas Emerg Nurs J 2011;14:120–8.
37. Patel H, Celenza A, Watters T. Effect of nurse initiated X-rays of the lower limb on patient transit time through the emergency department. Australas Emerg Nurs J 2012;15(4):229–34.
38. NSW Department of Health. Clinical Initiatives Nurse in Emergency Departments Education Program Resource Manual. Sydney: NSW Department of Health; 2011.
39. Taylor S, Taylor D, Jao K, et al. Nurse-initiated analgesia pathway for paediatric patients in the emergency department: a clinical intervention trial. Emerg Med Australas 2013;25:316–23.
40. Muntlin A, Carlsson M, Safwenberg U, et al. Outcomes of a nurse-initiated intravenous analgesic protocol for abdominal pain in an emergency department: a quasi-experimental study. Int J Nurs Stud 2011;48(1):13–23.

41. Cabilan C, Boyde M. A systematic review of the impact of nurse initiated medications in the emrgency department. Australas Emerg Nurs J 2017;20(2):53–62.
42. Brennan RJ, Bradt DA, Abrahams J. Medical issues in disasters. In: Cameron P, Jelinek G, Kelly A, et al, editors. Textbook of adult emergency medicine. 4th ed. Edinburgh: Elsevier; 2014. p. 841–84.
43. Australasian College for Emergency Medicine, Australian and New Zealand College of Anaesthetists, College of Intensive Care Medicine of Australia and New Zealand. Guidelines for transport of critically ill patients: Australasian College for Emergency Medicine; 2015. Available from: https://acem.org.au/getattachment/a7701840-29f2-4096-872a-b213bec75d9d/P03-Guidelines-for-Transport-of-Critically-Ill-Pat.aspx. [Accessed 2018].
44. Mackway-Jones K, editor. Major incident medical management and support: the practice approach at the scene. 3rd ed. Chichester: John Wiley; 2012.
45. Goldhill D, Gemmell L, Lutman D, et al. Interhospital Transfer http://www.aagbi.org/2009. Available from: http://www.aagbi.org/sites/default/files/interhospital09.pdf. [Accessed Dec 2014].
46. Kennedy MP, Gabbe BJ, McKenzie BA. Impact of the introduction of an integrated adult retrieval service on major trauma outcomes. Emerg Med J 2015;32(11):833–9.
47. Prabhudesai S, Kasala M, Manwani N, et al. Transport-related adverse events in critically-ill children: the role of a dedicated transport team. Indian Pediatr 2017;54(11):942–5.
48. Droogh JM, Smit M, Absalom AR, et al. Transferring the critically ill patient: are we there yet? Crit Care 2015;19(1):62.
49. Parmentier-Decrucq E, Poissy J, Favory R, et al. Adverse events during intrahospital transport of critically ill patients: incidence and risk factors. Ann Intensive Care 2013;3(1):10.
50. Wills CP, Young M, White DW. Pitfalls in the evaluation of shortness of breath. Emerg Med Clin North Am 2010;28:163–81.
51. Hore C, Roberts J. Respiratory emergencies: the acutely breathless patient. In: Fulde GFS, editor. Emergency medicine the principles of practice. Sydney: Elsevier; 2014.
52. Sarko J, Stapczynski J. Respiratory distress. In: Tintinalli J, Stapczynski J, Ma J, et al, editors. Emergency medicine; a comprehensive study guide. American College of Emergency Physicians. 8th ed. New York: McGraw-Hill; 2016.
53. Callahan JM. Pulse oximetry in emergency medicine. Emerg Med Clin North Am 2008;26:869–79.
54. Walkey A, Farber H, O'Donnel C, et al. The accuracy of the central venous blood gas for acid-base monitoring. J Intensive Care Med 2010;25(2):104.
55. National Asthma Council Australia. Australian Asthma handbook V1.3; 2018. Available from: www.asthmahandbook.org.au. [Accessed 11 Jan 2018].
56. Cyudlka R. Acute asthma in adults. In: Tintinalli J, Stapczynski J, Ma J, et al, editors. Emergency medicine; a comprehensive study guide. American College of Emergency Physicians. 8th ed. New York: McGraw-Hill; 2016.
57. National Asthma Council Australia. Asthma Management Handbook: Revised and updated 2014 2014. Available from: http:www.nationalasthma.org.au/cms/index.php. [Accessed May 2014].
58. Kelly A. Asthma. In: Cameron P, Jelinek G, Kelly A-M, et al, editors. Textbook of adult emergency medicine. 4th ed. Edinburgh: Elsevier; 2015.
59. Serrano-Pariente JPV. Near-fatal asthma: a heterogeneous clinical entity. Curr Opin Allergy Clin Immunol 2017;17(28):28–35.
60. National Asthma Council Australia. Rapid primary assessment of acuite asthma in adults and children. Australian Asthma Handbook V1.3 2017. Available from: www.asthmahandbook.org.au/acute-asthma/clinical/primary-assessment. [Accessed 11 Jan 2018].
61. Bates C, Cydulka R. Chronic obstructive pulmonary disease. In: Tintinalli J, Stapczynski J, Ma J, et al, editors. Emergency medicine; a comprehensive study guide. American College of Emergency Physicians. 8th ed. New York: McGraw-Hill; 2016.
62. Emerman C, Anderson E, Yealy D. Pneumonia and pulmonary infiltrates. In: Tintinalli J, Stapczynski J, Ma J, et al, editors. Emergency medicine: a comprehensive study guide. American College of Emergency Physicians. 8th ed. New York: McGraw-Hill; 2016.
63. Murrie J, Wu L. Factors influencing in-hospital mortality in community-acquired pneumonia: a prospective study of patients not initially admitted to the ICU. Chest 2005;127:1260–70.
64. Cullen L, Greenslade J, Hawkins T, et al. Improved Assessment of Chest pain Trial (IMPACT): assessing patients with possible acute coronary syndromes. Med J Aust 2017;207(5):195–200.
65. Mahler S. Chest pain. In: Tintinalli J, Stapczynski J, Ma J, et al, editors. Emergency medicine; a comprehensive study guide. American College of Emergency Physicians. 8th ed. New York: McGraw-Hill; 2016.
66. Hollander JDD. Acute coronary syndromes. In: Tintinalli J, Stapczynski J, Ma J, et al, editors. Emergency medicine; a comprehensive study guide. American College of Emergency Physicians. 8th ed. New York: McGraw-Hill; 2016.
67. Parsonage WA, Cullen L, Younger JF. The approach to patients with possible cardiac chest pain. Med J Aust 2013;199(1):30–4.
68. Whelan P, Whelan A. The approach to the patient with chest pain, dyspnoea or haemoptysis. In: Fulde GFS, editor. Emergency medicine: the principles of practice. Sydney: Elsevier; 2014.
69. Hofmann RJT, Lindahl B, Erlinge D, et al. Oxygen therapy in suspected acute myocardial infarction. N Engl J Med 2017;377(23):1240.
70. Chew DP, Scott SI, Cullen L, et al. National heart foundation of Australia and New Zealand: Australian clinical guidelines for the management of acute coronary syndromes 2016. Med J Aust 2016;205(3):128–33.
71. Australian Institute of Health and Welfare. Deaths. Canberra: Australian Institute of Health and Welfare; 2017.

72. Amsterdam EWN, Brindis R, Casey D. AHA/ACC Guideline for the management of patients with non-st-elevation acute coronary syndromes: executive summary. Circulation 2014;130(25).
73. Woo KC, Schnieder JI. High risk chief complaints 1: chest pain-the big three. Emerg Med Clin North Am 2009;27:685–712.
74. Prince L, Johnson G. Aortic dissection and related aortic syndromes. In: Tintinalli J, Stapczynski J, Ma J, et al, editors. Emergency medicine; a comprehensive study guide. American College of Emergency Physicians, 8th ed. New York: McGraw-Hill; 2011.
75. de Buriet KLP, Dennett E. Acute abdominal pain changes in the way we assess it over a decade. N Z Med J 2017;130(1463):39–44.
76. Gallagher EJ, Lukens TW, Colucciello SV, et al. Clinical policy: critical issues for the intial evaluation and management of patients presenting with a chief complaint of non traumatic abdominal pain. Ann Emerg Med 2000;36(4):406–15.
77. Kamin RA, Nowicki TA, Courtney DS, et al. Pearls and pitfalls in the emergency department evaluation of abdominal pain. Emerg Med Clin North Am 2003;21(1):61–72.
78. O'Brien C. Acute abdominal pain. In: Tintinalli JE, Stapczynski JS, Ma J, et al, editors. Tintinalli's emergency medicine: a comprehensive study guide. 8th ed. 2016.
79. O'Toole J. Abdominal pain: pathophysiology, etiology, diagnosis, and therapy (pain management in the ED). Top Emerg Med 2002;24(1):46–51.
80. McNamara R, Dean AJ. Approach to acute abdominal pain. Emerg Med Clin North Am 2011;29(2):159–73.
81. Dagiely S. An algorithm for triaging commonly missed causes of acute abdominal pain. J Emerg Nurs 2006;32(1):9.
82. Ozen O, Kiyan S. Views of emergency physicians working in university and state hospitals in Turkey regarding the use of analgesics in patients with acute abdominal pain. Ulus Travma Acil Cerrahi Derg 2016;22(2):175–83.
83. Chan K, Seow E. Approaches to abdominal pain. In: Cameron P, Jelinek G, Kelly A-M, et al, editors. Textbook of adult emergency medicine. 4th ed. Edinburgh: Elsevier; 2014.
84. Tillman K, Lee OD, Whitty K. Abdominal aortic aneurysm: an often asymptomatic and fatal men's health issue. Am J Mens Health 2013;7(2):163–8.
85. Gillet M. Aortic and vascular emergencies. In: Fulde GFS, editor. Emergency medicine: the principles of practice. 6th ed. Sydney: Elsevier; 2014.
86. Rubano E, Mehta N, Caputo W, et al. Systematic review: emergency department bedside ultrasonography for diagnosing suspected abdominal aortic aneurysm. Acad Emerg Med 2013;20(2):128–38.
87. Nshuti R, Kruger D, Luvhengo TE. Clinical presentation of acute appendicitis in adults at the Chris Hani Baragwanath academic hospital. Int J Emerg Med 2014;7(1):12.
88. Martin RKS. Acute appendicitis in adults: diagnostic evaluation UpToDate2017. Available from: www.uptodate.comacs.hcn.com.au/contents/acute-appenidicitis-in-adults-diagnostic-evaluation?sectionName=IMAGING&anchor=H612714599&source=see_link#H612714599. [Accessed 11 Jan 2018].
89. McDonald M, Wong C. Gastrointestinal emergencies. In: Fulde G, Fulde S, editors. Emergency medicine: the principles of of practice. 6th ed. Sydney: Elsevier; 2014.
90. Vallicelli C, Coccolini F, Catena F, et al. Small bowel emergency surgery: literature's review. World J Emerg Surg 2011;6(1):1.
91. Smolarek S, Shalaby M, Angelucci G, et al. Small bowel obstruction secondary to adhesions after open or laproscopic colorectal surgery. JSLS 2016;20(4).
92. Bordeianou L, Yeh DD. Overview of management of mechanical small bowel obstruction in adults UpToDate2017. Available from: https://www.uptodate.com.acs.hcn.com.au/contents/overview-of-management-of-mechanical-small-bowel-obstruction-in-adults?search=overview%20of%20management%20of%20mechanical%20bowel%20obstruction&source=search_result&selectedTitle=1~150&usage_type=default&display_rank=1. [Accessed 11 Jan 2018].
93. Alkatout I, Honemeyer U, Strauss A, et al. Clinical diagnosis and treatment of extopic pregnancy. Obstet Gynecol Surv 2013;68(8):571–81.
94. Sivalingam VN, Duncan WC, Kirk E, et al. Diagnosis and management of ectopic pregnancy. J Fam Plann Reprod Health Care 2011;37(4):231–40.
95. Tulandi T. Ectopic pregnancy: choosing a treatment. UpToDate2017. Available from: https://www.uptodate.com.acs.hcn.com.au/contents/ectopic-pregnancy-choosing-a-treatment?search=ectopic%20pregnancy%20choosing%20a%20treatment&source=search_result&selectedTitle=1~150&usage_type=default&display_rank=1. [Accessed 20 Jan 2018].
96. Kinlay S. Changes in stroke epidemiology, prevention, and treatment. Circulation 2011;124(19):e494–6.
97. Krock AB, Massaro L. Facilitating ED evaluation of patients with acute ischemic stroke. J Emerg Nurs 2008;34(6):519–22.
98. Whitely W, Emberson J, Lees K, et al. Risk of intracerebral haemorrhage with alteplase after acute ischaemic stroke: a secondary analysis of an individual patient data metaanalysis. Lancet Neurol 2016;15(9):925–33.
99. Nedeltchev K, Renz N, Karameshev A, et al. Predictors of early mortality after acute ischaemic stroke. Swiss Med Wkly 2010;140(17–18):254–9.
100. Stroke Foundation. Stroke symptoms: Stroke Foundation; 2018. Available from: https://strokefoundation.org.au/About-Stroke/Stroke-symptoms. [Accessed 2018].
101. Adams HP, Adams RJ, Brott M, et al. Guidelines for the early management of patients with ischemic stroke. Stroke 2003;34:1056–83.

102. Filho JMM. Initial assessment and management of acute stroke UpToDate2017. Available from: https://www.uptodate.com.acs.hcn.com.au/contents/initial-assessment-and-management-of-acute-stroke?search=initial%20assessment%20and%20management%20of%20acute%20stroke&source=search_result&selectedTitle=1~150&usage_type=default&display_rank=1. [Accessed 20 Jan 2018].
103. Pryor D, Chan A. Neurological emergencies. In: Fulde G, Fulde S, editors. Emergency medicine: the principles of practice. 6th ed. Sydney: Elsevier; 2014.
104. Uphaus T, Grings A, Groschel S, et al. Automatic detection of paroxysmal atrial fibrillation in patients with ischaemic stroke: better than routine diagnostic workup? Eur J Neurol 2017;24:990–4.
105. Goldstein LB, Adams R, et al. Primary prevention of ischemic stroke: a guideline from the American Heart Association/American Stroke Association Stroke Council (co-sponsored by the Atherosclerotic Peripheral Vascular Disease Interdisciplinary Working Group; Cardiovascular Nursing Council; Clinical Cardiology Council; Nutrition, Physical Activity, and Metabolism Council; the Quality of Care and Outcomes Research Interdisciplinary Working Group). Stroke 2006;37:1583–633.
106. Stroke Foundation. Clinical Guidelines for Stroke Management; 2017. Available from: http://brainfoundation.org.au/a-z-of-disorders/107-stroke#strokeaffectaustralians. [Accessed Jul 2018].
107. Hacke W, Kaste M, Bluhmki E, et al. Thrombolysis with alteplase 3 to 4.5 hours after acute ischemic stroke. N Engl J Med 2008;359(13):1317–29.
108. Del Zoppo GJ, Saver JL, Jauch EC, et al. Expansion of the time window for treatment of acute ischemic stroke with intravenous tissue plasminogen activator. A science advisory from the American Heart Association/American Stroke Association. Stroke 2009;40:2945–8.
109. Meehan TJ. Approach to the poisoned patient. In: Walls R, Hockberger RS, Gausche-Hill M, editors. Rosen's emergency medicine: concepts and clinical practice. 9th ed. Philadelphia: Elsevier; 2018. p. 1813–22.e2.
110. Murray L. Approaches to the poisoned patient. In: Cameron P, Jelinek G, Kelly A, et al, editors. Textbook of adult emergency medicine. 4th ed. Edinburgh: Elsevier; 2014. p. 951–1033.
111. World Health Organisation. Suicide Data: WHO; 2018. Available from: http://www.who.int/mental_health/prevention/suicide/suicideprevent/en/. [Accessed 2018].
112. Australian Institute of Health and Welfare. Australia's Health 2016. Canberra: AIHW; 2016.
113. Department of Health. Therapuetic Goods Administration: Australian Government; n.d. Available from: https://www.tga.gov.au/. [Accessed 2 April 2018].
114. Bailey GP, Najafi J, Elamin MEMO, et al. Delays during the administration of acetylcysteine for the treatment of paracetamol overdose. Br J Clin Pharmacol 2016;82(5):1358–63.
115. Roberts DM. Pesticides. In: Cameron P, Jelinek G, Kelly A, et al, editors. Textbook of adult emergency medicine. 4th ed. Edinburgh: Elsevier; 2014.
116. Ferri FFMD. Tricyclic antidepressant overdose; 2018, p. 1301.e9–e11.
117. Dowsett R. Corrosive ingestion. In: Cameron P, Jelinek G, Kelly A, editors. Textbook of adult emergency medicine. 4th ed. Edinburgh: Elsevier; 2014.
118. Bonney AG, Mazor S, Goldman RD. Laundry detergent capsules and pediatric poisoning. Can Fam Physician 2013;59(12):1295–6.
119. Hatten BW. Aspirin and nonsteriodal agents. In: Walls R, Hockberger RS, Gausche-Hill M, editors. Rosen's emergency medicine: concepts and clinical practice. 9th ed. Philadelphia: Elsevier; 2018. p. 1858–62.e1.
120. Green D, Graudins A. Salicylate. In: Cameron P, Jelinek G, Kelly A, editors. Textbook of adult emergency medicine. 4th ed. Edinburgh: Elsevier; 2014.
121. Graudins A. Paracetamol. In: Cameron P, Jelinek G, Kelly A, editors. Textbook of adult emergency medicine. 4th ed. Edinburgh: Elsevier; 2014.
122. Scott T, Foster T. Assessing carbon monoxide poisoning. Emerg Nurse 2013;20(10):14–19.
123. Welker K, Thompson TM. Pesticides. In: Walls R, Hockberger RS, Gausche-Hill M, editors. Rosen's emergnecy medicine: concepts and clinical practice. Philadelphia: Elsevier; 2018. p. 1947–56.e2.
124. Koutsogiannis Z. Iron. In: Cameron P, Jelinek G, Kelly A, et al, editors. Textbook of adult emergency medicine. 4th ed. Edinburgh: Elsevier; 2014.
125. Hoggett KA. Drugs of abuse. In: Cameron P, Jelinek G, Kelly A, editors. Textbook of adult emergency medicine. 4th ed. Edinburgh: Elsevier; 2014.
126. Minns AB, Clark RF. Substance abuse. In: Walls R, Hockberger RS, Gausche-Hill M, editors. Rosen's emergency medicine: concepts and clinical practice. 9th ed. Philadelphia, PA: Elsevier; 2018. p. 1823–8.e1.
127. Queensland Health, Royal Flying Doctor Service (Queensland section). Primary Clinical Care Manual. Cairns, Australia: The Rural and Remote Clinical Support Unit, Torres and Cape Hospital and Health Service; 2016. Available from: https://publications.qld.gov.au/dataset/27722ad1-4a1e-4a28-a3d7-bafea915bc00/resource/06f04fcb-6eb6-45eb-9770-c4a79a715b62/download/primary-clinical-care-manual-edition-9.pdf.
128. Royal Childrens' Hospital Melbourne. Clinical Practice Guidelines. Salicylate poisoning http://www.rch.org.au/2014. Available from: http://www.rch.org.au/clinicalguide/guideline_index/Salicylates_Posioning/. [Accessed Dec 2014].

129. Chiew AL, Fountain JS, Graudins A, et al. Summary statement. New guidelines for the management of paracetamol poisoning in Australia and New Zealand. Med J Aust 2015;03:215–18.
130. Buckley N. Carbon monoxide. In: Cameron P, Jelinek G, Kelly A, editors. Textbook of adult emergency medicine. 4th ed. Edinburgh: Elsevier; 2014.
131. Nelson LS, Hoffman RS. Inhaled toxins. In: Walls R, Hockberger RS, Gausche-Hill M, editors. Rosen's emergency medicine: concepts and clinical practice. Philadelphia: Elsevier; 2018. p. 1926–33.e2.
132. Hoyte C. Caustics. In: Walls R, Hockberger RS, Gausche-Hill M, editors. Rosen's emergency medicine: concepts and clinical practice. 9th ed. Philadelphia: Elsevier; 2018. p. 1890–4.e1.
133. Gummin DD. Hydrocarbons. In: Adams JG, Barton ED, Collings JL, et al, editors. Emergency medicine, clinical essentials. 2nd ed. Philadelphia: Saunders; 2013. p. 1299–307.
134. Osborne NJ, Cairns R, Dawson AH, et al. Epidemiology of coronial deaths from pesticide ingestion in Australia. Int J Hyg Environ Health 2017;220(2):478–84.
135. Little M, Murray L. Consensus statement: risk of nosocomial organophosphate poisoning in emergency departments. Emerg Med Australas 2004;16:456–8.
136. Isbister GK. Spider bite. In: Cameron P, Jelinek G, Kelly A, et al, editors. Textbook of adult emergency medicine. 4th ed. Edinburgh: Elsevier; 2015.
137. Hifumi T, Fujimi S, Yamagishi T, et al. Clinical characteristics of redback spider bites. J Intensive Care 2014;2(1):62.
138. Bryan SA, van Heezik Y, Vink CJ, et al. Invasive redback spiders (*Latrodectus hasseltii*) threaten an endangered, endemic New Zealand beetle (*Prodontria lewisii*). J Insect Conserv 2015;19(5):1021–7.
139. Thatcher L, Janes R. Latrodectism: case report of a katipo spider (*Latrodectus katipo*) bite and review of the literature. N Z Med J 2012;125(1351):92–4.
140. Isbister GK, Page CB, Buckley NA, et al. Randomized controlled trial of intravenous antivenom versus placebo for latrodectism: the second redback antivenom evaluation (RAVE-II) study. Ann Emerg Med 2014;64(6):620–8.e2.
141. Isbister GK, Sellors KV, Beckmann U, et al. Catecholamine-induced cardiomyopathy resulting from life-threatening funnel-web spider envenoming. Med J Aust 2015;203(7):302.
142. Seqirus. Funnel web spider antivenom product information. Available from: https://www.seqirus.com.au/docs/567/566/Funnel%20Web%20Spider%20Antivenom%20-%20approved%20Product%20Information%20v7_23%20Dec%202016.pdf. [Accessed 1 October 2018].
143. Welton RE, Dee D, Williams DJ. Snakes and latitude. Position 2016;80:28–9.
144. Australian Venom Research Unit. Snakebite in Australia: University of Melbourne; 2018. Available from: http://www.avru.org/health/health_snakes.html.
145. Sutherland S, Tibbals J. Australian animal toxins: the creatures, their toxins and care of the poisoned patient. 2nd ed. Melbourne: Oxford University Press; 2001.
146. Welton RE, Williams DJ, Liew D. Injury trends from envenoming in Australia, 2000-2013: envenoming injury Australia,2000–2013. Intern Med J 2016.
147. Welton RE, Liew D, Braitberg G. Incidence of fatal snake bite in Australia: a coronial based retrospective study (2000–2016). Toxicon 2017;131:11–15.
148. Isbister GK. Snakebite. In: Cameron P, Jelinek G, Kelly A, et al, editors. Textbook of adult emergency medicine. 4th ed. Edinburgh: Elsevier; 2015.
149. Avau B, Borra V, Vandekerckhove P, et al. The treatment of snake bites in a first aid setting: a systematic review. PLoS Negl Trop Dis 2016;10(10):e0005079.
150. White J, et al. Exotic snakebite. In: Cameron P, Jelinek G, Kelly A, editors. Textbook of adult emergency medicine. 4th ed. Edinburgh: Elsevier; 2015.
151. Nimorakiotakis V, Winkel KD. Prospective assessment of the false positive rate of the Australian snake venom detection kit in healthy human samples. Toxicon 2016;111:143–6.
152. Ratnayake I, Shihana F, Dissanayake DM, et al. Performance of the 20-minute whole blood clotting test in detecting venom induced consumption coagulopathy from Russell's viper (*Daboia russelii*) bites. Thromb Haemost 2017;117(3):500–7.
153. Berling I, Isbister G. Marine envenomations. Aust Fam Physician 2015;44(1–2):28–32.
154. Isbister GK, Seifert SA. Envenomation. 25th ed. 2016. p. 717–22.e2.
155. Murray L, Little M, Pascu O, et al. Toxicology handbook. 3rd ed. Chatswood: Elsevier; 2015.
156. Seymour JE. Are we using the correct first aid for jellyfish? Med J Aust 2017;206(6):249–50.
157. Little M, Fitzpatrick R, Seymour J. Successful use of heat as first aid for tropical Australian jellyfish stings. Toxicon 2016;122:142–4.
158. Pereira P, Seymour J. Marine injury, envenoming and poisoning. In: Cameron P, Jelinek G, Kelly A, et al, editors. Textbook of adult emergency medicine. 4th ed. Edinburgh: Elsevier; 2014.
159. Rathbone J, Franklin R, Gibbs C, et al. Review article: role of magnesium sulphate in the management of Irukandji syndrome: a systematic review. Emerg Med Australas 2017;29(1):9–17.

160. Perkins A. Marine poisonings, envenomations, and trauma. In: Bope ET, Kellerman RD, editors. Conn's current therapy 2018 e-book. Philadelphia: Elsevier; 2018. p. 1243–7.
161. Farrell H, Murray SA, Zammit A, et al. Management of ciguatoxin risk in Eastern Australia. Toxins (Basel) 2017;9(11):367.
162. Friedman MA, Fernandez M, Backer LC, et al. An updated review of ciguatera fish poisoning: clinical, epidemiological, environmental, and public health management. Mar Drugs 2017;15(3):72.
163. Feng C, Teuber S, Gershwin ME. Histamine (scombroid) fish poisoning: a comprehensive review. Clin Rev Allergy Immunol 2016;50(1): 64–9.
164. Meisenheimer E, Bevis Z, Tagawa C, et al. Drowning injuries: an update on terminology, environmental factors, and management. Curr Sports Med Rep 2016;15(2):91–3.
165. WHO. Drowning fact sheet World Health Organization; 2018. Available from: http://www.who.int/mediacentre/factsheets/fs347/en/. [Accessed 2018].
166. Brenner RA, Trumble AC, Smith GS, et al. Where children drown, United States, 1995. Pediatrics 2001;108(1):85–9.
167. Gaida F, Gaida J. Infant and toddler drowning in Australia: patterns, risk factors and prevention recommendations. J Paediatr Child Health 2016;52:923–7.
168. Kobusingye O. The global burden of drowning: Africa. In: Bierens J, editor. Handbook on drowning: prevention, rescue and treatment. Netherlands: Springer; 2003.
169. Martinez FE, Hooper AJ. Drowning and immersion injury. Anaesth Intens Care Med 2014;15(9):420–3.
170. Bernocchi P, Scalvini S, Tridico C, et al. Healthcare continuity from hospital to territory in Lombardy: TELEMACO project. Am J Manag Care 2012;18(3):e101–8.
171. Hasibeder W. Drowning. Curr Opin Anaesth 2003;16(2):139–45.
172. Middleton P. Drowning. Emergency medicine the principles of practice. 6th ed. Sydney: Elsevier; 2014.
173. Cantwell GP. Drowning. Medscape 2017. Available from: https://emedicine.medscape.com/article/772753-overview. [Accessed 2018].
174. Shepherd S. Submersion injury, near drowning; 2010. http://www.patient.co.uk/. Available from: http://www.patient.co.uk/doctor/Drowning-and-near-drowning.htm. [Accessed Dec 2014].
175. Handley AJ. Drowning. BMJ 2014;348:g1734.
176. Fiore M. Near drowning; 2009. Available from: http://www.emedicine.com/ped/topic2570.htm. [Accessed Dec 2014].
177. Chandy DWG, Dazl D, Grayzel J. Drowning (submersion injuries). UpToDate2017. Available from: https://www.uptodate.com.acs.hcn.com.au/contents/drowning-submersion-injuries?search=drowning%20submersion%20injuries&source=search_result&selectedTitle=1~74&usage_type=default&display_rank=1. [Accessed 18 Jan 2018].
178. Moon R, Long R. Drowning and near-drowning. Emerg Med 2002;14(4):377–86.
179. Brown D. Hypothermia. In: Tintinalli J, Stapczynski J, Ma J, et al, editors. Emergency medicine; a comprehensive study guide. American College of Emergency Physicians. 8th ed. New York: McGraw-Hill; 2016.
180. Lewis-Driver D. Hypothermia and hyperthermia. Emergency medicine: the principles of practice. 6th ed. Sydney: Elsevier; 2014.
181. Krantz M, Lowery C. Giant Osborne waves in hypothermia. N Engl J Med 2005;352(2):184.
182. Tsuei B, Kearney P. Hypothermia in the trauma patient. Injury 2005;35(1):7–15.
183. Hildebrand F, Giannoudis P, van Grievensen M, et al. Pathophysiologic changes and effects of hypothermia on outcome in elective surgery and trauma patients. Am J Surg 2004;187(3):363–71.
184. Ko C, Alex J, Jefferies S, et al. Dead? Or just cold: profound hypothermia with no signs of life. Emerg Med J 2002;19:478–9.
185. Zafren KMC. Accidental hypothermia in adults. UpToDate2017. Available from: https://www.uptodate.com.acs.hcn.com.au/contents/accidental-hypothermia-in-adults?search=accidental%20hypothermia&source=search_result&selectedTitle=1~150&usage_type=default&display_rank=1. [Accessed 11 Jan 2018].
186. LoVecchio F. Heat emergencies. In: Tintinalli J, Stapczynski J, Ma J, et al, editors. Emergency medicine; a comprehensive study guide. American College of Emergency Physicians. 8th ed. New York: McGraw-Hill; 2016.
187. Samarasinghe I, Wassertheil J. Mass casualty incidents, chemical, biological and radiological hazard contingencies. In: Fulde G, Fulde S, editors. Emergency medicine: the principles of practice. 6th ed. Sydney: Elsevier; 2014.
188. Advanced Life Support Group. Major incident medical management and support: the practical approach. 2nd ed. London: BMJ Books; 2002.
189. Emergency Management Australia. Australian emergency manuals series, Part 3. Emergency management practice, Vol. 1, Service provision; manual 2. Disaster medicine. Australian Government. 2nd ed. https://ema.infoservices.com.au/collections/handbook: Australian Emergency Management Institute; 2010.
190. Karam A. Radiological incidents and emergencies. In: Disaster nursing and emergency preparedness for chemical, biological and radiological terrorism and other hazards. 2nd ed. New York: Springer; 2007. p. 521–45.
191. Veenema TG, Benitez J. S. B. Chemical agents of concern. Disaster nursing and emergency preparedness for chemical, biological and radiological terrorism and other hazards. 2nd ed. New York: Springer; 2007. p. 483–505.
192. Varma DR, Guest I. The Bhopal accident and methyl isocyanate toxicity. J Toxicol Environ Health 1993;40(4):513–29.

193. Kumar V, Goel R, Chawla R, et al. Chemical, biological, radiological, and nuclear decontamination: recent trends and future perspective. J Pharm Bioallied Sci 2010;2(3):220–38.
194. Thornton R, Court B, Meara J, et al. Chemical, biological, radiological and nuclear terrorism: an introduction for occupational physicians. Occup Med (Lond) 2004;54(2):101–9.
195. Croddy E, Ackerman G. Biological and chemical terrorism: a unique threat. Disaster nursing and emergency preparedness for chemical, biological and radiological terrorism and other hazards. 2nd ed. New York: Springer; 2007. p. 365–89.
196. Pigott D, Kazzi Z. Biological agents of concern. Disaster nursing and emergency preparedness for chemical, biological and radiological terrorism and other hazards. 2nd ed. New York: Springer; 2007. p. 403–23.
197. Wessely S, Hyams KC. Editorials. Psychological implications of chemical and biological weapons. Long term social and psychological effects may be worse than acute ones. BMJ 2001;323:878.
198. Okumura T, Hisaoka T, Yamada A, et al. The Tokyo subway sarin attack – lessons learned. Toxicol Appl Pharmacol 2005;207(2 Suppl.):471–6.

Chapter 24

Trauma management

Catherine Bell, Kerstin Prignitz Sluys

KEY WORDS

abdominal trauma
burns
chest trauma
damage-control resuscitation
fractures
multitrauma
transport
trauma

Learning objectives

After reading this chapter, you should be able to:

- identify the benefits and limitations of an organised trauma system
- describe the rationale for a systematic approach to the patient who has sustained injuries
- discuss the benefits of appropriate management of the patient with serious injury and/or multitrauma
- describe the acute management of the patient with multiple serious fractures
- describe the acute management of patients with burn injuries, abdominal injuries and chest trauma
- describe the nurse's role in managing the trauma patient undergoing damage-control resuscitation.

Introduction

Injuries continue to be a major public health concern worldwide, whether measured by years of productive life lost, prolonged or permanent disability, or financial cost. In the Global Burden of Disease study,[1] it was estimated that 973 million people sustained injuries and warranted some type of healthcare annually, with 4.8 million dying from traumatic injuries: this accounted for 10% of the world's disease burden. Major causes of death were road traffic injuries (29%), suicides (18%), falls (12%) and interpersonal violence (9%). Of the people who sustained injuries, 56 million people were admitted to a hospital, of whom 22 million (39%) sustained fractures.

The epidemiology of injury differs with severity. The majority of injured patients requiring admission to an intensive care unit (ICU) are those with serious injuries associated with motor vehicles, motorbikes and pedestrian collisions. Falls, self-inflicted injuries and assaults are less common, but still lead to critical care admission. A significant proportion of injured patients admitted to critical care have experienced neurotrauma (see Chapter 17), while other common injuries include multiple fractures and injury to internal organs in the thorax and abdomen.

The systematic organisation of trauma systems, major changes in practice and delivery of time-critical interventions have made the traditional boundaries between pre-hospital emergency medical service and hospital-based emergency, surgery, radiology and intensive care services more seamless, improving the survival of trauma patients in recent years. Consequently, a greater number of patients with severe multiple injuries are now admitted to critical care units. These patients generally require complex nursing care, often for lengthy periods, both within the critical care unit and beyond. The common traumatic injuries that result in admission to adult critical care and the principles of management are outlined in this chapter. Paediatric trauma is covered in Chapter 27. The terms 'injury' and 'trauma' are used interchangeably in this text.

Trauma systems and processes

A trauma system is an integrated, organised approach to care delivery for injured patients from the site of the injury, to the appropriate hospital or trauma care facility with the capability to care for the patient through to rehabilitation and return to ideal functioning.[2,3] Trauma systems aim to save lives through preparedness and efficiency, that ensures patients gain access to appropriate levels of care in a timely, coordinated and cost-effective manner.[4] The operational components in a trauma system should include injury prevention, pre-hospital care, acute care facilities and post-hospital care, appropriate human resources and evaluation.[2,4]

While components of a trauma system should be similar, internationally each system is organised to suit the local requirements including their economic development and range of social structures present.[5] A regional, or exclusive system relates to dedicated care provided in a major trauma centre, whereas an inclusive trauma system encompasses all trauma-receiving hospitals within a defined area. Each service in an inclusive trauma system provides differing levels of service depending on their individual capabilities.[6] Exclusive models are suited to geographically small countries or regions with short transport times; consequently, these are frequently found in European countries.[5] Both systems consist of a public health model that is designed to reduce morbidity and mortality.

Dedicated care provided in a major trauma centre has been reported to improve outcomes in the USA, Canada, Australia and UK with an established relationship between trauma centre volume and outcomes, although inclusive trauma systems that have lower volume of trauma admissions have also demonstrated improved outcomes.[3]

Pre-hospital care

Pre-hospital care is a fundamental element of an organised trauma system with an agreed triage process at each step of the patient's journey. The elements of the pre-hospital system include:

1. emergency medical service (EMS) transport system, including paramedic, physician or nurse-led care
2. triage protocols and coordinated dispatch including communication between EMS and hospitals
3. appropriate transport platforms, and
4. agreed protocols for hospital designation, trauma bypass and inter-hospital transfer.[2,7]

Essential elements of pre-hospital care include a prompt response to injury, the implementation of basic life support (BLS) including airway, breathing, haemorrhage control, and transportation of the right patient to the right place in the right time.[8] In a systematic review, shorter response and transport times had a positive influence on mortality, although patients who had longer on-scene time also had improved survival odds, possibly related to the care delivered in the pre-hospital phase.[9] The level of evidence supporting these somewhat conflicting results was low. Consequently, the concepts of 'scoop and run' and 'stay and play' remain controversial and should not be considered in the context of transport distances, pre-hospital resources, and mechanism of injury (blunt vs penetrating) by the healthcare provider at the scene,[8] with time-critical interventions undertaken to allow safe transport and rapid transfer for ongoing management.[3]

One of the principles of trauma is the Golden Hour, which suggests that patient outcomes are improved when patients are transported to a designated trauma centre within an hour of injury.[7-9] This can be challenging to achieve depending on local resources, geographical considerations etc. and may also be injury-specific. For example, there is no evidence to support the principle for those with a traumatic brain injury (TBI), while there is support in those with haemorrhagic shock.[10]

Globally there is a wide range of pre-hospital trauma care, including non-existent, BLS provided by EMS, non-physician advanced life support (ALS),[11] physician and/or pre-hospital nurse ALS.[12] Within each system the skill level of the EMS providers can vary, with BLS providers able to initiate minimally invasive care and focus primarily on prompt transportation of the patient, and those with ALS skills able to provide advanced level interventions such as intubation, administration of intravenous fluids and medications.[13]

Transport of the critically ill trauma patient

As is suggested by the Golden Hour principle, trauma is a time-sensitive condition.[14] Transport of the trauma patient includes primary transport directly to the trauma centre, as well as secondary transport or retrieval from one healthcare facility to another for specialty services.

In most developed countries primary transportation of the injured patient is by road ambulance or helicopter.[7] However, injured people are also transported via civilian vehicle [14-16] or via emergency services vehicles, such as police cars,[17] from the scene.

The mortality associated with each modality of transport is widely debated. Victims of gunshot wounds (GSWs) in Germany and the USA had preferable outcomes when transported via either private or police vehicle when compared with those transported via EMS.[15,16] Similarly, the relative merits of ground-based versus helicopter EMS are controversial.[18] Although evidence is mixed, the benefits of helicopter transport appear to have greater evidence.[19,20]

Secondary transfer of trauma patients between healthcare facilities can occur via ground or air EMS. Air EMS is either helicopter or fixed wing depending on available services, distance and weather conditions. Secondary transfer of an injured person may occur for clinical reasons, such as specialist availability, the requirement for higher levels of care, or for non-clinical reasons such as bed availability. Factors that can influence the choice of transport vehicle for the trauma patient include:

- Nature of trauma
- Possible clinical impact of the transport environment
- Urgency of intervention
- Distances involved
- Number of retrieval personnel and volume of accompanying equipment
- Road transport times and road conditions
- Weather conditions and aviation restrictions
- Aircraft landing facilities
- Range and speed of vehicle.[5,21]

General principles related to the transport of critically ill and injured patients are covered in Chapter 23.

Trauma reception

Reception of the trauma patient at the emergency department (ED) is generally performed by the triage nurse, with patients managed in designated resuscitation areas and received by a trauma team.[7] In the severely injured patient, a multidisciplinary team receives the patient and commences assessment and treatment concurrently. In a mass-casualty incident, triage may be performed in the field. Despite documented benefits, such as shorter ED time, ED to computed tomographic imaging time, ED to operating room time and improved survival, having a trauma team is not universal, even within advanced trauma systems.[22]

In the ED, the trauma team receives the patient after a comprehensive, clear handover that is heard by the entire team. The importance of a handover from the paramedics cannot be overestimated.[23]

The formal process of triage provides a means of categorising patients based on threat to life, including rapid, standardised initial assessment and prioritisation. Although there are many different triage systems in use the most commonly used ones are the Manchester Triage Scale (MTS), the Canadian Triage Assessment Scale and the Australasian Triage Score (ATS).[24] The Canadian Triage Assessment Scale and the ATS are similar as they both use a time-to-treatment objective scale, while the MTS is an algorithm-based approach to decision making involving the selection from one of over 50 algorithms.[25] See Chapter 23 for further description of the ATS.

The triage nurse may be the first health care professional with contact with the family/next of kin. Consideration should be given to appropriate communication and meeting their needs.

Trauma teams

The purpose of the trauma team is to provide a coordinated and collaborative approach by relevant specialists to the injured patient in a designated resuscitation area. Despite the perceived benefits of having a trauma team they are not available in all hospitals. Some hospitals have developed two- or three-tiered activation criteria that incorporate information such as haemodynamic parameters, mechanism of injury, injuries sustained and age.[7] The pre-notification of arrival by the EMS and activation of the trauma team is an essential component of a well-organised trauma system (Table 24.1).[26] The trauma team consists of different members of specialty units such as emergency medicine, surgery, nursing, anaesthesia, intensive care and support staff, who all contribute to the assessment and management of the patient.[5,7,21] The efficiency of the team in undertaking resuscitation of the trauma victim may be influenced by the size of the team,[27] with some evidence suggesting that larger teams take longer to achieve key tasks.

The trauma team leader is responsible for overseeing the resuscitation of the injured person, including formulating a definitive plan and ensuring that additional investigations are undertaken. There are several elements that can affect the team's efficiency as well as clinical outcomes and as such the team leader role should include:

- Preparing the team
- Receiving handover
- Directing the team and responding to information
- Debriefing the team
- Talk with the patient's family/friend.[5,27]

Primary survey

Priorities of care are similar to those in all health settings and often based on Advanced Trauma Life Support (ATLS) principles outlined by the American College of Surgeons (see Chapter 23). The components of care will often occur simultaneously rather than sequentially and are designed to identify immediately life-threatening injuries, and treat them in a prioritised sequence, based on the patient's physiology at the time.[5]

TABLE 24.1
Criteria for activation of trauma team

PHYSIOLOGICAL CRITERIA	INJURY CRITERIA	MECHANISM	OTHER
Respiratory rate <10 or >30 per min	Penetrating injuries	Ejected from vehicle	Pregnancy
Systolic BP <100 mmHg (<75 mmHg for child)	Amputation	Fall >3 m	Age <16/>55
Oxygen saturation <90%	Suspected spinal injury	Explosion	Significant comorbidity
GCS <13	Burns >20%	Pedestrian impact >30 kph	All inter-hospital transfers
	Pelvic fracture	Prolonged extrication time	
	Significant injuries involving more than one body region		

Adapted from
Cameron P. Trauma. In: Cameron P, Jelinek G, Kelly A-M et al, editors. Textbook of adult emergency medicine. 4th ed. Elsevier; 2015, p. 71-162, Table 3.1.1.
Victoria T. Trauma Victoria: major trauma guidelines & education – Victorian State Trauma System. Victoria: Victorian Department of Health; 2018. Available: http://trauma.reach.vic.gov.au.

The evaluation of patients after trauma must be rapid, systematic and organised, and include:

- airway with cervical spine precautions
- breathing
- circulation with control of external haemorrhage
- disability, including brief neurological assessment
- exposure/environment, including prevention of hypothermia when removing clothing
- prevention of complications or further compromise.

Adjuncts used in the primary survey include continuous ECG monitoring, pulse oximetry, carbon dioxide (CO_2) monitoring (if indicated), and arterial blood gases (ABGs).[5]

Compromise to airway and breathing may result from direct injury, for example to the trachea, or indirectly through decreased level of consciousness. Compromise to circulation is usually a result of significant blood loss although it may occur as a result of injuries, such as cardiac contusions in chest trauma, or the patient's preexisting disease.

Secondary survey

Following primary survey and stabilisation of the life-threatening problems, patients should undergo a secondary survey (see Chapter 23). This is a systematic examination of the body regions to identify injuries that have not yet been recognised. It is essential that both the front and the back of the patient, as well as areas covered by clothing, are examined during this process. Consideration of the patient's history, both past medical history and mechanism of injury, if known, is important during the secondary survey.[5] Adjuncts to the secondary survey include diagnostic tests, such as additional X-rays, computed tomography (CT) scans, or angiography.

Tertiary survey

A tertiary survey should be conducted upon the arrival of trauma patients in the ICU, or soon after. The purpose of this third survey is to identify injuries that have not yet been detected, assess initial response to treatment and plan assessment and management strategies for future care.

The tertiary survey consists of another head-to-toe physical examination, assessment of the patient's condition in the context of his/her earlier condition and the treatment that has been administered, a full review of all diagnostic information gained so far, and acquisition of the patient's past health history if available. A systematic approach minimises the number of injuries that are not identified during the first 24 hours of care. It is also important to repeat the tertiary survey after the patient regains consciousness and begins to mobilise. Joint injuries may only become apparent during weight-bearing movements.

Radiological and other investigations

Initial radiological investigations will usually be performed in the ED using portable equipment. A radiographer is often a member of the trauma team that is activated on notification of the imminent arrival of a trauma patient. Radiological investigation is dependent on the type of injury sustained, but generally consists of an X-ray of the injured area/s if these include the chest, cervical spine or pelvis. Other X-rays at this stage are rarely beneficial, or rarely change the course of treatment.

If the patient is sufficiently stable after the secondary survey, more extensive investigation in the radiology department should be undertaken. This will include CT scans. It is essential that clinicians consider investigations carefully, to ensure that all necessary imaging is undertaken; for example, where a CT scan of the brain is required it is often prudent to also undertake a CT scan of the cervical spine. However, care should be taken to avoid investigations that will not change the planned treatment but may delay urgent interventions such as surgery. Required investigations will depend on the examinations undertaken as part of the secondary survey, the treatment that has already been administered and the current condition of the patient.

Furthermore, there may be significant implications of moving the patient on and off imaging tables for repeated imaging. The patient should be accompanied and monitored by appropriately skilled multidisciplinary clinicians during all transfers for investigation.

Focused assessment with sonography for trauma

Where abdominal trauma is suspected, a focused assessment with sonography for trauma (FAST) examination[28] is likely to be used as part of the secondary survey to determine whether free fluid is present in the abdominal cavity. The FAST exam is not designed to detect solid organ injuries, or injuries to the intestine, mesentery, diaphragm, or any retroperitoneal haemorrhage that may be associated with pelvic fractures; however, it has been shown to have a 73%–99% sensitivity when examining for free fluid.[28]

The abdomen is scanned in four zones:

- pericardial
- Morison's pouch (right upper quadrant, between the liver and kidney)
- splenorenal (left upper quadrant/perisplenic space, blood will usually collect around the spleen) and
- pelvis (the pouch of Douglas/rectovesicular space, blood usually pools behind the bladder).

A FAST scan generally takes 1–2 minutes when performed by an experienced, credentialled clinician. Findings are regarded as positive (fluid [blood] observed), negative or equivocal. Technical difficulties can be experienced with obese patients.[28] While a positive FAST is useful in identifying if a patient should receive urgent surgical intervention, a negative FAST does not rule out significant abdominal trauma. The FAST exam can produce a false positive result, particularly if there is misinterpretation of fluid-filled bowel as free fluid, or a false negative result if the scan is performed soon after the injury and the volume of free fluid is small.[28] Where a patient is undergoing a prolonged trauma resuscitation phase, there may be an indication to repeat the FAST after 20 minutes. The National Institute for Health and Care Excellence (NICE) released guidelines in 2016 recommending that FAST be omitted entirely if the patient is going to have CT imaging which is a more sensitive and specific test for intraabdominal injury; however, taking an unstable patient to the CT scan can result in catastrophe and delays in definitive management, in which case diagnosis should include physical examination, FAST and any radiographical imaging if time allows.[29] Diagnostic peritoneal lavage (DPL) is indicated when other methods of investigation (FAST, CT) are not available.[30]

Over recent years the extended focused assessment with sonography for trauma (E-FAST) has evolved in some EDs to evaluate the chest for either a pneumothorax or haemothorax, with reported sensitivity between 47% and 98%; however, the gold standard for evaluation of these injuries remains the CT scan.[31]

Common clinical presentations

Trauma generally occurs to a specific area of the body (e.g. the chest or the head) or consists of an injury caused by a specific external cause (e.g. burns). This section has been arranged according to these specific types of injury, including skeletal, chest, abdominal and burns. Specific considerations relating to penetrating injuries have been covered separately, although the majority of care for patients with penetrating injuries will follow the principles of the area of injury. For example, a patient with a penetrating injury of the abdomen will generally be cared for in the same way as all patients with abdominal trauma.

Patients with multi/poly-trauma will also be cared for according to the principles of care for each specific injury, although consideration of priorities is essential. Care should follow the common principles of airway, breathing and circulation as developed by the American College of Surgeons over 30 years ago,[5] hence concentrating on respiratory and circulatory compromise first, before the treatment of other injuries. The relative importance of other injuries, for example neurological trauma or skeletal trauma, will vary for each individual patient and will be dependent on the physiological impact of the injuries. Neurological and spinal cord injury are reviewed in Chapter 17.

Mechanism of injury

Mechanism of injury describes how energy from an external force is transferred to a person resulting in physical injury. Kinetic energy is energy in motion and can be classified as blunt or penetrating. The principles of kinetic energy associated with blunt trauma are generally those of acceleration and deceleration forces that can lead to shearing or compression injuries, while penetrating injury is proportional to the velocity of the object striking tissue and the associated energy dissipation leading to either permanent or temporary cavitation.[5] In addition to kinetic energy, there is thermal energy in the form of chemical agents, cold, heat and radiation. Injuries are also commonly classified based on intentionality. Unintentional injuries result typically from road traffic injuries, falls, fire and burn injuries, poisoning and drowning. Intentional injuries result from interpersonal violence (assault), suicide, and collective violence (war).[32]

The most common mechanisms of injury are either blunt or penetrating injury. The third, less common mechanism of injury is blast injury, usually as a result of explosions that can be related to industrial or recreational accidents or terrorist acts. The mechanisms of blast injuries include:

- primary blast injury – blast overpressure reaches the person and transmitted forces exert their effects on the body, causing direct tissue damage
- secondary blast injury – created by debris that is physically displaced by the blast overpressure
- tertiary blast injury – caused when the person is physically displaced by the force of the peak overpressure and blast winds leading to blunt traumatic injuries being sustained
- quaternary blast injury – miscellaneous blast injuries caused directly by the explosion including injuries such as burns, toxic substance exposure
- quinary blast injury – a hyperinflammatory state manifested by hyperpyrexia, diaphoresis, low central venous pressure (CVP) and positive fluid balance.[33]

The mechanism of injury is recognised as affecting both survival and requirements for admission to ICU.

Generic principles of management of the injured patient

Nursing care of trauma patients is characterised by the need to integrate practices directed towards limiting the impact of the injury, and healing injuries to multiple body areas in a complex process. The delivery of critical care services in a coordinated, multidisciplinary approach. This section outlines the principles of care relevant to all trauma patients, including positioning, mobilisation and damage-control resuscitation.

Positioning and mobilisation

Positioning and mobilisation can be a significant challenge, especially in those patients with multiple injuries that create competing needs. Positioning refers to the alignment and distribution of the patient in the bed, for example supine, Fowler, semi-recumbent or prone. In addition to these fundamental nursing postures, there is positioning of the limbs (i.e. elevated arms and legs). Mobilisation refers to the movement of joints by the patient, to shift from one place to another. This movement may be restricted to rolling within the bed, or moving out of the bed.

The principles of positioning and mobilisation are generally not different from those in other critically ill patients, and should incorporate the need to:

- promote the patient's comfort
- maintain the patient's and staff members' safety
- prevent complications
- facilitate delivery of care.

Difficulty in positioning and mobilisation is often experienced when there is concern for the stability of the patient's spine, in particular the cervical spine in the unconscious patient. Specific protocols such as the NEXUS criteria and the Canadian C-Spine Rule[34] are used for confirming the absence of injury to the cervical spine. These tools only evaluate the neck and depending on injury mechanism and patient assessment, motion restriction of the rest of the spine may be required. Patients are considered to be at extremely low risk of cervical spine injury if the following criteria are met:

- no midline cervical spine tenderness
- no focal neurological deficit
- no evidence of intoxication
- no painful distracting injuries
- no altered mental status.[35]

For patients who exhibit any of the above criteria, a clinical examination is unreliable and radiographic assessment is advised. The debate continues as to whether these protocols should be used in any patient who is unconscious, intoxicated or complaining of cervical soreness or abnormal neurology. The following principles should be incorporated into confirming the presence or absence of injury:[35,36]

- Obtain a detailed history of the injury wherever possible, including specific investigation of mechanisms of injury that might exert force on the cervical spine. A high index of suspicion should remain, particularly in the setting of injuries often associated with cervical spine injury, including craniofacial trauma, rib fractures, pneumothoraces and damage to the great vessels and/or trachea.
- Undertake plain X-rays of the full length of the spine, interpreted by a radiologist.
- Where any abnormality exists in clinical or radiological assessment, or the patient remains unconscious, a CT or MRI may be undertaken, and this must be reported by a radiologist.
- A correctly fitted rigid collar should remain in place only until the patient is appropriately reviewed and the chance of a cervical spine injury is eliminated. If a rigid collar is required for more than 4 hours, a semi-rigid collar e.g. Philadelphia, should be used.
- Maintain appropriate pressure area care to areas under the rigid collar as well as the usual pressure points until cervical clearance is gained.[23,37,38]

The practice of maintaining a patient in a rigid collar for days without active attempts to gain cervical clearance should be avoided at all costs. Adverse events of rigid cervical collars include:

- increased intra-cranial pressure related to pressure on neck veins
- unnecessary movement of unstable fractures that can occur with the fitting and application of a collar, discomfort and pain
- pressure injuries and tissue necrosis
- restricting mouth opening

TABLE 24.2
Spinal precautions[36]

ACTION	RATIONALE	AIM	METHOD
Head hold	To maintain the cervical spine in a neutral position during any position change	To prevent flexion, extension and lateral head tilting during any movement	1 Nurse holds head from head of bed – the head is held firmly by placing one hand around the patient's jaw with fingers spread to cup the jaw and hold the endotracheal tube as necessary. The forearm is used to support the side of the head 2 Nurse holds head from side of bed – nurse stands on side of bed that the patient will be rolled towards. One hand is placed firmly under the patient's occiput. Ensure nurse is in a position to support the weight of the head. The other hand holds the jaw and endotracheal tube as necessary. The patient is rolled onto the forearm of the nurse holding the head, which completes the biomechanical support for the head thus immobilising the cervical spine during the rolling
Log roll	To maintain the entire spine in anatomical alignment position during any position change	To prevent rotational torsion on the spinal column by minimising twisting of the craniocervical, cervicothoracic and thoracolumbar junctions of the spinal column	The patient is rolled in one smooth motion with assistants supporting the shoulder and pelvic girdles. Another assistant supports the legs so the patient moves in one plane The patient is rolled in one smooth motion with the nurse holding the head issuing the command to start and stop the manoeuvre

- difficulty swallowing, airway compromise and aspiration.[39]

The two methods available for moving the trauma patient are staff manual handling and lifting hoists. Generally, trauma patients can be log-rolled as frequently as required for nursing care (Table 24.2). Any restrictions to patient positioning and weight bearing due to injuries or physiological status must be considered through this process; it is essential that care be taken to prevent any worsening of injuries due to handling of the patient. Although the benefits of immobilisation of the cervical spine have not been demonstrated through research, it is a practice that is supported by years of cumulative trauma and triage clinical experience[37] and should be used to prevent worsening of injuries. Knowledge of the position restrictions for each limb, including all weight-bearing joints and the vertebrae, is imperative to avoid secondary iatrogenic injury. Certain injuries will impose position and mobility restrictions (Table 24.3).

Damage-control resuscitation

Uncontrolled posttraumatic bleeding is the leading cause of potentially preventable death, accounting for up to 40% of deaths related to trauma in the civilian setting.[40] In the last decade resuscitation of the haemorrhaging patient has undergone significant changes resulting in the concept of damage-control resuscitation (DCR). DCR refers to management bundles for resuscitation designed to rapidly identify the sources of bleeding, followed by immediate interventions to minimise blood loss, restore tissue perfusion and achieve haemodynamic stability.[41] DCR starts pre-hospital and continues intra-hospital through the emergency room, operating room and the ICU.

Pre-hospital time should be minimised and trauma patients in haemorrhagic shock should be transported directly to a hospital in a trauma system for surgical interventions.[41] The use of tourniquet is recommended on uncontrolled arterial bleeding from crushed extremity injuries, traumatic amputations, penetrating injuries and blast injuries and should be left in place until surgical control of the bleeding has been achieved.[42] Adequate ventilation, oxygenation and patent airway is of essence and normoventilation is recommended with a $PaCO_2$ of 5.0–5.5 kPa (35–40 mmHg) to avoid vasoconstriction, decreased cerebral blood flow and impaired tissue perfusion. Only in imminent cerebral herniation should hyperventilation-induced hypercapnia be used.[42] Intravenous morphine is recommended to be the first-line analgesic; the dose should be adjusted as needed to achieve adequate pain relief.[41,43]

Aggressive fluid replacement to maintain tissue oxygenation in haemorrhaging patients has been found to increase the hydrostatic pressure on wounds, dislodge blood clots, cause dilution of coagulation factors and hypothermia in the traumatised patient. To avoid the adverse effects of early aggressive volume replacement, DCR aims to achieve a lower than normal blood pressure called 'permissive hypotension'.[41] A target systolic blood pressure (SBP) of 80–90 mmHg is recommended, not as an end point but until surgical control of the

TABLE 24.3
Position and mobility restrictions in trauma patients

TYPE OF INJURY	RESTRICTIONS
Traumatic brain injury	• Nurse head up 15–30° • Side-lying as tolerated • Full tilt on bed if cervical spine not yet cleared of injury • Occasionally nursed flat if ICP problematic
Facial trauma	• Generally nurse in head-elevated position to reduce swelling, using either full bed tilt or back rest elevation
Chest trauma	• Nurse in varying positions from semi-Fowler to side-lying • Postural drainage (head down) usually beneficial if not contraindicated by other injuries (e.g. head or facial)
Abdominal trauma	• Nurse in varying positions from semi-Fowler to side-lying • Preferable to have some degree of hip flexion when lying supine to reduce abdominal suture line tension
Pelvic trauma	• Position restrictions are dependent on severity of fracture(s), use of external fixateurs and degree of stabilisation • Some patients may sit out of bed and ambulate with external pelvis fixateur in situ • Position restrictions require regular review, as changed or loss of fixation may affect recovery
Extremity trauma	• Significant position restrictions may include limb elevation, avoidance of side-lying or limited movement

ICP = intracranial pressure.

haemorrhage is obtained. In patients with severe TBI (GCS ≤8) and spinal injuries, permissive hypotension is contraindicated as an adequate perfusion pressure is essential for tissue oxygenation of the injured central nervous system (CNS). In these patients, a mean arterial blood pressure (MAP) above 80 mmHg should be maintained.[44] In acute life-threatening situations when blood pressure cannot be maintained by adequate volume resuscitation, vasopressors may also be required to maintain targeted arterial pressure. If the patient continues to have a poor response to fluid resuscitation cardiac dysfunction should be suspected and assessed promptly.[41]

The principles of DCR include:[45]

- minimisation of isotonic crystalloid
- permissive hypotension
- transfusion of a balanced ratio of blood products
- goal-directed correction of coagulopathy.

Upon admission to the hospital the initial assessment should focus on the bleeding using a combination of patient's physiological status, mechanism of injury, anatomical injury severity and the patient's response to initial DCR. The following bundle is used intra-hospital through the emergency room, operating room and the ICU.

Intra-hospital bundle[41]

- Full blood count, prothrombin time, fibrinogen, calcium, viscoelastic testing, lactate and/or base deficit and pH assessed within the first 15 minutes and monitored
- Immediate intervention applied in patients with haemorrhagic shock and an identified source of bleeding unless initial resuscitation measures are successful
- Immediate further investigation undertaken using FAST, CT or immediate surgery if massive intraabdominal bleeding is present in patients presenting with haemorrhagic shock and an unidentified source of bleeding
- Damage-control surgery applied if shock or coagulopathy are present
- DCR concept continued until bleeding source is identified and controlled
- Restrictive erythrocyte transfusion strategy (haemoglobin 7–9 g/dL).

Coagulopathy

About one-third of all bleeding trauma patients show signs of early acute coagulopathy upon arrival to hospital. These patients have a significant increase in multiple organ failure and death in comparison to patients with similar injuries in the absence of coagulopathy.[41] Early acute coagulopathy resulting from a combination of tissue injury, bleeding-induced shock, inflammatory changes and the activation of anticoagulant and fibrinolytic pathways is displayed in Fig. 24.1. The severity of the coagulopathy is affected by environmental and clinical interventions that result in or contribute to hypothermia, dilution from transfusion of crystalloids and blood products, acidosis, hypoperfusion and coagulation factor consumption. Brain injury and pre-hospital fluid administration is known to modify coagulopathy in addition to individual patient-related factors including age, genetic background, underlying disease and premedication such as oral anticoagulants and antiplatelet agents.[41]

Standard coagulation monitoring includes prothrombin time, activated partial thromboplastin time (APTT), platelet counts and fibrinogen. The international normalised ratio (INR) should be included in the measurement and repeated as required. Fibrinogen is the first coagulation factor to reach a critical low concentration

FIGURE 24.1 Schematic drawing of the factors, both preexisting and trauma related, that contribute to traumatic coagulopathy.

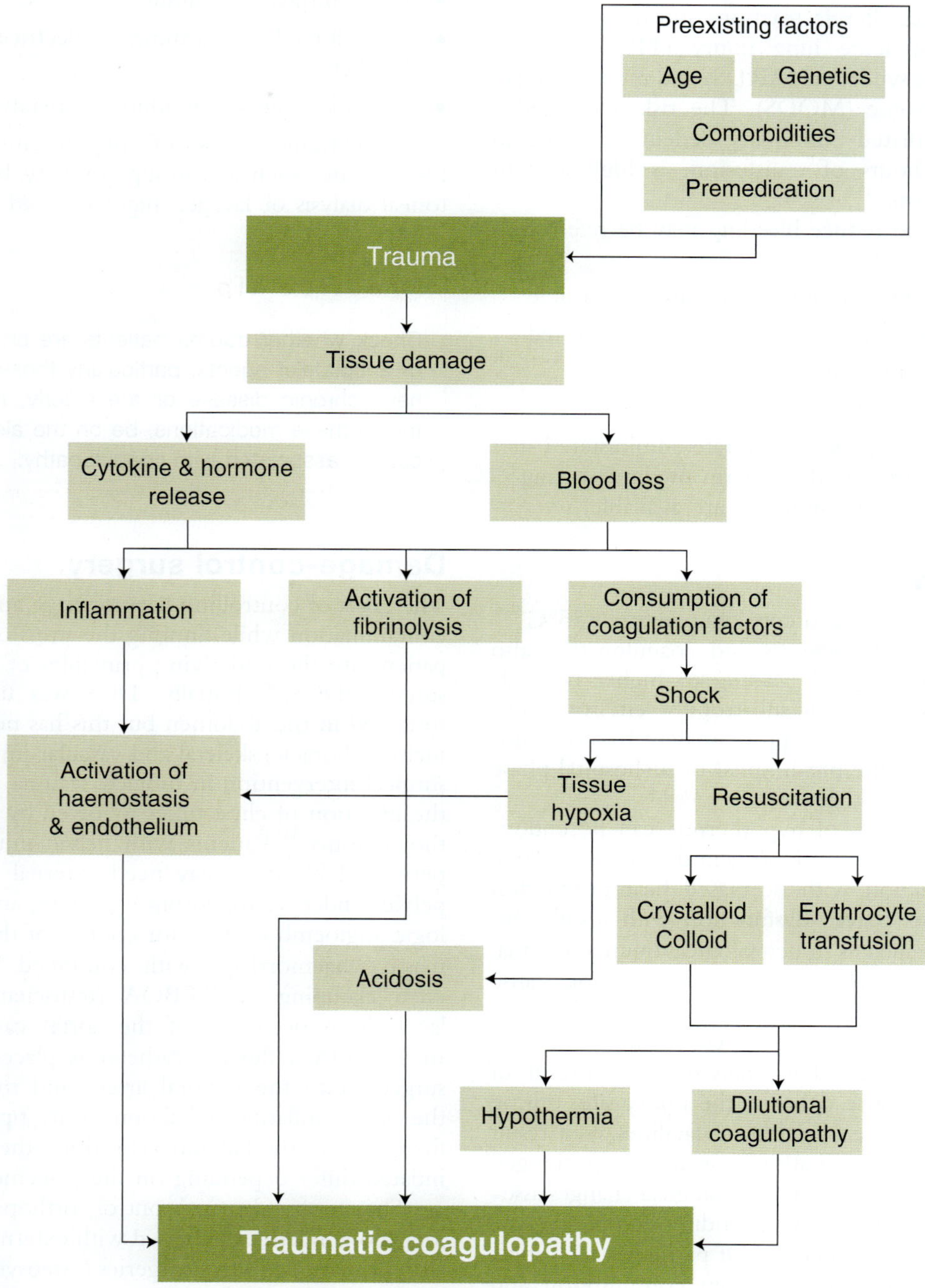

Reproduced from Rossaint R, Bouillon B, Cerny V et al. The European guideline on management of major bleeding and coagulopathy following trauma: fourth edition. Critical Care 2016;20:100.

during activation of coagulation in bleeding and studies have shown that early detection and prompt correction improve morbidity and mortality. Blood coagulation and fibrinolysis can be measured using traditional laboratories or a viscoelastic method (thrombelastography [TEG] or thromboelastometry [ROTEM]) preferably at bedside (point-of-care testing).[41]

Supplement of fibrinogen can be administered as fresh frozen plasma (FFP), cryoprecipitate, or fibrin concentrate.[45] Tranexamic acid prevents fibrinolysis and is recommended to be administered within 3 hours of injury.[46] Management of haemorrhage should be carefully monitored to ensure that blood transfusion is appropriate, as it is associated with significant risks, including overload, allergic reactions and trauma-related transfusion-related acute lung injury (TRALI), acute respiratory distress syndrome (ARDS) and multiple organ dysfunction syndrome (MODS). The risk for TRALI, inflammatory-mediated pulmonary oedema resulting in hypoxia within hours of transfusion, is highest with transfusion of plasma.[45]

Targeted care to reduce bleeding may be referred to as a *Coagulation bundle*:[41]

- Tranexamic acid administered as early as possible
- Acidosis, hypothermia and hypocalcaemia treated
- Fibrinogen maintained at 1.5–2 g/L
- Platelets maintained at >100 × 10^9/L
- Prothrombin complex concentrate administered in patients pre-treated with warfarin or direct-acting oral coagulants (until antidotes are available).

Hypothermia

Hypothermia is defined as a core temperature <35°C[47,48] and is associated with acidosis and coagulopathy, also known as the 'lethal triad' leading to higher morbidity and mortality. Even in sub-tropical environments, hypothermia is identified in approximately 10% of major trauma cases during the pre-hospital or in-hospital phase of care.[49,50]

Uncontrolled causes of hypothermia can be endogenous or accidental.[49,51,52] Endogenous causes include metabolic dysfunction with decreased heat production or central nervous system dysfunction with insufficient thermoregulation such as in neurological trauma. Dermal dysfunction, such as a burn, is another endogenous cause of hypothermia.

Accidental hypothermia can occur without thermoregulatory dysfunction, and generally occurs as a result of environmental exposure either at the injury site, during transport to, or between, healthcare facilities, as a result of aggressive fluid resuscitation[47] or during prolonged surgical procedures. The pathophysiological changes associated with hypothermia vary depending on the severity, and are outlined in Chapter 23. Of particular relevance, shivering leads to increased oxygen consumption and acidosis; platelet dysfunction leads to impaired clotting and fibrinolysis,[50,52] while haemorrhage reduces the circulating volume, which in turn may lead to a reduction in core body temperature and hypoperfusion of tissues. Hypoperfusion may cause hypoxia and subsequent production of lactic acid, which in turn slows the clotting cascade allowing haemorrhage to continue.[47] Studies have shown that these patients require more blood products and have an 80% increased risk of mortality.[41]

Measures to prevent and reduce hypothermia and the risk of hypothermia-induced coagulopathy include:

- removing wet clothing
- ensuring the patient is adequately covered to avoid additional heat loss
- warm intravenous fluids
- using forced air warming or electrical warming blankets
- increasing the surrounding temperature.

In extreme cases of hypothermia methods of re-warming, such as cardiopulmonary bypass and peritoneal dialysis or lavage, might be used.

> **Practice tip**
>
> Check whether trauma patients are on anticoagulant or antiplatelet agents, particularly those patients who have chronic disease or are elderly. If patients are taking these medications, be on the alert for complications associated with coagulopathy.

Damage-control surgery

The goals of controlling haemorrhage and prevention of contamination while limiting the stress of surgery to the patient are the underlying principles of damage-control surgery (DCS).[48] Initially, DCS was used for injuries sustained in the abdomen but this has now expanded to include thoracic, skeletal and vascular injuries.[53] The first surgical intervention in thoracic trauma with bleeding is the insertion of chest tubes followed by damage-control thoracotomy.[54] Patients with pelvic injuries and retroperitoneal bleeding may need external compression by pelvic binder, retroperitoneal packing and urgent radiologic angioembolisation for control of the bleeding.[55] In massive haemorrhage with continued bleeding, aortic cross clamping or REBOA (resuscitative endovascular balloon occlusion of the aorta) can be lifesaving. In REBOA a flexible catheter is placed by a vascular surgeon into the femoral artery and manoeuvred into the aorta, inflating a balloon at its tip to stop blood flow beyond the balloon. The times the balloon can be inflated differ depending on the placement.[56]

The term 'damage-control orthopaedics' includes long-bone fractures stabilised with external fixators rather than primary definitive surgeries (osteosynthesis) preventing patients from secondary procedure-related trauma. Definitive orthopaedic surgeries can be performed after 4 to 14 days when the patients have stabilised.[57]

Patients presenting with the following conditions are recommended for damage-control surgery:[41]

- Severely injured patients presenting with deep haemorrhagic shock, signs of ongoing bleeding and coagulopathy.
- Severely injured patients with coagulopathy, hypothermia (≤34°C), acidosis (pH ≤7.2), an inaccessible major venous injury with a need for

time-consuming procedures or concomitant injury outside the abdomen.

DCS consists of three stages. The first stage is a shortened resuscitative laparotomy for control of bleeding, control of contamination and restitution of blood flow. This is done rapidly and the abdomen is packed and temporarily closed, permitting angiographic embolisation if needed. The second stage is intensive care management including re-warming, correction of metabolic acidosis and coagulation disorders, optimising ventilation and haemodynamic status. To lower the risk of re-bleeding the removal of the packs is deferred for at least 48 hours. The third stage is the definite surgical repair that takes place when target physiological parameters have been achieved.[58]

Nursing a patient who undergoes DCS requires recognition of the principles and aims of the surgery, as well as flexibility in the care of the patient after the initial surgery but before definitive surgery. When the patient is admitted to the ICU postoperatively, the standard mechanisms for the treatment of hypothermia, acidosis and coagulopathy, as discussed above, should be implemented. After DCS, patients may also have an open abdomen with temporary dressings or skeletal fractures with external fixateurs in situ and may require multiple return trips to the operating room to achieve final closure.

Deep venous thrombosis (DVT) and pulmonary embolism (PE), collectively known as hospital-acquired venous thromboembolism (VTE) is a life-threatening complication with an incidence of up to 50% following multiple trauma related to immobility and the acute-phase response. PE is the third leading cause of death in those who survive beyond the third day. It is recommended that within 24 hours after bleeding has been controlled pharmacological thromboprophylaxis should be administered. This, in combination of the use of early mechanical thromboprophylaxis with intermittent pneumatic compression (IPC) or early mechanical thromboprophylaxis with anti-embolic stockings, may be applied.[41]

Skeletal trauma

Skeletal trauma involves injury to the bony structure of the body. Although skeletal injuries alone rarely result in the patient being admitted to critical care, damage to surrounding blood vessels and nerves, as well as potential complications such as fat embolism syndrome[59] and rhabdomyolysis, may cause the patient to become seriously ill. Patients with skeletal trauma who require admission to ICU include those with multiple injuries, severe pelvic fractures (often associated with significant blood loss), long bone fractures (often associated with fat embolism syndrome [FES]) and thoracic injuries such as flail segment. A small number of people with crush injuries that cause significant damage to muscles, often resulting in rhabdomyolysis, also require admission to the ICU.[60,61]

In Australia and the European Union approximately 50% of all trauma patients requiring admission to a hospital have fractures caused by falls and road traffic incidences.[62,63] More than 70% of all patients with major trauma need at least one surgical procedure, with survivors experiencing poor functional outcome or quality of life, especially those with lower limb injury.[60]

Pathophysiology

Bone is composed of an organic matrix as well as bone salts. The majority of the organic matrix is collagen fibres and the remainder is ground substance, a homogeneous gelatinous medium composed of extracellular fluid plus proteoglycans.[64,65] Calcium and phosphate are the primary ions in bone salts, although there are smaller amounts of magnesium, sodium, potassium and carbonate ions. These ions combine to form a crystal known as hydroxyapatite.

A fracture is simply defined as a break in the continuity of a bone and generally occur when there is force applied that exceeds the tensile or compressive strength of the bone. Fractures are classified as either complete or incomplete. A complete fracture is where the bone is broken all the way through, while incomplete fractures only involve part of the bone. Fractures are also classified according to the direction of the fracture line, and include linear, oblique, spiral and transverse fractures. Finally, fractures are classified as either open or closed, with those patients who sustain an open fracture having a higher risk of delayed healing or non-union compared with closed fractures. Loss of the haematoma that initiates the inflammatory phase of fracture healing and contamination leading to infection are causative influences behind delayed healing or non-union.[66]

A fracture causes disruption to the periosteum, blood vessels, marrow and surrounding soft tissue, resulting in a loss of mechanical integrity of the bone. When a fracture occurs, there is initial bleeding and soft tissue damage around the site, with haematoma formation within the medullary canal.[66] The healing sequence that follows a fracture depends on the type of fracture fixation that is used. When a fracture is fixed using a method that eliminates the interfragmentary gap and provides stability to the site, such as in screwing or wiring, primary healing takes place.[67] When a fracture is fixed in a manner that reduces but does not eliminate movement around the fracture site, secondary healing takes place.[67]

In primary healing, also referred to as direct union, the haematoma that initially formed is eliminated by the apposition of fracture ends during reduction. Once the bone ends are intact, osteoclasts form cutting cones that, in turn, form new haversian canals across the fracture gap.[64] These contain blood vessels that are essential to primary bone healing. By 5–6 weeks after the fracture, osteoblasts will fill the canals with osteons, which are the basic structure of the new bone. Although the bone is now formed, the strength and shape continues to develop over coming weeks. Clinical evaluation of whether a fracture has healed is based on both radiographic and clinical findings; however, associated injuries may confound the ability to use clinical criteria.[60,67]

In contrast to primary healing, secondary healing is characterised by an intermediate phase, where a callus of connective tissue is first formed and then replaced by bone.[64] The secondary healing phase begins with an inflammatory phase in which the haematoma clots and provides initial support, then inflammatory cells invade the haematoma to remove necrosed bone and debris. The reparative phase begins 1–2 weeks after the fracture and consists of immature woven bone being laid down and strengthened through a process known as mineralisation. The final remodelling stage consists of replacement of the woven bone by lamellar bone, through osteoblasts secreting osteoid that is mineralised and forms interstitial lamellae.[64] The remodelling of these structures occurs in response to appropriate levels of mechanical loading during this phase.[60]

Fat embolism

Fat embolism syndrome[66] may occur in patients who have experienced a fracture of a long bone, particularly if multiple fractures or fractures to the middle or proximal parts of the femur are experienced. Fractures to the pelvis can also lead to a fat embolism. Incidence of FES is low (<1%). FES consists of fat in the blood circulation associated with an identifiable pattern of clinical signs and symptoms that include hypoxaemia, neurological symptoms and a petechial rash.[61] Patients generally present 12–72 hours after they have experienced a relevant fracture and often require admission to a critical care unit for assessment and treatment, including mechanical ventilation.[68]

Internationally, there continues to be disagreement regarding the pathophysiological changes associated with FES, although there is general consensus on the following principles. It has been accepted that there is a mechanical component to the changes that take place in FES, where fat is physically forced into the venous system and causes physical obstruction of the vasculature.[68] Although marrow pressure is normally 30–50 mmHg, it can be increased up to 800 mmHg during intramedullary reaming (the process where the medullary cavity of the bone is surgically enlarged to fit a surgical implant such as a tibial nail), consequently reaching a pressure significantly above pressures throughout the vasculature.[68]

A second theory, associated with the biochemical changes that occur during trauma, proposes that trauma is associated with a higher level of circulating free fatty acids, which cause destabilisation of circulating fats and/or direct toxicity to specific tissues, including pulmonary and vascular endothelium.[68]

Rhabdomyolysis

Rhabdomyolysis is a potentially life-threatening condition and is caused by either acquired or inherited factors. Nine percent of cases occur as a result of trauma, 34% are due to substance abuse and 11% from medications.[69] Rhabdomyolysis is the breakdown of muscle fibres resulting in the distribution of the cellular contents of the affected muscle throughout the circulation, and occurs during the reperfusion of injured muscle. There are two phases of injury that are essential for the development of rhabdomyolysis: the first is when muscle ischaemia occurs and the second is with reperfusion of the injured muscle. The length of time that muscle is ischaemic affects the development of rhabdomyolysis, with periods of less than 2 hours generally not producing permanent damage whereas periods longer than 2 hours can result in irreversible anatomical and functional changes.[70] Presentation varies widely across patient groups and ranges from asymptomatic elevated creatinine kinase (CK) to life-threatening conditions with electrolyte disturbances, cardiac arrhythmias, acute renal failure and disseminated intravascular coagulation (DIC).[69,71]

Clinical manifestations

Common forms of skeletal trauma include the following:

- Long bone fractures – the long bones are the humerus, radius, ulna, femur, tibia and fibula. Fractures of these bones can carry a high level of morbidity, especially if they involve a joint such as a trimalleolar fracture of the ankle (distal tibia and fibula). In many cases definitive surgical management is required, with internal fixation.
- Dislocations – all joints are at risk of traumatic dislocation, depending on the mechanism of injury. Dislocations can be limb-threatening if they cause neurovascular compromise. Reduction of traumatic dislocation is a medical emergency.
- Open fractures (compound) – any break in the skin that communicates directly with the fracture is classified as an open fracture. Open fractures carry a high infection risk; irrigation and debridement should be performed within 24 hours.[72]
- Traumatic amputation – amputation refers to an avulsion in which the affected limb or body appendage is completely separated from the body. This can occur when a digit or extremity is sheared off by either mechanical or severing forces, for example amputation of a thumb by a bandsaw. Traumatic amputations vary in severity and ongoing compromise, with a clean-cut amputation more likely to be successfully reattached than a crushed extremity. Criteria that inform the surgical decision-making process include: the amount of tissue loss; location on the body at the connection site; damage to underlying and surrounding tissues, bones, nerves, tendons/muscles and vessels; and condition of the amputated part.
- Fractures of the pelvis – the pelvis is the largest combined bony structure in the body and serves

FIGURE 24.2 The classification of pelvic fractures.

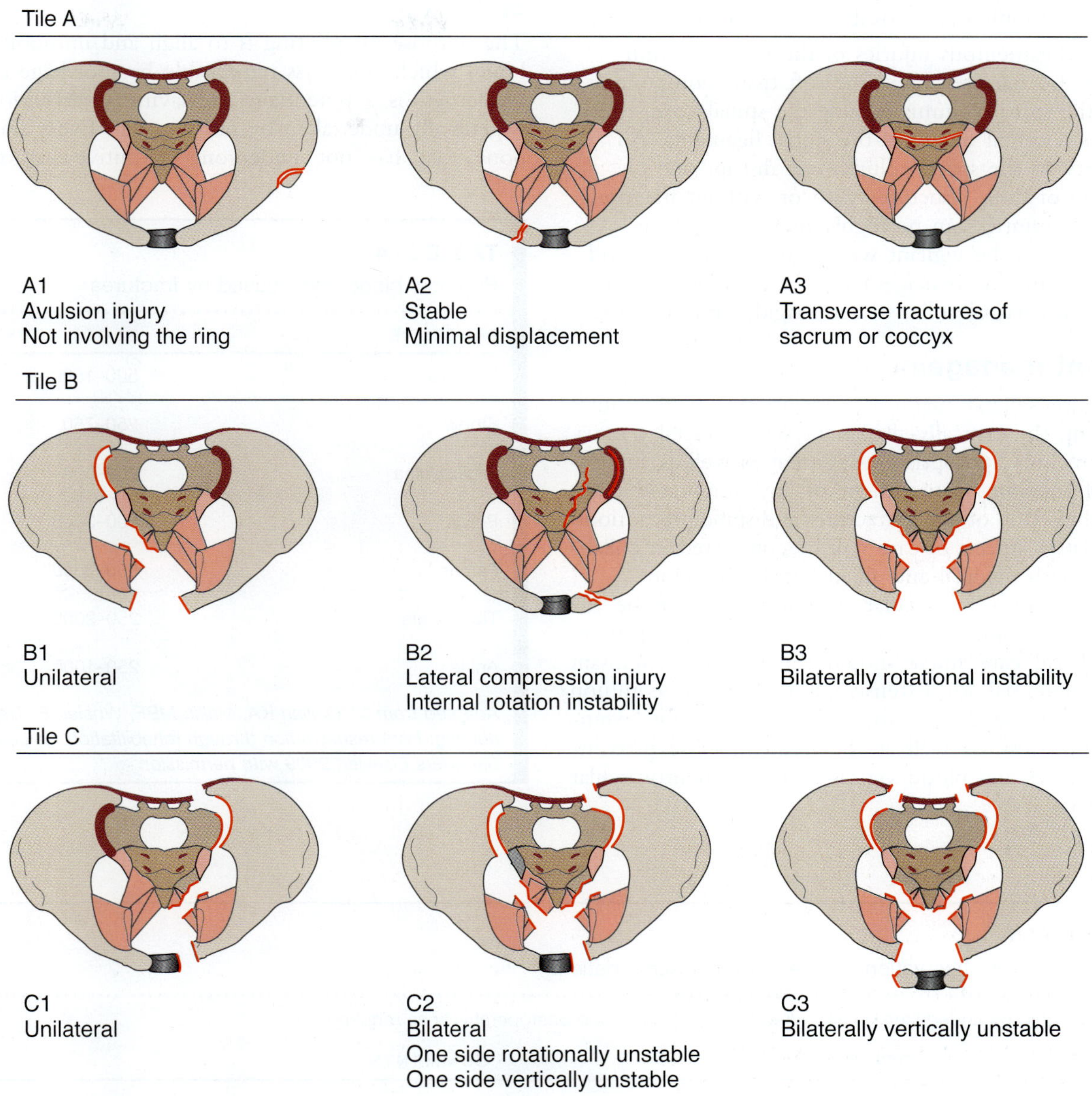

Ziran NM, Smith WR Pelvic fractures. In: Smith W, Stahel P, editors. Management of musculoskeletal injuries in the trauma patient. New York: Springer; 2014.
Gray A, Chandler H, Sabri O. Pelvic ring injuries: classification and treatment. Orthopaedics and Trauma 2018; 32(2): 80-90.

to provide an essential supporting framework for ambulation and protection of pelvic organs. Major blood vessels and nerves traverse the pelvic bones, supplying the lower limbs and pelvic organs. Therefore, injury to any part of the pelvis is serious. The three bones that comprise the pelvic ring are the two innominate bones (ilium and pubic rami) and the sacrum. Due to its reinforced structure, the amount of force required to fracture the pelvis is substantial. Fractures of the pelvis can affect one or both sides of the pelvis, and be stable or unstable. A variety of classification systems exist to describe the severity of pelvic fractures, the most common being the Tile classification (Fig. 24.2).

- Fractures of the spinal column (see also Chapter 17) – the spinal column includes all the bony components in the cervical, thoracic and lumbar vertebral regions. Fractures of the vertebra are common in trauma patients, but the actual incidence of fracture without spinal cord injury in multitrauma patients is not well described. Not all fractures cause vertebral column instability with the subsequent risk of spinal cord damage. A spinal column fracture will be diagnosed as mechanically stable or unstable and this will affect the positioning and possible activity of the patient.

- Discoligamentous injuries of the spinal column (see also Chapter 17) – the soft tissue components of the spinal column include the spinal cord, the intervertebral discs and the spinal ligaments. An injury to the spinal column can disrupt one or more of these structures with or without fracture. These injuries can be highly unstable, and the nurse must be vigilant with spinal precautions and the fitting and management of the patient requiring a rigid cervical collar or semi-rigid cervical collar.

Patient management

There are several major considerations for the nurse managing the critically ill patient with skeletal trauma. These include appropriate assessment as well as application of traction, management of any amputated parts, and stabilisation of pelvic fractures and spine precautions. These latter aspects of care will be conducted in collaboration with medical and allied health colleagues.

Bones are very vascular structures and can be the cause of substantial blood loss in the trauma patient. The critical care nurse should therefore be cognisant of the potential for extensive blood loss in common fractures (Table 24.4). Given the potential for extensive blood loss, as well as the frequent close proximity of nerves and blood vessels to bones, neurovascular assessment of the patient with skeletal trauma is essential (Table 24.5).

Splinting

The purpose of splinting is to align and immobilise the bone, which alone has remarkable haemorrhage control properties, is a potentially life-saving intervention and is generally undertaken by nursing staff. Every fractured bone that has not undergone definitive orthopaedic

TABLE 24.4
Potential blood loss caused by fractures

FRACTURE	BLOOD LOSS (ML)
Humerus	500–1500
Elbow	250–750
Radius/ulna	250–500
Pelvis	500–3000
Femur	500–3000
Tibia/fibula	250–2000
Ankle	250–1000

Adapted from McQuillan KA, Makic MBF, Whalen E. Trauma nursing: from resuscitation through rehabilitation. St Louis: Saunders Elsevier; 2009 with permission

TABLE 24.5
Neurovascular observations of the skeletal trauma patient

Note: should be undertaken on all injured limbs both pre- and postoperatively as required

OBSERVATION	PROCESS	COMMENTS
Skin colour	State the skin colour of the area inspected as it compares with the unaffected part NB: distal limb pulses may be difficult to palpate in the injured limb; a warm pink limb is a perfused limb	Pink: normal perfusion Pale: reduced perfusion Dusky, purple or cyanotic discolouration: usually indicating significantly reduced perfusion Demarcated: a distinct line where the skin colour changes to dusky (usually follows the vessel path)
Skin temperature to touch	State the ambient temperature of the skin to touch as it compares with normally perfused skin at room temperature	Normal: not discernibly cold to touch Reduced skin temperature indicates reduced perfusion
Voluntary movement	The patient should be able to move the non-immobilised distal part of any injured limb (i.e. fingers and toes of a plastered limb)	It is important to assess range of motion where that is possible, provided this will not aggravate the injury. Reduced movement may indicate compromise to either the nerve or blood supply to the limb
Sensation	The patient should be able to report normal sensation to touch	Sensation should be assessed in nerve distributions (i.e. all fingers and toes). Reduced sensation may indicate compromise to either the nerve or blood supply to the limb

management requires splinting. Examples of intermediate stabilisation of fractures include:

- Positioning of injured limbs – all patients who have a splint in situ may need to have it elevated to promote venous return and minimise tissue oedema. In the ICU the trauma patient will often be nursed flat, with the bed on tilt for a head-elevation position. In these circumstances, the injured dependent limb must be elevated on pillows. Care must be taken to ensure that elevation does not place pressure on any part of the limb; for example, a hand sack made from a pillowcase tied to an IV pole should not be used, as it places direct pressure on the path of the median nerve and can cause an iatrogenic neurapraxia.
- Wooden/air splints – are padded appliances that are strapped to the injured limb. Ideally, no patient should remain in wooden splints for longer than 4 hours, as pressure may build up on pressure points.
- Plaster backslab – limbs with fractures will often swell as a physiological response to injury; a plaster backslab composed of layered plaster of paris is the preferred treatment, as it accommodates swelling and can easily be loosened by nursing staff at any time of day. It is imperative that this be adequately padded within the limitations of providing structural support to the limb. Poorly made or ill-fitting backslabs can cause major complications, such as pressure sores or displacement of fractures.
- Traction – may be required as part of fracture management, and involves the application of a pulling force to fractured or dislocated bones. There are three types of traction:
  - skeletal, where traction pins are anchored into the bone (i.e. Steinmann pin)
  - skin, where the body is gripped, as in the use of slings and bandages
  - manual, applied by a clinician pulling on a body part, such as in the reduction of dislocation. It may also be applied to maintain the traction during such nursing care manoeuvres as log-rolling or repositioning of the traction.

The principles of traction are to achieve alignment of bones while preventing complications. Remember that incorrectly applied traction is painful and can exacerbate the injury. The following should guide management of the patient with traction:

1. The grip or hold on the body must be adequate and secure.
2. Provision for counter-traction must be made.
3. Minimise friction.
4. Maintain the line and magnitude of the pull, once correctly established.
5. Frequently check the apparatus and the patient to ensure that: 1) the traction set-up is functioning as planned; and 2) the patient is not suffering any injury as a result of the traction treatment.

Practice tip

No patient should remain in a wooden splint longer than 4 hours. Wooden splints must be changed to a resting backslab if prolonged splinting is required; this will maintain the injured limb in anatomical fracture alignment.

Traumatic amputations

Traumatic amputation is the separation of a limb or appendage from the body. During the pre-hospital phase any amputated body part should be wrapped in a clean or sterile (if available) cloth and placed in a plastic, waterproof bag inside an insulated cooler with ice. It is important that the ice does not come into direct contact with the amputated part. When managed using these principles, the amputated part may be viable for up to 6–12 hours before reattachment. Depending on any additional injuries, and the cardiovascular status of the patient, surgery for limb salvage will be scheduled as soon as possible.

Postoperative management will be guided by the type of surgery that was performed; specifically, whether or not amputation occurred. Principles of postoperative care include:

- appropriate positioning of the affected limb, usually based on surgical orders
- frequent neurovascular observations, particularly observing for reperfusion injury, which manifests as an acute compartment syndrome or vascular trashing of distal vessels from a clot
- implementing changes in treatment initiated in response to altered perfusion in a timely manner
- psychological support to assist the patient in dealing with the injury.

Practice tip

Where there are any signs of deterioration of the re-implanted part, communication should occur directly between the nursing staff and the surgical consultant to ensure timely implementation of changes to patient care to optimise salvage of the amputated part.

Practice tip

For patients with amputations, on arrival in the ED:

1. Inspect the amputated part.
2. Clean with 0.9% saline solution and return to a clean plastic bag wrapped in 0.9% saline-soaked gauze. Surround with ice in a thermal cooler.

FIGURE 24.3 Application of a pelvic binder.

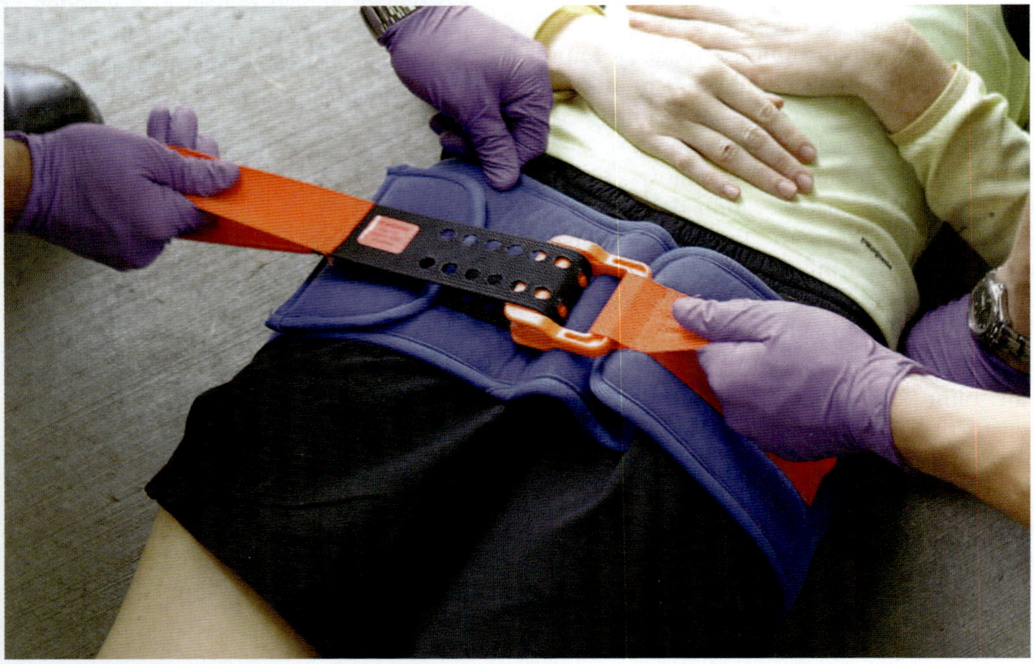

Courtesy Ferno Australia.

Pelvic stabilisation

Pelvic fractures occur in 5–16% of patients with blunt trauma and can be uncomplicated, requiring no surgical intervention, or they can be serious enough to be the primary cause of death from exsanguination.[73] The mortality rate from pelvic fracture ranges from 18% to 40% with death usually occurring within 24 hours of injury, frequently as a result of haemorrhage.[73] Appropriate assessment and management of pelvic fractures should encompass diagnostic evaluation, non-invasive pelvis stabilisation, abdominal evaluation, the requirement for surgical intervention and angiography.[74]

The initial management of the patient with a fractured pelvis involves assessment and splinting. Assessment should encompass the following two aspects:[75]

1. haemodynamic status – to identify signs of ongoing blood loss and determine fluid resuscitation requirements
2. stability of the pelvic ring – assessed via clinical examination and diagnostic imaging. Palpation and inspection of the anterior and posterior pelvis for signs of trauma, including tenderness in the conscious patient, is generally adequate.[75]

The orthopaedic surgeon may undertake further clinical assessments incorporating 'springing' of the pelvis, although it should be noted that this may aggravate the injury and cause additional bleeding. Nursing staff would not normally conduct such an assessment, unless under appropriate specialist guidance in a setting such as remote area trauma nursing or tele-health consultation.

Non-invasive pelvic binding, in the form of either a bedsheet or a proprietary pelvic binder, may make a significant impact on patient morbidity and mortality.[73,74] Such a manoeuvre will stabilise the pelvis and assist in approximating bleeding vessels, thereby assisting in haemostasis (Fig. 24.3).

Pelvic binders are temporary devices,[73-75] and ideally not left in situ for longer than 4 hours. If a patient is to remain in the binder longer than 4 hours, nursing staff must take care to minimise pressure. Conscious patients should be advised to report signs of increasing pressure, such as positional paraesthesia. Increasing abdominal swelling may indicate a need to reposition the binder. Position restrictions should be clarified by all members of the healthcare team, especially if the patient will be in the binder for a lengthy period. The patient may be able to be log-rolled and side-lie with a pelvic binder in situ. Release of a pelvic binder should be undertaken only with caution and as part of definitive care (e.g. within the operating theatre), with all relevant members (particularly the orthopaedic or trauma surgeon) of the healthcare team present.[75]

Invasive pelvic fixation uses an external fixateur (Fig. 24.4) to achieve pelvic stabilisation.[74,75] The application of an external bridging frame (either anterior or

FIGURE 24.4 External fixateur: pelvis.

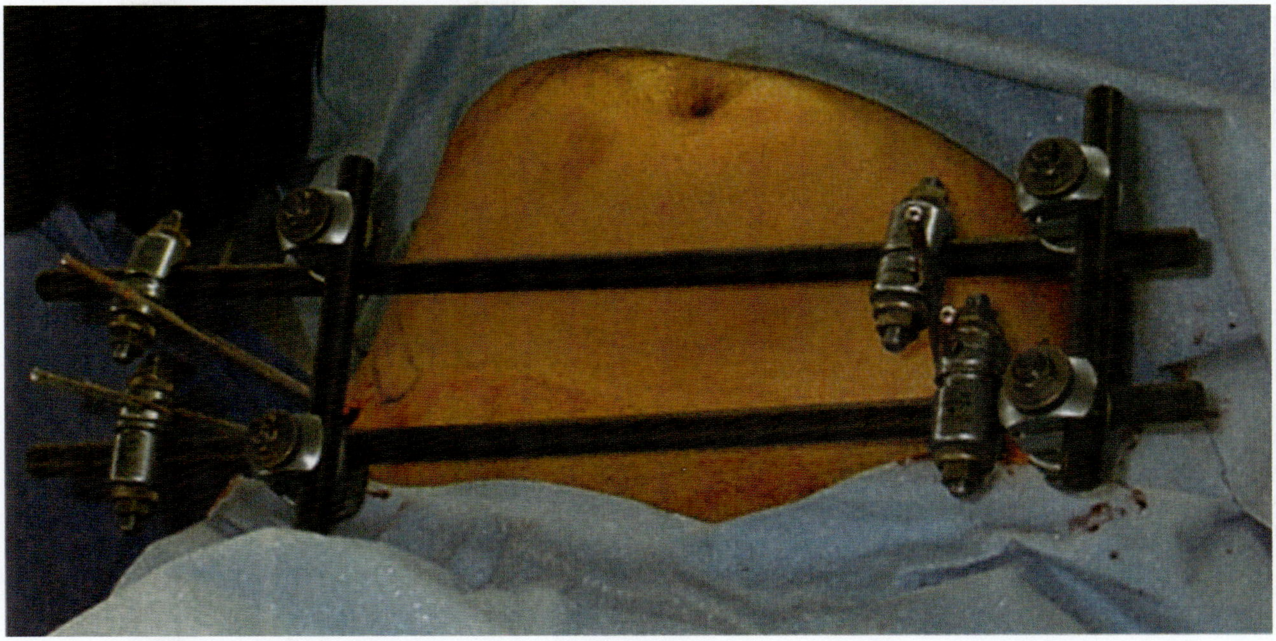

Source: Wiss DA. Master techniques in orthopaedic surgery: fractures. Wolters Kluwer; 2012.

posterior) to stabilise the pelvis may be an interim or definitive treatment measure that may be in situ for days or weeks. Patients in external fixation may be permitted to mobilise, although the extent of mobilisation will depend on the stability of the fracture. While the external fixateur is in place, the following nursing care is required:

- pin site care – usually cleaned with isotonic saline and left open unless there is a large amount of exudate, in which case the pin sites may be covered with dry absorbent dressing; care should be taken to identify gaping or stretched skin around the site, as this may require surgical intervention
- analgesia – based on patient reports of pain and taking into account planned activities such as mobilisation and physiotherapy
- mobilisation – based on stability of the pelvis, and in consultation with the surgeon
- patient education – particularly regarding the safety of the procedure and mobilisation and rehabilitation plans.

Pelvic embolisation involves interventional radiology to control haemorrhage in patients with pelvic fractures. Because of the large arteries that traverse the pelvis, arterial bleeding can be the cause of substantial blood loss in 10–20% of cases. The timing of embolisation, particularly in relation to stabilisation, remains controversial, and is dependent on the availability of appropriately trained staff and resources.[76]

Chest trauma

Chest trauma is recognised as a severe, potentially life-threatening form of injury that may require admission to critical care. In one review the higher the Abbreviated Injury Score (AIS) for thorax, the greater the likelihood that the injured patient will require admission to the intensive care, and intubation.[77]

Chest trauma represents approximately 10–15% of injuries that require admission to hospital[78] for more than 24 hours, with approximately 15% of those requiring admission to ICU.

In the severely injured patient approximately 50% will have an associated chest injury.[77] In 70–90% of patients who sustain a severe chest injury, associated injuries include the head, neck, spine, abdomen and limbs.[79]

Chest trauma is either blunt or penetrating in nature. The incidence of thoracic trauma varies, depending on the external cause of the injury and is reported to be 58–96% in those with blunt trauma,[21,80] often associated with road traffic crashes, work-related accidents, blast injuries in the military setting or mass terrorism.[78] The incidence of penetrating thoracic trauma is reported as between 4% and 41%.[80] Penetrating injuries can result in significant injury and are predominantly associated with knife-related crimes and GSWs, but can be associated with vehicle collisions and falls,[81] or as a result of blast injuries in which shrapnel is present.

The mortality rates for the injured person who sustains a chest injury is approximately 20–25% in those who survive to hospital,[21,82,83] which is likely related to the development of multi-organ failure[48] related to their thoracic injury.[78] Pre-hospital death is usually associated with injuries to the heart or major vessels.[84] Those who survive to hospital may still have life-threatening injuries that require immediate intervention and as such they require rapid assessment, diagnosis and treatment.[82]

Pathophysiology

The chest or thoracic cavity is made up of two structures; a bony cavity consisting of the ribs, sternum, scapulae and clavicles, and the muscular structure of the respiratory muscles and diaphragm. The organs contained in the chest include the lungs, airways, heart, blood and lymph vessels and oesophagus.

Chest trauma can be separated into injury to the thoracic structure, including the ribs and diaphragm; injury to the lung, airways and associated tissue; injury to the heart and associated tissue; or injury to the vascular or digestive system located in the chest. Physiological consequences of thoracic trauma are hypoxia, hypercarbia, and acidosis. Contusions, haematomas, and alveolar collapse, or changes in intrathoracic pressure related to injury can lead to hypoxia and metabolic acidosis. Hypercarbia is associated with insufficient ventilation and causes respiratory acidosis related to either changes in intrathoracic pressure relationships or by depressed levels of consciousness.[5] The other consequence is the combined effect on both the cardiovascular and respiratory functions due to hypovolaemia causing hypoperfusion and shock, generally related to blood loss.[78]

Chest trauma covers a broad array of injuries and severity, and ranges from relatively minor injuries (e.g. abrasions and fracture of a single rib) to major, immediately life-threatening injuries (e.g. cardiac rupture or tension pneumothorax).

Chest trauma includes the following:

- Rib fractures – a very common form of chest trauma, occurring in 10% of all trauma admissions,[82] often a source of severe pain and often associated with other injuries such as haemothorax, pneumothorax and pulmonary contusion.[5,84]
- Flail chest – occurs when a segment of the chest wall, usually as a result of multiple rib fractures, does not have bony continuity with the rest of the thoracic cage, resulting in a freely-moving section of the rib cage. It may also occur when there is costochondral separation of a single rib from the thorax.[5] In 80% of patients with a flail chest, ICU admission is required with >50% requiring mechanical ventilation.[2] The production of a flail segment is dependent on a number of factors, including the extent of adjacent soft tissue support. Usually such fractures occur in the anterior or lateral sections of the rib cage, where there is less muscle protection. The significant impact of this injury is paradoxical movement of the flail segment during spontaneous ventilation, so that when a patient inspires, the flail segment moves inwards with the negative intrapleural pressure instead of expanding with the rib cage.[84] In the mechanically ventilated patient this paradoxical movement may not be as evident.[2,84] Compromised respiratory function is caused by the increased work of breathing that this ineffective flail segment creates, as well as the contused lung that normally occurs underneath the flail segment[82] along with the severe pain and tenderness.[84]
- Diaphragmatic injuries – present in 1–6% of major thoracic injuries and generally occurs when there has been a significant rise in intraabdominal pressure,[83,84] usually with compression injuries. Diaphragmatic rupture occurs on the left side in three-quarters of cases. The right hemidiaphragm is thought to be congenitally stronger and protected by the liver.[5,83,84] When the rupture is sufficiently large, protrusion of the abdominal contents into the thoracic space is likely, resulting in respiratory compromise. Bilateral diaphragmatic injury is uncommon, with an incidence rate of approximately 5%.

Operations for other abdominal injuries may reveal a diaphragmatic tear, with the treatment being a direct repair.[5]

- Pulmonary contusion – bruising to the lung tissue, usually as a result of mechanical force.[7] This bruising is followed by diffuse haemorrhage and interstitial and alveolar oedema, resulting in impaired gas exchange due to shunting, and leading to hypoxia and increased oxygen requirements.[5,82–84] This injury is often associated with rib fractures; respiratory failure may develop over time rather than instantaneously.[5] Pulmonary contusions represents up to 75% of injured patients with significant blunt chest trauma. These contusions can be caused by motor vehicle accidents, high-velocity missile wounds or high-energy shock waves from explosions in the air and water.[84]
- Pneumothorax – the accumulation of air in the pleural space[2,5,84] which occurs with both blunt and penetrating mechanisms. A pneumothorax can be divided into three types: simple (or closed), communicating (or open) and tension. A simple or closed pneumothorax indicates that there is no communication with the atmosphere, and are generally caused by blunt chest trauma and result from a fractured rib puncturing the lung parenchyma; however, it may also occur when impact occurs at full inspiration and the glottis is closed, leading to increased intraalveolar pressure and subsequent rupture.[84] A communicating/open pneumothorax has an associated defect in the chest wall allowing air to flow in and out of the

wound.[82,84] This can also be described as a 'sucking chest wound'.[84]

Open pneumothoraces generally occur in the setting of penetrating trauma, where air is able to move from the external atmosphere to the pleural space during inspiration. If not all of the inspired air is able to escape during expiration, due to a tissue flap or similar obstruction covering the opening, the volume of the pneumothorax will gradually expand and cause collapse of the adjacent lung, with resultant hypoxaemia and hypercarbia.[5] Where air is not able to escape at all from the pleural space, this is referred to as a tension pneumothorax, and rapidly becomes a life-threatening event due to mediastinal displacement to the opposite side resulting in decreased venous return and compression of the opposite lung.[5,84]

With the use of imaging modalities such as CT scan, the phenomenon of occult pneumothorax (pneumothorax detected on CT scan that was not diagnosed on X-ray) has appeared.[82-87] A study by the American Association for the Surgery of Trauma (AAST) found that only 6% of occult pneumothoraces required treatment; the remainder should be monitored for progression.[2,82]

- Haemothorax – the accumulation of blood in the pleural space after blunt or penetrating chest trauma.[2,84] In blunt injuries the source of blood is most commonly from fractured ribs and adjacent lung laceration, although injury to the blood vessels or cardiac injuries may also be the cause. With penetrating injuries, haemothorax is related to direct injury to the lung, arteries, heart or major blood vessels in the thoracic cavity.[2] Breath sounds are usually reduced on the side of the haemothorax, percussion is noted to be dull rather than hyper-resonant unless it is a haemopneumothorax, and there may be evidence of tracheal deviation away from the affected side.[2] Small haemothoraces (<200 mL blood) may not be apparent on clinical or radiological investigation,[2,82,84] although respiratory compromise is likely to be present. Massive haemothorax is defined as more than 1500 mL and causes circulatory compromise from hypovolaemia, vena cava compression and hypoxaemia[83] and requires operative control of the bleeding.[2] Initial management of a haemothorax is the insertion of a chest tube to allow for drainage of the accumulated blood.[2,82] Optimal evacuation of residual clots and breakdown of adhesions and loculated effusions is important to prevent complications such as empyema or fibrothorax and can be achieved using a surgical approach in the later phase of care. In one study 80% of haemothoraces were visible on CT but not on CXR.[2]
- Cardiac trauma – ranging from relatively mild bruising of the heart muscle to rupture of the heart wall, septum or valves or damage to the coronary arteries.[5,82] The right side of the heart is most commonly injured, probably as a result of the anterior placement of this side of the heart in the thorax, although more than half the patients with a blunt cardiac trauma experience injury to multiple cardiac chambers.[86,87] Motor vehicle crashes account for 50% of blunt cardiac injuries, followed by pedestrians struck by vehicles, motorcyclists, and falls greater than 6 m.[5,84] The incidence of myocardial injury in blunt chest trauma ranges from 15% to 75%, so a high level of suspicion is necessary when assessing these patients.[78]
- Aortic injuries – injuries to the brachiocephalic, left subclavian or right subclavian branches of the aorta are associated with high mortality at the scene. Minor aortic injuries usually involve a small intimal tear with small peri-aortic haematoma, while significant injuries include the intima and full thickness of media with associated high risk of rupture.[83,84] Aortic transection and rupture is associated with >80% mortality within the first 30 minutes of injury;[82-84,87] those who do survive to hospital frequently have a significant injury. The mechanism of aortic injury is primarily believed to be shearing forces with motor vehicle crashes accounting for approximately 81% of the injuries.[83] Thoracic CT scan with IV contrast is the gold standard for diagnosis for those patients who survive to hospital, and of those up to 50% will die before repair of their aortic injuries can occur.[84] Currently thoracic endovascular aortic repair (TEVAR) is the recommended treatment if anatomically feasible.[83,87]
- Tracheobronchial injuries – tend to occur as a result of direct blunt trauma and in close proximity to the carina, but are relatively rare with an incidence rate between 0.85% and 2.8%.[5,78] Larger defects result in dyspnoea (with or without respiratory distress), pneumomediastinum, pneumothorax or subcutaneous emphysema,[87,88] while smaller injuries may initially go unnoticed. Many subtle presentations will manifest as either mediastinal air, separation in the tracheobronchial air column, respiratory tract deviation or as a specific location of separation on CT scan.[88] Negative CT scan should not preclude the consideration for a bronchoscopy if tracheobronchial trauma is still suspected.[5,87] Although major tracheobronchial injury in trauma is rare, it is associated with an 80% mortality pre-hospital.[87]

Clinical manifestations

Injuries to the thoracic cavity can manifest according to the structures and systems involved (Table 24.6). When multiple organs and systems are involved, the combined injuries pose an increased threat to life.

TABLE 24.6
Clinical manifestations of chest trauma

SYSTEM	MANIFESTATION	CLINICAL SIGNS AND SYMPTOMS
Respiratory • Airways • Lungs • Diaphragm	Any sign of respiratory compromise, noting that serial observations are an important indicator of imminent decompensation	Abnormal respiratory rate (<12 or >20 breaths/min) Abnormal chest wall movement, including asymmetrical chest wall expansion Reduced breath sounds Obstructed airway Hypoxia (<94%) Hypercarbia Apnoea Dyspnoea Haemoptysis Crepitus/surgical emphysema
Cardiovascular • Heart • Great vessels	Circulatory insufficiency resulting in decreased tissue perfusion	Abnormal heart rate (<60 or >100 beats/min) Arrhythmia In severe cases, pulseless electrical activity (see Chapter 11) Pulsus alternans Decreased cardiac output Lowered blood pressure (systolic <100 mmHg) Reduced peripheral perfusion Confusion and reduced consciousness level Interscapular or retrosternal pain
Gastrointestinal • Oesophageal rupture	Perforation and contamination of mediastinum	Crepitus Haemopneumothorax Pain – chest and abdominal Cough Stridor Bleeding Sepsis (late)
Systemic • Air embolism	May occur in response to injury of a vessel that traverses an air space; manifestations will vary depending on location and associated injuries	Varied depending on location, but may include: • Focal neurological sign • Cardiac deterioration

Patient management

Given the underlying structures of heart, lungs and great vessels, chest trauma can cause rapid deterioration in the patient. Ongoing and thorough assessment, particularly in relation to the signs and symptoms outlined in Table 24.6, is essential. Other essential aspects of care include patient positioning and management of pain relief.

Assessment

Initial assessment in the ED should be conducted on an ongoing basis, with formal documentation of these findings occurring every few minutes until stabilisation. The frequency of ongoing assessment will then be based on the patient's condition, but is likely to be needed every 15 minutes initially, reducing to hourly with transfer to the critical care unit. Signs of chest trauma that represent life-threatening emergencies include the following:

- Cardiac tamponade – as blood collects in the pericardium, the venous return to the heart is impeded, resulting in reduced cardiac output. Signs of cardiac tamponade include:
  - anxiety and agitation
  - elevated heart rate
  - muffled heart sounds
  - reducing pulse pressure, with falling systolic BP and rising diastolic BP
  - increased preload (CVP and/or PCWP)
  - distended neck veins
  - signs of reduced cardiac output, including lower level of consciousness, poor peripheral perfusion and reduced urine output.
- Tension pneumothorax – the lung/s collapse as the pleural space fills with air that cannot escape (Fig. 24.5). As the volume of air grows with each

FIGURE 24.5 Right tension pneumothorax.

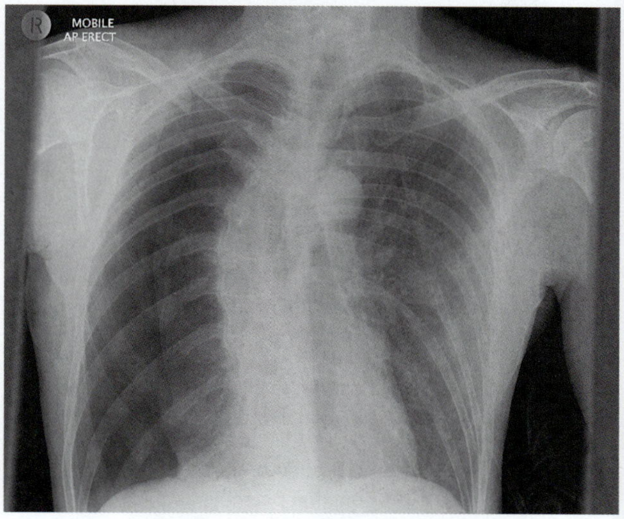

breath, the thoracic cavity contents are compressed or pushed against the opposite side of the chest. Signs of tension pneumothorax include:

- elevated heart rate
- increased respiratory rate
- hypotension
- decreased air entry, particularly over the affected lung
- tracheal deviation
- distended neck veins
- surgical emphysema.[5]

Practice tip

Unexplained hypotension in a patient with chest trauma may indicate a tension pneumothorax; an urgent chest X-ray is required for diagnosis.

Positioning

Early mobilisation of the patient with chest trauma is vital to prevent the complications of prolonged bed rest and immobility. Patients should be nursed side-to-side and in a variety of positions, including sitting upright. The extent to which the patient can be mobilised is dependent on other injuries. Patients should be mobilised to sit out of bed as soon as their injuries permit.

Care must be taken to accommodate the increased work of breathing that is associated with injuries to the lungs. Appropriate use of supplemental oxygen will assist the patient's exercise tolerance. Further, if the patient is mechanically ventilated, additional mechanical support (i.e. transient increase in pressure support) may be applied to assist the patient's exercise tolerance. Being unable to catch their breath is a terrifying experience that may result in increased anxiety for patients, and should be avoided wherever possible.

Pain relief

The principles of managing pain in chest trauma patients are similar to those for other patients, with effective pain management being a major determinant of maintaining adequate spontaneous breathing. Avoiding mechanical ventilation is a major goal in the less-severe group of chest trauma patients, so effective deep-breathing and coughing must be promoted. Pain relief will normally include IV opioids, but may also include intercostal or epidural analgesia and non-steroidal anti-inflammatory agents in selected patients (see Chapter 6). Non-pharmacological means such as the use of supplemental oxygen, breathing exercises, massage, relaxation and diversion techniques should also be considered. Providing and maintaining a comfortable posture for the patient that includes the elevation and support of injured limbs has remarkable analgesic properties. A confident, competent and efficient nurse who engenders trust from both the patient and family is very comforting.

Surgical management of injury

Surgical intervention in the chest trauma patient is generally limited to repair of tears and lacerations; for example, repair of vessel injuries including rupture, lung lacerations, heart injuries including lacerations and valvular injury. A ruptured diaphragm or oesophageal perforation will also be repaired surgically.

The emergency thoracotomy has proven beneficial in a select group of patients with penetrating trauma and less than 15 minutes of cardiopulmonary resuscitation; however, it is generally recognised as not providing benefit in patients with blunt chest trauma. While different techniques are used in different settings, the main access to the thoracic cavity is via a left thoracotomy, a midline sternotomy or a 'clam shell' incision. Initial assessment of the patient is used to determine the need for a thoracotomy in either the ED or the operating room. Nurses working in a trauma reception facility that has the capacity for emergency thoracotomy should be familiar with the equipment and process for this procedure. Postoperative nursing care of these patients should follow the same principles as for patients who have undergone routine cardiothoracic surgery.

Although not indicated in the unstable patient, the utilisation of video-assisted thoracoscopic surgery (VATS) in the relatively stable patient post-initial resuscitation allows for evacuation of clotted haemothorax or decortication of empyema. Surgical repair of rib fractures in the setting of flail chest is also being utilised in the trauma population; however, is not standard management globally.

Chest drainage

When injury to the pleura occurs, air or blood collects between the two layers of the pleura, causing collapse of the underlying area of lung and loss of the negative intrapleural pressure. Insertion of an intercostal catheter (ICC) drains the air and/or blood from between the pleura, resulting in reinstatement of the negative intrapleural pressure and reinflation of the underlying lung.

A central principle in the treatment of chest trauma is the use of the ICC[89] for chest drainage purposes. The principles of chest drainage include the following:

- The lungs are encased in a potential space. The visceral pleura attaches to the parietal pleura via surface tension, creating a negative intrapleural pressure and attaching the lung to the chest wall. During inspiration the rib cage moves out and the diaphragm contracts and moves down, increasing the size of the intrathoracic space. Air moves from an area of higher pressure in the environment to an area of lower pressure within the lungs along a pressure gradient.
- An ICC is inserted into the pleural space, passing between the ribs. The ICC is designed to drain both air and fluid as required.
- The drainage system and seal provide an ongoing means of removing air and/or fluid from the pleural space, while preventing air from the atmosphere entering via the ICC. If the traditional glass bottle system is being used, the seal is provided by placing the distal end of the ICC under water (usually 2 cm). The catheter should not be placed under excessive levels of water, as this creates resistance and will limit air and fluid escaping from the pleural space.
- Suction is often added to the drainage system to promote drainage of fluid.

Care of the chest trauma patient with intercostal drainage is directed towards ensuring sterility and patency of the system and assessing the amount and type of drainage, as well as the impact on the patient (Table 24.7). Additional considerations include the following:

- ICC may be positional, or alternatively haemo/pneumothoraces may be loculated. Repositioning of the patient may be necessary or consideration of replacing the existing catheter. The catheter should not be advanced into the pleural space once initial insertion is complete.
- Side-lying or lifting the patient, especially with a frame, may kink or disconnect the ICC.
- Surgical emphysema around the site of the ICC may dislodge the tip of the catheter out of the pleural cavity as the emphysema swells. Ongoing assessment, including a chest X-ray, is required to confirm the position of the ICC.
- Movement of the patient, including sitting upright, will assist with fluid drainage; the volume of drainage should be assessed after moving the patient.

TABLE 24.7
Assessment of chest drainage

CHARACTERISTIC	DESCRIPTION
Water seal	Ensure there is sufficient water in the water seal chamber
Bubbling	Continued bubbling indicates an air leak
Drainage	Observe the nature and volume of fluid exudate (NB: >1500 mL stat or 200/mL/h for 2–4 h; surgical exploration may be required)
Patency	Ensure the intercostal catheter is not blocked, remove any blood clots
Swinging	Oscillation of fluid in the ICC confirms patency, as this reflects the changes in intrapleural pressure with respiration; such oscillation should continue even when the lung has re-expanded
Suction	If suction is ordered, check the appropriate level is being delivered

- Monitoring of respiratory function should continue after removal of the ICC, along with consideration for repeat chest X-ray, to detect recollection of air or fluid.

Practice tip

Fresh, brightly-coloured blood drained from the ICC indicates continued active bleeding, while dark blood usually indicates older blood that has been resting in the pleural space for some time.

Ventilatory support

Ventilatory support is often required for patients with chest trauma (see Chapter 15 for general principles). The following specific considerations apply:

- Non-invasive ventilation – care should be taken based on associated injuries, with contraindications including fractured base of skull or facial fractures.
- Intubation – haemoptysis is relatively common in patients with lung injury, and care must be taken to ensure removal of blood clots from the endotracheal tube (ETT). Heated, humidified air and regular suctioning will assist with maintaining ETT patency.
- Airway injury – initiation of positive pressure ventilation in the chest trauma patient may identify

damage to a small airway that previously went unnoticed (damage to a large airway will usually have been detected early in the assessment phase). Treatment will depend on the severity and location of the rupture, but usually requires decompression of the pleura with an ICC, possibly surgical intervention and advanced respiratory support such as independent lung ventilation.

- Use of tracheostomy – this may be required for patients with injury to the trachea and is managed using the same principles as with any patient with a tracheostomy.

Allied health interventions

Physiotherapy is generally required for chest trauma patients. The primary aspects of care include chest physiotherapy, given the often-extended episodes of mechanical ventilation and bed rest that are required, as well as mobility exercises. Occupational therapy particularly offers benefits to the long-term ventilated patient in terms of diversional activity, while social work is often beneficial for patients with ongoing disability and financial and social problems. Early referral of selected patients to allied health professionals has the potential to significantly influence patient outcome.

Abdominal trauma

Abdominal trauma presents unique challenges to clinicians due to the abdominal cavity's high diversity of organs and structures. Approximately 20% of blunt trauma patients experience intraabdominal injury with high associated morbidity and mortality, generally related to haemorrhage or unrecognised injury;[21,30] hence the need for early, accurate diagnosis and treatment is paramount.

Road crashes account for most abdominal injuries and these are frequently associated with injuries to the thorax, head and extremities. Other blunt mechanisms of abdominal injury include falls, assaults and industrial accidents, while penetrating injuries are often associated with stabbing or GSWs.[30,90] Although GSWs are not as common as stabbing injuries, they do account for 90% of penetrating trauma mortality, especially in the USA.[90] The most commonly injured intraabdominal organs are the small intestine, liver and colon, with only a third of injuries penetrating the peritoneum; not all of those will require surgical intervention.[21] Indications for immediate exploration include hypotension, peritonitis and evisceration, otherwise serial examination may be sufficient.[91] In blunt abdominal trauma the spleen is the organ that is most commonly injured with the liver the second most common, while injury to the hollow viscous being relatively uncommon in comparison.[90,92]

Recent advances in diagnostic and treatment techniques for abdominal trauma have seen an increased emphasis on non-operative management for solid organ injury, with increased use of angio-embolisation. Non-operative management should be considered in haemodynamically stable patients, with an emphasis on close patient monitoring and regular laboratory examinations,[29,93] potentially including ICU or high dependency care.

Pathophysiology

The abdominal cavity consists of a range of tissues and organ structures, including musculoskeletal, solid and hollow organs, vessels and nerves. Musculoskeletal structures include the major abdominal muscle groups forming the abdominal wall, as well as the lumbar vertebrae and pelvis. Solid organs include the liver, spleen, pancreas, kidneys and adrenal glands (and ovaries in women). Hollow organs include the stomach, small and large intestines, gallbladder and bladder (and uterus in women). Finally, the vessels and nerves include a complex array of all abdominal blood vessels (arterial and venous), lymphatics and nerves including neural plexuses and the spinal cord. Traumatic abdominal injuries are classified as being extraperitoneal, intraperitoneal and/or retroperitoneal. Importantly, a patient can have any mix or multiples of these. The classification of injury guides clinical decision making.

The pathophysiology of abdominal trauma is largely related to the structure(s) injured. Careful serial assessments are essential to identify changing clinical manifestations. The most common clinical manifestation of abdominal trauma is haemorrhage[29] and/or signs of an acute abdomen, such as pain, tenderness, rigidity and bruising. Importantly, these are life-threatening signs and require immediate surgical intervention

The most significant sign of abdominal trauma in the conscious patient is thought to be pain,[91] although the injured person who presents with altered mental state from either a TBI, drugs, alcohol or metabolic disturbances cannot be assessed for pain.[29] Pain may be present immediately or the onset may be delayed. Other signs of abdominal injury include dizziness, nausea and vomiting, and dyspnoea related to irritation of the peritoneum or obstruction.[90] Inspection may elicit evidence of abrasions, bruising, obvious penetrating injury, distended abdomen or specific bruising that may raise the suspicion of a retroperitoneal injury.[21] Palpation may elicit pain, guarding, or distension of the abdomen which could be indicative of haemorrhage.[21] Auscultation can be used to note the presence or absence of bowel sounds, although this is a more significant sign if serial assessments are made.[21,30]

Where hollow viscus perforation has occurred, examination of the stable patient is important but often sub-optimal. Abdominal bruising reflective of a seatbelt pattern is reported to be associated with a 20–60% chance of intraabdominal injury and increases the risk of perforated bowel injury by a factor of 2.4. Bruising as an isolated finding with no associated pain or guarding raises suspicion but has a low risk of injury.[94] There is evidence that rear seat passengers have a higher incidence of intestinal injury, potentially as a result of seatbelts.[94] Other signs of abdominal trauma can be related to the structure that has been injured. For example, haematuria demonstrates trauma to some part of the urinary tract, including the kidneys.

A key aspect with any abdominal injury is that the superficial injury does not always reflect what lies below. For example, it is not possible to be certain of the trajectory that a bullet took after it passed through the skin.

Contusion/laceration

Sudden deceleration of moving body tissues can result in laceration or haemorrhage into the tissues (contusion). This is related to the tearing of the tissues that occurs due to inertia, or the tendency of tissues to resist changes in speed or direction (e.g. to keep moving forwards when the body has stopped moving, resulting in a tearing action to the tissues). Any structure in the abdomen is susceptible to this type of injury. Commonly, the liver and spleen are the worst-affected organs, largely related to a seatbelt injury in motor vehicle collisions. Laceration of a solid organ can be a minor injury that is appropriately monitored and managed conservatively or non-operatively; alternatively, a similar injury can lead to exsanguination (e.g. a liver laceration into the hilum that involves the inferior vena cava). Hollow viscus can be contused, as can the mesentery and peritoneum.

Perforation

Full-thickness injury, or perforation, to a hollow viscus organ is life-threatening. Perforation of the intestine can result in peritoneal soiling and ischaemic bowel. Small intestinal injuries constitute more than half of all blunt intestinal injuries with the second most common region being the colon; the left colon is more commonly injured in comparison to the right or transverse colon.[94] Full-thickness perforations are less common than serous or seromuscular tears.[94] The abdominal seatbelt sign – in other words, bruising across the anterior abdominal wall that follows the path of the lap and sash of the seatbelt – is a sentinel sign for hollow viscus perforation (see *Pathophysiology* above for more details). Importantly, patients with this type of abdominal trauma can present late (by days). If presenting late, the usual clinical manifestations are pain, peritonitis and sepsis, along with an associated increase in mortality and morbidity[21,92]

Secondary injury: abdominal compartment syndrome

The abdominal viscera are highly vascular and subject to vascular engorgement during massive fluid resuscitation. Where this occurs, there is an acute rise in intraabdominal pressure (IAP). Intraabdominal hypertension (IAH) was defined by the World Congress of Abdominal Compartment Syndrome as IAP less than 12 mmHg without physiological derangement, and abdominal compartment syndrome (ACS) was defined as IAP greater than 20 mmHg with new organ dysfunction or failure.[95] In severe cases, the IAP will rise to the point where cardiorespiratory function is compromised and if decompression does not occur the villi eventually rupture. This is a surgical emergency and the abdominal cavity requires decompression immediately; however, the resultant open abdomen is seen as a potential risk to life.[95] The incidence of ACS is difficult to determine because of the different assessment and measurement techniques used, but there is evidence of a decrease in the population with major torso trauma from 15% in the 1990s to 0–2% in 2011 following the introduction of guidelines to manage ACS in 2004.[95]

Clinical examination, looking for a distended and firm abdomen, is insensitive in the early stages of ACS and a high index of suspicion should be given to the patient who has an abdominal injury. Prediction of ACS is related to the pattern of injury (catastrophic blunt or penetrating injury with shock), pathophysiology (hypothermia, acidosis or coagulopathy), surgical approach of haemorrhage control, haemostatic resuscitation, and restriction of crystalloid administration.[95] See Chapter 20 for a detailed review of ACS including IAP monitoring and subsequent management.

Patient management

Recent trends have seen an increasing use of non-operative care of patients with abdominal injury. In these patients, monitoring for deterioration is essential, as is the ability to activate surgery and care for patients accordingly. Care of patients after abdominal trauma also includes effective diagnosis, surgical or radiological interventions, and associated care. DCS is now a mainstay in management.

With the high use of non-operative management techniques for solid organ injury, the role of monitoring of patients with abdominal trauma is pivotal. Nurses must be cognisant of the clinical signs of abdominal injury, especially haemorrhage, and act on these immediately (Table 24.8). Specific aspects of nursing care for patients after abdominal trauma include pain management, monitoring and postoperative care. Patients often experience severe pain as a result of both the primary trauma and any surgical intervention for repair (see Chapter 6).

Vital sign monitoring is a mainstay of nursing management in patients with abdominal trauma, and all patients should have appropriate monitoring (as outlined in trauma reception). It is also essential that patients receive a urinalysis after incurring abdominal trauma in order to identify trauma to the urinary system.

Where the patient has undergone a trauma laparotomy, postoperative care is standard as for any patient who has undergone an abdominal surgical procedure. The specific nursing care elements will depend on which organ has been injured and the surgical procedure undertaken. Careful attention must be paid to general nursing care elements for all patients (see Chapter 5).

Postoperative feeding and bowel care should be discussed with the healthcare team and plans made early

TABLE 24.8
Common signs of abdominal injury

SIGN	DESCRIPTION	SUSPECTED INJURY
Grey Turner's sign	Blueish discolouration of the lower abdomen and flanks 6–24 h after onset of bleeding	Retroperitoneal haemorrhage
Kehr's sign	Left shoulder tip pain caused by diaphragmatic irritation	Splenic injury, although can be associated with any intraabdominal bleeding
Cullen's sign	Bluish discolouration around the umbilicus	Pancreatic injury, although can be associated with any peritoneal bleeding
Coopernail's sign	Ecchymosis of scrotum or labia	Pelvic fracture or pelvic organ injury

Source: Wright JA. Seven abdominal assessment signs every emergency nurse should know. J Emerg Nurs. October 1997:446–50.

to avoid delays and adverse events such as constipation (see Chapter 19 for principles of feeding). A paralytic ileus is a common manifestation of the critically ill abdominal trauma patient. Ensuring that the gut is decompressed, with a functional enterogastric tube that is correctly positioned, is essential. Because constipation is a common problem, early intervention and implementation of a bowel care protocol for trauma should be considered (see Chapter 5).

Diagnosis in the trauma setting consists of a thorough clinical assessment, the potential use of FAST, DPL, abdominal CT and laparotomy or laparoscopy.

Clinical assessment may reveal clinical signs such as skin-bruising, lacerations, signs of abdominal rigidity and guarding. The various locations of clinical signs are clues to potential abdominal injury. The results of this phase of the investigation will determine what additional diagnostic tests are undertaken.

Diagnostic peritoneal lavage

DPL is a procedure that can be undertaken rapidly to assess for intraabdominal bleeding, although it is frequently only used where FAST or CT is not available.[31] DPL may be performed on a patient with unexplained persistent signs of shock (hypotension and tachycardia); where the abdominal clinical examination and FAST is inconclusive; or where there is a high index of suspicion of intraabdominal injury. DPL can identify the presence of haemorrhage with up to 98% accuracy but gives no indication of its source and can result in significant non-therapeutic laparotomy rates.[30,36] Disadvantages of DPL include:

- not organ-specific
- high false negative rate
- high level of invasiveness and associated complications
- inability to detect retroperitoneal, diaphragm or iatrogenic injuries
- potential interference with the interpretation of subsequent CT scans.[36]

Abdominal computed tomography

Abdominal CT is recognised as having high sensitivity and specificity in the setting of intraabdominal injury and is therefore accepted as a diagnostic mainstay, particularly for patients with blunt trauma who are haemodynamically stable, and may be useful in determining the disposition of the patient.[29] The main exception to this is where the results of a FAST examination are positive and the patient is taken to surgery urgently. The use of triple contrast abdominal CT in patients with either a penetrating or blunt injury has been found to have a sensitivity rate of 89–100%, for excluding surgically important injury and resulting in a decreased incidence of non-therapeutic laparotomy to 3%.[96] CT with intravenous contrast is a method of choice for evaluating wounds not identified as superficial.[90] With the advent of spiral or multi-detector CTs, the use of triple contrast abdominal CT was reassessed and a meta-analysis indicating 95% accuracy in predicting the requirement for a laparotomy, or for identifying the wound track, whether fragmentation has occurred, or for proving insight into what vascular structures may have been injured for those with penetrating abdominal injuries.[90,96] A pitfall for CT imaging occurs when the patient arrives at the scanner so quickly after the injury that major blood loss is not apparent and the extent of the injury is missed or underevaluated. A high index of suspicion in the setting of a negative CT and extensive abdominal trauma should remain, particularly if signs of shock develop.

Debate currently exists as to the role of oral contrast in the trauma patient who must remain supine and immobilised in a cervical collar. It is essential that nursing assessment for the risk of aspiration be conducted and strategies to manage the vomiting patient be planned. If patients have a wide-bore enterogastric tube in situ, consider aspirating this to reduce the risk of aspiration. Any supine patient given radiographic contrast should not be left unattended, and there should be sufficient staff available at short notice to roll the patient onto their side if he/she vomits. The healthcare team should discuss the risk of vomiting prior to ordering the test so that an informed decision can be made regarding the risk–benefit ratio on an individual case basis. Oral contrast has been demonstrated to be highly effective in revealing hollow viscus injury, and therefore has a place in the diagnostic evaluation of abdominal trauma, although it should be weighed against the increased time to diagnosis that may occur.[96]

Laparotomy/laparoscopy

The role and indications for diagnostic operations such as laparotomy/laparoscopy is well described in the literature,[5,29,30,90] and is essential to aid diagnosis (laparoscopy) and provide appropriate treatment to control haemorrhage and repair organ injury (laparotomy).[30] When this procedure is considered appropriate, rapid, but safe, transit to the operating room should be undertaken. As the consequences of missed or delayed diagnosis of abdominal injury can be catastrophic for the patient, opening the peritoneal cavity to exclude injury in selected cases is a necessity. The conversion rate to laparotomy is reported as 11.7% in penetrating injury and 22.9% in blunt abdominal trauma; however, it should be noted that there were limitations to this study in that the data was analysed retrospectively and that reproducibility may be dependent on the expertise in laparoscopic surgery at each healthcare institution.[97]

Indications for emergency laparotomy in blunt trauma include:

- peritonism
- free air under the diaphragm
- significant gastrointestinal haemorrhage
- hypotension with positive FAST scan
- increasing abdominal pain
- high grade solid organ injuries if embolisation is not available
- physiological deterioration.[5,21,29]

Indications for emergency laparotomy in penetrating trauma include:

- penetrating abdominal trauma + hypotension
- peritonism
- free air
- evisceration
- GSW traversing peritoneum.[5,21]

Embolisation

Interventional radiology is an option in the management of abdominal trauma. Via an arterial approach, the interventional radiologist can insert cannulae to identify arterial blushes (bleeders). Once identified, the vessel can be ligated via mechanical coiling or blocked chemically. Interventional radiology and embolisation assists in providing haemostasis in areas difficult to access by surgery, may prevent the need for re-operation in cases of suspected re-bleeding postoperative intervention, and may assist in providing non-operative management of high-grade solid organ injuries.[98] Post-identification of injury on CT scan, patients with vascular injuries are often managed with percutaneous selective embolisation rather than operatively.[99] The patient undergoing embolisation for the control of haemorrhage requires meticulous monitoring and an ability to respond immediately to hypovolaemic shock should the bleeding worsen.

Management of the patient with an open abdomen

In cases of severe abdominal trauma, the patient may be returned to the ICU with an open abdomen, covered with a temporary wound-closure system. There are various types of open abdominal dressings with negative pressure therapy techniques becoming the most extensively used. Negative pressure therapy prevents viscera-abdominal wall adherence, maintains medial fascial tension which assists with fascial closure rates, while also removing excess fluid and pro-inflammatory cytokines from the peritoneal space.[95] The principal aim of the dressing is to provide coverage for the contents of the peritoneum, or where there is a need for repeated opening of the abdomen. Ultimately, the aim is to close the skin as soon as possible, when the patient's physiological status normalises. It is possible for these abdominal dressings to cause a secondary ACS if they are too restrictive and monitoring for IAH should continue to ensure that this is recognised early.[100] Another challenge for the patient with the open abdomen is the potential for the development of enteroatmospheric fistulas, which can develop with the use of negative pressure therapy, and when fascial closure is not achieved, and there is a requirement for late reconstructive therapy.[95,100]

The primary aims of managing a patient with an open abdomen includes minimising complications of prolonged immobility, observing for signs of ongoing ACS, restoring the patient's physiology to normal and supporting the patient and family through a psychologically distressing time. Understandably, both the patient and their family can be distressed by the appearance of an open abdomen. There are no specific position restrictions for a patient with an open abdomen, but haemodynamic status is often labile so care must be taken with side-lying and hygiene care. Nutritional support is another aspect of recovery. Initiation of enteral nutrition has been found to lead to higher abdominal closure rates and a reduction of mortality in patients with an open abdomen.[100]

Splenic injuries

The spleen is the solid organ most commonly injured in blunt trauma with the degree of injury ranging from the small subcapsular haematoma to hilar

TABLE 24.9
Spleen injury scale

GRADE[a]	INJURY TYPE	DESCRIPTION OF INJURY
I	Haematoma	Subcapsular, <10% surface area
	Laceration	Capsular tear, <1 cm parenchymal depth
II	Haematoma	Subcapsular, 10–50% surface area
		Intraparenchymal, <5 cm in diameter
	Laceration	Parenchymal depth 1–3 cm not involving a trabecular vessel
III	Haematoma	Subcapsular, >50% surface area or expanding
		Ruptured subcapsular or parenchymal haematoma
		Intraparenchymal haematoma >5 cm or expanding
	Laceration	Parenchymal depth >3 cm or involving trabecular vessels
IV	Laceration	Laceration involving segmental or hilar vessels producing major devascularisation (>25% of spleen)
V	Laceration	Completely shattered spleen
	Vascular	Hilar vascular injury that devascularises spleen

[a]Advance one grade for multiple injuries, up to grade III.
Adapted from Olthof DC, van der Vlies CH, Scheerder MJ, et al. Reliability of injury grading systems for patients with blunt splenic trauma. Injury 2014;45(1):146–50 with permission.

devascularisation.[30,101] Its location (under the ribs) also makes it vulnerable to secondary injury from fractured ribs. Splenic injury should always be suspected in patients who have sustained a direct blow to the abdomen, as it is a large organ. The most common sign of splenic injury is pain over the left upper quadrant. There may be no changes to vital sign parameters until the patient has incurred significant circulating blood loss. Splenic injury is categorised in a scale consisting of five levels; this scale is designed to aid classification for management and research purposes[101] (Table 24.9). Complications associated with blunt spleen injury include significant bleeding after initial management. Pleural effusions, thrombocytopenia, splenic infarction, pneumonia and cyst formation can also occur after non-operative management or angio-embolisation.[91,101]

The spleen comprises more than 25% of the total lymphoid mass making it the largest lymphoid organ in the body with the primary function of assisting with immunity, especially against encapsulated organisms. Therefore, patients who have had a splenectomy are at risk of infections, particularly encapsulated organisms.[101] As these patients have a life-time increased risk of infection they require careful education surrounding the risks and the importance of follow up immunisations which should be in accordance with either the US Centre for Disease Control and Prevention(CDC) or professional organisations that assist with the prevention of disease.[101] These patients should be encouraged to seek medical attention promptly to decrease the risk of severe infection. The current recommendation for pre-discharge immunisations includes:

- pneumococcal vaccine
- meningococcal vaccines
- influenza vaccine.[101]

The patient may also be commenced on antibiotic prophylaxis and should be advised to wear a medi-alert disk or card and consult specialist travel advice when travelling.[101]

Liver injuries

As the largest abdominal solid organ traversing the midline, the liver is susceptible to injury from any external forces applied to the abdomen, for example seatbelt injuries and abdominal blows from an assault. The treatment of liver injuries is largely dependent on the nature of the injury or injuries to the liver itself, presence of concomitant injuries, premorbid status and overall injury severity. The treatment options may also be guided by the services and expertise that your health agency can offer the patient.

The liver is the second most commonly injured organ in blunt abdominal trauma, and has been the

TABLE 24.10
Liver injury scale

GRADE[a]		INJURY DESCRIPTION
I	Haematoma	Subcapsular, <10% surface area
	Laceration	Capsular tear, <1 cm parenchymal depth
II	Haematoma	Subcapsular, 10–50% surface area
		Intraparenchymal, <10 cm in diameter
	Laceration	Parenchymal depth 1–3 cm, <10 cm in length
III	Haematoma	Subcapsular, >50% surface area or expanding
		Ruptured subcapsular or parenchymal haematoma
	Laceration	Parenchymal depth >3 cm
IV	Laceration	Parenchymal disruption involving 25–75% of hepatic lobe or 1–3 Couinaud's segments within a single lobe
V	Laceration	Parenchymal disruption involving >75% of hepatic lobe or >3 Couinaud's segments within a single lobe
	Vascular	Juxtahepatic venous injuries; i.e. retrohepatic vena cava/central major hepatic veins
VI	Vascular	Hepatic avulsion

[a]Advance one grade for multiple injuries, up to grade III.
Source: Tominaga GT, Staudenmayer KL, Shafi S, et al. The American Association for the Surgery of Trauma grading scale for 16 emergency general surgery conditions: disease-specific criteria characterizing anatomic severity grading. J Trauma Acute Care Surg 2016;81(2):593–602.

most frequently missed injury in deaths from trauma.[30] Any injury to this highly vascular organ is serious and requires surgical review, especially in those patients with a high-grade injury and haemodynamic instability.[91] Liver injuries are graded using the six-level liver injury scale (Table 24.10).

Liver trauma is the most common cause of mortality related to abdominal trauma; however, this relates to the grading of the injury and associated injuries to other organs.[102] The majority, 80–85%, of injuries are low grade and can be managed non-operatively or with angio-embolisations, which enhances the success of non-operative management.[91] Non-operatively managed patients require close monitoring for signs of haemorrhage – surgical intervention at short notice should be available. Patients who sustain major liver trauma and uncontrolled bleeding with haemodynamic instability who proceed to laparotomy and DCS with early packing followed by angio-embolisation have shown significant decrease in overall and liver-specific mortality when compared with immediate definitive surgery.[102]

Early complications of liver injury relate to hypoperfusion or massive transfusions. Late complications of liver injury include infection, haematoma, bile leak and late haemorrhage.[30] Complications associated with angio-embolisation include hepatic necrosis, gallbladder necrosis, bile leak and abscess formation.[91]

Penetrating injuries

Penetrating trauma refers to the piercing of the skin by a foreign object, which is largely localised to a single body region. Exceptions to this may occur: for example, with firearm wounds if there are multiple bullet-entry wounds or multiple knife-stab sites. The most common examples include knife and GSWs, although solid objects such as fences, signposts and tools can cause penetrating trauma.

Caution must be taken when caring for patients with penetrating injury to prevent injury to staff. This is particularly important when the patient presents with a knife in situ or a large, protruding foreign object in their body. It should also be noted that some penetrating trauma occurs as a result of a criminal act, and it is essential to observe rules governing forensic evidence. Police should be notified by the senior clinician involved in providing care.

Clinical manifestations

The clinical manifestations of penetrating injuries are dependent on where in the body the penetrating injury has occurred, the underlying organs and the amount of force and dispersion caused by the injury. For example, a high-velocity bullet will cause substantial tissue damage in a wider area than only the bullet's track. The clinical manifestations of penetrating trauma can be divided into two broad types:

1. conspicuous – where the penetrating article is grossly visible (e.g. a shard of glass, a branch or a knife): care must be taken not to focus solely on the visible cause of injury but to continue to undertake a systematic trauma assessment
2. inconspicuous – where the penetrating article is not immediately visible and may become apparent only during the systematic trauma assessment of the patient (e.g. with GSWs and projectiles): in these injuries the visual signs on the external skin may not reflect the catastrophic injury underlying it (e.g. ventricle lacerations or serious vascular injury).

Patient management

Patients with penetrating injury will be cared for based on the severity and area of injury they have sustained. Surgical intervention is usually more urgent than that seen with blunt injury, as bleeding may be occurring from a ruptured organ or vessel either into a body cavity or externally. For this reason, the incidence of procedures such as laparotomy and thoracotomy is high in patients with a penetrating injury.

In Australia, Germany and many European countries the incidence of penetrating trauma represents a minority, unlike the USA where larger volumes of this type of trauma are experienced; as such management of this particular group can be challenging.[71]

In the emergency setting the following considerations are generally unique to the patient with a penetrating injury:

- Stabilise the foreign object. This may require padding and/or taping an object, for example a knife, to ensure minimal movement and prevent further damage until definitive care to remove the object.
- Care for the patient in a non-standard position. This will be dependent on how and where any foreign object is protruding from the body. For example, it may be necessary to care for a patient in the side-lying or prone position until the object is removed.
- Minimise volume resuscitation: this describes the practice of only resuscitating a patient sufficiently to maintain adequate perfusion to essential organs until definitive repair of the wound can be undertaken. Reduced volume of intravenous fluids may be associated with more favourable outcomes.[71]
- Provide psychosocial care of the patient and family. It is possible that patients with penetrating injury will need specific psychosocial care, particularly when the injury has occurred as a result of assault.

Burns

Burn injuries occur as a result of thermal, electrical, chemical, ionising radiation or friction injury and cause both local and systemic changes to a patient. The degree of injury depends on the source and the duration of contact.[103] An understanding of these changes will assist with planning appropriate care for this group of patients.

Burns can affect nearly every organ system and despite recent improvements in both shock and sepsis management, the patients have long-term morbidity and mortality associated with this injury type.[104] Patients who are admitted to specialised critical care services have been found to have an associated reduction in hospital mortality.[105,106] Recent trends in burn epidemiology suggest a downward trend in burn incidence in the majority of settings although these patterns are not consistent worldwide.[107]

Patients with burn injuries have unique challenges in regard to fluid resuscitation, metabolic stress, infections complicating burn recovery, along with abnormal drug pharmacology, severe pain, psychological stress, prolonged critical care and hospital stays, multiple surgical procedures, use of skin substitutes, and extensive rehabilitation.[103]

Burn injuries are highly variable and injuries affect all ages and social groups. In general terms, assessment is based on the size, depth and anatomical site of the injury, mechanism of injury and the presence of coexisting conditions. Burn injuries typically happen in the home or the workplace. The WHO reports that in high-income countries mortality has decreased due to a combination of prevention strategies and improvements in care; however, most of these changes have not been implemented completely in low and middle-income countries.[106] Outcomes for burns patients have improved with improvement of surgical treatment, intensive care management strategies and multidisciplinary team input.[105]

All patients with a serious burn injury should be referred to a specialised burns unit that is staffed and equipped appropriately to manage burns. The criteria for which patients require treatment in a specialised burns unit is outlined by associations such as the Australian and New Zealand Burns Association (ANZBA), the American Burns Association, the German Burn Society and the National Network for Burn Care in the United Kingdom (Box 24.1).[108-110]

Pathophysiology

The skin is the largest organ in the human body and accounts for 15% of its weight. The skin has multiple purposes, including protection from infection, regulation of body heat and function as a vapour barrier.

The skin consists of three layers, the epidermis, the dermis and subcutaneous tissue:

- Epidermis – the outer layer, composed of stratified epithelial cells that are metabolically active and provide a barrier that protect against infection, chemicals, and conserves moisture.[103] This layer is characterised by having regenerative ability.
- Dermis – the middle layer, composed of an outer papillary dermis and an inner reticular dermis,

BOX 24.1

Criteria for treatment in a specialised burn centre[106]

- Burns greater than 10% of total body surface area (TBSA)
- Burns to special areas: face, hands, feet, genitalia, perineum, major joints
- Full-thickness burns greater than 5% of TBSA
- Electrical burns
- Chemical burns
- Burns with an associated inhalation injury
- Circumferential burns of the limbs or chest
- Burns in the very young or very old
- Burns in people with preexisting medical disorders that could complicate management, prolong recovery or increase mortality
- Burns with associated trauma
- The possibility of non-accidental injury in children

Adapted from Australian and New Zealand Burns Association. Early management of severe burns (EMSB). Albany Creek: Australian and New Zealand Burns Association; 2013 with permission.

supplies nutrients to the epidermis as well as providing strength and flexibility to the skin. The dermis contains all the accessory structures including blood vessels, nerve endings, the sweat and sebaceous glands and the hair follicles.[103] The dermis has no regenerative ability, but because the glands, vessels and follicles are lined with epidermis, burns that involve this layer may still regenerate.

- Subcutaneous – the innermost layer, consists of adipose and connective tissue. This layer has no regenerative ability (Fig. 24.6).

Local changes

Once the cause of the burn has been removed response in the local tissues may lead to injury in deeper zones. Those local changes include the zones of coagulation, stasis and hyperaemia (Fig. 24.7) and the specific changes are outlined below.[111]

- Zone of coagulation: occurs at the point of maximum damage. Irreversible tissue loss occurs in this zone due to coagulation of the constituent proteins which requires debridement.
- Zone of stasis: the immediate area surrounding the necrosis has a moderate degree of insult with decreased tissue perfusion. The zone of stasis can either survive or go on to coagulative necrosis, and is associated with vascular damage and vessel leakage. Tissue in this zone is potentially salvageable if sufficient resuscitation is achieved to increase tissue perfusion. If insufficient resuscitation occurs, or if there are additional insults of hypotension, infection or oedema, tissue within this zone may convert to the zone of coagulation.
- Zone of hyperaemia: is the outermost zone. It experiences increased tissue perfusion as a result of local inflammatory response, which results in local vasodilation and an increase in vascular permeability. Tissue in this zone will usually recover, and is generally not at risk of further necrosis unless there are prolonged or severe periods of hypotension, infection or oedema.

FIGURE 24.6 Depth of burn.[111]

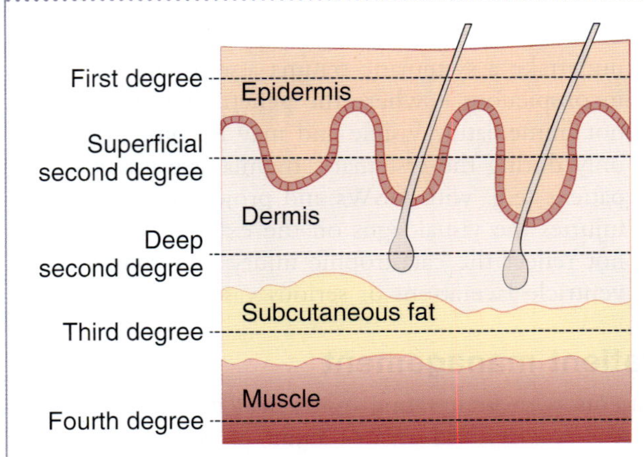

Source: Jeschke MGH, David N. Herndon. Sabiston Textbook of surgery. 20th ed. Elsevier; 2017.

FIGURE 24.7 Zone of burn damage.[111]

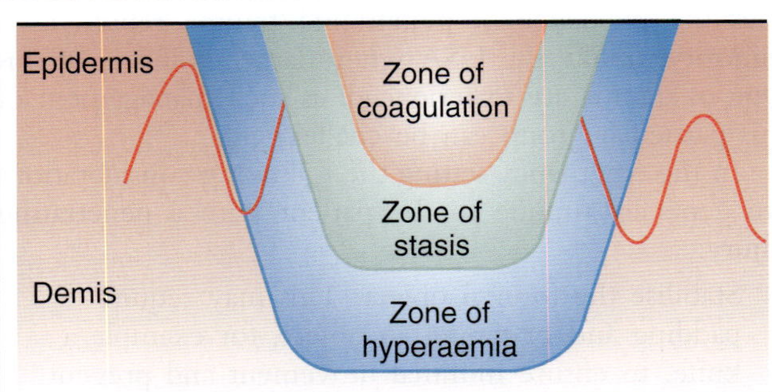

Source: Jeschke MGH, David N. Herndon. Sabiston Textbook of surgery. 20th ed. Elsevier; 2017.

Systemic changes

With a burn injury of >30% total burn surface area (TBSA), microcirculation vessel wall integrity is altered resulting in fluid and protein loss into the interstitium. The protein loss results in a reduction in osmotic pressure

FIGURE 24.8 Systemic changes that occur with burn injuries.[111]

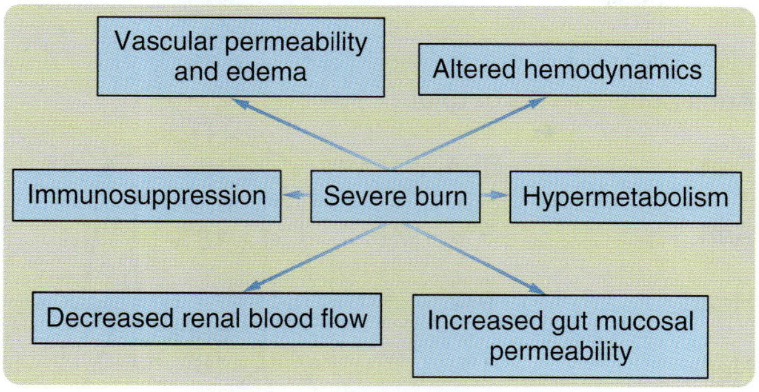

Source: Jeschke MGH, David N. Herndon. Sabiston Textbook of surgery. 20th ed. Elsevier; 2017.

that further insults circulating volume. Changes to the cardiovascular, respiratory, metabolic and immunological systems occur as a result of the release of cytokines and other inflammatory mediators in response to the injury (Fig. 24.8).[111]

Inhalation injury

Inhalation injury occurs in approximately 80% of fire-related deaths, with an overall mortality rate of 25–50% when patients require intubation for longer than a week.[111] Inhalation injury should be suspected in patients with facial burns, singed nasal hairs or eyebrows, wheezing or stridor, carbonaceous sputum, hoarseness, and anxiety.[103] Inhalation injury consists of three components that may occur independently but often occur simultaneously, and include heat injury to the upper airways, effects of smoke on the respiratory system and inhalation of toxic gases.[103,111] Bronchoscopic criteria for confirmation of an inhalation injury include airway oedema, inflammation, mucosal necrosis, soot or charring in the airway, tissue sloughing, and carbonaceous material in the airway.[103,111] This type of burn injury results in airway inflammation, pulmonary shunting, augmented microvascular pressure gradient and severe hypoxaemic respiratory failure. Other than traditional ventilation strategies extracorporeal life support could be considered as a respiratory support option although the evidence clarifying benefits and limitations is limited, largely due to the small sample sizes (extracorporeal life support is discussed further in Chapter 15).[112,113]

The specific changes are dependent on the types of substances inhaled at the time of injury. If coarse smoke particles are inhaled, these will primarily be deposited in the upper tracheobronchial tree, while fine smoke particles will usually be lodged in the alveoli. In carbon monoxide poisoning there is commonly mental status changes, varying from headache to coma, or the classic 'cherry red cyanosis', which may be obscured by soot or burns. Upper airway injury is characterised by progressive airway occlusion pharyngeal or supraglottic oedema and facial swelling and is generally identified in patients with early respiratory distress, stridor, or hypoxemia.[103] Injury to the lower airways causes chemical injury to the epithelium, which can progress to mucosal sloughing, mucous plugging, bronchiectasis, hypoxemia, and pneumonia, with clinical signs potentially not being evident in the first 72 hours.[103]

Clinical manifestations

The most prominent clinical manifestations of burn injury are the dermal signs of injury. Burn depth is classified by the degree of injury in the epidermis, dermis, subcutaneous fat, and underlying structures.[5]

1. Epidermal burns are painful, erythematous and blanch to touch. Skin is pink to red in colour, intact with an example being sunburn. Healing occurs within 7 days. Treatment is aimed at comfort using agents such as aloe, or simple pain relief such as oral non-steroidal anti-inflammatory agents.
2. Superficial partial-thickness burn injury involves the epidermal and superficial dermal layers caused by scald injuries and flash flame burns. Skin is erythematous, painful, blanches to touch and often blisters. This degree of burn injury will re-epithelialise in 7–14 days. After healing these burns may have a slight skin discoloration.[111]
3. Mid-dermal partial-thickness injuries extend a part way into the dermis. They have a large zone of damaged non-viable tissue extending into the dermis, with damaged but viable tissue at the base. Preservation of the damaged but viable tissue (particularly in the initial period following injury) is pivotal to preventing burn wound progression. As some of the nerve endings remain viable, pain is present but is less severe when compared with superficial burns. Similarly, as some of the capillaries remain viable, capillary return is present, albeit delayed. Skin appears pale and mottled, does not blanch but is painful to pin-prick.[111] Healing takes 2–5 weeks, often with severe scarring.
4. Deep partial-thickness burns extend into the deep dermal layer. The tissue is a characteristic pink to pale ivory in appearance. It can also have a blotchy red base due to extravasation of red blood cells. The underlying tissue does not blanch, and the hair is easily removed; sensation is reduced. These burns usually take in excess of 3 weeks to heal and are managed with surgical excision and closure.
5. Full-thickness burns destroy both layers of skin (epidermis and dermis) and may penetrate more deeply into underlying structures. Appearance is characterised by a hard, leathery eschar that is painless and black, white, or cherry red. These injuries require excision and skin grafting, otherwise these wounds heal by re-epithelialisation from the wound edges.[111]

Assessment of the TBSA of burns

The extent of injury is best described using the percentage of the TBSA that sustained burns. The measurement of burn surface area is important during the initial management of people with burns for estimating fluid requirements and determining the need for transfer to a burns service. Erythema should not be included when calculating burn area.

There are two frequently used methods that provide a reproducible estimation of the area of surface area burns. These are:

- Rule of nines – for the adult population, the most widely known and easily applied method of estimating TBSA is the 'rule of nines' (Fig. 24.9). The principle of this assessment method is that most areas of the body constitute 9% (or multiples of 9%) of the TBSA.[5,111]
- Palmar surface – the surface area of a patient's palm (including fingers) is about 1% TBSA. This method of estimating TBSA is yet to be validated. The palmar surface method can be used to estimate relatively small burns (<15% of total surface area) or very large burns (>85%, when unburnt skin is counted), but is inaccurate for medium-sized burns. This method is seen as crucial in evaluating burns of mixed distribution.[5,111]

FIGURE 24.9 Diagram of the 'rule of nines': (**A**) adult; (**B**) child.[111]

Adult body	% of total
Part	BSA
Arm	9%
Head	9%
Neck	1%
Leg	18%
Anterior trunk	18%
Posterior trunk	18%

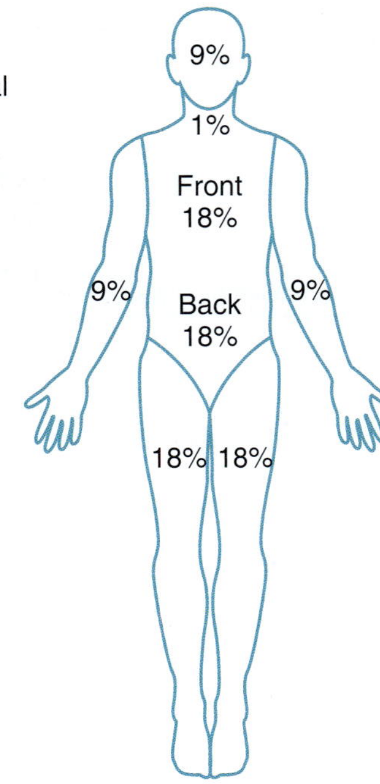

A

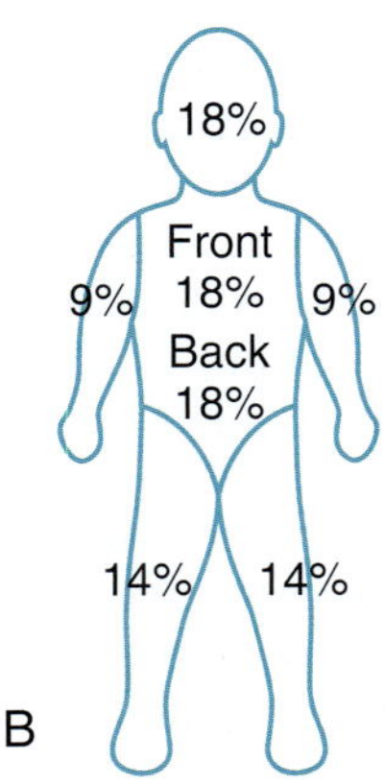

B

Child body	% of total
Part	BSA
Arm	9%
Head and neck	18%
Leg	14%
Anterior trunk	18%
Posterior trunk	18%

Source: Jeschke MGH, David N. Herndon. Sabiston Textbook of surgery. 20th ed. Elsevier; 2017.

Patient management

Care can be considered in four phases, including initial assessment, acute resuscitation, wound management, and rehabilitation.[103]

Initial assessment includes the immediate priorities of care (outlined below) and includes emergency principles, assessment and management of airway, breathing and circulation, and minimisation of hypothermia and hyperkalaemia.

Acute resuscitation is provided throughout the first 24 hours (Table 24.11). Care of the burn patient beyond that time will follow the general principles for critically ill patients, with additional considerations relating to wound care (discussed below).

Emergency principles of care

The principles of care once the danger has been removed, whether at the scene or in the ED, is to stop the burning process[103,111] and to cool the wound to minimise the burden of injury, using either running water, wet towels or saline-soaked gauze. Burns cooled for 20 minutes show greater re-epithelisation than other cooling times.[111,114] The wound and the patient should then be covered to reduce risk of hypothermia. Adequate analgesia must be provided early in patient care.

Airway

All patients with burn injury require supplemental oxygen. Facial burns or carbonaceous sputum (sputum with signs of smoke or charcoal) may indicate a burn injury to the airway. Upper airway obstruction may develop rapidly, and respiratory status continually monitored. A carboxyhaemoglobin of >10% within the first hour post-injury is strongly indicative of inhalation injury. Assume that carbon monoxide poisoning has occurred in patients trapped in enclosed areas, with caution required in interpreting oxygen saturation levels. Burns localised to the face and mouth cause more localised oedema and pose a greater risk for airway compromise. Classic signs of obstruction including stridor, dyspnoea and hoarse voice warrant immediate intubation and should be considered early as worsening oedema can make intubation difficult. Airway stability is mandatory for safe transfer.[5,111,114]

TABLE 24.11
Acute nursing care after burn injury (first 24 h)

ELEMENT OF CARE	MINOR BURN INJURY (<10%)	MAJOR BURN INJURY	CRITICALLY ILL
Fluid replacement	Generally not fluid loaded	Fluid replacement as per relevant formula	Major fluid replacement
Need for intubation and mechanical ventilation	Supplemental oxygen therapy. Only if airway burns are suspected or comorbidities require it	Supplemental oxygen therapy. Intubation and mechanical ventilation may be required with analgesia and in burns shock. Any airway burn in this group requires intubation	Mandatory
Respiratory and cardiovascular observations	Hourly TPR, BP, SpO_2 adapted according to patient status	Continuous ECG, SpO_2, temperature, urine output (hourly observations if not continuously monitored)	Continuous invasive haemodynamic, respiratory and urine output monitoring, including core temperature
Neurovascular observations	Assess neurovascular status of circumferential burns to chest and limbs (including fingers and toes)	Assess neurovascular status of circumferential burns to chest and limbs (including fingers and toes)	Assess neurovascular status of circumferential burns to chest and limbs (including fingers and toes)
Analgesia	Continuous, intermittent or patient-controlled (if patient capable) analgesia ± conscious sedation for dressings	Continuous intravenous analgesia ± conscious sedation for dressings	Continuous intravenous analgesia + sedation
Arterial blood gas, serum potassium; chloride and haemoglobin	Baseline and as indicated by patient's condition	Baseline and as indicated by patient's condition	Baseline and minimum 4-hourly depending on patient's condition, including temperature and ventilatory requirements
Haematology	Baseline and as indicated by patient's condition	Baseline and as indicated by patient's condition, noting that more frequent assessment will be needed if coagulopathy is present	Baseline and as indicated by patient's condition, noting that more frequent assessment will be needed if coagulopathy is present
Feeding	Oral intake should be monitored and encouraged	Enteral or oral intake should commence within 24 h of injury (NB: burns of >20% TBSA require enteral feeding)	Enteral feeding should commence within 24 h of injury
General burn dressings	Primary debridement undertaken by nursing staff with theatre debridement if indicated due to burn depth Burn escharotomy as indicated (unlikely unless circumferential injury)	Primary debridement undertaken by nursing staff with theatre debridement if indicated due to burn depth Burns escharotomy as indicated (likely with circumferential injury)	Primary debridement undertaken by nursing staff with theatre debridement if indicated due to burn depth Burns escharotomy as indicated (highly likely)

BP = blood pressure; ECG = electrocardiogram; SpO_2 = peripheral oxygen saturation; TBSA = total body surface area; TPR = temperature, pulse respiration.

Breathing

Carbonaceous pulmonary secretions are a hallmark of airway injury. Dyspnoea and tachypnoea are signs of respiratory distress, while pulmonary oedema will often ensue with airway burns.

Circulation

Evaluation of circulating blood volume can be difficult in severely burned patients, especially those who may have accompanying injuries. The massive interstitial and intracellular fluid shifts associated with acute burn injury will deplete circulating volume and result in shock if it remains uncorrected. Fluid resuscitation aims to prevent shock and to support organ function, while avoiding the complications of over- or under-administration of fluid. Fluid resuscitation should commence as indicated when there is >20% TBSA in adults.[114] Early intravenous cannulation (with two wide-bore cannulae) and the administration of high-volume fluids must begin immediately.[5,114] The initial fluid resuscitation guidelines have been updated by the American Burn Association to reflect concerns of over-resuscitation when using the traditional Parkland formula.[5] Crystalloid solution is recommended in the first 24 hours, with fluid administration titrated to patient response and should be delivered at 2 mL/kg/% TBSA based on the modified Parkland formula, over the first 24 hours commencing at the time of burn injury, with half the fluid administered within the first 8 hours and the remainder over the next 16 hours.

Fluid resuscitation should be guided by predetermined end points in combination with fluid volumes dictated by the formula. Precise end points for burns resuscitation remain debatable with urine output widely seen as the target for successful fluid replacement;[103] however, MAP targets and invasive haemodynamic monitoring parameters are also used to guide resuscitation end points.[115] The International Society for Burn Injuries[116] recommends titration of fluid resuscitation targeting a urine output of 0.3–0.5 mL/kg/h in adults and 1m/kg/h in children. Ideally urine output should be measured via indwelling catheters; however, this is not always practical in some geographical locations.[116]

The use of colloid solutions in the resuscitation of patients with burns remains controversial and there is limited evidence related to outcomes.[103,117] The evolution of 'fluid creep' has been reported due to over-resuscitation in the early phases of shock, which can result in complications such as acute lung injury, abdominal and extremity compartment syndrome, multi-organ failure and death.[103]

Patients with circumferential full-thickness burn injury may require escharotomies due to the extensive oedema and the inelasticity of burn eschar. Delayed capillary return, a cool limb and increased pain manifest earlier than loss of palpable pulse.

Invasive monitoring in the burns patient is controversial, as the relevant catheters often require insertion through a burn and therefore provide a portal of entry for infection. However, all serious burns patients require an indwelling catheter for monitoring. Relevance of other monitoring capability will be determined on an individual patient basis based on cardiovascular status, need for inotropic support, extent of the burn and potential for infection.

Minimising hypothermia

Treatment strategies, such as cooling the burn and administering high-volume fluid replacement, exposure of wounds following injury and during dressing changes, place the patient at high risk of hypothermia. Continuous temperature monitoring is essential, and strategies to maintain normothermia should be implemented immediately. Strategies include minimising exposure, warming fluids and warming the patient's environment. Warm blankets and heated humidified supplemental oxygen are valuable adjuncts along with consideration for invasive intravenous catheters with capability for warming or cooling, if available.

Hyperkalaemia

Cell destruction from the burn injury can result in high serum potassium levels, which should be monitored closely. Metabolic acidosis will exacerbate the hyperkalaemia, as intracellular exchange of hydrogen ions with potassium ions takes place.

Nutrition

Burns induce a hypermetabolic response which increases oxygen consumption, lipolysis and weight loss, which are proportional to burn size.[111] Supplemental feeding is mandatory and should commence as soon as possible following severe burn injuries, with recommendations that enteral nutrition be commenced within a few hours of injury.[103,111] Parenteral nutrition is another option, although it has been associated with increased complications and mortality in comparison to enteral feeding.[111] Adults with >20% TBSA and children with >10% TBSA are unable to meet their nutritional requirements orally.

The multitrauma burns patient

The combination of traumatic injury and burn injury often occurs in high-energy motor vehicle, industrial accidents or trauma associated with explosives. These patients present with a wide variety of severity and pattern, depending on the mechanism of injury. Treatment of many traumatic injuries takes priority over definitive burn care and early operation and repair is advised as fresh burns are initially thought to be free of bacteria.[103] Optimal management is achieved through balancing the conflicting treatment requirements for each injury as discussed below:[118]

- Spinal injury – if the patient has potential spinal injuries in addition to the burn, spinal precautions must be maintained; however, cervical collars should not be used over a burnt neck or upper chest due to the potential for swelling and subsequent restriction. If a collar is used, changing to an appropriate size as the swelling worsens or goes down is essential.
- Skeletal injury – skin traction cannot be used in a patient with burn injury; this will necessitate the use of an external fixateur, or early internal fixation which has an associated higher risk of infection.[118,119]

- Electrocution injuries – comprise approximately 4% of all reported burns,[120] are largely internal, and can cause devastating multiple internal injuries. The electrical current causes a burn at both the entry and exit sites. Burn care in this patient cohort is the same as other burn care, although early debridement may not demonstrate the deeper injury, thus serial debridement may be recommended to allow the wound time to declare itself before grafting occurs.[120] There are three types of electrical burn injury: true electrical injury by current flow, arc injury from the electrical arc as it passes from the source to an object, and a flame injury from ignition of clothing or surroundings.[120] All patients with confirmed or suspected high-voltage injury, must be admitted for close observation if they have, ECG changes, loss of consciousness, or concerns for extremity compartment syndrome. Close monitoring for cardiac damage and rhabdomyolysis is essential. Patients with low-voltage injuries and normal ECG can be discharged home if there are no other indications for admission.[120]

Secondary complications such as cataract formation or peripheral neurologic complications have been reported and require follow up.[120]

Burn dressings

Mitigating infection is the primary aim of good burns nursing. The greatest challenge is minimising the risk for cross-contamination, and patients should be nursed in a single room where possible. Burn dressings present a physical challenge, particularly when large areas of the body are affected.

The traditional burn dressing in the ICU is undertaken as a surgically clean technique. The following is a guide to specific aspects of burn management:

- Debridement – the excision of dead skin. Gentle scrubbing is generally used to remove loose tissue and burst blisters. Forceps and scissors may be required to lift and remove smaller areas of tissue. Extensive areas of debridement will usually be undertaken in the operating room.
- Blisters – small blisters should be left intact whereas large blisters may be aspirated or deroofed during debridement, although it should be noted that evidence regarding blister management is poor. Blisters over joints that are restricting movement should also be debrided.
- Escharotomy – an incision through the eschar, and does not involve opening muscle fascia. The escharotomy immediately relieves the compression and is a limb-/life-saving surgical manoeuvre. The escharotomy is dressed as a burn to prevent infection.
- Skin grafts – required to cover skin defects. They may be full-thickness or partial-thickness grafts, and may be harvested from the patient or obtained from a cadaver donor. Regardless of the type of skin graft, nursing care remains the same, with the aim being to maximise adherence. Specific nursing care of the graft site includes leaving the site intact and immobilising the graft site, applying the appropriate wound care regimen, preventing shearing injury to the graft site and minimising the risk for infection. With autografts, wound care will also be required for the donor site.[121]
- Skin substitutes – can be catagorised as either biological substitutes, synthetic substitutes or a combination of both. Synthetic skin substitutes are free from any risk of disease transmission; however, there are only a few available.[122] Some products are available to cover partial-thickness wounds that provide a moist environment that stimulates epithelialisation. These are best reserved for 'clean' wounds. Some products are able to act as full-thickness substitutes that provide wound closure, protection from mechanical trauma and bacteria and a vapour barrier.[122] Once the new dermis is created the substitute is removed.[121]

Summary

Care of the trauma patient presents the critical care nurse with multiple challenges. With the introduction of trauma systems, the outcome and survival of injured patients has improved dramatically. The severity of injury and patient outcome are dependent on effective pre-hospital care, resuscitation, definitive surgical management on arrival at the hospital and intensive care. Principles of resuscitation of the trauma patient are the same as for all patients, with a primary, secondary and tertiary survey being undertaken, and maintenance or correction of airway, breathing and circulation taking precedence. Prevention of the 'lethal triad' of acidosis, hypothermia and coagulopathy has the potential to significantly influence patient outcome. Consideration of the specific injury, with its resultant pathophysiological changes, is necessary to care effectively for patients with abdominal, chest, multiple or burn injuries. It is challenging work as trauma patients are largely a young and healthy population prior to injury and may experience significant ongoing compromise.

Case study

Peter, a 27-year-old man, was jogging at 06:00 when he was hit by a car at a pedestrian crossing and ejected 20 m. Initial GCS was 3, improved to 9 on EMS arrival, his breathing and pulse were present. He had an obvious open head injury, open right leg fractures and possible pelvic fracture.

Peter met the major trauma triage criteria and was transferred via road to a major trauma hospital. Trauma team activation occurred prior to Peter's arrival on arrival in the emergency department (ED). The team, including a trauma surgeon, trauma nurse leader, emergency doctor, orthopaedic surgeon, neurosurgeon, anaesthetist, specialist nurses and support staff, received handover and commenced primary survey.

EMS assessment and treatment included:

- Haemodynamically stable, unconscious GCS 3, SpO_2 95% on room air.
- IV cannula × 2 were inserted with 500 mL normal saline delivered. Peter received O_2 and morphine for pain, spinal immobilisation and splinting of leg and pelvis. C-spine collar removed as patient distressed.

ED assessment and treatment included:

- Fluctuating GCS, 8–12. Profoundly hypotensive, SpO_2 75%.
- Primary survey completed, including full blood count, clotting profile, ABG taken.
- Medical history of congenital blindness and deafness.
- Initial resuscitation included activation of massive transfusion protocol, insertion of arterial line, metaraminol for BP support and analgesia.
- Trauma series X-ray completed (chest, pelvis, R femur, R tibia/fibula).
- FAST +ve.
- ABG: acidotic, $Sp0_2$ 96%, K+ 4.9, glucose 17.4, lactate 4.5.

Duration in ED was 35 minutes.

Disposition from ED included:

- Initial operating theatre (OT) visit for emergency laparotomy – small bowel resection and diaphragm repair and post-stabilisation transported to Radiology for further scans.
- Post-CT scan patient proceeded to Angiography for embolisation prior to returning to theatre for insertion of intracranial pressure (ICP) monitoring. Intraoperatively noted increased ICPs.
- Repeat CT brain demonstrated increased subdural ≥ return to OT again for craniectomy, insertion of extraventricular (EVD) drain and application of external fixateur to leg and pelvis.

OT assessments and treatment included:

- Fluctuating haemodynamics, with ongoing acidosis, hypotension (SBP<95) and hypothermia over 10 h.
- Ongoing massive transfusion requirements: 20 units RBC, 13 units FFP, three pooled platelets, one pooled cryoprecipitate.

Total duration time 10 h.

Peter's injuries included: head (severe TBI), spine (C1/2 facet joint widening, T6 fracture), chest, abdomen, pelvis, upper and lower extremities, vascular injuries (bilateral internal carotid dissection and L vertebral artery dissection), bladder and ureteric injury.

Intensive care assessments and treatment included:

- Stable haemodynamics, including ongoing inotropic support and mechanical ventilation.
- First ABG demonstrated ongoing acidosis with a lactate 4.0; however, improved over first 4 h in ICU.
- Abdominal pressures measured via IDC: 20–24 mmHg.

- Hourly neuro observations and TBI protocol followed for management of ICPs. Haemodynamic parameters goals documented. GCS 3: pupils unreactive: ?preexisting. ICP <10 mmHg. Discussion with family on how to ask patient to open eyes (in context of being legally deaf and blind).
- Family meeting and update on injuries and prognosis provided by ICU medical and nursing staff along with support from Social Work with Auslan interpreters. Patient's sister nominated as emergency contact as patient's partner also deaf and blind.

Day 3 ICU, troponin 638, lactate 4.4.

- Ongoing abdominal assessment demonstrated increased abdominal distension, high nasogastric aspirates, decreasing urine output and rising lactate. Review by surgical team and returned to OT: subtotal colectomy and stoma formation, and flexible cystoscopy and retrograde pyelogram.
- Sedation and analgesia weaned off post-surgery for assessment of severity of TBI.
- Tertiary survey completed by Trauma unit and no further injuries identified.

Day 5: patient remained GCS 3 and MRI completed which demonstrated diffuse injury with likely dependent outcome.

Day 6: family meeting occurred. MRI report findings communicated with next of kin (NOK) and family. Patient had expressed wishes to be independent, which was reiterated by the entire family. Social work was present at the meeting as were staff from DonateLife due to availability of Auslan interpreters.

Day 10: Consent for Donation after Cardiac Death (DCD); however, did not meet criteria postextubation. Palliative care was involved with family and comfort care implemented. Corneal tissue donated, which restored sight to two people.

Within ICU the members of the multidisciplinary team that contributed to Peter's care included: nursing and medical, physiotherapists delivering ongoing respiratory assessment, passive limb movements and assessment for increasing tone in all limbs, Dietitian to assess nutritional requirements and provide total parenteral nutrition, pharmacist to provide parenteral nutrition formula and to assess previous medication history. Nursing care involved all aspects of hygiene, repositioning to prevent the development of pressure injuries or associated complications from injuries, interpretation of all blood results and escalation of abnormal levels, management of ventilation changes and assessment and management of TBI care and adjustment of treatment based on patient's physiological responses to interventions. Nursing staff provided support for the family when present, communication of changes and liaison with social work staff in organising family updates with interpreters.

Peter's care was complex and resource intensive, requiring the expertise and contribution of various clinical teams including the trauma, orthopaedic, vascular, neurosurgical and social work teams. Effective communication and consultation are essential to ensure optimal care.

Due to the family history of congenital blindness and deafness, communication for family meetings was challenging. Peter's partner was also blind and deaf from the same syndrome as were two of his three sisters. His eldest sister, who was not deaf or blind, was nominated as NOK due to the ability to contact her.

CASE STUDY QUESTIONS

1. Discuss the components of the 'DCR and surgery' and three stages in relation to this patient's initial presentation and disposition post-ED.
2. Discuss serial abdominal assessment in the intensive care environment and factors that may indicate hollow abdominal injury and contributing factors for the development of ACS in this patient.
3. Discuss factors for consideration in patients requiring massive blood transfusion.
4. Discuss the potential complications of vascular injuries for this patient and the observations that may indicate that vascular compromise has occurred. Vascular injuries are often managed non-operatively and patients are prescribed aspirin. Discuss the contraindications for this therapy in relation to Peter's injuries.
5. Describe the challenges for effective communication and assessment of GCS for Peter, including the entire patient journey with or without a TBI.

RESEARCH VIGNETTE

Hernandez MC, El Khatib M, Prokop L, Zielinski MD, Aho JM. Complications in tube thoracostomy: systematic review and meta-analysis. J Trauma Acute Care Surgery 2018; 85(2):410-416

Abstract

Background: Tube thoracostomy (TT) complications and their reported rates are highly variable (1-40%) and inconsistently classified. Consistent TT complication classification must be applied to compare reported literature to standardize TT placement. We aim to determine the overall TT related complication rates in patients receiving TT for traumatic indications utilizing uniform definitions.

Method: Systematic review and meta-analysis was performed assessing TT related complications. Comprehensive search of several databases (1975-2015) was conducted. We included studies that reported on bedside TT insertion (≥ 22 F) in trauma patients. Data were abstracted from eligible articles by independent reviewers with discrepancies reconciled by a third. Analyses were based on complication category subtypes: insertional, positional, removal, infection/immunologic/education and malfunction.

Results: Database search resulted in 478 studies; after applying criteria 29 studies were analyzed representing 4981 TTs. Injury mechanisms included blunt 60% [49-71], stab 27% [17-34], and gunshot 13% [7.8-10]. Overall median complication rate was 19% (95% CI, 14 - 24.3). Complication subtypes included insertional (15.3%), positional (53.1%), removal (16.2%), infection/immunologic (14.8%), malfunction (0.6%). Complication rates did not change significantly over time for insertional, immunologic, or removal p=0.8. Over time, there was a decrease in infectious related TT complications as well as an increase in positional TT complications.

Conclusions: Generation of evidence based approaches to improve TT insertion outcomes is difficult as a variety of complication classifications have been utilized. This meta-analysis of complications after TT insertion in trauma patients suggests that complications have not changed over time remaining stable at 19% over the past three decades.

Level of Evidence: III.

Critique

The status of TT complications in trauma patients has been summarised in this review. Complications of the procedure are underestimated with a significant risk of mortality, morbidity and cost. True rates of complications have been difficult to quantify due to the lack of universally standardised reporting making comparisons between hospitals and countries challenging. The authors specifically focused on the hypothesis that after using a uniformed classification of complications, the complication rates would show a consistent rate throughout time and that the majority of complications would be related to positional issues.

The database search yielded 478 studies, of these 29 (6%) fulfilled the inclusion criteria representing 4981 TT between 1978 and 2013. The authors used a validated classification system assigning complications from each of the 29 studies into separated categories representing complication subtype that were used in meta-analyses. The result in this study shows that one in five patients suffer from complications, the overall complication rate of 19% remained steady over time. A significant increase of positional complications was found whereas infectious complications decreased over time.

This study has several strengths. The authors describe a comprehensive literature search including design of a search strategy and the utilisation of library expertise with input from two of the authors. Three authors screened the abstracts from the search results through PRISMA guidelines (preferred reporting items for systematic and meta-analyses)[123] using the inclusion and exclusion criteria. The study used meta-analysis, a statistical process that summarises and combines data from multiple studies represented graphically in the study with blobbogram (forest plot). Publication bias was discussed.

There are also some shortcomings of this review. The database searching methods for knowledge synthesis could have used a search tool, e.g. PRESS 2015 Evidence-Based Checklist, to improve quality and comprehensiveness of the search and reduce errors. Furthermore, the study characteristics should have been more explicitly presented in the results, e.g. study size, follow-up period, country, detailed assessment of quality and citation.

TT placement is one of the most commonly performed procedures used in trauma patients for life-threatening emergencies such as the evacuation of haemothorax and prevention of the development of tension pneumothorax while promoting lung re-expansion and improve respiratory function. Overall, this review is a good example of a systematic review study demonstrating possibilities of translating knowledge into practice. Critical care nurses, using their clinical expertise, can prevent and identify complications through repeated clinical assessment and monitoring contributing to improving trauma patients' safety and outcome.

Learning activities

1. Describe potential complication subtypes associated with placement of TT and reflect on management of care, signs and symptoms, prevention and interventions in case problems arise.
2. Review your local guidelines for DCR and massive transfusion protocol. Reflect on the balance between timely and adequate resuscitation for patients, which saves lives, and the need to avoid blood product waste and morbidities associated with massive transfusion.
3. Discuss the benefits for the trauma patient with or without TBI of combining pharmacological thromboprophylaxis with mechanical thromboprophylaxis.
4. Outline the strengths and weaknesses of inclusive and exclusive trauma systems and the impact on staff training and management of the trauma patients in each.
5. Outline the components of a trauma system including discussion on the elements of pre-hospital system and key attributes of the Team Leader in the ED during resuscitation.

Online resources

American College of Surgeons, www.facs.org

Australian College for Emergency Medicine, www.acem.org.au

Australian and New Zealand Burn Association, www.anzba.org.au

Australian Trauma Society, www.traumasociety.com.au

Eastern Association for the Surgery of Trauma, www.east.org

European Society for Trauma and Emergency Surgery, www.esteonline.org

National Institute for Health and Care Excellence (NICE). Trauma, https://www.nice.org.uk/guidance/qs166

NSW Institute of Trauma and Injury Management, https://www.aci.health.nsw.gov.au/get-involved/institute-of-trauma-and-injury-management

NSW Trauma System, www.itim.nsw.gov.au/index.cfm

Royal Australasian College of Surgeons, www.surgeons.org

Society of Trauma Nurses, www.traumanurses.org

Trauma.org, an independent, non-profit organisation providing global education, information and communication resources for professionals in trauma and critical care, www.trauma.org

Trauma Victoria, www.trauma.reach.vic.gov.au

Victorian State Trauma System, www2.health.vic.gov.au

World Health Organization, www.who.int/topics/injuries/en/

Further reading

Cannon JW, Kahn MA, Raja AS, et al. Damage control resuscitation in patients with severe hemorrhage: a practice management guideline from the Eastern Association for the surgery of trauma. J Trauma Acute Care Surgery 2017;82(2): 605–17.

Mathews ZR, Koyfman A. Blast injuries. J Emerg Med 2015;49(2):573–87.

Rossaint R, Bouillon B, Cerny V, et al. European guideline on management of major bleeding and coagulopathy following trauma: fourth edition. Crit Care 2016;20(100):2–55. doi:10.1186/s13054-016-1265-x.

Skinner DV, Driscoll PA. ABC of major trauma. 4th ed. Chichester: Wiley; 2013.

References

1. Haagsma JA, Graetz N, Bolliger I, et al. The global burden of injury: incidence, mortality, disability-adjusted life years and time trends from the Global Burden of Disease study 2013. Inj Prev 2016;22(1):3–18.
2. Moore L, Champion H, O'Reilly G, et al. Impact of trauma system structure on injury outcomes: a systematic review protocol. Syst Rev 2017;6(1):12.
3. Lendrum RA, Lockey DJ. Trauma system development. Anaesthesia 2013;68(Suppl. 1):30–9.
4. Borgohain B, Khonglah T. Developing and organizing a trauma system and mass casualty management: some useful observations from the Israeli Trauma Model. Ann Med Health Sci Res 2013;3(1):85–9.
5. American College of Surgeons. ATLS student course manual: advanced trauma life support. 10th ed. Chicago: American College of Surgeons; 2018.
6. Lendrum R, Lockey D. Trauma system development. Anaesthesia 2013;68(s1):30–9.
7. Cameron PA, Gabbe BJ, Smith K, et al. Triaging the right patient to the right place in the shortest time. Br J Anaesth 2014;113(2):226–33.
8. Anand LK, Singh M, Kapoor D. Prehospital trauma care services in developing countries. Anaesth Pain Intensive Care 2013;17(1):65.
9. Harmsen A, Giannakopoulos G, Moerbeek P, et al. The influence of prehospital time on trauma patients outcome: a systematic review. Injury 2015;46(4):602–9.
10. Collopy K, Kivlehan S, Snyder S. Busting top trauma myths. Exploring best practices for prehospital trauma care. EMS world 2015;44(3):38–45.
11. Wisborg T, Castren M, Lippert A, et al. Training trauma teams in the Nordic countries: an overview and present status. Acta Anaesthesiol Scand 2005;49(7):1004–9.
12. Dagal A, Greer SE, McCunn M. International disparities in trauma care. Curr Opin Anaesthesiol 2014;27(2):233–9.
13. Rouse C, Hayre J, French J, et al. A traumatic tale of two cities: does EMS level of care and transportation model affect survival in patients with trauma at level 1 trauma centres in two neighbouring Canadian provinces? Emerg Med J 2017.
14. Aljerian N, Alhaidar S, Alothman A, et al. Association between the mode of transport and in-hospital medical complications in trauma patients: findings from a level-I trauma center in Saudi Arabia. Ann Saudi Med 2018;38(1):488–94.
15. Wandling MW, Nathens AB, Shapiro MB, et al. Association of prehospital mode of transport with mortality in penetrating trauma: a trauma system-level assessment of private vehicle transportation vs ground emergency medical services. JAMA Surg 2018;153(2):107–13.
16. Huber S, Crönlein M, von Matthey F, et al. Effect of private versus emergency medical systems transportation in trauma patients in a mostly physician based system-a retrospective multicenter study based on the TraumaRegister DGU®. Scand J Trauma Resusc Emerg Med 2016;24(1):60.
17. Debenham S, Fuller M, Stewart M, et al. Where there is no EMS: lay providers in emergency medical services care-EMS as a public health priority. Prehospital Disaster Med 2017;32(6):593–5.
18. Shaw JJ, Psoinos CM, Santry HP. It's all about location, location, location: a new perspective on trauma transport. Ann Surg 2016;263(2):413–18.
19. Brown JB, Gestring ML, Guyette FX, et al. Helicopter transport improves survival following injury in the absence of a time-saving advantage. Surgery 2016;159(3):947–59.
20. Thomas SH, Blumen I. Helicopter emergency medical services literature 2014 to 2016: lessons and perspectives, part 1 – helicopter transport for trauma. Air Med J 2017.
21. Victorian Department of Health. Trauma Victoria. Major trauma guidelines & education – Victorian State Trauma System; 2018. Available from: trauma.reach.vic.gov.au [Accessed 22 March 2018].
22. Tiel Groenestege-Kreb D, van Maarseveen O, Leenen L. Trauma team. Br J Anaesth 2014;113(2):258–65.

23. McCullough A, Haycock J, Forward D, et al. Early management of the severely injured major trauma patient. Br J Anaesth 2014;113(2):234–41.
24. Steiner D, Renetseder F, Kutz A, et al. Performance of the Manchester triage system in adult medical emergency patients: a prospective cohort study. J Emerg Med 2016;50(4):678–89.
25. Jeffries D. Triage acuity scales. In: Visser L, Monetjano AS, Grossman VA, editors. Fast facts for the traige nurse: an orientation and care guide in a nutshell. New York: Springer; 2015. p. 65–70.
26. Groenestege-Kreb DT, Van Maarseveen O, Leenen L. Trauma team. Br J Anaesth 2014;113(2):258–65.
27. Maluso P, Hernandez M, Amdur RL, et al. Trauma team size and task performance in adult trauma resuscitations. J Surg Res 2016;204(1):176–82.
28. Williams SRP, Phillips; Gharahbaghian, Laleh. The FAST and E-FAST in 2013: trauma ultrasonography. Crit Care Clin 2014;30(1):119–50.
29. Brenner M, Hicks C. Major abdominal trauma: critical decisions and new frontiers in management. Emerg Med Clin North Am 2018;36(1):149–60.
30. McArthur CL, Pieter HW. Abdominal and pelvic injuries. In: Bersten ADS, editor. Oh's Intensive care manual. 7th ed. Oxford: Elsevier; 2014. p. 807–13.
31. Akoglu H, Celik OF, Celik A, et al. Diagnostic accuracy of the Extended Focused Abdominal Sonography for Trauma (E-FAST) performed by emergency physicians compared to computed tomography. Am J Emerg Med 2017.
32. World Health Organization. Children's environmental health. Injuries: World Health Organization; 2018. Available from: http://www.who.int/ceh/risks/cehinjuries2/en/.
33. Wolf SJ, Bebarta VS, Bonnett CJ, et al. Blast injuries. Lancet 2009;374(9687):405–15.
34. Chandran A, Hyder AA, Peek-Asa C. The global burden of unintentional injuries and an agenda for progress. Epidemiol Rev 2010;32(1):110–20.
35. Ackland H Spinal clearance management protocol. Melbourne: Alfred Health; 2009. Available from: https://www.alfredhealth.org.au/contents/resources/clinical-resources/SpinalClearanceManagementProtocol_External.pdf; updated November 2009 [Accessed 25 February 2019].
36. Cameron P. Trauma. In: Cameron P, Jelinek G, Kelly A-M, et al, editors. Textbook of adult emergency medicine. 4th ed. Elsevier; 2015. p. 71–162.
37. Theodore N, Hadley MN, Aarabi B, et al. Prehospital cervical spinal immobilization after trauma. Neurosurgery 2013;72(suppl_3):22–34.
38. Newgard CD, Schmicker RH, Hedges JR, et al. Emergency medical services intervals and survival in trauma: assessment of the 'golden hour' in a North American prospective cohort. Ann Emerg Med 2010;55(3):235–46, e4.
39. Stanton D, Hardcastle T, Muhlbauer D, et al. Cervical collars and immobilisation: a South African best practice recommendation. Afr J Emerg Med 2017;7(1):4–8.
40. Bogert JN, Harvin JA, Cotton BA. Damage control resuscitation. J Intensive Care Med 2016;31(3):177–86.
41. Rossaint R, Bouillon B, Cerny V, et al. The European guideline on management of major bleeding and coagulopathy following trauma, 4th edn. Crit Care 2016;20(1):100.
42. Bulger EM, Snyder D, Schoelles K, et al. An evidence-based prehospital guideline for external hemorrhage control: American College of Surgeons Committee on Trauma. Prehosp Emerg Care 2014;18(2):163–73.
43. The National Institute for Health and Care Excellence (NICE). Major trauma: assessment and initial management. NICE guideline. London: NICE, 2016.
44. Berry C, Ley EJ, Bukur M, et al. Redefining hypotension in traumatic brain injury. Injury 2012;43(11):1833–7.
45. Chang R, Holcomb JB. Optimal fluid therapy for traumatic hemorrhagic shock. Crit Care Clin 2017;33(1):15–36.
46. CRASH-2 trial collaborators, Shakur H, Roberts I, et al. Effects of tranexamic acid on death, vascular occlusive events, and blood transfusion in trauma patients with significant haemorrhage (CRASH-2): a randomised, placebo-controlled trial. Lancet 2010;376(9734):23–32.
47. Moffatt SE. Hypothermia in trauma. Emerg Med J 2013;12:989–96.
48. Mylankal KJ, Wyatt MG. Control of major haemorrhage. Surg Oxford Int Ed 2010;28(11):556–62.
49. Frith D, Brohi K. The acute coagulopathy of trauma shock: clinical relevance. Surgeon 2010;8(3):159–63.
50. Langhelle A, Lockey D, Harris T, et al. Body temperature of trauma patients on admission to hospital: a comparison of anaesthetised and non-anaesthetised patients. Emerg Med J 2012;29(3):239–42.
51. Kheirbek T, Kochanek AR, Alam HB. Hypothermia in bleeding trauma: a friend or a foe? Scand J Trauma Resusc Emerg Med 2009;17(1):65.
52. Ireland S, Endacott R, Cameron P, et al. The incidence and significance of accidental hypothermia in major trauma – a prospective observational study. Resuscitation 2011;82(3):300–6.
53. Chovanes J, Cannon JW, Nunez TC. The evolution of damage control surgery. Surgical Clinics 2012;92(4):859–75.
54. O'Connor JV. Damage control thoracic surgery. J Cardiothor Trauma 2016;1(1):8.
55. Vaidya R, Waldron J, Scott A, et al. Angiography and embolization in the management of bleeding pelvic fractures. J Am Acad Orthop Surg 2018;26(4):e68.

56. Morrison JJ, Galgon RE, Jansen JO, et al. A systematic review of the use of resuscitative endovascular balloon occlusion of the aorta in the management of hemorrhagic shock. J Trauma Acute Care Surg 2016;80(2):324–34.
57. Caba-Doussoux P, Leon-Baltasar JL, Garcia-Fuentes C. Resines-Erasun C. Damage control orthopaedics in severe polytrauma with femur fracture. Injury 2012;43:S42–6.
58. Hsu JM, Pham TN. Damage control in the injured patient. Int J Crit Illn Inj Sci 2011;1(1):66.
59. Diercks DB, Mehrotra A, Nazarian DJ, et al. Clinical policy: critical issues in the evaluation of adult patients presenting to the emergency department with acute blunt abdominal trauma. Ann Emerg Med 2011;57(4):387–404.
60. Balogh ZJ, Reumann MK, Gruen RL, et al. Advances and future directions for management of trauma patients with musculoskeletal injuries. Lancet 2012;380(9847):1109–19.
61. Panteli M, Lampropoulos A, Giannoudis PV. Fat embolism following pelvic injuries: a subclinical event or an increased risk of mortality? Injury 2014;45(4):645–6.
62. EuroSafe. Injuries in the European Union: Summary of injury statistics 2012–2014 Amsterdam: Luxembourg Institute of Health; 2016, 6th edn. Available from: http://www.eurosafe.eu.com/key-actions/injury-data/reports.
63. Australian Institute of Health and Welfare (AIoHa). Injury; 2018. Available from: https://www.aihw.gov.au/reports-statistics/health-condition s-disability-deaths/injury/overview [Accessed 2018].
64. Little N, Rogers B, Flannery M. Bone formation, remodelling and healing. Surg Oxford Int Ed 2011;29(4):141–5.
65. Guyton ACH, John E. Textbook of medical physiology. 12th ed. Phildelphia: Saunders Elsevier; 2006.
66. Copuroglu C, Calori GM, Giannoudis PV. Fracture non-union: who is at risk? Injury 2013;44(11):1379–82.
67. Hak DJ, Fitzpatrick D, Bishop JA, et al. Delayed union and nonunions: epidemiology, clinical issues, and financial aspects. Injury 2014;45:S3–7.
68. Sinha P, Bunker N, Soni N. Fat embolism – an update. Curr Anaesth Crit Care 2010;21(5):277–81.
69. Zutt R, Van Der Kooi A, Linthorst G, et al. Rhabdomyolysis: review of the literature. Neuromuscul Disord 2014;24(8):651–9.
70. Bosch X, Poch E, Grau JM. Rhabdomyolysis and acute kidney injury. N Engl J Med 2009;361(1):62–72.
71. Wafaisade A, Paffrath T, Lefering R, et al. Patterns of early resuscitation associated with mortality after penetrating injuries. Br J Surg 2015;102(10):1220–8.
72. Srour M, Inaba K, Okoye O, et al. Prospective evaluation of treatment of open fractures: effect of time to irrigation and debridement. JAMA Surg 2015;150(4):332–6.
73. Chesser T, Cross A, Ward A. The use of pelvic binders in the emergent management of potential pelvic trauma. Injury 2012;43(6):667–9.
74. Langford JR, Burgess AR, Liporace FA, et al. Pelvic fractures: part 1. Evaluation, classification, and resuscitation. J Am Acad Orthop Surg 2013;21(8):448–57.
75. Walker J. Pelvic fractures: classification and nursing management. Nurs Stand 2011;26(10):49.
76. Eckroth-Bernard K, Davis JW. Management of pelvic fractures. Curr Opin Crit Care 2010;16(6):582–6.
77. Bayer J, Lefering R, Reinhardt S, et al. Thoracic trauma severity contributes to differences in intensive care therapy and mortality of severely injured patients: analysis based on the TraumaRegister DGU®. World J Emerg Surg 2017;12(1):43.
78. Fallouh H, Dattani-Patel R, Rathinam S. Blunt thoracic trauma. Surg Oxford Int Ed 2017;35(5):262–8.
79. Turkalj I, Petrović K, Stojanović S, et al. Blunt chest trauma: an audit of injuries diagnosed by the MDCT examination. Vojnosanit Pregl 2014;71(2):161–6.
80. Griwan M, Kumar S, Pal N. To study the etiology, pattern and short term outcome of chest injuries as prospective study. Int J All Res Educ Scientific Meth 2016;4(3):6–11.
81. Chowdhry TMF, Rathinam S. Penetrating injuries of the chest. Surg Oxford Int Ed 2017;35(5):255–61.
82. Biffl WL. Thoracic trauma. In: Vincent J-L, Abraham E, Moore FA, et al, editors. Textbook of critical care. 7th ed. Philadelphia: Elsevier; 2017. p. 1180–7.
83. Wiersema UF. Chest injuries. In: Bersten AD, editor. Oh's Intensive care manual. 7th ed. Oxford: Elsevier; 2014. p. 784–94, [Ch 77].
84. Raja AS. Thoracic trauma. In: Walls RM, Hockberger RS, Gausche-Hill M, et al, editors. Rosen's Emergency medicine - concepts and clinical practice. 9th ed. Philadelphia: Elsevier; 2018. p. 382–403.
85. Khan HS, Wadood A, Ayyaz M. Occult pneumothorax: what do we need to do? J Coll Physicians Surg Pak 2018;28(3):S31–2.
86. Marcolini EG, Keegan J. Blunt cardiac injury. Emerg Med Clin North Am 2015;33(3):519–27.
87. Platz JJ, Fabricant L, Norotsky M. Thoracic trauma: injuries, evaluation, and treatment. Surg Clin North Am 2017;97(4):783–99.
88. Altinok T, Can A. Management of tracheobronchial injuries. Eurasian J Med 2014;46(3):209.
89. Tricco AC, Tetzlaff J, Moher D. The art and science of knowledge synthesis. J Clin Epidemiol 2011;64.
90. Nichols JRP, Michael A. Abdominal trauma. In: Walls RM, Hockberger RS, Gausche-Hill M, et al, editors. Rosen's Emergency medicine: concepts and clinical practice. 9th ed. Philadelphia: Elsevier; 2018. p. 404–18.
91. Ingraham AP, Andrew B. Abdominal trauma. In: Vincent J-L, Edward A, Moore FA, et al, editors. Textbook of critical care. 7th ed. Philadelphia: Elsevier; 2017. p. 1188–90.
92. Mehta N, Babu S, Venugopal K. An experience with blunt abdominal trauma: evaluation, management and outcome. Clin Pract 2014;4(2):599.

93. Liagkos GT, Spyropoulos C, Tsourouflis G, et al. Successful non-operative management of blunt abdominal trauma in highly selective cases: a safe and effective choice. [Ulusal travma ve acil cerrahi dergisi]. Ulus Travma Acil Cerrahi Derg 2018;24(2):104–9.
94. Bège T, Brunet C, Berdah S. Hollow viscus injury due to blunt trauma: a review. J Visc Surg 2016;153(4):61–8.
95. Balogh ZJ, Lumsdaine W, Moore EE, et al. Postinjury abdominal compartment syndrome: from recognition to prevention. Lancet 2014;384(9952):1466–75.
96. Dreizin D, Munera F. Multidetector CT for penetrating torso trauma: state of the art. Radiology 2015;277(2):338–55.
97. Matsevych O, Koto M, Balabyeki M, et al. Trauma laparoscopy: when to start and when to convert? Surg Endosc 2018;32(3):1344–52.
98. Gamanagatti S, Rangarajan K, Kumar A. Blunt abdominal trauma: imaging and intervention. Curr Probl Diagn Radiol 2015;44(4):321–36.
99. Otsuka H, Sato T, Sakurai K, et al. Use of interventional radiology as initial hemorrhage control to improve outcomes for potentially lethal multiple blunt injuries. Injury 2018;49(2):226–9.
100. Burlew CC. Abdominal compartment sydrome and management of the open abdomen. In: Cameron JLC, Andrew M, editors. Current surgical therapy. 12th ed. Philadelphia: Elsevier; 2017. p. 1238–45.
101. Yorkgitis BK. Primary care of the blunt splenic injured adult. Am J Med 2017;130(3):365, e1–e5.
102. Tarchouli M, Elabsi M, Njoumi N, et al. Liver trauma: what current management? Hepatobiliary Pancreat Dis Int 2017;1.
103. Saffle JR. Critical Care Management of the severely burned patient. In: Parrillo JE, Dellinger RP, editors. Critical care medicine: principles of diagnosis and management in the adult. 4th ed. Philadelphia: Elsevier; 2014. p. 1177–98.
104. Ehrl D, Heidekrueger PI, Ninkovic M, et al. Effect of primary admission to burn centers on the outcomes of severely burned patients. Burns 2018.
105. Win TS, Nizamoglu M, Maharaj R, et al. Relationship between multidisciplinary critical care and burn patients survival: a propensity-matched national cohort analysis. Burns 2018;44(1):57–64.
106. World Health Organization. Fact Sheet. Burns; 2018. Available from: www.who.int/entity/mediacentre/factsheets/fs365/en/ [Accessed Jan 2018].
107. Smolle C, Cambiaso-Daniel J, Forbes AA, et al. Recent trends in burn epidemiology worldwide: a systematic review. Burns 2017;43(2):249–57.
108. NHS. National Burn Care Referral Guidance; 2012. Available from: https://www.britishburnassociation.org/wp-content/uploads/2018/02/National-Burn-Care-Referral-Guidance-2012.pdf.
109. Association ANZB. ANZBA Referral Criteria; 2013]. Available from: https://anzba.org.au/care/referral-criteria/ [Accessed 21 April 2018].
110. Association AB. Burn Center Referral Criteria; 2017. Available from: http://ameriburn.org/wp-content/uploads/2017/05/burncenterreferralcriteria.pdf.
111. Jeschke MGH, David N. Burns. Sabiston textbook of surgery. 20th ed. Philadelphia: Elsevier; 2017. p. 505–31.
112. Szentgyorgyi L, Shepherd C, Dunn KW, et al. Extracorporeal membrane oxygenation in severe respiratory failure resulting from burns and smoke inhalation injury. Burns 2018.
113. Chiu Y-J, Ma H, Liao W-C, et al. Extracorporeal membrane oxygenation support may be a lifesaving modality in patients with burn and severe acute respiratory distress syndrome: Experience of Formosa Water Park dust explosion disaster in Taiwan. Burns 2018;44(1):118–23.
114. Trauma Victoria. Major Trauma Guidelines & Education - Victorian State Trauma System. Victoria: Victorian Department of Health; 2018. Available from: http://trauma.reach.vic.gov.au.
115. Henschke A, Lee R, Delaney A. Burns management in ICU: quality of the evidence: a systematic review. Burns 2016;42(6):1173–82.
116. ISBI Practice Guidelines Committee, Steering Subcommittee, Advisory Committee. ISBI practice guidelines for burn care. Burns 2016;42(5):953–1021.
117. Eljaiek R, Heylbroeck C, Dubois M-J. Albumin administration for fluid resuscitation in burn patients: a systematic review and meta-analysis. Burns 2017;43(1):17–24.
118. Sheridan RL, Greenhalgh D. Special problems in burns. Surg Clin North Am 2014;94(4):781–91.
119. Bradshaw L, Wasiak J, Cleland H. Is operative management of fractures safe in the collocated burn and fracture injury? Injury 2015;46(6):1145–9.
120. Friedstat JB, David A, Levi, Benjamin. Chemical, electrical, and radiation injuries. Clin Plast Surg 2017;44(3):657–69.
121. Rowan MP, Cancio LC, Elster EA, et al. Burn wound healing and treatment: review and advancements. Crit Care 2015;19(1):243.
122. Wang Y, Beekman J, Hew J, et al. Burn injury: challenges and advances in burn wound healing, infection, pain and scarring. Adv Drug Deliv Rev 2018;123:3–17.
123. Moher D, Liberati A, Tetzlaff J, et al. Preferred reporting items for systematic reviews and meta-analyses: the PRISMA statement. Ann Intern Med 2009;151.

Chapter 25

Resuscitation

Trudy Dwyer, Jennifer Dennett

Learning objectives

After reading this chapter, you should be able to:

- identify the benefits of an international approach to resuscitation systems
- discuss the importance of basic life support in the context of advanced life support
- describe the safety precautions of defibrillation
- discuss the principles of therapeutic hypothermia
- discuss indications, actions and routes of administration of medications used in advanced life support
- outline the treatment algorithm for both shockable and non-shockable rhythms
- outline the nurse's role in facilitating family presence during an arrest.

KEY WORDS

advanced life support
capnography
cardiac arrest
cardiopulmonary resuscitation
out-of-hospital cardiac arrest
resuscitation
return of spontaneous circulation (ROSC)
sudden cardiac arrest

Introduction

The continuum of critical illness for an individual can span the period before and beyond hospital admission. Resuscitation is often required outside the critical care environment. The 'cardiac arrest' team has evolved to use a more proactive, early intervention approach, utilising a range of rapid response systems and instruments to detect deterioration in patients' clinical status (see Chapter 3). It is well recognised that improved outcomes from cardiac arrest are dependent on early recognition and initiation of the 'chain of survival'.[1] This chapter introduces the resuscitation systems and processes in both the pre-hospital and the in-hospital settings. The chain of survival provides a framework for the management of the person experiencing cardiac arrest and resuscitation in specific circumstances. The chapter expands on the final link in the chain, advanced life support, to outline advanced airway management, rhythm recognition, administration of medications and post-resuscitation care. Resuscitation involves many moral and ethical issues, such as family presence during resuscitation, deciding when to cease or initiate resuscitation and near-death experiences.

Cardiac arrest

Coronary heart disease (CHD) is the leading cause of death in most industrialised countries, with over half of these being due to sudden cardiac arrest (SCA).[2,3] Despite advances in CHD management, survival outcome figures from SCA remain poor with the survival rate reported to be between 6 and 12%.[4,5] Survival after SCA is dependent on the presenting rhythm, early defibrillation, effective cardiopulmonary resuscitation, early advanced life support and post-resuscitation care.[5,6] Traditionally, the presenting rhythm with the majority of witnessed SCAs was ventricular fibrillation (VF) hence bystander cardiopulmonary resuscitation and early defibrillation were the focus of resuscitation efforts.[2,6,7] But, over time the incidence of patients who have an out-of-hospital cardiac arrest (OHCA) presenting with VF is decreasing and those with shockable rhythm are increasing, possibly secondary to the modification of risk factors or interventions that shorten VF/ventricular tachycardia (VT) duration such as the use of cardiovascular drugs or implantable cardioverter-defibrillators.[8] Early interventions are now directed to uninterrupted CPR.

Incidence/aetiology of cardiac arrests

The prevalence of CHD varies worldwide; thus, estimates of the incidence of SCA are difficult to obtain.[9] There are many factors that contribute to cardiac arrest. In adults, the most common cause of cardiac arrest is a primary cardiac event,[10,11] with coronary artery disease accounting for up to 90% of all victims.[12,13] CHD is the most likely cause of death in those over 35 years of age, in comparison to non-cardiac causes such as drowning, acute airway obstruction or trauma for people less than 35 years of age.[13] While causes of cardiac arrest are numerous, most often it is associated with VF triggered by an acutely ischaemic or infarcted myocardium or primary electrical disturbance.[3] Causes of cardiac arrest may be separated into two categories, primary and secondary, as displayed in Table 25.1.

Acute myocardial infarction is the most common precursor to cardiac arrest. In victims of trauma, drug overdose and drowning, the predominant cause of cardiac arrest is asphyxia. Cardiac arrest in children is less common and even more rarely sudden,[14,15] with the common causes being trauma, congenital heart disease, long QT syndrome, drug overdose, hypoxia and hypothermia. The most common arrhythmia in infants is bradycardia; prognosis is especially poor if asystole is present.[14,16] Chest compression should be started if the pulse is less than 60/minute with poor perfusion.[16]

Pathophysiology

In SCA with cardiac origin, it is believed that myocardial ischaemia leads to ventricular irritability and the progression from VT to VF and ultimately asystole.[17] After the onset of VF (in animal studies), carotid arterial blood flow continues for approximately 4 min even in the absence of cardiac compressions, as coronary perfusion pressure (the pressure gradient between the aorta and the right atrium) falls over this period.[17] This initial phase is characterised by minimal ischaemic injury, and it is during this time that defibrillation is most likely to result in the restoration of a perfusing rhythm, while initiation of effective cardiac compressions will increase the coronary perfusion pressure.[17]

Progression of the cardiac arrest beyond four minutes results in accumulation of toxic metabolites, depletion of high-energy phosphate stores and the initiation of ischaemic cascades.[17] Increasing probability of irreversible cellular injury exists where a cardiac arrest extends for longer than 10 min, and the return of a spontaneous circulation during this period may initiate a reperfusion injury[17] (see Chapter 11 for further discussion).

TABLE 25.1
Causes of cardiac arrest

PRIMARY CAUSES	SECONDARY CAUSES
Acute myocardial infarction	Cessation of breathing
Cardiomyopathy	Airway obstruction
Electrical shock (low- and high-voltage)	Severe bleeding
Congenital heart disease (e.g. prolonged Q-T)	Hypothermia
Drugs	Hypoglycaemia
	Drug-induced proarrhythmia
	Metabolic disturbance
	Electrical disturbance
	Trauma
	Neuromuscular disease

Konstantopoulou A, Tsikrikas S, Asvestas D, et al. Mechanisms of drug-induced proarrhythmia in clinical practice. World J Cardiol 2013;5(6):175.

Resuscitation systems and processes

Since the rediscovery of the effectiveness of closed-chest CPR in 1960 and its subsequent widespread adoption, CPR has saved the lives of many, potentially ensuring years of productive life.[18] As CPR quickly became one of the most widely-used and researched procedures, voluntary coordinating bodies developed throughout the world. Organisations such as the European Resuscitation Council, the American Heart Association, the New Zealand Resuscitation Council, the Heart and Stroke Foundation of Canada, the Resuscitation Council of Southern Africa and the Australian Resuscitation Council established practice guidelines to improve standards in resuscitation, and coordinated resuscitation activities on a national basis.[19] The International Liaison Committee on Resuscitation (ILCOR), formed in 1992, promotes global discussion consistency of guidelines between these

FIGURE 25.1 Chain of survival.

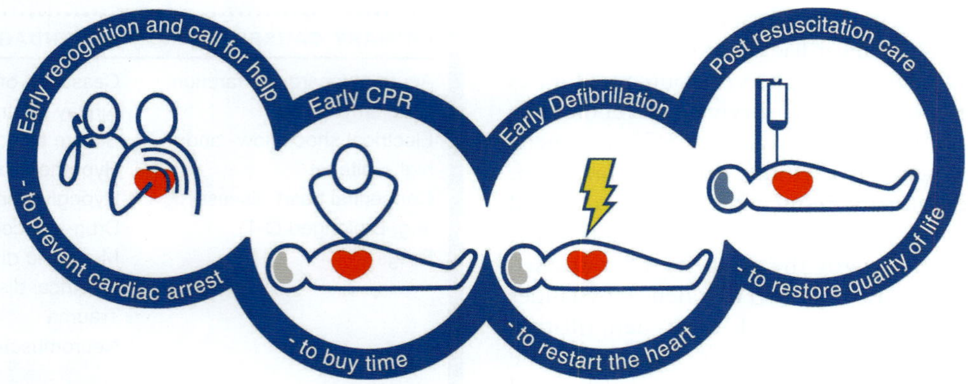

Perkins GD, Handley AJ, Koster RW, et al. European Resuscitation Council Guidelines for Resuscitation 2015: Section 2. Adult basic life support and automated external defibrillation. Resuscitation 2015; 95:81-99.

international resuscitation councils and provides a consensus mechanism for near continuous review of resuscitation science.[18]

Survival of arrests

Despite advances in resuscitation and technology, the survival to hospital discharge rates remain variable at around 5–10% for OHCA and 24% for in-hospital cardiac arrests (IHCA).[4,20] Factors associated with higher rates of mortality for adults are: age over 80 years, unwitnessed arrest, delays before commencing CPR, delayed defibrillation (pre-shock pauses) and delays prior to resumption of CPR (post-shock pauses) and non-ventricular tachycardia/fibrillation rhythm.[21] While the outcome statistics for children following IHCA are better than OHCA, only one-third of children with IHCA will survive to discharge with optimal neurological function.[15] Marked differences in the inclusion criteria and outcome definitions may, however, also explain the wide variations in survival rates from cardiac arrests. In recognition of these variations, international guidelines such as the Utstein guidelines[22] have been implemented to consistently document, monitor and compare OHCAs and in-hospital resuscitation.

In-hospital cardiac arrest survival to hospital discharge rates are reportedly around 18–33%, with survival to discharge reportedly higher in women and Caucasians. The majority of cardiac arrests occur on the general wards where patients are not monitored and the predominant presenting rhythms are VF/VT (17%) and asystole/pulseless electrical activity (PEA) (73%).[23] Many factors such as age, time of day, presence or absence of morbidity before or during the hospital admission, absence of 'not-for-resuscitation' orders, quality of the CPR, asystole and non-intensive care unit location contribute to the low in-hospital survival rates.[25,26]

Chain of survival

To optimise a person's chance of survival, the 'chain of survival' strategy has been developed,[27] which represents a sequence of events that must occur as quickly as possible: early recognition, early CPR, early defibrillation and post-resuscitation care (Fig. 25.1). These time-sensitive, sequential actions must occur to optimise a cardiac arrest victim's chances of survival. Communities with integrated links along this chain have demonstrated higher survival rates after OHCA than those with deficiencies in these links.[26]

Early recognition of cardiac arrest

The chain of survival begins with early recognition of a medical emergency and the activation of a rapid response system.[2,28] However, the chain of survival has not always been adequate when a cardiac arrest occurs in the hospital, from the point of view of early recognition, timeliness or availability of equipment or staff.[25,29] Two-thirds of IHCA are potentially avoidable, with up to 84% of all IHCA demonstrating evidence of deterioration in the 6–8 hours preceding the arrest.[30,31] There is variable evidence that the implementation of early warning systems, designed to facilitate early recognition of the deteriorating patient (Table 25.2),[32–35] or medical emergency team (MET) systems reduce hospital mortality, respiratory or cardiac arrests[3,36,37] (see Chapter 3 for further discussion). To further facilitate earlier activation of the rapid response teams, many hospitals have implemented systems for family and patients to directly escalate and activate a care process on a patient's behalf.[38]

Basic life support

When a patient is identified as in potential or actual arrest, a primary and secondary survey should be conducted in the DRSABCD sequence:[39]

TABLE 25.2
Early calling criteria[34,37]

AREA	ADULTS	CHILDREN	
		0–12 MONTHS	1–8 YEARS
Airway	Threatened	Threatened	Threatened
Breathing	All respiratory arrests RR <8 RR >27 SpO_2 <90%	All respiratory arrests RR <20 RR >50 Grunting respirations SpO_2 <90%	All respiratory arrests RR <15 RR >35 SpO_2 <90%
Circulation	All cardiac arrests PR <50 PR >130 Systolic BP <90	All cardiac arrests PR <100 PR >180 Systolic BP <50 Capillary return >4 seconds Marked pallor	All cardiac arrests PR <90 PR >160 Systolic BP <80
Neurology	Sudden fall in the level of consciousness (fall in the Glasgow Coma Scale score of ≥2 points) Repeated or prolonged seizures	Floppy Unresponsive Depressed conscious level Prolonged seizures	Floppy Unresponsive Depressed conscious level Prolonged seizures
Other	Any patient you are seriously worried about who does not fit the above criteria		

Note: these values are a guide and vary with different organisations.
BP = blood pressure; PR = pulse rate; RR = respiratory rate.

- **D**anger – check for danger (hazards or risks to safety).
- **R**esponsive – check for response (if responsive/unconscious).
- **S**end – send for help.
- **A**irway – open the airway. Airway assessment is undertaken to establish a patent airway while maintaining cervical spine support (if injury is suspected).
- **B**reathing – check breathing. Breathing includes the assessment and establishment of breathing, noting rate, pattern, chest movement and tissue oxygenation.
- **C**PR – start CPR. Give 30 chest compressions (almost 2 compressions/sec) followed by 2 breaths.
- **D**efibrillation – attach an automated external defibrillator as soon as available and follow its prompts.

Continue CPR until responsiveness and normal breathing return. Ideally, these interventions are performed simultaneously or in rapid sequence and will take no longer than 60–90 seconds to complete. This systematic approach correlates closely with the actions of health professionals when a patient collapses in the in-hospital environment (Fig. 25.2).

Airway

Recognition of airway obstruction includes listening for inspiratory (stridor), expiratory or grunting noises. The work of breathing can be assessed by the respiratory rate, intercostals, subcostal or sternal recession, use of accessory muscles, tracheal tug or flaring of the alae nasi. Nasal flaring is especially evident in infants with respiratory distress. Noisy breathing is obstructed breathing, but the volume of the noise is not an indicator of the severity of respiratory failure. Should obstruction to air flow be detected, then the airway should be opened using three manoeuvres: the head-tilt, chin-lift and jaw thrust. Assess a person's airway without turning them onto the side unless the airway is obstructed with fluid (vomit or blood) or submersion injuries.[39]

The airway of the infant differs from that of the older child or adult in that the infant has a large head and tongue and small mouth, and the larynx is narrower, shorter, more anterior and acutely angled[17] (see Chapter 27). The airway of an infant is also more cartilaginous and can be easily occluded when the neck is hyperextended; in addition, the large tongue can easily fall back to obstruct the pharynx.[40] Hence, the head of an infant should be maintained in the neutral position, whereas a child aged 1–8 years will require the 'sniffing position', with varying degrees according to age. The chin-lift and

FIGURE 25.2 Life support flow chart for the in-hospital patient.[36]

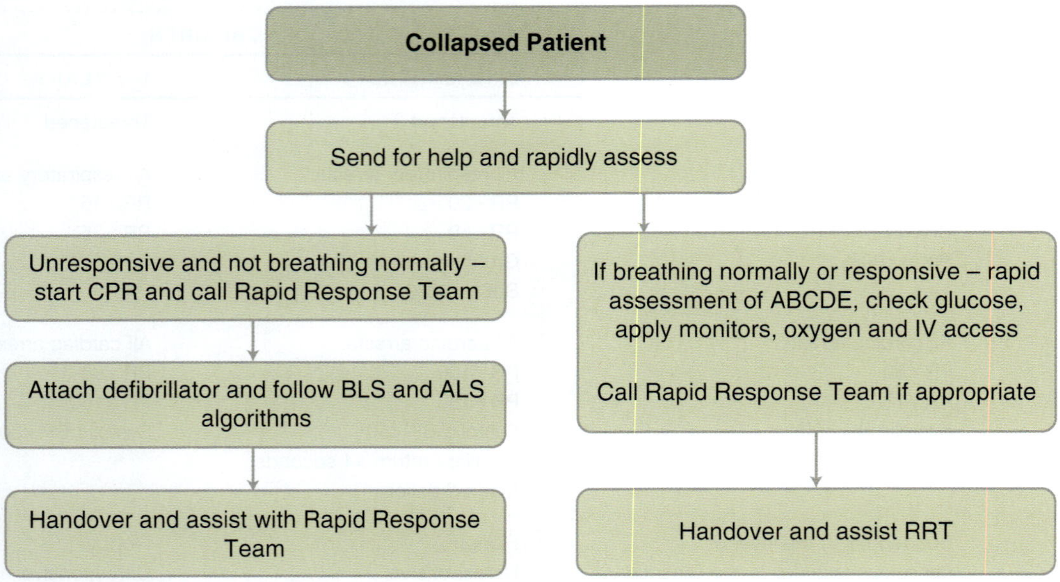

Adapted from European Resuscitation Council (ERC). Summary of the main changes in the Resuscitation Guidelines: ERC Guidelines 2015: ERC; 2015.

head-tilt manoeuvres may be used in children to obtain the appropriate positioning for age. Jaw thrust may be used if head-tilt/chin-lift is contraindicated.[40] Do not use the finger sweep to clear the airway of an infant, as this may result in damage to the delicate palatal tissues and cause bleeding, which can worsen the situation. Use of finger sweep can force foreign bodies further down into the airway.[40] Suction is more useful for removing vomitus and secretions.

Practice tip

In paediatric patients cuffed endotracheal tubes may be used in the short term.[40]

Breathing

To assess for the presence of breathing, look, listen and feel for breath sounds for no more than 10 seconds. If the person is unresponsive with absent or abnormal breathing, call for help and compressions should be commenced immediately. Agonal gasps are not to be considered as normal breathing. Typically, the arterial blood will remain saturated with oxygen for several minutes following the cardiac arrest and, as cerebral and myocardial cell oxygenation is limited more by the absence of cardiac output as opposed to the reduced PaO_2, effective compressions are more important than rescue breaths.[27]

Cardiopulmonary resuscitation

Cardiac compressions should be commenced if the victim is unconscious, unresponsive, not moving and not breathing normally. Where possible, change the person delivering the compressions every 2 min. Pulse check by lay rescuers and health professionals in basic life support (BLS) is not recommended. Assessment of effective chest compression by healthcare professionals may be made by continuous end tidal CO_2 ($ETCO_2$) monitoring. For CPR to be effective the patient should be flat, supine and on a firm surface. The chest should be compressed in the midline over the lower half of the sternum, which equates to the 'centre of the chest', at a depth of >5 cm (adults), 5 cm (children) and 4 cm (infants). Equal time should be spent in compression as spent on the release.[36] A rate of 100–120 compressions per minute for adults, infants and children, with the rate rising to 120/min for the newborn.[27,36] CPR should be initiated when the heart rate is <100 beats/min for the newborn,[14] and the small child and 40 beats/min for the large child. Performed correctly, external cardiac compressions (ECC) can produce a systolic blood pressure peak of 60–80 mmHg (in adults) and a cardiac output of 20–30% of normal.[27,41] With external chest compressions it takes time to reach optimal levels of coronary perfusion pressure and, ultimately, blood flow. Any interruption to chest compressions therefore decreases the coronary perfusion pressure and resultant blood flow, ultimately reducing survival.[42] After 30 compressions the airway should be opened and two breaths given.[43]

TABLE 25.3
CPR for adults, children and infants[1]

AGE	AIRWAY	COMPRESSION (CPR)	1 OR 2 PERSONS
Infants <1 year	Jaw support or chin-lift (no head-tilt)	Two fingers or two overlying thumbs on the lower end of the sternum with hands encircling the chest (preferred), 100–120 beats/min	30:2 PALS 15:2 (2 rescuers)
Younger child: 1–8 years	Head-tilt more than infants but less than adults	Heel of one hand, 100–120 beats/min	30:2 PALS 15:2 (2 rescuers)
Older child: 9–14 years	Head-tilt	Two hands, 100–120 beats/min	30:2 PALS 15:2 (2 rescuers)
Adult	Head-tilt	Two hands, 100–120 beats/min	30:2

PALS = paediatric advanced life support.

Survival potentially improves when an individual receives a higher number of chest compressions during CPR, even if the person receives fewer ventilations. Because of this, it is recommended that a 30:2 compression-to-ventilation ratio is used in adults, children and infants regardless of the number of rescuers, and 3:1 for neonates. Having noted this, in the advanced life support paediatric setting, the compression ratio changes to 15:2 and a ratio of 3:1 for the newborn with any number of rescuers (Table 25.3). The average person may not only be reluctant to initiate mouth-to-mouth resuscitation,[44] but will also take 8 seconds to deliver one breath.[45] When a rescuer is reluctant to perform rescue breaths, ECC without expired air resuscitation (EAR) should be encouraged, as the generally held belief is that ECC alone is better than no CPR at all.[46,47]

Evaluation during resuscitation

Maintenance of an effective cardiac output during CPR has traditionally been evaluated by palpating the carotid or femoral pulse in adults (brachial in children). However, neither lay-persons nor professionals can rapidly (in less than 10 sec) and accurately perform this step. Pulse checks are not recommended for evaluation after defibrillation until 2 min of CPR have been performed, regardless of the rhythm post-defibrillation.

The use of capnometry as a non-invasive technique for monitoring the effectiveness of CPR is recommended.[12] As the partial pressure of the $ETCO_2$ concentration correlates with pulmonary blood flow during CPR, the adequacy of resuscitation efforts is evaluated by measuring this parameter. $ETCO_2$ also correlates with cardiac output, return of spontaneous circulation (ROSC) and outcomes in cardiac arrest.[48,49] A mean $ETCO_2$ of 20 mmHg or above has been associated with survival from cardiac arrest, while a mean $ETCO_2$ <10 mmHg is associated with poor outcomes.[49] A rise in $ETCO_2$ during CPR may indicate the return of spontaneous circulation.[50] Having noted this, hyperventilation during CPR is not recommended and may be harmful. Clinical studies show that rescuers consistently hyperventilate patients during a cardiac arrest.[51]

Devices to augment compression

As ECC supplies only 30% of normal cardiac output[52] and 15% of normal cerebral blood flow, there is a great need to find ways to improve cardiac compression. While no circulatory adjunct is currently recommended, a few of the devices are outlined in Table 25.4.

Given the limited available information on the outcomes associated with use of any of these devices and the absence of evidence to demonstrate these devices are superior to conventional manual CPR, no device is currently recommended as a routine substitute for manual CPR.[20,53,54] There is, however, a growing incidence of the use of some of these devices in the pre-hospital environment and in situations where it is difficult to provide high-quality compressions such as during transport, prolonged cardiac arrests and cardiac catheter laboratories.[54] These devices should be used in a properly supervised program and the users should be well trained.[39,55]

Practice tip

CPR should commence if the patient is unconscious, unresponsive, not moving and not breathing, even if the patient is taking the occasional gasp.[40]

Defibrillation

While CPR has been associated with improved survival to discharge from hospital, it cannot be substituted for the definitive treatment of early defibrillation. It is thought that CPR will supply sufficient oxygen to the brain and heart until defibrillation is available. Ultimately, despite the most effective CPR, the single-most important cause of poorer prognosis in pulseless VT/VF cardiac arrests is a delay in electrical defibrillation.[3]

TABLE 25.4
Augment compression devices[53,56,57]

DEVICE	DESCRIPTION
Active compression–decompression (ACD-CPR)	• Utilises a small portable device to compress and decompress the chest ('plunger method') • Enhances ventilation and venous return by raising the negative intrathoracic pressure, which facilitates venous return, thus priming the heart for subsequent compressions[56]
Interposed abdominal compression (IAC) combined with CPR (IAC-CPR)	• Least technical device • The abdomen is compressed (midway between the xiphisternum and the umbilicus) alternately with the rhythm of chest compression • Rarely utilised method • Results in increased resistance in the descending aorta, thus raising the coronary perfusion pressure[57]
Non-invasive automated chest compression device (e.g. AutoPulse®)	• Utilises a load-distributing band (LDB) to compress the anterior chest • The device is built around a backboard that contains a motor[53] • The motor tightens or loosens LDB around the patient's chest

Precordial thump

A precordial thump is a single, sharp blow delivered with a clenched fist to the mid-sternum of a victim's chest from a height of 25–30 cm above the sternum.[7] The mechanical energy generated by the precordial thump may generate a few joules, and therefore is applied within the first few seconds of onset of a shockable rhythm, but it has a very low success rate at converting VF/VT to a perfusing rhythm.[58,59] Because of the very low success rate and the brief period for application, delivery of the thump must not delay accessing help or a defibrillator. A precordial thump may be used in monitored and witnessed VF/VT arrest while awaiting the arrival of the defibrillator.[36]

Electrical defibrillation

Defibrillation is the passage of a current of electricity through a fibrillating heart to simultaneously depolarise the mass of myocardial cells and allow them to repolarise uniformly to an organised electrical activity.[12]

> **Practice tip**
>
> For preterm infants, resuscitation should commence with low concentrations of oxygen and titrated (using a blender) minute by minute in response to the oxygen saturation.[19]

There are two types of external defibrillators: the manual external defibrillator and the automatic external defibrillator (AED). Most manual defibrillators have AED capacity. The AED can be either fully automatic or semiautomatic. The manual defibrillator requires the user to be able to immediately and accurately recognise arrhythmias and make the decision whether to initiate defibrillation or not. In comparison, the AED automatically detects and interprets the rhythm without relying on the user's recognition of arrhythmias. AEDs can be operated in both manual and semiautomatic mode. When using an AED, the user determines whether the person is unresponsive, not breathing and pulseless.[60] After checking for a pulse, the AED requires only four steps to operate: 1) turn power on; 2) place self-adhesive electrodes on a victim's chest; 3) rhythm analysis follows (hands-off period); 4) then (if advised by the machine) press the shock button. The AED will automatically interpret the cardiac rhythm and, if VF/VT is present, will advise the operator to provide a shock. This 'hands-off' period using the AED may result in significant interruptions to chest compressions and adversely impact patient survival. Health professionals with expertise in rhythm recognition may reduce the 'hands-off' period using a manual defibrillator.[61,62] The combined pre-shock and the post-shock pause ideally should be less than 5 seconds.[12] This can be achieved by continuing compressions while the defibrillator is charging and resuming chest compressions immediately after the delivery of the shock. Fully automatic defibrillators are programmed to assess the rhythm, charge the defibrillator and deliver shocks without user intervention.

To facilitate early defibrillation, ILCOR endorses the concept of non-medical individuals being authorised, educated and encouraged to use defibrillators.[12] This public access to early defibrillation has seen the placement of defibrillators on aircraft, in casinos and cricket grounds, with non-medical personnel such as police, flight attendants, security guards, family members and even children successfully initiating early defibrillation.[62] The effectiveness of training non-traditional out-of-hospital first responders to use the AED has improved survival to discharge rates.[20] Similarly, IHCA also occur in any area, and all healthcare workers should be capable of initiating early defibrillation.[12] While BLS does not have to include the use of adjunctive equipment, the use of AEDs by persons with education in their use is

TABLE 25.5

Factors contributing to the success or failure of defibrillation[69-72]

SUCCESS	FAILURE	PRECAUTIONS
• VF duration • Early defibrillation (if VF <3 min) • Initial CPR (if VF >3 min) • Presenting rhythm (VT/VF) • Paddle/pad size and placement • Use of self-adhesive pads	• Inadequate contact with the chest (excessive chest hair) • Faulty positioning of the paddles • Synchronise button in the 'on' position, flat battery or fractured lead • Positioning over bone/fat or breast tissue, chest size • Drying out of gel conduction pads • Patient factors: acidosis, hypoxia, electrolyte imbalance, drug toxicity, hypothermia • Time of respiration (best delivered at end-expiration) • PEEP and auto-PEEP (air-trapping) should be minimised • Paddles/electrodes too small (8–12 cm electrodes for adults)	• Place defibrillation electrodes at least 8 cm away from ECG electrodes, or implantable medical devices, pacemakers, vascular access devices • Remove medication patches, wipe the area before applying defibrillation electrodes • Do not defibrillate unless all clear of the bed/patient • Do not charge/discharge paddles in the air • Do not have the patient in contact with metal • Do not allow oxygen to flow onto the patient during delivery of the shock (at least 1 m from the patient) • Ensure the chest is dry • Do not use electrode gels and pastes as these can spread between the paddles and potentially spark

ECG = electrocardiogram; PEEP = peak end-expiratory pressure; VF = ventricular fibrillation; VT = ventricular tachycardia.

supported and should be taught. Fig. 25.2 outlines the integration of defibrillation with BLS.

Practice tip

When using the defibrillator in manual mode, limiting the pre-shock analysis pause to 5 seconds should improve survival.

For 90% of people in VF, return of a perfusing rhythm will occur after a single shock. However, it is rare that a pulse will be palpable with the perfusing rhythm; hence the immediate resumption of chest compressions in the post-shock period is supported.[12] Failure to successfully convert VF after the single-shock strategy may indicate the need for a period of effective CPR (30:2) for 2 minutes and rhythm re-analysis, followed by shock if indicated.[12] A single-shock strategy is now recommended for all patients in cardiac arrest requiring defibrillation for VF or pulseless VT.[39] Not all of the electrical energy delivered during defibrillation will traverse the myocardium. Table 25.5 outlines some of the common factors contributing to the success or failure of defibrillation. The optimum defibrillation energy level is that which sufficiently abolishes the arrhythmia to enable the return of an organised rhythm, with minimal myocardial damage.[12,63] Other biphasic energy levels may be used providing there is relevant clinical data for a specific defibrillator that suggests that an alternative energy level provides adequate shock success.[1,64] If the initial shock is unsuccessful, subsequent shocks should be delivered at the initial dose or higher energy levels may be selected.[12,65] In children, it is recommended 4 J/kg for the initial and subsequent shocks for both biphasic and monophasic defibrillators.[12] Standard adult AEDs and pads are suitable for use in children older than 8 years. Ideally, for children between 1 and 8 years, paediatric pads and an AED with paediatric capability should be used.[1,66] These pads are placed as per the adult methodology. If the AED does not have a paediatric mode or paediatric pads, the standard adult AED and pads can be used.[25] Defibrillation of infants less than 1 year of age is not recommended.[12]

The importance of early, uninterrupted chest compressions and early defibrillation are well promulgated in the ILCOR guidelines.[12] As the length of time from collapse is difficult to accurately estimate, it is imperative rescuers perform chest compressions until the defibrillator is both available and charged.[67,68]

Advanced life support

Basic life support provides about 20–30% of normal cardiac output and a fraction of inspired oxygen (FiO_2) of 0.1–0.16. Consequently, a significant number of patients rely on the provision of advanced life support (ALS) for survival. ALS extends BLS to provide the knowledge and skills essential for the initiation of early treatment and stabilisation of people post-cardiac arrest. Advanced skills traditionally include defibrillation, advanced airway management and the administration of resuscitation drugs. Algorithms for management of cardiopulmonary arrest (Figs 25.3 and 25.4) outline the two decision paths of therapy in ALS: 1) defibrillation and CPR for pulseless VT/VF (shockable) and 2) identifying

FIGURE 25.3 Advanced life support flow chart.[1]

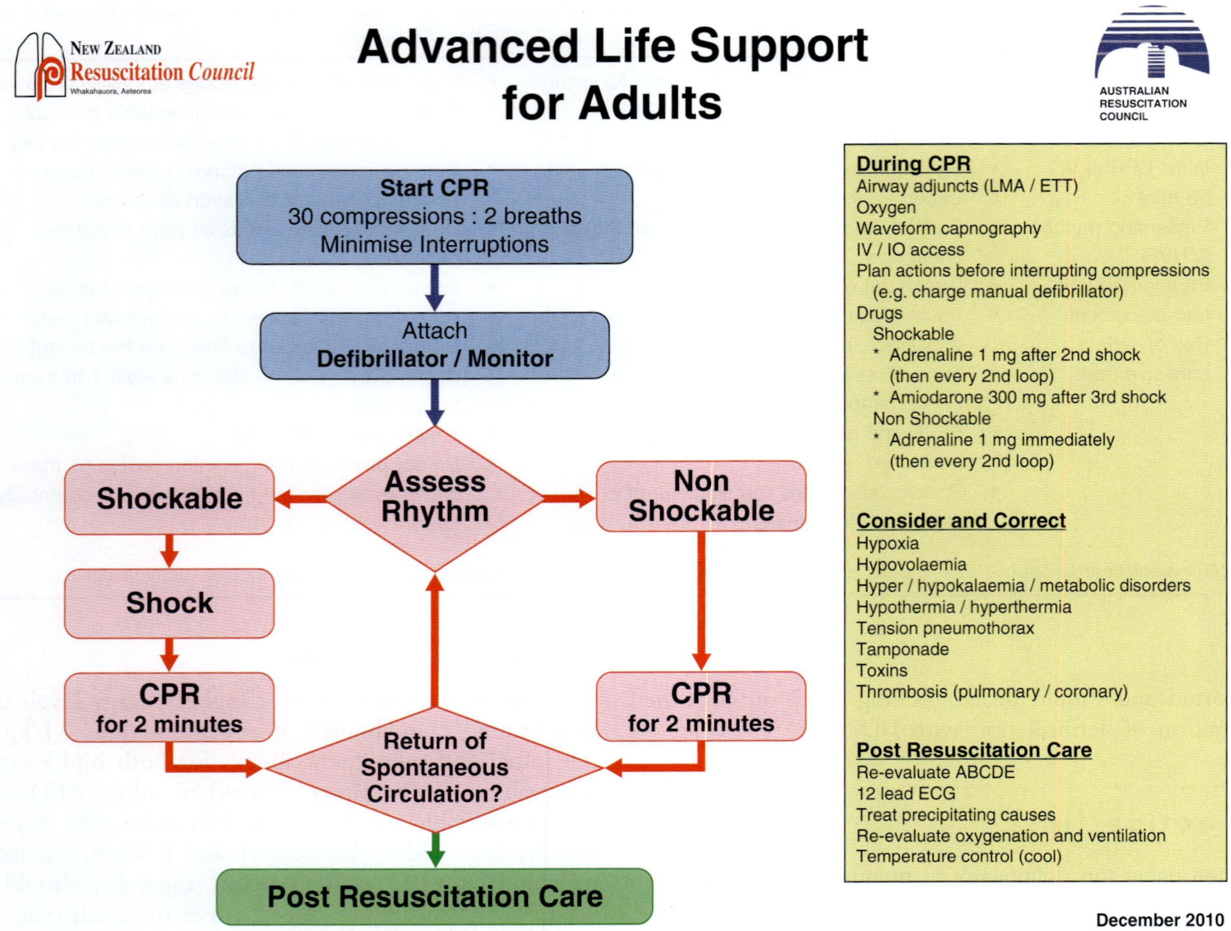

Australian resuscitation flow chart reproduced with permission. Australian and New Zealand Consensus on Resuscitation (ANZCOR). ANZCOR Guidelines. Victoria, Australia: Australian Resuscitation Council; 2016. http://www.resus.org.au. [Accessed April 2018].

and treating the underlying cause for non-VT/VF (non-shockable).

Advanced airway management

A person with signs of acute hypoxia should be administered oxygen at the highest possible concentration, including initially during CPR.[43] Oxygen should never be withheld for fear of adverse effects, as rescue breaths provide an inspired oxygen concentration of only 15–18%. The administration of oxygen alone does not result in adequate ventilation and, as such, the establishment of an effective airway is paramount. Airway management is essential in the performance of CPR, and may be administered using a variety of techniques. These may include: compression-only CPR with high-flow oxygen by face mask; bag–mask ventilation; insertion of a supraglottic airway device that does not require laryngoscopy or tracheal intubation.[73]

The choice of advanced airway adjunct is determined by the availability of equipment and experienced personnel[73] (see Table 25.6 and Chapter 15):

- oropharyngeal (Guedel's) airway
- nasopharyngeal airway
- laryngeal mask airway
- oesophageal tracheal combitube (Combitube)
- laryngeal tube (King airway)
- endotracheal intubation
- tracheostomy.

While the endotracheal tube (ETT) is considered the 'gold standard' for airway management in a cardiac arrest, as it protects the airway, assists effective ventilation, ensures delivery of high concentrations of oxygen and eases suctioning, no studies have found that ETT use during a cardiac arrest increases survival. It is vital

FIGURE 25.4 Advanced life support for infants and children flow chart.[1]

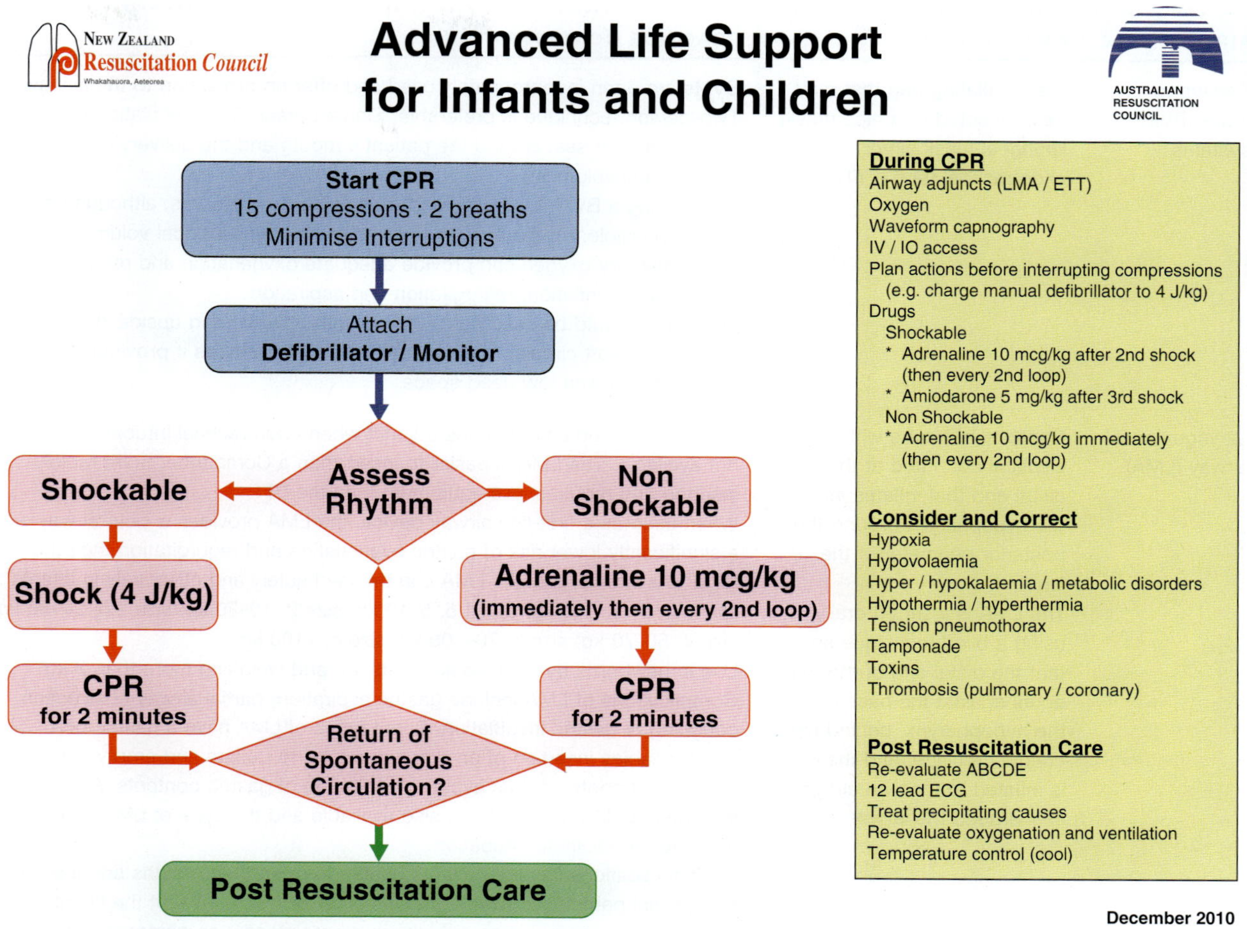

Australian resuscitation flow chart reproduced with permission. Australian and New Zealand Consensus on Resuscitation (ANZCOR). ANZCOR Guidelines. Victoria, Australia: Australian Resuscitation Council; 2016. http://www.resus.org.au. [Accessed February 2018].

TABLE 25.6

Adjuncts used during resuscitation[1,12,74-76]

AIRWAY TYPE	DESCRIPTION	PRACTICE CONSIDERATIONS
Oropharyngeal (Guedel's) airway	Conforms to the curve of the palate, moving the tongue forward away from the posterior pharyngeal wall. Sizes from 000–5	Incorrect size or placement may contribute to airway obstruction by pushing the tongue back into the pharynx. Unlike adult insertion, the insertion of the oropharyngeal airway in infants and young children is inserted right-way-up; a tongue depressor or laryngoscope should be used to aid insertion
Nasopharyngeal airway	Soft tube inserted into the nasopharynx	Use with caution in patients with head injuries With the exception of infant's head-tilt, jaw support or jaw thrust is still necessary when using either the oropharyngeal or the nasopharyngeal airway

Continued

TABLE 25.6
Adjuncts used during resuscitation—cont'd

AIRWAY TYPE	DESCRIPTION	PRACTICE CONSIDERATIONS
Bag–valve–mask (BVM) systems	A self-inflating bag that may be connected to a face mask, laryngeal mask airway or endotracheal tube (ETT)	BVMs are often inappropriately used and offer no protection to the airway. Two-person technique is preferable. Single-person BVM ventilation may result in a poor seal around the patient's mouth and the delivery of less than optimal tidal volumes[12] When using a BVM it is best performed using two rescuers, although not always possible, As the airway is not protected, smaller tidal volumes with supplementary oxygen can provide adequate oxygenation and reduce the risk of gastric inflation, regurgitation and aspiration The mask should be used right-way-up with children and upside-down with infants. The soft circular mask is preferred for infants, as it provides an excellent seal with low dead space
Laryngeal mask airway (LMA)	Consists of a tube with an elliptical cuff fitted at the distal end that inflates in the hypopharynx around the posterior perimeter of the larynx The LMA is inserted orally using a blind technique so that the distal end of the mask abuts against the base of the hypopharynx, behind the cricoid cartilage, and the cuff is inflated to form an airtight seal around the larynx	The LMA is used as a first-line adjunct when endotracheal intubation is not available. The LMA is easier to insert than a Combitube, more rapidly inserted and requires less equipment than the ETT When used as a first-line airway device, the LMA provides a clear airway with a significantly lower risk of gastric overinflation and regurgitation than the BVM[12] As with adults, the LMA can be used safely and effectively in infants[74] LMA: size 1 for <5 kg; size 1.5, 5–10 kg; size 2, 10–20 kg; size 2.5, 20–30 kg; size 4, 50–70 kg; size 5, 70–100 kg; size 6, >100 kg Use in newborns over 34 weeks gestation and weighing more than 2 kg[74] Complications of LMA include gastric aspiration, partial airway obstruction, coughing or gastric insufflation. Some types of LMA have a gastric port which enables insertion of an orogastric tube to deflate and empty the stomach of contents thus avoiding aspiration of gastric contents. An intubating LMA (Fastrach™) is also available and this type of LMA is used as a conduit to facilitate intubation Contraindications include patients unable to open their mouths adequately; pharyngeal pathology; airway obstruction at or below level of the larynx; low pulmonary compliance or high airway resistance; or increased risk of aspiration
Oesophageal–tracheal Combitube (ETC)	The ETC is a double-lumen airway with proximal and distal cuffs that is passed into the oesophagus	It is effective in maintaining an airway when performed by unskilled personnel and is a suitable alternative to tracheal intubation The ETC enables ventilation, whether it is positioned in the oesophagus or the trachea Only one size needed for most adults
Laryngeal tube (LT)	Airway tube with a small oesophageal cuff and a larger pharyngeal cuff. The distal tip is positioned in the upper oesophagus	Use is comparable to classic LMA and LMA ProSeal™[75]
i-gel®	The cuff of the i-gel is made of gel and does not require inflation	Very easy to insert with minimal training.[12] Enables continuous chest compression without interruption for ventilation[76]
Endotracheal tube (ETT)	During intubation, direct application of firm pressure to the cricoid cartilage is required to compress the oesophagus between the trachea and vertebral column and minimise/prevent regurgitation of gastric contents	Endotracheal intubation is a difficult skill to acquire and maintain In addition to routine clinical methods, ETT placement can be confirmed by either measurement of $ETCO_2$ or use of an oesophageal detector; the latter is more reliable in a non-perfusing rhythm (Class IIb) Immediate complications associated with intubation include oesophageal intubation; right main bronchi intubation; or ETT occlusion (kinking, sputum, cuff, blood)

that CPR is not interrupted for more than 10 seconds during attempts at endotracheal intubation. Waveform capnography or an oesophageal detector device should be applied to confirm the ETT placement.[12,73]

$ETCO_2$ should be used to monitor the quality of the CPR. Given the limitations noted in Table 25.6, a variety of adjunct airway/ventilation management devices are available, such as: bag–mask ventilation (BMV); supraglottic airways devices such as the laryngeal mask airway (LMA) and the classic laryngeal mask airway; the oesophageal–tracheal airway (Combitube); and the i-gel®. The benefit of the supraglottic airways devices is that they are easily inserted without interruption to chest compressions. Currently, there is no evidence to support the routine use of any particular advanced adjunct airway devices.[73] Healthcare professionals trained to use supraglottic airway devices (e.g. LMA) may consider their use for airway management during cardiac arrest and as a backup or rescue airway in a difficult or failed tracheal intubation.

Once an airway has been established, continue chest compressions, without interruption, and ventilate the lungs at a rate of approximately 6–10 ventilations a minute. Minimise the likelihood of excessive ventilation by delivering one breath during the relaxation phase of every 15th compression.[36] Ventilation adjuncts may include:

- a simple face mask with filter and oxygen connector (pre-intubation)
- bag–valve–mask systems
- ventilators.

If available, automated ventilators can be used. These may be set to deliver a tidal volume of 6–7 mL/kg at a rate of 10 breaths/min. The automated ventilator may be used with either the face mask or other adjunct airway devices.[16] Having noted this, there is currently no evidence to suggest that the use of automated ventilators during cardiac arrest is more beneficial than bag–valve–mask devices.[16]

Rhythms

There is an association between the initial cardiac arrhythmias and survival to discharge after SCA. Cardiac arrest rhythms can be divided into two subsets:

1. VF and pulseless VT (pVT)
2. non-VF/VT incorporating asystole and PEA.

The most common arrhythmias observed in SCA are pVT and VF, with 60–85% of all patients initially presenting with these lethal arrhythmias.[6] In-hospital PEA occurs as the initial rhythm in approximately 30–37% of cases[77,78] and the overall neurologically intact survival rate is 10%.[77] Asystole is the most common arrest arrhythmia in children (40% versus 35% in adults)[77] because their hearts respond to prolonged severe hypoxia and acidosis by progressive bradycardia leading to asystole.[12]

Ventricular fibrillation and pulseless ventricular tachycardia

As previously noted, the only intervention shown to unequivocally improve long-term survival after a ventricular fibrillation (VF) or pulseless ventricular tachycardia (pVT) arrest is prompt and effective BLS, uninterrupted chest compressions and early defibrillation.[12] VT and VF rhythms are displayed in Figs 25.5 and 25.6. Energy levels and subsequent shocks are equivalent for both VF and pVT.

Non-VF/VT

Non-VF/VT arrhythmias include PEA and asystole. PEA reflects dissociation between the heart's electrical and mechanical activities. It is important to note that PEA may present as any rhythm normally compatible with a pulse (e.g. sinus rhythm, sinus tachycardia/bradycardia). PEA is characterised by a stroke volume insufficient to produce a palpable pulse, despite adequate electrical activity.[79] Management of PEA includes identifying and correcting reversible causes, summarised as the four Hs and four Ts in Table 25.7.

Careful confirmation of asystole (Fig. 25.7) on two leads and the absence of a palpable pulse are essential when making the decision to manage asystole. When an in-hospital arrest has an initial rhythm of asystole, survival to discharge has been reported as 11%.[77]

Medications administered during cardiac arrest

Resuscitation drugs can be administered during a cardiac arrest using a variety of routes including peripheral and central veins or intraosseously. Administration by the

FIGURE 25.5 Ventricular tachycardia.

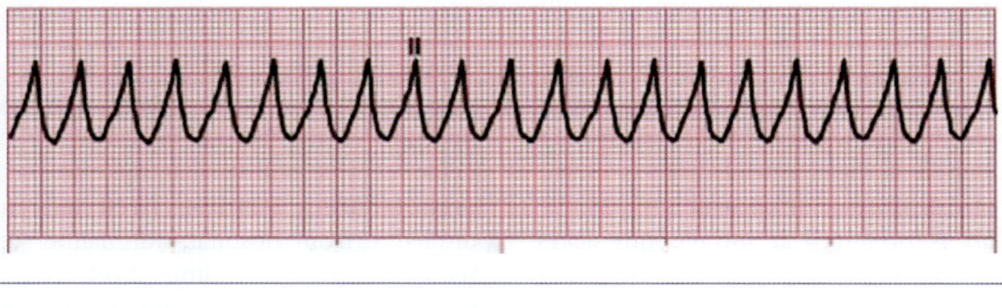

FIGURE 25.6 Ventricular fibrillation.

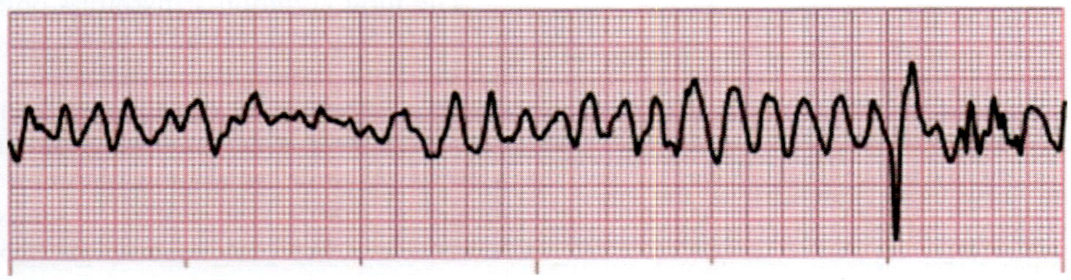

FIGURE 25.7 Asystole.

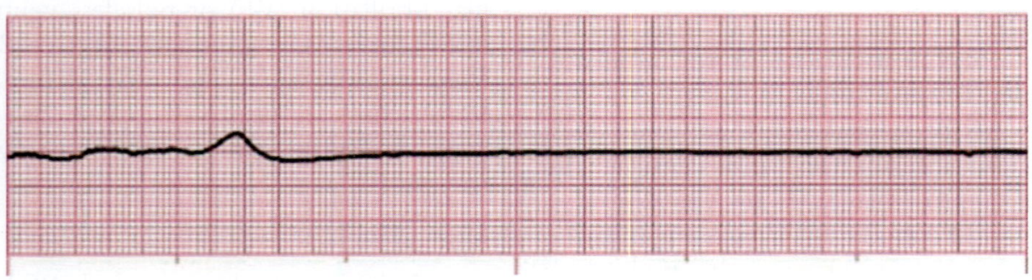

TABLE 25.7
Causes of pulseless electrical activity[1]

THE FOUR Hs	THE FOUR Ts
• Hypoxia	• Tamponade
• Hypovolaemia	• Tension pneumothorax
• Hypo/hyperthermia	• Toxins/poisons/drugs
• Hypo/hyperkalaemia and metabolic disorders	• Thrombosis: pulmonary/ coronary

central venous route remains the optimal method, but the decision to access peripheral versus central cannulation will depend on the skill of the operator. Peripheral venous cannulation is the quickest and easiest method; however, the patient in cardiac arrest may have inaccessible peripheral veins.[80] Should a decision be made to insert a central line during a cardiac arrest, this must not take precedence over defibrillation attempts, CPR or airway maintenance. Intravenous medications should be flushed with 20–30 mL (adults) of an isotonic solution followed by at least 1 min of continuous ECCs. Where there is difficulty accessing a peripheral vein, selected medications may be administered via an intraosseous route.[80] Tracheal administration of medication is no longer recommended as the dose delivered is unpredictable and the optimal dose is unknown.[80]

Intraosseous (IO) is preferred if intravenous access is not possible. Insertion sites include 1) proximal tibia (2–3 cm below the tibial tuberosity); 2) distal tibia (proximal to the medial malleolus); 3) distal femur (midline, 2–3 cm above external condyle; 4) proximal humerus; and 5) sternum. Intraosseous infusion involves the insertion of a metal needle using a drill into the bone marrow and provides a rapid, safe and reliable access to the circulation. The marrow sinusoids of long bones are a non-collapsible venous system in direct connection with the systemic circulation, allowing drugs to reach the central circulation as quickly as medications injected into central veins. Intraosseal access is safe and effective for use in patients of all age groups.[80] General blood specimens such as biochemistry values, blood cultures, haemoglobin and cross-match studies can also be taken from the marrow at cannulation.

Practice tip

Tibial and humerus intraosseous routes are as effective administering medications during CPR, reaching maximum blood concentrations in less than 2 min.

Vasopressors such as adrenaline (epinephrine) and vasopressin have been used as adjuncts in cardiac arrests to improve the success of CPR.[81-83] While there is no evidence that shows that the routine use of any vasopressor during a cardiac arrest will increase survival to discharge from hospital, adrenaline (epinephrine) is still recommended.[84] Findings from two randomised controlled trials have challenged the use of adrenaline in

OHCA.[82,85] While patients that receive adrenaline (epinephrine) demonstrate improved likelihood of ROSC[85] and 30-day survival than the use of placebo,[83] the chances of severe brain damage is almost doubled in the adrenaline group.[82]

The optimal dose of adrenaline (epinephrine) in the pre-hospital and in-hospital settings remains unclear. Current recommendations propose that adrenaline (epinephrine) 1 mg should be administered for VT/VF following the second shock and then every second loop thereafter. For asystole and PEA administer 1 mg of adrenaline (epinephrine) in the initial loop, then every second loop (Table 25.8).[1]

The optimal role and exact benefit of antiarrhythmic medications in cardiac resuscitation is yet to be fully elucidated, but they have very little, if any, role to play in the treatment of cardiac arrests.[12] The common antiarrhythmic drugs include amiodarone, magnesium, atropine and calcium (Table 25.8). Lignocaine is no longer recommended as first-line management in cardiac arrest. Amiodarone is the leading antiarrhythmic medication because its safety and efficacy have been demonstrated. If, after the third shock, the VT/VF has not reverted, a bolus injection of 300 mg of amiodarone is recommended and 150 mg for recurrent or refractory VT/VF. There is no evidence of improved survival with

TABLE 25.8
Medications used during resuscitation

ACTION	INDICATIONS	DOSE		ADVERSE EVENTS
		ADULTS	PAEDIATRIC	
Adrenaline (Epinephrine) is a catecholamine that increases aortic diastolic pressure and coronary artery perfusion by producing arteriolar vasoconstriction. It may facilitate defibrillation by improving myocardial blood flow during CPR. Traditionally the first-line medication for the treatment of VF and refractory VT, adrenaline (epinephrine) has not demonstrated improved outcomes after cardiac arrest and has been associated with post-resuscitation myocardial dysfunction	VF and pulseless VT resistant to the three initial counter shocks PEA and asystole	VF and pulseless VT: 1 mg after the second shock then after every second loop PEA and asystole: 1 mg in the initial loop, then every second loop	VF and pulseless VT: 10 mcg/kg after the second shock then after every second loop PEA and asystole: 10 mcg/kg immediately, then every second loop	Tachyarrhythmias; hypertension; coronary vasoconstriction; increased myocardial oxygen consumption
Amiodarone directly affects smooth muscle and blocks calcium channels and alpha-adrenergic receptors, resulting in coronary and peripheral arterial vasodilation and a reduction in afterload and systemic blood pressure	VT/VF refractory to three shocks Polymorphic VT and wide complex tachycardia of uncertain origin Control of haemodynamically stable VT when cardioversion unsuccessful (in the presence of LV dysfunction) Adjunct to electrical cardioversion of SVT Prophylaxis of recurrent VF/VT	Initial bolus dose: 300 mg in 20 mL dextrose. A further 150 mg could be considered for refractory cases *Periarrest:* an infusion of 15 mg/kg over 24 h may be commenced	Initial dose: 5 mg/kg bolus over 2 min, which may be repeated to a maximum of 300 mg *Periarrest:* IV infusion 5–15 mcg/kg/min as continuous infusion (max of 1.2 g in 24 h)	Vasodilation and hypotension, bradycardia, heart block May have negative inotropic effects Use with caution in renal failure Avoid use in torsades de pointes and other causes of prolonged Q-T

Continued

TABLE 25.8
Medications used during resuscitation—cont'd

ACTION	INDICATIONS	DOSE		ADVERSE EVENTS
		ADULTS	PAEDIATRIC	
Magnesium is a major intracellular cation resulting in smooth muscle relaxation and membrane stabilisation	Torsades de pointes with or without a pulse; cardiac arrest associated with digoxin toxicity Failure of defibrillation and adrenaline to reverse VF and pulseless VT Documented hypokalaemia or hypomagnesaemia	Bolus dose: 5 mmol *Periarrest:* may be followed by infusion of 20 mmol infused over 4 h	IV or IO bolus: 0.1–0.2 mmol/kg May be followed by an infusion of 0.3 mmol/kg over 4 hours	Hypotension with rapid administration Use with caution if renal failure present Muscle weakness, paralysis and respiratory failure Tachycardia and excitement
Calcium is essential to nerve and muscle impulse formation and excitation	Not recommended for routine administration in cardiac arrest. Consider administration for: hypocalcaemia, hyperkalaemia, overdose of calcium blockers	Bolus dose: 5–10 mL 10% calcium chloride (6.8 mmol)	0.2 mL/kg 10% calcium chloride, or 0.7 mL/kg 10% calcium gluconate via IV	Calcium is incompatible with a range of medications and may precipitate in IV lines Tissue necrosis with extravasation may occur
Sodium bicarbonate ($NaHCO_3$) is an alkaline agent that may be used to correct an acidosis. Routine administration of sodium bicarbonate for treatment of in-hospital and out-of-hospital cardiac arrest is not recommended	Correcting a metabolic acidosis (pH <7.1), or base deficit of ≤10 or after 15 min; preexisting hyperkalaemia; tricyclic antidepressant overdose and urinary alkalinisation in overdose; or hypoxic lactic acidosis	Bolus dose: 1 mmol/kg administered over 2–3 min. As $NaHCO_3$ is incompatible with many medications, it should be administered by a separate line or flushed before and after administration	0.5–1 mmol/kg via IV or IO administered over 2–3 min	Should not be routinely administered Alkalosis, hypernatraemia, hyperosmolality, paradoxical cerebral acidosis, depressed cardiac contractility and metabolic acidosis
Potassium is an electrolyte essential for cell membrane stabilisation that is occasionally used in ALS	Persistent documented VF, suspected hypokalaemia or hypomagnesaemia, and cardiac arrest associated with digoxin toxicity	Slow bolus: 5 mmol	0.03–0.07 mmol/kg via slow administration IV or IO *Periarrest:* 0.2 mmol/kg/h as a continuous infusion; dilute with at least 50 times its volume and mix well, as can be fatal 0.2–0.5 mmol/kg/h to a max of 1 mmol/kg if hypokalaemia severe but not immediately life-threatening	Hyperkalaemia with bradycardia, hypotension with possible asystole and extravasation may lead to tissue necrosis

ECC = external cardiac compression; IO = intraosseous; LV = left ventricular; PEA = pulseless electrical activity; SI = sinoatrial; SVT = supraventricular tachycardia; VF = ventricular fibrillation; VT = ventricular tachycardia.
Source: Adapted from Australian and New Zealand Consensus on Resuscitation (ANZCOR). ANZCOR Guidelines. Victoria, Australia: Australian Resuscitation Council. http://www.resus.org.au; 2018.

the use of atropine in a cardiac arrest with asystole or PEA.[23] Calcium chloride has little use in the management of arrhythmias unless caused by hyperkalaemia, hypocalcaemia or hypermagnesaemia, or an overdose of calcium channel-blocking drugs. Sodium bicarbonate is no longer administered routinely,[86] as it may cause hypernatraemia, hyperosmolality and intracellular acidosis from the rapid ingress of CO_2 generated from its dissociation. However, it is recommended if the cardiac arrest is associated with hyperkalaemia or tricyclic antidepressant overdose.[12]

There are insufficient data to support the routine use of magnesium in cardiac arrests,[84] except if torsades de pointes is suspected.[12,86] Thrombolytics should not be routinely administered in a cardiac arrest, but they may be considered in adults with proven or suspected pulmonary embolism or acute thrombotic aetiology.[12] Effective CPR should be continued for at least 60–90 min following the administration of the fibrinolytic medication as there is evidence of good neurological outcome and survival following extended periods of CPR in these situations.[50]

During the arrest, strategies should be initiated to prevent the development of serious periarrest arrhythmias. Whenever possible, arterial blood gases, serum electrolytes and a 12-lead ECG should be obtained to assist with determining the precise rhythm and appropriate medical interventions.[16] The presence or absence of adverse signs and symptoms will dictate interventions.

Interventions can broadly be divided into three options for immediate treatment:

1. antiarrhythmics (refer to *periarrest* in Table 25.8)
2. electrical cardioversion
3. cardiac pacing.

Common periarrest arrhythmias and interventions are covered in Chapter 11. Antiarrhythmic interventions such as medications, physical manoeuvres and electrical therapies may be proarrhythmic.[16] These proarrhythmic interventions alter the cardiac depolarisation and/or repolarisation, lengthening or shortening the QT and predisposing to fatal arrhythmias.[87]

Fluid resuscitation

Fluid resuscitation may be considered if hypovolaemia is suspected as a possible cause of the cardiac arrest. Sodium chloride (0.9%) or Hartmann's solution are recommended as a rapid infusion in the initial stages of resuscitation (at least 20 mL/kg). There is insufficient evidence to support or refute the routine administration of fluids during a cardiac arrest in the absence of hypovolaemia.[88]

Temporary cardiac pacing

During a cardiac arrest, temporary cardiac pacing may be required for sustained symptomatic bradycardia unresponsive to medical intervention. Two types of temporary cardiac pacing are utilised during a cardiac arrest: transvenous (invasive) and transcutaneous (external, non-invasive) pacemakers. As most current defibrillators have the capacity to pace, transcutaneous pacemakers are generally used in an arrest situation.

Ultrasound imaging

Ultrasound imaging has been shown to have some benefit in the detection and diagnosis of reversible causes of arrest including cardiac tamponade, pulmonary embolism, pneumothorax, aortic dissection or hypovolaemia. Placement of the probe at the sub-xiphoid position prior to stopping for planned rhythm assessment will facilitate views within 10 seconds and minimise chest compression interruptions.[20] While the use of imaging has not been shown to improve outcome, absence of heart motion on sonography during resuscitation is highly predictive of death.[20]

Special conditions

Although not common, there are some clinical presentations that require special considerations in a cardiac arrest scenario; these include pregnancy, electrical injuries and drowning. The principles of airway, breathing and circulation remain the same, but modifications must be made because of the physiological changes that occur.

Pregnancy

Researchers report that maternal mortality rates in the USA have either remained unchanged or increased in recent decades.[89] Precipitants included pulmonary embolism, sepsis, trauma, peripartum haemorrhage, amniotic fluid embolism, eclamptic seizure, congenital and acquired cardiac disease, myocardial infarction, subarachnoid haemorrhage, poisoning/self-harm and cerebral aneurysm.[90–94] The best outcome for both mother and the fetus is likely to be achieved by timely resuscitation or delivery by caesarean section in the setting of maternal cardiac arrest.[89,90]

The principles of airway, breathing and circulation remain the same, but modifications must be made because of the physiological changes that occur with normal pregnancy.[91] A number of factors may need to be considered when resuscitating a pregnant woman. If the fundus height is at or above the level of the umbilicus (approximately 20 weeks of gestational age), aortocaval compression may result in a fall in cardiac output of up to 25%.[92,94] During CPR, the mother may be placed in the left lateral tilt (15–30°)[93] or supine with a pillow under the right buttock, to displace the uterus from the inferior vena cava, facilitating venous return and cardiac output.[92–94] Often, the angle of the tilt is overestimated, potentially reducing the quality of the chest compressions.[94] The uterus may also be manually and gently displaced to the left to remove caval compression.[94] While ventilation-to-compression ratios remain the same for a pregnant woman, chest compression may be complicated by flaring of the ribs, raised diaphragm, obesity and breast hypertrophy.[91]

The superior displacement of stomach contents by the gravid uterus and a relaxed cardiac sphincter contribute to an increased risk of gastric aspiration in the pregnant woman.[91,95] Because of this increased risk, cricoid pressure should be applied until after the airway is protected by a cuffed tracheal tube.[94] Tracheal intubation should be attended to early, using a short-handled laryngoscope[95] or with a blade mounted at more than 90°,[94] as airway anatomy is altered with the larynx more anterior and superior, while the pharyngeal mucosa is slightly oedematous and friable.[94] A tracheal tube a size smaller than one normally chosen for a similar size non-pregnant woman may be used because of potential narrower airways secondary to oedema or swelling.[91] Defibrillation energy, drug doses and administration are in accordance with ALS guidelines.[94]

If maternal cardiac arrest occurs in the labour ward, operating room or emergency department and BLS and ALS measures are unsuccessful, the uterus should be emptied by surgical (scalpel) intervention within 4–5 min.[94] Maternal resuscitation may not be possible until the fetus is removed. Successful resuscitations have occurred after prompt surgical intervention.[94] Refer to Chapter 28 for additional information about critical illness and pregnancy.

Electrical injuries

Electrical burn injuries and lightning injuries are similar in that they occur infrequently, commonly cause widespread acute and delayed tissue damage and can arrest the heart and respiratory centre. Burn injuries are discussed in Chapter 24. This section focuses on the cardiac arrest situation. High-voltage electrocution is associated with a high incidence of cardiac abnormalities, including arrhythmias, prolongation of the QT interval, ST and T wave changes and myocardial infarction.[91] The most common cause of death with lightning injury is cardiac arrest due to VF or asystole or respiratory arrest.[96] Because of the potential for cardiac injuries, all patients should be admitted for cardiac monitoring after they experience a lightning strike.

A lightning strike may result in asystole followed by spontaneous return of circulation. If ventilation is initiated early and severe hypoxia does not ensue, a patient's chance of recovery should be better.[96] Initial response of BLS should always begin with D (danger), that is, avoidance of injury to the rescuer. Ensure that the environment is safe for rescuers by disconnecting the electrical supply, where possible, without touching the patient. Where high-voltage lines (power lines) are in contact with the person or the vehicle, no attempt should be made to extricate the person from the vehicle until the situation is deemed safe by an authorised electricity supply person. Once the environment is safe, commence BLS resuscitation. The neck and spine should be protected, as there may be trauma.

In lightning victims, emphasis is on the immediate resuscitation of those who appear unresponsive. Respiratory arrest may be prolonged due to paralysis of the medullary respiratory centre; if not corrected, cardiac arrest secondary to hypoxia ensues. Fixed, dilated pupils should not be used as a poor prognosis of outcome, as victims can benefit from prolonged resuscitation without major sequelae.[96]

Drowning

General issues in managing drowning presentations are discussed in Chapter 23. This section focuses on resuscitation of a cardiorespiratory arrest. Hypoxia and acute lung injury from drowning result in respiratory arrest that, if not corrected, may proceed to a cardiac arrest.[97] A patient's emotional state, associated diseases, previous hypoxia and water temperature all influence this progression.[91]

The primary goal of initial intervention is the relief of hypoxaemia[91] and restoration of cardiovascular stability.[97] Resuscitation of drowning victims follows BLS guidelines, with commencement as soon as practical. Rescue breathing may commence while the victim is still in the water, provided it is safe for the rescuer.[91] As drowning victims may have swallowed considerable amounts of water, vomiting and aspiration of gastric contents can be a major problem during resuscitation. To minimise the risks of inhalation, abdominal compression, the Heimlich manoeuvre and attempts to drain water from the lungs are not recommended. Instead, the victim should be placed on the side for the initial assessment of airway and breathing.[66] Cardiac arrest in these victims is secondary to hypoxia, so compression-only CPR is likely to be less effective and should be avoided.[91] Once experienced personnel arrive, ALS and administration of oxygen should be initiated. The principles of respiratory support and ventilation are discussed in Chapter 15, and treatment of the sequelae of a drowning victim is discussed in Chapter 23.

Extracorporeal CPR (eCPR)

Extracorporeal CPR (eCPR) is the provision of an artificial circulation via extracorporeal membrane oxygenation (ECMO) (see Chapter 15) in patients who have refractory cardiac arrest where the cause is potentially reversible. This rescue therapy is complex and is not universally available; however, ILCOR suggests that eCPR is increasingly being used in both out- and in-hospital cardiac arrest and may be considered in certain situations where implementation teams are available.[86]

Resuscitation teams

Resuscitation teams should be organised to ensure that the individual skills of each member are used effectively and efficiently.[98] The exact composition of the resuscitation team will vary between organisations, but generally the team should possess the following skills:[98]

- advanced airway management and intubation skills
- intravenous access skills including central venous access

- defibrillation and external pacing abilities
- medication administration skills
- post-resuscitation skills.

As members of a resuscitation team in the hospital generally do not work together but come from all areas of the hospital, the team should have a designated leader. The team leader gives direction and guidance, assigns tasks and makes clinical decisions without directly performing specific procedures.[16,98] The leader should engender the team's trust. Where leaders initiate structure within the arrest team, members not only work together better, they also perform the tasks of resuscitation more quickly and more effectively.[98] The leader nominates the roles of arrest team members. Roles of team members include airway management, chest compression, medication administration (including IV access), documentation of events and care of family members. The team leader should be responsible for post-resuscitation transfer, documentation, communicating with family members and healthcare professionals and debriefing of the team.[98]

The resuscitation scenario is both complex and stressful for all participants. Often, participants express feelings that too many people are involved, with no one person in control. Unfortunately, the concept of the multidisciplinary team, where all members' contributions are equally respected, is generally not evident in the literature.[99] In addition, while nurses already present at a cardiac arrest in the hospital setting may be willing and competent to perform CPR, they may be prevented from doing so because of the arrival of the cardiac arrest team.[100,101]

Post-resuscitation phase

The aim of post-resuscitation care is the maintenance of cerebral and myocardial perfusion and the return of a patient to a state of best possible health. Resuscitation does not cease with the return of spontaneous circulation (ROSC). However, ROSC after cardiac arrest does not always equate to a positive outcome for the patient. Mortality rates following IHCA vary between 67% and 71%.[102] This high mortality rate has been attributed to multiple organs that are involved with whole of body ischaemia during cardiac arrest. The reperfusion responses that occur following successful resuscitation are termed post-cardiac arrest syndrome.[102] Coordinated care and specific interventions initiated in the post-arrest phase can influence outcomes.[103] Control of body temperature, identification and treatment of acute coronary syndromes and optimisation of mechanical ventilation are a few of the targeted objectives of care.[1]

Targeted temperature management in adults after cardiac arrest

During cardiac arrest, prolonged global ischaemia coupled with inadequate reperfusion during the immediate post-resuscitation period can lead to severe cerebral hypoxic injury.[104] Targeted temperature as part of the post-cardiac arrest management provides significant survival benefit as well as improved cardiac and neurological function.[104–106] Several cooling techniques are described in Box 25.1.

BOX 25.1

Cooling techniques post-cardiac arrest[104,105,107]

External:

- Cooling blankets/pads, ice packs, wet towels, fanning, tents and cooling helmets

Internal:

- Transnasal evaporating cooling
- IV administration of cold saline or Hartmann's solution (15–30 mL/kg at 4°C over 30 min to achieve a 1.5°C fall in core temperature)
- IV heat-exchange device
- Peritoneal and pleural lavage (not generally used)

Targeted temperature cooling consists of the induction, maintenance and rewarming phases.[107] ILCOR recommends that unconscious adult patients with spontaneous circulation after a cardiac arrest should be cooled to maintain a targeted temperature between 32°C and 36°C for 12–24 hours with any initial rhythm.[104] It is important to note that shivering should be avoided, as should fever, for at least 72 hours.[106] Persistent hyperglycaemia following cardiac arrest has been associated with poor neurological outcome. Monitoring of blood sugar levels and treatment of hyperglycaemia (>10 mmol/L) with insulin is recommended in the post-cardiac arrest period.

Near-death experiences

With the rise in survival rates after a critical illness, there are increasing numbers of documented near-death experiences and out-of-body experiences.[108,109] While there is no single definition of this phenomenon, a near death has been described as 'a profound psychological event including transcendental and mystical elements, typically occurring to individuals close to death or in situations of intense physical or emotional danger'.[109] Experiences have typically included altered time perception, memories of light (described as brilliant, unusual or mystical), deceased relatives, out-of-body sensations, feelings of the presence of a deity, joy and peace.[110] While reported experiences are consistent, many of these studies are heterogeneous with targeted populations.[111] These experiences may vary between cultures: Euro-Americans may report a golden colour light whereas people from Tibet may report a clear light.[112] People report the experiences as pleasant, and they have resulted in positive life changes for the individual. After-effects of a near-death experience include absence of fear of death, a more spiritual view of life, less regard for material wealth and/or a heightened chemical sensitivity.[113] The incidence of near-death experiences after cardiac arrest is reported at 12–18%,[108] with the frequency generally being higher in people under 60 years of age.[113] Hence, an awareness of the incidence of near-death experiences and of the cultural differences and needs of the person with a reported near-death experience is essential post-cardiac arrest.[112] Chapter 7 provides more information about family and cultural care.

Special considerations

The chapter to this point primarily has focused on the physiological considerations of resuscitation to achieve the goal of preservation of cellular function. However, this outcome is only achieved in a minority of cases.[22–24] Decision making around the initiation of CPR and resuscitation interventions and the progression and termination of resuscitation involves a multitude of factors.

Family presence during an arrest

The practice of family members witnessing resuscitation has become more evident over time. This shift in practice has been attributed to increasing patient autonomy and the presence of family at a cardiac arrest in popular television shows. This has contributed to public support, and family members requesting – and expecting – to be present.[114,115] However, the issue of whether the family should be present during a cardiac arrest remains controversial. Proponents argue the importance of family being with loved ones during their last moments, as this shortens the period of grieving and provides closure. Indeed, professional resuscitation bodies recommend that family should be afforded the opportunity to be present.[114] However, translating these recommendations into practice varies among healthcare personnel and across cultures.[116] Commonly cited is a concern that the family may interrupt the work of the resuscitation team, the ethical and medicolegal implications or concern about offending the family.[117] Contrary to these beliefs, there is limited evidence that family interfere with the performance of the resuscitation team.[117,118]

Conflicting evidence exists as to the psychological effects of such an event on the family. Effects have been documented as ranging from no adverse effects[117] through to expressions of distress, haunting consequences and trauma.[117] Indeed, families with experience recommend and support family presence as they believe it was beneficial for their loved one and helped them to adjust to the family member's death.[114] Where families are provided the option of being present, a staff member should be identified to have sole responsibility of supporting the family and considering the needs of surrounding patients. In-patients who witness a resuscitation of another patient do find it a stressful experience and may require follow up care.[119] Chapter 7 is dedicated to family and cultural care, providing additional information about family support.

Ceasing CPR

The decision to cease CPR is often difficult; continuing CPR beyond 30 min without ROSC is usually futile unless the arrest was compounded by hypothermia, submersion in cold water, lightning strike, drug overdose or other identified and treatable conditions such as intermittent VF/VT.[16] Prolonging resuscitation for more than 60 min may be beneficial for a severely hypothermic, child victim of near-drowning. Pupillary signs should not be used as a predictor of outcome in infants and children, as 11–33% of children with non-reactive pupils have survived long-term after CPR.[17] It is important to have eliminated all causes as far as possible.

Termination of resuscitation is a multifactorial process, influenced by provider comfort and experience, patient prognosis and the patient's desires, wishes and values. Organisational issues such as the local culture, protocols, resources and guidelines will all impact on termination decisions. With scientific advances such as extracorporeal membrane oxygenation (ECMO) as a bridge for refractory VF and evidence-based protocols becoming more widely implemented, current impressions of termination decisions will change over time.[120,121] It is appropriate to invite suggestions from team members, to ensure that all members are comfortable with a decision to stop the resuscitation attempt.[16] Ultimately, terminating CPR is equivalent to a determination of death, and must be made by a doctor. In some out-of-hospital circumstances it may be the paramedical staff who make this decision to stop CPR, essentially terminating resuscitation.[122] Because of this need, termination of resuscitation guidelines have been developed for use in the out-of-hospital setting. One prospectively validated termination of resuscitation guideline is the 'basic life support termination of resuscitation rule' which may be adopted to guide the termination of pre-hospital CPR in adults.[25] This validated rule is described below.

In the pre-hospital setting stop CPR if:

- no ROSC

  and

- no shocks are administered

  and

- the arrest is not witnessed by emergency medical-services personnel.

Otherwise, the rule recommends transportation to the hospital, in accordance with routine practice.[123]

Legal and ethical considerations

Burgeoning technology in the 1960s enabled the support of oxygenation and circulation for people whose illnesses would have been lethal just a few years before. Enthusiasm for restoration of life led healthcare workers to routinely initiate CPR for all patients who died in hospital.[124] Unfortunately, this led to inappropriate resuscitation attempts and the realisation of the economic, medical and ethical burden to society when survivors had a resultant poor quality of life.[125,126] In the 1970s, growing concern about inappropriate application of CPR and patients' rights led authors to suggest means of forgoing resuscitation and involving patients in decision making. Traditionally, the decision to initiate or withhold CPR was often made by the treating medical team in the absence of the patient or family.[127,128]

Hospital personnel responded by developing procedures for withholding CPR through the documentation of 'do not attempt to resuscitate' orders, doctor's orders for life-sustaining treatment, advance directives or living wills[128,129] (see Chapter 4). For patients or their surrogates to meaningfully participate in decision making about CPR and limitation-of-treatment orders, they must have some understanding of survival rates and adverse effects associated with such interventions.[128] Consequently, much debate has ensued over the right of a person to forgo treatment.

Based on research findings, some propose that, while patients want to be involved in CPR decision making and want some form of advance directive, their knowledge is limited and often derived from television dramas.[128,130] Understanding of quality of life, morbidity and other outcomes after CPR strongly influences their preferences.[131,132] Most patients, and indeed healthcare workers, commonly hold unrealistic expectations of CPR success,[130] and will often reverse their preference for commencing CPR once they are informed of the true probability of survival, functional status and quality of life after resuscitation. When compared with the general public, survivors following cardiac arrest generally assess their quality of life as good 12 months post-arrest.[132] Regardless of this, healthcare workers continue to demonstrate a reluctance to discuss CPR options with patients.[133,134] Despite open discussion, variations in the timing of the orders, poor documentation and communication can result in CPR being inappropriately commenced.[129] Conversely, and contrary to medical and nursing opinions, some people choose CPR even when they have a terminal illness, coma or serious disability.[131]

Standardised orders for limitations on life-sustaining treatments (e.g. do not attempt to resuscitate) should be considered to decrease the incidence of futile resuscitation attempts and to ensure that adult patients' wishes are honoured. These orders should be specific, detailed, transferable across healthcare settings and easily understood. Processes, protocols and systems should be developed that fit within local cultural norms and legal limitations to allow providers to honour patients' wishes about resuscitation efforts.[25] With the exception of a zero-survival rate, there remains no formal consensus on 'do not attempt to resuscitate' decision-making practices or the termination of resuscitation. While researchers have attempted to develop prognostic indicators for cardiac arrest outcome, moralists would argue that the use of such prognostic tools alone reflects utilitarianism, and that they should never be used in isolation of the input of the patient and healthcare team.[135]

Summary

Outcomes for patients after in-hospital SCA remain poor. Successful management of a patient following SCA depends largely on the timely implementation of the chain of survival. Nurses should understand the role of the chain of survival in the resuscitation of the person following cardiac arrest. The chain emphasises the importance of early recognition and intervention, continuous uninterrupted compressions and the early use of the defibrillator as a BLS skill. Understanding when to start, when to continue and when to stop are equally important and are influenced by multiple factors. Including the patient's wishes in decision making is of utmost importance to ensure futile resuscitation attempts are avoided. Despite the plethora of research on the topic of resuscitation, there is much we still do not know.

Case study

Wednesday night in the intensive care unit (ICU): all beds are occupied, and the handover and allocation has occurred. Sam, an experienced ICU nurse, was the acting nurse unit manager (ANUM) for the shift and was also on for MET calls in the ward. This itself was not ideal, however. Due to sick leave where staff were not replaced, there had to be some doubling up of duties. Sam noted it could potentially be a busy night.

There was a MET call in one of the medical wards at 02:15. Sam and Louise (ICU registrar) grab the MET responder kit and together leave the ICU and travel to the ward. The medical ward was a 30-bed mixed ward, although mainly patients with respiratory conditions were admitted there. On arrival Sam and Louise were directed to a bathroom where they found the patient, Mr David Higgens, on the floor with two nurses assessing him.

Sam quickly commenced unpacking the MET gear and both he and Louise donned personal protective equipment. Louise asked for a handover. One nurse said Mr Higgens had got up to go to the bathroom and then she saw that the bathroom buzzer had been activated; when she arrived, Mr Higgens had slumped from the toilet to the floor. He was breathing but unconscious. Sam applied a SaO_2 probe and ECG leads and asked one of the nurses to apply the blood pressure cuff.

Mr Higgens was in rapid atrial fibrillation at a rate of 145, his oxygen saturations were 80%, respiratory rate 22 breaths/minute and laboured. The MET blood pressure cuff was too small to fit around his arm. Mr Higgens was extremely obese and on questioning the staff it was found that he weighed 170 kg.

After a few minutes a larger BP cuff was found, and the patient's blood pressure was 105/80 mmHg.

Sam had applied oxygen via a mask, noting the patient's observations (including glucose) and asking one of the ward nurses to be a scribe. Louise, in the meantime, was trying to put in intravenous (IV) access as Mr Higgens had no access (his IV cannula had been removed during the day due to looming phlebitis). During attempts at IV access Mr Higgens regained consciousness and was trying to sit up.

A HoverJack® mattress was called for to lift Mr Higgens from the floor of the bathroom and back onto his bed to enable nursing and medical staff to work in a safer environment. This took some time and one of the nurses on the ward left the scene to make the appropriate calls. The Hospital Coordinator had arrived at this time and was trying to determine the situation and what transfers needed to be made.

For a difficult 20 minutes Mr Higgens was placed on the HoverJack, lifted up and transferred back onto his bed. His vital signs were continuously monitored; an ECG showed that he was in rapid atrial fibrillation and had a left bundle branch block (LBBB), which was not new. Defibrillation pads were applied at this time. With the application of oxygen Mr Higgens's oxygen saturation levels increased to 88%. Meanwhile Louise was struggling to find IV access; she stopped at one point and did an arterial stab into Mr Higgens's left radial artery and that sample was couriered to the ICU for analysis.

The admission information on Mr Higgens was that he had presented with worsening shortness of breath and cardiac failure. Sam auscultated Mr Higgens's chest and reported that there were reduced breath sounds and course crackles to the midzones. Louise and Sam both continued to try and find IV access, to no avail. The following decisions regarding Mr Higgens were made:

1 Urgent transfer to the ICU was required
2 He required some form of access for resuscitation
3 He was in acute cardiac failure and acute pulmonary oedema was imminent
4 He required non-invasive (NIV) ventilation in the immediate short term.

Sam asked for an intraosseous drill to be brought to the ward from the emergency department which was closer than the ICU. When the drill arrived, Sam set it up with a bariatric needle (45 mm × 1.8 mm, 15 gauge) and primed the extension set with 2 mL of 2% lignocaine and attached a syringe to the set. A 20 mL syringe of saline was also drawn up. The IO dressing was also prepared. Louise located the appropriate location on Mr Higgens's leg (proximal anterior tibia) and prepared the area and then drilled into the bone. Once the give of the bone marrow was felt, Louise stopped drilling and removed the needle, she then attached the extension set with syringe and aspirated bone marrow fluid to confirm position, and then inserted the lignocaine via a slow push and followed it with the syringe of saline. The dressing was applied and an infusion of saline via an infusion pump was commenced at a slow rate to maintain access.

At this time a non-invasive ventilator arrived on the ward and Sam set it up initially with PEEP of 5 cm and pressure support of 5 cm (to enable Mr Higgens to get used to the pressure/flow and mask). The FiO_2 was set at 0.8.

The Hospital Coordinator reported to Sam and Louise that a bed in the ICU would be available in 15 minutes as the most stable patient who was ready for the ward was being transferred out. During these rather long 15 minutes the following occurred: 80 mg IO frusemide and 10 mg IO morphine were given, a 50 mg glyceryl trinitrate patch was applied, and the pressure support of the NIV was slowly turned up to 10 cmH_2O.

Louise phoned the ICU and asked that they prepare for central and arterial line insertions.

Finally, all was ready for transfer to ICU. Mr Higgens was transferred to the ICU at 04:00. On admission to the unit his cardiac rhythm suddenly changed to pVT. Mr Higgens was defibrillated at 200 joules and reverted to a sinus rhythm. CPR was immediately commenced post defibrillation. The NIV was removed and an LMA was inserted, and he was ventilated via a bag and valve with supplemental oxygen. After about 90 seconds Mr Higgens regained consciousness, his pulses were checked and it was confirmed that he had ROSC. The LMA was removed and NIV recommenced.

A central line and an arterial line were inserted and an indwelling urinary catheter, which drained 1500 mL of urine. Mr Higgens blood pressure improved now that he was in sinus rhythm and he was tolerating the NIV fairly well with his conscious state improving.

On investigation of his medical notes it was discovered that he had been in sinus rhythm with a LBBB, and the rapid atrial fibrillation was a new event. He was on a low dose of enoxaparin and this was increased to the therapeutic dose. His electrolytes were checked and topped up. He was loaded with amiodarone and commenced on an amiodarone infusion.

Once reasonably stable his medical notes were further investigated. His wife was phoned and updated on the emergency call and transfer. She said she would call her son to bring her into the hospital.

The observation chart was reviewed. It was seen that 6 h earlier Mr Higgens's HR and BP fell into the clinical review part of the chart; however, this was not actioned at the time. Mr Higgens remained in intensive care for 2 further days with intermittent non-invasive ventilation and treatment for cardiac failure prior to transfer to a step-down ward.

CASE STUDY QUESTIONS

1 What is the reasoning behind 2 min of compressions post-successful defibrillation?
2 What is the purpose of the track and trigger observation chart?
3 What is the first-line treatment for pulseless ventricular tachycardia and ventricular tachycardia with a pulse?
4 Why was 200 joules selected as the energy level for the first shock?
5 List the insertion sites for intraosseous access?
6 Why was lignocaine inserted into the IO prior to fluids and medications?

RESEARCH VIGNETTE

Hassankhani H, Zamanzade V, Rahmani A, Haririan H, Porter JE. Family support liaison in the witnessed resuscitation: a phenomenology study. Int J Nurs Stud 2017; 74:95-100

Background: Family-witnessed resuscitation remains controversial among clinicians from implementation to practice and there are a number of countries, such as Iran, where that is considered a low priority.

Objective: To explore the lived experience of resuscitation team members with the presence of the patient's family during resuscitation.

Design: The hermeneutic phenomenology.

Settings: The emergency departments and critical care units of 6 tertiary hospitals in Tabriz, Iran.

Participants: There were potentially 380 nurses and physicians working in the emergency departments and acute care settings of 6 tertiary hospitals in Tabriz. A purposive sample of these nurses and physicians was used to recruit participants who had at least 2 years of experience, had experienced an actual family witnessed resuscitation event, and wanted to participate. The sample size was determined according to data saturation. Data collection ended when the data were considered rich and varied enough to illuminate the phenomenon, and no new themes emerged following the interview of 12 nurses and 8 physicians.

Methods: Semi-structured, face-to-face interviews were held with the participants over a period of 6 months (April 2015 to September 2015), and Van Manen's method of data analysis was adopted.

Results: Three main themes emerged from the data analysis, including 'Futile resuscitation', 'Family support liaison', and 'Influence on team's performance'. A further 9 sub-themes emerged under the 3 main themes, which included 'futile resuscitation in end-stage cancer patients', 'when a patient dies', 'young patients', 'care of the elderly', 'accountable person', 'family supporter', 'no influence', 'positive influence', and 'negative influence'.

Conclusions: Participants noted both positive and negative experiences of having family members present during cardiopulmonary resuscitation. Welltrained and expert resuscitation team members are less likely to be stressed in the presence of family. A family support liaison would act to decrease family anxiety levels and to de-escalate any potentially aggressive person during the resuscitation. It is recommended that an experienced health care professional be designated to be responsible for explaining the process of resuscitation to the patient's family.

Critique

The concept of family presence during resuscitation (FPDR) is widely accepted by health professionals in western cultures and the general public expect to be invited when a family member requires resuscitation.[105,106] Its acceptance in other countries remains low. Findings from this Iranian study are consistent with observations from other studies conducted in Germany, Singapore, Turkey, Hong Kong, Saudi Arabia and Singapore where a general opposition to its implementation, relegating it a low priority during the resuscitation period is reported.[107]

Much of the literature collating evidence to understand barriers to FPDR implantation from a cultural perspective has used surveys. As individual attitudes and cultural variations do influence healthcare systems, Hassankhani et al sought to inform practice change and policy development by understanding the experiences of those involved. The choice of Heideggerian phenomenology as the methodology for the study was appropriate as it is a rich medium for understanding the experiences of those with prior exposure. As was the use of the hermeneutic cycle to analyse the data. While the authors touch on Van Manen's fundamental existentials, the application of these is not apparent in the paper, as would have been expected.

This was a purposive sample of emergency department nurses (n=12) and physicians (n=8) who had prior FPDR experience. This sampling method is appropriate in qualitative research as it provides access to participants who were able to provide information-rich information of the phenomenon of interest. To better understand the chance of a biased sample, the researchers should have reported how participants were recruited from the six tertiary sites in the first instance. The final sample consisted predominantly of male participants, which possibly reflects the health professional gender representation of the study population. A theme consistent in the FPDR literature is that nurses when compared with physicians hold more positive views; typically, the nurses in those studies have been female. Readers of this paper should consider the findings within the context that the predominant 'voice' of the participants in the study was male.

Three main themes emerged: *Futile resuscitation*, *Family support liaison* and *Influence on team's performance.* Participant voice within the latter two themes of *Family support liaison* and *Influence on team's performance* are generally consistent with existing literature, in that the presence of family support liaison will support the family in understanding the situation, particularly where the family has expectations that are at odds with the resuscitation team.

The emergence of *Futile resuscitation* as a dominant theme could be explained by the author's observation that Iranian physicians attempt resuscitation on all patients regardless of patient or family wishes. This absence of formal policy and guidelines means that staff values and preferences influenced their decision making regarding inviting family to be present and actual behaviour commencing, ceasing and, indeed, the duration of cardiopulmonary resuscitation. Participants reported that strong family ties, connections and emotional dependence on each other influence not only how family will respond, but also the extent to which health professionals will invite family to be present. In this study staff balanced the risks and benefits to justify their behaviour; for example, continuing CPR to meet the expectations of family or minimise risk of agitation of the family or litigation, or conversely to allow time for grieving. Developing formal policy will reduce family exclusion based on paternalistic or personal preference and these *Futile resuscitation* attempts, with, ultimately, improving the current low survival rate following resuscitation of just 7.2%. The aim of any qualitative study is not to generalise findings, rather it is to transfer the theoretical knowledge to other individuals, groups or situations. This study highlighted the cultural differences between Iranian and Western countries: an important observation to inform staff practices when supporting patients and their families who have emigrated from Iran. The findings also contribute extant literature on FPDR from a cultural perspective to facilitate the development and implementation of consistent FPDR practices that benefit the patient and family.

Learning activities

1 Discuss the benefits of compression-only CPR and conventional CPR with rescue breathing.

2 What is the rationale for targeted temperature management in adults after cardiac arrest?

3 Identify the stage in the ALS flow chart when amiodarone is given.

4 Explain the role of family and their contribution to early warning systems in the early detection of deterioration.

5 Identify two sites for administration of medications during a cardiac arrest and discuss the benefits and disadvantages of each site.

Online resources

American Heart Association (AHA), www.americanheart.org

Australian Resuscitation Council (ARC), www.resus.org.au

Center for Pediatric Emergency Medicine (CPEM), http://cpem.med.nyu.edu

European Resuscitation Council (ERC), www.erc.edu

International Liaison Committee on Resuscitation (ILCOR), http://www.ilcor.org/home/

New Zealand Resuscitation Council (NZRC), www.nzrc.org.nz

The Regional Emergency Medical Services Council of New York City, http://www.nycremsco.org/

Further reading

Hassankhani H, Haririan H, Porter JE, et al. Cultural aspects of death notification following cardiopulmonary resuscitation. J Adv Nurs 2018;74(17):1564–72.

Leidel BA, Kirchhoff C, Braunstein V, et al. Comparison of two intraosseous access devices in adult patients under resuscitation in the emergency department: a prospective, randomized study. Resuscitation 2010;81:994–9.

Xie A, Phan K, Tsai MY, et al. Venoarterial extracorporeal membrane oxygenation for cardiogenic shock and cardiac arrest: a meta-analysis. J Cardiothorac Vasc Anesth 2015;29(3):637–45.

References

1. Australian and New Zealand Consensus on Resuscitation (ANZCOR). ANZCOR Guidelines; 2018. Victoria, Australia: Australian Resuscitation Council. Online. Available from: http://www.resus.org.au. [Accessed April 2018].
2. Gräsner J-T, Bossaert L. Epidemiology and management of cardiac arrest: what registries are revealing. Best Pract Res Clin Anaesthesiol 2013;27(3):293–306.
3. Al-Khatib SM, Stevenson WG, Ackerman MJ, et al. AHA/ACC/HRS Guideline for management of patients with ventricular arrhythmias and the prevention of sudden cardiac death: a report of the American College of Cardiology/American Heart Association Task Force on Clinical Practice Guidelines and the Heart Rhythm Society. J Am Coll Cardiol 2017;2017:24390.
4. Gräsner J-T, Frey N. The best things to do – MTH and PCI after cardiac arrest? Resuscitation 2014;85(5):581–2.
5. Andrew E, Nehme Z, Wolfe R, et al. Long-term survival following out-of-hospital cardiac arrest. Heart 2017;103(14):1104–10.
6. Holmgren C, Bergfeldt L, Edvardsson N, et al. Analysis of initial rhythm, witnessed status and delay to treatment among survivors of out-of-hospital cardiac arrest in Sweden. Heart 2010;96:1826–30.
7. Wah W, Wai KL, Pek PP, et al. Conversion to shockable rhythms during resuscitation and survival for out-of hospital cardiac arrest. Am J Emerg Med 2017;35(2):206–13.

8. Berdowski J, Berg RA, Tijssen JGP, et al. Global incidences of out-of-hospital cardiac arrest and survival rates: systematic review of 67 prospective studies. Resuscitation 2010;81(11):1479–87.
9. Herlitz J, Engdahl J, Svensson L, et al. Can we define patients with no chance of survival after out-of-hospital cardiac arrest? Heart 2004;90(10):1114–18.
10. Australian Institute of Health and Welfare (AIHW). Australia's health 2012. Australia's health series no. 12; 2012. Canberra: AIHW. Online. Available from: http://www.aihw.gov.au/publication-detail/?id=10737422172.
11. Müller D, Agrawal R, Arntz H-R. How sudden is sudden cardiac death? Circulation 2006;114(11):1146–50.
12. Soar J, Nolan JP, Böttiger BW, et al. European resuscitation council guidelines for resuscitation 2015: section 3. Adult advanced life support. Resuscitation 2015;95:100–47.
13. Herlitz J, Svensson L, Engdahl J, et al. Characteristics of cardiac arrest and resuscitation by age group: an analysis from the Swedish Cardiac Arrest Registry. Am J Emerg Med 2007;25(9):1025–31.
14. Manley BJ, Owen LS, Hooper SB, et al. Towards evidence-based resuscitation of the newborn infant. Lancet 2017;389(10079): 1639–48.
15. Meert K, Telford R, Holubkov R, et al. Paediatric in-hospital cardiac arrest: factors associated with survival and neurobehavioural outcome one year later. Resuscitation 2018;124:96–105.
16. Kleinman ME, de Caen AR, Chameides L, et al. Part 10: pediatric basic and advanced life support: 2010 International Consensus on Cardiopulmonary Resuscitation and Emergency Cardiovascular Care Science with Treatment Recommendations. Circulation 2010;122(16 Suppl. 2):S466–515.
17. Frenneaux M. Cardiopulmonary resuscitation – some physiological considerations. Resuscitation 2003;58(3):259–65.
18. Olasveengen TM, de Caen AR, Mancini ME, et al. International consensus on cardiopulmonary resuscitation and emergency cardiovascular care science with treatment recommendations summary. Resuscitation 2017;121:201–14.
19. Perkins GD, Neumar R, Monsieurs KG, et al. The International Liaison Committee on Resuscitation – Review of the last 25 years and vision for the future. Resuscitation 2017;121:104–16.
20. Shuvy M, Morrison LJ, Koh M, et al. Long-term clinical outcomes and predictors for survivors of out-of-hospital cardiac arrest. Resuscitation 2017;112:59–64.
21. Perkins GD, Jacobs IG, Nadkarni VM, et al. Cardiac arrest and cardiopulmonary resuscitation outcome reports: update of the Utstein Resuscitation Registry Templates for Out-of-hospital Cardiac Arrest: a statement for healthcare professionals from a task force of the International Liaison Committee on Resuscitation and the American Heart Association Emergency Cardiovascular Care Committee and the Council on Cardiopulmonary, Critical Care, Perioperative and Resuscitation. Resuscitation 2015;96:328–40.
22. Kolte D, Khera S, Aronow W, et al. Gender and racial/ethnic differences in survival after cardiopulmonary resuscitation for in-hospital cardiac arrest. J Am Coll Cardiol 2014;63(12_S).
23. Nolan JP, Soar J, Smith GB, et al. Incidence and outcome of in-hospital cardiac arrest in the United Kingdom National Cardiac Arrest Audit. Resuscitation 2014;85(8):987–92.
24. Mallikethi-Reddy S, Briasoulis A, Akintoye E, et al. Incidence and survival after in-hospital cardiopulmonary resuscitation in nonelderly adults: US experience, 2007 to 2012. Circ Cardiovasc Qual Outcomes 2017;10(2):e003194.
25. Soar J, Mancini M, Bhanji F, et al. On behalf of the education, implementation, and teams chapter collaborators. Part 12: education, implementation, and teams: 2010 International Consensus on Cardiopulmonary Resuscitation and Emergency Cardiovascular Care Science with Treatment Recommendations. Resuscitation 2010;81:e288–330.
26. Meaney P, Bobrow B, Mancini M, et al. Cardiopulmonary resuscitation quality: improving cardiac resuscitation outcomes both inside and outside the hospital: a consensus statement from the American Heart Association. Circulation 2013;128(4):417–35.
27. Koster R, Baubin M, Bossaert L, et al. European Resuscitation Council Guidelines for Resuscitation 2010 Section 2. Adult basic life support and use of automated external defibrillators. Resuscitation 2010;81:1277–92.
28. McGaughey J, O'Halloran P, Porter S, et al. Early warning systems and rapid response to the deteriorating patient in hospital: a systematic realist review. J Adv Nurs 2017.
29. Smith GB. In-hospital cardiac arrest: is it time for an in-hospital 'chain of prevention'? Resuscitation 2010;81(9):1209–11.
30. Considine J, Botti M. Who, when and where? Identification of patients at risk of an in-hospital adverse event: implications for nursing practice. Int J Nurs Pract 2004;10(1):21–31.
31. Kause J, Smith G, Prytherch D, et al. A comparison of antecedents to cardiac arrests, deaths and emergency intensive care admissions in Australia and New Zealand, and the United Kingdom – the ACADEMIA study. Resuscitation 2004;62(3):275–82.
32. Sprogis S, Currey J, Considine J, et al. Physiological antecedents and ward clinician responses before medical emergency team activation. Crit Care Resusc 2017;19(1):50–6.
33. Le Lagadec D, Dwyer T. Scoping review: the use of early warning systems for the identification of in-hospital patient at risk of deterioration. Aust Crit Care 2017;30(4):211–18.
34. Prytherch DR, Smith GB, Schmidt PE, et al. ViEWS – Towards a national early warning score for detecting adult inpatient deterioration. Resuscitation 2010;81(8):932–7.
35. McNeill G, Bryden D. Do either early warning systems or emergency response teams improve hospital patient survival? A systematic review. Resuscitation 2013;84(12):1652–67.

36. Australian and New Zealand Consensus on Resuscitation (ANZCOR). ARC Guideline 11.1 – Introduction to and principles of in-hospital resuscitation: Australian Resuscitation Council; 2017. Available from: https://resus.org.au/guidelines/.
37. Smith GB, Prytherch DR, Meredith P, et al. The ability of the National Early Warning Score (NEWS) to discriminate patients at risk of early cardiac arrest, unanticipated intensive care unit admission, and death. Resuscitation 2013;84(4):465–70.
38. Guinane J, Hutchinson AM, Bucknall T. Patient perceptions of deterioration and patient and family activated escalation systems – a qualitative study. J Clin Nurs 2017;1–11.
39. Australian Resuscitation Council and New Zealand Resuscitation Council (ARC and NRZC). Australian Resuscitation Council, Airway: Guideline 4; 2014. Australian Resuscitation Council. Available from: http://www.resus.org.au.
40. Australian and New Zealand Consensus on Resuscitation (ANZCOR). ANZCOR Guideline 12.6 – Introduction to Paediatric Advanced Life Support Techniques in Paediatric Advanced Life Support; 2016. Available from: https://resus.org.au/guidelines/.
41. Wyckoff MH, Aziz K, Escobedo MB, et al. Part 13: neonatal resuscitation. Circulation 2015;132(18 Suppl. 2):S543–60.
42. Berg R, Saunders A, Kern K, et al. Adverse hemodynamic effects of interrupting chest compressions for rescue breathing during cardiopulmonary resuscitation for ventricular defibrillation cardiac arrest. Circulation 2001;104:2465–70.
43. Nolan J, Ornato J, Parr M, et al. Resuscitation highlights in 2016. Resuscitation 2017;114:A1–7.
44. Dwyer T. Psychological factors inhibit family members' confidence to initiate CPR. Prehosp Emerg Care 2008;12(2):157–61.
45. Assar D, Chamberlain D, Colquhoun M, et al. Randomised controlled trial of staged teaching for basic life support: skill acquisition at bronze stage. Resuscitation 2000;45:7–15.
46. Perkins GD, Handley AJ, Koster RW, et al. European Resuscitation Council Guidelines for Resuscitation 2015: section 2. Adult basic life support and automated external defibrillation. Resuscitation 2015;95:81–99.
47. Bobrow B, Spaite D, Berg R, et al. Chest compression-only CPR by lay rescuers and survival from out-of-hospital cardiac arrest. JAMA 2010;304(3):1447–54.
48. Touma O, Davies M. The prognostic value of end tidal carbon dioxide during cardiac arrest: a systematic review. Resuscitation 2013;84(11):1470–9.
49. Nolan JP. High-quality cardiopulmonary resuscitation. Curr Opin Crit Care 2014;20(3):227–33.
50. Paiva EF, Paxton JH, O'Neil BJ. The use of end-tidal carbon dioxide (ETCO2) measurement to guide management of cardiac arrest: a systematic review. Resuscitation 2018;123:1–7.
51. Park SO, Shin DH, Baek KJ, et al. A clinical observational study analysing the factors associated with hyperventilation during actual cardiopulmonary resuscitation in the emergency department. Resuscitation 2013;84(3):298–303.
52. Delguercio L, Feins N, Cohn J, et al. Comparison of blood flow during external and internal cardiac massage in man. Circulation 1965;31(Suppl. 1):171–80.
53. Li H, Wang D, Yu Y, et al. Mechanical versus manual chest compressions for cardiac arrest: a systematic review and meta-analysis. Scand J Trauma Resusc Emerg Med 2016;24(1):10.
54. Soar J, Nolan JP. Manual chest compressions for cardiac arrest – with or without mechanical CPR? Resuscitation 2014;85(6):705–6.
55. Wik L, Olsen J-A, Persse D, et al. Manual vs integrated automatic load-distributing band CPR with equal survival after out of hospital cardiac arrest. The randomized CIRC trial. Resuscitation 2014;85(6):741–8.
56. Luo X, Zhang H, Chen G, et al. Active compression-decompression cardiopulmonary resuscitation (CPR) versus standard CPR for cardiac arrest patients: a meta-analysis. World J Emerg Med 2013;4(4):266–72.
57. Babbs CF. The case for interposed abdominal compression CPR in hospital settings. Analg Resusc: Curr Res 2013;3:1.
58. Nehme Z, Andrew E, Bernard SA, et al. Treatment of monitored out-of-hospital ventricular fibrillation and pulseless ventricular tachycardia utilising the precordial thump. Resuscitation 2013;84(12):1691–6.
59. Pellis T, Kette F, Lovisa D, et al. Utility of pre-cordial thump for treatment of out of hospital cardiac arrest: a prospective study. Resuscitation 2009;80:17–23.
60. Dwyer T, Mosel Williams L, Jacobs I. The benefits and use of shock advisory defibrillators in hospitals. Int J Nurs Pract 2004;10(2):86–92.
61. Tomkins WGO, Swain AH, Bailey M, et al. Beyond the pre-shock pause: the effect of prehospital defibrillation mode on CPR interruptions and return of spontaneous circulation. Resuscitation 2013;84(5):575–9.
62. Husain S, Eisenberg M. Police AED programs: a systematic review and meta-analysis. Resuscitation 2013;84(9):1184–91.
63. Morrison LJ, Henry RM, Ku V, et al. Single-shock defibrillation success in adult cardiac arrest: a systematic review. Resuscitation 2013;84(11):1480–6.
64. Wang C-H, Huang C-H, Chang W-T, et al. Biphasic versus monophasic defibrillation in out-of-hospital cardiac arrest: a systematic review and meta-analysis. Am J Emerg Med 2013;31(10):1472–8.
65. Hess EP, Atkinson EJ, White RD. Increased prevalence of sustained return of spontaneous circulation following transition to biphasic waveform defibrillation. Resuscitation 2008;77(1):39–45.
66. de Caen AR, Kleinman ME, Chameides L, et al. Part 10: paediatric basic and advanced life support. Resuscitation 2010;81(Suppl. 1):e213–59.
67. Chan PS, Krumholz HM, Spertus JA, et al. Automated external defibrillators and survival after in-hospital cardiac arrest. JAMA 2010;304(19):2129–36.

68. Christenson J, Andrusiek D, Everson-Stewart S, et al. Chest compression fraction determines survival in patients with out-of-hospital ventricular fibrillation. Circulation 2009;120(13):1241–7.
69. Ristagno G, Li Y, Gullo A, et al. Amplitude spectrum area as a predictor of successful defibrillation. In: Anaesthesia and Pharmacology of Intensive Care Emergency Medicine APICE. Springer; 2011. p. 141–60.
70. Monteleone PP, Borek HA, Althoff SO. Electrical therapies in cardiac arrest. Emerg Med Clin North Am 2012;30(1):51–63.
71. Australian and New Zealand Consensus on Resuscitation (ANZCOR). ANZCOR Guideline 7 Defibrillation Australian Resuscitation Council. Online. Available from: https://resus.org.au/guidelines/. [Accessed February 2018].
72. Morley P. Cardiopulmonary resuscitation. In: Harley I, Hore P, editors. Anaesthesia: an introduction. 5th ed. East Hawthorn, Victoria: IP Communications; 2012. p. 174–89.
73. Soar J, Nolan JP. Airway management in cardiopulmonary resuscitation. Curr Opin Crit Care 2013;19(3):181–7.
74. Trevisanuto D, Cavallin F, Nguyen LN, et al. Supreme laryngeal mask airway versus face mask during neonatal resuscitation: a randomized controlled trial. J Pediatr 2015;167(2):286–91.e1.
75. Yamaga S, Une K, Kyo M, et al. Gas insufflation in the stomach during cardiopulmonary resuscitation using laryngeal tube ventilation in comparison with bag-valve-mask ventilation. Circulation 2012;126(Suppl. 21):A295.
76. Soar J. Which airway for cardiac arrest? Do supraglottic airways devices have a role? Resuscitation 2013;84(9):1163–4.
77. Morrison LJ, Neumar RW, Zimmerman JL, et al. Strategies for improving survival after in-hospital cardiac arrest in the United States: 2013 consensus recommendations. A consensus statement from the American Heart Association. Circulation 2013;127(14):1538–63.
78. Hellevuo H, Sainio M, Olkkola KT, et al. Ventricular fibrillation/tachycardia, pulseless electrical activity and asystole are equally common initial rhythms in in-hospital cardiac arrest due to cardiac reasons. Resuscitation 2014;85:S34.
79. Rosborough JP, Deno DC. Electrical therapy for post defibrillatory pulseless electrical activity. Resuscitation 2004;63(1):65–72.
80. Australian and New Zealand Consensus on Resuscitation (ANZCOR). ANZCOR Guideline 11.5 – Medications in Adult Cardiac Arrest: Australian Resuscitation Council; 2016. Available from: https://resus.org.au/guidelines/.
81. Mentzelopoulos SD, Zakynthinos SG, Siempos I, et al. Vasopressin for cardiac arrest: meta-analysis of randomized controlled trials. Resuscitation 2012;83(1):32–9.
82. Perkins GD, Ji C, Deakin CD, et al. A randomized trial of epinephrine in out-of-hospital cardiac arrest. N Engl J Med 2018;1–11.
83. Layek A, Maitra S, Pal S, et al. Efficacy of vasopressin during cardio-pulmonary resuscitation in adult patients: a meta-analysis. Resuscitation 2014;85(7):855–63.
84. Soar J, Callaway CW, Aibiki M, et al. Part 4: advanced life support: 2015 international consensus on cardiopulmonary resuscitation and emergency cardiovascular care science with treatment recommendations. Resuscitation 2015;95:e71–120.
85. Jacobs IG, Finn JC, Jelinek GA, et al. Effect of adrenaline on survival in out-of-hospital cardiac arrest: a randomised double-blind placebo-controlled trial. Resuscitation 2011;82(9):1138–43.
86. Neumar RW, Otto CW, Link MS, et al. Part 8: adult advanced cardiovascular life support: 2010 American Heart Association guidelines for cardiopulmonary resuscitation and emergency cardiovascular care. Circulation 2010;122(18 Suppl. 3):S729–67.
87. Pitcher D, Nolan J. Peri-arrest arrhythmias: Resuscitation UK; 2015. Available from: https://www.resus.org.uk/resuscitation-guidelines/peri-arrest-arrhythmias/.
88. Truhlář A, Deakin CD, Soar J, et al. European resuscitation council guidelines for resuscitation 2015: section 4. Cardiac arrest in special circumstances. Resuscitation 2015;95:148–201.
89. Clark SL, Christmas JT, Frye DR, et al. Maternal mortality in the United States: predictability and the impact of protocols on fatal postcesarean pulmonary embolism and hypertension-related intracranial hemorrhage. Am J Obstet Gynecol 2014;211(1):32.e1–9.
90. Lewis G. Saving mothers' lives: the continuing benefits for maternal health from the United Kingdom (UK) confidential enquires into maternal deaths; 2012. Semin Perinatol.
91. Idris AH, Bierens JJ, Perkins GD, et al. 2015 revised Utstein-style recommended guidelines for uniform reporting of data from drowning-related resuscitation: an ILCOR advisory statement. Resuscitation 2017;118:147–58.
92. Lipman S, Cohen S, Einav S, et al. The Society for Obstetric Anesthesia and Perinatology consensus statement on the management of cardiac arrest in pregnancy. Anesth Analg 2014;118(5):1003–16.
93. Australian and New Zealand Consensus on Resuscitation (ANZCOR). ANZCOR Guideline 11.10 – Resuscitation in special circumstances; 2011. Australian Resuscitation Council. Available from: https://resus.org.au/guidelines/.
94. Lavonas EJ, Drennan IR, Gabrielli A, et al. Part 10: special circumstances of resuscitation. Circulation 2015;132(18 Suppl. 2):S501–18.
95. Gupta S. Maternal cardiac arrest and resuscitation: some burning issues! J Obstet Anaesth Crit Care 2013;3(1):1.
96. Zafren K, Durrer B, Herry J-P, et al. Lightning injuries: prevention and on-site treatment in mountains and remote areas: official guidelines of the International Commission for Mountain Emergency Medicine and the Medical Commission of the International Mountaineering and Climbing Federation (ICAR and UIAA MEDCOM). Resuscitation 2005;65(3):369–72.
97. Layon AJ, Modell JH. Drowning: update 2009. Anesthesiology 2009;110(6):1390–401.
98. Yeung JHY, Ong GJ, Davies RP, et al. Factors affecting team leadership skills and their relationship with quality of cardiopulmonary resuscitation. Crit Care Med 2012;40(9):2617–21.
99. Hunziker S, Johansson AC, Tschan F, et al. Teamwork and leadership in cardiopulmonary resuscitation. J Am Coll Cardiol 2011;57(24):2381–8.

100. Jones L, King L, Wilson C. A literature review: factors that impact on nurses' effective use of the medical emergency team (MET). J Clin Nurs 2009;18(24):3379–90.
101. Dwyer T, Mosel Williams L, Mummery K. Defibrillation beliefs of rural nurses: focus group discussions guided by the theory of planned behaviour. Rural Remote Health 2005;5:322.
102. Rittenberger JC, Callaway CW. Post-cardiac arrest management in adults. UpToDate 2015;19:2015. Available from: https://www.uptodate.com/contents/post-cardiac-arrest-management-in-adults. [Accessed 1 February 2019].
103. Binks A, Nolan J. Post-cardiac arrest syndrome. Minerva Anestesiol 2010;76(5):362–8.
104. Donnino MW, Andersen LW, Berg KM, et al. Temperature management after cardiac arrest: an advisory statement by the advanced life support task force of the International Liaison Committee on Resuscitation and the American Heart Association Emergency Cardiovascular Care Committee and the Council on Cardiopulmonary, Critical Care, Perioperative and Resuscitation. Resuscitation 2016;98:97–104.
105. Nielsen N, Wetterslev J, Cronberg T, et al. Targeted temperature management at 33°C versus 36°C after cardiac arrest. N Engl J Med 2013;369(23):2197–206.
106. Aneman A, Cariou A, Nolan JP. Understanding temperature goals after cardiac arrest. Intensive Care Med 2017;1–4.
107. Polderman KH, Herold I. Therapeutic hypothermia and controlled normothermia in the intensive care unit: practical considerations, side effects, and cooling methods. Crit Care Med 2009;37(3):1101–20.
108. Agrillo C. Near-death experience: out-of-body and out-of-brain? Rev Gen Psychol 2011;15(1):1.
109. Greyson B. Getting comfortable with near death experiences. Missouri Med 2013;110(6):471.
110. Cassol H, Pétré B, Degrange S, et al. Qualitative thematic analysis of the phenomenology of near-death experiences. PLoS ONE 2018;13(2):e0193001.
111. Pistoia F, Mattiacci G, Sarà M, et al. Development of the Italian version of the Near-Death Experience Scale. Front Hum Neurosci 2018;12:45.
112. Belanti J, Perera M, Jagadheesan K. Phenomenology of near-death experiences: a cross-cultural perspective. Transcult Psychiatry 2008;45(1):121–33.
113. Cant R, Cooper S, Chung C, et al. The divided self: near death experiences of resuscitated patients – a review of literature. Int Emerg Nurs 2012;20(2):88–93.
114. Dwyer TA. Predictors of public support for family presence during cardiopulmonary resuscitation: a population-based study. Int J Nurs Stud 2015;52:1064–70.
115. Ong MEH, Chung WL, Mei JSE. Comparing attitudes of the public and medical staff towards witnessed resuscitation in an Asian population. Resuscitation 2007;73(1):103–8.
116. Lederman Z, Baird G, Dong C, et al. Attitudes of Singapore Emergency Department staff towards family presence during cardiopulmonary resuscitation. Clin Ethics 2017;12(3):124–34.
117. Jabre P, Belpomme V, Azoulay E, et al. Family presence during cardiopulmonary resuscitation. N Engl J Med 2013;368(11):1008–18.
118. Porter JE, Cooper SJ, Sellick K. Family presence during resuscitation (FPDR): perceived benefits, barriers and enablers to implementation and practice. Int Emerg Nurs 2014;22(2):69–74.
119. Fiori M, Latour JM, Los F. 'Am I also going to die, doctor?' A systematic review of the impact of in-hospital patients witnessing a resuscitation of another patient. Eur J Cardiovasc Nurs 2017;16(7):585–94.
120. Stub D, Bernard S, Pellegrino V, et al. Issues in establishing the refractory out-of-hospital cardiac arrest treated with mechanical CPR, hypothermia, ECMO and early reperfusion (CHEER) study. Heart Lung Circ 2012;21:S163.
121. Chen Y-S, Lin J-W, Yu H-Y, et al. Cardiopulmonary resuscitation with assisted extracorporeal life-support versus conventional cardiopulmonary resuscitation in adults with in-hospital cardiac arrest: an observational study and propensity analysis. Lancet 2008;372(9638):554–61.
122. Adams BD, Benger J. Should we take patients to hospital in cardiac arrest? BMJ 2014;349:5659.
123. Morrison LJ, Eby D, Veigas PV, et al. Implementation trial of the basic life support termination of resuscitation rule: reducing the transport of futile out-of-hospital cardiac arrests. Resuscitation 2014;85(4):486–91.
124. Lynn J, Gregory CO. Regulating hearts and minds: the mismatch of law, custom and resuscitation decisions. J Am Geriatr Soc 2003;51(10):1502–3.
125. Bossaert LL, Perkins GD, Askitopoulou H, et al. European Resuscitation Council Guidelines for Resuscitation 2015: section 11. The ethics of resuscitation and end-of-life decisions. Resuscitation 2015;95:302–11.
126. Salins NS, Pai SG, Vidyasagar M, et al. Ethics and medico legal aspects of 'not for resuscitation'. Indian J Palliat Care 2010;16(2):66.
127. Mills A, Walker A, Levinson M, et al. Resuscitation orders in acute hospitals: a point prevalence study. Australas J Ageing 2017;36(1):32–7.
128. Sritharan G, Mills AC, Levinson MR, et al. Doctors' attitudes regarding not for resuscitation orders. Aust Health Rev 2018;41(6):680–7.
129. Mockford C, Clarke B, Field R, et al. A systematic review of do-not-attempt-cardiopulmonary-resuscitation (DNACPR) orders: summarising the evidence around decision making and implementation. Resuscitation 2014;85:S85.
130. Harris D, Willoughby H. Resuscitation on television: realistic or ridiculous? A quantitative observational analysis of the portrayal of cardiopulmonary resuscitation in television medical drama. Resuscitation 2009;80(11):1275–9.

131. Yuen JK, Reid MC, Fetters MD. Hospital do-not-resuscitate orders: why they have failed and how to fix them. J Gen Intern Med 2011;26(7):791–7.
132. Smith K, Andrew E, Lijovic M, et al. Quality of life and functional outcomes 12 months after out-of-hospital cardiac arrest. Circulation 2015;131(2):174–81.
133. Sharma RK, Jain N, Peswani N, et al. Unpacking resident-led code status discussions: results from a mixed methods study. J Gen Intern Med 2014;29(5):750–7.
134. Hart J, Kerlin M. Interpreting 'Do not resuscitate': a cautionary tale of physician influence. Ann Am Thorac Soc 2017;14(4):491–2.
135. Gobert F, Le Cam P, Guérin C. Buying time to save a life: a 3-month 'call in the dark for awareness'. Intensive Care Med 2016;42(10):1634–6.

Chapter 26

Postanaesthesia recovery

Paula Foran, Ulrica Nilsson

KEY WORDS

anaesthesia
malignant hyperthermia
neuromuscular blockade
postanaesthesia care
postoperative complications
surgery

Learning objectives

After reading this chapter, you should be able to:

- describe the principles of immediate postoperative respiratory and cardiovascular management
- discuss the assessment and management of respiratory-related complications following surgery and general anaesthesia
- discuss the assessment and management of non-respiratory complications following surgery and general anaesthesia
- discuss the principles and possible complications of central neural blockade
- describe principles of managing postoperative pain
- discuss the signs, symptoms and treatment for anaesthetic complications such as malignant hyperthermia, inadvertent hypothermia and awareness under anaesthesia.

Introduction

In 1751, realising that postoperative patients were vulnerable, the first Post Anaesthetic Care Unit was created.[1] By the 1940s the importance of recovering from anaesthesia was recognised. Areas close to the operating theatre were created allowing patients leaving the operating theatre to be closely monitored for signs of respiratory failure so that appropriate management could be instituted.[1] Today, perianaesthesia nursing is recognised as a specialty in its own right and postgraduate education opportunities exist to support nurses to develop expertise in this area.

While surgical techniques and anaesthetic medications have changed exponentially, the primary purpose of immediate postanaesthesia/postoperative care, whether provided in the postanaesthesia care unit (PACU) or intensive care unit (ICU), has altered little in the last 70 years. The focus remains on critical evaluation and stabilisation of patients after surgery, with an emphasis on anticipation and prevention of complications arising from either the anaesthetic or the surgical procedure.[2] While this chapter is titled 'Postanaesthesia recovery', it is worth noting that patients are also recovering from their own specific surgical procedure, which may require specific assessment and management.

The Australian National Consensus Statement on essential elements for recognising and responding to clinical deterioration[3] reports that measurable physiological abnormalities occur prior to adverse events such as cardiac arrest and death and suggests that early recognition of changes in a patient's condition, followed by prompt and effective treatment, can minimise poor outcomes. While the mortality in surgical patients has fallen in the last decade, mainly due to effective recognition and treatment of patient deterioration, failures in this process are still occurring.[4] The understanding of such failures may be the driving force behind some patients being admitted to the ICU or high dependence unit following surgery, especially if they require ongoing high-level assessment and management. Postoperative patients who are not critically ill may also be recovered in ICU after hours, and it is this group of patients to which this chapter is directed. In this chapter a brief overview of nursing the patient in the period following surgery and anaesthesia is provided with the focus being on the recovery of non-critically ill patients.

In this chapter we will review anaesthesia and commonly used anaesthetic agents, postanaesthesia nursing care and assessment and management of specific postoperative complications. We acknowledge that postanaesthesia care nursing is a specialty in its own right and that this chapter will provide an overview. We encourage readers to refer to the end of this chapter for further reading about this specialty.

Introduction to anaesthesia

There are five components to anaesthesia. These include hypnosis, analgesia, muscle relaxation, sympatholysis and amnesia.[5] As a result of improvements in pharmacological agents used in anaesthesia, we now see patients emerging from anaesthesia in minutes rather than hours and, consequently, patients can be discharged from perianaesthesia care more quickly. Critical care nurses, whether they specialise in postanaesthesia recovery or not, need a thorough understanding of the pharmacology related to anaesthesia as this underpins patient assessment and management.

Phases of anaesthesia

There are four stages to anaesthesia that a critical care nurse should recognise and consider when undertaking patient assessment. The initiation of analgesia through to the loss of consciousness constitutes stage I, or the stage of analgesia. This is the lightest level of anaesthesia and, although there is sensory and mental depression, patients can often obey commands, breathe normally and maintain protective reflexes.[5] Stage II begins with loss of consciousness and ends when a regular breathing pattern starts and the eyelid reflex is lost. Also called the stage of delirium, stage II is characterised by excitement. Responses such as vomiting and laryngospasm can also occur in this stage, although with newer anaesthetic agents most patients move through this stage quite quickly.

Stage III, the stage of surgical anaesthesia, lasts from the time of onset of regular breathing to breathing cessation. Patients in stage III anaesthesia will not respond when a surgical incision is made. In stage III patients will have sensory depression, loss of recall, depressed reflexes and some evidence of skeletal muscle relaxation. In stage III anaesthesia swallowing, retching and vomiting reflexes disappear sequentially during induction and reappear in the same order during emergence from anaesthesia.[5]

During recovery from anaesthesia, if the patient is breathing using diaphragmatic muscles but does not have intercostal muscle involvement, they are likely still in stage III of anaesthesia. Lack of muscle tone, particularly in the jaw and abdomen, also suggests that the patient is in stage III anaesthesia. As the anaesthesia lightens, respiration will have a normal rate and rhythm.[5]

Stage IV of anaesthesia lasts from when respiration stops to failure of the circulatory system, hence is referred to as the stage of overdose. Determining the stage of anaesthesia cannot be done by assessing any single parameter.[5] Rather, all clinical signs should be considered in relation to the patient's clinical condition and the particular anaesthetic agent used.[5]

Anaesthetic agents

Once referred to as the 'art of anaesthesia', modern anaesthesia now rests firmly on scientific foundations; however, the practice still remains a mixture of science and art.[6] The aim of good anaesthesia is to provide the safest anaesthetic, in the lightest plane possible, which allows a given procedure to be performed while the patient is pain free. This is why other medications, such as muscle relaxants, will be given in conjunction with anaesthetic agents so that muscle relaxation can occur at a lighter stage of anaesthesia.

Non-opioid agents

Non-opioid intravenous agents include non-barbiturates, barbiturates and sedatives. Non-opioid drugs interact with gamma-aminobutyric acid (GABA), an inhibitory neurotransmitter in the brain, with the specific actions being drug dependent.

Non-barbiturates

Propofol is likely the most common non-barbiturate used clinically. Its unique pharmacological characteristics include quick onset, relatively short emergence time and minimal side effects, making propofol (2,6-diisopropylphenol) the most popular intravenous anaesthetic in use.[7] Propofol as a 1% solution is administered intravenously at a dose of 2–2.5 mg/kg for induction, although lower doses are used for older patients and those with hypovolaemia or cardiac disease.[7] As a single agent propofol is usually administered quickly (over 15 seconds) with unconsciousness occurring in about 30 seconds. With a half-life of 2–9 minutes, emergence from this drug is rapid and there are usually few effects on the central nervous system. If continuous infusion of propofol has been used for more than 12 hours, a longer recovery period can be expected.[7]

When administered, propofol can decrease cerebral blood flow, cerebral perfusion pressure and intracranial pressure. Blood pressure and cardiac output are also reduced and this can be more pronounced in those patients with compromised left ventricular function and hypovolaemia. The depressant effect of propofol on the respiratory system may result in airway and ventilatory support being required for those patients who are not already intubated and ventilated. Conflicting reports have been presented regarding the usefulness of propofol as an analgesic and antihyperalgesic agent thus more research will be required before this is unequivocally proven.[8]

> **Practice tip**
>
> Propofol administered to older adult patients can result in a significant drop in blood pressure. Therefore, this group of patients should be carefully monitored.

Etomidate is a short-acting hypnotic agent without any analgesic effects. Although not available in all countries, and not licensed for use in Australia, etomidate is used in many countries, especially for intubation of critically ill patients, mainly because of the minimal cardiovascular effects of the drug.[9] Etomidate causes only a slight increase in heart rate and slight decrease in blood pressure. Cardiac index and peripheral vascular resistance are not significantly influenced and the drug does not seem to be arrhythmogenic. Controversy does exist around the use of etomidate because it inhibits steroid synthesis with adrenal suppression lasing for 5–8 hours following a single dose.[10] Consequently etomidate should only be administered to select patients.

Barbiturates

Barbiturates as an intravenous anaesthetic agent have a long history, and thiopental sodium was used frequently until the 1990s but is used less frequently since the introduction of non-barbiturates such as propofol.[11] Previously, thiopental sodium was used in conjunction with other anaesthetics because it had poor analgesic properties. The disadvantages of thiopental sodium also include adverse effect on respiratory function, coughing, laryngospasm and bronchospasm. The highly alkaline pH of the drug could also contribute to tissue necrosis if extravenous administration occurred. Thiopental sodium also has antianalgesic properties at low doses, so patients recovering from surgery may have more pain and therefore be irritable and restless in the initial recovery phase.[7]

> **Practice tip**
>
> Obese patients administered thiopental sodium may have delayed wakening because the drug is highly fat soluble.

Inhalation anaesthesia

Assessing emergence from inhalation anaesthesia requires an understanding of the pharmacological effects of these agents, and an overview of their characteristics. A brief summary of these agents is provided in Table 26.1. These agents are essentially depressant drugs and some are more likely to affect myocardial and respiratory function than others. Because of respiratory depression, during recovery it is essential that patients are encouraged to continue taking deep breaths. The increased rate and depth of breathing can also assist with eliminating the agents into the atmosphere.

> **Practice tip**
>
> Encouraging deep breathing during the recovery period is essential to promote removal of inhalation gases.

Opioids

Opioids are an important agent in the anaesthetic process and the postoperative period, with their main purpose being to provide analgesia. Opioids also enhance the effectiveness of inhaled anaesthetics allowing lower doses to be provided. In the postoperative period, opioids are commonly administered to alleviate pain associated with the surgical process.

Opioids, whether they are natural or synthetic substances, bind to receptors producing a morphine-like or opioid agonist effect.[12] Opioid receptors include the mu (μ), delta (δ) and kappa (κ) receptors located in the central nervous system, mostly in the brainstem and spinal cord. The mu receptors, specifically the mu-1 receptors, are responsible for supraspinal analgesia effects when stimulated. When mu-2 receptors are stimulated hypoventilation, bradycardia, physical dependence, euphoria and ileus can occur.

Common opioid drugs used for pain relief in the postoperative period include morphine and fentanyl (Table 26.2), which remain cornerstone options for postoperative pain treatment.[13] Pethidine is no longer commonly used for long-term pain relief due to the accumulation of normeperidine over time, which can result in central nervous system toxicity.[14]

TABLE 26.1

Common inhalation anaesthetic agents[5]

AGENT	CHARACTERISTICS
Isoflurane	Reduces systemic arterial blood pressure and systemic vascular resistance Heart rate increased during recovery Produces respiratory depression Produces skeletal muscle relaxation in a dose-related fashion Does not sensitise the myocardium to catecholamines compared to halothane so fewer arrhythmias are observed Patient awakens 15–30 min following termination of anaesthetic gas but may be longer if surgery exceeds 45–60 min
Sevoflurane	Emergence from anaesthesia occurs in minutes Decreases blood pressure and systemic vascular resistance A respiratory depressant Does not increase risk of arrhythmias Can increase intracranial pressure in a dose-related manner
Desflurane	Extremely rapid emergence Dose-related decrease in blood pressure Low rate of cardiac arrhythmias Irritates respiratory tract and induces coughing May induce laryngospasm Almost totally eliminated by the respiratory system
Nitrous oxide	No side effects unless hypoxia is present Non-toxic and non-irritating Can be administered alone or in combination with other agents Diffusion hypoxia can occur when not enough nitrous oxide is removed from the lungs at the end of the surgical procedure

Source: Drain CB. Inhalation anesthesia. In: Odom-Forren J, editor. Perianesthesia Nursing: A Critical Care Approach. 7th ed. St. Louis: Elsevier; 2018.

TABLE 26.2

Opioid analgesics used for postoperative pain relief[13]

DRUG	DOSE[a]	ADVANTAGES	DISADVANTAGES
Morphine	IV: 4–10 mg Peak analgesic effect within 20 min; duration 2 h IM: 10 mg Onset of action approximately 20 min with peak effect in 45–90 min; duration of action 4 h	Minimal effect on heart rate/rhythm and blood pressure	Depresses respiratory rate and tidal volume Can cause orthostatic hypotension and syncope Can cause nausea and vomiting Causes histamine release
Fentanyl	IV: 1–2 mcg/kg OR 25–100 mcg PRN for analgesia Onset of action 4–6 min; peak effect within 5–15 min; duration 20–40 min IM: onset of action 7–15 min; duration 1–2 h	Has little or no hypotensive effect Usually does not cause nausea and vomiting	Delayed onset respiratory depression because of a secondary peak in the concentration of the drug occurs 45 min after apparent recovery Rapid IV administration can provoke bronchial constriction
Pethidine hydrochloride (meperidine hydrochloride)	IV: 25–50 mg every 3–4 h IM: 25–100 mg every 3–4 h IM: Onset of action 10 min; duration of action 2–4 h	Minimal cardiovascular effects although a transient increase in heart rate may occur with IV administration	May slow rate of respiration but this usually returns to normal within 15 min of IV injection Can cause histamine release Causes orthostatic hypotension

[a]Average recommended doses for adults. IM = intramuscular; IV = intravenous.

Source: Luo J MS. Postoperative pain management in the postanesthesia care unit: an update. J Pain Res 2017;10:2687–98.

Practice tip

Morphine is metabolised by the liver and the metabolites are excreted by the kidneys so the analgesic and sedating effects can be prolonged and potentially dangerous for patients with renal failure.

Practice tip

Pethidine (meperidine) is metabolised in the liver to normeperidine. Older adult patients have less tolerance to the central depressant effects of pethidine so this drug should be avoided or the dose limited to 25 mg.

Spinal and epidural opioid administration

Opioids can be administered as part of either spinal or epidural anaesthesia. In spinal anaesthesia, drugs are administered into the cerebral spinal fluid that surrounds the spinal cord, and puncture of the dura is required for this administration. In contrast with epidural administration, the drugs are delivered outside the dura.[15] Administration of morphine (0.1–0.2 mg) directly into the spinal fluid results in a maximal concentration within 5–10 min; the duration of action is 80–200 min. In contrast, a higher dose of morphine is required when administered into the epidural space (5 mg) with pain relief in effect within 30–60 min that can last up to 24 hours. Additional morphine can be administered via the epidural route if required to a maximum of 10 mg in 24 hours. Fentanyl and sufentanil can also be administered epidurally and are more suited for continuous infusion. When intrathecal or epidural opioids are administered, close observation of the patient, particularly respiratory and conscious state, is essential as there may be delayed respiratory depression. Caution should also be taken with additional opioid administration during the first 24 hours as the half-life of opioids administered via these routes is increased.

Opioid antagonists

Should opioid-induced respiratory depression occur in the postanaesthesia period, an opioid antagonist might be needed. Naloxone is a pure opioid antagonist that reverses the depressant effects of the drug and is usually administered in a titrated fashion, assessing patient response. A dose of 0.1–0.2 mg is usually sufficient. The onset of action is quick and occurs within 1–2 min of administration; the half-life is 30–80 min.[16] After 3–5 min, if reversal is still not achieved, additional doses of naloxone can be administered.[12]

Benzodiazepines and benzodiazepine antagonists

Benzodiazepines are sedatives that depress the limbic system and may cause some cortical depression.[7] They interact with GABA, the inhibitory neurotransmitter, causing decreased orientation through a hypnotic effect, retrograde amnesia, anxiolysis and skeletal muscle relaxation.[7] The hypnotic action of benzodiazepines is enhanced by the effects of opiates and barbiturates.

Midazolam is the most popular benzodiazepine used in anaesthesia and critical care and has a wide variety of uses including procedural sedation and induction of anaesthesia. While routine premedications are no longer given, midazolam can be used for some patients to allay anxiety[17] and is also an intraoperative adjunct to both inhalation and regional anaesthesia. Midazolam affects the benzodiazepine receptors in the central nervous system causing reduced anxiety and profound anterograde amnesia. Midazolam has a rapid onset of action – less than 60 seconds – with a peak effect seen within 2–5 min.[18] The duration of action is between 1 and 3 hours. Cardiovascular effects of midazolam include decreased blood pressure, increased heart rate and reduced systemic vascular resistance; thus it should be used with caution in patients with known myocardial ischaemia. In small doses midazolam is used as an antiemetic.[19]

Practice tip

Midazolam does not affect intracranial pressure and, therefore, can safely be used in patients with intracranial pathology or who are undergoing neurosurgery.

Although not commonly used, diazepam and lorazepam are longer-acting benzodiazepines that may be used for induction and as an adjunct to intravenous anaesthesia. Both diazepam and lorazepam have a longer half-life and delayed onset of effect compared to that of midazolam.[7] Diazepam has few cardiovascular depressant effects but is known to cause slight respiratory depression, an effect that is enhanced when it is administered at the same time as opiates.

If required, the pharmacological effects of benzodiazepines can be reversed. Flumazenil is a benzodiazepine agonist that should be administered intravenously in 0.1-mg increments to avoid rapid reawakening. The usual dose is 0.4 mg and the maximum amount administered should be no more than 1.0 mg.[7] The drug takes effect within 5 min of administration and has a duration of action between 1 and 2 hours.

Practice tip

Flumazenil has a shorter duration of action than most benzodiazepines so patients should be carefully assessed for resedation after the initial dose is administered. If signs of resedation are evident, additional flumazenil can be administered every 20 min to a maximum dose of 3.0 mg in a 1-hour period.

Non-specific effects of benzodiazepines can be reversed with the administration of physostigmine, an anticholinesterase that crosses the blood–brain barrier. Physostigmine inhibits acetylcholinesterase making increased amounts of acetylcholine available at the central nervous system receptors that are affected by benzodiazepines. Doses of 0.5–1.0 mg should be slowly administered in order to avoid cholinergic side effects.[7]

Butyrophenones

As sedative agents, butyrophenones such as haloperidol and droperidol produce a state of profound calm and immobility where the patient appears to be pain free and dissociated from their surroundings. Butyrophenone use in anaesthesia is, however, uncommon. Haloperidol is rarely used because of its long duration of action and high incidence of extrapyramidal side effects. Droperidol can be used on its own or in conjunction with fentanyl as part of a neurolept analgesic technique. Droperidol is also administered in small doses (0.625–1.25 mg intravenously) in the postoperative period to manage nausea and vomiting.[19]

> **Practice tip**
>
> Some patients who have received droperidol report feeling terrified and unable to express how they feel while also having an outward appearance of being very calm. It is important that in the postanaesthesia period support is provided to patients even if they appear calm.

In the postanaesthesia period, regular stimulation of the patient and encouragement of deep breathing is necessary as patients can drift back to sleep and have slow and/or shallow respirations. In some instances, patients who have received droperidol have become apnoeic.[7]

Neuromuscular blocking agents

Since the 1940s neuromuscular blocking agents have been used as pharmacological agents in anaesthesia. Although not all patients will require neuromuscular blockade during anaesthesia, these agents may be given to facilitate endotracheal intubation. Muscle relaxation is also indicated to facilitate some surgical procedures, such as abdominal surgery, in ophthalmic surgery to relax extraocular muscles, and to facilitate mechanical ventilation. Nurses who are responsible for the assessment and management of the postoperative patient should understand the physiology of neuromuscular transmission and mechanism of action of the various neuromuscular blocking agents that may be used in anaesthesia.

The neuromuscular junction has three components: the motor nerve fibre, the synaptic cleft and the motor end-plate of striated muscle (Fig. 26.1). Acetylcholine (ACh), a neurotransmitter that is deactivated by the cholinesterase family of enzymes, is stored and released from the presynaptic terminal and is the only neurotransmitter used in the somatic nervous system.[20] ACh receptors are located on the motor end-plate and, when bound to ACh, membrane channels open and this results in an influx of sodium ions causing depolarisation of the motor end-plate membrane. Potassium ions exit causing repolarisation, allowing the membrane potential to again

FIGURE 26.1 Neuromuscular junction.

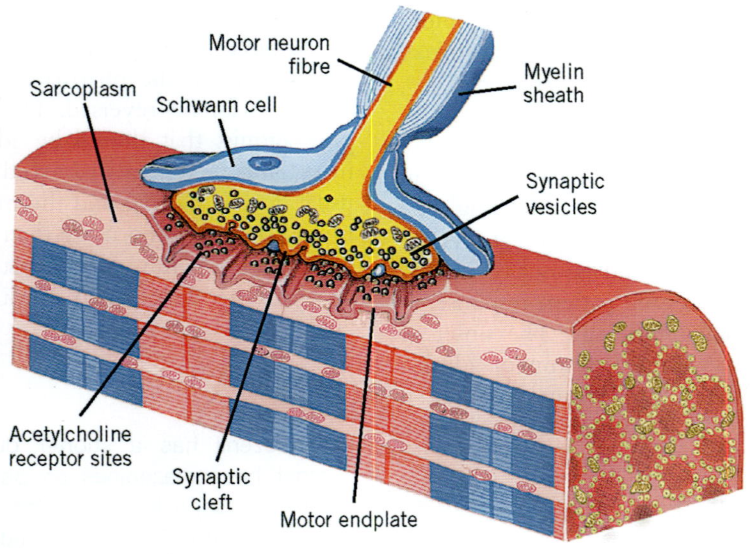

Adapted from Patton KT, Thibodeau GA. Anatomy and physiology. 7th ed. St Louis: Mosby; 2010, with permission.

become negative. These sequences allow muscle contraction to occur. ACh is broken down by acetylcholinesterase, which is present in the synaptic cleft, and is metabolised before the excited muscle returns to its resting state. The broken down ACh elements are then used for the manufacture of new ACh molecules in the nerve terminal ending.

Non-depolarising neuromuscular blocking agents

Non-depolarising neuromuscular blocking agents block the action of ACh at the postsynaptic receptor sites in the neuromuscular junction (Fig. 26.2) by competing with ACh at these binding sites and blocking neuromuscular transmission.[21] There are many different types of non-depolarising neuromuscular blocking agents.[22] Although the end effect of these agents is similar, their pharmacological effects differ in relation to onset of action, duration of effect and excretion (Table 26.3).

Residual neuromuscular block is a complication that can occur following use of neuromuscular blockade[23,24] and can result in adverse respiratory complications.[25] Pharmacological reversal of neuromuscular block can be used when the effects of the neuromuscular blocking agent remain present at the end of the surgery. Conventional reversal of neuromuscular blockade involves administration of an anticholinesterase. Anticholinesterase inhibits the action of cholinesterases that inactivate ACh, thus potentiating the effects of the neurotransmitter ACh, and helps restore skeletal muscle activity.[22,26] Anticholinesterases stimulate the muscarinic receptors and elicit side effects including bradycardia, arrhythmias, bronchospasm as well as nausea and vomiting. For this reason, antimuscarinic agents such as atropine or glycopyrrolate must be administered at the same time as the reversal agent.[22] The expanded array of neuromuscular blockade reversal agents now allows for fast and complete reversal and the reduction of postoperative complications from residual block.[26]

FIGURE 26.2 (**A**) Normal muscle contraction. (**B**) Neuromuscular blockade.[22]

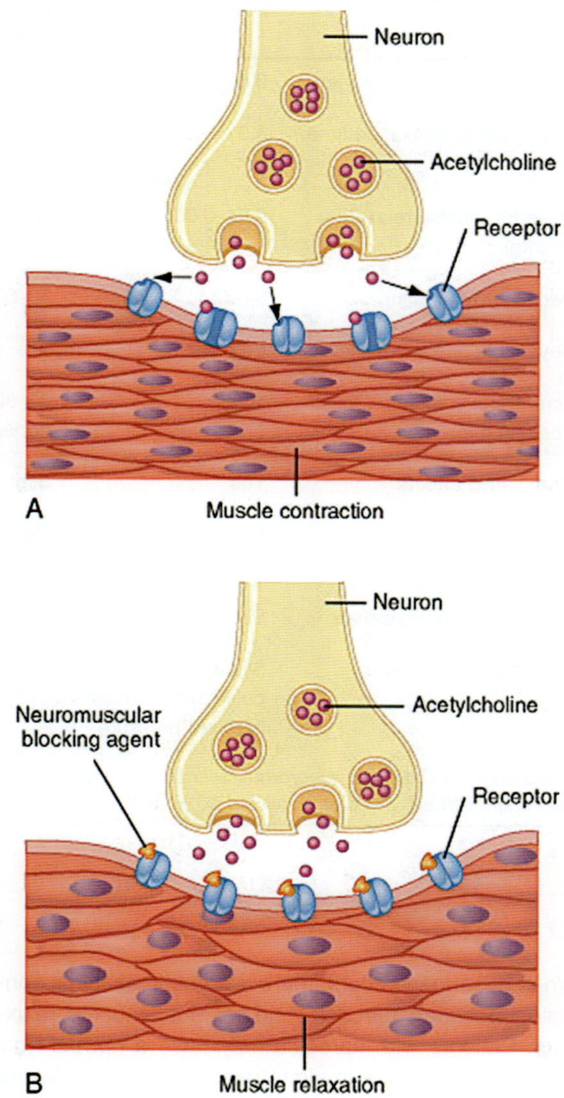

Adapted from Siedlecki SL. Pain and sedation. In: Carlson K, editor. Advanced critical care nursing. St Louis: Saunders; 2009, Figure 4-13, p. 79, with permission.

Practice tip

When patients return from surgery, review their anaesthetic record to see whether a neuromuscular blocking agent has been used and, if it was, whether a reversal agent was given.

If sugammadex is given to a female patient of childbearing years, and this patient was using a hormonal contractive agent, such as the contraceptive pill, vaginal ring, implant or intrauterine system or device, the patient should be advised to take additional contraceptive precautions for 7 days following sugammadex administration.[28]

Sugammadex is also used to reverse the effect of neuromuscular blockade, specifically when the agents rocuronium and vecuronium are used. Sugammadex is the first selective neuromuscular drug binding agent and reverses the effect of the neuromuscular blocking drugs through encapsulation. Hypersensitivity to sugammadex can occur within the first 5 minutes following administration and, as such, patients receiving this drug should be closely monitored for signs of drug-induced hypersensitivity.[27]

TABLE 26.3
Pharmacological overview of commonly used non-depolarising neuromuscular blocking agents[22]

	PANCURONIUM	VECURONIUM BROMIDE	ATRACURIUM BESYLATE	CISATRACURIUM BESYLATE	ROCURONIUM BROMIDE
Dose for intubation (mg/kg)	0.06–0.1	0.08–0.1	0.4–0.5	0.1–0.2	0.1
Intubation to relaxation time (min)	4.0	2.5–3.0	2.0–2.5	2.8–3.4	1.0–2.0
Dose for muscle relaxation (mg/kg)	0.04–0.08	0.05–0.06	0.2–0.5	2.5	0.6–1.0
Recovery time (min)	84–114	30–60	30–45	55–75	30–90
Reversible	Yes	Yes	Yes	Yes	Yes
Time to reversal (after initial dose, in min)	40–60	25–80 (dose-dependent)	20–35	10–15	5–10
Cumulative effects	Yes	Slight	No	No	No
Fasciculations and muscle soreness	No	None	No	No	No
Risk of histamine release	Slight to none	None	Minimal	No	No
Cardiovascular effects	Slight increase in pulse and increase in blood pressure	None	Few	None	None

Adapted from Drain CB. Neuromuscular blocking agents. In: Odom-Forren J, editor. Perianesthesia nursing: a critical care approach. 7th ed. St Louis: Elsevier; 2018, with permission.

Practice tip

When dyspnoea occurs, there is sometimes initial confusion between narcosis and residual muscle relaxants. Patients with narcosis may have a normal tidal volume but the rate is slow; residual muscle relaxant patients breathe very poorly due to a mechanical problem with their muscles of respiration but their respiratory effort is not impaired.

Depolarising neuromuscular blocking agents

Suxamethonium, also known as succinylcholine, is the only depolarising neuromuscular blocking agent used in anaesthesia. Suxamethonium is most often used in rapid sequence induction for the purpose of endotracheal intubation. Suxamethonium works at the site of the acetylcholine receptor and causes persistent depolarisation at the motor end-plate.[22] Patients administered suxamethonium demonstrate muscle fasciculations because of the sudden increase in acetylcholine at the motor end-plate.

A typical dose of suxamethonium is 0.5–1.5 mg/kg administered intravenously. The onset of action is rapid, usually within 30–60 seconds of administration. The very rapid onset of paralysis when using suxamethonium remains its true advantage as a patient can be intubated almost immediately. Suxamethonium administration can induce hyperkalaemia so its use in patients with electrolyte disorders, such as those with severe burns or diabetic ketoacidosis, is not recommended.[29] The duration of action of suxamethonium is relatively short as the drug is hydrolysed rapidly by plasma pseudocholinesterase. Paralysis associated with administration of suxamethonium usually only lasts 5–10 minutes. Some patients may have reduced pseudocholinesterase activity. This can be an acquired deficiency that might be associated with liver disease, severe anaemia, malnutrition, prolonged pyrexia, pregnancy and renal dialysis. Congenital deficiencies in pseudocholinesterase are relatively uncommon.

Practice tip

Patients with either acquired or congenital pseudocholinesterase deficiency may remain paralysed for prolonged periods of time and may require mechanical ventilation for up to 48 hours.

Factors influencing neuromuscular blocking agents

There are a number of factors that can influence neuromuscular blocking agents. Many of these include drug interactions and alterations in electrolyte balance (Table 26.4). Dehydration can also increase the sensitivity to skeletal muscle relaxants because of increased neuromuscular excitability, slowed renal function and drug excretion and increased plasma concentration of the relaxant. Acid–base balance can also influence neuromuscular blockade where acidosis and increased carbon dioxide levels result in a stronger effect of the neuromuscular blocking agent pancuronium.[22] Hypothermia can antagonise the effect of neuromuscular blocking agents, as with pancuronium, or can potentiate the effect as seen with suxamethonium. Prior to extubation of a patient following a relaxant anaesthesia, the anaesthetist may use 'train-of-four' where the level of neuromuscular block is assessed using a peripheral nerve stimulator.

Non-steroidal anti-inflammatory drugs

Non-steroidal anti-inflammatory drugs such as ketorolac and indomethacin can be used as analgesics in the postoperative period, although indomethacin is used much less frequently. Ketorolac has analgesic, anti-inflammatory and anti-pyretic actions and works by inhibiting the cyclooxygenase enzyme system, thereby decreasing prostaglandin synthesis. Ketorolac is administered by intramuscular or intravenous injection or given orally. An intramuscular dose of 30 mg as a loading dose can be followed by a further 15 mg after 6 hours. Ketorolac can also be used in conjunction with opioids for effective postoperative pain relief. The peak effect of ketorolac occurs in approximately 45–60 minutes so it can be administered approximately 1 hour before the end of the surgical procedure so that maximal pain relief occurs at emergence from anaesthesia.

Practice tip

The recommended dose range of ketorolac is 15–60 mg. Lower doses of ketorolac should be administered to older adults.

Dissociative anaesthetics

Ketamine is a dissociative drug that selectively blocks pain conduction and perception yet does not depress those parts of the central nervous system not involved in pain transmission and perception.[7] When patients are administered ketamine they experience profound analgesia and unconsciousness but respiratory function is usually unimpaired. Ketamine may also be considered a reasonable option in the management of severe acute episodes of asthma in children who failed to respond to standard therapy.[30] Ketamine also causes increased cerebral blood flow so should be avoided in those patients at risk of developing increased intracranial pressure.

Of particular importance to the nurse managing a postoperative patient who has received ketamine is an understanding that psychic aberrations can occur on emergence from anaesthesia. Patients can experience vivid dreaming with or without psychomotor activity. They can appear confused, irrational and have hallucinations. These effects can be managed by avoiding early verbal or tactile stimulation. If the patient does have augmented psychomotor responses and irrational behaviour, medications such as dexmedetomidine or a benzodiazepine can be administered.

Practice tip

Ketamine can be used as a sole anaesthetic agent for paediatric patients who appear to be less prone to psychic disturbances.

Drug interactions

Many patients undergoing anaesthesia will be taking medications in addition to those required for surgery and anaesthesia. Whenever two or more drugs are given to a patient there is a potential for drug interactions to occur (Box 26.1). Such interactions can have a potentially negative effect on the patient and knowledge of these interactions will help guide nursing assessment. Table 26.4 provides a summary of common medications and how these can interact with pharmacological agents used in surgery and anaesthesia.[31]

Practice tip

Some antibiotics such as gentamycin can potentiate non-depolarising muscle relaxants and make reversal of these agents more difficult.

Local and regional anaesthesia

Local anaesthesia works by blocking nerve conduction so that the patient does not feel painful stimuli. Local anaesthetics work by binding to sodium channels, preventing a conformational change and the influx of Na + and depolarisation slows, thus preventing depolarisation and transmission of the neuronal action potential.[32] A second mechanism may also cause disruption of the ion channel when local anaesthetic molecules are incorporated into the cell membrane (Fig. 26.3). The sensitivity to local anaesthetics depends on the nerve fibres, with sensitivity increased for the smaller nerve fibres. Myelinated fibres are also blocked before non-myelinated fibres, if they are of the same diameter. Assessment and management of the patient receiving local or regional anaesthesia is provided later in this chapter.

TABLE 26.4
Drug–drug interactions[31]

DRUG	INTERACTION	RESULT	MECHANISM
Antihypertensive drugs			
Propranolol	Inhalation anaesthetics	Bradycardia, hypotension	Additive effect
	Lignocaine	Enhanced negative inotropic effect	Propranolol reduces liver blood flow and lignocaine clearance
	Heparin	Myocardial depression	Heparin increases free fatty acids, which displace propranolol from plasma protein binding sites, leading to increased free propranolol
Lignocaine	Non-depolarising muscle relaxants	Increased duration of neuromuscular blockade	Synergistic effect
Digitalis	Suxamethonium / succinylcholine	Arrhythmias	Direct effect or caused by hyperkalaemia that can be induced by succinylcholine
	Thiazide diuretics	Increased potassium excreted by kidneys	Combined effect of two drugs on kidneys promotes potassium excretion
Quinidine	Digitalis	Can produce digitalis intoxication	Decreased digitalis clearance and increased concentration of digitalis
	Myasthenia gravis plus skeletal muscle relaxants	Postoperative respiratory depression	Blockade of acetylcholine receptors at neuromuscular postsynaptic membrane
Antibiotics			
Neomycin Streptomycin Dihydrostreptomycin Polymyxin A Polymyxin B Colistin Viomycin Paromomycin Kanamycin Lincomycin Gentamicin Tetracycline	Non-depolarising skeletal muscle relaxants	Potentiate non-depolarising muscle relaxants, respiratory depression	Neuromuscular blockade caused by reduction in amplitude of end-plate potential
Opioids			
Morphine Fentanyl Sufentanil Remifentanil	Inhalation anaesthetics	Potentiation, respiratory and cardiovascular depression	Depressant effects of inhalation anaesthetics and opioids are additive
Pethidine/meperidine	Inhalation anaesthetics	Potentiation, respiratory and cardiovascular depression	Depressant effects of inhalation anaesthetics and opioids are additive
	Enovid Norinyl	Birth control pill potentiates pethidine/meperidine	Excess female sex hormones with oral contraceptive therapy, which may slow metabolism of pethidine/meperidine
	MAOI	MAOI interacts with pethidine/ meperidine metabolite	Type I: seizures Type II: hypotension

TABLE 26.4
Drug–drug interactions—cont'd

DRUG	INTERACTION	RESULT	MECHANISM
Sympathomimetic amines			
Adrenaline	Inhalation anaesthetics	Cardiac arrhythmias	Anaesthetic agents may sensitise myocardium to endogenous and exogenous catecholamines
Electrolytes			
Increased extracellular potassium	Skeletal muscle relaxants	Increased resistance to depolarisation and greater sensitivity to non-depolarising muscle relaxants	Acute increase in extracellular potassium increases end-plate transmembrane potential, thus causing hyperpolarisation
Decreased extracellular potassium	Skeletal muscle relaxants	Increased effects of depolarising muscle relaxants and increased resistance to non-depolarising muscle relaxants	Acute decrease in extracellular potassium lowers resting end-plate transmembrane potential
Increased calcium levels	Non-depolarising skeletal muscle relaxants	Decreased response	Calcium increases release of acetylcholine and enhances excitation–contraction coupling mechanism
Magnesium ions	Muscle relaxants	Potentiation	Magnesium ions cause partial muscle relaxation by blocking release of acetylcholine
Calcium chloride	Digitalis	Additive effect on heart	High concentrations of calcium inhibit positive inotropic actions of digitalis and potentiate digitalis toxicity
Miscellaneous			
Frusemide Thiazide Ethacrynic acid	Non-depolarising skeletal muscle relaxants	Intensified neuromuscular block	Electrolyte imbalance (hypokalaemia)
Procaine Lignocaine	Non-depolarising and depolarising skeletal muscle relaxants	Enhanced neuromuscular blockade	Decreased end-plate potential
Lithium	Non-depolarising and depolarising skeletal muscle relaxants	Potentiated neuromuscular blockade	Lithium ions are substituted for sodium ions at presynaptic level
Chlorpromazine	Non-depolarising skeletal muscle relaxants	Enhanced neuromuscular blockade	Potentiation of neuromuscular blockade
All inhalation anaesthetics	Non-depolarising skeletal muscle relaxants	Augment block in dose-dependent manner	Central nervous system depression or presynaptic inhibition of acetylcholine
Insulin	Corticosteroids, oral contraceptives, loop and thiazide diuretics	Reduction in effects	Insulin antagonises effects
Hydrocortisone Dexamethasone Prednisone	Phenobarbital	Decreased effect of the steroids	Increased metabolism

Adapted from Nagelhout JJ. Basic principles of pharmacology. In: Odom-Forren J, editor. Perianesthesia nursing: a critical care approach. 7th ed. St Louis: Elsevier; 2018, with permission.

BOX 26.1

Monoamine oxidase inhibitors

The interaction of this class of drug with common anaesthetic agents is important to recognise. Although monoamine oxidase inhibitors (MAOI) are not as commonly used as in the past, many patients may still be prescribed these for management of depression. MAOIs inhibit N-demethylase and thus decrease the breakdown of pethidine/meperidine. A type I response to this drug interaction includes seizures, agitation, rigidity and hyperpyrexia. A Type II response includes hypotension, respiratory depression and coma.

Adapted from Rasool F, Ghafoor R, Lambert DG. Antidepressants and antipsychotics: anaesthetic implications. Anaesth Intensive Care Med 2014;15(7):314–17.

Practice tip

Administration of local anaesthetics results in loss of nerve function, and consequently pain, temperature, touch and proprioception are affected. Skeletal muscle tone is the last to be affected. This explains why patients may be able to feel touch but not pain after receiving local anaesthesia.

Assessment and management in the postoperative period

The postoperative recovery is divided into three stages: Early recovery, or phase I; Intermediate recovery, or phase II; and Late recovery, which may be referred to as phase III.[33] During phase I the patient is closely monitored in the PACU, high-dependency unit (HDU) or ICU until fully awake from anaesthesia and motor functions and protective reflexes are regained.[34]

FIGURE 26.3 Mechanism of action for local anaesthesia. (**A**) Transmission of the pain message to the central nervous system through depolarisation of the axon of a sensory nerve cell. (**B**) Blocking of the action potential in a sensory nerve cell through blocking of the sodium channel by local anaesthetic drugs.

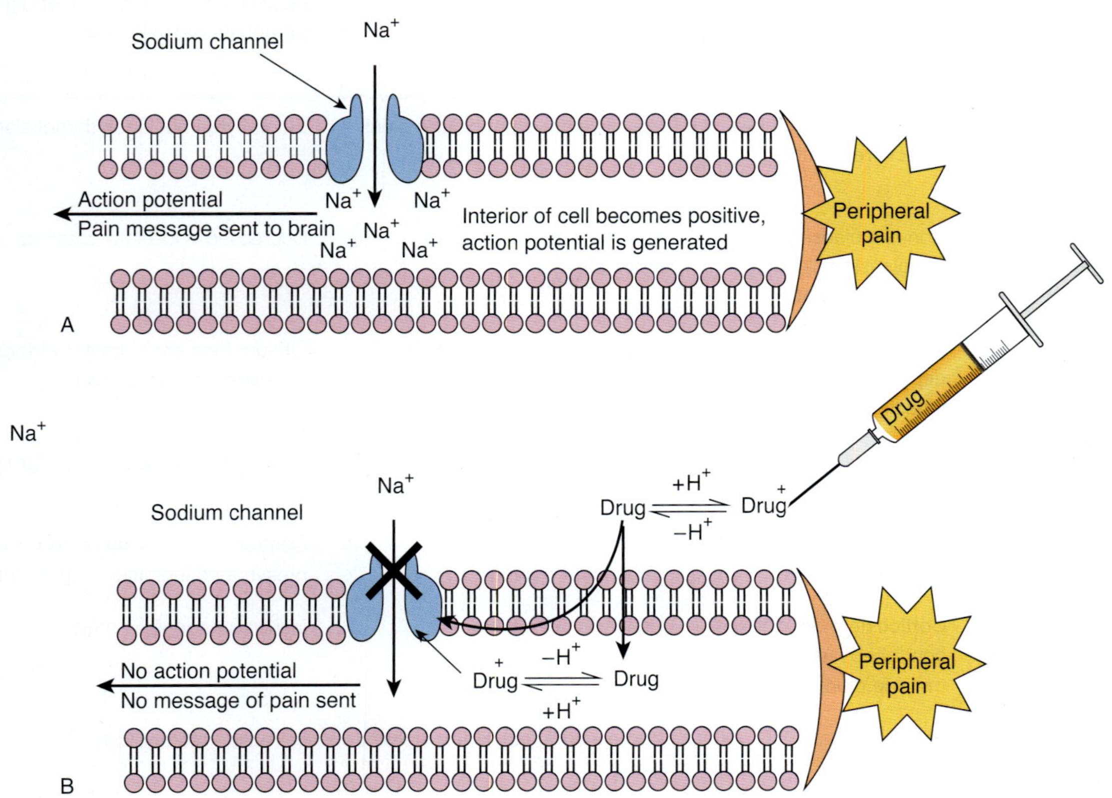

Adapted from Friel CJ, Eliadi C, Pesaturo KA. Local anesthetic use in perioperative areas. Perioperative Nurs Clin 2010;5:203–14, with permission.

When caring for a patient immediately after surgery, it is essential that the nurse has a full understanding of the possible complications of each individual procedure that has been performed. If a nurse is allocated a patient and they do not understand the surgical procedure they must ask, possibly at the time of anaesthetic handover, to gain an understanding of what complications might occur in their patient. It is beyond the scope of this text to discuss all possible procedural complications. However, some examples of specific complications include: water intoxication and/or sodium depletion in surgery that flushes large amounts of saline solution or water under pressure (e.g. transurethral resection of the prostate [TURP], endometrial ablation); upper airway obstruction following surgery under the muscle layer of the neck (thyroidectomy, parotid cyst); postpartum haemorrhage (post-lower uterine segment caesarean section) requiring assessment with fundal height measurements; specific vascular observations for patients following free flap surgery (deep inferior epigastric perforators [DIEP] or transverse rectus abdominis myocutaneous [TRAM]), not just observing for arterial vascularity but also venous engorgement; and cervical shock in gynaecological patients that causes both a fall in blood pressure and heart rate.

Anaesthetic handover

Handover is an important component that will help guide postoperative assessment and management. However, research suggests that postoperative patient handovers are typically fraught with technical and communication errors and, may provide the greatest opportunity to improve safety around surgery.[35] There is no standardised and agreed approach to handover; however, it is recognised that some form of standard process is required.[36] A formal handover will be provided by the treating anaesthetist to the nurse who will be caring for the patient at the time of transfer of care. The quality of the handover must be such that it allows the nurse to safely assume responsibility for the patient. It is important for nurses to understand this process, knowing what information needs to be gleaned from the handover as they accept responsibility for the patient's care. In some hospitals there is also a nursing handover from the perioperative nurse that may provide information about the surgical procedure, dressing, drain tubes and any notable intraoperative events. There are a variety of different handover tools available internationally, many of which incorporate similar elements. For example, the SBAR mnemonic is used to guide handover through discussion of the:

Situation
Background
Assessment
Recommendation.

The Australian and New Zealand College of Anaesthetists recommended the ISOBAR acronym, which represents:

Identification to ensure that the patient is correctly identified
Situation, including current clinical status and patient-centred care requirements
Observations – latest observations
Background and history
Assessment and **a**ctions to establish an agreed management plan
Responsibility and **r**isk management.[37]

Consistency in the handover method will help enhance its quality so it is important to know which approach is used in your hospital.

In the PACU it is common to use discharge criteria to assess the patient's readiness for transfer to a lower acuity nursing area. These are based on assessments using the patient baseline as a comparison, some are numeric based while others are not. The Aldrete scoring system is a commonly used numeric tool that assesses activity, respiration, circulation, consciousness and oxygen saturation using scoring points 0, 1 or 2, maximum total score 10, with 10 indicating the best possible condition.[38] Transition from the PACU to the phase II step-down unit requires a scoring of 9 or higher in the Aldrete scoring system (Table 26.5). Patients undergoing surgery with local anaesthesia usually proceed immediately to

TABLE 26.5
The modified Aldrete scoring system[38,39]

CRITERIA	POINT VALUE
Consciousness	
Fully awake	2
Arousable	1
Not responding	0
Oxygenation	
SpO_2 >94% on room air	2
SpO_2>90% on oxygen	1
SpO_2 <90% on oxygen	0
Mobility	
Able to move four extremities on command	2
Able to move two extremities on command	1
Able to move 0 extremities on command	0
Breathing	
Able to breathe deeply	2
Dyspnoea	1
Apnoea	0
Circulation	
Systemic BP ± 20% of the preanesthetic level	2
Systemic BP between 20% and 49% of the preanesthetic level	1
Systemic BP ± 50% of the preanesthetic level	0

Maximum score: 10; discharge score ≥ 9.
Source: Aldrete J, Kroulik D. A postanesthetic recovery score. Anesthesia & Analgesia 1970;49:924–34.

phase II recovery. In phase II recovery patients are still cared for at the day surgery unit or surgical ward but not monitored as closely as in phase I.[34]

Respiratory assessment and management

Immediately after surgery patients are susceptible to events that can compromise adequacy of ventilation and oxygenation, thus airway and respiratory management skills are fundamental for nursing staff caring for this group.[40] What differentiates non-critically ill postoperative patients from other ICU patients is the residual effects of anaesthesia medications that may include, but are not limited to, narcotics, sedatives, hypnotics, inhalational gases, muscle relaxants, intravenous fluids and blood products.[40] These medications can cause decreased rate and depth of breathing, which contributes to alveolar hypoventilation and consequently results in increased levels of carbon dioxide and decreased levels of oxygen in the blood. Anaesthetic agents can also contribute to blunted responses to carbon dioxide and an overall decrease in minute ventilation.[41] It is important to have a detailed knowledge and understanding of the respiratory system and how to assess the respiratory function of postanaesthesia patients. For a detailed discussion of respiratory assessment and monitoring, please refer to Chapter 13.

Assessment and management of the airway

One of the most common complications seen in the immediate postanaesthesia period is airway obstruction.[25] The depressant effects of anaesthesia can mean that the postoperative patient is not able to protect or maintain a patent airway. Signs that the patient might have an airway obstruction include increased respiratory effort, respiratory muscle retraction, abnormal breath sounds and signs of altered gas exchange. In many cases opening the airway by tilting the head backward and extending the neck (if not contraindicated) can help restore airway patency. Artificial airways may be used to prevent obstruction that occurs when the patient's tongue and epiglottis fall back on the posterior pharyngeal wall.

All airway complications are serious as they all, in some way or another, obstruct the airway to varying degrees and put the patient at risk of decreased oxygenation and possible hypoxia. These complications can be from an upper airway obstruction such as laryngeal spasm, subglottic oedema or lower airway obstruction such as bronchospasm and non-cardiogenic pulmonary oedema. They may result from a simple problem, such as poor mandibular positioning where the tongue falls back obstructing the airway, to a complete laryngeal spasm with no air entry.[25] Any of these problems can cause life-threatening hypoxia if not rectified immediately.

Some patients may leave the operating theatre with a supraglottic airway, for example a laryngeal mask or i-gel® and this can be removed once they are awake and able to open their mouth and maintain their own airway. Others may have an endotracheal tube in situ, which may be the reason for their transfer to ICU or HDU. In an intubated patient a systematic approach to determining whether the patient is ready to be extubated should be implemented and include assessing whether the patient is fully reversed, awake, cooperative and able to follow commands. The expanded landscape of neuromuscular blockade reversal drugs available today allows for a much faster and complete reversal of paralysis and this has considerably reduced postoperative complications due to residual block.[26] Reversal of non-depolarising muscle relaxants should be noted and the train-of-four assessed. The patient should be normothermic and, if airway oedema is suspected, an endotracheal tube leak test should be performed where the cuff is deflated and breathing assessed prior to tube removal. A medical officer needs to be available at extubation should immediate reintubation be required. Please refer to Chapter 15, *Ventilation and oxygenation management*.

Assessment and management of ventilatory capacity and oxygenation

The altered respiratory rate and depth that may occur as a result of anaesthesia require focused assessment and understanding of the ways in which anaesthetic agents can influence both ventilator capacity and oxygenation in the postoperative period. For accurate assessment of respiratory rate, measurement will need to be taken by observing respirations over a 1-minute period; this process makes it the vital sign that is most often neglected in clinical practice.[42] Recent research suggests that respiratory rate is considered an inferior vital sign to blood pressure, heart rate and temperature measurement.[43] Inaccurate assessment of respiratory rate continues despite recognition that it is considered to be the single most important vital sign in detecting patient deterioration.[42] Assessment of respiratory rate in the period following general anaesthesia is of particular importance as patients may have received several pharmacological agents, including neuromuscular blockade, narcotics and sedative agents, that could directly influence respiratory function. Respiratory rate and depth directly influence minute ventilation and gas exchange. Capnography can be used to assess end-tidal carbon dioxide measurements[44] while pulse oximetry will be used to assess oxygen saturation.[44] More accurate and detailed assessment of gas exchange requires arterial blood gas analysis. Depending on the nature of the surgical intervention, some patients may require a more detailed respiratory assessment that incorporates inspection, palpation, percussion and auscultation (see Chapter 13).

The use of oxygen therapy has been under some debate as it was previously believed that supplemental oxygen would aid in the elimination of anaesthetic gases and help meet increased oxygen demand associated with decreased blood volume or increased cellular metabolism.

> **Practice tip**
>
> Following a pneumonectomy, the post-pneumonectomy space fills with air and on chest X-ray the trachea should be midline. A chest tube is inserted and specific orders on clamping and releasing the drain are given by the surgeon. Unexpectedly rapid accumulation of fluid in the post-pneumonectomy space might indicate haemorrhage.

However, in recent years the free use of oxygen is being questioned as some believe that in patients with normal respiratory function and an oxygen saturation >94% on room air administration of supplemental oxygen may mask the symptoms of poor respiration function.[45] In contrast, the World Health Organization[24] has recommended that adult patients who have undergone general anaesthesia with endotracheal intubation for surgical procedures should receive supplemental oxygen at a fraction of inspired oxygen of 80% and, if feasible, that this continue for 2-6 hours postoperatively to reduce the risk of surgical site infections. In short, the free use of oxygen therapy should be replaced with a specific assessment of oxygen requirements for each individual patient.

Because respiratory effort can be compromised, almost all postoperative patients will receive supplemental oxygen, and with all patients the amount of oxygen received should be guided by the patient's clinical condition and assessment of arterial oxygen saturation. Oxygen therapy helps to wash out residual anaesthetic gases and provides a higher concentration of inspired oxygen for patients who may have residual effects of sedative and neuromuscular blocking agents causing hypoventilation. Patients who have had central neural blockade (epidural or spinal) or regional blocks will be assessed individually for oxygen requirements (see Chapter 13). Some patients may require respiratory support in the postoperative period and will remain intubated and ventilated for a period of time after surgery. If patients require ongoing mechanical ventilation, they may require admission to ICU. For a detailed understanding of patients requiring mechanical ventilation and ongoing respiratory support please refer to Chapter 15.

Cardiovascular assessment and management

In the postanaesthesia period assessment of cardiovascular function will be frequently undertaken with monitoring of blood pressure and heart rate. Detailed description of cardiovascular assessment is provided in Chapter 9. Postoperative patients are at risk of developing cardiovascular complications as they will have generally had some degree of blood loss, will have been administered anaesthetic medications, or have temperature changes that may have altered vascularity. For example, central neural blockage will cause vascular vasodilation and interference to the body's sympathetic responses, which can lead to hypotension. Conversely, hypertension can be present when patients experience pain.

Hypotension can be transient or more sustained. Transient hypotension can occur in relation to drug administration. Conversely, more sustained hypotension and the development of shock can occur in relation to blood loss or from an altered distribution of flow that occurs secondary to sympathetic blockade and vasodilation that can occur in regional anaesthesia. Decreased cardiac output might be seen in some patients and could be related to decreased preload that occurs in hypovolaemia or decreased cardiac output secondary to myocardial injury contractility as a result of either myocardial injury or cardiac output and vasodilatory states.[25,46] Shock is characterised by a decrease in blood pressure (20–30% decrease from the patient's baseline) and an increase in heart rate, and is not an uncommon occurrence in postoperative patients.[25] Cardiovascular compromise that results from blood and fluid loss can lead to hypovolaemic shock. Specific assessment and management strategies for the patient with shock are provided in Chapter 21.

> **Practice tip**
>
> Inadvertent hypothermia will cause vasoconstriction that may mask a low circulating blood volume.

Fluid and electrolyte balance

Postoperative patients are also particularly vulnerable to fluid and electrolyte imbalances due to the restrictions on fluid and electrolytes preoperatively, fluid loss during surgery, the patient's physical status and the associated stressors of surgery.[2] The normal bodily response to the stress of a surgical procedure is for the renal system to retain water and sodium.[2] For these reasons, the patient requires a full body assessment of their fluid and electrolyte status.[2] The primary goals of fluid management in the immediate postoperative phase are to maintain adequate intravascular volumes, left ventricular filling pressures, cardiac output, blood pressure and the delivery of oxygen to the tissues.[47] Normal concentrations of electrolytes and body fluids are vital to maintain the physiological function of all bodily systems.[47] The goals and strategies for volume replacement are patient-dependent and should take into consideration the preoperative condition of the patient, cardiovascular status and intraoperative fluid losses.[47]

Venous thromboembolism prophylaxis

Venous thromboembolism (VTE) prophylaxis is essential as postoperative deaths from deep vein thrombosis (DVT) and subsequent pulmonary embolism are not uncommon.[48] Unless there are specific contraindications, patients at high risk of developing VTE will require a pneumatic pressure device either commenced (as in the case of some orthopaedic surgeries where a tourniquet was used intraoperatively) or continued from the intraoperative phase. Thromboembolism deterrent anti-embolism stockings should be checked to ensure they are fitted correctly and anticoagulant medication must be ordered and administered. A preoperative screening tool for VTE can be used to guide practice and individual surgeons' preferences for VTE prophylaxis may be consulted.[49]

Pain assessment and management

Experiencing postoperative pain has been found to be the most common fear of surgical patients.[50] Despite this knowledge, extensive research and published guidelines for the management of postoperative pain, it continues to be inadequate.[14,51] Inadequate pain relief has been shown to alter the body's metabolic responses, which can delay recovery, extend hospital length of stay, increase morbidity rates and potentially lead to the development of a chronic pain state.[52] Conversely, effective pain control reduces postoperative complications, facilitates rehabilitation and provides a more rapid recovery from surgery.[52] For a detailed discussion on pain assessment and pain management please refer to Chapter 7. More information on pain medications is also provided in Chapter 7 and earlier in this chapter in the discussion on anaesthetic drugs. Specifically, a summary of opioid analgesics is provided in Table 26.2.

It is firmly believed that adequate pain relief requires more than one analgesic, and this approach is referred to as 'multimodal analgesia' and is considered an essential component of care.[51] Specific pain management techniques relevant to the postoperative period also include a mix of narcotic and non-narcotic analgesics, patient-controlled analgesia, central neural blockade and peripheral nerve blocks. Intravenous paracetamol (acetaminophen) has become a main feature of multimodal pain relief in moderate to severe pain[7] and also helps reduce nausea in postoperative patients.[53]

Tramadol is also an effective agent for pain relief. Tramadol binds to mu-opioid receptor and also inhibits the reuptake of serotonin and noradrenaline.[44] Tramadol can be administered intravenously and is also available in oral and rectal preparations. The primary advantage of tramadol is the relative lack of respiratory depression, an important consideration in the immediate postoperative period.[44] An oral controlled-release tablet containing both oxycodone-hydrochloride and the opioid antagonist naloxone is also available.[44] Research has showed promising results as lower doses of oxycodone-hydrochloride have been required in comparison to intravenous morphine in painful postoperative procedures.[54]

Two categories of non-steroidal anti-inflammatory drugs are available: non-selective, which inhibit both COX-1 and COX-2 pathways (ibuprofen, naproxen, ketorolac, diclofenac); and selective, which only inhibit COX-2 (celecoxib).[55] All of these analgesics add to the repertoire of multimodal pain relief.

Patient-controlled analgesia

Patient-controlled analgesia (PCA) is increasingly recognised as an ideal approach for managing postoperative pain due to its minimal pharmacokinetic and pharmacodynamic variability in individual patients.[14] PCA also provides significantly better analgesia and a superior patient satisfaction.[14] The patient is also able to anticipate activities such as rolling or coughing that are associated with increases in pain and is able to self-administer a narcotic bolus prior to the activity to manage any pain that might occur. Following a loading dose of analgesia, the PCA pump is programmed based on the patient's needs and the pharmacokinetics of the drug being administered. The parameters programmed into the PCA pump include the bolus dose and a lockout interval. This allows the patient to attain immediate analgesia with the lockout interval preventing acute increases in the amount of drug delivered.[51]

Regional anaesthesia

Regional anaesthesia is a broad term to describe nerve blocks that block a region, for example arm blocks or femoral blocks. Regional anaesthesia involves injecting a local anaesthetic near major nerve bundles. To improve accuracy of drug delivery, selected nerves can be located using ultrasound guidance or a nerve stimulator.[56]

Central neural blockade: epidural/spinal

Central neural blockade or neuraxial anaesthesia is a generic term for epidural, spinal, epidural–spinal or caudal anaesthesia,[32] which blocks pain during a surgical procedure. Many of the medications used in epidural or spinal anaesthesia can continue to provide pain relief in the postoperative period, with local anaesthetic agents having differing durations of action. Local anaesthetic agents with adrenaline may be given if a longer duration of action is required.[32] When intrathecal or epidural opioids are administered close observation of the patient, particularly the patient's respiratory rate and conscious state, are essential as there may be delayed respiratory depression. Despite our repertoire of pain management analgesics, postoperative pain remains one of the most common challenges for all healthcare professionals.[51]

Care of the patient following epidural or spinal anaesthesia requires an understanding of the possible complications associated with this type of anaesthesia. A wide range of complications can occur including high spinal block, hypotension, bradycardia, spinal and epidural haematoma, post-dural puncture headache, nausea and vomiting, urinary retention and transient neurological symptoms.[32] In addition to normal postoperative observations, continual assessment for possible complications should be maintained, including: observation of the

Practice tip

The two most popular positions for epidural and spinal blockade are the 'sitting position' where the patient rolls forward and pushes their back outward like an 'angry cat' and the 'lateral decubitus' position where the patient is in a lateral position assuming the 'fetal position'.[32] Both positions allow easier needle access between the vertebrae and are chosen by the anaesthetist. The most important factors that affect the level of neural blockade following spinal anaesthesia are the baricity of anaesthetic solution, drug dose, specific site of injection and the position of the patient at the time of insertion and immediately after injection.[57] Postoperatively, the patient may be seated.

Practice tip

Patients who have received a spinal blockade will have a greater motor block than those with an epidural. This is because the local anaesthetic is injected into the subarachnoid space with the cerebrospinal fluid where the spinal nerves are not myelinated, providing a denser motor block.

epidural catheter site for bleeding, catheter migration, swelling or redness; discussion with the patient regarding the onset of pain or tenderness at the catheter site; and protective care and observation of anaesthetised limbs.[32] Attention to pressure area care is essential, ensuring the patient is not lying on drain tubing or exposed to heat or cold packs while the block is still in effect as these will not be felt by the patient, thus increasing risk of injury.

High spinal block

Assessing dermatomes after spinal and epidural anaesthesia is important to identify exaggerated dermatome spread that can occur (Fig. 26.4).[44] Signs and symptoms may include dyspnoea, numbness or weakness in the upper extremities, nausea that often precedes hypotension and bradycardia.[44] Reduced doses of medications are necessary for select patients in whom a normal dose might be excessive. Blocking of the cardiac sympathetic fibres from T1–T4 may cause loss of chronotropic and inotropic drive and a fall in cardiac output, which results in hypotension and bradycardia requiring urgent medical attention.[44]

Practice tip

Elderly, pregnant, obese or very short patients may have excessive dermatome spread if administered normal doses of spinal or epidural anaesthesia.

FIGURE 26.4 Dermatomes.

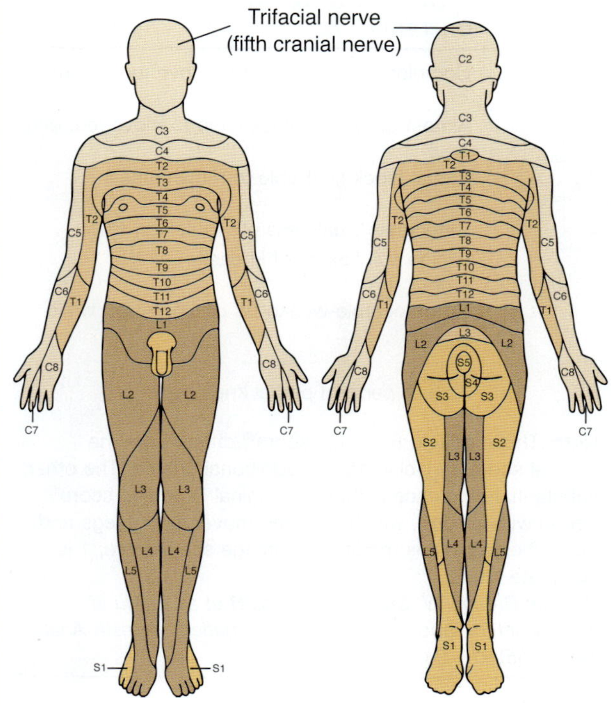

Adapted from Nagelhout J, Plaus K. Nurse anesthesia. 4th ed. St Louis: Saunders; 2010, with permission.

Careful assessment of dermatome levels must be performed. Ice is often used to assess sensory block as hot and cold pass on the same pathway as pain. Central neural blockade not only blocks sensory fibres but also motor function and sympathetic outflow. The level of muscle block can be assessed using the Bromage score (Table 26.6).

The level of differential blockade is judged by finding the level of sensory block with temperature sensitivity and recognising that the sympathetic block may be two or more segments higher. Motor blockade will be approximately two segments lower.[57] Sympathetic cardiac accelerator fibres arise from T1–T4 (at and above mid-nipple level). Close monitoring of heart rate and blood pressure should be initiated when the sensory block is sitting around T6 because of the potential for sympathetic outflow to be blocked.[57] A block at T1–T4 may produce profound bradycardia and hypotension from arterial dilation and venous pooling.[57] Consequently, a significant fall in cardiac output may occur without the body being able to compensate through the usual sympathetic responses. This change in patient condition should be treated as a medical emergency and treatment for shock implemented. Bradycardia can be treated with atropine and hypotension with fluid resuscitation therapy and/or vasopressors.[57] High spinal

TABLE 26.6
Modified Bromage score

SCORE	CRITERIA
1	Complete block (unable to move feet or knees)
2	Almost complete block (able to move feet only)
3	Partial block (just able to move knees)
4	Detectable weakness of hip flexion while supine (full flexion of knees)
5	No detectable weakness of hip flexion while supine
6	Able to perform partial knee bend

Note: This modified Bromage score[98] differs from the original score by including two additional criteria. The other substantial difference is that the original Bromage score[99] began with grade I, which was free movement of legs and feet, whereas in this modified Bromage scale score, 1 is complete block.
Source: Breen TW, Shapiro T, Glass B et al. Epidural anesthesia for labor in an ambulatory patient. Anesth Analg 1993;77(5):919–24.

blocks can affect respiratory muscles so ongoing assessment of respiratory function should be initiated and airway support provided as required.

Transient neurological symptoms

In administering a spinal or epidural anaesthetic a needle passes through the skin, subcutaneous tissues, muscle and ligaments. It is therefore not surprising that this procedure may cause varying degrees of tissue trauma such as bruising and localised inflammatory responses, with or without reflex muscle spasm. These muscle spasms may be responsible for postoperative backache,[57] which is usually mild and self-limiting. Backache can be treated with warm/cold packs or mild analgesics. Pain must be monitored carefully per the chance it may be an important clinical sign of more serious complications, such as epidural haematoma and abscess.[57]

Spinal or epidural haematoma

Both epidural and spinal haematomas are more likely to occur in patients who have abnormal coagulation levels, either disease-related or as a result of pharmacological therapies.[57] Consequently, coagulation studies must be performed prior to neuraxial anaesthesia being considered as changes in clotting profiles are an absolute contraindication to insertion of these blocks. Clotting status must also be performed prior to removal of the catheter and strict guidelines exist for removal in patients who are receiving prophylactic anticoagulants,[57] with recommendations specific to the anticoagulation medication used.

Epidural haematoma can lead to compression of the spinal nerves causing various degrees of irreversible damage. The symptoms of haematoma include sharp back and leg pain with a motor weakness and/or sphincter dysfunction.[57] Recognition of these symptoms can be delayed until after the effect of the anaesthesia has dissipated. In the event of such symptoms it is vital to call for immediate medical assistance. Rapid neurological imaging such as a computed tomography or magnetic resonance imaging scan should be performed to assess the location, size and extent of the haematoma as neurological outcomes are vastly improved if decompression occurs within 8–12 hours.[57]

Recent research reveals that epidural anaesthesia (compared with spinal anaesthesia) was found to be associated with a greater incidence of haematoma, and a much greater incidence of abscess.[59] It was also noted that there was a clear association between the adversity of outcome and the severity of the initial presentation, and the delay in surgical decompression, reinforcing early reporting of symptoms.[59]

Practice tip

Care must be taken when removing the epidural catheter as up to half of reported incidents of epidural haematoma are associated with catheter removal. Monitoring sensory observations after epidural removal is important to assess for complications, especially in those patients with abnormal clotting.

Post-dural puncture headache

Post-dural puncture headache is not an uncommon complication of interventional neuraxial blockade[60] and is the most common complication of spinal anaesthesia in the obstetric population.[61] If either a spinal or epidural needle accidentally tears the dura enough to cause cerebrospinal fluid (CSF) to leak out, this may cause a post-dural puncture headache. CSF is regenerated about 3–5 times over each day at a rate of approximately 0.3 mL per minute.[60] Although the exact mechanism of the headache is theoretical, experts believe that there appears to be a definitive relationship between the loss of CSF from the dural tear and the manifestation of symptoms and, put very simply, fluid loss disrupts the buoyancy of the brain.[60] Conservative management of this condition includes assisting the patient with full bed rest, maintaining adequate hydration and assisting the administering of prescribed medications such as analgesics and caffeine. An autologous blood patch/epidural blood patch may be fluoroscopically guided[61] or ultrasound-guided epidural blood patch can be used to manage post-dural puncture headaches.[62] This is done by taking approximately 10 mL of autologous blood and injecting it into the epidural space where the tear has occurred. The blood covers the area of dural puncture and prevents further leakage of CSF.[61]

Management of nausea and vomiting

Postoperative nausea and vomiting are a concern for patients and clinicians alike and affect as many as one-third of patients receiving anaesthesia. As the most undesirable postoperative complication, postoperative nausea and vomiting also can contribute to complications such as wound dehiscence, aspiration, increased intracranial pressure and increased cardiovascular demand. For some patients deep breathing, a cool cloth on the forehead and reassurance can help assist with nausea; however, for most postoperative patients, pharmacological interventions will be necessary. Common pharmacological agents for the management of nausea and vomiting are listed in Table 26.7.

Thermoregulation

The body has a highly sensitive system that provides a balance between heat production and heat loss. This consists of a complex feedback system that senses afferent messages, compares them to a central integrated set-point and sends reflex efferent messages to either cause vasoconstriction when the patient is cold or vasodilation when the patient is hot. Anaesthesia and the operating suite environment provide the perfect storm for the development of inadvertent hypothermia with the cold environment, exposure, opened body cavities, suppression of the thermoregulation centre and medications that cause vasodilation. Inadvertent or unplanned hypothermia is defined as a core temperature below 36°C[63] and is divided into three categories, mild (34–36°C), moderate (30–34°C) and severe (≤30°C).[64] Unlike the exposure hypothermia discussed in Chapter 23, inadvertent or unplanned hypothermia generally falls within the mild range but still has devastating consequences and is associated with increased mortality rates in postoperative patients.[65] Sequelae of this condition may include infection, sepsis, impaired wound healing, adverse cardiac events, shock, altered drug metabolism, impaired coagulation and increased postoperative discomfort.[65] In elective operations there was a fourfold increase in mortality and a doubled complication rate, with sepsis and stroke being the most increased.[65]

The pathophysiological effects of hypothermia include a left oxyhaemoglobin shift, increased oxygen requirements and the ability of vasoconstriction to mask a low circulating blood volume. Recognising these effects, nursing care should include rewarming the patient, providing supplemental oxygen and close monitoring of blood pressure during rewarming because of the potential for the patient to decrease their systolic blood pressure as vasoconstriction is reversed. Accurate temperature measurements reflecting the patient's core temperature are required and rewarming with external warming devices can be used (see Chapter 23).

> **Practice tip**
>
> During rewarming, patients with inadvertent hypothermia may initially decrease their body temperature before it starts to rise. This does not mean that the first temperature reading was inaccurate; rather, it is an indication of a phenomenon called 'after fall' that occurs when rewarming hypothermic patients.

Voiding and urinary retention

Urinary retention, inability to void, is a frequent postoperative complication which can result in bladder overdistension. Decreasing the risk for overdistension of the bladder is an important patient safety issue. The bladder damage is, to a large extent, an avoidable healthcare-related injury caused by inadequate bladder monitoring routines. The consequences for the patient include suffering from micturition problems, prolonged hospital stay, and increased costs to the patient and to society. Irreversible bladder damage greatly affects the patient's health-related quality of life and can imply lifelong inability to void, the need for

TABLE 26.7
Pharmacological interventions for postoperative nausea and vomiting[25]

DRUG (RECEPTOR SITE AFFINITY)	DOSE[a]	DURATION OF ACTION	ADVERSE EFFECTS	COMMENTS AND RECOMMENDATIONS FOR USE
Droperidol (dopamine)	Adult: 0.625–1.25 mg IV Paediatric: 20–50 mcg/kg IV (children ≥2 years)	12–24 h	Sedation, hypotension, EPS	Higher doses and doses that are repeated too soon can cause sedation, EPS and QT prolongation
Prochlorperazine (dopamine)	Adult: 5–10 mg IM or IV; 25 mg PR Paediatric:[b] 0.13 mg/kg IM; 0.2 mg/kg PO 2–3 times daily; 0.1 mg/kg 3–4 times daily PR	2–6 h IV, IM, PO; 12 h PR	Sedation, hypotension, EPS	Effective first-line agent

Continued

TABLE 26.7
Pharmacological interventions for postoperative nausea and vomiting—cont'd

DRUG (RECEPTOR SITE AFFINITY)	DOSE[a]	DURATION OF ACTION	ADVERSE EFFECTS	COMMENTS AND RECOMMENDATIONS FOR USE
Promethazine (dopamine, histamine, acetylcholine)	Adult: 6.25–25 mg IM, IV or PR Paediatric (≥2 years of age): 0.25–0.5 mg/kg IV, IM, PR[c]	4 h	Sedation, hypotension, EPS	Good for patients with motion sickness or undergoing surgery affecting vestibular apparatus
Diphenhydramine (histamine, acetylcholine)	Adult: 12.5–50 mg IM, IV Paediatric (≥2 years of age): 1 mg/kg IV or PO (maximum, 25 mg for <6 years of age)	4–6 hours	Sedation, dry mouth, blurred vision, urinary retention	Good for patients with motion sickness or undergoing surgery affecting vestibular apparatus
Metoclopramide (dopamine)	Adult: 10–20 mg IV Paediatric: 0.15–0.25 mg/kg	6–8 h	Sedation, hypotension, EPS	Increases gastric motility; good if nausea or vomiting is from gastric stasis; reduce dose to 5 mg in renal impairment; consider diphenhydramine to prevent EPS in children
Ondansetron (serotonin)	Adult: 4 mg IV; 4, 8 mg ODT or wafer Paediatric: 0.05–0.1 mg/kg	Up to 24 h	Headache, lightheadedness, constipation	Much more effective for vomiting than nausea; 2 mg may be sufficient to treat PONV in PACU
Granisetron (serotonin)	Adult: 1 mg IV over 30 s Paediatric: N/A	Up to 24 h	Headache, lightheadedness	Much more effective for vomiting than nausea
Palonosetron (serotonin)	Adult: 0.075 mg IV	24 h	Headache, constipation	Prolonged duration of action; given immediately before induction of anaesthesia
Hyoscine/ scopolamine (acetylcholine)	Adult: 1.5 mg transdermal patch Paediatric: N/A	72 h[d]	Sedation, dry mouth, visual disturbances, dysphoria, confusion, disorientation, hallucinations	Good for patients with motion sickness or undergoing surgery affecting vestibular apparatus; apply 4 h before exposure
Dexamethasone	Adult: 4–10 mg IV Paediatric: 0.5–1 mg/kg	Up to 24 h	Watch blood sugar in patients with diabetes; watch for fluid retention, especially in cardiac patients	Generally well tolerated in healthy patients; may take time (hours) to work – administer before induction of anaesthesia
Aprepitant	Adult: 40 mg PO 1–3 h before anaesthesia	Up to 24 h	Generally well tolerated	Oral prophylaxis only; caution with patients taking warfarin; can reduce effectiveness of oral contraceptives

[a]Unless otherwise indicated, paediatric doses should not exceed the adult dose for each antiemetic agent.
[b]Children weighing more than 10 kg or older than 2 years of age only. Change from IM to PO as soon as possible. With administration PR, dosing interval varies from 8–24 h depending on child's weight.
[c]Maximum of 12.5 mg in children younger than 12 years.
[d]Remove after 24 h when used to prevent or treat PONV. Instruct patient to wash the patch site and hands thoroughly.
ECG = electrocardiogram; EPS = extrapyramidal symptoms, such as motor restlessness or acute dystonia; IM = intramuscular; IV = intravenous; ODT = orally disintegrating tablets; PACU = postanaesthesia care unit; PO = orally; PONV = postoperative nausea and vomiting; PR = per rectum.
Adapted from O'Brien D. Postanesthesia care complications. In: Odom-Forren J. 7th ed. Perianaesthesia nursing: a critical care approach. St Louis: Elsevier; 2018, with permission.

TABLE 26.8
Urinary retention assessment

AMOUNT RETAINED	ACTION
100–150 mL	Assess again after 3 h
150–300 mL	Assess again after 2 h
300–400 mL	Assess again after 1 h
>400 mL	Intermittent, or indwelling catheter

daily intermittent self-catheterisation and a subsequent risk of chronic urinary tract infection.[66,67] Anaesthesia affects micturition in several ways. Spinal and epidural local anaesthetics block detrusor contraction and bladder sensation.[57] General anaesthetics cause bladder atony by interfering with the autonomic regulation of detrusor tone. Sedative-hypnotics and volatile anaesthetics suppress detrusor contraction and the micturition reflex. Overdistension occurs when bladder volumes exceed 500 mL and has a reported incidence of up to 44%.[67] The patient can experience discomfort and pain in the lower part of the abdomen, particularly upon palpation. Bladder distension can result in detrusor muscle damage, bladder atonia and chronic inability to void, with subsequent catheter-related problems and urinary tract infections.[68] To detect urinary retention a portable ultrasound scanner to monitor bladder volume is a non-invasive, safe and timesaving method. Action taken is dependent on the amount of urine which is retained in the bladder (Table 26.8).The gold standard of treatment for bladder distension is catheterisation and can be either intermittent, where the catheter is removed immediately after urine drainage is complete, or indwelling.[66]

The postoperative bariatric patient

The prevalence of obesity is increasing[69] and therefore management of the bariatric or obese patient in the postoperative period warrants detailed discussion. Bariatric patients undergoing anaesthesia will have particular needs in the postanaesthesia period, irrespective of the surgical procedure. For example, the higher incidence of cardiovascular disease means that careful electrocardiographic monitoring should be implemented during recovery from anaesthesia. Assessment of haemodynamic status is important, as it is with any postoperative patient, and accurate measurement of blood pressure is contingent on the use of appropriately sized blood pressure cuffs.

Bariatric patients are also at increased risk for resedation because many anaesthetic drugs are lipophilic and metabolised more slowly by obese patients. Because of increased respiratory compromise, opioid should be used with caution and multimodal treatments are encouraged including the use of non-steroidal anti-inflammatory agents, PCA, local anaesthesia or oral analgesia and the epidural route for analgesia.[70,71]

Specific assessment and management relative to the bariatric patient includes consideration for the prevention of venothromboembolism and pressure injuries. Proper fitting of compression stockings should be monitored so that a tourniquet effect of the stockings is avoided. Knowledge of the surgical procedure and intraoperative positioning will help guide assessment of the patient for signs of intraoperative pressure injury. Intravenous access should be monitored closely as initiating intravenous access can be challenging in this patient group.

The most important consideration in the postoperative period is the assessment of respiratory function. There is a direct correlation between the degree of obesity a patient suffers and the risk and rate of pulmonary complications.[70] Airway management may be difficult and hazardous due to anatomical features such as a large tongue and excessive pharyngeal and palatal soft tissue impairing vision and making mask ventilation awkward.

The dynamics of respiration are also altered in bariatric patients. There is a profound effect on the mechanics of the respiratory system with increased oxygen consumption and carbon dioxide production. Normocarbia is maintained by an increase in minute ventilation to expel increased carbon dioxide produced through metabolic activity of fat and the increased expenditure required for mobility and breathing.[72] Reduction in chest wall compliance also contributes to the increased work of breathing. Functional residual capacity may also decline particularly if the weight of the chest wall exceeds alveolar closing capacity, which results in small airway closure, ventilation perfusion mismatch and subsequent hypoxia.[72] Postoperatively, decreased lung function and capacity is expected for approximately 5 days and acute airway obstruction is more likely during this period.[72]

Provided cardiovascular stability is established it may be best to position obese patients sitting up. If the weight of the chest wall exceeds the closing capacity of the alveoli, the alveoli will collapse and desaturation will occur. By sitting the patient up, the weight of the chest wall is lessened, allowing greater tidal volume. If the patient is hypotensive, a discussion with medical staff would be required to assess which problem is worse; however, the 'banana' position (head up and feet up) may be required. It is essential to provide support for positioning to ensure upright sitting position is maintained. If edentulous, replace the teeth as these will assist in upper airway support.

Assessment and management of specific postoperative complications

Laryngospasm

Laryngospasm is an involuntary forceful spasm of the laryngeal musculature that is caused by stimulation of the superior laryngeal nerve.[73] It is more common in young paediatric patients than in adults, and is most common in infants 1–3 months old.[73] Laryngeal spasm can result in an incomplete or complete airway obstruction,[25,74] with the latter being more uncommon. Prevention of this condition includes extubating patients either deeply paralysed or fully reversed (but not in between) and causes include fluid or secretions on the vocal cords.

Treatment of laryngospasm includes gentle positive-pressure ventilation, forward jaw thrust and intravenous lignocaine (1–1.5 mg/kg) may be considered.[75] If hypoxia develops, paralysis with intravenous suxamethonium (0.5–1 mg/kg) or rocuronium (0.4 mg/kg) and controlled ventilation may be required.[73]

Signs and symptoms of laryngeal spasm include inspiratory stridor, dyspnoea, a distressed/sweating patient and on auscultation an upper airway noise can be heard. As postoperative patients generally have supplemental oxygen, these symptoms may or may not include a decrease in oxygen saturations in mild laryngeal spasm. Treatment of this condition will include sitting the patient up to facilitate ventilation, supplemental oxygen, gentle suctioning of the upper airway and providing airway support as required.[25,74] It is important to reassure the patient as anxiety can exacerbate the condition.

Non-cardiogenic pulmonary oedema

Pulmonary oedema may be defined simply as increased total lung water. Non-cardiogenic pulmonary oedema is where increased lung water occurs in the absence of a cardiac aetiology. In the postanaesthesia period non-cardiogenic pulmonary oedema can occur because of upper airway obstruction such as laryngospasm, bolus dosing with naloxone, reversal of neuromuscular blockade or significant hypoxia.[25] In young athletic males, non-cardiogenic pulmonary oedema may occur in relation to the generation of negative intrathoracic pressure during an upper airway obstruction as the diaphragm contracts against a closed or semi-closed glottis.[76] The severity of pulmonary oedema corresponds to the degree to which high negative inspiratory pressures are generated.[76] Symptoms usually occur within 1 hour of the upper airway obstruction, but may present as much as 6 hours later.[25] The patient may then develop sudden respiratory distress, tachypnoea, cough, shortness of breath, sudden decrease in oxygen saturation and the classic sign of pink frothy sputum.[25] Vital signs may or may not change.

Rapid diagnosis and treatment are essential to alleviate this respiratory complication. Treatment of this condition includes providing supplemental oxygenation. Continuous positive airway pressure can be used and, if the patient requires airway management, they may be intubated and mechanically ventilated with positive end-expiratory pressure.[25] For further information on oxygenation and caring for an intubated patient, please see Chapter 15.

Subglottic oedema/post-intubation croup

Subglottic oedema or post-intubation croup is a complication that occurs later than laryngospasm, but will almost always appear within 3 h following extubation.[73] Although this condition can occur in adults, it is most commonly seen in the 1–4-year-old age group.[25] The risk of developing subglottic oedema can be lessened in children by allowing a slight gas leak around the endotracheal tube.[73]

Signs and symptoms of subglottic oedema include inspiratory stridor, retractions, hoarseness, crowing respiration and a croup-like cough, and a patient who is apprehensive and restless. Humidified oxygen may help reduce airway swelling and nebulised racemic adrenaline can also help reduce subglottic oedema. If additional treatment is required, a helium–oxygen mixture can be used or dexamethasone administered.[25]

Bronchospasm

Bronchospasm is a lower airway obstruction, characterised by spasmodic smooth muscle contraction that causes narrowing of the bronchi and bronchioles.[25] Generally, bronchospasm will occur in patients with a preexisting pulmonary illness such as asthma or chronic obstructive pulmonary disease, but it may also develop in healthy patients in the presence of allergy, anaphylaxis or pulmonary aspiration. For this reason, if a patient without pulmonary pathology develops bronchospasm, a high degree of suspicion should be employed by the nurse to ensure that the underlying cause is not allergic or due to pulmonary aspiration.

Signs and symptoms of bronchospasm include coughing, distinct wheeze upon auscultation, noisy shallow respiration, chest retractions, use of accessory muscles, prolonged expiratory phase of respiration, hypertension and tachycardia. The nurse should sit the patient up, provide assisted oxygen, call for medical assistance and reassure the patient.

Initial management of this patient will include removal of the identified cause if possible,[25] and treatment will depend on the cause, specific symptoms and severity of the bronchospasm. This may include humidified oxygen, administration of a $beta_2$ adrenergic agonist, intubation and intermittent positive-pressure ventilation and perhaps antibiotics. Antihistamines and steroids may also be required.[25]

Aspiration pneumonitis

Mendelson syndrome, aspiration of gastric content that results in a severe pulmonary complication, was first reported in 1940s.[77] Preoperative patient preparation, including fasting, is aimed at minimising the risk of aspiration. Pregnant women, obese, patients with gastro-oesophageal reflux disease and non-fasting patients are all at increased risk of aspiration pneumonitis.[44]

Clinical progression after aspiration varies widely, from no and very mild symptoms to bronchopneumonia and possible development of acute respiratory distress syndrome.[44] The severity of progression is increased by several factors including the aspirate pH, quantity of aspirate and the presence of solid particles.[44] Symptoms include tachypnoea, tachycardia, cough and possible bronchospasm.[44] While this condition may be dramatic on onset it can also be insidious in nature. Bronchospasm that occurs in a healthy patient should be investigated further.[44]

Awareness under anaesthesia

Awareness under anaesthesia results from an imbalance between anaesthetic need and delivery and is an uncommon complication of anaesthesia, affecting only 0.1–0.2% of all surgical patients. Patients who have experienced awareness under anaesthesia report a perception of paralysis, being aware of conversations and surgical manipulations alongside feelings of helplessness, fear and pain. Depth of anaesthesia is assessed through monitoring of vital signs; however, in some patients this is unreliable.[78] There is growing evidence suggesting the awareness can lead to the development of posttraumatic stress disorder,[79] so appropriate management of patients with this condition is essential.

If a patient awakes from anaesthesia and tells you that they have suffered awareness under anaesthesia, comfort and support should be provided to the patient. Explain that the operation is over and that they are safe. The treating anaesthetist should be contacted immediately. It is important not to dismiss the patient's comments or contradict them in any way. Their report should be taken seriously and documented accurately in the patient's notes and through established hospital incident reporting systems.

Emergence delirium

Emergence delirium is a well-known phenomenon that may occur in the postoperative period.[80] In its milder form an awake patient may exhibit restlessness, disorientation, irrational conversations and inappropriate behaviour, and this may be referred to as emergence excitement.[25] Emergence delirium can also include symptoms such as hallucinations, hypersensitivity to external stimuli and hyperactivity, with the patient often screaming and thrashing.[80] On assessment the patient's eyes can appear glazed and they do not respond to verbal dialogue. Raised voices tend to worsen the situation so calm, confident reassurance is advised.

Children have a higher incidence, along with adults who have suffered a recent tragedy or bereavement, severe preoperative anxiety, a history of drug dependency or psychiatric illness or who have had certain medications including ketamine, droperidol, opioids, benzodiazepines, hyoscine (also known as scopolamine), atropine or large doses of metoclopramide.[25]

Clinical management of emergence delirium includes protecting the patient from self-injury, ensuring your own safety and calling for assistance. Patients should be assessed for hypoxia as a possible cause of the behaviour. If the cause of emergence delirium is known the cause should be treated. Sedation may be required.[25] Clinical evidence also suggests that emergence delirium is increasingly seen among military personnel who have seen active service.[81]

If you have prior knowledge that a patient is prone to emergence delirium, preparations can be made for their safe recovery by obtaining protective cot or bed sides to prevent injury, and ensuring appropriate human resources are available to help physically manage the patient if necessary.

Practice tip

Postoperative delirium often lasts about 20 minutes with the patient eventually falling back to sleep before waking with no recollections of the incident.

Delayed awakening

Time to emerge from anaesthesia is variable between patients, and may depend on a multitude of factors including the type of anaesthesia and length of surgery.[25] Occasionally, the time for a patient to awake may be slower than expected and this could be due to a plethora of factors.[25]

Delayed emergence may occur in a patient who was recovering in the ICU, or may be the reason for an admission to ICU. The most common cause of delayed awakening is prolonged effect from anaesthesia and associated medications, but it could also be due to metabolic complications including hypoglycaemia, hyponatraemia, hypocalcaemia, hypomagnesaemia, hypercarbia, hypoxia, hypothermia, hypovolaemia or neurological injury.[25] A full neurological assessment will be required[25] using the Glasgow Coma Scale. The primary management is always in support of airway, breathing and circulation, while the cause is sought.

Malignant hyperthermia

Malignant hyperthermia is a rare, catastrophic, often fatal syndrome that is triggered by volatile anaesthetic agents and suxamethonium.[82] It is an uncommon disorder with autosomal-dominant inheritance, involving abnormal skeletal muscle calcium metabolism.[82] Although its pathogenesis is relatively well understood, there is wide variability in the time of onset and the presentation of clinical signs and symptoms.[83] Most cases of malignant hyperthermia occur within 30 minutes of anaesthesia and therefore will be seen and treated in the operating suite, but some patients may have delayed symptoms up to 12 hours postoperatively.[84] In some circumstances the delayed onset has hindered timely recognition and treatment.[83] Patients presenting with febrile illness after surgery should be assessed for malignant hyperthermia. This is a particularly important consideration for those patients who are discharged home after surgery but re-present to the hospital emergency department.[85]

In malignant hyperthermia an intracellular skeletal muscle biochemical defect and exposure to trigger agents results in excessive amounts of calcium in the myoplasm released by the sarcoplasmic reticulum. The resultant high level of calcium causes intense skeletal muscle contraction, which in turn causes heat production, increased oxygen consumption and increased carbon dioxide production. Malignant hyperthermia is a cyclic process that liberates heat and produces lactic acid.[86] Cell membrane disruptions lead to potassium, phosphate, magnesium and myoglobin leakage into the extracellular fluid, which results in increased serum levels.[87] Early symptoms of malignant hyperthermia include tachycardia, tachypnoea, sweating, rise in end-tidal carbon dioxide levels, hyperthermia, skeletal muscle stiffness and possibly master muscle spasm.[81] Treatment of malignant hyperthermia is detailed in Box 26.2.

The treating medication, dantrolene sodium, is a skeletal muscle relaxant that decreases the amount of calcium released by the sarcoplasmic reticulum, thus reversing the pathophysiology of malignant hyperthermia. The dose of dantrolene sodium in malignant hyperthermia is 2.5 mg/kg given intravenously, regardless of age with no upper dose limit.[88] Dantrolene sodium when given intravenously has a half-life of 5 hours; some patients may require up to 30 mg/kg over 24 hours.[88] Because symptoms reoccur in 25% of patients[89] subsequent doses of dantrolene sodium are required,[90] usually as 1 mg/kg over 6 hours for the first 24–48 hours.

BOX 26.2

Management of malignant hyperthermia

- Stop trigger agents immediately.
- Administer 100% oxygen and hyperventilate.
- Call for help – press emergency bell.
- Contact the operating theatre to get specialised help from an anaesthetist.
- Obtain sodium dantrolene, the treating agent, and administer 2.5 mg/kg with no upper dose limit.
- Notify pharmacy department to replenish stores of sodium dantrolene.
- Use aggressive cooling to prevent the patient reaching the thermal critical level of >40.6°C.
- Assist in associated management of arrhythmias and electrolyte imbalance.
- Assess cardiac function, urine output and colour (urinary catheterisation may be required).

Adapted from with permission:
Hooper VD. Care of the patient with thermal imbalance. In: Odom-Forren J, editor. Perianesthesia nursing: a critical care approach. 6th ed. St Louis: Elsevier; 2013.
Hirshey Dirksen S, Van Wicklin S, Ledrut Mashman D et al. Developing effective drills in preparation for a malignant hyperthermia crisis. AORN 2013;97(3):330–52.

Practice tip

Sodium dantrolene must be reconstituted with sterile water because of compatibility issues. Reconstituted sodium dantrolene is very alkalotic (pH 9.5) so care must be taken to prevent extravasation. Patients receiving this drug should be monitored for thrombophlebitis.

Transferring care of the postoperative patient: discharge to an inpatient ward

Without question, the immediate postoperative period will require high quality, safe nursing care to detect and/or prevent serious complications.[91] Many factors affect the patient's response to anaesthesia and surgery, thus the length of stay for each patient will vary.[91]

For this reason, most PACUs have discharge criteria that involve a thorough assessment of the patient's vital signs, pain, conscious state, nausea and vomiting and escalation of care plan prior to patient discharge from the PACU.[91] These criteria are used to determine when a patient is ready to be discharged to the ward and can be used in the ICU when non-critically ill patients are in ICU recovering from anaesthesia (Table 26.9). Critically ill postoperative patients will have their discharge managed by the ICU clinician team.

TABLE 26.9
Discharge criteria for the postoperative patient

Conscious state	Conscious and able to respond appropriately to verbal stimuli
Respiratory function	Able to protect his or her own airway Has a cough reflex Respiratory rate must be greater than 12 breaths/min Oxygen saturation should be >94% on room air and assessed at least 10 min after oxygen discontinued Need for supplemental oxygen should be determined by medical team for those patients who do not have an oxygen saturation >94% on room air
Cardiovascular function	Vital signs need to be within normal limits and considered in relation to the patient's preoperative vital signs. Heart rate and blood pressure should be within 20% of preoperative
Temperature	Patient's core temperature should be between 36°C and 37°C
Pain	The patient should be pain free or have pain at a manageable level
Nausea and vomiting	The patient should be free from nausea and vomiting Patients with persistent nausea may return to the ward after liaison with medical staff and appropriate ongoing management in place
Wound care	Dressings should be dry and intact Drains should be labelled with amount, date and time. Drainage should be assessed to ensure excessive drainage is not present Women who have had a lower caesarean section will have their fundal height assessed. The fundal height should be equal to or less than the level of the umbilicus Per vaginal (PV) loss must be assessed in both gynaecological and obstetric patients ensuring that the blood loss in within normal limits
Neurological and neurovascular observations	Should be within normal limits
Documentation	Nursing documentation completed legibly in ink Ensure medical staff have written up appropriate notes and orders

Summary

In conclusion, patients who have received anaesthesia and undergone surgical procedures are vulnerable to a multitude of different complications. Although they may not be critically ill, patients who are transferred to the ICU immediately following surgery require close monitoring and observation. Respect for, and knowledge and understanding of, such complications will allow the nurse to provide a safer postoperative journey.

Case study

Mrs Mary Smith was a 69-year-old patient who presented to the ICU following coronary artery grafting surgery. Her past history included severe coronary artery disease and angina, and non-insulin dependent diabetes. She had had two previous unremarkable anaesthetics using volatile agents and no known family history of malignant hyperthermia.

Mrs Smith received a full relaxant general anaesthetic being induced with fentanyl, propofol and vecuronium, and anaesthesia was maintained with nitrous oxide and isoflurane. Mrs Smith had an uneventful operative period and was safely transferred to the ICU at 19:30 hours. She remained intubated and ventilated, with a plan for extubation the next morning if her condition was stable. She was in sinus rhythm with no ischaemic episodes.

At 19:50 hours, Mrs Smith developed tachycardia, became hypertensive and was noted to have an end-tidal CO_2 level rapidly rising from 36 mmHg to 59 mmHg. The nursing staff increased her ventilation rate and contacted medical staff, but the CO_2 levels continued to rise to 75 mmHg at 20:05 hours. It was then noted by the nursing and medical staff that the patient was hot to touch and was also suffering from muscular-skeletal stiffness.

At this point a diagnosis of malignant hyperthermia was made. An oesophageal temperature probe was inserted revealing a temperature of 39.2°C.

Sodium dantrolene was administered at 2.5 mg/kg (180 mg) at 20:15 hours with good effect. At 20:25 hours, the patient's temperature began to decrease, CO_2 was 45 mmHg, HR and BP were lower and skeletal muscle stiffness ceased.

Three additional dantrolene doses (1 mg/kg) were given every 6 hours. The remainder of the patient's stay was uneventful.

DISCUSSION

Malignant hyperthermia is at the forefront of thinking while the patient is in the perioperative environment, but once they leave the operating suite, it may be more difficult to diagnose and less easily understood. This patient had routine normal blood gases throughout the operation revealing that, while the condition was triggered by the volatile anaesthetic agents during the operation, the condition did not present itself until after the operation was complete. In research performed by Larach and colleagues,[92] 77 of 152 patients reported two previous unremarkable anaesthetics prior to their episode of malignant hyperthermia.[92]

Malignant hyperthermia is most likely to occur in the operating room; however, it can also present in the PACU and possibly up to 12 hours postoperatively, making this condition one that needs to be understood by intensive care nurses caring for postoperative patients.

CASE STUDY QUESTIONS

1 Describe the pathogenesis of malignant hyperthermia.
2 Discuss the risk factors for malignant hyperthermia in relation to the patient described in this case study.
3 What signs and symptoms did Mrs Smith present with and does a report of normal previous anaesthesia exclude patients from this condition?
4 Why is sodium dantrolene used in the treatment of malignant hyperthermia?
5 How can anaesthesia safely be provided to a patient who may be predisposed to developing malignant hyperthermia?

RESEARCH VIGNETTE

de Pater G, Florvaag E, Johansson S et al. Six years without pholcodine; Norwegians are significantly less IgE-sensitized and clinically more tolerant to neuromuscular blocking agents. Allergy 2017;72:813-19

Background: As a strong inducer of IgE antibodies to substituted ammonium ion epitopes (QAI), pholcodine (PHO) is a postulated cause of allergic anaphylaxis to neuromuscular blocking agents (NMBAs). Three years after withdrawal of PHO in Norway, a significant reduction in IgE sensitization and anaphylaxis reporting was seen.

Objective: Six-year follow-up study on the effects of PHO withdrawal on IgE sensitization and anaphylaxis reporting.

Methods: From 650 acute consecutive reports (2005–2013) to the Norwegian Network for Anaphylaxis under Anaesthesia (NARA), total number of reports on suspected anaphylactic reactions, number of reactions where NMBAs were administered, number of reactions where serum IgE antibodies (≥0.35 kUA/l) to suxamethonium (SUX) and PHO were present at time of reaction and anaphylaxis severity grades were retrieved. In addition, NMBA sales and prevalence of IgE sensitization to PHO and SUX among 'allergics' were monitored.

Results: From baseline period P0 (PHO on the market) through the first (P1) and second (P2), three-year periods after withdrawal, significant falls in total reports ($P < 0.001$) and reports with IgE antibodies to PHO ($P = 0.008$) and SUX ($P = 0.001$) at time of reaction were found. Total NMBA sales in P2 were 83% of P0, and SUX and rocuronium (ROC) together made up 86% of sales throughout the study. Five NMBA-related anaphylactic deaths occurred during P0 and P1 and, however, none during P2. Prevalence of IgE sensitization to SUX in 'allergics' fell to 0% at 4 and 5 years after withdrawal.

Conclusions: Six years after PHO withdrawal, the Norwegian population has become significantly less IgE-sensitized and clinically more tolerant to NMBAs.

Critique

Although a rare event, potentially catastrophic anaphylactic reactions may occur at any time during the perioperative period[93] either during surgery or immediately postoperatively in the PACU, or the high dependency unit or intensive care. The effective anticipation, prevention, and treatment of these reactions represent one of the greatest challenges for all nursing and medical staff who must work in a close cooperation, as a team, during these unexpected events.[93] Anaphylaxis is a life-threatening emergency that requires prompt recognition of signs and symptoms, early administration of adrenaline in adequate dosage, and aggressive fluid volume replacement.[94]

In 2011 and 2012, research was published by Florvaag and Johansson[95,96] indicating that there was a large difference in rates of anaphylaxis to neuromuscular blocking agents (NMBA) in Norway where it was high, compared with Sweden where anaphylaxis to NMBA was much lower.

In an attempt to understand this perplexing problem, researchers searched the homes of residents in both countries to try and identify sources of a tertiary or quaternary ammonium ion (QAI) that may have sensitised patients prior to anaesthesia and neuromuscular blocking agents.[96]

This exhaustive search revealed that the predominant difference was the availability and use of the over-the-counter cough suppressant pholcodine (PHO).[96] PHO was not available over-the-counter in Sweden, thus less widely used compared to Norway where its accessibility and use was much higher.[96] It was then postulated that the substituted ammonium ion structure of PHO was resulting in sensitisation and an increased reaction rate to NMBAs observed in Norway relative to Sweden.[96]

The subsequent 'Pholcodine hypothesis' was born and led to the voluntary withdrawal of the single PHO product on the market in Norway.[96] The data presented in the research discussed in this vignette shows that during the 6 years after removing PHO from the market in 2007, the Norwegian population has gradually become significantly less IgE-sensitised and clinically more tolerant to neuromuscular blocking agents.

Pholcodine is still freely available in other countries around the world, such as Australia and New Zealand, where this argument has been hindered by a lack of mandatory reporting of such serious anaphylactic reactions.[97] The Therapeutic Good Administration in Australia have cited a lack of reported cases as the reason for not supporting voluntary removal of over-the-counter PHO in Australia as they did in Norway.[97]

This research illustrates the power of research to make findings and subsequent changes to provide safer healthcare for our populations. It also highlights the importance of reporting of adverse events to allow such research and statistical analysis to be undertaken.

Learning activities

1. Subglottic oedema occurs mainly in young children but can also be observed in adults. Subglottic oedema may be observed as long as 3 hours postextubation. What signs and symptoms might you observe in the patient with subglottic oedema?
2. Anaphylaxis may be a life-threatening event with NMBA being significantly implicated in these occurrences. What is the name of the over-the-counter medication that was voluntarily withdrawn from Norway to reduce their statistics of anaphylaxis to NMBA?
3. Bariatric patients undergoing surgery warrant special consideration. What specific assessment might you undertake for this specific patient group?
4. What strategies could you use to manage emergence delirium?

Online resources

American Association of Nurse Anaesthetists, https://www.aana.com/

American Society of Anesthesiologists, www.asahq.org

American Society of PeriAnesthesia Nurses, www.aspan.org

Association of Anaesthetists of Great Britain and Ireland, www.aagbi.org

Association of PeriOperative Registered Nurses, www.aorn.org

Australian College of Operating Room Nurses, www.acorn.org.au

International Federation of Perioperative Nurses, http://www.ifpn.org.uk/

Operating Room Nurses Association of Canada, www.ornac.ca

Perioperative Nurses College of New Zealand Nurses Organisation, https://www.nzno.org.nz/groups/colleges_sections/colleges/perioperative_nurses_college

Practice guidelines for postanesthetic care: an updated report by the American Society of Anesthesiologists Task Force of Postanesthetic Care, www.guideline.gov/content.aspx?id=43896

Further reading

British Journal of Anaesthetic and Recovery Nursing.

Journal of PeriAnesthesia Nursing.

Odom-Forren J, editor. Drain's perianesthesia nursing: a critical care approach. 7th ed. St Louis: Elsevier; 2017.

Hamlin L, Davies M, Richardson-Tench M, et al. Perioperative nursing: an introduction. 2nd ed. Sydney: Elsevier; 2016.

References

1. American Society of Peri-Anesthesia Nurses. ASPAN's History Timeline 2012. Available from: http://www.aspan.org/AboutUs/History/tabid/3146/Default.aspx#Beginning.
2. Schick L. Assessment and monitoring of the perianesthesia patient. In: Odom-Forren J, editor. Perianaesthesia nursing: a critical care approach. 7th ed. St. Louis: Elsevier; 2018.
3. Australian Commission for Safety and Quality in Healthcare. National consensus statement: Essential elements for recognising and responding to clinical deterioration. Sydney: ACSQHC; 2010. p. 1- 20.
4. Helling T, Martin L, Martin M, et al. Failure events in transition of care for surgical patients. J Am Coll Surg 2014;218(April):723–31.
5. Drain CB. Inhalation anesthesia. In: Odom-Forren J, editor. Perianesthesia nursing: a critical care approach. 7th ed. St Louis: Elsevier; 2018.
6. Butterworth J, Mackey D, Wasnick J. The practice of anesthesiology. In: Butterworth J, Mackey D, Wasnick J, editors. Morgan and Mikhail's Clinical anesthesiology. 5th ed. New York: McGraw-Hill; 2013.
7. Drain CB. Nonopioid intravenous anesthetics. In: Odom-Forren J, editor. Perianesthesia nursing: a critical care approach. 7th ed. St Louis: Elsevier; 2018.
8. Kaye A, Chung K, Vadivelu N, et al. Opioid induced hyperalgesia altered with propofol infusion. Pain Physician 2014;17(2):225–8.

9. Cies J, Moront M, Parker J, et al. Use of etomidate for rapid sequence intubation (RSI) in pediatric trauma patients: a national survey. Crit Care Med 2013;41(12).
10. Flynn G, Shehabi Y. Pro/con debate: is etomidate safe in hemodynamically unstable critically ill patients? Crit Care 2012;16(4):227.
11. Yang HS, Kim T-Y, Bang S, et al. Comparison of the impact of the anesthesia induction using thiopental and propofol on cardiac function for non-cardiac surgery. J Cardiovasc Ultrasound 2014;22(2):58–64.
12. Drain CB. Opioid intravenous anesthetics. In: Odom-Forren J, editor. Perianesthesia nursing: a critical care approach. 7th ed. St Louis: Elsevier; 2018.
13. Luo J, Min S. Postoperative pain management in the postanesthesia care unit: an update. J Pain Res 2017;10:2687–98.
14. McKeen MJ, Quraishi SA. Clinical review of intravenous opioids in acute care. J Anesthesiol Clin Sci 2013;2.
15. Walets J, Kumar Z. Patient care during anaesthesia. In: Hamlin L, Davies M, Richardson-Tench M, et al, editors. Perioperative nursing - an introductory text. Sydney, Australia: Elsevier; 2016.
16. Howlett C, Gonzalez R, Yerram P, et al. Use of naloxone for reversal of life-threatening opioid toxicity in cancer-related pain. J Oncol Pharm Pract 2016;22(1):114–20.
17. Banchs RJ, Lerman J. Preoperative anxiety management, emergence delirium, and postoperative behavior. Anesthesiol Clin 2014;32(1):1–23.
18. Lu F, Lin J, Benditt DG. Conscious sedation and anesthesia in the cardiac electrophysiology laboratory. J Cardiovasc Electrophysiol 2013;24(2):237–45.
19. Gan TJ, Diemunsch P, Habib AS, et al. Consensus guidelines for the management of postoperative nausea and vomiting. Anesth Analg 2014;118(1):85–113.
20. Farooq K, Hunter JM. Neuromuscular blocking agents and reversal agents. Anaesth Intensive Care Med 2014;15(6):295–9.
21. Butterworth J, Mackey D, Wasnick J. Neuromuscular blocking agents. In: Butterworth J, Mackey D, Wasnick J, editors. Morgan and Mikhail's Clinical anesthesiology. 5th ed. New York: McGraw-Hill Medical; 2013.
22. Drain CB. Neuromuscular blocking agents. In: Odom-Forren J, editor. Perianesthesia nursing: a critical care approach. 7th ed. St Louis: Elsevier; 2018.
23. Belcher A, Leung S, Cohen B, et al. Incidence of complications in the post-anesthesia care unit and associated healthcare utilization in patients undergoing non-cardiac surgery requiring neuromuscular blockade 2005–2013: a single center study. J Clin Anesth 2017;43:33–8.
24. World Health Organization. Global guidelines on the prevention of surgical site infections. World Health Organization; 2016.
25. O'Brien D. Postanesthesia care complications. In: Odom-Forren J, editor. Perianaesthesia nursing: a critical care approach. 7th ed. St. Louis: Elsevier; 2018.
26. Minkowitz H, Valentine D. Real-world experience with neuromuscular blockade reversal. J Clin Anesth 2017;42.
27. Tsur A, Kalansky A. Hypersensitivity associated with sugammadex administration: a systematic review. Anaesthesia 2014.
28. Williams R, Bryant H. Sugammadex advice for women of childbearing age. Anaesthesia 2018;73(1):133–4.
29. Ben Salem C, Badreddine A, Fathallah N, et al. Drug-induced hyperkalemia. Drug Saf 2014;37(9):677–92.
30. Hendaus MA, Jomha FA, Alhammadi AH. Is ketamine a lifesaving agent in childhood acute severe asthma? Ther Clin Risk Manag 2016;12:273–9.
31. Nagelhout JJ. Basic principles of pharmacology. In: Odom-Forren J, editor. Perianesthesia nursing: a critical care approach. 7th ed. St. Louis: Elsevier; 2018.
32. Nagelhout J. Local anaesthesia. In: Odom-Forren J, editor. Perianaesthesia nursing: a critical care approach. St Louis: Elsevier; 2018.
33. Allvin R, Berg K, Idvall E, et al. Postoperative recovery: a concept analysis. J Adv Nurs 2007;57:552–8.
34. Ead H. Aldrete to PADSS: reviewing discharge criteria after ambulatory surgery. J Perianesth Nurs 2006;21:259–67.
35. Woersching J. Postoperative cognitive dysfunction after noncardiac and nonneurological surgery: an integrative review. AANA J 2017;85(1):17–27.
36. Segall N, Bonifacio A, Schroeder R, et al. Can we make postoperative patient handovers safer? A systematic review of the literature. Anesth Analg 2012;115(1):102–15.
37. Australian and New Zealand College of Anaesthetists. Statement on the Assistant for the Anaesthetist Background Paper. ANZCA [Internet]. 2016 B 14 April 2018. Available from: http://www.anzca.edu.au/documents/ps08-bp-2016.
38. Aldrete J, Kroulik D. A postanesthetic recovery score. Anesth Analg 1970;49:924–34.
39. Indian Journal of Anesthesia. Modified Aldrete Scoring System. 2009; 53(6):[654 p.]. Available from: http://www.ijaweb.org/viewimage.asp?img=IndianJAnaesth_2009_53_6_654_60239_t2.jpg.
40. Wright S. Assessment and management of the airway. In: Odom-Forren J, editor. Perianaesthesia nursing: a critical care approach. 7th ed. St. Louis: Elsevier; 2018.
41. Hedenstierna G. Oxygen and anesthesia: what lung do we deliver to the post-operative ward? Acta Anaesthesiol Scand 2012;56(6):675–85.
42. Subbe C. Failure to rescue: using rapid response systems to improve care of the deteriorating patient in hospital. Clin Risk 2013;19(1):6–11.
43. Cooper S, Cant R, Sparkes L. Respiratory rate records: the repeated rate. J Clin Nurs 2014;23(9–10):1236–8.
44. Foran P. Post-anaesthesia nursing. In: Hamlin L, Davies M, Richardson-Tench M, et al, editors. Perioperative nursing - an introductory text. Sydney, Australia: Elsevier; 2016.

45. Welle T, Basol R, Schneider N. Evaluating the need for routine supplemental oxygen in postoperative total joint replacement patients. J Perianesth Nurs 2013;28(1):21–5.
46. Anderson M, Watson G. Traumatic shock: the fifth shock. J Trauma Nurs 2013;20(1):37–43. Available from: http://eds.a.ebscohost.com.ezproxy-m.deakin.edu.au/ehost/detail?vid=4&sid=1306eb51-af87-4e3d-b582-06ca07c14ae3%40sessionmgr4002&hid=4202&bdata=JnNpdGU9ZWhvc3QtbGl2ZSZzY29wZT1zaXRl#db=ccm&AN=2012065447. [Accessed 16 July 2014].
47. Malina D. Fluid and electrolytes. In: Odom-Forren J, editor. Drains perianaesthesia nursing: a critical care approach. St Louis: Elsevier; 2018.
48. Department of Forensic Medicine Monash University. Victorian Institute of Forensic Medicine. Clinical Communiqué [electronic resource]: [Internet]. 2017; 4(1). Available from: http://vifmcommuniques.org/clinical-communique-volume-4-issue-1-march-2017/.
49. National Institute for Health and Clinical Excellence (NICE). Venous thromboembolism: reducing the risk for patients in hospital. NICE; 2010. p. 1–59. Available from: nice.org.uk/guidance/cg92.
50. Chan P, Skaggs DL, Sanders AE, et al. Pain is the greatest preoperative concern for patients and parents before posterior spinal fusion for adolescent idiopathic scoliosis. Spine 2017;42(21):1245–50.
51. Mitra S, Carlyle D, Kodumudi G, et al. New advances in acute postoperative pain management. Curr Pain Headache Rep 2018;22(35):1–11.
52. Samaraee A, Rhind G, Saleh U, et al. Factors contributing to poor post-operative abdominal pain management in adult patient: a review. Surgeon 2010;8:151–8.
53. Apfel CC, Turan A, Souza K, et al. Intravenous acetaminophen reduces postoperative nausea and vomiting: a systematic review and meta-analysis. Pain 2013;154(5):677–89.
54. Ruetzler K, Blome C, Nabecker S, et al. A randomised trial of oral versus intravenous opioids for treatment of pain after cardiac surgery. J Anesth 2014;28(4):580–6.
55. Pasero C. Pain management. In: Odom-Forren J, editor. Perianaesthesia nursing: a critical care approach. 7th ed. St. Louis: Elsevier; 2018.
56. Australian and New Zealand College of Anaesthetists. Types of anaesthesia. Melbourne: Australian and New Zealand College of Anaesthetists. Available from: http://www.anzca.edu.au/patients/types-of-anaesthestist. [Accessed 22 August 2014].
57. Butterworth J, Mackey D, Wasnick J. Spinal, epidural, and caudal blocks. In: Butterworth J, Mackey D, Wasnick J, editors. Morgan and Mikhail's Clinical anesthesiology. 5th ed. New York: McGraw-Hill Medical; 2013.
58. Weetman C, Allison W. Use of epidural analgesia in post-operative pain management. Nurs Stand 2006;20(44):54–64, quiz 6.
59. Bos E, Haumann J, de Quelerij M, et al. Haematoma and abscess after neuraxial anaesthesia: a review of 647 cases. Br J Anaesth 2018;120(4):693–704.
60. Shaparin N, Gritsenko K, Shapiro D, et al. Timing of neuraxial pain interventions following blood patch for post dural puncture headache. Pain Physician 2014;17(2):119–1125.
61. Karagucuchi M, Hashizume K, Watanabe K, et al. Fluoroscopically guided epidural blood patch in patients with postdural headache after spinal and epidural anesthesia. J Anesth 2011;25(3):450–3.
62. Gnaho A, Dubost C, Gentili M. Ultrasound-guided epidural blood patch. Praticien en Anesthesie Reanimation 2014;18(6):333–40.
63. Bernard H. Patient warming in surgery and the enhanced recover. Br J Nurs 2013;22(6):319–25.
64. Mulry D, Mooney B. Prevention of perioperative hypothermia. WIN 2012;20(2):26–7.
65. Billeter A, Hohmann S, Druen D, et al. Unintentional perioperative hypothermia is associated with severe complications and high mortality in elective operations. Surgery 2014;156(5):1245–52.
66. Joelsson-Alm E Bladder distension: aspects of a healthcare-related injury. Thesis; Department of Clinical Science and Education, Stockholm: Karolinska Institute; 2012.
67. Joelsson-Alm E, Nyman C, Lindholm C, et al. Perioperative bladder distension: a prospective study. Scand J Urol Nephrol 2009;43:58–62.
68. Darrah D, Griebling T, Silverstein J. Postoperative urinary retention. Anesthesiol Clin 2009;27:465–84.
69. Gurka M, Filipp S, DeBoer M. Geographical variation in the prevalence of obesity, metabolic syndrome, and diabetes among US adults. Nutr Diabetes 2018;8(1):1–8.
70. Clifford T. Care of the obese patient undergoing bariatric surgery. In: Odom-Forren J, editor. Perianaesthesia nursing: a critical care approach. St Louis: Elsevier; 2018.
71. Lloret-Linares C, Lopes A, Decleves X, et al. Challenges in the optimisation of post-operative pain management with opioids in obese patients: a literature review. Obes Surg 2013;23(9):1458–75.
72. Mendon J, Pereiraa H, Xaráa D, et al. Obese patients: respiratory complications in the post-anesthesia care unit. Rev Port Pneumol 2014;20(1):12–19.
73. Butterworth J, Mackey D, Wasnick J. Airway management. In: Butterworth J, Mackey D, Wasnick J, editors. Morgan and Mikhail's Clinical anesthesiology. 5th ed. New York: McGraw-Hill Medical; 2013.
74. Drain CB. The respiratory system. In: Odom-Forren J, editor. Drain's Perianaesthesia nursing: a critical care approach. 7th ed. St Louis: Elsevier; 2018.
75. Erb T, von Ungern-Sternberg B, Keller K, et al. The effect of intravenous lidocaine on laryngeal and respiratory reflex responses in anaesthetised children. Anaesthesia 2013;68:13–20.
76. Toukan Y, Gur M, Bentur L. Negative pressure pulmonary edema following choking on a cookie. Pediatr Pulmonol 2016;51(7):E25–7.

77. Ciardulli A, Saccone G, Anastasio H, et al. Less-restrictive food intake during labor in low-risk singleton pregnancies: a systematic review and meta-analysis. Obstet Gynecol 2017;129(3):473–80.
78. Russell IF. The ability of bispectral index to detect intra-operative wakefulness during isoflurane/air anaesthesia, compared with the isolated forearm technique. Anaesthesia 2013;68(10):1010–20.
79. Tasbihgou S, Vogels M, Absalom A. Accidental awareness during general anaesthesia – a narrative review. Anaesthesia 2018;73:112–22.
80. Read M, Maani C, Blackwell S. Dexmedetomidine as a rescue therapy for emergence delirium in adults: a case series. A A Case Rep 2017;9(1):20–3.
81. McGuire J. The incidence of and risk factors for emergence delirium in U.S. military combat veterans. J Perianesth Nurs 2012;27:236–45.
82. Chan T, Bulger T, Stowell K, et al. Evidence of malignant hyperthermia in patients administered triggering agents before malignant hyperthermia susceptibility identified: missed opportunities prior to diagnosis. Anaesth Intensive Care 2017;45(6):707–13.
83. Banek R, Weatherwax J, Spence D, et al. Delayed onset of suspected, malignant hyperthermia during sevoflurane anesthesia in an Afghan trauma patient: a case report. AANA J 2013;81(6):441–5.
84. Hommertzheim R, Steinke E. Malignant hyperthermia – The perioperative nurse's role. AORN J 2006;83(1):151–63.
85. Cain C, Riess M, Gettrust L, et al. Malignant hyperthermia crisis: optimizing patient outcomes through simulation and interdisciplinary collaboration. AORN J 2014;99(2):300–11.
86. Hooper VD. Care of the patient with thermal imbalance. In: Odom-Forren J, editor. Perianesthesia nursing: a critical care approach. 7th ed. St. Louis: Elsevier; 2018.
87. Hirshey Dirksen S, Van Wicklin S, Ledrut Mashman D, et al. Developing effective drills in preparation for a malignant hyperthermia crisis. AORN J 2013;97(3):330–52.
88. Seifert PC, Wahr JA, Pace M, et al. Crisis management of malignant hyperthermia in the OR. AORN J 2014;100(2):189–202, e1.
89. Mitchell-Brown F. Turn down the heat. Nursing 2012;42(5):39–44.
90. Nelson P, Litman R. Malignant hyperthermia in children: an analysis of the North American Malignant Hyperthermia Registry. Anesth Analg 2014;118(2).
91. Clifford T. Length of stay – discharge criteria. J Perianesth Nurs 2014;29(2):159–60.
92. Larach M, Gronert G, Allen G, et al. Clinical manifestation, treatment and complications of malignant hyperthermia in North America from 1987 to 2006. Anesth Analg 2010;110(2):498–507.
93. Mertes P, Florvaag E. Anaphylaxis in the operating theatre. Presse Med 2016;45(9):750–2.
94. Australian and New Zealand Anaesthetic Allergy Group. Australian and New Zealand Anaesthetic Allergy Group/Australian and New Zealand College of Anaesthetists Perioperative Anaphylaxis Management Guidelines. 2016.
95. Florvaag E, Johansson S. The pholcodine case. Cough medicines, IgE sensitisation, and anaphylaxis: a devious connection. World Allergy Organ J 2012;5:73–8.
96. Florvaag E, Johansson S, Irgens A, et al. IgE sensitization to the cough suppressant pholcodine and the effects of its withdrawal from the Norwegian market. Allergy 2011;66:955–60.
97. McAleer P, McNicol L, Rose M. Perioperative anaphylaxis: progress, prevention and pholcodine policy. Anaesth Intensive Care 2017;45(2):147–50.
98. Breen TW, Shapiro T, Glass B, et al. Epidural anesthesia for labor in an ambulatory patient. Anesth Analg 1993;77(5):919–24.
99. Bromage PR. Epidural analgesia. Philadelphia: WB Saunders; 1978.

Chapter 27

Paediatric considerations in critical care

Tina Kendrick, Anne-Sylvie Ramelet

Learning objectives

After reading this chapter, you should be able to:

- consider and anticipate the specific needs of critically ill infants, children and their families
- describe common conditions that lead to critical illness in infants and children
- apply and analyse age-appropriate assessment, monitoring and management of critically ill infants and children
- interpret age-appropriate parameters and care required by critically ill infants and children who require ventilation
- apply psychological and emotional care required by critically ill infants and children, and their families
- consider family as partners in their child's care and decisions.

KEY WORDS

airway obstruction
child development
gastrointestinal tract dysfunction
neurological dysfunction
paediatric intensive care
paediatric nursing
paediatric sepsis
paediatric trauma
paediatric ventilation
shock

Introduction

This chapter focuses on specific considerations for the care of critically ill infants and children experiencing, or at risk of experiencing, common life-threatening conditions. These include respiratory diseases common in the paediatric population, major trauma, shock and sepsis. It is aimed at the critical care nurse who encounters paediatric patients occasionally and, while not designed to meet all the needs of specialist paediatric critical care nurses, it provides a summary of the assessment, monitoring and care required by critically ill children. A systems approach has been used in this chapter for convenience, although paediatrics is a specialty defined by age rather than body systems.

Not only will children experience different patterns of illness and injury in comparison to adults, their behavioural and physiological responses to illness differ. It is important that the child's primary caregiver, who will usually be a parent (the term used throughout this chapter), is included in planning many aspects of care. While members of the critical care team are expert in management of critical illness, parents are generally the experts on their child. They can provide their child's health history and know how best to settle their child in addition to knowing what their 'normal' behaviours are. For these reasons, parents are valuable partners of the team and their concern should never be ignored or downplayed.

Children account for 8.3% of all intensive care unit (ICU) admissions in Australia and New Zealand, representing a figure of 1.8 admissions per 100,000 children, a slightly higher figure than in the UK (1.51/100,000).[1] 50% of these children required mechanical ventilation[1] compared with around 37.5% of adults in intensive care,[2] indicating a slight reduction in children requiring ventilation over the past 2 years.

The age distribution of children in ICUs has remained the same for many years, with 2016 Australian data showing that children under the age of 5 years represent just under 65.2% of admissions, with 56.8% of this age group under 12 months of age and 37.1% of all ICU admissions.[1] Boys make up almost 57.1% of children admitted to ICUs. Prolonged-stay patients have higher paediatric intensive care unit (PICU) mortality rate (up to 18.5%) and poor long-term outcomes with moderate-to-severe disability for 17.2%.[3]

Anatomical and physiological considerations in children

Children require age- and developmentally-appropriate care. An appropriate range of paediatric equipment is required to assess, monitor and treat all ages and sizes of infants and children. General considerations, based on differences between children and adults, are described with specific differences detailed using a systems approach. The terms 'infants' and 'children' are used throughout the remainder of this chapter. 'Infants' are aged up to 12 months, and 'children' are aged between 1 and 16 years. A number of general considerations, based on anatomical and physiological differences from adults, need to be considered for the critically ill child.

- Children and infants have increased surface area-to-volume ratio compared with adults, which leads to increased heat loss and insensible fluid losses, placing them at increased risk of developing hypothermia and dehydration. Providing an environment that maintains the infant and small child's body temperature is essential. Avoid exposing infants and children more than necessary; use warming blankets, open care systems for all newborns and infants under 4 kg, and overhead heaters when exposure is unavoidable. Temperature monitoring is required when using any heating devices to avoid iatrogenic thermal injury.
- Lower glycogen stores and increased metabolic rate predispose infants to hypoglycaemia. There are few standard doses in PICU. Medication doses and fluid requirements are calculated on age and kilograms of body weight. Weight of infants and children should therefore be estimated as accurately as possible. There are several length-based tapes that can be used to estimate weight and they outperform other methods of weight estimation.[4]
- Fluid requirements are based on body weight and aim to ensure adequate hydration while preventing fluid overload. Maintenance intravenous (IV) fluids for infants and young children typically require the addition of glucose. 0.9% sodium chloride is recommended for fluid boluses in paediatric resuscitation.[5,6] Table 27.1 provides a guide for fluid maintenance requirements of children based on body weight.
- Excluding the newborn period, normal values for all blood gas and serum electrolyte levels are the same as adult levels. Creatinine and urea levels will vary with age.

TABLE 27.1
Guide to maintenance fluids in healthy children

For each of the first 10 kg body weight: 100 mL/kg/day (approx. 4 mL/kg/h)
+ for each of the second 10 kg of body weight: 50 mL/kg/day (approx. 2 mL/kg/h)
+ for every subsequent kg of body weight: 20 mL/kg/day (approx. 1 mL/kg/h)

WEIGHT (KG)	ML/H	TOTAL ML/DAY
4	16	400
6	25	600
8	33	800
10	41	1000
12	46	1100
14	50	1200
16	54	1300
18	58	1400
20	62	1500
25	66	1600
30	75	1700
35	70	1800
40	79	1900
50	87	2100

Adapted and updated from Cavari Y, Pitfield AF, Kissoon N. Intravenous maintenance fluids revisited. Pediatr Emerg Care 2013; 29:1225–31.

Practice tip

To estimate weight, use the Broselow tape measure in the following way: 1) place the tape so the red arrow is positioned at the top of the child's head; 2) align the tape parallel to the side of the child, who must be lying in a supine position; 3) extend the legs straight; 4) bend the ankle so the toes are pointing straight up. Look at the weight in the coloured areas directly under the bottom of the foot.

Practice tip

If paediatric oxygen masks are not available, an adult-sized mask, including a partial non-rebreather mask, can be used in an emergency. Place the nose section under the child or infant's chin in the 'upside-down' position.

Central nervous system

Many central nervous system functions, such as locomotion and hand–eye coordination, take months to years to fully develop. Cerebral cortex functions are particularly underdeveloped, with myelination of all major nerve tracts continuing throughout infancy.[7] Consequently, assessment and management priorities will be dictated by the level of neurological maturity of the infant or child. The plasticity inherent in the brain of the infant may compensate for injury more readily than in older children and adults in some circumstances, with other areas of the infant's brain taking over function. Because the eight cranial bones are not yet fused, infants' skulls cope with both birth and ongoing growth, which is greatest in the first 2 years of life. In the first year, the cartilaginous sutures fuse at two points to form the posterolateral fontanelle. The larger anterior fontanelle closes during the second year as bone is laid down. By around 5 years of age, the sutures of the child's skull are completely fused.[8] However, the thinner skull will provide less protection to underlying tissues than the adult skull.

While slow rises in intracranial volume may be accommodated over time in children under 3 years of age, they will usually be accompanied by growing head circumference, making routine measurement of head circumference in children under 3 years of age an important assessment. However, the less rigid skull of the older child will not compensate for acute rises in intracranial volume, and the child will display symptoms of neurological compromise.[9] Normal ranges of intracranial pressure (ICP) and cerebral perfusion pressure (CPP) have not been formally studied in infants and children, but are presumed to be lower than in adults, reaching adult range by adolescence. Values that are commonly used to guide treatment are age-related and are displayed in Table 27.2.

TABLE 27.2
Target cerebral perfusion pressure (CPP) by age

AGE	DESIRABLE MINIMUM CPP
Infants under 1 year	45–50 mmHg
Children 1–10 years	>55 mmHg
Children over 10 years	>65 mmHg

Adapted from Allen BB, Chiu Y, Gerber LM, Ghaja J, Greenfield JP. Age-specific cerebral perfusion pressure thresholds and survival in children and adolescents with severe traumatic brain injury. Pediatr Crit Care Med 2014; 15:62-70.

Cardiovascular system

Infants produce both fetal and adult haemoglobin up to 6 months of age, when levels of fetal haemoglobin (approximately 60–70% to this point) fall rapidly and production of adult haemoglobin predominates[7]. Fetal haemoglobin allows greater amounts of oxygen to be carried for any given PaO_2 in utero and in infancy. Circulating blood volume per kilogram decreases with age; in the infant, circulating volume is approximately 85 mL/kg, with total body water accounting for 70% of body mass, adjusting to the adult values of 65 mL/kg and total body water of 60%.[7] The apex beat is heard at the fourth intercostal space, mid-clavicle and, by around 7 years of age, the left ventricle has grown and the apex beat can be heard at the fifth intercostal space, as in adults. An infant's cardiac output is approximately 500 mL/min, which, relative to body weight, is about twice that of an adult.[8] Heart rate is a major determinant of cardiac output in infants and young children, as there is limited ability to increase stroke volume. Tachycardia is an early sign of distress, but bradycardia is an ominous sign in infants and young children, as they are more dependent on a high heart rate to maintain cardiac output. In infants, bradycardia of 60/min and below requires resuscitation.

Arterial blood pressure should be appropriate for age, weight and clinical condition. Mean arterial pressure is generally used. Monitoring blood pressure using correct cuff sizes is important because incorrect cuff size is a common cause of inaccurate blood pressure readings in children. Diastolic blood pressure is recorded at Korotkoff sound 5 (K5); age-related parameters for mean blood pressure are displayed in Table 27.3.

Paediatric considerations for cardiovascular assessment

Cardiovascular assessment in children includes clinical parameters that are similar to those observed in adults.

TABLE 27.3
Age-related ranges for mean blood pressure

AGE	MEAN BP (MMHG)
Term	40–60
3 months	45–75
6 months	50–90
1 year	50–90
3 years	50–90
7 years	60–90
10 years	60–90
12 years	65–95
14 years	65–95

Adapted from NSW Clinical Excellence Commission. Between the flags standard paediatric observation charts. 2nd ed. Sydney: NSW Health; 2013.

The normal values are, however, age and weight dependent. Indirect evidence of poor systemic perfusion in infants may include:[10]

- feeding difficulties
- abdominal distension
- fluid imbalances
- temperature instability
- hypoglycaemia
- hypocalcaemia
- apnoea.

Neurological changes with poor systemic perfusion in children are irritability, then disorientation or lethargy. Clinical signs of reduced cardiac output, typically seen in shock, are similar to adults.[10] Age-related parameters for heart rate and respiratory rate are displayed in Table 27.4.

Respiratory system

The child's respiratory system, including airways, continues to mature until at least 8 years of age; therefore, the paediatric airway is described and managed differently from the adult's. Structural and mechanical differences predispose infants and young children to respiratory

TABLE 27.4
Age-related heart and respiratory rates

AGE	RESPIRATORY RATE 50TH CENTILE	RESPIRATORY RATE RANGE 10TH–90TH CENTILE	HEART RATE 50TH CENTILE	HEART RATE RANGE 10TH–90TH CENTILE
Birth–<3 months	35	27–47	142	123–165
3–<6 months	31	25–42	135	118–155
6-9 months	29	24–38	131	115–151
10–<12 months	28	23–36	127	111–150
12–<18 months	2	22–33	124	107–149
18–<24 months	25	21-31	120	103–145
2–<3 years	24	20-30	117	99–38
3–< 4 years	24	20–28	111	94–131
4–<6 years	23	20–27	105	88–126
6–<8 years	22	20–26	100	81–122
8–<12 years	20	18–24	94	77–116
12–<15 years	20	16–24	86	69–106
15–<16 years	20	16–23	83	66–103

Adapted from O'Leary F, Hayen A, Lockie, F, Peat J. Defining normal ranges and centiles for heart and respiratory rates in infants and children: a cross-sectional study of patients attending and Australian tertiary hospital paediatric emergency department. Arch Dis Child 2015;100: 733-737.

FIGURE 27.1 Anatomy of the adult airway.

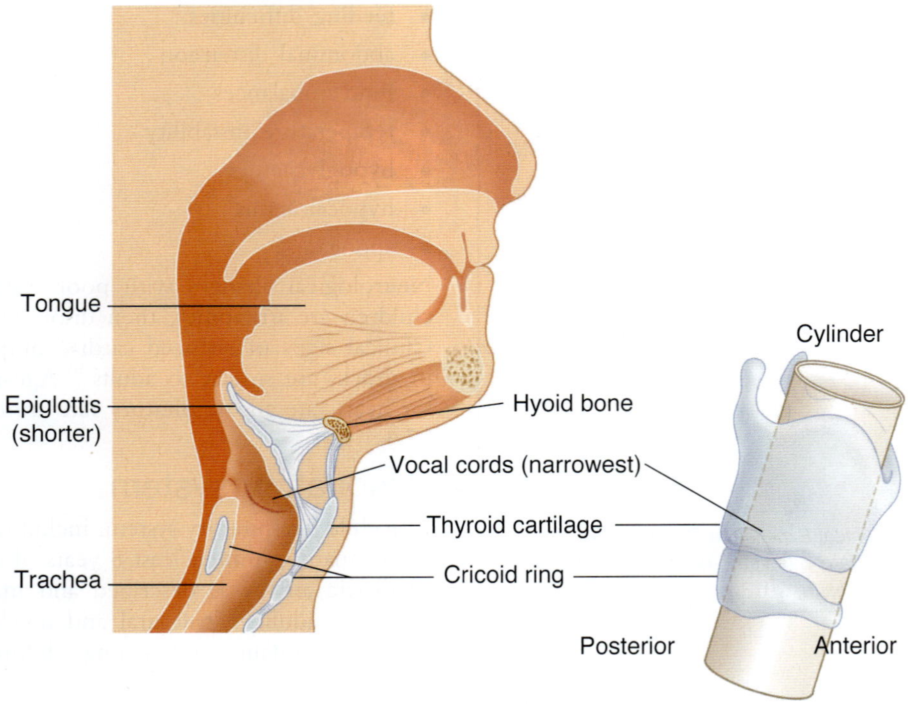

Courtesy Susan Gilbert.

compromise. Respiratory compromise leading to apnoea and even respiratory arrest is a relatively common occurrence in the paediatric population, although specific incidences of occurrence have not been determined.

The newborn's larynx is just one-third of the diameter of the adult larynx.[8] Narrow nasal passages, in combination with being obligatory nose-breathers up to 5–6 months of age, mean that infants may experience respiratory distress if nasal passages become oedematous or contain secretions such as mucus or blood. With the airway of an infant measuring around 6 mm in diameter at the level of the cricoid, obstruction is more likely. The paediatric airway is characterised and differentiated from an adult airway by the following features (Figs 27.1 and 27.2): [8]

- short maxilla and mandible
- large tongue
- floppy epiglottis
- shorter trachea
- more acute angle of airway, particularly notable when attempting to visualise with a laryngoscope
- a more cephalad larynx that moves distally as the neck grows
- a cricoid ring that is the narrowest portion of the airway
- smaller lower airways, less developed with fewer alveoli
- true alveoli not present until 2 months, with full complement developed by around 8 years of age
- little smooth muscle present in airways
- little collateral ventilation in airways, as the pores of Kohn and canals of Lambert are not fully developed until around 3 to 4 years of age.

Paediatric respiratory assessment

The thoracic cavity of infants and children is characterised by a thin chest wall that is highly compliant, with poorly developed intercostal and accessory muscles. The diaphragm is the most important muscle for infants and children in respiration, with abdominal muscles also used. The compliant chest wall prevents generation of high intrathoracic pressures, meaning that infants and young children are unable to significantly increase tidal volume; rather, they increase minute volume by breathing faster. This means that tachypnoea is a normal response to illness in infants and children, and a slowing respiratory rate in children may indicate impending collapse rather than clinical improvement.[11]

Assessing airway patency is important. Talking and crying indicate that the infant or child is maintaining their own airway. Adventitious airway noises in children

FIGURE 27.2 Anatomy of the paediatric airway.

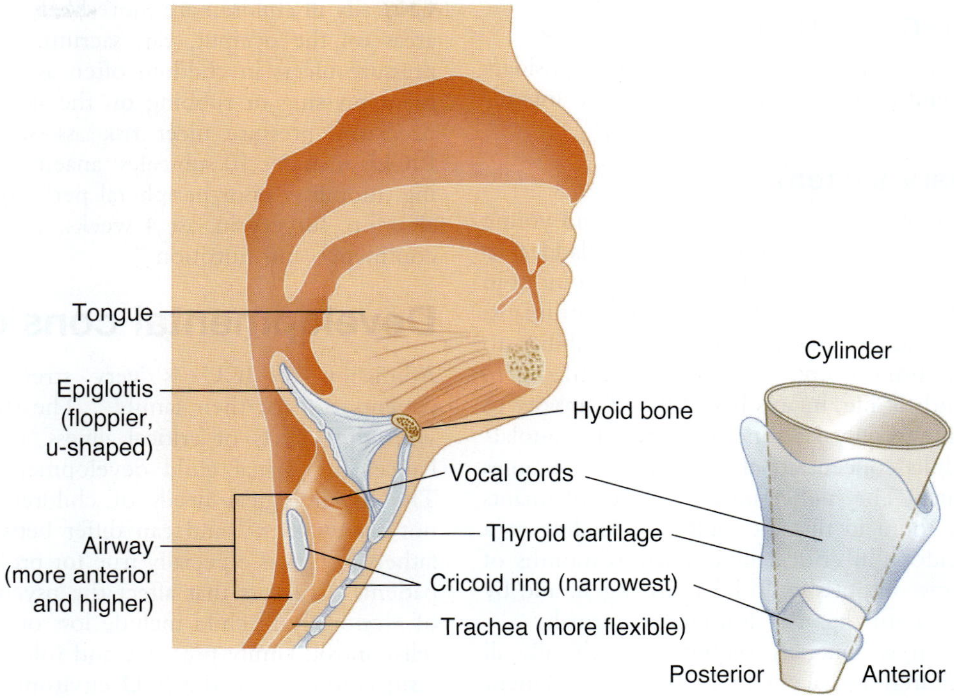

Courtesy Susan Gilbert.

include wheeze, stridor and grunting. In infants, grunting may be heard and is an attempt by the baby to produce positive end-expiratory pressure (PEEP). Infants and children who are grunting, gasping or unconscious need urgent assessment for possible endotracheal intubation.

Other observed signs of respiratory distress in infants and children up to about 8 years old include head bobbing in infants, nasal flaring and paradoxical chest movement observed in several locations on the chest and known as recessions. Recessions can be observed at the costal margin, or subcostal; between the ribs, or intercostal; at the sternum, or sternal; and at the trachea, called tracheal tug. Oral feeding is difficult for infants in moderate-to-severe respiratory distress due to limitations associated with sucking and breathing at the same time. In addition, tachypnoea greater than 60–80 breaths/min may lead to vomiting and aspiration, therefore enteral nutrition may not be possible initially, so consideration of intravenous therapy is essential.[12]

Diagnosis of an upper or lower respiratory illness may be made, using the history of the symptoms from the parent or the child when age-appropriate, in conjunction with physical assessment of the child. Assessment of the rate, rhythm, effort and pattern of breathing according to age as well as colour and agitation should be undertaken. Similar to how heart rate is used to increase cardiac output, children compensate to maintain oxygenation for some time by breathing more rapidly until they become fatigued, when they are likely to become hypoxic and ultimately apnoeic.

Gastrointestinal tract

There are few differences between the child's and adult's gastrointestinal tract (GIT) outside the neonatal period, although a palpable liver below the costal margin is a normal finding. It will be up to 3 cm below the costal margin in normal infants, decreasing to 1 cm by 4–5 years of age, and should no longer be palpable in adolescents. In the neonate, a relative pancreatic amylase deficiency means utilisation of starches is less effective. Fats are also absorbed less well, which is the reason why higher-fat milks such as cow's milk are not ideal for infants. Protein synthesis and storage is, however, enhanced in the neonate.[7]

As the infant liver is not completely mature at birth, gluconeogenesis is deficient, causing low and unstable blood sugar level in the first weeks of life. The infant is therefore reliant on fat stores until normal feeding is established.[8] Formation of plasma proteins and clotting factors are likely to be inadequate in the first weeks of life, thus all newborns in Australasia and many other areas of the world are given vitamin K shortly after birth to prevent bleeding. Blood glucose monitoring and provision of early nutrition are essential aspects of care, especially for infants. Children normally have increased metabolic demands to achieve growth but have fewer energy stores than adults.

Other systems and considerations

The following section presents the paediatric considerations of the genitourinary, musculoskeletal and integumentary systems.

Genitourinary system

The small developing pelvic bones of infants and young children cause adult pelvic organs, such as the bladder, to be located in the lower abdominal cavity. Urine output in children is calculated in mL/kg bodyweight/h. In infants with immature kidney function and limited ability to conserve water, urine output should be 1–2 mL/kg/h. In the first month of life, infants have limited capacity to concentrate urine to only 1.5 times their plasma osmolality, whereas adults concentrate their urine to 3–4 times plasma osmolality. The higher metabolic rate of infants produces twice the acid that an adult will, leading to a tendency to acidosis in critical illness.[7] By 6 months of age, normal urine output should be 1 mL/kg/h, and by adolescence 0.5–1 mL/kg/h is considered normal.

Catheterisation is generally required in critically ill infants and children for accurate hourly measurement of urine output. Where this is not possible, particularly where small sizes of indwelling catheters are not readily available, weighing nappies will provide an interim estimate of urine output. Inserting feeding tubes in place of a urinary catheter is not recommended.

> **Practice tip**
>
> Where catheterisation is not possible, nappies can be weighed to estimate urine output. Use an indelible marker to record the dry weight of a disposable nappy on the nappy itself. This weight is then subtracted from the nappy's wet weight to give an estimate of volume, with 1 g equivalent to 1 mL.

Musculoskeletal system

Children have less developed musculature than adults, with less protection from external forces that collide with the child. Conversely, a child's skeleton is more cartilaginous than adults and therefore more pliable. As a result, rib fractures rarely accompany chest trauma in children whereas lung contusions are common.[13] The skeleton in children changes from less cartilaginous in nature at infancy to complete ossification and adult features during adolescence, so daily calcium requirements increase over childhood and adolescence.[7]

Integumentary system

Infants have a thinner epidermis, dermis and subcutaneous tissue that will continue to mature. This results in a greater susceptibility to absorption of chemicals, injury from adhesive tapes and any shearing force and loss of water and heat, particularly in the newborn period.[8] Critically ill children are more likely to develop pressure areas on the occiput, ear, sacrum, heel or thigh with pressure ulcers in children often associated with equipment pressing or rubbing on the skin. The Glamorgan paediatric pressure ulcer risk assessment scale used in PICUs includes 10 subscales: anaemia, equipment pressing, mobility, poor peripheral perfusion, pyrexia, serum albumin, surgery in last 4 weeks, weight <10th centile, continence and nutrition.[14]

Developmental considerations

Admission to ICU is very stressful for paediatric patients and for their family.[15] The stressors, combined with the effects of critical illness, can lead to disturbances in normal child development and attachment. The psychological needs of children and families are not always met,[16] and can differ between mothers and fathers.[17] This is especially true for prolonged stay PICU patients.[18] Factors that affect the psychosocial wellbeing of a critically ill child include loss of usual routines and self-control; family presence and role; family and friends visit; comfort; and the ICU environment.

Knowledge and understanding of developmental psychology can help nurses assess and plan care for the critically ill child.[19] Identification of internal strengths, external supports and environmental modification can facilitate coping and reduce stress in these children.[20] Parental support is an important coping mechanism of infants and children during periods of stress. Strategies to facilitate coping in children of all ages include:

- facilitating parental presence at all times, including during invasive procedures and resuscitation[21]
- maintaining normal routines and rituals as much as possible, including story reading, bedtime routines and presence of favourite toys
- promoting sleep by reducing environmental noise[22]
- providing appropriate analgesia and sedation
- providing opportunities for play and activities unrelated to treatment.

Erikson's psychosocial theory is helpful for understanding childhood development.[23] Erikson's theory asserts that people experience eight 'psychosocial crisis stages' that significantly affect their development and personality. The first five stages are presented below.

Infants (stage 1)

The first year of life is concerned with developing a sense of trust, laying a foundation for all future relationships.[19] The affective exchanges between infant and the primary caregiver provide a foundation for neurological development and lead to the creation of neural networks (particularly in the right hemisphere) that will influence the infant's personality and relationships with others throughout life.[24] Generally, up to the age of 6 months, infants are able to cope with limited separation from their mothers; however, changes to usual routine create anxiety and stress. From about 6 to 18 months of age separation is the major fear, with changes to usual routine and environment resulting in anxiety. Therefore, critically ill infants require parental presence and maintenance of normal routines, including breastfeeding, as much as is practicable.

Toddlers (stage 2)

The toddler period, between 1 and 3 years of age, is a time for establishing autonomy and independence. Control over bodily functions, increasing ability to communicate, ability to view the self as separate from others and being able to tolerate brief separation from the mother are all developmental characteristics during this period. Toddlers tend to be egocentric in how they view the world, so illness, procedures and separation from parents may be perceived as punishment.[19] Their thinking processes include transduction, animism and ritual. Transductive thinking allows a child to link unrelated objects or events, such as separation and endotracheal suction if suction occurs after the parent leaves the room. Animism attributes lifelike traits to inanimate objects, so the ventilator may become a hissing monster, or monitoring leads may be trying to trap them. Many toddlers have varying levels of ritual or sameness, including always eating off the same plate or a security toy or blanket. Regression, or loss of recently acquired skills such as toileting, may also occur during critical illness, creating further distress. When caring for critically ill toddlers, encourage parental presence and maintain as many of the usual rituals and routines as possible to facilitate coping.

Pre-school children (stage 3)

Children from 3 to 5 years of age fall into the pre-school period of development. It is characterised by discovery, inventiveness, curiosity and the development of culturally and socially acceptable behaviour.[19] Pre-schoolers generally verbalise their needs reasonably well. While thought processes become less ritualistic and negative, pre-school children are still egocentric and experience emerging magical thinking; thus ideas about causality and linking events may be faulty. Fears, both real and imagined, are prevalent during this period.[25] For example, fears of monsters or being hurt may occur. They may also feel guilty as a result of illness. There is, however, greater understanding of the passage of time, so parents can leave the pre-schooler for defined short periods. Hospitalisation remains difficult, but pre-schoolers respond to anticipatory preparation and concrete explanations.[19]

School-age children (stage 4)

Children from 5 to 11 years are usually referred to as being of school age. This period represents a widening of the sphere of influence from parents/family to include the school environment and peers.[25] A transition from egocentric thinking to concrete operations occurs,[25] with children becoming more independent and achievement-oriented for their sense of self-worth. They understand that an object may change its appearance but retains its qualities. For example, if some water is poured into a differently shaped glass, the volume remains the same, even though its appearance has changed. In the ICU, school-aged children may have a distorted or fantasy-laden view, and will need concrete explanations. Sicker children are less able to cope with the ICU environment and are more likely to regress, which can have a significant impact on their sense of self-worth. Modesty and privacy are imperative at this age.[26] Preadolescence occurs between 10 and 11 years, and represents a time of turmoil and emotional upheaval.[25]

Adolescents (stage 5)

Adolescence is considered a time of transition from childhood to adulthood. It is typically represented by children aged 12–18 years, or teenagers. Internal changes relate to emotional upheaval, search for autonomy and transition of thought process from concrete to abstract, so they can imagine possible outcomes without actually experiencing them. External changes relate to physical changes, such as the emergence of secondary sex characteristics, with a related preoccupation with bodily functions and image.[19]

A goal in adolescence is to develop an integrated sense of self, achieved through managing the conflicting demands of family and peers. Peer identity is essential to psychological growth and development, as is the gradual shift from family to peer orientation. Peer groups provide a way for adolescents to self-evaluate and to bolster self-esteem. Adolescents also target authority figures with retaliation and defiance. Conversely, adolescents will seek out non-parental adults, such as a teacher or relative, to obtain approval and acceptance. Existing psychopathology in the adolescent negatively affect parental and peers' relationships as well as autonomy.[27] In this case, it is therefore important to adapt care of the adolescent and the family.

Family issues and consent

When children are admitted to an ICU, the whole family is affected by the hospitalisation. Parents' psychological reactions to their child's life-threatening situation include stress, anxiety and depression, but are not associated to illness type.[28] Around 25% of parents experiencing PICU hospitalisation of their child will show negative psychological outcomes after discharge.[29] Therefore, health professionals need to pay particular attention to parents who present those symptoms. Screening for psychological stress is warranted[30] and specialised psychological support may be required. Those whose child died in hospital need special support from nursing and medical staff[31] with follow-up consultations sometimes used.[32]

'Family-centred care' (FCC) provides a framework for the care of children and their family in hospital and is discussed in Chapter 8. Care based on an equal relationship between family and healthcare professionals, parental presence and participation in care, and open and honest information are recommended.[33] Critically ill children are particularly vulnerable to short- and long-term emotional and psychological sequelae, but parental presence and participation in care can make a difference.[34]

Parents need to feel involved in their child's care, and this includes the need for information, communication, understanding the child's illness and being part of the decision-making process.[35] Particular attention to communication should be paid to parents who are non-native language speakers with regular use of interpreters.[36] A partnership between staff and parents is the ideal situation, but parents often need to be reminded how to maintain the parental role and how they can effectively care for both their child's and their own psychological health.[37] Parents should be allowed to be present during potentially stressful situations such as endotracheal suction, cannulation and resuscitation if they choose to, providing adequate support from a nurse or another designated healthcare worker is given. Being present at the end of their child's life may help parents through their grieving process. Not allowing parents to be present during procedures is a form of paternalism that goes against the principle of patient and family-centred care (PFCC). Parents should, however, be informed of their right to leave if they wish.[38]

Consent and assent

Except for emergency treatment, parents or legal guardians need to consent to all aspects of medical care, including preventive, diagnostic or therapeutic measures for children. The legal age of consent differs between jurisdictions, but is 18 years in major European countries and some states of Australia. However, children also gain legal rights to agree for their own medical treatment, as they get older. Children aged ≥16 years can consent to medical treatment like adults in many countries, such as the UK, Switzerland, Germany, Belgium, France, Quebec, and Spain.[39,40] This is also the case in New South Wales and South Australia, where the legal age for consent is 14 and 16 years, respectively.[41] Informed assent is described as providing permission for procedures when a child is not legally authorised or lacks sufficient understanding to provide informed consent but has the emotional maturity and intellectual capacity to agree to procedures; this usually appears at around 12 years old.[42] To be considered competent, young people must be able to understand the nature of the decision as well as the consequences of making or not making the decision.[42] Whenever possible, it is recommended to obtain the child's assent for treatment or procedures. Children, even when deemed not competent, have the right to be informed and, when appropriate, to be asked for their permission. However, refusal of treatment by a child has no legal bearing when a parent has consented. Importantly, parents may also refuse to consent and, in that case, laws and legal mechanisms for resolving disputes may be used.[42] It should be noted that consenting to medical treatment differs from consenting to research participation; the legislation regarding the latter varies greatly across countries.[41,43]

Pain, sedation, delirium, and withdrawal

Critically ill infants and children are particularly exposed to painful procedures, invasive monitoring devices and treatments that require pain relief and sedation for their comfort. Nevertheless, deep sedation can result in developing delirium and benzodiazepine withdrawal, especially when high dose or prolonged administration is provided.[44] Unrelieved pain and delirium have been associated with short- and long-term physiological and psychological complications, including increased risk of mortality and morbidity.[45] Prevention of procedural pain is important not only to avoid pain-related complications and emotional trauma, but also to facilitate the procedure.[46] Optimal level of sedation varies for each patient and will be dependent on the underlying diagnosis and severity of illness. Evidence-based guidelines for best practice of analgesia and sedation, such as those for adults, have not been yet established for children. But an individualised sedation level targeted to the child's clinical status is recommended to help maintain children in a comfortable state without compromising haemodynamic and respiratory status, while minimising other undesirable effects of analgesics and sedatives.[47] Recent research has shown that targeted sedation that allows the administration of fewer sedatives and analgesics in ventilated children can be delivered safely and produces no long-term adverse outcomes.[48] Some children are difficult to sedate; preliminary work has shown those children require three or more sedation classes, have suspected delirium, and unplanned extubation and devices removal.[49] They often need other sedation adjuvants.[50]

When the provision of analgesics and sedatives is necessary to keep children comfortable, there is a risk for withdrawal of these drugs when given over a prolonged period of time and when receiving several sedative agents.[51] Prevalence rates of withdrawal syndrome in PICU patients receiving benzodiazepines and/or opioids for 5 or more days varied greatly between 20% and 85%, but tended to decrease in the last decade with rates below 50%.[51] New evidence suggests that prevention of withdrawal should be initiated as early as 3 days of treatment with opioids and sedatives.[52]

Delirium is highly prevalent in critically ill children (up to 30%).[53] The risks of developing delirium include administration of psychotropic agents, but are also associated with intellectual disability, mechanical ventilation and some organ failures.[53] Early screening for delirium is key to appropriate interventions and minimising the associated complications.[54]

Assessment

The assessment of pain, sedation, delirium, and withdrawal in children is particularly challenging, because all of these symptoms have overlapping behavioural cues.[55,56] Although several sources should be used to accurately assess pain in non-communicative children,[57] validated observation measurement tools remain the best methods and are recommended for use in daily practice to monitor and document pain intensity, level of sedation, presence of delirium, and signs of withdrawal.[55] To assess pain, the PICU Multidimensional Assessment Pain Scale (PICU-MAPS),[58] the COMFORT behaviour scale, and the modified Faces Legs Activity Cry Consolability (FLACC) scale are recommended. To assess non-pain-related distress, the COMFORT scale, the COMFORT behaviour scale, and the State Behavioural Scale (SBS) are the tools that have the strongest psychometric properties and clinical utility to evaluate the level of sedation in infants and children in ICU.[59,60] The evaluation of withdrawal should be performed when opioids and/or benzodiazepines are administered for 3–5 days and longer, using valid tools, such as the Withdrawal Assessment Tool (WAT-1)[61] and the Sophia Observation withdrawal Symptoms scale.[62] Finally, delirium can be assessed with the Paediatric Confusion Assessment Method-Intensive Care Unit (pCAM-ICU)[63] or the Sophia Observation withdrawal Symptoms-Paediatric Delirium scale (SOS-PD).[62]

Management

Painful procedures should be minimised when possible. Some non-pharmacological therapies have been shown to be beneficial alone in managing mild pain or in combination with drug therapy in infants and young children. These therapies include non-nutritive sucking (e.g. finger or pacifier) with or without sucrose for infants up to 4 months.[64] Recent evidence shows sweet solutions (24–30% sucrose and 25% glucose) have a positive analgesic effect in infants up to 12 months during immunisation and nasogastric tube insertion.[65] After 12 months there is no effect.[66] Music therapy shows decreased pain in postoperative children and can be indicated for clinical use.[67] Distraction can also be used.[68]

Pharmacological treatment in children is challenging as their drug responses differ from adults due to age-related differences. Therefore, pharmacological treatment of pain, sedation, and delirium should be tailored to the child's need and condition. Continuous opioid infusions are used at the lowest effective dose and minimum duration, based on regular pain assessment. Fentanyl boluses are not recommended in neonates as they may cause glottic and chest wall rigidity.[69] Although there is no consensus on sedation management, midazolam remains the first choice sedative for children, and if it fails adjuncts such as the α2-receptor agonists can be used.[46] Dexmedetomidine administered postoperatively in children demonstrated better analgesia and less shivering and agitation in PICU children than routine analgesia and sedation[70] and decreased the need for opioids.[71] The most frequent adverse effects reported with dexmedetomidine have been bradycardia in less than 3% of children[72] and hypotension,[73] but these effects can be resolved with dose reduction and careful monitoring.[73] The use of propofol remains off-label for children under 3 years and should be used with caution in children,[74] as it has been associated with sudden myocardial failure and death.[75] Prolonged infusion and/or short-term high dose are contraindicated.[46] Propofol has an acceptable safety profile and could be used in children for short-term procedural sedation via continuous infusion rather than boluses and under close monitoring of the airways.[74] Indications for the use of neuromuscular blocking agents in children, monitoring of the effects, and management are similar to adult practice.[44]

Upper airway obstruction

Upper airway obstruction is common in infants and young children for two major reasons: the anatomical size of the airway and the frequency of respiratory infections experienced in early childhood. Congenital structural abnormalities and infections as well as foreign body aspiration are the three categories of causes of upper airway obstruction in children.

General description and clinical manifestations

General indicators of respiratory distress will be present in a child suffering from upper airway obstruction. Specific clinical signs of upper airway obstruction in children include:

- a longer inspiratory phase with unchanged expiratory phase
- stridor on inspiration
- chest wall recessions
- lower respiratory rate
- in infants, head bobbing and nasal flaring
- hoarseness
- drooling of saliva.[76]

The aim is to assess the child without causing further distress as a crying, agitated child can further increase the degree of obstruction and work of breathing, leading to respiratory collapse.[77] Observing and listening to the child's symptoms without disturbing them will provide important clues about the level and degree of obstruction the child is experiencing. The Paediatric Assessment Triangle (PAT) is a useful and widely used tool to facilitate rapid assessment of the child's appearance, work of breathing and skin circulation.[78] Stridor indicates obstruction in the upper airway, while wheeze is suggestive of lower airway disease. When stridor is also associated with a barking cough, it is likely to be croup. A softer stridor in a child who looks systemically unwell may indicate epiglottitis. When a previously well child presents with a sudden onset of stridor, it is likely to indicate foreign body aspiration, and eliciting the history of a sudden choking episode can clarify the diagnosis.[76]

Congenital airway abnormalities

Congenital structural abnormalities of the airway are present at birth; depending upon severity of obstruction, they may take hours to months to become apparent. These include laryngomalacia, laryngeal web, tracheomalacia and vascular rings. These infants and children require referral to a specialist paediatric centre for ongoing management and, if they develop respiratory infections, are likely to become compromised much more easily than children with normal airways.

Laryngomalacia is the most common cause of stridor in the newborn period. Stridor is produced by flaccid, soft laryngeal cartilage and aryepiglottic folds that collapse into the glottis on inspiration.[79] An inspiratory stridor, usually high-pitched, will be present. It may be intermittent, may decrease when the patient is placed prone with the neck extended, may increase with agitation and is usually present from birth or the first weeks of life. The infant's cry is usually normal. Feeding problems may be associated with increased respiratory distress. Laryngoscopy confirms the laryngomalacia diagnosis. Treatment is supportive, with only a small proportion of infants requiring airway reconstructive surgery. Where respiratory distress interferes with feeding and growth, a tracheostomy may be indicated.[80]

A laryngeal web is made of membrane that typically spreads between the vocal cords, with an inspiratory stridor present soon after birth. Diagnosis is confirmed by laryngoscopy. Treatment involves lysis in the case of thin membranous webs whereas a tracheostomy may be required for a thicker fibrotic web.[81] Laryngeal webs can also develop after contracting illnesses such as diphtheria or after traumatic injuries in both children and adults.[82]

Tracheomalacia and tracheobronchomalacia involve malformed cartilage rings, with lack of rigidity and an oval shape to the lumen. Secondary tracheomalacia is associated with prolonged intubation and prematurity and presents within the first year of life.[83] Malacias are characterised by wheezing and stridor on expiration, with collapse of the tracheal or bronchial lumen. Diagnosis is confirmed by fluoroscopy and bronchoscopy, which demonstrate tracheal collapse on expiration. As the infant grows, cartilaginous development improves the airway by about 2 years of age, but a number of children will require airway stenting or reconstructive surgery.[83]

Vascular rings result from congenital malformations of the intrathoracic great vessels, resulting in compression of the airways.[84] Infants present with stridor at birth or within the first few weeks of life. Other symptoms include wheezing, cough, cyanosis, recurrent bronchopulmonary infections and dysphagia. Diagnosis may be confirmed by CT scan, MRI scan or endoscopy, which reveals indentations secondary to the extrinsic pressure of the vasculature.[84] The anatomy of the vascular malformations is determined by angiography. Treatment is surgical correction of the vascular malformation.[84]

Monitoring and diagnostics

Initial monitoring and diagnostic studies for infants and children with upper airway obstruction are ideally of a non-invasive nature, to avoid distress. Pulse oximetry is a non-invasive method of monitoring oxygenation. Arterial blood gases are performed only when absolutely necessary, as this may increase the child's distress and thus worsen the degree of obstruction. Continuous ECG monitoring is also indicated.

Lateral airway X-rays are unlikely to be helpful in the setting of croup and epiglottitis and, when they are likely to involve separating the child from a parent, are potentially harmful and not recommended.[85] When there is a less dramatic presentation of the infant or child, or when the diagnosis is not clear, as in the case of an inhaled foreign body, a chest X-ray may be diagnostic.

Practice tip

Close direct observation from a short distance away is an ideal nursing practice, accompanied by non-invasive monitoring. Ideally, the critical care nurse will be positioned to hear the child's stridor. Blood sampling, cannulation and other invasive procedures should be left until the airway has been secured, the child has been anaesthetised or airway obstruction is resolving.

Managing the paediatric airway

A child's airway may be managed in various ways. Simple positioning may be all that is required. Children will often assume an upright sitting position and may become more distressed if placed into the supine position; thus, when possible, the best position for an infant or child with upper airway obstruction may be sitting on their parent's lap. Because of the anatomy and physiology of the respiratory tract, avoid extending the head of infants. Chin-lift and jaw-thrust are useful airway adjuncts in children to maintain an airway and to facilitate use of a bag–valve–mask. It may be necessary to use an oropharyngeal airway or nasopharyngeal airway, laryngeal masks and endotracheal intubation in an unconscious or sedated infant.[77]

Intubation

Intubation may be required to manage airway obstruction.[77] The availability of a paediatric-specific endotracheal tube (ETT) with microcuff and markings to ensure correct placement below the glottis has seen the replacement in many settings of uncuffed ETTs with cuffed ETTs.[77] Cuffed ETTs facilitate ventilation when a leak is undesirable, including in the child with facial and airway burns,[86] for volume ventilation strategies, when using inhaled nitric oxide and for high-frequency ventilatory strategies such as oscillation ventilation. Equipment necessary for paediatric intubation is shown in Fig. 27.3. Fig. 27.4 shows a range of sizes of uncuffed ETTs, 2.5–5.5 mm, that should be available in 0.5-mm increments, while cuffed ETTs are now available in sizes from 3 mm through to 9 mm. Selecting the correct ETT size includes having the recommended tube size plus tubes that are 0.5 mm larger and smaller than calculated. For children over 1 year of age, several formulae exist to calculate appropriate tube sizes, but the age-based and the fifth fingernail width-based predictions of ETT size remain the most commonly used. Table 27.5 provides a guide for ETT sizes, suction catheter size and nasogastric tube size for infants and children.

FIGURE 27.3 Paediatric intubation equipment.

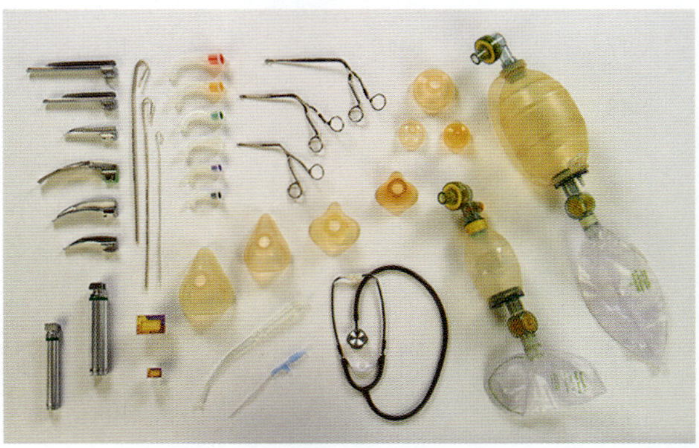

Courtesy Paul de Sensi.

FIGURE 27.4 Range of ETT sizes.

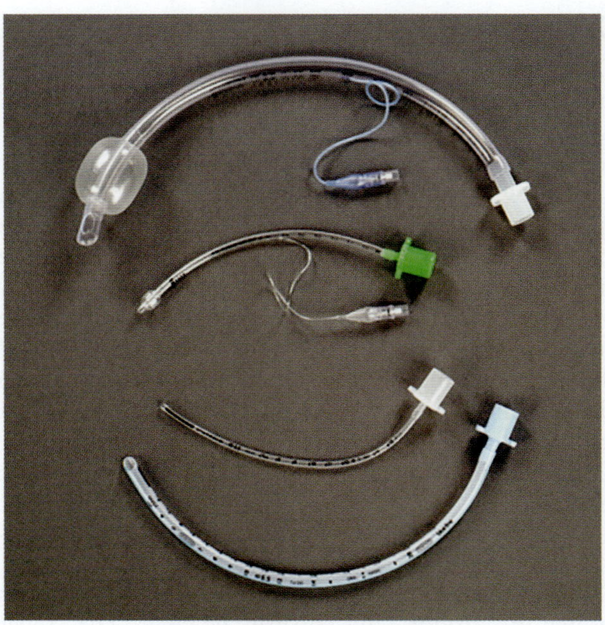

Courtesy Paul de Sensi.

Practice tip

To calculate ETT tube size and length, use the following guides from the 2016 Australian and New Zealand Resuscitation Guidelines:[5]

- for term newborns ≥3 kg: size 3.0 mm or 3.5 mm (uncuffed tubes) or 3.0 mm (cuffed tubes)
- for infant up to 6 months: size 3.5 mm or 4.0 mm (uncuffed tubes) or 3.5 mm (cuffed tubes)
- for infant 7–12 months: size 4.0 mm (uncuffed tubes) or 3.5 mm (cuffed tubes)
- for children over 1 year: uncuffed tubes, size (mm) = age (years)/4 + 4; cuffed tubes, size (mm) = age (years)/4 + 3.5.

Adapted from Australian Resuscitation Council. Techniques in paediatric advanced life support. Guideline 12.6. Melbourne: Australian and New Zealand Resuscitation Councils; 2016.[5]

The most common method used to intubate children is a modified rapid-sequence method. Rapid-sequence intubation is performed when the child may have a full stomach and is at risk of aspiration during intubation.[77] For children, the modification of technique involves bag–mask ventilation prior to intubation to prevent the occurrence of hypoxia.[87] It involves the practically simultaneous administration of sedative medication and a muscle relaxant immediately before intubation.[77] The main advantages of this method include avoidance of hypoxia, good airway visualisation with a relaxed jaw, open immobile vocal cords and elimination of all movement including gagging and coughing.[87] Careful consideration of appropriate induction agents is required for children with haemodynamic instability or a head injury/raised ICP as agents such as thiopentone, propofol and midazolam may not be appropriate or require dose modification.

Specific conditions affecting the upper airway

Bacterial and viral infections of the upper airway are common in children. Croup is the most common infection causing upper airway obstruction in children. Epiglottitis is now rarely seen since in countries

TABLE 27.5
Endotracheal tube (ETT) and nasogastric tube (NG) sizes for infants and children

AGE	WEIGHT (KG)	ETT SIZE (MM ID)	AT GUM (CM)	AT NOSE (CM)	ETT SUCTION CATHETER (FG)	GASTRIC TUBE (FG)
0	>3	2.5	6	7.5	5	6
0	3	3.0	8.5	10.5	6	8
0–3 months	3.5–5	3.5	9	11	6–7	8
3–12 months	6-9	3.5	10	12	6–7	8
1 year	10–12	4.0	11	14	8	8
2 years	13–14	4.5	12	15	8	10
3 years	14–15	4.5	13	16	8	10
4–5 years	16–19	5.0	14	17	8–10	12
6–7 years	20–23	5.5	1	19	10	12
8–9 years	24–29	6.0	16	20	10–12	12
10–11 years	30–37	6.5	17	21	12	14
12–13 years	38–49	7.0	18	22	12-14	16
14+ years	50–60	7.5	19	23	14	16
Adult	>60	8–9	20–21	24–25	14	16

FG = French gauge; ID = internal diameter.
Adapted from Shann F. Drug doses. 17th ed. Parkville: Royal Children's Hospital; 2017.

where immunisation against *Haemophilus influenzae* type b (Hib) was introduced into the immunisation schedule. However, epiglottitis has not disappeared, and it is important to distinguish epiglottitis from croup in order to initiate appropriate management.[88] Other less common infectious causes of upper airway obstruction seen in young children include bacterial tracheitis and retropharyngeal abscess. Diseases thought to have disappeared, such as Lemierre's syndrome and diphtheria, have not been completely eradicated with resurgences seen in recent years in both developed and developing countries.[89]

Infection of the lymphoid tissue around the nodes draining the nasopharynx, sinuses and eustachian tubes may cause pus to accumulate in the retropharyngeal space, leading to a retropharyngeal abscess. Presenting symptoms include history of upper respiratory tract infection (URTI), sore throat, fever, toxic appearance, meningismus, stridor, dysphagia and difficulty handling secretions.[85] Diagnosis is usually made on airway imaging or bronchoscopy.[90] Treatment involves surgical drainage and antibiotic administration. Short-term intubation may be required until swelling has resolved following surgery.

Croup

Croup (laryngotracheobronchitis) is the most common infective cause of upper airway obstruction in children aged 6 months to 6 years, with peak incidence at 2 years.[85,90] Croup is used to describe a set of symptoms caused by acute swelling causing obstruction in the upper airway (larynx, trachea and bronchi) from inflammation and oedema, caused mostly by the parainfluenza or influenza viruses, and is most commonly seen in winter months.[91] Recent advances in croup management have been responsible for a fall in the number of children requiring hospitalisation and intubation. Possible complications of croup include respiratory failure, respiratory arrest, hypoxic damage, secondary bacterial infection, acute pulmonary oedema, persistence or recurrence.[90]

Clinical manifestations

Croup is characterised by a barking or seal-like cough, inspiratory stridor and hoarse voice.[76] The severity of croup is assessed based on increased respiratory rate, increased heart rate, altered mental state, work

TABLE 27.6
Clinical features of croup and epiglottitis

	CROUP	EPIGLOTTITIS
Aetiology	Viral	Bacterial
Age	6 months–3 years	Infancy through adulthood
Onset	Subacute (over days)	Acute (over hours)
Fever	Mild (<38°C)	Severe (>38.5°C)
Cough	Present (often barking or seal-like)	May be present
Drooling	Absent	Present
Activity	Distressed	Lethargic
Colour	Pale/sick	Toxic
Obstruction	+++	+
Stridor	Inspiratory, high-pitched	Expiratory snore
Sore throat	Uncommon	Common
Position	Any	Tripod; sitting up
Course	Gradual worsening or improvement	Unpredictable; fatal if not treated
Season	Autumn–winter	Throughout the year

Adapted from Lee DR, Lee CH, Won YK et al. Clinical characteristics of children and adolescents with croup and epiglottitis who visited 146 Emergency Departments in Korea. Korean Journal of Pediatrics 2015; 58(10): 380-385.

of breathing and stridor. Stridor at rest is noted in moderate-to-severe croup and is often quite loud. If a child's stridor becomes softer but the work of breathing remains increased, it should be treated as an emergency as the obstruction may become more severe. The symptoms of croup are listed and compared with those of epiglottitis in Table 27.6. Diagnosis is made on physical assessment and the history of the illness.

Management

Management of croup depends on the severity of the upper airway obstruction. Children with moderate-to-severe croup should be given face-mask oxygen and allowed to adopt the position that they find most comfortable. Strategies such as positioning the child in a parent's lap and holding the face-mask close to their face may limit their distress and can have beneficial effects on oxygenation.[91]

Practice tip

If placement of a face-mask to deliver oxygen causes increased agitation and worsens respiratory distress in young children, have the parent hold the mask near their child's face and increase the flow rate. 'Blow-over' oxygen will increase oxygen saturation and, as the child settles, mask or nasal cannulae can be reintroduced.

The use of steroids in combination with nebulised adrenaline is responsible for significant improvement of symptoms in children within 12 hours of administration, abating the need for intubation in the vast majority of cases.[91] Nebulised adrenaline is efficacious in reducing airway inflammation, with effects seen within 5 minutes and lasting up to 2 hours. Although nebulisers can be repeated, the benefits lessen with subsequent treatments. Adrenaline does not alter the course of croup.

Epiglottitis

Epiglottitis is inflammation of the epiglottis, frequently involving surrounding structures, with the classic description of a swollen, cherry-red, softened and floppy epiglottis, which tends to fall backwards, obstructing the airway.[85] Obstruction also occurs circumferentially, from the oedematous, inflamed aryepiglottic folds surrounding the larynx. It is typically caused by Hib and, since the introduction of childhood immunisation programs to protect against Hib infection in many countries, the incidence has dropped significantly, with one major Australian centre reporting no cases for the previous 3 years.[76] Hib infection can cause meningitis, septicaemia, septic arthritis and cellulitis as well as epiglottitis. The disease process and development of major symptoms progress rapidly over a few hours and an untreated child may become acutely obstructed. A child will make a full recovery without sequelae if diagnosis and treatment are appropriate and timely. Supraglottitis has emerged in recent times as a more accurate description of a similar range of symptoms as epiglottitis, and has been linked with the herpes virus and other organisms, requiring treatment with aciclovir and vancomycin.[85]

Clinical manifestations

The child with epiglottitis presents looking unwell with a fever and is unable to swallow secretions, drooling saliva and refusing to talk or swallow. The child may maintain an upright position, usually leaning with the head extended, supporting a sitting position with the arms stretched out behind in what is known as the tripod position. Hypoxaemia is usually present. Sudden respiratory arrest followed by cardiac arrest can occur unpredictably. Cardiac arrest is likely to be asystolic in rhythm due to either vagal stimulation or hypoxia secondary to airway obstruction.[90]

Management

The most important aspect in the management of epiglottitis is rapid diagnosis and minimal handling of the child until an airway is in place. Children with epiglottitis require urgent intubation because acute airway obstruction followed by cardiac arrest is a potential hazard. Thus, the aim of nursing management at this time is to keep the child as calm as possible until the airway is secured.[92] The child should be nursed propped up with pillows or on a parent's lap while arrangements are made for intubation. Procedures such as cannulation and examination of the throat should be avoided until the child's airway is secure.[92]

Prophylaxis with antibiotics is required for families and household contacts if there is an infant under 12 months of age and/or a child in the household under the age of 5 years who is not fully immunised.

Foreign body aspiration

Aspiration of a foreign body into the upper airway is another relatively common cause of obstruction in children. Infants tend to swallow food items such as nuts and seeds, while toddler-aged children tend to swallow coins, teeth, etc.[93] An inhaled foreign body is likely to have a rapid onset with no previous symptoms. Sometimes the diagnosis is missed for days, weeks or even months, and the child's symptoms may be non-specific, such as a cough with or without blood-stained sputum.[93]

Clinical manifestations

Sudden onset of coughing, gagging and an audible stridor in a previously well infant or child is suggestive of an inhaled foreign body.[93] However, an accurate history – such as a recent coughing or choking episode – is the most sensitive factor in making a diagnosis of inhaled foreign body.

Patient management

Management will depend on the location and level of the aspirated foreign body, as it may have lodged in the pharynx, oesophagus, larynx, trachea or bronchial tree. Coughing is encouraged for mild airway obstruction.[5] Up to five back blows may be successful in dislodging the foreign body, which may be followed by up to five chest thrusts and back blows. Direct laryngoscopy and removal of a foreign body using Magill forceps may be required for an acute episode when back blows and chest thrusts have been unsuccessful. When the foreign body has lodged below the carina, diagnosis and definitive treatment usually consist of removal of the foreign body via a bronchoscopy under general anaesthesia.[93]

The child experiencing lower airway disease

Lower airway disease in children is a common reason for admission to ICU. Infants under 12 months usually present with bronchiolitis or pneumonia. Asthma is more common in older children, but infants nearing 12 months of age may develop asthma and there is often confusion between bronchiolitis and asthma at this age. Bronchiolitis and asthma are commonly seen in children, and the management of each condition is discussed below. National and worldwide clinical guidelines for these conditions have been developed and are continually updated.[94]

Bronchiolitis

Viral bronchiolitis in infancy is characterised by obstruction of the small airways, resulting in air trapping and respiratory distress in infants less than 12 months of age. It is the commonest severe respiratory infection in infancy, although the course is usually mild to moderate and is self-limiting, usually requiring no treatment.[95] Severe infection represents less than 5% of all cases and is usually associated with prematurity, infants under 3 months of age or congenital heart disease. Respiratory syncytial virus (RSV) causes 90% of bronchiolitis cases.[96] Other causative agents are parainfluenza virus types 1, 2 and 3, influenza B, adenovirus types 1, 2 and 5 and *Mycoplasma*. RSV invades the epithelial cells of the bronchioles, spreading via the creation of syncytia, which are created when host cell membranes fuse with neighbouring cells. This results in destruction of the epithelium and patches of necrosis. The debris associated with epithelial shedding and mucus production lead to small airway blockage and the clinical features of bronchiolitis.

In temperate regions of Australia and New Zealand most cases of bronchiolitis occur between late autumn and early spring, with a clear epidemic peak during the winter months and sporadic cases throughout the year.[97] There is a paradoxical relationship between the incidence of RSV and other viral pathogens causing bronchiolitis. RSV epidemics occur when other respiratory pathogen epidemics are diminishing, and vice versa.[97] The incidence rate of RSV infection varies between continents with rates as high as 225 per 1000 infants in the USA and 869/1000 infants in Australia.[98] The estimated RSV-related hospitalisation rates in Australia ranged from 2.2 to 4.5 per 1000/children less than 5 years of age to 8.7 to 17.4 per 1000/infants, with a total annual direct healthcare cost estimated to be up to 50 million dollars.[98] These figures are fairly similar to European figures.[99] There is also a higher incidence of bronchiolitis among indigenous children and those living in the most deprived regions of Australasia, and more severe illness when compared to non-indigenous people.[95] Younger children with one or more comorbidities are at higher risk of complications. RSV infection occurs throughout the year, with an annual peak during the winter months.[100]

When bronchiolitis occurs, the highest risk for hospitalisation is infants under 6 months of age, those with exposure to tobacco smoke and underlying conditions such as congenital heart disease, chronic lung and neurological diseases, prematurity and low socioeconomic group. Severe disease, requiring admission to a PICU, is associated with prematurity, particularly in infants with chronic lung disease or a history of ventilation in the newborn period and congenital heart disease.[101]

Clinical manifestations

Bronchiolitis is a clinical diagnosis, and non-isolation of a causative viral agent does not exclude the diagnosis. The typical clinical features of bronchiolitis start with URTI symptoms such as rhinorrhoea (runny nose) and an irritating cough. Within 3 days, the infant develops tachypnoea and respiratory distress, which may be mild, moderate or severe. An expiratory wheeze is often present with auscultation revealing fine to coarse widespread crackles. Fever is present in approximately 50% of infants. In very young, premature or low birth weight infants, apnoea is often the presenting symptom, which then develops into severe respiratory distress.[101] The clinical course of bronchiolitis is usually 7–10 days; however, the effects of severe illness may last much longer. Those who had tachypnoea of ≥70 breaths/min on the first of admission and low birth weight infants are at high risk for ICU admission.[102] Indications for intensive care admission are determined by local escalation policies but should be early.[101]

Assessment and patient management

A thorough history and assessment are important to provide a foundation for management of bronchiolitis. The infant with acute bronchiolitis requires hourly observations with continuous cardiorespiratory and oxygen saturation monitoring. Management of infants presenting with bronchiolitis depends on whether the symptoms are mild, moderate or severe, but it is largely supportive, as most pharmacological treatments are unproven. In general, management centres on supporting therapies, such as hydration and nutrition, oxygenation and maintaining vigilance for signs of deterioration that may require 1) respiratory support starting with heated humidified high-flow oxygen/air via nasal cannulae (HHFNC) in presence of hypoxia (oxygen saturation less than 92%) and moderate-to-severe recessions, 2) continuous positive airway pressure (CPAP), 3) in severe cases, mechanical ventilation. Prone positioning and minimising the impact of procedures on the infant are also important, especially in infants less than 3 months. Chest physiotherapy is not indicated and nasal suction not routinely recommended.[101]

Asthma

Asthma is a lower respiratory tract disease characterised by mucosal and immune system dysfunction. There is a complex interaction between bronchial wall cells, inflammatory mediators and the nervous system. The chronic inflammatory process causes narrowing of bronchial airways, thus obstructing airflow. This leads to episodes of wheezing, breathlessness and chest tightening that are usually reversible. In an acute episode of asthma, wheeze is not always audible, but a prolonged expiratory phase is an early sign.[103]

Development of childhood asthma results from a combination of genetic, environmental and socioeconomic risk factors.[104,105] Increasing prevalence of asthma over the past 20–30 years may be linked to a higher incidence of genetic predisposition, independent of environmental factors. Some studies identify links between asthma and various regions of the human genome, but the linkages are not consistent. Certain racial groups, such as African Americans, when compared with Americans of European origin, are also more likely to develop asthma and have complications, particularly those traditionally from tropical regions.[106] Once asthma has developed, there are triggers that may precipitate an attack. These include viral illnesses, particularly respiratory viruses; tobacco smoke exposure; house dust mites; exercise; pet hair; food; and environmental allergens.

Asthma is one of the commonest paediatric presentations to emergency departments (EDs)[107] and its worldwide prevalence is growing with differences among various populations.[108–110] The current disease rate is 8.4% in the USA,[111] 29.7% in the UK,[112] and 31% in Australia.[112]

Clinical manifestations

ICU admission is required when children present with respiratory failure due to an asthma exacerbation. These exacerbations can be due to viral infection and allergy, seasonal patterns, bacterial infections, environmental factors as well as psychological factors such as stress.[113] Other factors such as obesity and genetic predisposition may be important in reacting to beta$_2$ agonist therapy. These children exhibit clinical features associated with respiratory distress. Pulsus paradoxus, a phenomenon of palpable changes in blood pressure that occur with respirations, may also be present and can also be noted on plethysmography. Arterial blood gas analysis usually reveals a mild respiratory alkalosis and hypoxaemia initially; however, more severe asthma may show combined respiratory and metabolic acidosis and hypercapnia as the child tires and is unable to eliminate carbon dioxide.[113]

Patient assessment and management

Assessment of asthma severity is based on criteria such as the degree of respiratory failure as evidenced by cyanosis, length of sentences between breaths, retractions and hypoxia, as well as level of consciousness. There are many scores available to assist in determining the severity of asthma, including the National Asthma Campaign guidelines, the Pulmonary Index Score, the Respiratory Failure Score and the Modified Dyspnoea Scale. Whatever method is used, assessments should be frequent and response to treatment recorded. Severe asthma that worsens and/or does not respond to treatment warrants admission to a PICU.[108]

The broad aims of management of severe asthma include maintaining oxygenation, rapid bronchodilation and treating any cardiovascular compromise.[114] In children with severe asthma, hypoxaemia results from ventilation/perfusion (V/Q) mismatch due to lower airway obstruction, in addition to hypoventilation, hypercarbia and pulmonary vasoconstriction related to acidosis. Hypoxaemia can result in further bronchoconstriction, hypotension, systemically-reduced oxygen availability, increased myocardial oxygen consumption and neurological symptoms such as agitation, confusion or decreased level of consciousness. Bronchodilators may worsen hypoxaemia through worsening V/Q mismatch or bronchoconstriction, due to the hyperosmolarity of the nebulised solution. In addition, rapid changes to the compliance of the airways together with hyperexpanded lungs may result in airway collapse. Oxygen delivery is achieved by high-flow oxygen mask with a reservoir bag. All nebuliser therapy should be oxygen-driven. However, if hypoxaemia persists despite maximal bronchodilator therapy and oxygen administration, mask CPAP may be considered.

$Beta_2$ agonists, anticholinergics and steroids form the foundation of acute severe asthma management, but for children over 40 kg and those who have reached puberty it may be more appropriate to administer IV adrenaline. $Beta_2$ agonists act by relaxing bronchial smooth muscle, improving mucociliary transport and inhibiting mediator release. In severe to life-threatening asthma, inhaled short-acting $beta_2$ agonists combined with an anticholinergic is recommended as it improves lung function, decreases side effects such as nausea and tremor and decreases the risk for hospital admission if treated early.[115] Adverse effects of $beta_2$ agonist administration include hypokalaemia, tachycardia, tremors, agitation and hyperglycaemia. Mild lactic acidosis may also occur. Intravenous salbutamol infusion should be considered when there is severe, life-threatening asthma refractory to inhaled treatment. Inhaled salbutamol may be discontinued once IV infusion has commenced but should be re-established before ceasing the infusion. In acute severe episodes, salbutamol is usually given every 20 minutes; if there is little response, continuous nebuliser therapy may be required. In this instance, a feeding tube is inserted into the nebuliser and the chamber replenished as it empties. Anticholinergics, in combination with $beta_2$ agonists, improve lung function by augmenting the action of $beta_2$ agonists, blocking irritant receptors and bronchodilation of larger airways.[116]

Corticosteroids decrease airway inflammation, enhancing the effects of $beta_2$ agonists, and reduce mucus production. Oral and intravenous methods of administration are similarly efficacious. The effects of systemic steroids are apparent within 3–4 hours of administration, with maximal benefit achieved within 6–12 hours. There is little evidence to support giving inhaled steroids during an acute episode.

Magnesium sulfate promotes smooth muscle relaxation by inhibiting uptake of calcium. Intravenous magnesium sulfate has demonstrated efficacy in acute severe asthma, but there is modest benefit of inhaled magnesium sulfate combined with a $beta_2$ agonist.[117]

Intravenous aminophylline has shown some benefit with regard to improved lung function in severe asthma that is unresponsive to inhaled bronchodilators and steroids with the benefit being dependent of appropriate dosage. However, the currently recommended dosage may not be optimum in terms of safety and efficacy.[118] It is a bronchodilator, improving diaphragmatic contractility, and a central respiratory stimulant. However, the narrow therapeutic window and side effects of induced nausea and/or vomiting represent a non-negligible risk of complication; thus its use should be limited to managing asthma not responsive to other agents.[119]

Ventilation may be required when there is profound hypoxaemia, severe muscle fatigue or decreased level of consciousness.[103] However, as asthmatic children are at higher risk of complications such as barotrauma and air trapping, there is a higher risk of death associated with ventilation in this group of patients. Non-invasive positive pressure ventilation (NIV) is the first choice with some evidence that it rapidly corrects gas exchange abnormalities and assists with respiratory muscle fatigue.[120] The contraindications for NIV include: cardiac/respiratory arrest, severe encephalopathy, haemodynamic instability, facial surgery/deformity, high risk for aspiration, non-respiratory organ failure, severe upper gastrointestinal bleeding, unstable arrhythmia and upper airway obstruction.

Intubation may be necessary when signs of deterioration are present, such as elevated carbon dioxide levels, exhaustion, alteration of mental status, haemodynamic instability and refractory hypoxaemia.[121] Because of high airway pressures, a cuffed ETT should be used.

Children with acute asthma may have a raised metabolic rate and increased insensible losses, together with reduced oral intake. With increased intrathoracic pressure due to air trapping, even mild dehydration may compromise cardiac output. Therefore, adequate fluid replacement is necessary. In addition, pulmonary secretions will thicken and plug the airways if fluid intake is inadequate. IV fluids should be provided until the child's condition and oral intake improve.[121]

Nursing the ventilated child

Principals of mechanical ventilation were covered in Chapter 15. Issues such as gastric decompression, adequate analgesia and sedation and undertaking steps to prevent accidental extubation are similar to those for adults. Specific considerations for ventilating infants and children include:

- Most children are oxygenated before, during and after suctioning with 100% O_2. The child's clinical status is monitored throughout the procedure.

- Heated humidification is recommended in children although there is no evidence to suggest any type of humidification, but children have limited respiratory reserve and are prone to airway blockage.[122,123]
- Equipment should fit the child's size to avoid unnecessary dead space.
- Endotracheal suctioning should only be performed when clinically indicated[124] and normal saline instillation is not recommended.[122]
- To prevent iatrogenic atelectasis, the suction catheter size should be less than or equal to two-thirds the internal diameter of the ETT.
- Cuffed and uncuffed endotracheal tubes are appropriate for infants.[125] Suction pressure should be limited to 60 mmHg (8 kPa) for infants, and up to 200 mmHg (27 kPa) for adolescents. A suction regulator is useful to monitor the amount of applied negative pressure, as too much can result in atelectasis. As the patient's position affects ETT cuff pressure, it should be monitored and adjusted as required after mobilisation.
- Restraints may be required to limit the movement of the child, with the aim of preventing accidental extubation rather than maintaining the child in an immobile state. Restraints may be physical, such as arm boards or hand ties; or chemical, such as sedation.

A newly developed decision-making tool can assist nurses to make appropriate decisions to perform an endotracheal suction in children.[126]

Modes of ventilation

There are many modes of ventilation (see Chapter 15). This section includes information specifically related to paediatric ventilation. As with adults, arterial blood gases should be taken about 15–20 minutes after initiating mechanical ventilation.

Volume ventilation in children

Typically, volume ventilation is not used in infants under 5 kg due to the small tidal volumes, which risk being lost in the distensible tubing and leaking around the ETT. In addition, most volume ventilators do not have a constant fresh gas flow, so the infant must work harder to trigger a breath. Some of the newer models of ventilator have attempted to overcome these problems. Steps in beginning volume ventilation for a child are as follows:[122]

1. Set a tidal volume of 5 to 8 mL/kg. This is a protective lung strategy approach and can be increased if needed to a maximum of 9 to 10 mL/kg.
2. Set the rate at 20 breaths/min. This is lower than physiological for infants, but the slightly larger tidal volumes will compensate.
3. Set the FiO_2 at <0.6 and titrate according to oxygen saturation and blood gases.
4. Set the PEEP at 5 cmH_2O. This is slightly higher than physiological.
5. Set the trigger sensitive enough to allow the infant or child to trigger a breath without working too hard. If a continuous fresh gas flow is available, this is preferable. If autocycling occurs, decrease the trigger-setting sensitivity gradually until the autocycling stops.

Pressure ventilation in children

The pressure ventilation mode is most commonly used in infants weighing less than 5 kg or with children who have a large leak around an uncuffed ETT. Steps in beginning pressure ventilation for a child are as follows and should be based on arterial blood gases:[127]

1. set the peak inspiratory pressure (PIP) at 18–20 cmH_2O
2. set the PEEP at 4–6 cmH_2O (rarely exceeds 7 cmH_2O)
3. set the rate at 20 breaths/min
4. set the FiO_2 at <0.6 and titrate according to oxygen saturation and blood gases
5. set the trigger sensitivity to trigger a breath without auto-triggering. Most pressure ventilators have a constant fresh gas flow, which allows the child to breathe spontaneously without increased effort.

Non-invasive ventilation

NIV refers to ventilatory support without an artificial airway in the trachea (see Chapter 15). As in adults, NIV may be used to reduce the need for intubation in children. Its use in children is safe and effective for the treatment of acute respiratory failure, acute viral bronchiolitis, neuromuscular disease, and asthma.[36]

High-frequency oscillatory ventilation

High-frequency oscillatory ventilation (HFOV) uses supraphysiological ventilatory rates and tidal volumes less than anatomical dead space to accomplish gas exchange. Typical ventilator rates are 3–15 Hz or 180–600 breaths/min (1 Hz = 60 breaths). HFOV is primarily used in managing infants and children with diffuse alveolar or interstitial disease requiring high peak distending pressures. Goals include maximising alveolar recruitment, minimising barotrauma and providing adequate alveolar gas exchange.[128]

HFOV is delivered primarily by a specialised ventilator that uses a diaphragm piston unit to actively move gas into and out of the lung, and a non-compliant breathing circuit. A major difference between HFOV and other forms of ventilation is that there is active expiration with oscillation versus passive expiration for conventional ventilation. Unlike conventional ventilation, which uses bulk flow to deliver gas to the lungs, using smaller than dead space tidal volumes utilises the mechanisms of pendelluft, Taylor dispersion, asymmetrical velocity profiles, cardiogenic mixing and, to a very limited extent, bulk flow.[129] These are all terms used to describe the distribution of gas when rapid rates and tiny volumes are used.

Ventilation is dependent on amplitude (a determinant of tidal volume) much more than rate. With oscillation ventilation, lowering frequency (Hz) improves CO_2 removal. This is thought to occur because the oscillating diaphragm is able to move through a greater distance, thus increasing tidal volume by providing more inspiratory time and a longer expiratory time.

The principal determinants of oxygenation are the same as those for conventional ventilation. Therefore, as with conventional ventilation, the alveoli must be open and prevented from collapsing if hypoxaemia is to be corrected. HFOV theoretically achieves this through delivering a high mean airway pressure without imposing a large tidal volume, but there is insufficient evidence to promote its use over conventional ventilation in children and infants.[129]

Extracorporeal membrane oxygenation

Extracorporeal membrane oxygenation (ECMO) is an alternative method of providing ventilatory and/or cardiac support.[130,131] When used to support ventilation, ECMO allows the lungs to rest and heal. Ventilation settings are reduced to minimal to minimise the iatrogenic effects of positive pressure. There are two main methods of ECMO – venovenous and venoarterial. In venovenous ECMO, large-bore cannulas are placed in large veins, such as the internal jugular or femoral, but with the latter there is a risk for lower limb ischaemia. The use of distal arterial perfusion in paediatric femoral venoarterial ECMO reduces the risk of limb ischaemia.[132,133] Alternative placement of cannulas for venoarterial ECMO after heart surgery is the right atrium and aorta. Venoarterial ECMO allows support of both circulation and ventilation. Essentially, blood is drained from the 'venous' line, pumped through a membrane to oxygenate the blood and remove CO_2, then returned through a filter via the 'arterial' cannula.[134]

Children are considered for ECMO if they have potentially reversible lung or cardiac injury, or shock that has not responded to conventional therapies. Contraindications include irreversible brain or central nervous system (CNS) injury, immunodeficiency or severe coagulopathy. Long-term outcomes are mitigated with lower quality of life in ECMO patients compared with other PICU patients and mortality remains high.[135] ECMO centres need to maintain their competence by performing the procedure often.

The child experiencing shock

A detailed description of shock is given in Chapter 21, with specific paediatric considerations addressed here. Hypovolaemic and septic shock (also termed distributive shock) are the most common types of shock in children. Cardiogenic shock is rare and is seen mainly after open-heart surgery and severe myocarditis or untreated shock. The infant with an undiagnosed congenital heart defect, in particular lesions that rely on the ductus arteriosus – known as duct-dependent lesions – can present in shock in the first weeks of life as the duct closes.[136] As infants and children presenting in hypovolaemic shock are likely to respond to fluid resuscitation alone, they may not require transfer to a specialist paediatric centre. However, children presenting with septic shock or cardiogenic shock will require transfer to a specialist paediatric centre for ongoing management, and early contact should be made to initiate goal-directed therapy as soon as possible. Those children who do not respond to fluid volume alone will require invasive haemodynamic monitoring and possible pharmacological intervention. The development of shock in a hypovolaemic child is considered to indicate losses of at least 30 mL/kg.[137]

Sepsis is the leading cause of death in infants and children worldwide.[138-140] The mortality rate for septic shock in Westernised, resource-rich countries is reported to be between 2% and 10%.[139] In resource-limited countries, the mortality rate can be as high as 50%.[139] Over 26% of PICU deaths in the study period were attributable to sepsis.[141] A recent multicentre point prevalence study of sepsis in infants and children conducted across 128 sites and 26 countries found sepsis prevalence ranged from 6% to 23%, with mortality ranging from 11% to 40%.[142] Sepsis remains a significant source of critical illness and mortality globally in infants and children with some evidence suggesting the rate in children is increasing.[143] Early detection of sepsis in children has been the focus in many countries since failure to recognise is directly correlated with mortality. Recent work on inpatient sepsis deaths in children has revealed a similar trajectory as adults, namely refractory shock leading to death in the first 3 days, with later deaths after 3 days attributable to multiple organ dysfunction, and neurological and respiratory failure following treatment withdrawal.[138]

Causes of septic shock in infants and children are often different from those in adolescents and adults. The commonest infecting organisms are often age-related and are listed in Table 27.7. Meningococcal sepsis remains the leading cause of septic shock in developed countries such as Australia and New Zealand. In resource-limited countries, leading causes of fatal sepsis include diarrhoeal diseases, malaria, lower respiratory tract infections and HIV/AIDS.[140]

Clinical manifestations

There are many similarities between children and adults in the clinical manifestations of shock (see Chapter 21). When published it is likely that the new set of guidelines for children will similarly remove the emphasis previously placed on inflammatory response and incorporate organ dysfunction markers specific to children.[144]

TABLE 27.7
Organisms causing sepsis in newborns, infants and children

AGE GROUP	COMMON ORGANISMS CAUSING SEPSIS
Newborns	Group B beta-haemolytic streptococci Enterobacteriaceae (such as *E. coli*) *Listeria monocytogenes* Herpes simplex virus *Staphylococcus aureus* *Neisseria meningitidis*
Infants	*Haemophilus influenzae* *Streptococcus pneumoniae* *Staphylococcus aureus* *Neisseria meningitidis*
Children	*Staphylococcus aureus* *Neisseria meningitidis* *Streptococcus pneumoniae* Enterobacteriaceae

Adapted from Maloney PM. Sepsis and septic shock. Emerg Med Clin North Am 2013; 31:583–600.

Clinical features of evolving septic shock in children include:

- abnormal temperature (high or low)
- altered neurological status
- altered perfusion – peripheral vasodilatation *or* vasoconstriction with delayed capillary refill time – before hypotension develops
- abnormal white cell count – may be low in the neonate and then high in all other paediatric age groups
- abnormal heart rate and respiratory rate for age (high or low)
- two of the following: unexplained metabolic acidosis, increased lactate, oliguria.[145,146]

Systemic hypotension is not necessary to make the diagnosis of septic shock in children. Tachycardia in the absence of fever is a more reliable sign than hypotension, as up to 25% of the child's circulating volume may be lost before hypotension occurs. Hypotension is thus a late sign in children and may indicate late decompensated shock, particularly following fluid delivery.[10]

One other specific factor for children that is not relevant in the adult population is a higher risk of sepsis in preterm infants and in infants with cardiac defects or chronic lung disease.[140]

Patient assessment and diagnostics

Assessment of the child with shock is based on clinical assessment, with less reliance on biochemical testing than in adult shock.[137] Ideally, shock should be diagnosed before hypotension occurs. Hypothermia or hyperthermia and altered neurological status, which provides information about cardiac output and perfusion pressure, and peripheral vasodilation (warm shock) or vasoconstriction with capillary refill >3 seconds (cold shock) are clinical signs of shock in children.[146]

Careful respiratory and cardiovascular assessment is required, as described in this chapter and Chapters 11 and 13. Monitoring of children experiencing shock is the same as for adults (see Chapter 21). It consists of continuous monitoring of heart rate, SvO_2 saturation, quality of peripheral pulses, capillary refill, level of consciousness, temperature and urine output as indirect measures of cardiac output as well as serial blood gas, lactate and electrolyte analysis, with potential to use stroke index in children once admitted to ICU.[10,145,147] Diagnosis of septic shock can be difficult in children. When present, non-blanching rash is a specific sign of meningococcal septicaemia.[146]

> **Practice tip**
>
> As rash may be less visible in dark-skinned children, check soles of feet, palms of hands and conjunctivae in those children.

A certain proportion of children will present with non-specific symptoms or signs of infection, such as fever, vomiting, lethargy, irritability or headache and the conditions may be difficult to distinguish from other less serious infections.[146] Laboratory testing of samples of blood, urine, stool, sputum, cerebrospinal fluid and any obvious wounds or lesions is standard practice in adults and children.

Patient management

Early recognition of shock, institution of appropriate goal-directed therapy and targeting the causative agent remain the mainstays of managing septic shock in children as in adults. Goal-directed therapies such as oxygen therapy, fluid resuscitation, maintenance of acceptable blood pressure and institution of pharmacological treatment and other supportive treatments to achieve therapeutic goals are practised in managing shock in children, and are linked to better outcomes.[148,149]

Large amounts of fluid may be required by children despite peripheral oedema or absence of overt fluid loss.[146] The large African study – the FEAST trial[150] – demonstrated that fluid bolus of up to 40 mL/kg increased mortality in African children with sepsis; however, this study was conducted in a resource-poor environment without access to inotropes, biochemical testing or mechanical ventilation. Where access to inotropes and mechanical ventilation is readily available, aggressive fluid resuscitation and antibiotics in the first hour before development of hypotension is linked to improved mortality in children with hypovolaemic and septic shock.[138,142] Intravascular access in children can be difficult and umbilical venous access in newborns and intraosseous access in children can be used before the placement of central lines.[145] The use of the EZ-IO® (Vidacare Corporation, Texas) paediatric intraosseous needle set and driver system has become common in practice.[151] Other kinds of manually inserted intraosseous needles are available. Regardless of type, intraosseous needles all allow rapid access to the intramedullary capillary network, facilitating delivery of fluids, drugs and blood products. The preferred site in infants and children is the proximal tibia, 2–3 cm below the tibial tuberosity.[151] Once sited, a syringe must be attached to aspirate and ascertain correct placement. Fluid boluses can then be given via syringe into the intramedullary space with the aim of restoring circulating volume, which will in turn facilitate venous access with improvement of peripheral perfusion.[137]

Similarly to adults, after appropriate volume resuscitation has been given and symptoms of shock are not resolving or hypotension is developing, inotropes and vasopressors are recommended. Inotropic drugs that are recommended in children include adrenaline, noradrenaline and dopamine.[145] Vasodilators, including sodium nitroprusside or nitroglycerine, are used to recruit microcirculation; type III phosphodiesterase inhibitors are used to improve cardiac contractility.[145] ECMO may also be considered for a child who appears to be developing irreversible shock.[145] The use of hydrocortisone has not been shown to change outcome in septic shock in children.[142]

The child experiencing acute neurological dysfunction

There are many reasons why an infant or child can present with an acute episode of neurological dysfunction. Common presentations to an ICU include meningitis,[152] encephalitis, seizures and encephalopathy (see also Chapter 17). Assessment and recognition of the clinical features and management of the various causes of neurological dysfunction in children are the keys to achieving good outcomes.

Neurological assessment

To assess a child's level of consciousness, several different scales can be used. The Glasgow Coma Scale (GCS) is commonly used, but the Glasgow Coma motor subscore is more appropriate for children.[153] Another reliable scale is the Paediatric Full Outline of Unresponsiveness (FOUR) score; it includes four parameters (eye response, motor response, pupil reflexes and breathing) rated on a 0–4 scale, giving a possible score of between 0 (completely unresponsive) and 16.[154] The FOUR score and the GCS are both able to predict in-hospital morbidity and poor outcome at the end of hospitalisation.

Other neurological assessment parameters include:

- Pupils – assess size, reaction and symmetry.
- Posture – abnormal flexion posturing, often referred to as decorticate posturing, is a flexion response of the arms with either flexion or extension of the legs, while abnormal extension posturing, often referred to as decerebrate posturing, is an extension response of all limbs, where arms rotate externally. Both abnormal flexion and extension posturing in a previously normal child may indicate raised intracranial pressure.
- Meningism – this is indicated by neck stiffness in a child ≥ 2 years of age, and full/bulging fontanelle in an infant.[155]

Seizures

Seizures are covered in Chapter 17. The various aetiologies of seizures in children include febrile convulsions, CNS infection such as meningitis or encephalitis, metabolic imbalances, drugs, trauma or epilepsy. Seizures in children are common, with about 4–10% of children having an unprovoked seizure without recurrence.[156] Children between the ages of 6 months and 6 years are more likely to develop seizures.[157] Children, particularly those under 5 years, are at higher risk, as the developing brain has a lower threshold for seizures. Febrile convulsions occur in 2–5% of children, commonly between the ages of 6 months and 5 years.[158] They can be simple (generalised and occurs once in a 24-hour period and lasts less than 15 minutes), complex (focal or localised to a specific part of the body, lasts 15–30 min or recurrence within a 24-hour period), or develop into status epilepticus (lasts more than 30 min).

Patient management

Management of the paediatric patient with seizures is similar to management of the adult and include early administration of midazolam and barbiturate if first line treatment is refractory (see Chapter 17); there are, however, some specific paediatric considerations.

The paediatric patient who is suffering seizures is more susceptible than an adult to hypoglycaemia. Hypoglycaemia may lead to secondary brain injury during and after seizures. Blood sugar levels should always be checked in children suffering from seizures and intravenous fluids containing glucose administered.[159]

The care of the seizing or post-ictal child is generally supportive, and includes monitoring for signs of ongoing seizures, administration of appropriate anticonvulsants and regular assessment of neurological function. In young infants, seizures may be difficult to determine and may include stiffening, staring and lip smacking rather than obvious clonic activity. Continuous electroencephalogram monitoring is thus recommended for non-convulsive seizures.[160]

Meningitis

Meningitis is an acute inflammation of the meninges that usually develops over 1–2 days. A fulminant form of meningitis caused *Neisseria meningitidis*, responsible for invasive meningococcal disease (IMD) may develop over several hours. Organisms causing bacterial meningitis vary by age group. In infants under 3 months of age, group b *Streptococcus*, *E. coli*, *Streptococcus pneumoniae* and *Listeria* are the most likely agents. In children over 3 months of age meningococcus, *Haemophilus influenzae* type b and *Streptococcus pneumoniae* are more common.[161] The commonest causes of viral meningitis in infants and children include herpes simplex virus and the enteroviruses.[162] Tuberculous meningitis, while still rare, is becoming more common, particularly in immigrant families or those with recent travel to affected areas.[163] Bacterial meningitis continues to have a poorer outcome than other forms of meningitis, despite advances in therapy.[164]

Incidence

Data on the incidence of meningitis are limited to the major bacterial types, particularly for infants and children over 2 months of age. Hib, meningococcal and pneumococcal infections are all notifiable.[165] The mortality rate of meningococcal meningitis in children is lower than in adults (5% in children under 5 years of age versus 12%), and increases with associated sepsis.[166] However, IMD-related complications, such as hearing loss, occur more in children than in adults (21% versus 15%).[155] Neuropsychological follow-up of these children is recommended to better address their neuro-development.[167]

Meningococcus is the main cause of meningitis in children. Specific strains tend to be prevalent in different regions of the world, with serogroups (A, B, C, W-135, Y, and X) the current strains responsible for almost all invasive meningococcal disease.[155] In Europe, the Americas and Oceania serogroups B, C and Y have caused most cases. Serogroup A has been associated with the highest incidence (up to 1000 per 100,000 cases), causing large outbreaks of meningococcal disease in sub-Saharan Africa and Asia while serogroups W-135 and X have emerged more recently and are responsible for major disease outbreaks in sub-Saharan Africa.[168] Available vaccines differ around the world based on the prevalent strains, so recent overseas travel and place of vaccination should be obtained in the history.

The incidence of invasive pneumococcal disease has significantly dropped in developed regions such as Europe, North America and Australia since the introduction of routine vaccination and decreased hospitalisation rate.[169,170] An estimated prevalence rate of 11% is reported worldwide.[170] Risk factors include extreme prematurity, chronic lung disease, trisomy 21 (Down syndrome), diabetes and immunocompromised children.[170] Clinical manifestations or symptoms vary with the age of the child, duration of the illness and history of antibiotic use for the current illness. Case fatality ratio fluctuates between regions of the world (8.3%),[171] but is higher in developing countries (12–80%) with higher rates in low- and middle-income countries.[172]

Patient management

Initial management of the infant or child with meningitis includes assessment and management of the airway, breathing, circulation and disability. Rapid antibiotic therapy is recommended[173] and likely to decrease case fatality.[163] Once the initial resuscitation has been completed, consideration should be given to correcting any biochemical abnormalities. In particular, blood sugar level should be checked and corrected in the early management phase. Once meningitis is suspected, a lumbar puncture (LP) is generally performed to confirm diagnosis,[174] but if the child is haemodynamically unstable or has ongoing seizures, problems with ventilation or signs of raised intracranial pressure, the LP should be delayed and blood cultures obtained.[175]

Steroid use in meningitis has some benefit in reducing morbidity in adults,[161] but there is no evidence for its recommendation in children.[176] Infants and children with meningitis require intensive care management when there is a reduced level of consciousness, respiratory and/or circulatory compromise. The broad aims of management are to support ventilation and circulation, while preventing secondary brain injury. Regular assessment and monitoring of associated risks such as seizures, syndrome of inappropriate antidiuretic hormone secretion (SIADH) or cerebral salt wasting and sepsis is essential.

Encephalitis

The most common type of encephalitis in children is acute viral encephalitis, and the most common causative agent is herpes simplex virus (HSV).[177] Left untreated, HSV is almost uniformly fatal, with over half of survivors experiencing significant long-term morbidity. Other causes of encephalitis in children include:[178]

- enteroviruses (e.g. enterovirus 71, coxsackievirus, polio and echovirus)
- varicella zoster virus
- Epstein–Barr virus
- cytomegalovirus
- adenovirus
- rubella
- measles
- Murray Valley encephalitis (MVE) virus
- Kunjin virus.

Worldwide, the incidence of acute encephalitis ranges between 3.5 and 16 cases per 100,000 children.[178] Children under 1 year of age are at higher risk of developing encephalitis. Other risk factors include immune dysfunction and exposure to risk animals, or specific geographic location.

Encephalitis symptoms are similar to meningitis, but often with a much slower onset. Progressively worsening headache, fever and decreased level of consciousness or behavioural changes characterise encephalitis. Focal neurological signs and seizures may indicate involvement of the meninges or spinal cord.[179]

Patient management

Prompt administration of acyclovir is warranted to all patients with clinical symptoms suggesting encephalitis due to high mortality and morbidity rates.[165] Other viruses are also treated with acyclovir. Intensive care management involves supporting ventilation and managing neurological complications such as seizures and cerebral oedema. If the child is unconscious on presentation, the disease course will be more severe.

Gastrointestinal and renal considerations in children

Many critically ill infants and children are also at risk of developing complications involving the gastrointestinal tract (GIT). Although primary acute renal failure (ARF) is relatively rare in critically ill children, the incidence of renal impairment secondary to the underlying illness is recognised increasingly in children, although a paucity of prospective studies remains problematic. When paediatric Risk, Injury, Failure, Loss and End-stage kidney disease (pRIFLE) criteria were applied in a recent large study, the total incidence of kidney injury in PICU was 25%.[180] Identified risk factors for kidney injury include exposure to nephrotoxic medications and ECMO, organ dysfunction, and following congenital cardiac surgery.[181] Both primary and acquired kidney injury in children are associated with increased length of stay and increased mortality.[180] Consequently, continuous renal replacement therapy (CRRT) should be considered earlier in management than has previously been the case and is discussed in Chapter 18. Critically ill children experiencing, or at risk of developing, ARF will benefit from prompt transfer to a specialty PICU.

The child's GIT will need protection from developing ulceration and bleeding in critical illness. A potentially fatal complication, stress ulceration and bleeding, with studied incidence of around 10% in critically ill children.[182] Clinically significant bleeding causing haemodynamic instability or requiring transfusion is reported in about 1.6% of children in PICU.[182,183] The same treatments can be used in both children and adults, with no one agent, dose or regimen standing out as better for minimising bleeding and ulceration or leading to fewer complications such as pneumonia.[183]

Nutritional considerations

The aims of nutrition in critically ill children are two-fold. First, children are at particular risk of malnutrition because they are growing and have greater energy requirements for their weight and less storage capacity than adults. Second, children are at particular risk of developing protein–calorie malnutrition, which can lead to immunodysfunction, increased risk of infections, morbidity and death in those children with organ dysfunction.[184] Morbidity and mortality is also associated with malnutrition in children admitted to PICU – both obesity and underweight children are at risk.[185] Nutritional status should be monitored while in PICU.

Nutrition is also important in maintaining gut mucosa integrity, preventing the development of hypo- and hyperglycaemia, assisting with maintenance of immune function and in modulating the immune response as well as providing energy.[186] One barrier to achieving adequate nutrition for critically ill children is the fluid restrictions that are routine practice in the ICU, and both use of feeding protocol and liberalising fluids where possible to maximise enteral nutrition should be considered.[184]

When caring for critically ill infants and children, nutrition to support growth needs to be considered. Ideally, enteral feeding of critically ill children should commence within 12–24 hours of admission to ICU, but may not be achievable until the child is transferred to a specialist centre.[186] It may not be appropriate to commence feeds if the child requires transfer, surgery or intubation. A dietician should be consulted to advise on appropriate enteral feeding formulas for children, in addition to organising caloric supplementation of feeds.[187] The dietician can advise on handling of human milk while in hospital for breastfeeding mothers, who will need to express milk when the infant is not yet feeding orally or to provide milk for tube feeding. In addition, dieticians can assess the child's energy requirements and the amount of feed required to meet needs, as both under- and over-feeding have been identified as issues in PICU.[184,186,187] The evidence for additives in enteral feeding is not clear-cut in children, and therefore routine supplementation for critically ill infants and children is not common practice.

Intravenous therapy for children

Until enteral feeding is established, critically ill infants and children will require maintenance IV fluids. Traditionally, hypotonic fluids – fluids containing a concentration of sodium lower than normal serum sodium – have been administered as maintenance fluids. These included the hypotonic formulation of 0.225% sodium chloride with 3.75% glucose. In recent years this formulation has largely been replaced with 0.9% sodium chloride and 5% glucose, as iatrogenic hyponatraemia has been well documented.[188,189] Newborn infants up to around 1 month of age will require a higher concentration of glucose, up to 10%. It has been common paediatric practice to use only 500-mL IV bags in children for safety reasons; however, 1 L bags are more common. In the modern era across Westernised countries, use of volumetric IV pumps and burettes has been standard paediatric practice, although changes to larger volumes of IV formulations for children will need to be closely monitored.

The use of hypotonic fluids is under review in many countries, with increased level of monitoring of weight and serum electrolytes recommended. Hypotonic fluids are implicated in hospital-acquired hyponatraemia,[188] and, for critically ill children, the capacity to excrete additional free water is often impaired. In addition, some common conditions seen in the ICU increase secretion of antidiuretic hormone (ADH), including pain, nausea and infections of the CNS, the GIT, the lung and post-surgery, thus promoting the retention of water.[190] The risk of developing cerebral oedema is increased in children, who also have increased body tissue water content, and studies indicate that there is an increased risk of developing acute hyponatraemia leading to seizures.[190]

Infants and children generally require added glucose in IV fluids. In infants under 3 months, glucose concentration is increased to at least 5% and up to 10%. The addition of potassium chloride into maintenance fluids is common, particularly in fasting children, and requires serial monitoring of serum potassium. For fluid resuscitation in infants and children, the use of glucose-containing IV fluids is contraindicated, and 0.9% sodium chloride is the resuscitation fluid of choice across the life span, including in the delivery suite for newborn fluid resuscitation.[5]

Glucose control in children

The predisposition to hypoglycaemia in children has meant that aggressive treatment of hyperglycaemia is not commonplace in critically ill children. The most recently published study demonstrated no difference in outcome, but an increase in hypoglycaemia in the tight glucose control arm.[191] Hypoglycaemia is documented to occur more frequently in two groups of non-diabetic children: those requiring mechanical ventilation and those requiring inotropic support.[191] Monitoring for hypoglycaemia continues to be an important assessment parameter, particularly in sicker children who require ventilatory support, inotropic support and where enteral feeding may be contraindicated. Hypoglycaemia may be an indicator of worsening organ function; therefore, further research needs to focus on the safety of insulin therapy in the non-diabetic critically ill child before aggressive routine management of hyperglycaemia can be recommended.[191]

Liver disease in children

Acute liver failure is relatively rare in children. It arises as a primary problem in children from countries where viral hepatitis is endemic and is associated with paracetamol overdose and chronic liver disorders, toxins, autoimmune disease, malignancies, vascular and biliary tree malformations as well as unidentified causes.[192] Chapter 20 contains more detail on liver function and dysfunction. There are varying severities and forms of liver failure. Infants and children experiencing fulminant hepatic failure and hepatic encephalopathy, regardless of underlying cause, are critically ill, and require transfer to a specialist PICU for ongoing management and possible liver transplantation. Mortality rate is strongly linked with the development of cerebral oedema and intracranial hypertension, and is reported to be as high as 50% where cerebral oedema occurs.[192,193] Promising work with auxiliary liver transplant of partial livers and preservation of the native liver in predominantly older children with infections or toxic causes of their liver failure has demonstrated recovery of the native liver and subsequent withdrawal of immunosuppressive agents.[194] Many critically ill infants and children are at risk of developing some degree of liver dysfunction; therefore, liver function of all critically ill children requires careful monitoring and management. Clinical manifestations and management of infants and children with liver failure are similar to those of adults.

Paediatric trauma

Trauma is a leading cause of death in children and young adults in all developed countries; in the developing world it is second only to deaths from infections.[195] The approach to management of trauma in children is the same as in adults. See Chapter 24 for details on trauma systems and trauma management. While there has been some evidence from North America that specialist paediatric trauma centres produce better outcomes for children suffering traumatic injuries,[196] the largely spread-out and relatively small population distribution in Australia, New Zealand and many other countries means that children will often need to be treated initially in adult settings.

Incidence and patterns of injury in children

Injury is a leading cause of death in all children aged over 1 year across the world and represents half of all deaths in children 10 years and older.[140] Road traffic injuries, burns and drowning kill many children, while falls represent the leading cause of presentation to EDs worldwide.[140] Children who live in regional and rural areas have increased rates of traumatic injuries and deaths from trauma, as do children from lower socioeconomic backgrounds with crowded living conditions.[140]

Injury patterns in children differ from adults, with traumatic brain injury, blunt trauma and more diffuse injuries more common in children. There is a bimodal injury pattern associated with age, with peak incidence occurring in children aged 1–4 years and a second peak during adolescence and young adulthood, reflecting the different activities associated with each group.[197] Infants and young children have a decreased sense of danger and reduced ability to protect themselves, while adolescents have increased exposure to higher risk activities in conjunction with exposure to alcohol, drugs and motor vehicles.[198] Time of day and seasonal factors play a role in childhood injury, with children more likely to be injured at the end of the school day, and during summer months, when the incidence of drowning increases.[199]

Injury-related deaths in children are highest in the transport deaths category, followed by falls, drowning and assault.[200] Motor vehicle accidents involving children as passengers, pedestrians or cyclists are the commonest cause of injury in Australian children, with driveway injuries involving four-wheel drive or light commercial vehicles more likely to be fatal.[200] Trauma associated with the use of all-terrain vehicles, such as quad bikes, is becoming increasingly common, particularly in rural areas.[197] For children under 14, falling from one level to another, such as falling from a window, was the most common form of falls-related injury.[197]

Drowning is another leading cause of death in children, with more than 175,000 children drowning worldwide each year. In low- and middle-income countries across Southeast Asia and the Western Pacific, higher rates of drowning occur and are associated with playing, washing or collecting water from open bodies of water.[140] In wealthier countries such as Australia, drownings in this age group peak in the summer months and are more likely to be linked to recreational activities.[199] Boys outnumber girls in this category, with two-thirds being boys. Children under 5 years are more likely to drown by falling into backyard swimming pools while older children (5–14 years) drown during planned swimming or other recreational activities in pools and open waterways such as dams and rivers.[199]

In Europe, drowning is associated with lower socio-economic status, with a greater number of deaths by drowning in the poorer parts of eastern and southern Europe when compared to western Europe. In developing countries, the incidence remains high, with deaths from drowning having the highest mortality rate for all.[201]

Risk factors

The kinetic forces involved in injury are associated with a more diffuse injury pattern and a greater incidence of multiple trauma in children, as more of the child's body is subjected to the traumatic forces.[202] Children generally have less subcutaneous fat and musculature, providing less protection to the liver, kidneys and spleen, leading to a higher incidence of lung contusions and abdominal trauma.[202] In addition, the relatively large head size of the infant, particularly, and the child leads to a high incidence of head injury.

Primary survey and resuscitation

Initial stabilisation of children who have experienced a traumatic injury is likely to have occurred in the field. Once at the hospital, the primary survey is conducted to assess for, detect and stabilise the child with life-threatening injuries. Undertaking a primary survey and resuscitation uses the same structured approach in children and adults. Chapters 23 and 24 cover emergency presentations and trauma management; however, specific paediatric considerations are highlighted below.

Children sustaining trauma to the head, just as adults, are managed with cervical spine precautions including a collar, until the spine has been radiologically and clinically cleared.[198] A selection of paediatric collars should be available and the measuring guide used to ensure a good fit. As the collar can cause neck flexion in infants and small children, the child's torso may need to be elevated with a folded blanket to maintain a neutral neck position. The head and neck are usually immobilised, with head blocks (e.g. rolled towels) placed either side of the head to maintain in-line stabilisation and tapes applied to the forehead and chin to prevent movement. The combative, uncooperative child will not tolerate this, and the actions are likely to increase the child's agitation and movement. Critical care nurses can position themselves to maintain in-line stabilisation while talking and soothing the child or ideally, where parents are present, seek their assistance to console their child. Specific paediatric trauma boards are available that are designed to maintain the child's head in a neutral position.

Fluid resuscitation is a controversial area of practice in paediatric trauma, where therapies have been generally less well-studied than in adults. However, in a haemodynamically unstable child, including the child with a traumatic brain injury at risk of secondary brain injury from hypotension, fluid resuscitation of 20 mL/kg of 0.9% saline followed by reassessment is recommended.[203] If more than 20 mL/kg is required, immediate surgical assessment for bleeding is indicated.[203]

Exposure of the child, with temperature control, is necessary to assess the child completely for injuries. As hypothermia can develop quickly in children, overhead heating sources and blankets are ideally used to keep the child warm. Hypothermia in trauma patients is associated with increased risk for coagulopathy and mortality, as in adults, so providing warmth is essential paediatric trauma nursing care.[204] The child's right to privacy and dignity should also be considered and exposure minimised.

Secondary survey

Undertaking a secondary survey is similar in children and adults and is described in Chapters 23 and 24. Specific paediatric considerations are highlighted below.

In children, particularly those under 1 year of age, if injuries and the accompanying history do not seem to match, non-accidental injury should be considered and noted. History should be obtained from the child where possible, from any witnesses to the accident and from ambulance officers if they attended. Parents or caregivers will provide details of the child's past medical history, any medications and any known allergies.

Specific conditions

Specific injuries that are seen in children are discussed briefly under the headings of traumatic brain injury, chest trauma and abdominal trauma. Obtaining an accurate history of the accident or events leading up to an injury is useful in determining the type of injuries that children may have sustained. Regardless of aetiology, where a child has been involved in a motor vehicle accident (MVA) or sustained a fall, there are likely to be multiple injuries and the situation should be treated as such until other injuries have been considered and excluded.[204]

Traumatic brain injury

Traumatic brain injury (TBI) is a leading cause of deaths and injury worldwide in children. In developing regions such as Asia and Africa, TBI is increasing as the population has increased access to motor vehicles.[140] In Australia and other developed economies, children experience the greatest number of head injuries of any age group.[200,201] TBI is often associated with MVAs where the child is a vehicle occupant, a pedestrian or a cyclist, and with falls and with near-drowning. TBI is described in detail in Chapter 17.

Around 8% of all children aged 1–15 years of age who died in Australasian ICUs had sustained a TBI.[1] Age and gender are the most significant risk factors for TBI, with peak incidence in the 0–4-years group and in males.[1] Other factors to consider in children are the increased tendency of the immature brain of children to experience disruption of the blood–brain barrier and, unlike adults, for an increased cerebral blood volume to lead to cerebral oedema due to higher brain water content.[205]

While there are guidelines for the management of paediatric brain injury,[206] the limitations of the paediatric research evidence that underpinned these has led to reliance on less rigorous studies and ongoing dependence on extrapolation from adult research evidence.[206] Since the clinical manifestations of TBI in children are very similar to those in adults, management is also very similar. The practice of hyperventilation should be avoided as it is associated with regional cerebral ischaemia.[206]

The modified GCS for children has previously been described in this text and should be used when assessing children. Indications for ICP monitoring in children include all infants and children with a severe head injury, which equates to a GCS score of 8 or below that persists following adequate cardiopulmonary resuscitation, and those children who present with abnormal motor posturing and hypotension.[207] Combined with invasive haemodynamic monitoring, targeted therapy to manage both ICP and CPP remains an important part of treatment. While thresholds for treating intracranial hypertension in children have not been studied, it has been known since the 1980s that prolonged intracranial hypertension or high ICP levels will worsen outcome. An ICP of 20 mmHg is considered high in children, with 15 mmHg considered high in infants. ICPs of these values are the usual cut-off points and are likely to be treated with the aim of lowering ICP while maintaining an adequate CPP.[206] Target CPP for various ages is listed in Table 27.2.

Diagnosis

Diagnostic techniques and clinical management of children with TBI mirror those in adults[207] (see Chapter 17). The smaller size of children means that diagnostics such as mixed cerebral venous saturation and direct brain oxygen saturation are not yet common practice in paediatrics, with further work required in direct brain oxygen saturation to determine utility and parameters.[208] A high index of suspicion for spinal injuries in paediatric TBI should be maintained, as spinal cord injury without radiological abnormality on plain X-rays and CT is a feature of paediatric spinal injury.[205] While CT scans are available in more centres than MRI, they involve radiation exposure to the young spine and miss spinal cord injury without radiological abnormality. MRI is more effective in determining spinal cord injury than CT and, as it involves no radiation exposure, is the investigation of choice to determine spinal injury in children.[209]

Treatment

Several of the therapies used in the treatment of the child with severe head injury are controversial, as they have lacked sufficient scientific rigour when the small number of studies were evaluated to make clear, high quality evidence recommendations.[206] Essentially, treatment of TBI in children is identical to adult management: minimising intracranial hypertension and maintaining optimal CPP while preventing secondary injury from hypoxia, hypercarbia and hypotension while reducing the risk of iatrogenesis from treatment. Hyperglycaemia that persists beyond 48 hours of the injury is associated with a worse outcome;[210] however, studies are yet to be undertaken to determine whether this is modifiable with the use of tight glycaemic control.

Hypothermia has not been shown to make a difference in outcome in children with hypoxic-ischaemic brain injury as it has in newborns and adults. Moderate hypothermia (temperature maintained at 32–34°C) has been studied in children with disappointing results;[211] therefore, the current recommendation is that hypothermia should not be used for children with severe head injury outside of clinical trials.[211]

The use of decompressive craniectomy for early indications of herniation, ongoing neurological deterioration or development of intractable intracranial hypertension that is refractory to maximal treatment such as drainage of cerebrospinal fluid (CSF), sedation and barbiturates has demonstrated improved mortality and functional recovery for some children.[212]

Outcomes from TBI in children are associated with the severity of the initial injury and the presence and control of secondary brain injury, as in adults. Hypotension and hypoxia prior to hospital admission are strongly linked to mortality and poor functional outcome, with some emerging evidence that hypertension and hyperglycaemia in the first 24 hours may also predict poor outcomes at 1-year post-injury.[206]

Chest trauma

Thoracic injuries in children rarely occur in isolation with traumatic injuries and are often accompanied by head and neck injuries. There is some evidence that thoracic injuries are indicative of a more severe injury; they have been associated with higher mortality.[203] Injury to the heart and great vessels, in particular, is associated with higher mortality. The combination of head injury and thoracic injury is also known to have higher mortality. Most chest injuries in children are sustained as a consequence of MVAs.[13,213] The pattern of injury in children is predominantly one of blunt trauma. Lung contusions are the commonest thoracic injury seen in children.[13,213] As the ribcage is much more compliant in children, ribs are rarely broken, but they can damage underlying structures such as the lungs, so pulmonary contusions, pneumothorax and haemothorax are often seen. The clinical manifestations, approach to assessment, monitoring and management of children sustaining thoracic trauma are similar to those in adults, and are discussed in Chapter 24. Children with thoracic injuries are generally managed in a specialist trauma centre equipped to manage children.[203,213]

Abdominal trauma

Abdominal trauma in children is a leading cause of death when combined with head injury.[202] Blunt trauma from MVAs is the most common mechanism of injury, but bicycle handlebars may also inflict a significant injury. The liver and spleen are the most commonly injured organs in abdominal trauma and can usually be managed non-surgically in the haemodynamically stable child.[214] The abdominal organs are relatively large in children, with less musculature and a more compliant ribcage, meaning that there can be injury to underlying organs with no apparent external injury.[215] Blunt trauma is common, while penetrating injury is less common, resulting from gunshot and stab wounds. These injuries are associated with older children and adolescents, though a thinner body wall may result in greater underlying organ damage, particularly if the flank is penetrated.[215]

During the primary survey, the child's abdomen should be exposed and may reveal signs such as bruising from bicycle handles, tyre marks, abrasions or contusions. Abdominal distension is a less reliable sign in children, as distension may be from air that is swallowed from pain and crying. However, as in adults, the primary survey may not include the abdomen if other immediately life-threatening injuries are present, such as thoracic and/or head injuries. These injuries will take precedence, so it may not be until the secondary survey can be undertaken that abdominal injuries are considered. The monitoring and management of children sustaining abdominal trauma is very similar to that of adults,[214] and is discussed in Chapter 24.

More judicious use of CT scanning in paediatric centres is practised in relation to increased concerns regarding radiation exposure to children.[216] Clinical indicators will determine the need for a CT scan of the abdomen, including children with multiple injuries, gross haematuria with a minor injury and children with haemodynamic instability with no obvious source of blood loss. Diagnostic peritoneal lavage has largely ceased with the increasing utility of, and expertise with, focused ultrasound in trauma (FAST) in EDs, and the recent development of contrast-enhanced ultrasound is becoming a preferred investigation to detect injuries in the abdomen.[216] Monitoring of blood in urine is a simple, useful technique to detect bladder and kidney injuries. Management of abdominal trauma generally requires only haemodynamic and laboratory monitoring in conjunction with supportive therapies such as fluid replacement, monitoring of urine output and pain management with the aim of detecting signs of haemorrhage.[203]

Summary

Critically ill infants and children have several anatomical and physiological differences that predispose them to different types of critical illness when compared with adults. Children's relative physiological and psychological immaturity means that their needs may be different from adults when critically ill. Family support is important and parental presence should be allowed at all times. Patterns of disease may be different from adults – for example, a high incidence of respiratory illness and a predisposition to sustaining multiple trauma – but children have a lower incidence of sepsis, heart failure, liver failure and renal failure than adults. The need for specialised nursing and medical care as well as adapted equipment means that many critically ill children will require transfer to a specialist paediatric centre.

Case study

Caitlyn, a 6-year-old girl, arrived in the emergency department (ED) with ambulance paramedics. She is unconscious. Her mother, who has accompanied her, provided the following history:

Caitlyn was well when she went to school today. On returning home Caitlyn complained of painful legs, and her mother gave her oral ibuprofen. After this she wanted to use the bathroom, and was very wobbly, with her mother needing to help her to the bathroom. Caitlyn collapsed onto the floor with eyes rolling back while making some gurgling noises. Caitlyn was also incontinent of urine. After around 5 minutes, Caitlyn's mother called an ambulance as she was not responding.

Ambulance paramedics arrived 5 min later finding Caitlyn unconscious, eyes deviated upwards, not moving and with slow shallow breathing. Initial oxygen saturation was 72% and GCS assessed as 3. Paramedics administered a buccal dose of midazolam, provided oxygen via Hudson mask, and when Caitlyn appeared to stop breathing, they delivered bag–valve–mask assisted breaths and then placed a size 2 supraglottic airway based on weight of 19 kg (from mother). A peripheral IV cannula was inserted, and the paramedics administered a fluid bolus of Hartmann's solution and then transferred her to hospital with mother. Father, brother and grandmother drive to ED.

Caitlyn was transferred to the ED bed in a resuscitation bay at 16:40. ED first observations and examination showed: airway in situ, breathing inadequate initially, with hypoxia and hypercapnoea requiring bag–mask ventilation, hypotensive, clammy and pale, tachycardic and temperature 35.7°C. GCS 3, eyes deviated upwards, 5 mm, reacting sluggishly, jerky movements of L hand noted. Skin intact. Caitlyn appears slim and smaller than her age. Her mother tells you that her older brother is also smaller than many of his classmates.

A second cannula was sited for blood sampling and IV and bloods taken for multiple tests including blood gas and drug screen. IV levetiracetam is prepared and commenced. The emergency consultant found no other symptoms consistent with meningism. CT scan and Intensive Care are contacted for 1) urgent head CT; and 2) transfer to ICU post-CT scan.

Venous gas results show: pH 7.32, PO_2 65, PCO_2 67, HCO_3 24, BE –4, lactate 0.7, glucose 7.5.

IV antibiotics and antiviral are ordered and administered. Intensive care advice is sought regarding steroid – not given at this time. Nursing staff have set up for intubation, indwelling catheter (IDC) insertion and to administer IV fluids. On insertion of IDC Caitlyn became combative, making groaning sounds and attempting to push hands away from her face and to roll over. Medications are quickly given, Caitlyn ceases movements and oral intubation with a cuffed 4.5 mm ETT proceeds smoothly. IV infusions of muscle relaxants, morphine and midazolam are commenced, along with IV fluids at half maintenance rate. Chest X-ray shows good ETT placement, around 1 cm above the carina. Nasogastric (NG) tube is placed.

Caitlyn is then transferred to CT scan for head CT accompanied by the ED registrar, ED registered nurse (RN) and a senior ICU RN. The ED social worker accompanies Caitlyn's family to the ICU waiting room.

Caitlyn is transferred to ICU following CT scan at 18:30. She is placed on a ventilator, on synchronised intermittent mandatory ventilation (SIMV) volume support, rate 20, FiO_2 40%, tidal volume set to 7 mL/kg, inspiratory time of 0.8 seconds, PEEP 5 cmH_2O and generating peak pressure of 18–21 mH_2O. $ETCO_2$ is reading 34–39 mmHg, SpO_2 100% with good chest rise and equal air entry on auscultation. Vital signs are: HR 102, BP 95/55, MAP 68, RR 20, temperature 36.4^{0}C, capillary refill time 2 seconds.

The intensivist has discussed the CT findings with the radiologist and neurologist – a normal scan has been reported. Blood results including electrolytes, full blood count procalcitonin, liver function tests and drug screen are reported as normal, with no drugs detected. FiO_2 is weaned to 30%, and as Caitlyn is not initiating ventilated breaths, the rate is decreased to 15 and morphine and midazolam infusions reviewed.

The EEG technician completes an EEG which shows multiform epileptic activity. This disappears following the administration of a bolus of midazolam.

The plan overnight is to wean ventilation, morphine and midazolam and allow Caitlyn to wake up and the neurologist will conduct further tests in the morning. Caitlyn's mother will stay overnight with Caitlyn.

Need for antibiotics is questioned and then ceased. Anticonvulsants are prescribed regularly as per neurologist. NG feeds will not commence to facilitate morning extubation for Caitlyn following intensivist review.

Overnight Caitlyn's ventilation is weaned to CPAP 5 cmH_2O, pressure support 10 mH_2O, FiO_2 25% and she breathes at a rate of 13–18 breaths, generating tidal volumes of 5–7 mL/kg, $ETCO_2$ is 38–43 mmHg, SpO_2 95–98%. At times overnight Caitlyn has been waking and attempting to touch her ETT. Caitlyn's mother has spoken and sung to her, and she has quickly fallen asleep again. Morphine is ceased at 5 a.m. and planned to stop midazolam at 6 a.m. At 05:30, while her RN is emptying her IDC bag, Caitlyn wakes up, reaches for her ETT and self-extubates. Urgent medical review followed, and it is decided to observe Caitlyn's respiratory status without the ETT and administer low flow oxygen via nasal cannulae at 1 L/min, weaning as tolerated.

At 07:30 the intensivist examined her: resting comfortably, watching television with her mother, IV infusions ceased and IV fluids running. Vitals: HR 98, BP 90/52, RR 22, with SpO_2 97% in air, temp 36.7°C and requesting breakfast. The intensivist assessed her as ready for the ward following a further 2 hours of satisfactory observations postextubation, and that she could have some sips of water at around 11:30 before transfer.

Caitlyn was transferred to the ward at midday. Her diagnosis in the absence of infection, a normal CT scan and normal blood results is benign focal epilepsy. Caitlyn resumed her usual diet over the day. No further seizures were observed clinically and Caitlyn was discharged home with both parents the following morning. Discharge instructions included buccal medication as part of her home management plan, with appointments scheduled with the neurologist the following week and the paediatrician in 2 weeks.

CASE STUDY QUESTIONS

1. What are three important potential diagnoses to consider for Caitlyn on presentation?
2. Describe a preferred approach to intubation of a collapsed child. Calculate the appropriate ETT size for Caitlyn. Did Caitlyn have the correct size ETT placed for her age?
3. Caitlyn will be kept fasted for her first few hours in intensive care. Calculate her maintenance fluid requirements and consider the choice of IV fluids. Does she need to remain on her ½ maintenance fluid restriction?
4. How will you assess Caitlyn's level of sedation while she is intubated and ventilated?
5. Consider how you will explain the treatment and interventions Caitlyn is receiving in Intensive Care to her parents, 9-year-old brother and her grandmother?
6. Caitlyn self-extubated at around 5 a.m. Describe your immediate actions to this airway emergency. What criteria will you use to assess whether or not Caitlyn needs ongoing ventilatory support ± reintubation?

RESEARCH VIGNETTE

Rennick JE, Stremler R, Horwood L et al. A pilot randomized controlled trial of an intervention to promote psychological well-being in critically ill children: soothing through touch, reading, and music. Pediatr Crit Care Med 2018;19(7):e358-e366

Abstract

Objectives: To examine the feasibility and acceptability of a PICU Soothing intervention using touch, reading, and music.

Design: Nonblinded, pilot randomized controlled trial.

Setting: The PICU and medical-surgical wards of one Canadian pediatric hospital.

Patients: Twenty PICU patients age 2–14 years old and their parents, randomised to an intervention group (n = 10) or control group (n = 10).

Intervention: PICU Soothing consisted of: 1) parental comforting (touch and reading), followed by 2) a quiet period with music via soft headbands, administered once daily throughout hospitalization.

Measurements and main results: Acceptability and feasibility of the intervention and methods were assessed via participation rates, observation, measurement completion rates, semi-structured interviews, and telephone calls. Psychological wellbeing was assessed using measures of distress, sleep, and child and parent anxiety in the PICU, on the wards and 3 months post-discharge. Forty-four percent of parents agreed to participate. Seventy percent and 100% of intervention group parents responded positively to comforting and music, respectively. Most intervention group parents (70%) and all nurses felt children responded positively. All nurses found the intervention acceptable and feasible. Measurement completion rates ranged from 70% to 100%. Pilot data suggested lower intervention group child and parent anxiety after transfer to hospital wards.

Conclusions: PICU Soothing is acceptable and feasible to conduct. Results support the implementation of a full-scale randomized controlled trial to evaluate intervention effectiveness.

Critique

This study addresses an important issue that has been recognised as a research priority in paediatric intensive care: children's wellbeing. The authors have justified the study by highlighting the research gap in the population of interest: children admitted to intensive care. They rightly opted for a pilot randomised controlled trial, as there was no published data in that population, drawing hypotheses from neonatal research and general paediatrics. The non-blinded randomised controlled trial (RCT) pilot study aimed to determine to examine the feasibility and acceptability of the intervention and the study protocol to inform future implementation of a fully powered RCT. Feasibility and acceptability were assessed based on: 1) parent and child participation rates (≥70%); 2) semi-structured interviews with parents from the intervention group and nurses; 3) research assistant's recorded notes about children's, parents', and nurses' responses to the intervention. When the participation rate is a clear measurable acceptability outcome, the other two as described in the methods lack clarity. We understand, however, how feasibility was actually assessed in the results section. In addition to participation rate and reason for refusal, it included adherence to protocol (e.g. intervention delivery, rate of completion of the questionnaires and the diaries), perceptions of the different components of the intervention, and nurses' participation.

The procedure is particularly well described and as such could be easily replicated. Allocation to groups was randomly selected, including block randomisation to ensure equal age distribution in both groups. The intervention was provided once daily during the entire hospital stay, from 24 hours PICU admission to hospital discharge, which could have impacted on the dose of the intervention. We can see from the results, that participants in the intervention group had an average hospital length of stay of 7.4 days, compared with 5.7 days in the control group. This means that the intervention group participants received in total a higher 'dose' of soothing interventions than the control group. Inherent to the type of intervention tested, participants and researchers could not be blinded to the allocated groups. This introduces some measurement bias the authors acknowledged. The results are clearly reported and the discussion offers objective insights. The results suggest a larger, definitive trial may be feasible.

To evaluate the methodological quality of a pilot randomised controlled trial you can refer to the CONSORT statement: http://www.consort-statement.org/

Learning activities

The questions below relate to the following scenario.

As an experienced critical care nurse, you are called down from the ICU to review a 6-month-old infant (8 kg) in the paediatric ward with bronchiolitis, now day 4 of illness and day 2 of admission. The infant has increasing work of breathing and the paediatric nursing staff are concerned. The baby is lying flat in the bed, looks distressed, is crying and irritable with audible wheeze and moderate-to-severe respiratory distress and is receiving humidified high-flow oxygen therapy via nasal cannula. The baby's mother is present, looks tired and upset. Monitoring shows an oxygen saturation of 93%.

1 Consider your approach to assessing this infant. What are some immediate nursing interventions you could perform that may improve the baby's work of breathing while you perform your assessment?

2 What are the important aspects of history you need to consider before escalating treatment for this baby?

3 If you are thinking of escalating respiratory therapy, what options are available in your hospital? Where is the best place now for this baby to be nursed?

Online resources

Online weight-based maintenance fluid calculator from Royal Children's Hospital, Melbourne, https://www.rch.org.au/clinicalguide/forms/fluids-calculator/

OPENPediatrics is a free, open access online resource for the paediatric critical care community, https://www.openpediatrics.org

Further reading

Curley MAQ, Hasbani NR, Quigley SM, et al. Predicting pressure injury risk in pediatric patients: the Braden QD Scale. J Pediatr 2018;192:189–95.e2.

Gaillard-Le Roux B, Liet J-M, Bourgoin P, et al. Implementation of a nurse-driven sedation protocol in a PICU decreases daily doses of midazolam. Pediatr Crit Care Med 2017;18:e9–17.

Rimensberger PC. Pediatric and neonatal mechanical ventilation. Berlin: Springer-Verlag; 2015.

Uzark KC, Costello JM, DeSena HC, et al. Useful references in pediatric cardiac intensive care: the 2017 update. Pediatr Crit Care Med 2018;19(6):553–63.

References

1. ANZPIC Registry. Report of the Australian and New Zealand Paediatric Intensive Care Registry 2016. Melbourne, Australia: Centre for Outcome and Resource Evaluation; 2017.
2. ANZICS Centre for Outcome and Resource Evaluation. Report of the Australian and New Zealand Paediatric Intensive Care Registry 2016. Melbourne, Australia: Australian and New Zealand Intensive Care Society; 2016.
3. Namachivayam SP, Alexander J, Slater A, et al. Five-year survival of children with chronic critical illness in Australia and New Zealand. Crit Care Med 2015;43(9):1978–85.
4. Young KD, Korotzer NC. Weight estimation methods in children: a systematic review. Ann Emerg Med 2016;68(4):441–51.e10.
5. ANZCOR. Techniques in paediatric advanced life support. Guideline 126. Melbourne, Australia: Australian and New Zealand Resuscitation Councils; 2016.
6. Olasveengen TM, de Caen AR, Mancini ME, et al. 2017 international consensus on cardiopulmonary resuscitation and emergency cardiovascular care science with treatment recommendations summary. Resuscitation 2017;121:201–14.
7. Guyton AC, Hall JE. Fetal and neonatal physiology. Guyton and Hall Textbook of medical physiology. 13th ed. Philadelphia: Saunders; 2016. p. 1071–82.
8. Blackburn ST. Maternal, fetal and neonatal physiology: a clinical perspective. 5th ed. Maryland Heights: Elsevier Saunders; 2018.
9. Allen BB, Chiu Y, Gerber LM, et al. Age-specific cerebral perfusion pressure thresholds and survival in children and adolescents with severe traumatic brain injury. Pediatr Crit Care Med 2014;15(1):62–70.
10. Mathias B, Mira JC, Larson SD. Pediatric sepsis. Curr Opin Pediatr 2016;28(3):380–7.
11. Hammer J. Acute respiratory failure in children. Paediatr Respir Rev 2013;14:64–9.
12. Oymar K, Skjerven HO, Mikalsen IB. Acute bronchiolitis in infants: a review. Scand J Trauma Resusc Emerg Med 2014;22:22–3.
13. Reynolds SL. Pediatric thoracic trauma: recognition and management. Emerg Med Clin North Am 2018;36(2):473–83.
14. Kottner J, Kenzler M, Wilborn D. Interrater agreement, reliability and validity of the Glamorgan Paediatric Pressure Ulcer Risk Assessment Scale. J Clin Nurs 2014;23(7–8):1165–9.
15. Lopes-Junior LC, Rosa M, Lima RAG. Psychological and psychiatric outcomes following PICU admission: a systematic review of cohort studies. Pediatr Crit Care Med 2018;19(1):e58–67.

16. Zerden ML, Falkovich A, McClain EK, et al. Addressing unmet maternal health needs at a pediatric specialty infant care clinic. Womens Health Issues 2017;27(5):559–64.
17. Sood E, Karpyn A, Demianczyk AC, et al. Mothers and fathers experience stress of congenital heart disease differently: recommendations for pediatric critical care. Pediatr Crit Care Med 2018.
18. Marcus KL, Henderson CM, Boss RD. Chronic Critical illness in infants and children: a speculative synthesis on adapting ICU Care to meet the needs of long-stay patients. Pediatr Crit Care Med 2016;17(8):743–52.
19. Dunkel CS, Sefcek JA. Eriksonian lifespan theory and life history theory: an integration using the example of identity formation. Rev Gen Psychol 2009;13(1):13–23.
20. Roberts CA. Unaccompanied hospitalized children: a review of the literature and incidence study. J Pediatr Nurs 2010;25(6):470–6.
21. Oczkowski SJ, Mazzetti I, Cupido C, et al. The offering of family presence during resuscitation: a systematic review and meta-analysis. J Intensive Care 2015;3:41.
22. Kramer B, Joshi P, Heard C. Noise pollution levels in the pediatric intensive care unit. J Crit Care 2016;36:111–15.
23. Erikson EH. Identity and the life cycle. New York: Norton & Company; 1994.
24. Schore AN. Affect regulation and the origin of the self: the neurobiology of emotional development, Classic Edition. New York: Routledge Taylor & Francis; 2016.
25. Piaget J. The child's conception of the world: a 20th-century classic of child psychology. Maryland, USA: Rowman & Littlefield Publishers; 2007.
26. Hockenberry M, Rogers C, Wilson D. Wong's Essentials of pediatric nursing. 10th ed. St Louis: Mosby; 2016.
27. Meeus W. Adolescent psychosocial development: a review of longitudinal models and research. Dev Psychol 2016;52(12):1969–93.
28. Muscara F, McCarthy MC, Woolf C, et al. Early psychological reactions in parents of children with a life threatening illness within a pediatric hospital setting. Eur Psychiatry 2015;30(5):555–61.
29. Rennick JE. Advancing our understanding of the psychological impact of PICU hospitalization: is it time to pause and reflect? Pediatr Crit Care Med 2015;16(4):387–8.
30. McCarthy MC, Hearps SJ, Muscara F, et al. Family psychosocial risk screening in infants and older children in the acute pediatric hospital setting using the Psychosocial Assessment Tool. J Pediatr Psychol 2016;41(7):820–9.
31. Zimmermann K, Bergstraesser E, Engberg S, et al. When parents face the death of their child: a nationwide cross-sectional survey of parental perspectives on their child's end-of life care. BMC Palliat Care 2016;15:30.
32. Eggly S, Meert KL, Berger J, et al. A framework for conducting follow-up meetings with parents after a child's death in the pediatric intensive care unit. Pediatr Crit Care Med 2011;12(2):147–52.
33. Butler A, Copnell B, Willetts G. Family-centred care in the paediatric intensive care unit: an integrative review of the literature. J Clin Nurs 2014;23(15–16):2086–99.
34. Davidson JE, Aslakson RA, Long AC, et al. Guidelines for family-centered care in the neonatal, pediatric, and ddult ICU. Crit Care Med 2017;45(1):103–28.
35. Aronson PL, Shapiro ED, Niccolai LM, et al. Shared decision-making with parents of acutely ill children: a narrative review. Acad Pediatr 2018;18(1):3–7.
36. Zurca AD, Fisher KR, Flor RJ, et al. Communication with limited english-proficient families in the PICU. Hosp Pediatr 2017;7(1):9–15.
37. Ahlqvist-Bjorkroth S, Boukydis Z, Axelin AM, et al. Close Collaboration with parents intervention to improve parents' psychological well-being and child development: description of the intervention and study protocol. Behav Brain Res 2017;325(Pt B):303–10.
38. O'Connell K, Fritzeen J, Guzzetta CE, et al. Family presence during trauma resuscitation: family members' attitudes, behaviors, and experiences. Am J Crit Care 2017;26(3):229–39.
39. NHS. Consent to treatment 2018. Available from: https://www.nhs.uk/conditions/consent-to-treatment/children/.
40. Swiss Centre of Expertise in Human Rights (SCHR). La position de l'enfant face au traitement médical [Child's position in medical treatment] 2018. Available from: http://www.skmr.ch/frz/domaines/enfance/nouvelles/enfant_traitement_medical.html.
41. National Health and Medical Research Council. National Statement on Ethical Conduct in Human Research (2007). Canberra, Australia: Australian Government; 2007. Available from: https://www.nhmrc.gov.au/book/national-statement-ethical-conduct-human-research. [Accessed May 2015].
42. Grootens-Wiegers P, Hein IM, van den Broek JM, et al. Medical decision-making in children and adolescents: developmental and neuroscientific aspects. BMC Pediatr 2017;17(1):120.
43. Lepola P, Needham A, Mendum J, et al. Informed consent for paediatric clinical trials in Europe. Arch Dis Child 2016;101(11):1017–25.
44. Zuppa AF, Curley MAQ. Sedation, analgesia and neuromuscular blockade in pediatric critical care: overview and current landscape. Pediatr Clin North Am 2017;64(5):1103–16.
45. Patel AK, Bell MJ, Traube C. Delirium in pediatric critical care. Pediatr Clin North Am 2017;64(5):1117–32.
46. Baarslag MA, Allegaert K, Knibbe CAJ, et al. Pharmacological sedation management in the paediatric intensive care unit. J Pharm Pharmacol 2017;69(5):498–513.
47. Aydin SI, Ofori-Amanfo G, Ushay HM. Sedation and analgesia following pediatric heart surgery – less may be more. Crit Care Med 2018;46(1):170–2.

48. Watson RS, Asaro LA, Hertzog JH, et al. Long-term outcomes after protocolized sedation vs usual care in ventilated pediatric patients. Am J Respir Crit Care Med 2018.
49. Lebet RM, Asaro LA, Zuppa AF, et al. Face and content validity of variables associated with the difficult-to-sedate child in the paediatric intensive care unit: a survey of paediatric critical care clinicians. Aust Crit Care 2018.
50. Taffarel P, Bonetto G, Jorro Baron F, et al. Sedation and analgesia in patients on mechanical ventilation in pediatric intensive care units in Argentina. Arch Argent Pediatr 2018;116(2):e196–203.
51. Best KM, Wypij D, Asaro LA, et al. Patient, process, and system predictors of iatrogenic withdrawal syndrome in critically ill children. Crit Care Med 2017;45(1):e7–15.
52. da Silva PS, Reis ME, Fonseca TS, et al. Opioid and benzodiazepine withdrawal syndrome in PICU patients: which risk factors matter? J Addict Med 2016;10(2):110–16.
53. Ricardo Ramirez C, Alvarez Gomez ML, Agudelo Velez CA, et al. Clinical characteristics, prevalence, and factors related to delirium in children of 5 to 14 years of age admitted to intensive care. Med Intensiva 2018.
54. Norman S, Taha AA, Turner HN. Delirium in the critically ill child. Clin Nurse Spec 2017;31(5):276–84.
55. Harris J, Ramelet AS, van Dijk M, et al. Clinical recommendations for pain, sedation, withdrawal and delirium assessment in critically ill infants and children: an ESPNIC position statement for healthcare professionals. Intensive Care Med 2016;42(6):972–86.
56. Madden K, Burns MM, Tasker RC. Differentiating delirium from sedative/hypnotic-related iatrogenic withdrawal syndrome: lack of specificity in pediatric critical care assessment tools. Pediatr Crit Care Med 2017;18(6):580–8.
57. Krauss BS, Calligaris L, Green SM, et al. Current concepts in management of pain in children in the emergency department. Lancet 2016;387(10013):83–92.
58. Ramelet AS, Rees NW, McDonald S, et al. Clinical validation of the multidimensional assessment of pain scale. Paediatr Anaesth 2007;17(12):1156–65.
59. Ista E, van Dijk M, Tibboel D, et al. Assessment of sedation levels in pediatric intensive care patients can be improved by using the COMFORT 'behavior' scale. Pediatr Crit Care Med 2005;6(1):58–63.
60. Curley MA, Harris SK, Fraser KA, et al. State Behavioral Scale: a sedation assessment instrument for infants and young children supported on mechanical ventilation. Pediatr Crit Care Med 2006;7(2):107–14.
61. Franck LS, Scoppettuolo LA, Wypij D, et al. Validity and generalizability of the Withdrawal Assessment Tool-1 (WAT-1) for monitoring iatrogenic withdrawal syndrome in pediatric patients. Pain 2012;153(1):142–8.
62. Ista E, Te Beest H, van Rosmalen J, et al. Sophia Observation withdrawal Symptoms-Paediatric Delirium scale: a tool for early screening of delirium in the PICU. Aust Crit Care 2017.
63. Smith HA, Boyd J, Fuchs DC, et al. Diagnosing delirium in critically ill children: validity and reliability of the Pediatric Confusion Assessment Method for the Intensive Care Unit. Crit Care Med 2011;39(1):150–7.
64. Stevens B, Yamada J, Ohlsson A, et al. Sucrose for analgesia in newborn infants undergoing painful procedures. Cochrane Database Syst Rev 2016;(7):CD001069.
65. Chen S, Zhang Q, Xie RH, et al. What is the best pain management during gastric tube insertion for infants aged 0-12 months: a systematic review. J Pediatr Nurs 2017;34:78–83.
66. Harrison D, Yamada J, Adams-Webber T, et al. Sweet tasting solutions for reduction of needle-related procedural pain in children aged one to 16 years. Cochrane Database Syst Rev 2015;(5):CD008408.
67. Boric K, Dosenovic S, Jelicic Kadic A, et al. Interventions for postoperative pain in children: an overview of systematic reviews. Paediatr Anaesth 2017;27(9):893–904.
68. Matziou V, Chrysostomou A, Vlahioti E, et al. Parental presence and distraction during painful childhood procedures. Br J Nurs 2013;22(8):470–5.
69. Spence K, Henderson-Smart D, New K, et al. Evidenced-based clinical practice guideline for management of newborn pain. J Paediatr Child Health 2010;46(4):184–92.
70. Phan H, Nahata MC. Clinical uses of dexmedetomidine in pediatric patients. Paediatr Drugs 2008;10(1):49–69.
71. Zhu A, Benzon HA, Anderson TA. Evidence for the efficacy of systemic opioid-sparing analgesics in pediatric surgical populations: a systematic review. Anesth Analg 2017;125(5):1569–87.
72. Gong M, Man Y, Fu Q. Incidence of bradycardia in pediatric patients receiving dexmedetomidine anesthesia: a meta-analysis. Int J Clin Pharm 2017;39(1):139–47.
73. Su F, Hammer GB. Dexmedetomidine: pediatric pharmacology, clinical uses and safety. Expert Opin Drug Saf 2011;10(1):55–66.
74. Chidambaran V, Costandi A, D'Mello A. Propofol: a review of its role in pediatric anesthesia and sedation. CNS Drugs 2015;29(7):543–63.
75. Kang TM. Propofol infusion syndrome in critically ill patients. Ann Pharmacother 2002;36(9):1453–6.
76. Tibballs J, Watson T. Symptoms and signs differentiating croup and epiglottitis. J Paediatr Child Health 2010;47(3):77–82.
77. Schmidt AR, Weiss M, Engelhardt T. The paediatric airway: basic principles and current developments. Eur J Anaesthesiol 2014;31(6):293–9.
78. Horeczko T, Enriquez B, McGrath NE, et al. The Pediatric Assessment Triangle: accuracy of its application by nurses in the triage of children. J Emerg Nurs 2013;39(2):182–9.

79. Cooper T, Benoit M, Erickson B, et al. Primary presentations of laryngomalacia. JAMA Otolaryngol Head Neck Surg 2014;140(6):521–6.
80. Erickson B, Cooper T, El-Hakim H. Factors associated with the morphological type of laryngomalacia and prognostic value for surgical outcomes. JAMA Otolaryngol Head Neck Surg 2014;140(10):927–33.
81. Chen J, Shi F, Chen M, et al. Web thickness determines the therapeutic effect of endoscopic keel placement on anterior glottic web. Eur Arch Otorhinolaryngol 2017;274(10):3697–702.
82. Lennon P, Lang E, O'Dwyer T Acquired anterior laryngeal web in a shotgun injury. Irish Medical Journal [Internet]. 2015 March 18, 2018. Available from: http://hdl.handle.net/10147/558635.
83. Hysinger EB, Panitch HB. Paediatric tracheomalacia. Paediatr Respir Rev 2016;17:9–15.
84. Licari A, Manca E, Rispoli GA, et al. Congenital vascular rings: a clinical challenge for the pediatrician. Pediatr Pulmonol 2015;50(5): 511–24.
85. Davies I, Jenkins I. Paediatric airway infections. BJA Education 2017;17(10):341–5.
86. Hyland EJ, Harvey JG, Martin AJ, et al. Airway compromise in children with anterior neck burns: beware the scalded child. J Paediatr Child Health 2015;51(10):976–81.
87. Neuhaus D, Schmitz A, Gerber A, et al. Controlled rapid sequence induction and intubation - an analysis of 1001 children. Paediatr Anaesth 2013;23(8):734–40.
88. Lichtor JL, Roche Rodriguez M, Aaronson NL, et al. Epiglottitis: it hasn't gone away. Anesthesiology 2016;124(6):1404–7.
89. Byard RW. Diphtheria – 'The strangling angel' of children. J Forensic Leg Med 2013;20(2):65–8.
90. Pfleger A, Eber E. Management of acute severe upper airway obstruction in children. Paediatr Respir Rev 2013;14:70–7.
91. Tyler A, McLeod L, Beaty B, et al. Variation in inpatient croup management and outcomes. Pediatrics 2017.
92. Richards AM. Pediatric respiratory emergencies. Emerg Med Clin 2015;34(1):77–96.
93. Sink JR, Kitsko DJ, Georg MW, et al. Predictors of foreign body aspiration in children. Otolaryngol Head Neck Surg 2016;155(3):501–7.
94. The Global Initiative for Asthma. Global strategy for the diagnosis and management of asthma in children 5 years and younger: The Global Initiative for Asthma; 2011. Available from: http://www.ginasthma.org/index.asp.
95. O'Brien S, Wilson S, Gill FJ, et al. The management of children with bronchiolitis in the Australasian hospital setting: development of a clinical practice guideline. BMC Med Res Methodol 2018;18(1):22.
96. Mammas IN, Greenough A, Theodoridou M, et al. Current views and advances on paediatric virology: an update for paediatric trainees. Exp Ther Med 2016;11(1):6–14.
97. Hogan AB, Anderssen RS, Davis S, et al. Time series analysis of RSV and bronchiolitis seasonality in temperate and tropical Western Australia. Epidemics 2016;16:49–55.
98. Ranmuthugala G, Brown L, Lidbury BA. Respiratory syncytial virus – the unrecognised cause of health and economic burden among young children in Australia. Commun Dis Intell Q Rep 2011;35(2):177–84.
99. Cromer D, van Hoek AJ, Newall AT, et al. Burden of paediatric respiratory syncytial virus disease and potential effect of different immunisation strategies: a modelling and cost-effectiveness analysis for England. Lancet Public Health 2018;2(8):e367–74.
100. Dede A, Isaacs D, Torzillo PJ, et al. Respiratory syncytial virus infections in Central Australia. J Paediatr Child Health 2010;46(1–2):35–9.
101. Paediatric Research in Emergency Departments International Collaborative (PREDICT). Australasian bronchiolitis guideline. Melbourne: Paediatric Research in Emergency Departments International Collaborative (PREDICT); 2016.
102. Hasegawa K, Pate BM, Mansbach JM, et al. Risk factors for requiring intensive care among children admitted to ward with bronchiolitis. Acad Pediatr 2015;15(1):77–81.
103. Carroll CL, Sala KA. Pediatric status asthmaticus. Crit Care Clin 2013;29(2):153–66.
104. Marfortt DA, Josviack D, Lozano A, et al. Differences between preschoolers with asthma and allergies in urban and rural environments. J Asthma 2018;55(5):470–6.
105. Zhang J, Sun C, Liu W, et al. Associations of household renovation materials and periods with childhood asthma, in China: a retrospective cohort study. Environ Int 2018;113:240–8.
106. Cornell A, Shaker M, Woodmansee DP. Update on the pathogenesis and management of childhood asthma. Curr Opin Pediatr 2008;20(5):597–604.
107. Zhang Q, Lamichhane R, Diggs LA. Disparities in emergency department visits in American children with asthma: 2006-2010. J Asthma 2017;54(7):679–86.
108. Australian Institue of Health and Welfare. Asthma hospitalisation in Australia 2010-2011. Canberra: Australian Institue of Health and Welfare; 2013.
109. Delmas MC, Marguet C, Raherison C, et al. Les hospitalisations pour asthme chez l'enfant en France, 2002–2010. Arch Pediatr 2013;20(7):739–47.
110. Asher I, Pearce N. Global burden of asthma among children. Int J Tuberc Lung Dis 2014;18(11):1269–78.
111. Centers for Disease Control and Prevention. FastStats. Asthma Atlanta: Centers for Disease Control and Prevention; 2016. Available from: http://www.cdc.gov/nchs/fastats/asthma.htm. [Accessed September 2016].
112. Australian Centre for Asthma Monitoring. Asthma in Australia 2011. Canberra: Australian Institute of Health and Welfare; 2011. Available from: http://www.aihw.gov.au/publication-detail/?id=10737420159.

113. Asthma Management Handbook. Australian asthma handbook. Melbourne: the National Asthma Council Australia; 2017.
114. Nievas IFF, Anand KJS. Severe acute asthma exacerbation in children: a stepwise approach for escalating therapy in a pediatric intensive care unit. J Pediatr Pharmacol Ther 2013;18(2):88–104.
115. Indinnimeo L, Chiappini E, Miraglia Del Giudice M. Guideline on management of the acute asthma attack in children by Italian Society of Pediatrics. Ital J Pediatr 2018;6(44):1824–7288. (Electronic).
116. Travers AH, Milan SJ, Jones AP, et al. Addition of intravenous beta(2)-agonists to inhaled beta(2)-agonists for acute asthma. Cochrane Database Syst Rev 2012;(12):CD010179.
117. Knightly R, Milan SJ, Hughes R, et al. Inhaled magnesium sulfate in the treatment of acute asthma. Cochrane Database Syst Rev 2017;(11):CD003898.
118. Cooney L, Sinha I, Hawcutt D. Aminophylline dosage in asthma exacerbations in children: a systematic review. PLoS ONE 2016;11(8):e0159965.
119. Travers AH, Jones AP, Camargo CA Jr, et al. Intravenous beta(2)-agonists versus intravenous aminophylline for acute asthma. Cochrane Database Syst Rev 2012;(12):CD010256.
120. Yaman A, Kendirli T, Ödek Ç, et al. Efficacy of noninvasive mechanical ventilation in prevention of intubation and reintubation in the pediatric intensive care unit. J Crit Care 2016;32:175–81.
121. Papiris S, Manali E, Kolilekas L, et al. Acute severe asthma. Drugs 2009;69(17):2363–91.
122. Kneyber MCJ, de Luca D, Calderini E, et al. Recommendations for mechanical ventilation of critically ill children from the Paediatric Mechanical Ventilation Consensus Conference (PEMVECC). Intensive Care Med 2017;43(12):1764–80.
123. Gillies D, Todd DA, Foster JP, et al. Heat and moisture exchangers versus heated humidifiers for mechanically ventilated adults and children. Cochrane Database Syst Rev 2017;(9):CD004711.
124. Davies K, Monterosso L, Bulsara M, et al. Clinical indicators for the initiation of endotracheal suction in children: an integrative review. Aust Crit Care 2015;28(1):11–18.
125. Gupta R, Rosen D. Paediatric mechanical ventilation in the intensive care unit. BJA Education 2016;16(12):422–6.
126. Davies K, Bulsara M, Ramelet AS, et al. Reliability and criterion-related validity testing (construct) of the Endotracheal Suction Assessment Tool (ESAT©). J Clin Nurs 2018;27(9–10):1891–900.
127. Santschi M, Randolph AG, Rimensberger PC, et al. Mechanical ventilation strategies in children with acute lung injury: a survey on stated practice pattern*. Pediatr Crit Care Med 2013;14(7):e332–7.
128. Gupta P, Green JW, Tang X, et al. Comparison of high-frequency oscillatory ventilation and conventional mechanical ventilation in pediatric respiratory failure. J Am Med Assoc 2014;168(3):243–9.
129. Cools F, Offringa M, Askie LM. Elective high frequency oscillatory ventilation versus conventional ventilation for acute pulmonary dysfunction in preterm infants. Cochrane Database Syst Rev 2015;(3):CD000104.
130. Brown KL, Ichord R, Marino BS, et al. Outcomes following extracorporeal membrane oxygenation in children with cardiac disease. Pediatr Crit Care Med 2013;14(5, Suppl. 1):S73–83.
131. MacLaren G, Dodge-Khatami A, Dalton HJ, et al. Joint statement on mechanical circulatory support in children: a consensus review from the Pediatric Cardiac Intensive Care Society and Extracorporeal Life Support Organization. Pediatr Crit Care Med 2013;14(5 Suppl. 1): S1–2.
132. Schad CA, Fallon BP, Monteagudo J, et al. Routine use of distal arterial perfusion in pediatric femoral venoarterial extracorporeal membrane oxygenation. Artif Organs 2017;41(1):11–16.
133. Juo YY, Skancke M, Sanaiha Y, et al. Efficacy of distal perfusion cannulae in preventing limb ischemia during extracorporeal membrane oxygenation: a systematic review and meta-analysis. Artif Organs 2017;41(11):E263–73.
134. Maslach-Hubbard A, Bratton SL. Extracorporeal membrane oxygenation for pediatric respiratory failure: history, development and current status. World J Crit Care Med 2013;2(4):29–39.
135. Elias MD, Achuff BJ, Ittenbach RF, et al. Long-Term outcomes of pediatric cardiac patients supported by extracorporeal membrane oxygenation. Pediatr Crit Care Med 2017;18(8):787–94.
136. Strobel AM, Lu le N. The critically ill infant with congenital heart disease. Emerg Med Clin North Am 2015;33(3):501–18.
137. Weitz J. Fluid management in paediatric shock. Paediatr Child Health 2016;27(1):33–6.
138. Weiss SL, Balamuth F, Hensley J, et al. The epidemiology of hospital death following pediatric severe sepsis: when, why, and how children with sepsis die. Pediatr Crit Care Med 2017;18(9):823–30.
139. Khilanani A, Mazwi M, Paquette E. Pediatric sepsis in the global setting. Clin Pediatr Emerg Med 2014;15(2):193–203.
140. Global Burden of Disease Child and Adolescent Health Collaboration, Kassebaum N, Kyu HH, et al. Child and adolescent health from 1990 to 2015: findings from the global burden of diseases, injuries, and risk factors 2015 study. JAMA Pediatr 2017;171(6):573–92.
141. Schlapbach LJ, Straney L, Alexander J, et al. Mortality related to invasive infections, sepsis, and septic shock in critically ill children in Australia and New Zealand, 2002–13: a multicentre retrospective cohort study. Lancet Infect Dis 2015;15(1):46–54.
142. Weiss SL, Fitzgerald JC, Pappachan J, et al. Global epidemiology of pediatric severe sepsis: the sepsis prevalence, outcomes, and therapies study. Am J Respir Crit Care Med 2015;191(10):1147–57.
143. de Souza DC, Barreira ER, Faria LS. The epidemiology of sepsis in childhood. Shock 2017;47(1S Suppl. 1):2–5.

144. Schlapbach LJ, Javouhey E, Jansen NJG. Paediatric sepsis: old wine in new bottles? Intensive Care Med 2017;43(11):1686–9.
145. Davis AL, Carcillo JA, Aneja RK, et al. The American College of Critical Care Medicine clinical practice parameters for hemodynamic support of pediatric and neonatal septic shock: executive summary. Pediatr Crit Care Med 2017;18(9):884–90.
146. Prusakowski MK, Chen AP. Pediatric sepsis. Emerg Med Clin North Am 2017;35(1):123–38.
147. Ray S, Cvetkovic M, Brierley J, et al. Shock index values and trends in pediatric sepsis: predictors or therapeutic targets? A retrospective observational study. Shock 2016;46(3):279–86.
148. Fitzgerald JC, Weiss SL, Kissoon N. 2016 update for the Rogers' Textbook of pediatric intensive care: recognition and initial management of shock. Pediatr Crit Care Med 2016;17(11):1073–9.
149. Giuliano JS Jr, Markovitz BP, Brierley J, et al. Comparison of pediatric severe sepsis managed in US and European ICUs. Pediatr Crit Care Med 2016;17(6):522–30.
150. Maitland K, Kiguli S, Opoka RO, et al. Mortality after fluid bolus in African children with severe infection. N Engl J Med 2011;364(26):2483–95.
151. Bewick VJ. Intraosseous cannulation in children. Anaesth Intensive Care Med 2017;18(11):551–4.
152. Maoldomhnaigh OC, Drew RJ, Gavin P, et al. Invasive meningococcal disease in children in Ireland, 2001-2011. Arch Dis Child 2016;101(12):1125–9.
153. Fortune PM, Shann F. The motor response to stimulation predicts outcome as well as the full Glasgow Coma Scale in children with severe head injury. Pediatr Crit Care Med 2010;11(3):339–42.
154. Czaikowski BL, Liang H, Stewart CT. A pediatric FOUR score coma scale: interrater reliability and predictive validity. J Neurosci Nurs 2014;46(2):79–87.
155. Bosis S, Mayer A, Esposito S. Meningococcal disease in childhood: epidemiology, clinical features and prevention. J Prev Med Hyg 2015;56(3):E121–4.
156. Bonkowsky JL, Guenther E, Srivastava R, et al. Seizures in children following an apparent life-threatening event. J Child Neurol 2009;24(6):709–13.
157. Chen CY, Chang YJ, Wu HP. New-onset seizures in pediatric emergency. Pediatr Neonatol 2010;51(2):103–11.
158. Whelan H, Harmelink M, Chou E, et al. Complex febrile seizures – a systematic review. Dis Mon 2017;63(1):5–23.
159. Ghobadifar MA, Honar N, Jooya P, et al. Blood glucose level after febrile convulsion. Korean J Pediatr 2016;59(3):153–4.
160. Wilson CA. Continuous electroencephalogram detection of non-convulsive seizures in the pediatric intensive care unit: review of the utility and impact on management and outcomes. Transl Pediatr 2015;4(4):283–9.
161. Brouwer MC, McIntyre P, Prasad K, et al. Corticosteroids for acute bacterial meningitis. Cochrane Database Syst Rev 2015;(9):CD004405.
162. Rudolph H, Schroten H, Tenenbaum T. Enterovirus infections of the central nervous system in children: an update. Pediatr Infect Dis J 2016;35(5):567–9.
163. van Toorn R, Solomons R. Update on the diagnosis and management of tuberculous meningitis in children. Semin Pediatr Neurol 2014;21(1):12–18.
164. Christie D, Rashid H, El-Bashir H, et al. Impact of meningitis on intelligence and development: a systematic review and meta-analysis. PLoS ONE 2017;12(8):e0175024.
165. Maras Genc H, Uyur Yalcin E, Sayan M, et al. Clinical outcomes in children with herpes simplex encephalitis receiving steroid therapy. J Clin Virol 2016;80:87–92.
166. Schlapbach LJ, Straney L, Alexander J, et al. Mortality related to invasive infections, sepsis, and septic shock in critically ill children in Australia and New Zealand, 2002-13: a multicentre retrospective cohort study. Lancet Infect Dis 2015;15(1):46–54.
167. Briand C, Levy C, Baumie F, et al. Outcomes of bacterial meningitis in children. Med Mal Infect 2016;46(4):177–87.
168. Chang Q, Tzeng YL, Stephens DS. Meningococcal disease: changes in epidemiology and prevention. Clin Epidemiol 2012;4(1):237–45.
169. Alicino C, Paganino C, Orsi A, et al. The impact of 10-valent and 13-valent pneumococcal conjugate vaccines on hospitalization for pneumonia in children: a systematic review and meta-analysis. Vaccine 2017;35(43):5776–85.
170. Rose MA, Christopoulou D, Myint TT, et al. The burden of invasive pneumococcal disease in children with underlying risk factors in North America and Europe. Int J Clin Pract 2014;68(1):8–19.
171. Backhaus E, Berg S, Andersson R, et al. Epidemiology of invasive pneumococcal infections: manifestations, incidence and case fatality rate correlated to age, gender and risk factors. BMC Infect Dis 2016;16:367.
172. Maimaiti N, Ahmed Z, Md Isa Z, et al. Clinical burden of invasive pneumococcal disease in selected developing countries. Value Health Reg Issues 2013;2(2):259–63.
173. van de Beek D, Cabellos C, Dzupova O, et al. ESCMID guideline: diagnosis and treatment of acute bacterial meningitis. Clin Microbiol Infect 2016;22:S37–62.
174. Ramasamy R, Willis L, Kadambari S, et al. Management of suspected paediatric meningitis: a multicentre prospective cohort study. Arch Dis Child 2018;1468–2044. (Electronic).
175. Bargui F, D'Agostino I, Mariani-Kurkdjian P, et al. Factors influencing neurological outcome of children with bacterial meningitis at the emergency department. Eur J Pediatr 2012;171(9):1365–71.

176. Esposito S, Semino M, Picciolli I, et al. Should corticosteroids be used in bacterial meningitis in children? Eur J Paediatr Neurol 2013;17(1):24–8.
177. Garg M, Kulkarni S, Udwadia Hegde A. Herpes simplex encephalitis with thalamic, brainstem and cerebellar involvement. Neuroradiol J 2018;31(2):190–2.
178. Thompson C, Kneen R, Riordan A, et al. Encephalitis in children. Arch Dis Child 2012;97(2):150–61.
179. Song JL, Wang VJ. Altered Level of consciousness: evidence-based management in the emergency department. Pediatr Emerg Med Pract 2017;14(1):1–28.
180. Slater MB, Gruneir A, Rochon PA, et al. Risk factors of acute kidney injury in critically ill children. Pediatr Crit Care Med 2016;17(9):e391–8.
181. Vila Pérez D, Cambra FJ, Jordan I, et al. Prognostic factors in pediatric sepsis study from the Spanish Society of Pediatric Intensive Care. Pediatr Infect Dis J 2014;33(2):152–7.
182. Reveiz L, Guerrero-Lozano R, Camacho A, et al. Stress ulcer, gastritis and gastrointestinal bleeding prophyllaxis in critically ill pediatric patients: a systematic review. Pediatr Crit Care Med 2010;11(1):124–32.
183. Costarino AT, Dai D, Feng R, et al. Gastric acid suppressant prophylaxis in pediatric intensive care: current practice as reflected in a large administrative database. Pediatr Crit Care Med 2015;16(7):605–12.
184. Kyle UG, Lucas LA, Mackey G, et al. Implementation of nutrition nupport guidelines may affect energy and protein intake in the pediatric intensive care unit. J Acad Nutr Diet 2016;116(5):844–51, e4.
185. Bechard LJ, Duggan C, Touger-Decker R, et al. Nutritional status based on body mass index is associated with morbidity and mortality in mechanically ventilated critically ill children in the PICU. Crit Care Med 2016;44(8):1530–7.
186. Joosten K, van Puffelen E, Verbruggen S. Optimal nutrition in the paediatric ICU. Curr Opin Clin Nutr Metab Care 2016;19(2):131–7.
187. Wakeham M, Christensen M, Manzi J, et al. Registered dietitians making a difference: early medical record documentation of estimated energy requirement in critically ill children is associated with higher daily energy intake and with use of the enteral route. J Acad Nutr Diet 2013;113(10):1311–16.
188. McNab S, Ware R, Neville K, et al. Isotonic versus hypotonic solutions for maintenance intravenous fuid administration in children. Cochrane Database Syst Rev 2014;(12):CD009457.
189. McNab S, Duke T, South M, et al. 140 mmol/L of sodium versus 77 mmol/L of sodium in maintenance intravenous fluid therapy for children in hospital (PIMS): a randomised controlled double-blind trial. Lancet 2015;385(9974):1190–7.
190. Moritz ML, Ayus JC. Maintenance intravenous fluids in acutely ill patients. N Engl J Med 2015;373(14):1350–60.
191. Macrae D, Grieve R, Allen E, et al. A randomized trial of hyperglycemic control in pediatric intensive care. N Engl J Med 2014;370(2):107–18.
192. Kaur S, Kumar P, Kumar V, et al. Etiology and prognostic factors of acute liver failure in children. Indian Pediatr 2013;50(7):677–9.
193. Press CA, Morgan L, Mills M, et al. Spectral Eeectroencephalogram analysis for the evaluation of encephalopathy grade in children with acute liver failure. Pediatr Crit Care Med 2017;18(1):64–72.
194. Shanmugam NP, Al-Lawati T, Kelgeri C, et al. Auxiliary liver transplantation for acute liver failure. Indian Pediatr 2016;53(1):67–74.
195. Liu L, Oza S, Hogan D, et al. Global, regional, and national causes of child mortality in 2000-13, with projections to inform post-2015 priorities: an updated systematic analysis. [Erratum: Lancet 2015;385(9966):420], [Erratum: Lancet 2016;387(10037):2506; PMID: 27353684]. Lancet 2015;385(9966):430–40.
196. Sathya C, Alali A, Wales P, et al. Mortality among injured children treated at different trauma center types. JAMA Surg 2015;150(9):874–81.
197. Henley G, Harrison J. Hospitalised farm injury, Australia, 2010-2011 to 2014-2015.pdf. Canberra: Australian Institute of Health and Welfare, Flinders University; 2018. Report No.: INJCAT 189.
198. Kenefake ME, Swarm M, Walthall J. Nuances in pediatric trauma. Emerg Med Clin North Am 2013;31:627–52.
199. Royal Life Saving Society Australia. The national drowning report 2017. Sydney: Royal Life Saving Society Australia; 2017.
200. Henley G, Harrison J. Trends in injury deaths, Australia, 1999–00 to 2011–12. Canberra: Australian Institute of Health and Welfare Flinders University; 2017.
201. Sethi D, Aldridge E, Rakovac I, et al. Worsening inequalities in child injury deaths in the WHO European region. Int J Environ Res Public Health 2017;14(10):1128.
202. Hynick NH, Brennan M, Schmit P, et al. Identification of blunt abdominal injuries in children. J Trauma Acute Care Surg 2014;76(1):95–100.
203. Ahmed OZ, Burd RS. Management issues in critically ill pediatric patients with trauma. Pediatr Clin North Am 2017;64(5):973–90.
204. Kennedy AP, Scorpio RJ, Coppola CP. Assessment of the pediatric trauma patient: differences in approach. J Emerg Crit Care Med 2018;2(4):1–8.
205. Thurman DJ. The epidemiology of traumatic brain injury in children and youths: a review of research since 1990. J Child Neurol 2016;31(1):20–7.
206. Kochanek PM, Carney N, Adelson PD, et al. Guidelines for the acute medical management of severe traumatic brain injury in infants, children and adolescents. 2nd ed. Pediatr Crit Care Med 2012;13(Suppl.):S1–81.
207. O'Lynnger T, Shannon C, Le TM, et al. Standardizing ICU management of pediatric traumatic brain injury is associated with improved outcomes at discharge. J Neurosurg Pediatr 2016;17(1):19–26.

208. Okonkwo DO, Shutter LA, Moore C, et al. Brain oxygen optimization in severe traumatic brain injury phase-II: a phase II randomized trial. Crit Care Med 2017;45(11):1907–14.

209. Mahajan P, Jaffe DM, Olsen CS, et al. Spinal cord injury without radiologic abnormality in children imaged with magnetic resonance imaging. J Trauma Acute Care Surg 2013;75(5):843–7.

210. Chong S-L, Harjanto S, Testoni D, et al. Early hyperglycemia in pediatric traumatic brain injury predicts for mortality, prolonged duration of mechanical ventilation, and intensive care Stay. Int J Endocrinol 2015;2015:8.

211. Beca J, McSharry B, Erickson S, et al. Hypothermia for traumatic brain injury in children – A phase II randomized controlled trial. Crit Care Med 2015;43(7):1458–66.

212. Young AMH, Kolias AG, Hutchinson PJ. Decompressive craniectomy for traumatic intracranial hypertension: application in children. Childs Nerv Syst 2017;33(10):1745–50.

213. Skinner DL, Den Hollander D, Laing GL, et al. Severe blunt thoracic trauma: differences between adults and children in a level 1 trauma centre. S Afr Med J 2015;105(1).

214. Notrica DM. Pediatric blunt abdominal trauma: current management. Curr Opin Crit Care 2015;21(6):531–7.

215. Ghosh S, Shukla R, Mujalde V, et al. Pediatric blunt abdominal trauma – demography in a tertiary care set up of a developing nation. J Pediatr Surg Spec 2017;11(1):11–14.

216. Miele V, Piccolo CL, Galluzzo M, et al. Contrast-enhanced ultrasound (CEUS) in blunt abdominal trauma. Br J Radiol 2016;89(1061):20150823.

Chapter 28

Pregnancy and postpartum considerations

Wendy Pollock, Alison James

Learning objectives

After reading this chapter, you should be able to:

- identify the core physiological adaptations of pregnancy pertinent to critical care nursing
- describe the antenatal assessment that would be required when caring for a woman 28 weeks pregnant in ICU
- describe the priorities of management for a postpartum woman admitted to ICU with preeclampsia
- outline the standard postnatal care required by a woman in ICU, for the 48 hours following birth
- discuss the principles of cardiac arrest management during pregnancy
- consider the resources and equipment available in your workplace that are specifically required for the care of pregnant and postpartum women.

KEY WORDS

antenatal assessment
breastfeeding
critical illness in pregnancy
fetal wellbeing
postpartum care
obstetric haemorrhage
severe acute maternal morbidity
severe preeclampsia

Introduction

The admission of a pregnant or postpartum woman to an intensive care unit (ICU) can extend ICU staff beyond their comfort zone. Pregnant and postpartum women undergo substantial physiological adaptations. Nursing staff also need to consider the fetus and be aware of, and manage, obstetric conditions. This chapter provides an overview of the epidemiology of critical illness in pregnancy, describes the physiological adaptations of pregnancy and the puerperium, outlines some key medical conditions and their interaction with pregnancy and describes the major obstetric conditions that are associated with critical illness. Additionally, we include guidance on specific practices related to caring for pregnant and postpartum women in ICU. Research into critical care obstetrics is limited and at times the evidence being drawn on is dated, but still considered valid.

Epidemiology of critical illness in pregnancy

Most women experience a healthy, normal pregnancy and the development of critical illness associated with pregnancy is usually sudden and unexpected.

Approximately 1 in 370 births results in a maternal ICU admission, making up approximately 1% of the ICU population; more than three-quarters of admissions occur following the birth of the baby.[1,2] However, there are increasing numbers of women with comorbidities having children and this may lead to higher rates of ICU admission. For example, women with a BMI >50 kg/m^2 were over seven times more likely to be admitted to ICU than the general childbearing population.[3] Admission of a pregnant woman to ICU is infrequent and more likely to relate to a non-obstetric diagnosis such as pneumonia. Conversely, in postpartum women, a condition directly associated with pregnancy is more common, usually pre-eclampsia or obstetric haemorrhage.[1]

Pregnant and postpartum admissions to ICU are usually short with most lengths of stay less than 24 hours. There is variation in the threshold for admission to ICU as many women do not receive specific ICU interventions. In general, about one-third of women who experience severe acute maternal morbidity are admitted to ICU.[4] It is feasible that admission to ICU could be avoided by upskilling midwifery services to provide an intermediate level of care.[5] Furthermore, with early identification of clinical deterioration and timely, appropriate intervention, it is feasible that up to 40% of maternal ICU admissions are potentially preventable.[6] In developed countries, the mortality of pregnant and postpartum women admitted to ICU is relatively low at around 3% compared with the 15% mortality observed in the regular ICU population.[1]

Practice tip

Any maternal death or death of a woman during pregnancy or within 42 days of having been pregnant should be reported to the relevant authority, even if the pregnancy is not thought to have contributed to the cause of death.

Adapted physiology of pregnancy

The physiological changes that occur during pregnancy influence the majority of body systems (Table 28.1), commence shortly after conception and enable changes that facilitate fetal and uterine growth, and prepare the woman for birth and lactation. The physiological changes described in this chapter relate to women with singleton pregnancies who are not in labour. Where multiple pregnancy occurs, physiological adaptations may be exaggerated and labour brings further changes to the adapted physiology, such as increased cardiac output.[7] The normal physiological changes of pregnancy differ from woman to woman, depending on factors such as maternal age, health and genetic influences.[7] The uterus

TABLE 28.1
Key physiological changes in pregnancy

PARAMETER	CHANGE DURING PREGNANCY
CARDIOVASCULAR SYSTEM	
Heart rate	↑ 10–20 beats/min
Stroke volume	↑ 18–32%
Blood pressure	
Systolic	↓ 5–10 mmHg
Diastolic	↓10–25 mmHg
Cardiac output	↑ 30–50%
Systemic vascular resistance	↓ up to 40%
Central arterial and venous pressures	Unchanged
HAEMATOLOGICAL SYSTEM	
Blood volume	↑1200–1600 mL
Plasma volume	↑ 30–50%
Red blood cells	↑ 20–30%
White blood cells	↑ 100–300%
Platelets	Up to 20% decrease but count remaining within normal limits
Fibrinogen	↑ 100%
Serum albumin level	↓ 10–15%
RESPIRATORY SYSTEM	
Respiratory rate	Unchanged
Tidal volume	↑ 30–50%
Minute volume	↑ 40–50%
Oxygen consumption	↑ 15–20%
ARTERIAL BLOOD GAS ANALYSIS VALUES	
PaO_2	80–110 mmHg
$PaCO_2$	28–32 mmHg
pH	7.40–7.45
HCO_3^-	18–21 mmol/L
SaO_2	≥95%
Vital capacity	Unchanged
Functional reserve capacity	↓ 17–20% (from 1.7 L to 1.35 L)
Lung compliance	Unchanged
RENAL SYSTEM	
Glomerular filtration rate	↑ 40–50%
Serum urea and creatinine	↓
Urine output	Unknown
Proteinuria	<300 mg/day

and breasts undergo major changes during pregnancy and are described in detail in physiology and midwifery textbooks such as *Maternal, fetal, and neonatal physiology: a clinical perspective* and *Myles Textbook for midwives*.[8,9]

The puerperium (also referred to as the postnatal or postpartum period) commences after the placenta and membranes are expelled, when there is a sharp drop in the placental hormones including progesterone and oestrogens.[8] The puerperium is usually defined as 6 weeks, during which time the body systems gradually return to the pre-pregnant or near pre-pregnant state.[10] Lactation will become established where the mother chooses to breastfeed.

Haematological system

Blood volume and red cells

Total blood volume, plasma volume and red cell mass increase during pregnancy.[8] Plasma volume increases by 30–50% while the red cell mass increases by approximately 20–30%, causing a relative haemodilutional anaemia.[8,11] Maternal venous haematocrit will also be lower (34%) near term.[11] Overall, there will be an increase in total blood volume of 1200–1600 mL and this is required to accommodate the metabolic demands of the developing fetus, and prepares the woman for normal blood loss associated with birth (<500 mL).[8,11] Pregnant women are renowned for being able to maintain stable vital signs, with blood losses as much as 1500 mL, before acutely deteriorating.[12]

Blood clotting and haemostasis

Both elements of the haemostatic system (coagulation and fibrinolysis) activate during pregnancy. Pregnancy is termed a hypercoagulable state, due to an increase in clotting factors (e.g. VII, VIII, IX, X, XII), an increase in fibrinogen and fibrin degradation products and a decrease in some naturally occurring anticoagulants.[8] There is also venous stasis and microscopic vascular damage and combined, these factors comprise 'Virchow's triad'. Due to this triad of factors, both pregnant and postnatal women are at increased risk of venous thromboembolism (VTE).[13] The changes occurring to the haemostatic system are summarised in Table 28.2. Of note, gestational thrombocytopenia (defined as platelets of 80–150 × 10^9/L) occurs in 6–8% of healthy pregnant women and generally has no negative impact on the woman or fetus.[17]

TABLE 28.2
Haemostatic changes during pregnancy[14-16]

HAEMOSTATIC COMPONENT	CHANGES DURING PREGNANCY
PLATELETS	
Count	Unchanged
Lifespan	Unchanged
CLOTTING FACTORS	
Factors VII, VIII and IX,X, XII	Increased
Fibrinogen	Doubles by term
Other clotting factors	Mainly unchanged
FIBRINOLYSIS	
D-dimer level	Progressively increases during pregnancy By term, level >0.5 mg/L common

Cardiovascular system

Anatomical changes

The heart undergoes anatomical change during pregnancy including left ventricular hypertrophy by 12 weeks and increases in the cross-sectional areas of the aortic, pulmonary and mitral valves of 12–14%.[18] ECG changes may include atrial/ventricular ectopics, Q waves in lead II, III and AVF, ST-segment changes, T-wave inversion in lead III and left-axis shift of QRS.[19]

Heart rate, stroke volume and cardiac output

Peripheral vasodilation occurs from 5 weeks' gestation, stimulated by progesterone and endothelium-dependent factors including nitric oxide, which also vasodilates the placental vessels.[20-22] There is a subsequent 25–40% decrease in systemic vascular resistance (SVR).[23] The maternal heart rate increases by 10–20 beats/min, peaking in the third trimester.[8,24,25] Stroke volume increases between 18% and 32%, beginning as early as 8 weeks' gestation.[23,26,27] Cardiac output increases during the first and second trimesters, peaking at 30–50% over non-pregnant values towards the end of the second trimester (6–7 L/min), although this increase may not be linear.[23,26-28] The increase in cardiac output may manifest as early as 6 weeks' gestation and is a key adaptation.[8,29]

Blood pressure

Blood pressure begins dropping as early as 6-8 weeks of gestation, with the lowest levels recorded during the second trimester and returning to pre-pregnancy measurements near term (see Table 28.1).[23] The diastolic BP drops between 10 mmHg and 25 mmHg whereas the systolic BP remains more stable and may drop by 6–8%.[18,23] The decrease in blood pressure is attributed to widespread peripheral vasodilation occurring during pregnancy and the shunting of blood through the placenta.[18]

Aortocaval compression and supine hypotension

After 20 weeks of gestation, a woman lying flat on her back may experience supine hypotension, secondary to aortocaval compression, with reduction in venous return, cardiac output and placental blood flow.[30] Cardiac stroke

FIGURE 28.1 Manual displacement of the uterus to the left (one-handed and two-handed).

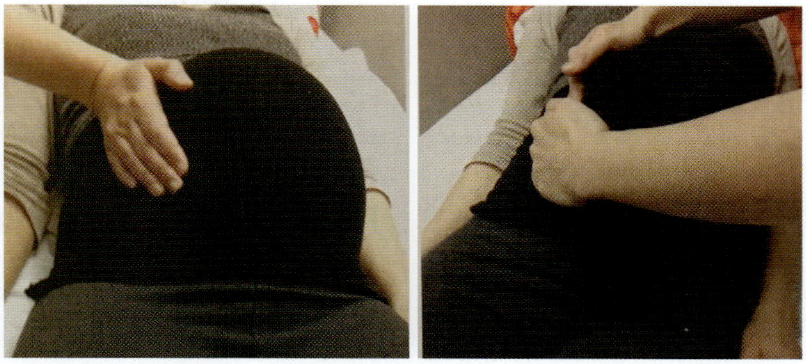

Source: C. Winter, et al, editors. Prompt course manual. 3rd ed. Cambridge University Press, 2017, p.31.

volume can be reduced by as much as 70% and a pregnant woman of ≥ 20 weeks gestation should not be nursed flat on her back.[22] A left lateral lying position of 15–30° results in improved maternal cardiac output and may be achieved with the use of a wedge/pillows, or tilted if on a theatre table or spinal board.[28] Left manual uterine displacement is advocated during CPR to facilitate optimal chest compressions (Fig. 28.1).[28,30]

Postpartum cardiovascular changes

Heart rate returns to pre-pregnancy levels by 10 days postpartum while blood pressure has normally returned to pre-pregnancy levels by term and does not change during the puerperium.[22] The first few days of the puerperium are associated with a significant diuresis, resulting in the haemoconcentration of blood. Therefore, the risk of thromboembolism is higher during the postpartum period than during pregnancy. Appropriate risk assessment and prophylactic measures should be implemented to reduce the risk of VTE.[13]

Post birth, cardiac output increases as approximately 500 mL of blood (no longer required by the fetus and placenta) is auto-transfused back into the maternal circulation.[27] At this point in the postpartum phase, stroke volume is increased, while the maternal heart rate is often slowed.[31] For most women, the immediate postpartum elevation in cardiac output only lasts 48 hours.[27] By 2 weeks postpartum, many haemodynamic parameters have returned to pre-pregnancy levels for most women, although some have been recorded as remaining above pre-pregnancy levels at 12 months postpartum, including cardiac output.[22,32]

Respiratory system

The respiratory system undergoes widespread adaptation from early pregnancy with effects on the airway through to gaseous exchange at the alveolar level evident, including variation to 'normal' parameters when interpreting arterial blood gas results. These changes support the increased metabolic demands of pregnancy.[33]

Changes to the upper airways and thorax

Normal physiological changes of pregnancy include generalised vasodilation of the upper airway vasculature, increased neck circumference due to fat deposition and an increase in mucosal oedema.[7,34] These physiological changes are thought to be responsible for the symptoms of rhinitis, nasal stuffiness and epistaxis that are more common in pregnancy.[7,34] Changes also occur to the chest wall, with relaxation of ligaments resulting in outward flaring of the lower ribs and a 50% increase in the subcostal angle.[8] The diameter and the circumference of the thorax increase by 2 cm and 5–7 cm, respectively.[8,33,34] These physical changes are thought to cause the diaphragm to rise by 4 cm, before there is additional pressure from the enlarging uterus.[33,34]

Respiratory muscle function does not change significantly during pregnancy and rib cage compliance is unaltered.[34] The functional residual capacity (FRC) is reduced by 10–30%, making the pregnant woman more vulnerable to hypoxaemia during any apnoeic period.[30,34,35] Chest X-ray interpretation is unchanged during pregnancy.[31] Overall, oxygen requirements increase by up to 33% at term.[30]

Changes to the physiology of breathing

From 5 weeks' gestation, multiple factors increase respiratory drive. Elevated progesterone levels are thought to lower the $PaCO_2$ threshold in the respiratory centre, resulting in hyperventilation.[36,37] Minute ventilation (MV) begins to increase soon after conception, peaking at 40–50% above pre-conception level at term (7.5–10.5 L/min).[18,36] The increase in minute ventilation is achieved by a 30–50% increase in tidal volume (e.g. an increase of 200 ± 50 mL at term), without any increase in respiratory rate.[18,36,38] Consequently, normal arterial blood gas values are different in pregnancy (Table 28.1). The reduced $PaCO_2$ level enables fetal CO_2 to cross the placenta for maternal excretion passively. PaO_2 normally increases by 10 mmHg, although the PaO_2 level is affected by posture, particularly as the pregnancy progresses.[39] Later in pregnancy the supine position can reduce PaO_2 by 10 mmHg when compared with the same woman in the sitting position.[40] The kidneys compensate for the lowered $PaCO_2$ by increasing bicarbonate excretion to maintain a normal pH.[39,41,42] Normal oxygen saturation in pregnancy has not been well investigated. It is likely to be 97–100% at sea level, with a healthy pregnant woman's saturation not dropping below 95% during moderate exercise.[38,43]

Hyperventilation of pregnancy is associated with a feeling of breathlessness in up to 70% of healthy pregnant women.[44] Consequently, distinguishing 'physiological dyspnoea' from 'pathological dyspnoea' (e.g. developing cardiomyopathy or pulmonary embolism) can present a challenge in pregnancy and requires careful investigation.[44]

Postpartum respiratory changes

Complete resolution of the spirometry and arterial blood gas changes occurring in pregnancy is accomplished by 5 weeks postpartum,[39] although the daily transition of these parameters over the first week postpartum is not known. One very old study reported that CO_2 levels took between 2 and 5 days to return to normal non-pregnant values postpartum.[45] Rapid changes to the $PaCO_2$ level will contribute to the development of acidaemia, which may be clinically relevant around the time of delivery or in the early postpartum phase if the woman has an active disease state or experiences a complication, such as severe postpartum haemorrhage.

Renal system

The smooth muscle of the renal pelvises, calyces, ureters and urethra dilate during early pregnancy due largely to the effects of progesterone. Each kidney lengthens by approximately 1–1.5 cm, due to dilation, associated mild hydronephrosis and increased vascularity.[7,18] Widespread dilation causes urinary stasis and increased likelihood of urinary tract infection.[8] Acute pyelonephritis is a common renal complication and is associated with preterm labour.[46]

Renal plasma flow increases by up to 80%.[47] The glomerular filtration rate (GFR) increases by 40–50%, peaking by the end of the first trimester, and may result in glycosuria and proteinuria.[46,47] Glycosuria does not accurately reflect blood sugar levels and is unhelpful in monitoring diabetes, as glucose excretion is increased up to 100 times above non-pregnant levels.[8] Proteinuria, up to 300 mg per 24 hours, is considered normal in pregnancy. Conversely, the high GFR results in lowered mean serum levels of both urea (3.2 mmol/L) and creatinine (44.2 micromol/L).[8] A plasma urea level exceeding 4.5 mmol/L and plasma creatinine level higher than 75 micromol/L should be viewed as abnormal and indicative of potential renal impairment requiring investigation.[48,49] There is a reduction in normal serum sodium level, from 140 to 136 mmol/L, and a reduction in plasma osmolality from 290 to 280 mOsmol/kg. These changes persist throughout pregnancy.[47,48]

Postpartum renal changes

The most significant postpartum renal change is the diuresis that occurs during the first 3 days. This diuresis serves to offload the additional blood volume that the woman has had circulating for the duration of the pregnancy. There has been little examination of 'normal urine output' with the standard 0.5 mL/kg/h reported as a minimum acceptable level; however, a true 'normal' level is likely to be closer to 0.8 mL/kg/h.[50] Creatinine levels are within the normal non-pregnancy range within 24 hours postpartum, while the lower urea levels remain for at least 48 hours.[49] The bladder returns to the pelvis in the early postpartum period as the uterus and other organs resume their pre-pregnancy position.

Gastrointestinal system and liver

The enlarging uterus pushes abdominal organs aside, making assessment and diagnosis of an acute abdomen difficult and changes landmarks for surgical incisions.[27,51] For example, the appendix is progressively displaced upwards and laterally from McBurney's point at the third month, reaching the level of the iliac crest by late pregnancy.[52] Pregnant women with prior abdominal surgery and adhesions are also more predisposed to intestinal obstruction.[53]

Due to the effects of progesterone and the mechanical presence of the enlarging uterus, there is delayed gastric emptying, decreased cardiac sphincter tone and raised intraabdominal pressure, which predisposes women to heartburn and increases their risk of aspiration.[8,27] Bowel peristalsis slows, from the effects of progesterone, commonly resulting in constipation; this slowing of peristalsis along with pressure from the gravid uterus on the pelvic vasculature also contribute to haemorrhoids.

Hepatobiliary changes in pregnancy

There is no significant increase in hepatic arterial blood flow during pregnancy. However, blood flow to the liver supplied by the portal vein doubles,[54] which may have an impact on oral medication metabolism. Changes in hepatic enzymes responsible for drug metabolism may alter the pharmacokinetics of some medications, e.g. higher plasma levels of midazolam. Serum albumin levels reduce to 30–40 g/L for the majority of pregnancy, with levels as low as 25 g/L normal during the second postpartum day.[49] This low albumin level reduces colloid osmotic pressure, contributing to the presence of oedema that is common in pregnancy.

The general smooth muscle vasodilation affects the hepatobiliary ducts, resulting in sluggish bile motility and delayed emptying of the gallbladder. These changes lead to an increased incidence of cholelithiasis and cholecystitis during pregnancy.[51]

Changes in white blood cells and the immune system

There is continued debate on whether pregnancy increases vulnerability to infection, secondary to some protective mechanism that prevents the woman's body from reacting to the fetus as a foreign body.[7] Pregnant women have increased innate immune system activity (non-specific response) and a lowered adaptive immune system (specific antibody response), with pregnant women more vulnerable to some infections, such as malaria and varicella.[55,56] Pregnant women are often in contact with small children and potentially have an increased exposure to various infections. The white blood cell number increases throughout pregnancy, peaking at around 30 weeks' gestation, when a normal level may be as high as 15–25 × 10^9/L.[9,49]

The placenta and membranes

Placental development

The placenta develops from the trophoblastic layer of the fertilised ovum and is completely formed and functioning 10 weeks following fertilisation. The chorionic villi attach to the uterine wall via the decidua. The result is an interface whereby maternal blood fills a space in which the nutritive villi float and are bathed in the maternal blood (Fig. 28.2). The blood drains back into the maternal circulation via maternal sinuses and the endometrial veins. Approximately 150 mL of maternal blood, replenished three to four times per minute, bathes the villi in the intervillous space.[9] The chorionic villi maximise the available surface area to optimise the exchange of products across the maternal–placental interface. By term, this surface area is said to be as large as 13 m^2.[57] Initially, four layers of cells separate the maternal blood from the fetal blood, reducing to three after 20 weeks' gestation; these cell layers are collectively referred to as the 'placental membrane' or 'placental barrier'.[57] Damage to villi, such as a threatened abortion or blunt trauma, can enable fetal haemoglobin and squames to enter the

FIGURE 28.2 The maternal–placental interface.

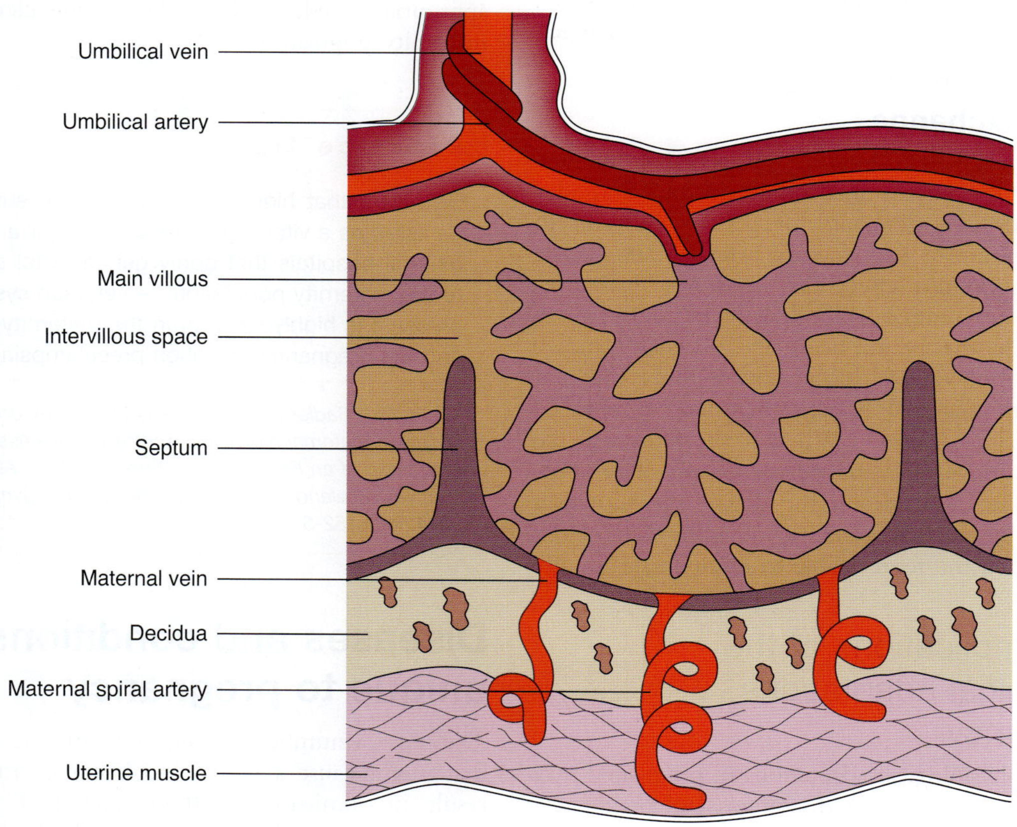

Reproduced from Marshall JE, Raynor MD, editors. Myles Textbook for midwives. 16th ed. Edinburgh: Elsevier; 2014.

maternal circulation, leading to rhesus isoimmunisation or, rarely, amniotic fluid embolism.

Functions of the placenta

The placenta provides six major functions to sustain the pregnancy and fetus: respiration, nutrition, storage, excretion, protection and endocrine.[9] Fetal lungs are filled with fluid and all oxygenation and removal of carbon dioxide must be provided via the placenta. Fetal haemoglobin has a slightly different structure to adult haemoglobin and has a higher affinity for oxygen. Both oxygen and carbon dioxide cross the placental membrane by simple diffusion. Nutrients are actively transported across the placental membrane, with the placenta able to select the substances needed by the fetus, even at the expense of the mother if necessary.[9] The placenta is able to store glucose by converting it to glycogen and reconverting it to glucose as required and also stores iron and some fat-soluble vitamins.

The placental membrane operates as a barrier between the maternal and fetal circulations and provides a limited protective function. Generally, few bacteria can cross the placenta, although viruses can cross readily. The placenta produces large volumes of hormones including progesterone, oestrogens, placental lactogen, chorionic gonadotropin, growth factors, cytokine vasoactive substances, placental growth hormone, thyrotropin and corticotropin.[8] The placenta does not have a nerve supply so all activities regulated by the placenta must be undertaken by other mechanisms, e.g. chemical, hormonal changes.

Impaired utero–placental gaseous exchange

Effective gas exchange across the placental membrane depends on sufficient maternal blood pressure and adequate O_2 and CO_2 gradients for passive diffusion to occur. In response to hypoxaemia, a fetal brain-sparing mechanism goes into effect that increases fetal arterial pressure and redirects blood delivery to the main organs, namely the brain, heart and adrenal glands.[58] This centralisation of fetal blood flow is more apparent in response to maternal hypoxaemia than to reduced utero–placental blood flow. Whether the fetus will die in utero or survive, and the degree of any neurological compromise, depends on the degree and duration of asphyxia, the recurrent nature of asphyxia and the degree to which the fetus is able to compensate for the asphyxia.

Clinical implications of the physiological adaptations of pregnancy

The normal physiological adaptations of pregnancy may explain the so-called 'minor discomforts' of pregnancy, including constipation, varicose veins, indigestion, breathlessness and fatigue. The adaptations influence the majority of body systems (see Table 28.1) and must be taken into consideration when monitoring physiological parameters, interpreting investigation results and planning treatment for the critically ill woman[59] (Table 28.3).

Recognition of clinical deterioration in pregnant and postpartum women

The physiological adaptations of pregnancy may make early recognition of clinical deterioration more challenging. For example, with 30–50% more cardiac output and 40–50% more circulating volume, substantial blood loss occurs before there are changes in vital signs, such as heart rate and blood pressure. Additionally, pregnancy and childbirth are considered normal life events in young, healthy women, and serious complications occur rarely, which can lead to complacency. The implementation of system-wide standards on the early recognition of clinical deterioration has resulted in a reduction of cardiac arrest-related admission to ICU.[60] Despite the UK Confidential Enquiry into Maternal Deaths recommending the use of maternity-modified early warning systems since 2007, agreed and universally accepted appropriate vital signs, taking into account the physiology of pregnancy, remain elusive for the maternity population.[61] However, pregnant and postpartum women do experience clinical deterioration in hospital with about 10% of Medical Emergency Team (MET) calls resulting in the women requiring admission to ICU.[62] Critical care nurses who attend maternity MET calls should be appropriately educated on the unique elements of the maternity population.

Practice tip

Be aware that high systolic blood pressure may not be listed as a vital sign criteria to trigger a MET call in general hospitals that apply generic vital sign criteria to the maternity population[63] – yet, high systolic blood pressure is highly relevant in the maternity population and the pregnancy condition preeclampsia.

Austin DM, Sadler L, McLintock C et al. Early detection of severe maternal morbidity: a retrospective assessment of the role of an Early Warning Score System. Australian and New Zealand Journal of Obstetrics and Gynaecology 2014;54(2):152-5.

Diseases and conditions unique to pregnancy

There are a number of conditions unique to pregnancy that might cause a woman to become critically ill and result in admission to ICU, including preeclampsia, obstetric haemorrhage, amniotic fluid embolism and peripartum cardiomyopathy. These conditions are discussed in detail below.

TABLE 28.3
Clinical relevance of physiological adaptations in pregnancy

EFFECTS OF THE NORMAL PHYSIOLOGY OF PREGNANCY	CLINICAL IMPLICATIONS
CARDIOVASCULAR SYSTEM	
Increased likelihood of: • venous stasis • varicose veins • deep vein thrombosis • haemorrhoids • swollen ankles	Consider use of thromboprophylaxis
Potential for aortocaval compression from about 20 weeks' gestation	Avoid nursing the woman flat on her back, e.g. tilt bed if unable to nurse woman on her side or use pillows/wedges to obtain a lateral tilt of 15°–30° but full left lying is best CPR and haemodynamic measurements should be done with a left lateral tilt. Manual displacement of the uterus is an alternative way to relieve aortocaval compression during CPR
Haemodynamic stability despite large blood loss Sudden deterioration	Be alert to subtle signs of haemodynamic compromise
RESPIRATORY SYSTEM	
Nasal passages more likely to bleed on instrumentation (e.g. nasal intubation, nasogastric insertion) More likely to bleed from the gums More prone to hypoxaemia during apnoea, e.g. when being intubated All pregnant women are considered to have a high-risk airway: • especially if the woman has preeclampsia • particularly if the woman is obese More likely to develop pulmonary oedema Diaphragm raised by about 5 cm	Nasal-tracheal intubation is not usually an option Have a doctor experienced with intubation on hand when a pregnant woman is being intubated Ensure that the artificial airway is protected and guard against accidental extubation Review the 'failed intubation' protocol in the ICU Pre-oxygenate with 100% O_2 prior to intubation or suctioning unless contraindicated Titrate fluid resuscitation carefully – especially in women with severe preeclampsia Check diaphragm location prior to ICC insertion for haemothorax/pleural effusion
GASTROINTESTINAL SYSTEM	
Pregnant women are more likely to: • aspirate • develop constipation • present with advanced signs and symptoms of acute abdomen, e.g. appendicitis, bowel obstruction Pregnant women have additional and specific nutritional needs	Maintain cricoid pressure, if instructed, throughout CPR and intubation until the person obtaining an artificial airway instructs its release Chart bowel actions and ensure a bowel management strategy is implemented Early consideration of non-obstetric causes of an acute abdomen Consult with a dietician early to ensure that the woman receives adequate nutrition during ICU admission
RENAL SYSTEM	
Progesterone and relaxin causes relaxation and dilation of smooth muscles Renal calyces and renal pelvis become distended Ureters and urethra are elongated, dilated and have reduced peristalsis Stasis of urine and increased risk of ascending infection Acute pyelonephritis is associated with preterm labour Bladder is displaced into the abdominal cavity after the first trimester	Minimise use of indwelling urinary catheter Renal impairment may be signified by lower serum urea and creatinine levels than in non-pregnancy Some glycosuria and proteinuria are normal in pregnancy The bladder is at risk of traumatic injury in the second and third trimesters

CPR = cardiopulmonary resuscitation; ICC = intercostal catheter.

Preeclampsia

The umbrella term 'hypertension in pregnancy' describes myriad conditions in pregnancy where hypertension is a major feature, with the definition for hypertension unchanged during pregnancy: systolic BP ≥140 mmHg and/or diastolic BP ≥90 mmHg. These hypertensive conditions include gestational hypertension, chronic hypertension and preeclampsia, which incorporates eclampsia and haemolysis-elevated liver enzymes and low platelets (HELLP) syndrome (Table 28.4). Comprehensive descriptions of these conditions and their management have been published by the UK's National Institute for Health and Clinical Excellence[64] and the Society of Obstetric Medicine Australia and New Zealand (SOMANZ).[65] Another useful resource is the California Maternity Quality Care Collaborative Preeclampsia Toolkit, available at https://www.cmqcc.org/resources-tool-kits/toolkits/preeclampsia-toolkit.[66]

Preeclampsia is a progressive, multisystem disorder consisting of variable clinical features related to endothelial dysfunction, which occurs in response to toxins released from the placenta. The indication for ICU admission is usually related to organ dysfunction.[67] Preeclampsia remains a leading cause of maternal death in both developed and developing countries.[68] It is the second most common condition associated with ICU admission in developed countries.

Aetiology

The placenta is strongly implicated in the cause of preeclampsia; its removal is the only definitive treatment for the condition. Theories explaining the pathophysiology of preeclampsia include immune maladaptation, abnormal trophoblast embedding, endothelial activation and excessive inflammatory response, and a genetic susceptibility. Additionally, it is postulated that there may be alternate pathophysiology for early-onset (<34 weeks) disease compared with later-onset disease (Box 28.1).[69] The contribution of each component and whether they are relevant in all cases of preeclampsia are not known.

Early-onset preeclampsia (<34 weeks) is associated with impaired remodelling of the uterine spiral arteries and abnormal placental implantation. It is thought that maternal–fetal immune maladaptation could be the main cause for this superficial placentation.[69] Placental flow defects are detected as early as 12 weeks in some women who go on to develop preeclampsia.[70] In late-onset preeclampsia (≥ 34 weeks), growth of the placental villi

TABLE 28.4
Definitions of conditions characterised by hypertension in pregnancy

TERM	DEFINITION
Hypertension in pregnancy	Systolic BP ≥ 140 mmHg and/or a diastolic BP ≥90 mmHg[65]
Chronic hypertension	Hypertension presenting in the first 20 weeks or that existed prior to the pregnancy without an apparent underlying cause[65]
Gestational hypertension	Hypertension arising after 20 weeks' gestation and resolving by 3 months postpartum No evidence of any other feature of the multisystem disorder preeclampsia[65]
Preeclampsia (also referred to as pregnancy-induced hypertension (PIH), toxaemia)	Hypertension after 20 weeks' gestation in combination with one or more of the following:[65] • Proteinuria >300 mg/24 h • Renal insufficiency: serum/plasma creatinine ≥0.09 mmol/L or oliguria (<80 mL in 4 hours) • Liver impairment: raised serum transaminases and/or severe epigastric/right upper quadrant pain • Neurological problems: convulsions (eclampsia), hyperreflexia with clonus, severe headaches with hyperreflexia, persistent visual disturbances, cerebral haemorrhage • Haematological disturbances: thrombocytopenia, DIC, haemolysis • Fetal growth restriction, placental abruption
Eclampsia	A form of severe preeclampsia Generalised tonic–clonic seizures, not caused by epilepsy or other disease, and occurring ≥20 weeks' gestation, during labour or in the postpartum
HELLP syndrome	A form of severe preeclampsia, although hypertension may not be present Diagnosis of HELLP syndrome is made by the presence of the following three criteria: 1 Haemolysis: characteristic peripheral blood smear and serum lactate dehydrogenase (LDH) >600 U/L or serum total bilirubin ≥1.2 mg/dL 2 Elevated liver enzymes: serum aspartate aminotransferase ≥70 U/L 3 Low platelet count: <100 × 10^9/L

DIC = disseminated intravascular coagulopathy; HELLP = haemolysis-elevated liver enzymes and low platelets.

BOX 28.1

Theories on the pathophysiology of preeclampsia[69]

Placentation and the immune theory of preeclampsia:

- Maternal–fetal (paternal) immune maladaptation
- Superficial abnormal placentation
- Impaired spiral artery remodelling

Placental debris hypothesis: syncytiotrophoblast shedding:

- Increased syncytiotrophoblast shedding
- Placental ischaemia and reperfusion with subsequent oxidative stress
- Increased circulating levels of inflammatory cytokines, corticotropin-releasing hormone, free-radical species and activin A

Endothelial activation and inflammation:

- Enhanced vascular sensitivity to angiotensin II and noradrenaline with vasoconstriction and hypertension
- A fall in production /activity of vasodilator prostaglandins, especially prostacyclin and nitric oxide

Genes, the genetic-conflict hypothesis and genetic imprinting:

- Susceptibility genes, many of which interact with the maternal cardiovascular or haemostatic system, or with the regulation of maternal inflammatory responses
- Early-onset (< 34 weeks) and late-onset (≥ 34 weeks) disease[71]
- Early-onset disease is underpinned by abnormal placentation – incomplete spiral artery remodelling
- Late-onset disease demonstrates a placenta that is stressed and beginning to fail as placental growth has reached its functional limits.
- Abnormal placental perfusion and release of angiogenic mediators (toxins) is the common outcome of both underlying causes

Source: Sibai B, Dekker G, Kupferminc M. Pre-eclampsia. Lancet 2005;365(9461):785–99.

have reached their functional limit resulting in intervillous hypoxia and leading to syncytiotrophoblast stress.[71] Placental ischaemia and reperfusion with subsequent oxidative stress have been regarded as major pathogenetic drivers in both pathways. Further, a number of anti-angiogenic factors are considered centrally responsible for the endothelial dysfunction and maternal organ injury.[71,72] The excessive systemic inflammatory response and associated endothelial dysfunction and enhanced vascular reactivity result in widespread vasospasm that precedes the onset of clinical signs, such as hypertension.[68] Other common clinical manifestations in preeclampsia include enhanced endothelial-cell permeability and platelet aggregation, explaining the increased likelihood of oedema and thrombosis.[69]

In summary, preeclampsia presents after 20 weeks' gestation, but the foundation for the disease may relate to abnormal placentation early in the first trimester.

Risk factors

A number of maternal characteristics are associated with an increased likelihood for the development of preeclampsia; these include:[69,73,74]

- nulliparity
- age ≥ 40 years
- preexisting medical conditions including diabetes, chronic hypertension, chronic renal disease, antiphospholipid antibodies
- preeclampsia in a prior pregnancy, particularly if it presented prior to 34 weeks
- family history of preeclampsia, particularly on the maternal side of the family
- multiple pregnancy, e.g. twins
- body mass index >25 prior to pregnancy
- time between pregnancies (>10 years).

High priority is placed on early and accurate diagnosis of preeclampsia. Although many studies have looked to predict which women will develop preeclampsia, no test, including biomarker measurements or ultrasound, has proven utility yet.[75] Identifying women at moderate-to-high-risk of preeclampsia is relevant though, as low-dose aspirin administered from 14–16 weeks' gestation, usually up to 37 weeks, has been shown to significantly reduce the development of the condition.[76] Improved understanding of risk factors and prediction of at-risk women, with the idea to prevent the development of preeclampsia, is a high-level current research area.

Incidence

The incidence of preeclampsia is reported to be 2–8%, with variations based on severity of the disease.[73] The incidence of eclampsia in developed countries has reduced since the routine use of magnesium sulfate has been adopted; in the UK, the rate is about three cases of eclampsia for every 10,000 births.[77] In Latin America the incidence of eclampsia is 17/10,000 births, while in Egypt it is 115/10,000 births.[78,79] However, there is variation in eclampsia even in high-income areas, considered to reflect the quality of care.[80] The incidence of HELLP syndrome is reported to be between 0.11% and 0.67% of all pregnancies.[81,82] Preeclampsia is one of the most common indications for ICU admission at approximately one ICU admission for every 1000 deliveries.[1,65]

Clinical presentation and diagnosis

The clinical presentation of preeclampsia is often subtle, resulting in delayed diagnosis and treatment. Common symptoms include feeling 'generally unwell', headache, heartburn, nausea and vomiting and oedema; all non-specific symptoms experienced by many pregnant women who do not have preeclampsia. Severe preeclampsia is associated with severe headache, hyperreflexia, visual disturbances, severe epigastric pain, right upper quadrant pain and, rarely, acute blindness. Diagnosis is made when the woman has hypertension (BP ≥140/90), in association with evidence of multisystem involvement (Box 28.2). Severe preeclampsia is diagnosed when the BP is ≥160/110, in association with multisystem involvement. Additionally, eclampsia and HELLP syndrome are considered severe variants of preeclampsia even if the woman is normotensive.

This clinical diagnosis has replaced the traditional triad of signs of hypertension, proteinuria and oedema, in accordance with increased understanding of the multisystem nature of the disease. Common investigations include urea, creatinine and electrolytes, full blood examination, liver function tests and spot urine protein/creatinine ratio. Additional tests, such as coagulation studies, may be required as indicated by the clinical condition. Intrauterine fetal growth restriction is a sign of placental involvement and timely investigation into fetal wellbeing will be indicated.

The presentation of preeclampsia is usually restricted to women ≥20 weeks' gestation unless they have a coexisting condition that is known to be associated with a <20 weeks presentation of preeclampsia including hydatidiform mole, multiple pregnancy, fetal triploidy, severe maternal renal disease or antiphospholipid antibody syndrome.[65] Importantly, preeclampsia should resolve within 3 months postpartum.

Most first eclamptic seizures occur during pregnancy (42–45%), with 19–24% during labour and 33–36% postpartum.[77] The majority of postpartum eclampsia occurs in the first 48 hours, although eclampsia may occur up to 2 to 3 weeks postpartum – even in women with no evidence of preeclampsia during pregnancy. Despite the nomenclature, eclampsia can occur without any preceding signs and symptoms of preeclampsia. In the UK Obstetric Surveillance System (UKOSS) eclampsia study, only 38% of women had established hypertension and proteinuria in the week preceding the eclamptic fit and 21% of women had no sign or symptom prior to the first eclamptic fit.[77] HELLP syndrome commonly presents during pregnancy with about 30% postpartum.[83] Most women admitted to ICU with a diagnosis of preeclampsia have usually delivered prior to transfer, and require support for complications of preeclampsia, e.g. acute kidney injury, disseminated intravascular coagulopathy (DIC), pulmonary oedema and fluid management. Once the placenta is delivered, most women improve within 24–48 hours; however, in particular, women with HELLP syndrome may experience a worsening of the condition in the first 48 hours postpartum. Uncontrolled hypertension remains a major concern and is associated with cerebral haemorrhage, one of the dominant causes of death in women with preeclampsia.

BOX 28.2

Diagnostic features of preeclampsia

Hypertension ≥140/90* accompanied by one or more of the following:

- Renal involvement:
  - Significant proteinuria: dipstick proteinuria subsequently confirmed by spot urine protein/creatinine ratio ≥30 mg/mmol or >300 mg protein in a 24-h urine collection
  - Serum or plasma creatinine ≥90 micromol/L
  - Oliguria (<80 mL/4 h)
- Haematological involvement:
  - Thrombocytopenia (<100 × 10^9/L)
  - Haemolysis
  - DIC
- Liver involvement:
  - Raised serum transaminases
  - Severe epigastric/right upper quadrant pain
- Neurological involvement:
  - Eclampsia
  - Hyperreflexia/sustained clonus
  - Severe headache
  - Visual disturbances (e.g. blurred vision, black spots)
  - Cerebral haemorrhage
- Cardiac involvement
  - Pulmonary oedema
- Placental involvement
  - Fetal growth restriction
  - Abruption

*Although hypertension is usually a component of diagnosis, it is not always present, especially in women with an atypical presentation, such as HELLP syndrome.

Adapted from

Lowe SA, Bowyer L, Lust K et al. The SOMANZ guideline for the management of hypertensive disorders of pregnancy 2014. Sydney: Society of Obstetric Medicine of Australia and New Zealand, 2014

Sibai B, Dekker G, Kupferminc M. Pre-eclampsia. Lancet 2005;365(9461):785–99.

Management priorities

The management of women with severe preeclampsia is focused on stabilising the woman's condition, optimal timing of delivery of the baby (and placenta) and preventing complications of the condition. Women with eclampsia and HELLP syndrome require the same treatments as other women with severe preeclampsia, even though they may or may not have the same degree of hypertension.[65,84]

Control of hypertension

Obtaining control of high blood pressure remains a priority not only to improve organ perfusion but to minimise the risk of cerebral haemorrhage.[29,85] Both systolic and diastolic pressures are important, and care should be taken to ensure a gradual lowering of blood pressure as a rapid drop can compromise fetal wellbeing. There is no evidence for the superiority of any specific antihypertensive, although there is some evidence that diazoxide may result in a potentially harmful rapid drop in the woman's blood pressure and that ketanserin may not be as effective as hydralazine.[86] Intravenous labetalol has replaced IV hydralazine as the most common drug used to treat very high blood pressure in many countries, though both are commonly used. Refractory hypertension may be treated with IV glyceryl trinitrate (GTN) or rarely, with nitroprusside. The UK NICE Quality Standard recommends a target BP of 140/90 if any organ damage is evident.[87]

Prevention and treatment of eclampsia

Eclampsia is a generalised tonic–clonic seizure in the setting of preeclampsia – though it may also be the first presenting sign with hypertension and proteinuria developing following the first seizure. Magnesium sulfate has received the most attention as an anticonvulsant in preeclampsia, with its mechanism of action thought to be connected to the release of prostacyclin from the endothelium, reversing the vasoconstriction that is the basis of the disease.[88,89] Magnesium is the anticonvulsant of choice to prevent and treat eclampsia and is superior to anticonvulsant drugs.[90] Magnesium has been shown to halve the likelihood of eclampsia.[90] A common magnesium regimen is:[68,90]

- give a 4 g IV loading dose over 15–20 min
- administer an ongoing infusion of 1 g/h
- give an additional 2–4 g IV loading dose over 10 min to treat a recurrent eclamptic seizure
- continue infusion until 24 hours following delivery or 24 hours following the last eclamptic fit, whichever occurs later.

Elevated serum magnesium levels can depress deep tendon reflexes and respiratory rate. Although clinical assessment may identify potentially toxic magnesium levels,[68,90] there is no consensus regarding the therapeutic serum magnesium required to prevent eclampsia. One author suggests a serum level of 2 mmol/L, but there is no rationale provided for this level.[91] Should a woman on a magnesium infusion experience an eclamptic seizure, the first drug of choice is more magnesium.

> **BOX 28.3**
>
> **Management of women with HELLP syndrome using steroids**
>
> The use of steroids has been evaluated in the management of HELLP syndrome in the belief that steroids may mitigate the severity of the disease. However, a *Cochrane Review* concluded that there was insufficient evidence to determine whether steroid use as a treatment for HELLP syndrome had a favourable outcome for mothers and babies, although steroids may be beneficial if an increase in platelet count was imperative.[94]

Otherwise, management of an eclamptic seizure is the same as any other generalised tonic–clonic seizure.

Optimal fluid management

Careful titration of intravenous fluid is required to optimise plasma volume and organ perfusion without causing pulmonary oedema.[92] Central venous pressure is universally accepted as unhelpful to guide fluid management in preeclampsia. Transthoracic echocardiography (TTE) has demonstrated impaired diastolic function in women with preeclampsia and TTE is advocated by some to guide fluid management.[93] See also Box 28.3.

Thromboprophylaxis

Preeclampsia is an independent risk factor for thromboembolic disease and due consideration must be made of the need for thromboprophylaxis (in the absence of any contraindications) for women in ICU.[95]

Betamethasone

When severe preeclampsia is diagnosed prior to 34 weeks' gestation, the woman is normally prescribed steroids to promote fetal lung maturity and surfactant production.[65]

Optimal timing of delivery

Women with severe preeclampsia can only be cured by delivery, regardless of gestation. Consequently, a woman with severe preeclampsia is usually stabilised (hypertension controlled and magnesium sulfate commenced) and arrangements made for delivery. Ideally, women <34 weeks' gestation should be transferred to a high-level referral obstetric centre prior to delivery.

Subsequent pregnancy and long-term cardiovascular health

Women who have experienced preeclampsia are eight times more likely to experience preeclampsia again in a subsequent pregnancy than women who did not experience preeclampsia in their first pregnancy.[74] It seems that earlier onset preeclampsia and more severe disease are related to risk of recurrence. Some treatments, e.g. low-dose aspirin, have shown benefit in reducing the likelihood of recurrence in select high-risk groups.[76] Importantly, women who have experienced preeclampsia are twice as likely to die from cardiovascular disease later in life, and thus preeclampsia is an important risk factor for cardiovascular disease development.[96]

Practice tip

Many maternity professionals abbreviate preeclampsia to PE. This can be very confusing given that, in other health care settings, the abbreviation PE usually stands for pulmonary embolism. Be clear in any notes that you make, and clarify when reading notes that have been given to you.

Obstetric haemorrhage

Obstetric haemorrhage is a generic term indicating that there is bleeding from the uterus or genital tract in a pregnant or postpartum woman. It may be used when a woman experiences early pregnancy bleeding, e.g. prior to 20 weeks' gestation, and also if she has experienced either antepartum (>20 weeks' gestation and prior to birth) or postpartum (after birth of the baby) haemorrhage. The past decade has seen an increase in both the incidence and severity of haemorrhage, with more women requiring a blood transfusion for postpartum haemorrhage than in the past.[97] Major obstetric haemorrhage is a common reason for postpartum women to be admitted to ICU at 0.7/1000 deliveries.[1] Unfortunately, there is no agreed terminology for major obstetric haemorrhage, for example maternal/obstetric, and massive/major/severe are often used interchangeably. Furthermore, definition of a 'major obstetric haemorrhage' is variable and may include >1500 mL blood loss, >2500 mL blood loss, drop of >4 g/L Hb, >4 units of red blood cells (RBCs) transfused within 4 hours, need for non-RBC blood products or >8 units of RBCs transfused within 24 hours. Regardless, major obstetric haemorrhage is often sudden and unexpected, and is frequently associated with an acute coagulopathy. Early recognition and treatment of major obstetric haemorrhage is vital to ensure the best outcome for mother and fetus. A repeated finding in maternal death reviews is a delay by obstetric providers in recognising the severity of haemorrhage and consequent deterioration in maternal condition.[85]

The common causes of antepartum and postpartum haemorrhage are described below with common management strategies presented at the end of the section.

Antepartum haemorrhage

The definition of antepartum haemorrhage (APH) varies around the world. In the UK, APH is defined as bleeding from the genital tract, occurring from 24 weeks of pregnancy and prior to the birth of the baby, while bleeding prior to 24 weeks' gestation, is classed as a threatened miscarriage.[98,99] Contrastingly, the Australian definition of APH is 'bleeding from the genital tract after the 20th week of pregnancy and before the onset of labour'.[100] APH occurs in 3–5% of all pregnancies and is a cause of maternal and fetal morbidity and mortality.[98,99] The two main known causes of APH are placental abruption and placenta praevia.[9] However, for many women, the cause of an APH may never be determined and this is designated antepartum haemorrhage of unknown origin.[99]

Placental abruption (or abruptio placentae)

Placental abruption is premature separation (i.e. before the birth of the baby) of a normally-sited placenta from the uterine wall, and has an incidence of 0.26–0.8%.[23,99] It results from bleeding into the decidua basalis of the placenta with haematoma formation and resultant placental separation.[33,101] Bleeding associated with placental abruption may be revealed (i.e. it is visible per vagina (PV)), and occurs when the placenta partially separates along an edge of the placenta.[102] However, bleeding may also be concealed (i.e. no blood loss is visible PV) where the centre part of the placenta detaches, leaving the placental edges attached.[33] A mixed placental abruption is said to occur where there is a combination of revealed and concealed bleeding.[9] Risk factors for placental abruption include previous abruption, preeclampsia, blunt trauma (e.g. car crash, domestic violence), a sudden reduction in uterine volume (e.g. after delivery of the first baby in a twin pregnancy), cocaine use and smoking.[99]

As the amount of visible blood loss may be disproportionate to the actual amount of bleeding that has occurred in placental abruption, careful assessment of maternal physiological parameters, clinical history, and assessment of fetal wellbeing is vital.[99] Placental abruption is often accompanied by abdominal pain, back pain where there is a posteriorly-situated placenta and contractions.[23] Mild abruptions may not have a detrimental impact on maternal or fetal wellbeing; however, close monitoring will be required during the initial stages as progress to moderate or severe abruption is possible.[23] Moderate abruptions (blood loss ≥ 1000 mL) are likely to necessitate urgent delivery by caesarean section, due to the presence of fetal distress and maternal physiological compromise.[33] Where a significant proportion of the placenta has separated and the abruption is severe, a woman may present with hypovolaemic shock, severe abdominal pain, a hard or woody uterus on palpation (couvelaire uterus), DIC and intrauterine fetal death.[33,101] Where fetal death has occurred, vaginal delivery may be advocated and in the majority of cases, only women with severe placental abruptions are admitted to ICU.

Placenta praevia

Placenta praevia occurs when part or the whole placenta is situated over (major) or alongside (minor) the cervical os. Placenta praevia has an incidence of 3% at term.[99,103]

BOX 28.4

Types of morbidly adherent placenta – commonly referred to as placenta accreta

- Placenta accreta: the placenta is abnormally adherent to the uterine lining
- Placenta increta: the placenta invades the uterine muscle (myometrium)
- Placenta percreta: the placenta grows through the myometrium and into adjacent structures, such as the bladder and ureters

Adapted from Oyelese Y, Smulian JC. Placenta previa, placenta accreta, and vasa previa. Obstet Gynecol 2006;107(4):927–41.

The lower uterine segment does not fully form until 28–32 weeks' gestation, and the shearing stress as the lower uterine segment forms may precipitate detachment of the placenta from the uterine wall causing maternal bleeding. Bleeding can occur at any time, is usually painless (unlike moderate/severe placental abruptions), and may be torrential. Placenta praevia is a main cause of APH, accounting for 30% of all cases.[103] Management is dictated by the estimated blood loss, maternal condition, fetal wellbeing and whether the bleeding is ongoing.

Morbidly adherent placenta – placenta accreta

Morbidly adherent placenta is a serious complication where the placental villi abnormally invade the myometrium; there are three types with increasing severity termed accreta, increta and percreta[8] (Box 28.4). The main risk factor for morbidly adherent placenta is anterior placenta praevia in a woman with a previous caesarean section.[104] In this event, screening for morbidly adherent placenta using ultrasound and/or MRI may be undertaken prior to elective caesarean section, although there is debate as to the most effective diagnostic method.[104] Placental tissue can be very invasive and may infiltrate local structures such as the bladder. Many women with morbidly adherent placenta undergo emergency hysterectomy at the time of caesarean section, as a means to remove the placenta and control bleeding.[104] Alternative management is to deliver the baby by caesarean section and leave the placenta in situ to be reabsorbed, where feasible to do so (conservative management).[98] Morbidly adherent placenta can cause catastrophic haemorrhage and maternal mortality; a coordinated multidisciplinary approach is required prior to delivery to minimise complications.[98,104]

Postpartum haemorrhage

Postpartum haemorrhage (PPH), a major cause of maternal death in developed and developing countries, is defined as ≥500 mL blood loss from the genital tract after the birth of the baby. The incidence and severity of PPH is increasing in developed countries.[105] PPH rates commonly sit at around 10% of all births although they may be as high as 25% in some jurisdictions.[97] As outlined earlier, severe PPH lacks an agreed definition. Consequently, the incidence of severe PPH varies depending on how it has been defined. Additionally, PPH is classified according to the timing of the haemorrhage in relation to the birth. Primary PPH occurs within the first 24 hours after birth whereas secondary PPH occurs from 24 hours up to 6 weeks following birth. Primary PPH is often caused by uterine atony, while secondary PPH is more likely to be associated with retained products and associated infection.

The causes of PPH are varied and have been classified by the 'four Ts': tone, tissue, trauma and thrombin (Box 28.5). The cause of PPH should be identified and targeted with specific management, in conjunction with the general principles of haemorrhage management.

BOX 28.5

Causes of postpartum haemorrhage characterised by the '4 Ts'

Tone:

- Uterine atony
- Functional or anatomical distortion of the uterus (e.g. bi-cornuate uterus, fibroids)

Tissue:

- Retained placental products
- Abnormal placenta

Trauma:

- Cervical and genital tract damage during delivery
- Uterine inversion

Thrombin:

- Coagulation disorders

Adapted from NSW Health. Maternity – prevention, detection, escalation and management of postpartum haemorrhage (PPH). Sydney: Department of Health, NSW; 2017.

Practice tip

Read a woman's operation report if she has a diagnosis of placenta accreta to identify the extent to which the placental tissue has invaded local structures, such as the bladder, ureters and bowel. For example, the bladder is often affected and a cystotomy may have been required to separate the placenta from the bladder.

Severe obstetric haemorrhage management priorities

The vast majority of women admitted to ICU with obstetric haemorrhage will be transferred following birth, and are thus postpartum on admission to ICU. As with any major haemorrhage (see Chapter 21), the principles of treatment are:

- restore an adequate circulating volume and maintain oxygen and perfusion to vital organs
- obtain haemostasis and correct coagulopathy
- prevent complications.

Maintaining circulating volume, oxygenation and perfusion

Haemodynamic instability following substantial blood loss is a frequent reason for admission to ICU.[106] Accurate estimation of blood loss is difficult as bleeding can be concealed, and blood loss may be mixed with amniotic fluid making accurate estimation a challenge, potentially leading to an underestimation of fluid resuscitation needs. Furthermore, peripartum women are at an increased risk of acute pulmonary oedema, which further complicates fluid resuscitation.[107,108] Standard resuscitation fluids, such as Hartmann's or normal saline, should be infused according to routine practice for the non-obstetric haemorrhage, remembering that large volumes of blood products may also be required.

> **Practice tip**
>
> Keep in mind the following:
>
> - Serum albumin levels decrease in normal pregnancy, with the lowest levels recorded in the early postpartum period[109]
> - Cardiac output remains elevated postpartum for the first few days at least
> - Central venous pressure (CVP) and pulmonary artery pressure (PAP) can be interpreted the same as for non-obstetric patients (as long as the woman does not have preeclampsia)

Achieving haemostasis and correct coagulopathy

Specific interventions to control bleeding include radiological arterial embolisation or balloon occlusion of the internal iliac arteries, uterine compression suture (e.g. B-Lynch suture), use of an intrauterine balloon tamponade (e.g. Bakri balloon) and emergency hysterectomy. Women may need to return to theatre for abdominal packing for ongoing 'ooze' that may continue after a hysterectomy. Many women with severe obstetric haemorrhage in ICU have developed DIC that requires treatment with the appropriate blood products.[110]

Patient blood management guidelines have been developed by the Australian National Blood Authority with Module 1 (critical bleeding), Module 4 (critical care) and Module 5 (obstetrics and maternity) of most relevance.[110-113] Fibrinogen is usually doubled by the end of pregnancy, and low fibrinogen levels are associated with increasing severity of PPH.[114] Fibrinogen concentrate for the treatment of PPH is of increasing interest although a recent study found that routine treatment with fibrinogen concentrate offered no benefit.[115] However, virtually all participants had a fibrinogen level of over 4 g/L at the time of randomisation. Point-of-care devices that examine the quality of the clot, such as thromboelastography (TEG) and rotational thromboelastometry (ROTEM), are frequently used in tertiary centres to guide management of obstetric haemorrhage. These point-of-care devices enable a more targeted approach to haemostatic resuscitation and have demonstrated a reduction in blood component usage with the use of fibrinogen concentrate.[116]

Recombinant factor VIIa has been used successfully in the management of severe obstetric haemorrhage and may be considered for use in the management of the bleeding woman in accordance with the massive transfusion protocol. Treatment is more likely to be effective if administered before the woman becomes hypothermic and acidotic.[117] Tranexamic acid has shown some benefit in the management of PPH and administration is recommended as soon as possible after the haemorrhage is recognised.[118] All maternity providers should have a 'massive transfusion protocol' that outlines action and escalation of care for massive bleeding.[113] Maternity adaptations from a standard massive transfusion protocol include: consideration for early triggering of the protocol given the common underestimation of blood loss and ability for the maternity patient to initially maintain haemodynamic stability despite large blood loss, aim to maintain a higher level of fibrinogen (>2.0 g/L) and avoidance of permissive hypotension while the uterus remains in situ.[113]

Preventing complications

Strategies to prevent the following complications should be implemented:

- Complications of major blood transfusion – these are similar in the obstetric patient as in the non-obstetric patient and include acid–base disturbance, transfusion-related acute lung injury (TRALI), hypocalcaemia, hyperkalaemia and hypothermia.
- Increased risk of thrombosis – particularly in the early postpartum period as the risk is exacerbated by lengthy theatre procedures, bed rest associated with ICU admission and following major haemorrhage with an associated massive blood transfusion. Suitable thromboprophylaxis should be considered as soon as feasible.
- Acute kidney injury – irreversible renal failure has been reported as a sequela of acute kidney injury following severe postpartum haemorrhage.[119] Routine monitoring and management of renal

impairment is required, keeping in mind that a pregnant patient has a lower urea and creatinine level than non-pregnant patients. Careful titration of fluid for renal purposes is needed due to the increased propensity for pulmonary oedema.

- Rh isoimmunisation – the potential to develop Rh isoimmunisation in Rh-negative women who have experienced antepartum haemorrhage should be considered.[120]
- Sheehan's syndrome – necrosis of the pituitary gland is a very rare complication of severe obstetric haemorrhage. While the syndrome may go undetected for many years, one of the earliest symptoms is a failure to establish lactation, due to the absence of prolactin secretion. Sheehan's syndrome can be prevented by maintaining adequate circulating volume, oxygenation and perfusion.

Use of intraoperative cell salvage for obstetric haemorrhage

The introduction of cell salvage in obstetrics was delayed in comparison to other surgeries for two key reasons: the theoretical risk of amniotic fluid embolism (AFE) and the risk of rhesus isoimmunisation.[121] Contemporary understanding suggests that AFE is more aligned with an anaphylactic reaction and, in practice, there has been no confirmed case of AFE following the use of cell salvage infusion.[122] Regardless, it is common practice to use a different suction device from the time of amniotic membrane rupture until after delivery (which is not re-used) with blood aspirated from the surgical field collected by the cell salvage device.[123] A leucocyte depletion filter should always be used during the reinfusion of salvaged maternal blood to filter any remaining foreign proteins.[121] Although safe, cell salvage is not recommended for routine use in women who are considered high risk for haemorrhage, as the vast majority of women do not haemorrhage and setting up cell salvage for all high-risk women is cost prohibitive.[124] Inability to predict who is likely to have a major haemorrhage and the time taken to set up cell salvage with suitable staff on hand means that cell salvage has a limited use for emergency management. Nevertheless, it remains a possible treatment for a small select group of women, such as those with placenta accreta. None of the currently available cell saver equipment is able to discern fetal from adult red blood cells and any present fetal cells are transfused to the woman. It is important for rhesus-negative women to have a post-infusion Kleihauer–Betke test to quantify the amount of fetal red cells in the maternal circulation to ensure that an adequate dose of anti-D immunoglobulin can be given to prevent isoimmunisation.

Amniotic fluid embolism

AFE is a rare and incompletely understood obstetric emergency that usually occurs during labour or pregnancy termination, or shortly after delivery. Traditional understanding of the condition was based around the notion that amniotic fluid entered the maternal blood stream via the endocervical veins or placental bed, with amniotic fluid, fetal cells, hair or other fetal debris functioning as an embolus, and resulting in the dramatic cardiorespiratory collapse seen with the condition. However, not all women diagnosed with AFE have evidence of fetal squames/amniotic fluid substances in the pulmonary vasculature and many women who do not develop AFE have fetal cells found in the maternal circulation.[125]

More recently, improved understanding of the mechanics of labour and the interaction of amniotic fluid and maternal blood, as well as the striking similarities between clinical and haemodynamic findings in AFE and both anaphylaxis and septic shock, have led to a belief that a common pathophysiological mechanism is likely to be responsible for all these conditions.[126] As AFE resembles an anaphylactic reaction to fetal material rather than an embolic event, the term 'anaphylactoid syndrome of pregnancy', instead of AFE, has been proposed.[126] The trigger for AFE is not well understood, although it is thought to be a fetal antigen (which may arise from amniotic fluid). It is possible that all labouring women are exposed to the fetal antigen, with those affected by AFE exhibiting a rare and abnormal maternal immune response.[125] One of the difficulties blocking improved understanding of AFE is the lack of a diagnostic test.

Regardless of the level of understanding, the abnormal mediator release gives rise to acute lung injury, resulting in acute dyspnoea and hypoxia and often the development of acute respiratory distress syndrome. Within 30 minutes of the antigen insult, there is evidence of severe pulmonary hypertension with acute right ventricular failure.[127] It is thought that inflammatory mediators are a more likely cause of pulmonary vasoconstriction, with physical obstruction to the pulmonary vasculature (embolism) not the main mechanism.[125,128] The left ventricular failure seen in AFE is considered a secondary response due to poor left ventricular filling pressures. Concomitantly, substances in the amniotic fluid trigger a profound consumptive coagulopathy.

Incidence and risk factors

The incidence of AFE is thought to be in the range of 2–8 women per 100,000 deliveries making it a very rare event.[129] However, the lack of a diagnostic test is a serious limiting factor for accurate determination of incidence, with geographical variation reported. AFE is more common in North America (1 in 15,200 deliveries) than in Europe (1 in 53,800 deliveries);[128] this may represent a true difference in incidence or reflect differences in clinical diagnosis or methods of case identification. Using similar definitions and case identification, the Australian and New Zealand (ANZ) incidence of AFE was 5.4/100,000 women giving birth, compared with 2.0/100,000 in the UK.[129,130] Similar numbers of women received cardiorespiratory resuscitation and survival rates were also similar, indicating that the higher rate in ANZ is real.

Diagnosis remains one of exclusion and there is a long list of differential diagnoses, including air or thrombotic pulmonary emboli, septic shock, cardiomyopathy, acute myocardial infarction, anaphylaxis, transfusion reaction, aspiration, placental abruption, eclampsia, uterine rupture, local anaesthetic toxicity and primary postpartum haemorrhage.[126] AFE remains a major contributor to maternal death, accounting for 5–15% of all maternal deaths in developed countries.[128,131]

Although controversy exists, the factors that have been proposed as contributing to an increased likelihood for AFE include:[125,126,128,129]

- induction of labour
- caesarean birth
- multiple pregnancy, e.g. twins
- maternal age ≥35 years
- forceps delivery
- placenta praevia, preeclampsia and placental abruption.

Given the rarity of AFE and the commonality of these potential risk factors, astute clinical assessment and early clinical suspicion based on the clinical presentation of the woman should be the focus for early identification and treatment.

Clinical presentation

The symptoms associated with AFE have been well described and usually comprise premonitory symptoms, such as restlessness, agitation and numbness/tingling prior to more severe maternal compromise, such as sudden onset hypotension, dyspnoea, hypoxia, altered mental status and haemorrhage.[128] Collapse of the maternal cardiovascular system leads to fetal distress as the placenta is deprived of maternal oxygen, quickly leading to fetal demise unless the fetus is delivered swiftly. Premonitory symptoms, shortness of breath and fetal distress have been reported as the early signs in the UK and ANZ studies.[129] Overall, haemorrhage and associated coagulopathy, hypotension and shortness of breath were the most commonly recorded symptoms.[129] Cardiac arrest was documented in 40% of cases and seizure in 15%. Haemorrhage and coagulopathy may not be immediately apparent; some women die before it develops. However, these clinical features usually develop in women who survive the initial insult.

Patient management

There is no specific treatment for AFE; all therapy is supportive with the aim to maintain adequate oxygenation and perfusion, control haemorrhage and correct any coagulopathy. Common interventions include:[129]

- urgent delivery of the fetus
- emergency hysterectomy to control postpartum haemorrhage
- admission to ICU, with associated support such as mechanical ventilation, nitric oxide and extracorporeal membrane oxygenation (ECMO).

A full range of blood components, including fresh frozen plasma, platelets and cryoprecipitate may be required to correct the coagulopathy. Transoesophageal echocardiography may be very helpful to guide fluid and inotrope management to optimise preload and enhance cardiac output. In developed countries, the mortality is 15–20%.[130]

Although it is possible for a woman to experience an AFE in a subsequent pregnancy, repeat AFE is thought to be unlikely as the trigger for AFE is specific to each fetus the woman carries. There have been a number of published case reports of women having a successful subsequent pregnancy and none reporting repeat AFE in the same woman.

Peripartum cardiomyopathy

Peripartum cardiomyopathy, sometimes referred to as postpartum cardiomyopathy, is an idiopathic cardiomyopathy frequently presenting with heart failure secondary to LV systolic dysfunction (LVEF <45%) towards the end of pregnancy or in the months following delivery, when other causes of heart failure have been excluded.[132] Peripartum cardiomyopathy is considered to be a dilated cardiomyopathy, resulting in a dilated left atrium and ventricle, and a reduced left ventricular ejection fraction (<45%).[133] Women commonly present with New York Heart Association class III or IV heart failure.[134] The incidence of peripartum cardiomyopathy varies widely from 1:100 in a small region of sub-Saharan Africa to 1:4000 in the USA, though many studies on peripartum cardiomyopathy were conducted on data that had been gathered retrospectively.[135,136] A prospective population-based study in the Netherlands found that 1 in 20,000 pregnancies required ICU admission for peripartum cardiomyopathy.[4]

The exact cause of peripartum cardiomyopathy is not well understood and a variety of factors have been implicated, including viral infection, autoimmune mechanisms, cytokine-mediated inflammation, increased myocyte apoptosis, increased oxidative stress, genetic disposition and/or cultural habits, and abnormal hormonal regulation.[133,137] More recently, it is postulated that oxidative stress cleaves the full-length, 23-kDa form of the hormone prolactin into an antiangiogenic, 16-kDa derivative.[138] Maternal mortality associated with peripartum cardiomyopathy is between 4-14%, with lower mortality in developed countries.[139] Studies show that approximately 20–40% of women recover their left ventricular function, usually within 6 months though it may take up to 2 years.[133,140] Women who never fully recover their cardiac function require ongoing medical management; a small proportion of women go on to require a mechanical-assist device and heart transplantation.

Patient management

Women with peripartum cardiomyopathy present with varying degrees of left heart failure. Signs and symptoms include dyspnoea, persistent cough, abdominal discomfort, palpitations and oedema and may be mistaken for 'discomforts of pregnancy' and lead to a delayed diagnosis. The diagnosis of peripartum cardiomyopathy is one of exclusion requiring systematic investigation to exclude both cardiac and non-cardiac differential diagnoses such as pulmonary embolism, acute myocardial infarction, severe preeclampsia and pneumonia.[141] Echocardiography is a useful diagnostic tool with a left ventricular end-diastolic diameter >60 mm predictive of poor recovery, as is a LVEF <30%.[133] When available, a cardiac MRI allows for better chamber volume and functional assessment and is a more sensitive tool to identify a left ventricular thrombus.[133]

The principles of managing acute heart failure in women with peripartum cardiomyopathy are no different to the management of heart failure from any other cause, and aim to reduce preload and afterload and to increase cardiac contractility (see Chapter 10 for a full description). Unfortunately, ACE inhibitors and angiotensin antagonists are contraindicated in pregnancy.

Bromocriptine, a relatively novel treatment for peripartum cardiomyopathy, is associated with increased left ventricular recovery and reduced morbidity and death.[142] Bromocriptine is directly able to reduce oxidative stress by blocking the release of prolactin.[143] For women with severe disease, bromocriptine should be considered as an adjunct treatment as soon as the diagnosis is made.[132] For women diagnosed with peripartum cardiomyopathy while pregnant, timing and mode of delivery are two other management decisions to be made. A multidisciplinary team, including cardiologist, obstetrician, anaesthetist and nursing/midwifery staff, should consider and plan for delivery dependent on maternal and fetal condition and the woman's known preferences. Ergometrine-containing drugs, used to contract the uterus post-delivery, are contraindicated because they cause vasoconstriction and the associated increase in afterload may be detrimental for maternal heart function. Synthetic oxytocin preparations are advised instead to prevent postpartum haemorrhage. Early consideration also needs to be given to thromboprophylaxis.[132] Finally, given the postulated role of prolactin in the aetiology of peripartum cardiomyopathy, there is debate about whether women should breastfeed. In milder cases when bromocriptine is not prescribed, it may be possible.[139]

Subsequent pregnancy

Family planning counselling is an important part of the care of women as they recover from peripartum cardiomyopathy.[139] After a diagnosis of peripartum cardiomyopathy, women have a 30% risk of relapse in any subsequent pregnancy.[140,144] Peripartum cardiomyopathy remains an important cause of maternal death, and this may occur in association with subsequent pregnancies.

Exacerbation of medical disease associated with pregnancy

Women with preexisting medical conditions pose additional challenges during pregnancy. Occasionally, pregnant and postpartum women are admitted to ICU with exacerbation of an underlying medical condition and two of the more common conditions, cardiac disease and asthma, are outlined in this section. Other conditions that result in ICU admission of pregnant or postpartum women include trauma, pneumonia and mental health disorders, and these are reviewed here.

Cardiac disease

Cardiac disease in pregnancy consists of women who have congenital heart disease and women who have acquired heart disease, such as rheumatic heart disease. The physiological adaptations of pregnancy can 'unmask' cardiac disease in women. Notably, only 17% of women who died of cardiac causes during 2009–2014 in the UK were known to have preexisting cardiac problems.[145]

Congenital heart disease

Congenital heart disease (CHD) refers to defects of the heart, or main vessels connected to the heart, which are present at birth. CHD is the most common serious birth defect, affecting about 1% of births.[146,147] Largely, the causes are unknown and attributed to factors within the maternal, fetal or placental environment; only 11% have a genetic diagnosis.[148] Most develop de novo and recognised risk factors for the development of CHD in the fetus include maternal obesity,[149] elevated blood glucose levels in the first trimester,[150] and low maternal vitamin D levels.[151] Some maternal medication also increases the likelihood of offspring CHD, such as selective serotonin reuptake inhibitors.[152]

Increasing numbers of those affected with CHD are surviving into adulthood with the greatest increase in survival benefit seen in people with severe disease.[153] The number of adults living with CHD is predicted to continue to grow, resulting in substantially higher clinical loads for adult CHD centres.[154] The risks women face in the pursuit of motherhood should not be overlooked[157,155] and include worsening cardiac function, arrhythmias and death. A tool to predict the likelihood of a cardiac complication associated with pregnancy has been developed for women with preexisting cardiovascular conditions to help guide pre-conception counselling and care (Table 28.5). Women with very severe disease are choosing to have children, such as those who have undergone Fontan procedures. While many women achieve motherhood, there is an increased likelihood of miscarriage, preterm birth and small babies.[156,157]

TABLE 28.5
Predicting risk of pregnancy for women with cardiovascular conditions

WHO RISK CLASS	CARDIOVASCULAR CONDITIONS	RISK OF PREGNANCY BY MEDICAL CONDITION

I	• Uncomplicated small or mild
	  ○ Pulmonary stenosis
	  ○ Patent ductus arteriosus
	  ○ Mitral valve prolapse
	• Successfully repaired simple lesions (atrial or ventricular septal defect, patent ductus arteriosus, anomalous pulmonary venous drainage)
	• Atrial or ventricular ectopic beats, isolated
		No detectable increased risk of maternal mortality and no/mild increase in morbidity

II	If otherwise well and uncomplicated: • Unoperated atrial or ventricular septal defect • Repaired tetralogy of Fallot • Most arrhythmias	Small increased risk of maternal mortality or moderate increase in morbidity
II or III	Depending on individual • Mild left ventricular impairment • Hypertrophic cardiomyopathy • Native or tissue valvular heart disease not considered WHO I or IV • Marfan syndrome without aortic dilatation • Aorta <45 mm in aortic disease associated with bicuspid aortic valve • Repaired coarctation	
III	• Mechanical valve • Systemic right ventricle • Fontan circulation • Cyanotic heart disease (unrepaired) • Other complex CHD • Aortic dilatation 40–45 mm in Marfan syndrome • Aortic dilatation 45–50 mm in aortic disease associated with bicuspid aortic valve	Significantly increased risk of maternal mortality or severe morbidity. Expert counselling required. If pregnancy is decided upon, intensive specialist cardiac and obstetric monitoring is needed throughout pregnancy, childbirth and the puerperium
IV	• Pulmonary arterial hypertension of any cause • Severe systemic ventricular dysfunction (LVEF < 30%, NYHA III-IV) • Severe mitral stenosis, severe symptomatic aortic stenosis • Marfan syndrome with aorta dilated >45 mm • Aortic dilatation >50 mm in aortic disease associated with bicuspid aortic valve • Native severe coarctation	Extremely high risk of maternal mortality or severe morbidity; pregnancy contraindicated. If pregnancy occurs termination should be discussed. If pregnancy continues, care as for Class III

CHD = congenital heart disease; LVEF = left ventricular ejection fraction; NYHA = New York Heart Association; WHO = World Health Organization.
Adapted from Regitz-Zagrosek V, Lundqvist CB, Borghi C et al. ESC guidelines on the management of cardiovascular diseases during pregnancy. Eur Heart J 2011;32:3147-97.

The combination of both cardiovascular and respiratory changes in pregnancy is poorly tolerated by some women, and cardiac disease in pregnancy still remains a leading cause of maternal death in developed nations.[131]

Rheumatic heart disease

Rheumatic heart disease (RHD) is the most frequently acquired heart disease and is a condition normally associated with developing countries.[158] One exception is Australia where Aboriginal people and Torres Strait Islanders in the Northern Territory have rates of RHD noted to be the highest in the world, and over 30 times higher than those of non-Indigenous Australians.[158] Similarly, in New Zealand, Maori and Pacific Islanders have a much higher incidence of RHD than New Zealanders of European ancestry. Refugee and immigrant women who have migrated from developing countries, such as in sub-Saharan Africa, also have a higher risk for RHD in pregnancy.

RHD is a delayed complication of acute rheumatic fever, and results from an untreated group A streptococcus bacterial throat or skin infection. There is progressive, structural heart damage that occurs after an initial episode of acute rheumatic fever. RHD usually begins with generalised carditis; then, as the disease advances, mitral valve insufficiency develops, although the aortic valve may also be affected. Valvular pathology includes restricted leaflet mobility, valvular prolapse, focal or generalised valvular thickening and abnormal subvalvular thickening, chordae tendineae or papillary muscle rupture and scarring, resulting in regurgitation and, rarely, stenosis.

Serial echocardiography throughout pregnancy by a skilled provider is essential to monitor maternal cardiac function and, specifically, valvular dynamics in women with RHD. Imaging can be technically challenging during pregnancy, and cardiac indices need to be aligned with the normal echocardiography pregnancy reference range.[159,160] The effect of RHD on pregnancy varies on the severity of the disease, with episodes of heart failure or arrhythmia leading to hospital admission.[160]

Acute myocardial infarction

Acute myocardial infarction (AMI), once rarely seen in association with pregnancy, is becoming more prevalent. Pregnancy has been reported to increase the risk of AMI 3–4-fold in same-age-matched non-pregnant women,[161] in part because coronary dissection is more common in association with a pregnancy.[162] The increasing incidence of AMI is also thought to be related to the changing demographics of the pregnant population, which now includes higher proportions of older women and women who are obese.[163]

In the maternity setting, symptoms of AMI or heart failure, such as clamminess, sweating, tachycardia, fatigue, anxiety, breathlessness and chest pain should not be dismissed without adequate investigation and due consideration of cardiovascular risk factors. Although 'breathlessness' may be a common symptom experienced by pregnant women, nocturnal dyspnoea, or breathlessness at rest, is not normal, even in the pregnant context. Similarly, heartburn, fatigue and dependent oedema may also indicate cardiovascular compromise. The UK maternal mortality report emphasises the need to obtain a diagnosis in pregnant women presenting with chest pain, as many women who died at home following an AMI had been sent home with no diagnosis.[145] In particular, ECGs, echocardiography, chest X-rays, cardiac enzymes (troponin) and computed tomographic pulmonary angiography should be attended as clinically indicated and investigations should not be denied to women who need them on the basis that they are pregnant.[145] Diagnosis of AMI in pregnancy is the same as for the non-pregnant patient, with troponin levels considered both reliable and accurate.[164,165] Percutaneous coronary angiography is suggested as the treatment of choice for coronary reperfusion, despite the risk of iatrogenic coronary dissection. There are limited data available to either support or refute the administration of thrombolytics such as tissue plasminogen activator in pregnancy and, due to the increased possibility of coronary dissection, they are not recommended.[160]

Other cardiac conditions

Rarely, spontaneous aortic dissection may occur in pregnant women with no preexisting cardiac disease.[166] Signs and symptoms of heart failure and complaints of chest pain must be investigated and not put down to the 'minor discomforts' of pregnancy. Given that the cardiac output is expected to increase 40–50% in a normal pregnancy, any cardiac condition resulting in poor left ventricular function and/or restricted left ventricular outflow is particularly associated with poor outcomes in pregnancy (Table 28.5).

Also relevant for the outcome of both mother and baby is whether any valvular disease has been repaired and whether a tissue or mechanical valve has been inserted. Use of anticoagulants is of particular concern during pregnancy, with warfarin contraindicated for use in pregnancy. However, the risk of thrombosis is relatively high in pregnant women and some women are advised to remain on warfarin despite the risk of associated congenital anomaly and the increased likelihood of miscarriage.[167]

Practice tip

Congenital and acquired cardiac disease can present for the first time during pregnancy, unmasked by the additional physiological requirements of pregnancy. Women with known preexisting disease may experience unpredictable deterioration in cardiac function.

Patient management

All women with cardiac disease are considered to have a 'high-risk' pregnancy and should receive maternity care by a multidisciplinary team including, as a minimum, obstetrician, midwife, cardiologist and anaesthetist.[168,169] The timing and location of delivery, choice of anaesthesia and delivery mode should each be discussed by the team with the woman, and planned well in advance. If a pregnant woman with cardiac disease is admitted to ICU, this multidisciplinary team should be consulted about her care. Priorities of care include:

- Pre-pregnancy counselling – this should allow a full and frank discussion about the likely risks of pregnancy for the individual and a discussion of treatment path. This is of particular importance for women who are on potentially teratogenic medication, such as warfarin or ACE inhibitors, and for women who may benefit from surgery or interventional treatment prior to conceiving. Additionally, women with CHD may require genetic counselling to determine the likelihood of CHD in any offspring.
- Diagnosis – standard investigations including chest X-ray, ECG, CT scan and MRI should be attended to as indicated by the clinical condition.

In general, diagnostic imaging of a critically ill woman should not be withheld due to concerns about the fetus, with abdominal shielding used whenever possible.[169]

- Heart failure – as was outlined in the section on peripartum cardiomyopathy, the principles of treatment for heart failure in pregnancy are the same as for the non-pregnant population.
- Arrhythmias – commonly used drugs include digoxin, lignocaine, flecainide, verapamil, sotalol, propranolol, adenosine and amiodarone; although limited studies exist in the pregnant population, all have been used safely and effectively during pregnancy.[170] Transient neonatal hypothyroidism has been described in women on amiodarone and monitoring of neonatal thyroid function is recommended.[171] For refractory rhythms or if the woman is haemodynamically unstable, cardioversion is considered a safe procedure during pregnancy.[168]
- Cardiac surgery – interventions such as valvuloplasty may be required. Open-heart surgery is only performed during pregnancy when the maternal condition is critical, for example coronary artery dissection or severe dysfunctioning valve, because of the high probability of fetal loss associated with the woman going on bypass. Standard care should be provided to a pregnant woman, with care to nurse the woman ≥20 weeks' gestation with a 15° left lateral tilt, to reduce the negative effects of aortocaval compression. Open-heart surgery and ECMO have been used successfully in pregnant women with good outcomes for some mothers and babies.[172,173]
- Thrombus prevention – is a priority in women with valvular disease/prosthetic valves, atrial fibrillation or dilated heart chambers at risk of thrombus formation, especially because of the normal hypercoagulopathy associated with pregnancy. Warfarin embryopathy, a recognised collection of developmental anomalies such as nasal hypoplasia and epiphysis stippling, is associated with warfarin use in the first trimester; consequently, warfarin use is contraindicated. However, pregnant women with mechanical valves experience unacceptably high rates of valve thrombosis and embolism when switched to heparin, and so many cardiologists consider the risks associated with the continued use of warfarin in pregnancy to be lower than the risks of stopping it. Therefore, a regimen that balances the risk of thrombosis with that of fetal loss or malformation and risk of haemorrhage should be implemented, with some variation of: stopping warfarin for the whole first trimester or from 6–12 weeks' gestation and then resuming until close to delivery; replacing warfarin with unfractionated or low-molecular-weight heparin for the whole pregnancy or continuing warfarin throughout pregnancy and replacing it with heparin for delivery only. Appropriate dosing schedules for heparin have not been confirmed with low-dose heparin considered inadequate and high doses of unfractionated heparin not researched.[174]
- Secondary prevention of RHD – monthly intramuscular (IM) penicillin, e.g. 1,200,000 units of benzylpenicillin, to minimise repeat acute rheumatic fever and associated further valve degeneration.[158]

Practice tip

When caring for a pregnant woman with cardiac disease or post-cardiac surgery, differences in normal haemodynamic and respiratory parameters in pregnancy must be considered.

Asthma

Asthma is the most common chronic health disease in pregnant women, affecting 4–8% of all pregnancies in the USA.[175] However, the incidence in Australia may be higher given the higher prevalence, 12–14%, of 'current asthma' in women of childbearing age.[176]

Course of asthma during pregnancy

The course of asthma during pregnancy is variable. Approximately one-third of women experience an improvement in asthma symptoms, one-third report no change and one-third experience exacerbation of asthma during pregnancy.[177] Very severe exacerbation of asthma during pregnancy requiring ICU admission is rare. A persisting problem in pregnant women with asthma is the reluctance to treat (by some doctors) and decreased medication compliance (by some women), based on concerns about the safety of medication during pregnancy, with a substantial number of asthma exacerbations in pregnancy associated with non-adherence to prescribed drugs.[178,179] Studies comparing medication use have shown pregnant women are also less likely to receive systemic corticosteroids than non-pregnant asthmatics.[178,180] The second and third trimesters are commonly the time when a worsening of asthma symptoms will develop, although women may have an improvement in symptoms for the last 4 weeks of a term pregnancy.[178] In one study only 20% of women with asthma had a written asthma plan during pregnancy.[181]

Effect of asthma on pregnancy

The relationship between asthma in pregnancy and adverse maternal and neonatal outcomes including pre-eclampsia, gestational diabetes, small-for-gestational-age neonates and preterm birth is inconsistent. The general belief is that poor maternal and neonatal outcomes are associated with poor asthma management and not a result of the treatment itself.[181]

Patient management

A pregnant woman admitted to ICU with asthma may be experiencing new-onset asthma or an exacerbation of preexisting asthma. Accurate diagnosis and evaluation of the disease is necessary and should involve the advice of a thoracic medicine specialist and an obstetrician, who will continue the care of the woman once discharged from ICU. Methacholine testing, used as a diagnostic tool for asthma, is contraindicated in pregnancy.[182] Treatment of severe asthma in pregnancy is no different to the treatment in non-pregnant patients (see Chapter 14), apart from the additional needs to monitor fetal wellbeing and consider the normal respiratory parameters in pregnancy (Table 28.6). Severe hypoxaemia places the fetus at risk and should be avoided; maternal SaO_2 should remain ≥95%. Peak flow measures are recommended to be used during pregnancy to assess and monitor the woman's condition, with the normal values unchanged in pregnancy.[182] The risks associated with current asthma medication use in pregnancy are far less than the risks associated with uncontrolled asthma, and the regular schedule of asthma medications should be prescribed in pregnancy according to asthma symptom level.[183] Likewise, none of the common drug categories, such as inhaled corticosteroids, long-acting beta-agonists and leukotriene-receptor antagonists, is contraindicated during lactation.[183] Influenza and pertussis vaccination during pregnancy is recommended for all women and is especially important in women with asthma.[184]

Special considerations

Any health condition resulting in ICU admission may occur in a pregnant woman. The more common of these include physical trauma, pneumonia and mental health disorders, and these are described in detail below. Drug and substance misuse in pregnancy can have harmful effects upon the woman, and her fetus. Substance misuse is complex, and may be interrelated with other factors such as domestic violence and mental health conditions, particularly in pregnancy. Obtaining a health history from a woman in the ICU setting may be challenging.

TABLE 28.6
Summary of management of acute exacerbation of asthma in pregnancy

1	$Beta_2$ agonist bronchodilator with one of the following: • Salbutamol MDI 4–8 puffs every 20 min up to 1 h, then every 1–4 h as needed • Salbutamol 2.5–5.0 mg nebulised every 20 min for 3 doses, then every 1–4 h as needed • Salbutamol continuous nebulisation 10–15 mg/h
2	Add anticholinergic therapy • Ipratropium bromide nebulised 0.5 mg every 20 min for 3 doses, then as needed, given simultaneously with salbutamol
3	Oxygen to maintain saturation >95%
4	Consider fetal monitoring if pregnancy has reached 2–28 weeks' gestation • Consult with specialist obstetrician for collaborative management and planning for delivery if relevant
5	Assess volume status – maintain euvolaemia and adequate maternal cardiac output
6	Initiate systemic glucocorticoids without delay for patients: • In severe exacerbation • Who are already on chronic oral glucocorticoids • Who have mild to moderate symptoms not responsive to steps 1–5 within the first hour
7	Adjunct therapies for patients not responding to above • Magnesium sulfate 2 g IV over 20 min (assess baseline serum magnesium level if renal insufficiency present) • Terbutaline 0.25 mg subcutaneously every 20 min for up to 3 doses
8	Consider intubation and mechanical ventilation • Plan early and obtain practitioner experienced in pregnant airway management • For patients in severe distress and not responsive to earlier treatment • When pH <7.35, arterial $PaCO_2$ >normal pregnancy range of 28–32 mmHg, or arterial PaO_2 <70 mmHg • Facilitate avoidance of hyperinflation by using a prolonged expiratory time and monitor intensely for hyperinflation • Titrate ventilation to achieve normal pH, normal pregnancy $PaCO_2$ 28–32 mmHg and normal PaO_2

Adapted from Bonham CA, Patterson KC, Strek ME. Asthma outcomes and management during pregnancy. Chest 2018;153:515-27.

If substance misuse is suspected, a toxicology screen may be useful to ensure the woman receives suitable care, management, support and referral to appropriate services for the remainder of the pregnancy.[185]

Trauma in pregnancy

The term 'trauma' refers to any accidental or intentional event resulting in injury. A systematic review suggests domestic violence/intimate partner violence and motor vehicle accidents (MVAs) are most prevalent reasons for pregnancy trauma.[186] The incidence of trauma in pregnancy is estimated to be in the range of 6–8% of all pregnancies and also includes slips/falls, burns, psychological and sexual abuse, toxicity, homicide and suicide.[187,188]

Domestic violence

Domestic violence is a complex public health issue. The overall prevalence of domestic abuse in pregnancy is unknown, although estimates range between 3% and 30% of women and vary from country to country.[189-191] Thirty percent of domestic violence begins during pregnancy and healthcare professionals should be trained to identify its signs and symptoms and screen women during routine maternity care.[191,192] The history regarding any injuries should be considered in relation to the presenting injury and likely mechanism of injury. A potential sign of domestic violence may be the woman seems evasive or reluctant to speak in front of her partner. Often, physical violence is directed towards the maternal abdomen.[187] Pregnancy-related violence is associated with low-birth-weight babies, APH, premature labour, fetal trauma, infection, maternal depression, posttraumatic stress disorder, attempted suicide and mortality.[193,194]

Motor vehicle trauma

Some pregnant women may believe there is no legal requirement to wear a seatbelt when pregnant and this places them and their fetus at increased risk of injury should they be involved in a MVA.[195] Preterm labour and stillbirth rates are reported to be higher for women who are unbelted.[196] Additionally, many pregnant women may not be informed on the correct positioning of a seatbelt during pregnancy, and incorrect positioning can increase the likelihood of placental abruption and additional injuries occurring[195] (Fig. 28.3). Uterine rupture has also been reported as a result of MVAs and can lead to fetal and maternal mortality if surgery is not undertaken promptly.[197]

Musculoskeletal injuries

Pregnancy hormones affect joints and ligaments, making them more lax and pliable. This explains why pregnant women are more likely to experience joint injury, pelvic instability, back pain and strained and dislocated joints. The altered centre of gravity caused by the enlarged maternal abdomen explains why pregnant women readily fall off ladders, for example, when decorating the nursery.

FIGURE 28.3 Positioning of a seatbelt during pregnancy. (**A**) Incorrect positioning. (**B**) Correct positioning.

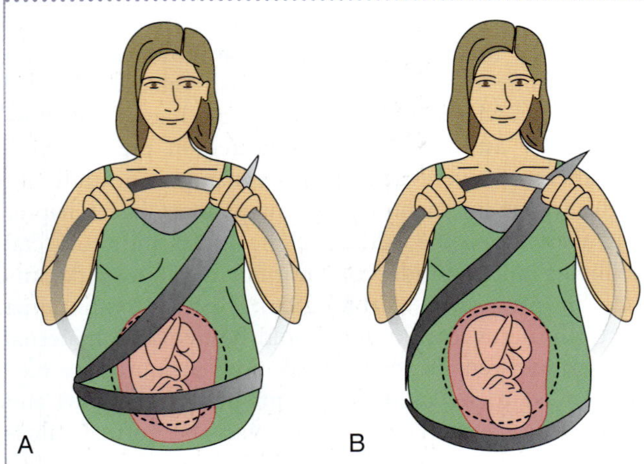

Source: Adapted from Brown HL. Trauma in pregnancy. Obstet Gynecol 2009;114(1):147–60. 10.1097/AOG.

Trauma management

The order of care should comprise the primary survey, followed by a fetal assessment and the secondary survey.[12] Trauma in pregnancy presents a number of challenges because of the anatomical and physiological adaptations that occur.[12] For example, if a chest drain is necessary to treat a haemothorax, use of the third or fourth intercostal space is recommended to accommodate the raised diaphragm.[12] Moreover, pregnant women may physiologically compensate for significant blood loss and then rapidly deteriorate. There is debate as to whether a Kleihauer–Betke test is performed to detect fetomaternal haemorrhage in all women who experience major/abdominal trauma, or only those who are rhesus negative.[198,199] Those women who are rhesus negative may require anti-D immunoglobulin.

Potential for perimortem caesarean section

Where a pregnant woman ≥20 weeks' gestation requires CPR, manual displacement of the uterus or left tilt must be employed during CPR and perimortem caesarean section commenced promptly.[25,200] (See section on *Modifications to basic and advanced life support* below.) If cardiotocography (CTG) monitoring is in progress, all leads must be removed before shocks are delivered.

Obstetric assessment in trauma

Consideration should be given to all women of childbearing age as to whether they may be pregnant.[201] Where a woman is obviously pregnant, an estimate of gestation can be made by measuring the symphysis fundal height. The height in cm equates approximately to the number of weeks' gestation, e.g. 22 cm = 22 weeks gestation, providing there is a singleton pregnancy and there are no pregnancy complications such as excess amniotic fluid (polyhydramnios) or fetal growth restriction.

All radiological investigations and imaging that are clinically indicated by the maternal condition should be initiated without delay over concerns for the fetus.[12,202] When possible and appropriate, a pelvic/abdominal lead shield may be used to protect the developing embryo/fetus.

Auscultation of the fetal heart using a hand-held Doppler is a quick method of assessing immediate fetal wellbeing. Subsequently, external cardiotocography (CTG) may be used to assess fetal wellbeing (see the section on fetal assessment). If there is likelihood of blunt trauma to the abdomen, a continuous external CTG should be undertaken for at least 4 hours, to identify fetal distress resulting from potential placental abruption.[187] An abdominal ultrasound is also usually performed to assess fetal wellbeing and may be useful in detecting free peritoneal fluid/maternal haemorrhage and placental abruption.[201] The bladder becomes an abdominal organ after 12 weeks of pregnancy and is prone to traumatic injury.

Pneumonia

Pneumonia in pregnancy is one of the more common reasons why a pregnant woman may be admitted to ICU. Although studies have shown that pregnant women are not more likely to contract pneumonia, the severity of pneumonia experienced by women in these studies has not been well examined.[203] Varicella pneumonia is more prominent in the pregnant population. It would appear from studies on pregnant women admitted to ICU and maternal death reports that severe community-acquired pneumonia in previously well women is a persisting concern in the pregnant population.

It is not fully understood why pregnant women may be vulnerable to severe pneumonia though the adaptations to the mechanics of breathing and changes in the immune response may be contributing factors.[203] Additionally, it has been postulated that pregnant women are among small children more often and may have an increased likelihood of exposure to infective agents. The treatment and management of pneumonia in pregnancy is no different to pneumonia in non-pregnant women: identify the causative organism and administer appropriate antibiotics or antiviral agents as indicated, maintain oxygenation and prevent complications (see Chapter 15). Assessment of fetal wellbeing and awareness of the changed respiratory parameters in pregnancy are the additional requirements.

Pregnancy and influenza

WHO has recommended since 2006 that all pregnant women receive the seasonal influenza vaccination, in recognition of the known increased risk that influenza poses during pregnancy and because vaccination during pregnancy is safe and confers immunity to the newborn for the first few vulnerable months. In developing countries, this policy has the potential to save the lives of many women and, in particular, their babies. In developed countries, maternal death caused by seasonal influenza is rare. However, the pandemic influenza, H1N1 09 (referred to as 'swine flu'), which swept across the world in 2009, demonstrated how vulnerable pregnant women are to influenza and emphasised the importance of influenza vaccination to prevent severe disease.

The H1N1 2009 flu epidemic killed seven pregnant/postpartum women in Australia and New Zealand in 3 months.[204] Over 60 women were admitted to ICU and a number of their babies died. Women in the second half of pregnancy were over 13 times more likely to be admitted to ICU with H1N1 influenza than non-pregnant women of childbearing age. Pregnant and postpartum women admitted to ICU with H1N1 influenza were particularly unwell, with 14% of women requiring ECMO.[205]

Mental health disorders

Mental health disorders during pregnancy and the postpartum consist of women with preexisting disease and women who develop signs and symptoms of mental health disease for the first time. The mental health disorder may be separate from the pregnancy or there may be a relationship between the pregnancy and the development of the disorder, such as postnatal depression.

Preexisting mental health disorders

The underlying principles of management of pregnant women with a preexisting mental health disorder are the same as for non-pregnant women: safety of the woman, stabilisation of the mental illness and empowerment of, and support for, the woman to make her own choices. A considerable additional challenge is maintaining stability of the mental health disorder if changes to medication are required due to potential teratogenesis or contraindication for use during pregnancy. Generally speaking, if the indication for treatment is unchanged, treatment should be continued during pregnancy.[206] Ideally, pre-conception counselling has occurred and the woman has commenced and stabilised on a medication regime considered safe for pregnancy, prior to becoming pregnant.

Pregnant women with preexisting mental health disorders may require admission to ICU due to acute deterioration in their mental health. This is most likely to be as a result of cessation or alteration of their regular medications.[207,208] Most relapses occur in the first trimester and many women who initially stop their medication recommence it during the pregnancy.[207] Routine care should be provided as clinically indicated, keeping in mind the additional requirements to monitor fetal wellbeing, conduct standard antenatal assessment and consider the impact of the physiological adaptations on treatments.

Mental health disorders related to pregnancy

Suicide related to unwanted pregnancy remains a cause of maternal death in developed countries, especially in adolescents and in women from cultures where childbirth outside of marriage is unacceptable.[131] Depression may arise during pregnancy (antenatal depression) although it is more likely to present during the postpartum period (postpartum depression). The most severe mental health disorder related to pregnancy is puerperal psychosis.

Puerperal psychosis

Puerperal psychosis is a rare mental health complication of pregnancy, said to occur in 1–2/1000 births.[209] The majority of cases occur in women with preexisting mental illness, such as bipolar disorder, with just 0.03/1000 deliveries occurring in women with no preexisting mental health disorder.[210] It usually presents within 2 weeks postpartum and is associated with an increased risk of suicide and infanticide.[211] Women with puerperal psychosis are frequently delusional, suffer hallucinations and require acute hospitalisation for treatment.

Postpartum depression

Postnatal depression is defined as a non-psychotic depressive illness; most definitions specify occurrence within 3 months postpartum although some specify a shorter period of only 1 month.[212,213] Risk factors include prior mental illness, poor social supports, relationship disharmony and recent life events.[212] Depression in the postpartum period raises treatment issues for the nursing mother and the developing infant.[212]

Early diagnosis and effective treatment are indicated. Self-harm in the first 12 months postpartum is a severe concern for women with serious depression. Care in the ICU is no different to that provided to other patients admitted with severe depression. Postnatal depression is not a contraindication to lactation, although some medication may be contraindicated. Medication should be prescribed as warranted on clinical grounds and may include antidepressants, hormonal treatment and psychological treatments.

Caring for pregnant women in ICU

Any pregnant woman in ICU is considered to be carrying an 'at-risk' fetus. This means that fetal wellbeing may be compromised and he/she is at risk of sustaining injury/suboptimal growth and development or death in utero. There are circumstances when the woman's clinical status would improve by delivery of the fetus, and times when the fetus needs to be delivered to increase the likelihood of its own survival. Consideration of both the maternal condition and fetal wellbeing contributes to the decision on when to deliver a fetus. Delivery prior to 24 weeks' gestation is only an option if the maternal condition is very critical and considered necessary to potentially save the woman's life; it is likely that the neonate's care in this instance would be palliative. Even though about half of babies born <24 weeks survive, they do so with a far higher risk of permanent disability.[210] Once gestation reaches 28 weeks, the neonate has more than a 90% chance of survival when cared for in a neonatal intensive care unit (NICU).[214]

Childbirth is a highly significant event in many cultures with associated specific practices and beliefs. These practices vary widely and, in particular, may relate to the pregnant woman, the birth event, the placenta, breastfeeding and the postpartum period[215] For general principles on culturally sensitive care see Chapter 7.

Obesity in pregnancy is associated with adverse outcomes for both the mother and the baby, with a dose-dependent relationship: the higher the BMI, the higher the likelihood of adverse outcomes.[216] This includes a seven-fold increased likelihood of admission to ICU for women with a BMI >50.[3] See Chapter 5 for general principles of caring for bariatric patients. From the maternity perspective, obesity in pregnancy poses difficulties in caring for women including determining fetal wellbeing, assessment of gestation and monitoring the progress of labour, and increased incidences of preeclampsia and gestational diabetes.[216] Lactation also proves more challenging to establish.[217] Additionally, thromboprophylaxis should be considered early, given the increased risk of thrombosis in pregnancy/postpartum, which is magnified further in obese women.

Mechanical ventilation of the pregnant woman

The provision of mechanical ventilation to a pregnant woman occurs rarely and there is little evidence to guide practice. Pregnancy is considered a 'high-risk airway' with the reported 'failure to intubate' rate about 1 in 250,[218] approximately eight times more likely than in the non-pregnant population. The physiological changes of pregnancy that contribute to the increased difficulty in intubation have already been described. Nasal intubation is not usually an option for pregnant women due to the risk of epistaxis. Women with preeclampsia may also have substantial pharyngeal oedema.

The principles of mechanical ventilation in pregnancy are the same as those for the non-obstetric population (see Chapter 15) with additional considerations as follows:

- Ensure target end points reflect the normal arterial blood gases (ABGs) for pregnancy.
- A small reduction in maternal oxygenation can severely impact on fetal oxygenation because of the left shift in the oxyhaemoglobin dissociation curve associated with fetal haemoglobin.[219]
- Permissive hypercapnia has not been evaluated in pregnancy (fetal carbon dioxide is higher than

the maternal level, given the gradient across the placental membrane).

- Normal tidal volumes in pregnancy are increased by up to 40–50% of non-pregnant values, although the mechanical provision of these larger tidal volumes with respect to volutrauma has not been examined; in practice, often respiratory rate is increased first and then increases in tidal volume are only used when necessary.[108]
- There is no evidence that delivery of the baby will improve the maternal respiratory state.[220]

Other, less common, methods to support gas exchange have been reported in the literature in the form of case studies. Of note, nitrous oxide, hyperbaric oxygen treatment and extracorporeal membrane oxygenators have all been used successfully to treat acute conditions, such as pulmonary embolism, in pregnant women.[221-223]

Practice tip

Remember that pregnancy is associated with a poor tolerance of short-term apnoea; for example during induction of anaesthesia and/or intubation, and pre-oxygenation is important.

Practice tip

Medical staff with experience in managing people with difficult airways should be present when a pregnant woman is intubated.

Fetal assessment

Fetal wellbeing will be reliant on the critically ill woman receiving the necessary treatment to promote physiological stability.[224] UK data shows the median gestation of pregnant women admitted to ICU is 25 weeks.[225] Fetal mortality in pregnant women admitted to ICU is often as high as 20–30%[226] and the assessment of fetal wellbeing in those who are critically ill may be used to guide decision making regarding the optimum timing of birth.

Methods of assessing fetal wellbeing include maternal monitoring of fetal movements, intermittent auscultation of the fetal heart (FH) rate using a Pinard stethoscope or hand-held Doppler, continuous external cardiotocograph (CTG) monitoring, ultrasound and fetal biophysical profiles.[227,228] The method(s) used will be dependent on gestation, length of stay on the ICU and the presence/absence of labour. Biophysical profiles use real-time ultrasonography to monitor fetal breathing, movements, tone and amniotic fluid volume.[228,229] Uterine artery Doppler flow measurements may be used in specific circumstances e.g. where the fetus is suspected to be small for gestational age.[229,230] Professionals interpreting fetal surveillance tests in the ICU must take into consideration the medications a woman is receiving as these may have an impact; for example, some maternal sedative medications may also sedate the fetus.

Cardiotocography

A traditional CTG monitor comprises a Doppler that records the FH rate and a pressure transducer that is placed fundally and detects uterine contractions. The FH and uterine activity are recorded on a timed graph (Fig. 28.4).

FIGURE 28.4 Normal CTG trace.

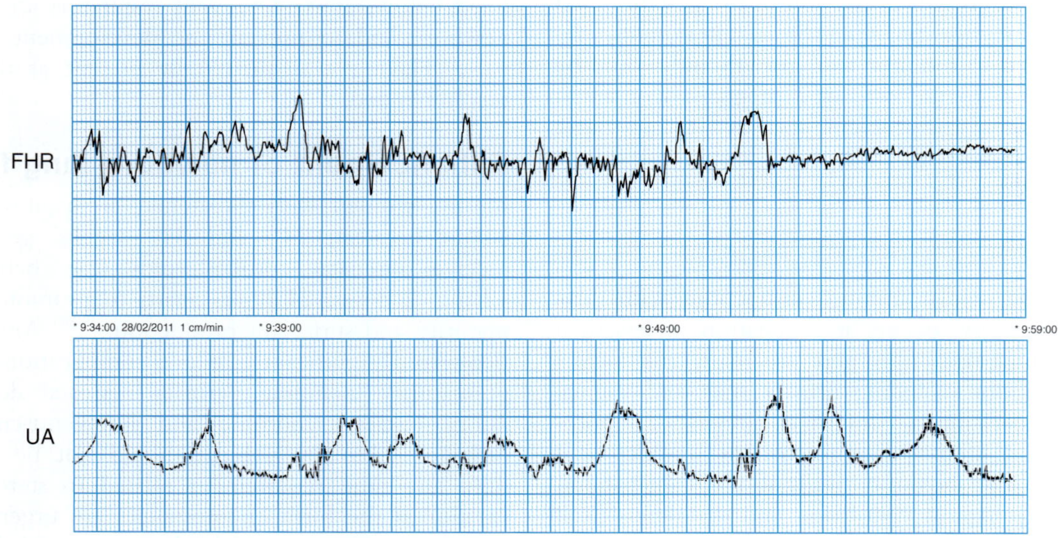

There have been reports of adverse outcomes where the maternal pulse, or recorded artefacts have mistakenly been interpreted as the FH.[231] Consequently, it is vital to differentiate between the FH and maternal pulse at commencement of the CTG, and at regular intervals during the CTG.[231]

There is debate regarding the earliest gestation at which a CTG should be done; ranges from 24 to 28 weeks are cited and depend upon the country, legal threshold for fetal viability and the interventions possible if a FH rate abnormality occurs.[232,233] The decision to commence a CTG at very early pregnancy gestations should be made by a senior obstetrician. CTG recordings are not predictive of longer-term fetal wellbeing and only provide information at the time the trace is recorded.

A normal FH rate is 110–160 beats/min with variability in the rate of ≥5 beats/min.[234] Other features recorded on a CTG include FH rate accelerations and/or decelerations plus the frequency of contractions. A CTG cannot be considered in isolation, but always as part of the overall clinical picture. Specialist obstetric hospitals may offer a CTG interpretation service for general hospitals without maternity staff to assist with interpretation of CTGs. The required frequency and duration of a CTG recording will vary according to the maternal clinical condition or diagnosis and whether the CTG recording is normal. For example, suspected placental abruption following blunt trauma may require 4 hours of continuous monitoring.[187] A CTG will also be recommended during and following elective cardioversion and many other procedures, as advised by the obstetric team.

Ultrasound

An ultrasound scan will measure core components of fetal anatomy, such as head circumference and femur length, to determine fetal size as well as quantify adequacy of amniotic fluid volume. Ultrasound is used to assess the adequacy of fetal growth in relation to the gestation and is used for biophysical profiling. Serial ultrasounds, e.g. weekly, are used to monitor fetal growth and would be a helpful adjunct to the care of a pregnant woman in ICU with a long-term problem, such as Guillain–Barré syndrome and those with additional obstetric risk factors such as intrauterine growth restriction.[235]

Recognition of preterm labour

Preterm labour, regular uterine contractions with dilatation of the cervix, occurs at a gestation of less than 37 completed weeks.[237,238] There are many risk factors for preterm labour including urinary tract and vaginal infections, preeclampsia, multiple pregnancy, polyhydramnios and lifestyle factors such as smoking and illegal drug taking.[9] In the critically ill pregnant patient, anaesthesia, mechanical ventilation and the illness itself may be related to the onset of preterm labour. Women may complain of pelvic pain, similar to period pain, or lower back pain, rather than the more typical abdominal pain associated with term labour. The pain has a cyclical pattern though, with complete pain relief in between contractions. For sedated women, be alert to any patient restlessness or increasing sedation requirements and ask for midwifery assistance to assess for the onset of labour. Placing a hand with firm pressure over the fundus will detect the presence or absence of uterine contraction.

Practice tip

The World Health Organization defines a livebirth as: 'The complete expulsion or extraction from its mother of a product of conception, irrespective of the duration of the pregnancy, which, after such separation, breathes or shows any other evidence of life – e.g. beating of the heart, pulsation of the umbilical cord or definite movement of voluntary muscles – whether or not the umbilical cord has been cut or the placenta is attached.'[236-238] Whether a stillborn baby needs to be registered as a birth and a death varies according to the jurisdiction. For example, in Australia and New Zealand all births need to be registered if the gestation is ≥ 20 weeks or, if the gestation is not known, the birthweight is more than 400 g, while in the UK the stillbirth needs to be registered if the gestation is ≥ 24 weeks' gestation.

Preparation for preterm birth

Preterm birth occurs at a gestation of less than 37 completed weeks. If it is anticipated that a pregnant woman in ICU is likely to give birth prematurely, cohesive planning between the ICU, obstetric and neonatal teams is paramount to achieve the best outcomes. In particular, medication administration, as outlined below, aims to prevent respiratory disease in the newborn and to prevent the development of cerebral palsy. Having a neonatologist present at the birth is recommended.

Enhancement of newborn lung function

Ideally, women with threatened or diagnosed preterm labour between 24^{+0} and 34^{+6} weeks' gestation will receive antenatal corticosteroids (e.g. betamethasone 12 mg, 2 doses, 24 hours apart) to promote fetal lung maturity and surfactant production.[239,240] Antenatal corticosteroids significantly reduce complications related to prematurity including perinatal/neonatal death, respiratory distress syndrome and intraventricular haemorrhage.[241] However, birth should not be delayed to fulfil any time requirement related to steroid administration if the birth circumstances are urgent, as some benefit is seen even if birth occurs <24 hours after a single dose.[240] Antenatal corticosteroids are not contraindicated in women with diabetes, but close monitoring of the blood glucose levels and the need for increased insulin requirements must be taken into consideration.

Fetal neuroprotection

The administration of magnesium sulfate to a woman who is 24^{+0}–29^{+6} weeks gestation with a viable fetus, in preterm labour (or planned to deliver within 24 hours), has been shown to reduce the likelihood of cerebral palsy developing in the infant.[239,242] Neuroprotection with magnesium sulfate may also be considered for women up to 33^{+6} weeks gestation.[239,243] A common regimen is 4 g IV loading dose over 20–30 min followed by a continuous infusion at 1 g/h for 24 hours or until birth (whichever is sooner).[239] However, the 'best' dosage regimen has not been determined.[244,245] Maternal monitoring must include regular checking of the deep tendon reflexes. High doses of magnesium may lead to toxicity, manifesting initially as loss of the deep tendon reflex.

Prevention of rhesus disease

During pregnancy, a small amount of fetal blood can enter the maternal circulation. If the mother is Rh-negative and the fetus is Rh-positive, the mother produces antibodies against the rhesus D (RhD) antigen on her baby's red blood cells.[8] During this, and subsequent pregnancies, the anti-D antibodies are able to pass across the placenta to the fetus and, if the level is sufficient, cause destruction of rhesus D-positive fetal red blood cells, leading to the development of rhesus disease. The disease ranges from mild to severe, and the consequences for the fetus can include varying degrees of anaemia, hydrops fetalis or death. Management of rhesus disease is outlined in Table 28.7.

Most rhesus disease is prevented by treating all pregnant women who are RhD negative with anti-D, termed routine antenatal anti-D prophylaxis. The woman is given an IM injection of anti-D immunoglobulin, which destroys any RhD-positive fetal red blood cells in her circulation before the maternal immune system recognises them and produces anti-D antibodies. Administration of 625 IU of anti-D immunoglobulin to all rhesus D-negative pregnant women at 28 and 34 weeks comprises routine care in Australia and New Zealand.[246] Anti-D is also given when potential sensitising events occur, such as first trimester miscarriage/ectopic pregnancy and second or third trimester APH, MVA and fetal death.[246,247] Another dose of anti-D is given within 72 hours following birth, if the cord blood of the baby is found to be rhesus D-positive.[246,247] In the UK, some providers use non-invasive prenatal testing, which involves testing maternal blood for fetal DNA to ascertain whether the fetus' genotype is rhesus D-positive or negative, thereby reducing the number of women who require treatment.[248]

TABLE 28.7
Management of rhesus disease

BLOOD TESTS AND MANAGEMENT	RATIONALE
Kleihauer–Betke test or flow cytometry	Confirms that fetal blood has passed into the maternal circulation, also estimates the amount of fetal blood that has passed into the maternal circulation
Indirect Coombs test	Screens maternal blood for anti-D antibodies that may pass through the placenta and cause haemolytic disease of the newborn
Quantitative analysis of maternal anti-RhD antibodies	An increasing titre level suggests fetal rhesus disease
FETAL BLOOD (OR UMBILICAL CORD BLOOD) TESTS	
Direct Coombs test	Confirms that maternal anti-D antibodies are present in the fetal/newborn circulation
Full blood count	Haemoglobin level and platelet count to assess for anaemia
Bilirubin	Both total and indirect

Practice tip

The dose of anti-D immunoglobulin depends on the amount of fetal blood cells detected in the maternal blood using the Kleihauer–Betke test. The more fetal cells present, the higher the dose of anti-D required.

Glucose management in pregnancy

Pregnancy is associated with changes to carbohydrate and fat metabolism in order to provide adequate nutrients to the fetus during pregnancy.[249] Some of the pregnancy hormones, including human placental lactogen, contribute to a progressive insulin resistance as the hormone levels increase throughout the pregnancy. Glucose readily crosses the placenta while insulin does not. If the mother has persistently high glucose levels, from either preexisting diabetes or gestational diabetes, the fetus may be large for gestational age (macrosomic) and develop hyperinsulinaemia.[250] Additionally, hyperglycaemia is associated with poor obstetric and neonatal outcomes including congenital anomalies, birth trauma, caesarean birth, preeclampsia, newborn respiratory distress syndrome and stillbirth.[250] Recommended capillary blood glucose level targets for women with diabetes are <5.3 mmol/L fasting and <6.4 mmol/L 2 hours after a meal.[247] Although hyperglycaemia is associated with adverse obstetric and neonatal outcomes, hypoglycaemia should also be avoided.[251]

Modifications to basic and advanced life support

Generally, all standard basic and advanced life support algorithms can be used with only minor adaptations for the pregnant and postpartum woman[12] (Box 28.6). For women over 20 weeks' gestation, left lateral displacement of the uterus is paramount to ensure CPR is as effective as possible. Regardless, it is very difficult to obtain adequate perfusion during CPR of an obviously pregnant woman and arrangements should be made for an emergency caesarean section (termed perimortem caesarean section (PMCS)) or forceps delivery (where appropriate), as soon as resuscitation commences. The general rule is that PMCS should proceed if there is no response to 4 minutes of CPR (the 4-minute rule), with birth of the baby occurring in the next minute, although this timescale is under debate.[28,200,252] A difficult intubation should be anticipated and an experienced individual should be available to intubate the trachea wherever possible.[253] Transfer to an operating theatre for PMCS leads to unnecessary delay and is not advised.[12,200] The list of obstetric conditions that may have precipitated the arrest should be considered and specific treatment instigated.[12] Cardiac arrest in pregnancy is a rare event (1:36,000 maternities) and the chance of a successful resuscitation will be influenced by factors that include the place of arrest (home versus hospital) and delay in commencing PMCS.[200]

Sepsis associated with pregnancy

Maternal sepsis can occur at any time during pregnancy and postpartum and from any cause. Common obstetric-related events include termination of pregnancy, spontaneous miscarriage, prolonged rupture of membranes, caesarean and vaginal birth and mastitis, and non-obstetric-related events include urinary tract infection and pyelonephritis, and respiratory tract infection. The most common organism responsible for maternal sepsis resulting in death is Lancefield group A *Streptococcus* (also known as *Streptococcus pyogenes*).[85] Notable in the review of maternal deaths from sepsis is the rapidity with which some women succumbed. The septic course is often insidious and women may appear deceptively well before suddenly collapsing, often with little or no warning.[85] Although there is no research evaluating the Surviving Sepsis Campaign guidelines in the maternity setting, they are recommended for use.[85,254] The Sepsis Obstetric Score was developed and validated for use in the emergency department to predict likelihood of ICU admission.[255] The Society of Obstetric Medicine of Australia and New Zealand has developed guidelines for the identification and management of sepsis in pregnancy.[256] They recommend use of an obstetric-modified quick Sequential Organ Failure Assessment score. Management of sepsis is described in Chapter 21.

BOX 28.6

Maternal modified cardiac arrest algorithm

Anticipate a difficult airway.

Women with an obviously gravid uterus, e.g. >20 weeks' gestation:

- To relieve aortocaval compression and enable more effective CPR, manually displace the uterus towards the left
  - Alternatively, use a wedge to position the woman in a left lateral tilt
- Call for immediate obstetrician attendance when the arrest is activated
- Remove any internal or external fetal monitors if present
- Prepare for a potential emergency caesarean section
- Aim for delivery within 5 min of onset of resuscitative efforts
- Continue all elements of resuscitation effort during and after caesarean section

Consider and treat any possible contributing factors:

- If the woman is on a magnesium infusion, cease and consider administration of calcium chloride 10 mL in 10% solution or calcium gluconate 30 mL in 10% solution to treat hypermagnesaemia
- Haemorrhage with or without DIC; assess for hypovolaemia and treat appropriately but cautiously
- Placental abruption/praevia if the woman is in the second half of pregnancy
- Uterine atony if the woman is postpartum
- Embolism, e.g. pulmonary, amniotic fluid
- Anaesthetic complications, e.g. high spinal block
- Cardiac disease, e.g. preexisting or new
- Preeclampsia
- Sepsis

Adapted from Vanden Hoek TL, Morrison, LJ, Shuster M et al. Part 12: Cardiac arrest in special situations: 2010 American Heart Association guidelines for cardiopulmonary resuscitation emergency cardiovascular care. Circulation 2010;122(18 Suppl 3):S829–61.

Medication administration in pregnancy

Many drugs used in the critical care environment have not been researched for safe use in pregnant or lactating mothers. There are two key periods when consideration of drug therapy is paramount: during the first trimester when embryo/fetal malformations may occur and immediately prior to delivery as the newborn baby may be adversely affected, e.g. sedated and unable to spontaneously breathe. The decision to administer various medications is often a balance between the benefit of administering the drug to the pregnant woman and the risk of not administering the drug.

There are a number of anatomical, physiological, cellular and molecular changes in pregnancy that affect the pharmacokinetic and pharmacodynamic mechanisms of drugs administered during pregnancy.[257] These include reduced serum protein levels (altered protein binding capacity), increased circulating volume (potential for dilution), delayed gut motility (potential for increased gut absorption), increased GFR (potential for increased excretion) and changes to maternal drug-metabolising enzymes (difficult to predict metabolism pattern of regular drugs).[258] Standard adult doses may be inadequate or toxic during pregnancy due to the adapted physiology of pregnancy.[253] There is a lack of information on efficacy, safety, teratogenicity and pharmacokinetics in pregnancy as drug trials routinely exclude pregnant women.[259]

Potential for teratogenesis

A teratogen is any agent that increases the incidence of a congenital anomaly.[9] The major organs are developed by 10 weeks' gestation; however, the recommendation is to avoid any teratogenic drug throughout the first trimester (14 weeks).[9] Some medications exert an adverse effect in the second or third trimesters of pregnancy, such as ACE inhibitors (fetal anuria and stillbirth), indomethacin (potential premature closure of the ductus arteriosus) and selective serotonin uptake inhibitors (neonatal withdrawal syndrome).[9] Medical staff prescribing drugs and nursing staff administering them should each check the potential impact of the medication in pregnancy, and consult a pharmacist when possible.

Administered immediately prior to delivery

Apart from effects on the structural development of the fetus in the first trimester, the other key time for consideration of drug administration is immediately prior to delivery. Common sedative agents such as midazolam, morphine, fentanyl and propofol cross the placenta readily and exert an action on the fetus.[260-262] Consequently, even mature term babies may be born sedated and require assistance with breathing. Planning for delivery of a pregnant woman in ICU should include the involvement of a paediatrician/neonatologist or the local newborn emergency transport service (NETS) if no paediatricians are on site.

Therapeutic routine drug therapy in pregnancy

For women admitted to ICU for prolonged periods, for example those with Guillain–Barré syndrome, consideration may be given to routine therapeutic medication in pregnancy. For example, folic acid (400 mcg daily) is recommended pre-conception and throughout the first trimester to prevent neural tube defects.[9] Similarly, iron and vitamin D supplementation may be indicated dependent on blood levels. Vitamin D deficiency is common, yet often unrecognised in critically ill patients.[263] Maternal vitamin D deficiency is associated with childhood asthma and increased risk of osteoporotic fracture in their offspring.[264] Due attention should be paid to a pregnant woman's nutritional status in ICU as poor nutrition during pregnancy is associated with poor birth outcomes and pregnancy is associated with increased nutritional requirements.[265]

Caring for postpartum women in ICU

Women admitted to ICU during the postpartum period are often separated from their newborn, possibly even transferred to another hospital, and may not see their baby for days, until discharged from ICU.[266] Specific care that should be provided to the postpartum woman includes postpartum observations, assistance to establish lactation as required and support to early nurturing of a mother–infant bond. Finally, attention to the psychological needs of both the woman and her partner is an important part of care.

Routine postpartum observations

Ongoing surveillance of a postpartum woman is essential in addition to any ad hoc visits provided by a midwife. Routine maternity observations include assessment of the fundus, PV loss and perineum, assessment of the breasts and nipples, consideration of deep vein thrombosis and thromboprophylaxis and evaluation of her psychological wellbeing and transition to motherhood (Box 28.7).

Uterine involution

Uterine 'involution' is the process by which the uterus returns to its near-normal size, tone and position. The vagina, ligaments of the uterus and muscles of the pelvic floor also return to their pre-pregnant state during the involution process. During this process, the lining of the uterus is cast off in the lochia, more commonly referred to as PV loss, and is later replaced by the new endometrium.[8] Following birth, and post-expulsion of the placenta, the muscles of the uterus constrict the blood vessels, so the blood circulating within the uterus is dramatically decreased.[8] Redundant muscle, fibrous and elastic tissue is disposed of – the phagocytes of the blood stream deal with this – but the process is usually

BOX 28.7

Routine postnatal observations

- Examination of breasts, looking for signs of engorgement, mastitis, cracked nipples
- Height, depth and texture of fundus, to ensure involution is happening
- Lochia, inspection of PV loss
- Examination of perineum/wound for signs of healing
- Examination for signs of deep vein thrombosis; thromboprophylaxis is often indicated in a postpartum ICU woman
- Micturition and bowels; to ensure bowel and urinary pattern returning to normal

incomplete, and some elastic tissue remains and the uterus will never fully return to the pre-pregnant state.[9]

The rate of involution is measured by the rate of descent of the uterine fundus (the top of the uterus) in relation to either the umbilicus or the symphysis pubis. Important markers include:

- At day 1 postnatal, the height of the fundus is usually at or just below the umbilicus.
- There is a steady decrease in size of around 1 cm per day.
- By postnatal day 10 the uterus may not be palpable above the symphysis pubis.[9]

The rate of involution varies and may be slower in multiparous women, where there is infection, retained placental tissue and when birth has been by caesarean section.[8] Where deviations from normal have occurred (e.g. caesarean section, atonic postpartum haemorrhage, uterine infection), regular uterine palpation will be required to monitor whether the uterus remains well contracted.[267]

A normally contracted uterus feels firm on palpation; as you palpate the fundus to locate the top and feel the texture of the uterus, you cannot push your fingertip into the tissue of the uterus. A so-called boggy uterus is one that is not contracted properly (atonic) and the fundus does not feel firm on palpation. Reasons for a 'boggy uterus' include uterine atony, retained tissue/membrane/clots or a full bladder that is impeding the uterine nerve stimulus to contract. The uterus responds well to tactile stimulation, and the first treatment for a 'boggy uterus' is to 'rub-up' the fundus. This involves palpating the top of the uterus and literally giving it a rub. The uterus will usually respond and you will feel it tighten and become harder. Such an action may result in a small gush of PV loss. On some occasions, a drug that causes the uterus to contract (uterotonic), such as oxytocin, may be needed to promote uterine contraction. If the uterus does not contract properly, the vessels that supplied the placental bed will not be closed off by the uterine muscle contraction (called the living ligatures) and the woman will continue to bleed.[9]

Practice tip

Uterotonics, drugs that cause the uterus to contract, are usually stored in the refrigerator; for example, Syntocinon, Syntometrine.

Practice tip

Many midwives document fundal height by finger widths in relation to the belly button. For example, two finger widths below the belly button would be notated by 2F ↓⊙.

Lochia and perineal care

The changes in the appearance of the lochia are described in three stages: lochia rubra, serosa and alba.[264] Lochia rubra consists of blood coming chiefly from the placental site. Three or 4 days post-delivery the lochia changes to a pinky-brownish colour and is called lochia serosa. Seven days post-delivery the lochia changes to yellowish in appearance; this is called lochia alba. Normal lochia is not offensive in odour but the amount and duration of blood loss will vary between women.[269] Offensive lochia with or without maternal pyrexia may indicate a uterine infection (postpartum endometritis). High and low vaginal swabs for culture and sensitivity, and the commencement of antibiotic cover, should be initiated. Offensive lochia coupled with sub-involution of the uterus may require ultrasound to exclude retained placental tissue.[268]

Regular assessment of the PV loss is required in the early postpartum phase. Generally, this includes 1–2-hourly checks if the PV loss is relatively heavy (pad soaked within 1–2 hours) for the first day, progressing to 4-hourly checks on day 2, with further reductions in observation frequency based on clinical condition. Check the fundus and PV loss regularly enough to detect any excessive blood loss or loss of uterine tone. The colour and volume of PV loss is usually documented along with any pad changes. Weighing pads to quantify PV loss is preferable to describing the loss as 'mild', 'moderate' or 'severe'.

The perineum should be examined daily or more frequently, as dictated by clinical circumstances. A vulval haematoma/varicosities may be present and require obstetric assessment. For women who have had a vaginal birth, review the medical notes to ascertain if perineal trauma was sustained or an episiotomy performed. Examine perineal wounds and/or sutures for signs of infection or wound breakdown and ensure the area is kept clean. Ice packs applied to the perineum may help relieve swelling and discomfort.[267]

Increased potential for deep vein thrombosis

Most postpartum women admitted to ICU are likely to fulfil the criteria that recommend medical thromboprophylaxis.[95,267] Routine postpartum care involves examining the legs for signs of deep vein thrombosis (DVT) and appropriate use of thromboembolic stockings, sequential compression devices and thromboprophylaxis as required.[95]

Breast care and breastfeeding

Breastfeeding provides many health benefits for mothers and their babies and should be facilitated whenever possible in the ICU.[267]

Initiation and establishment of lactation

The establishment and maintenance of lactation are complex hormone-mediated processes termed lactogenesis and galactopoiesis.[8] The physiological trigger for the establishment of lactation is a fall in progesterone combined with maintained levels of prolactin and cortisol.[270] During the initial postnatal period colostrum is produced and this contains high levels of protein, immunologic and growth factors.[271] The normal timing for milk to 'come in' is between 3 and 4 days post-delivery.[272,273] Of note, the drug dopamine may hinder lactation, as it inhibits prolactin secretion.[273] It is unlikely that the severity of maternal illness plays much of a role in the initial capacity to produce milk; anecdotally, 100 mL of breast milk has been expressed 4-hourly from a postpartum woman on ECMO. The initial regularity of hand expression or breastfeeding and milk removal provide the stimulus to produce milk.

Throughout pregnancy, the breasts develop and are capable of producing colostrum from 16 weeks onwards.[8] Ideally, the first breastfeed should occur within an hour of birth.[274] However, there is some debate regarding how crucial the first 24–48 hours are for the successful establishment of lactation as in some cultures, colostrum is considered poisonous and breastfeeding is withheld for 2–3 days.[275] These women go on to successfully breastfeed and so too do many women recovering from illness with suboptimal breast expression in the first day or two postpartum. However, for women wanting to breastfeed, early and frequent expression is likely to help establish lactation and set up a positive cycle.

Hand expression is also used when babies are premature, there are problems with attachment, the mother is ill, or mother and baby are in different locations.[276] Box 28.8 outlines the principles of hand expressions and Fig. 28.5 the process. Frequent, short expression of the breasts is more effective than prolonged infrequent expressing, and night expression is also important because prolactin, the hormone required to stimulate milk secretion, is produced in greater quantities overnight.[274,277] Breast pumps (hand or electric) may be helpful for women where long-term expression is required.[277] To promote successful milk expression, measures including relaxation, holding or seeing a photograph of the baby and massaging the breasts may be employed.[277] Overall, the two main factors that support the establishment of lactation are breast stimulation (infant suckling or hand/pump expression) and milk removal. In a positive feedback

BOX 28.8

Principles of expressing breast milk

How often should I express?

Generally speaking, women are recommended to express 2–3-hourly. This may be difficult to achieve in the ICU environment. Clinicians should aim for at least 6 times per 24 h including at least once overnight.

Hand express or machine express?

It is recommended to use hand expression only in the first few days with use of a machine reserved for when the milk has come in. Always start and finish the expression by hand, as hand expression provides a better stimulus for milk production than the machine does, and promotes release of the 'let-down' reflex which will assist with milk flow and removal. Expressing by hand or machine should not be painful.

Storage and transport of expressed milk

The most useful container for collection of expressed colostrum is a 2- or 5-mL syringe and a sterile plain specimen container for small volumes of milk. Label the container with the woman's name, date and time of collection. Use a new container for each expression. Breast milk must be stored in a refrigerator and may be frozen. A 'cooler bag' with ice packs should be used to transport the milk from ICU to where the baby is being cared for.

FIGURE 28.5 How to hand express.

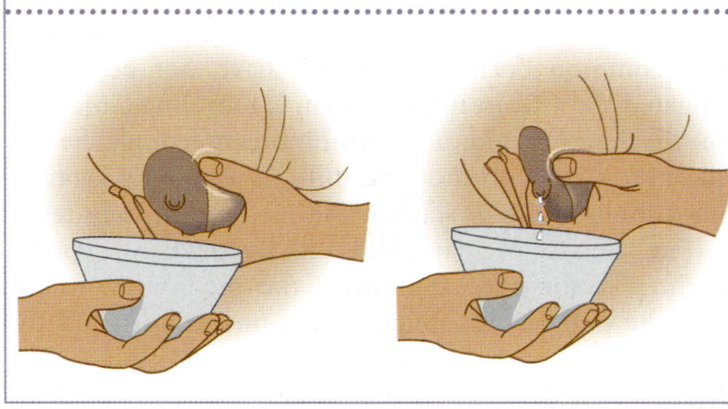

loop, the more often milk is removed from the breast, the more milk will be produced.[8]

If the mother's intention was to formula feed, or if the baby has died, then the lactation process may be suppressed. In practice, this means providing no stimulation to the breasts (i.e. no hand expression). Although used in the past, medications are rarely used to influence this process. With no breast expression, some women may still experience milk 'coming in' at or after day 4 postpartum and comfort measures may assist if the breasts become very uncomfortable. Cold compresses may be of use and it is important for the critical care nurse to observe for signs like reddened hot areas on the breast that may be an indication of mastitis.

Breast care

A woman's breasts should be assessed at least twice a shift to assess their condition and identify signs of complications, such as mastitis. Assess all women, regardless of whether they are breastfeeding or not. The breasts are usually soft although as the milk comes in, they may become engorged and tender to touch. A localised area that is red and painful may be indicative of mastitis, which results from poor attachment and insufficient emptying of milk from the breast.[278] Mastitis is sometimes accompanied by flu-like symptoms and may require treatment with antibiotics. The nipples should be inspected for cracks and soreness if the woman is using a breast pump or breastfeeding. Good positioning and attachment of the baby at the breast are vital for successful breastfeeding and will minimise the incidence of cracked nipples.[274] Colostrum (or milk once it has come in) may leak from the nipples and can be gently applied over the nipples to promote healing.[279]

Medication administration and lactation

Many drugs are safe to use in breastfeeding, although most common critical care drugs have not been well evaluated.[280,281] Even if the woman is receiving a medication that is contraindicated during breastfeeding, she can still express (and discard) the milk to establish lactation, unless she is likely to stay on the medication long term.

The safety of the expressed milk for the baby depends on three factors; the amount of the medication in the milk, the oral bioavailability of the medication, and the ability of the infant to metabolise the medication.[282] The gestation and condition of the infant are relevant as the function of the gut, liver and kidney varies with maturity and illness. Consequently, advice from the baby's neonatologist or paediatrician can help determine whether the neonate can receive the expressed breast milk, or whether it should be discarded. Breast milk is of particular importance to preterm infants as it reduces the likelihood of necrotising enterocolitis developing.[283]

Perinatal mental health

Major emotional changes take place in the majority of women during the puerperium, but there is wide variation in the impact these changes have. The 'baby blues' are thought to occur 2–3 days post-birth, and are characterised by emotional lability (mood swings), thoughts of inadequacy, concern for the baby and last up to 2 weeks.[284] It is estimated that the baby blues are experienced by up to 80% of women.[284] It is also recognised that women can suffer posttraumatic stress disorder (PTSD) following childbirth, highlighting the importance of healthcare professionals attending to women's psychological needs during an episode of critical illness.[285]

The family unit

Maternal admission to ICU often separates the mother from her newborn and may also be associated with a period of heavy sedation/loss of consciousness. Thus, the woman may not be able to recollect the birth process and will often not have seen her baby before being transferred to ICU.

Promoting maternal–infant attachment

Promoting maternal–infant attachment depends on the condition of both the mother and her baby, and their physical locations. The best-case scenario is that the baby is able to 'room in' with the mother for periods of time in ICU. Skin to skin contact is recommended as it has many benefits for both mother and baby including a calming effect for both, neonatal temperature regulation and stimulation of the lactation hormones.[286] Alternatively, organising for either the baby to visit the mother in ICU or the mother, if well enough, to visit the baby in NICU is often feasible. Physically seeing and touching the baby is likely to be an important step for the mother. Newer technologies, like Skype, are used in some ICUs to enable the mother to see her baby in a different hospital and to watch significant events, such as the first bath.

The use of diaries, one about the mother's condition and one about the baby's progress, complete with photos, visitor and clinician entries, is another strategy that may be useful to promote maternal–infant attachment. The first few days following birth are often a blur for the mother with little recollection of events. It is also common to have photographs of the baby for the mother to look at, and clinicians keep in touch with the nursery where the baby is being cared for and give the mother regular updates on the baby's condition.

Caring for the partner and other family members

The partner is likely to be shocked and distressed by the sudden and severe illness of the mother. The partner may also be torn between two ICUs, with the newborn admitted to NICU in one hospital and the mother in ICU in another hospital.[266] This situation is further compounded if there are other children to consider. Usual strategies such as explanation, open visiting and social work support are important.

Summary

Intensive care management of pregnant and postpartum women is challenging for a variety of reasons including, but not limited to, the presence of the fetus, physiological adaptations of pregnancy and due to clinical conditions that are unique to the obstetric population. ICU staff are often not educationally prepared to provide midwifery care and there may be difficulty in obtaining midwifery and obstetric consultation. Importantly, childbirth is viewed as a normal, healthy event in our society and is usually a cause of celebration. A life-threatening event associated with childbirth may seem more overwhelming due to this context. The best outcomes for both the mother and her baby will result from collaborative and coordinated care between maternity and critical care service providers.

Case study

Ann Jones is coming from the birth suite. She is a 32-year-old woman who has just had her first baby. Ann was admitted to the birth suite feeling generally unwell at 33 weeks' gestation. She was a primipara with no past or current medical/obstetric history of note, though she reported having severe indigestion for a day and a headache for 6 hours. She also reported intermittent abdominal pains for several hours. On examination shortly after admission, Ann was found to be in advanced labour. Her BP was 185/110 with 4+ protein in her urine. She was hyperreflexic with four beats of clonus.

The midwife handing over explained that Ann had a rapid labour and normal birth 45 min after being admitted to the birth suite. Her third stage of labour was uneventful and her placenta appeared complete. She had an estimated blood loss of 250 mL. Her baby girl, Florence, was born in good condition but required admission to the neonatal unit for prematurity.

Ann's initial blood results showed: haemoglobin 109 g/L, platelets, 85×10^9, creatinine 99 micromol/L, ALT 740 IU/L, AST 690 IU/L and total bilirubin 32 micromol/L. She was diagnosed with HELLP syndrome (Haemolysis, Elevated Liver enzymes and Low Platelets). Ann received the following medications while on the Labour ward:

- IV Syntocinon 5 IU slow bolus (for active management of third stage of labour)
- IV magnesium sulfate 4 g bolus followed by a 1 g/h maintenance infusion
- Bolus doses of IV labetalol and a continuing maintenance infusion at 80 mg/h
- IV Hartmann's restricted to 80 mL/h via infusion pump.

Despite the labetalol infusion Ann's blood pressure remained labile, peaking at 170/110 and the obstetric team decided that Ann required transfer to the ICU where arterial line monitoring could be initiated. Just as you were settling Ann in, she suffered an eclamptic seizure lasting 2 min. Four hours later she was diagnosed with pulmonary oedema and required IV Lasix and CPAP.

CASE STUDY QUESTIONS

1. What is the significance of epigastric pain in a woman who has severe preeclampsia/HELLP syndrome?
2. Outline the management of an eclamptic seizure, including the recommended medication.
3. Discuss the importance of controlling raised blood pressure in pregnancy.
4. What nursing assessment should be undertaken and documented for Ann?
5. Explain the most likely reason why Ann has developed pulmonary oedema?
6. Soon after arrival in the ICU, Ann informs you she wishes to breastfeed. What advice and support can be provided on the ICU?

RESEARCH VIGNETTE

Beckett VA, Knight M, Sharpe, P. The CAPS Study: incidence, management and outcomes of cardiac arrest in pregnancy in the UK: a prospective, descriptive study. BJOG 2017;124 (9):1374-81

Abstract

Objective: To describe the incidence, risks, management and outcomes of cardiac arrest in pregnancy in the UK population, with specific focus on the use of perimortem caesarean section (PMCS).

Design: A prospective, descriptive study using the UK Obstetric Surveillance System (UKOSS).

Setting: All UK hospitals with maternity units.

Population: All women who received basic life support in pregnancy in the UK between 1 July 2011 and 30 June 2014 (n = 66).

Methods: Prospective case identification through UKOSS monthly mailing.

Main outcome measures: Cardiac arrest in pregnancy, PMCS, maternal death.

Results: There were 66 cardiac arrests in pregnancy, resulting in an incidence of 2.78 per 100 000 maternities (1:36000; 95% CI 2.2–3.6). In all, 28 women died (case fatality rate 42%); 16 women arrested solely as a consequence of obstetric anaesthesia, 12 of whom were obese. Basic and advanced life support were rapidly delivered. Those who died were more likely to have collapsed at home. Perimortem caesarean section was performed in 49 women, 11 in the emergency department. The time from collapse to PMCS was significantly shorter in women who survived (median interval 3 versus 12 min, P = 0.001). Forty-six of 58 babies were born alive; 32 babies to surviving mothers and 14 to women who died.

Conclusion: Cardiac arrest is rare in the pregnant UK population, however, nearly a quarter of cases are precipitated by obstetric anaesthesia, suggesting an opportunity to reduce the incidence further. Maternal survival rates of 58% were achieved with timely resuscitation, including PMCS, delay in which was associated with maternal death. Inpatient arrests were associated with higher survival rates than arrests that occurred outside the hospital setting.

Critique

This study was undertaken to provide contemporary data on maternal cardiac arrest rates in the UK and to determine the number of women who had PMCS; this intervention improves maternal cardiac output and may bring about spontaneous circulation.

The UKOSS data collection process was familiar to the nominated professionals responsible for completing the monthly reporting cards. When a maternal cardiac arrest was reported, detailed information was collected by follow-up questionnaire. The authors do not state whether the questionnaire was piloted before distribution, but the questionnaire is available on www.npeu.ox.ac.uk/ukoss/dcf for review.[287] Up to five follow-up reminders were sent.

A clear definition of maternal cardiac arrest was presented at the outset of the study; 'any woman who had received BLS [basic life support] during pregnancy'. However, this definition was altered in the third year of study to include women who required BLS in the first 24 hours post-birth. This change was instigated after it was identified that some cardiac arrests occurred in the immediate postpartum period, but deterioration leading up to these occurred while women were still pregnant. Piloting of the reporting cards may have negated the need to change the study inclusion criteria part way through the study period.

The results are clearly reported and take into consideration the change in definition of cardiac arrest. The statistical tests used are clearly stated and the denominator data used for calculating the incidence of maternal cardiac arrest were based on National statistics.

The incidence of cardiac arrest during pregnancy is reported at 2.8 per 100,000 maternities, whereas for the final year of the study (which included 25 cardiac arrests in the first 24 hours post birth), a rate of 6.3 per 100,000 maternities is reported. However, despite stating that the Intensive Care National Audit and Research Centre gather data on 'all individuals receiving chest compressions and/or defibrillation', there was no strategy to identify potentially missed cases. Of note, only six women were <20 weeks' gestation and UKOSS identification prior to 20 weeks may be suboptimal. The reason for death was available for 21 (75%) of the 28 women. Complications of obstetric anaesthesia accounted for 16 pregnancy deaths and included intubation difficulties (n=3), collapse following epidural top ups (n=3) and total spinal anaesthesia (n=10). Twelve women who died due to anaesthetic-related causes had a BMI ≥30. When women were assessed to have more than one cause of death, both were reported. Forty-five of the women who collapsed were admitted to an ICU and of these, 12 died.

It was determined that basic and advanced life support (ALS) were instigated in a timely manner for both the women who died and those who survived. The researchers attribute this to the annual multidisciplinary training undertaken by professionals who provide maternity care in the UK.

The place of collapse influenced maternal survival rates, with more women surviving in the hospital setting compared with those who collapsed at home ($P < 0.001$). PMCS was performed for 49 women and those who were not moved prior to PMCS had higher survival rates; 72% versus 36%. However, some women required transfer to hospital or had return of spontaneous circulation. Overall, seven women had unnecessary moves prior to PMCS and of these, three died. Manual displacement of the uterus was performed for four women during CPR, while 21 women had left pelvic tilting and the researchers suggest that this is an area where further education and training may be beneficial.

In relation to fetal outcome, more babies survived when PMCS was performed within 5 min, compared to > 5 min (96% versus 70%). Moreover, neonatal outcome was worse when the mother did not survive.

Overall, the researchers acknowledge the strengths of this study include its prospective nature and the well-established UKOSS reporting mechanisms already in place. A drawback is the change of definition for cardiac arrest after 2 years of data collection, although the results section clearly differentiates between pregnancy and early postnatal cardiac arrests.

The ongoing importance of annual BLS/ALS training is reinforced, with left manual displacement of the uterus during CPR and timely PMCS advocated. Clinical areas providing care for pregnant women (e.g. ICU) should have appropriate equipment available for PMCS. Prospective research examining the hours leading up to maternal collapse may identify failure to rescue situations and opportunities for prevention.

Learning activities

1. Identify four causes of maternal collapse during pregnancy.
2. Discuss the physiological adaptations of pregnancy that must be considered when managing a cardiac arrest in a woman who is 33 weeks' pregnant.
3. Outline why pregnant/postnatal women are at greater risk of developing venous thromboembolism compared with the non-pregnant general population.
4. Identify the maternity-specific resources and equipment in your workplace. For example, are their maternity-specific modifications in your ALS protocol, do you have a wedge on your resuscitation trolley, what policies and procedures do you have in place to support the care of a maternity patient?

Online resources

Australasian Maternity Outcomes Surveillance System (AMOSS), www.amoss.com.au

California Maternity Quality Care Collaborative; www.cmqcc.org

Cardiac Society of Australia and New Zealand, www.csanz.edu.au/resources/

National Institute for Health and Clinical Excellence, NICE guidelines for the management of asthma, https://www.nice.org.uk/guidance/ng80

Perinatal and Maternal Mortality Review Committee (PMMRC),www.hqsc.govt.nz/our-programmes/mrc/pmmrc/

Royal Australian and New Zealand College of Obstetricians and Gynaecologists, www.ranzcog.edu.au/Statements-Guidelines

Royal College of Obstetricians and Gynaecologists, www.rcog.org.uk/guidelines

Society of Obstetric Medicine of Australia and New Zealand (SOMANZ), www.somanz.org/guidelines.asp

UK Confidential Enquiry into Maternal Death, www.npeu.ox.ac.uk/mbrrace-uk/programme-of-work

Further reading

Belfort M, Saade G, Foley MR, et al, editors. Critical care obstetrics. 5th ed. Oxford: Wiley-Blackwell; 2010.

Foley M, Strong T, Garite T, editors. Obstetric intensive care manual. 5th ed. Columbus: McGraw-Hill Education; 2018.

Impey L, Child T. Obstetrics and gynaecology. 5th ed. Chichester: Wiley Blackwell; 2017.

Van de Velde M, Scholefield H, Plante L, editors. Maternal critical care: a multidisciplinary approach. New York: Cambridge University Press; 2013.

Winter C, Crofts J, Draycott T, et al, editors. PROMPT practical obstetric multi-professional training. 3rd ed. Cambridge: Cambridge University Press; 2017.

References

1. Pollock W, Rose L, Dennis C-L. Pregnant and postpartum admissions to the intensive care unit: a systematic review. Intensive Care Med 2010;36:1465–74.
2. Harrison DA, Penny JA, Yentis SM, et al. Case mix, outcome and activity for obstetric admissions to adult, general critical care units: a secondary analysis of the ICNARC Case Mix Programme Database. Crit Care 2005;9(Suppl. 3):S25–37.
3. Sullivan EA, Dickinson JE, Vaughan GA, et al. Maternal super-obesity and perinatal outcomes in Australia: a national population-based cohort study. BMC Pregnancy Childbirth 2015;15(1):322.
4. Zwart JJ, Dupuis JRO, Richters A, et al. Obstetric intensive care unit admission: a 2-year nationwide population-based cohort study. Intensive Care Med 2010;36(2):256–63.
5. Hazelgrove JF, Price C, Pappachan VJ, et al. Multicenter study of obstetric admissions to 14 intensive care units in southern England. Crit Care Med 2001;29(4):770–5.
6. Lawton B, MacDonald EJ, Brown SA, et al. Preventability of severe acute maternal morbidity. Am J Obstet Gynecol 2014;210(6):557.e1–6.
7. Norwitz E, Robinson J. Pregnancy-induced physiologic alterations. In: Belfort M, Saade G, Foley MR, et al, editors. Critical care obstetrics. 5th ed. Oxford: Wiley-Blackwell; 2010. [Chapter 4].
8. Tucker Blackburn S. Maternal, fetal and neonatal physiology: a clinical perspective. St Louis: Elsevier; 2018.
9. Marshall JE, Raynor MD, editors. Myles Textbook for midwives. 16th ed. Edinburgh: Elsevier; 2014.
10. National Institute for Health and Care Excellence. Postnatal care. London: NICE; 2015.
11. Hytten F. Blood volume changes in normal pregnancy. Clin Haematol 1985;14(3):601–12.
12. Paterson-Brown S, Howell C, editors. Managing obstetric emergencies and trauma. The MOET course manual. 3rd ed. Cambridge: Cambridge University Press; 2014.
13. Royal College of Obstetricians and Gynaecologists. Thrombosis and embolism during pregnancy and the puerperium, the acute management of (Green-top Guideline No. 37b). London: RCOG; 2015.
14. Uchikova EH, Ledjev II. Changes in haemostasis during normal pregnancy. Eur J Obstet Gynecol Reprod Biol 2005;119(2):185–8.
15. Paniccia R, Prisco D, Bandinelli B, et al. Plasma and serum levels of D-dimer and their correlations with other hemostatic parameters in pregnancy. Thromb Res 2002;105(3):257–62.
16. Szecsi PB, Jorgensen M, Klajnbard A, et al. Haemostatic reference intervals in pregnancy. Thromb Haemost 2010;103(4):718–27.
17. Burrows RF, Kelton JG. Incidentally detected thrombocytopenia in healthy mothers and their infants. N Engl J Med 1988;319(3):142–5.
18. Yanamandra N, Chandraharan E. Anatomical and physiological changes in pregnancy and their implications in clinical practice. In: Chandraharan E, Arulkumaran S, editors. Obstetric and intrapartum emergencies: a practical guide to management. Cambridge: Cambridge University Press; 2012.
19. Sunitha M, Chandrasekharappa S, Brid SV. Electrocardiographic Qrs axis, Q wave and T-wave changes in 2nd and 3rd trimester of normal pregnancy. J Clin Diagn Res 2014;8(9):BC17.
20. Mabie W, DiSessa T, Crocker L, et al. A longitudinal study of cardiac output in normal human pregnancy. Am J Obstet Gynecol 1994;170(3):849–56.

21. Lyall F, Robson SC, Bulmer JN. Spiral artery remodeling and trophoblast invasion in preeclampsia and fetal growth restriction: relationship to clinical outcome. Hypertension 2013;62(6):1046–54.
22. Clapp J, Capeless E. Cardiovascular function before, during, and after the first and subsequent pregnancies. Am J Cardiol 1997;80(11):1469–73.
23. Creasy R, Resnik R, Iams J, et al. Creasy and Resnik's Maternal-fetal medicine. Principles and practice. 7th ed. Philadelphia: Elsevier Saunders; 2013.
24. Hunter S, Robson SC. Adaptation of the maternal heart in pregnancy. Br Heart J 1992;68(6):540–3.
25. Nevo O, Soustiel JF, Thaler I. Maternal cerebral blood flow during normal pregnancy: a cross-sectional study. Am J Obstet Gynecol 2010;203(5):475.e1–6.
26. Meah VL, Cockcroft JR, Backx K, et al. Cardiac output and related haemodynamics during pregnancy: a series of meta-analyses. Heart 2016;102(7):518–26.
27. Hill CC, Pickinpaugh J. Physiologic changes in pregnancy. Surg Clin North Am 2008;88(2):391–401.
28. Winter C, Crofts J, Draycott T, et al, editors. PROMPT Practical Obstetric multi-Professional Training course manual. 3rd ed. Cambridge: Cambridge University Press; 2017.
29. Tan EK, Tan EL. Alterations in physiology and anatomy during pregnancy. Best Pract Res Clin Obstet Gynaecol 2013;27(6):791–802.
30. Jeejeebhoy FM, Zelop CM, Lipman S, et al. Cardiac arrest in pregnancy: a scientific statement from the American Heart Association. Circulation 2015;132(18):1747–73.
31. Duvekot J, Peeters L. Maternal cardiovascular hemodynamic adaptation to pregnancy. Obstet Gynecol Surv 1994;48(12):S1–4.
32. Robson S, Dunlop W, Moore M, et al. Haemodynamic changes during the puerperium: a Doppler and M-mode echocardiographic study. BJOG 1987;94(11):1028–39.
33. Rankin J, editor. Physiology in childbearing with anatomy and related biosciences. Edinburgh: Elsevier; 2017.
34. Hegewald MJ, Crapo RO. Respiratory physiology in pregnancy. Clin Chest Med 2011;32(1):1–13.
35. Archer G, Marx G. Arterial oxygen tension during apnoea in parturient women. Br J Anaesth 1974;46(5):358–60.
36. Crapo R. Normal cardiopulmonary physiology during pregnancy. Clin Obstet Gynecol 1996;39(1):3–16.
37. Jensen D, Duffin J, Lam Y, et al. Physiological mechanisms of hyperventilation during human pregnancy. Respir Physiol Neurobiol 2008;161(1):76–86.
38. Langford E, Khwanda A, Langford K. Oxygen saturation response to exercise in healthy pregnant women: a simple protocol and normal range. Obstet Med 2010;3(2):65–8.
39. Templeton A, Kelman G. Maternal blood-gases, (PAO2-PaO2): physiological shunt and VD/VT in normal pregnancy. Brit J Anaesth 1976;48(10):1001–4.
40. Prodromakis E, Trakada G, Tsapanos V, et al. Arterial oxygen tension during sleep in the third trimester of pregnancy. Acta Obstet Gynecol Scand 2004;83(2):159–64.
41. MacRae D, Palavradji D. Maternal acid–base changes in pregnancy. BJOG 1967;74(1):11–16.
42. Andersen G, James G, Mathers N, et al. The maternal oxygen tension and acid–base status during pregnancy. BJOG 1969;76(1): 16–19.
43. Richlin S, Cusick W, Sullivan C, et al. Normative oxygen saturation values for pregnant women at sea level. Prim Care Update Ob Gyns 1998;5(4):154–5.
44. LoMauro A, Aliverti A. Respiratory physiology of pregnancy: physiology masterclass. Breathe 2015;11(4):297–301.
45. Boutourline-Young H, Boutourline-Young E. Alveolar carbon dioxide levels in pregnant, parturient and lactating subjects. BJOG 1956;63(4):509–28.
46. Matuszkiewicz-Rowińska J, Małyszko J, Wieliczko M. Urinary tract infections in pregnancy: old and new unresolved diagnostic and therapeutic problems. Arch Med Sci 2015;11(1):67–77.
47. Cheung KL, Lafayette RA. Renal physiology of pregnancy. Adv Chronic Kidney Dis 2013;20(3):209–14.
48. Davison J. The kidney in pregnancy: a review. J Royal Soc Med 1983;76(6):485–501.
49. Klajnbard A, Szecsi P, Colov N, et al. Laboratory reference intervals during pregnancy, delivery and the early postpartum period. Clin Chem Lab Med 2010;48(2):237–48.
50. Mackenzie M, Woolnough M, Barrett N, et al. Normal urine output after elective caesarean section: an observational study. Int J Obstet Anesth 2010;19(4):379–83.
51. Bouyou J, Gaujoux S, Marcellin L, et al. Abdominal emergencies during pregnancy. J Visc Surg 2015;152(6 Suppl.):S105–15.
52. Baer J, Reis R, Arens R. Appendicitis in pregnancy: with changes in position and axis of the normal appendix in pregnancy. JAMA 1932;98(16):1359–64.
53. Augustin G, Majerovic M. Non-obstetrical acute abdomen during pregnancy. Euro J Obstet Gynecol Reprod Biol 2007;131(1):4–12.
54. Nakai A, Sekiya I, Oya A, et al. Assessment of the hepatic arterial and portal venous blood flows during pregnancy with Doppler ultrasonography. Arch Gynecol Obstet 2002;266(1):25–9.
55. Miller E. Changes in serum immunity during pregnancy. Am J Human Biol 2009;21(3):401–3.
56. Rogerson S, Hviid L, Duffy P, et al. Malaria in pregnancy: pathogenesis and immunity. Lancet Infect Dis 2007;7(2):105–17.

57. Kingdom J, Huppertz B, Seaward G, et al. Development of the placental villous tree and its consequences for fetal growth. Eur J Obstet Gynecol Reprod Biol 2000;92(1):35–43.
58. Low J. Fetal asphyxia and brain damage. Fetal Matern Med Rev 2001;12(2):139–58.
59. Talbot L, Maclennan K. Physiology of pregnancy. Anaesth Intensive Care Med 2016;17(7):341–5.
60. Jones D, Bhasale A, Bailey M, et al. Effect of a national standard for deteriorating patients on intensive care admissions due to cardiac arrest in Australia. Crit Care Med 2018;46(4):586–93.
61. Smith GB, Isaacs R, Andrews L, et al. Vital signs and other observations used to detect deterioration in pregnant women: an analysis of vital sign charts in consultant-led UK maternity units. Int J Obstet Anesth 2017;30:44–51.
62. Crozier TM, Galt P, Wilson SJ, et al. Rapid response team calls to obstetric patients in a busy quaternary maternity hospital. Aust N Z J Obstet Gynaecol 2018;58(1):47–53.
63. Austin DM, Sadler L, McLintock C, et al. Early detection of severe maternal morbidity: a retrospective assessment of the role of an Early Warning Score System. Aust N Z J Obstet Gynaecol 2014;54(2):152–5.
64. National Collaborating Centre for Women's and Children's Health. UK). National Institute for Health and Clinical Excellence: guidance. Hypertension in pregnancy: the management of hypertensive disorders during pregnancy. London: RCOG Press; 2010.
65. Lowe SA, Bowyer L, Lust K, et al. SOMANZ guidelines for the management of hypertensive disorders of pregnancy 2014. Aust N Z J Obstet Gynaecol 2015;55(5):e1–29.
66. Druzin M, Shields L, Peterson N, et al Preeclampsia toolkit: improving health care response to preeclampsia (California Maternal Quality Care Collaborative Toolkit to Transform Maternity Care). Developed under contract #11-10006 with the California Department of Public Health; Maternal, Child and Adolescent Health Division; 2013. Available from: https://www.cmqcc.org/resources-tool-kits/toolkits/preeclampsia-toolkit.
67. Roberts JM, Redman CWG. Pre-eclampsia: more than pregnancy-induced hypertension. Lancet 1993;341(8858):1447–51.
68. Steegers EAP, von Dadelszen P, Duvekot JJ, et al. Pre-eclampsia. Lancet 2010;376(9741):631–44.
69. Sibai B, Dekker G, Kupferminc M. Pre-eclampsia. Lancet 2005;365(9461):785–99.
70. Plasencia W, Maiz N, Bonino S, et al. Uterine artery Doppler at 11 + 0 to 13 + 6 weeks in the prediction of pre-eclampsia. Ultrasound Obstet Gynecol 2007;30(5):742–9.
71. Redman C, Sargent I, Staff A. IFPA Senior Award Lecture: making sense of pre-eclampsia–two placental causes of preeclampsia? Placenta 2014;35:S20–5.
72. Kaitu'u-Lino TJ, Tuohey L, Ye L, et al. MT-MMPs in pre-eclamptic placenta: relationship to soluble endoglin production. Placenta 2013;34(2):168–73.
73. Duckitt K, Harrington D. Risk factors for pre-eclampsia at antenatal booking: systematic review of controlled studies. BMJ 2005;330(7491):565–72.
74. Bartsch E, Medcalf KE, Park AL, et al. Clinical risk factors for pre-eclampsia determined in early pregnancy: systematic review and meta-analysis of large cohort studies. BMJ 2016;353.
75. Henderson JT, Thompson JH, Burda BU, et al. Preeclampsia screening: evidence report and systematic review for the us preventive services task force. JAMA 2017;317(16):1668–83.
76. Rolnik DL, Wright D, Poon LC, et al. Aspirin versus placebo in pregnancies at high risk for preterm preeclampsia. N Engl J Med 2017;377(7):613–22.
77. Knight M. Eclampsia in the United Kingdom 2005. BJOG 2007;114(9):1072–8.
78. Vigil-De Gracia P, Rojas-Suarez J, Ramos E, et al. Incidence of eclampsia with HELLP syndrome and associated mortality in Latin America. Int J Gynaecol Obstet 2015;129(3):219–22.
79. Mahran A, Fares H, Elkhateeb R, et al. Risk factors and outcome of patients with eclampsia at a tertiary hospital in Egypt. BMC Pregnancy Childbirth 2017;17(1):435.
80. Schaap TP, Knight M, Zwart JJ, et al. Eclampsia, a comparison within the International Network of Obstetric Survey Systems. BJOG 2014;121(12):1521–8.
81. Abraham KA, Connolly G, Farrell J, et al. The HELLP syndrome, a prospective study. Ren Fail 2001;23(5):705–13.
82. Weinstein L. Preeclampsia/eclampsia with hemolysis, elevated liver enzymes, and thrombocytopenia. Obstet Gynecol 1985;66(5):657–60.
83. Haram K, Svendsen E, Abildgaard U. The HELLP syndrome: clinical issues and management. A review. BMC Pregnancy Childbirth 2009;9(1):8.
84. Vigil-De Gracia P. Pregnancy complicated by pre-eclampsia-eclampsia with HELLP syndrome. Int J Gynaecol Obstet 2001;72:17–23.
85. Centre for Maternal and Child Enquiries (CMACE). Saving mothers' lives: reviewing maternal deaths to make motherhood safer: 2006-2008. The Eighth Report on Confidential Enquiries into Maternal Deaths in the United Kingdom. BJOG 2011;118(Suppl. 1):1–203.
86. Duley L, Meher S, Jones L. Drugs for treatment of very high blood pressure during pregnancy. Cochrane Database Syst Rev 2013;(7):CD001449.
87. National Institute for Clinical Excellence. Hypertension in pregnancy. Quality statement 3: Antenatal blood pressure targets London: NICE; 2017. Available from: https://www.nice.org.uk/guidance/qs35/chapter/Quality-statement-3-Antenatal-blood-pressure-targets.
88. Young BC, Levine RJ, Karumanchi SA. Pathogenesis of preeclampsia. Annu Rev Pathol 2010;5(1):173–92.

89. Sontia B, Touyz RM. Role of magnesium in hypertension. Arch Biochem Biophys 2007;458(1):33–9.
90. The Magpie Trial Group. Do women with pre-eclampsia, and their babies, benefit from magnesium sulphate? The Magpie Trial: a randomised placebo-controlled trial. Lancet 2002;359(9321):1877–90.
91. Rugarn O, Carling Moen S, Berg G. Eclampsia at a tertiary hospital 1973-99. Acta Obstet Gynecol Scand 2004;83(3):240–5.
92. Smith C, Phelan J. Determinants for invasive monitoring in severe preeclampsia. Contemp Obstet Gynaecol 1986;109–24.
93. Dennis AT, Castro JM. Transthoracic echocardiography in women with treated severe pre-eclampsia. Anaesthesia 2014;69(5):436–44.
94. Woudstra DM, Chandra S, Hofmeyr GJ, et al. Corticosteroids for HELLP (hemolysis, elevated liver enzymes, low platelets) syndrome in pregnancy. Cochrane Database Syst Rev 2010;(9):CD008148.
95. Royal College of Obstetricians and Gynaecologists. Reducing the risk of venous thromboembolism during pregnancy and the puerperium (Green-top Guideline No. 37a). London: RCOG; 2015.
96. Brown M, Best K, Pearce M, et al. Cardiovascular disease risk in women with pre-eclampsia: systematic review and meta-analysis. Eur J Epidemiol 2013;28(1):1–19.
97. Flood M, McDonald SJ, Pollock W, et al. Incidence, trends and severity of primary postpartum haemorrhage in Australia: a population-based study using Victorian Perinatal Data Collection data for 764 244 births. Aust N Z J Obstet Gynaecol [Internet] 2018;0(0). Available from: https://obgyn.onlinelibrary.wiley.com/doi/abs/10.1111/ajo.12826.
98. Royal College of Obstetricians and Gynaecologists. Antepartum haemorrhage (Green–top Guideline No. 63). London: RCOG; 2011. (updated 2014).
99. Varouxaki N, Gnanasambanthan S, Datta S, et al. Antepartum haemorrhage. Obstet Gynecol Reprod Med 2018;28(8):237–42.
100. van Altvorst MEWA, Chan EHY, Taylor RS, et al. Antepartum haemorrhage of unknown origin and maternal cigarette smoking beyond the first trimester. Aust N Z J Obstet Gynaecol 2012;52(2):161–6.
101. Giordano R, Cacciatore A, Cignini P, et al. Antepartum haemorrhage. J Prenat Med 2010;4(1):12–16.
102. Hladky K, Yankowitz J, Hansen WF. Placental abruption. Obstet Gynecol Surv 2002;57(5):299–305.
103. Raj S, Kaur A, Grover S, et al. Maternal and perinatal outcome in antepartum hemorrhage – a clinical study. J Adv Med Dent Sci Res 2018;6(8):53–8.
104. American College of Obstetricians and Gynecologists. Placenta accreta spectrum. Obstetric Care Consensus No. 7. Obstet Gynecol 2018;132:e259–75. Available from: https://www.acog.org/Clinical-Guidance-and-Publications/Obstetric-Care-Consensus-Series/Placenta-Accreta-Spectrum.
105. Knight M, Callaghan W, Berg C, et al. Trends in postpartum hemorrhage in high resource countries: a review and recommendations from the International Postpartum Hemorrhage Collaborative Group. BMC Pregnancy Childbirth 2009;9(1):55.
106. Lapinsky S, Kruczynski K, Seaward G, et al. Critical care management of the obstetric patient. Can J Anaesth 1997;44(3):3259.
107. Huang WC, Chen CP. Pulmonary edema in pregnancy. Int J Gynaecol Obstet 2002;78(3):241–3.
108. Campbell L, Klocke R. Implications for the pregnant patient. Am J Respir Crit Care Med 2001;163(5):1051–4.
109. Klajnbard A, Szecsi PB, Colov NP, et al. Laboratory reference intervals during pregnancy, delivery and the early postpartum period. Clin Chem Lab Med 2010;48(2):237–48.
110. Chamberlain G, Steer P. ABC of labour care: obstetric emergencies. BMJ 1999;318(7194):1342–5.
111. National Blood Authority. Patient blood management guidelines. Module 1 Critical Bleeding/Massive Transfusion. Canberra: National Blood Authority; 2011. Available from: https://www.blood.gov.au/pbm-guidelines.
112. National Blood Authority. Patient blood management guidelines. Module 4 Critical Care. Canberra: National Blood Authority; 2013.
113. National Blood Authority. Patient blood management guidelines. Module 5 Obstetrics and Maternity. Canberra: National Blood Authority; 2015.
114. Cortet M, Deneux-Tharaux C, Dupont C, et al. Association between fibrinogen level and severity of postpartum haemorrhage: secondary analysis of a prospective trial. Br J Anaesth 2012;108(6):984–9.
115. Wikkelsø AJ, Edwards HM, Afshari A, et al. Pre-emptive treatment with fibrinogen concentrate for postpartum haemorrhage: randomized controlled trial. Br J Anaesth 2015;114(4):623–33.
116. Mallaiah S, Barclay P, Harrod I, et al. Introduction of an algorithm for ROTEM-guided fibrinogen concentrate administration in major obstetric haemorrhage. Anaesthesia 2015;70(2):166–75.
117. Phillips L, McLintock C, Pollock W, et al. Recombinant activated factor VII in obstetric hemorrhage: experiences from the Australian and New Zealand Haemostasis Registry. Anesth Analg 2009;109(6):1908–15.
118. Shakur H, Roberts I, Fawole B, et al. Effect of early tranexamic acid administration on mortality, hysterectomy, and other morbidities in women with post-partum haemorrhage (WOMAN): an international, randomised, double-blind, placebo-controlled trial. Lancet 2017;389(10084):2105–16.
119. Wang HY, Chang CT, Wu MS. Postpartum hemorrhage complicated with irreversible renal failure and central diabetes insipidus. Ren Fail 2002;24(6):849–52.
120. Fung Kee Fung K, Eason E, Crane J, et al. Prevention of Rh alloimmunization. J Obstet Gynaecol Can 2003;25(9):765–73.
121. Allam J, Cox M, Yentis SM. Cell salvage in obstetrics. Int J Obstet Anesth 2008;17(1):37–45.
122. Khan KS, Moore PA, Wilson MJ, et al. Cell salvage and donor blood transfusion during cesarean section: a pragmatic, multicentre randomised controlled trial (SALVO). PLoS Med 2017;14(12):e1002471.

123. King M, Wrench I, Galimberti A, et al. Introduction of cell salvage to a large obstetric unit: the first six months. Int J Obstet Anesth 2009;18(2):111–17.
124. Khan KS, Moore P, Wilson M, et al. A randomised controlled trial and economic evaluation of intraoperative cell salvage during caesarean section in women at risk of haemorrhage: the SALVO (cell SALVage in Obstetrics) trial. Health Technol Assess 2018;22(2):1.
125. Clark SL. Amniotic fluid embolism. Obstet Gynecol 2014;123(2 Pt 1):337–48.
126. Tuffnell DJ, Slemeck E. Amniotic fluid embolism. Obstet Gynecol Reprod Med 2014;24(5):148–52.
127. Shechtman M, Ziser A, Markovits R, et al. Amniotic fluid embolism: early findings of transesophageal echocardiography. Anesth Analg 1999;87(6):1456.
128. Conde-Agudelo A, Romero R. Amniotic fluid embolism: an evidence-based review. Am J Obstet Gynecol [Internet] 2009;201(5):e1–13.
129. Knight M, Tuffnell D, Brocklehurst P, et al. Incidence and risk factors for amniotic-fluid embolism. Obstet Gynecol 2010;115(5): 910–17.
130. McDonnell N, Knight M, Peek MJ, et al. Amniotic fluid embolism: an Australian-New Zealand population-based study. BMC Pregnancy Childbirth 2015;15(1):1.
131. AIHW, Johnson S, Bonello M, et al. Maternal deaths in Australia 2006–2010, Maternal Death Series no. 4. Cat. no. PER 61. Canberra: AIHW; 2014.
132. Bauersachs J, Arrigo M, Hilfiker-Kleiner D, et al. Current management of patients with severe acute peripartum cardiomyopathy: practical guidance from the Heart Failure Association of the European Society of Cardiology Study Group on peripartum cardiomyopathy. Eur J Heart Fail 2016;18(9):1096–105.
133. Sliwa K, Hilfiker-Kleiner D, Petrie MC, et al. Current state of knowledge on aetiology, diagnosis, management, and therapy of peripartum cardiomyopathy: a position statement from the Heart Failure Association of the European Society of Cardiology Working Group on peripartum cardiomyopathy. Eur J Heart Fail 2010;12(8):767–78.
134. Sliwa K, Fett J, Elkayam U. Peripartum cardiomyopathy. Lancet 2006;368(9536):687–93.
135. Pearson GD, Veille J-C, Rahimtoola S, et al. Peripartum cardiomyopathy: National Heart, Lung, and Blood Institute and Office of Rare Diseases (National Institutes of Health) workshop recommendations and review. JAMA 2000;283(9):1183–8.
136. Ntusi N, Mayosi B. Aetiology and risk factors of peripartum cardiomyopathy: a systematic review. Int J Cardiol 2009;131:168–79.
137. Cruz MO, Briller J, Hibbard JU. Update on peripartum cardiomyopathy. Obstet Gynecol Clin North Am 2010;37(2):283–303.
138. Hilfiker-Kleiner D, Struman I, Hoch M, et al. 16-kDa Prolactin and bromocriptine in postpartum cardiomyopathy. Curr Heart Fail Rep 2012;9(3):174–82.
139. Sliwa K, Petrie MC, Hilfiker-Kleiner D, et al. Long-term prognosis, subsequent pregnancy, contraception and overall management of peripartum cardiomyopathy: practical guidance paper from the Heart Failure Association of the European Society of Cardiology Study Group on Peripartum Cardiomyopathy. Eur J Heart Fail 2018;20(6):951–62.
140. Fett JD, Sannon H, Thélisma E, et al. Recovery from severe heart failure following peripartum cardiomyopathy. Int J Gynaecol Obstet 2009;104(2):125–7.
141. Egan DJ, Bisanzo MC, Hutson HR. Emergency department evaluation and management of peripartum cardiomyopathy. J Emerg Med 2009;36(2):141–7.
142. Hilfiker-Kleiner D, Haghikia A, Berliner D, et al. Bromocriptine for the treatment of peripartum cardiomyopathy: a multicentre randomized study. Eur Heart J 2017;38(35):2671–9.
143. Hilfiker-Kleiner D, Sliwa K. Pathophysiology and epidemiology of peripartum cardiomyopathy. Nat Rev Cardiol 2014;11(6):364–70.
144. Hilfiker-Kleiner D, Meyer GP, Schieffer E, et al. Recovery from postpartum cardiomyopathy in 2 patients by blocking prolactin release with bromocriptine. J Am Coll Cardiol 2007;50(24):2354–5.
145. Knight M, Nair M, Tuffnell D, et al. Saving lives, improving mothers' care – Surveillance of maternal deaths in the UK 2012–14 and lessons learned to inform maternity care from the UK and Ireland confidential enquiries into maternal deaths and morbidity 2009–14. Oxford: National Perinatal Epidemiology Unit, University of Oxford; 2016.
146. van der Linde D, Konings EEM, Slager MA, et al. Birth prevalence of congenital heart disease worldwide: a systematic review and meta-analysis. J Am Coll Cardiol 2011;58(21):2241–7.
147. Leirgul E, Fomina T, Brodwall K, et al. Birth prevalence of congenital heart defects in Norway 1994-2009 – a nationwide study. Am Heart J 2014;168(6):956–64.
148. Hoang TT, Goldmuntz E, Roberts AE, et al. The Congenital Heart Disease Genetic Network Study: cohort description. PLoS ONE 2018;13(1):e0191319.
149. Persson M, Cnattingius S, Villamor E, et al. Risk of major congenital malformations in relation to maternal overweight and obesity severity: cohort study of 1.2 million singletons. BMJ 2017;357.
150. Helle EIT, Biegley P, Knowles JW, et al. First trimester plasma glucose values in women without diabetes are associated with risk for congenital heart disease in offspring. J Pediatr 2018;195:275–8.
151. Koster MPH, van Duijn L, Krul-Poel YHM, et al. A compromised maternal vitamin D status is associated with congenital heart defects in offspring. Early Hum Dev 2018;117:50–6.
152. Nembhard WN, Tang X, Hu Z, et al. Maternal and infant genetic variants, maternal periconceptional use of selective serotonin reuptake inhibitors, and risk of congenital heart defects in offspring: population based study. BMJ 2017;356.

153. Silversides CK, Marelli A, Beauchesne L, et al. Canadian Cardiovascular Society 2009 Consensus Conference on the management of adults with congenital heart disease: executive summary. Can J Cardiol 2010;26(3):143–50.
154. Bracher I, Padrutt M, Bonassin F, et al. Burden and impact of congenital syndromes and comorbidities among adults with congenital heart disease. Int J Cardiol 2017;240:159–64.
155. Rao S, Ginns JN. Adult congenital heart disease and pregnancy. Semin Perinatol 2014;38(5):260–72.
156. Cauldwell M, Steer PJ, Bonner S, et al. Retrospective UK multicentre study of the pregnancy outcomes of women with a Fontan repair. Heart 2017.
157. Zentner D, Kotevski A, King I, et al. Fertility and pregnancy in the Fontan population. Int J Cardiol 2016;208:97–101.
158. RHD Australia (ARF/RHD writing group), National Heart Foundation of Australia and the Cardiac Society of Australia and New Zealand. The Australian guideline for prevention, diagnosis and management of acute rheumatic fever and rheumatic heart disease. 2nd ed. Casuarina: Menzies School of Health Research; 2012.
159. Mesa A, Jessurun C, Hernandez A, et al. Left ventricular diastolic function in normal human pregnancy. Circulation 1999;99(4):511–17.
160. van Hagen IM, Cornette J, Johnson MR, et al. Managing cardiac emergencies in pregnancy. Heart 2016.
161. James AH, Jamison MG, Biswas MS, et al. Acute myocardial infarction in pregnancy: a United States population-based study. Circulation 2006;113(12):1564–71.
162. Elkayam U, Havakuk O. Pregnancy-associated coronary artery dissection: a therapeutic dilemma. J Am Coll Cardiol 2018;71(4):469–70.
163. Merrigan O. Diagnosing and treating acute myocardial infarction in pregnancy. Br J Nurs 2009;18(21):1300–4.
164. Firoz T, Magee LA. Acute myocardial infarction in the obstetric patient. Obstet Med 2012;5(2):50–7.
165. Bush N, Nelson-Piercy C, Spark P, et al. Myocardial infarction in pregnancy and postpartum in the UK. Eur J Prev Cardiol 2013;20(1):12–20.
166. Koul AK, Hollander G, Moskovits N, et al. Coronary artery dissection during pregnancy and the postpartum period: two case reports and review of literature. Catheter Cardiovasc Interv 2001;52(1):88–94.
167. Sadler L, McCowan L, White H, et al. Pregnancy outcomes and cardiac complications in women with mechanical, bioprosthetic and homograft valves. Br J Obstet Gynaecol 2000;107(2):245–53.
168. Canobbio MM, Warnes CA, Aboulhosn J, et al. Management of pregnancy in patients with complex congenital heart disease: a scientific statement for healthcare professionals from the American Heart Association. Circulation 2017.
169. Regitz-Zagrosek V, Lundqvist CB, Borghi C, et al. ESC Guidelines on the management of cardiovascular diseases during pregnancy. Eur Heart J 2011;32:3147–97.
170. Yankowitz J. Fetal effects of drugs commonly used in critical care. In: Dildy GA, Belfort M, Phelan D, et al, editors. Critical care obstetrics. 4th ed. Malden: Blackwell Science; 2004. p. 612–19.
171. Bartalena L, Bogazzi F, Braverman LE, et al. Effects of amiodarone administration during pregnancy on neonatal thyroid function and subsequent neurodevelopment. J Endocrinol Invest 2001;24(2):116–30.
172. Arnoni RT, Arnoni AS, Bonini RCA, et al. Risk factors associated with cardiac surgery during pregnancy. Ann Thorac Surg 2003;76(5):1605–8.
173. King PT, Rosalion A, McMillan J, et al. Extracorporeal membrane oxygenation in pregnancy. Lancet 2000;356(9223):45–6.
174. Chan WS, Anand S, Ginsberg JS. Anticoagulation of pregnant women with mechanical heart valves: a systematic review of the literature. Arch Intern Med 2000;160(2):191–6.
175. Kwon H, Belanger K, Bracken M. Asthma prevalence among pregnant and childbearing-aged women in the United States: estimates from national health surveys. Ann Epidemiol 2003;13(5):317–24.
176. Australian Centre for Asthma Monitoring. Asthma in Australia 2008. AIHW Asthma Series no.3. Canberra: Australian Institute of Health and Welfare; 2008.
177. Juniper E, Newhouse M. Effect of pregnancy on asthma: a critical appraisal of the literature. In: Schatz M, Zeiger RS, editors. Asthma and allergy in pregnancy and early infancy. New York: Marcel Dekker; 1993. p. 223–49.
178. Hardy-Fairbanks AJ, Baker ER. Asthma in pregnancy: pathophysiology, diagnosis and management. Obstet Gynecol Clin North Am 2010;37(2):159–72.
179. Gluck JC, Gluck PA. The effect of pregnancy on the course of asthma. Immunol Allergy Clin North Am 2006;26(1):63–80.
180. Murphy VE, Gibson P, Talbot PL, et al. Severe asthma exacerbations during pregnancy. Obstet Gynecol 2005;106(5):1046–54.
181. Robijn AL, Jensen ME, Gibson PG, et al. Trends in asthma self-management skills and inhaled corticosteroid use during pregnancy and postpartum from 2004 to 2017. J Asthma 2018;1-22.
182. Cydulka RK, Emerman CL, Schreiber D, et al. Acute asthma among pregnant women presenting to the emergency department. Am J Respir Crit Care Med 1999;160(3):887–92.
183. Schatz M, Dombrowski MP. Asthma in pregnancy. N Engl J Med 2009;360(18):1862–9.
184. National Asthma Council Australia. Australian asthma handbook version 1.2. South Melbourne: National Asthma Council Australia; 2016.
185. Steven G, Whitworth M, Cox S. Substance misuse in pregnancy. Obstet Gynaecol Reprod Med 2014;24(10):309–14.
186. Mendez-Figueroa H, Dahlke JD, Vrees RA, et al. Trauma in pregnancy: an updated systematic review. Am J Obstet Gynecol 2013;209(1):1–10.

187. Murphy NJ, Quinlan JD. Trauma in pregnancy: assessment, management, and prevention. Am Fam Physician 2014;90(10):717–22.
188. Huls CK, Detlefs C. Trauma in pregnancy. Semin Perinatol 2018;42(1):13–20.
189. Van Parys A-S, Verhamme A, Temmerman M, et al. Intimate partner violence and pregnancy: a systematic review of interventions. PLoS ONE [Internet] 2014;9(1). Available from: https://doi.org/10.1371/journal.pone.0085084.
190. Garcia-Moreno C, Jansen H, Ellsberg M, et al. World Health Organization Multi-country study of women's health and domestic violence against women. Initial results on prevalence, health outcomes and women's responses. Geneva: WHO; 2005.
191. Almeida FSJ, Coutinho EC, Duarte JC, et al. Domestic violence in pregnancy: prevalence and characteristics of the pregnant woman. J Clin Nurs 2017;26(15–16):2417–25.
192. National Institute for Health and Care Excellence. Domestic violence and abuse. Public health guideline [PH50]. London: NICE; 2016. Available from: https://www.nice.org.uk/guidance/ph50.
193. Van Parys AS, Verstraelen H, Roelens K, et al. Maternal intensive care: a systematic literature review. Facts Views Vis ObGyn 2010;2(3):161–7.
194. Gharacheh M, Azadi S, Mohammadi N, et al. Domestic violence during pregnancy and women's health-related quality of Life. Glob J Health Sci 2016;8(2):27–34.
195. Sirin H, Weiss H, Sauber-Schatz E, et al. Seat belt use, counseling and motor vehicle injury during pregnancy: results from a multi-state population-based survey. Matern Child Health J 2007;11(5):505–10.
196. Vladutiu CJ, Marshall SW, Poole C, et al. Adverse pregnancy outcomes following motor vehicle crashes. Am J Prev Med 2013;45(5):doi:10. 1016/j.amepre.2013.06.018.
197. Chibber R, Al-Harmi J, Fouda M, et al. Motor-vehicle injury in pregnancy and subsequent feto-maternal outcomes: of grave concern. J Matern Fetal Neonatal Med 2015;28(4):399–402.
198. Queensland Clinical Guidelines. Trauma in pregnancy. Document Number MN14.31-V1-R19. Queensland Health; 2014.
199. Royal College of Obstetricians and Gynaecologists. Guidelines Research Services. Guidelines. Kleihauer test in antepartum haemorrhage (query bank). London: RCOG; 2011.
200. Beckett V, Knight M, Sharpe P. The CAPS Study: incidence, management and outcomes of cardiac arrest in pregnancy in the UK: a prospective, descriptive study. BJOG 2017;124(9):1374–81.
201. Brown H. Trauma in pregnancy. Obstet Gynecol 2009;114(1):147–60.
202. Jain V, Chari R, Maslovitz S, et al. Guidelines for the management of a pregnant trauma patient. J Obstet Gynaecol Can 2015;37(6):553–74.
203. Goodnight WH, Soper DE. Pneumonia in pregnancy. Crit Care Med 2005;33(10 Suppl.):S390–7.
204. ANZIC Influenza Investigators, Australasian Maternity Outcomes Surveillance System. Critical illness due to 2009 A/H1N1 influenza in pregnant and postpartum women: population based cohort study. BMJ 2010;340:c1279.
205. Webb SA, Pettila V, Seppelt I, et al. Critical care services and 2009 H1N1 influenza in Australia and New Zealand. N Engl J Med 2009;361(20):1925–34.
206. Klinger G, Merlob P. Selective serotonin reuptake inhibitor induced neonatal abstinence syndrome. Isr J Psychiatry Relat Sci 2008;45(2):107–13.
207. Cohen LS, Altshuler LL, Harlow BL, et al. Relapse of major depression during pregnancy in women who maintain or discontinue antidepressant treatment. JAMA 2006;295(5):499–507.
208. Kulkarni J. Special issues in managing long-term mental illness in women. Int Rev Psychiatry 2010;22(2):183–90.
209. VanderKruik R, Barreix M, Chou D, et al. The global prevalence of postpartum psychosis: a systematic review. BMC Psychiatry 2017;17(1):272.
210. Tschinkel S, Harris M, Le Noury J, et al. Postpartum psychosis: two cohorts compared, 1875-1924 and 1994-2005. Psychol Med 2007;37:529–36.
211. Sharma V, Mazmanian D. Sleep loss and postpartum psychosis. Bipolar Disord 2003;5(2):98–105.
212. Craig M, Howard L. Postnatal depression. BMJ Clin Evid 2009;2009.
213. Wylie L, Hollins Martin CJ, Marland G, et al. The enigma of post-natal depression: an update. J Psychiatr Ment Health Nurs 2010;18(1):48–58.
214. Chow S. Report of the Australian and New Zealand Neonatal Network 2011. Sydney: Australian and New Zealand Neonatal Network; 2013.
215. Selin H, Stone PK, editors. Childbirth across cultures: ideas and practices of pregnancy. London, New York: Springer; 2009.
216. Martin A, Krishna I, Ellis J, et al. Super obesity in pregnancy: difficulties in clinical management. J Perinatol 2014;34.
217. Catalano PM, Shankar K. Obesity and pregnancy: mechanisms of short term and long term adverse consequences for mother and child. BMJ 2017;356.
218. McDonnell NJ, Paech MJ, Clavisi OM, et al. Difficult and failed intubation in obstetric anaesthesia: an observational study of airway management and complications associated with general anaesthesia for caesarean section. Int J Obstet Anesth 2008;17(4):292–7.
219. Cousins L. Fetal oxygenation, assessment of fetal well-being, and obstetric management of the pregnant patient with asthma. J Allergy Clin Immunol 1999;103(2, Suppl. 1):S343–9.
220. Lapinsky SE, Rojas-Suarez JA, Crozier TM, et al. Mechanical ventilation in critically-ill pregnant women: a case series. Int J Obstet Anesth 2015;24(4):323–8.

221. Bugge JF, Tanbo T. Nitric oxide in the treatment of fulminant pulmonary failure in a young pregnant woman with varicella pneumonia. Eur J Anaesthesiol 2000;17:269–72.
222. Silverman JA, Barrett J, Callum JL. The appropriateness of red blood cell transfusions in the peripartum patient. Obstet Gynecol 2004;104(5 Pt 1):1000–4.
223. Plotkin JS, Shah JB, Lofland GK, et al. Extracorporeal membrane oxygenation in the successful treatment of traumatic adult respiratory distress syndrome: case report and review. J Trauma 1994;37(1):127–30.
224. Gaffney A. Critical care in pregnancy – Is it different? Semin Perinatol 2014;38(6):329–40.
225. Intensive Care National Audit & Research Centre. Female admissions (aged 16–50 years) to adult, general critical care units in England, Wales and Northern Ireland reported as 'currently pregnant' or 'recently pregnant'. Report from the Intensive Care National Audit & Research Centre. London; 2013.
226. Keizer JL, Zwart JJ, Meerman RH, et al. Obstetric intensive care admissions: a 12-year review in a tertiary care centre. Eur J Obstet Gynecol Reprod Biol 2006;128(1):152–6.
227. Mangesi L, Hofmeyr GJ, Smith V, et al. Fetal movement counting for assessment of fetal wellbeing. Cochrane Database Syst Rev 2015;(10):Art. No.: CD004909, doi:10.1002/14651858.CD004909.pub3.
228. American College of Obstetricians and Gynecologists. Practice bulletin no. 145: antepartum fetal surveillance. Obstet Gynecol 2014;124(1):182–92.
229. Everett TR, Peebles DM. Antenatal tests of fetal wellbeing. Semin Fetal Neonatal Med 2015;20(3):138–43.
230. Royal College of Obstetricians and Gynaecologists. Small-for-gestational-age fetus, investigation and management (Green-top Guideline No. 31). London: RCOG; 2014.
231. Medicines and Healthcare products Regulatory Agency. Fetal monitor/cardiotocograph (CTG) - adverse outcomes still reported 2010. Available from: https://www.gov.uk/drug-device-alerts/medical-device-alert-fetal-monitor-cardiotocograph-ctg-adverse-outcomes-still-reported.
232. Afors K, Chandraharan E. Use of continuous electronic fetal monitoring in a preterm fetus: clinical dilemmas and recommendations for practice. J Pregnancy [Internet] 2011;7. Article ID 848794. Available from: http://dx.doi.org/10.1155/2011/848794.
233. Grivell RM, Alfirevic Z, Gyte GML, et al. Antenatal cardiotocography for fetal assessment. Cochrane Database Syst Rev 2015;(9): CD007863.
234. Nageotte MP. Fetal heart rate monitoring. Semin Fetal Neonatal Med 2015;20(3):144–8.
235. Walker KF, Thornton JG. Advanced maternal age. Obstet Gynecol Reprod Med 2016;26(12):354–7.
236. World Health Organization. Health statistics and information systems. Maternal mortality ratio (per 100000 live births). Geneva: WHO; 2018 Available from: http://www.who.int/healthinfo/statistics/indmaternalmortality/en/.
237. New Zealand Ministry of Health. Report on maternity 2015. Wellington: Ministry of Health; 2017.
238. Australian Institute of Health and Welfare. Australia's mothers and babies 2015 – in brief. Perinatal statistics series no. 33. Cat no. PER 91. Canberra: AIHW; 2017.
239. National Institute for Health and Care Excellence. Preterm labour and birth, NICE guideline [NG25]. NICE; 2015.
240. Royal College of Obstetricians and Gynaecologists. Antenatal Corticosteroids: Guidelines for the use by RCOG. London: RCOG; 2016-2017. Available from: https://dailyrounds.org/library/antenatal-corticosteroids-guidelines-for-the-use-by-rcog.
241. Roberts D, Brown J, Medley N, et al. Antenatal corticosteroids for accelerating fetal lung maturation for women at risk of preterm birth. Cochrane Database Syst Rev 2017;(3):CD004454.
242. Shepherd E, Salam RA, Middleton P, et al. Antenatal and intrapartum interventions for preventing cerebral palsy: an overview of Cochrane systematic reviews. Cochrane Database Syst Rev 2017;(8):CD012077.
243. De Silva DA, Synnes AR, von Dadelszen P, et al. MAGnesium sulphate for fetal neuroprotection to prevent Cerebral Palsy (MAG-CP) – implementation of a national guideline in Canada. Implement Sci 2018;13(1):8.
244. Bain E, Middleton P, Crowther CA. Different magnesium sulphate regimens for neuroprotection of the fetus for women at risk of preterm birth. Cochrane Database Syst Rev 2012;(2):CD009302, doi:10.1002/14651858.CD009302.pub2.
245. Vilchez G, Dai J, Lagos M, et al. Maternal side effects & fetal neuroprotection according to body mass index after magnesium sulfate in a multicenter randomized controlled trial. J Matern Fetal Neonatal Med 2018;31(2):178–83.
246. Royal Australian and New Zealand College of Obstetricians and Gynaecologists. Guidelines for the use of Rh (D) immunoglobulin (Anti-D) in obstetrics in Australia. C-Obs 6. Melbourne: RANZCOG; 2015.
247. National Institute for Health and Care Excellence. Routine antenatal anti-D prophylaxis for women who are rhesus D negative. Technology appraisal guidance [TA156]. London: NICE; 2008.
248. National Institute for Health and Care Excellence. High-throughput non-invasive prenatal testing for fetal RHD genotype. Diagnostics guidance [DG25]. London: NICE; 2016.
249. Zeng Z, Liu F, Li S. Metabolic adaptations in pregnancy: a review. Ann Nutr Metab 2017;70(1):59–65.
250. Wilmot EG, Mansell P. Diabetes and pregnancy. Clin Med (Northfield Il) 2014;14(6):677–80.
251. National Institute for Health and Care Excellence. Diabetes in pregnancy: management from preconception to the postnatal period. Clinical Guideline NG3. London: NICE; 2015.
252. Benson MD, Padovano A, Bourjeily G, et al. Maternal collapse: challenging the four-minute rule. EBioMedicine 2016;6:253–7.

253. Zieleskiewicz L, Chantry A, Duclos G, et al. Intensive care and pregnancy: epidemiology and general principles of management of obstetrics ICU patients during pregnancy. Anaesth Crit Care Pain Med 2016;35(Suppl. 1):S51–7.
254. Bamfo JE. Managing the risks of sepsis in pregnancy. Best Pract Res Clin Obstet Gynaecol 2013;27(4):583–95.
255. Albright CM, Has P, Rouse DJ, et al. Internal validation of the sepsis in obstetrics score to identify risk of morbidity from sepsis in pregnancy. Obstet Gynecol 2017;130(4):747–55.
256. Bowyer L, Robinson HL, Barrett H, et al. SOMANZ guidelines for the investigation and management sepsis in pregnancy. Aust N Z J Obstet Gynaecol 2017;57(5):540–51.
257. Malek A, Mattison DR. Drug development for use during pregnancy: impact of the placenta. Expert Rev Obstet Gynecol 2010;5(4):437–54.
258. Hodge LS, Tracy TS. Alterations in drug disposition during pregnancy. Expert Opin Drug Metab Toxicol 2007;3(4):557–71.
259. Scaffidi J, Mol B, Keelan J. The pregnant women as a drug orphan: a global survey of registered clinical trials of pharmacological interventions in pregnancy. BJOG 2017;124(1):132–40.
260. Bacon RC, Razis PA. The effect of propofol sedation in pregnancy on neonatal condition. Anaesthesia 1994;49(12):1058–60.
261. Kopecky EA, Ryan ML, Barrett JFR, et al. Fetal response to maternally administered morphine. Am J Obstet Gynecol 2000;183(2):424–30.
262. Littleford J. Effects on the fetus and newborn of maternal analgesia and anesthesia: a review. Can J Anaesth 2004;51(6):586–609.
263. Lee P, Eisman JA, Center JR. Vitamin D deficiency in critically ill patients. N Engl J Med 2009;360(18):1912–14.
264. Camargo CA Jr, Rifas-Shiman SL, Litonjua AA, et al. Maternal intake of vitamin D during pregnancy and risk of recurrent wheeze in children at 3 y of age. Am J Clin Nutr 2007;85(3):788–95.
265. Abu-Saad K, Fraser D. Maternal nutrition and birth outcomes. Epidemiol Rev 2010;32:5–25.
266. Ray JG, Urquia ML, Berger H, et al. Maternal and neonatal separation and mortality associated with concurrent admissions to intensive care units. CMAJ [Internet] 2012;184(18):e956–62.
267. National Institute for Health and Care Excellence. Postnatal care up to 8 weeks after birth. Clinical guideline 37. London: NICE; 2006. (updated 2015).
268. Sherman D, Lurie S, Frenckle E, et al. Characteristics of normal lochia. Am J Perinatol 1999;16(8):399–402.
269. Fletcher S, Grotegut CA, James AH. Lochia patterns among normal women: a systematic review. J Womens Health 2012;21(12):1290–4.
270. Truchet S, Honvo-Houéto E. Physiology of milk secretion. Best Pract Res Clin Endocrinol Metab 2017;31(4):367–84.
271. Ballard O, Morrow AL. Human milk composition: nutrients and bioactive factors. Pediatr Clin North Am 2013;60(1):49–74.
272. Neville MC, Allen JC, Archer PC, et al. Studies in human lactation: milk volume and nutrient composition during weaning and lactogenesis. Am J Clin Nutr 1991;54(1):81–92.
273. Grattan DR. Behavioural significance of prolactin signalling in the central nervous system during pregnancy and lactation. Reproduction 2002;123(4):497–506.
274. World Health Organization. Infant and young child feeding: model chapter. Geneva: WHO; 2009.
275. Morse J, Jehle C, Gamble D. Initiating breastfeeding: a world survey of the timing of postpartum breastfeeding. Int J Nurs Stud 1990;27(3):303–13.
276. Johns HM, Forster DA, Amir LH, et al. Prevalence and outcomes of breast milk expressing in women with healthy term infants: a systematic review. BMC Pregnancy Childbirth 2013;13(1):212.
277. Becker GE, Smith HA, Cooney F. Methods of milk expression for lactating women. Cochrane Database Syst Rev 2016;(9):CD006170.
278. Crepinsek MA, Crowe L, Michener K, et al. Interventions for preventing mastitis after childbirth. Cochrane Database Syst Rev 2010;(8):CD007239.
279. Dennis C-L, Jackson K, Watson J. Interventions for treating painful nipples among breastfeeding women. Cochrane Database Syst Rev 2014;(12):CD007366.
280. Hotham N, Hotham E. Drugs in breastfeeding. Aust Prescr 2015;38(5):156–9.
281. Committee on Ethics. Ethical considerations for including women as research participants. Committee Opinion No. 646. American College of Obstetricians and Gynecologists. Obstet Gynecol 2015;126:e100–7. Available from: https://www.acog.org/Clinical-Guidance-and-Publications/Committee-Opinions/Committee-on-Ethics/Ethical-Considerations-for-Including-Women-as-Research-Participants.
282. Hale T. Medications in breastfeeding mothers of preterm infants. Pediatr Ann 2003;32(5):337–47.
283. Sullivan S, Schanler RJ, Kim JH, et al. An exclusively human milk-based diet is associated with a lower rate of necrotizing enterocolitis than a diet of human milk and bovine milk-based products. J Pediatr 2010;156(4):562–7, e1.
284. Jones I, Shakespeare J. Postnatal depression. BMJ 2014;349.
285. de Graaff L, Honig A, van Pampus M, et al. Preventing post-traumatic stress disorder following childbirth and traumatic birth experiences: a systematic review. Acta Obstet Gynecol Scand 2018;97(6):648–56. doi:10.1111/aogs.13291.
286. UNICEF UK. The baby friendly initiative. Skin to skin contact. 2018. Available from: www.unicef.org.uk.
287. Knight M, Kurinczuk JJ, Tuffnell D, et al. The UK Obstetric Surveillance System for rare disorders of pregnancy. BJOG 2005;112(3):263–5.

Chapter 29

Organ donation

Debbie Friel, Anne Flodén

KEY WORDS

brain death
consent
coroner
designated officer
next of kin
organ donation
organ donor
organ donor advocacy
organ recipient
organ retrieval
professional ethics
transplant

Learning objectives

After reading this chapter, you should be able to:

- differentiate between coma and brain death
- differentiate between the different types of living and deceased donation practices
- differentiate informed and presumed consent to organ donation
- understand the process of donor identification and referral in the critical care setting
- be aware of best practice for the consent-seeking process including cultural considerations
- understand the principles of donor management in the critical care setting
- understand the donor family care throughout the organ and tissue donation process.

Introduction

Organ transplantation is an established method of lifesaving and cost-effective treatment that offers severely ill people a chance of survival. The lack of organs for transplant purposes is a global problem. Long periods on the waiting list for organ transplantation may result in patients deteriorating or dying before they get the opportunity to receive a transplant. Although Australia is a world leader in successful transplant outcomes the waiting list for transplantation remains at around 1400 people every year.[1]

In the USA, over 116,000 people are waiting for a transplantation, and approximately 20 individuals die each day while waiting.[2] In the member states of the European Union (EU), more than 60,000 patients are waiting for an organ transplantation, and 11 of those die each day because there was no organ available.[3] Regarded as an experimental procedure until the 1980s, today transplantation is the best lifesaving treatment for end-stage organ failure and is performed in 112 countries all over the world.[1] The potential of organ rejection limited the number of transplants performed until the early 1980s when the medical advances in the prevention of rejection led to more successful transplants and an increase in demand.[2,4]

Allografts are transplanted organs or tissues from one person (living or deceased) to another person. The first successful human-to-human transplant of any kind was a corneal transplant performed in Moravia (now the Czech Republic) in 1905.[1] Transplantation surgery commenced in Australia in 1911, with a pancreas transplant in Launceston General Hospital, Tasmania.[2] The first successfully transplanted human organ was performed in 1954 at the Peter Bent Brigham Hospital in Boston and was a living kidney donation between identical twins. By the late 1960s, transplantation of liver, heart and pancreas became successful while transplantation of lungs and intestines began in the 1980s.

It took many decades to progress to solid organ transplantation. In 1968 Harvard Medical School produced a report on the 'hopelessly unconscious patient'. This report noted that life support could be withdrawn from patients diagnosed with 'irreversible coma' or 'brain death' (terms they used interchangeably) and that, with appropriate consent, the organs could be removed for transplantation.[5] The committee's primary concern was to provide an acceptable course of action to permit withdrawal of mechanical ventilator support for the purpose of organ donation for human transplantation. In 1981, a USA President's Commission declared that individual death depended on either irreversible cessation of circulatory and respiratory functions or irreversible cessation of all functions of the entire brain. The consequent *Uniform Determination of Death Act* referred to 'whole brain death' as a requirement for the determination of brain death.[5,6] Similar laws were adopted internationally: in Europe, Spain got their law defining brain death in 1979 and in Sweden the law came in 1988. The law that defined brain death and enabled heart-beating retrieval was enacted in New Zealand in 1964 and in Australia from 1982. Legislation heralded the establishment of formal transplant programs.[1] The success of transplantation in the current era as a viable option for end-stage organ failure is primarily due to the discovery of the immunosuppression agent cyclosporin A.[7] This chapter discusses the processes and clinical implications of living and deceased organ and tissue donation, within a critical care nursing context. It describes critical care nurses' role in the multidisciplinary team and the management of the donor and their family.

Donation and consent systems

There are currently two general systems of approach to seeking consent for living and deceased organ and tissue donation in operation around the world. Some countries (e.g. Spain, Singapore and Austria) have legislated an 'opt out', or presumed consent, system where eligible persons are considered for organ retrieval at the time of their death if they have not previously indicated their explicit objection[1,8] (Table 29.1). In Australia, New Zealand, the USA, the UK and most other common-law countries, the approach is to 'opt in', with specific consent required from the potential donor's next of kin.[1] In Australia people can indicate an intent for consent to organ donation on the Australian Organ Donor Register (AODR) administered by the Australian Government Department of Human Services.[9,10] In Singapore, the Human *Organ Transplant Act* of 1987 combines a presumed consent system with a required consent system for the Muslim population.

TABLE 29.1
Overview of law of consent systems by country[1]

COUNTRY	TYPE OF CONSENT	YEAR AND DESCRIPTION
Australia	Informed consent	1982, donor registry since 2000
Austria	Presumed consent	1982, non-donor register since 1995
Belgium	Presumed consent	1986, combined register since 1987, families informed and can object to organ donation
Bulgaria	Presumed consent	1996, in practice, consent from family required
Canada	Informed consent	1980
Croatia	Presumed consent	2000, family consent always requested
Cyprus	Presumed consent	1987
Czech Republic	Presumed consent	1984
Denmark	Informed consent	1990, combined register since 1990, previously presumed consent
Estonia	Presumed consent	No date identified

TABLE 29.1
Overview of law of consent systems by country—cont'd

COUNTRY	TYPE OF CONSENT	YEAR AND DESCRIPTION
Finland	Presumed consent	1985
France	Presumed consent	1976, non-donor register. Changed legislation in 2017, including withdrawal of the families' possibility to override the wishes of the deceased
Germany	Informed consent	1997
Greece	Presumed consent	1978
Hungary	Presumed consent	1972
India	Informed consent	1994
Ireland	Informed consent	Follows UK legislation
Israel	Presumed consent	1953
Italy	Presumed consent	1967, combined register since 2000, families consulted before retrieval
Japan	Informed consent	1997
Korea	Informed consent	2000
Latvia	Presumed consent	No date identified
Lithuania	Informed consent	No date identified
Luxemburg	Presumed consent	1982
The Netherlands	Informed consent	1996, combined register since 1998
New Zealand	Informed consent	1964
Norway	Presumed consent	1973, families consulted and can refuse
Poland	Presumed consent	1990, non-donor register since 1996
Portugal	Presumed consent	1993, non-donor register since 1994
Romania	Informed consent	1998, combined register since 1996
Singapore	Presumed consent	1987, informed consent for Muslim population
Slovak Republic	Presumed consent	1994
Slovenia	Presumed consent	1996
Spain	Presumed consent	1979, in practice, consent required from families
Sweden	Presumed consent	1996, families can veto consent if wishes of the deceased are not known; combined register since 1996
Switzerland	Informed consent	1996, some cantons have presumed consent laws
Turkey	Presumed consent	1979, in practice, written consent required from family
UK	Informed consent	1961, donor register since 1994
USA	Informed consent	1968, donor registers in some states

Note: A combined register is a register of consent and refusal.

The informed consent laws of Japan and Korea are two of the most recent to come into force, in 1997 and 2000 respectively; before then, only living donation and donation after cardiac death were possible.[10]

Types of donations

Organ and tissue donation includes retrieval of organs and tissues both after death and from a living person. Donations from a living person include regenerative tissue (blood and bone marrow) and non-regenerative tissue (cord blood, kidneys, liver (lobe/s), lungs (lobe/s), femoral heads). The implications of consent are different for each type of requested tissue. For example, the collection of bone marrow and the retrieval of a kidney, the lobe of a liver or lung are invasive procedures that could potentially risk the health and wellbeing of the donor.[11] In contrast, donation of a femoral head could be the end-product of a total hip replacement, where the bone is otherwise discarded. Similarly, cord blood from the umbilical cord is discarded if not retrieved immediately after birth.

After cardiac death, many people can still be donors for eyes, heart valves and cardiac tissue, long bones, pelvis, tendons, ligaments and skin.[12] It is after confirmation of brain death that the 'traditional' organs of the heart, lungs, liver, kidneys, pancreas, intestine and tissues can be retrieved, as well as tissues, including eyes. In Australia in 2010 a national protocol for the reintroduction of Donation after Cardiac Death (sometimes referred to as non-beating heart donation or donation after circulatory death) was introduced. This enables the potential donation of lungs, kidneys, liver and sometimes pancreas, along with tissues and eyes.[1] In 2014, hands and faces were added to the organ transplant list in the USA.[13] Known as vascularised composite allotransplantation (VCA), it is the transplantation of a vascularised body part containing multiple tissue types as an anatomical/structural unit. And protocols for this are determined by individual agencies with no international guidelines yet developed.[14]

Organ donation and transplant networks

The donation and transplantation process in many countries, including Australia and New Zealand, the USA and European countries, is a nationally coordinated network in the healthcare system.

International perspectives

From an international perspective, donation and transplantation networks have collaborated to develop consensus on donation and transplantation protocols. As such, the World Health Organization (WHO) Guiding Principles on Human Cell, Tissue and Organ Transplantation have been established to apply to both living and deceased donation[15] (Table 29.2).

Many countries internationally, including Australia, have responded with the adoption of reform initiatives to improve organ and tissue donation rates for transplantation, including:

1. An appropriate legal and ethical framework
2. A national coordinating body
3. Hospital-based clinical donation specialists
4. Specialist training for clinical staff in management of the deceased donation process and family donation conversations
5. Implementation of a clinical governance framework that supports quality assurance and audit of hospital clinical practice and governance of the donation process
6. Financial support to donor hospitals to ensure that costs related to donor management are not a barrier to donation
7. Media engagement and national community awareness and education
8. International cooperation to share best practice.[1]

Regulation and management

In Australia, quality processes involved in organ and tissue retrieval and transplant are governed by the Therapeutic Goods Administration and State Government law.[1,8,16] Other countries have similar agencies that regulate the standards for healthcare products including organ and tissue donation.[12] In Australia, the process of potential donor identification and management in critical care is directed by the Australian and New Zealand Intensive Care Society (ANZICS) (Box 29.1).[5,17] Donor criteria and organ allocation is regulated by the Transplantation Society of Australia and New Zealand (TSANZ). Donor and recipient data are collated by the Australia and New Zealand Organ Donation Registry (ANZOD Registry) and published on an annual basis.[18] The laws governing organ donation in New Zealand and Australia take the form of legislated Acts covering the use of human tissue both before and after death which differ between states.[1] These laws enable a person to choose to be a donor, and organ donation can proceed unless that wish is reversed or the family does not consent. If the deceased's wishes are not apparent, consent for organ donation rests with the next of kin.

In 1977, the Australian Law Reform Commission addressed the absence of a definition of death in Australian law, recommending that a statutory definition of death should be introduced. They recommended that death be defined as:

1. irreversible cessation of all function of the brain of the person; or
2. irreversible cessation of circulation of blood in the body of the person.[1,5]

Tissue donation is also very tightly regulated in all of Australia and New Zealand. In Australia, the

TABLE 29.2
World Health Organization (WHO) Guiding Principles on Human Cell, Tissue and Organ Transplantation[1,16]

Guiding Principle 1	Cells, tissues and organs may be removed from the bodies of deceased persons for the purpose of transplantation if: (a) any consent required by law is obtained, and (b) there is no reason to believe that the deceased person objected to such removal
Guiding Principle 2	Physicians determining that a potential donor has died should not be directly involved in cell, tissue or organ removal from the donor or subsequent transplantation procedures; nor should they be responsible for the care of any intended recipient of such cells, tissues and organs
Guiding Principle 3	Donation from deceased persons should be developed to its maximum therapeutic potential, but adult living persons may donate organs as permitted by domestic regulations. In general living donors should be genetically, legally or emotionally related to their recipients. Live donations are acceptable when the donor's informed and voluntary consent is obtained, when professional care of donors is ensured and follow-up is well organized, and when selection criteria for donors are scrupulously applied and monitored. Live donors should be informed of the probable risks, benefits and consequences of donation in a complete and understandable fashion; they should be legally competent and capable of weighing the information; and they should be acting willingly, free of any undue influence or coercion
Guiding Principle 4	No cells, tissues or organs should be removed from the body of a living minor for the purpose of transplantation other than narrow exceptions allowed under national law. Specific measures should be in place to protect the minor and, wherever possible, the minor's assent should be obtained before donation. What is applicable to minors also applies to any legally incompetent person
Guiding Principle 5	Cells, tissues and organs should only be donated freely, without any monetary payment or other reward of monetary value. Purchasing, or offering to purchase, cells, tissues or organs for transplantation, or their sale by living persons or by the next of kin for deceased persons, should be banned. The prohibition on sale or purchase of cells, tissues and organs does not preclude reimbursing reasonable and verifiable expenses incurred by the donor, including loss of income, or paying the costs of recovering, processing, preserving and supplying human cells, tissues or organs for transplantation
Guiding Principle 6	Promotion of altruistic donation of human cells, tissues or organs by means of advertisement or public appeal may be undertaken in accordance with domestic regulation. Advertising the need for or availability of cells, tissues or organs, with a view to offering or seeking payment to individuals for their cells, tissues or organs, or, to the next of kin, where the individual is deceased, should be prohibited. Brokering that involves payment to such individuals or to third parties should also be prohibited
Guiding Principle 7	Physicians and other health professionals should not engage in transplantation procedures, and health insurers and other payers should not cover such procedures, if the cells, tissues or organs concerned have been obtained through exploitation or coercion of, or payment to, the donor or the next of kin of a deceased donor
Guiding Principle 8	All health care facilities and professionals involved in cell, tissue or organ procurement and transplantation procedures should be prohibited from receiving any payment that exceeds the justifiable fee for the services rendered
Guiding Principle 9	The allocation of organs, cells and tissues should be guided by clinical criteria and ethical norms, not financial or other considerations. Allocation rules, defined by appropriately constituted committees, should be equitable, externally justified, and transparent
Guiding Principle 10	High-quality, safe and efficacious procedures are essential for donors and recipients alike. The longterm outcomes of cell, tissue and organ donation and transplantation should be assessed for the living donor as well as the recipient in order to document benefit and harm. The level of safety, efficacy and quality of human cells, tissues and organs for transplantation, as health products of an exceptional nature, must be maintained and optimized on an ongoing basis. This requires implementation of quality systems including traceability and vigilance, with adverse events and reactions reported, both nationally and for exported human products
Guiding Principle 11	The organization and execution of donation and transplantation activities, as well as their clinical results, must be transparent and open to scrutiny, while ensuring that the personal anonymity and privacy of donors and recipients are always protected

Source: Reprinted from World Health Organisation (WHO), Guiding Principles on Human Cell, Tissue and Organ Transplantation. www.who.int/transplantation/Guiding_PrinciplesTransplantation_WHA63.22en.pdf.

BOX 29.1

Medical management of the potential donor[3,6,17]

Referral

- Refer all potential organ donors to the local state DonateLife agency or the regional organ procurement organisation, even if uncertain of medical suitability. Criteria for suitability change over time and may vary according to recipient circumstances (i.e. if someone is on the critical list).

Medical management

- Maintain MAP >70 mmHg: maintain euvolaemia, if required administer vasopressor agents (e.g. noradrenaline and/or vasopressin 5–2.5 U/h).
- Maintain adequate organ perfusion (monitor urine output, lactate), consider invasive haemodynamic monitoring.
- Monitor electrolytes (Na^+, K^+) every 2–4 h and correct to normal range
- Suspected diabetes insipidus (UO >200 mL/h, rising serum sodium): administer desmopressin (DDAVP) (e.g. 4 mcg IV in adults) and replace volume loss with 5% dextrose or sterile water for infusion (via CVAD only, observing closely for signs of haemolysis).
- Treat hyperglycaemia (Actrapid infusion): aim for blood glucose 5–8 mmol/L.
- Keep temp >35°C. Pre-emptive use of warming blankets is advised as hypothermia may be difficult to reverse once it has developed.
- Provide ongoing respiratory care (suctioning when needed, positioning/turning, PEEP, recruitment manoeuvres).
- Maintain haemoglobin >80 g/L.

Hormone replacement therapy

The use of hormonal replacement therapy remains controversial and it is infrequently used in Australia. Some centres use it in the setting of persistent haemodynamic instability (despite volume resuscitation and low-dose inotropes) and/or if cardiac ejection fraction <45%. Typical regimens include:

- liothyronine (triiodothyronine) (T3) – 4 mcg IV bolus, then 3 mcg/h by IV infusion
- arginine vasopressin (AVP) – 0.5–4.0 U/h to maintain MAP 70 mmHg
- methylprednisolone – 15 mg/kg IV single bolus.

CVAD: central venous access device.

Commonwealth statutory body is the Therapeutic Goods Administration (TGA)[16] and in New Zealand, the statutory body is the Medicines and Medical Devices Safety Authority (MEDSAFE).

Internationally, a dual approach to consensus has evolved: an international governmental response coordinated by the World Health Assembly and World Health Organization (WHO), and a professional response formulated through collaboration with international societies led by The Transplantation Society and the International Society of Nephrology.[15]

In 2014, the Department of Service Delivery and Safety at the World Health Organization consulted with 20 independent experts from all six WHO regions across the world to establish a global agreement on the clinical criteria in the determination of death. As a result, a 'brain death' algorithm was proposed to determine 'neurological arrest', when the traditional cardiocirculatory criteria of death cannot be applied.[19] This algorithm identified the three general components of the process, including:

- the basic requirements that must exist for triggering the algorithm
- the clinical examination and diagnosis
- confirmatory testing to ensure irreversibility.[20]

Professional education

Health professional education in organ and tissue donation has been cited a key initiative in increasing the donor rate globally.[21] The Transplant Procurement Management (TPM) program is an international collaboration that provides training education in organ donation and transplantation for health professionals across over 100 countries, with the aim of increasing the quantity, quality and effectiveness of organ and tissue donation for transplantation through a variety of training initiatives. To date, over 14,000 healthcare professionals working across multiple disciplines in organ donation and transplantation have undertaken training through the program.[22] In Australia, the Australian Organ and Tissue Authority (AOTA) provides funding to each Donate Life Agency across all states and territories in Australia to offer a Professional Education Package (PEP) for all clinicians involved in all aspects of organ and tissue donation and transplantation.[1] The PEP package was developed with collaboration from agencies in both Europe and the USA and has been adopted internationally.

Identification of organ and tissue donors

The four main factors that directly influence the number of multi-organ donations are:

- incidence of brain death
- identification of potential donors (both cardiac death and brain death donors)

- brain death confirmation and informed consent for donation
- donor management after brain death.

Brain death

The incidence of brain death is the first factor and has traditionally determined the size of the potential organ donor pool. Diagnosis of brain death is now widely accepted, and most developed countries have legislation governing the definition of death and the retrieval of organs for transplant.[17,23]

The most common cause of brain death has changed from traumatic head injury to cerebrovascular accident, which has implications for the organs and tissues retrieved. Donors are older and often have cardiovascular and other comorbidities.[24] If organs and tissues are not going to be retrieved for transplantation, there is no legal requirement to confirm brain death if treatment is deemed futile.[5]

Brain death is observed clinically only when the patient is supported with artificial ventilation, as the respiratory reflex lost due to cerebral ischaemia will result in respiratory and cardiac arrest. Artificial (mechanical) ventilation maintains oxygen supply to the natural pacemaker (SA node) of the heart, which functions independently of the central nervous system. Brain death results in hypotension due to loss of vasomotor control of the autonomic nervous system, loss of temperature regulation, reduction in hormone activity and loss of all cranial nerve reflexes. Table 29.3 lists the conditions commonly associated with brain death, but not all people who have progressed to brain death exhibit all of the conditions. Irrespective of the degree of external support, cardiac standstill will occur in a matter of hours to days once brain death has occurred.[3,6,24]

TABLE 29.3
Conditions associated with brain death[6,26]

CONDITION	INCIDENCE
Hypotension	81%
Diabetes insipidus	53%
Disseminated intravascular coagulation	28%
Arrhythmias	27%
Cardiac arrest	25%
Pulmonary oedema	19%
Hypoxia	11%
Acidosis	11%

Testing methods

The aim of testing for brain death is to determine irreversible cessation of brain function.[25] Testing does not demonstrate that every brain cell has died but that a point of irreversible ischaemic damage involving cessation of the vital functions of the brainstem has been reached. There are a number of steps in the process, the first being the observation period. With the exception of a hypoxia-ischaemic brain injury that has been treated with therapeutic hypothermia, where an observation period of 24 hours is required following rewarming to 35°C,[5] an observation period of at least 4 hours from onset of observed no response is required. This must be documented before the first set of testing commences, in the context of a patient being mechanically ventilated with a Glasgow Coma Scale score of 3, non-reacting pupils, absent cough and gag reflexes and no spontaneous respiratory effort.[5] Second step is to consider the preconditions (Box 29.2). Once the observation period has passed (during which the patient receives ongoing treatment) and the preconditions have been met, formal testing can occur.[25]

Practice tip

Family presence during brain death testing may assist their comprehension of brain death. If this is possible, assign a support person to be with the family to assist in explaining and interpreting the testing process.[26]

The Association of Organ Procurement Organizations in the USA provides information and facts covering the organ donation process e.g. donor management and declaration of brain death.[6] The *Guide to the quality and safety of organs for transplantation* by the Council of Europe provide recommendations on brain death declaration according to the best practices usually applied at the European level. The guidelines state that the brain death declaration should be based on scientific and nationally agreed criteria, including that the

BOX 29.2

Preconditions of brain death testing[6]

- Known diagnosis of injury and coma is consistent with progression to brain death.
- Exclude involvement of drugs.
- Exclude metabolic causes for coma (e.g. severe electrolyte or endocrine abnormalities).
- Exclude hypothermia (core temperature greater than 35°C).
- Systolic BP >80 mmHg.
- Confirm neuromuscular conduction.

TABLE 29.4
Clinical brain death testing[6,28]

TEST	CRANIAL NERVES/ NEUROLOGICAL FUNCTION	TEST TECHNIQUE	OUTCOME
1 Response to painful stimuli	Trigeminal V (sensory), facial VII (motor)	Stimulus within the cranial nerve distribution (e.g. firm pressure over supraorbital region)	If reflex is absent, the patient will not grimace or react
2 Pupillary response to light	Optic II, oculomotor III	Using torch	If reflex is absent, the pupils are fixed: may or may not be dilated
3 Corneal reflex	Trigeminal V (sensory), facial VII (motor)	Using wisp of cotton wool to touch the cornea	If reflex is absent, the eyes will not react or blink
4 Gag reflex	Glossopharyngeal IX, vagus X	Using a tongue depressor on the oropharynx or moving ETT	If reflex is absent, there is no gag or pharyngeal response
5 Cough reflex	Glossopharyngeal IX, vagus X	Using suction catheter down ETT to deliberately stimulate the carina	If reflex is absent, there is no cough response
6 Oculovestibular reflex	Vestibulocochlear VII, oculomotor III, abducens VI	Checking first that both tympanic membranes are intact or not obstructed; then slowly irrigating both ears with 50 mL iced water while eyes are held open	If reflex is absent, the eyes remain fixed rather than deviating towards the stimulus
7 Apnoea test	Medullar respiratory centre	Last test to be performed when all other reflexes have proven to be absent. The patient is preoxygenated on 100% O_2, an ABG analysis is performed to ascertain the baseline CO_2, then the patient is disconnected from mechanical ventilation but supplied with oxygen via catheter or T piece; the patient is observed for signs of respiratory effort	The period of time disconnected from the ventilator must be long enough for the arterial CO_2 level to rise to a threshold high enough to normally stimulate respiration, i.e. an arterial CO_2 >60 mmHg and an arterial pH of <7.30
8 Oculocephalic reflex (doll's eyes)	Ocular function and internuclear pathway in brainstem for cranial nerves III, IV, VI; labyrinthine semicircular canals, otoliths and neck muscle proprioceptors	Although not a formal component of brain death testing, this reflex may be tested as routine practice. The test must not be performed if an unstable cervical spine is suspected. Holding the eyes open, rotate the head from side to side, observing the position of the eyes	If the reflex is absent, the eyes will move with the head and do not move within their orbit, indicating significant brainstem injury

ABG = arterial blood gas; CO_2 = carbon dioxide; ETT = endotracheal tube.

determination of death and the time of declaration of death stay under the legal responsibility of the physician in charge and address some key points for the clinical diagnosis of brain death, similar to the ones presented for the Australian context.[1,2] Formal testing for brain death, in Australia, is undertaken using either clinical assessment or cerebral blood flow studies.[5] Assessment of the brainstem involves assessment of the cranial nerves and the respiratory centre. The most common approaches to testing are described in Table 29.4. Brain death is confirmed if there is no reaction to stimulation of these reflexes, with the respiratory centre tested last and only if the other reflexes are absent. The tests may be done consecutively, but not simultaneously, with no fixed interval between the two sets of clinical tests required, except in specific age-related criteria.[5]

If the preconditions outlined in Box 29.2 are unable to be verified, brain death can be confirmed using cerebral blood flow imaging to demonstrate absent blood flow to the brain. Both contrast angiography and radionuclide scanning can be used to confirm brain death. Contrast angiography can be performed by direct injection of contrast into both carotid arteries and one or both of the vertebral arteries, or via the vena cava or aortic arch. Brain death is confirmed when there is no blood flow above the carotid siphon. A radionuclide scan is performed by administering a bolus of short-acting isotope intravenously or by nebuliser while imaging the head using a gamma camera for 15 minutes. No intra-cranial uptake of isotope confirms absent blood flow to the brain.[27] If brain death is confirmed, the time of death is recorded as the time of certification of the testing result (i.e. at the completion of the second set of clinical tests, or the documentation of the results of the cerebral blood flow scan).[5]

Identification of a potential multi-organ donor

The second factor influencing the number of actual organ donors is identification of a potential donor. A potential donor is defined in this situation as a patient who is suspected of, or is confirmed as, being brain dead. Inclusion and exclusion criteria for organ and tissue donation are constantly being reviewed and refined, and may also be dependent on the critical waiting list of patients.[2,6,14]

When considering the medical suitability of potential organ donors, advice can be sought 24 hours a day, 7 days a week, from respective state and territory organ donation agencies in Australia as well as in most countries (see *Online resources*).

The WHO critical pathway for deceased donation provides a reportable uniformity in the approach to deceased donation. The pathway is a tool for a systematic approach to the organ donation process, and how to assess the potential of deceased donation.[15,29]

Seeking consent

The third factor influencing the possibility for organ donations is brain death confirmation and consent for donation.[30] Consent is sought for individual organs and tissues, rather than a 'global' approach. If granted, the individual organs/tissues are recorded on the consent form or named if the consent is being recorded over the telephone; only those organs/tissues granted will be retrieved. Common practice in Australia and New Zealand is for the treating medical staff either to initiate or at least to be involved in approaching the next of kin after death has been confirmed.[5] Contacting the next of kin to seek consent is part of the duty of care to patients who may have indicated their wish to be a donor at the time of their death.[5,30] Offering the option of organ donation is also considered part of the duty of care to the family.[5,31] Three elements are involved when approaching a family regarding the option of organ donation:

1. their knowledge, beliefs and attitudes
2. their in-hospital experience
3. any beliefs and biases of health professional/s conducting the approach.[32-34]

The outcome of an approach cannot be predicted or anticipated. A large UK study demonstrated that clinical staff were incorrect 50% of the time when asked to predict the response of next of kin.[32]

Attitudes to organ donation are influenced by spiritual beliefs, cultural background, prior knowledge about organ donation, views on altruism and prior health experiences.[32] Next of kin consider two aspects associated with existing attitudes and knowledge: the decision maker(s)' own thoughts and feelings and the previous wishes and beliefs of the person on whose behalf they are making the decision.[32] There is evidence of a link between consent rates and prior knowledge of the positive outcomes of organ donation.[28,32,35] Several other studies found that consent rates improved when conversations about brain death and organ donation were separated, were held in a private setting and when an organ donation professional/ trained requestor was involved.[32,33,35]

Delivery of relevant information

An important consideration for all health professionals is that family members may have a diminished ability to receive and understand information because of their stress and psychological responses at this time of family crisis.[31,32,36] As interviews held with the family are the foundation of the entire organ donation and transplant process, the discussion about brain death must be clear and emphatic, using language free of medical terminology, and include an explanation of the physical implications.[36] Diagrams, analogies, and written materials have been suggested as useful aids for enhancing understanding by next of kin.[28] One approach is to describe brain death as like a jigsaw puzzle with a piece missing, to illustrate the relationship of the brain to the rest of the body. Opportunities for staff to train and role-play this scenario with programs like TPM and the European Training Program on Organ Donation in Europe (see *Online resources*) improve the likelihood of meeting the needs of families.[3,22,32]

As the time of confirmation of brain death is the person's legal time of death, multiple family conversations may occur with the family to discuss their options and associated implications. Options are to: 1) cease ventilation and allow cardiac standstill to occur; or 2) maintain ventilation and haemodynamic support to explore and potentially facilitate viable organ and tissue donation. The retrieval process must be fully explained to ensure an informed decision, but not to overload the next of kin.[28,32] Table 29.5 lists some aspects of the organ donation process that ought to be included in such a discussion. As information given to a family contains both good news and bad news it is suggested to start with the positive news – the benefits of donation, the right of the family to refuse consent (legislation differs between countries) and the lack of cost – and then move to the less positive news – the reality of the surgical intervention and the lack of guarantee that the organs will be transplanted.[1] Families frequently gain solace from

TABLE 29.5
Information about the organ donation process and retrieval to assist in informed decision making[1,35]

DECISION	ISSUES
Ensure that the next of kin (NOK) have understanding of:	• Brain death • Time of death • Eventual organ failure if kept ventilated in critical care • The two options: to immediately cease ventilation or organ donation
If they choose to donate:	• They will not be with the donor at time of cardiac arrest • Donor will remain in critical care, monitored and ventilated until going to theatre for retrieval • Explain the organ retrieval surgery, including the presence of an anaesthetist to monitor the haemodynamics and ventilation • Explain to the family that the person no longer feels any pain, so an anaesthetic is not given • Discuss which organs and tissue would be potentially medically suitable for retrieval for transplant • NOK can give specific consent; they are not obliged to grant global consent • Only named organs and tissues with consent are retrieved • Advise expected length of process • Explain reason for bloods being taken and stored • Advise that a coordinator will be present through the entire process • Explain how the donor will look after the retrieval • Organ donation will not delay funeral plans • Explain consent form • Provide copy of consent form • Explain privacy implications of the relevant Human Tissue Act, for donor family and transplant recipients • Explain reasons why donation may not proceed • Explain that organs may be transplanted some distance away • In the event of an abnormality/diseases, organs will not be retrieved • Explain consent for research: offer copy of research page • The site designated officer (or equivalent) will also sign the consent form
If coroner's case:	• Coroner's consent required • Police identification required • Autopsy? Brain retrieval? • Deceased will go to the coroner's mortuary after retrieval • Explain contact with coroner's court
If organs are retrieved and not able to be transplanted:	• Offer options. Will be returned and placed with donor, or disposed of as medical waste
Support services:	• Offer viewing of patient or a telephone call after the retrieval • Offer lock of hair and/or handprint • Provide contact details of coordinator • Provide printed information • Explain other support services available
Follow-up information:	• Outcome of retrieval • Recipient outcomes • Written material and letters • Counselling services • Availability of transplant coordinator to answer questions

the positive aspects of donation, of helping or reducing the suffering of other families. Of note, a best practice approach aims to assist the family to make the decision that is 'right' for them and does not necessarily result in gaining consent.[35]

Meetings with the family

Identifying who the appropriate family members are to meet with in relation to organ donation is a first consideration, and then the process by which the discussions will be held needs to be considered, including

TABLE 29.6
Definition of next of kin for children and adults in Australian (Queensland) law[4,6]

DONOR	ORDER OF SENIORITY	RELATIONSHIP
Child	1	Parent
	2	Adult sibling (over 18 years)
	3	Guardian (immediately before death)
Adult	1	Spouse or de facto (at time of death)
	2	Adult offspring (over 18 years)
	3	Parent
	4	Adult sibling (over 18 years)

cultural aspects which differ internationally.[1,8] Meetings with family to discuss organ donation and ascertaining the donors wishes is a sensitive and difficult conversation. Healthcare professionals aim to balance respect for a family's decision regarding organ donation with the knowledge of the list of patients awaiting transplant and the associated burden of illness while maintaining objectivity in family discussions.[36]

In Australia the definition of next of kin for adults and children is listed in strict order (Table 29.6). In New Zealand there is no hierarchy of next of kin, with the definition including a surviving spouse or relative.[5] In both countries, the next of kin can override the known wishes of the deceased regarding consent, but experience shows that the family rarely disagree if the wishes of the deceased are known, regardless of their own personal beliefs.[5] The right to override a known wish to donate or not differs between countries depending on their law. Internationally, there are various cultural differences within populations (including religious perspectives) to consider with regard to the approach for organ donation.[1] Further discussions regarding culturally appropriate communication can be found in Chapter 7.

The timing, location, content and process of discussions with the family are all important considerations. An effective protocol for communicating with the family of a potential donor must include: 1) frequent and honest updates on the patient's prognosis; 2) clear explanation of brain death; 3) the decoupling of the brain death and organ donation conversations[28,32,34] until the family accepts that the patient is dead;[37] 4) conversations held in a private and quiet setting;[28,32,34] and 5) involvement of an organ donation professional with a clear definition of roles.[32]

There is compelling evidence that the meeting confirming diagnosis of brain death should be held separately or decoupled from the conversation about the option of organ and tissue donation.[32] In reality, the pace and flow of discussions should be assessed on a case-by-case basis, as there may be circumstances when the discussion about organ donation is appropriately held prior to the confirmation of death.[5,32]

Staff roles, delineation and involvement

Staff involved in the explanation of brain death must have a clear understanding of brain death, and have practised explaining it themselves before attempting to explain it to a family.[28,32] Ideally, requestors are specifically trained in the approach of requesting organ and tissue donation and have completed some form of formal education, for example TPM. Additionally, having the organ donor coordinator present to answer specific questions raised by the family assists in the process.[5] The process of organ and tissue donation in critical care is significant for all concerned. When death is confirmed it marks the end of an episode that has been catastrophic for both patient and loved ones, and a potentially stressful and exhausting experience for staff.[3,36] Approaching a potential donor family is a multidisciplinary team effort, and guidelines encourage treating medical staff to continue their involvement with patient and family after brain death is confirmed, for continuity of care.[5] The individual physician's or nurse's willingness to act, to respect, represent and safeguard the (potential) donor's will and wishes in these situations is termed *organ donor advocacy,* and is built on the professional ethics and its demand to make decisions of the best actions for the patient/donor. The concept of *attitudes toward organ donor advocacy,* developed by Flodén, is theoretically anchored in the framework of patient advocacy.[38,39] In the situation of organ donation, participation in the donation process and caring for the potential or actual organ donor can be viewed as advocacy activities (i.e. respecting the potential or actual organ donor's rights, representing or speaking up for his/her wishes as well as the relatives' points of view in the organ donation decision-making process).[38,39] Nursing staff involvement in the process of organ and tissue donation is central and intrinsic, including the practicalities of the process, and care of the potential donor and family during the decision-making process.[34] Donor families have identified nurses as being the most helpful health professionals in providing information and emotional support.[5,28]

A holistic approach to supporting families in critical care may also include involvement of social workers, pastoral care workers and other allied health professionals.[40] Often these health professionals have been working with the family for a number of days and act as confidants and a resource for information on issues such as implications of a coronial enquiry and a religious denomination's stance on organ donation. Most major religions are supportive of organ and tissue donation for transplant and would instruct the family to make the decision that they felt was correct.[1,41]

In many countries there are organ donation coordinators that act as a resource and are invited into critical care when appropriate.[3,41,42] A professional who is an expert in donation and has the time to spend with the family may be the best person to undertake an approach to a potential donor family.[34,41]

Practice tip

The multidisciplinary team involved in the process of organ donation is not limited to staff within the ICU. In order for the donor's wishes to become a reality and provide organ and tissues for transplantation the following disciplines are involved:[1]

- medical
- nursing
- allied health
- pastoral care
- operational services
- administration
- police service
- coroner's and magistrate's office
- designated officer.

Adapted from the DonateLife website, http://www.donatelife.gov.au.

Role of designated specialists

In most countries, senior medical staff eligible to certify brain death using brain death criteria must be appointed by the governing body of their health institution, have relevant and recent experience and not be involved with transplant recipient selection.[18] In many countries, the most common medical specialties appointed to the role are intensivists and neurologists.[18] Appointed medical staff confirming brain death must also act independently, must be appropriately qualified and suitably experienced in the care of such patients.[5,43] Medical staff should not be involved in treating the recipient of the organ to be removed but rather be a specialist in charge of the clinical care of the patient.[14,43]

Role of designated officers

Similarities between Australia and international practice extend to the role of the 'designated officer' whereby an executive level appointment within the institution is afforded the power to authorise a non-coronial postmortem and the removal of tissue from a deceased person for transplant or other therapeutic, medical or scientific purposes;[5] and to to protect healthcare consumers. This officer must be satisfied that all necessary inquiries have been made and any necessary consent has been obtained before granting authority. Medical, nursing and administrative staff can be appointed to the role, but they must not act in a case if they have had clinical or personal involvement in the donor's case.[5] International guidelines on ethics, access and safety in tissue and organ transplantation are published by the WHO.[44]

Role of coroner and forensic pathologists

Because of the nature of their death, many donors are subject to coronial inquiry. In this case, permission to undertake organ and tissue retrieval is sought from the respective forensic pathologist and coroner according to local policy and procedure as part of the consent-seeking process. The coronial system is very supportive of donation for transplant and, in 2012, 43% of the Australian and 50% of New Zealand multi-organ donors were coroner's cases.[18]

Consent indicator databases

The most influential factor to affect family unit decision making is the existence of an advance care directive or prior indication of consent.[28,32] This information has eased decision making and preserved patient autonomy,[28,32] enabling wishes of the patient to be followed even when family decision makers would have made the opposite decision.

Cultural competence

With large cultural mixes in many countries, best practice for approaching a family includes openness and awareness of what information the family member(s) may need to make their decision. As significant differences also exist within various cultural groups, expectations of responses cannot be stereotyped.[45] When healthcare professionals are unsure of how a family may perceive a situation, it is best to ask, as acknowledgment of expectations and needs can lead to improved communication.[28,32,] Importantly, the most significant differences between potential donor families are socioeconomic and educational factors, rather than cultural or racial background.[46,47] Therefore, individual assessment must guide the approach by health professionals. Cultural aspects of critical care nursing practice are discussed in Chapter 7.

Organ donor care

Understanding the brain death physiology and the importance of time management is critical in the management of a potential organ donor. Those patients who have sustained traumatic brain injuries can deteriorate rapidly following brain death, exhibiting severe physiological instability requiring vigilant monitoring and specialised treatment to stabilise and maintain organ perfusion. This is a time of great distress for families with the patient's death usually the result of a sudden, unexpected illness or injury, and therefore discussion surrounding organ and tissue donation must be undertaken in a sensitive manner by skilled requestors who possess a strong professional commitment to the quality of the process.[5,46]

Ideally, the time between brain death and organ retrieval should be minimised to ensure an optimal outcome for transplant recipients. Therefore, the focus of medical management changes from ensuring brain perfusion to maintaining good organ perfusion for transplantation.[35,46] Early referral, application of recognised management protocols and collaboration between the donation centre and retrieval teams are paramount. Donor family care forms a crucial part of the process, with up-to-date and accurate information essential to ensure the bereavement process is managed appropriately.

Referral of potential donor

If consent is granted, the donor referral process usually commences immediately. The longer the time delay, the more likely that organ failure-related complications will occur.[14] In 2016, the median time from brain death confirmation to the commencement of organ retrieval was 21.6 hours in Australia and 15.1 hours in New Zealand.[18]

The referral process is consistent across international organisation, including North America, Europe and the UK, and begins with hospital-based specialists and donor coordinators collating the past and present medical, surgical and social history of the potential donor, and relaying this information to the relevant transplant units.[49,50] (Table 29.7). In Australia, a National Electronic Donor Record was introduced in 2014, enabling secure and rapid relay of information to transplant units as opposed to individual transplant unit telephone calls to relay information. Using this information, transplant teams allocate the organs to the most suitable and appropriate recipient/s. If the transplant team does not have a suitable recipient, the offer is extended to another team in Australia or New Zealand on rotation using Transplant Society of Australia and New Zealand (TSANZ) guidelines.[14] Similarly, referral practices through LifeNet in the USA and the NHS referral network in the UK ensure all potential donors are identified and referred early for appropriate management and to ensure opportunity for organ and tissue donation is honoured.[49,50]

Tissue typing and cross-matching

A vital component of the assessment and referral process is tissue typing, cross-matching and virology testing of the potential donor's blood. Blood is taken from an arterial or central line of the potential donor and sent to the relevant accredited laboratory (Table 29.8). Tissue typing identifies the human leucocyte antigen (HLA) phenotype from the genes on chromosome 6. The HLA molecules control actions of the immune system to differentiate between 'self ' and foreign tissue, and initiate an immune response to foreign matter. As a transplanted organ will always be identified as foreign tissue by the recipient's body, immunosuppressive drugs are used to suppress the immune response. A cross-match is routinely used to predict the level of this response. Lymphocytes from the potential donor are added to the potential

TABLE 29.7
Donation referral information[15,41,46]

SECTION	DETAILS
Personal details	Address, phone number, sex, age, height, weight, race, religion, build, occupation
Current admission details	Dates and time of hospital admission, intubation, critical care admission Other trauma or significant event
Declaration of brain death	Cause of death, time, date, method of testing
Consent details	Which organs, designated officer details, coroner's details, police details, who gave consent, which databases accessed
Donor history	Family, medical, surgical, travel, social and sexual history
Blood results	Blood group, biochemistry and haematology on admission and within past 12 h, microbiology, gas exchange
Test results	Chest X-ray including lung field measurements, ECG, echocardiogram, bronchoscopy, sputum
Haemodynamics	BP, MAP, HR, CVP, temperature
Admission history	Cardiac arrest, temperature, renal function, nutrition, drug and fluid administration
Physical examination	Scars, trauma, needle marks, tattoos, etc

BP = blood pressure; CVP = central venous pressure; ECG = electrocardiogram; HR = heart rate; MAP = mean arterial pressure.

TABLE 29.8
Blood tests required for organ donation[6,15]

MEASUREMENT REQUIRED	TEST
Serology	• HIV I and II • HTLV 1 antibody • Hepatitis B sAg • Hepatitis B sAb • Hepatitis B core Ab • Hepatitis C sAb • CMV (IgG) • EBV (in some settings) • Syphilis (in some settings) • Toxoplasma IgG and IgM (in some settings) • HSV (in some settings)
NAT screen (nucleic acid test)	• HIV NAT Screen • HCV NAT Screen
Tissue typing	• Cross-matching with the blood of potential recipients of relevant ABO

Ab = antibody; CMV = cytomegalovirus; EBV = Epstein–Barr virus; HCV = hepatitis C virus; HIV = human immunodeficiency virus; HSV = herpes simplex virus; HTLV = human T-lymphotropic virus; IgG = immunoglobulin G; IgM = immunoglobulin M; NAT = nucleic acid testing; sAb = surface antibody; sAg = surface antigen.

recipient's serum to test whether the recipient has an antibody that is specific to the donor's HLA antigens. A positive cross-match reaction, where the recipient's serum destroys the donor's cells, is a contraindication for transplantation.[14,41]

Practice tip

Organ and tissue transplantation are associated with the potential for the transmission of some infectious diseases and malignant conditions. In the process of organ and tissue donation and transplantation this risk is balanced against the recipients waiting and their urgency.

Adapted from Transplant Society of Australia and New Zealand.

Donor management

The fourth factor influencing the number of actual organ donors is the clinical management that the donor and family receive after confirmation of death. The aim of donor management is to support and optimise organ function until organ retrieval commences, while maintaining dignity and respect for the donor and support for the family. All aspects of intensive care unit (ICU) treatment, apart from brain-oriented therapy, should continue until it is certain that organ donation will not occur.[5] Medical management of potential donors is detailed in Box 29.1.

Retrieval surgery

Organ retrieval surgery occurs in the hospital where the donor has been managed in the ICU (often following transfer from a regional or rural hospital), with the local operating theatre staff integral to the process. The donor is transferred to theatre after routine preoperative checks and documentation is completed, including death certification and consent for organ and tissue retrieval. All documentation, particularly consent, is viewed by all members of the retrieval surgical team before surgery commences.[35] Depending on which organs are to be retrieved, the retrieval teams will be tasked to abdominal organs and thoracic organs, and will bring most of their specialised equipment with them. An anaesthetist monitors haemodynamics, ventilation and administers medications, which may include a long-acting muscle relaxant given prior to the surgical procedure, to prevent interference in the surgical process by spinal reflexes, only after consultation with the retrieval team.[41] No other anaesthetic agents are administered. The local scrub staff will work with the visiting surgical teams, and the DonateLife donor coordinator will be present to document the procedure and outcomes, fulfil any family wishes in regard to theatre and act as a resource for all staff present.

Surgery may take 4–5 hours depending on the extent of the retrieval; cross-clamp will occur once the surgeons have identified all the various anatomical points. The aorta is cross-clamped with vascular clamps below the diaphragm and at the aortic arch, the heart is stopped and ventilation is ceased. Retrieval teams administer a cold perfusion fluid with an electrolyte mix specific to the organs being retrieved, and remove the organs. Organs are bagged with sterile ice and perfusion fluid and transported by the retrieval teams to the transplanting hospitals. The donor's surgical wound, from the sternal notch to the pubis, is closed by the surgeons in a routine manner and dressed with a surgical dressing. If the donor is not a coroner's case, the remaining lines, catheter and drains are removed according to local policy, the patient is washed and arrangements are made to transfer the patient to a location for family viewing or to the mortuary. Musculoskeletal tissue and retinal retrieval can occur after the solid organ retrieval in theatre or later in the mortuary.[14]

Donor family care

Supportive care of a donor family begins from the time their family member is admitted to hospital and continues beyond organ retrieval in all international organ donation agencies.[51] In addition to personal factors such as cultural background, family dynamics, coping skills and prior experiences with loss that may influence the grieving process, the family of an organ and tissue donor will be dealing with a number of unique factors. Death of their family member was possibly sudden and unexpected; brain death can be difficult to understand when people look as if they are asleep rather than dead; having the option of organ donation may mean making a decision on behalf of the person if his/her wishes were not known; and the process of organ donation means they will not be with the person when their heart stops.[33] Further information about specific cultural groups and general considerations for tailoring discussions to the family's background can be found in Chapter 7.

Practice tip

Prior to family meetings regarding organ donation it is beneficial for staff to go over their roles and the potential conversation that might occur. Providing an opportunity for staff debriefing, operational reviews and documenting staff involved in the donation and retrieval process is also important, particularly in regional or rural settings where cases may be infrequent and the community is smaller, facilitating collaboration with the organ retrieval teams.

Donor families benefit from emotional and physical support throughout and after the organ donation process. In critical care units, this support can include open visiting times, privacy for meetings, clear and precise information and regular contact with the attending clinical team, support personnel and the DonateLife donor coordinator. After organ retrieval, ongoing care can include contact with a bereavement specialist, written material, telephone support, private or group counselling and correspondence from recipients.[1] Internationally, organ donation agencies identify the importance of family support and follow-up in developing trust and providing comfort during and after the donation decision, and provide aftercare programs for the families of organ donors through a variety of follow-up support services[1,32,36,52] (see *Online resources*). Involvement of trained personnel with a donor family through this process can positively influence the family's grief journey.[1,41]

The National Donor Family Support Service operates through the DonateLife Network and is a nationally consistent program of support provided to cadaveric organ and/or tissue donor families. All families whose next of kin are identified as possible donors are offered end-of-life support including bereavement counselling at the time, whether or not the potential donor proceeds to donation.[1]

Donation after cardiac death

Donation after cardiac death (DCD), also known as non-heart-beating donor (NHBD) and in some instances as donation after circulatory death, provides a solid organ donation option for a patient who has not progressed and is not likely to progress to brain death. Prior to brain death legislation, donation after cardiac death was the source of cadaveric kidneys for transplant.[13,41,53,54] Four categories of potential DCD donors, known as the Holland–Maastricht categories, have been identified:

1 dead on arrival (uncontrolled)
2 failed resuscitation (uncontrolled)
3 withdrawal of support (controlled)
4 arrest following brain death (uncontrolled).[48]

DCD programs around the world are being re-established, with successful retrieval and transplant of kidneys, livers and lungs.[1,48,55] The AOTA has developed a national DCD protocol that outlines an ethical process that respects the rights of the patient and ensures clinical consistency, effectiveness and safety for both donors and recipients.[1] Internationally, in some countries, DCD accounts for a large number of deceased organ donors compared to heart-beating donors.[56] The WHO has estimated that the current transplant rate addresses only 10% of the need globally for organ transplants[57] and several countries now have well-developed protocols in DCD, including UK, Ireland, Spain and several other European countries.[58] The Donation after Circulatory Death Registry is maintained by the International Society for Heart and Lung transplantation.[59]

Identification of a potential DCD donor

Using lessons learned from multi-organ donor programs, the aims of a successful DCD program are to maintain dignity for the donor at all times, provide the donor family with support and information and limit warm ischaemia time[55,59] (time from withdrawal of ventilation and treatment to confirmation of death to commencement of infusion of cold perfusion fluid and/or organ retrieval). Longer warm ischaemia time potentiates the risk of irreparable hypoxic damage to the organ.[41] As noted above, Holland–Maastricht category 3 is the only option that can be controlled and possibly regulate warm ischaemia time. A potential category 3 DCD donor is a person ventilated and monitored in critical care about whom a decision has already been made that further treatment is futile, and current interventions are to be withdrawn. Clinical suitability assessment for organ retrieval replicates a multi-organ donor, with medical, surgical and social history, virology and organ function information collected. Legal requirements of the consent-seeking process also reflect those of a multi-organ donor. Potential donor families are informed that retrieval may not occur due to a number of factors, including the length of time from treatment withdrawal to cardiac standstill.[35,41,54,60]

Retrieval process alternatives

Withdrawal of treatment for a potential category 3 DCD patient can occur in critical care or in the operating theatre, depending on which organs are planned for retrieval. Death is determined by cessation of circulation, with recommendations that the ECG is not monitored (electrical activity can persist for many minutes following cessation of circulation), but an arterial line is used to determine the time of cessation of circulation.[5] If withdrawal occurs in critical care, an intraabdominal catheter may be inserted via the femoral artery after cardiac standstill to infuse cold perfusion fluid into the abdominal cavity. If the lungs are to be retrieved, perfusion fluid may be infused via bilateral intercostal catheters.[53] The patient is then transferred to theatre for organ retrieval. When withdrawal of treatment occurs in theatre, a catheter is not required and retrieval may commence after the patient is declared deceased (cessation of circulation for greater than 2 min). If the patient does not die during the window of time available for organ retrieval, they are transferred back to ICU.[1]

Tissue-only donor

People confirmed as dead using cardiac criteria can be tissue donors. Eyes (whole and corneal button) are retrieved for cornea and sclera transplant. Musculoskeletal tissue is used for bone grafting (long bones of arms and legs, hemipelvis), urology procedures and treatment of sport injuries (ligaments, tendons, fascia and meniscus). Heart valves (bicuspid, tricuspid valves, aortic and pulmonary tissue) are used for heart valve replacement and cardiac reconstruction. Skin (retrieved from the lower back and buttocks) is used for the treatment of burns.[1]

Identification of a potential tissue-only donor

The most influential aspect for tissue donation is early notification of the potential donor's death to the relevant tissue bank, ideally within hours of the person's death. All deceased persons can be considered potential donors, with assessment for clinical suitability on a case-by-case basis. As noted earlier, there is no expectation that treating clinicians will be required to make that decision or make the approach to the next of kin. In general, once the death notification has been received, the determining factors are age, cause of death, time elapsed since death, virology results and presence of infection. The legal requirements of the consent-seeking process mirror those of the multi-organ donor.

After checking medical suitability and the relevant consent indicator database, a coordinator from the tissue bank or other trained personnel approach the next of kin with the option of tissue retrieval.[1] After tissue retrieval, every effort is made to restore anatomical appearance. Wounds are sutured closed and covered with surgical dressings, limbs given back their form, and eye shape is restored with the lids kept closed with eye caps.[1,32] Support requirements for families of tissue-only donors share many aspects of programs provided for families of multi-organ donors. A sensitive approach, provision of adequate information to assist informed decision making, offers of bereavement counselling and follow-up information of recipient outcomes are evidence-based strategies of successful programs.[1,34]

Summary

An overview of organ donation has been provided in this chapter. In several countries, including Australia and New Zealand, opt-in systems of giving consent for organ and tissue donation are in place but in other countries, such as Singapore and Spain, opt-out systems are used. After death has been confirmed or is impending in the case of DCD, the option of organ and tissue donation is given to the next of kin and information from a consent indicator database is sought to determine the wishes of the person. Each person is assessed on a case-by-case basis to determine medical suitability for organ and tissue retrieval for transplant. The treating clinicians are not expected to make this decision, but their involvement and care are vital. Support and information are available around the clock from the respective donor agencies and tissue banks. Donor family care commences at the time of the family member's admission and continues as required with structured bereavement programs specific to donor family care. The intent to be an organ and tissue donor can be indicated by people when alive or by the next of kin after death.

Three 'types' of organ or tissue donor are identified including the multi-organ and tissue donor (after brain death has been confirmed),[61] the organ and tissue donor after cardiac death, and the tissue-only donor (after cardiac death). Four factors have been identified that directly influence the number of multi-organ donations internationally and include the incidence of brain death, the identification of potential donors, brain death confirmation and gaining consent for donation and, finally, the management of the donor after the confirmation of brain death.

There is evidence to address each factor, but each case needs to be approached on a case-by-case basis. The medical suitability for every potential donor is assessed individually at the time of the person's death, and support and guidance from donor agencies and tissue banks are available at all times. Internationally, priority is given to providing care and support of the potential and actual donor family and, as part of this, regular routine follow-up and debriefing opportunities for all staff involved are important to manage stress reactions or other concerns.

Case study

DAY 1

Lucy, a 16-year-old high school student had been preparing breakfast with her mother at 07:20 on a Wednesday morning when she suddenly developed an intensely painful headache, and collapsed in the kitchen. Her mother described the event as occurring very rapidly over a period of less than 5 minutes. She immediately called an ambulance and placed Lucy in a recovery position as she had a pulse and was shallow breathing.

Paramedics arrived on scene in under 7 min and immediately intubated and ventilated Lucy for transfer to a regional hospital. On arrival to the emergency department 14 min later, Lucy was assessed by a multidisciplinary team with vital signs documented at 07:48: Glasgow Coma Score (GCS) 3, BP 150/120 mmHg, heart rate (HR) 56, SaO_2 94%.

Lucy had been intubated on scene and exhibited no respiratory effort or reaction to painful stimuli. Lucy had a single IV line with N/saline at 84 mL/h and a second large bore IV access was established, and she was escorted to radiology for urgent cerebral computerised tomography (CT), outlining a grade V subarachnoid haemorrhage (SAH).

Lucy was immediately admitted to the ICU at 09:30 for assessment with further line placements of arterial and central line insertion. Haemodynamic status remained unchanged, with pupils unequal, ventilated (synchronised intermittent mandatory ventilation [SIMV], respiratory rate 18, tidal volume 350 mL, positive end-expiratory pressure [PEEP] 5), with no sedation or paralysing agents, afebrile 35.7°C.

A family interview was conducted to inform Lucy's mother (her only kin) of her current condition with the Intensive Care Consultant, registrar, bedside nurse and social worker. Lucy's mother was supported by a close friend during the interview and understood her daughter's poor prognosis. She raised the question of her daughter's eligibility for organ donation as they had recently discussed this with Lucy preparing for her driving licence. Lucy's mother agreed to talk to the hospital donor coordinator.

Initial brain stem death tests were performed at 12:20, just over 4 hours from the first observation of potential brain death, revealing no reflex responses, fixed dilated pupils, and PCO_2 of 70 with apnoea. A second set of testing was performed at for 14:30 with confirmed brainstem death. The hospital donor coordinator contacted the state-based DonateLife coordinator and a further family conference with Lucy's mother and support person was held and Lucy's mother gave consent for organ retrieval to occur with the exception of eye tissue.

The regional coordinator commenced the referral documentation in collaboration with the ICU medical and nursing teams and briefed all staff in the management of the process including family care, physiological management and multidisciplinary involvement including staff from the emergency department and operational services teams. Coroner's consent was granted following police identification with Lucy's mother, and blood collected and sent for virology, tissue typing and cross-matching. Lucy's full medical history and admission documentation were collected for referral. Nursing and medical care of Lucy with physiological management continued with Lucy's mother remaining at the bedside throughout.

The state DonateLife organ donor coordinator advised transplant teams would arrive onsite by 22:00 for retrieval of solid organs including heart, lungs, liver and kidneys and were oriented to the regional hospital and supported by the operational services staff. Operating theatre setup commenced with teams providing all the necessary instrumentation and Lucy was transferred for the retrieval procedure at 23:20. Lucy's mother insisted on waiting at the family room in ICU and was supported throughout by her support person, social worker and local donor coordinator.

DAY 2

At 03:45, retrieval was complete with teams transported to the airport for return to their respective hospitals to complete the transplantation procedure for matched recipients. Lucy's body was returned to a private room in the ICU by the bedside nurse and donor coordinator and prepared for viewing by her mother at 04:30. Lucy's mother sat with her daughter over the next 2 hours along with her support person. The donor coordinator provided bereavement support contacts and information and advised that she would be contacted by the state coordinator to advise of the transplant outcomes if she wished.

At 06:30 the donor coordinator and social worker debriefed all staff involved in both the ICU and operating theatre and completed all documentation.

DAY 3

At 10:00, as arranged, the state donor coordinator rang Lucy's mother to let her know the outcomes of the transplant procedures and brief recipient details, and followed this with a phone call to the regional donor coordinator to inform hospital staff and advise of follow-up letters arriving within a few days to provide an update.

CASE STUDY QUESTIONS

1. Reflect on the professional responsibility of Organ Donor Advocacy and consider how this applies in the care of an organ donor and their next of kin.
2. Identify the priorities of care of the donor in ensuring optimal management for transplantation success.
3. Analyse the effectiveness of healthcare professional attitudes and education in the management of the organ donation process including consent.

RESEARCH VIGNETTE

Oczkowski SJW, Centofanti JE, Durepos P et al. Organ donation in the ICU: a document analysis of institutional policies, protocols, and order sets. Intensive Crit Care Nurs 2018;45:58-65

Abstract

Objective: To better understand how local policies influence organ donation rates.

Research methodology/design: We conducted a document analysis of our ICU organ donation policies, protocols and order sets. We used a systematic search of our institution's policy library to identify documents related to organ donation. We used Mindnode software to create a publication timeline, basic statistics to describe document characteristics, and qualitative content analysis to extract document themes.

Setting: Documents were retrieved from Hamilton Health Sciences, an academic hospital system with a high volume of organ donation, from database inception to October 2015.

Findings: We retrieved 12 active organ donation documents, including six protocols, two policies, two order sets, and two unclassified documents, a majority (75%) after the introduction of donation after circulatory death in 2006. Four major themes emerged: organ donation process, quality of care, patient and family-centred care, and the role of the institution. These themes indicate areas where documented institutional standards may be beneficial.

Conclusion: Further research is necessary to determine the relationship of local policies, protocols, and order sets to actual organ donation practices, and to identify barriers and facilitators to improving donation rates.

Critique

This document analysis of ICU organ donation policies and protocols aims to provide better understanding of how local policies influence organ donation rates. In total 12 documents were identified that were relevant to the ICU. All documents used were uploaded on the academic hospital system covering one region and used in one ICU, in Canada. The study is interesting and acknowledges the importance of standardised guidelines. The results explore four major themes, and these themes are applicable in the organ donation process in general: organ donation process; quality of care, patient and family-centred care, and the role of the institution. A limitation of the study is that the documents used came from only one ICU in Canada. Due to this selection, the results may not be readily transferable to other ICUs. Additionally, it is not possible to understand the extent to which the vested interests of the authors who wrote the initial documents could be accounted for in the document analysis. The authors conclude that documentation is an important part of the donation process; however, how this conclusion was reached is not evident. The documents used were described as focusing on the process itself and not on the outcome. Therefore, no conclusions can be drawn related to the program effectiveness and its impact on the organ donation rates. Overall, this paper recognises the importance to standardise and improve the care of organ donors in the ICU, and to theoretically identify key areas to consider when developing guidelines to describe and influence clinical practice throughout the organ donation process.

Learning activities

1. What four factors have been identified as directly influencing the number of multi-organ donations, including the incidence of brain death?
2. What are the effects of the interdisciplinary international education program (TPM) for donor coordinators and transplant coordinators?
3. What are the professional accountabilities of the critical care staff in the identification of the potential organ donor?
4. What is the definition of the concept *attitudes toward organ donor advocacy*?
5. Describe the different existing systems (internationally) for achieving consent to organ donation?
6. What is the aim of donor management and how is it regulated?
7. Describe factors throughout the organ and tissue donation process that influence the grieving process for the family.

Online resources

Achieving Comprehensive Coordination in Organ Donation throughout the European Union (ACCORD), www.accord-ja.eu

Association of Organ Procurement Organizations (AOPO), www.aopo.org

Australia and New Zealand Cardiothoracic Organ Transplant Registry, www.anzcotr.org.au

Australia and New Zealand Dialysis and Transplant Registry (ANZDATA), www.anzdata.org.au

Australia and New Zealand Liver Transplant Registry, www.anzltr.org

Australia and New Zealand Organ Donation Registry (ANZOD), www.anzdata.org.au

Australian and New Zealand Intensive Care Society (ANZICS), www.anzics.com.au

Australian Bone Marrow Registry, www.abmdr.org.au/

Australian College of Critical Care Nurses (ACCCN), www.acccn.com.au

Australian Corneal Graft Registry, www.flinders.edu.au/medicine/sites/ophthalmology/clinical/the-australian-corneal-graft-registry.cfm

Australian Organ Donor Register (AODR), https://www.humanservices.gov.au/individuals/services/medicare/australian-organ-donor-register?utm_id=9

Australasian Transplant Coordinators Association (ATCA), www.atca.org.au

Coalition on Donation, www.shareyourlife.org

DonateLife, www.donatelife.gov.au

Donation and Transplant Institute, http://tpm-dti.com/

Donor Tissue Bank of Victoria, www.vifm.org

European Society for Organ Transplantation, www.esot.org

European Training Program on Organ Donation (ETPOD), etpod.il3.ub.edu

Eye Bank Association of Australia and New Zealand, http://www.ebaanz.org/

Eye Bank of South Australia, http://www.flinders.edu.au/medicine/sites/ophthalmology/clinical/eyebank.cfm

Gift of Life, www.giftoflife.on.ca

Global Observatory on Donation and Transplantation (GODT), www.transplant-observatory.org

International Registry in Organ Donation and Transplantation (IRODaT), www.irodat.org

Japan Organ Transplant Network, www.jotnw.or.jp

Lions Corneal Donation Service, https://www.cera.org.au/community/lions-eye-donation-service/

Lions Eye Bank (WA), https://www.lei.org.au/

MESOT: The Middle East Society for Organ Transplantation, www.mesot-tx.org

Multi Organ Harvesting Aid Network Foundation, www.mohanfoundation.org

NATCO, The Organization for Transplant Professionals, www.natco1.org

New Zealand National Transplant Donor Coordination Office, www.donor.co.nz

Organ Procurement and Transplantation Network, optn.transplant.hrsa.gov

Perth Bone and Tissue Bank, https://www.pluslife.org.au/

Professional Education Packaqe (PEP), www.donatelife.gov.au/professional-education-package

Queensland Tissue Bank, http://www.donatelife.gov.au/eye-and-tissue-banks

The Transplantation Society (TTS), www.tts.org

Transplant News Network, www.centerspan.org

Transplant Nurses' Association (TNA), www.tna.asn.au

Transplantation Society of Australia and New Zealand (TSANZ), www.tsanz.com.au

United Network for Organ Sharing (UNOS), www.unos.org

World Health Organization, www.who.int/transplantation/en

Further reading

Australian College of Critical Care Nurses. ACCCN position statement on organ and tissue donation and transplantation; 2009. https://www.acccn.com.au/about-us/position-statements.

Declaration of Istanbul. http://www.declarationofistanbul.org/.

European Commission. Organ donation and transplantation. Special Eurobarometer 333a. Belgium: European Commission; 2010 ec.europa.ed/public_opinion/archives/ebs/ebs_333a_en.pdf.

National Health and Medical Research Council (NHMRC). National protocol for donation after cardiac death; 2010. http://www.donatelife.gov.au.

Rudge C, Mateasanz R, Delmenica FL, et al. International practices of organ donation. Br J Anaesth 2012;108:48–55.

Russ GR. Organ donation in Australia: international comparisons. http://www.donatelife.gov.au.

World Health Organization. Global glossary on organ donation. http://www.who.int/transplantation/activities/GlobalGlossaryonDonation Transplantation.pdf?ua=1.

References

1. Australian Government Organ and Tissue Authority. DonateLife. Organ and Tissue Authority; 2018. Available from: http://www.donatelife.gov.au. [Accessed May 2018].
2. United Network of Organ Sharing (UNOS). 2017. Available from: http://www.unos.org. [Accessed May 2018].

3. Council of Europe. Guide to the quality and safety of organs for transplantation, 6th edn; 2016. Available from: https://www.esot.org/news/latest-news/guide-quality-and-safety-organs-transplantation-6th-edition. [Accessed June 2018].
4. Barker CF, Markmann JF. Historical overview of transplantation. Cold Spring Harb Perspect Med 2013;3:a014977. Available from: http://perspectivesinmedicine.cshlp.org/content/3/4/a014977.full. [Accessed April 2018].
5. Australian and New Zealand Intensive Care Society (ANZICS). The ANZICS statement on death and organ donation, edn 3.2. Melbourne: ANZICS; 2013. Available from: http://www.anzics.com.au. [Accessed May 2018].
6. Association of Organ Procurement Organizations (AOPO), Association of Organ Procurement Organizations. 2018. Available from: http://www.aopo.org/wikidonor/. [Accessed May 2018].
7. Colombo D, Ammirati E. Cyclosporine in transplantation – a history of converging timelines. J Biol Regul Homeost Agents 2011;25(4):493–504.
8. Queensland Government. Transplantation and Anatomy Act; 1979 (Qld) s. 4 (Australia). Available from: https://www.legislation.qld.gov.au/view/html/inforce/current/act-1979-074. [Accessed August 2018].
9. Australian Department of Human Services. Australian Organ Donor Register; 2018. Available from: https://www.humanservices.gov.au. [Accessed May 2018].
10. Kim JR, Elliott D, Hyde C. The influence of sociocultural factors on organ donation and transplantation in Korea: findings from key informant interviews. J Transcult Nurs 2004;15(2):147–54.
11. Abouna G. Ethical issues in organ and tissue transplantation. Exp Clin Transplant 2003;2:125–38.
12. Suguitan GA, Cabanayan-Casasola RA, Danguilan RA, et al. Outcomes of referrals for deceased organ donation to the government organ procurement organisation. Transplant Proc 2014;46:1074–6.
13. US Department of Health & Human Services. Organdonor.gov; 2018. Available from: http://organdonor.gov. [Accessed May 2018].
14. The Transplantation Society of Australia and New Zealand Inc (TSANZ). Clinical guidelines for organ transplantation from deceased donors; 2018. Available from: https://www.tsanz.com.au/organallocationguidelines/index.asp. [Accessed May 2018].
15. World Health Organization (WHO). Guiding principles on human cell, tissue and organ transplantation; 2010. Available from: http://www.who.int/transplantation/Guiding_PrinciplesTransplantation_WHA63.22en.pdf. [Accessed May 2018].
16. Therapeutic Goods Administration. 2018. Available from: https://www.tga.gov.au. [Accessed May 2018].
17. McKeeown DW, Bonser RS, Kellum JA. Management of the heartbeating brain-dead organ donor. Br J Anaesth 2012;108(Suppl. 1):i96–107.
18. Australia and New Zealand Organ Donation Registry (ANZOD). Registry report; 2017. Available from: http://www.anzdata.org.au/anzod/v1/AR-2017.html. [Accessed May 2018].
19. Rudge C, Matesanz R, Delmonico FL, et al. International practices of organ donation. Br J Anaesth 2012;108:i48–55.
20. Shemie SD, Hornby L, Baker A, et al. International guideline development for the determination of death. Intensive Care Med 2014;40(6):788–97.
21. Radunz S, Juntermanns B, Heuer M, et al. The effect of education on the attitude of medical students towards organ donation. Ann Transplant 2012;17(1):140–4.
22. Donation Transplant Institute (DTI). 2018. Available from: http://tpm-dti.com/. [Accessed May 2018].
23. Escudero D, Valentín MO, Escalante JL, et al. Intensive care practices in brain death diagnosis and organ donation. Anaesthesia 2015;70:1130–9.
24. Arbour RB. Brain death: assessment, controversy and confounding factors. Crit Care Nurse 2013;33(6):27–46.
25. Gardiner D, Shemie S, Manara A, et al. International perspective on the diagnosis of death. Br J Anaesth 2012;108(S1):i14–28.
26. Tawil I, Brown LH, Comfort D, et al. Experiences of the families concerning organ donation of a family member with brain death. Iran J Nurs Midwifery Res 2014;19(3):323–9.
27. Zuckier LS. Radionuclide evaluation of brain death in the post-McMath era. J Nucl Med 2016;57:1560–8.
28. Birtan D, Arslantas MK, Dincer PC, et al. Effect of interviews done by intensive care physicians on organ donation. Transplant Proc 2017;49(3):396–8.
29. Domínguez-Gil B, Delmonico FL, Shaheen FAM, et al. The critical pathway for deceased donation: reportable uniformity in the approach to deceased donation. Transpl Int 2011;24:373–8.
30. Marck CH, Neate SL, Skinner MR, et al. Factors relating to consent for organ donation: prospective data on potential organ donors. Intern Med J 2015;45(1):40–7.
31. Organ and Tissue Authority. National Study of Family Experiences of Organ and Tissue Donation Wave 1 – 2010 and 2011; 2014. Available from: http://www.donatelife.gov.au. [Accessed May 2018].
32. Hulme W, Allen J, Manara AR, et al. Factors influencing family consent rate for organ donation in the UK. Anaesthesia 2016;71:1053–63.
33. Jawoniyi OO, Gormley K. How critical care nurses' roles and education affect organ donation. Br J Nurs 2015;24(13):698–700.
34. Yousefi H, Roshani A, Nazari F. Experiences of the families concerning organ donation of a family member with brain death. Iran J Nurs Midwifery Res 2014;19(3):323–9.
35. Citerio G, Cypel M, Dobb G, et al. Organ donation in adults: a critical care perspective. Intensive Care Med 2016;42(3):305–15.
36. Oroy A, Stromskag KE, Gjengedal E. Approaching families on the subject of organ donation: a phenomenological study of the experience of healthcare professionals. Intensive Crit Care Nurs 2013;29:202–11.

37. Lustbader D. Organ donation: practicalities and ethical conundrums. Am J Crit Care 2014;23(1):81–4.
38. Forsberg A, Lennerling A, Fridh I, et al. Attitudes towards organ donor advocacy among Swedish intensive care nurses. Nurs Crit Care 2015;20(3):126–33.
39. Flodén A, Lennerling A, Fridh I, et al. Development and psychometric evaluation of the instrument: Attitudes Towards Organ Donor Advocacy Scale (ATODAS). Open Nurs J 2011;5:65–73.
40. Australian College of Critical Care Nurses. ACCCN Position Statement (2012) on Organ and Tissue Donation and Transplantation: The roles of critical care nurses and the critical care units and the provision of critical care education; 2012. Available from: https://www.acccn.com.au/documents/item/18. [Accessed August 2018].
41. Mercer L. Improving the rates of organ donation for transplantation. Nurs Stand 2013;27(26):35–40.
42. Gomez MP, Perez B, Manyalich M. International registry in organ donation and transplantation – 2013. Transplant Proc 2014;46:1044–8.
43. New Zealand Human Tissue Act. Organ donation and transplantation; 2008. Available from: https://www.health.govt.nz/our-work/hospitals-and-specialist-care/organ-donation-and-transplantation Section 2, www.health.govt.nz. [Accessed May 2018].
44. World Health Organisation. Clinical criteria for the determination of death WHO technical expert consultation; 2017. Available from: http://apps.who.int/iris/bitstream/handle/10665/254737/WHO-HIS-SDS-2017.5-eng.pdf;jsessionid=F4FABF517E526CCBFF075D29729EEF3B?sequence=1. [Accessed May 2018].
45. Randhawa G. Death and organ donation: meeting the needs of multiethnic and multifaith populations. Br J Anaesth 2012;108(Suppl.):i88–91.
46. Irving MJ, Tong A, Jan S, et al. Factors that influence the decision to be an organ donor: a systematic review of the qualitative literature. Nephrol Dial Transplant 2012;27(6):2526–33.
47. Wong LP. Factors limiting deceased organ donation: focus groups' perspective from culturally diverse community. Transplant Proc 2010;42:1439–44.
48. Thuong M, Ruiz A, Evrard P, et al. New classification of donation after circulatory death donors definitions and terminology. Transpl Int 2016;29:749–59.
49. East Cheshire NHS Trust. Operational policy for organ donation and required referral; 2016. Available from: http://www.eastcheshire.nhs.uk/About-The-Trust/policies/O/Operational%20Organ%20Donation%20Policy%20and%20Required%20Referral%20ECT2566.pdf. [Accessed May 2018].
50. LifeNet Health. Early referral; 2018. Available from: https://www.lifenethealth.org/transplant-services-opo/healthcare-professionals/collaborative-donation-process/early-referral. [Accessed May 2018].
51. Nebraska Organ Recovery. Aftercare of the donor family; 2018. Available from: http://www.nedonation.org/donation-guide/organ/aftercare-of-the-donor-family. [Accessed May 2018].
52. Kim HS, Yoo YS, Cho OH. Satisfaction with the organ donation process of brain dead donors' families in Korea. Transplant Proc 2014;46(10):3253–6.
53. Levvey B, Griffiths A, Snell G. Non-heart beating organ donors: a realistic opportunity to expand the donor pool. Transplant Journal of Australasia 2004;13(3):8–12.
54. Rady M, Verheijde JL, McGregor J. Organ procurement after cardiocirculatory death: a critical analysis. J Intensive Care Med 2008;23(5):303–12.
55. Andrews PA, Burnapp L, Manas D. Summary of the British Transplantation Society guidelines for transplantation from donors after deceased circulatory death. Transplantation 2014;97(3):265–70.
56. Manara AR, Murphy PG, O'Callaghan G. Donation after circulatory death. Br J Anaesth 2012;108(S1):i108–21.
57. Manyalich M, Nelson H, Francis D. The need and opportunity for donation after circulatory death worldwide. Curr Opin Organ Transplant 2018;23(1):136–41.
58. Neyrincka A, Van Raemdonck D, Monbaliud D. Donation after circulatory death: current status. Curr Opin Anaesthesiol 2013;26:382–90.
59. Cypel M, levvey B, Van Raemdonck D, et al. International society for heart and lung transplantation donation after circulatory death registry report. J Heart Lung Transplant 2015;34(10):1278–82. doi:10.1016/j.healun.2015.08.015.
60. Morrissey PE, Monaco AP. Donation after circulatory death: current practices, ongoing challenges, and potential improvements. Transplantation 2014;97(3):258–64.
61. Bernat JL. Controversies in defining and determining death in critical care. Nat Rev Neurol 2013;9:165–73.

Appendix A

Practice standards for specialist critical care nurses

DOMAIN	NO.	STANDARD	NO.	ELEMENT
Professional Practice The standards in this domain relate to the professional, legal and ethical responsibilities of critical care nurses and include knowledge of the legal implications of critical care nursing practice, accountability for practice and the ability to interpret unfamiliar situations in a legal and ethical sense. The standards also include awareness and protection of the rights of patients and their families	1	Functions within professional and legal parameters of critical care nursing practice	1	Applies a knowledge of relevant legislation, professional standards, policies and procedures to critical care nursing practice
			2	Observant of the legal implications of actions taken within the critical care team and fulfils the duty of care in clinical practice
			3	Recognises and responds to unsafe or unprofessional practices by reporting appropriately
			4	Applies the required legal and ethical framework of recording information in the critical care setting
			5	Contributes to formation of policies and protocols to ensure safe patient outcomes
	2	Protects the rights of patients and their families	1	Applies knowledge of, and advocates for, the rights of patients and their families in critical care settings
	3	Demonstrates accountability for nursing practice	1	Accepts responsibility for own actions
			2	Makes complex and informed independent decisions within own level of competence and scope of practice
	4	Demonstrates and contributes to ethical decision making	1	Demonstrates an accurate knowledge of contemporary ethical issues underpinning critical care nursing and complies with the profession's code of ethics and code of conduct
			2	Contributes to multidisciplinary ethical discussion and decision-making processes/framework within the critical care setting

Continued

DOMAIN	NO.	STANDARD	NO.	ELEMENT
Provision and Coordination of Care This domain relates to essential nursing practices that establish and sustain a holistic nurse-patient-family relationship that optimises the wellbeing of the patient and family. The standards include an ability to address the physiological, psychological, physical, emotional and spiritual needs of the patient and family, as well as to optimise the physical and non-physical environment	5	Provides patient- and family-centred critical care	1	Involves the patient and family as active participants in the process of care
			2	Practises with cultural sensitivity and awareness of social factors to enhance patient and family wellbeing
			3	Personalises the patient care environment
			4	Meets the comfort needs of patients and their families
			5	Establishes, maintains and concludes therapeutic interpersonal relationships with patients and their families
	6	Promotes optimal comfort, wellbeing and safety in a highly technical environment that is often unfamiliar to patients and families	1	Ensures a safe environment for patients, families and staff by identifying, minimising or eliminating risks
	7	Manages and coordinates the care of a variety of patients	1	Organises workload to meet planned and unplanned patient care needs to ensure optimal patient outcomes
			2	Negotiates and delegates care to optimise between nurses' scope of practice and the complexity of care for individual patients
			3	Optimises delivery of care through the effective use of human and physical resource management
	8	Manages therapeutic interventions	1	Acts on assessment findings to appropriately initiate, monitor and manage therapeutic interventions
			2	Applies specialised knowledge in the use of critical care technologies
Critical Thinking and Analysis This domain relates to applying specialised knowledge for clinical problem solving. Integrated clinical decision making provides a foundation for the application of research evidence to practice. The domain reflects the capacity of the critical care nurse to respond to planned and unanticipated changes in patient care and to recognise the need for advanced assessment, planning and application of specialised knowledge to deliver evidence-based care	9	Applies integrated patient assessment and interpretive skills to achieve optimal patient outcomes	1	Gathers, analyses and integrates data from a variety of sources and acts on the significance of findings to formulate an individualised plan of care
	10	Develops and manages a plan of care to achieve desired outcomes	1	Formulates and implements an integrated plan of care incorporating specialised knowledge to achieve desired patient outcomes
			2	Assesses effectiveness of nursing care to achieve desired outcomes and reviews plan accordingly
			3	Anticipates, evaluates and responds effectively to physiological deterioration and emergency situations
	11	Evaluates and responds effectively to changing situations	1	Initiates pre-emptive interventions in order to avoid complications
			2	Analyses alterations in physiological parameters and intervenes appropriately
			3	Anticipates, evaluates and responds effectively to physiological deterioration and emergency situations
	12	Engages in and contributes to evidence-based critical care nursing practice	1	Maintains an informed position in relation to current research studies and incorporates evidence-informed practice into critical care setting
			2	Promotes and participates in quality activities to improve critical care patient outcomes

DOMAIN	NO.	STANDARD	NO.	ELEMENT
Collaboration and Leadership The standards in this domain relate to the leadership and education role displayed by the specialist critical care nurse and integral part played by experienced critical care nurses in the professional development of peers, students and less experienced staff	13	Collaborates with the critical care team and other health professionals to achieve desired outcomes	1	Establishes and maintains collaborative and constructive relationships with colleagues in critical care and the broader healthcare team
			2	Acts as an advisor beyond the walls of the critical care environment
	14	Acts to enhance the professional development of self and others	1	Assesses own abilities and engages in activities to enhance personal and professional development
			2	Identifies and assists in meeting the learning needs of others
			3	Actively participates in promoting the profession of critical care
	15	Contributes toward a supportive environment for all members of the healthcare team	1	Initiates strategies to support colleagues and facilitates resolution of situations that may impact on the wellbeing of others

Appendix **B**

Normal laboratory values

Blood analysis: parameters, applications and normal ranges

PARAMETER	APPLICATION	NORMAL RANGE
Adrenocorticotrophic hormone (ACTH)	Aetiology of corticosteroid abnormality	<10 pmol/L
Albumin	Hydration, nutrition status, protein-related disorders and liver disease	32–45 g/L
Alkaline phosphatase (ALP)	Hepatobiliary or bone disease	Neonates/paediatrics: 0 days to <1 week (80–380) U/L 1 week to <4 weeks (120–550) U/L 4 weeks to <26 weeks (120–650) U/L 26 weeks to <2 years (120–450) U/L 2 years to <6 years (120–370) U/L 6 years to <10 years (120–440) U/L Males: 10 years to <14 years (130–530) U/L 14 years to <15 years (105–480) U/L 15 years to <17 years (80–380) U/L 17 years to <19 years (50–220) U/L 19 years to <22 years (45–150) U/L 22 years to <120 years (30–110) U/L Females: 10 years to <13 years (100–460) U/L 13 years to <14 years (70–330) U/L 14 years to <15 years (50–280) U/L 15 years to <16 years (45–170) U/L 16 years to <22 years (35–140) U/L 22 years to <120 years (30–110) U/L
Alanine aminotransferase (ALT)	Liver damage	Neonate: <50 U/L Adult: <35 U/L
Amylase	Acute pancreatitis	Varies based on laboratory method (25–130 U/L) GCUH[1]
Anion gap	Aetiology of metabolic acidosis	8–16 mmol/L (4–13 mmol/L if K not included)
Aspartate aminotransferase (AST)	Liver damage	Neonates: <80 U/L Adults: <40 U/L
Base excess (arterial blood)	Metabolic component of acid–base disorders	(–3) to (+3) mmol/L

PARAMETER	APPLICATION	NORMAL RANGE
Bicarbonate (HCO_3^-)	Acid–base disorders, particularly metabolic component	Neonates/paediatrics: 0 days to <1 week (15–28) mmol/L 1 week to <2 years (16–29) mmol/L 2 years to <10 years (17–30) mmol/L 10 years to <18 years (20–32) mmol/L Adults: 18 years to <120 years (22–32) mmol/L
Bilirubin	Hepatobiliary disease and haemolysis	Total: <20 micromol/L Direct: <7 micromol/L
Calcium (Ca^{2+})	Hyper/hypocalcaemia	Neonates/paediatrics: 0 days to <1 week (1.85–2.80) mmol/L 1 week to <26 weeks (2.20–2.80) mmol/L 26 weeks to <2 years (2.20–2.70) mmol/L 2 years to <18 years (2.20–2.65) mmol/L Adults: 18 years to <120 years (2.10–2.60) mmol/L Calcium corrected for albumin: 18 years to <120 years (2.10–2.60) mmol/L Ionised calcium: 18 years to <120 years (1.16–1.30) mmol/L
Carboxyhaemoglobin	Carbon monoxide exposure	0.2–2.0% of total haemoglobin normally, up to 8.5% in heavy smokers
Chloride (Cl^-)	Causes of acid–base disturbance	Neonates/paediatrics: 0 days to <1 week (98–115) mmol/L 1 week to <18 years (97–110) mmol/L Adults: 18 years to <120 years (95–110) mmol/L
Cholesterol	Lipid status	Total: ≤4.0 mmol/L (recommended by NHF) HDL: 1.0–2.2 mmol/L (females) 0.9–2.0 mmol/L (males) Therapeutic targets: >1.0 mmol/L LDL: 2.0–3.4 mmol/L Therapeutic targets: <2.5 mmol/L
Creatinine kinase (CK)	Diagnosis of myocardial damage	Neonate: 70–380 U/L Adult female: 30–180 U/L Adult male: 60–220 U/L
Creatine kinase MB isoenzyme (CKMB)	Diagnosis of myocardial damage	CKMB 0–1 U/L; 0–5% of the total CK
Creatinine (Cr)	Renal function, particularly glomerular filtration	Neonates/paediatrics: 0 days to <1 week (22–93) micromol/L 1 week to <4 weeks (17–50) micromol/L 4 weeks to <2 years (11–36) micromol/L 2 years to <6 years (20–44) micromol/L 6 years to <12 years (27–58) micromol/L Adult males: 12 years to <15 years (35–83 micromol/L) 15 years to <19 years (50–100 micromol/L) 19 years to <60 years (60–110 micromol/L) Adult females: 12 years to <15 years (35–74 micromol/L) 15 years to <19 years (38–82 micromol/L) 19 years to <60 years (45–90 micromol/L)

Continued

PARAMETER	APPLICATION	NORMAL RANGE
Glucose	Hyper/hypoglycaemia	Fasting: 3.0–5.4 mmol/L Random: 3.0–7.7 mmol/L
Iron	Iron deficiency or overload	Varies according to laboratory method
L-lactate	Metabolic acidosis	Fasting arterial blood: 0.3–0.8 mmol/L Fasting venous blood: 0.3–1.3 mmol/L
Lactate dehydrogenase (LDH)	Assessment of liver disease	120–250 U/L (method and age-dependent) Normal range for adults
Magnesium (Mg)	Hypomagnesaemia	Neonates/paediatrics: 0 days to <1 week (0.60–1.00) mmol/L 1 week to <18 years (0.65–1.10) mmol/L Adults: 18 years to <120 years (0.70–1.10) mmol/L
Myoglobin (serum)	Detection of muscle damage	<55 mcg/L
Osmolality	Suspected poisoning with some substances, e.g. alcohol, methanol	Neonates: 270–290 mmol/kg Adults: 275–295 mmol/kg
Phosphate (PO_4)	Renal failure, hyper-/hypoparathyroidism metabolic bone disease	Neonate/paediatrics: 0 days to <1 week (1.25–2.85) mmol/L 1 week to <4 weeks (1.50–2.75) mmol/L 4 weeks to <26 weeks (1.45–2.50) mmol/L 26 weeks to <1 year (1.30–2.30) mmol/L 1 year to <4 years (1.10–2.20) mmol/L 4 years to <15 years (0.90–2.00) mmol/L 15 years to <18 years (0.80–1.85) mmol/L Adults: 18 years to <20 years (0.75–1.65) mmol/L 20 years to <120 years (0.75–1.50) mmol/L
Potassium (K^+)	Hyper/hypokalaemia	Neonates/paediatrics: 0 days to <1 week (3.8–6.5) mmol/L 1 week to <26 weeks (4.2–6.7) mmol/L 26 weeks to <2 years (3.9–5.6) mmol/L 2 years to <18 years (3.6–5.3) mmol/L Adults: 18 years to <120 years (3.5–5.2) mmol/L
Protein	Used in conjunction with albumin to calculate globulin, diagnosis of protein- and nutrition-related disorders	Neonate: 40–75 g/L Child <2 years: 50–75 g/L Adults: 60–80 g/L
Sodium (Na^+)	Fluid and electrolyte status	Neonates/paediatrics: 0 days to <1 week (132–147) mmol/L 1 week to <18 years (133–144) mmol/L Adults: 18 years to <120 years (135–145) mmol/L
Triglyceride	Lipid status	<2.0 mmol/L (fasting)
Troponin I or troponin T	Myocardial infarction	Normally not detected
Urea	Renal function	Neonates: 1.0–4.0 mmol/L Adults: 3.0–8.0 mmol/L

Haematology: parameters, applications and normal values

PARAMETER	APPLICATION	NORMAL VALUE
Activated clotting time (ACT)	Heparin therapy	Varies based on product in use
Activated partial thromboplastin time (APTT)	Coagulopathy and monitoring of heparin therapy	Varies based on laboratory methods, usually 25–35 seconds
Antithrombin III (AT III)	Investigation of venous thromboembolism	Varies based on laboratory method Functional (guide only): 80–120% of activity in pooled normal plasma Immunoassay (guide only): 0.2–0.4 g/L
Bleeding time	Assessment in some bleeding disorders, e.g. von Willebrand's disease	For investigation of bleeding risk, please refer to coagulation profile, platelet function analyser (PFA), platelet aggregometry
D-dimers	Indication of recent or ongoing fibrinolysis, possibly indicating disseminated intravascular coagulation (DIC)	Varies based on laboratory method
Haemoglobin (Hb)	Anaemia	Children 6–59 months: ≥ 110 g/L Children 5–11 years: ≥ 115 g/L Children 12–14 years: ≥ 120 g/L Non-pregnant women (≥ 15 years): ≥ 120 g/L Pregnant women: ≥ 110 g/L Men (≥ 15 years): ≥ 130 g/L
International normalised ratio (INR)	Oral anticoagulant therapy	Varies according to clinical indication. Typically 2.0–3.0, although a target of up to 4.5 may be used in those with a mechanical heart valve
Packed cell volume (PCV) (also referred to as haematocrit)	Anaemia	Infant (3 months): 0.32–0.44 Child (3–6 years): 0.36–0.44 Child (10–12 years): 0.37–0.45 Adult (female): 0.37–0.47 Adult (male): 0.40–0.54
Plasminogen	Investigation of tendency towards clotting, e.g. venous thromboembolism	50–150%
Platelet count	Excessive or inappropriate bleeding	150–400 310^9/L
Prothrombin time (PT)	Detection of coagulation factor deficiencies due to vitamin K deficiency	Varies based on laboratory Reagent-dependent; prothrombin time generally 11–15 seconds
Red cell count (RCC)	Anaemia	Neonate/paediatrics: Term cord blood: $4.0–6.0 \times 10^{12}$/L 3 months: $3.2–4.8 \times 10^{12}$/L 1 year: $3.6–5.2 \times 10^{12}$/L 3–6 years: $4.1–5.5 \times 10^{12}$/L 10–12 years: $4.0–5.4 \times 10^{12}$/L Adults: Female: $3.8–5.8 \times 10^{12}$/L Male: $4.5–6.5 \times 10^{12}$/L
Thrombin time (TT)	Acquired or inherited disorders of haemostasis	Varies based on laboratory method, but usually 14–16 seconds
White cell count (WCC)	Infection or inflammatory disease	Neonate: $6.0–22.0 \times 10^9$/L Child (1 year): $6.0–18.0 \times 10^9$/L Child (4–7 years): $5.0–15.0 \times 10^9$/L Child (8–12 years): $4.5–13.5 \times 10^9$/L Adult: $4.0–10.0 \times 10^9$/L

Blood gases: parameters and normal values

PARAMETER	NORMAL VALUE
ARTERIAL	
pH	7.36–7.44 (36–44 nmol/L)
Partial pressure of oxygen (PaO_2)	11.0–13.5 kPa (80–100 mmHg) (varies with age)
Partial pressure of carbon dioxide ($PaCO_2$)	4.6–6.0 kPa (35–45 mmHg)
Oxygen saturation (SaO_2)	>94%
VENOUS	
pH	7.34–7.42
Partial pressure of oxygen (PvO_2)	37–42 mmHg
Partial pressure of carbon dioxide ($PvCO_2$)	42–50 mmHg
Oxygen saturation (SvO_2)	>70%

Urine analysis: parameters, applications and normal values

PARAMETER	APPLICATION	NORMAL VALUE
Albumin	Diabetic nephropathy, renal disease	Normal: <30 mg albumin/g creatinine Microalbuminuria: 30–300 mg albumin/g creatinine Macroalbuminuria: >300 mg albumin/g creatinine
Calcium	Renal calculi	2.5–7.5 mmol/24 h Fasting spot urine: Males: 0.04–0.45 mol/mol creatinine Females: 0.10–0.58 mol/mol creatinine
Chloride	Identification of site of chloride loss in electrolyte disturbance	Dependent on intake, but usually 100–250 mmol/24 h
Cortisol (free)	Adrenocortical hyperfunction	100–300 nmol/24 h
Creatinine clearance	Glomerular filtration rate	>70 mL/min in a young adult, typically falling approx. 0.5 mL/min per year at ages over 30 years
Magnesium	Urinary magnesium loss	2.5–8.0 mmol/24 h (related to daily intake)
Myoglobin	Suspected rhabdomyolysis	Not normally detected
Osmolality	Renal disease, syndrome of inappropriate antidiuretic hormone, polyuric syndromes	50–1200 mmol/kg
Potassium	Differentiation of renal potassium loss from other causes of hypokalaemia	40–100 mmol/24 h (related to daily intake)
Protein	Renal disease	<150 mg/24 h During pregnancy: <250 mg/24 h

PARAMETER	APPLICATION	NORMAL VALUE
Sodium	Causes of hyponatraemia	In hyponatraemia or hypovolaemic shock without acute tubular necrosis, urine sodium should be <20 mmol/L and fractional excretion of sodium should be <1.5% If extracellular fluid volume and plasma sodium are normal, urine sodium should equal intake minus non-renal losses, typically 75–300 mmol/24 h
Urea	Renal function, occasionally assessment of nitrogen balance in patients receiving parenteral nutrition	420–720 mmol/24 h

Reference

1. The Royal College of Pathologists of Australasia. RCPA manual – online. ISSN 1449-8219. Available from: https//www.rcpa.edu.au/Manuals/RCPA-Manual. [Accessed 10 May 2019].

Glossary of terms

ablation. Therapy designed to destroy tissues that generate or sustain arrhythmias.

Aboriginal. Refers to both Aboriginal and Torres Strait Islander peoples.

actigraph. Used for measuring movement, in particular to measure the quantity of sleep.

action potential. The electrical activity developed in a muscle or nerve cell during activity.

acute coronary syndrome (ACS). A broad spectrum of clinical presentations, spanning ST-segment elevation myocardial infarction through to an accelerated pattern of angina without evidence of myonecrosis.

acute respiratory distress syndrome. An acute syndrome of rapid onset in which the patient has evidence of hypoxia and non-cardiogenic pulmonary oedema.

acute respiratory failure. Occurs when there is a reduction in the body's ability to maintain either oxygenation or ventilation, or both.

advance directives. A method to document preferences about an individual's future healthcare should situations arise where they are no longer competent to make decisions.

advanced life support. The provision of effective airway management, ventilation of the lungs and production of circulation by means of techniques additional to those of basic life support. These techniques may include, but are not limited to, advanced airway management, tracheal intubation, intravenous access/drug therapy and defibrillation.

adverse event. An injury or event that is due to healthcare management and results in temporary or permanent harm to patients.

afterload. The load imposed on the muscle during contraction, and translates to systolic myocardial wall tension.

allograft. A tissue graft from a donor of the same species as the recipient but not genetically identical.

anabolism. The chemical process by which complex molecules, such as peptides, proteins, polysaccharides, lipids and nucleic acids, are synthesised from simpler molecules.

anastomosis. A surgical connection between two structures.

anhidrosis. Absence of sweating.

antepartum haemorrhage. Any bleeding from the genital tract after 20 weeks' gestation and before the birth of the baby.

anterior cord syndrome. Spinal cord injury to the motor and sensory pathways in the anterior parts of the spine; thus patients are able to feel crude sensation, but movement and detailed sensation are lost in the posterior part of the spinal cord.

anxiety. A disorder characterised by excessive concern or worry with difficulty controlling the level of concern, and with irritability, restlessness and disturbed sleep.

arterial blood gas. An arterial blood sample taken to assess pH, bicarbonate, oxygen and carbon dioxide levels, and other electrolytes.

asterixis. Abnormal tremor, especially in the hands.

asthma. A lower respiratory tract disease characterised by mucosal and immune system dysfunction. The chronic inflammatory process causes narrowing of bronchial airways, obstructing airflow leading to episodes of wheezing, breathlessness and chest tightening.

auscultation. The action of listening to sounds from the heart, lungs or other organs, typically with a stethoscope.

automatic tube compensation. A feature available on some ventilators in which the ventilator employs an algorithm to increase airway pressure to overcome the resistance of the artificial airway during inspiration.

autonomic dysreflexia. Dysfunctions of the autonomic nervous system characterised by abnormalities in heart rate, respiratory rate, systolic blood pressure and increased muscle tone and temperature. Other characteristics include decerebrate (extensor) or decorticate (flexor) posturing, and profuse sweating.

axon. Part of the neuron that transmits information to other neurons.

backwards upwards right pressure manoeuvre. A technique where pressure is applied to mobilise the thyroid cartilage in the sequence backwards (towards the spine) and to the right side in order to help visualise the vocal cords and assist with intubation.

beneficence. To do good; promoting the wellbeing of another person.

best interests. Acting in a way that optimally promotes good for the individual and is a principle for making decisions about healthcare.

biphasic. Pattern of electrical flow where the current reverses direction in the middle of the waveform, flowing first from one electrode pad, through the heart, to the second electrode pad, and then from the second pad through the heart to the first.

birth. The complete expulsion or extraction from its mother of a baby of at least 20 weeks' gestation or, if gestation is unknown, weighing at least 400 g, who is either born alive or stillborn.

birth weight. The first weight of the baby (stillborn or live born) obtained after birth.

bronchiolitis. Obstruction of the small airways, resulting in air trapping and respiratory distress, generally seen in infants less than 12 months of age.

Brown–Séquard syndrome. Injury to the left or right side of the spinal cord. Movements are lost below the level of injury on the injured side, but pain and temperature sensation are lost on the opposite side of injury.

business case. A management tool used to outline the clinical needs (who, what, when, where and how) and their implications, such as the expected financial return on investment.

caesarean section/birth. Operative birth through an abdominal incision.

capnography. Monitoring of expired carbon dioxide.

caput medusa. The appearance of distended and engorged paraumbilical veins that radiate from the umbilicus across the abdomen.

cardiac arrest. Cessation of heart action recognised by the absence of response, absence of normal breathing and absence of movement.

cardiac pacing. The delivery of an electrical impulse to either or both the atria and ventricles to initiate or maintain normal cardiac electrical activity.

cardiopulmonary resuscitation. Comprises those techniques used to minimise the effects of circulatory arrest and to assist the return of spontaneous circulation, including the technique of rescue breathing combined with external chest compressions.

care bundle. A set of evidence-based interventions or processes of care, applied to selected patients in order to ensure appropriate, standardised care.

catabolism. The convergent process, in which many different types of molecules are broken down into relatively few types of end products.

central cord syndrome. Injury to the centre of the cervical spinal cord, producing weakness, paralysis and sensory deficits in the arms but not the legs.

cerebral microdialysis. A tool for investigating the metabolic status of the injured brain. The microdialysis probe is inserted into the cerebral tissue where substances in the extracellular fluid surround the semipermeable membrane at the tip of the catheter. Following equilibration of the tissue metabolites with the perfusion fluid, the dialysate can be analysed for concentrations of products of energy metabolism (glucose, lactate, pyruvate) as indicators of hypoxia and ischaemia.

cerebral oedema. Increased brain water content.

cerebral spinal fluid. An ultrafiltrate of blood plasma composed of 99% water, making it close to the composition of the brain extracellular fluid.

cerebrovascular resistance. The amount of resistance created by the cerebral vessels, which is controlled by the autoregulatory mechanisms of the brain.

chemoreceptor. A sensor that responds to change in chemical composition in the blood.

chemosis. Conjunctival oedema, often associated with positive pressure ventilation, positive end-expiratory pressure or prone positioning.

child. 'Young child' is aged between 1 and 8 years and 'older child' is aged between 9 and 14 years inclusive.

chronic heart failure (CHF). Refers to a complex syndrome distinguished by a number of characteristics, particularly shortness of breath or fatigue, that occur at rest or on exertion. It is also characterised by objective evidence of cardiac dysfunction or structured cardiac abnormalities that impair the left ventricle from filling with or ejecting blood to meet the body's demands.

clinical decision making. The cognitive processes and strategies that nurses use when utilising data to make clinical decisions regarding patient assessment and care.

clinical practice guideline. Statements about appropriate health care for specific clinical circumstances.

coagulopathy. Disorder of the clotting mechanism of the blood, which can be caused by preexisting disease, medications, pathophysiological conditions such as hypothermia and acidosis or current treatment such as massive blood transfusion.

cognitive dysfunction. Associated with problems remembering, solving problems, thinking and making decisions.

coma. A state of unresponsiveness from which the patient cannot be aroused by verbal and physical stimuli to produce any meaningful response; therefore, coma implies the absence of both arousal and content of consciousness.

complementary therapies. Treatments that have not been considered part of standard Western medicine but that are increasingly being used in combination with standard medical treatments. These may include therapies for pain, such as massage and relaxation techniques, and some nutritional therapies.

conduction. The process by which electrical activity is directly transmitted through cells when there is a difference of electrical potential between adjoining regions, without movement of the tissue.

contact activation pathway. Previously termed the 'intrinsic' coagulation pathway.

continuous lateral rotation therapy. An intervention in which the patient is rotated continually, on a specialised bed, through a set number of degrees; it helps to relieve pressure areas and can significantly improve oxygenation. It is also known as kinetic bed therapy.

contractility. The force of ventricular ejection, or the inherent ability of the ventricle to perform external work, independent of afterload or preload.

coronary heart disease or coronary artery disease. A narrowing of the small blood vessels that supply blood and oxygen to the heart.

counterpulsation. Rapid inflation of the intra-aortic balloon catheter at the onset of diastole of each cardiac cycle and then deflation immediately before the onset of the next systole.

critical care nursing. Specialised nursing care of critically ill patients who have an immediate life-threatening or potentially life-threatening illness or injury.

critically ill patients. Patients who have an immediate life-threatening or potentially life-threatening illness or injury causing compromise to the function of one or more organs.

cross-clamp. The act of clamping the aorta to achieve a controlled arrest of the heart, ceasing blood flow to all organs, and commencement of infusion of cold perfusion fluid during organ retrieval surgery. Marks the beginning of cold ischaemic time.

croup (laryngotracheobronchitis). A set of symptoms caused by acute swelling causing obstruction in the upper airway (larynx, trachea and bronchi) from inflammation and oedema and is most commonly seen in winter months.

cultural safety. Involves effective nursing practice whereby patients and their families determine that their cultural needs have been met and that they feel safe. Effective nursing practice requires nurses to reflect on their own cultural location and how this may influence the way in which they interact with patients from another culture. In addition to ethnically related culture, culture is defined broadly to include age, generation, gender, sexual orientation, socioeconomic status, migrant experience, occupation, religious or spiritual beliefs and disability.

cytotoxic/histotoxic anoxia. The inability to use oxygen, even when available.

cytotoxic oedema. Cellular swelling, usually of astrocytes in the grey matter, which is generally seen after cerebral ischaemia caused by cardiac arrest or minor head injury.

damage-control surgery. A four-stage surgical approach that involves rapid initial control of haemorrhage and contamination, usually with packing and temporary closure, followed by ongoing resuscitation in the ICU and reoperation for definitive repair and reconstruction.

dendrite. Part of the neuron that receives positive or negative charges from other neurons.

donation after cardiac death. A solid organ donation option for a patient who has not progressed and is not likely to progress to brain death. It is also known as non-heart-beating donor and donation after circulatory death.

depolarisation. The electrical state in an excitable cell where the inside of the cell becomes less negative relative to the outside.

depression. Characterised by feeling sad or having low or negative mood. People may experience a lack of interest in activities, feel slowed down or have difficulties thinking, concentrating or making decisions.

eclampsia. A severe variant of preeclampsia, characterised by tonic–clonic seizures that are not caused by any preexisting disease or other identifiable causes, e.g. epilepsy, cerebral haemorrhage.

electroencephalography. The recording of electrical activity by sensors along the scalp produced by the firing of neurons within the brain.

embolism. Obstruction of an artery, typically by a blood clot or an air bubble.

encephalitis. Inflammation of the brain substance.

endotracheal tube. An artificial airway used in critical care settings to enable delivery of mechanical ventilation and clearance of airway secretions.

enzyme. Substance produced by a living organism that acts as a catalyst to bring about a specific biochemical reaction.

epiglottitis. Inflammation of the epiglottis, frequently involving surrounding structures, with the classic description of a swollen, cherry-red, softened and floppy epiglottis, which tends to fall backwards, obstructing the airway.

ethics. The study of rational processes to inform a course of action in response to a particular situation where conflicting options exist.

evidence-based nursing. The conscientious, explicit and judicious use of research-based information in making decisions about care delivery to individuals or groups of patients.

extracorporeal membrane oxygenation. A therapy in which blood is removed from the patient and oxygenated in an artificial membrane before being returned to the patient, i.e. circulation of blood outside the body provides total artificial support of cardiac and pulmonary function.

family. Those closest to the person in knowledge, care and affection, including the immediate biological family; the family of acquisition (related by marriage or contract); and the family of choice and friends (not related biologically or by marriage or contract).

family-centred care. Incorporates planning, delivery and evaluation of health care that is governed by mutually beneficial partnerships among healthcare providers, patients and families.

fidelity. Keeping promises; honouring contracts and commitments.

flaccid areflexic paralysis. Paralysis that is characterised by an absence of reflexes and lack of muscle tone.

general anaesthesia. A drug-induced state where the patient will not respond to stimuli, including pain.

gestation. The estimated gestational age of the baby in completed weeks using all available obstetric information (clinical estimation, ultrasound, cycle length etc), counting from the first day of the woman's last menstrual period. Commonly recorded as $35^{+2}/40$, indicating that the gestation is 35 weeks and 2 days.

gravidity. The total number of pregnancies a woman has had, including the index pregnancy, regardless of the outcome (therefore including spontaneous and induced abortions and any stillborn or live born infants).

Guillain–Barré syndrome. An immune-mediated disorder resulting from generation of autoimmune antibodies and/or inflammatory cells that cross-react with epitopes on peripheral nerves and roots, leading to demyelination or axonal damage or both, and autoimmune insult to the peripheral nerve myelin.

gynaecomastia. Benign enlargement of the breast tissue in males.

health-related quality of life. How an individual's health status may influence how they assess their quality of life.

haemodynamic monitoring. The measurement of pressure, flow and oxygenation within the cardiovascular system.

heart failure with preserved ejection fraction (HFpEF). Refers to impaired diastolic filling of the left ventricle. There may or may not be impaired systolic dysfunction.

heart failure with reduced ejection fraction (HFrEF). Refers to inability of the heart to contract in systole.

HELLP syndrome. A severe variant of preeclampsia characterised by haemolysis, elevated liver enzymes and low platelets.

high-frequency oscillatory ventilation. A mode of ventilation that delivers small breaths at a very high respiratory rate (between 300 and 420) to maintain alveolar opening and facilitate carbon dioxide elimination.

homeostatic. The tendency of the body to seek and maintain a condition of balance or equilibrium within its internal environment.

hypercapnoeic respiratory failure. Also known as type II respiratory failure (or failure to ventilate), presents with a high PaCO as well as a low PaO.

hypoxaemic respiratory failure. Also known as type I respiratory failure (or failure to oxygenate), presents with a low PaO and a normal or low PaCO.

icterus. Jaundice.

indigenous person. Aboriginal or Torres Strait Islander person of Australia, or Maori person of New Zealand.

induction of labour. Procedure performed for the purpose of initiating and stimulating the process of labour. This may include the artificial rupture of the membranes and/or the use of uterine stimulating medication.

infant. A person less than approximately 1 year of age.

infant death. The death of an infant occurring within 1 year of birth.

intra-aortic balloon pump (IABP). Mechanical assistance for a failing heart based on the principles of diastolic augmentation and systolic unloading by counterpulsation of a balloon in the aorta.

intracranial hypertension. A sustained intracranial pressure of >15 mmHg.

intracranial pressure. The pressure exerted by the contents of the brain within the confines of the skull. Normal ICP is 0–10 mmHg.

jugular venous oximetry. Jugular venous catheterisation used to collect data on oxygen-based variables such as jugular venous oxygenation, cerebral oxygen extraction and arteriovenous difference in oxygen, which can indicate changes in cerebral metabolism and blood flow.

justice. Fair, equitable and appropriate treatment in light of what is due or owed to an individual.

laryngotracheobronchitis. Also known as croup; a set of symptoms caused by acute swelling causing obstruction in the upper airway (larynx, trachea and bronchi) from inflammation and oedema and is most commonly seen in winter months.

live birth. The birth of an infant, regardless of maturity or birth weight, who breathes or shows any other signs of life after being born.

magnetic resonance imaging. An imaging technique that uses the characteristic of hydrogen protons, which function like tiny spinning magnets, to generate images of the brain and body.

malignant hyperthermia. A severe reaction to anaesthetic agents which can cause muscle rigidity, breakdown of muscle fibres, high temperature, tachycardia and acidosis; if untreated, it can be life-threatening.

mechanical circulatory support. Partial or total cardiovascular support devices such as IABP, ventricular assist devices and total artificial hearts.

medical futility. Treatment with no apparent benefit to the patient.

meningitis. Inflammation of the pia and arachnoid layers of the meninges.

monophasic. Pattern of electrical flow where the current, throughout the pulse, flows in one direction, from one electrode pad through the heart to the other electrode pad.

morality. The norms widely shared by a community or among members of a professional group about what is 'right' or 'wrong' about human conduct, the widely held views then forming stable social consensus.

multigravida. A woman who is pregnant for the second or subsequent time.

multipara. A woman who has had more than one pregnancy resulting in a live birth or stillbirth.

murmur. A low continuous background noise.

myasthenia gravis. An autoimmune disorder caused by autoantibodies against the nicotinic acetylcholine receptor on the postsynaptic membrane at the neuromuscular junction, which is characterised by weakness and fatigue in voluntary muscles.

myelin sheath. A lipid–protein casing that covers the neuron and provides protection to the axon, speeding the transmission of impulses along the nerve cells.

myocardial infarction. Myocardial cell death due to prolonged ischaemia.

near-infrared spectroscopy. A non-invasive method of monitoring continuous trends of cerebral oxygenated and deoxygenated haemoglobin by utilising an infrared light beam transmitted through the skull.

negligence. A legal term where the provider owed a duty of care to the recipient; they failed to meet that duty; the recipient sustained damages as a result; and the provider should have reasonably foreseen that these damages would occur.

neonatal death. The death of a live born infant, within 28 days of birth, whose birth weight was at least 400 g or of at least 20 weeks' gestation.

neonate. An infant in the first minutes to hours following birth.

neuroglia. The non-neuronal cells of the nervous system that are 10–50 times more prevalent than the number of neurons.

neuron. A specialised cell in the nervous system comprised of a dendrite, cell body (also known as soma) and axon.

neurotransmitter. A chemical messenger used by neurons to communicate in one direction with other neurons.

neurally adjusted ventilatory assistance. A type of ventilation that uses diaphragmatic movement to trigger gas flow and breath delivery.

non-maleficence. Doing no harm and maximising possible benefits while minimising possible harm.

non-technical skills. Cognitive, social and personal skills that complement technical skills and contribute to safe and efficient task performance.

nullipara. A pregnant woman who has not had a prior birth of an infant of 20 weeks' gestation or more.

open disclosure. Telling the truth to the patient or family about what and how an adverse event has occurred.

palmar erythema. Reddening of the skin on the palmar aspects of the hands.

parity. Number of previous pregnancies resulting in live birth or stillbirth.

partogram. Birth suite chart that records maternal and fetal monitoring during labour, and the progress of labour, e.g. strength and frequency of contractions, fetal descent.

parturient. Pregnant woman; of or relating to giving birth.

patient dependency. An approach to quantify the care needs of individual patients, classifying patients into groups requiring similar nursing care.

patient safety. Reduction of the risk of unnecessary harm to patients to an acceptable level.

perinatal death. A stillbirth or neonatal death.

person-centred care. Emphasis on the individual nature of the person with the illness that promotes the perception (and reality) of equal power and a shared partnership between the person and healthcare provider/s.

placenta accreta. Abnormal adherence of the placenta to the uterine wall.

placenta praevia. The placenta is partially or wholly implanted in the lower uterine segment on either the anterior or posterior wall.

polysomnography. The continuous recording of various physiological variables during sleep; these variables typically include brain wave activity, eye movement and muscle tone.

post-intensive care syndrome. Term given to a range of physical and emotional health issues that patients may experience after discharge from intensive care.

postpartum. After birth. The postpartum period is normally classified as the 6 weeks following birth, when the woman's body returns to the pre-pregnancy state.

postpartum haemorrhage. ≥500 mL blood loss from the genital tract following birth. It is categorised as primary, within the first 24 hours following birth, or secondary, from 24 hours to 6 weeks postpartum.

posttraumatic amnesia. A disorder after brain injury reflecting the time elapsed from injury until recovery of full consciousness and the return of ongoing memory.

posttraumatic stress disorder. A response to either experiencing or witnessing a traumatic event. People may present with a range of symptoms including reliving the event, nightmares and/or flashbacks, avoidant behaviours, intrusive thoughts or images and intense distress.

preeclampsia. A multisystem pregnancy disorder resulting from widespread vasospasm that is often characterised by hypertension and proteinuria.

preload. The load imposed by the initial fibre length of the cardiac muscle before contraction (i.e. at the end of diastole).

primigravida. A woman pregnant for the first time.

primipara. A woman who has had one pregnancy resulting in a live birth or stillbirth.

pseudocholinesterase deficiency. An inherited abnormality in the pseudocholinesterase enzyme that results in slower metabolic degradation of the depolarising neuromuscular blocking agent suxamethonium (succinylcholine).

pulse oximetry. The measurement of peripheral arterial oxygen saturation.

quality monitoring. Measurement of and responses to the incidence and patterns of adverse events.

quality of life. How a person evaluates or views their life. There are many aspects of life that people used to assess its quality such as social, economic, spiritual, and psychological and health.

rapid response system. System developed to recognise and provide emergency response to patients who experience acute deterioration.

regional anaesthesia. An umbrella term used to describe injection of local anaesthetic in the vicinity of major nerve bundles supplying specific body areas to produce nerve blocks, epidural and spinal blocks.

repolarisation. The process by which the membrane potential of a neuron or muscle cell is restored to the cell's resting potential.

research participant. Individual (or group of living individuals) about whom a researcher conducting research obtains data through intervention or interaction with that person or their identifiable private information.

resuscitation. Preservation or restoration of life by the establishment and/or maintenance of airway, breathing and circulation, and related emergency care.

return of spontaneous circulation (ROSC). Resumption of sustained perfusing cardiac activity associated with significant respiratory effort after cardiac arrest.

root cause analysis. A detailed method to investigate an adverse event whereby the system and processes that contributed to the event are examined in an effort to identify system or process improvements to prevent the event from reoccurring.

safety culture. The product of individual and group values, attitudes, perceptions, competencies and patterns of behaviour that determine the commitment to, and the style and proficiency of, an organisation's health and safety management.

seizure. An abrupt discharge of ions from a group of neurons resulting in epileptic activity. Seizures are classified depending on how they start: as partial or focal seizures; generalised or full body seizures involving both cerebral hemispheres; or partial seizures with secondary generalisation.

sensory overload. A prolonged overstimulus of the senses that can result from excessive or prolonged periods of noise, light, odours and touch from both equipment and personnel.

situational awareness. An individual's awareness and understanding of information that is relevant to their current environment and task.

skill mix. The ratio of caregivers with various skills, training and experience in a clinical unit.

somnolence. A state of unconsciousness from which the patient can be fully awakened.

spider angiomata. Swollen blood vessels slightly beneath the surface of the skin. There is usually a central red spot with extensions moving outward like a spider web.

spontaneous breathing trial. A technique in which the patient is removed from the ventilator to see if they are able to breathe unassisted by the mechanical ventilator.

spontaneous vaginal birth. Birth without intervention in which the baby's head is the presenting part.

status epilepticus. Enduring seizure activity that is not likely to stop spontaneously. Traditionally defined as 30 minutes of continuous seizure activity, it has been changed to 5 minutes or 2 or more seizures without full recovery of consciousness between the seizures.

stillbirth. The birth of an infant weighing at least 400 g or of at least 20 weeks' gestation, which shows no signs of life after birth.

stupor. A state of unconsciousness from which the patient can be awakened to produce inadequate responses to verbal and physical stimuli.

tissue factor pathway. Previously termed the 'extrinsic' coagulation pathway.

transcranial Doppler. A safe and reliable ultrasound technology for measuring cerebrovascular blood velocities and evaluating cerebral circulation and haemodynamics.

transformational leadership. A style of leadership characterised by developing a shared vision, inspiring and communicating, valuing others, challenging and stimulating, developing trust and enabling others.

traumatic brain injury. Heterogeneous pathophysiological process from a mixture of diffuse and focal lesions on the brain because of the mechanism of injury. It can range in severity from concussion through to post-coma unresponsiveness.

values. The beliefs and attitudes that individuals hold about what is important and that therefore influence individual actions and decision making.

vasogenic oedema. Extracellular brain oedema from increased capillary permeability.

venous thromboembolism. A term used to reflect both deep vein thrombosis and pulmonary embolism.

ventilator-associated pneumonia. A form of hospital-acquired pneumonia that occurs in patients who are mechanically ventilated.

ventricular assist device (VAD). Full or partial ventricular assistance provided by an implanted device.

veracity. Telling the truth; full and honest disclosure so that individuals can weigh up the risks and benefits of treatments.

warm ischaemia. Time taken from withdrawal of ventilation and treatment to the confirmation of death of a donation after cardiac death (DCD) donor to the commencement of infusion of cold perfusion fluid and/ or organ retrieval.

Index

Page numbers followed by "*f*" indicate figures, "*t*" indicate tables, and "*b*" indicate boxes.

C

E

F

G

H

O

P

S